PATHOLOGY

Implications for the Physical Therapist

PATHOLOGY

Implications for the Physical Therapist

SECOND EDITION

Catherine Cavallaro Goodman, MBA, PT

Faculty Affiliate
School of Pharmacy and Allied Health Sciences
Department of Physical Therapy
University of Montana
Missoula, Montana

Medical Multimedia Group, Medical Writer
Missoula, Montana

Kenda S. Fuller, PT, NCS

ABPTS Board Certified Specialist in Neurologic Physical Therapy
Physical Therapist, South Valley Physical Therapy, P.C.
Denver, Colorado

Clinical Instructor, Physical Therapy Program
University of Colorado Health Sciences Center
Denver, Colorado

Affiliate Faculty, Physical Therapy Program
Regis University
Denver, Colorado

William G. Boissonnault, MS, PT

Assistant Professor
University of Wisconsin–Madison
Program in Physical Therapy
Madison, Wisconsin

Assistant Professor
University of St. Augustine Center of Health Sciences
St. Augustine, Florida

Clinical Assistant Professor, Department of Rehabilitation Sciences
University of Tennessee–Memphis College of Allied Health Sciences
Memphis, Tennessee

Adjunct Faculty, Massachusetts General Hospital
Institute of Health Professions
Boston, Massachusetts

Instructor, Krannert Graduate School of Physical Therapy
University of Indianapolis
Indianapolis, Indiana

SAUNDERS
An Imprint of Elsevier

SAUNDERS
An Imprint of Elsevier

The Curtis Center
Independence Square West
Philadelphia, Pennsylvania 19106

PATHOLOGY: IMPLICATIONS FOR THE PHYSICAL THERAPIST

NOTICE

Physical Therapy is an ever-changing field. Standard safety precautions must be followed, but as new re-search and clinical experience broaden our knowledge, changes in treatment and drug therapy may become necessary or appropriate. Readers are advised to check the most current product information pro-vided by the manufacturer of each drug to be administered to verify the recommended dose, the method and duration of administration, and contraindications. It is the responsibility of the licensed prescriber, relying on experience and knowledge of the patient, to determine dosages and the best treatment for each individual patient. Neither the publisher nor the author assumes any liability for any injury and/or damage to persons or property arising from this publication.

Previous edition copyrighted 1998

ISBN-13: 978-0-7216-9233-3
ISBN-10: 0-7216-9233-8

Acquisitions Editor: Andrew Allen
Developmental Editor: Peg Waltner
Publishing Services Manager: Linda McKinley
Project Manager: Rich Barber
Designer: Julia Dummitt

GW/QWD

Printed in The United States

Last digit is the print number: 9 8 7 6

CONTRIBUTORS

JOHN R. CORBOY, MD
Associated Professor and Vice Chairman of Neurology
Director, University of Colorado Multiple Sclerosis Center
University of Colorado Health Sciences Center

ALLAN GLANZMAN, PT, PCS, ATP
Clinical Specialist
Children's Seashore House
Children's Hospital of Philadelphia
Philadelphia, Pennsylvania

SHARON M. KONECNE, M.H.S., P.T.
National Oncology Rehabilitation Consultant and Lecturer
Clinician Denver Visiting Nurses Association
Affiliate Faculty Physical Therapy Program
Regis University
Denver, Colorado
Lecturer Physical Therapy Program
University of Colorado
Denver, Colorado

MICHAEL B. KOOPMEINERS, MD (FIRST EDITION)
Associate Professor
University of St. Augustine for Health Sciences
St Augustine, Florida

Medical Director
WorkSite Health
Health Partners
Minneapolis, Minnesota

BONNIE LASINSKI, PT
Lymphedema Therapy
Woodbury, New York

JAMES J. LASKIN, PT, PHD
Assistant Professor
Department of Physical Therapy, School of Pharmacy and
  Allied Health Sciences
The University of Montana
Missoula, Montana

D. MICHAEL MCKEOUGH, PT, PHD
Shenandoah University, Program in Physical Therapy
Winchester, Virginia

JIM MIEDANER, MS, PT (FIRST EDITION)
Associate Director, Physical Therapy Department
University of Wisconsin Hospital and Clinics
Madison, Wisconsin

TERRY RANDALL, MS, PT, OCS, AT, C (FIRST EDITION)
Somerset Physical Therapy
Somerset, Kentucky

MARCIA B. SMITH, PT, PHD
Associate Professor
Rehabilitation Medicine
Physical Therapy Education Program
University of Colorado Health Sciences Center
Denver, Colorado

TERESA E. KELLY SNYDER, MN, RN, CS
Clinical Specialist in Medical-Surgical Nursing
Associate Professor of Nursing
Montana State University
Bozeman, Montana

STEVEN H. TEPPER, PT, PHD
Shenandoah University, Program in Physical Therapy
Winchester, Virginia

PAMELA UNGER, PT
Community General Hospital
Center for Wound Management
Reading, Pennsylvania

CHRIS L. WELLS, PHD, PT, CCS, ATC
University of Maryland Medical Systems
Department of Physical Therapy
Baltimore, Maryland

Assistant Professor
Graduate School of Physical Therapy
Slippery Rock University
Slippery Rock, Pennsylvania

PATRICIA S. WINKLER
South Valley Physical Therapy
Assistant Professor
Department of Physical Therapy
Regis University
Denver, Colorado

REVIEWERS

W.B. BEKEMEYER, MD
Critical Care, Pulmonology, and Internal Medicine
Western Montana Clinic
Missoula, Montana

KATHERINE S. BIGGS, PT, MS
Supervisor, Department of Rehabilitation Service
Yale New Haven Hospital
New Haven, Connecticut

JAMES A. BIRKE, PhD, PT
Director Rehabilitation Services
Louisiana State University Health Sciences Center
Diabetes Foot Program
Baton Rouge, Louisiana

MARVIN BORIS, MD
Clinical Professor of Pediatrics
Cornell University School of Medicine
New York, New York
Medical Director
Lymphedema Therapy
Woodbury, Long Island, New York

MARY C. BOURGEOIS, PT, CCS
Beth Israel Deaconess Medical Center
Coordinator Outpatient Cardiopulmonary Physical Therapy
Home Care Rehabilitation Services
Boston, Massachusetts

PEG BROWNLEE, RPH
Director, Pharmacy Technician Program
University of Montana- Missoula, College of Technology
Missoula, Montana

J. A. CAIN, MD
Missoula, Montana

MICHELLE CAMERON, PT, OCS
Health Potentials
Oakland, California

JOSEPH P. CAVORSI, MD
Vascular and General Surgery, Medical Director
The Center for Advanced Wound Care
West Lawn, Pennsylvania

MERYL COHEN, MS, PT, CCS
Instructor
University of Miami School of Medicine,
    Division of Physical Therapy
Coral Gables, Florida
Adjunct Instructor
Massachusetts General Hospital Institute
    of Health Professions
Boston, Massachusetts

DAVE CULP, BSN, RN
Missoula County Health Department
Missoula, Montana

LIANNE M. DELANEY, RN, BSN, CIC
Infection Control Coordinator
St. Patrick Hospital
Missoula, Montana

ANTHONY L. DOERR, MD
Adult and Pediatric Urology
Community Medical Center
Missoula, Montana

MAUREEN DONOHOE, PT, PCS
Alfred I duPont Hospital for Children
Wilmington, Delaware

MEREDITH E. DRENCH, PhD, PT
Director, Adaptive Health Associates, Inc.
East Greenwich, Rhode Island

MARY LOU GALANTINO PhD, PT
Associate Professor
Richard Stockton of New Jersey Program
    in Physical Therapy
Pomona, New Jersey
Garden State Infectious Disease Clinic,
    Early Intervention Program (EIP)- HIV Clinic
Voorhees, New Jersey
University of Pennsylvania – Philadelphia,
    Chronic Pain and Alternative Therapy
Rehabilitation Medicine Department
Philadelphia, Pennsylvania

BRANT GOODE, RN, C
Communicable Disease Intervention Specialist
Missoula City-County Health Department
Missoula, Montana

ANNE HARTLEY, BPHE, DIP ATM, CAT(C), DOMP
Sheridan College, Sports Injury Management Program
Oakville, Ontario

Susan J. Herdman, PT, PhD
Professor
Department of Rehabilitation Medicine and Otolaryngology
Emory University School of Medicine
Atlanta, Georgia

Hollis Herman, MS, PT, OCS
Healthy Women
Cambridge, Massachusetts

Marcia M. Herrin, EdD, MPH, RD
Co-Director, Eating Disorders Prevention, Education
 and Treatment Program
Dartmouth College
Hanover, New Hampshire

Ellen Hillegass, MMSc, PT, CCS
Georgia State University
Department of Physical Therapy
College of Health Sciences
Atlanta, Georgia

Elizabeth Greenslade Hockey, MEd, PT
Department of Rehabilitation Services
University Hospitals of Cleveland
Cleveland, Ohio

Carole L. Johnson, PT, PhD
Fall City, Washington

Zoher F. Kapasi, PhD, PT
Assistant Professor
Division of Physical Therapy
Department of Rehabilitation Medicine
Emory University
Atlanta, Georgia

Karen G. Kendall, PT, CWS
Medical Center for Continuing Education
Gulf Breeze, Florida

Guenter Klose, LMT
Director/Certified Instructor
Klose-Norton Training & Consulting
Red Bank, New Jersey

Harriett Baugh Loehne, PT, CWS
Wound Care Clinical Educator
Archbold Wound Care Center Program
Archbold Medical Center
Thomasville, Georgia

Louis Marzella, MD, PhD
Food and Drug Agency
Bethesda, Maryland

Mary Massery, PT
Owner, Massery Physical Therapy
Adjunct Faculty, Northwestern University
Glenview, Illinois

Leonard N. Matheson, PhD, CVE
Director, ERIC Human Performance Laboratory
Assistant Research Professor
Program in Occupational Therapy
Washington University School of Medicine
St. Louis, Missouri

Matt Maxwell, MD
International Heart Institute of Montana
Missoula, Montana

R.G. Murney, MD
Western Montana Clinic
Missoula, Montana

Lee B. Nelson, MS, PT
Clinical Professor
Department of Physical Therapy
University of Vermont
South Burlington, Vermont

Cynthia E. Neville, PT
Progressive Step Rehabilitation Services
Jacksonville Beach, Florida

Patricia O'Brien, MD
Associate Professor of Medicine
University of Vermont
College of Medicine
South Burlington, Vermont

Donna S. Oldfield, PT
Gulf States Hemophilia Diagnostic
 and Thrombophilia Center
University of Texas – Houston Medical School
Houston, Texas

Lucinda Pfalzer, PhD, PT, FACSM
Professor and Associate Director
Physical Therapy Department
School of Health Professions and Studies
University of Michigan – Flint
Flint, Michigan

Susan Polich, MT (ASCP), PT, MEd
Assistant Clinical Professor
Physical Therapy Department
Northeastern University
Boston, Massachusetts

William A. Reynolds, MD, MACP
Endocrinologist
Staff Physician – Western Montana Clinic (retired)
Clinical Professor Emeritus, University of Washington
Missoula, Montana

George Risi, MD
Infectious Disease Clinician
Missoula, Montana

JUDY L. SCHMIDT, MD, FACP
Board Certified in Hematology, Oncology & Internal
  Medicine
Community Physician Center
Missoula, Montana

KEVIN M. SCHOENBERGER, PT (RETIRED)
Primary Children's Medical Center
Salt Lake City, Utah

WILLIAM J. SCHWARZ, PT
Massapequa Park, New York

LANA SINEATH, PT, RN
Medical University of South Carolina (MUSC)
Medical Center
Charleston, South Carolina

WAYNE STUBERG, PT, PhD, PCS
Associate Professor and Director
Physical Therapy, Brace Place & Motion Lab
Munroe-Meyer Institute
Omaha, Nebraska

CARRIE SUSSMAN, PT
Sussman Physical Therapy
Member Of the APTA Integumentary Guide Practice
  Patterns Panel
National Pressure Ulcer Advisory Panel
Torrance, California

VALERIE WANG, PT
St. Luke's Rehabilitation Institute
Spokane, Washington

MITCHEL A. WOLTERSDORF, PhD, PT
Wesley Rehabilitation Hospital
Midwest Brain Function Clinic
Wichita, Kansas

Dedicated to the wonderful staff members at WB Saunders Company.
This edition especially goes to thank Julie Lawley for her many years of dedication
in the Permissions department.

CCG

To the next generation: Joshua, Jacob, Eliya, Becky, Brandee, and Paul.

WGB

To my many patients who suffer the effects of neurological dysfunction.
You have been my inspiration to learn, and you have taught me so much
about how to live my life.

KSF

FOREWORD

*B*eing a physical therapist has two special joys. One is seeing the progress that our patients make each day in our care. Another is the satisfaction found in knowing and growing with our colleagues. This text epitomizes both of these joys for me.

Pathology: Implications for the Physical Therapist represents an important contribution to the quality of care that we provide to our patients. Knowledge of the pathology of disease has always stood as one of the fundamental prerequisites to safe and effective health care practice. By understanding principles of pathology, we can put names to the problems we find in our patients. These names, or diagnoses, allow us to then classify our patients to lead to effective interventions with maximum outcome.

With the development and application of the disablement model, physical therapists, along with others, have been able to place pathology in its appropriate context. Rather than seeing pathology as the primary, and perhaps single, basis for understanding and naming illness, the disablement model places pathology as the initiation of a cascade of affects that can lead to impairments, functional limitations, disability, and handicap. Physical therapists recognize that we also name these impairments and functional limitations in diagnosing and classifying our patients.

Catherine Goodman, William Boissonnault, and Kenda Fuller set their presentation of pathology in this context. This text not only provides the basis for our conversations with other health care practitioners about our patients, but it also frames that conversation in the clinical decisions that we, as physical therapists, make about and with our patients. We must understand pathology and the changes it induces in our patients, and then we must use this knowledge to help us make accurate diagnoses that lead to accurate prognoses about the ability of our patients to benefit from our interventions. The format of this text, with its grounding in the disablement model, its presentation of pathology, the addition of the medical and surgical management of patients with specific pathology, and, finally, special implications for physical therapists, provides students and clinicians alike with the basis for our clinical decisions. In addition, the authors provide extensive text and journal references so that readers can seek the evidence that supports the authors' contentions.

The authors' concern about the quality of our care is imbued throughout the text. Because of this concern, the authors' attention to detail, and the application of the disablement model, the text offers us an important and useful tool to improve our patient care. It can be used successfully by students, faculty, and clinicians as a reference for patient care, helping them to experience the true joy providing the best possible physical therapy care to their patients.

This text has also given me the opportunity to experience the second joy to be found in our field. Physical therapy continues to grow and expand, but it remains a closely-knit group, offering many opportunities for development of a true community, with all of the interrelationships found in a community of colleagues. I have had the great pleasure to meet and interact with almost all of the authors and reviewers of this text. They continually impress me with their professional expertise and their dedication to improving physical therapy. Bill Boissonnault has provided important leadership in the area of orthopedic physical therapy through his clinical care, teaching, and professional activities. But I take special pride in my professional relationship with Catherine Cavallaro Goodman. I first met Cat many years ago when she was a student and I was a teacher and her advisor in the physical therapy program at the University of Pennsylvania. In the intervening years, we have each taken a different path. How wonderful it is to have these paths occasionally intertwine, to be able to point with pride and joy to her many contributions to our field, and to see the excitement, enthusiasm, and expertise she brings to her writing and teaching.

Physical therapy is truly a source of joy and excitement for those of us blessed to be part of this profession. *Pathology: Implications for the Physical Therapist* offers us one more opportunity to strengthen the quality of the care we provide our patients. I am confident that readers will agree with me that this is indeed cause for celebration. May they all enjoy the contribution of this text to our profession!

Laurita M. Hack, PT, MBA, PhD, FAPTA

PREFACE

The community of physical and occupational therapists has responded to this text in an overwhelmingly positive way. Although many health care professionals from a variety of backgrounds will find this an appropriate text for study and reference, whenever possible, the terminology and concepts of the Guide to Physical Therapist Practice (referred to as the Guide), developed by the American Physical Therapy Association, have been integrated into this second edition.

The Guide was developed as an expert consensus document by panels of clinicians and then reviewed by over 1000 therapists across the country. Three conceptual models are integrated throughout the Guide: the (Nagi) Disablement Model, the Integration of Prevention and Wellness Strategies, and the Patient/Client Management Model.

The Disablement Model extends the scope of the medical model of disease with its primary emphasis on diagnosis and treatment of disease by placing the focus on the functional consequences of disease. Both the medical model and the Disablement Model are reflected in this text. Diagnosis and treatment of disease in this text are presented following the medical model along with the Disablement Model's assessment of the impact of acute and chronic conditions on the functioning of specific body systems (impairments) and basic human performance (functional limitations).

Thus the reader will see terminology reflective of these two models such as "etiology," "pathogenesis," "diagnosis," and "prognosis" from the traditional medical model and "impairments," "interventions," "desired outcomes," and "functional limitations" from the Disablement Model.

The Guide includes a section of specific diagnostic groups referred to as Preferred Practice Patterns that represent the major body systems and are designed to facilitate a systems approach to patient/client management. The Practice Patterns are described in four sections: musculoskeletal, neuromuscular, cardiovascular/pulmonary, and integumentary. We were unable to place all diseases included just within these four categories. Rather, this text continues to follow a medical model in its presentation of diseases because the therapist will encounter multiple medical co-morbidities that extend beyond the four categories of preferred practice patterns outlined in the Guide.

Although therapists do not usually devise intervention strategies for primary systemic conditions, they must be aware of the impact that such diseases may have on the rehabilitation process. Therapists play an important role in disease prevention and health promotion so whenever possible, risk factor reduction and prevention strategies are a part of the discussion surrounding each disease.

In addition to integrating information from the APTA's Guide and updating scientific and medical information, this second edition continues to offer details about the clinical impact of diseases and "dis-eased" body systems on clinical interventions. Whenever possible, a new special section on the role of exercise and each condition or pathology is included to reflect the current understanding of the importance of exercise as a primary intervention for many diseases. The key strength of this text continues to be the Special Implications for the Therapist, whether the therapist is a student with that first client or a seasoned clinician of many years.

Catherine Cavallaro Goodman

ACKNOWLEDGMENTS

We wrote the first edition of this text without the benefit of e-mail and only Internet access to the National Library of Medicine. We were naïve in the undertaking! Now that we know better and are armed with the benefits of electronic communication, there are many people who deserve our thanks and praise. First, to the reviewers who gave their time and expertise without financial reward ... your names are in lights on the Reviewers page! Special thanks to the physical therapy community across the United States and those closer to home in our own communities for their ongoing support of this project.

We offer thanks to those people and organizations who shared their slides, handouts, notes, abstracts, poster presentations, and other resources with us... and to all who contributed to the formation of the *Guide to the Physical Therapist Practice*.

A special thanks to all the physicians who answered questions, reviewed materials, responded to countless phone calls and e-mail requests for information; to Nola Rodahl Levison, RN, PT for her invaluable and extensive research assistance; and to Rick Aldred for keeping my computer system up and running and answering the same technology questions over and over.

The lymphatic chapter (Chapter 12) is dedicated by the chapter author (Bonnie Lasinski) to the late Dr. John Ross Casley-Smith and to Dr. Judith Casley-Smith—pioneers in the field of lymphology, dedicated teachers, tireless patient advocates, mentors, and friends. Special thanks to Drs. Marvin Boris and Stanley Weindorf; Denise Tucker, PTA; Maureen Brady, PTA; Sharon Betz, PTA; Elena Reicher PTA; Kristine Belardo, PTA; Candis Glasgow Yarde, PTA; and Allan Goldblatt, PA for their tireless efforts to improve the care for individuals living with lymphedema. A heartfelt thanks goes to the chapter reviewers Marvin Boris, MD; Patricia O'Brien, MD; Lee Nelson, PT; and Guenter Klose, LMT for their time and suggestions. To my editor, Catherine Goodman – Thank you for believing in this project and for your constant encouragement and support. Finally, to my family, Paul, Matthew, and Andrew, for their patience and support.

Thanks go to the staff of St. Patrick Hospital, Missoula, Montana, especially the medical library staff, Marianne Farr and Kathy Murphy for seeing us through two editions of this text now.

Peg Waltner, our developmental editor for both editions ... it isn't true that you can't get help like you used to ... Peg's contribution to this text (and therefore to our profession) is outstanding.

To all at South Valley Physical Therapy for allowing me (Kenda Fuller) to leave the country to work on the manuscript and for questions answered during the preparation.

And always, to our families for standing by our sides, sometimes day and night, putting aside their time schedules, and contributing intangible love and support. To Cliff Goodman, especially, the "snack sultan," "captain of the cuisine," and the "garden guru": thanks for two entire summers of grocery shopping, errands, meal preparations, and family care from top to bottom, not to mention great sex on the side.

To these people and to the many others who remain unnamed but not forgotten, we say thank you. Your support and encouragement have made this text possible.

Catherine Cavallaro Goodman
William G. Boissonnault
Kenda S. Fuller

CONTENTS

Section III Pathology of the Musculoskeletal System

CHAPTER 1

INTRODUCTION TO CONCEPTS OF PATHOLOGY

CATHERINE C. GOODMAN

PATHOGENESIS OF DISEASE

Pathology is defined as the branch of medicine that investigates the essential nature of disease, especially changes in body tissues and organs that cause or are caused by disease.[31] *Clinical pathology* in medicine refers to pathology applied to the solution of clinical problems, especially the use of laboratory methods in clinical diagnosis. *Pathogenesis* is the development of unhealthy conditions or disease, or more specifically, the cellular events and reactions and other pathologic mechanisms that occur in the development of disease.

This text examines the pathogenesis of each disease or condition—that is, the progression of each pathologic condition on both its cellular level and clinical presentation whenever signs and symptoms are manifested. For the therapist, clinical pathology has a different meaning regarding the effects of pathologic processes (i.e., disease) on the individual's functional abilities and limitations. The relationship between impairment and functional limitation is the key focus in therapy.

To this end, we have incorporated practice patterns, outlined in the *Guide to Physical Therapist Practice,* which was developed by the American Physical Therapy Association[3] as an expert consensus document. Three conceptual models are integrated throughout the *Guide:* the (Nagi) Disablement Model, the Integration of Prevention and Wellness Strategies, and the Patient/Client Management Model. The Disablement Model extends the scope of the medical model of disease with its primary emphasis on diagnosis and treatment of disease by placing the focus on the functional consequences of disease. Both the medical model and the Disablement Model are reflected in this text. Diagnosis and treatment of disease are presented after the medical model, along with the Disablement Model's assessment of the impact of acute and chronic conditions on the functioning of specific body systems (impairments) and basic human performance (functional limitations).

Using these tools and this revised definition of clinical pathology, we ask the following: *How does this particular disease or condition affect this person's functional abilities and functional outcome? What precautions should be taken when someone with this condition is exercising? Should vital signs be monitored during therapy for this disease? How will that information affect the treatment plan or intervention?*

Each individual client must be evaluated on the basis of the clinical presentation in conjunction with the underlying pathology. For example, the person with osteoporosis may require joint mobilization, but this technique must be modified for the presence of osteoporosis. The individual with cardiac valvular disease may need a different exercise program than that prescribed for a healthy athlete. The adult with musculoskeletal symptoms of thoracic spine pain, muscle spasm, and loss of thoracic motion who has a primary medical diagnosis (e.g., posterior penetrating ulcer) will be unaffected by therapy techniques.

The *Guide* includes a section of specific diagnostic groups referred to as *Preferred Practice Patterns* that represent the major body systems and are designed to facilitate a systems approach to patient/client management. The Practice Patterns are described in four sections: musculoskeletal, neuromuscular, cardiopulmonary, and integumentary. It is not possible to place all diseases included just within these four categories at this time. The therapist will encounter multiple medical comorbidities that extend beyond the four categories of preferred practice patterns outlined in the *Guide.* However, therapists will not be devising intervention strategies for liver disease, for example, but must be aware of the impact that such diseases may have on the rehabilitation process. The most likely practice patterns associated with each disease or disorder discussed are presented in the *Special Implications for the Therapist* boxes. These patterns may vary with each episode of care, depending on clinical presentation.

Advances in medicine have resulted in a population with greater longevity but also with a more complex pathologic picture. Orthopedic and neurologic conditions are no longer present as singular phenomena; they often occur in a person with other medical pathology. We must be knowledgeable of the impact other conditions and diseases have on the individual's neuromusculoskeletal system, and the necessary steps must be taken to provide safe, effective treatment. Specific therapy interventions are not the focus of this text but whenever possible, risk factor reduction strategies are offered, since risk factors are a part of the discussion surrounding each disease and therapists play an important role in disease prevention and health promotion.

CONCEPTS OF HEALTH AND ILLNESS

◆ Health

Many people and organizations have attempted to define the concept of health but no universally accepted definition has been adopted. A dictionary definition describes health in terms of an individual's ability to function normally in society.

1

Some definitions characterize health as a disease-free state or condition. The World Health Organization[36] has defined *health* as a state of complete physical, mental, and social well-being and not merely as the absence of disease or infirmity. All of these definitions present health as an either/or circumstance, meaning an individual is either healthy or ill.

Health is more accurately viewed as a continuum on which wellness, on one end, is the optimal level of function and illness, on the other, may be so unfavorable as to result in death. Health is a dynamic process that varies with changes in interactions between an individual and the internal and external environments. This type of definition recognizes health as an individual's level of wellness. Health reflects a person's biologic, psychologic, spiritual, and sociologic state. The *biologic* or physical state refers to the overall structure of the individual's body tissues and organs, and to the biochemical interactions and functions within the body. The *psychological* state includes the individual's mood, emotions, and personality. The *spiritual* aspect of health addresses the individual's religious needs, which may be affected by illness or injury. The *sociologic* or social state refers to the interaction between the individual and the social environment. A high level of wellness or holistic health is achieved when the biopsychosocial needs of a person are met.

◆ Illness

Definition.   *Illness* is often defined as sickness or deviation from a healthy state, and the term has a broader meaning than disease. *Disease* refers to a biologic or psychologic alteration that results in a malfunction of a body organ or system. Disease is usually a term used to describe a biomedical condition that is substantiated by objective data, such as elevated temperature or presence of infection (as demonstrated by positive blood cultures). Illness is the perception and response of the person to not being well. Illness includes disturbances in normal human biologic function and personal, interpersonal, and cultural reactions to disease. Disease can occur in an individual without he or she being aware of illness and without others perceiving illness. However, a person can feel very ill even though no obvious pathologic processes can be identified.[15]

Acute Illness.   *Acute illness* usually refers to an illness or disease that has a relatively rapid onset and short duration. The condition often responds to a specific treatment and is usually self-limiting, although exceptions to this definition are numerous (see Chapter 7). If no complications occur, most acute illnesses end in a full recovery, and the individual returns to the previous level of functioning. *Subacute* refers to a condition or illness that is somewhat acute (i.e., between acute and chronic). Chronic conditions sometimes flare up and may be referred to as *subacute*.

Acute illnesses usually follow a specific sequence, or stages of illness, from onset through recovery. The first stage involves the experience of physical symptoms (e.g., pain, shortness of breath, fever); cognitive awareness (i.e., the symptoms are interpreted to have meaning); and an emotional response, usually one of denial, fear, or anxiety.

Subsequent stages of an acute illness may include assumption of a sick role as the person recognizes the problem as being sufficient to require contact with a health care professional. If the illness is confirmed, the individual continues in the sick role; if it is not confirmed, a return to normalcy may occur or the person may continue to seek health care to identify the illness. A stage of dependency* occurs when the person receives and accepts a diagnosis and treatment plan. Depending on the severity of the illness, the individual may give up independence and control and assume a more dependent sick role. During this stage, sick people often become more passive and concerned about themselves. Most people move to the final stage of recovery or rehabilitation. During this stage, the individual gives up the sick role and resumes more normal activities and responsibilities. Individuals with long-term or chronic illnesses may require a longer period to adjust to new lifestyles.

Chronic Illness.   Chronic illness describes illnesses that include one or more of the following characteristics: permanent impairment or disability, residual physical or cognitive disability, or the need for special rehabilitation and/or long-term medical management. Chronic illnesses and conditions may fluctuate in intensity as acute exacerbations occur that cause physiologic instability and necessitate additional medical management (e.g., diabetes mellitus, fibromyalgia, rheumatoid arthritis). A person who has exacerbations of chronic illness may progress through the stages of illness described in the previous section.

Psychologic Aspects.   The most important factor influencing psychologic reactions to illness is the premorbid (before illness) psychologic profile of the affected person. For example, a person with a dependent-type personality may become very dependent, perhaps seeking unusually great amounts of advice or reassurance from the health care specialist or expecting attention beyond that required for the degree of illness present. A narcissistic (self-centered) person may be particularly concerned about the need to take medication or the loss of the ability to work. The stoic person (indifferent to or unaffected by pain) may have difficulty admitting to being sick at all.

Other factors that affect a person's psychologic reaction include the extent of the illness and the particular symptoms that develop. Extremely mild disease may have little effect, whereas completely unexpected and debilitating illness may be very distressing. A common reaction to any illness is fear or anxiety related to the loss of control over one's own body. Denial is an unconscious defense mechanism that allows a person to avoid painful reality as long as possible. Denial can be a natural part of the process of dealing with illness, which culminates in acceptance.

Noncompliance with treatment may have a psychologic basis (e.g., denial: "There is nothing wrong with me, so I do not need medical treatment."), but it may also occur as a result of previous experience. For example, noncompliance with prescribed corticosteroid therapy may be based on aversion to side effects experienced during use of this drug during previous disease flare. With chronic autoimmune diseases (e.g., connective tissue diseases), denial may continue for years as a

---

*This type of dependency in the psychologically and emotionally balanced person represents awareness, acceptance, reliance on diagnosis, and care beyond self-help. This definition of dependency differs from dependency associated with dependent personality disorder, in which the affected person lacks self-confidence or the ability to function independently, and allows others to assume responsibility for his or her care.

coping mechanism for the individual who continues to decline in physical functional capacity.

It is important to recognize that psychologic or psychiatric symptoms such as impairment of memory; personality changes (e.g., paranoia); loss of impulse control; or mood disorders (e.g., persistent depression or elation) can have a functional or organic basis. Functional symptoms occur without significant physical dysfunction of brain cells, whereas organic symptoms can be caused by abnormal physiologic changes in brain tissue. An example of a functional symptom is depression that is considered to be the psychologic consequence of a general medical condition (e.g., myocardial infarction).

Organic symptoms occur as a direct physiologic consequence of a medication (see Table 2-14) or medical condition (see Table 2-12). For example, onset of corticosteroid-induced psychologic symptoms are often dose-related, and subside as the corticosteroids are tapered. Another example of an organic basis for symptomatology is the person with systemic lupus erythematosus (SLE) who experiences symptoms of organic mental disorders secondary to SLE-mediated vasculitis, called *lupus cerebritis*, or the person with end-stage liver disease who develops hepatic encephalopathy when toxic substances in the blood, such as ammonia, reach the brain.

◆ Disability Classifications[19,23]

Disability is a large public health problem in the United States affecting an estimated 54 million people who report disabling conditions. Prevalence* of disability is higher among women than among men and is reported highest among people 65 years and older. One of the national health goals for 2010 is to eliminate health disparities among different segments of the population, including among people with disabilities. National estimates of disability range from 15% to 20% for adults over the age of 18 years but these figures are most likely underestimated and do not account for severity or duration of disability.[13] The World Health Organization (WHO) has identified 483 disabilities related to 107 diseases and injuries most common throughout the world and has introduced the concept of disability-adjusted life years (DALY) to estimate the cost of a lost year of healthy life. The WHO is seeking to quantify not just the number of disabilities but also the impact of disability on a population.[37]

Physical Disability
World Health Organization Model.   The WHO[38] has developed an International Classification of Impairments, Disabilities, and Handicaps (ICIDH) to provide a conceptual framework for standardization of data and monitoring of chronic and disabling conditions. The ICIDH clarifies the concepts common to rehabilitation and further defines impairments, disability, and handicap.

Impairment is any loss or abnormality of psychologic, physiologic, or anatomic structure or function (e.g., range-of-motion limitations, decreased strength or muscle performance, edema, lack of sensation). Impairments can be temporary or permanent and are considered to occur at the organ level.

Another example is proprioceptive loss in an extremity, resulting in decreased sensory input to the central nervous system.

Disability is any restriction or lack of ability to perform an activity in a normal manner or within the normal range. A person's disability status or activity restriction describes how the impairment affects activities at work or home or participation in sports. The disability resulting from an impairment in proprioception might be excessive weight shift away from the affected extremity. The person may be at greater risk of falling. Not all disease leads to impairment, and not all impairment leads to disability. For example, diabetes can result in impairment (e.g., diminished circulation), but not all people with diabetes sustain a disability (e.g., vision loss or amputation).[14]

A *handicap* is a disadvantage for an impaired or disabled individual that limits or prevents the fulfillment of normal life roles. An example of a handicap would be the inability to be independently mobile in the community due to lack of stability required in the diverse environmental situations encountered there.

Nagi Model.   A second system often used by health care professionals to classify the impact of disease or trauma is the Nagi health status model.[30] The Nagi model differs from the ICIDH in the use of the terms functional limitation and disability (Table 1-1). Nagi proposed that functional limitations were the result of impairments and consisted of an individual's inability to perform the tasks and roles that constitute usual activities for that individual. According to the Nagi model, *disability* is defined as the patterns of behavior that emerge over long periods of time when functional limitations cannot be overcome to create normal task performance or role fulfillment.

Cognitive Disability.[35]   Problems such as mental illnesses like depression, alcoholism, schizophrenia and cognitive impairments, although responsible for only about 1% of deaths, are seriously underestimated sources of disabilities that account for 11% of the world's disease burden.[37] These conditions are often undiagnosed and although therapists cannot diagnose these impairments, recognizing the deficits is important. Only cognitive disability is discussed in this section; common mental illnesses are discussed in Chapter 2. Five types of cognitive deficit are associated with specific areas of brain damage and linked to possible causes that may be barriers to successful treatment (Table 1-2).

TABLE	1-1	o

Disability Classifications

ICIDH MODEL	NAGI MODEL
Disease	Disease
Impairment	Impairment
Disability	Functional limitations
Handicap	Disability

Data from Fuller K, Huber L: Improving postural control through integration of sensory inputs and visual biofeedback, *Top Stroke Rehabil* 1:32–47, 1995.
ICIDH, International Classification of Impairments, Disabilities, and Handicaps.

Prevalence measures all cases of a condition (new and old) among those at risk for developing the condition. Measures of prevalence are made at one point in time (e.g., on a specific day). *Incidence* is the number of new cases of a condition in a specific period of time (e.g., 6 months or 1 year) in relation to the total number of people in the population who are "at risk" at the beginning of the period.

TABLE	1-2

Types of Cognitive Deficits

TYPE	LESION	ETIOLOGIC FACTORS	THERAPIST STRATEGIES
Decreased executive functions	Right hemisphere lesion, frontal lobe damage	Car accidents, whiplash injuries, exposure to organic solvents, HIV/AIDS complications, Korsakoff's disease, Parkinson's disease, craniotomy	More active role in maintaining treatment program, educating family and client's employer, and teaching self-monitoring skills; include pacing in treatment regimen; use home trainers; closely monitor all clinic activities; teach time management techniques; include client in group activities; do not take socially inappropriate behavior personally
Poor complex problem solving	Diffuse and/or global cortical damage	Exposure to occupational toxins, postsurgical anoxia, stroke, hydrocephalus, small-vessel disease associated with hypertension	Fragment treatment program into small pieces and reassemble pieces into coherent whole when each has been well learned; turn the new into the familiar through repetition; reduce complexity of treatment components; avoid abstract visual aids and abstract verbal explanations
Slowed information processing	Diffuse cortical or subcortical system damage, reticular activating system of the brainstem	Alcohol abuse, drug abuse, exposure to toxins, developmental delays, traumatic brain injury	Slow the rate of presentation; remove environmental distractors; do not speak loudly as though client were hearing impaired; simply present one type of information at a time, making sure the client understands you before you move on
Memory deficits	Temporal lobe damage	Alcohol abuse, temporal lobe injuries, seizures, traumatic brain injury, exposure to toxins, age-related deterioration	Make certain that no learning or emotional disorder is involved; use external aids and multichannel approaches to improve retention of information; determine which aid or approach works best for each individual
Learning disabilities	Unclear	Unknown, possibly traumatic birth or genetic predisposition, early acquired brain damage, metabolic abnormalities	Avoid written material unless it is appropriate to the person's reading level; use nonverbal modes of communication

Modified from Woltersdorf MA: Beyond the sensorimotor strip, *Clin Manage* 12:63-69, 1992.
HIV, human immunodeficiency virus; *AIDS*, acquired immunodeficiency syndrome.

Executive functions may be described as cortical functions involved in formulating goals and in planning, initiating, monitoring, and maintaining behavior.[25] *Behavior* is defined here in its broadest terms to include not only overt motor behavior but also affective and social behavior. A person with executive function deficits typically appears inert or apathetic. Clinically, these clients typically have a right hemisphere lesion and apraxia, unilateral neglect, or both. When frontal lobe damage occurs, the effects of impaired executive functions may be attributed to depression. Although the two may occur simultaneously, depression is usually characterized by a lack of energy, whereas impaired executive functions are demonstrated by a lack of involvement.

Complex problem solving may be described as the effective handling of new information. Impaired problem solving results in concrete thinking, inability to distinguish the relevant from the irrelevant, erroneous application of rules, and difficulty generalizing from one situation to another. For example, when a client learns how to accomplish wheelchair transfers and then generalizes that information to various settings (bed to chair, chair to toilet, chair to car, in hospital, at home), he or she is using new information in complex problem-solving.

Information processing involves the speed with which information travels from one part of the brain to another and the amount of information assimilated at that speed.[25] Whereas complex problem-solving has to do with the orchestration of information, information processing involves the efficient transfer of information. As a result of genetic, environmental, and educational factors, some people are more proficient processors than others. As a result of trauma, some people may lose processing ability and speed. Noise levels, external sensory stimulation (e.g., presence of other people and other activities), and presentation of more than one kind of information at a time (e.g., providing a written home program then discussing the time of the next appointment) are examples of distractions to people with reduced information processing abilities.

Memory deficits result from a failure to store or retrieve information. Before it can be determined that the person is experiencing a memory lapse, it must be established that the material was learned in the first place. Memory problems typically are acquired rather than developmental. Depression may masquerade as memory loss, but the depressed person is usually less attentive or interactive with the environment and therefore registers (or learns) less. For example, a client may appear to be suffering from a memory dysfunction when, in fact, the decreased attention span is a result of depression that has reduced learning.

Learning disability occurs in a person with normal or near-normal intelligence as difficulty acquiring information in specific domains, such as spelling, arithmetic, reading, and visual-spatial relationships. Therapists most commonly encounter learning disabilities manifested as noncompliance with written treatment programs, repeated tardiness or absence for treatment sessions, and an overly anxious approach to the physical symptoms that have brought the client to the therapist in the first place.

Special Implications for the Therapist   1-1

DISABILITY CLASSIFICATIONS

Physical Disability

The *APTA Guide to the Physical Therapist Practice*[3] was developed for clinical use by physical therapists as an expert consensus document. Panels of clinicians were involved in the first step of formulating the *Guide,* and then more than 1000 therapists across the country participated in reviewing the document. Three conceptual models are integrated throughout the *Guide:* the (Nagi) Disablement Model, the Integration of Prevention and Wellness Strategies, and the Patient/Client Management Model.

The Disablement Model moves away from the medical model of disease (i.e., primary emphasis on diagnosis and treatment of disease) and places the focus on the functional consequences of disease. Both the medical model and the Disablement Model are reflected in this text. Diagnosis and treatment of disease in this text is presented after the medical model along with the Disablement Model's assessment of the impact of acute and chronic conditions on the functioning of specific body systems (impairments) and basic human performance (functional limitations).

Thus the reader will see terminology reflective of these two models such as *etiology, pathogenesis, diagnosis,* and *prognosis* from the traditional medical model and *impairments, interventions, desired outcomes,* and *functional limitations* from the Disablement Model.

Cognitive Disability

Although therapists cannot diagnose cognitive deficits, the therapist's evaluation and clinical observations may help identify cognitive deficits that might interfere with treatment. Appropriate referral is always recommended when problems beyond our expertise are suspected. Specific rehabilitation and training strategies for people with cognitive disabilities are available.[35] ∎

◆ Theories of Health and Illness[8]

Germ Theory.   Many theories exist as to the cause of illnesses. In the latter part of the nineteenth century, Louis Pasteur took medicine out of the Dark Ages. It was not "bad air" or "bad blood" that caused diseases like malaria and yellow fever but pathogens transmitted by mosquitoes. Pasteur's germ theory promoted our understanding of infectious disease and helped reduce deaths from infection. Pasteur proposed that a specific microorganism was capable of causing an infectious disease. Infections such as poliomyelitis; tuberculosis; human immunodeficiency virus (HIV) associated with acquired immunodeficiency syndrome (AIDS); or legionellosis (legionnaire's disease) are caused by a known agent. Once the causative agent is identified, specific treatment methods can be determined.

Pasteur's germ theory has been labeled *Germ Theory, Part I* and has been expounded on by today's biologists in what is referred to as *Germ Theory, Part II.* Taken from Darwin's description of how an organism and its environment fit together, it is now restated that the success of an organism is relative to competing organisms. According to this theory, genetic traits that may be unfavorable to an organism's survival or reproduction do not persist in the gene pool for very long. Natural selection, by its very definition, weeds them out in short order. By this logic, any inherited disease or trait that has a serious impact on fitness must fade over time because the genes responsible for the disease or trait will be passed on to fewer and fewer individuals in future generations. Common illnesses that cannot be linked to genetics or to some hostile environmental element (including lifestyle) must have some other explanation.

The current germ theory suggests that diseases present in human populations for many generations that still have a substantial negative impact may have an infectious origin. Chronic diseases of the late twentieth century that have been considered hereditary, environmental, or multifactorial may in fact be caused by an infectious pathogen. For example, *herpes viruses* have been linked to multiple sclerosis, Kaposi's sarcoma, B-cell lymphomas, Burkitt's lymphoma, and several other forms of cancer. *Helicobacter pylori,* found in the stomachs of a third of adults in the United States, causes inflammation of the stomach lining and can result in ulcers. In most cases, these ulcers can be cured in less than a month with antibiotics. The lymphoid tissue of the stomach can produce a low-grade gastric lymphoma under the influence of this bacterium. Early reports indicate that the lymphoma is cured in

50% of cases by resolving the *H. pylori* infections, which may mark the first time in medical history that cancer has been cured with an antibiotic.[1]

Heart disease is now being linked to *Chlamydia pneumoniae*, a newly discovered bacterium that causes pneumonia and bronchitis. Several studies have now shown that people who have had a heart attack have high levels of antibodies to *C. pneumoniae* and that about 50% of adults in the United States carry these antibodies.[27,29] Regardless of whether this finding supports an infectious cause for the development of atherosclerosis and subsequent coronary artery disease remains a topic of intense research at this time. See Chapter 7 for further discussion of the relationship between infectious pathogens and chronic diseases.

The Germ Theory, Part II also hypothesizes that clinical depression or mental illness such as schizophrenia may have an underlying infectious basis given how common these conditions are in the general population. According to Germ Theory proponents, natural selection should have eliminated any genes for these conditions to ensure survival and reproduction. No one has found a depression virus or a schizophrenia virus yet but research continues in this area. The germ theory cannot explain all diseases, and other more complex theories have been postulated.

Biomedical Model. The biomedical model explains disease as a result of malfunctioning organs or cells. Within this model, conditions can be classified as diseases if they have a recognized cause, if a change occurs in structure or function of an organ, and if a consistently identifiable group of signs and symptoms are apparent. The biomedical model focuses on cause-and-effect relationships but does not take into account psychosocial components of disease, such as varying reactions to a disease due to age, lifestyle, personality, and compliance with therapy.

Neither the germ theory nor the biomedical model can explain the widespread increase in noninfectious chronic diseases that affect modern civilizations. In the past, the high death rate from epidemics of infectious diseases meant that many people did not live long enough for chronic illnesses to develop, especially those that occur with aging. With the development of penicillin in 1928 and the subsequent development of other antibiotics, people in the twentieth century have had reduced mortality from infectious disease. Heart disease and cancer have become the center of focus—ailments that plague modern industrialized nations.

Multicausal Theory. It is now recognized that lifestyle, diet, and stress response contribute to the development of diseases, and treatment interventions are focusing more on the relationship of the individual with his or her external and internal environment. Multicausal theories have been proposed to take into account the many additional factors associated with health and the development of illness (Fig. 1-1). Many of these variables are discussed further in Chapter 3.

Homeostasis Theory. Homeostasis theories developed in the nineteenth century continue to be expanded on through the twenty-first century. Homeostasis is the body's ability to maintain its internal environment in a constant state of equilibrium despite external influences that promote imbalance. Homeostasis begins at the cellular level in that the cell re-

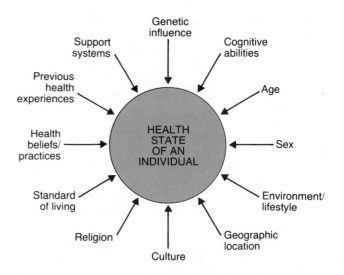

FIGURE 1-1 Multiple variables influence the health and illness of an individual. (From Ignatavicius DD, Workman ML, and Mishler MA: *Medical-surgical nursing: across the health care continuum*, ed 3, Philadelphia, 1999, WB Saunders.)

ceives nutrients, oxygen, water, and essential minerals from the environment. It uses these resources to generate energy, maintain its own integrity, and contribute to the body's internal stability. The body's ability to maintain temperature, blood pressure, and levels of fluid and electrolytes, serum glucose, blood oxygen, and carbon dioxide within a given range are examples of dynamic homeostasis that begins at the cellular level. External stimuli can alter the body's equilibrium or homeostasis. External demands may exceed the capacity of the cell to adapt, resulting in a permanent disequilibrium and injury or illness. *Injury* occurs when the cells or tissues have been required to adapt beyond their limitations. Like a muscle that has exceeded its ability to stretch, has ruptured, and is no longer able to contract, cells can be irreparably damaged and unable to return to the original steady state. Illness is the result of an imbalance in the body's (cell's) ability to regulate the internal environment. The concept of fight or flight to explain the body's reactions to emergencies was added to the homeostasis theory and continues to be used today to explain homeostasis as a dynamic equilibrium designed to maintain a steady state.

General Adaptation Syndrome. The general adaptation syndrome continued to build on the homeostasis theory and concept of fight or flight by describing a response to stress that, regardless of diagnosis, has common symptoms, such as appetite loss, weight loss, myalgias, and fatigue. The entire body responds to stress in an attempt to maintain or adapt through the autonomic and central nervous systems. If the demand or stress continues, the adaptive capacity of the body can be exceeded, and disease may result. This theory suggests that stress causes disease by placing excessive demands on the body, which in turn produces high levels of adaptive hormones, such as glucocorticoids, which reduce inflammation, and mineralocorticoid hormones, which regulate electrolyte and water metabolism. These hormones lower the body's resistance to disease and cause organ damage. When stress is continuous, the adaptive capacity of the body may be exceeded and disease (or even death) may result.

Psychosocial Theory.   Psychosocial theories of disease attempt to integrate physiologic, psychologic, and social factors to explain disease. An individual's degree of resistance to microbes depends largely on how well he or she is coping to internal and external stresses. Resistance to infectious disease, allergies, and possibly cancer depends on a well-functioning immune system. People who cope poorly with stress have significantly impaired immune responses, as manifested by a diminished activity level in natural killer cells. These are a special type of leukocyte that destroy viruses and cancer cells without having previously encountered them. Biopsychosocial concepts as they relate to health are discussed more fully in Chapter 2.

Psychoneuroimmunology Theory.   As new research added important information, the psychosocial theory has been modified to become the Psychoneuroimmunology (PNI)* Model first described in the 1980s. PNI is the study of the interactions among behavior and neural, endocrine, enteric, and immune system function. Illness was once thought of as the result of a breakdown within the immune system alone but immune function is now recognized as the integrative defense mechanism of multiple systems. This theory has outlined the influence of the nervous system on immune and inflammatory responses and how the immune system communicates with the neuro-endocrine systems. This information is very relevant in understanding host defenses and injury/repair processes. Further, the integration of the hypothalamic-pituitary-adrenal axis and the neuro-endocrine-enteric axis has a biologic basis first discovered in the late 1990s. Physiologically adaptive processes occur as a result of these biochemically based mind-body connections.

Candace Pert,[32] formerly a molecular biologist at the National Institutes of Health (NIH) made a groundbreaking discovery when she identified the biologic basis for emotions (neuropeptides and their receptors). This new understanding of the interconnections between the mind and body goes far beyond our former understanding of psychosomatic or psychosocial theories of health and illness. It is now known that these chemical messengers (sometimes referred to as *peptides, neuropeptides, ligands, neurotransmitters, or information molecules*) move through the blood stream to every cell of the body. When these chemicals find body cells that have receptors that attract them like magnets, they attach and make significant changes in that cell structure and organ system. These information molecules are the messengers the body uses to communicate between all the major body systems. For example, both the digestive (enteric) system and the neurologic system communicate with the immune system via these peptides. These three systems can exchange information and influence one another's actions.

Knowledge of PNI sheds new light on many of the previously postulated theories of health and illness, whereas understanding dysfunctions in the PNI system may highlight a wide variety of system disorders and diseases. For example, explaining how the body maintains homeostasis through autonomic temperature regulation (Homeostasis Theory) will now have an added dimension when considering the role of these information molecules or understanding that the sympathetic nervous system controls cardiovascular and immune functions, hormones control energy balance, and neurohormones control salt and fluid balance (General Adaptation Syndrome) via the interactions of the PNI. Continued research in this area has brought new information to light about the effects of variables such as stress and coping, personality, mental status, socioeconomic status, and work and family life and their role in the outcome of surgery or the development and progression of disease, morbidity, and mortality (e.g., Multicausal Theory, Psychosocial Theory).[6,20,30,33]

◆ Genetic Aspects of Disease

In addition to research on the biopsychosocial aspects of diseases, a great deal of recent research has gone into the genetic aspects of diseases. The completion of the Human Genome Project, combined with advances in technology, has enabled researchers to begin identifying the actual genes that encode particular disorders. It may be possible in the near future to treat altered gene structure (called *gene therapy*) to attempt to cure or control previously incurable diseases. The laboratory studies and advances in the collection of immune cells made it possible to begin clinical trials of gene therapy in the early 1990s. The recent explosion in biotechnology has advanced the field of genetic testing, a necessary component in the genetic treatment of diseases and disorders.

The Human Genome Project

Researchers have deciphered the genetic code by sequencing the 3.1 billion chemical subunits of deoxyribonucleic acid (DNA) and mapping their location in the 23 pairs of chromosomes in all cells. This work represents a scientific revolution referred to as the *Human Genome* Project. The goals of this project have been to identify all human genes, map the genes' locations on chromosomes, and ultimately provide detailed information from the genetic coding about how the genes function. Interestingly, 99.99% of the genome is the same across the human population, regardless of race or ethnic origin. Individual variations can increase the risk of disease as some people can become more vulnerable to bacteria, viruses, toxins, and chemicals, but the Human Genome Project dispels many previously held beliefs about biologically based racial differences.

Knowing the order in which these chemical units are arranged on each strand of DNA does not tell where the genes are located within the genome, the specific function of each gene in the sequence, or which genes make which proteins. In medicine, sequences will provide a basis for the study of susceptibility to disease, the pathogenesis of disease and the development of new preventative and therapeutic approaches. Additionally the completion of the human genome project has enhanced the widespread use of prenatal diagnosis, DNA

---

*The point is made by those who founded the research in this area that PNI is a misnomer because it reveals only part of the process and redundantly includes the brain as psycho and neuro, leaving out the powerful impact of the endocrine system.[32] The literature refers to this theory by a variety of names such as neuroendocrine immunology, neurogastroimmunology, psychoimmunonology, and is seemingly dependent on the system under investigation.

---

*Genome, meaning to produce, refers to the complete set of genes in the chromosomes of each cell of a specific organism or in this case the human genome. A genome map is the graphic representation of the locations of genes in a genome. The human genome map locates 5264 markers for genes and has led to the discovery of 223 genes linked to more than 200 diseases. The mouse genome map locates 7377 markers on 20 chomosomes.[5]

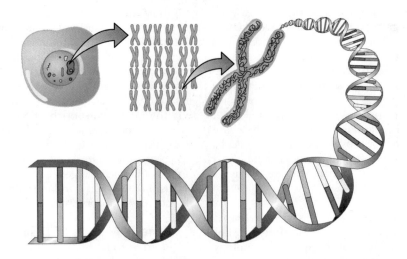

FIGURE   **1-2**   Schematic diagram of deoxyribonucleic acid (DNA). Inside the nucleus of nearly every cell in the body, a complex set of genetic instructions, known as the *human genome* is contained on 23 pairs of chromosomes. Chromosomes are made of long chains of a chemical called *DNA*, packaged into short segments called *genes*. Every cell of every human body contains a copy of the same DNA. Genes contain instructions to direct all body functions written in a molecular language. This molecular language is made up of four letters; each letter represents a molecule on the DNA: *a*denine, *c*ytosine, *g*uanine, *t*hymine. The As, Cs, Gs, and Ts form in triplets, constituting a code; each triplet of letters instructs the cell to attach to a particular amino acid (e.g., TGG attaches to amino acid tryptophan). Amino acids combined together form proteins. If the DNA language becomes garbled or a word is misspelled, the cell may make the wrong protein or too much or too little of the right one—mistakes that often result in disease.

chip technology, and will make it possible to analyze a sample of DNA collected from saliva. Drugs designed and prescribed to accommodate individual differences in metabolism may be possible from the data derived from this project. All of these areas of interest will be the substance of future studies.

Information about the genes is made available immediately on the Internet to scientists, clinicians, librarians, educators, and the general public. The cataloging and filing of this information is under the auspices of the Cancer Genome Anatomy Project (CGAP). By bringing together all the information about active or silent genes in a specific tumor-type, CGAP will help scientists make progress in the fight against cancer.*

Gene Therapy.[24]   Genes are the chemical messengers of heredity. Some 70,000 to 130,000 human genes are composed of DNA molecules along a double helix and carry instructions for synthesizing every protein that the body needs to function properly (Fig. 1-2). Their order determines the function of the gene. Genes determine everything from appearance to the regulation of everyday life processes (e.g., how efficiently we process foods, how effectively we fight infection).

DNA is composed of different combinations of molecules called *nucleic acids*. The sequence of nucleic acids provides instructions for assembling amino acids, which are the basic structural units of proteins (Fig. 1-3). A change in the normal DNA pattern of a particular gene is called a *mutation*. Some illnesses are caused by a tiny change in the DNA of just one gene, whereas others are caused by major changes in the DNA of multiple genes.

Most illnesses, including most cases of cancer, are caused by acquired mutations. Acquired mutations arise during normal daily life, usually during the process of cell division. Each day the body replaces thousands of worn-out cells. Some genetic errors are inevitable as old cells replicate and pass DNA flaws along to replacement (daughter) cells. When all goes well, daughter cells recognize these mutations and repair them, but the repair mechanism can fail or be disabled by environmental toxins and diet. Although acquired mutations can be passed on to daughter cells, they cannot be inherited.

More specifically, gene therapy (also known as *human genetic engineering*) is the process in which specific malfunctioning cells are targeted and repaired or replaced with corrected genes. Essentially, DNA is used like a drug, allowing it to replace or repair defective genes. It is hoped that the altered cells will yield daughter cells with healthy genes; these offspring cells will help eliminate the diseased cells. Alternately, cells can be genetically altered to contain a toxin-producing suicide gene to treat some cancers.[26]

Research is ongoing into such cures for a wide variety of hereditary disorders and diseases caused by aging (Box 1-1); some diseases such as hemophilia are being studied as a good model for gene therapy. Gene therapy for the treatment of diseases in children before birth is being actively pursued at many medical centers using animal models. In utero gene therapy (IUGT) could be beneficial for those with genetic diseases if gene therapy is performed before symptoms are manifested.[39]

Gene insertion has been used to successfully treat humans with inoperable coronary artery disease. Researchers injected a gene that makes a protein called *vascular endothelial growth factor* (VEG-F) into the hearts of candidates with severe chest

---

*The data are available on the Web at http://www.nhgri.nih.gov.

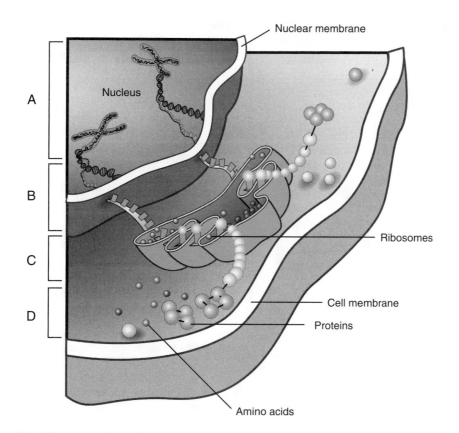

FIGURE   **1-3** The chain of events from DNA; this is how the DNA directs the cell. **A,** Ribonucleic acid (RNA) receives instructions from the DNA code in the chromosomes. **B,** The RNA travels from the nucleus to link up with ribosomes (protein-making units). **C,** Instructions from the code contained within the DNA are used by the RNA-ribosome complex to assemble amino acids. **D,** Cellular function is now directed by proteins containing the amino acids.

pain caused by ischemia that could not be corrected with bypass surgery or angioplasty. Tests suggest that once installed, the gene produces blood vessel-promoting proteins for 2 or 3 weeks (enough to grow a permanent new blood supply) before ceasing to work. The heart actually sprouts tiny new blood vessels (therapeutic angiogenesis) too small to be seen but with improved blood flow to the heart readily demonstrated.[21,34] Investigations continue to examine gene therapy strategies to deliver genes coding for the angiogens.

Gene therapy may take a number of different approaches. The original design was to inject one or more genes into the person to replace those that are absent or not functioning properly. A second approach called *small-molecule therapy* injects a small molecule (i.e., a drug) to modify the function of one or more genes in the body that is making a normal product but just too much or too little of it.

Other approaches include transferring a gene into cancer cells to sensitize them to drugs[17] or restoring immune function in HIV by transferring a therapeutic gene into target cells, rendering them resistant to HIV replication. Infusion of protected cells may limit virus spread and delay AIDS disease progression. Efforts are underway to deliver antiviral genes to hematopoietic stem cells to ensure a renewable supply of HIV-protected cells for the life of the individual.[11,12]

Some obstacles to gene therapy must be overcome before this procedure is considered a viable treatment option. Examples include finding appropriate harmless viral vectors to carry the normal gene to the target cells that do not provoke an immune response against them as foreign invaders or cause toxic side effects, engineering the transplanted genes to be efficient and effective, and finding ways to modify retrovirus vectors so they can carry the genes into nondividing cells (presently, genes can only be delivered to actively dividing cells when delivered by retrovirus vectors).

Ethical concerns have also been raised about the use of human genetic engineering for purposes other than therapy (e.g., eugenics). These include the use of genes to improve ourselves cosmetically; increase intelligence (a gene has been discovered that seems to make mice more intelligent); accomplish ethnic cleansing ("designer babies" genetically engineered before birth); or cause permanent changes in the gene pool. Some researchers are advocating the use of human genetic engineering for the treatment of serious diseases only.[4]

Gene Testing.   The new and rapidly expanding field of genetic testing holds great promise for detecting many devastating illnesses long before their symptoms become apparent. Such testing identifies people who have inherited a faulty gene that may (or may not) lead to a particular disorder. In the last 15 years, such predictive tests have been developed for more than 200 of the 4000 diseases thought to be caused by inherited gene mutations. The result has been earlier monitoring, preventive treatments, and in some cases, planning for long-term care.

BOX 1-1

Potential Uses of Gene Therapy*

Adenosine deaminase (ADA) deficiency
Acquired immunodeficiency syndrome (AIDS)
Alzheimer's disease
Arthritis
Cancer (not all forms)
Chronic pain
Congenital heart defects
Cystic fibrosis
Diabetes mellitus
Familial hypercholesterolemia
Heart disease
Hemophilia
Hepatitis
Hepatocellular carcinoma (liver cancer)
Huntington's disease
Liver failure
Marfan Syndrome
Mesothelioma
Muscular dystrophy (Duchenne)
Neurofibromatosis
Peripheral vascular disease
Schizophrenia
Severe combined immunodeficiency (SCID)
Sickle cell anemia

*This is only a partial list of diseases or disorders being studied and compiled from research reported but should give the reader an idea of the broad and varied applications of genetic manipulation.

However, gene testing is not without its difficulties. For example the presence of a particular mutation does not mean that illness is inevitable, making the interpretation of test results a highly complex task. The psychologic implications of predictive testing must be considered. Determining who is a candidate for testing remains to be determined. Inheritance accounts for a limited number of diseases suggesting that genetic testing should be reserved for people with a strong family history of the particular disease. Safeguards and protocols are not always in place before testing has found its way into general practice. For these reasons, it has been recommended that predictive testing should be confined to research or clinical settings where skilled counseling is available.

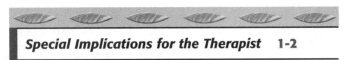

Special Implications for the Therapist 1-2

GENETIC ASPECTS OF DISEASE

As scientists strive to unravel the complex etiologic factors of diseases like obesity, diabetes, and cardiovascular disease through the use of molecular and genetic tools now available, understanding the interaction and influence of environmental factors such as exercise on gene expression and function has taken on increasing importance.

The Genome Project emphasizes the importance of other factors in disease susceptibility when genetic differences are eliminated. For example, regular exercise has been shown to improve glucose tolerance, control of lipid abnormalities, diabetes mellitus, hypertension, bone density, immune function, psychologic function, sleep patterns, and obesity, with the greatest benefits realized by sedentary individuals who begin to exercise. Responses to exercise interventions are often highly variable among individuals and research has indicated that response to exercise may be mediated or influenced in large part by variation in genes.[10]

The study of acute and chronic effects of exercise on the structure and function of organ systems is now a field of research referred to as *exercise science*. During the last 30 years, exercise-related research has rapidly transitioned from an organ to a subcellular/molecular focus. It is expected that genetic research will be focused on translating fundamental knowledge into solving the complexities of a number of degenerative diseases influenced heavily by activity/inactivity factors such as cardiopulmonary disease, diabetes mellitus, obesity, and the debilitating disorder associated with aging.[7] ∎

Other ethical issues and privacy concerns must also be settled such as the potential use of genetic testing to screen job applicants or to qualify for insurance coverage.

HEALTH PROMOTION AND DISEASE PREVENTION

The first set of national health targets was published in 1979 in Healthy People: The Surgeon General's Report on Health Promotion and Disease Prevention. *Healthy People 2000* was released in 1990 as a management tool with goals to reduce mortality, increase independence among older adults, reduce disparities in health among different population groups, and achieve access to preventive health services.

This program has become an ongoing comprehensive program of public health planning now called *Healthy People 2010* that is a tremendously valuable asset to all who work to improve health. *Healthy People 2010* (available at http://health.gov/healthypeople/) has a series of objectives to bring better health to all people in this country and to eliminate disparities among different segments of the population. These include differences that occur by gender, race or ethnicity, education or income, disability, residence in rural localities, and sexual orientation. More about these programs will be discussed in Chapter 2. This program has a built-in means to measure progress toward achieving 10-year targets across a broad range of health behaviors and outcomes.

◆ Health Promotion

Health promotion as a concept and as an active process is built on the principles of self-responsibility, nutritional awareness, stress reduction and management, and physical fitness. Health promotion is not limited to any particular age group but rather extends throughout the life span from before birth (e.g., prenatal care) through old age. Health promotion programs that encompass the entire life span are applicable to people of both genders and all socioeconomic and cultural backgrounds, to those who have no health problems, and to those with chronic illnesses and disabilities. Many types of health promotion programs are in existence, such as health screening, wellness, safety, stress management, or support groups for specific diseases.

◆ Disease Prevention

It has been recognized that preventing disease is more cost-effective than treating disease, and this has therefore been addressed by greater numbers of health care professionals. Preventive medicine as a branch of medicine is categorized as primary, secondary, or tertiary.

Primary prevention is geared toward removing or reducing disease risk factors, for example, by maintaining adequate levels of calcium intake and regular exercise as a means of preventing osteoporosis and subsequent bone fractures or by giving up or not starting smoking to reduce multiple causes of morbidity. Use of seat belts, helmets by motorcyclists and bicyclists, and immunizations are other examples of primary prevention strategies.

Secondary prevention techniques are designed to promote early detection of disease and to employ preventive measures to avoid further complications. Examples of secondary prevention include skin tests for tuberculosis or screening procedures such as mammography, colonoscopy, or routine cervical Papanicolaou smear.

Tertiary prevention measures are aimed at limiting the impact of established disease (e.g., radiation or chemotherapy to control localized cancer). Tertiary prevention involves rehabilitation and may end when no further healing is expected. The goal of tertiary prevention is to return the person to the highest possible level of functioning and to prevent severe disabilities.

Special Implications for the Therapist   1-3

HEALTH PROMOTION AND DISEASE PREVENTION

The practice of physical and occupational therapies is becoming increasingly complex. Rapid changes in the health care system are placing increased pressure on therapists for effective and efficient management of clients amidst high client turnover. Diagnosis, prediction of prognosis, intervention, and client-family education must be done quickly and accurately. The integration of examination, evaluation, diagnosis, prognosis, and intervention (including health promotion and prevention education) are important parts of the routine client management.[22]

In many hospitals, decreased acute care length of stay (LOS) means that physical and occupational therapists are being consulted or called on to treat clients earlier in the course of the hospitalization to help prevent secondary complications of immobility. Additionally, many individuals seeking physical and occupational therapy services have extensive medical histories requiring careful evaluation.

Understanding the diseases, surgeries, and medications frequently encountered in practice is necessary for safe and appropriate interventions and establishing a reasonable prognosis. The *APTA Guide to the Physical Therapist Practice*[3] describes the components that make up the history portion of an exami-

nation. These components include the investigation of a client's coexisting health problems such as illnesses, surgeries, and medications that have implications for health promotion, disease prevention, and direct treatment interventions.[9]

Role in Secondary and Tertiary Care[3]

Physical and occupational therapists play major roles in secondary and tertiary care. Clients with musculoskeletal, neuromuscular, cardiopulmonary, or integumentary conditions are often treated initially by another health care practitioner and are then referred to the therapist for secondary care. Therapists provide secondary care in a wide range of settings from hospitals to preschools.

Tertiary care is provided by therapists in highly specialized, complex, and technologically based settings (e.g., transplant services, burn units, emergency departments) or when supplying specialized services (e.g., to clients with spinal cord lesions or closed-head trauma) in response to requests for consultation made by other health care practitioners.

Role in Prevention and Wellness[3]

Physical and occupational therapists are involved in prevention and wellness activities, screening programs, and the promotion of positive health behavior. These initiatives decrease costs by helping clients achieve and restore optimal functional capacity; minimize impairments, functional limitations, and disabilities related to congenital and acquired conditions; maintain health and thereby prevent further deterioration or future illness; and create appropriate environmental adaptations to enhance independent function.

Prevention is not confined to a single form of presentation but rather takes one of three forms: primary, secondary, or tertiary. Primary prevention involves preventing disease in a susceptible or potentially susceptible population through general health promotion. Secondary prevention is comprised of decreasing duration of illness, severity of disease, and sequelae through early diagnosis and prompt intervention. Tertiary prevention includes limiting the degree of disability and promoting rehabilitation and restoration of function in clients with chronic and irreversible diseases.

The beneficial role of prescriptive exercise for health and disease has been documented many times and in many ways. When prescribed appropriately, exercise, including cardiovascular training, endurance training, and strength training, is effective for developing fitness and health, for increasing life expectancy, for the prevention of injury and disease, and for the rehabilitation of impairments and disabilities (Box 1-2). Prescriptive exercise programs to develop and maintain a significant amount of muscle mass, endurance, and strength contributes to overall fitness and health. Exercise plays a significant role in reducing risk factors associated with disease states (e.g., osteoporosis, diabetes mellitus, heart disease), the risk of falls and associated injuries, and the morbidity associated with chronic disease.[18]

Although not as abundant, the evidence also suggests that involvement in regular exercise can provide a number of psychologic benefits related to preserved cognitive function, alleviation of depression symptoms and behavior, and an improved concept of personal control and self-direction. It is important to note that while participation in physical activity may not always elicit increases in the traditional markers of physiologic performance and fitness in older adults (e.g., $VO_{2\,max}$, body composition, blood pressure changes), it does improve health as mea-

BOX 1-2

Benefits of Exercise

Increased cardiovascular functional capacity, decreased myocardial oxygen demand

Reduced mortality in people with coronary artery disease

Favorable change in metabolism of carbohydrates and lipids, including an increase in level of high-density lipoproteins

Improved hemodynamic, hormonal, metabolic, neurologic, and respiratory function

Improves immune function (stressful or excessive exercise can have the opposite effect)

Facilitates biorhythms and thermoregulation; prevents insomnia

Favorable effect on fibrinogen levels in older men

Increased sensitivity to insulin

Increase bone density; prevent osteoporosis

Greater strength and flexibility; maintain muscle mass

Improve postural stability; reduce falls

Improved psychologic functioning, self-confidence, and self-esteem

Reduction in some type A behaviors

Modified from American Heart Association: Recommendations: benefits of exercise, and guidelines for becoming—and remaining—active, *J Musculoskel Med* 14(5):60-65, 1997.

sured by a reduction in disease risk factors and improved functional capacity and quality of life in the aging population.[2]

As always when planning treatment intervention, including client education, the therapist must take into consideration the comorbidities and pathologic processes present. This requires identification of lifestyle factors (e.g., amount of exercise, stress, weight) that lead to increased risk for serious health problems, identification of risk factors for disease or injury, and performance of screening examinations (e.g., osteoporosis, skin cancer).

As a final reminder, the study and understanding of basic mechanisms of disease physiology and pathokinesiology along with the identification of lifestyle or risk factors are necessary but insufficient guides for clinical practice. Many variables affect the relationships among pathology, impairments, and disability. Attention must be paid to the psychosocial, educational, and environmental variables that modify client outcomes.[16] ■

REFERENCES

1. Agaki T: Gastric mucosa-associated lymphoid tissue lymphoma and Helicobacter pylori infection: evaluation of antibiotic treatment, *Intern Med* 39(4):273-274, 2000.
2. American College of Sports Medicine (ACSM): Position stand: exercise and physical activity for older adults, *Med Sci Sports Exerc* 30(6):992-1008, 1998.
3. American Physical Therapy Association: Guide to physical therapist practice, *Phys Therap* 77:1163-1650, 1997.
4. Anderson WF: Gene therapy: the best of times, the worst of times, *Science* 288(5466):627-629, 2000.
5. Anderson KN, Anderson LE, Glanze WD: *Mosby's medical, nursing, and allied health dictionary*, ed 5, St Louis, 1998, Mosby.
6. Balbin EG, Ironson GH, Solomon GF: Stress and coping: the psychoneuroimmunology of HIV/AIDS, *Baillieres Best Pract Res Clin Endocrinol Metab* 13(4):615-633, 1999.
7. Baldwin KM: Research in the exercise sciences: where do we go from here? *J Appl Physiol* 88(1):332-336, 2000.
8. Black JM: Theories of health and illness. In Black JM, Matassarin-Jacobs E, editors: *Medical-surgical nursing*, ed 6, Philadelphia, 2000, WB Saunders.
9. Boissonnault WG: Prevalence of comorbid conditions, surgeries, and medication use in a physical therapy outpatient population: a multicentered study. *J Orthop Sports Phys Ther* 29:506-525, 1999.
10. Bray MS: Genomics, genes, and environmental interaction: the role of exercise, *J Appl Physiol* 88(2):788-792, 2000.
11. Bridges SH, Sarver N: Gene therapy and immune restoration for HIV disease, *Lancet* 345(8947):427-432, 1995.
12. Cairns JS, Sarver N: New viral vectors for HIV vaccine delivery, *AIDS Res Hum Retroviruses* 14(17):1501-1508, 1998.
13. Center for Disease Control and Prevention (CDC): State specific prevalence of disability among adults, *MMWR* 49(31):711-714, 2000.
14. Clifton DW: Tolerated treatment well may no longer be tolerated, *PT Mag* 3:24-27, 1995.
15. Coe R: *Sociology of medicine*. New York, 1970, McGraw-Hill.
16. Duncan PW: Evidence-based practice: a new model for physical therapy, *PT Mag* 12(12):44-48, 1996.
17. Evrard A et al: Enhancement of 5-fluorouracil cytotoxicity by human thymidine-phosphorylase expression in cancer cells: in vitro and in vivo study, *Int J Cancer* 80(3):465-470, 1999.
18. Feigenbaum MS, Pollock ML: Prescription of resistance training for health and disease, *Med Sci Sports Exerc* 31(1):38-45, 1999.
19. Fuller K, Huber L: Improving postural control through integration of sensory inputs and visual biofeedback, *Top Stroke Rehab* 1:32-47, 1995.
20. Greer S: Mind-body research in psychooncology, *Adv Mind Body Med* 15(4):236-244, 1999.
21. Hamawy AH et al: Cardiac angiogenesis and gene therapy: a strategy for myocardial revascularization, *Curr Opin Cardiol* 14(6):515-522, 1999.
22. Jensen GM et al: Expert practice in physical therapy, *Phys Therap* 80(1):28-44, 2000.
23. Jette AM: Functional disability and rehabilitation of the aged, *Top Geriatr Rehab* 1:1-7, 1986.
24. Johns Hopkins Medical Letter: What your genes can and can't tell you 11(12):4-5, 2000.
25. Lezak M: *Neuropsychological assessment*, New York, 1983, Oxford University Press.
26. Link CJ et al: Cellular suicide therapy of malignant disease, *Oncologist* 5(1):68-74, 2000.
27. Maas M et al: Detection of chlamydia pneumoniae within peripheral blood monocytes of patients with unstable angina or myocardial infarction, *J Infect Dis* 181(Suppl 3):S449-451, 2000.
28. Mausch K: Psychoimmunology and disease based on certain research results, *Psychiatr Pol* 33(2):231-239, 1999.
29. Muhlestein JB: Chronic infection and coronary artery disease, *Med Clin North Am* 84(1):123-148, 2000.
30. Nagi SZ: Disability and rehabilitation, Columbus, Ohio, 1969, Ohio State University Press.
31. O'Toole M, editor: *Miller-Keane encyclopedia and dictionary of medicine, nursing, and allied health*, ed 6, Philadelphia, 1997, WB Saunders.
32. Pert C: *Molecules of emotion: the science behind mind-body medicine*, New York, 1998, Touchstone (Simon and Schuster).
33. Petry JJ: The role of the mind and emotions of patient and surgeon in the outcome of surgery, *Plast Reconstr Surg* 105(7):2636-2637, 2000.
34. Rosengart TK, Patel SR, Crystal RG: Therapeutic angiogenesis: protein and gene therapy delivery strategies, *J Cardiovasc Risk* 6(1):29-40, 1999.
35. Woltersdorf MA: Beyond the sensorimotor strip, *Clin Management* 12:63-69, 1992.
36. World Health Organization: Constitution of the World Health Organization, *Chron World Health Organization*, Geneva, Switzerland, 1947.
37. World Health Organization: *Global burden of disease and injury report*, Geneva, Switzerland, 1997.
38. World Health Organization: International classification of impairments, disabilities, and handicaps: a manual of classification relating to the consequences of disease, Geneva, Switzerland, 1990.
39. Zanjani ED, Anderson WF: Prospects for in utero human gene therapy, *Science* 285(5436):2084-2088, 1999.

CHAPTER 2

BIOPSYCHOSOCIAL-SPIRITUAL CONCEPTS RELATED TO HEALTH CARE

CATHERINE C. GOODMAN

OVERVIEW

The biomedical model has governed the thinking of most health practitioners for the past three centuries holding to the premise that all illness can be explained based on disorder and disease of bodily anatomy and physiologic processes. This model assumes that psychologic, social, and spiritual influences are independent of the disease process. By contrast, the biopsychosocial model of health and illness supports the idea that biologic, psychologic, and social variables are key factors in health and illness. The mind and body cannot be separated since they both influence the state of health. The biopsychosocial model emphasizes health and illness, rather than considering illness as a deviation of the healthy state.

During the 1980s, the medical model was influenced by a movement toward what was then called *holistic health,* the notion that the physical, mental, social, and spiritual aspects of a person's life must be viewed as an integrated whole. Since that time, it has become well established that social support plays a key role in promoting health, decreasing susceptibility to disease, and facilitating recovery from illness or injury.

During the 1990s, basic scientists and clinicians have continued to recognize the healing potential of faith, spirituality, and religious beliefs and started to consider the complex biopsychosocial-spiritual phenomena associated with disease, illness, and injury. Multidisciplinary team and managed care approaches to such conditions address the needs of the client in terms of the emotional and psychologic impact, social and spiritual needs, and comprehensive biologic picture that goes beyond medication and surgical intervention as the primary forms of medical treatment (see Fig. 1-1).

PERSONAL HEALTH CARE AND PREVENTIVE MEDICINE

◆ Variations in Client Populations

Healthy People 2010 (see Chapter 1) recognizes the need for all Americans to benefit from advancements in quality of life and health, regardless of race, ethnicity, gender, geographic location, disability status, income, spiritual orientation, or educational level. Recognizing variations in client populations is important in helping all health care professionals to provide health-promoting and preventive programs.

Sociodemographics

Sociodemographic information and results of the 2000 census have provided us with a composite picture of America never before so broad based or so complete. Americans are more diverse ethnically with an estimated ethnic racial mix of 72% white, 12% black, 12% Hispanic,* and 4% Asian and Pacific Islander. By the year 2020 the number of people of Asian descent will double from 10 million to 20 million, and by 2050, whites will comprise only 53% of the U.S. population. Rapid population shifts to the mountain states and resurgent growth in suburbs have changed the urban/rural configurations.

More than 70% of all rural counties gained population in the last decade. Finally, the percentage of Americans who are married continues to drop most recently from 58.1% of those age 15 and older in 1992 to 56.4% in 1998.[192] Since the census was completed, new reports indicate that the percentage of single heads of households (52%) has now surpassed married households.

Health Status

The health status of the United States is a description of the health of the total population using information that is representative of most people living in this country.† Health status of a nation can be measured by birth and death rates, life expectancy, quality of life, morbidity from specific diseases, risk factors, the use of ambulatory care and inpatient care, accessibility of health personnel and facilities, financing of health care, health insurance coverage, and many other factors.

The leading causes of death are often used to describe the health status of a nation. For example, in the United States, obesity, alcoholism, sedentary lifestyle, and tobacco use have contributed significantly to the most common causes of morbidity and mortality in 2000, compared with the year 1900 when infectious diseases ran rampant in the United States and worldwide and topped the leading causes of death. One century later, with the control of many infectious agents and the increasing age of the population, chronic diseases top the list (Table 2-1).

Life expectancy is edging up, infant mortality is the lowest ever, and firearm deaths among children have dropped, al-

---

*The American Hispanic population is made up of two groups, the Puerto Ricans and the Chicanos. Chicanos include Mexican-American, Latin-American, Latin, Latino, and Mexican people.

†However, it must be noted that our current epidemiologic system does not keep data on people who do not obtain treatment; no universal registry is available in the United States.

TABLE	2-1

The Five Leading Causes of Death in the United States and Associated Modifiable Risk Factors

CAUSE OF DEATH (1900)	CAUSE OF DEATH (2000)
Pneumonia, influenza	Heart disease
	Tobacco use
	Elevated serum cholesterol
	High blood pressure
	Obesity
	Diabetes mellitus
	Sedentary lifestyle
Tuberculosis	Malignant neoplasms
	Tobacco use
	Improper diet
	Alcohol
	Occupational and environmental
	exposures
Heart disease	Cerebrovascular disease
	High blood pressure
	Tobacco use
	Elevated serum cholesterol
Diarrhea, enteritis	Chronic obstructive pulmonary disease
	Tobacco use
	Occupational and environmental
	exposures
Stroke	Accidental Injuries
	Motor vehicle accidents; seat belt
	nonuse; air travel accidents
	Cycle helmet nonuse
	Alcohol and other substance abuse
	Poisoning, drowning
	Falls, fires
	Firearms
	Occupational hazards

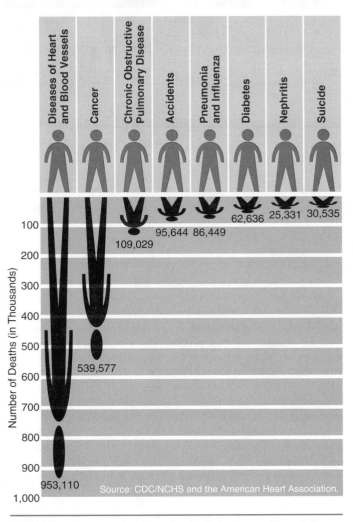

FIGURE   2-1   Deaths from the leading causes, United States. The total for Diseases of Heart and Blood Vessels represents the combined total for the categories Heart Diseases and Cerebrovascular Disease in Table 2-1. (From Centers for Disease Control and Prevention (CDC) and American Heart Association: *Death from the leading causes: still number one*, Pub No 55-0533, Dallas, 2000, American Heart Association.)

though unintentional injuries remains the leading cause of death for children of all ages. Heart disease, cancer, and stroke remain as the top three causes of death in America, although the death rates for all three are declining (Fig. 2-1). Mortality from human immunodeficiency virus (HIV) infection has declined by 47% in the United States (worldwide mortality now exceeds malaria and ranks as one of the top five causes of death), whereas obesity and diabetes have become major concerns for health care providers. Additionally, teen smoking and drug use are higher than ever before.

Deaths, permanent disability, and unnecessary suffering from medical errors are an escalating problem that remains largely unreported. According to the Institute of Medicine[103] medical errors kill upward of 44,000 people in United States hospitals each year. Statistics are not available for similar errors in other health-related settings such as same-day surgery, outpatient clinics, retail pharmacies, nursing homes, and in-home care. Deaths from medication errors that occur both in and out of hospitals (more than 7000 annually) exceed those caused by injuries in the workplace.

Geographic Variations

The concept of "community" as it relates to where individuals live geographically and the characteristics of that place has a definite impact on the status of people's health. For example, based on statistics pertaining to crime, divorce, population density, unemployment, and average commuting time, the most stressful cities and jobs have been identified as well as the least stressful locations and occupations.[121] Other factors such as urban pockets of minority groups (usually associated with increased levels of poverty); access to fresh fruits and vegetables (or lack thereof); and even local smoking ordinances contribute to the geographic variations people experience that can impact their health.[160]

The geographic and political climates of countries also play a role in determining how people live and the health problems that commonly develop. A half century ago a few physicians cultivated an interest in diseases that seemed to have strict geographic boundaries. As a result, a discipline called *geographic pathology* developed. Geographic pathology was concerned with diseases endemic (present in a community at all times) to certain areas of the world, most often parasitic and infectious diseases that seemed unique to individual geographic regions. A component called *occupational disease* was added with the discovery that chemical agents are mediators of a variety of tissue changes, and with the recognition that many of these causative agents are environmental contaminants. Disease caused by contaminants was included to constitute the field of *environmental pathology*. For further discussion, see Chapter 3.

One other issue related to geographic variations is the fact that treatment for a single medical condition can vary significantly from one geographic location to another. Rates and types of surgical procedures differ from one geographical location to another, depending on the prevailing health care system; physician and hospital preferences (not client preferences or needs); and where the physician was trained.[28,157]

Race and Ethnicity

In the past, it was believed that race or ethnic background predisposed people to certain diseases and chronic conditions. However, during the last 50 years, "race" has been scientifically disproved—that is race is not a real, natural phenomenon. Data about human variation comes from studies of genetic variation, which are clearly quantifiable and replicable. Genetic data show that no matter how racial groups are defined, two people from the same racial group are as different as two people from any two different racial groups. The American Anthropological Association suggests that race and ethnicity categories should be consolidated into one, using the term *ethnic group* rather than race or ethnicity for collection of scientific and/or demographic data.[1]

Current information about biologic and genetic characteristics of various groups (e.g., blacks, Hispanics, Native Americans, Alaskan Natives, Native Hawaiians, or Pacific Islanders) does not explain the health disparities experienced by these groups. These differences are believed to be the result of the complex interaction among genetic variations, environmental factors, and specific sociocultural and health behaviors.

Data indicate that some conditions are more prevalent in certain groups; for example, nonwhite people (black, Native Americans, and Asians) are three times more likely to die of hypertension than whites of the same age group. In the past, causes of death were identified that together accounted for more than 80% of mortality in nonwhite people, including cancer; cardiovascular disease and stroke; chemical dependency; cirrhoses; diabetes; homicides, suicides, and accidents; and infant mortality.[73] Other conditions that are peculiar to ethnic or racial groups include Tay-Sachs disease (Jewish people of northeastern European origin are most susceptible); cystic fibrosis (incidence is highest in whites and rare in Asians); and sickle cell anemia, which affects blacks, especially Africans.

Research is now focusing on factors beyond race or ethnicity (e.g., access to health care, language differences, place of birth, residential segregation, socioeconomic status, access to adequate nutrition) that can help explain the great disparities in death rates among groups of Americans. For example, statistics show a broad gap between the death rates for blacks and whites, but blacks differ more from each other than they do from whites.[65] Whites living in higher socioeconomic areas have lower mortality rates than whites living in predominantly black areas for all age groups, and elderly blacks living

in black areas (despite their less favorable socioeconomic status) have lower mortality rates for all causes than those living in white areas.[66]

Although cancer death rates are declining nationally, ethnic groups and medically underserved populations have a higher incidence and lower survival rate. Racial differences in the surgical treatment of blacks as compared with whites have been documented.[20] Available education and health care resources are not accessible to minorities and rural residents with limited financial means. Routine programs such as anti-smoking campaigns and cancer screening (e.g., breast, prostate, or colon) tend to be focused on affluent Americans who are better educated and can afford regular medical care.[102]

Age and Aging

Age and gender play important roles in the development of most diseases. Age often represents the accumulated effects of genetic and environmental factors over time. Today life expectancy at birth is 78.5 years for women, compared with 48 years at the turn of the last century, and 71.8 years for men and is expected to continue increasing for both genders. Whites and blacks have similar life expectancies at age 65, but a higher death rate exists among younger blacks. Once adults reach age 65, men can expect to live an additional 15.8 years, and women can expect an additional 17.6 years. Individuals 75 years of age can be expected to live an average of 11 more years for a total of 86 years.[191]

A dramatic extension of longevity has occurred in the last 100 years. In 1900, people over age 65 years constituted 4% of the U.S. population. By 1988, that proportion was up to 12.4%, and it is predicted that by 2025, one third of all Americans will be age 65 or older, and 30% of the over-65 population will be nonwhite by 2050, representing an even greater cultural diversity among the aging.[18] The most rapid population increase over the next decade will be among those over age 85. Additionally, almost 80% of those born today will live to see a 65th birthday. This aging trend of the U.S. population is reflected in the kinds of clients and problems therapists will treat in the coming decades.

Research has produced dramatic advancements in children's health that have an impact on adulthood. The long-term benefits of childhood intervention to prevent adult disease are documented. For example, preventing osteoporosis in the aging adult begins by providing necessary dietary calcium intake during bone development and calcification in childhood. Preventing tobacco-related cancer and lung diseases begins with educating children about the risks of initiating smoking. Healthy People 2010 is leading the country in trying to develop effective and economic self-management strategies and interventions for children and families to prevent disease and improve health.

As the young and the aging continue garnering attention, teenagers are falling between the cracks of medical care. Prenatal and well-child prevention programs have boosted the care given to the under-12 age group, but most physicians do not categorize teenagers as adults and may not be adequately addressing the needs of this group. Adolescents as a group are the primary users of illicit drugs, tobacco, and alcohol and comprise the largest group with unwanted pregnancies, abortions, and sexually transmitted diseases. Preventive health care and intervention among this age group are the next targets for the Healthy People 2010 campaign.

Finally, the older adult can be assessed for modifiable risk factors that contribute to functional decline. Slow gait, short-acting benzodiazepine use, depression, low exercise level, and obesity are significant modifiable predictors of functional decline in both vigorous and basic activities. Weak grip predicts functional decline in vigorous activities, whereas long-acting benzodiazepine use and poor visual acuity predict decline in basic activities. Known nonmodifiable predictors of functional decline include age, education, medical comorbidity, cognitive function, smoking history, and presence of previous spine fracture.[172]

Gender

Increasingly, research efforts are finding that the differences between men and women go far beyond the reproductive organs to affect every physiologic function and organ in the body, including the aging process. Striking physiologic differences exist between men and women. For example, it has been known that women's hearts beat faster, but it is now recognized that the configuration and activity of the cardiac cell membrane functions differently between the genders. Men's brains are larger than women's, but women have more brain cells. Diagnostic scanning shows that different areas of the brain light up in response to an identical task between men and women. Age-related changes that differ in men and women are just now coming to the forefront of science.

Until the late twentieth century, evidence for gender bias, usually against women, was evidenced in three areas: (1) the historical use of public monies to fund research predominantly in men, (2) perpetuation of the view in medicine that the 70-kg man is the norm for representing all humans in medicine, and (3) use of federal funds through Medicare to provide better reimbursement for conditions more prevalent in men compared with those more prevalent in women.[40]

The National Institutes of Health (NIH) issued guidelines in 1990 requiring the inclusion of women and minorities in all NIH-sponsored clinical research and revised these guidelines in 1994 to require analysis of clinical trial outcomes by gender. Although most clinical studies since that time have included women as study subjects, only a small percentage of research findings are analyzed by gender.[193] New studies evaluating differences between the genders regarding a variety of factors are currently underway.[86]

Gender-based biology has demonstrated major gender differences in such things as risk factors, response to medications, response to surgical procedures, and response to treatment. Men are less likely than women to seek medical care and practice preventive medicine, and men are less likely to have a primary care physician. Some gender differences may represent either environmental or genetic factors. Diseases with rates of occurrence that differ between men and women may reflect lifestyle or environmental differences or anatomic and hormonal differences.

It is clear now that men and women experience different patterns of disease. For example, women are twice as likely as men to contract a sexually transmitted disease (STD) and 10 times more likely to contract the human immunodeficiency virus (HIV) in particular during unprotected sex with an infected partner; women smokers are more likely to develop lung cancer than men who smoke; women are more likely to have a second heart attack within a year of the first, and nearly one half of men but only one third of women survive 1 year after a heart attack; women constitute 80% of those who have bone loss (osteoporosis) severe enough to increase fracture risk significantly; women have higher blood alcohol levels than men after both consume the same amount; and women tend to regain consciousness after anesthesia more quickly than men.[99] Additionally, the incidence of health risks to women, such as depression, anxiety, alcoholism, and eating disorders, is increasing.

Men, however, face some unique health challenges. They die an average of 5 years earlier than women, develop heart disease a decade earlier, and are more likely to participate in dangerous jobs and recreational activities. Men are two times more likely than women to die from unintentional injuries and four times more likely to die from firearm-related injuries. Gender expectations play a role in response to health issues in most cultures in the United States. The familiar male stereotype, which places a high value on stoicism and self-reliance, may make asking for medical help a sign of weakness. Males are expected to show less expression of pain than females, and in most cultures, men will be less expressive in describing pain. In some cultures, male children are held in higher regard than female children and are more likely to receive any necessary care and follow-up prescribed. Additionally, researchers are now examining whether people are more vulnerable to environmental and biologic challenges during periods of critical biochemical change than in times of relative quiescence. For example, are social, biologic, or psychologic changes that affect health influenced during hormonal fluctuations associated with puberty, premenstrual cycles, pregnancy, and menopause, compared with other periods in a woman's life cycle?

Previously, it was taught that few differences between men and women exist in response to exercise, so few adjustments were made when prescribing exercise for the female as opposed to the male. New research results document significant differences that exist in neuroendocrine, metabolic, and cardiovascular counter-regulatory responses in men and women to prolonged moderate exercise. How these differences will affect exercise programs or recommendations remains to be determined.[52] It is important to match the intensity of the exercise to the capacity of the individual. When training heart rate has not been determined through prescreening exercise testing, an exercise protocol should progress in slow stepwise increments.

◆ Variations in Lifestyle

More than half of deaths from the leading causes in the United States (see Table 2-1) result from behavioral and lifestyle factors such as diet, exercise, smoking, and substance abuse. More than any other intervention, changing behavior and lifestyle could help prevent death, enhance the quality of life, and reduce the escalating costs of treating chronic illnesses.[32] Although heart disease remains the number one cause of death in the U.S. adult population, the cardiac death rate has been reduced by 52% over the last two decades as a result of changes in diet and lifestyle.

Variations in lifestyle influencing clients' perceptions of health care may occur as a result of cultural, religious, socioeconomic, or even age factors. Although clinical manifestations of a disease or condition are essentially the same across cultures, how a person (or family member) responds or interprets the experience can vary. This phenomenon of response based on cultural influence is called *cultural relativity*—that is, behavior must be judged first in relation to the context of the culture in which it occurs. For example, some groups consider health as a function of luck (good or bad), whereas others see health problems as a punishment for bad behavior and good health as a reward for good behavior.

Health and disease must be evaluated in the context of the other cultural variables present but often unseen. Cultural beliefs of some people result in practices that can bring about seemingly unexplainable signs and symptoms. For example, herbal and home remedies may be used in combination with prescribed medications that can alter the medication's intended effect. The person who takes an antacid medication combined with baking soda as a home remedy can overload the body with sodium and develop fluid imbalances (see Chapter 4).

Cultural factors may also prevent illness. For example, people belonging to religious faiths that forbid drinking or smoking have lower cancer rates than the general population. Religious beliefs related to health must be recognized and respected. Research to study the effects of religiosity as a predictor of outcome in a variety of disorders is beginning to draw definitive conclusions about the efficacy of prayer, religious practices and activities, and philosophical orientation toward health.[16,116,181.] Research suggests that one of the principle reasons people are attracted to alternative medicine is that they find many of these therapies in keeping with their personal beliefs.[17]

Generational differences are seen among groups such as the Matures (born from 1900 to 1946); the baby boomers (born from 1946 to 1964); the Generation X-ers (born from 1965 to 1979); and finally, the Millennials (born from 1980 to 1999). Many people born before 1946 tend to assume a passive role in their own health and in receipt of health care by accepting whatever happens to them and whatever treatment is outlined. However, baby boomers have grown up questioning authority, and their offspring are even more likely to consider themselves consumers asking for treatment rationales, seeking second opinions, and combining allopathic treatment with alternative medicine (e.g., naturopathy, aroma therapy, acupuncture, or massage therapy).

The most adverse influence on health is socioeconomic status, with a higher percentage of low-socioeconomic class members experiencing health-related problems than any other group. Adults with higher incomes tend to experience better health and can expect to live more than 3 years longer than those in the lowest income bracket. The percentage of people in the lowest income families reporting limitation in activity caused by chronic disease is three times that of people in the highest income families.[93] Lack of health insurance coverage and/or access to quality health care may result in delayed or postponed diagnosis and treatment of health problems. Differences in attitudes toward health have been found to be greater between social classes than between races or ethnic groups. Ninety percent of all health care dollars is spent on extraordinary care in the last 2 to 3 years of life. This style of death-based medicine assigns the greatest financial and professional resources to treating the diseases of aging.[113]

The homeless have become one of the fastest growing populations in need of health care in the United States. Traditionally, the homeless consisted primarily of older, single men, often alcoholics, but now this group includes families and children who are runaways or adolescent throwaways. Declining public assistance, a shortage of affordable rental housing, and an increase in poverty are additional contributing factors to the rise in homelessness. Although estimates of homeless people vary, the National Coalition for the Homeless[152] report that on any given night, 700,000 Americans are homeless and up to 2 million homeless people are reported in a year's time. This number includes an estimated 100,000 children in the United States who are homeless; more than half are under age 5.

Adverse experiences in childhood are linked to the development of physical problems later including alcoholism, drug and/or tobacco addiction or addictions, obesity, fibromyalgia, or other autoimmune disorders. Children who have been exposed to four or more adverse experiences in childhood are more likely to have attempted suicide and to have had multiple sex partners, increasing their risk of sexually transmitted diseases. Dangerous or apparently counterproductive behaviors can serve a purpose (e.g., coping mechanism, barrier against social contact). The strong relationship between exposure to abuse or household dysfunction during childhood and multiple risk factors for several of the leading causes of death in adults are beginning to be recognized in the health care setting.[10,71] Healthy People 2010 has set goals of primary prevention of adverse childhood experiences and improved treatment of exposed children to reduce self-destructive behaviors such as smoking among adolescents and adults.

Other risk factors in lifestyle affecting health status and health care are considered individually modifiable and include personal habits such as rest and sleep; diet, including calcium, fat, and fiber intake; level of activity and exercise (fitness); stress and coping ability; substance abuse; high-risk sexual activity; travel; and environmental or occupational status. Individual modifying factors (IMFs) of lifestyle and environment moderate how a person responds to and/or tolerates medical treatment, as well as therapy intervention by the physical or occupational therapist.

The gay and lesbian population comprises a diverse community with disparate health concerns. Major health issues for gay men are HIV/AIDS and other sexually transmitted diseases, substance abuse, depression, and suicide. Gay male adolescents are two to three times more likely than their peers to attempt suicide. Some evidence suggests lesbians have higher rates of smoking, obesity, alcohol abuse, and stress than heterosexual women. The issues surrounding personal, family, and social acceptance of sexual orientation can place a significant burden on mental health and personal safety.[93]

Special Implications for the Therapist   2-1

VARIATIONS IN LIFESTYLE: ADAPTING TREATMENT INTERVENTION TO THE INDIVIDUAL

In the final decades leading to the twenty-first century, the demographics of the United States have changed rapidly, bringing with it biopsychosocial-spiritual variables that affect the episode of care seen in a therapist's practice, especially health care issues centered around minorities and economic variables. The therapist's role in education and prevention has never been more important as we come to understand the effect individual modifying (risk) factors have on pathology and

Continued

recovery. A biopsychosocial-spiritual model is essential because risk factors correlate with result, especially in chronic disease/disorders.

Race, culture, religion, and ethnicity are important factors in an individual's response to pain, disability, and disease. It is essential to remember that people of any culture may deal with pain, impairment, movement dysfunctions, and disability differently than expected. The culturally sensitive health professional must screen for cultural practices such as fasting or the use of alternative remedies, document these practices, and notify the physician. This is especially important for the client who may have a medical condition (e.g., diabetes mellitus, hypertension) that could be compromised by these practices.

Illness, especially life-threatening illness, often results in feelings of loss of control. Control; modes of control (e.g., passive acceptance, positive yielding or acceptance, or assertive control); and the desire for control are considered important variables that may influence physiologic function and health outcomes. Balancing active and yielding control styles and matching control strategies to client control styles and preferences may lead to optimal psychosocial adjustment and quality of life in the face of life-threatening illnesses.[24,30] Some cultures have a very conservative view of physical contact requiring a modified approach to the hands-on or manual therapist. In all situations where control may be an issue, the rationale and specifics for direct intervention must be clearly communicated and acceptable to the client.

In any setting, it is important for therapists to be aware of their own attitudes and values regarding lifestyle choices; responses to pain, illness, and disability; and health practices. It may be beneficial to adapt the individual intervention program to ethnic practices and beliefs. Health care education may be most effective if provided without trying to change the individual's or family's longstanding beliefs. Knowing what is needed to effectively rehabilitate an individual does not assure success unless provided within a cultural and socioeconomic framework acceptable to the individual or family. Language barriers make health care literature unavailable to many individuals who do not speak English and who require an interpreter (often unavailable) or for whom English is a second language, especially if English is spoken but not read. Keeping an open mind, asking questions, and respecting cultural differences are other ways to improve health care quality and delivery among minority groups.

In the past, studies examining personal factors to treatment failure have focused primarily on the client, not on the practitioner.[31] Taking a closer look at ourselves and understanding certain psychologic concepts such as transference, countertransference,* or direction of care (whether toward the client or therapist) can help the health professional become more effective, efficient, and consistent in the delivery of health care.[32,33]

These issues may be especially important to examine for the therapist who has had adverse childhood experiences that remain unresolved. This is especially important when interviewing clients about their childhood (and current) experiences, including a history of abuse or alcoholism or whether a family member was murdered or committed suicide. If people share their emotionally painful past with a trusted health care provider it can start the healing process for the client but potentially bring up difficulties for the therapist. In such a situation, the therapist may want to refer the client to another therapist. Sidestepping the client's personal issues or ignoring them will likely result in the client's continued visits to offices and clinics with a variety of physical problems that have psychologic roots (see the section on Somatization in this chapter).

The Americans with Disabilities Act of 1990 was designed to improve access to health care among people with disabilities, but barriers still exist for many people in receiving full age-appropriate primary care services. Disabled individuals, especially disabled women age 65 and older often do not receive appropriate primary care. The more severe the disability, the less likely a person is to receive adequate care and undergo health screening.[34] The therapist can be very instrumental in assessing the disabled person's access to important screening and prevention services, advocate for the care of the disabled, encourage these people to become their own advocates for health care, and conduct research on people with disabilities.

Therapists are increasingly faced with addressing the needs of the homeless who often experience frostbite, poor nutrition and hygiene, fatigue, mental illness, and a host of other minor medical problems. Many have additional secondary diagnoses (e.g., diabetes mellitus, hypertension, peripheral vascular disease, HIV, previous or present untreated orthopedic injuries) that complicate rehabilitation services. A third of the homeless clients have histories of past (and current) alcohol addiction and substance abuse.[35] ∎

Substance Abuse

Substance abuse is defined as the excessive use of mood-affecting chemicals (Box 2-1) that are a potential or real threat to either physical or mental health. Substance abuse has become increasingly prevalent in American society among people of every age, social, economic, professional, and educational status. The reasons for this phenomenon are multifactorial including personality characteristics, genetic influences, peer pressure, parental and cultural influences, nonadaptive coping skills, and as a means of self-treatment in posttraumatic stress disorder, a syndrome with symptoms resulting from past trauma outside normal human experience.

The origin of early age onset substance use disorder (SUD), classified as a psychiatric illness, is also considered complex and multifactorial, possibly involving genetic and environmental interactions beginning at conception. Alterations in somatic and neurologic maturation in the presence of adverse environmental variables result in behavioral dysregulation identified at first as difficult temperament in infancy, progressing to conduct problems in childhood and substance use in early adolescence, and eventually leading to severe SUD by young adulthood.[186]

Substance abuse may take the form of both addiction and habituation leading to psychologic craving or dependence, tolerance* and physiologic dependence accompanied by

---

Transference is defined as the unconscious transfer of emotions and beliefs about significant others such as parents onto an unsuspecting party, usually an authority figure such as a health care provider. *Countertransference* is the authority figure's reciprocal transfer of emotions and beliefs that do not belong to the client.

---

*The central nervous system adapts to the continued presence of a substance by compensating for its effect in a process referred to as tolerance. As a result, the person has to take increased quantities of the substance to obtain the same effect or to feel normal. This phenomenon leads to physical dependence and pathologic organ changes.

BOX 2-1

Mood-Affecting Chemicals*

Tobacco
Alcohol (wine, beer, liquor)
Caffeine-containing substances:
- Coffee
- Black tea
- Some carbonated beverages
- Medications, including many over-the-counter (OTC) medications
- Chocolate
- Prescription drugs
- Illicit drugs (e.g., hallucinogens, cocaine, marijuana)
- OTC medications

---

*These are listed in order of societal impact.

---

withdrawal symptoms† when use is discontinued. These substances become necessary to help the individual function normally. The addiction may lead to a lifestyle (e.g., prostitution, theft, violent crime) that puts the person at considerable risk for illness, disease, and injury.

Incidence.   Substance abuse is associated with violence, injury, and HIV infection and is estimated to be a factor in half of all highway fatality accidents. Varying center-based statistics show that 25% to 50% of all people with spinal cord injury (SCI) have substance abuse problems compared with an estimated 10% of the general population. The statistics for alcohol and drug use at the time of injury are as high as 68% to 80%. Among a sample of people admitted to one center, nearly half of all people who sustained an SCI were intoxicated when injured; although many newly admitted clients with SCI reduce or eliminate alcohol use during their hospitalization, 56% resume drinking after 1 year.[148]

Alcoholism is the most common drug abuse problem in the United States affecting more than 15 million Americans, including the adolescent and aging populations. The frequency of binge drinking among college students has increased dramatically in the last decade with an increase in the number of alcohol-related injuries, property damage, and disruption.[196] Alcohol-related deaths outnumber deaths related to drugs four to one and alcohol is a factor in more than half of all domestic-violence and sexual assault cases. Alcohol slows reaction time and impairs judgment, making it a leading cause of all types of accidents including 40% of all automobile accidents and a large percentage of accidents that occur on the job.[109] Alcoholism is extremely prevalent yet underdiagnosed among adults with symptomatic terminally ill cancer.[36]

The injection of illicit drugs has played a central and expanding role in the HIV/AIDS epidemic. The proportion of new AIDS cases attributable to this risk factor has doubled in the last decade; approximately 30% of people reported with AIDS have injection drug use as their recorded risk behavior. Injection drug use is especially important in the HIV/AIDS epidemic among women and children and represents the major route for heterosexual and perinatal transmission of HIV.[78]

Cigarette smoking and the use of tobacco products is the single most preventable cause of disease and death in the United States. Smoking results in more deaths each year in the United States than AIDS, alcohol, cocaine, heroin, homicide, suicide, motor vehicle crashes, and fires combined. Tobacco-related deaths number more than 430,000 per year among U.S. adults and direct medical costs attributable to smoking total at least $50 billion per year. Thirty-six percent of adolescents and approximately 24% of adults are current smokers. Every day, an estimated 3000 young people start smoking. Almost half of all adolescents who continue smoking regularly will die from a smoking-related illness. Following years of steady decline, rates of smoking among adults appear to have leveled off in the 1990s. Smoking appears to be more highly correlated with low income, formal education less than 12 years, military personnel, and specific groups such as Native Americans and Alaskan Natives. Men have only somewhat higher rates of smoking than women within the total U.S. population.[93]

Aging and Substance Abuse.   Alcohol is by far the most serious drug problem among the elderly or aging population. Many older people view alcohol problems in a moral context associated with feelings of shame and weakness, which prevents them from seeking help. An older adult is at greater risk for difficulties with alcohol than a young person for several reasons. Both total body water and lean body mass are reduced as a person ages. Even though ethanol metabolism is not decreased in the older adults (unless an underlying condition causes it), blood alcohol levels are less diluted and thus higher in the older person than in the younger person when both are given equivalent amounts determined by body surface area. Thus the same person as he or she ages can achieve higher blood alcohol levels with no increase in the amount ingested, all other factors remaining constant. Illness, malnutrition, the administration of other hepatotoxic drugs, or drugs that require breakdown in the liver may all increase an elderly person's sensitivity to alcohol.

Many over-the-counter (OTC) liquid cold remedies, mouthwashes, and cough syrups contain alcohol, which the aging person may consume as a substitute for drinking. Signs and symptoms of alcohol abuse may occur, but the person denies alcohol intake. Further questioning may be necessary to uncover these hidden problems with alcohol.

The older person is even more vulnerable to the detrimental effects of alcohol on cognitive function than the younger person. These effects on cognitive function occur even with light social drinking and are similar to those associated with aging. Alcohol can mimic or exacerbate cognitive changes linked both with normal aging and Alzheimer's disease.

Sleep disorders are common among older people leading to the use of alcohol and other sedative or hypnotic drugs as chemical management for insomnia. Alcohol does act to decrease sleep latency (the time between falling asleep and the first rapid eye movement [REM] period), which increases with age, but it also tends to further reduce REM and stages 3 and 4 of non-REM sleep, which is already decreased in older

---

†Withdrawal is the pattern of physical responses that appears when regular drug use is discontinued. When a physically dependent person abruptly stops consumption, signs and symptoms of withdrawal occur. Most withdrawal reactions produce an effect opposite to that of the ingested substance (e.g., a depressant causes hyperactivity during withdrawal).

adults. The net result is a virtual elimination of the restful and restorative portions of the sleep cycle. This can be further complicated by alcohol withdrawal occurring during sleep with the accompanying sympathetic discharge and arousal.

Abuse of sedative-hypnotics, taken either for sleep or anxiety, is a common form of drug abuse among the elderly. Complications of these drugs may be related to the development of toxic levels from the long half-lives of these compounds along with their slow metabolic breakdown in the elderly. Slowed response, hypersomnia, and increasing confusion are sometimes thought to relate to aging when actually they are symptoms of toxic drug levels. Withdrawal symptoms may occur when the medication is abruptly discontinued as a result of hospitalization or other change in life circumstances. Symptoms can be severe and may include tachycardia, hyperthermia, hypertension, altered mental states, seizures, and opisthotonos (severe spasm of the body backward into extension). The withdrawal is often not recognized or diagnosed immediately.

Caffeine is included as a substance because it is a chemical stimulant and the most common behaviorally active drug that can result in physical dependence. The most common source of dietary caffeine among the aging is coffee with average consumption around 200 mg/day. Caffeine is distributed essentially only through lean body mass. Because of the greater proportion of adipose tissue to lean body mass in older humans, a dose of caffeine may result in a higher plasma and tissue concentration in older adults compared with younger individuals. Responses to caffeine may be greater in older adults at doses in the 200 to 300 mm range, and the preponderance of data suggest that caffeine has a greater impact on calcium metabolism and bone in older people.[134]

Although smoking is less prevalent in older adults, older smokers are at greater risk because they have smoked longer, tend to be heavier smokers, and are more likely to already have smoking-related illnesses.[146]

Pathogenesis. In recent years it has been discovered that dopamine, a neurotransmitter plays a pivotal role in substance dependence by activating channels in the brain that register feelings of arousal, reward, and satisfaction. It is thought to be instrumental in enabling us to identify actions that pay off so that we can duplicate them. Many substances that create dependence influence dopamine levels. They may stimulate dopamine release, attach to dopamine receptors, or alter the way dopamine receptors respond. Whatever the pathway, the effect of heightened stimulation of neurons in the reward channel is the same.

For people who become drug dependent, the pathway becomes more deeply ingrained with each use and becomes linked with cues evoking drug use such as smells; location (e.g., smoky bar, abandoned house); paraphernalia used to prepare and administer the drug; or certain companions. When a person who is substance dependent encounters a use-associated cue, a spontaneous and overwhelming desire for the substance occurs, triggered by a dopamine release in the brain. These chemical pathways appear to be present even after years of abstinence, making relapses common, along with a new understanding that substance dependence is a chronic medical condition and not a weakness of will.

Illicit drug use or narcotic abuse may damage neurotransmitter receptor sites; the subsequent imbalance produces symptoms that may mimic other psychiatric illnesses such as agitated depression or amphetamine (speed)-induced seizures or paranoia. Repeated stimulation of the brain, called *kindling,* increases susceptibility to focal brain activity with minimal stimulation until the individual experiences spontaneous effects without the use of chemicals. The effects of kindling may be manifested as mood swings, panic, psychosis, and occasionally seizures. Behavioral effects are also noted such as poor work performance, job loss, pathologic lying, truancy, paranoia and aggression, violence, marital problems, or erratic behavior. Nonspecific signs such as red eyes; fatigue; signs of upper respiratory infection, especially cough; heart palpitations; avoidance of eye contact; confusion; or evidence of trauma may be present.

Caffeine appears to work not by speeding us up but by keeping us from slowing down. Each time brain cells fire, adenosine is produced that functions as an "off" switch, keeping neural activity in check. Caffeine binds with receptors on cell walls that normally respond to adenosine, overriding the switch so it cannot be turned down. Caffeine along with other stimulants such as cocaine and amphetamines mimic the stress response affecting the cardiovascular system and stimulating the sympathetic nervous system to increase production of adrenaline, causing the effects listed in Table 2-2.

Caffeine in toxic amounts (more than 250 mg/day or 3 cups of caffeinated coffee) may also produce additional symptoms. High daily doses of caffeine in excess of the equivalent of 5 cups of coffee may increase the chance of miscarriage or fetal growth retardation, although it is possible that some of this risk is due to confounders such as cigarette smoking and alcohol use.[114] No data support a link between caffeine and cancer, and no evidence exists showing that caffeine increases the risk of fibrocystic breast changes. However, cigarettes have been linked to fatal breast cancer. Overall, moderate amounts of caffeine are considered safe, but women are cautioned against substituting coffee for milk or ingesting more than moderate amounts of caffeine during pregnancy or while breast-feeding.

Alcohol and the addictive effects of alcohol may be caused by an enzyme protein kinase C-epsilon (PKC-epsilon) in the brain responsible for creating a desire to drink. It may be that the channels in the gamma-aminobutyric acid (GABA) neurotransmitter system in the brain causing chemical and electrical changes in neurons are kept open longer than normal by alcohol. This effect results in increased responsiveness to the signals leading to feelings of pleasure, calmness, or sleepiness. Studies involving mice show that in the absence of PKC-epsilon, alcohol makes the GABA receptor system even more sensitive. Inhibiting this enzyme may remove the rewarding effects of alcohol affected by GABA.[95]

There is no longer any question that women are more vulnerable to the effects of alcohol than men. Women produce substantially less of the gastric enzyme alcohol dehydrogenase, which breaks down ethanol in the stomach. As a result, women absorb 75% more alcohol into the bloodstream. Women have a smaller proportion of total body water than men (51% versus 65%), so the alcohol in the blood is less diluted, producing higher blood levels. Women feel the effects of alcohol sooner and more intensely than do men. Similarly, women and older adults of either gender have less water in their tissues than men of comparable height and build. Because alcohol is soluble in water, it tends

TABLE	2-2

Specific Effects and Adverse Reactions to Substances

	CAFFEINE	CANNABIS	DEPRESSANTS	NARCOTICS	STIMULANTS	TOBACCO
Examples:	Coffee, black tea, chocolate, some soft drinks	Marijuana Hashish	Alcohol Sedatives Tranquilizers	Heroin Opium Morphine Codeine	Cocaine, crack Amphetamines	Cigarettes, cigars, pipe smoking, smokeless tobacco products
Effects:	Nervousness Irritability Agitation Sensory disturbances Tachypnea Urinary frequency Sleep disturbances relieves, then increases fatigue Muscle tension Headaches Intestinal disorders Enhances pain perception Heart palpitation Vasoconstriction (heart) Vasodilation (head) Miscarriage, decreased birthweight (daily high doses)	Short-term memory loss Decreased concentration Sedation Tachycardia Euphoria Increased appetite Relaxed inhibitions Fatigue Paranoia Psychosis[34] Ataxia, tremor Paresthesias	Vasodilation Fatigue Depression Altered pain perception Blurred vision Slurred speech Decreased concentration Decreased coordination and motor reaction times Altered behavior Clammy skin Slow, shallow breathing Cognitive impairment Coma (overdose)	Euphoria, hallucinations Drowsiness Dizziness Respiratory depression GI symptoms	Increased alertness Excitation Euphoria Increased pulse rate Increased blood pressure Increased risk of myocardial infarction Insomnia Loss of appetite Agitation, increased body temperature, hallucinations, convulsions, death (overdose)	Increased heart rate Vasoconstriction (e.g., impotence, macular degeneration) Decreased O_2 to heart Increased risk of atherosclerosis, thrombosis, stroke Increased risk of respiratory disease (e.g., bronchitis, pneumonia, emphysema, COPD) Increased risk of cancer: • Leukemia • Cervical • Esophagus • Laryngeal • Lung • Kidney • Oropharyngeal • Pancreas • Stomach • Bladder Loss of appetite Poor wound healing Osteoporosis Increased risk of diabetes mellitus Back pain, spinal disk disease

to dissolve more slowly in older adults and women than in young men, causing intoxication after fewer drinks and longer-lasting effects.

Clinical Manifestations and Health Impact.   Alcohol and illicit drug use are associated with child and spousal abuse; sexually transmitted diseases, including HIV infection; teen pregnancy; school failure; motor vehicle crashes; escalation of health care costs; low worker productivity; and homelessness. Alcohol and illicit drug use can result in substantial disruptions in family, work, and personal life.

People who use and abuse illicit drugs, any substances mentioned in Box 2-1, or any combination of these substances have special health care needs. Specific effects and adverse reactions depend on the drug type (see Table 2-2). Death can

occur in anyone as a result of interaction between depressants such as alcohol combined with certain medications. Nicotine addiction in tobacco use requires daily use of tobacco products to maintain nicotine levels in the brain, primarily to avoid the negative effects of nicotine withdrawal but also to modulate mood. Nicotine dependence is the single most common psychiatric diagnosis in the United States, and substance abuse, major depression, and anxiety disorders are the most prevalent psychiatric comorbid conditions associated with nicotine dependence. Additionally, regular tobacco users exhibit altered levels of stress, arousal, and impulsivity.[27] The many respiratory diseases directly attributable to tobacco are discussed in Chapter 14.

Heavy drinking is associated with an increased risk of several cancers (e.g., mouth, esophagus, pharynx, liver, pancreas).[88] The link between alcohol ingestion and breast cancer remains unclear with studies reporting contrary findings, but most researchers are convinced that alcohol increases breast cancer risk.[120,210] If alcohol consumption and breast cancer are associated, researchers speculate that this is caused by alcohol's influence on the metabolism of estrogen. Additionally, prolonged exposure to high levels of estrogen over a lifetime has been linked to increased breast cancer risk.

Pregnant women are advised to avoid alcohol because no safe level has been identified. Even as little as one drink per day has been shown to cause teratogenic effects in offspring (e.g., developmental abnormalities). Drinking early in pregnancy and binge drinking are associated with the greatest risk to offspring. The most severe consequences are referred to as *fetal alcohol syndrome* (FAS), which is characterized by prenatal or postnatal growth retardation; central nervous system disturbance with neurologic abnormalities, behavioral dysfunction, intellectual impairment, and structural abnormalities (e.g., microcephaly); and a characteristic face with elongated midface, thin upper lip, and flattened maxilla. Research to identify how alcohol triggers neurodegeneration suggests that the destruction of millions of neurons in the developing human brain could explain the reduced brain mass and associated dysfunction.[101]

Medical Management. Substance abuse of any kind requires an overall treatment program including counseling, education, behavior modification, and for some substances, pharmacologic help. The addiction to substances is considered a biochemical disorder that can be arrested by altering behavior; success depends on compliance with treatment regimens. In the rehabilitation of SCI and traumatic brain-injured (TBI) clients, pain may be undertreated, causing some clients to turn to other, sometimes illicit, drugs to self-medicate. Timely, effective intervention for pain control is the goal in treatment before substance abuse becomes a problem.

Of the estimated 48 million adult smokers in the United States, approximately 16 million attempt to stop smoking cigarettes for at least 24 hours annually; another 2 to 3 million attempt to stop but cannot abstain for 24 hours. However, 1.2 million people do stop smoking each year, often without the behavioral and pharmacologic aids now available for smoking cessation. The number of pharmacologically assisted quit attempts per year jumped from 1 to 2 million to approximately 7 million, corresponding with the availability of nicotine gum and the nicotine patch as OTC products. Pharmacologic interventions double the success rates and all health care workers are encouraged to recommend smoking cessation to all clients while providing appropriate treatment referral.[43,45]

Prevention is the key to any successful substance abuse program. The American Medical Association has released guidelines recommending that all people over age 60 be screened and treated for substance abuse problems. The Healthy People 2010 (see Chapter 1) goals for substance abuse are to reduce substance abuse to protect the health, safety, and quality of life for all, especially children; to increase tobacco cessation rates; and to increase pregnant women's rate of abstinence from alcohol from 86% in 1997 to 94% in 2010.

Special Implications for the Therapist 2-2

SUBSTANCE ABUSE

Preferred Practice Patterns
4A: *Primary Prevention/Risk Factor Reduction for Skeletal Demineralization (Alcohol and tobacco use/abuse)*
5E: *Impaired Motor Function and Sensory Integrity Associated with Acute or Chronic Polyneuropathies (Alcohol-related)*
6A: *Primary Prevention/Risk Factor Reduction for Cardiopulmonary Disorders (All substances but especially cocaine and tobacco products)*
6B: *Impaired Aerobic Capacity and Endurance Secondary to Deconditioning Associated with Systemic Disorders (All substances but especially tobacco products)*
7A: *Primary Prevention/Risk Factor Reduction for Integumentary Disorders (Injection drug use, tobacco use and delayed wound healing, spinal cord injury [SCI] population)*

Substance abuse can impair or slow the rehabilitation process, especially delaying wound healing. The client using any substances discussed in this section should be encouraged to reduce (eliminate if possible) intake of these chemicals during the rehabilitation process.* Not only will the healing process accelerate, but levels of perceived pain can be reduced when these substances are eliminated.

However, many people who seek medical attention for seemingly unrelated conditions fail to disclose their use of alcohol or other substances. As part of the assessment process, therapists can screen for the presence of chemical substances by asking about the use of prescribed drugs, over-the-counter drugs and self-prescribed drugs such as nicotine, caffeine, alcohol, or street drugs. It may be helpful to assess the behavioral impact of substance abuse by asking, "Are you concerned about your chemical use? Do you have a pattern of cutting back or stopping the use of a substance but then restarting it? Has anyone around you raised concern about your chemical use?" An appropriate final question may be "Do you take (use) any drugs or substances that you haven't told me about yet?" Specific interviewing techniques are provided in more appropriate sources.[53-56] The National Council on Alcoholism and Drug Dependence (http://www.ncadd.org or [800] NCA-CALL) also has a self-test available for assessing the signs of alcoholism.

If the client reports the use of substances, the therapist may want to ask whether the person has discussed this with his or her physician or other health care personnel. Encourage the client to seek medical attention or inform the individual that you plan to discuss this as a medical problem with the physician. You can take the approach that this situation is no different from a case of undiagnosed or untreated angina. The client's health is impaired by the use and abuse of substances, and therapy will not be effective as long as the person is under the influence of chemicals.

---

*Primary intervention or care for the chemically dependent person is essential. However, the realistic picture is more often one of a person who has a pattern of substance abuse and either denies the problem or admits failure in the past. For example, people who smoke or chew tobacco and have repeatedly tried to quit most commonly admit failure.

With the SCI and traumatic brain injury (TBI) population, the therapist must be alert to any suspicious signs or symptoms of substance abuse (see Clinical Manifestations). More than half of all people with SCI or TBI incurred their disabilities while under the influence of drugs or alcohol; some studies report as much as 80%.[36] It is estimated that two thirds of people with disabilities who abuse drugs and/or alcohol did so before their injury and many turn to substance use afterward to cope with life changes caused by the disability. Medical professionals should also be observant for excessive sleeping and unusual symptoms such as muscular inflammation and myopathies, which can occur with the use of street drugs.

The health care professional is cautioned against actively or passively encouraging the use of substances out of an attempt to normalize socialization or out of a sense of compassion or pity. This concept is termed *entitlement* and may take the form of subtle agreement with the use of substances or even actively participating with the client (e.g., going out for a few drinks together, providing marijuana and getting "stoned" together). The concept of moderation is acceptable for some people, but for anyone with a past history or current use of substances, the best advice health care professionals can offer is to avoid all substances at all times. The risk of dangerous interactions with medications or further injury from the effects of these chemicals is too great to offer anything but abstinence as an acceptable treatment goal.[36]

Tobacco

Healthy People 2010 has targeted tobacco use as one of its focus areas with the goal of reducing illness, disability, and death related to tobacco use and exposure to secondhand smoke. Smoking has been shown to be the leading cause of preventable illness and death in the United States. Cigarette smoking is a risk factor for many medical disorders including skin diseases, pulmonary disorders, insulin resistance and diabetes mellitus, and cardiovascular disease.

Smoking may especially exacerbate circulatory problems leading to foot amputation in people with diabetes. The detrimental effects of cigarette smoking on wound healing and peripheral circulation are well documented. This population generally has a lower oxygen supply to the lower extremities because they are subject to advanced atherosclerosis. Since good oxygen supply is required for wound healing in soft tissue, it is imperative that people with a history of diabetes and smoking, now presenting with pressure ulcers or other foot complications, receive adequate arterial blood supply to the lower extremities (see Chapters 9 and 10).

Heavy smoking is commonly associated with chronic alcohol abuse and both addictions have a negative influence on bone formation, probably the result of defective osteoblastosis. Women who smoke are at significantly higher risk of developing osteoporosis late in life and subsequent bone fractures compared with nonsmokers.[57,58] (See Special Implications for the Therapist: Osteoporosis, Chapter 23.)

The relationship between smoking and pain has also been documented including an association with the incidence and prevalence of back pain in all ages.[59,60] A link between smoking and back pain in occupations requiring physical exertion was also established possibly as a result of smoking-related reduced oxygen perfusion and malnutrition of tissues in or around the spine causing these tissues to respond inefficiently to mechanical stresses.[61] Study findings may have implications for targeting at-risk groups for back care education or intervention programs.[62]

The effects of tobacco use (see Table 2-2) have a direct impact on the client's ability to exercise and must be considered when starting a treatment intervention or exercise program. Smokers are more likely than nonsmokers to suffer fractures, sprains, and other physical injuries even at an early age; these detrimental effects of smoking on injuries appear to persist at least several weeks after cessation of smoking.[63] In addition to the overall effects of nicotine, inhaled nicotine has additional pulmonary effects. The combination of smoking and coffee ingestion raises the blood pressure of hypertensive clients about 15/33 mm Hg for as long as 2 hours,[64] requiring careful monitoring of vital signs during exercise.

A clear need to increase the frequency of smoking cessation advice and counseling for all tobacco users is evident. However, the difference in receipt of advice to quit among racial/ethnic groups may be influenced by social or cultural factors. For example, among older Hispanic and Asian-American adults, language barriers may affect the lower rates of receiving advice to quit or in understanding the advice. Health care providers should offer culturally appropriate or tailored interventions for racial/ethnic populations.[42]

In 1996 the American Physical Therapy Association endorsed the Agency for Health Care Policy and Research's Clinical Practice Smoking Cessation Guideline. This has been superseded by a new, updated *Tobacco Cessation Guideline* released by the Public Health Service on June 27, 2000. The Guidelines recommend that every client who smokes or uses tobacco products* should be advised on the known dangers of tobacco use and increased success of smoking cessation programs. The therapist is often in a unique position as the health care professional that the client feels most comfortable with and able to trust for supportive education. Explaining some of the immediate and long-term benefits of smoking cessation may be helpful (Table 2-3). Whenever possible, clients who smoke should be encouraged to stop smoking or at least reduce tobacco use before surgery and when recovering from wounds or injuries resulting from trauma (including surgery) or disease.[65] The National Cancer Institute ([800] 4-CANCER) provides educational materials for health professionals that contain practical steps toward stopping smoking. All smokers trying to quit should be encouraged to use a medication approved by the Food and Drug Administration, either nicotine replacement therapy (gum, inhaler, nasal spray, or patch) or a nonnicotine pharmacologic aid (e.g., bupropion [see Table 2-15]).[52]

Depressants

Alcohol; barbiturates; and similarly acting sedatives, hypnotics, and antianxiety agents are central nervous system depressants. Approximately 30% of hospitalized people, including older adults, are alcohol abusers, and many traumatic injuries occur as a result of excessive alcohol consumption. Alcohol addiction, a prevalent problem in the acute care setting, often remains hid-

Continued

---

*Tobacco products includes pipe smoking, cigars, and smokeless tobacco, the latter available in two different forms: snuff and chewing tobacco. Snuff, a fine grain tobacco, comes in cans or pouches. Users take a "pinch," "dip," or "quid," and place it between the lower lip or cheek and gum and suck on it. Chewing tobacco comes in pouches in the form of long strands of tobacco that, when used, are commonly called "plugs," "wads," or "chew." All tobacco products have dangerous adverse risks and are associated with increased risk of developing various cancers (see Table 2-2).

den until withdrawal symptoms appear. Alcohol withdrawal manifests itself with a wide range of symptoms that usually begin 3 to 36 hours after the last drink. The person may present with tremulousness; motor hyperactivity; anxiety and hyperalertness; irritability and agitation; diaphoresis; tachycardia; hypertension (to 200/100 mm Hg or higher); pounding headache; abdominal cramping; anorexia; nausea; vomiting; or diarrhea. Withdrawal may be accompanied by behavioral manifestations (e.g., aggression, uncooperative actions) or physiologic complications such as electrolyte disorders, dehydration, polyneuropathy, or myopathy.[66] Whenever the therapists observes a cluster of these signs or symptoms, nursing or medical staff should be contacted to confirm the possibility of alcohol withdrawal and to discuss the implications for that individual in a therapy setting.

Alcohol affects many body systems (Fig. 2-2), but the effects on the neurologic and musculoskeletal systems are of particular interest to therapists. Alcoholic polyneuropathy is a degenerative process involving mutliple nerves and occurs as a result of nutritional deficiencies associated with chronic alcoholism. It occurs most frequently between ages 40 and 70 and develops slowly over a long period. Some people with neuropathies are asymptomatic but neurologic assessment usually reveals varying degrees of motor, reflex, and sensory loss, which typically occur in the feet before the hands, moving distal to proximal. Sensory disturbances usually appear first and are described as tingling, pricking, burning, or numbing sensations. Safety precautions are very important for people with diminished sensation (see Table 11-22). Calf muscles may be tender to the touch and diminished sensation and weak muscles may result in a wide-stance gait.

Alcohol ingestion may damage skeletal muscle, resulting in subclinical, acute, or chronic alcoholic myopathy. The pathologic process is the same as in alcoholic cardiomyopathy (see Chapter 11). *Acute alcoholic myopathy* is a syndrome of muscle pain, tenderness, and edema occurring after acute excesses of alcohol ingestion. The proximal muscles of the extremities, the pelvic and shoulder girdles, and the muscles of the thoracic cage are most commonly affected. Symptoms may subside in 1 to 3 weeks with cessation of alcohol use but may recur with repeated alcohol ingestion. Treatment consists of a well-balanced diet with supplemental vitamins and abstinence from alcohol. *Chronic alcoholic myopathy* is characterized by muscle weakness and wasting involving the same muscle groups described in acute alcoholic myopathy. Onset is slow and insidious with no history of pain or tenderness. Treatment intervention is the same as for acute alcoholic myopathy.

Prolonged use of excessive alcohol contributes to three known skeletal complications: a syndrome of nontraumatic hip osteonecrosis, deficient bone metabolism leading to osteomalacia and osteoporosis, and an increased incidence of fractures and other injuries secondary to trauma and falls. Impaired coordination due to high blood alcohol levels is a contributing factor to falls.

Saturday night palsy, an injury to the radial nerve in the spiral groove, may occur during deep sleep in intoxicated persons. Prolonged compression of the radial nerve results in paralysis of the extensor muscles of the wrist and fingers. The nerve may be injured at or above the elbow; its purely motor posterior interosseous branch, supplying the extensors of the wrist and fingers, may be involved immediately below the elbow, but then sparing of the extensor carpi radialis longus occurs so that the wrist can still be extended. The triceps muscle is spared because of its more proximal nerve supply (see Chapter 38).

Stimulants

The use of chemical stimulants such as caffeine, cocaine, and amphetamines has a direct effect on the central nervous system and may enhance a person's perception of pain. Pain can be relieved by reducing the daily intake of these chemicals, but care must be taken to avoid the withdrawal syndrome (e.g., symptoms of headache, lethargy, fatigue, muscle pain, and stiffness). The negative effects of caffeine on TBI are also problematic for the therapist working with the agitation often present in this group. Caffeine may also act on the dopaminergic system of the brain, indirectly enhancing neurotransmission of dopamine and masking the symptoms of Parkinson's disease. Higher caffeine intake is associated with a significantly lower incidence of Parkinson's disease.[67]

The combination of exercise and caffeine can cause elevated blood pressure, especially for people with high blood pressure or healthy people with a family history of hypertension. People who know they have high blood pressure should avoid caffeine for at least 2 hours before a workout or strenuous rehabilitation session.[68] For more detailed information on the effects of caffeine see Gupta and Gupta, 1999 or Spiller, 1998.[69,70]

Cocaine significantly increases the risk of having a heart attack in the first hour after using it and this risk applies to people who are otherwise at low risk.[71] The role that exercise may have in this phenomenon remains unknown, but given the ability of cocaine to increase pulse rate and blood pressure, therapists must monitor vital signs to prescreen all clients in a rehabilitation or exercise program. People taking stimulants such as cocaine and amphetamines are easily provoked into aggressive, violent behavior. A calm approach is essential, and realistic goals for client behavior and rehabilitation are important.

Injection Drug Use

Injection drug use is associated with a high rate of skin and soft tissue infections from the use of unsterile intravenous and subcutaneous injection (skin popping). This factor, combined with the presence of pathogenic microorganisms on the skin, results in a wide range of clinical problems from simple cellulitis and abscess to life-threatening necrotizing fasciitis and septic thrombophlebitis. The clinical appearance is often atypical and subtle because of longstanding damage to the skin and to venous and lymphatic systems, resulting in underlying lymphedema, hyperpigmentation, scarring, and regional lymphadenopathy. The therapist may observe redness, warmth, and tenderness with tender inguinal or axillary lymph nodes. Skin ulcers resulting from skin popping consisting of low-grade foreign body granulomatous inflammation and necrosis are common and easily become superinfected requiring local wound care, occasionally requiring skin grafting.[40]

Cannabis

The effects of cannabis derivatives usually last a few hours and with repeated use, less of the drug is needed to produce the same effects. The agent persists in the body as an active metabolite as long as 8 days after use, so less of the drug is needed to produce the same effects during this time. As with any substance, clients are encouraged to eliminate the use of cannabis derivatives during the rehabilitation process. Relapse or worsening of symptoms in people with a history of psychologic disorders occurs with the use of cannabis. ■

TABLE   2-3

Benefits of Smoking Cessation

TIME SINCE LAST CIGARETTE	BENEFIT
20 minutes	Vital signs return to person's baseline normal level (blood pressure, pulse, temperature)
8 hours	Oxygen levels increase; carbon monoxide levels decrease
1 day	Risk of myocardial infarction (heart attack) decreases
2 days	Increased ability to smell and taste; nerve endings begin repair
2 weeks-3 months	Improved circulation and lung function; reduced shortness of breath, improved exercise capacity
1-9 months	Cilia in lungs regenerate improving movement of secretions; reduced coughing and sinus congestion; decreased fatique and increased energy levels
1 year	Risk of coronary heart disease reduced to one-half that of a smoker
5 years	Risk of lung cancer reduced by 50%; reduced risk of cerebrovascular accident (stroke); risk of oropharyngeal cancer (mouth, throat) reduced to one-half that of a smoker
10 years	Lung cancer death rate corresponds to nonsmoker's rate; risk of other tobacco-related cancers reduced
15 years	Risk of coronary heart disease equals that of a nonsmoker

American Cancer Society, 2000 (www.cancer.org/)

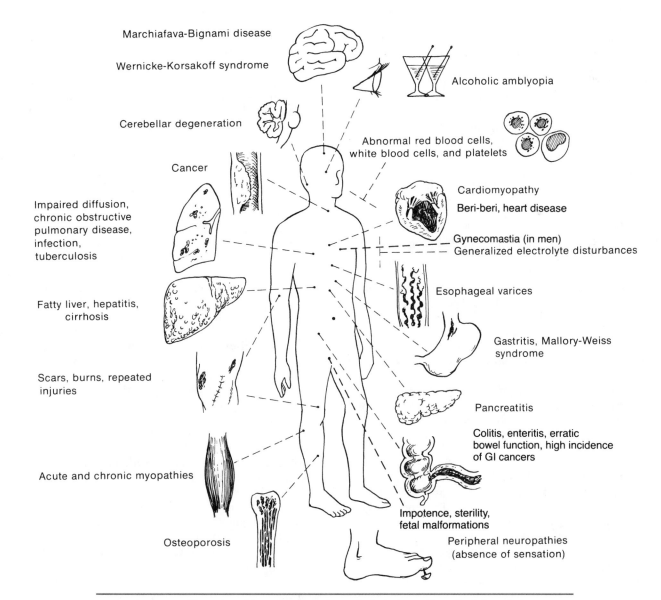

FIGURE   2-2   Clinical problems resulting from alcohol abuse. Not all of the conditions pictured in this figure are discussed in this text. (From Kneisl CR: Nursing care of clients with substance abuse. In Black JM, Matassarin-Jacobs E, editors: *Luckmann and Sorensen's medical-surgical nursing,* ed 4, Philadelphia, 1993, WB Saunders.)

Eating Disorders

Eating disorder is the general term used to describe an obsession with food and weight including anorexia nervosa, bulimia nervosa, and binge-eating disorders. According to the Harvard Eating Disorders Center,[92] more than five million people in the United States experience eating disorders.

The cause of eating disorders is unknown, although it is likely that a variety of factors (e.g., biologic, psychologic, sociocultural) affect whether an individual may develop an eating disorder. Typically, an underlying dissatisfaction with body image exists that is based on the faulty belief that weight, shape, or thinness is the primary source of self-worth and value. Risk factors associated with eating disorders include female gender (although an estimated 10% of eating disorder cases now occur in boys and men); personality traits (e.g., perfectionist, rigid, risk-avoidance); dieting; personal or family history of obesity, drug and/or alcohol abuse, depression, sexual abuse or other forms of trauma, or eating disorders; and elite athletic performance.

Up to 20% of women with type 1 diabetes mellitus have some kind of eating disorder; this in turn predisposes them to further complications with glucose control. The treatment of diabetes mellitus greatly emphasizes weight control, dietary habits, and food. This focus, combined with stress, poor self-esteem, and altered body image that can result from any chronic illness, contribute to the risk of eating disorders in this population.

Several groups of athletes are at greater risk for eating disorders. This includes women who participate in sports that emphasize the importance of low body weight, such as distance running; sports in which judging is based on aesthetic criteria, such as gymnastics and figure skating; and sports where being lean improves performance such as gymnastics or diving. Men at risk are those who participate in sports that use weight classes, such as wrestling and rowing. Horse-racing jockeys of both genders also exhibit these behaviors.[185]

Whereas eating disorders is considered an illness, *disordered eating* is a reaction to life situations or a habit that can be changed with education, self-help, or nutritional counseling. Disordered eating does not include persistent thinking and altered behaviors centered around body, food, and eating and does not lead to health, social, school, or work problems as is common with eating disorders. Disordered eating may lead to transient weight changes or nutritional problems but rarely causes major medical complications.

Eating disorders can be treated successfully. Overall, degrees of response range along a continuum. With good treatment, 70% of people with eating disorders can be cured. However, it may take years, and the chances of relapse on the road to recovery is as high as 30%.

Anorexia Nervosa.
Anorexia nervosa is a refusal to eat. It is characterized by severe weight loss in the absence of obvious physical cause and is attributed to emotions such as anxiety, irritation, anger, and fear. This condition is characterized by distorted thinking, including a fear of becoming obese despite progressive weight loss, accompanied by the perception that the body is fat when it is underweight. The person may use laxatives, diuretics, fasting, exercise, and self-induced vomiting to achieve additional weight loss. The effects of starvation have psychologic, emotional,

and physical sequelae, and medical complications that may lead to death.

Anorexia nervosa has been characteristically observed in adolescent and young adult females from middle- and upper-class families, often at or near the onset of menstruation (menarche), but this has spread now to include younger girls, boys, and all economic classes. An increased incidence of anorexia occurs among sports participants, especially sports that emphasize leanness such as gymnastics, wrestling, diving, figure skating, and distance running and in ballet dancers. Anorexia occurs in men in approximately 5% to 10% of cases; it is suspected that this figure is a low estimate, since it is likely that more males experience anorexia than what is made aware to health professionals.

Although attributed to psychologic and emotional factors (e.g., the need for control is a common variable; fear of growing up; fear of sexuality; rejection of self), the cause of anorexia remains unknown. During the past several decades, single-factor causal theories have been replaced by the view that anorexia nervosa is a multifactorial biopsychosocial disorder (Fig. 2-3). Specific early experiences and family influences may create intrapsychic conflicts that determine the psychologic predisposition. The challenges and conflicts of pubertal endocrine changes (biologic factors) may initiate the disorder. Social factors, such as the American cultural obsession with thinness, reinforce the pursuit of thinness. The cumulative effect leads to dieting (a known risk factor for eating disorders) and other means of weight loss. This in turn results in malnutrition and starvation neurosis. The vicious circle of psychologic dysfunction fostering further dieting and psychologic denial becomes established and may lead to death.

Clinical Manifestations.
Besides the obvious lack of appetite and refusal to eat with weight loss, other signs and symptoms may occur as a result of starvation, vomiting, and chronic laxative or diuretic abuse (Box 2-2). These practices also lead to alternating periods of dehydration and "rebound" excessive water retention observed as swelling or reported as "puffiness" in the fingers, ankles, and/or face. Edema is usually noticed most immediately after vomiting and laxative abuse has been stopped. Normalization of food intake and discontinuation of the purging practices will gradually reduce the wide swings in water balance, but the individual often becomes so alarmed at the sudden weight gain or swelling that they repeat the cycle by returning to vomiting or laxatives.[79] Starvation seriously compromises cardiac functioning and when combined with electrolyte disturbances may result in life-threatening arrhythmias. Mitral valve prolapse (MVP) may occur secondary to starvation-induced decrease in left ventricular volume (see Special Implications for the Therapist: Mitral Valve Prolapse in Chapter 11).

Brain scans are abnormal in more than half of all anorexia cases and in some cases of bulimia nervosa. In both eating disorders, this condition appears to reverse itself with renourishment.[188] Loss of body fat results in cessation of menstrual cycle (amenorrhea), hypothermia (cold intolerance), and the subsequent development of lanugo (the fine hair sometimes seen on the body of the newborn infant). Behavioral symptoms are listed in Table 2-4.

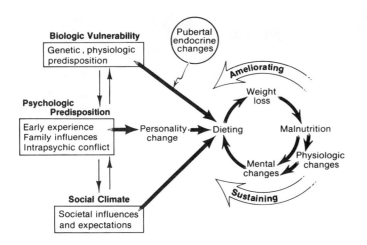

FIGURE 2-3 Biopsychosocial model for anorexia nervosa. See text discussion. (From Lucas AR: Toward an understanding of anorexia nervosa as a disease, *Mayo Clin Proc* 56:254, 1981.)

Bone density is decreased in anorexic and bulimic women, possibly resulting from estrogen deficiency, low intake of nutrients, low body weight, early onset and long duration of amenorrhea, low calcium intake, reduced physical activity, and hypercortisolism. This type of reduced bone density is associated with a significantly increased risk of fracture even at a young age.[87] A new term has been coined (female athlete triad) to describe the combination of disordered eating, amenorrhea, and osteoporosis, a situation that often goes unrecognized and untreated.[171]

Medical Management. Diagnostic criteria may be taken from the American Psychiatric Association's *Diagnostic and Statistical Manual of Mental Disorders, Fourth Edition*[*55] (DSM-IV-TR) (Box 2-3). Various laboratory tests may be performed to evaluate hormone levels in men and women and imaging studies may include a dual-energy x-ray absorptiometry scan to evaluate bone density.

No universally accepted treatment for anorexia nervosa exists. Treatment can be difficult and lengthy if the eating disorder becomes entrenched or if medical complications exist. Treatment may include behavior therapy, demand feeding, behavioral contracts, psychotherapy, family therapy, nutritional counseling, and correction of nutritional status, which may require hospitalization. Hospitalization is indicated if the body weight or body mass index (BMI) drops below a certain minimum (e.g., less than 16 BMI for adults), treatment-resistant bingeing occurs, or vomiting and/or laxative abuse persist.[11] As mentioned, starvation-induced cardiac failure and death are possible.

Estrogen replacement, although beneficial in treating bone loss in menopause, has not been proven to prevent progressive osteopenia in people with anorexia. Recovery from this condition is associated with improved bone density.[115,165] Researchers continue to investigate this issue with varied results and recommendations.[37,110]

---

*The term *mental disorder* unfortunately implies a distinction between mental and physical when, in fact, much physical is in mental disorders and much mental is in physical disorders. The problem raised by the term *mental disorders* has been much clearer than its solution, and the term persists for lack of an appropriate substitute.[55]

BOX 2-2

Physical Complications of Eating Disorders

Electrolyte disturbances
Edema and dehydration
Cardiac abnormalities:
- Bradycardia
- Tachycardia
- Hypotension
- Ventricular arrhythmias
- Mitral valve prolapse (MVP)
- Cardiomyopathy (ipecac use)
- Cardiac failure
Kidney dysfunction
Neurologic abnormalities:
- Cerebral atrophy
- Seizures
- Muscular spasms (tetany)
- Peripheral paresthesia
Endocrine dysfunction:
- Cold intolerance, hypothermia
- Hair loss, growth of lanugo (fine hair)
- Dry, yellow skin
- Brittle nails
- Constipation
- Fatigue
- Diabetes insipidus
- Menstrual dysfunction (amenorrhea)
- Reproductive dysfunction (infertility, prenatal complications)
- Osteoporosis/bone fracture
- Sleep disturbance
Proximal muscle weakness (ipecac use):
- Abnormal muscle biopsy
- Abnormal electromyography
- Gait disturbance
Gastrointestinal disturbances:
- Hypertrophy of salivary glands/facial swelling
- Esophagitis
- Abdominal pain/bloating
- Diarrhea/constipation
- Rectal bleeding
Dental deterioration/discoloration
Finger clubbing
Anemia
Emotional/psychologic disturbance:
- Depression
- Anxiety
- Irritability
- Mood swings
- Personality changes

More needs to be done in the areas of prevention, early detection, and early treatment of eating disorders. Education efforts should be focused on girls in early middle school or junior high because of the rapid bone formation during puberty that will be necessary for the rest of their lives. Several national organizations provide valuable educational and preven-

TABLE 2-4

Common Behavioral Symptoms of Eating Disorders

SYMPTOMS	ANOREXIA NERVOSA*	BULIMIA NERVOSA*	BINGE EATING DISORDER
Excessive weight loss in relatively short period of time	+	−	−
Continuation of dieting although bone-thin	+	−	−
Dissatisfaction with appearance; belief that body is fat, even though severely underweight	+	−	−
Unusual interest in food and development of strange eating rituals	+	+	−
Eating in secret	+	+	+
Obsession with exercise	+	+	−
Serious depression	+	+	+
Bingeing (consumption of large amounts of food)	−	+	+
Vomiting or use of drugs to stimulate vomiting, bowel movements, and urination	−	+	−
Bingeing but no noticeable weight gain	−	+	−
Disappearance into bathroom for long periods of time to induce vomiting	−	+	−
Abuse of drugs or alcohol	−	+	+
Self-esteem based on weight and shape	+	+	+

*Some individuals experience anorexia and bulimia and have symptoms of both disorders.
Modified from Hoffman L: *Eating disorders*, National Institutes of Health, NIH Publ No 93-3477, Bethesda, Md, January 1993.

BOX 2-3

Diagnostic Criteria for Anorexia Nervosa

A. Refusal to maintain body weight at or above a minimal normal weight for age and height or failure to make expected weight gain during period of growth, leading to body weight 15% below that expected.

B. Intense fear of gaining weight or becoming fat, even though underweight

C. Disturbance in the way in which one's body weight, size, or shape is experienced (e.g., the person claims to feel fat even when emaciated and believes that one area of the body is too fat even when obviously underweight; undue influence of body weight or shape on self-evaluation; or denial of the seriousness of the current low body weight)

D. In menstruating females, absence of at least three consecutive menstrual cycles when otherwise expected to occur (primary or secondary amenorrhea); a woman is considered to have amenorrhea if her periods occur only after hormone (e.g., estrogen) administration

Modified from American Psychiatric Association: Diagnostic and statistical manual of mental disorders-text revision, ed 4, (DSM-IV-TR), Washington, DC, 2000, The Author.

tion information (Eating Disorders Awareness and Prevention EDAP:http://www.edap.org; National Association of Anorexia Nervosa and Associated Disorders: http://www.anad.org). Women identified as meeting the criteria for the female athlete triad should not be disqualified from athletic participation but rather provided with appropriate education and treatment intervention.

Bulimia Nervosa. Bulimia nervosa is characterized by episodic binge eating (consuming large amounts of food at one time) followed by purging behavior such as self-induced vomiting, fasting, laxative and diuretic abuse, and excessive exercising. Before the 1970s, this disorder was relatively uncommon but since that time, its incidence has increased to exceed that of anorexia.

Risk factors are the same as for anorexia nervosa, and the bulimic person has a preoccupying pathologic fear of becoming overweight despite the fact that she or he is usually within normal weight standards. The individual is usually aware that the eating pattern is abnormal, and self-recrimination is frequent. In contrast to people with anorexia nervosa who restrict food as a means of gaining control over problems, people with bulimia react to distress by the binge-purge cycle. For many people with bulimia, the binge-purge cycle is initiated by a period of starving or extreme dieting to lose weight. Periods of normal eating may occur, but the pattern of fasting or bingeing will resume at some point in time.

The exact cause of bulimia nervosa is unknown although low tryptophan levels (precursor to serotonin) have been implicated. Several theories include a primary neurologic dysfunction, an electrical disorder similar to epilepsy, disturbance in the appetite and satiety center of the hypothalamus, and a learned behavior for dealing with stress and unpleasant feelings. A vicious circle of depression, overeating to feel better, vomiting and purging or fasting and exercising to maintain normal weight, and subsequent depression perpetuates this disorder.

Clinical Manifestations. In contrast to individuals with anorexia nervosa who are severely undernourished, the person with bulimia nervosa may appear to be of normal weight or even overweight. The effects of bulimia nervosa are similar to self-induced vomiting in anorexia nervosa: erosion of the tooth enamel and subsequent dental decay, irritation of the throat and esophagus, fluid and electrolyte imbalances, and rectal bleeding associated with laxative abuse. Binge eating results in abdominal distention and pain until relieved by vomiting or laxative use. Other symptoms may include mood changes, secretiveness, impulsive behaviors, sleep difficulties, and obsession with food and exercise (see Table 2-4). An increasing number of reports of seasonal mood fluctuations (e.g., seasonal affective disorder [SAD], discussed later in this chapter) are associated with bulimia nervosa. This connection is likely due to a common neurobiologic abnormality in the serotonergic dysfunction common to both disorders.[82]

Medical Management.   The DSM-IV provides diagnostic criteria for this condition. Treatment is also similar to the intervention recommended for anorexia, including psychotherapy, family therapy, and self-help groups. Pharmacotherapy may include selective serotonin reuptake inhibitors (SSRIs) such as Prozac, Zoloft, Fluvox, and Paxil. Treating bulimia with antidepressant drugs to increase serotonin levels may decrease the number of binge episodes and eases the depression associated with bulimia.

Binge-Eating Disorder.   Bingeing, sometimes referred to as *compulsive overeating*, has been defined as eating an unusual amount of food in a discrete period (e.g., within any 2-hour period) while feeling out of control (i.e., being unable to stop eating or control what or how much is eaten). It occurs as a normal consequence of restrictive eating or dieting. Usually, the binge eater is waiting too long between meals and snacks, avoiding certain types of food (usually considered high in calories and/or fat), or is not obtaining the necessary caloric or nutrient needs. A fear of weight gain underlies this eating disorder, but purging by the use of laxatives or induced vomiting is not typical.

Binge-eating differs from bulimia nervosa in that the person binge-eating does not engage in compensatory behaviors (e.g., vomiting, diuretics, laxatives, fasting). It differs from overeating by normal individuals in that during binge-eating, the food is eaten more rapidly than normal, the person eats until uncomfortably full, eats large amounts when not feeling physically hungry, and experiences feelings of embarrassment by how much is being eaten or disgust with oneself. Guilt and depression are often part of the behavioral characteristics.

Binge-eating disorder is possible to overcome with cognitive-behavioral therapy in a self-help format. This method of treatment has been shown to be the most effective for this disorder.[199]

Special Implications for the Therapist   2-3

EATING DISORDERS

Preferred Practice Patterns
4A: Primary Prevention/Risk Reduction for Skeletal Demineralization
4B: Impaired posture
4C: Impaired muscle performance (especially with malnutrition and fluid and electrolyte disturbances)

6A: Primary Prevention/Risk Factor Reduction for Cardiovascular/Pulmonary Disorders
6B: Impaired Aerobic Capacity/ Endurance Associated with Deconditioning
7A: Primary Prevention/Risk Reduction for Integumentary Disorders (malnutrition)

Women with eating disorders may be relatively open about severely restrictive dieting, but they are usually less likely to spontaneously offer information about purging or the use of exercise to compensate for eating. Denial of the illness is quite common among individuals with eating disorders, and interview techniques to obtain information are often unsuccessful. Establishing a strong therapeutic relationship characterized by genuineness, acceptance, honesty, and warmth is a prerequisite to eliciting accurate information. The therapist should be aware that people with eating disorders may be very resistant or very ambivalent about seeking counseling, nutritional guidance, or direct intervention of any kind.

Anorexia Nervosa
Rehabilitation may be required for the person with anorexia to regain muscle mass lost as a result of low-calorie diets, malnutrition, bingeing, and purging. It is important for the therapist to be aware of the physical side effects of previously diagnosed anorexia. Vital sign instability can be severe, including orthostatic hypotension, irregular and decreased pulse, and bradycardia and hypothermia, which can result in cardiac arrest. Heart rate must be monitored and maintained within safe limits during exercise. Profound heart abnormalities have been observed during exercise and can be associated with sudden death. Electrolyte imbalance and dehydration, fatigue, muscle weakness, and muscle cramping are physical complications associated with starvation, self-induced vomiting, and purgative abuse. Poor nutritional status and dehydration also contribute to easy bruising and poor wound healing (see Chapter 4).

Posture is often poor because of the loss of upper body muscle mass. Exercise tolerance may be low and endurance reduced significantly as a result of malnutrition. Clients may be resistive to exercise or may engage in excessive exercise to vent or work off their feelings and to burn up caloric intake. Consulting with other members of the health care team such as psychologists and psychiatrists can help in providing a behavioral approach to physical therapy and especially to an exercise program (Box 2-4).

After entering a recovery program or during hospitalization, a graduated exercise program may be introduced when clinically safe. Any exercise program must be adjusted for bone density and cardiac status, and laboratory values must be monitored for signs of dehydration, low white blood cell count, or anemia (see Chapter 39). Exercise is not recommended if the body weight is below a BMI of 18. Strenuous exercise programs such as aerobics are not introduced until the person is in a maintenance weight range and then only if the client is medically stable.

The health care provider must also remain aware of the possibility of undiagnosed eating disorders in any population group, especially preadolescents, adolescents, and young adults. The therapist may notice the presence of a painless swelling of the salivary glands and accompanying facial swelling during a head and neck examination. A musculoskeletal problem can be an indication of an eating disorder. Overuse injuries such as shin splints, tendinitis, stress fractures, or hip or back pain can occur from excessive ex-

Continued

ercise; the individual may continue to exercise despite fatigue, weakness, and pain. Early detection and prompt referral to an appropriate center with expertise in treating this illness is essential.

Bulimia Nervosa

Bulimia contributes to problems associated with fluid depletion and temperature regulation. For people who use vomiting to purge and abuse laxatives or diuretics, significant dehydration and potassium loss are quite frequent. The immediate outcome of such behavior is usually muscle cramping, including irregular heartbeat as the heart muscle cramps); fatigue; and low blood pressure on standing. In such situations, the therapist should delay intervention until electrolyte levels are within normal limits and encourage fluid intake and reduced activity level. In the more extreme condition, motor incoordination, confusion, and disorientation may be observed requiring medical attention.

Most deadly among the forms of purging is the abuse of ipecac, an emetic (a syrup that induces vomiting) used to treat poison victims. Many people who try it once find it so unpleasant that they avoid further use, but repeated use can cause toxic levels in the body producing myopathy with arm or leg weakness, or affecting the heart and causing sudden death. ■

Obesity

Definition. *Obesity* is medically defined as weight greater than 20% of desirable weight for adults of a given gender, body structure, and height. This definition may be somewhat misleading, since obesity by dictionary definition is an excessive accumulation of fat in the body. A person's body weight may be in excess of the normal range according to a height and weight chart, but if no excess body fat is evident, that person is not considered obese (bariatric is a medical term for obese). A more precise definition has been suggested: overweight describes someone who weighs 10% more than his or her optimum weight; obese individuals weigh 15% more, and grossly obese persons weigh 20% or more above the optimum weight for height and body type. (See Diagnosis in this section for other forms of measurement of body fat or obesity.)

Incidence. Obesity is now so common within the world's population that it is beginning to replace undernutrition and infectious diseases as the most significant contributor to ill health. It is second only to cigarette smoking as a leading cause of preventable death in the United States and contributes to 500,000 deaths annually. More than half of adult Americans are overweight or obese and more than half of this population is overweight with associated medical conditions.[155] The U.S. Department of Health and Human Services reports that one out of every five children is obese and the obesity rates have increased 147% from 1971 to 1994 among children ages 6 to 11.[44]

Etiologic Factors. The cause of obesity remains unknown, and the mechanisms that control homeostasis are not completely understood. A growing body of evidence suggests that some forms of obesity are more likely the result of biochemical defects rather than consumption of excess calories.[174] After a 40-year search, scientists have found three genes linked to obesity (ob, neuropeptide Y [Npy], and the Beacon gene). Npy and the Beacon gene produce a protein that stimulates the appetite, whereas the ob gene

---

BOX | **2-4**

Behavioral Goals and Guidelines for Eating Disorders

- Obtain an accurate exercise history.
- Determine the person's target heart rate and teach how and why it is important to monitor heart rate during exercise.
- Develop a well-rounded program of exercise, including stretching exercises, breathing techniques, light weights for upper extremity toning, aerobic exercise, and cooldown.
- Convey to the person that the treatment or exercise plan is to help and protect the person's overall health status and is not meant to control the person.
- Instruct each person on how to determine the appropriate frequency, intensity, and duration of each component of exercise. Monitor daily and weekly amounts of exercise using a chart or written record and use this tool to help the person develop a consistent and appropriate level of exercise.
- Make clear upper limits on number of repetitions and/or sets, since a tendency to overexercise exists.
- Encourage the client whenever possible to make decisions about the treatment plan; this will help provide a sense of control and increase self-confidence.
- Discern the person's attitude toward exercise and consistently encourage recognition of exercise as part of the overall health plan, not just as a means of losing weight.
- Exercise is only one tool for stress relief; encourage each individual to develop alternative ways of expressing feelings.
- Modifying thought patterns and changing behavior is a slow process. Encouragement and support are essential. Reinforce even small steps and successes.
- Watch for signs of dissociation (e.g., glazed look or faraway expression) and assist the person to remain aware of the effect of exercise on the physical body; paying attention to the physical discomfort helps prevent working through fatigue, striving for the runner's high, overexercising, and overuse injuries.
- Avoid making value judgments about the client's body or physical condition. When the client makes comments such as "I lost/gained a pound this week" or "I cannot believe how fat my arms are," do not react or judge by saying, "You are not supposed to be weighing yourself" or "You are not fat at all!" Seek professional guidance to handle such situations.

---

produces a protein (leptin) that switches off the appetite. In some obese people, the body does not respond to leptin; in others, the Beacon gene is working in overdrive, producing too much appetite-stimulating protein.[49] Preliminary studies show that the Beacon gene is the same across various regions and ethnicities.

Despite the new discoveries about single-gene mutations resulting in obesity, most cases of obesity are more likely the result of subtle interactions of several related genes with environmental factors, which favor the net deposition of calories as fat resulting in obesity. The increasing rates of obesity cannot be exclusively explained by changes in the gene pool, although genetic variants that were previously silent are now being triggered by the high availability of energy- and fat-dense foods and by the increasingly sedentary lifestyle of modern societies.[132,147]

The dramatic increase in size and weight of children may be the result of prenatal exposure to chemicals that have hormonal effects (e.g., dichloroethane [DDE], a product of the insect-killer DDT and polychlorinated biphenyl [PCB], a liquid electric insulator). Although these toxic environmental contaminants were banned in the United States in the 1970s, residents continue to carry both chemicals in their bodies and continued absorption is possible as a result of their use in other countries that have not banned their use. Studies are underway to identify more specifically how prenatal exposures at background levels may affect body size at puberty.[84]

Other causes of obesity may include depression; smoking cessation; endocrine and metabolic disturbances, which are uncommon and may actually occur secondary to the obesity; polycystic ovary syndrome; low set-point (obese people may have a genetically predetermined preferred body weight); delayed puberty; and failure of aging people to adjust food intake to lowered metabolism and diminished activity. Yo-yo dieting, or weight cycling with fluctuations of body weight produced by repeated cycles of weight loss and gain, appears to contribute to the inability to lose weight on a long-term basis.

Pathogenesis.   The pathogenesis of obesity is not understood. Several theories explain the physiology of obesity. The most obvious cause of obesity is an excessive intake of calories in proportion to the expenditure of calories. Inactivity and a high-fat, low-carbohydrate diet with excess intake of refined sugar are contributing factors to excess adipose tissue and weight gain. Low-fat diets can be high in calories and have a similar indirect effect of weight gain.

Accumulating evidence indicates that obesity is a central nervous system–mediated neuroendocrine dysfunction, since the central nervous system plays a key role in the regulation of food intake and energy balance. This evidence includes findings that either spontaneous genetic mutations or targeted gene deletions that impair central nervous system signaling cause disrupted food intake and body-weight control.[26] Researchers are studying the highly complex process of signaling molecules (see Chapter 1) involved in the regulation of food intake and how inherited or acquired defects in the function of these hormonal and neuropeptide signaling pathways contribute to obesity.[175,206]

The *Metabolic Syndrome* theory is another hypothesis involving the neuroendocrine system and suggests that hormonal dysfunction affecting the hypothalamic-pituitary-adrenal axis results in a complex series of events. Stress stimulates daily, periodic elevations of cortisol secretion and results in impaired cortisol secretion, prolonged stimulation of the sympathetic nervous system, and subsequent hypothalamic arousal. The net effect of this neuroendocrine-endocrine cascade is poorly regulated cortisol secretion, insulin resistance, elevated blood pressure, and visceral accumulation of body fat (central obesity).[29]

The sodium (Na^+)/potassium (K^+)/adenosine triphosphatase (ATPase) pump is believed to play a major role in the development of obesity. This enzyme pump transports sodium out of the cell and potassium into the cell at the expense of cellular energy in the form of adenosine triphosphate (ATP). Obese people have fewer ATPase pumps than the nonobese; the obese person uses less energy and expends fewer calories, keeping a state of equilibrium within the body.

The *fat cell* or *adipose cell theory* postulates that some people have an excessive number of fat cells (adipocytes) and the size of the fat cells is increased. The *lipoprotein lipase (LPL) theory* suggests that LPL (the enzyme that helps fat to be deposited in adipocytes) is elevated in obese persons and weight reduction stimulates even more production of LPL, causing fat cells to return to their hypertrophic size.

Clinical Manifestations.   The outward signs and symptoms of obesity are readily observable (excess body fat), but the effects and complications of obesity are less easily identified at onset. Obesity is associated with significant increases in both morbidity and mortality and is associated with three leading causes of death: cardiovascular disease, cancer, and diabetes mellitus.

More specifically, shortness of breath; atherosclerosis (hyperlipidemia) and high blood pressure; cardiomyopathy; increased susceptibility to infectious diseases, fatigue, menstrual disorders and infertility; and psychologic disturbances such as irritability, loneliness, depression, binge eating, and tension can be linked to obesity. Other complications may include nephrotic syndrome and renal vein thrombosis, other thromboembolic disorders, digestive tract diseases such as gallstones and reflux esophagitis, obstructive sleep apnea and subsequent pulmonary compromise with decreased gas exchange, vital capacity, and expiratory volume.

Type 2 diabetes mellitus (formerly, non-insulin-dependent) is often associated with obesity. Excessive food intake stimulates hyperinsulinemia. Through a negative-feedback mechanism, excessive insulin levels decrease the number of insulin receptor sites on adipose cells. The decrease in insulin receptor sites decreases the amount of glucose that can enter the cells. This promotes high blood levels of glucose. The excess glucose is stored as glycogen in the liver or as triglycerides in adipose cells, thereby enhancing hypertrophy and hyperplasia of fat cells in the already obese person. Weight reduction does reverse this process.

Diet accounts for about 35% of all cancers[8]; obesity is a known risk factor for hormone-related cancers such as breast, cervical, endometrial, and liver cancer in women and prostate, colon, and rectal cancer in men.[7,117] As discussed, dietary patterns (highly processed and refined foods without fiber) in combination with physical inactivity contribute to obesity and metabolic consequences. Nutritional modulation of growth-enhancing and differentiating hormones is discussed further in Chapter 8.

Medical Management

Diagnosis.   In most cases, physical examination is sufficient to detect excess body fat and also provides an assessment of the degree and distribution of body fat, overall nutritional status, and signs of secondary causes of obesity. Pediatricians are using new growth charts that now also calculate BMI (Table 2-5) as a better predictor of risk for being overweight. In the adult population, the physician must rule out lipedema, a symmetrical "swelling" of both legs, extending from the hips to the ankles, caused by deposits of subcutaneous adipose tissue (see discussion, Chapter 12).

Using calipers (the pinch test) to measure subcutaneous fat is one way to determine the presence of obesity. A fold of skin and subcutaneous fat from various body locations (e.g., midbiceps, midtriceps, and subscapular or inguinal areas) greater

TABLE	2-5

Body Mass Index to Determine Obesity Classification

CLASSIFICATION	BODY MASS INDEX (BMI)* (kg/m²)
Anorexia	<17.5
Underweight	17.5-19.9
Normal	20-24.9
Overweight	25-29.9
Obese	30-40
Severely obese	>40

*To calculate your BMI using pounds (lbs) and inches (in), multiply your weight (lbs) × 700 and divide the product by your height in inches squared. For example, if you weigh 155 lbs, 155 × 700 = 108,500. Now calculate your height in inches squared; for example, if you are 5 ft 8 in or 68 in tall, your height squared is $68^2 = 4624$; therefore 108,500 divided by 4624 = 23.4. This is considered within the normal classification.
NOTE: You can easily calculate BMI on the internet at http://www.nhlbisupport.com/bmi/.

than 1 inch indicates excessive body fat, although measuring with accuracy is a problem with this test. This measurement is taken into consideration along with body type and height.

Other procedures include electrical devices using light rays to measure the change in body composition as people progress through a weight loss program and relative weight (measured body weight (the desirable weight × 100) and BMI (measured body weight in kilograms [kg] (height in meters squared [m²]; see Table 2-5). BMI has replaced the old height/weight tables, although some criticism remains that BMI is not a valid indication of obesity, especially for people who are very muscular or very tall. It has, however, become the standard measure in studies evaluating health risk.

Treatment.   Many nutritionists involved in promoting the overall health of Americans question the need for weight loss in overweight or obese people who are not in the high risk BMI category. Some suggest that weight loss is not necessary for the healthy overweight or moderately obese person.[94] A multidisciplinary approach with emphasis on weight loss maintenance should be directed toward anyone with BMIs of 30 and above and for those people with a BMI in the 25 to 29 range who have associated health problems. Such a treatment program includes moderate calorie intake, behavior modification, exercise, and social support.

Medications for obesity are widely available OTC and by prescription. The use of pharmacologic agents to inhibit appetite and increase metabolic rate is highly controversial and provides, at best, only a short-term benefit. Researchers continue to look for drugs that can prevent or alter the physiology of obesity. Surgical treatment (referred to as *bariatric surgery*) may be considered for some obese people if serious attempts to lose weight have failed, BMI is greater than 40 kg/m², and complications of obesity are life-threatening.

Prognosis.   Little progress has been made in the successful treatment of obesity, especially when therapy is confined to dietary measures alone. The death rate increases in

proportion to the degree of obesity and in the presence of complications. For example, among the cardiovascular problems associated with obesity, hypertension in combination with obesity increases the risk for development of cerebrovascular disease, specifically cerebral thrombosis. Weight loss alters conditions associated with obesity and even moderate weight loss in an obese person (i.e., 10 to 20 pounds [lbs]) provides substantial changes in risk factors. Following weight loss in the obese, a decrease in blood pressure usually occurs with a regression of left ventricular hypertrophy, total and high-density lipoprotein (HDL) cholesterol are favorably changed, and glucose tolerance improves in those with type 2 diabetes mellitus. The addition of exercise to a comprehensive program of caloric reduction and behavior modification can improve results. Regular exercise can maximize body composition change and increase the probability of maintaining weight loss.

Patterns of fat distribution are important in determining the risk factor of obesity. Visceral fat within the abdominal cavity is more hazardous to health than subcutaneous fat around the abdomen. Upper body obesity around the waist and flank is a greater health hazard than lower body obesity marked by fat in the thighs and buttocks. People who are obese with high waist-to-hip ratios (greater than 1.0 in men and 0.8 in women) have a significantly greater risk of diabetes mellitus, stroke, coronary heart disease, and early death than equally obese people with lower ratios. Waist circumference alone has also been designated as an independent predictor of health risks and may replace the waist-to-hip measurement as a predictor of increased risk. For women, weight-related health risks increase when the waist measurement is 35 inches or more; for men, this figure is 40 inches or more.

Although the connection between obesity (BMI greater than 30) and coronary heart disease is well established, it remains unknown whether a similar link exists for mild overweight. A recent study has shown that even people (specifically women in this study) whose BMI at midlife (30 to 55 years of age) was between 23 and 24.9 had a 50% higher risk of heart attack compared with those whose BMI was under 20. Women whose BMI was greater than 29 had a 3.6 times greater risk of heart attack compared with the leanest group.[198]

Special Implications for the Therapist   **2-4**

OBESITY

Preferred Practice Patterns
Integument: 7A, 7B, and 7C. Primary prevention/risk factor reduction of integumentary disorders; impaired integument secondary to superficial or partial-thickness skin involvement (pressure ulcer prevention).
Various musculoskeletal patterns may be observed depending on clinical presentation.
Cardiopulmonary: 6A and 6B. Primary prevention/risk factor reduction for cardiopulmonary disorders; impaired aerobic capacity and endurance secondary to deconditioning

Problems associated with obesity commonly seen in a therapy program include back pain; arthritis; biomechanical dysfunction affecting the hips, knees, and ankle/foot; skin breakdown;

and cardiopulmonary compromise. Obesity is a known risk factor in the development of type 2 diabetes mellitus often accompanied by diabetic neuropathy, foot ulcerations, and neuropathic fractures (see discussion on Diabetes Mellitus in Chapter 10).

For the therapist, working with the obese person poses a definite risk to good health. Using proper body mechanics, careful planning for transfers, and obtaining adequate help are essential during any hands-on therapy.

Prevention

Prevention and screening programs for adults and children are being advocated by Healthy People 2010 toward the goal of promoting health and reducing chronic disease associated with diet and weight. Our role in prevention and wellness, including screening programs and health promotion, is discussed in Chapter 1 and presented in detail in the *Guide to Physical Therapist Practice* (2001). Therapists can be involved in hypertension and obesity screening as suggested by the Surgeon General because regular exercise is an important component toward physical and mental well-being and prevention of the comorbidities associated with obesity.

Since obesity is often associated with an increased prevalence of cardiovascular risk factors, graded exercise testing may be indicated before prescribing an exercise program. Even morbidly obese people can be evaluated on the treadmill with some modification in the testing protocol such as beginning with slow walking without treadmill elevation, followed by gradual increases in speed to achieve maximal exertion. Submaximal exercise testing overcomes many of the limitations of maximal exercise testing and may be applicable to this population.[101,102]

Exercise

Prescribing exercise for obese people follows the principles used with healthy people (Box 2-5), including modifications for mechanical limitations, awareness of potential hazards of exercise (Box 2-6), and awareness of the greater heat intolerance of the obese. Some equipment modifications may be necessary if the client is too large to use a stationary bicycle or exceeds the manufacturer's recommended weight capacity. For example, the client can pedal some stationary bikes while seated in a chair behind the bike.

A higher incidence of exercise-related injury exists among the obese that requires extra caution in the first few weeks. Recommendations include adequate warm-up and stretching, and progressive increases in intensity, frequency, and duration. Severe obesity contributes to back pain and back injury and affects foot mechanics, which can lead to foot and ankle problems. Selection of appropriate footwear with possible orthotic devices that provide heel support or compensatory foot pronation is recommended to make exercise safer and more comfortable.[103]

Aerobic exercise with a frequency of four times a week to produce significant weight loss is recommended because it provides the greatest caloric expenditure per minute of training. However, the frequency required is the reason most exercise programs fail for obese people, so compliance and caloric expenditure are the early goals toward achieving a habit of regular exercise rather than an immediate increase in aerobic endurance. Developing an exercise program the person likes and can complete over time is the initial focus. Finding the right match may take some time and several unsuccessful attempts.

Moreover, studies indicate that improved fitness through regular physical activity reduces cardiovascular morbidity and mortality for overweight individuals even if they remain overweight. The ultimate goal for the exercising obese person is to make a life-long commitment to achieving reasonable energy expenditure through routine physical activity.[104] The American College of Sports Medicine (ACSM) (1998a)[105] presents the benefits of low-intensity, short-duration regular exercise.

The influence of body weight on exertion and lower-extremity trauma may support an initial program of stationary cycling. Aquatic exercise programs can be an important part of reducing strain on joints by providing nonweight-bearing exercise for the obese person. Resistive exercises and weightlifting can be structured to produce aerobic gains by using a circuit style with low resistance, multiple repetitions, and short rests between sets. For most individuals, caloric expenditure with traditional strength-training techniques is not as great as with circuit lifting or aerobic conditioning, but strength training does use calories and can increase lean body mass.[106,107]

Behavior modification focusing on routine daily activities requiring no special equipment and involving only simple lifestyle changes may be the only type of physical activity that is continued for any length of time. For example, less reliance on vehicular transportation, parking a distance from the destination, avoiding elevators and using stairs, delivering messages within the work structure rather than telephoning, and walking 10 minutes during lunch are useful and easily accommodated suggestions for increasing energy expenditure. ∎

BOX **2-5**

Strategies to Facilitate Successful Exercise Programs

- Ask the client if he or she is currently exercising regularly (or was before illness or injury). Provide a brief description of benefits that the person could achieve from such a program.
- Stress exercise benefits of improving health rather than achieving weight loss.
- Allow the person to respond to the recommendation for an exercise program. Encourage the person to verbalize any thoughts or reactions to your suggestions.
- Determine whether the person believes that an exercise program will benefit him or her personally. Help the individual to set personal goals for exercise.
- Elicit from the client a statement accepting an exercise program.
- Be aware of any cultural or philosophical beliefs the person may have regarding exercise.
- If resistance to the idea of an exercise program is encountered, give the person an opportunity to list potential barriers to exercise. Ask the person to suggest ways to overcome potential barriers.
- Whenever possible, provide a written (preferably just pictures because of the potential of undisclosed illiteracy) of the proposed exercise program. Review progress and reward attempts, successes, and progression of the exercise program.
- Make it fun to foster a lifestyle approach characterized by long-term adherence.

BOX | 2-6

Potential Hazards of Exercise for the Obese Person

Precipitation of angina pectoris or myocardial infarction
Excessive rise in blood pressure
Aggravation of degenerative arthritis and other joint problems
Ligamentous injuries
Injury from falling
Excessive sweating
Skin disorders, chafing
Hypohydration and reduced circulating blood volume
Heat stroke or heat exhaustion

From Skinner JS: *Exercise testing and exercise prescription for special cases: theoretical basis and clinical application*, ed 2, Philadelphia, Lea & Febiger, 1993.

Domestic Violence

Violence is a term that encompasses a broad range of maltreatment including one or more of the following: physical violence, sexual violence, threats of physical and/or sexual violence, stalking, and psychologic/emotional abuse. No clear profile is available of the type of person who may be in an abusive relationship; pregnant women and women with disabilities are as much at risk as the able-bodied person. Domestic violence occurs across all races and socioeconomic groups.

Domestic violence or domestic abuse has reached epidemic proportions in the United States. Each year a reported 3 to 4 million women are physically assaulted or raped, as are a smaller unknown number of men, including older adults. An estimated 900,000 violent crimes against women committed by an intimate partner (spouse/partner, ex-spouse/ex-partner, friend, or boyfriend) are reported annually; the number of homicides remains unknown, but the National Institute for Occupational Safety and Health (NIOSH) reports that homicide is the leading cause of death for women at work.[153] Reports of elder abuse vary from 200,000 to nearly 2 million. The exact incidence is unknown. Complaints include cold food; lack of privacy; physical, sexual, and verbal abuse; neglect; and poor care. A significant number of the homebound elderly are also victims of passive judgment, arising from a lack of knowledge, time, or ability to cope with the problems of a dependent elder. Currently, data systems for monitoring and responding to violence against women across the United States are nonexistent.

Clinical manifestations of domestic violence are many and varied (Table 2-6). Therapists are most likely to see manifestations of abuse, which must be distinguished from accidental injuries by the location; pattern (e.g., gags leave lesions at the corners of the mouth, rope burns or pressure lines may appear where a restraint has been applied around the neck, wrists, or ankles; hair loss; circular burns); presence of multiple lesions; and the failure of new lesions to appear during hospitalization or after removal from the home or caretaker. The therapist should make every effort to obtain the client's permission to photograph physical evidence for immediate or perhaps later use in documentation.

Children may demonstrate any of the physical and/or behavioral signs listed, in addition to some manifestations

more common in children. Signs of passive neglect can be difficult to detect, and older adults are often reluctant to report mistreatment, fearing nursing home placement. Those at high risk of domestic violence include women between ages 17 and 28; women who are single, divorced, separated, or planning separation or divorce; women who have a history of abuse as a child or who witnessed abuse as a child; women who use alcohol or drugs or who have partners who use alcohol or drugs; and women whose partners are possessive or easily jealous.

Special Implications for the Therapist   2-5

DOMESTIC VIOLENCE

Preferred Practice Patterns
May vary depending on physical manifestations (e.g., musculoskeletal injuries, somatoform disorders, genitourinary disorders, central nervous system trauma [see Table 2-6])

Domestic violence often remains undetected and goes unreported. The therapist is able to develop a trusting relationship with clients and may become the first professional to identify the problem. During the therapy interview, the question, "Were you or have you been assaulted or hit?" can elicit the underlying cause for the injury or presenting symptoms.* Some sources advocate asking every client whether violence, assault, or rape has occurred, although ongoing debate occurs over this issue as it relates to the person's perceived sense of safety and willingness or ability to continue in rehabilitation. It may be necessary to ask this question later after the therapist has developed rapport with the client.

Questions should be asked with sensitivity and compassion but also directly and specifically. For example, if an injury seems questionable or the client presentation is suspicious of abuse, the therapist may ask, "Were you hit, kicked, or pushed? Can you tell me anything else about your situation?" A series of questions can be used as an abuse assessment screening.

In the case of the nonverbal client, the therapist may have to rely solely on physical manifestations of suspected abuse. Many good resources are available to help the therapist develop a screening and intervention program for domestic violence.[109-113]

Many aging adults subjected to abuse are cared for at home by family members who are at least age 50 and unprepared physically, emotionally, or financially for the added responsibility. Neglect is often not intentional or willful but rather the result of lack of information or misjudgment. Spouses may also physically abuse their partners. The home health therapist is often in the best position to evaluate or screen for potential mistreatment. Questions asked by the therapist in any setting or comments made by the client may reveal the need for further evaluation by the physician, social worker, or visiting nurse.

The health care professional should be familiar with community services available for the battered person whose safety is at risk. The therapy department should have pocket-sized

---

Assault is defined as a physical or verbal attack. Many people who have been physically struck, pushed, or kicked do not consider the action an assault, especially if inflicted by someone they know. Therefore it may be necessary to use some other word besides assaulted.

cards with phone numbers of appropriate agencies to provide a suspected or known victim of domestic violence. Local hospitals may have a consultant or domestic violence task force available to provide assistance once the problem has been identified. Telephone numbers for local shelters or hotlines should also be posted where the information can be obtained easily, such as the women's bathroom, where the victim can go unaccompanied by the perpetrator. Some facilities even provide a telephone in the restroom with directions on how to contact a local agency for help.

Since it is not always possible to recognize signs of abuse, therapists should approach intervention involving physical touch with clear instructions for all clients. Many important guidelines in the treatment of children and adults with a history of abuse are available in the resources previously listed. Additionally, the American Physical Therapy Association (APTA) has available *Guidelines for Recognizing and Providing Care for Victims of Child Abuse.*[14]

Any reasonable suspicion of child abuse must be reported as mandated by law in all 50 states of the United States.

Failure to do so can result in a civil and/or criminal penalty. Reporting a potential abusive situation in the case of an adult client must be approached with extreme caution and is not recommended if it puts the victim at risk. The therapist can make recommendations but must not push the client into making a decision; many people have been killed as a result of the perpetrator responding violently to intervention. The victim is the best person to know when it is safe to leave or obtain outside help.

Finally, it is important to remain aware of the signs of potential violence in the therapist's workplace. Experts on predicting violent behavior advise trusting your instincts and practice self-protection.[53] Notify local law enforcement personnel, hospital security, manager, or supervisor when experiencing any indication or intuition of danger. All facilities should have protocols in place to provide a safe and healthful workplace free of violence. Employers should provide written policies on violence in the workplace and provide employee training, proper staffing, and follow-up for any incidents. ■

TABLE   2-6

Clinical Manifestations of Domestic Violence

PHYSICAL	BEHAVIORAL	CHILDREN
Injuries (head, neck, chest, breast abdomen):	Hyperventilation	Diaper burn; severe diaper "rash"
Contusions	Multiple vague or nonspecific complaints	Genital bleeding
Lacerations	Sleep disturbances, insomnia	Developmental delays
Fractures	Self-destructive behaviors:	Enuresis
Head, neck, or face trauma:	Mood and appetite disorders	Discipline problems; angry outbursts
Dysphagia (from choking)	Alcohol and/or substance abuse	Tactile defensiveness
Hearing loss	Suicide ideation or attempts	Death
Ocular motor dysfunction	Self-mutilation	
Vestibular dysfunction	Social isolation, interpersonal distrust	
Recurrent sinus infections	Depression, anxiety, decreased sexual libido	
Temporomandibular joint pain/dysfunction	Poor work or school performance	
Deviated septum (broken nose)	Confusion (older adult)	
Bruises, burns, welts	Frequent physician or emergency department visits; frequent physician changes; frequently missing therapy appointments	
Headaches, somatopain disorders, chronic pain disorders, PTSD		
Gastrointestinal disturbance/symptoms	Bringing all the children to every appointment or always being accompanied by spouse or partner	
Poor nutrition and/or hygiene		
Pressure ulcers	Overuse of prescription drugs	
Sexual assault:		
Anuresis (urine retention)		
Dyspareunia (difficult or painful coitus)		
Recurrent genitourinary infections		
Temporomandibular pain/dysfunction		
Infertility		
Central nervous system:		
Subdural hematoma (blunt trauma or shaking)		
Retinal hemorrhage (shaking)		
Subarachnoid hemorrhage (shaking)		
Cerebral infarction (secondary to cerebral edema)		

Variations in Physical Activity and Exercise

Poor eating habits and a sedentary lifestyle are major risk factors for disease. Hypercholesterolemia, obesity, and muscular atrophy are only a few of the potential results of inactivity leading to atherosclerosis, constipation, hypertension, cardiorespiratory disorders, and some cancers. Much has been learned in the last decade about the adaptability of various biologic systems and the ways that regular physical activity and exercise can influence them. Participation in regular physical activity (both aerobic and strength training) is an effective intervention modality to reduce and/or prevent a number of functional declines associated with aging and to elicit a number of favorable responses that contribute to healthy aging.[30] (Box 2-7).

The effect of training intensity, psychosocial variables influencing exercise, and the breadth of emotional benefit from physical activity has not been fully determined, although studies in this area are ongoing.[74,50] Other research to determine the potential links between oxidative stress and physical activity/exercise in the aging adult is ongoing. Exercise, especially when performed strenuously, is associated with increased free radical formation (see Fig. 5-2), damaging key cellular components.[162] This is important in the older adult where the balance between beneficial and potentially harmful effects of exercise is influenced by sedentary lifestyle, nutritional deficiencies, and co-morbidities that can all deplete the individual's antioxidant reservoir.

Aging adults face additional problems of deconditioning or loss of balance and stability as a result of disease or illness. The most successful exercise programs take into consideration the person's functional capacity, medical status, and personal interests. Some helpful strategies for facilitating an exercise program (whether for a specific body part or as an overall fitness program) are listed in Box 2-7.

The importance of exercise in the prevention and rehabilitation of individual diseases is documented throughout this book. Even though the benefits of exercise are becoming widely known, most Americans remain sedentary. It is estimated that less than 10% of sedentary adults will begin an exercise program in a given year, and long-term adherence remains poor among those who do attempt to exercise regularly. About 50% of people discontinue exercise during the first year of practice.[56,158] Gender does not appear to be a significant predictor of exercise compliance.[58]

Exercise may be contraindicated in some conditions, and orthopedic problems are a common reason for noncompliance with an exercise program. Other barriers include increased demands at work or home, travel requirements, scheduling conflicts, illnesses, and disability. The risks and benefits of exercise among people with disabilities remain unknown. As people with disabilities live longer, the need for addressing long-term health issues, assessing the risk for secondary disability, and prescribing exercise from the perspective of disease prevention while reducing the risk for injury is needed.[51]

The therapist is often involved in the use of exercise as a treatment intervention, which may either follow the lifestyle approach to intervention based on the individual's motivational readiness and preferences for integrating physical activity into daily routines or a more structured approach (e.g., frequency, intensity, duration) in relation to diseases and chronic conditions. Whenever possible, specific information related to these aspects of exercise are included in Special Implications

---

BOX **2-7**

Biopsychosocial Benefits of Regular Activity and Exercise

Reduce/prevent functional declines associated with aging

Maintain/improve cardiovascular function; enhance submaximal exercise performance; reduces risk for high blood pressure; decreases myocardial oxygen demand

Aids in weight loss and weight control

Improved function of hormonal, metabolic, neurologic, respiratory, and hemodynamic systems

Alteration of carbohydrate/lipid metabolism resulting in favorable increase in high-density lipoproteins

Strength training helps to maintain muscle mass and strength, especially in the aging group

Reduces age-related bone loss; reduction in risk for osteoporosis

Improved flexibility, postural stability, and balance; reduction in risk of falling and associated injuries

Psychologic benefits (e.g., preserves cognitive function, alleviates symptoms/behavior of depression, improves self-awareness, promotes sense of well-being)

Reduction in disease risk factors

Improves functional capacity

Improves immune function (excessive exercise can inhibit immune function)

Reduces age-related insulin resistance

Reduces incidence of some cancers (e.g., colon, breast)

Contributes to social integration

Improves sleep pattern

American College of Sports Medicine (ASCM) Position Stand: Exercise and physical activity for older adults, *Med Sci Sports Exerc* 30(6):992-1008, 1998.

for the Therapist boxes in this chapter. The reader is referred to more basic texts for the underlying rationale related to exercise and disease.[4,124,177]

Psychologic Risks of Exercise

Few psychologic problems are associated with exercising, but some people become obsessed, even fanatical, about exercise. Any interruption in their exercise routine or schedule causes anger, irritability, and depression. Some people even become addicted to exercise, and certain clinical problems (e.g., anorexia nervosa, obsessive-compulsive personality disorder) are associated with excessive exercise.

Special Implications for the Therapist   **2-6**

VARIATIONS IN PHYSICAL ACTIVITY AND EXERCISE

Exercise as an intervention modality must be individually prescribed. When prescribed appropriately, exercise training is effective for developing fitness and health, preventing injury and disease, and rehabilitating injuries. Specific information on exercise training protocols for the healthy individual, aging adult, and individual with chronic illness or disease is readily available.[127-130]

The Addicted Exerciser

The therapist should be alert to the occasional client who becomes addicted to exercise. Clinical characteristics of such a person may include training to the exclusion of other important activities, dysphoria (depression accompanied by anxiety; disquiet) or panic when the exercise schedule is disrupted, exercising against medical advice, exercising more than once a day, and exercising to decrease or maintain an excessively low body weight (see the section on Anorexia Nervosa in this chapter). On the whole the challenge of achieving adherence to a regular exercise program far outweighs concern about the occasional person who becomes obsessed with habitual exercise. ■

STRESS, COPING, AND ADAPTATION

Stress

Definition and Overview.   *Stress* is a collective term used to describe the many social (e.g., change in job, residence, or marital status); psychologic (e.g., anxiety, fear of the unknown); and physiologic (e.g., blood loss, anesthesia, pain, immobility, infection) factors that cause neurochemical changes within the body. Stress and other emotional responses are components of complex interactions of genetic, physiologic, behavioral, and environmental factors that affect the body's ability to remain or become healthy or to resist or overcome disease. Regulated by nervous, endocrine, and immune systems, stress exerts a powerful influence on other bodily systems with important implications for the initiation or progression of cancer, cardiovascular disease, HIV, autoimmune diseases, and other illnesses.[24]

Holmes and Rahe[96] first developed the notion that personal or work-related life changes as a source of stress can eventually lead to disease. Their findings rank ordered major life change events, giving each event an assigned number to represent units of stress that could be totaled and scored. Today, a better measure of the impact of stress on an individual is through an assessment of behavioral responses (Box 2-8). As with any assessment tool, the key is to look for any new onset of behavioral symptoms (i.e., developed over the last 6 weeks to 6 months) that correlate with the onset or exacerbation of neuromusculoskeletal symptoms. Some people may score in the higher ranges normally, depending on their personality type (e.g., Type A) and temperament and not necessarily as a stress response to external circumstances.

The body's response to any stress, whether caused by events perceived as positive or negative, is to mobilize its defenses to maintain homeostasis (Table 2-7). The success of the stress response in maintaining homeostatic balance is determined by biobehavioral factors such as a person's age; gender; physical condition; coping mechanisms; health-enhancing or -impairing behaviors (e.g., diet, exercise, tobacco use, exposure to sunlight); and the duration of the stress.[160]

TABLE	2-7

Stress and Stress-Related Components

STRESS FACTORS	STRESS RESPONSE	SYMPTOMS OF STRESS
Situational	Increased heart rate and blood pressure	Hypertension
Poor social support (e.g., family, friends, coworkers)	Changes in respiratory system	Chest pain
Exposure to safety hazards	Release of glucose, adrenaline	Headache
Recent life changes (e.g., death of a parent, child or partner; family separation; pregnancy or birth; change in job or housing; retirement or being fired; heavy debt; sexual difficulties)	Redirection of blood supply (brain, muscles)	Myalgia, arthralgia, fibromyalgia
	Decrease in blood clotting time	Allergic responses
	Dilation of pupils	Gastrointestinal symptoms
Environmental	Contraction of the spleen	Depression, anxiety, panic attacks
Physical work environment; noise, lighting, temperature	Increased sweat production	Discouragement, boredom
Exposure to chemicals, dust, pathogens	Decreased peristalsis and gut function	Eating disorder
Rotating shift work (regularly changing work hours)	Decreased immune response (chronic stress)	Prolonged fatigue (chronic, fatigue syndrome)
Psychologic		Poor work or school performance; errors in judgment
Personality traits (e.g., aggressive, hostile Type A behavior)		Sleep disturbance
Lack of faith, spirituality, or religious practices		
Relationship or work conflict, work-family conflict, high job demands/low control		
History of abuse (physical, psychologic, emotional, sexual)		
Physical		
Sleep disturbances and/or sleep deprivation		
Chemical or biologic triggers (e.g., foods, poor nutrition, caffeine)		
Medical events, change in personal health, injury		
No exercise or excessive exercise		

BOX 2-8

The Stress Questionnaire

Mostly Yes	Mostly No	Question
_____	_____	1. Have you been feeling uncomfortably tense lately?
_____	_____	2. Are you engaged in frequent arguments with people close to you?
_____	_____	3. Is your social life satisfactory?
_____	_____	4. Do you have trouble sleeping?
_____	_____	5. Do you feel lethargic about life?
_____	_____	6. Do many people annoy or irritate you?
_____	_____	7. Do you have constant cravings for candy and other sweets?
_____	_____	8. Is your cigarette or alcohol consumption way up?
_____	_____	9. Are you becoming addicted to soft drinks or coffee?
_____	_____	10. Do you find it difficult to concentrate on your work?
_____	_____	11. Do you often grind your teeth?
_____	_____	12. Are you increasingly forgetful about little things like mailing a letter?
_____	_____	13. Are you increasingly forgetful about big things like appointments and major errands?
_____	_____	14. Are you making too many trips to the restroom?
_____	_____	15. Have people commented lately that you do not look well (or "good")?
_____	_____	16. Do you get into verbal fights with people too frequently?
_____	_____	17. Have you been involved in more than one fight lately?
_____	_____	18. Do you have a troublesome number of tension headaches?
_____	_____	19. Do you feel nauseated much too often?
_____	_____	20. Do you feel light-headed or dizzy almost every day?
_____	_____	21. Do you have churning sensations in your stomach too often?
_____	_____	22. Are you in a big hurry all the time?
_____	_____	23. Are far too many things bothering you?
_____	_____	24. Do you often feel tired and exhausted for no particular reason?
_____	_____	25. Do you have difficulty shaking colds or other infections?

Scoring

0-7	*Mostly Yes answers:* You seem to be experiencing a normal amount of stress
8-17	*Mostly Yes answers:* Your stress level seems high. Become involved in some kind of stress management activity.
18-25	*Mostly Yes answers:* Your stress level appears much too high. Discuss your stress level with a mental health professional or visit your family physician (or both).

From DuBrin AJ: *Fundamentals of organizational behavior: an applied approach,* Cincinnati, Ohio, 1997, South-Western College Publishing.

Risk Factors.   A growing consensus among stress researchers is to understand the relationship between stress and illness outcomes, so the factors that modify or mediate the relationship must be identified. Although stressors may produce temporary physiologic and psychologic changes, most stressors are not followed by long-term illness. A stressor may produce an extreme reaction in one person but no reaction in another, or the same stressor may produce variable reactions in the same individual at different times. This suggests that factors exist that alter the responses to stressors.

One factor that can alter a stress response is the environment, such as social support, which tends to buffer individuals from the potentially negative effects of stressors. Those people with strong social supports live longer and have a lower incidence of physical illness. Several large studies have established that women feel stress more than men do at comparable life stages and in similar circumstances. Women's catecholamines and blood pressure tend to remain elevated long after the end of the workday, whereas the men's start to decline as soon as they leave work.[75,98] Other potential factors are listed in Table 2-7.

Negative life events, especially work-related are associated with depressed mood and mental strain but not with elevation of biologic risk factors such as elevated blood pressure and serum lipids. Depressed mood and mental strain are related to increased tobacco consumption in labor workers and increased alcohol consumption in professional workers.[167] Although many factors causing stress have been studied, the ability to predict a stress response in any given individual remains poor.

Pathogenesis.   Research supports a strong correlation between chronic stress response and the manifestation of various disorders (Box 2-9) but a direct link has not been estab-

BOX 2-9

Stress-Related Conditions and Diseases

Allergic and hypersensitivity diseases
Anorexia nervosa
Asthma
Bulimia nervosa
Cancer
Cerebrovascular accident
Connective tissue disease
Crohn's disease (regional enteritis)
Emphysema
Gastrointestinal ulcers
Headache
Hypertension
Infections
Irritable bowel syndrome
Myocardial infarction
Obesity
Peripheral vascular disease
Sexual dysfunction
Tuberculosis
Ulcerative colitis

   At one time, it was thought that a direct link could be established between stress events and illness or between personality type and illness. At that time, it was not uncommon to hear professionals speak of a colitis, ulcer, or stroke personality. However, none of these theories have held up under investigation. At this time, only personality (angry, hostile type A behavior) has been *directly* linked with (heart) disease (see Chapter 11).

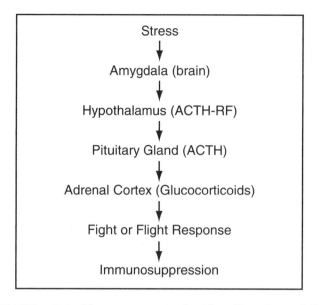

FIGURE 2-4 The stress response algorithm. (From Bancroft B: Immunology simplified, *Semin Perioperative Nurs* 3:70-78, 1994.)

lished. The body's response to stress is a complex combination of biologic and behavioral mechanisms that are regulated by the neurohormonal axis. How stress produces disease is frequently debated, and the exact pathophysiologic mechanism remains unknown. The stress response has been associated with a variety of physiologic changes that may be postulated as mediators in the development of disease. The hypothalamic-pituitary axis, the autonomic nervous system, and the catecholamine response are often cited as stress-sensitive systems. These and other neurologic and endocrine systems may be important factors in the chain of events leading to cardiovascular, gastrointestinal, endocrine, and other stress-related disorders.

   Recently, significant amounts of information have become available on how the stress response systems interact in combination with a proposed neuroendocrine-neuroimmune stress response to affect autoimmunoregulation. Findings that link immune and neuroendocrine function may provide explanations of how the emotional state or response to stress can modify a person's capacity to cope with infection, inflammation, or cancer and influence the course of autoimmune disease. For example (Fig. 2-4 and 2-5; see Fig. 10-2), in response to a stress impulse, the amygdala in the brain signals the hypothalamus to release adrenocorticotropic hormone–releasing factor (ACTH–RF). This stimulating hormone causes ACTH (corticotropin) to be released from the pituitary gland. ACTH

is the major hormone regulator of the body's adaptive response to stress and the physiologic stimulus for the release of stress hormones (e.g., adrenaline, noradrenaline, cortisol) from the adrenal glands (target organ). These powerful hormones and glucocorticoids (cortisol) create within the body the fight-or-flight response. This cascade of events can lead to hypercortisolism and inappropriately elevated catecholamines, resulting in immunosuppression (i.e., decreased numbers of lymphocytes [white blood cells]) and antibodies and thus increasing vulnerability to infectious diseases including viral-induced cancers and other diseases.[106]

   Studies of the hypothalamic-pituitary-adrenal (HPA) axis as a potential psychobiologic mediator of these effects are underway.[23] Understanding the biochemical mechanisms underlying stress may permit the development of pharmacologic strategies to treat chronic stress and possibly prevent the development of stress-related disorders. In 1995, researchers identified a peptide known as *prepro-TRH178-199* that had been shown to reduce the secretion of corticotropin, or ACTH, by 50%. Administration of this corticotropin release–inhibiting factor (CR–IF) in animal studies before exposure to stress revealed significantly reduced levels of ACTH and other hormones elevated in response to stress. This peptide also decreased fear and anxiety-related behaviors. Ongoing studies continue to look for ways to use this peptide for therapeutic purposes.[59]

   Another theory holds that certain kinds of stress are consistently likely to produce given physiologic responses, and, consequently, specific pathologic states. The impact of stress on cells directly or indirectly, causes protein denaturation, and elicits a stress response. A cell with normal anti-stress mechanisms may be able to withstand stress if the intensity is not beyond that which will cause irreversible protein damage. Age-related degenerative disorders with protein deposits in various tissues may be an example of the physiologic result of this type of stress.[127]

   Still another viewpoint is that stress is nonspecific and that personal factors such as conditioning and heredity determine

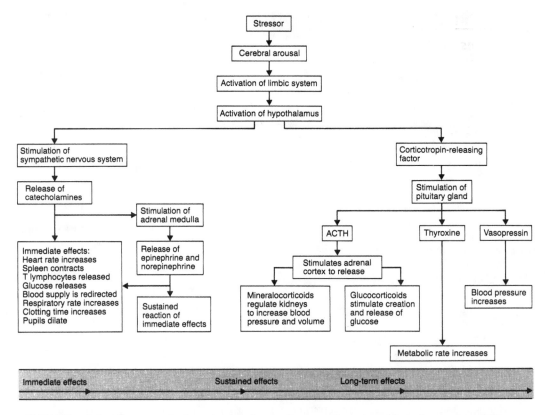

FIGURE **2-5**   The general adaptation syndrome. See text discussion. (From Ignatavicius DD, Workman ML, Mishler MA: Medical-surgical nursing, ed 2, Philadelphia, 1995, WB Saunders)

which organ system, if any, will be affected by a variety of stressors. A given individual may have a specific susceptible organ that will be the target of a variety of stresses; thus some people are gastrointestinal reactors; others are cardiac or muscle tension reactors. Familial patterns may account for the hereditary factor determining which organ system is affected. Low back pain, abdominal pain, and migraine headaches affecting adults often also occurred in the parents. Finally, stress may be viewed as a nonspecific force that exacerbates existing disease states.

Stress can play a key role in psychogenic pain (i.e., pain believed to be caused by emotional factors rather than the result of physiologic dysfunction). Although psychogenic pain begins without a physical basis, repeated severe stress most likely alters the complex physiology of pain transmission, modulation, and perception. When the psychogenic effects of stress, anxiety, fear, and anger produce painful alterations in physiology, this is referred to as *psychophysiologic pain*. For example, stress can produce chronic excessive muscle contraction with resultant ischemia, and pain with eventual functional impairment. For further discussion see the Psychophysiologic Disorders section in this chapter.

Clinical Manifestations.   Therapists often treat people with neuromusculoskeletal dysfunction, especially head, neck, and back pain without an identified point of injury or cause. Stress, reaction to stress, and posttraumatic stress disorder are common causes of physical manifestations treated by the therapist. Muscle tension and pain, restlessness, irritability, fatigue, increased startle reaction, breath holding, hyperventilation, tachycardia, palpitations, and sleep distur-

bances are some of the more common symptoms reported to the therapist (see Table 2-7). Clients often self-medicate using chemical (alcohol, nicotine, drugs) or food substances; the alert therapist may help assist the client by facilitating treatment intervention for this aspect of the person's stress response.

Recent studies provide clear and convincing evidence that chronic psychosocial stress contributes significantly to the pathogenesis and exacerbation of coronary artery atherosclerosis, whereas acute stress induces ovarian dysfunction, hypercortisolism, and accelerated atherosclerosis. Acute stress triggers myocardial ischemia, stimulates platelet function, increases blood viscosity, and causes coronary vasoconstriction in the presence of underlying atherosclerosis (coronary heart disease).[170]

Some individuals also experience exaggerated heart rate and blood pressure responses to psychologic stress. Emotionally responsive individuals report less satisfaction with social support and higher levels of perceived daily stress, anxiety, and depressive symptoms. Psychosocial traits that have been linked to cardiovascular disease may be associated with more marked cardiovascular activation occurring in response to negative emotions experienced throughout the day.[39] Researchers hypothesize the exaggerated systemic vascular resistance responses during stress may be caused by endothelial dysfunction. This association may help explain the growing evidence of a relationship between stress hemodynamics and cardiovascular disease risk. It is postulated that the interplay between the sympathetic nervous system and the endothelium accounts for the regulation or dysfunction of vascular tone.[178]

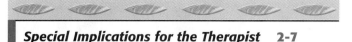

Special Implications for the Therapist 2-7

STRESS

Preferred Practice Patterns
Other patterns associated with additional variables (e.g., substance use/abuse, posttraumatic stress disorder, side effects of medications) may be observed
Musculoskeletal 4B: Impaired posture; 4C: Impaired muscle performance

The therapist may be called on to assist the client in reducing the physical impact of stress on the body as well as providing a means of physical or emotional control. *Progressive muscle relaxation (PMR)*, breathing exercises, physical activity and exercise, and biofeedback are the primary tools used in therapy to teach the client effective stress-reducing techniques. Since stress commonly causes muscle tension, producing somatic symptoms such as headaches and neck and back pain, control of muscle tension appears to help reduce the physical effects of such tension as well. PMR involves the alternate tensing and relaxing of all major muscle groups, usually in sequential steps. It is easy to teach and inexpensive.

Breathing exercises can be helpful in restoring normal respiration by providing moments of deep breathing because the person in a stressful situation tends to breathe shallowly or even unconsciously holds his or her breath. Teaching diaphragmatic breathing skills and suggesting ways clients can remember to check their breathing (e.g., whenever the telephone rings, setting their watches to beep on the hour, at every stop sign when in an automobile) can aid in reducing the chest and upper body muscle tension and diaphragmatic tension and dysfunction that accompanies altered breathing patterns.

Physical activity and exercise is only one of the behavioral and psychologic therapies recommended for the treatment of selected clients, such as those with coronary disease. Exercise, particularly when combined with a weight loss program can lower both resting and stress-induced blood pressure levels and produce a favorable hemodynamic pattern for the treatment of hypertension.[144]

Exercise training along with type A behavior* modification, psychologic counseling, smoking cessation, and dietary modification are all considered important in the overall holistic treatment approach to many people. For example, aerobic exercise has been found to consistently attenuate (weaken or reduce) the psychophysiologic responses to stress, particularly in type A personalities.[145] Type A beliefs may predispose individuals to health problems through impaired interactions with their interpersonal environment,[147] as will mechanisms that increase cardiovascular and neuroendocrine responses.[148] In this particular population, aerobic training blunts their cardiovascular and adrenal response to stress.

Although physical exercise may be considered a stressor itself, significant differences are apparent in the way the body responds to exercise versus the way the body responds to a mental stressor. A key difference is between the diastolic and systolic blood pressure responses. Exercise results in a rise in the systolic pressure and possibly a small increase in diastolic pressure, whereas mental stress produces a significant increase in both diastolic and systolic blood pressures. Blood vessels dilate during physical exercise to increase the blood supply to the muscles. During this vasodilation the diastolic blood pressure tends to stabilize or increase mildly, whereas during mental stress, the muscles may isometrically contract (muscle tension), but no substantial movement of the body by the muscles and no metabolic reason for vasodilation occurs. Decreased vagal activity may contribute to the exaggerated diastolic blood pressure reactivity to mental stress.[149]

Biofeedback can be an effective means of training people to reverse the subtle changes in blood pressure, muscle tension, and heart rate that accompany a stress-induced somatic response. Biofeedback involves using electronic instrumentation to signal selected somatic changes. Surface electrodes are sensitive to small changes in the electrical activity of the muscles, signaling to the client by way of sound or sight the need to practice physiologic quieting techniques (e.g., visualization, imagery, deep breathing). ∎

Anxiety Disorders

Anxiety is defined as a generalized emotional state of fear and apprehension usually associated with a heightened state of physiologic arousal such as elevation in heart rate and sweat gland activity. The most common anxiety disorders encountered in the therapy practice include adjustment disorder with anxious mood; general anxiety disorder; posttraumatic stress disorder (PTSD); panic disorder; and obsessive-compulsive disorder (OCD). Somatic symptoms referable to the autonomic nervous system or to a specific organ system (e.g., chest pain, dyspnea, palpitations, paresthesias) often occur. Anxiety can become self-generating because the symptoms reinforce the reaction, causing a spiral effect. Stimulants such as caffeine, cocaine or other stimulant drugs, or medications containing caffeine, or stimulants used in treating asthma can also trigger anxiety disorders and contribute to this spiral effect.

The *adjustment disorder* is usually a temporary phenomenon in response to a stressor such as a traumatic injury (e.g., SCI, cerebrovascular accident, total body burns); change in family system due to debilitation of the wage earner; or a known organic condition such as a pulmonary embolus with a life-threatening status. During the adjustment phase, the person gathers resources to maintain self-worth, acceptance, and ability to cope. For some people, the adjustment stage becomes more of a maladjustment stage, in which case the person remains unable to come to terms with fear, disbelief, anger, guilt, or depression and remains hampered by the disease's real or perceived impairment. When viewed by the client as an unpredictable, variable, and disabling condition, chronic illnesses such as chronic obstructive pulmonary disease (COPD) or multiple sclerosis are often associated with such an adjustment disorder.

General anxiety disorders are marked by a focus on physical or emotional pain; the person either notices pain more or interprets pain as being more significant than a nonanxious per-

---

*A behavior pattern associated with the development of coronary heart disease, characterized by excessive competitiveness and aggression and a fast-paced lifestyle. Persons exhibiting type A behavior are constantly struggling to accomplish ill-defined or broadly encompassing goals in the shortest time possible. This type of behavior has been shown to be as significant as other risk factors in the development of coronary artery disease and myocardial infarction when accompanied by hostility associated with anger.[146] The opposite type of behavior, exhibited by people who are relaxed, unhurried, and less aggressive, is called type B.

son would. Disability, pain behavior such as limping and grimacing, and medication-seeking may develop. Symptoms may present as physical, behavioral, cognitive, or psychologic (Table 2-8).

Posttraumatic stress disorder (PTSD), a condition once thought to be limited to combat veterans as a result of situations that were considered outside the range of usual human experience* is now recognized as a stress disorder that can occur at any age, including childhood. Characteristic symptoms usually begin within the first 3 months after exposure to an extreme traumatic stressor. This may involve direct personal experience of an actual or threatened death or serious injury; other threat to one's physical integrity; or witnessing of an event that involves death, injury, or threat to someone else. The person's response to the event involves intense fear, helplessness, or horror (or in children, disorganized or agitated behavior).

Traumatic events that are experienced may include military combat; violent personal assault (sexual assault, physical attack, robbery, mugging); being kidnapped or taken hostage; terrorist attack; torture; incarceration as a prisoner of war or in a concentration camp; natural or man-made disasters; experiencing a significant medical event (e.g., cardiac arrest and resuscitation); or being diagnosed with a life-threatening illness. For children, sexually traumatic events may include developmentally inappropriate sexual experiences without threatened or actual violence or injury.

A delay of months, or even years, may occur before symptoms appear. The person with PTSD experiences persistent symptoms of anxiety, increased arousal, or hypervigilance not present before the trauma. These symptoms may include difficulty falling or staying asleep, exaggerated startle response, or difficulty concentrating on or completing tasks. Children may also exhibit various physical symptoms such as headaches and stomachaches. Other associated conditions can exist, such as panic disorder, agoraphobia, obsessive-compulsive disorder, social phobia, specific phobia, major depressive disorder, somatization disorder, and substance abuse disorders.

After a traumatic event, people often report using substances to relieve their symptoms of anxiety, irritability, and depression. Alcohol may relieve these symptoms because drinking compensates for deficiencies in endorphin activity after a traumatic experience. Within minutes of exposure to a traumatic event an increase occurs in the level of endorphins in the brain, which remain elevated and help numb the emotional and physical pain of the trauma. After the trauma is over, endorphin levels gradually decrease, and this may lead to a period of endorphin withdrawal that can last from hours to days, producing emotional distress and contributing to the symptoms of PTSD. Because alcohol use increases endorphin activity, drinking after trauma may be used to compensate for this endorphin withdrawal and thus avoid the associated emotional distress.[139,194]

Panic disorder is characterized by periods of sudden, unprovoked, intense anxiety with associated physical symptoms lasting a few minutes to less than 2 hours. Initial panic attacks may develop during a period of extreme stress, or fol-

TABLE	2-8

Symptoms of Anxiety and Panic Attacks

Physical	Behaviorial	Cognitive
Increased sighing respirations	Hyperalertness	Fear of losing one's mind
Increased blood pressure	Irritability	Fear of losing control
Tachycardia	Uncertainty	
Shortness of breath	Apprehensiveness	
Dizziness	Difficulty with memory or concentration	
Lump in throat	Sleep disturbance	
Muscle tension		
Dry mouth		
Diarrhea		
Nausea		
Clammy hands		
Sweating		
Pacing		
Chest pain*		

*Chest pain associated with anxiety accounts for more than half of all emergency room admissions for chest pain. The pain is substernal, a dull ache which does not radiate, and is not aggravated by respiratory movements, but *is* associated with hyperventilation and claustrophobia.

lowing surgery, a serious accident, illness, or childbirth. The premenstrual period is one of heightened vulnerability. Panic disorder may be due to an inherently unstable autonomic nervous system, coupled with cognitive distress. Worrisome signs and symptoms such as marked dyspnea; tachycardia; palpitations; headaches; dizziness; paresthesias (nose, cheeks, lips, fingers, toes); choking; smothering feelings; nausea; and bloating are associated with feelings of alarm and a sense of impending doom. Recurrent sleep panic attacks (not nightmares) occur in about 30% of panic disorders. Residual sore muscles are a consistent finding after the panic attack; the person with sleep panic attacks awakens feeling fatigued, stiff, and sore.

Obsessive-compulsive disorder (OCD) is characterized by obsessions (constantly recurring thoughts such as fear of exposure to germs) and compulsions (repetitive actions such as washing the hands hundreds of times a day). The motivating force behind such behaviors was thought to be the need to maintain control, but the fact that some people with OCD respond well to specific medications suggests the disorder may have a neurobiologic basis. Most clients do not mention the symptoms or the disorder (if diagnosed) and must be asked about their presence and effect on the person's life and rehabilitation. Major depression is present in two thirds of cases of OCD. A person is not considered to have OCD unless the obsessive and compulsive behaviors are extreme enough to interfere with daily activities.

People with OCD should not be confused with a much larger group of individuals who are sometimes considered compulsive because they hold themselves to a high standard of performance in their work and even in their recreational (or rehabilitation) activities. Compulsive exercising sometimes accompanied by bulimia or other eating disorders can interfere with the rehabilitation process.

---

*Researchers are now examining the long-term health status of those people in dangerous occupations such as firefighters and police officers..

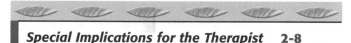

Special Implications for the Therapist   2-8

ANXIETY DISORDERS

Although clients with panic disorder may fear exercise, panic attacks during exercise are rare. Recognizing that our clients may experience anxiety or panic in reaction to our intervention, our actions, and the treatment environment is important. If a client experiences a panic attack during therapy, reassurance and distraction often work well to help the person move through the episode. Hyperventilation may be an accompanying symptom requiring intervention. A paper bag is used for rebreathing in such instances.

Recognizing risk factors and signs and symptoms of previously undiagnosed anxiety disorders can result in referral to a physician or mental health professional and can provide the client with beneficial treatment. Medications can provide significant relief from the symptoms of anxiety disorders in more than half of all cases. Combining physical therapy with behavioral therapy can often accelerate both the physical and psychologic rehabilitation process. Sufficient evidence now exists for the effectiveness of regular exercise as a direct intervention for anxiety disorders.[117,152] The exact mechanism whereby exercise reduces symptoms of anxiety has not been determined; differing psychologic and physiologic mechanisms have been proposed.

The therapist must remain alert to the possibility of suicide or alcohol abuse sometimes combined with dependence on sedatives. Suspicion of either should be reported to the case manager, counselor, or physician (see the section on Suicide in this chapter). Clients with obsessive-compulsive tendencies must be given specific guidelines for any home program prescribed. Specific limits for numbers of repetitions must be provided, including the strict admonishment to avoid checking their pain or loss of motion to see if any improvement has occurred. ∎

Psychophysiologic Disorders

Psychophysiologic disorders, also referred to as *psychosomatic disorders*, are any disorders in which the physical symptoms may be caused or exacerbated by psychologic factors. Common examples include migraine headaches, low back pain, gastric ulcer, or irritable bowel syndrome. Previously, it was believed that psychologic factors caused these conditions. More recently, the existing lack of certainty about the actual role of psychologic factors in causing these conditions has led researchers to suggest that psychologic factors are more likely to be contributory to physical conditions.

Psychophysiologic disorders are generally characterized by subjective complaints that exceed objective findings, symptom development in the presence of psychosocial stresses, and physical symptoms involving one or more organ systems. This category includes somatoform disorder, malingering, psychogenic pain disorder, and factitious disorder. Although malingering is not a true psychiatric disorder, it is included in this section, since it can occur across many domains.

Somatoform Disorder.

Somatoform disorder is the presence of physical symptoms that suggest a medical condition causing significant impairment in social, occupational, or other areas of functioning. The physical symptoms associated with somatoform disorders are not intentional or under voluntary control, which differentiates it from factitious disorder and malingering. Somatoform disorders are characterized more by symptoms, suffering, and disability than by consistently demonstrable tissue abnormality. It has been suggested that the somatoform disorders all involve the same pathophysiologic dysregulation and blunting of the central nervous system's response to stress, but the exact mechanism remains unknown.[48]

Although discrete pathophysiologic causes may ultimately be found in these disorders, these people's experiences are exacerbated by a self-perpetuating, self-validating cycle in which the symptoms are incorrectly attributed to serious abnormality. Four psychosocial factors propel this cycle of symptom amplification: (1) the belief that one has a serious disease; (2) the expectation that the condition is likely to get worse; (3) the sick role, including the effects of litigation and potential compensation; and (4) the portrayal of the condition as catastrophic and disabling.[22]

Somatic distress and medically unexplained symptoms have always been endemic to daily life but the social and cultural characteristics in each era have shaped the expression, interpretation, and attribution of these symptoms. Similar constellations of symptoms acquire different diagnostic labels and are attributed to different causes in different time periods. Although the somatic syndromes are not new, people who have these syndromes today differ from those several decades ago by being less relieved by negative findings on medical examination and less responsive to explanation, reassurance, and palliative treatment. Variables that may account for this change include decline in the authority of physicians and public certainty of or agreement with medical opinion, mass media reporting that these conditions are epidemics with sensational portrayal of individual sufferers, strong advocacy groups that mobilize public opinion and shape public policy, and the increasing litigious society in which we live with class actions seeking to attribute liability and fault for these conditions.[22]

People who are unable to cope with emotional problems or conflicts may develop physical symptoms as a means of coping, because it may be easier to accept physical symptoms as a cause of unhappiness or conflict than to admit to an underlying emotional or psychologic cause. The disorder is characterized by vague, multiple, recurring physical complaints that have no biologic or physiologic cause. This disorder was previously included in the group of psychologic conditions called *hysterical neurosis* (conversion type).

The term *somatoform disorder* is often used interchangeably with somatization disorder, but in fact, somatoform disorder includes six distinct conditions, namely somatization disorder, undifferentiated somatoform disorder, conversion disorder, pain disorder, hypochondriasis, and body dysmorphic disorder.

Specific symptoms of somatization disorder (Briquet's syndrome) (Box 2-10) may include double or blurred vision, food sensitivity, abdominal pain or bloating, bowel problems, vomiting, fainting, headaches, back pain, chest pain or palpitations, nonexertional dyspnea, painful menstruation, muscle aches or joint pain, or sexual indifference. These symptoms are often presented in a dramatic and exaggerated way, but the person is vague about the exact nature of the symptoms. Depression and anxiety are often key components of this disorder, but it is often difficult to determine which condition is the cause and which is the effect. The person will consult with multiple physicians and receive a variety of treatment approaches, often including multiple surgeries, with apparent unsuccessful outcome.

The term *functional somatic syndrome* refers to several related somatization disorders that have developed more recently and have acquired major sociocultural and political dimensions. These include multiple chemical sensitivity, the sick building syndrome, repetition stress injury, chronic whiplash, chronic Lyme disease, the side effects of silicone breast implants, candidiasis hypersensitivity, the Gulf War syndrome, food allergies, mitral valve prolapse, and hypoglycemia.[22] These individuals often have a strong sense of assertiveness and embattled advocacy with respect to their condition, whereas at the same time, the medical world may devalue and dismiss them because of lacking epidemiologic or pathophysiologic support for these syndromes.

Undifferentiated somatoform disorder is characterized by unexplained physical complaints lasting at least 6 months that are below the threshold for a diagnosis of somatization disorder. The most common complaints are chronic fatigue, loss of appetite, or gastrointestinal or genitourinary symptoms that cannot be fully explained by any known general medical condition. Physical symptoms or impairment are beyond what would be expected from the history, physical examination, or laboratory findings.

Hypochondriasis is marked by a preoccupation with one's health and exaggeration of normal sensations and minor complaints into a serious illness. Hypochondriasis is focused on a single illness, unlike somatization, which is accompanied by multiple complaints. With hypochondriasis, symptoms are amplified and the client is hyperresponsive to the treatment administered, especially in the therapy setting. No amount of reassurance can convince the person that he or she is healthy; hypochondriasis is often common in panic disorders.

Somatoform pain disorder is another type of somatization disorder frequently encountered in the therapy setting. Pain disorder is characterized by pain as the predominant focus of clinical attention, but psychologic factors have an important role in the onset, severity, exacerbation, or maintenance of this disorder.[55] This condition may be viewed as (1) pain disorder associated with psychologic factors; (2) pain disorder associated with a general medical condition; and (3) pain disorder associated with both psychologic factors and a medical condition. Both acute and chronic forms of somatoform pain disorder can occur. Chronic pain associated with a known medical condition (e.g., neoplasm, diabetic polyneuropathy, postoperative pain) is discussed in the next section, Chronic Pain Disorders.

Body dysmorphic disorder is a particular type of somatization disorder often encountered in people who have undergone amputation or extensive surgery or had burns with significant scarring and those with weight control problems.[202] A preoccupation with the imagined or exaggerated defect in personal appearance often occurs.

Conversion is a psychodynamic phenomenon rather than a behavioral response to illness or injury and is quite rare in the chronically disabled population. Conversion is defined as a transformation of an emotion into a physical manifestation. It can occur at any age and has many possible causes but the un-

---

BOX 2-10

Diagnostic Criteria for Somatization Disorder

A. A history of many physical complaints beginning before age 30 years that occur over a period of several years and result in treatment being sought or significant impairment in social, occupational, or other important areas of functioning.

B. Each of the following criteria must have been met, with individual symptoms* occurring at any time during the course of the disturbance:

  1. *Four pain symptoms:* A history of pain related to at least four different sites or functions (e.g., head, abdomen, back, joints, extremities, chest, rectum, during menstruation, during sexual intercourse, or during urination)

  2. *Two gastrointestinal symptoms:* A history of at least two gastrointestinal symptoms other than pain (e.g., nausea, bloating, vomiting other than during pregnancy, diarrhea, or intolerance of several different foods)

  3. *One sexual symptom:* A history of at least one sexual or reproductive symptom other than pain (e.g., sexual indifference, erectile or ejaculatory dysfunction, irregular menses, excessive menstrual bleeding, vomiting throughout pregnancy)

  4. *One pseudoneurologic symptom:* A history of at least one symptom or deficit suggesting a neurologic condition not limited to pain (conversion symptoms such as impaired coordination or balance, paralysis or localized weakness, difficulty swallowing or lump in throat, aphonia, urinary retention, hallucinations, loss of touch or pain sensation, double vision, blindness, deafness, seizures; dissociative symptoms such as amnesia; or loss of consciousness other than fainting)

C. Either (1) or (2):

  1. After appropriate investigation, each of the symptoms in criterion B cannot be fully explained by a known general medical condition or the direct effects of a substance (e.g., a drug of abuse, a medication)

  2. When a related general medical condition exists, the physical complaints or resulting social or occupational impairment are in excess of what would be expected from the history, physical examination, or laboratory findings

D. The symptoms are not intentionally produced or feigned (as in factitious disorder or malingering).

*Symptoms are listed in the approximate order of their reported frequency.
Modified from American Psychiatric Association: *Diagnostic and statistical manual of mental disorders-text revision,* ed 4 (DSM-IV-TR), Washington, DC, 2000, The Author.

derlying basis is an unresolved psychologic conflict. The person is unable to verbally express an emotion (considered threatening or unacceptable) and expresses a physical symptom instead. Conversion symptoms are peripheral and anesthetic, most commonly presenting as paralysis of the limbs or loss of vision without physical explanation or findings.

Psychophysiologic symptoms associated with conversion occur when anxiety activates the autonomic nervous system (an unconscious, unintentional process), resulting in tachycardia, hyperventilation, and vasoconstriction. Other symptoms may include hysterical pain response (excessive pain without organic cause) and symptoms related to voluntary motor or sensory functioning, referred to as pseudoneurologic. Motor symptoms or deficits include localized weakness or paralysis; impaired coordination or balance; aphonia (loss of voice); difficulty swallowing or a sensation of a lump in the throat; and urinary retention. Sensory changes include loss of touch or pain sensation; double vision; blindness; deafness; and hallucinations. Seizure or convulsions may also occur. No cause or disease can explain the distribution of such symptoms; the physician must carefully differentiate conversion symptoms from physical disorders with unusual presentations such as multiple sclerosis.

Psychogenic Pain Disorder.

Psychogenic pain is often ill-defined, and its anatomic distribution depends more on the person's concepts of disease and dysfunction than on the actual course of the clinical disease. The client presents with multiple unrelated symptoms, and the fluctuations in the course of symptoms are determined more by crises in the person's psychosocial life than by physical changes.

Factitious Disorder.

Factitious disorder is characterized by signs and symptoms that are predominantly psychological or physical for the purpose of gaining primary or secondary gain. *Primary gain* describes the attention received from health care personnel and *secondary gain* refers to undeserved financial gain or other external benefits from the deception.[55] Disease simulation represents a spectrum of behavior that ranges from relatively common and benign (e.g., pleading illness to avoid an unwanted social obligation) to rare and malignant forms (e.g., Munchausen's syndrome).

When an individual presents with a medical condition in an attempt to get admitted to (or to stay in) a hospital, the disorder is referred to as *Munchausen's syndrome*. A parent may fabricate an illness in a child so that treatment can be given to satisfy a somatoform disorder in the parent. If the adult is inducing an illness in a child (or children) or feigning a disorder, the condition is referred to as *Munchausen syndrome by proxy* (MSBP). The person's motivation is often unclear; often the client is already involved in some way with the health care profession (e.g., works in a physician's office). Adolescents often feign illness or injury to receive attention they feel they lack at home.

Today, a condition referred to as *Munchausen by Internet* exists, whereby "virtual" factitious disorders are presented over the Internet through formats such as chat rooms and newsgroups. In any form of this disorder, the symptoms are determined by the person's medical knowledge, sophistication, and imagination and result in mortality in 10% of MSBP victims.[69] This condition is currently considered a form of child abuse and not a mental disorder.[70]

Symptoms intentionally produced do not count toward a diagnosis of somatoform disorder, but factitious or malingering symptoms are often mixed with other nonintentional symptoms, resulting in a diagnosis of somatoform disorder and a factitious disorder or malingering. In factitious disorder, the motivation is to assume the sick role and to obtain medical evaluation and treatment, whereas in malingering, more external incentives are apparent, such as financial compensation, avoidance of duty, evasion of criminal prosecution, or obtaining drugs.

Malingering.[204]

Malingering is a psychosocial variable defined as a conscious or willful and deliberate feigning or exaggeration of the symptoms of an illness or injury to obtain a consciously desired end.[12] It is included in the DSM-IV-TR,[55] but as a V-code since it is not a true psychiatric disorder. It must be differentiated from factitious disorder, since the latter is the purposeful creation or exaggeration of symptoms for the purpose of primary gain (e.g., emotional needs as in assuming the sick role for the nurturing benefits derived), but unlike malingering, factitious disorder never includes any external rewards. Malingering must be differentiated from the psychiatric somatoform disorders, since the person in both situations can appear to produce nonphysiologic and/or inconsistent responses. Again, the somatoform disorders are unconsciously driven and have no external stimuli, whereas malingering is consciously created for some external gain.

The base rate for medico-legal contexts (e.g., personal injury, malpractice, disability claims, and worker's compensation) varies from 24% to 48% in the literature depending on the client populations under review.[83] Individuals who are identified as conscious symptom magnifiers are malingering if a chance for external gain exists. Unconscious symptom magnifiers (i.e., no external gain) may be depressed, finding some other means of expressing a need for help, or have some other psychiatric diagnosis (e.g., illness behavior or somatization disorder). In some cultures (e.g., Middle Eastern, Latin), acting out one's illness is sanctioned and can appear as hysteria or malingering.

Clinical manifestations of malingering vary depending on the client. Physical malingering may take the form of trying to look like less range of motion or less strength is available than is actually present; sensory malingering may present as heightened pain (more than is really present); cognitive malingering may appear as though more damage from traumatic brain injury (TBI) occurred than is really present. PTSD is a common complaint after mild TBI in those individuals who are considered malingerers. Emotional malingerers act more depressed from the injury than is really the case. A person can demonstrate malingering in any of these categories, singly or in combination.

Personality Disorder.[203]

A personality disorder is a fixed and maladaptive interpersonal style that often causes social and/or occupational impairment. Personality disorders are distinct and separate from personality types. Some personality types may not blend well together and therefore create conflicts, but personality disorders do not blend with anything. They begin to emerge in late adolescence and may appear to diminish or become less obvious with age because people learn with experience how to adapt to social situations.

Individuals with personality disorders are unable to respond to various people and situations according to the demands of the moment but rather tend to respond in the same way, lacking the social, interpersonal, and occupational problem-solving tools that allow optimal flexibility in hectic or changing situations. Personality disorders are ego-syntonic—that is, they do not cause distress in the person who has them. This differs from somatoform disorders, for which an essential criterion is distress to the involved individual. Pointing out that a person has a personality disorder is usually unproductive, as people with this disorder do not believe they have a problem but more likely that *you* have a problem.

The DSM-IV-TR lists 12 personality disorders, but not all are seen in a physical or occupational therapy setting. Several types are rarely seen in a therapy practice (e.g., paranoid, antisocial, obsessive compulsive), whereas others are not usually a problem (e.g., histrionic, dependent). The therapist is most likely to find it difficult working with borderline, narcissistic, and passive-aggressive personality types. *Borderline personality disorder* is known for a pervasive instability of identity, interpersonal relationships, and mood. They can be supportive and inviting one minute and vicious and attacking the next. *Narcissistic personality disorder* is known for grandiose behavior, being critical in the evaluation of others, and a lack of empathy. This person may have an exaggerated sense of self-importance, demanding special treatment with a sense of entitlement. *Passive-aggressive personality disorder* has been renamed *negativistic personality disorder* and involves passive resistance to social expectations and demands for performance. This is the person who arrives late or does not show up for the next appointment, loses the independent program sheet, agrees to do something and then "forgets," or writes down the wrong appointment time to avoid complying with the authority of the therapist.

Medical Management

Diagnosis.   With all psychophysiologic disorders, the physician must rule out general medical conditions characterized by vague, multiple, and confusing somatic symptoms, such as hyperparathyroidism, acute intermittent porphyria, multiple sclerosis, or systemic lupus erythematosus. The onset of multiple physical symptoms late in life is almost always due to a general medical condition. Psychiatric disorders must be ruled out as well.

Several criteria must be met before a somatoform disorder can be established (Table 2-9; see Box 2-10). For all psychophysiologic disorders (somatoform disorders, psychogenic pain disorder, factitious disorder), a remarkable absence of findings in laboratory test results support the subjective report of symptoms. Likewise, the physical examination is remarkable for the absence of objective findings to fully explain the many subjective symptoms. Extensive medical testing carries the risk for iatrogenesis and reinforces the belief that a biomedical basis exists for the condition. The use of evidence-based guidelines is recommended in determining the appropriate extent of medical evaluation and the frequency with which medical tests are repeated.

Detecting exaggeration does not automatically indicate that the individual is malingering[105] and the differential diagnosis of malingering includes factitious disorder, the somatoform disorders, the dissociative disorders, and specific medical conditions without somatoform disorder.[126] Factitious disorders are differentiated from malingering by the goal that motivates the individual's behavior. The only apparent goal in factitious illness is to gain the sick role; the goal in malingering is to gain rewards such as compensation or to avoid the unwanted such as military service or jail.[201]

TABLE	2-9

Somatoform Disorders

DISORDER	PRESENTATION	CRITERIA
Somatization disorder (Briquet's syndrome)	Multiple focal symptom focus	Begins before age 30, extends over a period of years, characterized by a combination of pain, gastrointestinal, sexual, or pseudoneurologic symptoms
Undifferentiated somatoform disorder	Diffuse symptom focus	Unexplained physical complaints that are below the threshold for the diagnosis of somatization disorder; complaints must be present for at least 6 months
Hypochondriasis	Single symptom focus	Preoccupation with the fear of having, or the idea that one has, a serious disease based on the person's misinterpretation of body symptoms
Somatoform pain disorder	Pain is the predominant focus	Pain the prime complaint with psychologic factors having an important role in the onset, worsening, or maintenance of the disorder
Body dysmorphic disorder	Body part distortion	Preoccupation with an imagined or exaggerated defect in physical appearance
Conversion disorder	Motor/sensory symptoms	Involves unexplained symptoms affecting voluntary motor or sensory functions that mimic a general medical or neurologic condition; psychologic factors are associated with the presentation of the symptoms

Modified from Woltersdorf MA: Hidden disorders: psychological barriers to treatment success, *Phys Ther* 3:58-66, 1995.

Treatment. Medical management of psychophysiologic disorders requires a collaborative alliance between the health care provider and the client making restoration of function (rather than elimination of symptoms) the goal of treatment. Accordingly, treatment approach may vary depending on the clinical presentation and client profile. Medical management is currently comprised of palliative treatment (often including physical therapy), cognitive-behavioral therapy, antidepressants, or other pharmacologic treatment. The individual may seek alternative therapies, which may benefit them, but empirical data on these interventions are not yet available.

Prognosis. The course of psychophysiologic disorders varies with each type of disorder. Within the somatoform disorders, somatization disorder and undifferentiated somatoform disorder are chronic and unpredictable and rarely remit. Conversion is often of short duration, and hospitalized individuals have remission within 2 weeks in most cases. A good prognosis for conversion is associated with acute onset, presence of clearly identifiable stress at the time of onset, a short interval between onset and the initiation of treatment, above-average intelligence, and symptoms of paralysis, aphonia, and blindness. Poor prognostic indicators include symptoms of tremors and seizures.

Pain disorders resolve relatively quickly when associated with an acute episode, but a wide range of variability exists in the course of chronic pain (see Chronic Pain Disorders in this chapter). Hypochondriasis is usually chronic, but can remit completely, especially in the absence of a personality disorder and the absence of a secondary gain. Body dysmorphic disorder often has a continuous course once it is diagnosed. Symptoms are almost always present, although the intensity may vary over time.

The course of psychogenic pain disorder or factitious disorder may be limited to one or more brief episodes, but it is more often of a chronic nature with a lifelong pattern of hospitalization. In the case of malingering, painful symptoms and movement dysfunction resolve completely when the court case involved has been completed or the possibility of financial gain has been eliminated.

Special Implications for the Therapist   2-9

PSYCHOPHYSIOLOGIC DISORDERS

Preferred Practice Patterns
Patterns will vary depending on clinical presentation of (real or feigned) signs and symptoms and the presence of impaired function.

The therapist's practice is often comprised of individuals with somatoform disorders, personality disorders, malingering, or other psychophysiologic disorders. The health care professional who can communicate a willingness to consider all aspects of illness, whether physiologic or psychological, can foster a trusting relationship with the client. Such an attitude promotes client self-disclosure and a reliance on confidentiality. The presence of these diagnoses frequently requires behavioral and treatment modifi-

cations. As with all psychologically based illnesses, the therapist is encouraged to practice in cooperation with the other team members, especially when behavioral or psychologic approaches are the basis of medical treatment.

Somatoform Disorders

Somatoform disorders can account for 80% of all physician visits and make up a large portion of clients in a therapy setting. Personality disorders, although rare in the general population, are common in the medical arena and especially in the physical therapist's practice when medical treatment has been unsuccessful in improving their physical complaints. Somatoform clients are often described as whiners and can have a bewildering array of symptoms, all of which are highly resistant to improvement through therapy or other medical or psychologic treatment.

The essential markers for the somatoform disorders are the absence or inadequacy of physical findings, insatiable complaints, excessive social and occupational consequences, preoccupation with problems, and lack of obvious secondary or material gain. This is not to say that adopting the (sometimes enjoyable) sick role has no gain associated with it—just not material or monetary gain. However, somatoform disorders can coexist with a concurrent physical illness, emphasizing the need for ongoing evaluation.

These persons often seek treatment from several physicians concurrently, which may lead to complicated and sometimes hazardous combinations of treatment (polypharmacy). Frequent use of medications may lead to side effects and substance-related disorders. The therapist is encouraged to maintain close communication with the physician(s) if either of these situations is suspected or discovered.

Working with individuals who have somatoform disorders places the therapist at risk for personal and professional burnout. To preserve one's sanity and maintain a professional perspective, people with somatoform disorders must be identified. It may be helpful to affirm that somatic symptoms are not imaginary or feigned and describe the process of amplification whereby sociocultural and psychologic stresses amplify symptoms and hinder recovery. Such a discussion can help give clients an explanatory model that focuses on processes and functioning rather than on structural or biomedical abnormalities. At the same time, the therapist should discourage the client from assuming the sick role, minimize alarming expectations about the clinical course, and avoid making distressing symptom attributions.

Intervention includes the identification and alleviation of factors that amplify and perpetuate the person's symptoms and cause functional impairment. A discussion of current psychosocial stressors may be helpful, but the therapist should not become more than a therapist for them. Therapists trained in the therapeutic interventions that enable the person to move toward a state of physical and emotional well-being (e.g., somatoemotional release, myofascial release, craniosacral therapy) may find clinical success with some individuals. The individual with a somatoform disorder are "sick" out of a need to assume the patient role or to better handle stress in their lives. Confronting him or her about the condition may only increase the problems (unconsciously) and exacerbate symptoms. It is better to stay supportive, conservative, and treat only what is objectively found and not what is subjectively reported.[204]

A brief summary of the somatoform disorders and possible clinical strategies are provided in Tables 2-9 and 2-10.

Continued

The reader is referred to articles on these topics written specifically for the health care professional for more specific details.[22,55,128,202,203,205]

Factitious Disorder

In the case of a factitious disorder involving Munchausen's syndrome, the Munchausen's syndrome by proxy (MSBP) parent fosters a close relationship with the medical team and pushes for findings not supported by the physical examination or laboratory tests. The perpetrator may even convince the therapy staff of the need for support in obtaining invasive diagnostic procedures. The health care professional should be observant of the following red flags: (1) a parent with little formal education or training who has extensive knowledge of the child's medical condition, (2) a history of repeated hospitalizations or trips to the emergency department accompanied by an apparent lack of concern on the part of the parent, (3) inconsistent medical history, (4) clinical presentation does not fit the history and/or does not match any neuromuscular or musculoskeletal pattern of symptoms, (5) the child's condition develops only when left alone with the parent in question. Any of these findings requires a consultation with the physician.

Malingering

The high base rate of malingering after events or incidents that lead to litigation (e.g., accidents, workman's compensation, disability claims, malpractice claims) requires assessment by the therapist. A therapist cannot rely on any single test to determine malingering; therefore a collection of information must be gleaned, which documents consistent (or inconsistent) history; congruence of clinical presentation with known pathologic process (e.g., symptoms last longer than the expected time for physiologic healing, symptoms are out of proportion for the type of injury); test scores and measurements, including observations regarding effort, motivation, inconsistent behavior; and a host of other variables.

Documentation of findings is important in all cases of suspected malingering. The therapist does not make the determination or diagnosis of malingering but provides complete objective data for the client's record. This is important given the potential for a lawsuit against the therapist. Discussion of findings with the physician is essential because systemic disorders can masquerade as neuromusculoskeletal symptoms and can present with the same mismatching of disproportionate symptoms for the injury or pathology.

If the physician has ruled out the possibility of an underlying systemic disorder accounting for the client's clinical manifestations, then the best approach is to discuss the therapist's concerns with the client over the lack of effort and/or inconsistent findings that have no apparent clinical meaning. The therapist should avoid confrontation or directly labeling the person as a malingerer but should remain focused on objective data and functional limitations.

Personality Disorder

Personality disorders cannot be "fixed" but rather should be approached by the therapist with an eye to self-protection and self-preservation while avoiding being taken advantage of by the client. This can be accomplished through awareness and understanding of the disorder involved. It is helpful to identify those people who can be helped and keep them focused on their physical needs. The therapist with realistic expectations who offers consistent professional help in his or her area of expertise will fare well. People with somatoform disorders and personality disorders cannot be helped unless they actually allow it. The therapist should be familiar with specific strategies for each personality disorder.[203] ■

Chronic Pain Disorders

Definition and Overview.   Chronic pain has been recognized as pain that persists past the normal time of healing.[33] This may be less than 1 month, or more often, more than 6 months. The International Association for the Study of Pain has settled on 3 months as the dividing line between acute and chronic pain.[142] Chronic pain appears to be often associated with depressive disorders, whereas acute pain appears to be more commonly associated with anxiety disorders. The associated mental disorders may precede the pain disorder (and possibly predispose the individual to it), co-occur with it, or result from it.[55]

The International Association for the Study of Pain has proposed a five-axis system for categorizing chronic pain (Table 2-11) that has been in use for the last 15 years. This disease-based (etiologic) classification approaches pain according to (1) anatomic region, (2) organ system, (3) temporal characteristics of pain and pattern of occurrence, (4) person's statement of intensity and time since onset of pain, and (4) etiologic factors. This five-axis system focuses primarily on the physical manifestations of pain but provides for comments on the psychologic factors on both the second axis where the involvement of a mental disorder can be coded and on the fifth axis where possible etiologic factors include psychophysiologic and psychologic ones.

An alternate classification scheme has been proposed based on the possible mechanisms of pain and the accompanying physiologic characteristics (e.g., transient pain such as a pinprick, tissue injury pain, nervous system injury pain). This mechanism-based classification model is the result of the dramatic growth in the understanding of the molecular, cellular, and system's mechanisms responsible for nociception and pain.[208] A mechanism-based classification could provide the basis for more reliable and valid tools for treatment and clinical investigation. Such an approach may lead to specific pharmacologic, surgical, or physical therapy interventions for each identified mechanism involved in a particular syndrome. For example, groups of people with the same symptom but not necessarily the same disease (e.g., herpetic neuralgia versus diabetic neuropathy) could possibly be treated with a single drug effective across a variety of etiologies.[207] This approach to the assessment and treatment of chronic pain has not been validated yet, and further testing is under way.

Incidence.   Chronic pain disorders can occur at any age and are relatively common. For example, it is estimated that in any given year, 10% to 15% of adults in the United States have some form of work disability due to back pain alone. Females appear to experience certain chronic pain conditions such as headaches and musculoskeletal pain more often than do males.[55]

Etiologic Factors.   Chronic pain disorders can be psychologically based (somatoform pain disorder); the result of a

TABLE	2-10

Clinical Strategies for Somatoform Disorders

DISORDER	PROBLEM	SOLUTION
Personality disorders	Rigid, inflexible, interpersonal style that has no correlation to the current personal relationship or needs of the setting of the moment	*Do:* Focus on the physical needs of the client, remind self that you are not there to satisfy all the needs of the client, remain professional, document objectively any troublesome exchanges. *Don't:* Try to be a friend, ever take any client's response personally, allow emotions to creep into your documentation.
Somatization disorder	Bewildering array of physical complaints that exceed findings	*Do:* Keep accurate records of all physical findings, assess regularly, mention his or her progress often, focus on what you can change (stiffness) and avoid what you cannot (nausea), praise his or her strengths. *Don't:* Tell the client that it is "in his or her head," even if you are right; don't confront the obvious contradictions.
Undifferentiated somatoform disorder	Diffuse, ambiguous complaints	*Do:* Assess for physical findings only. *Don't:* Become more than a therapist for them; refer appropriately.
Hypochondriasis	Intense, single-symptom focus	Same as somatization disorder.
Somatoform pain disorder	Pain, pain, pain	*Do:* Remember pain cannot be measured directly, focus on the indirect effects of pain, have a multidisciplinary approach, demand regular improvement and set criteria early in treatment for what improvement looks like. *Don't:* Get angry with your clients, confront their inconsistencies; document objectively and unemotionally.
Body dysmorphic disorder	Excessive concerns about appearances	*Do:* Focus on a client's strengths, stay upbeat, downplay any undue attention to the actual area of disfigurement. *Don't:* Have the client talk about his or her feelings about the body part in question, tell him or her they are being unreasonable, say you know how they feel.
Conversion disorder	Motor/sensory inconsistencies	Same as somatization disorder.

Modified from Woltersdorf MA: Hidden disorders: psychological barriers to treatment success, *PT Magazine* 3(12):58-66, 1995.

general medical condition; or a mixture of both. Among the most common general medical conditions associated with chronic pain are various *musculoskeletal conditions* (e.g., disk herniation, osteoporosis, osteoarthritis or rheumatoid arthritis, myofascial syndromes); *neuropathies* (e.g., diabetic neuropathies, postherpetic neuralgia); and *malignancies* (e.g., metastatic lesions in bone, tumor infiltration of nerves).[55] The most common chronic pain conditions encountered by the therapist are listed in Box 2-11. Chronic pain may be a form of self-defense as a result of domestic violence or abuse. (See the section on Somatoform Disorders and Domestic Violence in this chapter.)

Chronic postoperative pain occurs in a small percentage of people after some procedures such as tumor resection and subsequent regrowth or invasion of the chest wall; mastectomy with pain from interruption of the intercostobrachial

nerve (branches from the brachial plexus to the thoracic region); surgical amputation followed by phantom limb pain; and chemotherapy when associated with neuropathies producing painful dysesthesias (abnormal sensations) of the feet and hands.

Physiologic, Psychologic, and Behavioral Response.
Physiologic responses to chronic pain depend in part on the persistent (e.g., low back pain) or intermittent (e.g., migraine headache) nature of the pain. Intermittent pain produces a physiologic response similar to that of acute pain, whereas persistent pain allows for physiologic adaptation (e.g., normal heart rate, blood pressure, and respiratory rate). The traditional view conceptualizes pain as being directly associated with the extent of physical pathology. However, since people report pain in the absence of physical pathology and individ-

TABLE	2-11

Classification of Chronic Pain

Axis I: Regions
Head, face, and mouth
Cervical region
Upper shoulder and upper limbs
Thoracic region
Abdominal region
Low back: lumbar spine, sacrum, and coccyx
Lower limbs
Pelvic region
Anal, perineal, and genital region
More than three major sites

Axis II: Systems
Nervous system (central, peripheral, and autonomic) and special senses; physical disturbance or dysfunction
Nervous system (psychological and social)
Respiratory and cardiovascular systems
Musculoskeletal system and connective tissue
Cutaneous and subcutaneous and associated glands (breast, apocrine, etc.)
Gastrointestinal system
Genitourinary system
Other organs or viscera (e.g., thyroid, lymphatic, hemapoietic)
More than one system

Axis III: Temporal Characteristics of Pain: Pattern of Occurrence
Not recorded, not applicable, or not known
Single episode, limited duration (e.g., ruptured aneurysm, sprained ankle)
Continuous or nearly continuous, nonfluctuating (e.g., low back pain, some cases)
Continuous or nearly continuous, fluctuating severity (e.g., ruptured intervertebral disk)
Recurring irregularly (e.g., headache, mixed type)
Recurring regularly (e.g., premenstrual pain)

Axis III:—cont'd
Paroxysmal (e.g., tic douloureux)
Sustained with superimposed paroxysms
Other combinations
None of the above

Axis IV: Person's Statement of Intensity: Time Since Onset of Pain*
Not recorded, not applicable, or not known

Mild	≤1 mo
	1-6 mo
	>6 mo
Medium	≤1 mo
	1-6 mo
	>6 mo
Severe	≤1 mo
	1-6 mo
	<6 mo

Axis V: Etiologic Factors
Genetic or congenital disorders (e.g., congenital dislocation)
Trauma, operation, burns
Infective, parasitic
Inflammatory (no known infective agent), immune reactions
Neoplasm
Toxic, metabolic (e.g., alcoholic neuropathy, anoxia, vascular, nutritional, endocrine), radiation
Degenerative, mechanical†
Dysfunctional (including psychophysiologic)‡
Unknown or other
Psychologic origin (e.g., conversion hysteria, depressive hallucination)

*Determine the time at which pain is recognized retrospectively as having started even though the pain may occur intermittently. Grade for intensity in relation to the level of the current pain problem.
†For example, a lumbar puncture headache would be mechanical.
‡For example, migraine headache, tension headache, or irritable bowel syndrome; syndromes where a pathophysiologic alteration is recognized are also included. Emotional causes may or may not be present.
Modified from Merskey H, editor: Classification of chronic pain: scheme for coding chronic pain diagnoses, *Pain* (suppl 3):S10-S11, 1986.

uals demonstrate objective physical pathology without symptoms, along with cases of low association between impairments and disability, it is suggested that factors other than physical pathology contribute to reports of pain. Behavioral, cognitive, and affective factors have direct effects on the report of pain, adaptation to the pain, and response to treatment, as well as indirect effects by influencing sympathetic nervous system and neurochemical factors associated with nociception.[189]

At the same time, the presence of chronic pain can be associated with significant behavioral and psychologic changes. A constellation of life changes that produces altered behavior in the individual and that persists even after the cause of the pain has been eradicated make up the *chronic pain syndrome*. Painful symptoms out of proportion to the injury or that are not consistent with the objective findings may be a red flag indicative of systemic disease or a psychogenic pain disorder. This can be differentiated from a chronic pain syndrome in that the syndrome is characterized by multiple complaints, excessive preoccupation with pain or physical symptoms, and often, excessive drug use. The person exhibiting symptoms of a chronic pain syndrome may isolate himself or herself socially from other people and be fatigued, tense, fearful, and depressed. Chronic pain cases do occur in which a diagnosis is finally made (e.g. spinal stenosis or thyroiditis) and the treatment is specific and not one of pain management alone.

BOX 2-11

Chronic Pain Conditions

Arthritis
Persistent neck/back pain
Neuralgias
Peripheral neuropathies
Peripheral vascular disease
Causalgia
Chronic regional pain syndrome (CRPS), formerly reflex
    sympathetic dystrophy (RSD)
Hyperesthesia
Myofascial pain syndrome
Fibromyalgia syndrome
Phantom limb pain
Cancer
Postoperative pain
Spinal stenosis

Two polarizing stereotypes about how men and women cope differently with pain have been put forth over the years: (1) women are more likely to seek medical help and (2) men are more stoic about their pain and will avoid consulting a physician. Researchers studying all types of chronic pain are currently collecting data on how men and women approach pain. Does it matter if the pain is due to a chronic condition like fibromyalgia syndrome versus the pain associated with a life-threatening disease such as metastatic cancer? Are men and women treated differently by the medical profession when their major symptom is pain? How do men and women respond to post-surgical pain? Thus far, numerous studies have found that the role of gender in chronic pain may be less important than psychologic and behavioral responses. In other words, gender does not appear to factor into how well people adapt to their chronic pain condition as much as coping mechanisms and strategies.[190]

People with chronic pain often are depressed, have sleep disturbances, and may become preoccupied with the pain. People with chronic pain often attempt to maintain their former lifestyle to appear as normal as possible, even denying pain and engaging in activities that exacerbate their painful symptoms. They may not report the full extent of their pain, for fear of being labeled a complainer or hypochondriac. The need to hide the pain conflicts with the need to have someone understand the pain. The result is emotional and psychologic conflicts. (See the section on Coping and Adapting later in this chapter.)

Symptom Magnification Syndrome.

Symptom magnification syndrome (SMS) is defined as a self-destructive, socially reinforced behavioral response pattern consisting of reports or displays of symptoms which function to control the life of the sufferer.[135,137] At the present time, SMS is not listed in the DSM-IV. It is likely that in the future, SMS will be categorized as a somatoform disorder, possibly a variant of somatoform pain disorder of a chronic nature.

Leonard N. Matheson first coined the term in 1977 to describe people whose symptoms have reinforced their self-destructive behavior—that is, the symptoms have become the predominant force in the client's function, rather than the physiologic phenomenon of the injury determining outcome (unless physiologic changes occur leading to deconditioning). Conscious symptom magnification is referred to as malingering, whereas unconscious symptom magnification is labeled illness behavior or somatoform disorder.

SMS can fall into several categories and the reader is referred to Matheson (1991)[136] for an in-depth understanding of this syndrome. The following three signs indicate that a client may be exhibiting symptom magnification:

1. Ineffective strategy for balancing symptoms against activities.
2. Client acts as if the future cannot be controlled because of the presence of symptoms; limitation is blamed on symptoms: "My [back] pain won't let me..."
3. Client may exaggerate limitations beyond those that are reasonable in relation to the injury; client applies minimal effort on maximum performance tasks and overreacts to loading during objective examination.

Updated research on the identification of SMS has focused on screening for less than full effort performance during a functional capacity evaluation. Most methods of identification are not significant predictors of the syndrome and even the best methods frequently lead to misclassification.[138]

Medical Management

Diagnosis.   The clinical evaluation of pain currently involves identification or diagnosis of the primary disease/etiologic factor considered responsible for producing/initiating the pain; placing the individual within a broad pain category, typically nociceptive, inflammatory, or neuropathic pain; and then identifying the anatomic distribution, quality, and intensity of pain. In conjunction with the proposed five-axis system for categorizing chronic pain (see Table 2-11), the physician may use the diagnostic criteria outlined in DSM-IV-TR (Box 2-12).

A newer approach to the problem of chronic pain is being evaluated in which the pain itself is considered the disease, and instead of emphasizing or categorizing the client on the basis of diagnosing the primary disease, an attempt is made to identify the mechanisms responsible for the pain. Although identifying the disease is essential, especially when disease-modifying treatment is possible (e.g., acute herpes zoster, diabetes, tumor), the vast majority of people with persistent or chronic pain cannot be treated for the disease or pathology and/or the injury is not reversible (e.g., peripheral/segmental nerve lesions, brachial avulsion, spinal cord injury, post-stroke central pain).[208]

Valid criteria for assessing malingering and symptom embellishment do not exist, thereby requiring careful clinical judgment on the part of the physician and all other health care professionals.[187]

Prognosis.   A wide range of variability exists in the course of chronic pain. In most cases, symptoms persist for many years, but function can improve when the individual follows a self-management program (usually prescribed by a therapist in conjunction with other health care professionals). Participation in regularly scheduled physical activity, exercise, and outside activities such as volunteer or paid work should be a part of the program whenever possible.

BOX **2-12**

Diagnostic Criteria for Pain Disorder

A. Pain in one or more anatomic sites is the predominant focus of the clinical presentation and is of sufficient severity to warrant clinical attention.
B. The pain causes clinically significant distress or impairment in social, occupational, or other important areas of functioning.
C. Psychologic factors are judged to have an important role in the onset, severity, exacerbation, or maintenance of the pain.
D. The symptom or deficit is not intentionally produced or feigned (as in factitious disorder or malingering).
E. The pain is not better accounted for by a mood, anxiety, or psychotic disorder and does not meet criteria for dyspareunia.

Modified from American Psychiatric Association: Diagnostic and statistical manual of mental disorders-text revision, ed 4 (DSM-IV-TR), Washington, DC, 2000, The Author.

Special Implications for the Therapist   **2-10**

CHRONIC PAIN DISORDERS

Preferred Practice Patterns
Musculoskeletal and Neuromuscular patterns may be present, depending on the underlying etiologic factors or pain mechanism present (e.g., myofascial syndrome, neuropathy) and the degree of impairment or disability.

It is counterproductive to speculate about whether the client's pain is real. Current data on the prevalence of malingering in cases of chronic pain are not consistent, and no reliable method for detecting malingering among those individuals diagnosed with chronic pain is available.[199] Pain is real to the person, and acceptance of the pain as part of the clinical picture places the therapist in alliance with the client toward mutually acceptable goals. Focusing on improving functional outcomes rather than on reducing the pain should be the underlying direction in therapy.

Chronic anxiety and depression may produce heightened irritability, overreaction to stimuli, and a heightened awareness of the symptoms. The person may become preoccupied with the details of anatomic function and how each movement or external event affects the symptoms. This self-focus must be redirected toward improving function and differs from the overdramatization of the discomfort sometimes helpful in alleviating the problem in certain cultures. The cornerstone of a unified approach to chronic pain syndrome is a comprehensive behavioral program. Whenever possible, the therapist should reinforce the behavioral approaches used by the other members of the team. Some general guidelines are outlined in Box 2-13.

Pain may lead to inactivity and social isolation, which in turn can lead to additional psychologic problems (e.g., depression) and a reduction in physical endurance that results in fatigue and additional pain.[78] People whose pain is associated with severe depression and those whose pain is related to a terminal illness, most notably cancer, appear to be at increased risk for suicide (see the discussion on suicide in this chapter).

Symptom Magnification
Health care providers should recognize that we often contribute to symptom magnification syndrome by focusing on the relief of symptoms, especially pain, as the goal of therapy. Reducing pain is an acceptable goal for some clients, but for those who experience pain after their injuries have healed, the focus should be restoration, or at least, improvement of function. Instead of asking if the client's symptoms are better, same, or worse, it may be more appropriate to inquire as to functional outcomes, for example, what can the client accomplish at home that she or he was unable to attempt at the beginning of treatment, last week, or even yesterday? Materials and courses on symptom magnification and functional capacity evaluations are available. ■

◆ Mood Disorders

Many of the earlier models of mental disorders, their causes, and their neural substrates have been disproved. The concept that abnormal levels of one or more neurotransmitters could explain the pathogenesis of depression or schizophrenia appears to be too simple of a model. The notion that a single gene can cause mental disorders or behavioral variations has been replaced by a complex genetic picture in which multiple genes act in concert with nongenetic factors to produce a risk of mental disorder. Current investigations are seeking to find a model that can explain the complex patterns of disease transmission within families and explain the expression of risk genes during brain development and of their function.[100]

Psychoneuroimmunology (PNI) studies are attempting to determine and define the links among neural activity, the endocrine system, and altered immune responses in people with depressive disorders. Although the literature indicates some type of relationship exists between these systems, the exact mechanisms remain unknown.[104,111]

Depression
Definition and Overview.   Depression in psychiatric terms is a morbid sadness, dejection, or a sense of melancholy, distinguished from grief, which is a normal response to a personal loss.[55] Mild, sporadic depression is a relatively common phenomenon experienced by almost everyone at some time, referred to as the common cold of emotions. Depression is the most commonly seen mood disorder within a therapy practice, often associated with other physical illnesses (Table 2-12). Depression is a normal response to (not a cause of) pain, which may influence the client's ability to cope with pain. Although anxiety is more apparent in acute pain episodes, depression occurs more often in clients with chronic pain. When the pain is relieved, the depression usually disappears.

Mood disorders can be classified into three broad types: major depressive disorder, organic mood disorder, and bipolar illness (manic depression). The most common type of depression observed is *major depressive disorder* encompassing several conditions including depression, dysthymia, and SAD. Major depressive disorder can occur as a single isolated episode lasting weeks to months or intermittently throughout a person's life. This type of depression may be seen as an adjustment disorder with depressive mood and occurs as a result of external circumstances (e.g., environmental stress, loss, or trauma). Profound depression may be an illness itself, considered as an

Behavioral Goals and Guidelines for Chronic Pain Syndrome

Identify and eliminate pain reinforcers.

Decrease drug use.

Use positive reinforcers that shift the focus from pain.

Concentrate on abilities, not disabilities.

Avoid the concept of cure: concentrate on control of pain and improved function.

Avoid discussion of pain except as arranged by the team (e.g., only during monthly reevaluation, only with a designated team member).

Use a home program to focus on function and functional outcome (e.g., self-help tasks within capabilities).

The client should keep a log of accomplishments so that progress can be measured and remembered.

Measure success by what the individual client can accomplish, not based on others' success.

Take one day at a time. Direct energy toward solving today's problems rather than focusing on the future.

Avoid negative reinforcers such as sympathy and attention to symptoms, especially pain.

Encourage tolerance to increasing activity levels.

Gradual progress is better than quick results with increased symptoms.

Teach the client how and when to ask for and accept help when necessary. Do not offer help or yield to the demands of someone who does not need help.

---

affective or anxiety disorder, or it may be symptomatic of another psychiatric disorder such as schizophrenia.

Organic mood disorder is also biologically based; structural changes in the brain associated with disease (e.g., multiple sclerosis) or brain trauma (e.g., left-sided cerebrovascular accident, traumatic brain injury) can cause depressive reactions, either on a short-term or recurring basis (see Table 2-12). Anticonvulsant medications such as valproic acid (Depakote) and carbamazepine (Tegretol) are often effective, especially in the TBI population.

Bipolar disorder or *manic depressive disorder* is characterized by cyclical mood swings that often include intense outbursts of high energy and activity, elevated mood, a decreased need for sleep, and a flight of ideas (mania) followed by extreme depression (Table 2-13); each may last from days to months, switching back and forth quickly or with normal periods in between. Bipolar disorder manifests itself as a manic episode with or without depression (bipolar I), severe depression and only mild mania (bipolar II), or frequent alterations of mood extremes (rapid cycling). Heightened creativity and creative talent are sometimes associated with both phases of bipolar disorder.

Incidence and Prevalence.

Major depressive disorder is the most common adult psychiatric disorder beginning at any age with an average onset in the mid-20s, although it appears to be occurring at earlier ages for those born in the last decade. In the United States, an estimated 15 million people are di-

agnosed with mild to severe depression. Epidemiologic data from diverse cultures indicate the lifetime prevalence of major depression is twice as high in women as in men.[54] Rates in men and women are highest in the 25- to 44-year-old age group, although rates increase again in older adults. Bipolar disorder can occur at any age but fully half of all cases begin before age 20, affecting men and women equally.

Etiologic and Risk Factors.

Predisposing factors for the development of depression may be genetic, familial, biologic, or psychosocial (e.g., childhood history of sexual abuse, battery and rape during adulthood, other recent stressful life events, socioeconomic status, raising children without support). Given the fact that bipolar disorder occurs in families, research is focusing to identify a genetic basis. Linkage studies have implicated chromosome 18 or 21, but this has not yet been proven.[151,166]

Depression may occur in association with medical or chronic illness or surgical procedures. Medical illness is the most consistently identified factor associated with the presence of late-life depression (see Table 2-13). A newly described condition called *vascular depression* accounts for 30% to 40% of all depression in people over the age of 65 and in people with a history of diabetes, hypertension, atherosclerosis, and angioplasty or bypass surgery. It appears to be a biologic alteration rather than a chemical one with black holes (lacunes) observed in the basal ganglia representing cerebral ischemia or silent strokes.[118] Major depression is considered a risk factor for cardiac morbidity and mortality; treating depression to reduce cardiac disease is under investigation.[41]

Depression may occur as a result of medications, especially sedatives, hypnotics, cardiac drugs, antihypertensives, steroids (Table 2-14); alcohol or drug abuse, especially cocaine dependence; or exposure to heavy metals or toxins (e.g., gasoline, paint, organophosphate insecticides, nerve gas, carbon monoxide, carbon dioxide); this type of depression may be labeled substance-induced mood disorder.[11] Other causes of depression among the general population include prenatal and postpartum depression occurring in approximately 20% of all pregnancies and SAD, a dysfunction of circadian rhythms that occurs more commonly in the winter as a result of decreased exposure to sunlight.

Pathogenesis.

Researchers have examined several theories of pathogenesis based on etiologic factors. These include biochemical mechanisms, neuroendocrine mechanisms, sleep abnormalities, genetics, and psychosocial factors. Recent study of the *biochemical basis* of depression has centered on two primary neurotransmitters: norepinephrine and serotonin. Depression is associated with levels of norepinephrine, dopamine, and serotonin that are either produced in inadequate amounts or the receptor sites are not functioning properly; mania results from excessive levels of norepinephrine and dopamine. As demonstrated in animal models, antidepressant drugs decrease the sensitivity of postsynaptic receptors by blocking the reuptake of the neurotransmitters into nerve endings. This change occurs 1 to 3 weeks after treatment, correlating with the delay seen clinically in the effectiveness of antidepressants.

Neuroendocrine abnormalities, such as in the limbic hypothalamic-pituitary-adrenal axis, have been implicated in the cause of depression, prompting a search for a reliable

---

TABLE 2-12

Physical Conditions Commonly Associated With Depression

Cardiovascular
Atherosclerosis
Hypertension
Myocardial infarction
Angioplasty or bypass surgery

Central Nervous System
Parkinson's disease
Huntington's disease
Cerebral arteriosclerosis
Stroke
Alzheimer's disease
Temporal lobe epilepsy
Postconcussion injury
Multiple sclerosis
Miscellaneous focal lesions

Endocrine, Metabolic
Hyperthyroidism
Hypothyroidism
Addison's disease

Endocrine, Metabolic—cont'd
Cushing's disease
Hypoglycemia
Hyperglycemia
Hyperparathyroidism
Hyponatremia
Diabetes mellitus
Pregnancy (post-partum)

Viral
Acquired immunodeficiency syndrome
Hepatitis
Pneumonia
Influenza

Nutritional
Folic acid deficiency
Vitamin B_6 deficiency
Vitamin B_{12} deficiency

Immune
Fibromyalgia
Chronic fatigue syndrome
Systemic lupus erythematosus
Sjögren's syndrome
Rheumatoid arthritis
Immunosuppression (e.g., corticosteroid
   treatment)

Cancer
Pancreatic
Bronchogenic
Renal
Ovarian

Miscellaneous
Pancreatitis
Sarcoidosis
Syphilis
Porphyria
Corticosteroid treatment

TABLE 2-13

Clinical Manifestations of Bipolar Disorder

MANIA	DEPRESSION
Excessive high or euphoric feelings	Persistent sad, anxious, or empty mood
Sustained period of behavior different from usual	Feelings of hopelessness or pessimism
Increased energy, activity, restlessness, racing thoughts, and rapid talking	Feelings of guilt, worthlessness, or helplessness
Decreased need for sleep	Loss of interest or pleasure in ordinary activities, including sex
Unrealistic beliefs in one's abilities and powers	Decreased energy, feeling fatigued, or being slowed down
Extreme irritability and distractibility	Difficulty concentrating, remembering, making decisions
Uncharacteristically poor judgment	Restlessness or irritability
Increased sexual drive	Sleep disturbances
Abuse of drugs, particularly cocaine, alcohol, and sleeping medications	Loss of appetite and weight, or weight gain
Obnoxious, provocative, or intrusive behavior	Chronic pain or other persistent bodily symptoms that are not caused by physical disease
Denial that anything is wrong	Thoughts of death or suicide; suicide attempts

Modified from National Institute of Mental Health: *Bipolar disorder: manic-depressive illness,* NIMH Pub No (ADM) 89-1609, Rockville, Md, 1989.

serum abnormality that could be used as a depression test. Some examples of possible abnormalities include oversecretion of cortisol, suppressed nocturnal secretion of melatonin, and decreased prolactin production in response to tryptophan administration. A known association exists between hormonal variations such as low testosterone levels in men and basal levels of follicle-stimulating hormone (FSH) and luteinizing hormone (LH) in women and some depressions.

Sleep abnormalities are consistently associated with depression, including decreased REM latency (the time between falling asleep and the first REM period); longer first REM period; less continuous sleep; and early morning awakenings. Animal studies have shown that many antidepressants can reset the internal clock. Whether these sleep abnormalities represent causes or effects of depression remains unknown.

Genetic-based pathogenesis is suspected for bipolar depression based on a clear familial pattern and chromosomal linkage studies. Evidence exists that the key gene involved in the transmission of bipolar disease is X-linked. A familial pattern in the development of major depressive disorder is also evident, since this type of depression occurs up to three times more often in first-degree biologic relatives of people with this disorder.

TABLE	2-14

Drugs Commonly Associated With Depression

Psychoactive Agents
Amphetamines
Cocaine
Benzodiazepines
Barbiturates
Neuroleptics

Antihypertensive Drugs
β-Blockers, especially propranolol (Inderal)
α_2-Adrenergic antagonists
Methyldopa (Aldomet)
Hydralazine (Apresoline)

Analgesics
Salicylates
Propoxyphene (Darvon, Darvocet-N)

Analgesics—cont'd
Pentazocine (Talwin)
Morphine
Meperidine (Demerol)

Cardiovascular Drugs
Digoxin (Lanoxin)
Procainamide (Pronestyl)
Disopyramide (Norpace)

Anticonvulsants
Phenytoin (Dilantin)
Phenobarbital

Hormonal Agents
Corticosteroids
Oral contraceptives
Anabolic steroids

Miscellaneous
Alcohol, illicit drugs
Histamine H_2 receptor antagonists, especially cimetidine (Tagamet)
Metoclopramide (Reglan)
Levodopa (Dopar, Larodopa)
Nonsteroidal anti-inflammatory drugs
Antineoplastic agents
Disulfiram (Antabuse)
Cytokines (interferons)

Psychosocial factors, such as life events and perceived stress, are clearly associated with depression, but it is difficult to establish whether they cause depression or merely determine when a susceptible person will experience depression. Episodes of major depressive disorder often follow a severe psychosocial stressor such as the death of a loved one or divorce. Psychosocial events as stressors may play a more significant role in the precipitation of the first or second episodes of major depressive disorder but less of a role in the onset of subsequent episodes. People hospitalized for any reason are particularly susceptible to feelings of depression and a sense of loss and despair.

Clinical Manifestations.   Depressed mood and loss of interest in usually pleasurable activities are the hallmarks of depression (see Table 2-13). More than 95% of depressed people report decreased energy, even for minor daily tasks. The inability to accomplish new or challenging activities often results in occupational or school dysfunction; 90% report having problems with concentration and memory. Difficulty concentrating and marked forgetfulness is particularly common in depressed older adults and is called *pseudodementia*.

People with mood disorders, particularly depressive disorders, may present with somatic complaints, most commonly headache, gastrointestinal disturbances, or unexplained pain (Box 2-14) (see earlier discussion under Somatoform Disorders). Depression is also associated with elevated heart rate and reduced heart rate variability, which are known risk factors for cardiac disease.[41,184] Other mental disorders often co-occur with major depressive disorder such as anxiety, substance-related disorders, panic disorder, obsessive-compulsive disorder, anorexia nervosa, bulimia nervosa, and borderline personality disorder.

Almost 80% of depressed people report problems with sleep, including early morning and frequent nocturnal awakenings. Among older adults, depression is often the cause of sleep disturbances, but it may only be the first symptom of systemic illness. Often depression by itself or linked with acute confusion, falling, incontinence, or syncope signify underlying disease requiring medical referral.

BOX	2-14

Somatic Symptoms Associated with Depression*

Weakness	Tinnitus
Headaches	Dry skin
Joint pain (arthralgia)	Sexual dysfunction
Muscle pain (myalgia)	Flushing
Excess perspiration	Slurred speech
Dizziness	Chest pain
Dry mouth or excessive salivation	Amenorrhea,
Rapid breathing	polymenorrhea
Blurred vision	Difficulty with urination
Constipation	

*Refers to nonmedicated persons and is listed in order of decreasing prevalance.

Bipolar disorder may be characterized by elation (mania), but mania is often accompanied by anxiety, intense irritability, or an uncomfortable feeling of being too energized. People with bipolar disorder may have bursts of creativity and productivity when they are manic, but they are more likely to be impulsive and make reckless decisions.

Medical Management
Diagnosis.   Depression is often underrecognized and undertreated; primary care physicians detect only 33% to 50% of depressed outpatients. More than 50% of people with depression present with somatic complaints or masked depression. Instead of telling the physician or health care worker, "I am sad and depressed," they are more likely to report physical symptoms such as abdominal pain, headaches, joint pain, fatigue, sleep disturbance, or any of the somatic symptoms listed in Box 2-14. The application criteria based on the DSM-IV-TR (2000)[78] remain problematic with as

many as 50% of people with depressive symptoms being un-classified using these diagnostic criteria.

The diagnosis of manic episodes associated with bipolar disorder has been difficult, relying on reports of the person's behavior during a manic episode as described in Table 2-13. Driven behaviors such as late-night telephone calls, impulsive sexual liaisons, pathologic gambling, and excessively flamboyant dress and behavior are also characteristic. New neuroimaging studies available in some areas are making it possible to identify those people with biochemical changes associated with depression.

The physician will use the history, laboratory findings, and physical examination to determine whether the depression is a mood disorder due to a general medical condition (i.e., the direct physiologic consequence of a medical condition such as multiple sclerosis, stroke, or hypothyroidism) or if the depression is considered to be the psychologic consequence of having the general medical condition (e.g., myocardial infarct). No etiologic relationship between the depression and the medical condition may be evident. The medical management of general medical conditions with accompanying major depressive disorder is more complex, with a less favorable prognosis than just the medical condition alone.

Treatment. Treatment for major depression includes psychosocial therapy, pharmacotherapy, and electroconvulsive therapy. Shock therapy (electroconvulsive therapy [ECT]) remains a viable treatment tool for depression. ECT uses an electrical stimulus to provoke a controlled seizure inside the brain to affect the brain in the same ways as antidepressants. It is a painless and safe procedure used for depressed people with dementia who do not improve with antidepressant therapy[164] or who are severely suicidal, self-mutilating, catatonic, or unable to eat or function. National trials are under way to study the use of a vagal nerve stimulator, originally used to control epilepsy, with severe depression that is resistant to medications. The device, implanted under the clavicle with direct attachment to the vagus nerve sends electrical pulses to the brain and improves mood. In the case of SAD, light therapy is indicated along with lifestyle changes such as attention to nutrition and exercise.

Bipolar disorders are treated with various medications (psychopharmacology) including antipsychotics (e.g., risperidone/Risperdal, olanzapine/Zyprexa); anticonvulsants (seizure medication such as divalproex/Depakote); and antidepressants (SSRIs), which are often combined with a mood stabilizer such as lithium carbonate. Some people choose to suffer the extremes of this disorder to avoid losing the creative edge that can occur when the medication balances the mood swings. Some programs advocate a predetermined plan of action to put in place if and when warning signs (called *prodromes*) of mania or depression develop. This may help delay or prevent the onset of acute mania.

Complementary therapies have gained increasing popularity as people seek out alternative strategies to cope with depression. Research is limited, but some evidence exists to support the beneficial effects of exercise; herbal therapy (Hypericum perforatum/St. John's wort, S-adenosyl-L-methionine/SAM-e); and to a lesser extent, acupuncture and relaxation therapies.[62]

Prognosis. Depression is a chronic relapsing disorder associated with high morbidity and mortality; the severity of the initial depressive episode appears to predict persistence.[182] Adolescent-onset depressive disorder may carry an increased risk for poor outcome.[199] Chronic general medical conditions are also a risk factor for more persistent episodes. Up to 15% of people diagnosed with this mood disorder die by suicide. Epidemiologic evidence also suggests a fourfold increase in death rates in people with major depressive disorder who are over age 55 years; from 1980 to 1992 the suicide rate among individuals age 65 and older increased by 9%. In the same time span, the suicide rate for men and women age 80 to 84 increased 35%.[150] People with this condition admitted to nursing homes may have a markedly increased likelihood of death in the first year. Finally, considerable research investigates whether treating depression will improve medical prognosis in people who have a depressive disorder and a history of coronary artery disease or who have suffered an acute myocardial infarction.[42]

Special Implications for the Therapist 2-11

DEPRESSION

Preferred Practice Patterns
4A: *Primary Prevention/Risk Factor Reduction for Skeletal Demineralization*
6A: *Primary Prevention/Risk Factor Reduction for Cardiopulmonary Disorders*

Depression occurs in more than 50% of people with Parkinson's disease and strokes. In these and other clients, the therapist may detect early signs of depression such as pessimistic statements about the illness and its prognosis (poor in the individual's mind) and passive noncompliance during therapy with minimal or no compliance in following a home program or in following (performing) postoperative or rehabilitative exercises.

If the therapist suspects the possibility of depression, baseline information can be obtained and provided to the physician when referring that client. Screening (not diagnostic) tests such as the Beck Depression Index (BDI)[192]; McGill Pain Questionnaire[193]; the Multidimensional Pain Inventory (MDI)[194]; and the Geriatric Depression Scale[195] are noninvasive, easy to administer, and do not require interpretation that is outside the scope of a therapist's practice. Asking for permission to discuss symptoms of depression (or other mood or psychiatric disorders) with the referring practitioner or other appropriate health care professional is recommended; in the case of a minor, parental consent may be needed.

When depression is noted, it should be included as a problem in the care plan; the team can then develop strategies to help the person. A client who is not progressing in rehabilitation and who is moderately or severely depressed but not receiving intervention for the depression may need to delay rehab until the depression is under control. Under these circumstances, the therapist should not hesitate to refer a client for evaluation and treatment.

The client with mood disorders may cry easily and often for no apparent reason. Such a situation can be handled by offering reassurance and redirecting the person's attention toward the instructions, activity, or other more positive topics. Using the acronym PLISSIT* may help provide the therapist with some direction early on in the intervention: **P**ermission: Acknowledge the presence of the depression and give the person permission to feel depressed. **L**imited **i**nformation: "Of course you are feeling down. You broke your hip, it hurts, and you cannot get around." Again, this acknowledges and validates the person's experience. **S**pecific **s**uggestions: For example, knowing that depression often causes the person to avoid social contact and seek isolation, which then contributes to the depression, encourage the person to make telephone contact with at least one person every day or listen to upbeat music every morning and evening or make arrangements to exercise with someone else (even if only for 10 minutes once a week). Intensive **t**herapy: The client is referred to appropriate specific therapy from other trained professionals. For the client already taking antidepressants or other medication, the PLISSIT model may be inappropriate because the therapist may be observing "breakthrough" symptoms when the depression (or mania) breaks through the medicinal barrier. This type of situation requires medical reevaluation.

Depression may also lead to anger observed as outbursts of hostility, attempts to sabotage treatment efforts, or blame for the injury placed on the work site or employer. Sometimes the client sees the therapist as an extension of the employer and carries over anger into the rehabilitation process. The therapist can persist in asking questions and actively listening without communicating judgment when the client expresses despair, anger, or negative feelings. The therapist can offer encouragement by pointing out improvements in symptoms or function (see Special Implications for the Therapist: Coping and Adapting in this chapter).

Although the physician must differentiate between pseudo-dementia of depression and dementia in the aging, the therapist's observations may be helpful toward this end. For example, characteristically, a person with dementia who does not know the answer to a question becomes tangential, changing the subject or resorting to confabulation. In contrast, a person with depression gives up easily and responds by saying, "I don't know." With some encouragement and extra time, the depressed person often makes an appropriate response, but the person with dementia moves further from the topic with each comment. People with depression commonly have global memory loss, whereas dementia results in loss of recent memory but retention of detail for remote memory. It is possible for dementia and depression to coexist.

Additionally, a recent study has reported that depression is a risk factor for osteoporosis, especially among the aging population and for men.[197] Researchers do not know how depression might cause a loss of bone mineral density, but increases in the stress hormone cortisol could account for some of the loss. The therapist's intervention for people who are experiencing major depression should include fracture prevention.

Exercise and Depression

Physical activity and exercise has a known benefit in the management of mild-to-moderate mental health diseases, especially depression and anxiety. The exact physiologic mechanism

for this effect remains unknown, but researchers attribute aerobic exercise with the release of endorphins from the pituitary gland. Endorphins, which are neuropeptides, improve our mood and relieve pain. They also reduce the levels of cortisol in the bloodstream; cortisol is linked to stress and depression. Additionally, exercise appears to increase the sensitivity of serotonin neurotransmitter receptors much the same way that antidepressant drugs and therapies release serotonin to help a person relax or sleep.

Increased aerobic exercise or strength training has been shown to reduce mild-to-moderate depressive symptoms significantly in people less than 60 years although habitual physical activity has not been shown to prevent the onset of depression. Studies of older adults and adolescents with depression have been limited but physical activity and exercise appear beneficial in these populations as well.[153] Numerous studies have shown that resistance training (weight lifting) can be both safe and appropriate for even the frailest individual, many of whom cannot take antidepressants because of the side effects.

In some cases, exercise can alleviate depression immediately, independent of achieving fitness, although some evidence exists that exercise must be continued to remain effective.[198] Exertion appears to increase the levels of various neurotransmitters (e.g., dopamine and serotonin) in the same direction as antidepressants. Earlier research reporting that exercise increases levels of b-endorphins (believed to be low in depressed people) is being reevaluated now that more highly specific radioimmunoassay tests are available.[199]

Medications

Psychotropic drugs used to affect mood, behavior, and mental function include antidepressants, antianxiety, and antipsychotics. Antipsychotics are often used in long-term care settings to help normalize disturbances of thought. The therapist must be aware of anyone taking these medications because of the extrapyramidal effects or movement disorders commonly observed with their use. Dystonias, sustained abnormal postures, and disruption of movement due to muscle tone alterations can develop within 5 days of administration. Other common extrapyramidal effects may include restlessness, anxiety, or pacing (akathisia) and Parkinson-like symptoms. Long-term use of antipsychotics can result in permanent involuntary choreoathetoid muscle movements of the face, jaw, and extremities.

For the client taking tricyclic antidepressants (TCAs), heart rate during peak exercise should be monitored (see Appendix B) because the anticholinergic effect of these medications significantly increases heart rate. Drugs used to treat mood disorders may cause a number of other side effects as a result of increased norepinephrine levels such as dry mouth, blurred vision, urinary retention, constipation, palpitations, and orthostatic hypotension (Table 2-15). The last can be the source of dizziness and fainting, increasing the risk of falls and accidents, especially in older adults. Older adults taking TCAs are at greater risk for heat stroke, especially in the summer. These people are not able to adjust easily to ambient air temperatures, which may affect their exercise program or pool therapy. Since some of these medications' side effects are dose-related, the therapist should encourage the client to report any symptoms to the prescribing physician.

The therapist may observe the breakthrough symptoms mentioned earlier when the depression, mania, personality changes, or psychosis break through the medicinal barrier, or alternately, symptoms may occur when the individual decides to

Continued

---

*Although PLISSIT was developed as a model for sexual health interventions,[196] this same concept can be applied to depression.

stop taking the prescribed medication without notifying a health care professional. Symptoms related to TCA withdrawal can occur immediately or up to 48 hours after withdrawal and can continue for as long as 14 days. Withdrawal symptoms may include mood fluctuations, sleep disturbance, gastrointestinal distress, palpitations, dry mouth, or tremors. Withdrawal from TCAs must be monitored by the physician; if the therapist is aware that the client has decided to discontinue use of these (or other) medications without physician approval, appropriate counsel should be offered. Anyone demonstrating breakthrough symptoms must be referred to the prescribing physician. ∎

◆ Coping and Adapting

People react to a stressful event using coping mechanisms, also called *relief behaviors*. Behavioral or cognitive coping mechanisms are used to resolve, reduce, or replace the level of stress, depression, and anxiety. When the stress is resolved, accepted, or changed, adaptation occurs, implying that a sense of equilibrium is restored to the person disordered by stress.

The body also has coping mechanisms, referred to as the *generalized adaptation response* to stressors with multiple physiologic events (see Fig. 2-5). The first stage is the alarm stage or fight-or-flight response when the autonomic nervous system activates the body's involuntary responses such as hormone secretions, metabolism, and fluid regulation. Once the body recognizes continued threat, physiologic forces are mobilized to maintain an increased resistance to stressors and return to a state of homeostasis. Chronic resistance eventually causes damage to the involved systems as the body enters a stage of exhaustion, possibly resulting in diseases of adaptation or stress-related diseases (see Box 2-9).

The process of coping with chronic pain, trauma, or illness is ongoing. Each change in the downward course of the illness requires new and painful acceptance of the disease and its limitations. Behavioral or cognitive coping may be adaptive (e.g., talking or reading about the problem, prayer or seeking God) or maladaptive, such as denial and distancing or the use of alcohol or drugs. When a person is unable to mobilize the necessary resources to manage stress, death from disease may result or suicide may be the final step to conflict resolution.

TABLE **2-15**

Side Effects of Antidepressants

DRUG CLASS	TRICYCLIC ANTIDEPRESSANTS (TCA)	SELECTIVE SEROTONIN REUPTAKE INHIBITORS (SSIs)	MONAMINE (MAO) INHIBITORS
Examples:	Amitriptyline (Elavil/Endep) Amoxapine (Asendin) Desipramine (Norpramin, Pertofrane) Doxepin (Adapin, Sinequan) Imipramine (Janimine, Tofranil)	Citalopram (Celexa) Fluoxetine (Prozac) Fluvoxamine (Luvox) Paroxetine (Paxil) Sertraline (Zoloft)	Phenelzine (Nardil) Tranylcypromine (Parnate) Selegiline (Deprenyl)
Function:	Increase norepinephrine and serotonin levels	Block reuptake of serotonin resulting in higher circulating levels of active serotonin	Inactive MAO, the enzyme responsible for degradation of norepinephrine and serotonin

Effects:	Anticholinergic effects
	  Dry mouth
	  Blurred vision
	  Nausea, vomiting
	  Abdominal bloating
	  Constipation
	  Confusion (older adults)
	Heart arrhythmia
	Tachycardia
	Orthostatic hypotension
	  Low blood pressure, sudden drop
	  Dizziness
	  Weakness
	Sedation/drowsiness
	Sleep disturbance/nightmares
	Sexual dysfunction
	Weight gain
	Fine tremor (older adults)
	Skin rash/photosensitivity
		Nervousness/jitteriness
		Gastrointestinal distress
		  Appetite loss
		  Nausea
		  Diarrhea
		Headache
		Insomnia/sleep disturbance
		Sexual dysfunction
			Hypertensive crisis
			Postural hypotension
			Insomnia
			Headache
			Anemia
			Hyperreflexia
			Muscle weakness, tremors
			SIADH-like syndrome
			Sexual dysfunction
			Gastrointestinal disturbance

BOX 2-15

Risk Factors for Suicide

Past history of attempted suicide
Suicidal ideation, talking about suicide, determining a suicide method
Mood disorders or mental illness:
- Clinical depression, especially manic depressive illness
- Schizophrenia
- Personality disorders, especially borderline and antisocial
Substance abuse
Circumstantial risk factors: stressful life events (see Table 2-7)
Exposure to suicide or suicidal behavior, especially in adolescents and young adults
Genetic predisposition/family history of suicidal behaviors
Decreased levels of serotonin
Availability of firearms (most common method of completed suicide)
Gender (males are five times more likely to commit suicide)
Age (under age 40 or over age 80)

Courtesy of the American Foundation for Suicide Prevention, New York, 2000 (http://www.afsp.org; (888) 333-AFSP).

Suicide

Overview and Incidence.
Suicide is by far the most devastating outcome of depression, but people commit suicide who are not clinically depressed, as do people with significant mood disorders who do not end their lives. At least 500,000 people attempt suicide annually and approximately 1 in 10 are successful, making suicide the eighth leading cause of adult deaths, second or third among youths in the United States, and second among college students. Between 25% and 50% of people with manic-depressive illness attempt suicide at least once. Most people who kill themselves have a treatable mental disorder but do not seek medical care because of social stigma or financial limitations. Many who do see a physician are misdiagnosed. New research in the area of the biologic basis for depression and suicide may result in better care and fewer deaths in the future.

Etiologic and Risk Factors.
Great progress has been made in identifying the clinical, genetic, social, and biochemical factors that contribute to suicidal behavior. Positron emission tomography (PET) is now being used to pinpoint biologic markers commonly found in people who are at greatest risk of attempting or completing suicide.[131,133] These imaging studies show impaired metabolic activity in the prefrontal cortex of the brains of people who have attempted suicide, compared with depressed individuals who have not attempted suicide. The prefrontal cortex is the area of the brain involved in mood regulation. An important factor in setting an individual's threshold for acting on suicidal impulses is brain serotonergic function; serotonin is the neurotransmitter that keeps impulsive and aggressive behaviors in balance. People who are both impulsive or aggressive and depressed have a much higher likelihood of attempting suicide. Studies continue to examine the relationship of these (and other) variables. Indicators of suicide risk are listed in Box 2-15. In addition to these risk factors, males are five times more likely to

take their own lives, and suicide rates are highest for young people under 25 and white men over age 80.

Pathogenesis.
Although the signaling and functional roles of serotonin have been implicated in the psychopathology of suicide, the exact physiologic phenomenon remains unknown. Fewer serotonin transporter sites with local reduction of serotonin binding may be associated with the predisposition to act on suicidal thoughts.[130,131]

Medical Management.
New diagnostic neuroimaging now offers an opportunity to visualize serotonin function in a more direct way than has previously been available. Although this technology may provide the possibility of timely therapeutic intervention in people at high risk for suicide, it is not available everywhere. Major depression can be treated pharmacologically although it is often undertreated, even in the presence of a history of suicide attempt. Some suicide attempts may be preventable if diagnosed early and treated adequately. The need for psychoeducation for health professionals and the public is evident.[204]

Special Implications for the Therapist   2-12

COPING AND ADAPTING

Clients often present with somatic symptoms with an underlying psychosocial basis (see the section on Psychophysiologic Disorders in this chapter). It is not easy for people to make necessary changes (or they would have done so long ago), and denial often obscures the picture. Patience is a vital tool for the therapist working with clients who are having difficulty adjusting to the stress of illness and disability or the client who has a psychologic disorder. Relaxation, breathing, and exercise techniques are helpful in reducing the reaction to stressful events. Studies have confirmed that exercise reduces stress, whether it originates in the brain, the hormonal system, or the immune system and is an important intervention modality (see the section on Immunology and Exercise in Chapter 6). The health care provider also assists the client in recognizing physical responses to stress and teaches how to use these stress-reducing techniques early in the stressful situation or event.

The therapist may need to develop personal coping mechanisms when working with clients who have chronic illnesses or psychologic disturbances. Preexisting character issues or the presence of psychologic problems in a client (e.g., anxiety, panic disorder, depression) can create obstacles to rehabilitation or prevent progress. Recognizing psychologically problems over conditions that are the direct result of organic dysfunction, such as disease or traumatic injury, assists the therapist in coping with clients who are hostile, ungrateful, adversarial, noncompliant, or negative. As part of the treatment team, a psychiatrist, psychologist, or counselor can assist other members of the health care team to better understand individual clients, thereby reducing the therapist's stress and maximizing the client's recovery. Knowing what to say when a client becomes provocative, insulting, or angry is an important coping mechanism for the ther-

Continued

apist (see Special Implications for the Therapist: Psycho-physiologic Disorders in this chapter).

Other basic techniques for coping with anxious, depressed, angry, or otherwise psychologically compromised clients may include reassurance and education, cognitive restructuring, and operant conditioning. Reassurance can be provided by letting the person know that his or her experience is normal and by providing education about the condition and outlining the steps to recovery. Cognitive restructuring guides the client to focus on active coping behaviors and improving function instead of focusing on physical symptoms and pain. Reinforcing positive active behaviors and ignoring pain-related behaviors is called operant conditioning (see Box 2-13).

Suicide

Treatment of depression (whether pharmacologic or psychotherapy) does not change or alleviate symptoms immediately; most drugs used to treat depression require 3 to 4 weeks before a true mood-elevating effect is perceived. The physical symptoms of sleep and appetite disturbances, fatigue, and agitation are the first to improve with medication. Cognitive symptoms such as low self-esteem, guilt, uncertainty, pessimism, and suicidal thoughts resolve more slowly.

Side effects of antidepressant medications are common and may affect multiple systems. The therapist should be alert to any mention of these and encourage the affected person to continue taking the prescribed medications and to contact his or her physician before discontinuing or tapering dosage.

The therapist may be able to offer some practical suggestions such as an over-the-counter artificial saliva spray for dry mouth; an education and prevention and management program for orthostatic hypotension (see the section on Postural Hypotension in Chapter 11); or reduced caffeine intake for people experiencing tremor.

Although some severely depressed people lack the energy necessary to complete an impulsive act such as suicide, close observation is required during the early weeks of pharmacologic treatment. As energy is restored but before a stable elevation of mood is achieved, the individual is at increased risk for suicide. All suicidal thoughts and acts must be taken seriously and responded to appropriately. Three fourths of all suicide victims give some warning of their intentions to a friend or family member. Most older adults who commit suicide have contact with a health care professional (usually their primary care physician) in the month before killing themselves; 40% are in contact with their physicians sometime in the week before taking their own lives.[205] Observe for changes in client mood, such as calmness or tranquility in a formerly hostile, angry, or depressed client. Such a behavior change may be a prelude to a suicidal event.

Comments such as, "I won't be seeing you again," or "My family would be better off without me" may be a form of suicidal communication. Do not hesitate to ask whether a person is considering suicide or even if he or she has a plan or particular method in mind. Do not attempt to argue someone out of suicide but rather, let that person know that you care and understand and that depression can be treated. Avoid the temptation to offer reasons for living such as, "You have so much to live for," "You have come so far to throw your life away," or "Your suicide will hurt your family; think about them." People who are suicidal may also be manipulative; therefore, therapy staff members need to be aware of and

manage their own feelings while empathizing with the client's point of view. When in doubt, report concerns to the appropriate resource (e.g., physician or counselor when one is involved). ■

REFERENCES

1. AAA (American Anthropological Association): Recommendations to the Census Bureau and Office of Management and Budget for 2010, (www.ameranthassn.org/), 2000.
2. ACSM's (American College of Sports Medicine) *Guidelines for exercise testing and prescription*, ed 5, Philadelphia, 1995, Williams & Wilkins.
3. ACSM (American College of Sports Medicine): Position stand: The recommended quantity and quality of exercise for developing and maintaining cardiorespiratory and muscular fitness, and flexibility in healthy adults, *Med Sci Sports Exerc* 30(6):975-991, 1998a.
4. ACSM's (American College of Sports Medicine) resource manual for guidelines for exercise testing and prescription, ed 3, Philadelphia, 1998b, Williams & Wilkins.
5. Adams WL: Screening for problem drinking in older primary care patients, *JAMA* 276(24):1964-1967, 1996.
6. Altarac M, Gardner JW, Popovich RM et al: Cigarette smoking and exercise-related injuries among young men and women, *Am J Prev Med* 18(3 suppl 1):96-102, 2000.
7. American Cancer Society. Cancer Facts. New York, Author, 1986.
8. American Institute for Cancer Research: Food, Nutrition and the Prevention of Cancer: A Global Perspective, Washington, D.C., 1997.
9. American Physical Therapy Association: Guide to physical therapist practice, *Phys Ther* 77:1163-1650, 1997.
10. Anda RF, Croft JB, Felitti VJ et al: Adverse childhood experiences and smoking during adolescence and adulthood, *JAMA* 282(17):1652-1658, 1999.
11. Anderson AE, Bowers W, Evans K: Inpatient treatment for anorexia nervosa. In Garner DM, Garfinkel PE, editors: *Handbook for treatment for eating disorders*, New York, 1997, Guilford, pp. 327-353.
12. Anderson KN, Anderson LE, Glanze WD: *Mosby's medical, nursing, & allied health dictionary*, ed 5, St. Louis, 1998, Mosby.
13. Annon JS: The PLISSIT model: A proposed conceptual scheme for the behavioral treatment of sexual problems, *J Sex Educ Ther* 2:1-15, 1976.
14. APTA: Guidelines for recognizing and providing care for victims of child abuse, Alexandria, Va, 2000, American Physical Therapy Association.
15. Astin JA, Anton-Culver H, Schwartz CE et al: Sense of control and adjustment to breast cancer: the importance of balancing control coping styles, *Behav Med* 25(3):101-109, 1999a.
16. Astin JA, Harkness E, Ernst E: The efficacy of "distant healing": a systematic review of randomized trials, *Ann Intern Med* 132(11):903-910, 2000.
17. Astin JA, Shapiro SL, Lee RA et al: The construct of control in mind-body medicine: implications for healthcare, *Altern Ther Health Med* 5(2):42-47, 1999b.
18. Avers D: Challenges 2000: Geriatrics, *PT Magazine* 8(1):43-46, 2000.
19. Babyak M, Blumenthal JA, Herman S et al: Exercise treatment for major depression: maintenance of therapeutic benefit at 10 months, *Psychosom Med* 62(5):633-638, 2000.
20. Bach PB, Cramer LD, Warren JL et al: Racial differences in the treatment of early-stage lung cancer, *N Engl J Med* 341(16):1198-1205, 1999.
21. Barry HC, Eathorne SW: Exercise and aging, *Med Clin North Am* 78(2):357-376, 1994.
22. Barsky AJ, Borus JF: Functional somatic syndromes, *Ann Intern Med* 130(11):910-921, 1999.
23. Bauer ME, Vedhara K, Perks P et al: Chronic stress in caregivers of dementia patients is associated with reduced lymphocyte sensitivity to glucocorticoids, *J Neuroimmunol* 103(1):84-92, 2000.
24. Baum A, Posluszny DM: Health psychology: mapping biobehavioral contributions to health and illness, *Annu Rev Psychol* 50:137-163, 1999.
25. Beck AT, Ward CH, Mendelson M et al: An inventory for measuring depression, *Arch Gen Psychiatry* 4:561-571, 1961.

26. Benoit S, Schwartz M, Baskin D et al: CNS melanocortin system involvement in the regulation of food intake, *Horm Behav* 37(4):299-305, 2000.

27. Bergen AW, Caporaso N: Cigarette smoking, *J Natl Cancer Inst* 91(16):1365-1375, 1999.

28. Birkmeyer JD, Sharp SM, Finlayson SR et al: Variation profiles of common surgical procedures, *Surgery* 124(5):917-923, 1998.

29. Bjorntorp P, Rosmond R: Neuroendocrine abnormalities in visceral obesity, *Int J Obes Relat Metab Disord* 24 (suppl 2):S80-85, 2000.

30. Blain H, Vuillemin A, Blain A et al: The preventive effects of physical activity in the elderly, *Presse Med* 29(22):1240-1248, 2000.

31. Blumenthal JA, Wei J: Psychobehavioral treatment in cardiac rehabilitation, *Cardiol Clin* 11:323-331, 1993.

32. Blumenthal SJ: Critical women's health issues in the 21st century, *JAMA* 283(5):667, 2000.

33. Bonica JJ: *The management of pain*, Philadelphia, 1953, Lea & Febiger.

34. Brown SA, Tapert SF, Granholm E et al: Neurocognitive functioning of adolescents: effects of protracted alcohol use, *Alcohol Clin Exp Res* 24(2):164-171, 2000.

35. Bruckner J, Trenouth J: The story of physical therapy at Boston's Barbara M. McInnis House, *PT Magazine* 8(1):50-53, 2000.

36. Bruera E: The frequency of alcoholism among patients with pain due to terminal cancer, *J Pain Symptom Manage* 10(8):599-603, 1995.

37. Bruni V, Dei M, Vicini I et al: Estrogen replacement therapy in the management of osteopenia related to eating disorders, *Ann NY Acad Sci* 900:416-421, 2000.

38. Bush K: The AUDIT alcohol consumption questions (AUDIT-C): an effective brief screening test for problem drinking, Ambulatory Care Quality Improvement Project (ACQUIP). Alcohol Use Disorders Identification Test, *Arch Intern Med* 158(16):1789-1795, 1998.

39. Carels RA, Blumenthal JA, Sherwood A: Emotional responsivity during daily life: relationship to psychosocial functioning and ambulatory blood pressure, *Int J Psychophysiol* 36(1):25-33, 2000.

40. Carnes M: Health care in the U.S.: is there evidence for systematic gender bias? *WMJ* 98(8):15, 17-19, 25, 1999.

41. Carney RM, Freedland KE, Stein PK et al: Change in heart rate and heart rate variability during treatment for depression in patients with coronary heart disease, *Psychosom Med* 62(5):639-647, 2000.

42. Carney RM, Freedland KE, Veith RC et al: Can treating depression reduce mortality after an acute myocardial infarction? *Psychosom Med* 61(5):666-675, 1999.

43. CDC (Centers for Disease Control and Prevention): Cigarette smoking among adults—United States, 1998, *MMWR* 49(39):881-884, 2000a.

44. CDC (Centers for Disease Control and Prevention): Health Statistics (www.cdc.gov), 2000b.

45. CDC (Centers for Disease Control and Prevention): Use of FDA-approved pharmacologic treatments for Tobacco Dependence–United States, 1984-1998, *MMWR* 49(20):665-668, 2000c.

46. Chan L: Do Medicare patients with disabilities receive preventive services? A population-based study, *Arch Phys Med Rehabil* 80(6):642-646, 1999.

47. Clark TJ, McKenna LS, Jewell MJ: Physical therapists' recognition of battered women in clinical settings, *Phys Ther* 76(1):12-19, 1996.

48. Clauw DJ, Chrousos GP: Chronic pain and fatigue syndrome: overlapping clinical and neuroendocrine features and potential pathogenic mechanisms, *Neuroimmunomodulation* 4:134-153, 1997.

49. Collins G: New gene linked to obesity. Presentation at the Conference of the European Society for the Study of Diabetes, Jerusalem, Israel, September 2000.

50. Cooper KH: The Cooper Institute for Aerobic Research, 2000 (www.cooperaerobics.com).

51. Cooper RA, Quatrano LA, Axelson PW et al: Research on physical activity and health among people with disabilities: a consensus statement, *J Rehabil Res Dev* 36(2):142-154, 1999.

52. Davis SN, Galassetti P, Wasserman DH et al: Effects of gender on neuroendocrine and metabolic counterregulatory responses to exercise in normal man, *J Clin Endocrinol Metab* 85(1):224-230, 2000.

53. de becker G: *The gift of fear: survival signals that protect us from violence*, New York, 1999, Dell Publishing (Random House).

54. Desai HD, Jann MW: Major depression in women: a review of the literature, *J Am Pharm Assoc* (Wash) 40(4):525-537, 2000.

55. *Diagnostic and statistical manual of mental disorders*, ed 4 [DSM–IV-TR], Washington, DC, 2000, American Psychiatric Association.

56. Dishman RK, Sallis JF, Orentstein DR: The determinants of physical activity and exercise, *Public Health Rep* 100:158-171, 1985.

57. Dunbar-Jacob J: Contributions to patient adherence: is it time to share the blame? *Health Psychol* 12:91-93, 1993.

58. Emery CF, Hauck ER, Blumenthal JA: Exercise adherence or maintenance among older adults: 1-year follow-up study, *Psychol Aging* 7:466-470, 1992.

59. Engler D, Redei E, Kola I: The corticotropin-release inhibitory factor hypothesis: a review of the evidence for the existence of inhibitory as well as stimulatory hypophysiotropic regulation of adrenocorticotropin secretion and biosynthesis, *Endocr Rev* 20(4):460-500, 1999.

60. Ensel WM, Lin N: Age, the stress process, and physical distress: the role of distal stressors, *J Aging Health* 12(2):139-168, 2000.

61. Eriksen W, Natvig B, Bruusgaard D: Smoking, heavy physical work and low back pain: a four-year prospective study, *Occup Med* (London) 49(3):155-160, 1999.

62. Ernst E, Rand JI, Stevinson C: Complementary therapies for depression: an overview, *Arch Gen Psychiatry* 55(11):1026-1032, 1998.

63. Evans WJ: Exercise training guidelines for the elderly, *Med Sci Sports Exerc* 31(1):12-17, 1999.

64. Ewing JA: Detecting alcoholism. The CAGE questionnaire, *JAMA* 252(14):1905-1907, 1984.

65. Fang J, Madhavan S, Alderman MH: The association between birthplace and mortality from cardiovascular causes among black and white residents of New York City, *N Engl J Med* 335(21):1545-1551, 1996.

66. Fang J, Madhavan S, Bosworth W et al: Residential segregation and mortality in New York City, *Soc Sci Med* 47(4):469-476, 1998.

67. Feigenbaum MS, Pollock ML: Prescription of resistance training for health and disease, *Med Sci Sports Exerc* 31(1):38-45, 1999.

68. Feldman DE, Rossignol M, Shrier I et al: Smoking. A risk factor for development of low back pain in adolescents, *Spine* 24(23):2492-2496, 1999.

69. Feldman MD: Munchausen by Internet: detecting factitious illness and crisis on the Internet, *South Med J* 93(7):669-672, 2000.

70. Feldman MD, Eisendrath SJ, editors: *The spectrum of factitious disorders*, Washington, D.C., 1996, American Psychiatric Publishing, Inc.

71. Felitti VJ, Anda RF, Nordenberg D et al: Relationship of childhood abuse and household dysfunction to many of the leading causes of death in adults. The Adverse Childhood Experiences (ACE) Study, *Am J Prev Med* 14(4):245-258, 1998.

72. Fishbain DA, Cutler R, Rosomoff HL et al: Chronic pain disability exaggeration/malingering and submaximal effort research, *Clin J Pain* 15(4):244-274, 1999.

73. Fleury K: Profile of the Native American. Bureau of Indian Affairs, Washington, D.C., 1994.

74. Fox KR: The influence of physical activity on mental well-being, *Public Health Nutr* 2(3A):411-418, 1999.

75. Fox ML, Dwyer DJ, Ganster DC: Effects of stressful job demands and control on physiological and attitudinal outcomes in a hospital setting, *Acad Manage J* 36(2):289-318, 1993.

76. Fredrikson M, Blumenthal JA: Serum lipids, neuroendocrine, and cardiovascular responses to stress in healthy Type A men, *Biol Psychol* 34:45-58, 1992.

77. Freestone S, Ramsay LE: Effect of coffee and cigarette smoking on the blood pressure of untreated and diuretic-treated hypertensive patients, *Am J Med* 73:348-353, 1982.

78. Friedland G: HIV disease in substance abusers: treatment issues. In Sande MA, Volberding PA, editors: *The medical management of AIDS*, Philadelphia, 1999, WB Saunders, pp. 575-591.

79. Garner DM, Garfinkel PE: *Handbook of treatment for eating disorders*, ed 2, New York, 1997, Guilford Press.

80. Geissler CA, Miller DS, Shah M: The daily metabolic rate of the postobese and the lean, *Am J Clin Nutr* 45:914-920, 1989.

81. Georgiades A, Sherwood A, Gullette EC et al: Effects of exercise and weight loss on mental stress-induced cardiovascular responses in individuals with high blood pressure, *Hypertension* 36(2):171-176, 2000.

82. Ghadirian AM, Marini N, Jabalpurwala S et al: Seasonal mood patterns in eating disorders, *Gen Hosp Psychiatry* 21(5):354-359, 1999.

83. Giuliano A, Barth J, Hawk G et al: In McCaffrey R, Williams A, Fisher J, editors: *The practice of neuropsychology: meeting challenges in the courtroom*, New York, 1997, Plenum Press, pp. 22-23.

84. Gladen BC, Ragan NB, Rogan WJ: Pubertal growth and development and prenatal and lactational exposure to polychlorinated biphenyls and dichlorodiphenyl dichloroethane, *J Pediatr* 136(4):490-496, 2000.

85. Goldberg MS, Scott SC, Mayo NE: A review of the association between cigarette smoking and the development of nonspecific back pain and related outcomes, *Spine* 25(8):995-1014, 2000.

86. Greenberger P: The women's health research coalition: a new advocacy network, *J Women's Health Gend Based Med* 8(4):441-442, 1999. The Society for the Advancement of Women's Health Research is a nonprofit, nonpartisan organization committed to improving the health of women through research and can be viewed at www.womenshealth.org/.

87. Grinspoon S, Miller K, Coyle C et al: Severity of osteopenia in estrogen-deficient women with anorexia and hypothalamic amenorrhea, *J Clin Endocrin Metab* 84(6):2049-2055, 1999.

88. Gronbaek M, Becker U, Johansen D et al: Type of alcohol consumed and mortality from all causes, coronary heart disease, and cancer, *Ann Intern Med* 133(6):411-419, 2000.

89. Gupta BS, Gupta U: *Caffeine and behavior*, Boca Raton, Fla., 1999, CRC Press.

90. Harbach H, Hell K, Gramsch C et al: Beta-endorphin (1-31) in the plasma of male volunteers undergoing physical exercise, *Psychoneuroendocrinology* 25(6):551-562, 2000.

91. Hartley TR, Sung BH, Pincomb GA et al: Hypertension risk status and effect of caffeine on blood pressure, *Hypertension* 36(1):137-141, 2000.

92. Harvard Eating Disorders Center: Information about eating disorders (www.hedc.org), 2000.

93. Healthy People 2010: Understanding and improving health. U.S. Department of Health and Human Services. Bethesda, Maryland, 2000 (http://web.health.gov/healthypeople/).

94. Herrin M, Parham E, Ikeda J et al: Alternative viewpoint on National Institutes of Health Clinical Guidelines, *J Nutr Educ* 31(2):116-118, 1999.

95. Hodge CW, Mehmert KK, Kelley SP et al: Supersensitivity to allosteric GABA(A) receptor modulators and alcohol in mice lacking PKC epsilon, *Nat Neurosci* 2(11):997-1002, 1999.

96. Holmes TH, Rahe RH: The Social Adjustment Rating Scale, *J Psychosom Res* 11:213-218, 1967.

97. Hopper JL, Seeman E: The bone density of female twins discordant for tobacco use, *N Engl J Med* 330:387-392, 1994.

98. (HWHW): Harvard Women's Health Watch: Gender and stress 7(2):1, 1999a.

99. (HWHW): Harvard Women's Health Watch: Gender differences in disease 6(5):5, 1999b.

100. Hyman SE: The genetics of mental illness: implications for practice, *Bull World Health Organ* 78(4):455-463, 2000.

101. Ikonomidou C: Ethanol-induced apoptotic neurodegeneration and fetal alcohol syndrome, *Science* 287(5455):1056-1060, 2000.

102. Intercultural Cancer Council: Cancer rates higher in minorities, 2000 (http://icc.bcm.tmc.edu/).

103. Institute of Medicine: *To Err is Human: Building a Safer Health System*. Washington D.C., 2000, National Academy Press, National Academy of Sciences (www4.nationalacademies.org).

104. Irwin M: Immune correlates of depression, *Adv Exp Med Biol* 461:1-24, 1999.

105. Iverson GL, Binder LM: Detecting exaggeration and malingering in neuropsychological assessment, *J Head Trauma Rehabil* 15(2):829-858, 2000.

106. Jessop DS: Stimulatory and inhibitory regulators of the hypothalamo-pituitary-adrenocortical axis, *Baillieres Best Pract Res Clin Endocrinol Metab* 13(4):491-501, 1999.

107. Jiang W, Hayano J, Coleman ER et al: Stability over time of circadian rhythm of variability of heart rate in patients with stable coronary artery disease, *Am J Cardiol* 72:551-554, 1993.

108. Johnson C: Handling the hurt: physical therapy and domestic violence, *PT Magazine* 5(1):52-64, 1997.

109. Johns Hopkins: Health After 50—When alcohol and aging don't mix, 10(12):4-5, 1999.

110. Karlsson MK, Weigall SJ, Duan Y et al: Bone size and volumetric density in women with anorexia nervosa receiving estrogen replacement therapy and in women recovered from anorexia nervosa, *J Clin Endocrinol Metab* 85(9):3177-3182, 2000.

111. Kaye J, Morton J, Bowcutt M et al: Stress, depression, and psychoneuroimmunology, *J Neurosci* 32(2):93-100, 2000.

112. Kerns RD, Turk DC, Rudy TE: The West Haven-Yale Multidimensional Pain Inventory, WHYMPI, *Pain* 23:345-356, 1985.

113. Klantz RM: *LEXCORE now underway: a model for the implementation of longevity diagnostic elements in the anti-aging medical practice*, Anti-aging Medical News, American Academy of Anti-aging Medicine, Chicago, Spring 2000.

114. Klebanoff MA, Levine RJ, DerSimonian R et al: Maternal serum paraxanthine, a caffeine metabolite, and the risk of spontaneous abortion, *N Engl J Med* 341(22):1639-1644, 1999.

115. Klibanski A, Biller BM, Schoenfeld DA et al: The effects of estrogen administration on trabecular bone loss in young women with anorexia nervosa, *J Clin Endocrin Metab* 80(3):898-904, 1995.

116. Koenig HG, Larson DB: Use of hospital services, religious attendance, and religious affiliation, *South Med J* 91(10):925-932, 1998.

117. Kopelman PG: Obesity as a medical problem, *Nature* 404(6778): 635-643, 2000.

118. Krishnan KR: Depression as a contributing factor in cerebrovascular disease, *Am Heart J* 140(4[2]):70-76, 2000.

119. Kuehl K, Elliot DL, Goldberg L: Predicting caloric expenditure during multistation resistance exercise, *J Appl Sport Sci* 4:63-67, 1990.

120. Kuper H, Ye W, Weiderpass E et al: Alcohol and breast cancer risk: the alcoholism paradox, *Br J Cancer* 83(7):949-951, 2000.

121. Langway L: The best cities, *Ladies Home Journal* 155(11):209-216, 1998.

122. Lavernia CJ, Sierra RJ, Gomez-Marin O: Smoking and joint replacement: resource consumption and short-term outcome, *Clin Orthop* 367:172-180, 1999.

123. Lebowitz B: Decade of the brain, National Alliance for the Mentally Ill (NAMI), Arlington, Va., Summer 1997.

124. Leutholtz BC, Ripoll I: *Exercise and disease management*, Boca Raton, Fla., 1999, CRC Press.

125. Levangie PK: Association of low back pain with self-reported risk factors among patients seeking physical therapy services, *Phys Ther* 79(8):757-766, 1999.

126. LoPiccolo CJ, Goodkin K, Baldewicz TT: Current issues in the diagnosis and management of malingering, *Ann Med* 31(3):166-174, 1999.

127. Macario AJ, Conway de Macario E: Stress and molecular chaperones in disease, *Int J Clin Lab Res* 30(2):49-66, 2000.

128. Maestri A: PT for patients with psychiatric disorders, *PT Magazine* 4(7):54-57, 1996.

129. Mann JJ: Role of the serotonergic system in the pathogenesis of major depression and suicidal behavior, *Neuropsychopharmacology* 21(suppl 2):99S-105SS, 1999.

130. Mann JJ, Huang YY, Underwood MD et al: A serotonin transporter gene promoter polymorphism (5-HTTLPR) and prefrontal cortical binding in major depression and suicide, *Arch Gen Psychiatry* 57(8): 739-740, 2000.

131. Mann JJ, Oquendo M, Underwood MD et al: The neurobiology of suicide risk: a review for the clinician, *J Clin Psychiatry* (suppl 60)2:7-11, 18-20, 113-116, 1999.

132. Martinez D, Mawlawi O, Hwang D et al: Positron emission tomography study of pindolol occupancy of 5-HT(1A) receptors in humans: preliminary analyses, *Nucl Med Biol* 27(5):523-527, 2000.

133. Martinez JA: Body-weight regulation: causes of obesity, *Proc Nutr Soc* 59(3):337-345, 2000.

134. Massey LK: Caffeine and the elderly, *Drugs Aging* 13(1):43-50, 1998.

135. Matheson LN: Symptom magnification casebook, Anaheim, Calif. Employment and Rehabilitation Institute of California, 1987.

136. Matheson LN: Symptom magnification syndrome structured interview: rationale and procedure, *J Occup Rehabil* 1:43-56, 1991.

137. Matheson LN: Work capacity evaluation: systematic approach to industrial rehabilitation. Anaheim, Calif. Employment and Rehabilitation Institute of California, 1986.

138. Matheson L, Bohr P, Hart D: Use of maximum voluntary effort grip strength testing to identify symptom magnification syndrome in persons with low back pain, *J Back Musculoskel Rehab* 10:125-135, 1998.

139. McFarlane AC: Posttraumatic stress disorder: a model of the longitudinal course and the role of risk Factors, *J Clin Psychiatry* (suppl 61)5: 15-20, 2000.

140. McInnis KJ: Exercise and obesity, *Coron Artery Dis* 11(2):111-116, 2000.

141. Melzack R: The McGill pain questionnaire: major properties and scoring methods, *Pain* 1:277-299, 1975.

142. Merskey H, editor: Classification of chronic pain: descriptions of chronic pain syndromes and definitions of pain terms, *Pain* (suppl 3): S5, 1986.

143. Messier SP, Davies AB, Moore DT et al: Severe obesity: Effects on foot mechanics during walking, *Foot Ankle Int* 15:29-34, 1994.

144. Mittleman MA, Maclure M, Sherwood JB et al: Triggering of myocardial infarction onset by episodes of anger (abstract), *Circulation* 89:936, 1994.

145. Mittleman MA, Mintzer D, Maclure M et al: Triggering of myocardial infarction by cocaine, *Circulation* 99(21):2737-2741, 1999.

146. MMWR (Morbidity and Mortality Weekly Report): Receipt of advice to quit smoking in Medicare managed care—United States 1998, *MMWR* 49(35):797-801, 2000.

147. Mokdad AH, Serdula MK, Dietz WH et al: The continuing epidemic of obesity in the United States, *JAMA* 284(13):1650-1651, 2000.

148. Moore D: Personal communication. Substance Abuse Resources and Disability Issues (SARDI), Wright State University School of Medicine, Dayton, Ohio, 2000.

149. Myers JN: Exercise testing. In Shankar K: *Exercise prescription*, Philadelphia, 1999, Hanley & Belfus, Inc., pp. 73-96.

150. NAMI (National Alliance for the Mentally Ill): www.nami.org Arlington, Virginia, 2000.

151. Nancarrow DJ, Levinson DF, Taylor JM et al: No support for linkage to the bipolar regions on chromosomes 4p, 18p, or 18q in 43 schizophrenic pedigrees, *Am J Med Genet* 96(2):224-227, 2000.

152. National Coalition for the Homeless: Fact Sheet. Washington, D.C., 1999 www.nch.ari.net.

153. National Institute for Occupational Safety and Health. Division of Safety Research. Violence in the workplace: risk factors and prevention strategies. Cincinnati (OH): Department of Health and Human Services DHHS (NIOSH) Pub. No. 96-100, 1996.

154. Neufeld B: SAFE questions: overcoming barriers to the detection of domestic violence, *Amer Fam Phys* 53(8):2575-2580, 1996.

155. NIDDKD (National Institute of Diabetes and Digestive Kidney Diseases): Overweight, obesity, and health risk. National Task Force on the Prevention and Treatment of Obesity, *Arch Intern Med* 160(7):898-904, 2000.

156. Noonan V, Dean E: Submaximal exercise testing: clinical application and interpretation, *Phys Ther* 80:782-807, 2000.

157. O'Connor GT, Quinton HB, Traven ND et al: Geographic variation in the treatment of acute myocardial infarction: the Cooperative Cardiovascular Project, *JAMA* 281(7):627-633, 1999.

158. Oldridge NB: Compliance and exercise in primary and secondary prevention of coronary heart disease: a review, *Prev Med* 11:56-70, 1982.

159. Oquendo MA, Malone KM, Ellis SP et al: Inadequacy of antidepressant treatment for patients with major depression who are at risk for suicidal behavior, *Am J Psychiatry* 156(2):190-194, 1999.

160. Paluska SA, Schwenk TL: Physical activity and mental health: current concepts, *Sports Med* 29(3):167-180, 2000.

161. Pfalzer L: University of Michigan-Flint: Flint, Michigan. Personal communication, 2000.

162. Polidori MC, Mecocci P, Cherubini A et al: Physical activity and oxidative stress during aging, *Int J Sports Med* 21(3):154-157, 2000.

163. Potter CN: He just bumps into things: recognizing and reporting signs of child abuse, *PT Magazine* 8(4):52-62, 2000.

164. Rao V, Lyketsos CG: The benefits and risks of ECT for patients with primary dementia who also suffer from depression, *Int J Geriatr Psychiatry* 15(8):729-735, 2000.

165. Robinson E, Bachrach LK, Katzman DK: Use of hormone replacement therapy to reduce the risk of osteopenia in adolescent girls with anorexia nervosa, *J Adolesc Health* 26(5):343-348, 2000.

166. Rojas K, Liang L, Johnson EL et al: Identification of candidate genes for psychiatric disorders on 18p11, *Mol Psychiatry* 5(4):389-395, 2000.

167. Rose G, Bengtsson C, Dimberg L et al: Life events, mood, mental strain and cardiovascular risk factors in Swedish middle-aged men. Data from the Swedish part of the Renault/Volvo Coeur Study 48(5):329-336, 1998.

168. Rosenblatt DE, Cho KH, Durance PW: Reporting mistreatment of older adults: the role of physicians, *JAGS* 44(1):65-70, 1996.

169. Ross GW, Abbott RD, Petrovitch H et al: Association of coffee and caffeine intake with the risk of Parkinson disease, *JAMA* 283(20): 2674-2679, 2000.

170. Rozanski A, Blumenthal JA, Kaplan J: Impact of psychological factors on the pathogenesis of cardiovascular disease and implications for therapy, *Circulation* 99(16):2192-2197, 1999.

171. Sanborn CF, Horea M, Siemers BJ et al: Disordered eating and the female athlete triad, *Clin Sports Med* 19(2):199-213, 2000.

172. Sarkisian CA, Liu H, Gutierrez PR et al: Modifiable risk factors predict functional decline among older women: a prospectively validated clinical prediction tool. The Study of Osteoporotic Fractures Research Group, *J Am Geriatr Soc* 48(2):170-178, 2000.

173. Sasche DS: Delirium tremens, *AJN* 100(5):41-42, 2000.

174. Schwartz MW, Seeley RJ: The new biology of body weight regulation, *J Am Diet Assoc* 97:54-58, 1997.

175. Schwartz MW, Woods SC, Porte D et al: Central nervous system control of food intake, *Nature* 404(6778):661-671, 2000.

176. Schweiger U, Weber B, Deuschle M et al: Lumbar bone mineral density in patients with major depression: evidence of increased bone loss at follow-up, *Am J Psychiatry* 157(1):118-120, 2000.

177. Shankar K: *Exercise prescription*, Philadelphia, 1999, Hanley & Belfus, Inc.

178. Sherwood A, Johnson K, Blumenthal JA et al: Endothelial function and hemodynamic responses during mental stress, *Psychosom Med* 61 (3):365-370, 1999.

179. Selzer ML: A self-administered Short Michigan Alcoholism Screening Test (SMAST), *J Stud Alcohol* 36(1):117-126, 1975.

180. Slemenda CW: Cigarettes and the skeleton, *N Engl J Med* 330:430-431, 1994.

181. Sloan RP, Bagiella E, VandeCreek L et al: Should physicians prescribe religious activities? *N Engl J Med* 342(25):1913-1916, 2000.

182. Solomon DA, Keller MB, Leon AC et al: Multiple recurrences of major depressive disorder, *Am J Psychiatry* 157(2):229-233, 2000.

183. Spiller GA: *Caffeine*, Boca Raton, Fla., 1998, CRC Press.

184. Stein PK, Carney RM, Freedland KE et al: Severe depression is associated with markedly reduced heart rate variability in patients with stable coronary heart disease, *J Psychosom Res* 48(4-5):493-500, 2000.

185. Stone D: Eating disorders in athletes: spotting early hallmarks, *J Musculoskel Med* 16(8):443-444, 1999.

186. Tarter R, Vanyukov M, Giancola P et al: Etiology of early age onset substance use disorder: a maturational perspective, *Dev Psychopathol* 11(4):657-683, 1999.

187. Thimineur M, Kaliszewski T, Sood P: Malingering and symptom magnification: a case report illustrating the limitations of clinical judgment, *Conn Med* 64(7):399-401, 2000.

188. Touyz SW, Beumont PJV: Neuropsychological assessment of patients with anorexic and bulimia nervosa. In Touyz SW, Bryne D, Gilandas A, editors: *Neurophyschology in clinical practice*, New York, 1994, Academic Press.

189. Turk DC: The role of psychological factors in chronic pain, *Acta Anaesthesiol Scand* 43(9):885-888, 1999.

190. Turk DC, Okifuji A: Does sex make a difference in the prescription of treatments and the adaptation to chronic pain by cancer and noncancer patients? *Pain* 82(2):139-148, 1999.

191. U.S. Census Bureau: Statistical Brief: Sixty-five plus in the United States. Economics and Statistics Administration, U.S. Department of Commerce, May 1995.

192. U.S. Census Bureau: U. S. Demographics, 2000 (www.census.gov/).

193. Vidaver RM, Lafleur B, Tong C et al: Women subjects in NIH-funded clinical research literature: lack of progress in both representation and analysis by sex, *J Womens Health Gend Based Med* 9(5):495-504, 2000.

194. Volpicelli J, Balaraman G, Hahn J et al: The role of uncontrollable trauma in the development of PTSD and alcohol addiction, *Alcohol Res Health* 23(4):256-262, 1999.

195. Watkins PL, Ward CH, Southard DR et al: The Type A belief system: Relationships to hostility, social support, and life stress, *Behav Med* 18:27-32, 1992.

196. Wechsler H, Lee JE, Kuo M et al: College binge drinking in the 1990s: a continuing problem. Results of the Harvard School of Public Health 1999 College Alcohol Study, *J Am Coll Health* 48(5):199-210, 2000.

197. Weissman MM, Wolk S, Goldstein RB et al: Depressed adolescents grown up, *JAMA* 281(18):1707-1713, 1999.

198. Willett WC, Manson JE, Stampfer MJ et al: Weight, weight change, and coronary heart disease in women: risk within the 'normal' weight range, *JAMA* 273:461-465, 1995.

199. Wilson GT, Fairburn CG, editor: Binge-eating: nature, assessment, and treatment, New York, 1996, Guilford Press.

200. Windham GC, Von Behren J, Waller K et al: Exposure to environmental and mainstream tobacco smoke and risk of spontaneous abortion, *Am J Epidemiol* 149(3):243-247, 1999.

201. Wise MG, Ford CV: Factitious disorders, *Prim Care* 26(2):315-326, 1999.

202. Woltersdorf MA: Beyond the sensorimotor strip, *Clin Manage* 12:63-69, 1992.

203. Woltersdorf MA: Hidden disorders: psychological barriers to treatment success, *PT Magazine* 3(12):58-66, 1995.

204. Woltersdorf MA: Personal communication. Wesley Rehabilitation Hospital, Midwest Brain Function Clinic, Wichita, Kansas, 2000.

205. Woltersdorf MA: Transference: Whistling in the dark, *PT Magazine* 2(1):60-65, 1994.

206. Woods SC, Schwartz MW, Baskin DG et al: Food intake and the regulation of body weight, *Annu Rev Psychol* 51:255-277, 2000.

207. Woolf CJ, Bennett GJ, Doherty M et al: Towards a mechanism-based classification of pain? *Pain* 77:227-229, 1998.

208. Woolf CJ, Decosterd I: Implications of recent advances in the understanding of pain pathophysiology for the assessment of pain in patients, *Pain* (suppl 6): S141-S147, 1999.

209. Yesavage JA: The geriatric depression scale, *J Psychiatr Res* 17(1):37-49, 1983.

210. Zhang Y, Kreger BE, Dorgan JF et al: Alcohol consumption and risk of breast cancer: the Framingham Study revisited, *Am J Epidemiol* 149(2):93-101, 1999.

space heaters; stoves; pilot lights; gas ranges; mothballs; cleaning fluids; glues; photocopiers; formaldehyde in foam, glues, plywood, particleboard, carpet backing, and fabrics; and infectious and allergic agents such as dust mites, cockroaches, bacteria, fungi, viruses, and pollen. Toxic chemicals found in every home, from drain cleaners to furniture polish, are three times more likely to cause respiratory distress than airborne pollutants. The National Pollution Control Center estimates that the average home has approximately 62 different chemicals and that more than 2 million poisonings involving children age 6 and younger occur every year in the United States. Older children and adults account for another 900,000 poisonings.

Radon, a product of the breakdown of radium, poses an environmental risk because of its carcinogenic, especially lung cancer, properties. Exposure is predominantly naturally occurring rather than generated by human polluters and is present in poorly ventilated homes in the form of an odorless gas. Other sources include radioactive waste and underground mines; exposure to tobacco smoke multiplies the risk of concurrent exposure to radon.[52,61]

Outdoor air pollution has long been associated with clinically significant adverse health effects. Although exposure to air pollution is classified separately as indoor and outdoor, the concept of total personal exposure, whether exposure occurs in the home, office, outdoors at home or at work, in a car, movie theater, and so on, is relevant to every individual. People considered especially susceptible to air pollution include cigarette smokers, older adults, infants and young children, and people with chronic obstructive pulmonary disease (COPD) or coronary heart disease (CHD).

Carbon monoxide (CO), an odorless, tasteless, and colorless gas, is a common environmental pollutant from automobile exhaust emissions; the use of liquefied petroleum gas (LPG)-powered forklifts in inadequately ventilated warehouses and production facilities; fires; and in some areas, home heating systems (e.g., the incidence of CO poisoning in homes with faulty furnaces has become an increasing problem, especially in the Midwest). Inexpensive CO monitoring devices have helped identify many previously undetected cases of high levels of CO in private homes.

CO is commonly recognized for its toxicologic characteristics, especially central nervous system (CNS) and cardiovascular effects. CO combines 240 times more quickly with hemoglobin (or myoglobin affecting muscles) than does oxygen, so when carbon dioxide is bound to hemoglobin, its oxygen-carrying capacity is decreased. In the presence of CO, oxygen is not released normally by the blood, resulting in tissue hypoxia. Tissue hypoxia has serious functional consequences for organ systems that require a continuous supply of oxygen, such as the brain and the heart. Exposure to CO also causes impaired visual acuity, headache, nausea, vomiting, fatigue, seizures, behavioral change, and ataxia. In addition, when tissue partial pressure of oxygen is low, CO binds to intracellular hemoproteins such as myoglobin, inhibiting its function and thereby affecting muscle function. More severe CO poisoning can produce metabolic acidosis, pulmonary edema, coma, and death. The classic clinical findings of cherry-red lips and nail bed cyanosis due to the bright-red color of carboxyhemoglobin (COHb) may occur if the COHb concentration is above 40%, but this is rarely observed.

Other air pollutants include smog, a combination of smoke and fog that develops when car exhaust fumes containing nitrous oxides and hydrocarbons are photochemically oxidized.* Nitrogen dioxide and ozone are toxic byproducts of this reaction. Ozone is also produced in the welding process when oxygen is ionized. Both of these byproducts are toxic to the respiratory tract, damaging ciliated endothelial cells lining bronchioles and impairing the mucociliary clearance mechanism. The very young, very old, heavy smokers, or those with preexisting lung disease are at increased risk in the presence of these toxins.

Acid rain caused by the interaction of sulfur dioxide and nitrogen oxides in the atmosphere forms fine sulfate and nitrate particles transported by wind currents over long distances through the air. Outdoor sulfate and nitrate particles penetrate indoors and can be inhaled deep into the lungs. The northeastern United States experiences the greatest levels of acid and sulfate aerosols (up 25% of the breathable particles) during the spring and summer months.[39,88] No known correlation exists between elevated levels of these fine particles and bronchoconstrictive disorders such as asthma, emphysema, and bronchitis.

As part of the Clean Air Act of 1990, the EPA has set air quality standards to protect sensitive population groups from air pollutants. The Clean Air Act regulates oxide emissions, making these particles less available to react with volatile organic compounds that form ozone. Healthy People 2010 has set goals to reduce the proportion of people exposed to air that does not meet the EPA's standards for ozone and to reduce the proportion of nonsmokers exposed to environmental tobacco smoke. Preliminary research on pollutants indicates that biofiltration technology used to clean up airborne waste stream removes 94% of total hazardous air pollutants. Scientists are working to identify microbes that will clean up more difficult-to-remove pollutants.[32]

Water pollution in the form of contamination of drinking water by toxic chemicals has become widely recognized as a public health issue since the late 1970s. Increased monitoring since then has shown that many pesticides and industrial chemicals can be detected in drinking water. The EPA, in conjunction with public health officials and the drinking water industry (e.g., Partnership for Safe Water), have worked diligently to survey and reduce waterborne-disease outbreaks, chemical contamination from leached industrial waste chemicals, and toxins released into recreational and drinking water.[6]

Food as a pollutant is one of the major environmental agents to which people are exposed. In many documented cases, reversible and irreversible human and ecological damage has occurred as a result of pollution-induced food contamination. As scientific and epidemiologic information accumulates, society is questioning to what degree these technologies and byproducts contribute to the steadily rising incidence of certain cancers, autoimmune and other chronic diseases, birth defects, and other health problems for which the cause is not well understood. Pesticide residues in food, hormone residues, food irradiation (a method of preservation and protection from mi-

---

*Ozone and nitrogen, the components of smog, result from the action of sunlight on the products of vehicular internal combustion engines. Automobiles and trucks emit unburnt hydrocarbons and nitrogen dioxide. Ultraviolet irradiation of these compounds leads to complex chemical reactions that produce ozone, various nitrates, and other organic and inorganic compounds constituting smog.

crobial contamination), genetically modified foods, and food additives and preservatives are major consumer concerns. For example, pesticides that are not registered or are restricted for use in the United States can be imported in fruits, vegetables, and seafood produced abroad. Environmental quality is a global concern as increasing numbers of people and products cross national borders, transferring health risks such as infectious diseases and chemical hazards.

Contaminated soil is often the main source of chemical exposure for humans, and an active interchange of chemicals occurs between soil and water, air, and food. Direct contact and ingestion of soil are important exposure pathways, and inhalation of volatile compounds or dust must also be considered. The movement of contaminants through soil is very complex, some moving rapidly and others slowly, eventually reaching and contaminating surface or ground water, on which people rely for drinking and other purposes.

Asbestos continues to be a significant occupational hazard. Abatement workers employed to remove asbestos in buildings wear protective clothing to decrease exposure but still are considered at risk. Long latency (exposure occurring 30 or more years ago continues to affect former workers) and long-term, low-level exposure to the presence of indoor asbestos remain risk factors. See Chapter 14 for a discussion of asbestosis.

Manmade vitreous fibers containing mineral wool, glass wool or fiber, and ceramic fiber have replaced asbestos in the workplace. The nonoccupational exposure to manmade minerals does not put consumers at substantial risk; health issues related to these materials mainly occur among workers with long duration of exposure. Clinical consequences are similar to those of asbestos, including pulmonary fibrosis, bronchogenic carcinoma, mesothelioma, and possibly other types of cancers.

Polyvinyl chloride (PVC), a type of plastic made flexible through the addition of a chemical is used in a variety of products* including medical solutions stored in PVC medical devices such as saline bags. Concern exists over the possibility of chemical plasticizers leaching into the solutions used long-term by certain populations including people on dialysis, individuals with hemophilia, or neonates exposed at critical points in development. Additionally, measured changes in the acidity of intravenous (IV) solutions in PVC packaging have been reported.[90] Dioxin, a byproduct of PVC plastics manufacturing was declared a carcinogen by the EPA in June 2000. Dioxin accumulates in fatty tissues of mammals and fish. The observed toxicities of these chemicals have resulted in the request for PVC-free medical devices and reduction of environmental contamination with these compounds to the lowest possible.[50,92]

Fire and pyrolysis† directly affect two million people annually who are treated for burns, including civilians and firefighters. The most common type of injuries is in the category of smoke inhalation and respiratory problems followed by lacerations, contusions, and falls. Death can occur as a result of smoke inhalation and myocardial infarction. See Occupational Burns in this chapter.

Waste from solid, hazardous, and incinerator byproducts are not likely to be encountered directly in a therapy practice. However, the effects of exposure to medical/infectious waste may be more problematic. Standard precautions for handling all medical/infectious waste are available (see Chapter 7 and Appendix A).

Heavy Metals

Heavy metals such as lead, arsenic, and mercury actually fall under the chemical agents category but are mentioned separately here because of their former prevalence and uniqueness as classical occupational and environmental hazards. Environmental concerns are shifting, and attention to lead, mercury, arsenic (and asbestos) exposure is waning in the face of continued high production volume chemical development, toxicology testing, issues centered around environmental justice, and others.[53]

Lead poisoning is on the decline in the United States as a result of federal initiatives to end the use of lead in gasoline, lead solder in the seams of food cans (beware of foods in cans manufactured outside the United States), and lead-based paints in homes. However, the ingestion of lead paints found in older residential neighborhoods and exposure to lead dust particles during home renovation projects remains a continuing problem among the pediatric population. Likewise dust and soil containing lead particles too small to see expose children who are more likely to be on the ground or outside and who engage in more hand-to-mouth activities. Other risk factors for children include age under 6 years, low income, and urban dwelling. Adults are more likely to be exposed to lead in the manufacture of brass, batteries, bullets, solder, or glass; furniture refinishing; home renovations; stained-glass or pottery making; and prolonged exposure to the burning of metallic wick candles (e.g., home use, restaurant, religious, or ceremonial).[67,87]

Lead is particularly toxic to infants and children for several reasons, including (1) the blood-brain barrier is immature before the age of three, allowing lead to ender the brain more readily; (2) ingested lead has a 40% bioavailability in children, compared with 10% in adults; (3) and the behavioral hand-to-mouth habits previously mentioned. Lead is stored in the body predominantly in bone, but may adversely affect many organ systems, including the central nervous, gastrointestinal, hemopoietic, reproductive, and renal systems. Serum levels once thought to be safe have been shown to be associated with intelligence quotient (IQ) deficits, behavioral disorders, slowed growth, and impaired hearing. The impairment of cognitive function begins to occur at levels greater than 10 micrograms/100 ml, even though clinical symptoms are not apparent; serum levels are required for diagnosis.

Arsenic is used in the manufacture of glass, pesticides, and wood preservatives and has been found to contaminate water, beer, and seafood. Arsenic binds to tissue proteins and is concentrated in the liver, skin, kidney, nervous system, and bone, with bone being affected to a lesser extent than lead. The symptoms of acute inorganic arsenic poisoning may include severe burning of the mouth and throat, abdominal pain, nausea, vomiting, diarrhea, hypotension, and muscle spasms. In severe cases, cardiomyopathy, jaundice, renal impairment, red cell hemolysis, ventricular arrhythmias, coma, seizures, and intestinal hemorrhage are seen. Chronic arsenic poisoning is characterized by an irregular dusky pigmentation and hyperkeratosis of the skin that looks like raindrops on a dusty road. Painful dysesthesia in the hands and feet, bone marrow depression,

---

*Vinyl chloride production has doubled in the last 20 years, with current production of 27 million tons per year worldwide.

†Pyrolysis, or incomplete combustion, of wood releases many highly toxic compounds that can react with other organic substances to produce new toxic and irritant chemicals. Incomplete combustion and fire-fighting water also produce highly acidic aerosols. Smoldering or partially controlled fires release many toxic products.

transverse white striae of the nails, altered mentation, and occasionally garlicky perspiration odor may occur. Cancer of the skin and lungs has been associated with arsenic poisoning, but the mechanisms responsible for arsenic carcinogenesis have not been established. Increasing evidence indicates that arsenic acts at the level of tumor promotion by modulating the signaling pathways responsible for cell growth.[85]

Mercury is widespread and persistent in the environment. Exposures to women of childbearing age are of great concern because a fetus is highly susceptible to adverse effects. Exposure to hazardous levels of mercury can cause permanent neurologic (e.g., mental retardation, cerebral palsy, seizures) and kidney impairment. Elemental or inorganic mercury is released into the air or water where it accumulates in animal tissues and increases in concentration through the food chain. The U.S. population primarily is exposed by eating fish but mercury is also used in electrical products, as a fungicide, and in dental amalgams.*

Although mercury is poorly absorbed from the gastrointestinal tract, mercury vapor is well absorbed through the lungs and from the gut. Mercury poisoning causes irritation of the mouth and pharynx and is accompanied by vomiting, dehydration, abdominal cramps, and bloody diarrhea. Death can occur from acute renal failure. Chronic exposure to mercury may cause additional symptoms of gingivitis, speech defects, tremor, and chronic personality disorder called the *Mad Hatter syndrome*, characterized by unusual shyness, labile affect, and decline in intellect. Mercury poison affects the nervous system, resulting in dysarthria, ataxia, paresthesias, and constricted visual fields.

The long-term strategy for reducing exposure to mercury is to lower mercury concentrations in fish by limiting mercury releases into the atmosphere from burning mercury-containing fuel and waste and other industrial processes. EPA regulations for waste incineration have resulted in decreased air emissions of mercury in the last two decades and this trend is expected to continue. The Food and Drug Administration (FDA) advises that pregnant women and those who may become pregnant should not eat shark, swordfish, king mackerel, and tile fish known to contain elevated levels of mercury.[60] Additional information is available at http://www.fda.gov/bbs/topics/ANSWERS/2001/advisory.html.

Xenoestrogens/Xenobiotics.

Xenoestrogens are also part of chemical environmental exposure but are discussed separately because of their unique place as a hazardous agent. In the early 1970s, scientists from around the world met together to discuss the cumulative efforts of researchers investigating various endangered species. Together they identified that exposure to petrochemicals (previously called *xenoestrogens* but now referred to as *xenobiotics*, meaning "foreign to life") as the underlying cause of dwindling births in these species. Petrochemicals such as pesticides and insecticides are the primary xenobiotics and constitute substances totally foreign to nature—that is, they are not found in the natural world but rather are synthesized chemicals. Other petrochemicals are present in commonly used items or products such as

emollients in lotions and creams, spreaders in salad dressing, carpet glues, paints, solvents, automobile gasoline, plastics, and a multitude of other common household objects. Researchers concluded that the effect of these residues is selective to the reproductive systems of the developing fetuses so that exposure in the developing fetuses resulted in infertility or sterility. Since that time, it has been recognized that these chemicals can affect other systems including the thyroid, immune function, and nervous system.

The effect of these chemicals has been to create what is referred to as an *estrogen-dominant environment* because the chemicals have estrogenic activity. The effect of this estrogen dominance on humans (men and women although women are more susceptible) is the subject of intense scrutiny by scientists and researchers. This biologic phenomenon may be linked to autoimmune dysfunction, increased body fat, decreased sex drive and sperm production, altered blood clotting, early menarche, zinc deficiency associated with prostate dysfunction, endometriosis, and headaches associated with fluid retention. Researchers are in agreement that such compounds in high doses may cause developmental, reproductive, and tumorigenic effects, but controversy remains regarding the risks associated with xenoestrogens under low exposure that are considered more realistic and how to assess the interaction of exogenous compounds with the endocrine system and its complex regulation.[24]

Physical Agents.

Physical agents are the source of much environmental damage. The long-term effects of exposure to *electromagnetic radiation* or electromagnetic fields (EMF), including radiofrequency and microwave, ultraviolet light, x-ray, and gamma rays remains under intense scrutiny. Ionizing radiation is the result of electromagnetic waves entering the body and acting on neutral atoms or molecules with sufficient force to remove electrons, creating an ion. The most common sources of ionizing radiation exposure in humans are accidental environmental exposure and medical, therapeutic, or diagnostic irradiation.

All living material is vulnerable to ionization by high-energy radiation because the disruption of atoms joined into molecules producing ions and free radicals (see Chapter 5 and Fig. 5-2) can result in further biochemical damage, including somatic effects such as cell death, and genetic effects, including reproductive effects and cancer. Radiation-induced changes can cause genetic mutations and structural rearrangements in chromosomes that can be transmitted from generation to generation.[9,94] A wide range of other adverse health effects have been attributed to ionizing radiation, including visual, thermal, behavioral, CNS, and auditory effects; effects on the blood-brain barrier; and immunologic, endocrinologic (including effects on biorhythm), hematologic, developmental, and cardiovascular effects.

Exposure to nonionizing radiation (i.e., the electromagnetic wave does not have enough energy to strip an atom of its electron) occurs most commonly as a result of the use of a wide variety of industrial and electronic devices (e.g., microwave

---

*Dental fillings still contain mercury as other materials have not been developed that are as strong or as long lasting. Despite consumer concerns about mercury exposure from dental fillings, clients and dental personnnel are at greatest risk when amalgams are removed. The aerolization during removal creates greater mercury exposure than the hardened and intact filling in the mouth. It is advised that amalgams only be removed when the filling (or tooth) is no longer intact, rather than to eliminate mercury exposure. Dental personnel are at greatest risk for this type of repeated exposure.

---

*Chemical compounds from plastic wrap surrounding food or covering dishes used in a microwave can leach into the foods and affect the body. Packaging and plastic wraps that contain polyethylene are preferred for use in the microwave, since these do not have plasticizers (materials that make the wrap more pliable). Containers meant for cold foods such as margarine or whipped topping should also be avoided for microwave use, since these containers can melt, dispersing some of their components into the food.

ovens,* scanning lasers in stores, high-intensity lamps, video display terminals (VDTs), scanning radar, electronic antitheft surveillance). Considerable speculation has gone on around the world that long-term exposure to electromagnetic fields is correlated with the development of breast cancer, leukemia, miscarriage, and neurodegenerative diseases such as Alzheimer's, Parkinson's, and amyotrophic lateral sclerosis.[38] The unexplained high incidence of breast cancer in industrialized nations is suspected as being linked to electric power generation and consumption. The proposed biologic mechanism is the inhibition of melatonin caused by the products of electric power generation, EMFs, and light at night, but this has not been proved and further investigation is warranted.[14,18]

Most exposures to electromagnetic interference are transient and pose no threat to people with pacemakers and implantable cardioverter defibrillators; however, magnetic resonance imaging (MRI) and prolonged exposure to EMFs is contraindicated in anyone who is pacemaker dependent.[72] Concerns that cellular telephone radiation is linked to brain tumors or causes a variety of serious problems (e.g., genetic damage, pacemaker or implantable cardioverter defibrillator disruption, interference with heart/lung monitors, compromise to the blood-brain barrier) have not been substantiated or proven clinically important.[93] Further studies are needed to account for longer induction periods, especially for slow-growing tumors with neuronal features.[23,63,99] The only health hazard of cell phones that has been confirmed is the increased risk of having an accident while driving. Likewise, a previous concern that living in close proximity to power lines was correlated to cancer has not been proved[12,86] nor have reports linking VDTs to miscarriages been substantiated.[54]

However, considerable evidence suggests that EMFs affect sleep and therefore affect mood, behavior, and cognitive abilities.[83] Exposure to EMFs has been suggested as the cause of a condition referred to as *electrosupersensitivity/screen dermatitis* in susceptible people using VDTs or artificial light. Cutaneous problems (e.g., itch, heat sensation, pain, erythema, papules, pustules) and symptoms from internal organs (e.g., the heart) have been reported in association with EMFs. From the results of recent studies it is clear that EMFs affect mast cells releasing inflammatory substances such as histamines that result in these symptoms. Mast cells are also present in the heart tissue, and data from studies made on interactions of EMFs with cardiac function have demonstrated changes present in the heart after exposure to EMFs. However, the exact significance or cause of these changes remains unknown.[34]

Vibration is divided into two types: whole-body vibration (WBV) and hand-arm vibration (HAV). Truck, bus, and boat drivers, helicopter operators, heavy equipment operators, miners, and others are at increased risk for WBV. Major clinical concerns of WBV exposure are chronic back pain and degenerative disk diseases, visual and vestibular changes, and circulatory and digestive system disorders.[10,36,58] The risk for increased spinal loading and physiologic changes associated with WBV can be reduced by vibration damping, good ergonomic design, reducing exposure, and reducing other risks such as lifting.[73] Vibration-induced white finger disease is the most common example of an occupational injury caused by vibration of the hands. This condition occurs secondary to use of hand tools such as power saws, grinders, sanders, pneumatic drills, jackhammers, and other equipment used in construction, foundry work, machining, and mining. Interestingly, the use of WBV called vibration exercise (VE) is a new neuromuscular training method being used in athletes to increase the mechanical power output of muscles and improve neuromuscular efficiency; VE is also being investigated for the prevention and treatment of osteoporosis.[13,57,77]

Heat stress exceeding human tolerance can result in heat disorders (e.g., stroke, exhaustion, cramps, dehydration, prickly heat) and heat illnesses (e.g., chronic heat exhaustion, reduced heat tolerance, anhidrotic heat exhaustion), some of which are fatal. In a therapy setting, the groups of people most likely to experience heat stress include older adults during temperature extremes, industrial workers, fire fighters, outdoor sports participants, agricultural workers, pregnant women, people taking mood-altering drugs (i.e., they lose touch with their environment). Additionally, antidepressants such as tricyclic antidepressants affect the body's ability to respond to temperature changes.

High-altitude environment (8000 to 14,000 feet) is characterized by atmosphere with decreasing partial pressure of oxygen and decreasing temperature. Hypoxia (reduced availability of oxygen to the body) appears to be the underlying cause of most of the physiologic changes of elevated altitude. Acute altitude sickness includes acute mountain sickness, high-altitude pulmonary edema, and high-altitude cerebral edema. These three probably represent a continuum of disease, but each has different symptom complexes, pathogenesis, and slightly different treatment interventions. People with cardiopulmonary and other diseases (e.g., sickle cell disease) are at increased risk for worsening of the medical disorder and possibly at increased risk for acute altitude illnesses with ascent to high altitudes. Aviation and aerospace illnesses are rarely encountered by the therapist and are beyond the scope of this book.

◆ Risk Factors

Environmental pathogenesis requires an understanding of latency, the concept that a hazardous or toxic agent may initiate a series of internal reactions that do not manifest as overt disease for many years or even decades as the body strives to maintain a state of optimal health or homeostasis. Many factors such as route of exposure (e.g., inhalation, ingestion, absorption through the skin); magnitude or concentration (dose) of exposure; duration (e.g., minutes, hours, days, lifetime); and frequency (e.g., seasonal, daily, weekly, monthly) play into the development of progressive and overt disease. Likewise, personal factors that vary from one person to another may affect pathogenesis and must be considered. These include age, gender, ethnicity, nutritional status, personal habits and lifestyle, genetic makeup and host susceptibility, and the strength of individual defense mechanisms. The host-agent-environment interactions are immensely complex and poorly understood at this time.

◆ Pathogenesis

Once a hazardous substance is released into the environment, it may be transported and transformed in a variety of complex ways. For example, a chemical may be modified by the environment before entering the body; transformed by chemical or biochemical processes; or undergo vaporization, diffusion, dilution, or concentration by physical or biologic processes. Plants and animals may accumulate small doses of a chemical agent and bioconcentrate them to the degree that they become hazardous when consumed by humans.

All cells respond to a variety of different adverse environmental stimuli with a cellular defense response now commonly referred to as the stress response. Molecules released by the cells in response to stress (e.g., hyperthermic shock, radiation, toxins, viral infections) are called *heat shock* or *stress proteins*. Increased levels of these proteins after a cellular injury from any of the environmental hazardous agents seem to act as molecular chaperones that facilitate the synthesis and assembly of new reparative proteins. Cells that produce high levels of stress proteins seem better able to survive ischemic damage; stress proteins may be influential in certain immunologic responses and may also be a requirement for cells to recover from a metabolic insult. This finding may lead to further research investigating the role of pharmacology in raising the levels of stress proteins to provide additional protection to injured tissues and organs. Such a therapeutic approach could have other applications outside environmental medicine such as to reduce tissue damage from surgery-induced ischemia or to help protect isolated organs used for transplantation, which often experience ischemia and reperfusion injury.[29]

Some people once sensitized to chemicals, develop increasingly severe reactions to more and more chemicals at smaller and smaller concentrations. The allergic response that occurs does not appear to be a typical response, perhaps suggesting altered immune system modulation. Immunologists have also discovered a possible connection between stress proteins and autoimmune disease, which may lead to preparations of specific protective vaccines.[19,97]

◆ Clinical Manifestations

An environmental illness may manifest in a variety of ways. The illness may present as a newly developed clinical syndrome or an aggravation or change in a preexisting condition. The EPA[28] identifies the following seven categories of human health effects from hazardous exposures:

1. *Carcinogenicity:* Can cause cancer
2. *Heritable genetic and chromosomal mutations:* Can cause mutations in genes and chromosomes that will be passed on to the next generation, such as caused by ionizing radiation
3. *Developmental toxicity:* Can cause birth defects or miscarriages
4. *Reproductive toxicity:* Can damage the ability of men and women to reproduce
5. *Acute toxicity:* Can cause death from even short-term exposure to the lungs, through the mouth, or the skin
6. *Chronic toxicity:* Can cause long-term damage other than cancer, such as liver, kidney, or lung damage
7. Neurotoxicity: Can harm the nervous system by affecting the brain, spinal cord, or nerves

Local toxicities from exposure to environmental agents can occur such as ocular damage; mucous membrane complaints (eye, nose, and throat irritation); chemical burns to skin; noise-induced hearing loss; and vestibular disorders. Systemic toxicities can involve any organ system (Table 3-1). The clinical syndrome may mimic a wide range of psychiatric, metabolic, nutritional, inflammatory, and degenerative diseases. Over the last 15 years, a new syndrome of environmental symptoms associated with chemicals has been observed both in the United States and in European countries called *multiple chemical sensitivity (MCS)*. MCS is characterized by a chronic condition with symptoms that recur reproducibly in response to low levels of exposure to a wide variety of substances (e.g., multiple unrelated chemicals) and improve or resolve when irritants are removed. Recently, an additional requirement for MCS has been added: symptoms occur in multiple organ systems.[20] Two to four times as many cases of MCS exist among Gulf War veterans compared with undeployed controls[75] (see the section on Gulf War Syndrome in this chapter).

Objective physical findings and consistent laboratory abnormalities or biomarkers associated with MCS are typically nonexistent, leading some of the medical community to call this condition *idiopathic environmental intolerance (IEI)*, a psychosomatic or neuropsychiatric disorder. Reported symptoms include fatigue, headaches, weakness, malaise, decreased attention/concentration, memory loss, disorientation, confusion, and mood changes. The treatment focus of this philosophy is to overcome the affected individual's belief in a toxicogenic explanation for the symptoms,[89] whereas other health care professionals are calling for accurate diagnostic assessment, agreement on the use of specific questionnaires, clinical and technical diagnostic procedures, and prospective clinical studies of people with MCS, comparative groups, experimental approaches.[3] All in all, the concept of MCS has ignited considerable controversy in the fields of medicine, toxicology, immunology, allergy, psychology, and neuropsychology.[49]

Neurotoxicity.   Of particular interest to the therapist may be the effects of hazardous or toxic agents on the nervous system. Neurologic symptoms are common presenting symptoms in people seen by occupational and environmental health professionals. Cognitive difficulties, headaches, fatigue, dizziness, and limb paresthesias are often experienced, but these are nonspecific and seldom point to a single disease or cause. Many toxins manifest as a nonspecific syndrome of distal sensorimotor impairment that is indistinguishable from the neuropathy due to common systemic diseases (e.g., diabetes mellitus, vitamin B_6 deficiency, alcoholism, uremia). Toxins such as lead have a striking predilection for motor fibers and usually produce minimal sensory symptoms.

Neurologic symptoms that appear immediately after acute exposure are usually due to the physiologic effects of the specific (usually chemical) agent. These symptoms subside with cessation of exposure and elimination of the compound from the body. By contrast, delayed neurologic disorders are generally a result of pathologic alterations of the nervous system. Symptoms appear in a subacute manner over days or weeks after short-term exposure. In the case of long-term exposure, symptoms may appear insidiously and progress over many weeks or months. Recovery can be expected after cessation of exposure, but the recovery is slow and depends on the extent of neuronal damage; the half-life of the chemical (i.e., continued exposure until the drug is out of the system); and the adverse effects of chelates used in the chemotherapy of metal poisoning.

Neurotoxicants do not cause focal (asymmetrical) neurologic syndrome. Neurotoxins reach the nervous system by the systemic route and cause neurologic symptoms and deficits in a diffuse and symmetrical manner resulting in polyneuropathy. Any significant asymmetry in the presentation, such as weakness or numbness affecting one limb or one side of the body, is not likely to be attributed to neurotoxicity. Multiple neurologic syndromes are possible from a single toxin. Although the effects of neurotoxins are symmetrical, neurons from different parts of the nervous system react differently to the agent.

TABLE 3-1

Systemic Manifestations of Toxicity

Optic	Optic nephropathy, optic neuritis, optic atrophy	Central nervous system	Sensorimotor polyneuropathies (mild to severe weakness)
Integument	Atopic dermatitis		Muscular fasciculations and weakness
	Urticaria		Reduced or absent reflexes
	Pain, itching, erythema		Cranial neuropathy
	Pustules, papules		Prominent autonomic dysfunction
	Chemical burns		Encephalopathy
Cardiovascular	Cardiac arrhythmia		Cerebellar ataxia
	Coronary artery disease	Hematopoietic system	Aplastic anemia
	Hypertension		Hemolytic anemia
	Myocardial injury		Myelodysplastic syndromes
	Nonatheromatous ischemic heart disease		Multiple myeloma
	Peripheral arterial occlusive disease		Toxic thrombocytopenia
Respiratory system	Airway inflammation and hyperreactivity		Porphyria
	Bronchitis	Immune system	Allergic disease
	Asthma		Allergic rhinitis
	Hypersensitivity pneumonitis		Bronchial asthma
	Pneumoconiosis		GI allergy (food)
	Interstitial fibrosis		Anaphylaxis
	Asbestosis		Autoimmune diseases
	Silicosis		Neoplasia
	Granuloma formation	Reproductive system	Menstrual disorders
	Diffuse alveolar damage		Altered fertility or infertility
Gastrointestinal (GI tract)	Cancer		Spontaneous abortion or stillbirth
Liver	Acute or subacute hepatocellular injury		Birth defects, low birth weight
	Cirrhosis		Cancer
	Angiosarcoma		Reduced libido or impotence
	Carcinoma		Altered or reduced sperm production
	Hepatitis		Premature menopause
Kidney and urinary tract	Acute renal disease		
	Chronic renal failure		
	Tubulointerstitial nephritis		
	Nephrotic syndrome		
	Rapidly progressive glomerulonephritis		

Toxic polyneuropathy affects the distal limbs first, reflecting the greater vulnerability of the longest nerve axons. Sensory disturbances are usually reported as a tingling or burning sensation distributed in a stocking-and-glove pattern (see Fig. 38-5). The toes and the feet are affected first; hand symptoms are seldom present during the early stage. Involvement of the motor nerve fibers, if present, manifests first as atrophy and weakness of the intrinsic foot and hand muscles, bilaterally. More severe cases may present with footdrop or wristdrop, reflecting degeneration of motor axons to the lower leg and forearm muscles.

Neuropathic pain is commonly encountered in people with peripheral neuropathies regardless of the cause. In other words, pain patterns associated with chemically induced peripheral neuropathies do not differ significantly from the clinical picture of pain associated with neuropathy of other causes. Often this pain bears little relationship to the severity of neuropathy and may intensify during a period of recovery, or it may remit paradoxically as the neuropathy progresses, often with further loss of sensation. Pain is not a reliable indicator of neurologic progression or recovery.

◆ Medical Management

Clinical assessment may include assessing the details of exposure and correlating them with the medical condition. Various testing procedures may be developed on the basis of the historical information provided by the client. The clinical presentation, environmental history, and results of laboratory tests assist the physician in demonstrating a correlation between exposure and the clinical manifestations. Nerve conduction velocity (NCV) studies and electromyography (EMG) are the primary tools for the laboratory evaluation of neuromuscular disorders. A toxic polyneuropathy is characterized by a diffuse and relatively symmetrical pattern of NCV abnormalities.

Removal from exposure and decontamination of the exposed victim is essential in the treatment of exposure-linked toxicity. Specific intervention protocols depend on the agent involved (e.g., pesticide poisoning requires symptom-specific therapy such as IV anticonvulsants to halt a seizure; antihistamines are used for allergic reactions); the particular organ system involved; and the presenting pathologic condition.

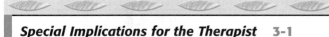

Special Implications for the Therapist   3-1

ENVIRONMENTAL MEDICINE

Preferred Practice Patterns
Various patterns may apply depending on the system(s) involved and the corresponding clinical manifestations (see Table 3-1).
5B: Impaired Motor Function and Sensory Integrity Associated With Nonprogressive Disorders of the Central Nervous System: aquired in adolescence or adulthood (hypoxia, vestibular disorders)
5E: Impaired Motor Function and Sensory Integrity Associated with Acute or Chronic Polyneuropathies

Environmental Hazards

Given the context of industrial, occupational, and environmental medicine and the single overriding factor of latency, health care professionals must view each client's health status holistically, as a composite of the individual's total life experience. Whenever symptoms present in the absence of a clearly identifiable history or cause, the client's past medical history must be carefully reviewed. An occupational history includes dates of employment, a list of current and longest-held jobs, average hours worked per week, exposure to potential hazards in the workplace, common illnesses in coworkers, and personal protective equipment worn (or not worn) on the job. Any information elicited by the therapist but unknown to the physician must be documented and reported.

Air Pollution

Vigorous exercise outdoors, which increases the dose of pollution delivered to the respiratory tract, should be avoided during periods of ambient air pollution.[31,79] Health care providers can reasonably advise all clients, especially anyone with respiratory disorders but also athletes in training,[76] to stay indoors during pollution episodes.

Respiratory protective equipment (RPE) has been developed for use in the workplace to minimize exposure to toxic gases and airborne particles. Many of these devices, particularly those likely to be most effective, add to the work of breathing and are not well tolerated by some people, especially those with respiratory disease. Much remains unknown about the efficacy of RPE and concerns have been raised about the risk of dangerous carbon dioxide accumulation within the device, proper fit and inward leakage, resistance to airflow as the filter load increases, and individual breathing rates and filter replacement schedules. Research to answer these questions is necessary before specific recommendations can be made for the general population as well as for individuals with known respiratory disease.

Studies on the efficacy of high efficiency-filter air cleaners have been shown to improve airway hyperresponsiveness and decrease peak flow amplitude in people with allergic asthma (studies to date have centered on children) who are sensitized and exposed to pets.[95] Future studies are needed to develop biologic markers to identify more accurately people who have a clinical improvement after allergen eviction.

Carbon Monoxide

The main symptoms of carbon monoxide (CO) poisoning are dizziness, headache, nausea, weakness, and tachypnea, followed at higher amounts by loss of consciousness, coma, convulsions, and death. As CO binds to hemoglobin to form carboxyhemoglobin the reduced capacity of the blood to deliver oxygen to the tissues results in increased frequency of coronary heart disease and arrhythmias and stresses the immune system.[37,44,82] Acute myonecrosis (death of individual muscle fibers) has been associated with CO poisoning. Clinical studies of people and heart disease have been carried out to evaluate the effects of CO exposure on exercise capacity. During exercise, persons with coronary artery disease experience a decreased time to occurrence of myocardial ischemia when exposed to CO compared to healthy subjects.[1, 2]

Neurologic recovery in people with mild to moderate CO poisoning is good. The prognosis after severe poisoning is variable and correlates with the extent and duration of the insult. Short-term memory impairment, depression, and syndromes related to lesions of the basal ganglia are well known. A syndrome of delayed neurologic deterioration occurs in about 10% of victims of serious CO intoxication. Risk factors for the delayed syndrome include age older than 40 years, prolonged exposure, and abnormalities of the brain on computed tomography (CT).[71]

Lead

The brain is the target of lead toxicity in children, but adults usually present with manifestations of peripheral neuropathy. Typically, the radial and peroneal nerves are affected resulting in wristdrop and footdrop, respectively. Anyone presenting with vague or nonspecific symptoms of myalgias, paresthesias, arthralgias accompanied by fatigue, irritability, lethargy, abdominal discomfort, poor concentration, headaches, tremors, and known risk factors may be suffering from lead poisoning. Pica (compulsive chewing on nonnutritive objects such as dirt, paint or plaster, clay) observed in children may be associated with lead toxicity and must be evaluated. Lead anemia and lead nephropathy may also occur. (See the section on Neurotoxicity in this chapter.) For more information, contact the National Lead Information Center Clearinghouse (800) 424-5323) or for hotline help at (800) 532-3394.

Vibration

Tools can be modified to reduce some of the dangerous levels of vibration. Grip kits provide grips that can be applied easily to any type of tool and dampening products made of sorbothane reduce shock and vibration.

Heat Stress

Muscle cramps and distal extremity edema, dehydration, and electrolyte imbalance are the most commonly observed phenomena associated with heat stress in a therapy practice. The implications surrounding these adverse effects are discussed fully in Chapter 4.

High Altitude

Many issues are related to altitude change (e.g., effects on fetal size and development, ultraviolet intensity with increases in altitude, sympathetic nervous system changes during acclimatization, air pollution at higher elevations, physiologic changes and pathologic conditions occurring in military and

Continued

aerospace personnel) that are being researched and reported in the literature. These are beyond the scope of this text. Implications here are confined to the more common issues in a therapy practice related to exercise capacity.

Chronic exposure to high altitude is known to result in changes in the mechanisms regulating oxygen delivery to the contracting muscles, but the underlying cause of changes in exercise capacity associated with high altitude is not completely understood.[35] The primary effect of altitude on exercise capacity is through effects on the cardiovascular system, with a decrease in maximum oxygen consumption (VO_{2max}) and a decrease in maximum heart rate. Studies of oxygen saturation during submaximal exercise in natives of high-altitude areas compared with individuals born at sea level and acclimated to high altitudes suggest that oxygen saturation during exercise may be influenced by adaptation during growth and development and larger lung volume and pulmonary diffusion capacity for oxygen in the native high-altitude population.[15] With continued exposure to increased altitude, exercise capacity does seem to improve, but never reaches that attained at sea level for the native sea level population.[80] People with congestive heart failure or coronary artery disease are more likely to be symptomatic at high altitudes. Those with either of these conditions are likely to experience reduced exercise capacity.[45,62]

Mild sensory neuropathy may also occur at high altitudes both as part of the burning feet/burning hands syndrome (distal limb burning and tingling paresthesias) associated with chronic mountain sickness and as a separate entity among control groups studied. This condition resolves with low-altitude sojourn (even for high-altitude natives), suggesting that a mechanism of altered axonal transport may be involved. Additionally, reduced thickness of microvessels observed implies that adaptive structural changes to hypobaric hypoxia may also occur in peripheral nerve and are similar to those reported in other tissues of high altitude natives.[91]

Neurotoxicity

Litigation and other potential sources of secondary gains often complicate environmental or occupational exposures that result in neurologic disorders. Psychologic factors may have profound effects on the client's perception of neurologic symptoms, even in those people with genuine organic disease. Emotional issues must be recognized and addressed throughout the rehabilitation process.

Coasting is the phenomenon of continuing clinical progression of neurologic deficits after removal of the offending toxin. Weakness or sensory deficits of these neuropathies often worsen for as long as 4 to 5 months after cessation of exposure, reflecting the delayed neuronal death or degeneration induced by the toxin.

Neurologic recovery is facilitated by the plasticity of the nervous system (i.e., its ability to adapt to injury). Peripheral sensory and motor nerve fibers have a remarkable capacity to regenerate after removal of the neurotoxin. Although the neurons in the central nervous system lack the ability to multiply, surviving neurons may eventually take over the function of degenerated neurons and partially restore neurologic function. Physical and occupational therapy is beneficial during the recovery time to facilitate this process. When given sufficient time (18 to 24 months), partial clinical improvement is demonstrable in the majority of cases. ■

OCCUPATIONAL INJURIES AND DISEASES

A total of 5.7 million nonfatal injuries and illnesses were reported in private industry work during 1999, resulting in a rate of 6.3 cases per 100 equivalent full-time workers. Overall incidence rates for injuries and illnesses show a decline in the last decade. Healthy People 2010 continues to maintain and work toward the goal of preventing injuries and illnesses by developing effective safety strategies. Injury rates are generally higher for mid-size establishments employing 50 to 249 workers than for smaller or larger establishments, although this does not hold within certain industry divisions.[11]

Risk factors for musculoskeletal occupational injury have been identified by OSHA. If workers are exposed to two or more of these factors (Box 3-2) during their shift, this signals increased risk requiring preventive intervention. Additionally, in April 2000, Congress adopted the Senior Citizens' Freedom to Work Act allowing retired seniors to continue working without losing their Social Security benefits. The growing silver collar work force (adults of the baby boom generation working past the age of 65) may represent a unique risk factor, since aging is associated with a progressive decrement in various components of physical work capacity, including aerobic power and capacity, muscular strength and endurance, flexibility and coordination, and the tolerance of thermal stress.[81] Aging may thus contribute to additional workplace injuries and accidents.

Other risk factors in the general population may include psychosocial stress, gender, and personality. For example, psychosocial stress increases the physical demands of lifting for people with certain personality traits, making those people more susceptible to spine-loading increases and suspected low-back disorder risk.[55]

◆ Ergonomics

Derived from the Greek terms *ergon*, meaning work, and *nomos*, meaning law, *ergonomics* is the study of work and of the relationship between humans and their working and physical environment (i.e., the science of fitting the job to the worker). Over the last two decades, ergonomics has become a branch of industrial engineering that seeks to maximize productivity by minimizing worker discomfort and fatigue. Ergonomics is an interdisciplinary field of study that integrates engineering, medicine, and physical and behavioral management sciences and addresses issues arising from the interaction of humans in an increasingly technologic society. As a field of study, ergonomics deals with job design, work performance, health and safety, stress, posture, body mechanics, biomechanics, anthropometry (measurement of body size, weight, and proportions in relation to the task requirements), manual material handling, equipment design, quality control, environment, workers' education and training, and employment testing.

Humans have limitations arising from factors such as gender differences; differences in size, weight, and body proportions; aging; physical fitness and lifestyle choices; diet; stress; and pain and injury. Our abilities (and limitations) combined with the necessary acquired skills, determine how well we perform our daily tasks. Ergonomics helps people recognize their abilities and limitations for safe and effective performance within the environment. Work environments are often de-

BOX 3-2

Risk Factors for Occupational Injury

Worker Characteristics

Age
Psychosocial stress
Gender
Personality
Physical fitness, including aerobic capacity, endurance, strength, flexibility, range of motion
Health status, including lifestyle and presence of pregnancy or disease(s) such as chronic fatigue, fibromyalgia, Raynaud's, diabetes, arthritis, coronary artery disease
Individual anatomy and physiology (e.g., body capacity versus job requirements, tissue resilience, functional reach)
Work experience and training

Occupational Risk Groups*

Manufacturing (e.g., assembly line work, meat packing, automobile plants)
Health care workers, especially in hospitals, nursing and personal care facilities
Lumber and building material retailing
Trucking (over the road) and ground courier (e.g., United Parcel Service, Federal Express)
Sawmills, planing mills, millwork
Construction
Computer operators (keyboarding)
Crude petroleum and natural gas extraction
Retail store clerks and cashiers, especially grocery stores
Musicians
Agriculture production
Beauty salons

Work Site Factors

Lighting, temperature, noise
Poor workstation ergonomics
Poor ergonomic practices; inadequate injury prevention training

Work Site Factors—cont'd

Vibration
Overtime, irregular shifts, length of workday; recovery time between shifts
Infrequent or no breaks during work shift
Continuing to work when injured or hurt (voluntarily or involuntarily)

Task-Specific Factors

Performance of the same motions or motion pattern every few seconds for more than 2 hours at a time (repetition)
Fixed or awkward work postures for more than a total of 2 hours (e.g., overhead work, twisted or bent back, bent wrist, kneeling, stooping, or squatting)
Use of vibrating or impact tools or equipment for more than a total of 2 hours
Unassisted manual lifting, lowering, or carrying of anything weighing more than 25 lbs more than once during the work shift
Piece rate or machine-paced work for more than 4 hours at a time
Using hands/arms instead of available tool(s)
Improper positioning or use of tools
Static or awkward postures
Contact stress (placing the body against a hard or sharp edge)

For the Health Care Worker*

Performing manual orthopedic techniques
Assisting clients during gait activities
Working with confused or agitated clients
Unanticipated sudden movements or falls by client
Treating a large number of clients in one day

*From Cromie JE, Robertson, VJ, Best MO: Work-related musculoskeletal disorders in physical therapists: prevalence, severity, risks, and responses, *Phys Therap* 80(4):336-351, 2000.

signed without adequate consideration for the people who will use them. Inadequate workplace design can contribute to stress, injury, pain, job-related impairments, and disabilities, and subsequently, lost productivity. If products are designed without considering the human factor, health and safety hazards can occur.

A substantial body of validated scientific research and other evidence (epidemiologic, biomechanical, pathophysiologic studies) support the positive outcomes of ergonomic programs.[65,66] The evidence strongly supports two basic conclusions: (1) a consistent relationship exists between musculoskeletal disorders and certain workplace factors, especially at higher exposure levels; and (2) specific ergonomic interventions can reduce these injuries and illnesses.

Ergonomic Certification.   Certification as an ergonomist practitioner is available through two national boards: Board of Certified Professional Ergonomists (BCPE) and the Oxford Research Institute (ORI). Previously, board certification in professional ergonomics accredited engineering ergonomists through a certification examination. Today, psychologists, therapists, and others have joined engineers in the pursuit of ergonomics as a career. A new branch of ergonomists, rehabilitation ergonomists, are health care professionals who in addition to functioning as an ergonomist practitioner, also use knowledge of the relationship between pathology and work to match the demands of the job to the capacity of the worker. Rehabilitation ergonomists work with people who do not fit the normal standards but require modification to safely and productively perform their job or task. Concentrating on improved safety focuses on physiologic improvement, which in turn increases productivity.

A wide range of private certification programs are available to the health care professional seeking training and certification as an ergonomist. The Occupational Injury Prevention and Rehabilitation Society (OIPRS) supports the accreditation of therapists through BCPE and ORI but recognizes other programs that meet the minimum criteria for certification as an ergonomist. These criteria and a listing of ergonomic certification options for therapists are available.[43]

◆ Occupational Injuries

The most common occupational injuries referred to as *musculoskeletal disorders (MSDs)* involve cumulative trauma disorders caused by prolonged static positioning while using force (e.g., exerting constant force with the thumb pressed in while holding a computer mouse or constant gripping of tools or handles) and forceful repetition of work (repetitive strain injury) while using incorrect muscle groups or posture (e.g., keyboarding, meat cutting, or repetitive lifting and turning). The use of the term *strain* may be a misnomer as the symptoms occur in response to static muscle overload or maintenance of constrained postures rather than repetitive or dynamic muscle load.

Back injuries account for 60% of all work-related cases, whereas upper extremity injuries account for a majority of the remaining percentage. Seventy percent of the repeated trauma cases are in manufacturing industries.[11] The shift in the United States economy to service industries such as nursing homes, in which staff members are required to perform heavy lifting, has contributed significantly to the number of back injuries.[51] Other commonly sustained workplace injuries include eye injuries, hearing impairment, fractures, amputations, and lacerations severe enough to require medical intervention.

Musculoskeletal Disorders. MSDs encompass both cumulative trauma disorders (CTDs) and repetitive strain injuries (RSI) and are more accepted terminology in the fields of ergonomics and occupational medicine, although the use of CTD and RSI is still often used in the literature. *Work-related musculoskeletal disorders (WMSDs)* are defined as injury or disorder of the muscles, tendons, ligaments, cartilage, or spinal discs as diagnosed by a health care professional, resulting in a positive physical finding sufficient to require medical intervention and/or days away from work or assignment (i.e., an "OSHA-recordable" injury). MSDs do not include injuries resulting from slips, trips, falls, or accidents. The disorder must be directly related to the employee's job and specifically connected to activities that form the core or a significant part of the job (e.g., a poultry processor might report tendinitis, but a back injury while changing the water bottle occasionally would not be covered).[70]

WMSDs account for more than a third of all occupational injuries that are serious enough to result in days away from work. Back injuries and carpal tunnel syndrome (CTS) are the most prevalent, most expensive, and most preventable MSDs. Each year more than 100,000 women experience work-related back injuries that cause them to miss work. It is estimated that 300,000 injuries and $9 billion in worker's compensation can be saved with improved industry safety and ergonomic practices.

CTS accounts for more days away from work than any other workplace injury. In addition to workers who spend hours at the computer, carpal tunnel syndrome has been reported in meat packers, assembly line workers, jackhammer operators, athletes, physical and occupational therapists, and homemakers. Women comprise 70% of the CTS cases and 62% tendinitis cases that are serious enough to warrant time off work.[69] This finding may be due to occupational, physical, and physiologic differences. For example, CTS is associated with pregnancy and rheumatoid arthritis, a condition that affects women more often than men. In both genders, CTS can be associated with other medical conditions such as thyroid problems, liver disease, multiple myeloma, and diabetes, as well as to other musculoskeletal disorders that may or may not be work-related (see Table 38-X). For all work-related CTS, poor worksite design, poor posture and body mechanics, and industrial equipment and computers that take out the automatic pauses of work must be evaluated as possible contributors. For in depth discussion of CTS, see Chapter 38.

Workers suffering from MSDs, especially upper extremity MSDs (UEMSDs), may experience decreased grip strength and range of motion, impaired muscle function, and inability to complete ADLs. Symptoms are persistent (although intermittent, they return and progress over time) and most commonly include pain (e.g., headache, neck, back, shoulder, wrist, hip, knee); burning sensation, numbness, and/or tingling (hands or feet); Raynaud's phenomenon; and myalgias and arthralgias with spasm, stiffness, swelling, or inflammation. Neural tissues at the cervical spine, carpal tunnel, cubital tunnel, or thoracic outlet can be compressed as a result of the swelling associated with the biomechanical microtrauma. The individual may perceive weakness and drop objects or have difficulty with handwriting. Common MSDs/UEMSDs are listed in Box 3-3.

A predictable sequence of events leads up to MSDs of a repetitive nature or those caused by static postures (e.g., some

---

BOX **3-3**

Common Work-Related Musculoskeletal Disorders

Carpal tunnel syndrome
Carpet layers' knee
Cubital tunnel syndrome
de Quervain's disease
Epicondylitis (medial or lateral tennis elbow)
Focal hand dystonia
Hand-arm vibration syndrome
Herniated spinal disc
Pronator syndrome
Radial tunnel syndrome
Raynaud's phenomenon
Rotator cuff syndrome
Sciatica
Tenosynovitis (finger flexors or extensors; trigger finger)
Tension neck syndrome, thoracic outlet syndrome, cervical radiculopathy
Ulnar nerve syndrome

tasks such as prolonged writing or typing at a keyboard require cocontraction of the agonists and antagonists). Fatigue and the inability to recover from fatigue brought on by additional hours and pressured deadlines, combined with emotional stress and improper posture, improper use of tools, or an ergonomically inadequate work station results in muscle soreness. Over time and without intervention or a change in the contributing factors, the body strains to keep up, and pain develops followed by injury or trauma. In the case of tendinitis or focal hand dystonia, it is possible that a sensory problem rather than just a motor problem occurs caused by a dysfunction in corticol sensory processing.[17] Evidence suggests that aggressive sensory discriminative training complemented by traditional exercises to facilitate musculoskeletal health can improve sensory processing and motor control.[16]

Special Implications for the Therapist   3-2

OCCUPATIONAL INJURIES

Preferred Practice Patterns

4B: Impaired Posture

4C: Impaired Muscle Performance

4E: Impaired Joint Mobility, Motor Function, Muscle Performance, and Range of Motion Associated With Localized Inflammation

4F: Impaired Joint Mobility, Motor Function, Muscle Performance, Range of Motion, or Reflex Integrity Secondary to Spinal Disorders (disk herniation, nerve root compression, synovitis, and tenosynovitis)

4G: Impaired Joint Mobility, Muscle Performance, and Range of Motion Associated With Fracture (Patterns 4I, 4J, and 4K may also apply depending on the outcome of the injury.)

5F: Impaired Peripheral Nerve Integrity and Muscle Performance Assoicated with Peripheral Nerve Injury

5H: Impaired Motor Function, Peripheral Nerve Integrity, and Sensory Integrity Associated With Nonprogressive Disorders of the Spinal Cord (nerve root compression due to lumbar radiculopathy; orthopedic or spinal instability)

Therapists often play a significant role in the prevention (e.g., work site analysis and workstation redesign) and rehabilitation of occupational injuries. When conducting a job analysis, the therapist evaluates job duties and environmental factors that put physical stress on the worker; stressors most typically include force (any weight that is lifted, pushed, or carried); repetition; and posture. The therapist will assess the amount of force needed to produce the necessary work, the number of repetitions, and the postural tolerances required by the job. These variables are evaluated for both newly developing programs or job tasks and in industrial rehabilitation programs for cases of work conditioning and work hardening, a fairly recent innovation in rehabilitation specifically geared toward reemployment for previously injured or impaired workers. Unlike conventional programs, work conditioning/hardening does not focus on such goals as symptom reduction or increased physical capacity.

Through graded work simulations conducted in a realistic industrial or office setting, injured people rebuild physical and psychologic fitness to work.[56]

Quantifying the requirements for each job is essential in both prevention and return to work situations. Therapists can provide analysis and management of injury-related job hazards, injury prevention training; examination/evaluation management of musculoskeletal disorders (MSDs); development of job/task alterations; and return-to-work program planning.[5] Specific ways to prevent work-related MSDs (WMSDs) are available.[70] Therapists also need to modify traditional intervention strategies for prevention and treatment of injuries in the silver collar work force previously mentioned. Although older workers may have lower injury rates than younger workers, their injuries are likely to be more severe and their recovery time longer. Therapists can assist industries and job sites to adapt job duties accommodating for age-related conditions such as reduced muscle strength and motion. Providing ergonomically correct work sites and work areas, implementing diagnostic and training programs to prevent specific conditions (e.g., carpal tunnel syndrome [CTS], tendinitis, back injuries), and instituting wellness programs to include home- or gym-based exercise programs and organized stretch/walk breaks will help keep all employees, particularly seniors, in good health and injury free.[7]

Finally, interventions employed by therapists can lead to WMSDs among themselves although little is known about this segment of the population. A summary of prevalence, severity, risks, and responses associated with MSDs in physical therapists suggests that therapists at greatest risk are more inexperienced therapists (more than 50% have their first episode as a student or in their first 5 years of practice); those in neurology and rehabilitation; and those performing manual orthopedic techniques. Researchers have demonstrated that knowledge of ergonomics, injury, and intervention strategies is not associated with a reduced risk of injury among therapists. Further research is needed to identify aspects of therapy practice that place the therapist at greatest risk and ways to reduce that risk.[22] ∎

◆ Occupational Burns

Of the more than one million fire fighters employed in the United States, 300,000 are career firefighters. The rate of injury and death occurring on the fireground or while responding to or returning from an incident has declined since the late 1980s with the mandatory use of gloves, self-contained breathing apparatus (SCBA), and full personal protective clothing. National trends for firefighter injuries are sprain/strain- and stress-related. Over 50 percent of all injuries involve overexertion, lifting, pulling, or carrying hose and equipment. Studies support the long-standing assertion that the number of firefighters responding to a fire is a factor that affects injuries.[96]

Aside from the acute injurious effects of fire, clinicians must be alert to the pathophysiologic changes associated with exposure to heat and smoke and to the chronic sequelae, both physical and psychologic (Table 3–2). In addition to the management of burns and trauma, it is necessary to evaluate clients for all acute systemic effects of exposure to smoke, heat, or toxic substances; recognize toxic effects that may be obscured by more serious traumatic effects; be alert for delayed consequences; and recognize acute and chronic exposure and

TABLE **3-2**

Types of Fire-and-Rescue–Related Acute and Chronic Injury

ACUTE	CHRONIC
Lacerations, contusions	Chronic cardiovascular
Falls (including on site and	disease
from moving apparatus)	Chronic respiratory disease
Burns (superficial, deep, internal)	Noise–induced hearing loss
Dermal reactions to toxicants	Posttraumatic stress disorder
Eye irritation, injuries, and burns	Physical disability
Smoke inhalation	Hepatitis C
• Sore throat, hoarseness, cough	
• Exacerbated asthma	
• Dyspnea, tachypnea, wheezing	
• Headaches	
• Cyanosis	
Cardiovascular strain	
Musculoskeletal trauma	
Heat stress and fatigue	
Neuropsychiatric effects	
Renal damage	
Death (motor vehicle accidents,	
falls, asphyxiation, burns)	

Modified from NIOSH Fire Fighter Fatality/Injury Investigation Reports (http://www.cdc.gov/niosh/firehome.html, 2001).

BOX **3-4**

Asthma-Triggering Substances in the Health Care Setting

Latex (primarily latex gloves)
Glutaraldehyde (sensitizing agent used in cold sterilization)
Ammonia and chlorine (cleaning and disinfecting solutions)
Dust and irritating particles in the air (construction and remodeling projects)
Mold and fungus (carpeting, ceiling tiles exposed to water)
Perfumes, scented personal care products worn by clients/patients, coworkers, visitors
Isocyanate (a class of extremely hazardous substances found in orthopedic casting materials)
Pharmaceutical drugs (e.g., psyllium, rifampin, penicillin, tetracycline)
Formaldehyde used in specimen preparation

From Bain EI: Perils in the air: Avoiding occupational asthma triggers in the workplace, *AJN* 100(6):88, 2000.

health effects due to toxic chemicals in smoke, especially among firefighters.

Carbon monoxide is always present at fires. Smoldering fires with incomplete combustion of burning material can lead to significant levels of carbon monoxide. For this reason firefighters are required to wear SCBA at every incident. Respiratory responses of firefighters while wearing SCBA will reduce their breathlessness during exercise (exertion on the job).[25]

◆ Occupational Pulmonary Diseases

Materials inhaled in the workplace can lead to all the major chronic lung diseases except those due to vascular disease. Exposure in office buildings and hospitals is now included as a known workplace-related cause of disease. Identifying this source of illness is important because it can lead to cure and prevention for others.[8] Disorders caused by chemical agents are classified as (1) pneumoconioses, (2) hypersensitivity pneumonitis, (3) obstructive airway disorders, (4) toxic lung injury, (5) lung cancer, and (6) pleural diseases. These conditions are discussed more fully in Chapter 14.

Asbestos and other silicates such as kaolin, mica, and vermiculite can cause *pneumoconiosis*. Asbestos-induced diseases cause lung inflammation and fibrosis as a result of activation of alveolar macrophages. Coal worker's pneumonoconiosis is another parenchymal lung disease caused by inhalation of coal dust. *Hypersensitivity pneumonitis* has many other names (e.g., extrinsic allergic alveolitis, farmer's lung, detergent worker's lung) and is characterized by a granulomatous in-

flammatory reaction in the pulmonary alveolar and interstitial spaces. Silicosis is a parenchymal *toxic lung disease* caused by inhalation of crystalline silica, a component of rock and sand. Workers at risk include miners, tunnellers, quarry workers, stonecutters, sandblasters, foundry workers, glass blowers, and ceramic workers.

Occupational asthma or work-related asthma (WRA) (*airway obstruction*) is asthma that is attributable to, or is made worse by, environmental exposures (e.g., inhaled gases, dusts, fumes, or vapors) in the workplace. The air in health care institutions may contain irritating and sensitizing chemicals and particles that can cause or aggravate asthma (Box 3-4). WRA has become the most prevalent occupational lung disease in developed countries, is more common than is generally recognized, and can be severe and disabling. The reactions can be immediate or delayed, sometimes hours after leaving the workplace. Identification of workplace exposures causing and/or aggravating the asthma and appropriate control or cessation of these exposures can often lead to reduction or even complete elimination of symptoms and disability.[33]

OSHA requires employers to provide a safe and healthy work environment free from recognized hazards. In addition, the Americans with Disabilities Act of 1990 requires employers to accommodate workers with asthma. Suspected episodes of WRA should be documented including symptoms, suspected exposures, visits to health services, and similar symptoms reported by other employees. Many effective and appropriate substitutions and controls are available that can be incorporated to eliminate or prevent airborne and topical exposures.[4]

◆ Occupational Cancer

It is estimated that 30% to 40% of the population in the industrialized world will develop malignant disease during their lifetime. Various studies have attributed cancer in humans to environmental causes (e.g., exposure to arsenic is associated with increased risk of skin, urinary bladder, and respiratory tract cancers; chronic exposure to ultraviolet light is associated with skin cancer; vinyl chloride is associated with liver cancer; dry cleaning solvents are associated with kidney and liver cancer and non-Hodgkin's lymphoma) but research is ongoing to assess combined genetic and environmental contributions to risk.[84,98]

Alteration or mutation in the genetic material (deoxyribonucleic acid [DNA]) may occur as a result of exposure to carcinogenic chemicals or radiation. Both experimental animal models of cancer and the study of human cancers with known causes have revealed the existence of a significant interval between first exposure to the responsible agent and the first manifestation of a tumor. This period is referred to as the *induction period*, latency period, or induction-latency period. For humans, the length of the induction-latency period varies from a minimum of 4 to 6 years for radiation-induced leukemias to 40 or more years for some cases of asbestos-induced mesotheliomas. For most tumors, the interval ranges from 12 to 25 years; such a long period may easily obscure the relationship between a remote exposure and a newly discovered tumor. In the future, individuals with a high environmental risk of developing cancer may benefit from immune stimulation as a means of cancer prevention by inducing specific immunity through the use of vaccines.[30] Individual cancers and their treatment are discussed in organ-specific chapters in this text; see also Chapter 8.

◆ Acute Radiation Syndrome

Acute radiation syndrome is caused by brief but heavy exposure of all or part of the body to ionizing radiation. The radiation disrupts chemical bonds, which causes molecular excitation and free radical formation. Highly reactive free radicals react with other essential molecules such as nucleic acids and enzymes, and this in turn disrupts cellular function. The clinical presentation and severity of illness depend on many factors including volume of tissue treated, the dosage (fractionation), and other independent variables. Tissues with the most rapid cellular turnover are the most radiosensitive and include reproductive, hematopoietic, and gastrointestinal tissues. See previous section on Physical Agents in this chapter; see also the section on Radiation Injuries in Chapter 4.

◆ Occupational Infections

Occupational infections are diseases caused by work-associated exposure to microbial agents, including bacteria, viruses, fungi, and protozoa. Occupational infections are distinguished by the fact that some aspect of the work involves contact with a biologically active organism. Occupational infection can occur after contact with infected people, as in the case of health care workers; infected animal or human tissue, secretions, or excretions, as in laboratory workers; asymptomatic or unknown contagious humans, as happens during business travel; or infected animals, as in agriculture (e.g., brucellosis). Tuberculosis, herpes simplex and herpes zoster (shingles), hepatitis, and acquired immunodeficiency syndrome (AIDS) are the most likely occupational infections encountered in a therapy practice.

◆ Occupational Skin Disorders

Accounting for 20% of all cases of occupational disease in the United States, 61,000 new cases of occupational skin disease are reported each year. It is likely that many cases of work-related skin disorders are underreported, since it is often not a life-threatening condition and never diagnosed or treated. The health care industry reports 4000 cases of skin illness each year, but the highest rates are in agriculture and manufacturing. Dermatoses are more prevalent in some states such as California and Florida; contact dermatitis from plants, especially in combination with sunlight, and chemicals such as pesticides or fertilizers is common among agricultural workers. Other agents in the workplace include irritating chemicals such as solvents, cutting oils, detergents, alkalis, and acids. Arsenic and tar products can increase the risk of cancer either alone or in combination with sunlight.

Contact dermatitis (acute, chronic, or allergic) is the most common of occupational skin disorders, but other types include contact urticaria; psoriasis; scleroderma; vitiligo (areas of depigmentation); chloracne (Fig. 3-1); actinic skin damage known as farmer's skin or sailor's skin; cutaneous malignancy; and cutaneous infections. Skin cancer is an important occupational illness and is most often the result of excessive exposure to ultraviolet light; farmers, fisherman, roofers, and road workers who continuously work in the sun are at greatest risk. For further discussion of specific skin disorders, see Chapter 9.

Latex Rubber Allergy.   During the past 10 years, the incidence of natural latex allergy (NLA or LA) has dramatically increased, possibly aided by the introduction of standard precautions and subsequent increased occupational exposure. It occurs predominantly in certain high-risk groups (Box 3-5); the estimated prevalence in health care workers varies widely (2.8% to 18%), and studies do not always distinguish between those who are positive in an assay for latex-specific IgE and those with clinical allergy.[74] The prevalence of LA in the general population ranges from 0.1% to 1.0%, compared with as

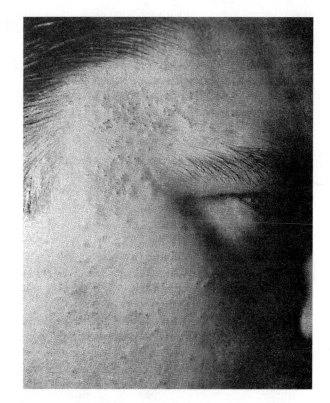

FIGURE   3-1 Chloracne. (From Raffle PAB, Adams PH: *Hunter's diseases of occupations*, ed 8, London, 1994, Edward Arnold.)

BOX 3-5

Risk Factors for Latex Allergy

Repeated or frequent exposure to latex products via one or more of the following:
- Repeat or frequent catheterization or other urologic procedure(s)
- Occupation
  Health care workers (dentist, nurses, surgeons, laboratory or operating room technicians, therapists, especially wound care specialists)
  Rubber or latex industry workers
  Doll manufacturing workers
  Occupation requiring gloves (hair stylist, food handler, gardener or greenhouse worker, housekeeper)
- Immunocompromised individuals
- Individuals with spina bifida or myelomeningocele
- Spinal cord injury (presence of indwelling urinary catheter)
- History of multiple surgeries
- Individuals (including children) receiving home mechanical ventilation
- (Personal or family history of eczema, asthma or atopy (allergies), including food allergies*

*Cross-reactivity occurs between latex and avocado, kiwi fruit, papayas, chestnuts, brazil nuts, tomatoes, and bananas, probably because latex proteins are structurally homologous with other plant proteins. Clinically, perioral itching and local urticaria occur; rarely food-induced anaphylactic shock occurs.

high as 60% for those with spina bifida or other chronic medical conditions associated with repeated exposure to latex.[64]

This occupational sensitivity to natural latex rubber (NLR) (i.e., latex proteins and in some cases, the associated cornstarch glove powder serves as a carrier for the allergenic proteins from the NRL) has resulted in the following three types of reactions:

1. Immediate hypersensitivity (Type I hypersensitivity; IgE-mediated) with urticaria (hives); watery eyes; rhinitis; respiratory distress; and asthma or skin rash, which can spread from the hands, up the arms, and to the face (it can also cause swelling of the lips, eyes, ears, and larynx (laryngeal edema can prevent the person from speaking).
2. Irritation or irritant contact dermatitis manifested as dry, crusty, hard bumps, sores, and horizontal cracks on the skin (Fig. 3-2)
3. Mild-to-severe allergic contact dermatitis (delayed Type IV hypersensitivity; cell-mediated)

The first two reactions are related to mechanical and chemical exposure, whereas LA is caused by sensitization to the proteins in natural rubber latex. These responses occur when items containing latex touch the skin, mucous membranes (eyes, mouth, nose, genitals, bladder, or rectum), or open areas. Once sensitized, some health care workers are at risk for severe systemic allergic reactions, which can be fatal in some cases.

The two major routes of exposure include dermal exposure and inhalation exposure. NRL protein absorption is enhanced when perspiration collects under latex clothing articles (e.g., elastic waistbands and leg bands in underwear). Just the elim-

ination of wearing latex gloves has not been successful in eliminating latex sensitization, since latex allergens are airborne. Exposure by the respiratory route occurs when the NRL protein becomes airborne, especially since glove powder becomes airborne, acting as a carrier for the NRL protein when gloves are donned or removed. Latex-induced rhinitis and occupational asthma are new forms of occupational illness secondary to airborne latex allergens in operating rooms, intensive care units, and dental suites. Anyone with latex allergies should be treated as the first case of the day, whether in the operating room or in a therapy department to avoid latex in the air and to avoid introducing any latex from clothes or materials from previous contacts.

Special Implications for the Therapist   3-3

LATEX RUBBER ALLERGY

Preferred Practice Patterns
7A: Primary Prevention/Risk Factor Reduction for Integumentary Disorders
7B: Impaired Integumentary Integrity Secondary to Superficial Skin Involvement
Possible patterns related to latex-induced asthma: 6B, 6C, 6F, 6G, 6H, 6I

All clients should be screened for known latex allergy (LA) or risk factors on admission. It is not enough to ask if someone is allergic to latex; risk factors and past medical history must be assessed. This is especially important, as anaphylaxis could be the first sign of LA.

Should anyone in the rehabilitation or therapy department develop symptoms in association with the use of latex gloves, emergency medical care may be required. The presence of hives, perioral itching, respiratory distress, watery eyes, and facial swelling may indicate a type I hypersensitivity and requires immediate medical attention. In a hospital setting, a physician can be paged immediately; other locations may require an emergency medical team (calling 9-1-1 or an emergency medical service). Check with the facility for incident report requirements. For the health care worker with a known sensitivity, a medical-alert bracelet should be worn, and the individual should have autoinjectable epinephrine (EpiPen) for use if another reaction occurs. Anyone experiencing the first reaction should not ignore the symptoms; further episodes must be avoided by developing a latex-safe environment and using nonlatex medical products.

All clients with myelomeningocele are to be treated as if latex allergic. The therapist, family members, and caregivers must avoid using toys, feeding utensils, pacifiers, nipples, or other items made of latex that the infant or child might put in the mouth. Parents must be advised to read all labels and avoid all items containing latex. If no indication of latex content is evident, the manufacturer should be contacted for verification before purchase or use of the item. More information on this topic is available at the Web site Exceptional Parent (http://www.eparent.com/toys/latex.htm) or Latex Allergy News ([860] 482-6869 or htttp://www.latexallergyhelp.com).

A latex-safe environment may be required for complete recovery for people with LA and is essential for all pediatric cases

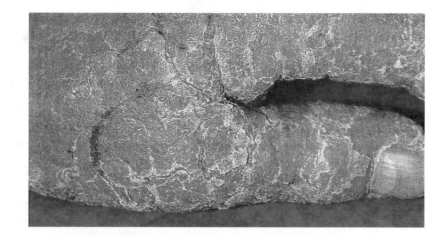

FIGURE   **3-2**   Rubber glove dermatitis. (From Raffle PAB, Adams PH: *Hunter's diseases of occupations*, ed 8, London, 1994, Edward Arnold.)

and anyone with known LA. A latex-safe environment, including the operating room, is described as one in which no latex gloves are used by any personnel, no direct client contact with latex devices (e.g., catheters, condoms, adhesives, tourniquets, and anesthetic equipment) occurs; and all medical and patient/client care items have been assessed for latex and labeled. Hand washing before donning and after removing gloves must be carried out at all times with special care given to using a pH-balanced soap and rinsing well to remove all residue. All medical products containing natural rubber latex that could come in contact with clients must be labeled. Keep in mind that many latex-free supplies have packaging that contains latex (glue), and those workers in the production or packaging of these products may have worn latex gloves. No latex balloons should be allowed in health care facilities; crash carts should be latex free. Personnel in the therapy department must be aware of the many items in the department that contain latex and replace these with latex-free products or a latex-free barrier (Table 3-3). Almost all equipment, supplies, and personal protective equipment is available in latex-free form, although not by all manufacturers. Complete guidelines for prevention and protection are available through the American Nurses Association at (800) 274-4ANA.

Several potential sources of powder-free, natural hypoallergenic latex gloves may be tolerated by latex-sensitive individuals, but no single replacement glove has been found for all people affected. Cotton liners or barrier creams can be effective interventions. Vinyl gloves are generally less protective than latex and more prone to tearing. Some of the new synthetic materials such as nitrile, neoprene, and thermoplastic elastomer offer equal or superior barrier protection and durability and are a reasonable alternative to latex or vinyl, offer better protection than latex types when handling lipid-soluble substances and chemicals, and are reasonably priced.[78] However, like latex, synthetic glove products can cause allergic reactions because they may contain chemical additives similar to those found in latex since both are manufactured using the same process called vulcanization. Additionally, synthetic gloves also provide a poorer fit than their latex counterpart and come with environmental concerns (e.g., the production and disposal of vinyl gloves releases toxic substances such as dioxins into the environment).

Glove specifications (e.g., leak defect rate; American Society for Testing and Materials [ASTM] specifications for length, width, tensile strength, thickness; powder particulate weight per glove, protein levels) are available and should be examined by each health care provider according to facility or client based use.[100] For more information, see NIOSH Alert: Preventing Allergic Reactions to Natural Rubber Latex in the Workplace (800-35-NIOSH) or OSHA: Technical Information Bulletin—Potential for Allergy to Natural Rubber Latex Gloves and Other Natural Rubber Products (http://www.osha-slc.gov/html/hotfoias/tib/TIB19990412.html) or call (202) 693-1999. ■

◆ Military-related Diseases

Seven diseases (asthma, laryngitis, chronic bronchitis, emphysema, and three eye ailments) have been identified by the Department of Veterans Affairs for compensation as a result of exposure to toxic chemicals during World War II. Survivors of the Vietnam War who have been exposed to a dioxin (TCDD) contained in the herbicide mixture Agent Orange (aerial-sprayed in Vietnam to defoliate jungles from 1962 to 1971) may be at risk for the development of soft tissue sarcoma; non-Hodgkin's lymphoma; Hodgkin's disease; respiratory and prostate cancers; diabetes and hyperinsulinemia; a skin-blistering disease; chloracne (see Fig. 3-1); and preterm birth, intrauterine growth retardation, infant death, and spina bifida among offspring. Considerable debate and long-term investigative studies continue to center around the potential effects of Agent Orange.[21,26,42,48] More recently, a group of symptoms presented by participants in the Gulf War have been identified. Amyotrophic lateral sclerosis (ALS), or Lou Gehrig's disease, has been identified among these military personnel. The U.S. government confirmed this link in December 2001. Anyone seeking more information about either Agent Orange or the Gulf War Syndrome can contact the Gulf War/Agent Orange Helpline at (800) PGW-VETS.

Gulf War Syndrome

Overview.   Regardless of whether an actual Gulf War syndrome (GWS) exists, it remains a hotly debated topic. According to the Centers for Disease Control and Prevention (CDC), Americans who served in the Persian Gulf War are significantly more likely than others to experience more than

| TABLE | 3-3 | | |

Potential Sources of Latex in a Therapy Department

ITEM	REPLACEMENT ITEM	ITEM	REPLACEMENT ITEM
Personal Protective Equipment		***Equipment/Supplies—cont'd***	
Gloves (sterile and nonsterile)	Nitrile, neoprene, or thermoplastic elastomer examination gloves		Theraband Latex Free
			Latex-free CANDO exercise band (SPRI)
Goggles			Use free weights that are not covered with materials containing latex
Hair covers			
Respirators			
Rubber aprons		Exercise mats	Cover with sheet or blanket
Shoe covers		Foam rubber lining splints, braces	Line with cloth, felt
Surgical masks		Mini trampoline	
		Positioning supports and pads of foam rubber without complete coverings	Cover with stockinette
Equipment/Supplies			
Bandages			
Casting material			
Crash cart			
Crutch and walker handgrips	Cover with stockinette	Reflex hammer	Cover with latex-free plastic bag
Crutch axillary pads	Cover with stockinette	Rubber bands	String, paper clips
Dressings		Shoe orthotics	
Elastic netting	Band Net Latex Free (Western Medical, Ltd.)	Stethoscope tubing	Cover with gauze or premade cover
	Stretch Net: Latex Safe (DeRoyal)	Sphygmomanometer	Cover cuff or extremity with gauze
	The Net Works (Wells Lamont Medical)		
Electrode pads, especially disposable TENS		Tape (all kinds)	Cover skin first with gauze; tape over gauze
Exercise balls	Cover ball with a towel	Toys; toys made from latex gloves	
Exercise bands	Use the following latex-free brand:	Vascular stockings	
	REP Band (Magister Corporation)	Wheelchair cushions	Cover with cloth
		Wheelchair tires	Propel with leather or cloth gloves

Courtesy of Harriett B. Loehne, P.T., C.W.S., 2001.

a dozen disorders known generically as GWS. The CDC does not term this phenomenon GWS but reports that people who went to the Persian Gulf are experiencing problems (referred to as *Persian Gulf illness* or *PGI*) that those who did not go are not experiencing. However, the Department of Defense does not support the existence of this illness, reporting only that the results of medical examinations of 10,000 veterans and family members affected revealed multiple illnesses with overlapping symptoms.[47]

Incidence and Clinical Manifestations. Of the 700,000 troops dispatched to the Persian Gulf between August 1990 and June 1991, as of January 2001, more than 100,000 veterans have filed with the federal registry reports of symptoms that include (in order of frequency) fatigue, skin rash, headache, muscle and joint pain, memory loss, shortness of breath, sleep disturbances, diarrhea and other gastrointestinal symptoms, and depression. CDC data show that the GWS affects 27% of veterans compared with 2% of nonveterans. Fatigue has been reported to affect 54% of Gulf War veterans compared with 16% of non–Gulf War veterans.

Etiologic Factors. No single cause has been identified, but possible factors include chemical or biologic weapons used on allied forces, insecticides, oil well fires in Kuwait, nerve agents from the demolition of Iraqi chemical weapons, parasites, pills protecting against nerve gas, and inoculations against petrochemical exposure administered by the military that had unexpected side effects or reacted with one another to create adverse symptoms. In 1993, the Birmingham, Ala. Veterans Administration Center was designated as a national pilot center to study the possible neurologic effects of exposure to environmental agents in the Persian Gulf. Other designated environmental hazards research centers are located in Boston; East Orange, N.J.; and Portland, Ore.

Pathogenesis. The pathogenesis for Gulf War Syndrome remains unknown but researchers are investigating the similarities between the underlying mechanisms of chronic fatigue syndrome, fibromyalgia, migraine headaches, and the Gulf War Syndrome. MRI studies of veterans with different Gulf War syndromes have biochemical evidence of neuronal damage in different distributions in the basal ganglia and brainstem supporting the theory of neurologic toxicity related to chemically induced injury to dopaminergic neurons in the basal ganglia.[40,41]

A new theory referred to as *toxicant-induced loss of tolerance (TILT)* has been suggested. Drug addition and multiple chemical intolerance (abdiction) appear to be polar opposites (addiction characterized by craving and dependency, abdiction characterized by aversion); however, when compared side-by-side, common underlying mechanisms are observed. Both addiction and chemical intolerance involve a fundamental breakdown in innate tolerance, resulting in an amplification of various biologic effects, particularly withdrawal symptoms. Although addicts seek further exposures to avoid unpleasant withdrawal symptoms, chemically intolerant individuals avoid exposure to reduce unpleasant symptoms. The question of whether addictive drugs and environmental pollutants initiate an identical pathogenic process with triggered symptoms and cravings remains under investigation.[58]

Medical Management.   No specific intervention beyond management and symptomatic measures exists for PGI. Focusing on triggering events rarely helps define treatment for people with syndromes like GWS. Understanding the entire spectrum of illnesses from chronic fatigue syndrome to fibromyalgia to GWS in light of treatment must be the means to developing multidisciplinary treatment programs for affected people that includes allopathic, naturopathic, and alternative treatment.

REFERENCES

1. Adir Y et al: Effects of exposure to low concentrations of carbon monoxide on exercise performance and myocardial perfusion in young healthy men, *Occup Environ Med* 56(8):535-535, 1999.
2. Alfred EN: Short-term effects of carbon monoxide exposure on the exercise performance of subjects with coronary artery disease, *N Engl J Med* 321:1426, 1989.
3. Altenkirch H: Multiple chemical sensitivity (MCS)—differential diagnosis in clinical neurotoxicology: a German perspective, *Neurotoxicology* 21(4):589-597, 2000.
4. Bain EI: Perils in the air: avoiding occupational asthma triggers in the workplace, *AJN* 100(6):88, 2000.
5. Bainbridge D: OSHA standards call for ergonomics in the workplace, *PT Magazine* 9(1):61, 2001.
6. Barwick RS et al: Surveillance for waterborne-disease outbreaks—United States, 1997-1998, *MMWR* 49(4):1-21, 2000.
7. Bassett J: Silver collar workers seek silver dollar paychecks, *ADVANCE Physical Therap PT Assist* 12(2):9-10, 2001.
8. Beckett WS: Occupational respiratory diseases, *NEJM* 342(6):406-413, 2000.
9. Bertam JS: The molecular biology of cancer, *Mol Aspects Med* 21(6):167-223, 2000.
10. Betts GA et al: Neck muscle vibration alters visually-perceived roll after unilateral vestibular loss, *Neuroreport* 11(12):2659-2662, 2000.
11. Bureau of Labor Statistics: Workplace injuries and illnesses in 1999, January 2001. Available at http://stats.bls.gov/oshhome.htm.
12. Boorman GA et al: Magnetic fields and mammary cancer in rodents: a critical review and evaluation of published literature, *Radiat Res* 153 (5 Pt 2):617-626, 2000.
13. Bosco C et al: Hormonal responses to whole-body vibration in men, *Europ J Appl Physiol* 81(6):449-454, 2000.
14. Brainard GC, Kavet R, Kheifets LI: The relationship between electromagnetic field and light exposures to melatonin and breast cancer risk: a review of the relevant literature, *J Pineal Res* 26(2):65-100, 1999.
15. Brutsaert TD et al: Higher arterial oxygen saturation during submaximal exercise in Bolivian aymara compared to Europeans born and raised at high altitude, *Am J Phys Anthropol* 113(2):169-181, 2000.
16. Byl NN, McKenzie A: Treatment effectiveness for patients with a history of repetitive hand use and focal hand dystonia: a planned, prospective follow-up study, *J Hand Ther* 13(4):289-301, 2000.
17. Byl NN et al: A primate model for studying focal dystonia and repetitive strain injury: effects on the primary somatosensory cortex, *Phys Ther* 77(3):269-284, 1997.
18. Caplan LS, Schoenfeld ER, O'Leary ES et al: Breast cancer and electromagnetic fields—a review, *Ann Epidemiol* 10(1):31-44, 2000.
19. Clark JI, Muchowski PJ: Small heat-shock proteins and their potential role in human disease, *Curr Opin Struct Biol* 10(1):52-59, 2000.
20. Consensus Statement: Multiple chemical sensitivity: a 1999 consensus, *Arch Environ Health* 54(3):147-149, 1999.
21. Cranmer M et al: Exposure to 2,3,7,8-tetracholorodibenzo-p-dioxin (TCDD) is associated with hyperinsulinemia and insulin resistance, *Toxicol Sci* 56(2):431-436, 2000.
22. Cromie JE, Robertson VJ, Best MO: Work-related musculoskeletal disorders in physical therapists: prevalence, severity, risks, and responses, *Phys Ther* 80(4):336-351, 2000.
23. Dalton R: From cell phones to brain cells, *Nature* 406(6796):552, 2000.
24. Degen GH, Bolt HM: Endocrine disruptors: update on xenoestrogens, *Int Arch Occup Environ Health* 73(7):433-441, 2000.
25. Donovan KJ, McConnell AK: Do fire-fighters develop specific ventilatory responses in order to cope with exercise whilst wearing self-contained breathing apparatus? *Eur J Appl Physiol Occup Physiol* 80(2):107-112, 1999.
26. Downey DC: Porphyria and chemicals, *Med Hypotheses* 53(2):166-171, 1999.
27. Eis D: Clinical ecology—an unproved approach in the context of environmental medicine, *Zentralbl Hyg Umweltmed* 202(2-4):291-330, 1999.
28. Environmental Protection Agency: Categories of released chemicals reported to the toxic release inventory, 1998.
29. Fan LK et al: Hsp72 induction: a potential molecular mediator of the delay phenomenon, *Ann Plast Surg* 44(1):65-71, 2000.
30. Forni G et al: Immunoprevention of cancer: is the time ripe? *Cancer Res* 60(10):2571-2575, 2000.
31. Foster WM et al: Bronchial reactivity of healthy subjects: 18-20 h post-exposure to ozone, *J Appl Physiol* 89(5):1804-1819, 2000.
32. Frazer L: The trickle-down theory of cleaner air, *Environ Health Perspect* 108(4):178-180, 2000.
33. Friedman-Jimenez G et al: Clinical evaluation, management, and prevention of work-related asthma, *Am J Ind Med* 37(1):121-141, 2000.
34. Gangi S, Johansson O: A theoretical model based upon mast cells and histamine to explain the recently proclaimed sensitivity to electric and/or magnetic fields in humans, *Med Hypotheses* 54(4):663-671, 2000.
35. Green H et al: Human skeletal muscle exercise metabolism following an expedition to Mount Denali, *Am J Physiol Regul Integr Comp Physiol* 279(5):R1872-1879, 2000.
36. Griefahn B, Brode P, Jaschinski W: Contrast thresholds and fixation disparity during 5-Hz sinusoidal single- and dual-axis (vertical and lateral) whole-body vibration, *Ergonomics* 43(3):317-332, 2000.
37. Gold DR et al: Ambient pollution and heart rate variability, *Circulation* 101(11):1267-1273, 2000.
38. Grigor'ev IG: Delayed biological effect of electromagnetic fields action, *Radiats Biol Radioecol* 40(2):217-225, 2000.
39. Gwynn RC, Burnett RT, Thurston GD: A time-series analysis of acidic particulate matter and daily mortality and morbidity in the Buffalo, New York region, *Environ Health Perspect* 108(2):125-133, 2000.
40. Haley RW et al: Effect of basal ganglia injury on central dopamine activity in Gulf War syndrome, *Arch Neurol* 57(9):1280-1285, 2000.
41. Haley RW et al: Brain abnormalities in Gulf War syndrome: evaluation with 1H MR spectroscopy, *Radiology* 215(3):807-817, 2000.
42. Hardell L, Eriksson M, Axelson O: Agent Orange in war medicine: an aftermath myth, *Int J Health Serv* 28(4):715-724, 1998.
43. Heller A: Becoming a board certified ergonomist, *ADVANCE Phys Therap PT Assist* November 27, 2000, pp 11-12, 26. Reprints available at (800) 355-5627 (ext 446).
44. Herbert R et al: Occupational coronary heart disease among bridge and tunnel officers, *Arch Environ Health* 55(3):152-163, 2000.

45. Hultgren HN: High-altitude medical problems. In Rubenstein E, Federman DD, editors: *Scientific American medicine,* New York, 1992, Scientific American.

46. Institute of Medicine: *Review of the health effects in Vietnam veterans of exposure to herbicides: third biennial update* (Proj No HPDP-H-99-05-A), Washington, DC, 2001, National Academy of Science. Available at http://www4.nas.edu.

47. Joseph S: *No unique illness afflicts Gulf veterans* (news release), Washington DC, August 2, 1995.

48. Kramarova E et al: Exposure to Agent Orange and occurrence of soft-tissue sarcomas or non-Hodgkin lymphomas: an ongoing study in Vietnam, *Environ Health Perspect* 106 Suppl 2(9):671-678, 1998.

49. Labarge XS, McCaffrey RJ: Multiple chemical sensitivity: a review of the theoretical and research literature, *Neuropsychol Rev* 10(4):183-211, 2000.

50. Larsen JC, Farland W, Winters D: Current risk assessment approaches in different countries. *Food Addit Contam* 17(4):359-369, 2000.

51. Lavelle M: Burdened by old age: the hazards of toiling in the service economy, *US News World Rep* 126(19):69, 1999.

52. Lee ME et al: Radon-smoking synergy: a population-based behavioral risk reduction approach, *Prev Med* 29(3):222-227, 1999.

53. Lewis PG: Occupational and environmental medicine: moving the factory fence or hedging our bets? *Occup Med* (London) 50(4):217-220, 2000.

54. Marcus M et al: Video display terminals and miscarriage, *J Am Med Womens Assoc* 55(2):84-88, 105, 2000.

55. Marras WS et al: The influence of psychosocial stress, gender, and personality on mechanical loading of the lumbar spine, *Spine* 25(23):3045-3054, 2000.

56. Matheson LN: Work hardening for patients with back pain, *J Musculoskel Med* 10:53-63, 1993.

57. Mester J, Spitzenfeil P, Schwarzer J: Biological reaction to vibration—implications for sport, *J Sci Med Sport* 2(3):211-226, 1999.

58. Miller CS: Toxicant-induced loss of tolerance, *Addiction* 96(1):115-137, 2001.

59. Miyazaki Y: Adverse effects of whole-body vibration on gastric motility, *Kurume Med* 47(1):79-86, 2000.

60. Morbidity Mortality Weekly Report: Blood and hair mercury levels in young children and women of childbearing age—United States, 1999, *MMWR* 50(08):140-143, 2001.

61. Morbidity Mortality Weekly Report): Radon testing in households with a residential smoker—United States, 1993-1994, *MMWR* 48(31):683-686, 1999.

62. Morgan BJ: The patient with coronary heart disease at altitude: observations during acute exposure to 3100 meters, *J Wilderness Med* 1:147, 1990.

63. Muscat JE et al: Handheld cellular telephone use and risk of brain cancer, *JAMA* 284(23):3001-3007, 2000.

64. Nakamura CT et al: Latex allergy in children on home mechanical ventilation, *Chest* 118(4):1000-1003, 2000.

65. National Academy of Sciences: *Work-related musculoskeletal disorders: the research base,* Washington, DC, 1998, The Academy.

66. National Institute of Occupational Safety and Health: *Ergonomics: effective workplace practices and programs,* Washington DC, 1997. Available at http://www.osha.gov.

67. Nriagu JO, Kim MJ: Emissions of lead and zinc from candles with metal-core wicks, *Sci Total Environ* 250(1-3):37-41, 2000.

68. O'Brien M: *Making better environmental decisions: an alternative to risk assessment,* Cambridge, Mass, 2000, MIT Press.

69. Occupational Safety and Health Administration: *One size doesn't fit all approach* (OSHA national news release), USDL 99-333, November 22, 1999. Available at http://www.osha.gov/media/oshnew.

70. Occupational Safety and Health Administration: *Preventing work-related musculoskeletal disorders,* Month 1999. Available at http://www.osha-slc.gov.

71. Piantadosi CA: Physical, chemical, and aspiration injuries of the lung. In Goldman L, Bennett JC, Cecil RL, editors: *Cecil textbook of medicine,* ed 21, Philadelphia, 2000, WB Saunders.

72. Pinksi SL, Trohman RG: Interference with cardiac pacing, *Cardiol Clin* 18(1):219-239, 2000.

73. Pope MH, Wilder DG, Magnusson ML: A review of studies on seated whole-body vibration and low-back pain, *Proc Inst Mech Eng* 213(6):435-446, 1999.

74. Pridgeon C et al: Assessment of latex allergy in a health care population: are the available tests valid? *Clin Exp Allergy* 30(10):1444-1449, 2000.

75. Proctor SP: Chemical sensitivity and gulf war veterans' illnesses, *Occup Med* 15(3):587-599, 2000.

76. Pyne DB et al: Training strategies to maintain immunocompetence in athletes, *Int J Sports Med* 21 Suppl 1(6):S51-S60, 2000.

77. Rittweger J, Beller G, Felsenberg D: Acute physiologic effects of exhaustive whole-body vibration exercise in man, *Clin Physiol* 20(2):134-142, 2000.

78. Russell-Fell RW: Avoiding problems: evidence-based selection of medical gloves, *Br J Nurs* 9(3):139-146, 2000.

79. Salvi S et al: Acute inflammatory responses in the airways and peripheral blood after short-term exposure to diesel exhaust in healthy human volunteers, *Am J Respir Crit Care Med* 159(3):702-709, 1999.

80. Schneider A et al: Peripheral arterial vascular function at altitude: sea-level natives versus Himalayan high-altitude natives, *J Hypertens* 19(2):213-222, 2001.

81. Shephard RJ: Age and physical work capacity, *Exp Aging Res* 25(4):331-343, 1999.

82. Sheps DS: Production of arrhythmias by elevated carboxyhemoglobin in patients with coronary artery disease, *Ann Intern Med* 113:343, 1990.

83. Sher L: The effects of natural and man-made electromagnetic fields on mood and behavior: the role of sleep disturbances, *Med Hypotheses* 54(4):630-633, 2000.

84. Shields PG, Harris CC: Cancer risk and low-penetrance susceptibility genes in gene-environment interactions, *J Clin Oncol* 18(11):2309-2315, 2000.

85. Simeonova PP, Luster MI: Mechanisms of arsenic carcinogenicity: genetic or epigenetic mechanisms? *J Environ Pathol Toxicol Oncol* 19(3):281-286, 2000.

86. Sliwinska-Kowalska M: Environmental exposure to electromagnetic fields and the risk of cancer, *Med Pr* 50(6):581-591, 1999.

87. Sobel HL, Lurie P, Wolfe SM: Lead exposure from candles, *JAMA* 284(2):180, 2000.

88. Spengler JD et al: Health effects of acid aerosols on North American children: air pollution exposures, *Environ Health Perspect* 104(5):492-499, 1996.

89. Staudenmayer H: Psychological treatment of psychogenic idiopathic environmental intolerance, *Occup Med* 15(3):627-646, 2000.

90. Story DA, Thistlewaite P, Bellomo R: The effect of PVC packaging on the acidity of 0.9% saline, *Anaesth Intensive Care* 28(3):287-292, 2000.

91. Thomas PK, King RH, Feng SF et al: Neurological manifestations in chronic mountain sickness: the burning feet-burning hands syndrome, *J Neurol Neurosurg Psychiatry* 69(4):447-452, 2000.

92. Tickner JA et al: Health risks posed by use of Di-2-ethylhexyl phthalate (DEHP) in PVC medical devices: a critical review, *Am J Ind Med* 39(1):100-111, 2001.

93. Tri JL et al: Cellular phone interferes with external cardiopulmonary monitoring devices, *Mayo Clin Proc* 76(1):11-15, 2001.

94. Trosko JE: Human health consequences of environmentally-modulated gene expression: potential roles of ELF-EMF induced epigenetic versus mutagenic mechanisms of disease, *Bioelectromagnetics* 21(5):402-406, 2000.

95. van der Heide S, van Aalderen WM, Kauffman HF: Clinical effects of air cleaners in homes of asthmatic children sensitized to pet allergens, *J Allergy Clin Immunol* 104(2 Pt 1):447-451, 1999.

96. Vatter MJ: The impact of staffing levels and fire severity on injuries, *Fire Engin* 152(8), August 1999. Available at http://www.fe.pennwell.net.com.

97. Weigl E et al: Heat shock proteins in immune reactions, *Folia Microbiol* 44(5):561-566, 1999.

98. Weinberg CR, Umbach DM: Choosing a retrospective design to assess joint genetic and environmental contributions to risk, *Am J Epidemiol* 152(3):197-203, 2000.

99. White B: Life, hazardous; cell phones, not so much, *Sci Am* 284(1):14, 2001.

100. Worthington K: Seeking the perfect fit: alternatives to latex gloves, *AJN* 100(8):88, 2000.

CHAPTER 4

PROBLEMS AFFECTING MULTIPLE SYSTEMS

CATHERINE C. GOODMAN AND TERESA E. KELLY SNYDER

OVERVIEW

Many conditions and diseases seen in the rehabilitation setting can affect multiple organs or systems (Box 4-1). With the kinds of multiple co-morbidities and multiple system impairments encountered in the health care arena, the therapist must go beyond a systems approach and use a biopsychosocial-spiritual approach to client management. Chronic diseases and multiple system impairment require such an approach because risk factors correlate with health outcome; early intervention and intervention results are correlated with improved outcome. Individual modifying (risk) factors (IMF) such as lifestyle variables and environment affect pathology and modify how a person responds to health, illness, and disease. For example, adverse drug reactions are correlated with increasing age and obesity, whereas fitness level has a profound impact on recovery from injury, anesthesia, and illness.

Additionally, a single injury, disease, or pathologic condition can predispose a person to associated secondary illnesses. For example, refer to the victim of a motor vehicle accident from Chapter 5 (see Special Implications for the Therapist: Cell Injury, 5-1) who suffers a traumatic brain injury and concomitant pelvic fracture and then develops pneumonia and pulmonary compromise, subsequently experiencing a myocardial infarction. This type of clinical scenario involving multiple cell injuries and comorbidities is not uncommon. Also consider the medically complex person who needs a splint. The therapist must first review laboratory values (see Chapter 39) to determine albumin levels (nutritional status) and platelet levels (potential for bleeding); perform a skin assessment (see Chapter 9); and consult with both nursing staff and the nutritionist before providing an external device that could create skin breakdown and add to an already complex case.

Although medical conditions encountered in the clinic or home health care setting are discussed individually in the appropriate chapter, the health care provider must understand the systemic and local effects of such disorders. This chapter provides a brief listing of the systemic effects of commonly encountered pathologic conditions and a basic presentation of acid-base and fluid and electrolyte imbalances. The scope of this test does not allow for an in-depth discussion of each condition or disease and its related multiple systemic effects.

The importance of using the *Guide to Physical Therapist Practice* (2001)[41] is recognized throughout this text. However, identifying preferred practice patterns in multisystem disorders depends on the presenting signs and symptoms and their influence on individual function and the rehabilitation process. For this reason, specific practice patterns are not listed with each section. The reader is referred to individual chapters discussing the underlying pathology or directly to *The Guide*.

SYSTEMIC EFFECTS OF PATHOLOGY

◆ Systemic Effects of Acute Inflammation

Acute inflammation can be described as the initial response of tissue to injury, particularly bacterial infections and necrosis, involving vascular and cellular responses. Local signs of inflammation (e.g., redness, warmth, swelling, pain, and loss of function) are commonly observed in the therapy setting. Local inflammation can lead to abscesses, when excessive suppuration (formation of pus); chronic inflammation; and the formation of adhesions occur. Systemic effects of acute inflammation include fever, tachycardia, and a hypermetabolic state. These effects produce characteristic changes in the blood, such as elevated serum protein levels (C-reactive protein, serum amyloid A, complement, and coagulation factors) and an elevated white blood count (leukocytosis).[42] For a complete discussion of inflammation and its effects, see Chapter 5.

◆ Systemic Effects of Chronic Inflammation

Chronic inflammation is the result of persistent injury, repeated episodes of acute inflammation, infection, cell-mediated immune responses, and foreign body reactions. The tissue response to injury is characterized by accumulation of lymphocytes, plasma cells, and macrophages (mononuclear inflammatory cells) and production of fibrous connective tissue (fibrosis).* The associated fibrosis causes progressive tissue damage and loss of function. Systemic effects of chronic inflammation may include low-grade fever, malaise, weight loss, anemia, fatigue, leukocytosis, and lymphocytosis (caused by viral infection).[17] Inflammatory activity can be detected by the erythrocyte sedimentation rate (ESR). In general, as the disease improves, the ESR decreases.

---

*Fibroblasts and small blood vessels, along with collagen fibers synthesized by fibroblasts, constitute fibrosis. Grossly, fibrotic tissue is light gray and has a dense, firm texture that causes contraction of the normal tissue.

BOX 4-1

Conditions That Affect Multiple Systems

Autoimmune disorders
Burns
Cancer
Cystic fibrosis
Congestive heart failure (CHF)
Connective tissue diseases:
- Rheumatoid arthritis
- Progressive systemic sclerosis (scleroderma)
- Polymyositis
- Sjögren's syndrome
- Systemic lupus erythematosus
- Polyarteritis nodosa

Endocrine disorders (e.g., diabetes, thyroid disorders)
Environmental and occupational diseases
Genetic diseases
Infections (e.g., tuberculosis, human immunodeficiency virus [HIV])
Malnutrition or other nutritional imbalance
Metabolic disorders
Multiple organ dysfunction syndrome (MODS)
Renal failure (chronic)
Sarcoidosis
Shock
Trauma
Vasculitis

◆ Systemic Factors Influencing Healing

In addition to local factors that affect healing (e.g., infection, blood supply, extent of necrosis, presence of foreign bodies, protection from further trauma or movement), a variety of systemic factors influence healing as well (see Box 5-4). Systemic factors may include general nutritional status, especially protein and vitamin C; psychological well-being; presence of cardiovascular disease, cancer, hematologic disorders (e.g., neutropenia), systemic infections, and diabetes mellitus; and whether the person is undergoing corticosteroid or immunosuppressive therapy.[52]

Healing in specific organs varies according to the underlying cause and site of the injury. For example, myocardial infarctions heal exclusively by scarring, and the heart is permanently weakened. A cerebrovascular accident (CVA), or stroke, may cause permanent disability, and healing occurs by the formation of nervous tissue (e.g., astrocytes, oligodendrocytes, and microglia) rather than by collagenous scar formation; this process is called *gliosis*.

In other organs, effective tissue regeneration depends primarily on the site of injury. Necrosis of only parenchymal (functional visceral) cells with retention of the existing stroma (framework or structural tissue) may permit regeneration and restoration of normal anatomy, whereas necrosis that involves the mesenchymal framework (connective tissue, including blood and blood vessels) usually results in scar formation (e.g., as in hepatic cirrhosis). For further discussion, see Chapter 5.

◆ Consequences of Immunodeficiency

Immunodeficiency diseases are caused by congenital (primary) or acquired (secondary) failure of one or more functions of the immune system, predisposing the affected individual to infections that a noncompromised immune system could easily resist. The therapist is more likely to encounter individuals with acquired (rather than congenital) immunodeficiency from nonspecific causes, such as those that occur with viral and other infections; malnutrition; alcoholism, aging; autoimmune diseases; diabetes mellitus; cancer, particularly myeloma, Hodgkin's lymphoma, and non-Hodgkin's lymphoma; chronic diseases; steroid therapy; cancer chemotherapy and radiation therapy.[36]

Predisposition to opportunistic infections, resulting in clinical manifestations of those infections, is the primary consequence of immunodeficiency. Selective B-cell deficiencies predispose an individual to bacterial infections. T-cell deficiencies predispose to viral and fungal infections. Combined deficiencies, including acquired immunodeficiency syndrome (AIDS), are particularly severe because they predispose to many kinds of viral, bacterial, and fungal infections.

◆ Systemic Effects of Neoplasm

Malignant tumors, by their destructive nature and uncontrolled cell proliferation and spread, produce many local and systemic effects. Locally, the rapid growth of the tumor encroaches on healthy tissue, causing destruction, necrosis, ulceration, compression, obstruction, and hemorrhage. Pain may or may not occur, depending on how close tumor cells, swelling, or hemorrhage occurs to the nerve cells. This process also occurs locally at metastatic sites. Pain may occur as a late symptom as a result of infiltration, compression, or destruction of nerve tissue. Secondary infections often occur as a result of the host's decreased immunity and can lead to death.[96]

The person with a malignant neoplasm often presents with systemic symptoms such as gradual or rapid weight loss, muscular weakness, anorexia, anemia, and coagulation disorders (granulocyte and platelet abnormalities). Continued spread of the cancer may lead to bone erosion or liver, gastrointestinal (GI), pulmonary, or vascular obstruction. Other vital organs may be affected; in the brain, increased intracranial pressure by tumor cells can cause partial paralysis and eventual coma. Hemorrhage caused by direct invasion or necrosis in any body part leads to further anemia or even death if the necrosis is severe.

Advanced cancers produce cachexia (wasting) as a result of tissue destruction and the body's nutrients being used by the malignant cells for further growth. Multiple mechanisms may be involved in this process, including release of cytokines such as tumor necrosis factor (also called *cachectin*). Paraneoplastic syndromes (see Chapter 8) are produced by hormonal mechanisms rather than by direct tumor invasion. For example, hypercalcemia can be caused in cases of lung cancer by the secretion of a peptide with parathyroid hormone, and polycythemia can be caused by the secretion of erythropoietin by renal cell carcinoma. Neuromuscular disorders such as Eaton-Lambert syndrome, polymyositis/dermatomyositis, and hypertrophic pulmonary osteoarthropathy are other examples of paraneoplastic syndromes that can occur as a systemic effect of neoplasm (see Tables 8-4 and 8-5).

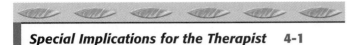

Special Implications for the Therapist   4-1

SYSTEMIC EFFECTS OF PATHOLOGY[20,21]

Medical advances, the aging of America, the increasing number of people with multisystem problems, and the expanding scope of the therapist's practice require that the therapist anticipate, assess, and manage the manifestations of disease and pathology. Physical and occupational therapists are primary health care professionals who focus on maximizing functional capacity and physical independence by optimizing healthy active lifestyles and community-based living.

Interventions to maximize oxygen transport (e.g., mobilization, positioning, breathing control, exercise) should be an important focus even in people who are acutely and critically ill. Enhancing oxygen transport centrally and peripherally minimizes the potential for more risky, invasive procedures. At the same time, many therapy interventions elicit an exercise stimulus that stresses an already compensated oxygen transport system. Exercise is now recognized as a prescriptive intervention in pathology that has indications, contraindications, and side effects. These factors necessitate careful and close monitoring of cardiopulmonary status, especially in the person with multisystem involvement.

Hematologic abnormalities require that the results of the client's blood analysis and clotting factors be monitored so that therapy intervention can be modified to minimize risks. Individualized treatment programs are developed for each person addressing the special needs of that client and the family, responding to physical, psychologic, emotional, and spiritual needs. The reader is encouraged to review an excellent article[20] for an additional in-depth discussion of specific implications for physical therapy management in systemic disease. ■

ADVERSE DRUG REACTIONS

Drugs were once developed through a hit or miss process whereby researchers would identify a compound and test it in cells and animals to determine its effect on disease. When a compound appeared to be successful, it was often tested in humans with little knowledge of how it worked or what side effects it might have.

Today, biochemists know much more about disease processes and work at the molecular level designing drugs to interact with specific molecules. Disease modifying anti-rheumatic drugs (DMARDs), selective estrogen receptor modulators (SERMs), and cyclooxygenase enzyme COX-2 inhibitors are examples of such "designer drugs." Drugs in the future will have greater molecular specificity possibly even with the ability to accommodate genetic differences in individual's metabolism. Despite these advances, adverse drug reactions still remain a significant problem in the health care industry today.

Definition and Overview.   *Adverse drug reactions (ADRs)* are defined as unwanted and potentially harmful effect(s) produced by medications or prescription drugs. The term usually excludes nontherapeutic overdosage such as accidental exposure or attempted suicide. *Side effects* are usually defined as

predictable pharmacologic effects that occur within therapeutic dose ranges and are undesirable in the given therapeutic situation. Overdosage toxicity is the predictable toxic effect that occurs with dosages in excess of the therapeutic range for a particular person.[35]

ADRs are classified as *mild* (no antidote, therapy, or prolongation of hospitalization necessary); *moderate* (change in drug therapy required), although not necessarily a cessation of therapy; may prolong hospitalization or require special treatment); *severe* (potentially life–threatening, requires discontinuation of the drug and specific treatment of the adverse reaction); and *lethal* (directly or indirectly leads to the death of the person).

Incidence.   Although it is recognized that ADRs are not uncommon, the exact incidence among ambulatory or outpatient clients remains undetermined. Specific studies have been conducted to determine the rate of ADR-related admissions to hospitals or the rate of ADRs associated with immunizations. Current statistics remain unclear regarding actual morbidity and mortality; various studies report anywhere from 14,000 to 200,000 ADR deaths occur annually in the United States.

Etiologic and Risk Factors.   Definite risk factors for experiencing a serious ADR can include age (over age 75, younger for some pharmaceuticals); gender; ethnicity (occurring most often in older adult white women); concomitant alcohol consumption; new drugs; number of drugs; dosages; concomitant use of herbal compounds[18]; duration of treatment; noncompliance (e.g., unintentional repeated dosage); small stature; and presence of underlying conditions (e.g., hepatic or renal insufficiency).[12,15,70]

Of all the risk factors, age has the most prevalent effect in the aging American population. A number of factors that affect the distribution of drugs are altered by age. A decrease in lean body mass and an increase in the proportion of body fat results in a decrease in body water. As a result, water-soluble drugs (e.g., morphine) have a lower volume of distribution that speeds up onset of action and raises peak concentration. High peak concentrations are associated with increased toxicity. On the other hand, lipid-soluble drugs are distributed more widely, have a delayed onset of action, and accumulate with repeated dosing. Aging adults are also at risk for drug accumulation because of changes in both metabolism and elimination.

With advanced age, functional liver tissue diminishes and hepatic blood flow decreases. Consequently, the capacity of the liver to break down and convert drugs and their metabolites declines. This may be exacerbated by other changes such as age-related reduction in renal mass and blood flow, the accompanying decline in glomerular filtration and tubular reabsorption rates, and other conditions such as dehydration, cancer, heart failure, and cirrhosis. Additionally, drugs commonly prescribed for older clients, such as the calcium-channel blockers verapamil and diltiazem and the anti-gout drug allopurinol further slow drug metabolism, potentially contributing to toxicity and adverse drug reactions. The drugs most commonly associated with ADRs in the aging are listed in Table 4-1. Halothane (anesthesia)–induced hepatic necrosis and anaphylactic reaction to penicillin are among the most common fatal reactions. The risk of fatal reaction is increased in older adults taking multiple drugs.

TABLE 4-1

Drugs That Most Commonly Cause Adverse Drug Reactions in the Aging

Digoxin	Sedative-hypnotics
Aminoglycoside antibiotic	Warfarin (Coumadin)
Anticoagulants (heparin and warfarin)	Antacids
Insulin overdose	Oral hypoglycemics
Steroid-induced GI bleeding	Digoxin
Aspirin	
Tranquilizers (phenothiazines)	

BOX 4-2

Common Signs and Symptoms of Adverse Drug Reactions in the Aging

Restlessness
Orthostatic hypotension (dizziness, decreased blood pressure, falls)
Depression
Confusion
Loss of memory
Constipation
Incontinence
Extrapyramidal syndromes (e.g., parkinsonism, tardive dyskinesia)

ADRs may be dose-related (predictable drug injury) or non–dose-related (unpredictable or idiosyncratic drug injury). Dose-related effects may include drug toxicity from overdose, variations in pharmaceutical preparations, preexisting liver disease, presence of co-morbidities such as renal or heart failure, or drug interactions. Non–dose-related effects may occur as a result of hypersensitivity, resulting in acute anaphylaxis or delayed hypersensitivity or other nonimmunologic idiosyncratic reactions, according to individual susceptibility. Cardiac or pulmonary toxicity may occur as a result of the irradiation and immunosuppressive drugs given to prepare recipients for organ transplantation or for any type of cancer. Some of the more common specific target organs and effects are listed in Table 4-2.

Clinical Manifestations.   Rashes, fever, and jaundice are common signs of drug overdosage toxicity. Older adults may develop ADRs that are clearly different from those seen in younger persons (Box 4-2).[73] Early symptoms of salicylate intoxication include tinnitus, deafness, disequilibrium, drowsiness, and a moderate delirium.[70] Digitalis toxicity is a life-threatening condition that may present with systemic or cardiac manifestations (see Table 11-4) (see the section on Chemotherapy in this chapter).

Medical Management.   Differentiating an ADR from underlying disease requires a thorough history, especially when a symptom appears 1 to 2 months after a medication regimen has been started. Monitoring blood cell counts and levels of liver en-

zymes; electrolytes; blood urea nitrogen (BUN); and creatinine is indicated for certain drugs. Digoxin and other cardiotropic drugs cause arrhythmias that require electrocardiogram (ECG) monitoring. With dose-related ADRs, dose modification is usually all that is required, whereas with non–dose-related ADRs, the drug therapy is usually stopped and reexposure avoided.

Special Implications for the Therapist   4-2

ADVERSE DRUG REACTIONS

Knowing when a person is having an ADR to medication or experiencing disease or illness symptoms is not always easily distinguished. Knowing about potential drug effects and using a drug guide to look up potential side effects is a good place to start. If the therapist suspects medication or drug-related signs or symptoms, several observations can be made and reported to the physician, such as correlation between the time medication is taken and length of time before signs and symptoms appear (or increase). Additionally, family members can be asked to observe whether the signs or symptoms increase after each dosage. Interpretation of drug-related or disease-induced signs and symptoms is beyond the scope of a therapist's practice, but the therapist can identify when these clinical manifestations are interfering with rehabilitation and make the necessary referral for evaluation.

Exercise and Drugs

Exercise can produce dramatic changes in the way drugs are absorbed, distributed, localized, transformed, and excreted in the body (pharmacokinetics). The magnitude of these changes is dependent on the characteristics of each drug (e.g., route of administration, chemical properties) and exercise-related factors (e.g., exercise intensity, mode, and duration). A single exercise session can cause sudden changes in pharmacokinetics that may have an immediate impact on people who exercise during therapy. Exercise training can also produce changes in pharmacokinetics, but these tend to occur over a longer period and cause a slower and fairly predictable change in a person's response to certain medications. A detailed description of the effects of exercise, physical agents, and manual techniques on drug bioavailability is available.[14,74]

For the most part, drugs administered locally by transdermal techniques or by subcutaneous or intramuscular injection are potentially absorbed more with increased systemic bioavailability in the presence of exercise, local heat, or massage of the administration site. In addition, allergic and potentially fatal anaphylactic drug reactions are mediated by exercise. The therapist should always consider the possibility that anyone in therapy taking drugs may have an altered response to those drugs as a result of interventions used in therapy.[80] ■

◆ Nonsteroidal Antiinflammatory Drugs

Nonsteroidal antiinflammatory drugs (NSAIDs) are a heterogeneous group of drugs that are useful in the symptomatic treatment of inflammation; some appear to be most useful as analgesics. NSAIDs are commonly used postoperatively for discomfort; for painful musculoskeletal conditions, especially among the older adult population; and in the treatment of inflammatory rheumatic diseases. These medications may con-

TABLE   4-2

Target Organs and Effects of Adverse Drug Reactions

Heart
Arrhythmia
Cardiomyopathy
  Adriamycin
Myocardial infarction
  Oral contraceptives
Orthostatic hypotension

Lung
Alveolitis and interstitial fibrosis
  Nitrofurantoin
  Busulfan
  Bleomycin
Asthma
  Aspirin
  Propranolol
Pneumonia
  Corticosteroids
  Immunosuppressants (See Table 4-6)

Gastrointestinal Tract
Gingival hyperplasia
  Phenytoin (Dilantin)
Gastritis and peptic ulcer
  Steroids
  Aspirin
  Other NSAIDs
Pseudomembranous colitis
  Broad-spectrum antibiotics

Liver
Fatty change
  Corticosteroids
  Tetracycline
  Aspirin (pediatrics: Reye's syndrome)
Cholestatic jaundice
  Phenothiazines
  Anabolic-androgenic steroids
Hepatitis
  Halothane
  Isoniazid
Massive necrosis
  Halothane
  Acetaminophen (overdose)

Liver—cont'd
Adenoma
  Oral contraceptives

Fetal Injury
Phocomelia
  Thalidomide
Vaginal carcinoma
  Diethylstilbestrol
Discoloration of teeth
  Tetracycline
Multiple congenital anomalies
  Antineoplastic agents
  Phenytoin
  Sodium warfarin

Kidneys
Acute interstitial nephritis
  Methicillin
  Other antibiotics
  Contrast dye for imaging studies
Acute tubular necrosis
  Gentamicin
  Amphotericin B
Chronic interstitial nephritis and
  papillary necrosis
Phenacetin
Acetaminophen
Aspirin, other NSAIDs

Endocrine System
Adrenocortical atrophy
  Corticosteroids

Skeletal System
Osteoporosis, avascular necrosis
  Coricosteroids

Nervous System
Central
  Intracranial hemorrhage
  Warfarin; heparin; Lovenox (enoxaparin)
  Cerebral infarction
  Oral contraceptives

Nervous System—cont'd
Central—cont'd
  Pseudodementia
  Benzodiazepines
  Narcotics

Peripheral
Neuropathy
  Vinblastine, vincristine (antineoplastic
  agents)

Blood and Bone Marrow
Anemias
  Penicillins
  Cephalosporins
  Methyldopa
  Antimalarial drugs
  Sulfonamides
  Nitrofurantoin
  Methotrexate
  Phenytoin
  Antineoplastic agents
Thrombocytopenia
  (See Table 13-6)
Deep vein thrombosis
  Tamoxifen
  Raloxifen
  Estrogen
  Megate

Skin
Urticaria
  Penicillins
  Contrast dye for imaging studies
Erythema nodosum
  Sulfonamides
  Oral contraceptives

Ears, Nose, Throat (ENT)
Deafness
  Aminoglycosides (Gentamicin)

Eyes
Asthma induced by β-blockers used for
  glaucoma

NSAIDs, Nonsteroidal antiinflammatory drugs.

sist of over-the-counter (OTC) preparations such as acetylsalicylic acid (ASA), or aspirin; other salicylates and ibuprofen (e.g., Advil, Motrin, Nuprin, Medipren, Rufen); or prescription drugs (Table 4-3).

The incidence of significant adverse reactions to NSAIDs is low. However, the widespread use of readily available OTC NSAIDs results in a substantial number of people being affected. Older adults are especially susceptible and more commonly use these medications. The more commonly occurring side effects of NSAIDs are stomach upset and stomach pain, possibly leading to ulceration. Most susceptible individuals are people age 65 years or older, especially those with a history of ulcer disease. Side effects are generally dose-related, but other risk factors include taking NSAIDs longer than 3 months, taking high-dose or multiple NSAIDs, and receiving corticosteroid therapy at the same time.[13]

NSAIDs are associated with a wide spectrum of potential clinical toxicities, which occur most often in the GI tract; central nervous system (CNS); hematopoietic system; kidneys; skin; and liver (Table 4-4). NSAIDs limit the capacity of the kidneys

TABLE	4-3

Nonsteroidal Antiinflammatory Drugs*

GENERIC NAME	BRAND NAME
Prescription	
celecoxib	Celebrex
diclofenac sodium	Voltaren
diflunisal	Dolobid
etodolac	Lodine
fenoprofen calcium	Nalfon
flurbiprofen	Ansaid
ibuprofen	Motrin (prescription strength)
indomethacin	Indocin
ketoprofen	Orudis, Oruvail
ketorolac tromethamine	Toradol (short-term use only)
meclofenamate sodium	Meclomen
mefenamic acid	Ponstel
nabumetone	Relafen
naproxen	Naprosyn, Anaprox, Anaprox DS, EC
oxaprozin	Daypro
phenylbutazone	Butazolidin
piroxicam	Feldene
rofecoxib	Vioxx
sulindac	Clinoril
tolmetin sodium	Tolectin
Over-the-Counter (OTC)	
aspirin	Anacin, Ascriptin†, Bayer†, Bufferin†, Ecotrin†, Excedrin†
ibuprofen	Advil, Motrin, Nuprin, Ibuprofen, various generic store brands
ketoprofen	Actron, Orudis KT
naproxen sodium	Aleve, various generic store brands

Modified from Goodman CC, Snyder TE: *Differential diagnosis in physical therapy*, ed 3, Philadelphia, 2000, WB Saunders.
*The listing of these drugs does not imply endorsement.
†These all have "extras" in them besides aspirin but are known as aspirin products.

to respond to ischemic stress, inhibit renal prostaglandin production, and decrease renal blood flow and clearance. These effects result in an accelerated tendency for damage in people with preexisting cardiorenal disease or dehydration, or in the aging kidney.[91] Slow-acting antirheumatic drugs such as gold and penicillamine are well known for renal toxic effects, which resolve once the drug has been discontinued.

NSAIDs are potent reversible platelet inhibitors. Aspirin is the most powerful agent, because its effects on platelets are irreversible; a single dose of aspirin impairs clot formation for 5 to 7 days, and two aspirin can double bleeding time. To varying degrees, all NSAIDs can cause sodium retention and edema in susceptible people.[48] NSAIDs may also attenuate (weaken or lessen) the antihypertensive effects of diuretics; beta-blockers; angiotensin-converting enzyme (ACE) inhibitors; and other antagonists.* This adverse influence on blood pressure is a matter of public health concern as

*Research has indicated that verapamil, a calcium-channel blocker, is unaffected by concomitant administration of ibuprofen or naproxen and may therefore offer some advantage in maintaining control of blood pressure in persons who regularly take NSAIDs.[77]

TABLE	4-4

Possible Systemic Effects of Nonsteroidal Inflammatory Drugs

SITE	SYMPTOM
Gastrointestinal	Indigestion, abdominal pain
	Gastroesophageal reflux
	Exacerbate peptic ulcers
	GI hemorrhage and perforation
	Nausea, vomiting, diarrhea, constipation
Hepatic	Cholecystic hepatitis
	Transaminase elevation
Renal	Dysuria
	Hematuria
	Cystitis
	Analgesic nephropathy:
	• Acute renal necrosis
	• Chronic interstitial nephritis
	• Fluid/electrolyte disorders
	• Nephrotic syndrome
Hematologic	Thrombocytopenia
	Neutropenia
	Hemolytic anemia
	Red cell aplasia
	Prolonged bleeding time
Cardiovascular	Blunt action of cardiovascular drugs (e.g., diuretics, ACE inhibitors, beta-blockers)
	Possible influence on blood pressure
	Increase fluid retention
	Isolated lower extremity edema
	Congestive heart failure (for those on diuretics with cardiovascular risk factors)
Musculoskeletal	Suppression of cartilage repair and synthesis
	Bone marrow failure (aplastic anemia)
Cutaneous	Skin reactions and rashes
	Pruritus
	Urticaria (hives), sweating
	Dry mucous membranes
Respiratory	Bronchospasm
	Pneumonitis, rhinitis
Central nervous system	Headache
	Dizziness, lightheadedness
	Insomnia
	Personality change
	Depression
	Aseptic meningitis
	Tinnitus
	Confusion (elderly treated with indomethacin, naproxen, ibuprofen), memory loss
Opthamologic	Blurred vision, decreased acuity
	Corneal deposits

ACE, Angiotensin-converting enzyme.

12 million adults in the United States are concurrently treated with NSAIDs and antihypertensive drugs.[91]

New (second generation) NSAIDs known as COX-2 inhibitors (Celebrex, Vioxx) have completed clinical trials. These NSAIDs are now being distributed for use in cases of people experiencing somatic pain from osteoarthritis and/or rheumatoid arthritis (RA). Like all NSAIDs, COX-2 inhibitors relieve pain by blocking the enzyme cyclooxygenase, which is required for the production of inflammatory prostaglandins (chemical mediators of pain) during acute tissue damage. COX-2 inhibitors bypass the mechanism that harms the stomach lining reportedly reducing the severe GI toxicity associated with older NSAIDs. COX-2 inhibitors are no more effective at relieving pain or inflammation than other NSAIDs, and complications can occur especially in anyone over age 60, those with other chronic diseases, smokers, people with a prior history of ulcers, and those using other NSAIDs or cortisone derivatives.

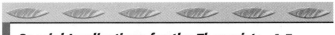

Special Implications for the Therapist   4-3

NONSTEROIDAL ANTIINFLAMMATORY DRUGS

The therapist is advised to observe for any side effects or adverse reactions to NSAIDs especially among older adults; those taking high doses of NSAIDs for long periods (e.g., for rheumatoid arthritis); those with peptic ulcers, renal or hepatic disease, congestive heart failure, or hypertension; and those treated with anticoagulants. NSAIDs have antiplatelet effects that can be synergistic with the anticoagulant effects of drugs such as warfarin (Coumadin). Easy bruising and bleeding under the skin may be early signs of hemorrhage.

Ulcer presentation without pain occurs more often in older adults and in those taking NSAIDs. Often, people who take prescription NSAIDs also take Advil or aspirin. Combining these medications or combining these medications with drinking alcohol increases the risk for development of peptic ulcer disease.[70] Any client with GI symptoms should report these to the physician. Musculoskeletal symptoms may recur after discontinuing NSAIDs, owing to the masking effects of antiinflammatory agents and the fact that they do not prevent tissue injury or affect the underlying disease process.[63,66] Once the drug is discontinued, painful musculoskeletal symptoms caused by underlying ulcer disease may return.

NSAIDs produce significant increases in blood pressure, averaging 5 mm Hg and should be avoided in people with borderline blood pressures or who are hypertensive.[57] All NSAIDs are renal vasoconstrictors with the potential of increasing blood pressure, resulting in increased fluid retention, especially lower-extremity edema, as the body conserves sodium and water. NSAIDs also reduce the antihypertensive effects of beta-blockers and angiotensin-converting enzyme (ACE) inhibitors and should generally be avoided in people receiving these cardiac medications. Interaction between most NSAIDs and loop and thiazide diuretics reduces the effects of the diuretic and may lead to a worsening of congestive heart failure in a person predisposed to this condition.[34]

It is important to check blood pressure the first few weeks of therapy and to periodically check thereafter to identify any adverse blood pressure response to the combination of NSAIDs, antihypertensive agents, and increased activity. In addition,

TABLE	4-5

Major Immunosuppressants

DRUGS	INDICATIONS FOR USE
Azathioprine (Imuran)	Renal transplantation (antirejection) Bone marrow transplantation Severe rheumatoid arthritis
Corticosteroids (see Box 4-3)	Various inflammatory conditions Cancer Bone marrow, tissue, and organ transplantation (antirejection) Autoimmune diseases
Cyclsporine (CSA or CYA; Neoral, Sandimmune)	Organ transplantation (antirejection)
Cyclohosphamide (Cytoxan, Neosar, Procytox)	Lymphoma, leukemia, other cancers (antineoplastic alkylating agent) Autoimmune diseases
Methotrexate	Cancer (antineoplastic): • Acute lymphocytic leukemia • Lymphosarcoma • Head, neck, breast, lung cancer Rheumatoid arthritis (antimetabolite for inflammatory condition)
Mycophenolate mofetil (Cellcept)	Renal transplantation (antirejection)
Rapamune (Sirolimus (SRL), rapamycin)	Renal transplantation (antirejection)
Tacrolimus (Prograf, FK-506)	Organ transplantation (antirejection)

NSAIDs may potentiate digoxin toxicity and potassium abnormalities in people who have renal disease and reduce renal clearance of digoxin and increase plasma concentration in anyone with reduced renal function. ■

◆ Immunosuppressants

Immunosuppressants work by decreasing bone marrow production of white blood cells (WBCs) or by selectively inhibiting components of the immune response. Most immunosuppressants (Table 4-5) are used for organ transplants to prevent rejection, with autoimmune diseases, or for neoplasms. Usually, intensive immunosuppression is required only during the first few weeks after organ transplantation or during rejection crises. Subsequently, the immune system accommodates to the graft and can be maintained with relatively small doses of immunosuppressive drugs with fewer adverse effects.

Immunosuppression may lead to CNS complications either directly (e.g., cyclosporine-induced CNS lesions) or indirectly (e.g., increased susceptibility to infectious agents, many of which, such as fungi and viruses, involve the CNS). Neurologic (and other) effects associated with immunosuppression are listed in Table 4-6. The severity of neurologic symptoms seems to be correlated to the serum level of cyclosporine and to the degree of nephrotoxicity (uremia and hypomagnesemia associated with renal failure affect both the central and peripheral nervous systems). The pathogenetic

---

TABLE 4-6

Potential Adverse Effects of Immunosuppression*

Central Nervous System	*Cancer—cont'd*
Confusion, altered mental status, psychosis	Lymphomas
Insomnia	Kaposi's sarcoma
Severe headache	Renal neoplasm
Cortical blindness, other visual disturbances	Hepatobiliary tumors
Quadriplegia (spasticity, paresis, ataxia)	Vulva/perineum tumors
Stroke	*Other*
Tremors	Leukopenia, invection (primary effect of immunosuppression)
Seizures	Reactivation of latent viruses (herpes simplex, varicella zoster, cytomegalovirus)
Coma	
Peripheral Nervous System	Thrombocytopenia (bruising, bleeding)
Neuropathy	Diabetes mellitus
Paresthesia	Hepatotoxicity
	Cardiomyopathy
Musculoskeletal	Hirsuitism
Decreased bone density, osteoporosis	Gingival hyperplasia
Myopathies	Renal failure (albuminemia, hematuria, proteinuria)
	Gastrointestinal (GI) distress
Cancer	Hypertension
Squamous cell carcinoma	Peripheral edema
Leukemia	Electrolyte imbalances

*See Table 4-8.

mechanism of cyclosporine toxicity is not yet understood. Current research suggests vasogenic edema as a possible underlying mechanism. This may explain the complete recovery of brain lesions (and symptoms) observed on magnetic resonance imaging (MRI) when the drug is withdrawn.[22] Temporary peripheral neuropathy and paresthesias may result in varying combinations and degrees of weakness in the intrinsic muscles of the hands and feet; wristdrop or footdrop may result.

Cyclophosphamide, methotrexate, and azathioprine may be used in the management of severe, active RA. The dosage used to treat RA is much lower than that used to treat cancer. Likewise, the side effects are fewer than those associated with doses to treat cancer. In cases of inflammatory conditions resistant to corticosteroids, immunosuppressive agents such as cyclophosphamide, chlorambucil, and azathioprine may be used.

The most serious adverse reactions to immunosuppressants are renal failure (e.g., albuminuria, hematuria, proteinuria) and hepatotoxicity. A substantial risk of secondary infection is possible, because all immunologic reactions are suppressed; overwhelming infection is the leading cause of death in transplant recipients.[5] An increase in certain kinds of malignancy occurs with long-term use of immunosuppressants, including squamous cell carcinoma, certain leukemias, and lymphoma. Other risks of immunosuppression include reactivation of latent herpesviruses (cytomegalovirus, herpes simplex virus, vari-

cella-zoster virus). The most common side effects are mouth sores (oral *Candida* infection and/or herpes simplex); gum hyperplasia; tremors; and headache.

Special Implications for the Therapist 4-4

IMMUNOSUPPRESSANTS

Careful handwashing is essential before contact with any client who is immunosuppressed. If the therapist has a known infectious or contagious condition, he or she should *not* work with the immunosuppressed client (see Table 7-6). Both client and therapist can wear a mask in the presence of an upper respiratory infection.

Peripheral neuropathies and subsequent functional impairment can be addressed by the therapist while the client waits for resolution of these side effects. Upper extremity splinting (e.g., cock-up splint for the hand) may be appropriate, or an ankle-foot orthosis to prevent falls and assist in continued and safe ambulation may be provided.[9] (See the section on Cancer and Exercise in Chapter 8.) ■

◆ Corticosteroids

Naturally occurring corticosteroids are hormones produced by the adrenal cortex; synthetic equivalents can be prescribed as medication. All hormones, whether produced by the adrenal cortex or produced elsewhere, are steroid-based with similar chemical structures but quite different physiologic effects. Generally, they are divided into *glucocorticoids* (cortisol, or hydrocortisone, cortisone, and corticosterone), which mainly affect carbohydrate and protein metabolism and the immune system; *mineralocorticoids* (aldosterone, desoxycorticosterone, corticosterone), which regulate electrolyte and water metabolism; and *androgens* (androsterone and testosterone), which cause masculinization. See Box 4-3 for a list of commonly prescribed synthetic corticosteroids. Mineralocorticoids are given for adrenal insufficiency or adrenogenital syndrome.

Glucocorticoids are used to decrease inflammation in a broad range of local or systemic conditions (Box 4-4), for immunosuppression (see previous section on Immunosuppressants), and as an essential replacement steroid for adrenal insufficiency. Some products may be given for allergy, adrenal insufficiency (e.g., Addison's disease), or cerebral edema. Therapists most often see people who have received prolonged, systemic corticosteroid therapy in the treatment of cancer; organ, tissue, and bone marrow transplants; collagen diseases (e.g., systemic lupus erythematosus, scleroderma); rheumatic diseases; and respiratory diseases (e.g., asthma).

Corticosteroids are also used to control several different types of pain, including chronic nonmalignant pain. Of particular use to people with cancer is the ability of corticosteroids to treat bone pain associated with metastasis, malignant epidural cord compression, superior vena cava syndrome, bowel obstruction, and cerebral edema (secondary to brain tumors). Corticosteroids are also indicated for painful lymphedema, pain caused by obstruction of a hollow viscus or by

BOX **4-3**

Commonly Prescribed Corticosteroids

Betamethasone (Celestone)
Cortisone (Cortistan)
Desoxycorticosterone (Topicort)
Dexamethasone (Decadron)
Fludrocortisone (Florinef acetate)
Hydrocortisone sodium succinate (Solu-Cortef)
Methylprednisolone (Medrol)
Paramethasone acetate (Haldrone)
Prednisolone (Delta-Cortef)
Prednisone (Deltasone)
Triamcinolone (Aristocort)

BOX **4-4**

Therapeutic Use of Corticosteroids

Adrenal insufficiency
Alcoholic hepatitis
Allergic disorders
Asthma (oral agents)
Autoimmune disorders:
• Rheumatic fever
• Systemic lupus erythematosus
Blood dyscrasia:
• Idiopathic thrombocytopenic purpura
• Acquired hemolytic anemia
Chronic obstructive disease (oral agents)
Chronic active hepatitis
Giant cell arteritis
Gout (unresponsive to other drugs)
Hypopituitarism
Immunosuppression
Inflammatory bowel disease:
• Regional enteritis (Crohn's disease)
• Ulcerative colitis
Myocarditis
Neoplastic diseases (e.g., myeloma or bone metastases, Hodgkin's disease, lymphoma, acute lymphoblastic leukemia)
Nephritis
Pericarditis
Pruritus
Psoriasis
Rheumatic diseases (e.g., rheumatoid arthritis, ankylosing spondylitis)
Sarcoidosis
Shock (e.g., acute adrenal insufficiency)
Systemic lupus erythematosus
Topical dermatologic therapy (skin disorders)
Transplantation (immunosuppression)

organ capsule distention, and neuropathic pain caused by compression of or infiltration of peripheral nerve structures.[72]

Anabolic-Androgenic Steroids

Anabolic-androgenic steroids (AASs), or anabolic steroids, synthetic derivatives of the hormone testosterone, are most commonly used in a nonmedical setting to develop secondary male characteristics (androgenic function) and to build muscle tissue (anabolic function). The use of anabolic steroids to enhance physical performance by athletes has been declared illegal by all national and international athletic committees. Even so, an estimated one million individuals in the United States alone are current or past nonmedical users of AASs. Administration of these compounds can be orally (25%); intramuscularly (50%); or by injection (25%).[75] One survey reports the average age at first-time use is 14 years with a significant number of children (15%) taking an AAS before the age of 10.[83]

Studies indicate that adolescent AAS users are significantly more likely to be males and to use other illicit drugs, alcohol, and tobacco. Student athletes are more likely than nonathletes to use an AAS, and football players, wrestlers, weightlifters, and body builders have a significantly higher prevalence rate than students not engaged in these activities.[4]

The use of this type of steroid is illegal and potentially unsafe, unless given under the direction of a licensed physician; most of these drugs cannot even be prescribed legally but are still obtained from other athletes, physicians, and coaches.[83] Athletes tend to take doses that are 10, 100, or even 1000 times larger than the doses prescribed for medical purposes. They cycle the drugs before competition, a technique known as *stacking*, alternately tapering the dosage upward and downward before a competitive event. Human growth hormone has been used alone and in combination with anabolic steroids to further enhance athletic performance. Human growth hormone is synergistic with anabolic steroids and is very difficult to detect using current drug screening methods.[79]

Misuse of supraphysiologic doses of AASs for nonmedical reasons has been linked with serious side effects such as hypertension, ischemic heart disease, acute myocardial infarction, hypertrophic cardiomyopathy, sudden and premature death, hepatic coma, and non-Hodgkin's lymphoma.[69,85] Homicides, suicides, poisonings, and other accidental deaths associated with AAS use have been attributed to impulsive, disinhibited behavior characterized by violent rages, mood swings, and/or uncontrolled drug intake.[87] Shared use of multidose vials, dividing drugs using syringes, and elevated sexual risk behavior associated with effects of AAS use on sex drive or due to a risk-taking personality trait among AAS users are potential routes for HIV and hepatitis infection.[61]

Medical uses for AASs (testosterone and growth hormones such as oxandrolone, a synthetically derived testosterone that promotes muscle mass and reverses catabolic processes) are being investigated as a result of the recent physiologic evidence that anabolic steroids may be used in the pharmacologic intervention against losses in lean body mass associated with age, disease, trauma, and burn injury.[82,95]

Growth factors are being looked toward as the next step forward in providing more efficient and effective nutritional support to catabolic or wasted individuals. If a direct link can be found between androgens, androgen receptors, and increases in skeletal muscle mass, anabolic hormone supplementation may also find a place in the treatment of chronic obstructive pulmonary disease (COPD); spinal cord injury (SCI); cachexia associated with advanced cancer and cancer treatment; human immunodeficiency virus (HIV); and chronic renal disease.[6,10,51]

Other researchers have demonstrated another important use of anabolic steroids in the treatment of acute and chronic wounds (including burns) by increasing appetite and promoting weight gain when combined with a high-protein diet.[24,25] Another current use of testosterone in women combines a small amount of testosterone with estrogen in postmenopausal women with a loss of libido. The use of testosterone in aging men to prevent loss in muscle mass and strength is also being investigated.

Adverse Effects of Corticosteroids*

Corticosteroids are far superior to NSAIDs as effective antiinflammatory agents, but long-term use to sustain the benefits of these drugs is accompanied by an increased risk of side effects and adrenal suppression.[93] Additionally, their long-term use as an antiinflammatory agent is not warranted, because steroids neither cure nor alter the natural course of disease. Long-term use of corticosteroids is necessary for adrenal insufficiency.

The most common adverse effects of corticosteroids include change in behavior (e.g., insomnia, euphoria); GI irritation; metabolic reactions (e.g., hypokalemia, hyperglycemia); and sodium and fluid retention with edema formation (Table 4-7); adverse reactions are dose-related. The most serious side effects of steroid use are the masking of inflammation, GI tract ulceration, and development of diabetes mellitus.

Severe adrenal insufficiency may follow sudden withdrawal of the medication. During or after steroid withdrawal, especially in the presence of infection or other types of stress, the person may experience vomiting, orthostatic hypotension, hypoglycemia, restlessness, anorexia, malaise, and fatigue. These symptoms should be reported to the physician. In the rehabilitation setting, it is important to know the effects of corticosteroids on skin and connective tissue; the musculoskeletal, GI, and cardiovascular systems; and the liver.

Effects on the skin and connective tissue include excessive hair growth (hirsutism); thinning of the subcutaneous tissue accompanied by splitting of elastic fibers with resultant red or purple striae (stretch marks); and ecchymoses (bruising). Glucocorticoids alter the response of connective tissue to injury by inhibiting collagen synthesis, which is why these agents are used to suppress manifestations of the collagen diseases. Clients who are taking steroids experience delayed wound healing with decreased wound strength, inhibited tissue contraction for wound closure, and impeded epithelization. Fortunately, vitamin A has been shown to reverse the healing impairments caused by steroids.[49]

Effects of hydrocortisone in physiologic quantities on the musculoskeletal system include smooth muscular contraction, but in large doses it causes muscle weakness and atrophy due to inhibi-

---

*Generally, glucocorticoids cause fluid imbalances, and mineralocorticoids cause electrolyte imbalances. However, mineral corticosteroids are used minimally (e.g., for adrenal insufficiency or adrenogenital syndrome). Most adverse effects seen by the clinical therapist will be related to glucocorticosteroids. Adverse effects of anabolic steroids primarily occur in an athletic or sports-training setting.

TABLE	4-7

Possible Adverse Effects of Prolonged Systemic Corticosteroids

SYSTEM	SYMPTOM
Metabolic	Increased glucose/protein metabolism
	Stimulates appetite, weight gain
	Electrolyte and fluid imbalance
	Fluid retention/edema
	Potassium loss (hypokalemia)
	Calcium loss (hypocalcemia)
	Corticosteroid withdrawal syndrome
	Growth retardation (children)
Endocrine	Diabetes
	Hirsutism (hair growth)
	Cushing's syndrome (hypercortisolism)
	See Figs. 10-5 through 10-7
Cardiovascular	Hyperlipidemia, accelerated atherosclerosis
	Increased blood pressure
Hematologic	Thrombocytopenia (bruising, bleeding)
	Immune system
Immune system	Increased risk of opportunistic infections
	Masking infection
Musculoskeletal	Increases muscle catabolism (degenerative myopathy, muscle wasting)
	Tendon rupture
	Other musculoskeletal injuries
	Osteoporosis
	Osteonecrosis, avascular necrosis of femoral head
	Bone fractures
Gastrointestinal	Peptic ulcer disease
Nervous system	*Central:* Change in behavior (insomnia, euphoria)
	Psychosis, depression
	Reversible dementia
	Benign intracranial hypertension
	Brain atrophy
	Autonomic: ANS dysfunction
	Peripheral Nervous System: Peripheral neuropathy
Ophthalmologic	Cataracts, glaucoma
Integument	Acne
	Striae (stretch marks)
	Alopecia (baldness or hair loss)
	Bruising, hematomas
	Skin atrophy, delayed wound healing

---

tion of protein synthesis. Specifically, because of the glucocorticoid receptor sites that exist in skeletal muscle, muscle is one of the target organs for corticosteroids. The resulting decreased oxidative metabolism, enhanced glucose synthesis, and inhibited protein synthesis leads to muscle wasting. The glucocorticoid action reduces the uptake of amino acids by skeletal muscle and inhibits amino acid incorporation into proteins. The overall effect is a negative nitrogen balance resulting in increased protein wasting, weight loss, muscle atrophy, and myopathy.[43]

TABLE	4-8

Functional Classifications of Corticosteroid-Induced Myopathy

LEVEL	FUNCTION
Advanced	Person has difficulty climbing stairs
High	Person cannot rise from a chair
Intermediate	Person cannot walk without assistance
Low	Person cannot elevate extremities or move in bed

Modified from Askari A, Vignos PJ, Moskoweitz RW: Steroid myopathy in connective tissue disease, *Am J Med* 61:485-492, 1976.

Corticosteroid-induced myopathies are characterized by loss of muscle substance and focal myositis. Histologically, atrophy of type IIb-muscle fibers occurs after prolonged treatment with higher doses of glucocorticoids, although atrophy is not confined to these fast fibers. Steroid-induced myopathy is also characterized by increased variation in diameter of fibers with increased amounts of connective tissue in between fibers.[23]

Steroid-induced myopathia may be acute or chronic. Recovery from acute corticosteroid-induced myopathy can occur with dose reduction; improvement in strength may occur within 2 to 3 weeks; complete resolution may take much longer. Chronic steroid myopathia primarily affects the proximal musculature of the lower and upper extremities, leading to proximal muscle weakness, although ventilatory muscle weakness (including the diaphragm) and quadriceps weakness have been documented to indicate the effect on other musculature.[23,32] Recovery from chronic myopathy (with cessation of drug) may take from 1 to 4 months up to 1 to 2 years, depending on the underlying diagnosis before treatment with corticosteroids (e.g., organ transplantation requiring lifetime administration of corticosteroids). Four functional classifications of muscle weakness can occur in people with corticosteroid-induced myopathy (Table 4-8).

Use of corticosteroids for longer than 6 months results in osteoporosis from altered resorption of calcium (hypocalcemia); inhibition of osteoblast collagen synthesis, elevation of parathormone levels that amplify osteoclastic bone resorption, and enhanced renal excretion of calcium. Users of anabolic steroids may experience an increased susceptibility to tendon strains and injuries, especially biceps and patellar tendons, because muscle size and strength increase at a rate far greater than tendon and connective tissue strength. Adolescent steroid use may lead to accelerated maturation and premature epiphyseal closure.[84] Long-term exposure to corticosteroids increases the risk of avascular necrosis, which often requires orthopedic intervention (e.g., total hip replacement).

Effects on the GI tract, liver, and cardiovascular system include peptic ulcer, especially in people with RA; decreased clotting function leading to subsequent bruising and hematomas, and hypertension, hypervolemia, edema, and congestive heart failure, respectively. Any person receiving corticosteroids should also consider taking a GI protective drug (e.g., Prilosec, a proton pump inhibitor).

Special Implications for the Therapist   4-5

CORTICOSTEROIDS

Inflammation and Infection

In the rehabilitation setting, large doses of steroids are administered early in the treatment of traumatic brain-injured (TBI) and in some spinal cord-injured (SCI) clients to control cerebral or spinal cord edema. Suppression of the inflammatory reaction in people who are given large doses of steroids may be so complete as to mask the clinical signs and symptoms of major diseases, perforation of a peptic ulcer, or spread of infection. In the orthopedic population, local symptoms of pain or discomfort are also masked, so the therapist must exercise caution during evaluation or treatment to avoid exacerbating the underlying inflammatory process.

Increased susceptibility to the infections associated with impaired cellular immunity and the decreased rate of recovery from infection associated with corticosteroid use requires careful infection control. Special care should be taken to avoid exposing immunosuppressed clients to infection, and everyone in contact with that person should follow strict handwashing policies (see Special Implications for the Therapist: Control of Transmission, in Chapter 7). Some facilities recommend that people with a WBC count of less than 1000 mm³ or a neutrophil count of less than 500 mm³ wear a protective mask (see Table 8-11). Therapists should ensure that anyone who is immunosuppressed is provided with equipment that has been disinfected according to standard precautions (see Appendix A).

Depending on the therapy intervention planned, the therapist may schedule the client according to the timing of the medication dosage. For example, with a chronic condition such as adhesive capsulitis, the goal may be to increase joint accessory motion, which requires more vigorous joint mobilization techniques. Masking local painful symptoms may help the client remain relaxed during mobilization procedures. When pain can be predicted (i.e., pain is brought on by treatment intervention), the drug's peak effect should be timed to coincide with the painful event. For nonopioids, such as corticosteroids (including NSAIDs), the peak effect occurs approximately 2 hours after oral administration. However, in a condition such as shoulder impingement syndrome, teaching the client proper positioning and functional movement to avoid painful impingement may require treatment without the maximal benefit of medication. The therapy session could be scheduled for a time just before the next scheduled dosage. If back pain occurs in a person who is receiving corticosteroids, diagnostic measures should be undertaken to rule out osteoporosis or compression fracture.

Intensive Care Setting

It is generally well accepted that prolonged treatment (8 to 14 days) with glucocorticoids (animal studies) at either moderate or high doses results in a reduction of both diaphragm muscle mass and force production. The results of at least one study[32] indicate that short-term, high doses of glucocorticoids result in a decrease in body and diaphragm mass and a decrease in diaphragm force production. These findings support clinical observations of individuals in intensive care units who experience difficulty weaning from the ventilator or inability to clear lung secretions. Applying current knowledge of the benefits of exercise in recovery from

Continued

myopathic and contractile changes due to glucocorticoid use can guide the therapist in providing this population with effective therapeutic interventions toward improved outcomes.

Intraarticular Injections

Occasionally, intraarticular injections of corticosteroids are necessary to control acute inflammation in a joint that is otherwise uncontrollable. Such injections can provide prolonged relief and improve the client's mobility and function. The rationale for use in the joint is to suppress the synovitis, because no evidence currently indicates that intraarticular injections retard the progression of erosive disease. Intraarticular injections must be carefully selected, and no single joint should have more than three or four injections before other procedures are pursued.[66]

Most steroid injections are accompanied by an anesthetizing agent such as lidocaine or bupivacaine, which usually provides immediate pain relief, although the antiinflammatory may require 2 to 3 days to take effect. During this time, the client should be advised to continue using proper supportive positioning and avoid movements that would otherwise aggravate the previous symptoms. Some controversy remains as to whether the person can bear weight on the joint for several days after the injection; a less conservative approach permits nonstrenuous activity. Vigorous exercise may speed resorption of the steroid from the joint and reduce the intended effect. Intraarticular injection of corticosteroid may also result in pigment changes that are most noticeable among dark-skinned people.

Exercise and Steroids

The harmful side effects of glucocorticoid steroids can be delayed or reduced in their severity by physical activity; regular exercise (aerobic or fitness); strength training; and proper nutrition. Unfortunately, these clients are often too sick to engage in exercise at all, much less at a level of intensity that would reverse myopathy. Whenever possible, the therapist can help emphasize the importance of exercise, especially activities that produce significant stress on the weight-bearing joints (e.g., walking; jogging is not usually recommended), to decrease the calcium loss from long bones that is attributable to prolonged steroid use. It is essential to consult with the client's oncologist before initiating aerobic exercise, especially in clients who have received high-dose chemotherapy or radiation to the thoracic region, as cardiac and pulmonary toxicity can occur. (See the sections on Radiation Injuries and Chemotherapy in this chapter.)

Glucocorticoid-induced changes in body composition in heart transplant recipients occur early after transplantation. However, 6 months of specific exercise training restores fat-free mass to levels greater than before transplantation and dramatically increases skeletal muscle strength. Resistance exercise, as a part of a strategy to prevent steroid-induced myopathy should be initiated early after transplantation[8] (see Chapter 20).

Strength training or stair exercise is one way to maintain the large muscle groups of the legs, which are most affected by the muscle-wasting properties of corticosteroids. The treatment plan should also include closed-chained exercises to prevent shearing forces across joint lines and to allow for normal joint loading, prevention of vertebral compression fractures, and education about proper body mechanics during functional activities.[43,86]

Client education about the importance of proper footwear and choice of exercise surfaces is important for the individual receiving long-term corticosteroid therapy. For the person at risk of avascular necrosis of the femoral head, exercising the surrounding joint musculature in a non–weight-bearing position may be required.

Monitoring Vital Signs

Long-term use of corticosteroids may result in electrolyte imbalances (e.g., hypokalemia, metabolic alkalosis, sodium and fluid retention, edema, hypertension), which necessitates monitoring of vital signs during aerobic activity because of the demand placed on the cardiovascular system in conjunction with these adverse effects. (See the section on Guidelines for Activity and Exercise in Appendix B.)

Laboratory Values

The therapist can monitor protein wasting (whether caused by prolonged corticosteroid-use or other factors such as malnutrition or exercise levels that are beyond the client's physiologic capabilities) by checking certain laboratory values. An elevation in the percentage of blood creatinine (see Table 39-11), accompanied by changes in muscle enzymes (e.g., creatine kinase [CK-MM]), may be present if protein wasting is severe. A decrease in serum albumin and serum total protein (see Table 39-15) may also occur.

Steroids, Nutrition, and Stress

People taking steroids may be advised to increase their dietary intake of potassium to counteract the loss of potassium in the urine, or to take antacids so as to decrease gastric irritation.[45] Protein intake is recommended for muscle growth to offset steroid-induced catabolism. Corticosteroids stimulate gluconeogenesis and interfere with the action of insulin in peripheral cells, which may result in diabetes mellitus or may aggravate existing conditions in diabetes. Regular blood glucose monitoring is recommended to detect steroid-induced diabetes mellitus. Some facilities establish exercise protocols based on blood glucose levels. Exercise is not recommended for people with blood glucose levels greater than 300 mg/dL without ketosis or greater than 250 mg/dL with ketosis.[2]

Clients taking replacement glucocorticoids (e.g., for Addison's disease) may need to increase the required dosage during stressful situations (e.g., emotional stress, dental extractions, minor surgery, upper respiratory infections). Temporary mineralocorticoid dosage increases may also be indicated if the client receiving replacement mineralocorticoid experiences profuse diaphoresis for any reason (strenuous physical exertion, heat spells, fever).[38] Either of these situations requires physician evaluation.

Psychologic Considerations

Corticosteroid use can result in a range of mood changes from irritability, euphoria, and nervousness to more serious depression and psychosis. Insomnia is often also a reported problem during corticosteroid therapy. The intensity of changes in mood may depend on the dosage administered, the sensitivity of the individual, and the underlying personality. When intense changes are observed, the physician should be notified so that an adjustment in dosage can be made.

Chronic corticosteroid use may alter a person's body image because of changes in adipose tissue distribution, thinning of skin, and development of stretch marks. The classic characteristics of a cushingoid appearance may develop, including a moon-shaped face; enlargement of the supraclavicular and cervicodorsal fat pads (buffalo hump); and truncal obesity (see Figs. 10-5 to 10-7). Some people may be extremely self-conscious about these cosmetic changes, and others may be emotionally devastated by them; caution is required in discussing assessment findings with the client. These cosmetic changes do reverse when the drug is discontinued slowly.

The therapist needs to be aware of the affected individual's coping abilities. Treatment intervention can include educating the individual about traditional stress-management techniques. Therapists can facilitate psychosocial support by contacting social work and clinical nurse specialists to integrate programs such as survivorship support groups and image consultants.

Anabolic Steroids

Therapists working with athletes, especially adolescent athletes, may observe signs and symptoms of (nonmedical, illegal) anabolic steroid use, including rapid weight gain (10 to 15 lb in 3 weeks); elevated blood pressure and associated edema; acne on the face, upper back, and chest; alterations in body composition, with marked muscular hypertrophy; and disproportionate development of the upper torso along with stretch marks around the back and chest. After prolonged anabolic steroid use, jaundice may develop.

Other signs of steroid use include needle marks in the large muscle groups, development of male pattern baldness; gynecomastia (breast enlargement); and frequent hematoma or bruising. Abscesses from injection use may also develop. Among females, secondary male characteristics may develop, such as a deeper voice, breast atrophy, and abnormal facial and body hair. Irreversible sterility can occur (females being affected more than males), and menstrual irregularities may develop in women.

Changes in personality may occur; the athlete may become more aggressive or experience mood swings and psychologic delusions (e.g., believe he or she is indestructible). "Roid rages," characterized by sudden outbursts of uncontrolled emotion, may be observed. The therapist who suspects an athlete may be using anabolic steroids should report findings to the physician. The therapist may consider approaching that person to discuss the situation. Testing for elevated blood pressure may provide an opportunity for evaluation of anabolic steroid use. Information as to the long-term adverse effects of anabolic steroids should be provided as part of the education process for all athletes. The therapist or trainer can provide healthy and safe strength training, stressing the importance of nutrition and proper weight-training techniques. ■

◆ Radiation Injuries

Definition and Overview.   Radiation therapy, or radiotherapy, is the treatment of disease (usually cancer) by delivery of radiation to a particular area of the body. Radiation therapy is one of the major treatment modalities for cancer used in approximately 60% of all cases of cancer (see Chapter 8). Radiotherapy is used in the local control phase of treatment but has both direct and indirect toxicities associated with its use. Radiation reactions and injuries are the harmful effects (acute, delayed, or chronic) to body tissues of exposure to ionizing radiation.

Etiologic and Risk Factors.   Localized radiation therapy for acne (no longer considered appropriate management); enlarged thymus; or tumors (e.g., skin cancer or leukemia) accounts for most instances of radiation injury. Whole-body irradiation occurs with nuclear reactor accidents or nuclear explosions; it is also administered before bone marrow transplantation. Other risk factors include environmental exposure (e.g., to radon, which causes lung cancer; ultraviolet sunlight which causes skin cancer); atomic bomb survivors were found to have breast cancer, leukemia, and thyroid cancer; and radium dial painters were found to have breast and oral cancer.

Pathogenesis.   Radiation therapy uses high-energy ionizing radiation to kill cancer cells. Ionizing radiation interacts with nuclear deoxyribonucleic acid (DNA) directly or indirectly to stop cellular reproductive capacity. The radiation causes the breakage of one or both strands of the DNA molecule inside the cells, thereby preventing their ability to grow and divide. Although cells in all phases of the cell cycle can be damaged by radiation, normal cells are usually better able to repair the DNA damage, but irradiation can cause injury of susceptible normal cells. Ionizing radiation causes radiolysis of water and the production of hydroxyl radicals (OH). These radicals will lead to membrane damage and breakdown of structural and enzymatic proteins resulting in cell death. Often arterioles supplying oxygenated blood are damaged, resulting in inadequate nutritional supply leading to ischemia and death of the irradiated tissues. Irradiation also causes damage to nucleic acids and may result in gene mutations, possibly leading to neoplasia years later (see the section on Mechanisms of Cell Injury in Chapter 5).

Clinical Manifestations.   Immediate and delayed effects of radiation (the latter caused by excessive doses) listed in Table 4-9 vary with radiation site, dose, fraction, and time (see Table 8-8). Radiotherapy and chemotherapy most severely affect rapidly reproducing tissue (e.g., GI mucosa, mucous membranes, bone marrow stem cells). In general, most side effects will not begin before a week to 10 days after the first treatment. The severity of side effects depends on many factors including volume of tissue treated; total dose; daily dose (fractionation) of therapy; method of treatment; and certain individual factors (e.g., age, baseline pulmonary function before therapy, concomitant administration of chemotherapeutic agents).

Side effects vary from individual to individual, but typically continue throughout the course of treatment and for several weeks after the last treatment. Chronic changes can occur over a longer period of 6 to 18 months and delayed effects may not occur for several decades. When the radiation administered is a large fraction or a large total dose or when the radiation field includes sites of active bone marrow (e.g., sternum, iliac crests, long bones), hematopoiesis is altered, and bone marrow suppression can occur. This can lead to infection, bleeding, and anemia.

The fetus is very sensitive to radiation. Pregnant women or those who suspect they may be pregnant must avoid all possible exposure to sources of radiation. Congenital anomalies after intrauterine exposure, especially if it occurs during early pregnancy or 2 to 12 weeks postconception during organ development, may include microcephaly, growth and mental retardation, hydrocephalus, spina bifida, blindness, cleft palate, and club foot. Later development of cancer, especially leukemia and thyroid cancer are most often reported when the fetus is exposed to a source of radiation.[90]

TABLE 4-9

Immediate and Delayed Effects of Ionizing Radiation*

IMMEDIATE	DELAYED (CHRONIC) EFFECT
Anorexia, nausea, vomiting, diarrhea	Skin scarring, delayed wound healing
Urinary dysfunction	Telangiectasis (vascular lesion)
Skin toxic effects	Cataract
Erythema	Myelopathy (spinal cord dysfunction)
Edema	Cerebral injury
Dryness, itching	Obliterative endarteritis
Epilation or hair	Pericarditis
loss at roots	Endocrine dysfunction (cranial radiation)
Destruction of	Fibrosis
fingernails	Hepatitis
Epidermolysis	Intestinal stenosis
(loose skin)	Nephritis
Xerostomia	Malignancy
(dry mouth)	Skin cancer (squamous cell)
Stomatitis	Leukemia
(inflammation of	Thyroid
mouth mucosa)	Amenorrhea, menopause
	Decreased fertility (both sexes)
	Decreased libido (females only)
	Radiation plexopathy (brachial, lumbosacral, or pelvic plexus)
	Lymphedema
	Bone marrow suppression (anemia, infection, bleeding)

*The health care professional must remember that some of the delayed effects of radiation, such as cerebral injury, pericarditis, pulmonary fibrosis, hepatitis, intestinal stenosis, other GI disturbances, and nephritis, may be signs of recurring cancer. The physician should be notified by the affected individual of any new symptoms, change in symptoms, or increase in symptoms.

Radiation Syndromes

Although the side effects of radiation just described are common, an acute radiation sickness syndrome occasionally develops causing hematopoietic syndrome, GI syndrome, or cerebral syndrome (fatal). This condition is a systemic reaction that occurs most often when the therapy is given in a large dose or high fraction rate to large areas over the abdomen; it occurs less often when radiotherapy is given over the thorax, and rarely when it is given over the extremities. Thoracic radiation may result in pericarditis and pneumonitis, which can progress to pulmonary fibrosis weeks, or even months, after radiation treatments have ended. Radiation esophagitis can cause difficulty swallowing and severe pain with eating and swallowing. Prevention of radiation esophagitis is extremely important since its presence can significantly impair nutritional intake. Medications such as amifostine (Ethyol) are used just before the onset of therapy, and Carafate, Nilstat, and tetracycline, along with other soothing agents, are used during treatment.[7]

Radiation Enterocolitis

Radiation therapy is often used for cancer of the bladder, prostate, rectum, colon, and female genital organs. With in-creasing doses of radiation, the rate of cell loss from the intestinal villi exceeds the reproductive capacity, resulting in reduced total epithelial surface and reduced absorption. The symptoms of radiation enteritis are the same as those of chronic intestinal obstruction (e.g., abdominal pain, distention, and spasm; reflexive vomiting associated with pain; constipation; constitutional symptoms; dehydration). Radiation colitis is manifested by bleeding and diarrhea.

Radiation Lung Disease

The lung is a radiosensitive organ that can be affected by external beam radiation therapy. The pulmonary response is determined by the volume of lung radiated, the dose and fraction rate of therapy, and enhancing factors such as concurrent chemotherapy, previous radiation therapy in the same area, and simultaneous withdrawal of corticosteroid therapy.[11]

Symptomatic radiation lung injury occurs in about 5% to 15% of clients treated with megavoltage therapy for carcinoma of the lung, and 5% to 35% of clients treated for mediastinal lymphoma.

The two phases of pulmonary response to radiation are an acute phase (radiation pneumonitis) and a chronic phase (radiation fibrosis). *Radiation pneumonitis* usually occurs 2 to 3 months (range, 1 to 6 months) after completion of radiotherapy. It is often asymptomatic with only a small scar to the affected tissue. Sometimes, in more serious cases, it is characterized by insidious onset of dyspnea, persistent dry cough, chest fullness or pain, weakness, and fever.[60]

Pulmonary function studies reveal reduced lung volumes, reduced lung compliance, hypoxemia, reduced diffusing capacity, and reduced maximum voluntary ventilation. Treatment is symptomatic and consists of administration of cough suppressants. Acute respiratory failure is treated appropriately when present. Although no proof is evident that corticosteroids are effective in radiation pneumonitis, prednisone is prescribed immediately, with early tapering of dosage. Radiation pneumonitis usually resolves in 2 to 3 months.

Pulmonary radiation fibrosis occurs in nearly all clients who receive a full course of radiation therapy for cancer of the lung or breast. Pulmonary fibrosis occurs approximately 6 to 12 months after resolution of radiation pneumonitis, although radiation fibrosis can develop without radiation pneumonitis. Most people are asymptomatic, but progressive dyspnea may develop slowly. No specific therapy is necessary, and corticosteroids have no value.[53] In approximately 1% of the people who receive pulmonary radiation treatment, idiopathic interstitial fibrosis develops, leading to death.[71]

Cutaneous Effects of Radiation

Although all body systems can be affected by radiation, the skin is the system at greatest risk for acute injury, including open, weeping wounds and alterations in the mucosal integrity.* Radiotherapy increases the mitotic production of basal cells in the skin, upsetting the balance between cell reproduction and cell destruction. Cellular breakdown in the epidermis results in an inflammatory process similar to a sunburn that can occur during the course of therapy but generally resolves 2 to 4 weeks after the completion of treatment. Soothing and lubricating lotions/creams (e.g., aloe-vera,

*This is also true for GI and genitourinary mucosa.

Aquaphor) are usually used in the treatment and prevention of radiation-related skin reactions.[7]

First-degree reactions resemble sunburn and can destroy hair roots, causing the hair to fall out. *Second-degree* reactions, also called *dry desquamation*, produce bright-red erythema. Sweat glands and hair follicles are damaged and the hair falls out, which may be irreversible. *Third-degree* reactions, also called *moist desquamation*, are characterized by a dark purple color and possible formation of blisters and ulcers. If the area is exposed to air, scabbing can occur over the exposed area. *Fourth-degree* reactions (rare) occur as a result of radiation overdose. The tissue is dysvascular, and the capillary beds are fibrosed with loss of sensation and characterized by tissue necrosis.

Radiation-induced skin ulcers that develop 10 to 20 years after radiation treatment for cancer are being treated in the therapist's practice.[54] Until now, these ulcers have been extremely difficult to close, much less heal, and are usually exquisitely painful. Although these chronic wounds appear to be resistant to healing, researchers are reporting beneficial effects on impaired wound healing of this type using a low intensity laser irradiation that promotes angiogenesis of the dermal vessels.[78]

Another type of radiation-induced skin injury is the *radiation recall reaction*. Radiation recall reactions are inflammatory skin reactions that occur in a previously irradiated site, during the administration of certain chemotherapeutic drugs (e.g., dactinomycin, Adriamycin, methotrexate). Months and even years may pass from the time of the initial radiation therapy to the onset of this reaction. A more immediate reaction (within 2 to 3 days) often occurs after the initiation of chemotherapy and is usually characterized by a mild, sunburned appearance. However, in some cases, it can be more severe and can occur in tissues other than the skin (e.g., mucous membranes, lung, esophagus, GI tract, and heart) causing more significant problems for the affected person.[59]

Effects of Radiation on Connective Tissue

Radiation therapy, especially teletherapy, is well known to cause significant long-term or chronic effects on the connective tissue. Acute irradiation toxicity is less likely because connective tissue has a slower turnover or reproductive rate and striated muscle tolerates relatively high doses of radiation. Late changes such as fibrosis, atrophy, and contraction of tissue can occur to any area irradiated (e.g., lungs, bladder) but especially to collagen tissue. In growing bones and limbs, irradiation can cause profound and irreversible changes resulting in limb length discrepancies requiring orthopedic surgical correction.

Fibrosis of connective tissue can result in edema, decreased range of motion, and functional impairment. Radiation of the pelvic cavity often causes dense pelvic adhesions that may cause painful motion restrictions and more rarely, plexopathy. Subsequently, these effects lead to soft tissue fibrosis, resulting in decreased range of motion, pain, and in some cases, lymphedema.

The fibrotic effect of radiation on the circulatory and lymphatic system is typically seen in a loss of elasticity and contractility of the irradiated vessels that are required to transport the blood, lymph, and waste products from the area of the body being exposed.[3] These types of effects can be minimized by sparing lymphatics from the radiation por-

tal, but presently, up to 30% of breast cancer survivors in the United States develop lymphedema sometime in their lifetime. It is important to remember that lymphedema may not be a side effect of radiation but rather a sign of advanced progressive metastases associated with cancer recurrence. Lymphedema can develop when lymphatic overload contributes to systemic congestion; a medical differential diagnosis is required.

Effects of Radiation on the Nervous System

Injury of the nervous system can also occur as a complication of excessive radiation dosage to tissue. Both acute and subacute transient symptoms may develop early, but progressive, permanent, and often disabling nervous system damage may not be evident for months to years after radiation therapy. Acute encephalopathy consisting of headache; nausea and vomiting; somnolence (sleepiness); and progressive neurologic signs may develop after the first or second dose of radiation. This condition becomes less severe as the radiation therapy continues if dexamethasone (a corticosteroid) is used before and during whole brain radiation. Early-delayed radiation encephalopathy occurs in the first 2 to 4 months after therapy and results in cognitive impairments. Some form of cognitive impairment is very common with radiation of the nervous system, especially when the brain is irradiated.

Early-delayed radiation myelopathy (functional disturbance or pathologic change in the spinal cord) follows radiation therapy to the neck or upper thorax and is characterized by Lhermitte's sign (an electric shocklike sensation radiating down the back and into the legs on flexion of the neck). This syndrome may be seen early during treatment to the cervicothoracic spinal cord and resolves spontaneously 2 to 4 months after the completion of therapy. Dexamethasone, used before and during radiation to reduce edema surrounding an entrapped nerve that is causing nerve root compression, can help with symptom reduction. Late-delayed radiation damage to the nervous system may appear months to years after treatment, including brachial neuropathy after radiation for breast or lung cancer and Brown-Séquard syndrome (weakness and proprioceptive sensory loss on one side of the body and loss of pain and temperature sensation on the other side, leading to eventual paraplegia) after radiation for extraspinal tumors (e.g., Hodgkin's disease).

The incidence of brachial plexopathy after radiation therapy has been reduced significantly with improved treatment, but women who were given large daily fractions of postoperative telecobalt therapy to the axillary, supraclavicular, and parasternal lymph node regions 30 years ago have shown a progression of both prevalence and severity of the late effects these many years later.[47] Today, with improved irradiation techniques (e.g., matching fields, maintaining the client's position between fields, and avoiding overlapping fields that can cause hot spots), the overall incidence is about 0.5% of all cases of irradiated breast cancer. Some concern exists that this complication could increase in numbers with the more conservative surgery and radical radiotherapy now employed in early breast cancer, but it is too soon to examine epidemiologic data.[40] Plexopathy can be caused by cancer recurrence or new cancer onset rather than the effects of irradiation and must be differentially diagnosed by a physician.

Lower extremity plexopathy is also possible when the pelvic area is irradiated. Clinical manifestations of radiation-induced plexopathy appear to be a result of fibrosis around the nerve trunks and include paresthesias (100%); hypesthesia (74%); progressive weakness; decreased reflexes; and pain (approximately 50%). The peripheral nerves in younger women seem more vulnerable, but this is a clinical observation that has not yet been documented with empirical evidence. Currently, no curative treatment is available, although therapeutic intervention can achieve significant pain control and improved strength and function in the affected limb.[40] Comprehensive lymphedema management may be required in cases of lymphedema (see Chapter 12).

Medical Management.   Treatment of systemic reactions is symptomatic and supportive. Often radiation treatment is delayed during the time that treatment is administered for the systemic reaction. When radiation dosage levels are sufficient to cause damage to GI mucosa, bone marrow, and other vital tissues, blood and platelet transfusions, antibiotics, fluid and electrolyte maintenance, and other supportive medical measures may be used.

Prognosis depends on the dose, the rate at which it was received, and its distribution within the body. Researchers continue to work to improve control rates while limiting biophysiologic destruction, reducing comorbidities, and improving survival. For the last 30 years, researchers have investigated ways of combining chemotherapy and radiation with various cancers to improve on the results with radiation therapy alone. Recently, clinical trials have focused on decreasing the toxicity of radiotherapy through dose modifications and conformal field arrangements.[33,55] Serial hematologic studies are helpful in monitoring the person's status.

Special Implications for the Therapist   4-6

RADIATION

Radiation Hazard for Health Care Professionals

People who receive external radiation do not give off radiation to those who come in contact with them. Internal implants can present some hazards to others as long as the implant is in place. Pregnant staff members should avoid all contact with the internally radiated client. When administering direct care, staff members should plan interventions so that each task can be accomplished as quickly as possible. Distance provides some protection; therefore it is advisable to use positions that place the staff person as far away from the radioactive implant as possible. For example, if the implant is in the pelvis, the caregiver might stand at the head or foot, not the side, of the bed.

The use of protective lead aprons or portable shields may be recommended according to the hospital protocol. Each staff member is encouraged to know and follow the recommended policies and procedures for the given institution. A film badge or ring badge worn on the outside of any protective devices or clothing of the caregivers records the cumulative dose of radiation received and is used to monitor exposure over a period. When removed, this badge should be stored in a location where no additional radiation exists.

Some sources of radiation (e.g., iodine 131, phosphorus 32) are excreted in body fluids (e.g., urine, sweat, tears, saliva) for several days after administration to the client. These clients are placed in strict radioactive isolation during hospitalization and treatment. All articles used by the client, such as urinals, toothpicks, tissues, and bed linens, are considered as a possible radiation hazard. Disposal of all such items should follow hospital protocol. Good quality examination gloves made of latex or a strong synthetic material (not vinyl) are adequate for general care, although the use of two sets of gloves is recommended when in direct contact with body fluids deemed radioactive. Careful removal and disposal of any personal protective equipment worn by the therapist must be done according to radiation safety instructions posted. Thorough handwashing after glove removal is essential.[97]

Postradiation Therapy

For the client who is in the process of receiving external radiation therapy, handwashing before treating the client is essential to protect him or her from infection. Skin care precautions include the following:

- Avoid topical use of alcohol or other drying agents, lotions, gels, oils, or salves; do not wash away markings for target area.
- Avoid positions in which the client is lying on the target area.
- Avoid exposure to direct sunlight, heat lamps, or other sources of heat, including thermal modalities.

Radiation to the low back may cause nausea, vomiting, or diarrhea because the lower digestive tract is exposed to the radiation.[64] Radiation of the pelvic cavity often causes dense pelvic adhesions that can cause painful motion restrictions. The therapist's role in the postradiation treatment of these clients is to increase range of motion and provide stretching exercises. Early, aggressive intervention by the therapist is essential to prevent or minimize restrictive scarring.

Some effects of radiation on the nervous system can develop as late as 1 year after treatment, although radiation plexopathy can develop many years after exposure to the radiation doses used 20 or 30 years ago. Anyone with neurologic signs or symptoms of unknown cause must be questioned about past medical history (cancer, heart disease) and the possibility of prior radiation treatment, keeping in mind that progressive disease or a vascular event can also cause an acute or subacute neurologic event. The physician must rule out cancer recurrence in anyone with a previous history of cancer and evaluate for the presence of some other cause of new onset neurologic signs and symptoms.

Postradiation Infection

Signs and symptoms of infection are often absent because the immunosuppressed person cannot mount an adequate inflammatory response. Fever may be the first and only sign of infection. Swelling, redness, and pus are absent in infected tissue. The therapist must observe very carefully for any sign of infection, anemia, or bleeding and other signs of thrombocytopenia (see Chapter 13).

Radiation Therapy and Exercise

Radiation and chemotherapy can cause permanent scar formation in the lungs and heart tissues, whereas drug-induced cardiomyopathies can contribute to limitations in cardiovascular function (see the sections on Chemotherapy and Exercise in this chapter, Cancer and Exercise in Chapter 8, and Tables 8-11, 39-6, and 39-7). Both of these variables require monitoring of vital signs whenever working with people who are recovering or in remission from cancer treatments. Clients should be taught to monitor their own vital signs including pulse rate, respiratory rate, perceived exertion rate (PER), which is not to exceed 15 to 17 for moderate intensity training or submaximal testing, and observe for early signs of cardiopulmonary complications of cancer treatments such as dyspnea, pallor, excessive perspiration or fatigue during exercise. Self-monitoring of blood pressure and pulse oximetry may be warranted in some cases.[31]

Low- to moderate-intensity aerobic exercise (e.g., self-paced walking) during the weeks of radiation treatment can help manage treatment-related symptoms by improving physical function and lowering reported levels of fatigue, anxiety, depression, and sleep disturbance.[62,81] A successful aerobic training protocol for a client with cancer should include client education, an exercise evaluation, and an individualized exercise prescription. Ideally, these components of cancer treatment should begin when the person receives the diagnosis. Current guidelines recommend that clients should be advised not to exercise within 2 hours of chemotherapy or radiation therapy as increases in circulation may increase the effects of the treatments.[39] Guidelines for choosing an exercise test and prescribing an exercise prescription are available[1,31]

Additionally, it is very important that the client carry out careful, daily stretching during and after radiation treatment. Postradiated tissue can tear when stretching. Therapist and client must observe for blanching of the skin and avoid stretching beyond that point. Stretching must be continued for 18 to 24 months postradiation as the fibrotic process continues for that amount of time.[71] ■

◆ Chemotherapy

Systemic chemotherapy plays a major role in the management of the 60% of malignancies that are not curable by regional modalities. As with radiation therapy, chemotherapy acts by interfering with cell division by chemically interacting with DNA. Chemotherapy may be used to cure cancer, to palliate or stabilize disease as preliminary therapy before bone marrow transplantation, or as adjuvant therapy. The principal goal of chemotherapy is to destroy malignant cells without harming normal cells or the host. However, most chemotherapeutic agents are nonspecific and therefore affect both malignant and normal cells.[76]

The patterns of toxicity of some commonly used cytotoxic drugs are outlined in Table 4-10 (see Table 8-7). Certain agents cause breaks in the integrity of the oral and GI mucosa, which provide openings for normal flora (bacteria normally present in the gut) to invade the bloodstream. This loss of mucosal integrity from chemotherapy or radiation therapy predisposes the GI tract to invasion by bacteria, fungi, or viruses. People who have received anthracycline antibiotics (e.g., doxorubicin) as part of a chemotherapeutic regimen may develop cardiac toxic effects (e.g., arrhythmias, conduction disturbances).

Myelosuppression (inhibits bone marrow production of blood cells and platelets) as a result of specific chemothera-

TABLE	4-10

Major Toxicities of Commonly Used Cancer Chemotherapeutic Agents

SHORT-TERM EFFECT	LONG-TERM EFFECT
Nausea, vomiting	Leukemia
Diarrhea, constipation	Cardiac involvement
Alopecia (hair loss)	(see text)
Myelosuppression	Pulmonary fibrosis
Anemia	Hemolytic-uremic syndrome
Leukopenia (infection)	Peripheral neuropathy
Thrombocytopenia (bleeding)	Premature menopause,
Hypersensitivity	sterility
Tissue necrosis (vesicants/blisters)	Encephalitis (cognitive
Stomatitis	impairment)
Renal failure	
Hemorrhagic cystitis	
Ileus	
Hepatotoxicity (acute or chronic)	

peutic agents or drug combinations is the primary factor that predisposes the individual to infection and/or bleeding.[92] With increased dosages or more frequent administration of drugs, more profound and prolonged myelosuppression may occur.[7] However, the use of prophylactic antibiotics and colony-stimulating factors (granulocyte-colony stimulating factor [G-CSF] and/or granulocyte-macrophage colony–stimulating factor [GM-CSF]) has helped dramatically in the prevention of infection and control of myelosuppression.

Fluid and electrolyte imbalances associated with the use of chemotherapy are discussed later in this chapter. Dyspnea and fatigue are the most common signs that a chemotherapeutic drug is becoming cardiotoxic. Delayed-onset cardiac toxicity as a result of chemotherapeutic agents may appear as a chronic cardiomyopathy. Other cardiac problems that may develop include acute or chronic pericarditis, conduction disturbances, accelerated and radiation-induced coronary artery disease, and valvular dysfunction. The development of accelerated atherosclerosis associated with cardiothoracic radiation can lead to coronary ischemia and myocardial infarction in a premature manner. Diseases of particular concern are those that require radiation therapy for large mediastinal masses (e.g., Hodgkin's disease).

Pulmonary toxicity from chemotherapy is relatively uncommon but potentially fatal. Renal toxicity is dependent on the specific chemotherapeutic agent used and may be acute, reversible, or irreversible with chronic renal failure as the end result. Hemorrhagic cystitis occurs in approximately 10% of the people who receive standard chemotherapy and in as many as 40% in those individuals receiving high-dose chemotherapy for bone marrow transplantation. Acute or chronic hepatoxicity is possible because the majority of chemotherapeutic agents are metabolized in the liver. Veno-occlusive disease of the liver, hepatic fibrosis, and cirrhosis are potential side effects of various chemotherapeutic agents administered.[76]

CHEMOTHERAPY

The period during chemotherapy administration is critical for each client who may be susceptible to spontaneous hemorrhage and infection. The usual precautions for thrombocytopenia (see Chapter 13) and infection control must be adhered to strictly. The importance of strict handwashing technique with an antiseptic solution cannot be overemphasized. The therapist should be alert to any sign of infection and report any potential site of infection, such as mucosal ulceration or skin abrasion or tear (even a hangnail). Check skin for petechiae, ecchymoses, chemical cellulitis, and secondary infection.

Neuropathy can occur as a result of the neurotoxic effects of chemotherapy (e.g., vincristine, vinblastine). For the immobile client, prevention of pressure ulcers through client and family education and positioning with appropriate protection (e.g., footboard to prevent footdrop, protective coverings, such as sheepskin and eggshell foam) are also important. For the mobile client, safety standards must be followed during ambulation because of weakness and numbness of the extremities.

Drug-induced mood changes ranging from feeling of well-being and euphoria to depression and irritability may occur; depression and irritability may also be associated with the cancer. Knowing these and other potential side effects of medications used in the treatment of cancer can help the therapist better understand client reactions during rehabilitation or therapy intervention.

Chemotherapy and Exercise[27]

Fatigue is a common and severe problem of many individuals undergoing chemotherapy or chemoradiotherapy to the extent that some people are unable to carry out usual daily activities (see the section on Radiation Therapy and Exercise in this chapter). Additionally, other effects of treatment such as anemia, corticoid-induced myopathy, and cardiotoxicity can severely affect a person's functional ability. Erythropoietin (e.g., Epogen/procrit), a biologic modifier (hormone), can be used to control the rate of red blood cell (RBC) production and thereby manage the anemia caused by reduced erythropoietin production associated with myelosuppression. For those clients with symptomatic anemia, follow precautions as outlined (see the section on Anemia in Chapter 13).

Bone marrow suppression is a common and serious side effect of many chemotherapeutic agents (and can be a side effect of radiation therapy in some instances). It is extremely important to monitor the hematology values in clients receiving these treatment modalities. Before any type of vigorous exercise or rehabilitative treatment is initiated, laboratory values should be monitored (see Table 8-11).

Research has shown that people recovering from high-dose chemotherapy should not be instructed to rest but should increase physical activity to reduce fatigue and improve physical performance.[31] An optimal balance of rest and physical exercise is essential in the successful treatment of these symptoms.[27,28,94] Results indicate that 6 weeks of endurance training consisting of low to moderate levels of aerobic exercise (walking for 30 minutes daily on a treadmill after an interval-training program) yielded a significant improvement of physical perfor-

mance and a reduction of fatigue, along with an improved mood and reduced mental stress while undergoing chemotherapy.[29] Additionally, no reported increases in chemotherapy-related complications were associated with an endurance-training program. ∎

SPECIFIC DISORDERS AFFECTING MULTIPLE SYSTEMS

◆ Vasculitic Syndromes

Vasculitis is a term that applies to a diverse group of diseases characterized by inflammation in blood vessel walls. The primary forms of vasculitis encountered in a therapy practice include giant cell (temporal) arteritis, polyarteritis nodosa, hypersensitivity vasculitis, Kawasaki disease, and thromboangiitis obliterans. These are discussed in greater detail in Chapter 11. Because the pathogenesis of most forms of vasculitis remains poorly understood and cases of vasculitis show great variability, it may not be possible to apply a specific disease label to such cases. Such instances of vasculitis may be diagnosed as *systemic vasculitis*.

Blood vessels of different sizes in various parts of the body may be affected by vasculitis, causing a wide spectrum of clinical manifestations. The inflammation often causes narrowing or occlusion of the vessel lumen and produces ischemia of the tissues that are supplied by the involved vessels. The inflammation may weaken the vessel wall, resulting in aneurysm or rupture. Major symptoms of small blood vessel vasculitis are skin lesions that may be accompanied by fever, malaise, and myalgia. Conditions characterized by this type of small-vessel involvement include temporal arteritis, Sjögren's syndrome, connective tissue disorders, chronic active hepatitis, ulcerative colitis, malignancies, biliary cirrhosis, and infections such as bacterial endocarditis.

Vasculitis may occur either as a primary disease or as a secondary manifestation of other illnesses such as RA, childhood dermatomyositis, systemic lupus erythematosus, mixed connective tissue disease, and systemic sclerosis. The next section contains a more detailed description of rheumatoid vasculitis; the other conditions are discussed elsewhere in the text.

◆ Rheumatoid Arthritis

Considering the multiple systemic processes that occur in RA, the condition might be more appropriately termed *rheumatoid disease*. Although RA is best known as a disease affecting synovial tissue, extraarticular rheumatoid nodules can appear at almost any body site, including the pleura, pericardium, and parenchyma of any organ. Serositis (inflammation of the serous membrane) can also involve the heart and lungs (see Table 26-4).

Certain autoimmune disorders appear to be associated with RA, most notably fibrosing alveolitis and Sjögren's syndrome. The chronic immune stimulation that occurs in people with RA can give rise to amyloidosis, Felty's syndrome (splenic disease), or lymphadenopathy. Other extra-articular conditions that can occur with RA include anemia, osteopenia, and cardiac or renal involvement; the extraarticular features of RA are more common in men.

Rheumatoid vasculitis is the least frequent extraarticular manifestation of RA, but because the vasculitic lesions can cause infarction or dysfunction in major organs, including the brain, vasculitis is associated with considerable morbidity and mortality. Vasculitis usually develops when joint disease is relatively quiet; early onset in the course of RA is associated with a poor prognosis. (See Collagen Vascular Disease in Chapter 11.)

Clinical features of systemic rheumatoid vasculitis are diverse, because any size blood vessel may be involved anywhere in the body. Skin ulcers and unexplained weight loss are clues to vasculitis. The most common findings are cutaneous lesions such as nail-edge infarctions (see Fig. 26-12), rashes, and skin ulcers. Skin ulcers usually develop suddenly as deep, punched-out lesions at sites that are unusual for venous ulceration, such as the dorsum of the foot or the upper calf. Peripheral neuropathies (mononeuritis multiplex) present with sensory symptoms of paresthesia or numbness and motor impairment (e.g., weakness in the muscles supplied by the affected nerve). Systemic manifestations of rheumatoid vasculitis may include unexplained weight loss, anorexia, and malaise. Malaise may be related to the widespread release of cytokines (substances released by lymphocytes with various immunologic functions) and may be accompanied by fatigue, low-grade fever, and night sweats. Individuals with severe RA who experience any of these symptoms should be referred to the physician for further evaluation.

Anemia in the presence of RA is usually proportional to the disease severity, and it resolves as RA is brought under control. Iron deficiency is often caused by GI bleeding as a result of therapy with NSAIDs or inadequate food intake, especially in people with systemic illness. The anemia is treated by controlling the underlying RA, and the therapist should follow special precautions related to anemia until the disease is under control (see Special Implications for the Therapist: Anemia in Chapter 13).

Osteopenia may result from general immobility, but it may also be an inherent part of RA. Initially, areas around the joints are affected. With long-standing disease, osteoporosis may become generalized and can lead to fractures after minimal stress. Management with corticosteroids increases the incidence of osteoporosis and related complications.

◆ Systemic Lupus Erythematosus

Lupus erythematosus is a chronic inflammatory disorder of the connective tissues that appears in two forms: discoid lupus erythematosus (DLE), which affects only the skin, and systemic lupus erythematosus (SLE), which affects both multiple organ systems and the skin and can be fatal. SLE may involve every organ system, but cardiovascular, renal, or neurologic complications are prevalent. Like RA, SLE is characterized by recurring remissions and exacerbations, which are especially common during the spring and summer. SLE affects women eight times as often as men, increasing to 15 times as often during childbearing years. (For further discussion of DLE see Chapter 9; see Chapter 6 for discussion of SLE.)

◆ Systemic Sclerosis

Systemic sclerosis, also known as progressive systemic sclerosis (PSS); scleroderma; and the CREST (**C**alcinosis, **R**aynaud's phenomenon, **E**sophageal dysmotility, **S**clerodactyly, and **T**elangiectasia) syndrome is a diffuse connective tissue disease characterized by fibrotic, degenerative, and occasionally inflammatory changes throughout the body. Most commonly affected sites include the skin, blood vessels, synovial membranes, skeletal muscles, and internal organs, especially the esophagus, GI tract, thyroid, heart, lungs, and kidneys. It affects women more than men, especially between ages 30 and 50 years. Approximately 30% of people with PSS die within 5 years of onset. (See Chapter 9 for discussion of this condition; see Chapter 14.)

◆ Tuberculosis

Tuberculosis (TB) is an acute or chronic infection caused by *Mycobacterium tuberculosis*. Although the primary infection site is the lung, mycobacteria commonly exist in other parts of the body; this is referred to as *extrapulmonary tuberculosis*. The extrapulmonary sites may include the renal system; skeletal system (osteomyelitis; vertebral TB is known as *Pott's disease*); GI tract, meninges (tuberculous meningitis); and genitals. Extrapulmonary tuberculosis occurs with greatly increased frequency in people with HIV infection (see Chapter 14 for more on pulmonary tuberculosis; see Chapter 24 for more on tuberculous spondylitis [Pott's disease]).

◆ Sarcoidosis

Sarcoidosis is a multisystem disorder characterized by the formation of granulomas, a formation of inflammatory cells (e.g., mononuclear inflammatory cells or macrophages), usually surrounded by a rim of lymphocytes. These granulomas may develop in the lungs, liver, bones, or eyes (see Table 14-16) and may be accompanied by skin lesions (see Fig 14-18). In the United States, sarcoidosis occurs predominantly among blacks, affecting twice as many women as men. Acute sarcoidosis usually resolves within 2 years. Chronic, progressive sarcoidosis, which is uncommon, is associated with pulmonary fibrosis and progressive pulmonary disability (see Chapter 14 for a complete discussion of this condition.)

◆ Multiple Organ Dysfunction Syndrome

Overview.   Care of critically ill people has progressed significantly during the last 50 years. Significant advances have been made in the care of shock, acute renal failure, acute brain injury, and acute respiratory failure, and more people are surviving these conditions. However, despite these advances, progressive deterioration of organ function may occur in people who are critically ill or injured. People often die of complications of disease, rather than from the disease itself. Multiple organ dysfunction syndrome (MODS) is often the final complication of a critical illness; it accounts for many deaths in noncoronary intensive care units.

Definition and Etiologic and Risk Factors.   MODS, formerly called *multiple organ failure syndrome (MOFS)*, is the progressive failure of two or more organ systems after a very severe illness or injury. Although sepsis and septic shock are the most common causes,[98] infection is not necessary to its development. MODS also can be triggered by persistent inflammatory processes, necrosis, severe trauma, pulmonary contusion, major surgery, multiple blood transfusions, burns, circulatory shock, acute pancreatitis, acute renal failure, and adult respiratory distress syndrome (ARDS).

Systemic inflammatory response syndrome (SIRS), formerly called *sepsis syndrome*, characterizes the clinical manifestations of hypermetabolism (e.g., increased temperature, heart rate, and respirations) present in many clients with

MODS.[49] Because it is a response to tissue insult or injury, SIRS is present in many individuals admitted to a critical care unit (CCU).

After an initial insult or injury, other factors can increase a person's chances of developing MODS/SIRS, including inadequate or delayed resuscitation; age over 65 years; alcoholism; diabetes; surgical complications (e.g., infection, hematoma formation); bowel infarction; or the previous existence of organ dysfunction (e.g., renal insufficiency).

Pathogenesis. The physiologic changes in MODS/SIRS are complex and incompletely understood at this time. In response to illness or traumatic injury, the neuroendocrine system activates stress hormones (e.g., cortisol, epinephrine, norepinephrine, endorphins) to be released into the circulation, whereas the sympathetic nervous system is stimulated to compensate for complications such as fluid loss and hypotension. Because of the initial insult and subsequent release of mediators, three major plasma enzyme cascades are activated with the overall effect of massive uncontrolled systemic immune and inflammatory responses. This hyperinflammation and hypercoagulation perpetuates edema formation, cardiovascular instability, endothelial damage, and clotting abnormalities. At the same time, initial oxygen consumption demand increases, because the oxygen requirements at the cellular level increase. Flow and oxygen consumption are mismatched because of a decrease in oxygen delivery to the cells caused by maldistribution of blood flow, myocardial depression, and a hypermetabolic state. Tissue hypoxia with cellular acidosis and impaired cellular function result in multiple organ dysfunction characteristic of MODS.[68]

Clinical Manifestations. A clinical pattern in the development of MODS has been well established. After the precipitating event, low-grade fever, tachycardia, dyspnea, SIRS, and altered mental status develop. The lung is the first organ to fail, resulting in ARDS (see Chapter 14). Between 7 and 10 days, the hypermetabolic state intensifies, GI bacteremia is common, and signs of liver and kidney failure develop. During days 14 to 21, renal and liver failures progress to a severe status and the GI and immune systems fail, with eventual cardiovascular collapse. Ischemia and inflammation are responsible for the CNS manifestations.

Protein metabolism is also affected, and amino acids derived from skeletal muscle, connective tissue, and intestinal viscera become an important energy source. The result is a significant loss of lean body mass.

Medical Management. Prevention and early detection and supportive therapy are essential for MODS, as no specific medical treatment exists for this condition. A way to halt the process, once it has begun, has not yet been discovered. Pharmacologic treatment may include antibiotics to treat infection, inotropic agents (e.g., dopamine, dobutamine) to counteract myocardial depression, and supplemental oxygen and ventilation to keep oxygen saturation levels at or above 90%. Fluid replacement and nutritional support are also provided. The recent development of monoclonal antibodies to modulate or inhibit the immune and inflammatory responses may lead to more specific pharmacologic treatment.[50]

MODS is the major cause of death (usually occurring between days 21 and 28) after septic, traumatic, and burn in-

juries. If the affected individual's condition has not improved by the end of the third week, survival is unlikely. The mortality rate of MODS is 60% to 90% and approaches 100% if three or more organs are involved, sepsis is present, and the individual is older than 65 years.

Special Implications for the Therapist **4-8**

MULTIPLE ORGAN DYSFUNCTION SYNDROME

Only the critical care or burn unit therapist will encounter the client with MODS/SIRS. The hypermetabolism associated with this condition is accompanied by protein catabolism, primarily of skeletal muscle and visceral organs. Lean body mass can be significantly depleted in 7 to 10 days, necessitating skin precautions and skin care. ∎

FLUID AND ELECTROLYTE IMBALANCES*

Observing clinical manifestations of fluid or electrolyte imbalances may be an important aspect of client care, especially in the acute care and home health care settings. Identifying clients at risk for such imbalances is the first step toward early detection. Although the causes of fluid and electrolyte imbalance are many and varied, generally, any disease process or injury, medication, medical treatment, dietary restrictions, and imbalance of fluid intake with fluid output can disrupt fluid and electrolyte balance.[88] The most common causes of fluid and electrolyte imbalances in a therapy practice include burns, surgery, diabetes mellitus, malignancy, acute alcoholism, socioeconomic status, and the various factors affecting the aging adult population (Box 4-5). See further discussion Common Causes of Fluid and Electrolyte Imbalances in this chapter.

◆ Aging and Fluid and Electrolyte Balance
The volume and distribution of body fluids composed of water, electrolytes, and nonelectrolytes vary with age, gender, body weight, and amount of adipose tissue. Throughout life, a slow decline occurs in lean body or fat-free mass with a corresponding decline in the volume of body fluids. Only 45% to 50% of the body weight of aging adults is water compared with 55% to 60% in younger adults. This decrease represents a net loss of muscle mass and a reduced ratio of lean body weight to total body weight and places older people at greater risk for water-deficit states.

The effects of increasing age on homeostatic mechanisms controlling fluid and electrolyte status are complex and not clearly understood. For example, it is clear that older adults do not respond to thirst and are at risk of dehydration but the ex-

---

*This is a brief presentation of the normal homeostatic processes of fluid and electrolyte balance. The interactions of these systems and how they maintain fluid and electrolyte balance and acid-base regulation are beyond the scope of this text. For a more in-depth study of these and other concepts presented in this text, the reader is referred to Guyton AC, Hall JE: *Textbook of medical physiology,* ed 10, Philadelphia, 2000, WB Saunders.

Factors Affecting Fluid and Electrolyte Balance in the Aging

Acute illness (fever, diarrhea, vomiting)
Bowel cleansing for GI diagnostic testing
Change in mental status
Constipation
Decreased thirst mechanism
Difficulty swallowing
Excessive sodium intake:
- Diet
- Sodium bicarbonate antacids (e.g., Alka-Seltzer)
- Water supply or water softener
- Decreased taste sensation (increased salt intake)
Excessive calcium intake:
- Alkaline antacids
Immobility
Laxatives (habitual use for constipation)
Medications:
- Antiparkinsonian drugs
- Diuretics
- Propranolol
Tamoxifen (breast cancer therapy)
Sodium-restricted diet
Urinary incontinence (voluntary fluid restriction)

act mechanism for this change remains unknown. The normal ranges for serum electrolytes such as sodium, potassium, and chloride in healthy older adults do not change significantly with increasing age, but the balance is fragile and more easily disturbed when taking medications, when under extreme psychologic or emotional stress, or in women who are perimenopausal.[56] Age-related renal changes may also contribute to the fragility of fluid and electrolyte imbalances in the older adult, especially when renal and membrane changes associated with hypertension are present.

◆ Fluid Imbalances

Overview.   Approximately 45% to 60% of the adult human body is composed of water, which contains the electrolytes that are essential to human life (see the section on Electrolytes in this chapter). This life-sustaining fluid is found within various body compartments, including the intracellular (within cells); interstitial (space between cells); intravascular (within blood vessels); and transcellular compartments.* The fluid in the interstitial and intravascular compartments comprises approximately one third the total body fluid, called the *extracellular fluid* (ECF). Fluid found inside the cells accounts for the remaining two thirds of total body fluid, called the *intracellular fluid* (ICF).

The cell membrane is water permeable with equal concentrations of dissolved particles on each side of the membrane

---

*Fluid in the transcellular compartment is present in the body but is separated from body tissues by a layer of epithelial cells. This fluid includes digestive juices, water, and solutes in the renal tubules and bladder, intraocular fluid, joint–space fluid, and cerebrospinal fluid.

maintaining equal volumes of ECF and ICF and preventing passive shifts of water. Passive shifts occur only if an inequality occurs on either side of the membrane in the concentration of solutes that cannot permeate the membrane. Water can also move with sodium ion movement.

The following five types of fluid imbalances may occur: (1) ECF volume deficit (ECFVD); (2) ECF volume excess (ECFVE); (3) ECF volume shift; (4) ICF volume excess (ICFVE); and (5) ICF volume deficit (ICFVD). A simpler approach to this subject is to view fluid shifts in terms of intravascular or extravascular movement. Movement from the vascular space to the extravascular areas and vice versa takes place easily and is the first mechanism of extracellular movement. *Increased intravascular fluid* results in congestive heart failure, increased pulse, and increased respiration. *Decreased intravascular fluid* results in decreased blood pressure, increased pulse, and increased respirations. However, *increased extravascular fluid* may cause edema, ascites, or pleural effusion. *Decreased extravascular fluid* results in decreased skin turgor and fatigue. The material in this section is presented on the bases of three broad categories: fluid deficit, fluid excess, and fluid shift (see Chapter 12).

Etiologic Factors and Pathogenesis.   Maintaining constant internal conditions (homeostasis) requires the proper balance between the volume and distribution of ECF and ICF to provide nutrition to the cells, allow excretion of waste products, and promote production of energy and other cell functions. Maintenance of this balance depends on the differences in the concentrations of ICF and ECF fluids, the permeability of the membranes, and the effect of the electrolytes in the fluids.

A fluid imbalance occurs when either gains or losses of body fluids and electrolytes cause fluid deficit or a fluid excess. Sodium is the major ion that influences water retention and water loss. A deficit of body fluids occurs with either an excessive loss of body water or an inadequate compensatory intake. The result is an insufficient fluid volume to meet the needs of the cells. It is manifested by dehydration (Box 4-6); hypovolemia such as blood or plasma loss; or both. Severe fluid volume deficit can cause vascular collapse and shock.

An *excess* of water occurs when an overabundance of water is in the interstitial fluid spaces or body cavities (edema) or within the blood vessels (hypervolemia). A *fluid shift* occurs when vascular fluid moves to interstitial or intracellular spaces or interstitial or intracellular fluid moves to vascular fluid space. Fluid that shifts into the interstitial space (i.e., fluid not in the vascular compartment) and remains there is referred to as *third-space fluid*. Third-space fluid is commonly seen in a therapy practice as a result of altered capillary permeability secondary to tissue injury or inflammation, but the most common cause is liver disease. Decreased serum protein (albumin) associated with liver disease and/or states of malnutrition result in third-space fluid.

Other areas called *potential spaces* can fill with fluid in the presence of inflammation or fluid imbalances. Examples of potential spaces include the peritoneal cavity fluid (e.g., ascites) and the pleural cavity (e.g., pleural effusion).

Clinical Manifestations.   *Fluid volume deficit* (FVD) is most often accompanied by symptoms related to a decrease in cardiac output, such as decreased blood pressure, increased pulse, and orthostatic hypotension. FVD can occur from loss of blood (whether obvious hemorrhage or occult GI bleed-

BOX **4-6**

Clinical Manifestations of Dehydration

Absent perspiration, tearing, and salivation
Body temperature (subnormal or elevated)
Confusion
Disorientation; comatose; convulsions
Dizziness when standing
Dry, brittle hair
Dry mucous membranes, furrowed tongue
Headache
Incoordination
Irritability
Lethargy
Postural hypotension
Rapid pulse
Rapid respirations
Skin changes:
• *Color:* gray
• *Temperature:* cold
• *Turgor:* poor
• *Feel:* Warm, dry if mild; cool, clammy if severe
Sunken eyeballs
Sunken fontanel (children)

person. A fluid balance record is kept on any individual who is susceptible or already experiencing a disturbance in the balance of body fluids. In addition, medical evaluation of clinical signs and laboratory tests are helpful in the assessment of a person's hydration status. Laboratory tests may include serum osmolality, sodium, hematocrit, and blood urea nitrogen (BUN) measurements (see the section on Laboratory Values in Chapter 39).

Serum osmolality measures the concentration of particles in the plasma portion of the blood. Osmolality increases with dehydration and decreases with overhydration. Serum sodium is an index of water deficit or excess; an elevated level of sodium in the blood (hypernatremia) would indicate that the loss of water from the body has exceeded the loss of sodium such as occurs in the administration of osmotic diuretics, uncontrolled diabetes insipidus, and extensive burns. Hematocrit increases with dehydration and decreases with excess fluid. BUN serves as an index of kidney excretory function; BUN increases with dehydration and decreases with overhydration (see Table 39-11).

Treatment is directed to the underlying cause; in the case of fluid volume deficit, the aim is to improve hydration status. This may be accomplished through replacement of fluids and/or electrolytes by oral, nasogastric, or intravenous (IV) means, including tube feeding or parenteral hyperalimentation, which is administered via a venous catheter, usually inserted into the superior vena cava.

ing); loss of plasma (burns, peritonitis); or loss of body fluids (diarrhea, vomiting, diaphoresis, lack of fluid intake), resulting in dehydration. Hypernatremia occurs if the body fluid loss is a loss of body water without solute components (e.g., diabetes insipidus). Most often, however, body fluid losses contain both body water and its solute components. The affected individual experiences symptoms of thirst, weakness, dizziness, decreased urine output, fever, weight loss, and altered levels of consciousness (i.e., confusion, coma). Significant decreases in systolic blood pressure (less than 70 mm Hg) result in symptoms of shock and require immediate medical treatment and possibly life-sustaining emergency management.

Fluid volume excess (FVE) is primarily characterized by weight gain and edema of the extremities. With intravascular FVE, other clinical manifestations include dyspnea, engorged neck and hand veins, and a bounding pulse. In the early stages, if the fluid is in the third space (interstitial fluid between cells), the person may not exhibit any of these symptoms.

Fluid shift from the vascular to the extravascular (interstitial) spaces (e.g., burns, peritonitis) is manifested by signs and symptoms similar to fluid volume deficit and shock, including skin pallor, cold extremities, weak and rapid pulse, hypotension, oliguria, and decreased levels of consciousness. When the fluid returns to the blood vessels, the clinical manifestations are similar to those of fluid overload such as bounding pulse, engorgement of peripheral and jugular veins, and an increased blood pressure. The jugular pulse is not normally visible. If the jugular pulse is noted 2 cm above the sternal angle when the individual sits at a 45-degree angle, it may be a sign of fluid overload.

Medical Management. The ECF is the only fluid compartment that can be readily monitored; clinically, the status of ICF is inferred from analysis of plasma and the condition of the

Special Implications for the Therapist 4-9

FLUID IMBALANCES

Monitoring Fluid Balance

Fluid balance is so critical to physical well-being and cardiopulmonary sufficiency that fluid input and output records are often maintained at bedside. The therapist may be involved in maintaining these records, which also include fluid volume lost in wound drainage, GI output, and fluids aspirated from any body cavity. Body weight may increase by several pounds before edema is apparent. The dependent areas manifest the first signs of fluid excess. Individuals on bed rest show sacral swelling; people who can sit on the edge of the bed or in a chair for prolonged periods tend to show swelling of the feet and hands.[19]

Water and fluids should be offered often to older adults and clients with debilitating diseases to prevent body fluid loss and hypernatremia. However, increasing fluid intake in clients with congestive heart failure or severe renal disease is usually contraindicated. Caffeinated fluids and alcohol can increase water loss, thereby increasing the serum sodium level; these beverages should be avoided to prevent fluid loss due to this diuretic effect.[45] Water is the preferred fluid for hydration except in athletic or marathon race situations, which require replacement of electrolytes.[37]

Dehydration

Dehydration (water deficit) degrades endurance exercise performance, and physical work capacity is diminished even at marginal levels of dehydration (defined clinically as a 1% loss of body weight through fluid loss). Alterations in VO_{2max} occur with a 2% or more deficit in body water loss. Greater body water deficits are associated with progressively larger reductions in physical work capacity. Dehydration results in larger reductions in physical work capacity in a hot environment (e.g., aquatic or outdoor setting), as compared with a thermally neutral environment. Prolonged exercise that places large demands on aerobic metabolism is more likely to be adversely affected by dehydration than is short-term exercise.[16]

Core body temperature increases predictably as the percentage of dehydration increases. The heart rate increases about 6 beats/minute for each 1% increase in dehydration. This is not true for older adults who may have limited rate changes with increased activity. Older individuals with hypovolemia cannot compensate as easily with an increased heart rate like younger people can, so shock is more difficult to treat. In addition, aging individuals are often being treated with cardiac medications such as beta-blockers or Digoxin that block or inhibit a rapid heart rate and limit rate changes with increased activity. Heart transplant recipients also have a unique situation as the heart has been denervated (see Special Implications for the Therapist: Heart Transplantation in Chapter 20).

Individuals exercising in the heat, including aquatic exercise, should be encouraged to drink water in excess of normal desired amounts. When exercise is expected to cause an increase of more than 2% in dehydration, target heart rate modifications are necessary.[58] Severe losses of water and solutes can lead to hypovolemic shock. It is important for the therapist to be aware of possible fluid losses or water shifts in any client who is already compromised by advanced age or by the presence of an ileostomy or tracheostomy that results in a continuous loss of fluid. Because the response to fluid loss is highly individual, it is important to recognize the early clinical symptoms of fluid loss (see Box 4-6) and to carefully monitor clients who are at risk (e.g., observe for symptoms, monitor vital signs). People at risk for profound and potentially fatal fluid volume deficit, as in severe and extensive burns, should be assessed frequently and regularly for mental acuity and orientation to person, place, and time.

Skin Care
Careful handling of edematous tissue is essential to maintaining the integrity of the skin, which is stretched beyond its normal limits and has a limited blood supply. Turning and repositioning the client must be done gently to avoid friction. A break in or abrasion of edematous skin can readily develop into a pressure ulcer. Client education may be necessary in the proper application and use of anti-embolism stockings, lower-extremity elevation, and the need for regular exercise. Clients should be cautioned to avoid crossing the legs, putting pillows under the knees, or otherwise creating pressure against the blood vessels.[30,65] ■

◆ Electrolyte Imbalances
Overview.   Electrolytes are chemical substances that separate into electrically charged particles, called *ions*, in solution. This process allows the ions in the body fluids to conduct an electrical charge necessary for metabolic activities and essential to the normal function of all cells. The electrolytes that consist of positively charged ions, or *cations*, are sodium (Na^+); potassium (K^+); calcium (Ca^{2+}); and magnesium (Mg^{2+}). Those that consist of negatively charged ions,

or *anions*, are chloride (Cl^+); bicarbonate (HCO_3^-); and phosphate (PO_4^{3-}).

Concentration gradients of sodium and potassium across the cell membrane produce the membrane potential and provide the means by which electrochemical impulses are transmitted in nerve and muscle fibers. *Sodium* affects the osmolality of blood and therefore influences blood volume and pressure and the retention or loss of interstitial fluid. Sodium imbalance affects the osmolality of the extracellular fluid and is often associated with fluid volume imbalances. Adequate *potassium* is necessary to maintain function of the sodium-potassium pump, which is essential for the normal muscle contraction-relaxation sequence. Imbalances in potassium affect muscular activities, notably those of the heart, intestines, and respiratory tract, and neural stimulation of the skeletal muscles.

Calcium influences the permeability of cell membranes and thereby regulates neuromuscular activity. Calcium plays a role in the electrical excitation of cardiac cells and in the mechanical contraction of the myocardial and vascular smooth muscle cells. An imbalance in calcium concentrations affects the bones, kidneys, and GI tract. Conditions that can cause movement of calcium from the bones into the extracellular fluid (e.g., bone tumors, multiple fractures, osteoporosis) can cause hypercalcemia. (Other causes of hypo- or hypercalcemia are listed in Table 4-11.)

Magnesium, an important intracellular enzyme activator, exerts physiologic effects on the nervous system, which resemble the effects of calcium. Magnesium plays a role in maintaining the correct level of electrical excitability in the nerves and muscle cells by acting directly on the myoneural junction. Magnesium depresses acetylcholine release at synaptic junctions; when concentrations of Mg^{2+} in the plasma are altered then associated changes also occur in the concentration of Ca^{2+}. Magnesium imbalances affect parathyroid hormone (PTH) function and if severe, can change or impair end-organ response to PTH. Neuromuscular irritability results from hypomagnesemia (e.g., poor diet, chronic alcohol abuse, diuretic use, prolonged diarrhea) and magnesium excess (rare but occurs with renal failure or the overuse of magnesium-containing antacids) causes neuromuscular depression affecting the musculoskeletal and cardiac systems.[67]

Etiologic and Risk Factors.   An electrolyte imbalance exists when the serum concentration of an electrolyte is either too high or too low. Stability of the electrolyte balance depends on adequate intake of water and the electrolytes and on homeostatic mechanisms within the body that regulate the absorption, distribution, and excretion of water and its dissolved particles. Bodily fluid loss associated with weight loss, excessive perspiration, or chronic vomiting and diarrhea are the most common causes of electrolyte imbalance. Many other conditions can interfere with these processes and result in an imbalance (see Table 4-11).

Oxygen deprivation is accompanied by electrolyte disturbances, particularly loss of potassium, calcium, and magnesium from cells when cellular death ensues (see the section on Cell Injury in Chapter 5). Myocardial cells deprived of necessary oxygen and nutrients lose contractility, thereby diminishing the pumping ability of the heart. Diuretics also can produce mild to severe electrolyte imbalance. These factors explain the careful observation of specific electrolyte levels in the cardiac client.

TABLE	4-11

Causes of Electrolyte Imbalances

	RISK FACTORS FOR IMBALANCE		RISK FACTORS FOR IMBALANCE
Potassium		Hypernatremia—cont'd	Excess adrenocortical hormones (Cushing's syndrome)
Hypokalemia	Dietary deficiency (rare)		IV administration of high-protein, hyperosmotic tube feedings and diuretics
	Intestinal or urinary losses as a result of diarrhea or vomiting (anorexia, dehydration), drainage from fistulas, overuse of gastric suction	**Calcium**	
		Hypocalcemia	Inadequate dietary intake of calcium and inadequate exposure to sunlight (Vitamin D) necessary for calcium use
	Trauma (injury, burns, surgery): damaged cells release potassium, are excreted in urine		Impaired absorption of calcium from intestinal tract (severe diarrhea, overuse of laxative, and enemas containing phosphates; phosphorus tends to be more readily absorbed from the intestinal tract than calcium and suppresses calcium retention in the body)
	Chronic renal disease		
	Medications such as potassium-wasting diuretics, steroids, sodium-containing antibiotics		
	Alkalosis		
	Hyperglycemia		
	Cushing's syndrome, primary aldosteronism, severe magnesium deficiency		Hypoparathyroidism (injury, disease, surgery)
Hyperkalemia	Conditions that alter kidney function or decrease its ability to excrete potassium		Severe infections or burns
			Overcorrection of acidosis
	Intestinal obstruction that prevents elimination of potassium in the feces		Pancreatic insufficiency
			Renal failure
	Addison's disease		Hypomagnesemia
	Chronic heparin therapy, lead poisoning, insulin deficit	Hypercalcemia	Hyperparathyroidism, hyperthyroidism, adrenal insufficiency
	Trauma: crush injuries, burns		Tumors (bone, lung, stomach, and kidney)
	Acidosis		Multiple fractures
Sodium			Excess intake of calcium (excessive antacids), excess intake of vitamin D, milk alkali syndrome
Hyponatremia	Inadequate sodium intake (low-sodium diets)		
	Excessive intake or retention of water (kidney failure and heart failure)		Osteoporosis, immobility, multiple myeloma
			Thiazide diuretics
	Excessive water loss and electrolytes (vomiting, excessive perspiration, tap-water enemas, suctioning, use of diuretics)		Sarcoidosis
		Magnesium	
		Hypomagnesemia	Decreased magnesium intake or absorption (chronic malnutrition, chronic diarrhea, bowel resection with ileostomy or colostomy, chronic alcoholism, prolonged gastric suction, acute pancreatitis, biliary or intestinal fistula, diuretic therapy)
	Loss of bile (high in sodium) as a result of fistulas, drainage, GI surgery, and suction		
	Trauma (loss of sodium through burn wounds, wound drainage from surgery)		
	IV fluids that do not contain electrolytes		
	Adrenal gland insufficiency (Addison's disease) or hyperaldosteronism		Excessive loss of magnesium (diabetic ketoacidosis, severe dehydration, hyperaldosteronism and hypoparathyroidism, diuretic therapy)
	Cirrhosis of the liver with ascites		
	SIADH: brain tumor, cerebrovascular accident, pulmonary disease, neoplasm with ADH production, medications	Hypermagnesemia	Chronic renal and adrenal insufficiency
			Overuse of antacids and laxatives containing magnesium
Hypernatremia	Decreased water intake (comatose, mentally confused, or debilitated client)		Severe dehydration (resulting oliguria can cause magnesium retention)
	Water loss (excessive sweating, diarrhea, failure of kidney to reabsorb water from urine)		Overcorrection of hypomagnesemia
			Near-drowning (aspiration of sea water)
	ADH deficiency (diabetes insipidus)		

Modified from Horne M, Bond E: Fluid, electrolyte, and acid-base imbalances. In Lewis S, Heitkemper M, Dirksen S, editors: *Medical-surgical nursing: assessment and management of clinical problems*, ed 5, St Louis, 2000, Mosby.
GI, gastrointestinal; *IV*, intravenous; *SIADH*, syndrome of inappropriate antidiuretic hormone; *ADH*, antidiuretic hormone.

TABLE **4-12**

Clinical Features of Various Electrolyte Imbalances

	SYSTEM DYSFUNCTION	
Potassium Imbalance	**HYPOKALEMIA**	**HYPERKALEMIA**
Cardiovascular	Dizziness, hypotension, arrhythmias, ECG changes, cardiac arrest (with serum potassium levels 2.5 mEq/L)	Tachycardia and later bradycardia, ECG changes, cardiac arrest (with levels >7.0 mEq/L)
GI	Nausea and vomiting, anorexia, diarrhea, abdominal distention, paralytic ileus or decreased peristalsis	Nausea, diarrhea, abdominal cramps
Musculoskeletal	Muscle weakness and fatigue, leg cramps	Muscle weakness, flaccid paralysis
Genitourinary	Polyuria	Oliguria, anuria
Central nervous system (CNS)	Malaise, irritability, confusion, mental depression, speech changes, decreased reflexes, respiratory paralysis	Hyperreflexia progressing to weakness, numbness, tingling, and flaccid paralysis
Acid-base balance	Metabolic alkalosis	Metabolic acidosis
Calcium Imbalance	**HYPOCALCEMIA**	**HYPERCALCEMIA**
CNS	Anxiety, irritability, twitching around mouth, laryngospasm, convulsions, Chvostek's sign, Trousseau's sign	Drowsiness, lethargy, headaches, depression or apathy, irritability, confusion
Musculoskeletal	Paresthesia (tingling and numbness of the fingers), tetany or painful tonic muscle spasms, facial spasms, abdominal cramps, muscle cramps, spasmodic contractions	Weakness, muscle flaccidity, bone pain, pathologic fractures
Cardiovascular	Arrhythmias, hypotension	Signs of heart block, cardiac arrest in systole, hypertension
Gastrointestinal (GI)	Increased GI motility, diarrhea	Anorexia, nausea, vomiting, constipation, dehydration, polydipsia
Other	Blood-clotting abnormalities	Renal polyuria, flank pain, and, eventually, azotemia
Sodium Imbalance	**HYPONATREMIA**	**HYPERNATREMIA**
CNS	Anxiety, headaches, muscle twitching and weakness, convulsions	Fever, agitation, restlessness, convulsions
Cardiovascular	Hypotension; tachycardia; with severe deficit, vasomotor collapse, thready pulse	Hypertension, tachycardia, pitting edema, excessive weight gain
GI	Nausea, vomiting, abdominal cramps	Rough, dry tongue; intense thirst
Genitourinary	Oliguria or anuria	Oliguria
Respiratory	Cyanosis with severe deficiency	Dyspnea, respiratory arrest, and death (from dramatic rise in osmotic pressure)
Cutaneous	Cold clammy skin, decreased skin turgor	Flushed skin; dry, sticky mucous membranes
Magnesium Imbalance	**MAGNESEMIA**	**HYPERMAGNESMIA**
Neuromuscular	Hyperirritability, tetany, leg and foot cramps, Chvostek's sign (facial muscle spasms induced by tapping the branches of the facial nerve)	Diminished reflexes, muscle weakness, flaccid paralysis, respiratory muscle paralysis that may cause respiratory impairment
CNS	Confusion, delusions, hallucinations, convulsions	Drowsiness, flushing, lethargy, confusion, diminished sensorium
Cardiovascular	Arrhythmias, vasomotor changes (vasodilation and hypotension), occasionally, hypertension	Bradycardia, weak pulse, hypotension, heart block, cardiac arrest

Clinical Manifestations.   In a therapy practice, paresthesias, muscle weakness, muscle wasting, muscle tetany, and bone pain are the most likely symptoms first observed with electrolyte imbalances (Table 4-12). (See the Clinical Manifestations section under Common Causes of Fluid and Electrolyte Imbalances in this chapter.)

Medical Management.   Potassium, calcium, and to a lesser extent, magnesium imbalances are reflected on ECG. Values for sodium or chloride can be measured in plasma. A sweat test for sodium and chloride levels can be done if cystic fibrosis is suspected. Elevated values in the presence of a family history or clinical findings of cystic fibrosis are diagnostic.

Intracellular levels of electrolytes cannot be measured; therefore all values for electrolytes are expressed as serum values. Serum values for electrolytes are given as milliequivalents per liter (mEq/L) or milligrams per deciliter (mg/dL) (see Table 39-8). As with fluid imbalances, the underlying cause of electrolyte imbalances must be determined and corrected.

Special Implications for the Therapist 4-10

ELECTROLYTE IMBALANCES

Encourage adherence to a sodium-restricted diet prescribed for clients. The use of OTC medications for people on a sodium-restricted diet should be approved by the physician. Encourage activity altered by rest periods. Monitor for worsening of the underlying cause of fluid or electrolyte imbalance and report significant findings to the nurse or physician. If dyspnea and orthopnea are present, teach the client to use a semi-Fowler position (head elevated 18 to 20 inches from horizontal with knees flexed) to promote lung expansion. Frequent position changes are important in the presence of edema; edematous tissue is more prone to skin breakdown than is normal tissue.

Older adults have frequent problems with hypokalemia most often associated with the use of diuretics. Assessment for signs and symptoms of electrolyte imbalance must be ongoing, and changes need to be reported immediately. Decreased potassium levels can result in fatigue, muscle cramping, and cardiac dysrhythmias, usually manifested by an irregular pulse rate or complaints of dizziness and/or palpitations. Fatigue and muscle cramping increase the chance of musculoskeletal injury. Observing for accompanying signs and symptoms of fluid and electrolyte imbalances will help promote safe and effective exercise for anyone with the potential for these disorders.

With appropriate medical therapy, cardiac, muscular, and neurologic manifestations associated with electrolyte imbalances can be corrected. Delayed medical treatment may result in irreversible damage or death. ∎

◆ Common Causes of Fluid and Electrolyte Imbalances

The exact mechanisms of fluid and electrolyte imbalances are outside the scope of this text. A brief description of the common causes and overall clinical picture encountered in a therapy practice is included here.

Burns, surgery, and trauma may result in a fluid volume shift from the vascular spaces to the interstitial spaces. Tissue injury causes the release of histamine and bradykinin, which increases capillary permeability, allowing fluid, protein, and other solutes to shift into the interstitial spaces. In the case of burns, the fluid shifts out of the vessels into the injured tissue spaces, as well as into the normal (unburned) tissue. This causes severe swelling of these tissues and a significant loss of fluid volume from the vascular space, which results in hypovolemia. Severe hypovolemia can result in shock, vascular collapse, and death. In the case of major tissue damage, potassium is also released from the damaged tissue cells and can enter the vascular fluids, causing hyperkalemia.

In an attempt to treat shock, large quantities of fluid are administered intravenously to maintain blood pressure, cardiac output, and renal function. After 24 to 72 hours, capillary permeability is usually restored and fluid begins to leave the tissue spaces and shift back into the vascular space. If renal function is not adequate, the accumulation of fluid used for treatment and fluid returning from the tissue spaces into the vascular space can cause fluid volume overload. Fluid overload can then cause congestive heart failure.

Diabetes mellitus (Type 1) may result in a condition called *diabetic ketoacidosis*, as a result of overproduction of ketone bodies and the accompanying metabolic acidosis that occurs (see discussion, Chapter 10). As the pH of the blood decreases (acidosis), the accumulating hydrogen moves from the extracellular fluid to the intracellular fluid. Movement of hydrogen into the cells promotes the movement of potassium out of the cells and into the extracellular fluid. As the potassium enters the vascular space, the plasma potassium levels increase. However, since severe diuresis is also occurring, the accumulated potassium is quickly excreted in the urine. As a result, severe potassium losses occur (hypokalemia), which unless treated immediately, cause life-threatening cardiac dysrhythmias.

Malignant tumors can produce remote effects as a result of impaired hormonal regulation of body water and electrolytes. Production of these hormones is not regulated by normal suppression feedback loops; consequently, the ectopic hormone* continues to be released by the tumor, often causing life-threatening electrolyte imbalances. The generally accepted theory that accounts for the production of ectopic hormones is faulty genetic regulation by the malignant tumor itself.[46] One example of this phenomenon is the ectopic production of antidiuretic hormone (ADH) by lung carcinomas resulting in severe water retention.

Tumor-induced imbalances can affect the CNS and cause neurologic syndromes referred to as *paraneoplastic syndromes* (see Chapter 8). The neurologic syndromes are generally produced by cancer stimulation of antibody production.[89] For example, cancer cells produce antibodies that impair presynaptic calcium-channel activity, which hinders the release of acetylcholine. In the Lambert-Eaton myasthenic syndrome (LEMS), autoantibodies directed against the presynaptic calcium channels at the neuromuscular junction cause impaired release of acetylcholine from the presynaptic nerve terminals, resulting in muscle weakness.[44]

A more local effect of malignancy occurs when metastases to the skeletal system produce hypercalcemia from the osteolysis of bone. The treatment of malignancies also can create fluid and electrolyte imbalances such as occurs with hormonal treatment for breast cancer (tamoxifen); hyponatremia and hypokalemia may also result from nausea and vomiting caused by chemotherapy, and hyponatremia from water intoxication may occur in association with the use of certain chemotherapeutic drugs (e.g., vincristine and cyclophosphamide).

Alcohol withdrawal and *eating disorders* are also associated with physiologic changes that can include electrolyte imbalances. See discussion of each individual condition, Chapter 2.

---

*Hormone that arises at or is produced at an abnormal site or in a tissue where it is not normally found.

BOX **4-7**

Clinical Manifestations of Fluid/Electrolyte Imbalance*

Skin changes:
- Poor skin turgor
- Changes in skin temperature

Neuromuscular irritability:
- Muscle fatigue
- Muscle twitching
- Muscle cramping
- Tetany

CNS involvement:
- Changes in deep tendon reflexes
- Convulsions
- Depression
- Memory impairment
- Delusions
- Hallucinations

Edema

Changes in vital signs:
- Tachycardia
- Postural hypotension
- Altered respirations

*Only signs and symptoms most likely to be seen in a therapy practice are included here.

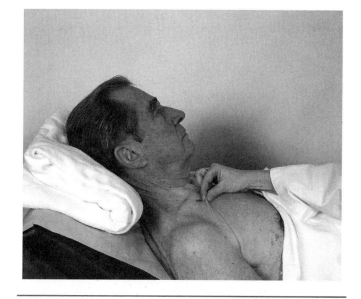

FIGURE **4-1** Testing skin turgor (normal resiliency of a pinched fold of skin). Turgor is measured by the time it takes for the skin and underlying tissue to return to its original contour after being pinched up. If the skin remains elevated (i.e., tented) for more than 3 seconds, turgor is decreased. Normal turgor is indicated by a return to baseline contour within 3 seconds when the skin is mobile and elastic. Turgor decreases with age as the skin loses elasticity; testing turgor of some older persons on the forearm (the standard site for testing) is less valid due to decreased skin elasticity in this area. (From Jarvis C: *Physical examination and health assessment*, ed 3, Philadelphia, 2000, WB Saunders.)

Clinical Manifestations. The effects of a fluid or electrolyte imbalance are not isolated to a particular organ or system (Box 4-7). Symptoms most commonly observed by the therapist may include skin changes; neuromuscular irritability (muscle fatigue, twitching, cramping, or tetany); CNS involvement; edema; and changes in vital signs, especially tachycardia and postural (orthostatic) hypotension (see Box 11-8).

Skin changes include changes in skin turgor and alterations in skin temperature. In a healthy individual, pinched skin will immediately fall back to its normal position when released, a measure of skin turgor. In a person with fluid volume deficit (FVD) such as dehydration, the skin flattens more slowly after the pinch is released, and may even remain elevated for several seconds referred to as *tenting* of tissue (Fig. 4-1). Tissue turgor can vary with age, nutritional state, race, and complexion and must be accompanied by other signs of FVD to be considered meaningful. Skin turgor may be more difficult to assess in older adults owing to reduced skin elasticity compared with that of younger clients. Skin temperature may become warm and flushed as a result of vasodilation (e.g., in metabolic acidosis) or pale and cool due to peripheral vasoconstriction compensating for hypovolemia.

Neuromuscular irritability can occur as a result of imbalances in calcium, magnesium, potassium, and sodium. (See Chapter 23 for discussion of osteoporosis associated with calcium loss.) Specific signs of neuromuscular involvement associated with these imbalances occur because of increased neural excitability, specifically increased acetylcholine action at the nerve ending, resulting in lowering of the threshold of the muscle

membrane. Tetany (continuous muscle spasm) is the most characteristic manifestation of hypocalcemia. The affected person may report a sensation of tingling around the mouth (circumoral paresthesia) and in the hands and feet, and spasms of the muscles of the extremities and face. Less overt signs (latent tetany) can be elicited through Trousseau's sign (Fig. 4-2); Chvostek's sign (Fig. 4-3); and changes in deep tendon reflexes (DTRs) (Table 4-13). Many other factors can produce abnormalities in DTRs requiring the therapist to evaluate altered DTRs in light of other clinical signs and client history.

Nervous system involvement may occur in the peripheral system (hyperkalemia) or the CNS (hypocalcemia). CNS manifestations of hypocalcemia may include convulsions, irritability, depression, memory impairment, delusions, and hallucinations. In chronic hypocalcemia, the skin may be dry and scaling, the nails become brittle, and the hair is dry and falls out easily.

Hypokalemia seen in a therapy practice can be associated with diuretic therapy; excessive sweating, vomiting, or diarrhea; diabetic acidosis; trauma; or burns. It is also accompanied by muscular weakness that can progress to flaccid quadriparesis. The weakness is initially most prominent in the legs, especially the quadriceps; it extends to the arms, with involvement of the respiratory muscles soon after.[67] Finally, a condition called *rhabdomyolysis* (disintegration of striated muscle fibers with excretion of myoglobin in the urine) can occur with potassium or phosphorus depletion.

Edema, defined as an excessive accumulation of interstitial fluid (fluid that bathes the cells), may be either localized or

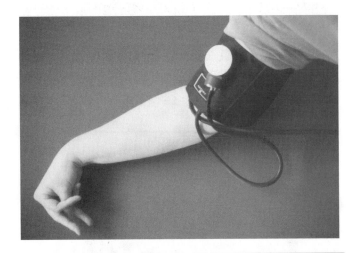

FIGURE 4-2 Carpopedal attitude of the hand, a form of latent tetany associated with hypocalcemia, is called *Trousseau's sign*. This can be tested for by inflating a blood pressure cuff on the upper arm to a level between diastolic and systolic blood pressure and maintaining this inflation for 3 minutes. A positive test results in the carpal spasm shown here. (From Ignatavicius DD et al: *Medical-surgical nursing across the health care continuum*, ed 3, Philadelphia, 1999, WB Saunders.)

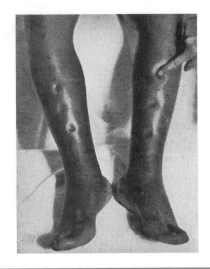

FIGURE 4-4 Severe, bilateral, dependent, pitting edema occurs with some systemic diseases, such as congestive heart failure and hepatic cirrhosis. (From Delp MH, Manning RT: *Major's physical diagnosis: an introduction to the clinical process*, ed 9, Philadelphia, 1981, WB Saunders.)

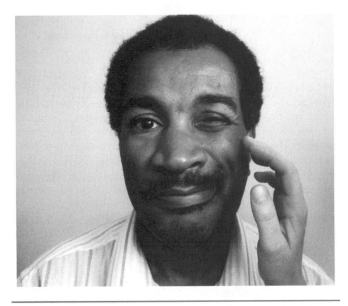

FIGURE 4-3 To check for *Chvostek's sign*, tap the facial nerve above the mandibular angle, adjacent to the ear lobe. A facial muscle spasm that causes the person's eye and upper lip to twitch, as shown, confirms tetany. (From Ignatavicius DD et al: *Medical-surgical nursing across the health care continuum*, ed 3, Philadelphia, 1999, WB Saunders.)

TABLE	4-13

Changes in Deep Tendon Reflexes Associated With Fluid/Electrolyte Imbalance

INCREASED (HYPERACTIVE)	DECREASED (HYPOACTIVE)
Hypocalcemia	Hypercalcemia
Hypomagnesemia	Hypermagnesemia
Hypernatremia	Hyponatremia
Hyperkalemia	Hypokalemia
Alkalosis	Acidosis

generalized. Generalized edema may be characterized by shortness of breath, ankle swelling that subsides after lying down, nocturia, and orthopnea. Other manifestations of generalized edema may include decreased urinary output; weight gain; bounding or arrhythmic pulse; labored, shallow, and increased respiratory rate; distended neck veins at 45 degrees elevation of the head; changes in venous and arterial blood pressure; and abnormal laboratory findings (e.g., electrolytes, serum creatinine, blood urea nitrogen, hemoglobin, and hematocrit). Pulmonary edema results from excessive shifting of fluid from the vascular space into the pulmonary interstitium and air spaces. When edema forms as a result of salt retention, the clinical picture is usually one of pitting edema (Fig. 4-4).

Vital sign changes, including pulse, respirations, and blood pressure, may signal early development of fluid volume changes. Decreased blood pressure and tachycardia are usually the first signs of the decreased vascular volume associated with FVD as the heart pumps faster to compensate for the decreased plasma volume. Irregular pulse rates and dysrhythmias may also be associated with magnesium, potassium, or calcium imbalances.

Orthostatic hypotension is another sign of volume depletion (hypovolemia). Moving from a supine to standing position causes an abrupt drop in venous return, which is normally compensated for by sympathetically mediated cardiovascular adjustments. For example, in the healthy individual, increased peripheral resistance and increased heart rate maintain car-

TABLE	4-14

Assessment of Fluid and Electrolyte Imbalance

Area	Fluid Excess/Electrolyte Imbalance	Fluid Loss/Electrolyte Imbalance
Head and neck	Distended neck veins, facial edema	Thirst, dry mucous membranes
Extremities	Dependent edema, pitting, discomfort from weight of bed covers	Muscle weakness, tingling, tetany
Skin	Warm, moist, taut, cool feeling when edematous	Dry, decreased turgor
Respiration	Dyspnea, orthopnea, productive cough, moist breath sounds	Changes in rate and depth of breathing
Circulation	Hypertension, jugular pulse visible at 45-degree sitting angle, atrial arrhythmias	Pulse rate irregularities, arrhythmia, postural hypotension, tachycardia
Abdomen	Increased girth, fluid wave	Abdominal cramps

Modified from Briggs J, Drabek C: Fluid and electrolyte imbalance. In Phipps WJ, Sands J, Marek J, editors: *Medical-surgical nursing: concepts and clinical practice*, ed 5, St Louis, 1999, Mosby, p. 420.

diac return. Blood pressure is unaffected or characterized by a small decrease in systolic pressure, and the diastolic pressure may actually rise a few millimeters (mm) of mercury. In contrast, for the person with FVD, systolic pressure may fall 20 mm Hg or more, accompanied by an increase in the pulse rate greater than 15 beats/minute.[46] The decreased volume results in compensatory increases in pulse rate as the heart attempts to increase output in the face of decreased stroke volume. As fluid volume depletion worsens, blood pressure becomes low in all positions due to loss of compensatory mechanisms and autonomic insufficiency. Conditions such as diabetes, associated with autonomic neuropathy, can also produce orthostatic blood pressure and pulse changes (see the section on Orthostatic Hypotension in Chapter 11).

Special Implications for the Therapist   4-11

ASSESSMENT OF FLUID AND ELECTROLYTE IMBALANCE

Assessment of fluid and electrolyte balance is based on both subjective and objective findings (Table 4-14). At the bedside or in the home health care setting, the therapist must be alert to complaints of headache, thirst, and nausea and changes in dyspnea, skin turgor, and muscle strength. More objective assessment of fluid and electrolyte balance is based on fluid intake, output, and body weight. (See Special Implications for the Therapist: Fluid Imbalances and Electrolyte Imbalances in this chapter.) ■

ACID-BASE IMBALANCES

Normal function of body cells depends on regulation of hydrogen ion concentration (H^+) so that H^+ levels remain within very narrow limits. Acid-base imbalances occur when these limits are exceeded and are recognized clinically as abnormalities of serum pH (i.e., the measure of acidity or alkalinity of blood). Normal serum pH is 7.35 to 7.45. Cell func-

tion is seriously impaired when pH falls to 7.2 or lower or rises to 7.55 or higher (see the section on Laboratory Values in Chapter 39).

Three physiologic systems act interdependently to maintain normal serum pH: immediate buffering of excess acid or base by the *blood buffer systems*; excretion of acid by the *lungs* (occurs within hours); and excretion of acid or reclamation of base by the *kidneys* (occurs within days). The four general classes of acid-base imbalance are respiratory acidosis, respiratory alkalosis, metabolic acidosis, and metabolic alkalosis. Table 4-15 summarizes these four imbalances (see Table 39-9).

Acidosis refers to any pathologic process causing a relative excess of acid in the body. This can occur as a result of accumulation of acid or depletion of the alkaline reserve (bicarbonate content, HCO_3^-) in the blood and body tissues. *Acidemia* refers to excess acid in the blood and does not necessarily confirm an underlying pathologic process. The same distinction may be made between the terms *alkalosis* and *alkalemia*; alkalosis indicates a primary condition resulting in excess base in the body. Although efforts have been made to standardize acid-base terminology, these terms are often used interchangeably.

Incidence.   The incidence of acid-base imbalances in hospital settings is high. Acid-base imbalances are often related to respiratory and/or metabolic problems typical of the critically ill or injured individual. Some people have more than one acid-base imbalance at the same time.

Clinical Manifestations.   A guide to the clinical presentation of acid-base imbalances is shown in Table 4-15. Besides the major distinguishing characteristics of acid-base imbalance described in this chapter, potassium excess (hyperkalemia) is associated with both respiratory and metabolic acidosis, and neuromuscular hyperexcitability is associated with both respiratory and metabolic alkalosis.[19]

Medical Management
Diagnosis.   The blood test used most often to measure the effectiveness of ventilation and oxygen transport is oxygen saturation. However, this test only provides information about the levels of arterial oxygen and does not provide information about carbon dioxide level or pH. A more comprehensive procedure is the arterial blood gas (ABG) test (see Table 39-21).

TABLE   4-15

Overview of Acid-Base Imbalances

MECHANISM	ETIOLOGIC FACTORS	CLINICAL MANIFESTATIONS	TREATMENT
Respiratory Acidosis			

Hypoventilation	Acute respiratory failure
	COPD
	Neuromuscular disease
	  Guillain-Barré
	  Myasthenia gravis
	Respiratory center depression
	  Drugs
	    Barbiturates
	    Sedatives
	    Narcotics
	    Anesthetics
	  CNS lesions
	    Tumor
	    Stroke
	Inadequate mechanical ventilation
		Hypercapnia, restlessness, disorientation, confusion, sleepiness, visual disturbances, headache, flushing, dyspnea, cyanosis, decreased deep tendon reflexes, hyperkalemia, palpitations, pH <7.35, $Paco_2$ >45 mm Hg	Treat underlying cause; support ventilation; correct electrolyte imbalance

Excess carbon dioxide production	Hypermetabolism
	  Sepsis
	  Burns
	Total parenteral nutrition
	Enteral feeding (gastrostomy)		

Respiratory Alkalosis			

Hyperventilation	Hypoxemia
	 Pulmonary embolus
	 High altitude
	Impaired lung expansion
	  Pulmonary fibrosis
	  Ascites
	  Scoliosis
	  Pregnancy*
	Congestive heart failure
	Stimulation of respiratory center
	  Anxietyhyperventilation syndrome
	  Bacterial toxins (sepsis)
	  Ammonia (hepatic failure)
	  Salicylates (aspirin overdose)
	  CNS trauma
	  CNS tumor
	  Excessive exercise
	  Extreme stress
	  Severe pain
	Mechanical overventilation
		Tachypnea, hypocapnea, dizziness, difficulty concentrating, numbness and tingling, blurred vision, diaphoresis, dry mouth, muscle cramps, carpopedal spasms, muscle twitching and weakness, hyperreflexia, arrhythmias, pH >7.45, $PaCO_2$ <35 mm Hg, hypokalemia, hypocalcemia (see Table 4-12)	Treat underlying cause; increase carbon dioxide retention (rebreathing, sedation)

Metabolic Acidosis			

Acid excess	Renal failure (acid retention)
	Diabetic or alcoholic ketoacidosis
	Lactic acidosis
	Starvation
	Ingested toxins
	  Aspirin
	  Antifreeze
		Hyperventilation (compensatory), muscular twitching, weakness, malaise, nausea, vomiting, diarrhea, headache, hyperkalemia (cardiac arrhythmias), pH <7.35, Hco_3^-, <22 mm Hg, $Paco_2$ normal or slightly decreased, coma (death)	Treat underlying cause, correct electrolyte imbalance $NaCO_3$

Base deficit	Severe diarrhea (HCO_3 loss) Renal failure (inability to reabsorb HCO_3)		

TABLE	4-15—cont'd

Overview of Acid-Base Imbalances

MECHANISM	ETIOLOGIC FACTORS	CLINICAL MANIFESTATIONS	TREATMENT
Metabolic Alkalosis			

Fixed acid loss (with base excess)	Hypokalemia
	    Diuresis
	    Steroids
	Vomiting
	Nasogastric suctioning
		Hypoventilation (compensatory); dysrhythmias, nausea, prolonged vomiting, diarrhea, confusion, irritability, agitation, restlessness, muscle twitching, cramping, hypotonia, weakness, Trousseau's sign, paresthesias, seizures, coma, hypokalemia, hypocalcemia, pH >7.45, $PaCO_2$ normal or slightly increased	Treat underlying cause; administer potassium chloride

Excessive HCO_3^- intake	Peptic ulcer
	    Milk-alkali syndrome
	    Excessive intake of antacids
	Overcorrection of acidosis
	Massive blood transfusion		

Metabolic Alkalosis			
Excessive HCO_3^- resorption	Hyperaldosteronism Cushing's disease		

COPD, chronic obstructive pulmonary disease; *ARDS*, adult respiratory distress syndrome; *PaCO₂*, partial pressure of carbon dioxide; *NaCO₃*, sodium bicarbonate; *HCO₃⁻*,
*In the third trimester of pregnancy, the hormone progesterone also stimulates respiration.

This measurement is important in the diagnosis and treatment of ventilation, oxygen transport, and acid-base problems. The test measures the amount of dissolved oxygen and carbon dioxide in arterial blood and indicates acid-bases status by measurement of the arterial blood pH. The pH is inversely proportional to the hydrogen ion concentration (H^+) in the blood. Therefore, as the hydrogen ion concentration (H^+) increases (acidosis), the pH decreases; as the hydrogen ion concentration (H^+) decreases (alkalosis), the pH increases.

The PCO_2 is a measure of the *partial pressure of carbon dioxide* in the blood. PCO_2 is termed the *respiratory component* in acid-base measurement because the carbon dioxide level is primarily controlled by the lungs. As the carbon dioxide level increases, the pH decreases (respiratory acidosis); as the carbon dioxide level decreases, the pH increases (respiratory alkalosis).

Treatment. Treatment in acid-base imbalances is directed toward the underlying cause and correction of any coexisting electrolyte imbalance. For example, respiratory infections contributing to ventilatory failure are managed with appropriate antibiotic therapy. Use of pharmaceutical agents that depress the respiratory control center is minimized. Dialysis may be indicated in renal failure or overdose of toxins. Respiratory support may be required via hydration, pulmonary hygiene, oxygen therapy, and possibly, continuous mechanical ventilation.

◆ Respiratory Acidosis

Respiratory acidosis is nearly always due to hypoventilation and subsequent retention of carbon dioxide. In a therapy setting, respiratory acidosis is most commonly observed in the population with COPD whenever the diaphragm is impaired

(e.g., Guillain-Barré syndrome, myasthenia gravis, chest wall deformities); secondary to burns; and as a result of lesions of the CNS (e.g., tumor, stroke, muscular dystrophy).

The respiratory system has an important role in maintaining acid-base equilibrium. In response to an increase in the hydrogen ion concentration in body fluids, the respiratory rate increases, causing more carbon dioxide (CO_2) to be released from the lung. Anything that impairs this carbon dioxide (CO_2) exhalation causes the CO_2 to accumulate in the blood, where it unites with water to form carbonic acid (H_2CO_3), decreasing the blood pH. In addition, the kidneys begin to excrete more acid and retain more bicarbonate to further correct the acid imbalance.

Respiratory acidosis can be acute, due to a sudden failure in ventilation, or chronic, as with long-term pulmonary disease (e.g., COPD). In the *acute* episode, the blood buffer systems cannot compensate to restore the acid-base balance because normal blood circulation and tissue perfusion are impaired. The lungs and kidneys are little help because the lungs are malfunctioning and the kidneys require more time to compensate than the acute condition permits. *Chronic* respiratory acidosis results from gradual and irreversible loss of ventilatory function. Although there is increased retention of carbon dioxide, the kidneys have time to compensate by retaining bicarbonate and thereby maintaining a pH within tolerable limits. However, if even a minor respiratory infection develops, the person is subjected to a rapidly developing state of acute acidosis, because the lungs cannot remove more than a minimal amount of carbon dioxide.

Clinical Manifestations. Acute respiratory acidosis produces CNS disturbances that reflect changes in the pH of cerebrospinal fluid (CSF) rather than increased carbon dioxide levels in cerebral circulation. Effects range from restlessness, confusion, and apprehension to somnolence (sleepiness), with a fine or flapping tremor (see the section on Asterixis in Chapter 16), or coma. The person may report headaches and shortness of breath with retraction and use of accessory muscles. On examination, deep tendon reflexes may be depressed. This disorder may also cause cardiovascular abnormalities, such as tachycardia, hypertension, atrial and ventricular arrhythmias, and, in severe acidosis, hypotension with vasodilation (bounding pulses and warm periphery).

◆ Respiratory Alkalosis

Respiratory alkalosis, the opposite of respiratory acidosis, occurs as a result of a loss of acid without compensation, most commonly when the lungs excrete excessive amounts of carbon dioxide (hyperventilation). Conditions associated with respiratory alkalosis fall into the following two categories:

1. *Pulmonary*, caused by hypoxemia in early stage pulmonary problems (e.g., pulmonary edema, pulmonary embolism, pneumonia, and acute asthma) and by overuse of a mechanical ventilator
2. *Nonpulmonary*, which includes anxiety; hysteria; pain; hypoxia; fever; high environmental temperature; pregnancy; poisoning; early cerebral vascular accident (CVA); and CNS disease (see Table 4-15).

Clinical Manifestations. The cardinal sign of respiratory alkalosis is deep, rapid breathing, possibly exceeding 40 breaths/minute (much like the Kussmaul's respirations that characterize diabetic acidosis) (see Table 4-15). Such hyperventilation usually leads to CNS and neuromuscular disturbances such as dizziness or light-headedness (due to below-normal carbon dioxide levels that decrease cerebral blood flow); inability to concentrate; tingling and numbness of the extremities and around the mouth; blurred vision; diaphoresis; dry mouth; muscle cramps; carpopedal (wrist and foot) spasms; twitching (possibly progressing to tetany); and muscle weakness. Severe respiratory alkalosis may cause cardiac arrhythmias, convulsions, and syncope.

◆ Metabolic Acidosis

Metabolic acidosis is an accumulation of acids or a deficit of bases, usually resulting from an accumulation in the blood of acids (e.g., ketone bodies and lactic acid or in the presence of renal impairment, phosphoric or sulfuric acids). This type of acidosis can occur with an acid gain (e.g., diabetic ketoacidosis, lactic acidosis, poisoning, renal failure) or bicarbonate loss (e.g., diarrhea) (see Table 15-2). Specific etiologic factors are listed in Table 4-15. *Ketoacidosis* occurs when insufficient insulin for the proper use of glucose results in increased breakdown of fat. This accelerated fat breakdown produces ketones and other acids. Although the body attempts to neutralize these increased acids, the plasma bicarbonate (HCO_3^-) is used up. In the case of *renal failure*, the failing kidney cannot rid the body of excess acids and cannot produce the necessary bicarbonate to buffer the acid load that is accumulating in the body. *Lactic acidosis* occurs as excess lactic acid is produced during strenuous exercise or when oxygen is insufficient for proper use of carbohydrate, glucose, and water. *Severe diarrhea* depletes the body of highly alkaline intestinal and pancreatic secretions.[67]

Clinical Manifestations. The symptoms of metabolic acidosis can include muscular twitching, weakness, malaise, nausea, vomiting, diarrhea, and headache (see Table 4-15). Compensatory hyperventilation may occur as a result of stimulation of the hypothalamus as the body attempts to rid itself of excess hydrogen through increased ventilation and subsequent excretion of carbonic acid. As the acid level goes up, these symptoms progress to stupor, unconsciousness, coma, and death. The breath may have a fruity odor in the presence of acetone associated with ketoacidosis.

◆ Metabolic Alkalosis

Metabolic alkalosis occurs when either an abnormal loss of acid or excess accumulation of bicarbonate occurs. This condition is associated with hypokalemia (potassium deficiency) commonly seen in hospitalized clients secondary to taking certain medications (e.g., diuretics, steroids). Postoperative loss of acids through vomiting or gastric suctioning may also result in metabolic alkalosis. In the outpatient setting, excessive use of antacids and milk (milk alkali syndrome) may occur in people with peptic ulcers associated with NSAIDs. Other causes are listed in Table 4-15.

Clinical Manifestations. Signs and symptoms occur as the body attempts to correct the acid-base imbalance, primarily through hypoventilation. Respirations are shallow and slow as the lungs attempt to compensate by building up carbonic acid stores. Clinical manifestations may be mild at first, with muscle weakness, irritability, confusion, and muscle twitching (see Table 4-15). If untreated, the condition progresses and the person may become comatose, with possible convulsive seizures and respiratory paralysis.

◆ Aging and Acid-Base Regulation

The normal aging process results in decreased ventilatory capacity and loss of alveolar surface area for gas exchange; thus older adults are prone to respiratory acidosis due to hypoventilation and to respiratory alkalosis due to hypoxemia and subsequent hyperventilation. Older adults are often taking multiple medications for hypertension or cardiovascular disease; these drugs may contribute to hypokalemia (potassium deficiency) and metabolic alkalosis. Respiratory compensation in these conditions can be compromised, owing to the structural and functional changes mentioned. Decreased cardiac output in the aging person diminishes renal perfusion and glomerular filtration.[35] Aldosterone is less effective in older adults, as is ammonia buffering. These changes limit renal compensation for respiratory imbalances and place the individual at higher risk for metabolic imbalance.[73,88]

Special Implications for the Therapist 4-12

ACID-BASE IMBALANCES

The therapist must observe clients at risk for acid-base imbalance for any early symptoms. This is especially true for people with known pulmonary, cardiovascular, or renal disease; clients in a hypermetabolic state such as occurs in fever, sepsis, or burns; clients receiving total parenteral nutrition or enteral tube feedings that are high in carbohydrate; mechanically ventilated clients; clients with insulin-dependent diabetes; older clients whose age-related decreases in respiratory and renal function may limit their ability to compensate for acid-base disturbances; and clients with vomiting, diarrhea (see Table 15-2), or enteric drainage.[73] Specific reference values in acid-base disorders are listed in Tables 4-15 and 39-9.

Client and family education in the prevention of acute episodes of metabolic acidosis, particularly diabetic ketoacidosis, is essential. A fruity breath odor from rising acid levels (acetone) may be detected by the therapist treating someone who has uncontrolled diabetes. The therapist should not be hesitant to ask the client about this breath odor, as immediate medical intervention is required for diabetic ketoacidosis. Dehydration occurs rapidly as a result of severe hyperglycemia. A rising pulse rate and a drop in blood pressure are critical (and often, late) indicators of a fluid volume deficit due to dehydration.

Safety measures to avoid injury during involuntary muscular contractions are the same as for convulsions or epileptic seizures. Vigorous restraint can cause orthopedic injuries as the muscles contract strongly against resistance. Placing padding to protect the person is a key to prevention of injury.

Measures that facilitate breathing are essential to client care during respiratory acidosis. Frequent turning, coughing, and deep breathing exercises to encourage oxygen-carbon dioxide exchange are beneficial. Postural drainage, unless contraindicated by the client's condition, may be effective in promoting adequate ventilation.

In the case of respiratory hyperventilation, rebreathing carbon dioxide in a paper sack is helpful, as is encouraging the individual to hold the breath. Oxygen may be given to reduce respiratory effort and the resultant blowing off of carbon dioxide in the person who has anoxia caused by pulmonary infection or congestive heart failure. Individuals with COPD may retain carbon dioxide; the use of oxygen is contraindicated in these clients, as it can further depress the respiratory drive, causing death.

Any client receiving diuretic therapy must be monitored for signs of potassium depletion (e.g., postural hypotension, muscle weakness, and fatigue; see Table 4-12) and alkalosis (see Table 4-15). Decreased respiratory rate may be an indication of compensation by the lungs, but the physician must make this assessment. Signs of neural irritability, such as Trousseau's sign (see Fig. 4-2), may be seen when taking blood pressure measurements, and they are helpful in detecting early stages of tetany due to calcium deficiency. ■

REFERENCES

1. ACSM (American College of Sports Medicine): ACSM guidelines for exercise testing and prescription, ed 6, Baltimore, 2000, Lippincott Williams and Wilkins.
2. American Diabetes Association: Clinical practice recommendations 2000, *Diabetes Care* 23(Suppl 1):S1-116, 2000.
3. Augustine E: Oncology section of the APTA position statement—physical therapy: management of lymphedema in patients with a history of cancer, *Rehabil Oncol* 18(1):9-12, 2000.
4. Bahrke MS et al: Risk factors associated with anabolic-androgenic steroid use among adolescents, *Sports Med* 29(6):397-405, 2000.
5. Bartucci M: Management of persons with organ/tissue transplants. In Phipps W, Sands J, Marek J, editors: *Medical-surgical nursing concepts and clinical practice*, ed 6, St Louis, 1999, Mosby.
6. Bauman WA and Spungen AM: Metabolic changes in persons after spinal cord injury, *Phys Med Rehabil Clin N Am* 11(1):109-140, 2000.
7. Bender C, Yasko J: Nursing management, cancer. In Lewis S, Heitkemper M, Dirksen S, editors: *Medical-surgical nursing: assessment and management of clinical problems*, ed 5, St Louis, 2000, Mosby.
8. Braith RW et al: Resistance exercise prevents glucocorticoid-induced myopathy in heart transplant recipients, *Med Sci Sports Exerc* 30(4):483-489, 1998.
9. Bushbacher L: Rehabilitation of patients with peripheral neuropathies. In Braddom R, editor: *Physical medicine and rehabilitation*, ed 2, Philadelphia, 2000, WB Saunders.
10. Casaburi R: Skeletal muscle function in COPD, *Chest* 117(Suppl 1):267S-271S, 2000.
11. Cho L, Glatstein E: Radiation injury. In Fauci A et al, editors: *Principles of internal medicine*, ed 14, New York, 1998, McGraw-Hill.
12. Chyka P: How many deaths occur annually from adverse drug reactions in the United States? *Am J Med* 109:122-130, 2000.
13. Ciccone C: Geriatric pharmacology. In Guccione A, editor: *Geriatric physical therapy*, ed 2, St Louis, 2000, Mosby.
14. Ciccone C: Introduction: pharmacology, *Physical Therapy* 75:342-351, 1995.
15. Cohen J: Avoiding adverse reactions: effective lower-dose drug therapies for older patients, *Geriatrics* 55: 54-56, 59-60, 63-64, 2000.
16. Cohen R, Moelleken B: Disorders due to physical agents. In Tierney L, McPhee S, Papadakis M, editors: *Current medical diagnosis and treatment*, ed 39, New York, 2000, Lange Medical Books/McGraw-Hill.
17. Cotran R, Kumar V, Collins T: Acute and chronic inflammation. In Cotran R, Kumar V, Collins T, editors: *Robbins pathologic basis of disease*, ed 6, Philadelphia, 1999, WB Saunders.
18. Dantas F, Rampes H: Do homeopathic medicines provoke adverse effects? A systematic review, *Br Homeopath J* 89(Suppl):S35-8, 2000.
19. Dean E: Monitoring systems in the intensive care unit. In Frownfelter D, Dean E, editors: *Principles and practice of cardiopulmonary physical therapy*, ed 3, St Louis, Mosby, 1996.
20. Dean E: Oxygen transport deficits in systemic disease and implications for physical therapy, *Physical Therapy* 77(2):187-202, 1997.
21. Dean E et al: Cardiovascular/cardiopulmonary physical therapy sinks or swims in the twenty-first century: addressing the health care issues of our time, *Physical Therapy* 80(12):1275-1278, 2000.
22. Debaere C et al: Diffusion-weighted MRI in cyclosporin A neurotoxicity for the classification of cerebral edema, *Eur Radiol* 9(9):1916-1918, 1999.
23. Decramer M, de Bock V, Dom R: Functional and histologic picture of steroid-induced myopathy in chronic obstructive pulmonary disease, *Am J Respir Crit Care* 153(6 Pt 1):1958-1964, 1996.
24. Demling RH, DeSanti L: Closure of the "non-healing wound" corresponds with correction of weight loss using the anabolic agent oxandrolone, *Ostomy Wound Manage* 44(10):58-68, 1998.
25. Demling RH, DeSanti L: Oxandrolone, an anabolic steroid, significantly increases the rate of weight gain in the recovery phase after major burns, *J Trauma* 43(1):47-51, 1997.
26. Dimeo FC: Exercise programs for cancer patients during chemo- and radiotherapy. In L'Esprit Rehabilitation Centers Symposium: *Cancer rehabilitation: the multidisciplinary integration of traditional and "whole person" care*, Montreal, Canada, January 21-23, 2000, The Symposium.
27. Dimeo FC et al: Effects of aerobic exercise on the physical performance and incidence of treatment-related complications after high-dose chemotherapy, *Blood* 90:3390-3394, 1997.
28. Dimeo FC, Rumberger BG, Keul J: Aerobic exercise as therapy for cancer fatigue, *Med Sci Sports Exercise* 30:475-478, 1998.
29. Dimeo FC et al: Effects of physical activity on the fatigue and psychological status of cancer patients during chemotherapy, *Cancer* 85(10):2273-2277, 1999.
30. Dirksen S: Integumentary system. In Lewis S, Heitkemper M, Dirksen S, editors: *Medical-surgical nursing: assessment and management of clinical problems*, ed 5, St Louis, 2000, Mosby.
31. Drouin J, Pfalzer LA: Moderate intensity aerobic exercise for the person with cancer. In Wruble E, editor: *Acute care perspectives*, Robbinsville, N.J., spring 2001, Acute Care Section—APTA.
32. Eason JM et al: Detrimental effects of short-term glucocorticoid use on the rat diaphragm, *Physical Therapy* 80(2):160-167, 2000.
33. Eifel PJ: Chemoradiation for carcinoma of the cervix: advances and opportunities, *Radiat Res* 154(3):229-236, 2000.

34. Eisenhauer L et al: *Clinical pharmacology and nursing management,* ed 5, Philadelphia, 1998, JB Lippincott.

35. Felsenthal G, Lehman J, Stein B: Principles of geriatric rehabilitation. In Braddom R, editor: *Physical medicine and rehabilitation,* ed 2, Philadelphia, 2000, WB Saunders.

36. Fine N, Scallion L: Hodgkins disease. In Miaskowski C, Buchsel P, editors: *Oncology nursing: assessment and clinical care,* St Louis, 1999, Mosby.

37. Finn S, Scherer R: Seizure after exercise in the heat: recognizing life-threatening hyponatremia, *Physician Sports Med* 28:61, 62, 65-67, 2000.

38. Fitzgerald P: Endocrinology. In Tierney L, McPhee S, Papadakis M, editors: *Current medical diagnosis and treatment,* ed 39, New York, 2000, Lange Medical Books/McGraw-Hill.

39. Gerber LH: Cancer rehabilitation: the bridge to cross between organ and organism. In L'Esprit Rehabilitation Centers Symposium: *Cancer rehabilitation: the multidisciplinary integration of traditional and "whole person" care,* Montreal, Canada, January 21-23, 2000, The Symposium.

40. Gudas S: Shoulder rehabilitation post surgery and irradiation: brachial plexopathy. In L'Esprit Rehabilitation Centers Symposium: *Cancer rehabilitation: the multidisciplinary integration of traditional and "whole person" care,* Montreal, Canada, January 21-23, 2000, The Symposium.

41. American Physical Therapy Association: *Guide to physical therapist practice,* ed 2, Alexandria, Va, 2001, The Association.

42. Guyton A, Hall J: *Textbook of medical physiology,* ed 10, Philadelphia, 2000, WB Saunders.

43. Haas L: Endocrine problems. In Lewis S, Heitkemper M, Dirksen S, editors: *Medical-surgical nursing: assessment and management of clinical problems,* ed 5, St Louis, 2000, Mosby.

44. Hammerstad J: Strength and reflexes. In Goetz C, Pappert E, editors: *Textbook of clinical neurology,* ed 1, Philadelphia, 1999, WB Saunders.

45. Heitkemper M: Upper gastrointestinal problems. In Lewis S, Heitkemper M, Dirksen S, editors: *Medical-surgical nursing: assessment and management of clinical problems,* ed 5, St Louis, 2000, Mosby.

46. Horne M, Bond E: Fluid, electrolyte and acid base imbalances. In Lewis S, Heitkemper M, Dirksen S, editors: *Medical-surgical nursing: assessment and management of clinical problems,* ed 5, St Louis, 2000, Mosby.

47. Johansson S et al: Brachial plexopathy after postoperative radiotherapy of breast cancer patients-a long term follow-up, *Acta Oncol* 39(3):373-382, 2000.

48. Karch A: *2001 Lippincott's nursing drug guide,* Philadelphia, 20001, JB Lippincott.

49. Keller K, Fenske N: Uses of vitamins A, C and E and related compounds in dermatology: a review, *J Am Acad Dermatol* 39(4 Pt 1): 611-625, 1998.

50. Kim PK, Deutschman CS: Inflammatory responses and mediators, *Surg Clin North Am* 80: 885-894, 2000.

51. Kopple JD: Therapeutic approaches to malnutrition in chronic dialysis patients: the different modalities of nutritional support, *Am J Kidney Dis* 33(1):180-185, 1999.

52. Lewis S: Inflammation and infection. In Lewis S, Heitkemper M, Dirksen S, editors: *Medical-surgical nursing: assessment and management of clinical problems,* ed 5, St Louis, 2000, Mosby, 2000.

53. Lichter A: Radiation therapy. In Abeloff M et al, editors: *Clinical oncology,* ed 2, New York, 2000, Churchill-Livingstone.

54. Loehne H: Personal communication. Winston-Salem, NC, 2000.

55. Ludin A, Macklis RM: Radiotherapy for pediatric genitourinary tumors. Its role and long-term consequences, *Urol Clin North Am* 27(3):553-562, 2000.

56. Lye M: Disturbances of homeostasis. In Talis R, Fillit H, Brocklehurst JC, editors: *Brocklehurst's textbook of geriatric medicine and gerontology,* ed 5, New York, 1998, Churchill Livingstone.

57. Massie B: Systemic hypertension. In Tierney L, McPhee S, Papadakis M, editors: *Current medical diagnosis and treatment,* ed 39, New York, 2000, Lange Medical Books/McGraw-Hill.

58. McArdle W, Katch F, Katch V: *Exercise physiology: energy, nutrition and human performance,* ed 4, Philadelphia, 2000, Lippincott Williams and Wilkins.

59. McDonald C, Muglia J, Vittorio C: Alopecia and cutaneous complications. In Abeloff M, Armitage J, Lichter A, Niederhuber J: *Clinical oncology,* ed 2, New York, 2000a, Churchill-Livingstone.

60. McDonald S, Garrow G, Rubin P: Pulmonary complications. In Abeloff M, Armitage J, Lichter A, Niederhuber J, editors: *Clinical oncology,* ed 2, New York, 2000b, Churchill-Livingstone.

61. Midgley SJ et al: Risk behaviors for HIV and hepatitis infection among anabolic-androgenic steroid users, *AIDS Care* 12(2):163-170, 2000.

62. Mock V et al: Effects of exercise on fatigue, physical functioning, and emotional distress during radiation therapy for breast cancer, *Oncology Nurs Forum* 24(6):991-1000, 1997.

63. Moncur C, Williams HG: Rheumatoid arthritis: status of drug therapies, *Physical Therapy* 75: 61-75, 1995.

64. National Cancer Institute: *Radiation therapy and you,* Bethesda, MD, 1997 US Department of Health and Human Services.

65. Nicol N, Ruszkowski A: Integumentary problems. In Lewis S, Heitkemper M, Dirksen S, editors: *Medical-surgical nursing: assessment and management of clinical problems,* ed 5, St Louis, 2000, Mosby.

66. Nicholas J, Lennard T: Joint and soft tissue injection techniques. In Braddom R, editor: *Physical medicine and rehabilitation,* ed 2, Philadelphia, 2000, WB Saunders.

67. Okuda T, Kiyoshi K, Papadakis M: Fluid and electrolyte disorders. In Tierney L, McPhee S, Papadakis M, editors: *Current medical diagnosis and treatment,* ed 39, New York, 2000, Lange Medical Books/McGraw-Hill.

68. Papathanasoglou E et al: Does programmed cell death (apoptosis) play a role in the development of multiple organ dysfunction in critically ill patients: a review and theoretical framework, *Critical Care Medicine* 28:537-542, 2000.

69. Parssinen M et al: Increased premature mortality of competitive power-lifters suspected have used anabolic agents, *Int J Sports Med* 21(3):225-227, 2000.

70. Percy L, Fang M: Geriatric rheumatology, geropharmacology for the rheumatologist, *Rheumatic Dis Clin North Amer* 26:1-21, 2000.

71. Pfalzer L: *Personal communication,* Physical Therapy Department, School of Health Professions and Studies, Flint, Mich, 2000, University of Michigan-Flint.

72. Portenoy R, McCaffery M: Adjuvant analgesics. In McCaffery M, Pasero C, editors: *Pain: clinical manual,* ed 2, St Louis, 1999, Mosby.

73. Priebe H: The aged cardiovascular risk patient, *Br J Anaesth* 85:763-778, 2000.

74. Reents S: *Sport and exercise pharmacology,* Champain, Ill, 2000, Human Kinetics.

75. Rich JD et al: The infectious complications of anabolic-androgenic steroid injection, *Int J Sports Med* 20(8):563-566, 1999.

76. Rieger PT, Escalante CP: Complications of cancer treatment. In Boyer K et al: *Primary care oncology,* Philadelphia, 1999, WB Saunders.

77. Sajadieh A et al: Nonsteroidal anti-inflammatory drugs after acute myocardial infarction, DAVIT Study Group, Danish Verapamil Infarction Trial, *Am J Cardiol* 83(8):1263-1265, 1999.

78. Schindl A et al: Low intensity laser irradiation in the treatment of recalcitrant radiation ulcers in patients with breast cancer, *Photodermatol Photoimmunol Photomed* 16(1):34-37, 2000.

79. Schnirring L: Growth hormone doping: the search for a test, *Physician Sportsmed* 28:16-18, 2000.

80. Shaddick N: The natural history of exercise-induced anaphylaxis: survey results from a 10-year follow-up study, *J Allergy Clin Immunol* 104:123-127, 1999.

81. Segar ML et al: The effect of aerobic exercise on self-esteem and depressive and anxiety symptoms among breast cancer survivors, *Oncol Nurs Forum* 25(1):107-113, 1998.

82. Sheffield-Moore M: Androgens and the control of skeletal muscle protein synthesis, *Ann Med* 32(3):181-186, 2000.

83. Stilger VG, Yesalis CE: Anabolic-androgenic steroid use among high school football players, *J Community Health* 24(2):131-145, 1999.

84. Sturmi J, Diorio D: Sports pharmacology, *Clinics Sports Med* 17:261-281, 1998.

85. Sullivan ML, Martinez CM, Gallagher EJ: Atrial fibrillation and anabolic steroids, *J Emerg Med* 17(5):851-857, 1999.

86. Sullivan P, Markos P: Ambulation: a framework of practice applied to a functional outcome. In Guccione A, editor: *Geriatric physical therapy,* ed 2, St Louis, 2000, Mosby.

87. Thiblin I, Lindquist O, Rajs J: Cause and manner of death among users of anabolic androgenic steroids, *J Forensic Sci* 45(1):16-23, 2000.

88. Thompson L: Physiological changes associated with aging. In Guccione A, editor: *Geriatric physical therapy,* ed 2, St Louis, 2000, Mosby.

89. Tunkel R et al: Physical rehabilitation. In Abeloff M et al: *Clinical oncology,* ed 2, New York, 2000, Churchill-Livingstone.

90. Varricchio C, editor: *A cancer source book for nurses*, ed 7, Atlanta, 1997, American Cancer Society.

91. Whelton A: Nephrotoxicity of nonsteroidal anti-inflammatory drugs: physiologic foundations and clinical implications, *Am J Med* 106(5B):13S-24S, 1999.

92. Wilkes G, Ingwersen K, Burke M: *1999 oncology nursing drug handbook*, Boston, 1999, Jones and Bartlett.

93. Wilson B, Shannon M, Stang C: *Nursing drug guide*, Upper Saddle River, NJ, 2001, Prentice-Hall.

94. Winningham ML: The role of exercise in cancer therapy. In Watson R, Eisinger M, editors: *Exercise and disease*, Boca Raton, Fla, 1992, CRC Press.

95. Wolfe R et al: Testosterone and muscle protein metabolism, *Mayo Clin Proc* 75(Suppl):S55-59, 2000.

96. Workman M, Visovsky C: Cancer pathophysiology. In Miaskowski C, Buchsel P, editors: *Oncology nursing: assessment and clinical care*, St Louis, Mosby, 1999.

97. Worthington K: Guarding against radiation exposure, *AJN* 100(5):104, 2000.

98. Young L: Sepsis syndrome. In Mandell G, Bennett J, Dolin R, editors: *Principles and practice of infectious diseases*, ed 5, Philadelphia, 2000, Churchill Livingstone.

CHAPTER 5

INJURY, INFLAMMATION, AND HEALING

STEVEN H. TEPPER AND D. MICHAEL MCKEOUGH

*P*athology is defined as the structural and functional changes in the body caused by disease or trauma. Understanding the normal structure and function of the tissues is required before the discussion of pathology. The organization of the material presented in this chapter parallels the process underlying pathology—that is, cell injury and the factors causing this injury, inflammation as a secondary response to cell injury, and tissue healing, the third step of the process toward homeostasis.

Recent knowledge showing the influences of the nervous system on immune and inflammatory responses and how these contribute to the healing and repair process composes a new area of science called *psychoneuroimmunology* (see Chapters 1 and 6). It is now clear that mast cells, T cells, neutrophils, and monocytes can directly alter tissue physiology through the release of mediators and cytokines. The role of nerve-immune interactions in regulation and tissue healing is just beginning to be revealed and will continue to enhance our understanding of and intervention in injury, inflammation, and recovery.[2,3]

CELLULAR AGING

The ability of a cell to resist microorganisms or to recover from injury or inflammation is dependent in part on the underlying state or health of the cells. Age-related changes at the cellular level are present but remain difficult to measure or quantify; researchers are working toward finding satisfactory biomarkers of aging at the cellular level.* The recent research on telomeres, the structure at the end of chromosomes is revealing clues about a cell's life span and its relationship to human aging and many illnesses associated with aging. Because of the close association between telomere dysfunction and malignancy, both pathologists and clinicians expect this molecule to be a useful malignancy marker.[21]

Various components of cells (e.g., mitochondria, ribosomes, cell membrane) are subject to changes associated with aging. Mitochondrial deoxyribonucleic acid (DNA) is considered a prime target for age-related changes. DNA has to replicate and maintain itself to preserve the primary genetic message. This takes place through division, which can result in alterations of the genetic code by anything that can damage DNA (e.g.,

physical, chemical, or biologic factors; spontaneous mutations of genes; exposure to radiation). Anything that can alter the information content of the cell can cause changes in function and affect the ability of the cell to maintain homeostasis.

Age-associated deterioration in cells leads to tissue or organ deficiencies and ultimately to the expression of aging or disease. The most well described age-associated change in the subcellular structure (lysosomes) of postmitotic cells, especially neurons and cardiac myocytes, is the presence of a component called *lipofuscin*, an aging-pigment granule that is found in high concentrations in old cells. The explanation for the increase of lipofuscin with age and the effects of these intracellular deposits on function remains unknown. It is suspected that pressure from this pigmented lipid on the cell nucleus may interfere with cellular function.

The aging process is often associated with impaired wound healing, but the cellular and molecular mechanisms implicated are not completely understood.[43] More than 300 theories exist that explain the aging phenomenon from a cellular level. Many of these theories originate from the study of changes that accumulate with time. In organs that are composed of cells that cannot regenerate, such as those of the heart and brain, the wear-and-tear hypothesis may account for the decline in function of these organs. Other factors may also play a role, such as the influence of genetics suggested by the genetic hypothesis (i.e., that aging is a genetically predetermined process) (see Chapter 1).

The free radical theory of aging is the most popular and widely tested and is based on the chemical nature and wide presence of free radicals causing DNA damage and cellular oxidative stress as it relates to the aging process (see the section on Mechanisms of Cell Injury: Chemical Factors in this chapter). Recently, the discovery of the telomere has added an additional theory for the molecular mechanisms that lead to senescence: the telomere aging clock theory, which suggests that the telomere acts as a molecular clock signaling the onset of cell senescence. Normal human cells will not divide forever but eventually enter a viable nondividing state (senescence). The progressive accumulation of senescent cells contributes to, but does not exclusively cause, the aging process. Cell senescence acts as an anticancer mechanism to control the potential for cellular proliferation[38,68] (see Chapter 8).

Pathologic changes associated with aging vary from individual to individual but usually consist of reduced functional reserve caused by atrophy of tissue or organ. Resistance to infection declines with age and pathologic processes such as atherosclerosis result in increased cardiovascular and cere-

---

*Two difficulties exist in the study of cellular aging: (1) current research techniques are not accurate enough to measure decline in function of specific cellular components and (2) human studies in vivo are obviously very limited; using animal models may not accurately reflect aging in human tissues.

brovascular injuries or death. Studies have shown that considerable potential exists for improving aerobic capacity by training. This observation has cellular implications. For example, mitochondria of cardiac and skeletal muscle cells improve function under appropriate training conditions. If changes in diet, exercise, treatment with hormones, or compounds such as antioxidants (see Fig. 5-2) are able to modify damage by reactive oxygen species and the body can reestablish cellular norms, then this information has great implications for the various cellular and molecular theories about aging and our approach to the aging process.[18]

CELL INJURY

The structural and functional changes produced by pathology begin with injury to the cells that make up the tissues. Mild injury produced by stressors leads to sublethal alterations of the affected cells, whereas moderate or severe injury leads to lethal alterations. After cell injury, the body reacts by initiating the process of inflammation. The amount, type, and severity of the inflammatory reaction are dependent on the amount, type, and severity of the injury. Inflammation is responsible for the removal of the injurious agent, removal of cellular debris, and the initiation of the healing process. The healing process occurs to allow restoration of structure and function whenever possible. To achieve complete restoration of function, regeneration of the damaged tissue must occur. Often, regeneration of the tissue is not possible, and the body must settle for tissue repair by nonfunctional, connective tissue (fibrosis, scar tissue). This connective tissue helps maintain structural integrity but has none of the functional properties of the original cells and tissues. Understanding cell injury, inflammation, and tissue healing will serve as a solid foundation for the other topics presented in this text.

◆ Mechanisms of Cell Injury
Cells may be damaged by a variety of mechanisms. The most important mechanisms are listed in Box 5-1. Each of these mechanisms leads to either a reversible (sublethal) or irreversible (lethal) injury. Whether the injury is reversible is dependent on the cell's ability to withstand the derangement of homeostatic mechanisms and its adaptability (i.e., ability to return to a state of homeostasis). Reversing the injury and achieving homeostasis is determined by a combination of factors including the mechanism of injury, length of time the injury is present without intervention, and the severity of the injury.

BOX 5-1

Mechanisms of Cell Injury

Ischemia (lack of blood supply)	Nutritional factors
Infectious agents	Physical factors
Immune reactions	Chemical factors
Genetic factors	

Ischemia
At the level of tissue or organ, ischemia is blood flow below the minimum necessary to maintain cell homeostasis and metabolic function. This can be due to a reduction in flow or an increase in metabolism of the tissue beyond the capability of the arterial vascular system. Insufficient blood flow results in a critical reduction in oxygen delivery to the tissue that is partial (hypoxia) or total (anoxia); a decreased delivery of nutrients; and decreased removal of waste products from the tissue. The lack of oxygen leads to loss of aerobic metabolism. The resulting reduction in adenosine triphosphate (ATP) synthesis leads to accumulation of ions and fluid intracellularly. The cells swell and their function is compromised (see the section on Reversible Cell Injury in this chapter).

Hypoxia or anoxia may occur under many circumstances including obstruction of the respiratory tree (e.g., suffocation secondary to drowning); inadequate transport of oxygen across the respiratory surfaces of the lung (e.g., pneumonia); inadequate transport of oxygen in the blood (e.g., anemia); or an inability of the cell to use oxygen for cellular respiration (e.g., chemical poisoning).[16] Ischemia is usually the result of arterial lumen obstruction and narrowing caused by atherosclerosis and/or an intravascular clot called a *thrombus*. Ischemia, resulting in myocardial infarction and stroke (lack of blood flow to the heart or brain, respectively), can cause death of tissue (necrosis) and accounts for two of the three leading causes of mortality in industrialized nations.

Infectious Agents
Infectious agents such as bacteria, viruses, mycoplasmas, fungi, rickettsiae, protozoa, prions, and helminths (see Chapter 7) may also cause cell injury or death. Bacterial and viral agents are responsible for the vast majority of infections. Bacterial infections cause cell injury primarily by invading tissue and releasing exotoxins and endotoxins that can cause cell lysis and degradation of extracellular matrix and aid in the spread of the infection. Injury can also result from the inflammatory/immunologic reactions induced by bacteria in the host. For example, exotoxins may be released by clostridial organisms that cause gas gangrene, tetanus, and botulism. *Clostridium tetani*, for example, releases an exotoxin that is preferentially absorbed by the alpha motor neurons and delivered into the central nervous system (CNS). Once inside the CNS the exotoxin crosses the synapse of the anterior horn cell and interferes with release of inhibitory neurotransmitters. This disruption of homeostasis eventually causes the activation of motor neurons that in turn causes involuntary muscular contractions (tetanus).[58]

When microorganisms or their toxins are present in the blood, a condition called *sepsis* can occur. Endotoxins released from gram-negative bacteria induce the synthesis of cytokines (extracts of normal leukocytes such as tumor necrosis factor [TNF] and interleukins [ILs]) that are responsible for many of the systemic manifestations of sepsis (see Table 5-5). In sepsis, endothelial cell damage, loss of plasma volume, and maldistribution of blood flow result in hypovolemia. Cardiovascular collapse may ensue and lead to a condition called *septic shock*. The detection of an infectious agent initiates an inflammatory reaction designed to contain and inactivate the pathogen but the magnitude of this defensive response by the host may also cause cellular or tissue destruction in the infected area.

Viruses kill cells by one of two mechanisms (Fig. 5-1) and are the consequence of complete redirection of the cell's biosynthesis towards viral replication. The first is a direct cytopathic effect usually found with ribonucleic (RNA) viruses. These viruses kill from within by disturbing various cellular processes or by disrupting the integrity of the nucleus and/or plasma membrane. Virally encoded proteins become inserted into the plasma membrane of the host cell (forming a channel) and alter the permeability of the cell membrane to ions. The resulting loss of the ionic barrier leads to cell swelling and death. DNA type viruses also kill cells through an indirect cytopathic effect by integrating themselves into the cellular genome. These viruses encode the production of foreign proteins, which are exposed on the cell surface and recognized by the body's immune cells. Immunocompetent cells such as the T lymphocyte recognize these virally encoded proteins inserted into the plasma membrane of host cells and attack and destroy the infected cell. When the immune system is compromised or if the number of invading microorganisms overwhelms the immune system, disease (and the symptoms of illness) occurs.

Immune Reactions

The mechanisms by which the immune system can lead to cell injury or death include antibody attachment, complement activation, and activation of the inflammatory cells (e.g., neutrophils, macrophages, T and B lymphocytes, mast cells, basophils). Although the immune system normally functions in defense against foreign antigens, sometimes the system becomes overzealous in its activity leading to hypersensitivities ranging from a mild allergy to life-threatening anaphylactic reactions or autoimmune disorders (attacking oneself).

Cell injury and disease can be caused by the immune system in numerous ways. For example, allergies are caused by the presence of high numbers of a specific antibody-E (IgE) on the surface of specialized cells (mast cells and basophils, which release histamine), resulting in mild, moderate, or severe allergic reactions. Examples of mild reactions include the runny nose and watery eyes caused by a mild allergic response. Moderate reactions include severe hypoxia caused by asthmatic bronchoconstriction, and severe reactions include the potentially life-threatening circulatory collapse seen in anaphylaxis (a whole-body allergic reaction). The presence of what would normally be considered optimal ratios of antigen to antibody in the circulation may lead to damage of filtration in the kidney because of excess deposition of antigen-antibody complexes in the glomeruli. Cross reactivity between foreign and host antigens may lead to injury of cardiac valves due to cross-reaction between streptococcal and myocardial antigens such as occurs in rheumatic fever. The chronic persistence of a foreign antigen by a foreign body or microorgan-

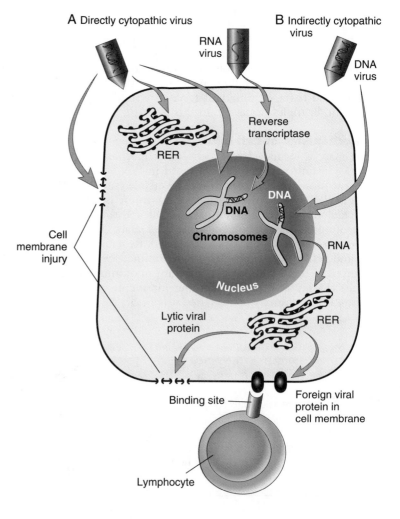

FIGURE   **5-1**   Mechanisms of cell destruction by viruses. **A,** Direct cytopathic effect: RNA virus inserts itself in a receptor on the cell membrane and is brought into the cell. The RNA virus is altered into DNA by reverse transcriptase. The DNA within the nucleus of the cell forms various types of RNA that allows for protein synthesis in the rough endoplasmic reticulum (RER). The protein formed inserts itself into the cell membrane forming a channel that allows ions and extracellular fluid to enter, leading to cell lysis (directly killing the cell). **B,** Indirect cytopathic effect mediated by immune mechanisms: DNA virus inserts itself in a receptor on the cell membrane and is brought into the cell. The DNA virus within the nucleus of the cell forms various types of RNA that allows for protein synthesis in the rough endoplasmic reticulum (RER). This foreign viral protein inserts into the cell membrane and becomes a neoantigen. This neoantigen will be recognized by the T lymphocytes that will react to and kill (indirectly) the infected cell. (Damjanov I: *Pathology for the health-related professions,* ed 2, Philadelphia, 2000, WB Saunders.)

ism that cannot be cleared by the body may lead to a specific type of chronic inflammatory reaction called a *granuloma* (e.g., tuberculosis). Finally, sensitization to endogenous antigens can lead to type 1 diabetes mellitus (DM) due to destruction of islet cells by T lymphocytes sensitized by islet antigens released during an antecedent viral infection.

Genetic Factors

Genetic alterations lead to cellular injury or death by three primary means: (1) alterations in the structure or number of chromosomes that induce multiple abnormalities, (2) single mutations of genes that cause changes in the amount or functions of proteins, and (3) multiple gene mutations that interact with environmental factors to cause multifactorial disorders. These genetic alterations can be severe enough to cause fetal death in utero resulting in spontaneous abortion. Some may cause congenital malformations, whereas others do not manifest pathologic alterations until midlife such as Huntington's chorea. Down syndrome is an example of an alteration in the number of chromosomes that results in multiple abnormalities. This condition, caused by the abnormal presence of a third chromosome in the twenty-first pair, includes cardiac malformations, increased susceptibility to severe infections, mental retardation, and increased risk of leukemia and Alzheimer's dementia. Sickle cell anemia, low-density lipoprotein (LDL) receptor deficiency, and alpha-antitrypsin deficiency are examples of single gene mutations. In the case of alpha-antitrypsin deficiency, the deficiency in a protease inhibitor causes enhanced degradation of elastic tissue surrounding the alveoli of the lungs, which in turn leads to emphysema. Examples of multiple gene mutations that can cause disease include hypertension and type 2 diabetes mellitus (DM). In type 2 DM, obesity and other environmental factors induce the expression of the diabetic genetic trait.

Nutritional Factors

Imbalances in essential nutrients can lead to cell injury or cell death. For example, deficiencies of essential amino acids interfere with protein synthesis. Synthesis of proteins is required to replace cell proteins lost through normal catabolism, growth, and in preparation for cell replication. Cell replication is essential for the healing processes after cell injury and the replacement of cells lost through normal turnover. The consequence of protein malnutrition is a condition called *kwashiorkor*; marasmus, another form of malnutrition, is a consequence of generalized dietary deficiency. These two diseases are still leading causes of death in impoverished countries. In many industrialized countries, excessive nutrient intake leads to obesity and its many complications. Nutritional imbalance can also occur as a result of abnormal levels of either vitamins or minerals. These nutrients function as cofactors for biosynthetic reactions or are essential components of proteins or membranes; their deficiency usually affects selected cells or tissues. For example, a deficiency of iron leads to anemia, and the presence of excessive amounts of iron in the tissue can cause damage by the formation of free radicals. Also, vitamin C (ascorbic acid) deficiency can be associated with a wide range of connective tissue symptoms (Box 5-2). Frank deficiencies of ascorbate are uncommon in the United States, although certain population groups may be at increased risk for deficient intake sometimes referred to as *biochemical scurvy* (Box 5-3).

BOX **5-2**

Connective Tissue Symptoms Associated with Vitamin C Deficiency

Reduced collagen tensile strength (scurvy)
Altered capillary structure (petechiae and hemorrhage)
Osteopenia (bone pain and pathologic fractures)
Skin and gum lesions
Impaired skin and wound healing (decreased collagen formation, lack of scar formation, impaired vascularization)
Bilateral femoral neuropathy
Muscle weakness
Joint pain and effusions
Edema

From Bucci LR: *Nutrition applied to injury rehabilitation and sports medicine,* Boca Raton, Fla, 1995, CRC Press.

BOX **5-3**

Risk Factors for Vitamin C Deficiency

Inadequate food intake (anorexia, chronic dieters, older adults, bedridden individuals)
Malabsorption syndromes
Moderate to severe physical injury or emotional stress
Pregnancy and lactation
Use of tobacco products (smoking or chewing)
Obesity
Alcoholism
Rheumatoid arthritis
Kidney dialysis (hemodialysis or peritoneal dialysis)
Diabetes mellitus
Oral contraceptives
Drugs or medications (e.g., salicylates, corticosteroids, tetracycline)

From Bucci LR: *Nutrition applied to injury rehabilitation and sports medicine,* Boca Raton, Fla, 1995, CRC Press.

Physical Factors

Trauma and physical agents may also lead to cell injury and/or death. Blunt trauma caused by motor vehicle accidents is a leading killer in the United States. Massive brain contusions, injury to internal organs and soft tissues, and blood loss may lead to immediate mortality. Survivors may succumb to infections and multiple organ failure. Repair of injuries to soft tissue, skeletal and muscular systems, and internal organs often requires prolonged periods of rehabilitation. Penetrating trauma inflicted by a variety of weapons can result in multiple complications.

Extremes of physical agents such as temperature, radiation, and electricity may damage cells. Generalized increases in body temperature (hyperthermia) or reduction in body temperature (hypothermia) can lead to cell injury; high or low tissue temperatures can cause tissue injury or death (see Chapter 9). With increased temperature, the resulting morbidity and mortality is dependent on the severity of the burn and the total surface area that was burned. Markedly reduced temperatures may induce the freezing of tissue (frostbite). Ice crystals in cellular tissue rupture the cell membrane, which leads to cell death.

Irradiation for the treatment of cancer can cause injury of susceptible normal cells. Ionizing radiation causes radiolysis of water and the production of hydroxyl radicals (^-OH). These radicals will lead to membrane damage and breakdown of structural and enzymatic proteins resulting in cell death. Often arterioles supplying oxygenated blood are damaged resulting in inadequate nutritional supply leading to ischemia and death of the irradiated tissues. Irradiation also causes damage to nucleic acids and may result in gene mutations possibly leading to neoplasia years later.

Chemical Factors

Toxic substances cause chemical injury. These substances can be divided into two categories: those that can injure cells directly and those that require metabolic transformation into the toxic agent. Examples of chemicals that injure cells directly are heavy metals such as mercury that binds to and disrupts critical membrane proteins and a number of toxins and drugs such as alkylating agents used in chemotherapy. Alkylating agents such as nitrogen mustards induce cross linking of DNA and inactivation of other essential cellular constituents. Carbon tetrachloride and acetaminophen are examples of inert substances that must be metabolized to reactive intermediates to cause cell injury. Taken in large amounts, most medications can be toxic, and many are even lethal. Suicide by drug overdose is a common example of drug-induced chemical toxicity.

An important mechanism of cell injury and disease is the production of reactive oxygen species sometimes referred to as the *formation of free radicals*. A variety of normal and pathologic reactions can lead to the activation of oxygen by the sequential addition of one electron at a time (Fig. 5-2). For example, the body's natural process of using oxygen and food to produce energy can create free radicals as a byproduct of these functions. These unpaired electrons are reactive and commonly bind to oxygen for stabilization. The oxygen then binds to hydrogen for stabilization. This series of reactions generated by normal cellular metabolism results in a phenomenon referred to as *oxygen toxicity* and yields superoxide (O_2^-), hydrogen peroxide (H_2O_2), and hydroxyl radical (^-OH). These forms of reactive oxygen are referred to as *oxygen radicals*, which are toxic to cells. The cellular enzymes always scavenging the body to protect cells from this type of injury normally inactivate these radicals and convert the radical back to usable oxygen. However, if produced in excess (a situation referred to as *oxidative stress*), these radicals can become the mechanism of cell injury and subsequent cell death. Free radicals have been considered central to the damaging effects that can lead to degenerative conditions such as heart disease, cataracts, premature aging, and perhaps even cancer.

Reactive oxygen species or free radical formation occur as a result of many events such as prolonged exercise; exposure to high levels of oxygen, irradiation, ultraviolet or fluorescent light, pollutants, and pesticides (airborne or in food); drug overdose; and the reperfusion injury that is induced by the restoration of normal blood flow after a period of ischemia such as occurs during organ transplantation or after a myocardial infarction. Free-radical toxicity may also be the underlying cause of degeneration of neurons located in the *substantia nigra* leading to the loss of dopamine necessary for the normal control of movements that produces the abnormal movements seen in Parkinson's disease.[13]

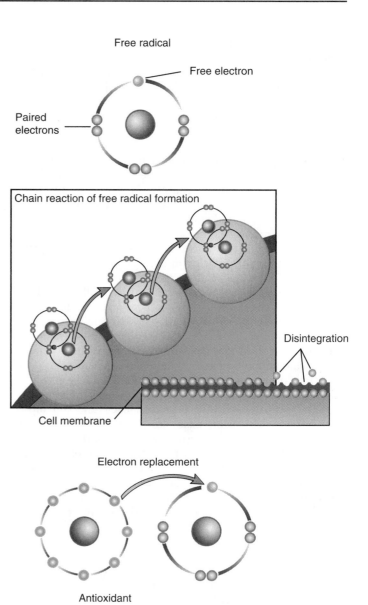

FIGURE **5-2** The oxidative process. Normal metabolic processes and a variety of other extrinsic factors such as pollution, poor nutrition, and exposure to toxic chemicals can result in the formation of free radicals when normal oxygen atoms lose one of their four paired electrons. The resulting unstable atom attempts to replace the missing electron by "stealing" an electron from a healthy cell creating another unstable atom (free radical) and setting off a chain reaction referred to as *oxidation*. Oxidation as a byproduct of metabolism damages cell membranes leading to intrinsic cellular damage, a part of the normal aging process. Free radical damage (oxidation) is believed to alter the way cells encode genetic information in the DNA and may contribute to a variety of diseases and disorders. Antioxidant molecules freely give up an electron to stabilize the oxygen atom without becoming unstable and without initiating a chain reaction.

A variety of enzymatic and nonenzymatic defense mechanisms are present within cells to detoxify reactive oxygen species and protect the cells from this type of injury. Researchers are finding a variety of uses for natural antioxidants in combating the effects of aging and disease. For example, vitamin E effectively scavenges several types of free radicals and other reactive species in lipid membranes and other lipid concentrations, making it a potentially effective antioxidant (able to neutralize the free radical before damage occurs) in preventing LDL cholesterol from adhering to the walls of arteries. In the case of the prostate, lycopene, the compound that makes tomatoes red, is a potent antioxidant potentially effective in promoting prostate health.[31,44] Adequate folate intake has been shown to reduce the risk of breast cancer associated with alcohol consumption by providing bioactive compounds to counteract the formation of oxidative compounds.[30,72]

Multiple trials are ongoing to investigate oxidation, its effect on cellular injury, aging, and disease (e.g., cancer, heart disease, cataracts) and the use of antioxidants found naturally in food and plants to combat oxidative stress, thereby preventing or possibly modifying diseases at the cellular level. Animal and human studies have confirmed that regular, moderate physical activity and exercise strengthens the antioxidant defense system, whereas intense or prolonged, strenuous exercise (especially in a person who has a sedentary lifestyle) constitutes an oxidative stress.[26,52,54]

◆ Reversible Cell Injury

Alteration in a cell's functional environment, either acute or chronic, produces a stress to the cell's ability to attain or maintain homeostasis. The extent to which the cell is able to alter mechanisms and regain homeostasis in the altered environment is considered an adaptation by the cells or tissues. When the cell is unable to adapt, injury can occur. A sublethal or reversible injury occurs if the stress is sufficiently small in magnitude or short enough in duration that the cell is able to recover homeostasis after removal of the stress.

Cells react to injurious stimuli by changing their steady state to continue to function in a hazardous environment. Reversible (sublethal) injury caused by any of the mechanisms of cell injury listed in Box 5-1 is a transient impairment in the cell's normal structure or function. Normal cell structure and function can return after removal of the stressor or injurious stimulus (Fig. 5-3). Acute reversible injury causes an impairment of ion homeostasis within the cell and

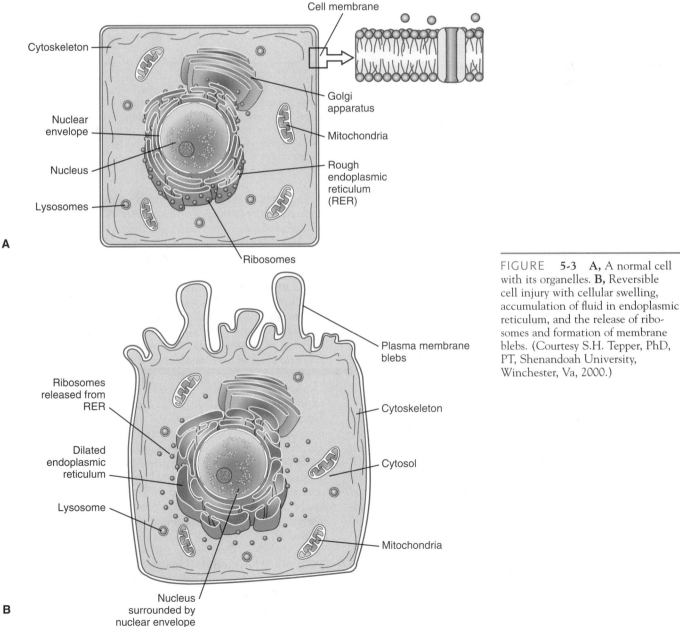

FIGURE 5-3 **A,** A normal cell with its organelles. **B,** Reversible cell injury with cellular swelling, accumulation of fluid in endoplasmic reticulum, and the release of ribosomes and formation of membrane blebs. (Courtesy S.H. Tepper, PhD, PT, Shenandoah University, Winchester, Va, 2000.)

leads to increased intracellular levels of sodium and calcium. An influx of interstitial fluid into the cell accompanies these ionic shifts and causes increased cell volume (swelling). Swelling occurs within the cytosol (liquid medium of the cytoplasm) and within organelles such as mitochondria and the endoplasmic reticulum. Swollen mitochondria generate less energy. Thus instead of oxidative adenosine triphosphate (ATP) production, the cell reverts to less efficient anaerobic glycolysis, which results in excessive production of lactic acid. The pH of the cell becomes acidic, which slows down the cell metabolism, resulting in further cellular damage. The injured cell forms plasma membrane *blebs* that can seal off and detach from the cell surface. In severely injured cells, ribosomes detach from the rough endoplasmic reticulum (RER) and a decrease in the number of polysomes occurs. These changes lead to reduced protein synthesis by the affected cells and the cycle of damage can continue. However, if the cell nucleus remains undamaged and the energy source is restored or the toxic injury is neutralized, the cell is able to recover and pump the ions and excess fluid back out. The swelling disappears and the cell is returned to the original steady state constituting a reversible cell injury.

Cellular Adaptations in Chronic Cell Injury

When a sublethal stress remains present over a period, stable alterations (adaptations) take place within the affected cells, tissues, and organs. Adaptation enables the cells to function in an altered environment and thereby avoid injury. Characteristics of cell adaptation such as change in size, number, or function increase the cell's ability to survive. In many, but not all cases, these changes benefit the function of the parent organ or structure within which the cell resides. These changes are potentially reversible; common cellular adaptations include atrophy, hypertrophy, hyperplasia, metaplasia, and dysplasia (Fig. 5-4).

Atrophy is a reduction in cell and organ size. Atrophy can occur with vascular insufficiency, reduction in hormone levels, malnutrition, immobilization, pain limiting function, and chronic inflammation. Atrophy, involving the entire body, may occur with aging and is referred to as *physiologic atrophy*. Bone loss, thymus involution, muscle wasting, and brain cell loss are examples of either tissue or organ atrophy associated with aging. Pathologic atrophy occurs as a result of some of the mechanisms of cell injury listed in Box 5-1 such as ischemia, inadequate nutrition, or physical factors. For example, ischemia of the viscera results in atrophied organs; cancer or malnutrition can result in cachexia, a general wasting of the body; and spinal cord injury results in atrophy of the affected muscles.

Hypertrophy is an increase in the size of the cell and organ. Hypertrophy can occur when increased functional demands are placed on the cells, tissue, or organs and with increased hormonal input (e.g., exercise stress can induce skeletal muscle hypertrophy). Pure hypertrophy only occurs in the heart and striated muscles, as these organs consist of cells that cannot divide. Hypertrophy of the heart is a common pathologic finding that occurs as an adaptation of heart muscle to an increased workload. Specifically, hypertrophy of the left ventricle is a typical complication of hypertension. Increased blood pressure requires that the heart produce more force to eject the blood. The additional force is produced by hypertrophy of muscle fibers in the left ventricle.

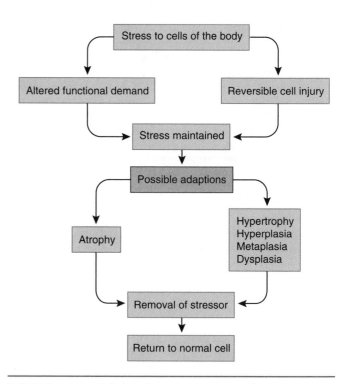

FIGURE **5-4** Cellular adaptations and reversible cell injury in response to stress. When the body is under persistent stress leading to either reversible cell injury or altered functional demand, the tissues adapt. Adaptations could include atrophy, hypertrophy, hyperplasia, metaplasia, or dysplasia. All of these changes are reversible with removal of the stressor. (Courtesy S.H. Tepper, PhD, PT, Winchester, Va, Shenandoah University, 2000.)

Hyperplasia is an increase in the number of cells leading to increased organ size. Tissues can divide and in the presence of excessive functional demands, these tissues increase in cell number. Pure hyperplasia typically occurs because of hormonal stimulation (e.g., prolonged estrogen exposure causes the endometrium of the uterus to become thick) or chronic stimulation (e.g., persistent pressure on the skin induces hyperplasia and the formation of a callous). Some hyperplasia has no discernible cause and may represent early neoplasia. Hypertrophy and hyperplasia often occur together such as in the case of prostate enlargement and obstruction of the urethra and bladder. The result is an increase in size and number of smooth muscle cells in the wall of the urinary bladder.

Metaplasia is a change in cell morphology and function resulting from the conversion of one adult cell type into another. For example, in smokers, portions of the respiratory tract change from ciliated pseudostratified columnar epithelium into stratified squamous epithelium leading to a thickening of the respiratory epithelium and loss of the functional clearance of mucous and debris along the respiratory tree. Dysplasia is an increase in cell numbers that is accompanied by altered cell morphology and loss of histologic organization. Considered to be a preneoplastic alteration, dysplasia can be found in areas that are chronically injured and undergoing hyperplasia or metaplasia.

Intracellular Accumulations or Storage

Intracellular accumulations are increases in the storage of lipids, proteins, carbohydrates, or pigments within the cell that occur as a result of an overload of various metabolites or exogenous material. These accumulations can also be caused by metabolic disturbances altering cell function. For example, when the liver is sublethally injured, lipid (triglyceride) accumulates within the hepatocyte. This lipid accumulation occurs when a reduction in protein synthesis occurs as a result of disaggregation of the ribosomes from the rough endoplasmic reticulum as previously discussed. Hepatocytes normally produce our endogenous lipoproteins. With sublethal damage to hepatocytes (e.g., alcohol abuse), a lack of protein shell formation occurs so that lipoproteins cannot be packaged and transported to the plasma. As a result, lipids remain within the hepatocyte, causing the characteristic "fatty liver" found in alcoholics.

◆ Irreversible Cell Injury

If the injurious or stressful stimulus is of sufficient magnitude or duration or if the cell is unable to adapt, the cell will be irreversibly injured. Irreversible cell injury is synonymous with cell death. Hallmarks of lethally injured cells include alterations in the cell nucleus, mitochondria, and lysosomes, and the rupture of the cell membrane. Damage to the nucleus can present in three forms: pyknosis, karyorrhexis, and karyolysis. Nuclei undergo clumping or pyknosis, a degeneration of the cell as the nucleus shrinks in size and the chromatin condenses to a solid mass. The pyknotic nuclei can fragment, a process termed *karyorrhexis,* or it can undergo dissolution, (karyolysis). Mitochondria lose their membrane potential and become unable to synthesize ATP leaving the cell without the necessary energy production for cell function. Morphologically, irreversibly injured mitochondria appear swollen, contain large lipid-protein aggregates called *flocculent densities,* and may also contain dense crystalline deposits of calcium (Fig. 5-5).

After cell death, lysosomes release their digestive enzymes within the cytoplasm of the cell, initiating enzymatic degradation of all cellular constituents, a process that may be aided by enzymes released from inflammatory cells. The active process of degradation of dead cells is called *necrosis.* Enzymes help dissolve the dead tissue, making it easier for phagocytic cells to remove the dead tissue in preparation for healing by repair (laying down of a collagenous tissue scar) or regeneration (regrowth of parenchymal tissue). Dead cells release their contents into the extracellular fluid, eventually making their way into the cir-

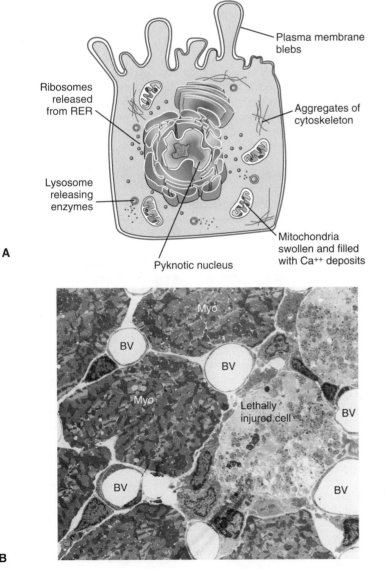

Plasma membrane blebs

Ribosomes released from RER

Aggregates of cytoskeleton

Lysosome releasing enzymes

Mitochondria swollen and filled with Ca++ deposits

Pyknotic nucleus

A

Myo

BV

BV

Myo

Lethally injured cell

BV

BV

BV

B

FIGURE **5-5** Irreversible cell injury: ultrastructural alterations in an irreversibly killed cell. **A,** Mitochondria are nonfunctional and filled with flocculent densities. Lysosomes are releasing their digestive enzymes. The nucleus is condensing upon itself (pyknosis). (Courtesy S.H. Tepper, PhD, PT, Shenandoah University, Winchester, Va, 2000.) Membrane breakdown allows intracellular enzymes to be released into the interstitial area. **B,** Electron micrograph of lethally injured cardiomyocytes next to healthy viable cardiomyocytes (Myo). Note lethally injured cells to the right of the Myo are swollen, mitochondria are filled with flocculent densities, there is a loss of myofilaments, and mononuclear phagocytic cells are beginning to remove these dead cells. BV, *blood vessel. Original magnification* × 1500. (From Tepper SH, Anderson PA, Mergner WJ: Recovery of the heart following focal injury induced by dietary restriction of potassium, *Path Res Prac* 186(2):265-285, 1990.)

TABLE	5-1

Types of Necrosis

TYPE	CAUSE	EFFECT	AREA OF INVOLVEMENT
Coagulative	Ischemia (lack of blood supply)	Cell membrane is preserved; nucleus undergoes pyknosis and karolysis (dissolution); organelles dissolve	Solid internal organs (e.g. heart, liver, kidneys) Dry gangrene (extremities)
Caseous ("cheesy")	*Mycobacterium tuberculosis* (TB); seen with other fungal infections	Cell membrane is destroyed; debris appears cheeselike and does not disappear by lysis but persists indefinitely; damaged area is walled off in a fibrous calcified area forming a granuloma	Lungs, bronchopulmonary lymph nodes, skeletal bone (extrapulmonary TB)
Liquefactive	Pyogenic bacteria (e.g., *Staphylococcus aureus*)	Death of neurons releases lysosomes that liquefy the area, leaving pockets of liquid and cellular debris (abscess or fluid-filled cavity); shapeless, amorphous debris remains	Brain tissue (e.g., brain infarct); skin, wound, joint infections Wet gangrene (extremities)
Fatty necrosis	Acute pancreatitis, abdominal trauma	Formation of calcium soaps by the release of pancreatic lipases	Abdominal area
Fibrinoid	Trauma in blood vessel wall	Plasma proteins accumulate; cellular debris and serum proteins form pink deposits	Blood vessels (tunica media, smooth muscle cells)

culation where they can be measured as clinically useful signs of cell injury. For example, levels of aspartate aminotransferase (AST); creatine kinase (CK); and lactate dehydrogenase (LDH) are typically elevated in the serum of people with myocardial infarct or viral hepatitis (see Tables 39-13 to 39-15).

Types of Necrosis

Dead tissue becomes morphologically distinguishable from healthy tissue only after the process of necrosis begins with the dissolution of irreversibly injured cells within living tissue. Removal of this dead tissue is essential for healing to take place. Histologically, several different types of necrosis are recognized (Table 5-1) with some additional subcategories. For example, gangrene caused by bacterial infection and associated with tissue ischemia (peripheral vascular disease) may form coagulative necrosis (dry gangrene) or liquefactive necrosis (wet gangrene). The fermentation reactions caused by certain bacterial pathogens may cause the formation of gas bubbles in the infected tissue. In muscle necrosis, one of the causative agents is *Clostridium perfringens*. The term used to describe this condition is *clostridial myonecrosis* or gas gangrene (see Chapter 7).

Pathologic Tissue Calcification

Calcification is the deposition of calcium salts, primarily calcium phosphate, in body tissues. Normally, 99% of all calcium is deposited in the teeth and bone matrix to ensure stability and strength; the remaining 1% is dissolved in body fluids such as blood or within skeletal muscle. Two types of pathologic calcification are evident. The first type is dystrophic calcification, the deposition of calcium salts in an area of dead tissue. Classic examples of dystrophic calcification include tuberculosis and atherosclerosis. With tuberculosis, calcification occurs in the granulomas (accumulations of macrophages and connective tissue) that may be found in lymph nodes or in the lung parenchyma and may be seen on radiograph. In the case of atherosclerosis, vessels damaged by the deposition of cholesterol may become calcified. Calcifications within the vessel wall lead to a reduction in elasticity of the vessel.

The second type of calcification is metastatic calcification. This type occurs with hypercalcemia (increased blood calcium levels; see Chapter 4) in living tissue. The normal absorption of calcium is facilitated by parathyroid hormone and vitamin D. When there are increased levels of parathyroid hormone in the blood (e.g., hyperparathyroidism), an increased accumulation of calcium in the pulmonary alveoli, renal tubules, thyroid gland, gastric mucosa, and arterial walls interfering with normal organ function.

Special Implications for the Therapist   5-1

CELL INJURY: MULTIPLE CELL INJURIES

The concepts discussed in this first section on cell injury are essential for understanding the pathogenesis of a variety of acute illnesses the therapist may see as a primary practice pattern. Often, multiple episodes of care with complex cases involving comorbidities occur in clinical practice. For example, the victim of a motor vehicle accident experiencing a traumatic brain injury (TBI) and concomitant pelvic fracture may develop pneumonia and pulmonary compromise, subsequently experiencing a myocardial infarction. The therapy staff following this client from the intensive care unit (ICU) through rehabilitation to a home health service setting and possibly as an outpatient can better meet the needs of such an individual during the healing process by understanding these concepts of injury and recovery.

TBI often occurs during motor vehicle accidents. With direct trauma to the head, brain tissue can be lethally damaged by two means (primary and secondary injury). Depending on the nature, direction and magnitude of forces applied to the skull, primary injury to the brain may be of any or all of the following types: (1) local brain damage occurs at the site where the brain impacts the skull (coup injury) and the site opposite impact (countrecoup injury); (2) polar brain damage occurs at the tips (poles) of the frontal, temporal, and occipital lobes and the undersurface of the frontal and temporal lobes when the brain moves inside the skull, (3) diffuse axonal injury (DAI) occurs throughout the subcortical white matter (and brainstem if the magnitude of force is great enough) with sufficient shear force to injure axons. Secondary injury is usually the result of hypoxic-ischemic injury (HII) caused by cerebral edema. Because the soft and pliable brain is enclosed within the rigid skull, abnormal brain fluid dynamics caused by cerebral edema result in increased intracranial pressure (ICP). Signs and symptoms of increased ICP include headache, loss of sense of smell, obtunded consciousness, and loss of consciousness. Even a mild increase in ICP is sufficient to cause death of neural tissue due to inadequate profusion. Moderate and severe increases in ICP can cause brain tissue to shift position or herniate from one chamber into another. Intracranial hematomas (epidural, subdural, and intracerebral) are another source of secondary brain damage. Passive imaging techniques (e.g., computed axial tomography [CAT] and magnetic resonance imaging [MRI]) are useful to visualize the structural changes that occur with TBI, whereas active imaging techniques (e.g., electroencephalogram [EEG], positron emission tomography [PET], and evoked potentials) are useful to visualize physiologic changes that occur with TBI.

Open wounds and fracture are common sequelae associated with motor vehicle accidents. In this case the pelvic fracture resulted from the mechanical force distributed through the pelvis during a motor vehicle accident. Fractures are often diagnosed by radiograph. When a bone is fractured, its normal blood supply is disrupted. Osteocytes (bone cells) die from the trauma and the resulting ischemia. Bone macrophages remove the dead bone cells and damaged bone. A precursor fibrocartilaginous model growth of tissue occurs before the laying down of primary bone, eventually followed by the laying down and remodeling on normal adult bone. This process from fracture to full restoration of the bone will take weeks to months depending on the type of fracture, location, vascular supply, health, and age of the individual.

In this example, if the myocardium is subjected to ischemia for a sufficient duration, the myocytes become irreversibly injured. A cascade of physiologic and anatomic changes leads to the death of myocardial cells. Coagulative necrosis ensues, followed by acute inflammation and finally repair by scar tissue formation. Coagulative necrosis begins with the release of lysosomal enzymes that cause dissolution of the normal structural relationships found within myocytes. The dead cells attract acute inflammatory cells that phagocytize the necrotic debris and release growth factors. The growth factors initiate the proliferation of blood vessels (angiogenesis) and fibroblasts resulting in the eventual production of a collagenous scar (Fig. 5-6).

Signs and symptoms correlate with the different stages of lethal cell injury and differ according to the organ or structure(s) involved. During acute myocardial infarction, the individual usually experiences angina, shortness of breath, sweating, and nausea. These symptoms of physiologic stress are caused by the release of histamines, bradykinins, and prostaglandins such as substance P from the lethally injured myocytes. An electrocardiogram (ECG) reveals ST segment elevation and Q waves over the affected area. The person is also at an increased risk for life-threatening dysrhythmias due to the loss of electrical conductivity of lethally injured myocytes and disrupted conductivity (irritability) of the adjacent cells. If a significant percentage of the myocardium is infarcted, cardiogenic shock or congestive heart failure may ensue. Cytoplasmic enzymes or proteins (e.g., creatine kinase [CK-MB])

Time Period

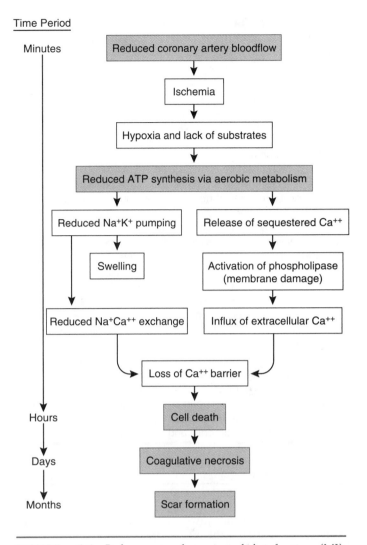

FIGURE 5-6 Pathogenesis of a myocardial infarction (MI). With reduction in coronary artery blood flow (CABF) due to a thrombus formation, ischemia results in a reduction of aerobic metabolism. Irreversible cell injury occurs followed by necrosis of the heart tissue. Release of intracellular enzymes (CK-MB; troponin) from the dead heart tissue serve as biochemical markers in the early diagnosis of MI (see Table 39-13 and 39-14). In the following weeks, healing occurs by repair, the formation of a connective tissue scar. (Courtesy S.H. Tepper, PhD, PT, Shenandoah University, Winchester, Va, 2000.)

are released from the dead cells. Normally, the plasmalemma is impermeable to these large molecules and contains them within the confines of the cytoplasm. After lethal injury the plasmalemma is broken down by the actions of phospholipases, and these molecules are released from inside the cell. A number of cytoplasmic proteins are released into the interstitial area and are taken up by adjacent lymphatic vessels and finally enter the bloodstream. Lactate dehydrogenase (LDH), CK-MB, and troponin (see Tables 39-13 and 39-14) are clinically relevant for diagnosis and assessment of the severity of a myocardial infarction.

The therapist must understand the process of injury and repair to the brain, pelvic bones, and myocardium (or other involved organs and/or structures) as appropriate client care is determined by the different stages of this process. For example,

Continued

recovery from TBI tends to follow the progression outlined by the Rancho Los Amigos Levels of Cognitive Function (LOCF) (see Table 32-1). In general, intervention is directed by the person's current Rancho level. During Rancho levels I to III primary goals involve increasing tolerance of activities including intervention, tolerating upright posture, and increasing interaction with the environment. During levels IV to VI the emphasis shifts to increasing physical and cognitive endurance. During levels VII and VIII intervention focuses on the skills necessary to reenter the community.

Following fracture of bone, a period of immobilization usually occurs to remove longitudinal stress. This period allows for the phagocytic removal of necrotic bone tissue and the initial deposition of the fibrocartilaginous callus. As the fracture heals as revealed by radiograph, gradual progression of stress is applied. Mobilization of this individual will occur depending on the type of fixation used on the pelvis. For example, if an external fixation is applied for fracture stabilization, mobilization can occur almost immediately within tolerance of the person's symptoms.

The highest risk of death during the first hours after myocardial infarction stems from dysrhythmias. Rupture of the myocardium is possible during days 3 to 10 after a transmural myocardial infarction (from outside epicardium to inside endocardium). The risk of these events dictates that exercise during this time must not subject damaged cells to excessive stress. Proper mobilization of the individual soon after infarction may decrease the likelihood of succumbing to the negative effects of bedrest but may be complicated by variables such as pelvic fracture, pneumonia, and the TBI in this case. ■

INFLAMMATION

◆ Definition

In contrast to cell injury, which occurs at the level of single cells, inflammation is the coordinated reaction of body tissues to cell injury and cell death that involves vascular, humoral, neurologic, and cellular responses. Regardless of the type of cell injury or death, the inflammatory response follows a basically similar pattern. Due to all of the factors described above, inflammation occurs only in living organisms.

The functions of the inflammatory reaction are to inactivate the injurious agent, to break down and remove the dead cells, and to initiate the healing of tissue. The key components of the inflammatory reaction are: (1) blood vessels; (2) circulating blood cells; (3) connective or interstitial tissue cells (fibroblasts, mast cells, and resident macrophages); (4) chemical mediators derived from inflammatory cells or plasma cells; and (5) specific extracellular matrix constituents, primarily collagen and basement membranes.*

Inflammation of sudden onset and short duration is referred to as *acute inflammation*, whereas inflammation that does not resolve but persists over time is called *chronic inflammation*.

---

*Basement membranes are thin, sheetlike structures deposited by endothelial (cells that line the heart, blood vessels, lymph vessels, and serous body cavities) and epithelial cells (cells that cover the body and viscera) but are also found surrounding nerve and muscle cells. They provide mechanical support for resident cells and function as a scaffold for accurate regeneration of preexisting structures of tissue. Basement membrane tissue also serves as a semipermeable filtration barrier for macromolecules in organs such as the kidney and the placenta and act as regulators of cell attachment, migration, and differentiation. The major constituents are collagen type IV and proteoglycans.

◆ Acute Inflammation

Normally, inflammation has a protective role and is generally beneficial to the body. However, inflammation, whether in the acute or chronic stage (and with all of its components), can be detrimental, causing damage and even death to adjacent healthy tissue. In the acute stage, the inflammatory stimulus acts on blood cells and plasma constituents. Chemical mediators are produced that alter vascular tone and permeability. These mediators also cause the accumulation of plasma proteins, fluid (edema), and blood cells in the injured site (Fig. 5-7). The clinical manifestations of this inflammatory reaction are redness, swelling, increased temperature, pain, and decreased function of the affected site (Table 5-2). Accompanying clinical findings include increased muscle tone or spasm and loss of motion or function. Cyriax describes two components of passive movement testing that also suggest acute inflammation: a spasm end feel and pain reported before resistance is noted by the practitioner as the limb is moved passively.[15] If movement testing suggestive of acute inflammation persists, inflammation becomes chronic with proliferation of blood vessels and connective tissue components.

Vascular Alterations

Acute inflammation can last from a few minutes (e.g., redness and swelling from scratching your skin) to a few days (e.g., after an open cut on the finger), during which time a series of vascular events occurs. After an injury that disrupts the integrity of a vessel wall, the small arteries supplying blood to the area undergo vasoconstriction. This is mediated by a neural reflex and results in a slowing down of blood flow to the affected area. At the same time, the blood flowing into the surrounding tissue exerts pressure on the damaged vessels, compressing them from outside. The slowdown of the blood flow promotes aggregation of platelets, which leads to the formation of a blood clot resulting in a reduction in the amount of blood loss.

In the case of an injury that does not disrupt the integrity of the blood vessel wall but does cause tissue injury, the temporary neurally mediated constriction of arterioles is followed by a more sustained and overriding vasodilation, resulting in an increased blood flow to the affected area. The increased blood volume raises hydrostatic pressure, and an increased loss of protein-poor fluid occurs from the vasculature into the injured tissue.

TABLE	5-2

Four Cardinal Signs/Symptoms of Inflammation

Sign	Precipating Events
Erythema	Vasodilation and increased blood flow
Heat	Vasodilation and increased blood flow
Edema	Fluid and cells leaking from local blood vessels into the extravascular spaces
Pain	Direct trauma; chemical mediation by bradykinins, histamines, serotonin; internal pressure secondary to edema; swelling of the nerve endings

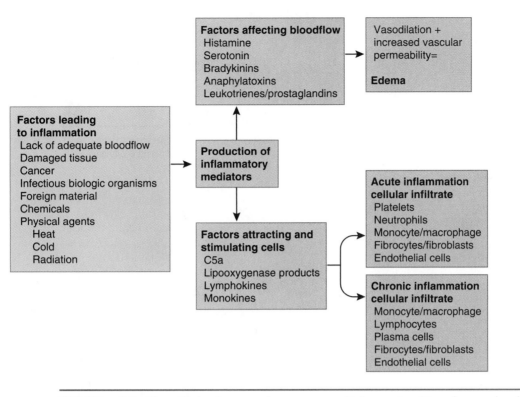

FIGURE   **5-7**   Contributing factors and components of inflammation. Note the vascular alterations associated with factor affecting blood flow (vasoactive mediators) leading to edema and the factors attracting and stimulating cellular alterations (chemotactic factors) resulting in acute (and sometimes) chronic inflammation. (Courtesy S.H. Tepper, PhD, PT, Shenandoah University, Winchester, Va, 2000.)

At this stage, clinical manifestations include redness (erythema) and warmth of the injured area due to the increased blood flow. The leakage of protein-poor fluid (transudate) from the vasculature into the interstitial spaces is called *transudation** and causes the affected area to appear swollen (Fig. 5-8). When fluid transudates or leaks from blood vessels and accumulates inside an anatomic space such as the pleural, pericardial, or peritoneal cavities or the joint space, these accumulations are called effusions. Effusion is a more general term referring to the escape of a fluid and can either be a transudate or an exudate. Exudates occur when an increase in capillary permeability allows proteinaceous fluid and/or cells to leak out primarily through openings created between adjacent endothelial cells in the capillaries or venules (Fig. 5-9). Exudate contains much more protein than transudate. Exudate may also contain inflammatory phagocytic cells that occur in response to necrotic tissue and or an infection. Protein-rich fibrinous (stringy) material found within some blisters or pus are sometimes identified as exudates. Various types of exudate are evident, depending on the stage of inflammation and its cause (Table 5-3). Removal of the fluid for analysis is required when differentiating between transudates and exudates and helps establish a specific diagnosis.

Sometimes exudates are described by visual appearance (e.g. serosanguinous exudate, a fluid containing erythrocytes or red blood cells [RBCs]).

The time of onset of the vascular reaction to injury varies. Mild injuries may induce an increase in vascular permeability that occurs very soon after injury and resolves in a few minutes. In this case, the anatomic site responsible for the leak is the capillary/venule.[47] The leak occurs because endothelial cells lining the lumen of the capillary/venules actively contract and open up their intercellular junctions. This increase in vascular permeability allows proteins to shift from the plasma into the interstitium, causing a greater attraction and retention of fluid in this area. The increase in vascular permeability caused by the injury may be delayed for some time and may persist for days such as the delayed reaction seen in tissue injury caused by ultraviolet light (sunburn) or irradiation (radiation therapy); typically, the vascular leak begins a few hours after exposure to the sun. In severely injured tissues (e.g., trauma or extensive burns), all vascular structures may be directly injured and become leaky instantly.

Leukocyte Accumulations

An important consequence of the exudation of protein and fluid from the vasculature is the engorgement of vessels with blood cells. This causes a slowing or cessation of blood flow in the affected vessels, a phenomenon called *stasis*. During stasis, the leukocytes (white blood cells [WBCs]) accumulate and adhere to the endothelial cells of blood vessel walls at the site of injury in a process called margination. Inflammatory medi-

---

*Transudation, the passage of fluid through a membrane or tissue surface occurs as a result of a difference in hydrostatic pressure, primarily in conditions in which there is protein loss and low protein content (e.g., left ventricular failure, cirrhosis, nephrosis). Typically, transudate is thin and watery, containing few blood vessels or other large proteins. The terms *transudate, exudate, effusion,* and *edema* are often used interchangeably, although each of these has its own clinical significance.

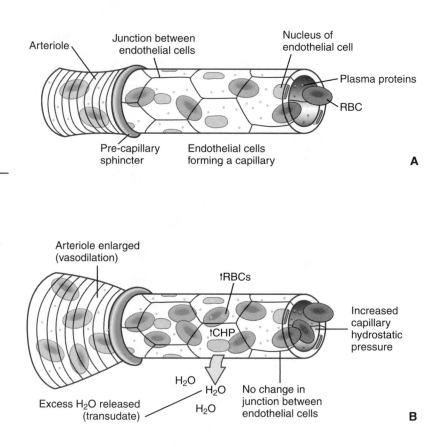

FIGURE 5-8 Normal capillary **(A)** reveals endothelial cells connected by tight junctions limiting flow of plasma proteins into the interstitium. With mild injury **(B)** vasodilation results in increased capillary hydrostatic pressure pushing more water into the interstitial area (transudate). (Courtesy S.H. Tepper, PhD, PT, Shenandoah University, Winchester, Va, 2000.)

ators cause an increased expression of specific glycoproteins called *adhesion molecules* on the surface membrane of leukocytes and endothelial cells. These adhesion glycoproteins, by adhering to each other, function as receptors and counter-receptors. The adhesion glycoproteins are the glue that binds the leukocytes to each other and to the endothelium of venules and capillaries.

The binding of leukocytes to receptors on endothelial cells of venules is the first step in the migration of leukocytes from the vasculature to the interstitial tissues. This process initiates the circulation of leukocytes through the extravascular space in normal conditions and the infiltration of leukocytes into the site of inflammation. In the following stage, the leukocytes actively migrate out of the vessels, passing through the vascular walls without damaging the blood vessels and entering the interstitial space in a process called *diapedesis*, or oozing (Fig. 5-10). The continued migration of leukocytes in interstitial space is directed by a chemical trail created by a concentration gradient of one of many possible attractants. The attractants are called *chemotactic agents,* and the process of locomotion is called chemotaxis. In other words, leukocytes are attracted to and accumulate at the site of an inflammatory reaction in response to a chemical stimulus.

The presence of leukocyte accumulations in tissue or fluid specimens is diagnostic of an inflammatory process. The predominant cell type found in a specimen identifies the type of inflammation and/or its duration and its original stimulus (see Table 39-4). Typically, during acute inflammation, neutrophils predominate (neutrophilia). Neutrophils inhibit bacterial growth by releasing lactoferrin, a protein that binds with iron thus preventing microorganisms from using iron for growth and development. Neutrophils also demonstrate direct cyto-

toxic activity toward viruses, fungi, and bacteria by releasing defensin, which are peptides with natural antibiotic activity. If the inflammatory stimulus subsides, the neutrophils rapidly die out as their life span (after extrusion from the circulation) is approximately 24 hours; they are replaced by monocytic/macrophage cells responsible for cleaning up the cellular debris left after neutrophils have done their job. Certain inflammatory stimuli can induce a sustained neutrophil response (e.g., first defense against pyogenic bacteria), a predominantly lymphocytic response (e.g., fight tumor cells or respond to viruses), or an eosinophilic response (e.g., plays a role in asthma and allergies or attacks parasites).

In addition to the types of WBCs present, the total and differential counts of the leukocytes in the circulating blood are also very important diagnostic tools (see Table 39-4). An increased number of circulating leukocytes (leukocytosis) is often an indication of an active inflammatory reaction (typically to an infection or tissue injury). A decreased WBC count (leukopenia) can, for example, be seen in certain types of infections and is an indicator of grave prognosis in severe systemic infections (sepsis).

The main function of the leukocytes recruited to the affected tissue is to remove or eliminate the injurious stimulus. Leukocytes achieve this function by releasing enzymes and toxic substances that kill, inactivate, and degrade microbial agents, foreign antigens, or necrotic tissue. Leukocytes also take up these materials by phagocytosis and release growth factors necessary for healing or regeneration (see Fig. 5-15).

In addition to the role played by blood vessels in inflammation, a contribution is made from a system of thin-walled channels formed by endothelial cells with loose junctions. These channels are called *lymphatics* and ultimately drain into the subclavian vein via the thoracic duct (see Fig. 12-8).

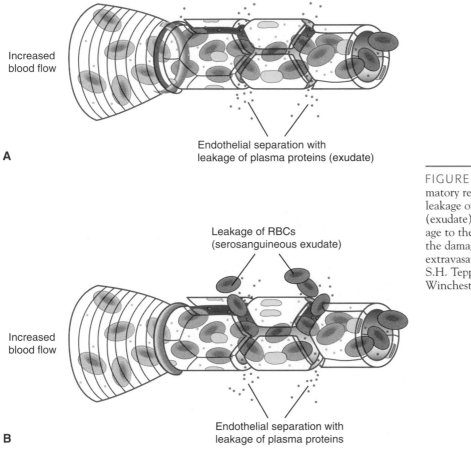

FIGURE   **5-9 A,** With a more severe inflammatory response, endothelial cells separate causing leakage of plasma proteins into the interstitium (exudate). This accentuates the edema. **B,** With damage to the endothelial cells, the separation between the damaged cells may allow even erythrocytes to extravasate (serosanguineous exudate). (Courtesy S.H. Tepper, PhD, PT, Shenandoah University, Winchester, Va, 2000.)

TABLE	5-3

Inflammatory Exudates

TYPE	APPEARANCE	SIGNIFICANCE
Hemorrhagic; sanguinous	Bright red or bloody; presence of red blood cells (RBCs)	Small amounts expected after surgery or trauma. Large amounts may indicate hemorrhage. Sudden large amounts of dark red blood may indicate a draining hematoma
Serosanguinous	Blood-tinged yellow or pink; presence of RBCs	Expected for 48 to 72 hours after injury or trauma to the microvasculature. A sudden increase may precede wound dehiscence (rupture or separation)
Serous	Thin, clear yellow, or straw-colored; contains albumin and immunoglobulins	Occurs in the early stages of most inflammations; common with blisters, joint effusion with rheumatoid arthritis, viral infections (e.g., skin vesicles caused by herpesvirus); expected for up to 1 week after trauma or surgery. A sudden increase may indicate a draining seroma (pocket of serum within tissue or organ)
Purulent	Viscous, cloudy, pus; cellular debris from necrotic cells and dying neutrophils (PMNs)	Usually caused by pus-forming bacteria (streptococci, staphylococci) and indicates infection. May drain suddenly from an abscess (boil)
Catarrhal	Thin, clear mucus	Seen with inflammatory process within mucous membranes (e.g., upper respiratory infection)
Fibrinous	Thin, usually clear; may be yellow or pink, tinged, or cloudy	Occurs with severe inflammation or bacterial infections (e.g., strep throat, pneumonia); does not resolve easily; can cause fibrous scarring and restriction (e.g., constrictive pericarditis)

Modified from Black J: Wound healing. In Black JM, Matassarin-Jacobs E, editors: *Luckmann and Sorensen's medical-surgical nursing*, ed 5, Philadelphia, 2000, WB Saunders.

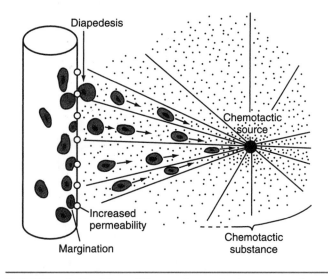

FIGURE 5-10 Many different chemical substances in the tissues cause both neutrophils and macrophages to move through the capillary pores in a process called *diapedesis* and toward the area of tissue damage by *chemotaxis*. Chemotaxis depends on the concentration gradient of the chemotactic substance. The concentration is greatest near the source, which directs the unidirectional movement of the white blood cells. Chemotaxis is effective up to 100 micrometers away from an inflamed tissue. Since almost no tissue area is more than 50 micrometers away from a capillary, the chemotactic signal can easily move vast numbers of WBCs from the capillaries into the inflamed area. (Guyton AC, Hall JE: *Textbook of medical physiology,* ed 10, Philadelphia, 2000, WB Saunders.)

These channels in physiologic conditions help drain fluid and protein from the interstitium thereby reducing edema. They also serve as a conduit for the removal of certain leukocytes and inflammatory stimuli.[65] The movement of the phagocytic cells into the lymphatic vessels allows presentation of the engulfed material to immunocompetent cells located in the lymph nodes. Hyperplasia of immunocompetent cells (T and B lymphocytes) in the lymph nodes leads to an enlargement of the nodes called lymphadenopathy. During the process of removing infectious agents, lymphatics and their lymph nodes may become actively inflamed. Clinically, the inflamed lymphatics may appear as red streaks under the epidermis and may be painful to palpation; this condition is called *lymphangitis* (see Chapter 12).

Chemical Mediators of Inflammation

A large number of chemical mediators are responsible for the vascular and leukocyte responses generated by the cells involved in an acute inflammatory response. These mediators are either released from inflammatory cells (cell-derived) or are generated by the action of plasma protease (plasma derived). Mediators of inflammation are multifunctional and have numerous effects on blood vessels, inflammatory cells, and other cells in the body. Some of their primary effects in the inflammatory response include vasodilation or vasoconstriction, modulation of vascular permeability, activation of inflammatory cells, chemotaxis, cytotoxicity, degradation of tissue, pain, and fever. These mediators include histamine, serotonin, bradykinin, the complement system, platelet activating factors, arachidonic acid derivatives (e.g., prostaglandins, leukotrienes), and cytokines (Table 5-4).

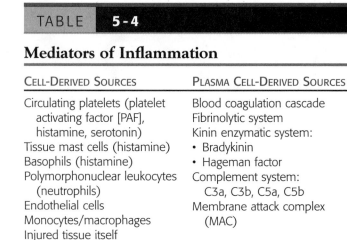

TABLE	5-4

Mediators of Inflammation

CELL-DERIVED SOURCES	PLASMA CELL-DERIVED SOURCES
Circulating platelets (platelet activating factor [PAF], histamine, serotonin)	Blood coagulation cascade
	Fibrinolytic system
	Kinin enzymatic system:
Tissue mast cells (histamine)	• Bradykinin
Basophils (histamine)	• Hageman factor
Polymorphonuclear leukocytes (neutrophils)	Complement system: C3a, C3b, C5a, C5b
Endothelial cells	Membrane attack complex (MAC)
Monocytes/macrophages	
Injured tissue itself	
Arachidonic acid derivatives (prostaglandins, leukotrienes)	
Cytokines (TNF, IL-1)	

Histamine. Histamine is synthesized and stored in granules (for quick availability and release) of mast cells, basophils, and platelets. Histamine causes endothelial contraction leading to the formation of gaps, which increase blood vessel permeability and allow fluids and blood cells to exit into the interstitial spaces (vascular leak). Histamine's effect occurs quickly but is short lived, as it is inactivated in less than 30 minutes. Histamine is also a potent vasodilator and bronchoconstrictor. Serotonin is another mediator released from platelets; it induces vasoconstriction, but its effect is usually overridden by the vasodilator action of histamine.

Platelet Activating Factor. Leukocytes and other cells on stimulation also synthesize three classes of inflammatory mediators that are derived from phospholipids (the major lipids present in cell membranes). The first of these mediators is an acetylated lysophospholipid named platelet-activating factor (PAF). The other two classes of mediators are derived from a fatty acid (arachidonic acid) of membrane phospholipids and are called *prostaglandins* and *leukotrienes.* All three of these lipid mediators have potent and wide-ranging inflammatory activities. In addition, these mediators have hormone-like functions that modulate physiologic responses and induce pathology in a variety of organ systems.

PAF was so-named because it was first found to induce platelet activation and secretion. PAF is now known to be a potent activator of cells such as smooth muscle cells, endothelial cells, and leukocytes by receptor binding and intracellular signaling mechanisms. As a consequence, PAF can induce the aggregation of leukocytes and leukocyte infiltration in tissues and can profoundly affect vasomotor tone and permeability.[62] PAF can potentiate (increase or strengthen) the activity of other inflammatory mediators.

Arachidonic Acid Derivatives. The synthesis of prostaglandins and leukotrienes begins with the cleavage (splitting) of arachidonic acid from membrane phospholipids by the action of the phospholipase (Fig. 5-11). Once this step is completed, either a cyclooxygenase (COX) enzyme or a lipoxyge-

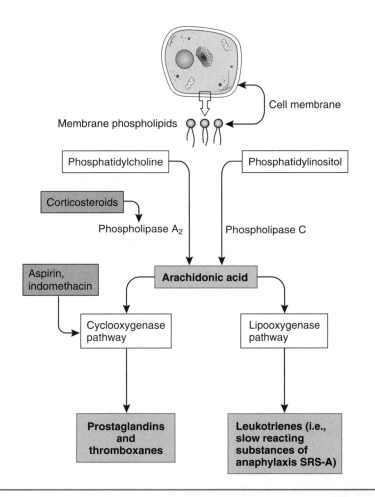

FIGURE   **5-11**   Production of prostaglandins and leukotrienes from damaged cell membranes. Note sites for pharmacologic (aspirin and prednisone) interventions. (Courtesy S.H. Tepper, PhD, PT, Shenandoah University, Winchester, Va, 2000.)

nase enzyme further metabolizes the arachidonic acid. The cyclooxygenase pathway leads to the production of several types of prostaglandins that modulate vasomotor tone and platelet aggregation (e.g., thromboxane is a strong platelet aggregator and vasoconstrictor, whereas prostacyclin [PGI$_2$] is a strong platelet inhibitor and vasodilator). Clinically, prostaglandins are also important because they are mediators of the fever and pain responses associated with inflammation.[13] The lipoxygenase pathway leads to the production of leukotrienes. Leukotrienes occur naturally in leukocytes and produce allergic and inflammatory reactions similar to those of histamine. They are extremely potent mediators of immediate hypersensitivity reactions and inflammation, producing smooth muscle contraction, especially bronchoconstriction, increased vascular permeability, and migration of leukocytes to areas of inflammation. They are thought to play a role in the development of allergic and autoimmune disease such as asthma and rheumatoid arthritis. Certain leukotrienes (C4, D4, E4) are collectively known as SRS-A (a slow-reacting substance of anaphylaxis), the name given when their potent bronchoconstrictor activity was discovered; they also cause leakage of fluid and proteins from the microvasculature.

The importance of the arachidonic acid metabolites in the inflammatory process is made evident by the excellent clinical response to treatment of acute and chronic inflammatory con-

ditions with drugs that block the production of arachidonic acid (corticosteroids) or inhibit the enzyme and block the production of prostaglandins cyclooxygenase (nonsteroidal antiinflammatory drugs [NSAIDs] such as aspirin or the newer COX-2 inhibitors). These antiinflammatory medications are commonly used for people with somatic pain or inflammatory conditions, especially rheumatoid arthritis.

Cytokines.   Leukocytes also produce polypeptide substances called *cytokines* (see Chapter 6) that have a wide range of inflammatory actions affecting either the cytokine-producing cells themselves (autocrine effects) or adjacent cells (paracrine effects). Cytokines also have a number of systemic "hormonal" inflammatory effects. Two important cytokines with overlapping functions are interleukin-1 (IL-1)* and tumor necrosis factor (TNF). TNF is thought to be capable of inducing most of the actions of IL-1 with the exception of activation of lymphocytes.

IL-1 has a number of local actions that promote the inflammatory reaction and a number of systemic actions that induce metabolic, hemodynamic, and hematologic alterations

---

*As many as 15 ILs are now identified. Most ILs direct other cells to divide and differentiate, each interleukin acting on a particular group of cells that have receptors specific for that interleukin.

(Table 5-5). These alterations are discussed in some detail because of their importance in the clinical and laboratory diagnosis of inflammation. IL-1 causes fever by raising the production of prostaglandins in the hypothalamus and thereby resetting the threshold of temperature-sensitive neurons. Fever, in turn, raises the systemic metabolism and increases the systemic consumption of oxygen by approximately 10% for each degree Celsius of body temperature elevation. As a result, a decrease in systemic vascular resistance occurs thereby producing hypotension and an increase in cardiac output to increase the flow of blood and the delivery of oxygen to various organs. These hemodynamic changes are characteristic of severe systemic infections and a febrile condition.

IL-1 also causes characteristic changes in blood chemistry. Albumin and transferrin levels are decreased while levels of coagulation factors, complement components, C-reactive protein, and serum amyloid A increase. These changes occur because IL-1 alters the rate of synthesis of these proteins by the liver. IL-1 also increases the number of neutrophils and decreases the number of lymphocytes in the circulation.

The Blood Coagulation, Fibrinolytic, and Complement Systems.   Plasma proteins produce chemical inflammatory mediators by the enzymatic activity of proteases on plasma proteins. Plasma proteases are enzymes that act as a catalyst in the breakdown of proteins. These plasma protein systems are the blood coagulation and fibrinolytic, kinin enzymatic, and the complement systems. All of these systems

---

TABLE	5-5

Actions of Cytokines: Interleukin-1 and Tumor Necrosis Factor

Local
> Stimulates leukocyte adhesion to endothelium
> Modulates the coagulation cascade
> Stimulates production and/or secretion of inflammatory mediators (including IL-1 itself)
> Activates fibroblasts, chrondrocytes, osteoclasts

Systemic
Metabolic
> Induces fever
> Increases body metabolism
> Decreases appetite
> Induces sleep
> Induces adrenocorticotrophic hormone (ACTH) release to secrete corticosteroids
> Nonspecific resistance to infection

Hemodynamic
> Causes hypotension
> Hypovolemia (sepsis)

Hematologic
> Changes blood chemistry (see text)
> Activates endothelial, macrophage, and resting T cells
> Increases neutrophils in circulation
> Decreases lymphocytes in circulation
> Stimulates synthesis of collagen and collagenases

---

can become activated by contact with byproducts of cell injury or foreign materials. Examples include contact with components of denuded vascular endothelial cells revealing their underlying basement membrane, which occurs with trauma to the vessel wall and contact with bacterial endotoxins. The key plasma protein in the activation sequence of these systems is clotting factor XII also known as *Hageman factor*.

The blood coagulation system (Fig. 5-12) is formed, in part, by plasma proteins. When bleeding occurs, a series of enzymes are activated sequentially to generate the enzyme thrombin, which converts the plasma protein fibrinogen to fibrin, the essential component of a blood clot. Fibrin forms a meshwork at bleeding sites to stop the bleeding and trap exudate, microorganisms, and foreign materials, keeping this content contained in an area where eventually the greatest number of phagocytes will be found. This localizing effect prevents the spread of infection to other sites and begins the process of healing and tissue repair.

The fibrinolytic system (designed to dissolve these clots) is activated by the conversion of plasminogen to the enzyme plasmin (also known as *fibrinolysin*, which means "to loosen"). Plasmin splits or divides fibrin and lyses the blood clots. Both the coagulation and the fibrinolytic systems are activated in inflammation and function together in a system of checks and balances to preserve vascular function. The products of fibrin degradation are chemotactic for leukocytes and increase vascular permeability. The kinin enzymatic system is also activated by Hageman factor and functions to produce bradykinin. Bradykinin is a mediator that causes dilatation and leakage of blood vessels and induces pain.

The complement system is composed of a group of plasma proteins that normally lie dormant in the blood, interstitial fluid, and mucosal surfaces. Then, through a series of enzymatic reactions, several plasma protein fragments (C3a, C3b, C5a, C5b)* are formed that are potent inflammatory mediators. These components are also active in immunologic processes. The complement system is activated by microorganisms or antigen-antibody complexes causing four events to occur that promote inflammation: (1) vasodilates the capillaries, which increases blood flow to the area; (2) facilitates the movement of leukocytes into the area by chemotaxis; (3) coats the surfaces of microbes to make them vulnerable to phagocytosis; (4) formation of a membrane attack complex (MAC).

Complement activation can follow one of two pathways, the classic or the alternate pathway; each pathway produces the same active complement components. The products of the complement system bind to particles of foreign material, microorganisms, or other antigens, coating them to make them vulnerable to phagocytosis by leukocytes, a process called *opsonization*. Activation of the complement cascade by either pathway also results in the formation of the MAC. The MAC is inserted in cell membranes of the microorganism where it creates an opening (pore or channel) in the cell membrane, leading to influx of sodium and extracellular fluid eventually leading to its lysis (Fig. 5-13). For example, in he-

---

*In the nomenclature used for the complement system, each complement component (C) is designated by a number (1 to 9). The individual subunits that make up each component are designated by a letter. For example the first component of complement is designated C1. C1 is made up of three subunits that are designated C1q, C1r, and C1s. The protein fragments that are generated from the proteolytic degradation of complement components are also identified by a letter (a, b).

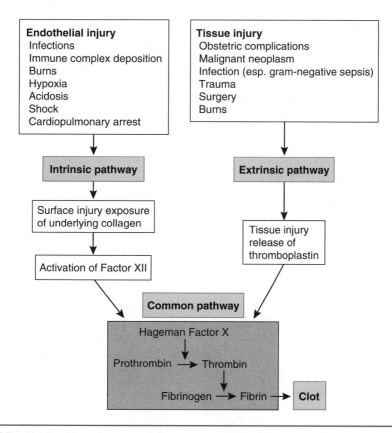

FIGURE   **5-12**   Clinical causes of the activation of a clotting cascade, intrinsic and extrinsic pathways of activation, and the mechanism by which both pathways lead to the formation of fibrin threads, or clot. (Courtesy S.H. Tepper, PhD, PT, Shenandoah University, Winchester, Va, 2000.)

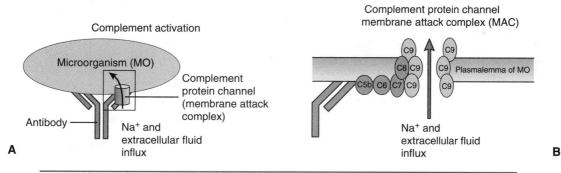

FIGURE   **5-13**   **A,** When an antibody attaches to an antigen (foreign protein) on a microorganism (MO), the antibody-antigen stimulates plasma derived complement proteins to attach and form the membrane attack complex (MAC). **B,** This MAC forms a channel through the membrane of the invading cell and allows ions and extracellular fluid to enter causing cytolysis (death of the microorganism). (Courtesy S.H. Tepper, PhD, PT, Shenandoah University, Winchester, Va, 2000.)

molytic anemia, MAC bores holes in the cell membrane of RBCs causing their destruction.

The plasma protease systems (blood coagulation, fibrinolytic, kinin enzymatic, and complement systems) are interconnected at several steps. This arrangement serves to amplify the stimulus for the inflammatory reaction as a balance mechanism. For example the activation of the plasma protein Hageman factor can initiate both the coagulation (blood clotting) and the kinin systems (produces bradykinin causing dilation and vascular leakage). The kinin system can in turn activate the fibrinolytic system by producing plasmin (splits or

divides fibrin and lyses blood clots). Plasmin then can activate the complement system and further amplify these protease loops by activating Hageman factor, once again starting the cycle (Fig. 5-14).

Phagocytosis.   One of the most important functions of the inflammatory reaction is to inactivate and remove the inflammatory stimulus and to begin the process of healing. The process of ingestion (phagocytosis) of microorganisms, other foreign substances, necrotic cells, and connective tissue constituents by specialized cells (phagocytes) is important in

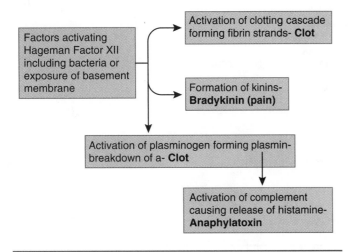

FIGURE   5-14   Clot formation. Revealed in this figure are the mechanisms for activating both the intrinsic and the extrinsic pathways for clot formation. Either of the above pathways leads to activation of the Hageman Factor XII that results in the formation of a fibrin clot. (Courtesy S.H. Tepper, PhD, PT, Shenandoah University, Winchester, Va, 2000.)

achieving this goal. Although phagocytosis could be considered the next step in the process of acute inflammation (as a separate section after the section on Chemical Mediators of Inflammation), it is included here as part of the section on Chemical Mediators because the chemical mediators are what attract phagocytic cells to the area for removal of the dead tissue or microorganisms. After ingestion by phagocytic cells, microorganisms are killed or inactivated, and necrotic debris is removed to allow tissue healing to proceed. The most important phagocytes involved in the inflammatory and healing reactions are neutrophils, monocytes, or when found in tissues of the body, macrophages. Macrophages have different names depending on their location (e.g., histiocytes in the skin, osteoclasts in bone, and microglial cells in the CNS).

The mechanism of phagocytosis is well understood. Phagocytosis is facilitated by the coating (opsonization) of particles to be ingested by IgG antibody or by the C3b component of complement. These opsonins bind to specific receptor sites located on the cell surface of neutrophils and macrophages. This receptor binding initiates a process of transmembrane signaling allowing calcium influx that activates cytoskeletal proteins within the cell. These cytoskeletal structures allow the movement of cell membranes that is necessary for phagocytosis.

The internalization of the opsonized particle begins by the enfolding of the cell surface membrane (see Fig. 5-15). The membrane folds surround the particle to be ingested and seal it within a pouch that separates it from the cell surface and becomes an intracellular vacuole called the *phagosome*. The phagosomes fuse with lysosomes (containing digestive materials and bactericidal components) and acquire enzymes and other substances that allow the killing and degradation of microorganisms and other ingested materials. Many neutrophils (e.g., polymorphonuclear neutrophils [PMNs]) die in their battle with bacteria. Dead and dying leukocytes, mixed with tissue debris and lytic enzymes form a viscous yellow fluid known as *pus*. Inflammations identified by their pus formations are called *purulent* or *suppurative* (see Table 5-3).

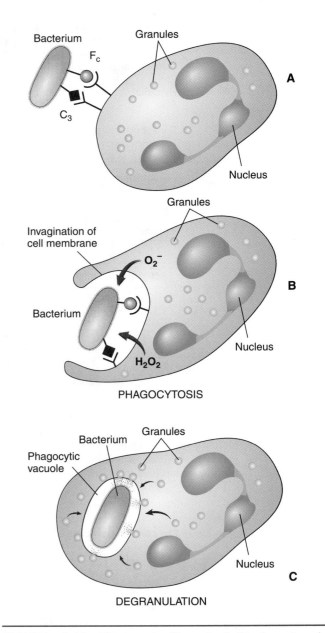

PHAGOCYTOSIS

DEGRANULATION

FIGURE   5-15   Phagocytosis of bacteria. **A,** The bacterium that was opsonized (coated with IgG and complement [C3]) binds to the Fc and complement receptors on the surface of the leukocytes. **B,** Engulfment of the bacterium into an invagination of surface membrane is associated with an oxygen burst and formation of oxygen radicals that are bactericidal and thus kill the bacterium. **C,** Inclusion of the bacterium into a phagocytic vacuole is associated with the fusion of the vacuole with lysosomes and specific granules of the leukocyte. The contents of the lysosomes and specific granules are bactericidal and contribute to final inactivation and degradation of the bacterium. The cytoplasm of the leukocyte becomes devoid of granules in a process referred to as degranulation of leukocytes. (From Damjanov I: *Pathology for the health-related professions*, ed 2, Philadelphia, 2000, WB Saunders.)

◆ Chronic Inflammation

As described, acute inflammation follows injury and once the injurious agent is removed, acute inflammation subsides. If little necrosis is present and replacement of lost parenchymal cells is possible, restitution of normal structure and function of the tissue occurs. In the presence of extensive necrosis or if re-

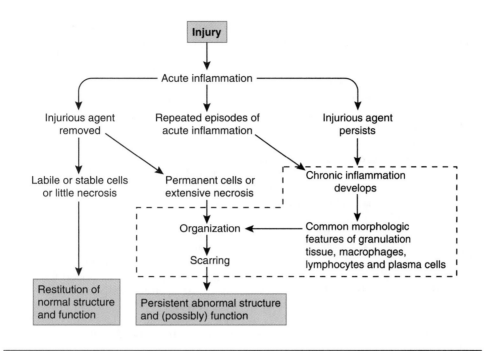

FIGURE 5-16 Overview following tissue injury: acute inflammation, chronic inflammation, and the likely healing process. (Courtesy S.H. Tepper, PhD, PT, Shenandoah University, Winchester, Va, 2000.)

generation of parenchymal cells is not possible (e.g., heart, central, or peripheral nervous system cells), the inflammatory reaction becomes chronic. Chronic inflammation also develops if the injurious agent persists for a prolonged period; if repeated episodes of acute inflammation occur in the same tissue over time; or if low-grade, persistent immune reactions are occurring (Fig. 5-16).

The hallmark of chronic inflammation in a tissue is the accumulation of macrophages, lymphocytes, and plasma cells (see Fig. 5-7). The macrophage accumulation is the result of chemotaxis of monocytes (precursors to macrophages) to the area of injury. Macrophages modulate lymphocyte functions and promote growth of endothelial cells and fibroblasts by the release of growth factors. Eosinophils may also be present, particularly if allergic reactions or parasite invasions are involved.

Granulation tissue made up of proliferating endothelial cells and fibroblasts is also seen in areas of chronic inflammation. Granulation tissue can be seen in well-healing, open wounds. Inspection of the wound site reveals red "beefy" tissue with pinpoint red dots (new capillaries) and a granular surface composed of newly formed collagen. Certain diseases cause the formation of a specific type of chronic inflammation called a *granuloma*. The granuloma is a microscopic (less than 2 mm in diameter) aggregate of macrophages often surrounded by lymphocytes. Most of the macrophages are flattened "epithelioid" in appearance and some may fuse together, giving rise to large cells with multiple nuclei (Langerhans' and foreign body giant cells). The presence of granulomatous inflammation is clinically important because it aids in the diagnosis of the injurious stimulus. Tuberculosis, a disease caused by *Mycobacterium tuberculosis*, classically causes granulomas or tubercles in this condition with a central focus of caseous necrosis. The presence of a foreign body (e.g., a suture) is another common cause of granulomatous inflammation.

Chronic inflammation can contribute to the healing of injured tissue but usually not the full return of function. The proliferation of endothelial cells reconstitutes the vasculature in the injured tissue, whereas proliferation of fibroblasts and the production of collagens and proteoglycans (polymers that form the gel between collagen fibrils) reconstitute the extracellular matrix. Together, these constituents make up the granulation tissue and lead to the formation of a connective tissue scar. This process is regulated by growth factors derived from macrophages, platelets, and plasma.

Special Implications for the Therapist   5-2

INFLAMMATION

Inflammation, which involves all of the processes described in this section, can also damage adjacent healthy tissue. The role of the therapist is important in limiting inflammation and its consequences. For example, chronic activation of inflammatory cells can cause tissue injury such as occurs with rheumatoid arthritis. This disease illustrates how the inflammatory mediators discussed are activated and how this process leads to clinical manifestations observed in a therapy practice. Inflammatory activity can be detected by the erythrocyte sedimentation rate (ESR). The therapist can review laboratory values (see Table 39-2) to assess systemic factors; in general, as the inflammation improves, the ESR decreases. Systemic effects of acute and chronic inflammation are discussed previously (see Chapter 4).

Clinical Example

The majority of people with rheumatoid arthritis produce rheumatoid factor, an antibody that is made against the person's

Continued

own antibodies of the immunoglobulin G (IgG) class. In this case the IgG antibody actually functions as an antigen (Ag) capable of inducing an immune response. This antibody-to-antibody attachment can occur in the joint space where it leads to the formation of large antibody-antigen (Ig-Ag) aggregates. Ig-Ag complexes stimulate complement activation by the classic pathway and to the formation of the strongly chemotactic cleavage products C3a and C5a. These products attract neutrophils, which then release free radicals (see Fig. 5-2) and enzymes that degrade the joint cartilage, prostaglandins, and leukotrienes that amplify the inflammatory reaction. The Ig-Ag complex is phagocytosed by synovial-lining cells that are stimulated to release collagen-degrading enzymes, prostaglandins, and IL-1. Lymphocytes contribute to the acute reaction by the production of rheumatoid factor and are responsible for the evolution of a chronic inflammatory reaction by producing cytokines that attract and activate macrophages. The macrophages produce cytokines such as IL-1 that further amplify the inflammatory reaction by attracting more neutrophils and lymphocytes and by stimulating the synthesis and release from fibroblasts, chondrocytes, and osteoclasts of enzymes that degrade cartilage and bone.

Clinically, the joints affected by the inflammatory process appear red, swollen, and are painful; a low-grade fever may also be present. Very prominent is joint stiffness that is relieved by activity. With disease progression, damage to the joints occurs, with loss of cartilage, narrowing of the joint space, and resorption of bone evident on radiograph. These changes are associated with a decrease in the range of motion of the affected joints. In later stages, obvious joint deformities develop that are accompanied by muscle wasting. Antiinflammatory agents such as aspirin and corticosteroids are effective in providing symptomatic relief and in slowing the progression of the disease.

The inflammatory process associated with rheumatoid arthritis may also affect other organ systems (see Table 26-4). Foci of chronic inflammation can develop in muscles, tendons, blood vessels, nerves, and various organs of the body (e.g., heart and lungs). In the skin, these foci cause the deposition of connective tissue called *subcutaneous nodules*.

Exercise and Inflammation

Exercise and physical training definitely influence the concentration of immunocompetent cells in the circulating pool, the proportional distribution of lymphocyte subpopulations, and the function of these cells in relation to tissue injury and infection. However, the extent of these changes and their clinical significance remains a topic for intense study at this time.[51] The mechanisms of exercise-associated muscle damage and the initiation of the inflammatory cytokine cascade are further discussed in Chapter 6 (see the section on Exercise and the Immune System). ∎

TISSUE HEALING

The process of tissue healing begins soon after tissue injury or death and occurs either by regeneration (regrowth of original tissue) or by repair (formation of a connective tissue scar). The inflammatory cells that are recruited from the blood circulation begin the healing process by breaking down and removing the necrotic tissue. This is accomplished primarily by phagocytes that secrete degradative enzymes and also phagocytose the cellular debris, connective tissue fragments, and plasma proteins present in the dead tissue.

◆ Synthesis of Extracellular Matrix

After the removal of the dead tissue, the healing process undertakes the repair of the tissue defect that remains. Tissue repair begins within 24 hours of the injury with the migration of fibroblasts from the margins of the viable tissue into the defect caused by the injury. The fibroblasts proliferate and synthesize and secrete proteins such as fibronectin, various proteoglycans and elastin, and several types of collagen. The function of these proteins is to reconstitute the extracellular matrix and provide a scaffolding-like framework for the developing endothelial and parenchymal cells.

Fibronectin

Fibronectin has numerous functions in wound healing, the most important of which are the formation of scaffold, the provision of tensile strength and the ability to "glue" other substances and cells together. It is one of the earliest proteins to provide the structural support that stabilizes the healing tissue. Plasma proteins that leak from inflamed vessels are the first source of fibronectin for the healing tissue. Plasma-derived fibronectin binds to and stabilizes fibrin, a protein that makes up the blood clots that are present in the injured tissue.

Fibronectin binds together several types of proteins present in the extracellular matrix and can also bind to debris, such as DNA material derived from necrotic cells, thereby acting as an opsonin to facilitate phagocytosis during the breakdown of necrotic tissue. Fibronectin is also responsible for attracting fibroblasts and macrophages by chemotaxis to the healing tissue. The stimulated fibroblasts, in turn, secrete more fibronectin. Fibronectin binds to proteoglycans and collagens and this binding further stabilizes the healing tissue. The importance of fibronectin can be seen as researchers seek to explain the lack of a functional healing response in the anterior cruciate ligament (ACL) after injury. Studies focusing on the signaling pathways and on binding to fibronectin for specific tissues such as the ACL may yield improved prevention and intervention strategies in the future.[63,71]

Proteoglycans and Elastin

Proteoglycans, proteins containing carbohydrate chains and sugars are secreted in abundance by fibroblasts early during the tissue repair reaction. Proteoglycans bind to fibronectin and to collagen and help stabilize the tissue that is undergoing repair. Proteoglycans also retain water and aid in the hydration of the tissue being repaired. Once the tissue is healed, proteoglycans contribute to the organization and stability of collagen and create an electrical charge that gives basement membranes the property of functioning like molecular sieves. Fibroblasts also synthesize and secrete elastin, a protein that becomes cross-linked to form fibrils or long sheets that provide tissues with elasticity.

Collagen

Collagen is the most important protein to provide structural support and tensile strength for almost all tissues and organs of the body. The different types of collagen give stability to healing tissue; the word collagen is derived from the Greek and means *glue producer*. Collagen is a fibrous protein molecule consisting of three chains of amino acid coiled around each other in a triple helix (Fig. 5-17). At least 18 collagen types have been identified.[14,50] Each collagen type has a specialized function (Table 5-6). The amino acid makeup of the collagen molecule and the manner in which the mole-

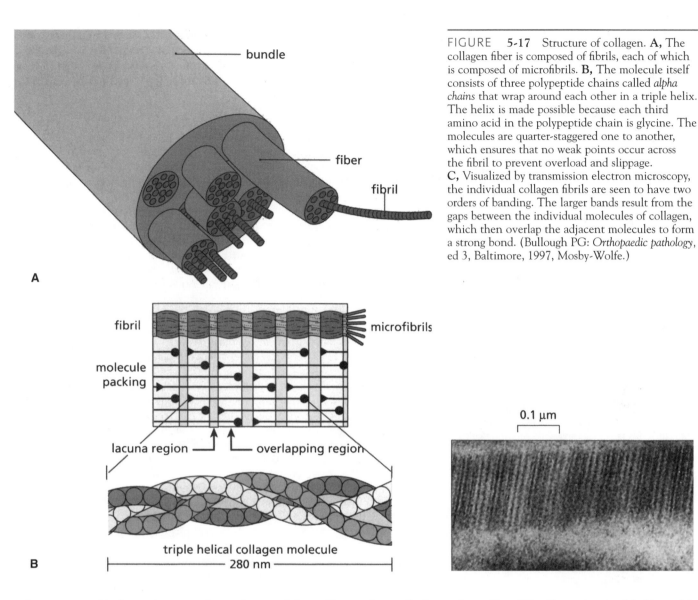

A

B

triple helical collagen molecule
— 280 nm —

C

0.1 µm

FIGURE **5-17** Structure of collagen. **A,** The collagen fiber is composed of fibrils, each of which is composed of microfibrils. **B,** The molecule itself consists of three polypeptide chains called *alpha chains* that wrap around each other in a triple helix. The helix is made possible because each third amino acid in the polypeptide chain is glycine. The molecules are quarter-staggered one to another, which ensures that no weak points occur across the fibril to prevent overload and slippage. **C,** Visualized by transmission electron microscopy, the individual collagen fibrils are seen to have two orders of banding. The larger bands result from the gaps between the individual molecules of collagen, which then overlap the adjacent molecules to form a strong bond. (Bullough PG: *Orthopaedic pathology,* ed 3, Baltimore, 1997, Mosby-Wolfe.)

cules are assembled together vary for each one of the collagen types.

The differences in organization and composition account for the structural properties of each collagen type. For example, collagen organized in unidirectional or parallel bundles contributes to the strength of tendons, in random arrangement collagen provides flexibility of the skin and rigidity of bone, organized at right angles collagen allows transmission of light in the cornea and vitreous, and collagen laid down in a tubular fashion contributes to the elasticity of the blood vessels. Some collagen molecules are assembled into progressively thicker and stronger filamentous structures, allowing the molecules to become cross-linked. These cross-links impart tensile strength to collagen fibers and prevent slippage of molecules past one another when under tension. The structural stability of the extracellular matrix is primarily a consequence of collagen and the extent of cross-linking.[12]

Type I collagen, the most common form, is assembled as a thick bundle that is structurally very strong and can be found in all body tissues where it forms bundles together with other collagen types. Type I collagen is the main component of mature scars and is also predominant in strong tissues such as tendons and bones. Type II collagen is assembled into thin supporting filaments and is the predominant collagen type found in cartilaginous tissue. Type III collagen is assembled into thin filaments that make tissues strong and pliable. It contains interchain disulfide bonds or bridges not found in type I or II and comprises the collagen type first deposited in wound healing (i.e., fresh scars). This type of collagen accounts, in part, for the plasticity of skin and blood vessels. Type IV collagen is not assembled into fibers. Together with other proteins, it forms the basement membrane to which epithelial, endothelial, and certain mesenchymal cells are anchored.

During the initial stages of tissue repair, fibroblasts secrete large amounts of type III collagen, which provides support for the developing capillaries. Within a few days after the tissue injury, type III collagen is degraded by enzymes secreted by fibroblasts and other cells and is replaced by newly synthesized type I collagen. Type I collagen is the main component of the scar tissue that remains after repair is completed. This type I collagen enhances wound tensile strength.

Mutations in the genes for collagen cause a wide spectrum of diseases of bone, cartilage, and blood vessels, including *osteogenesis imperfecta,* a variety of chondrodysplasias, Alport syndrome, the Ehlers-Danlos syndrome, and more rarely, some forms of osteoporosis, osteoarthritis, and familial aneurysms. Current research is finding that aberrant collagen cross-linking and increased collagen synthesis is present in some malignan-

TABLE 5-6

Types of Collagen

TYPE	LOCATION
Type I	Predominant structural collagen of the body; constitutes 80% to 85% of dermal collagen; prominent in mature scars, tendon, bone, and dentin
Type II	Predominant component of hyalin cartilage (e.g., outer ear, end of nose, joint); not present in skin; found in nucleus pulposus
Type III	Prominent in vascular and visceral structures (e.g., blood vessels, gastrointestinal tract, liver, uterus) but absent in bone and tendon; constitutes 15% to 20% of dermal collagen; abundant in embryonic tissues; first collagen deposited in wound healing
Type IV	Found in basement membranes (base of epithelial, endothelial, and mesenchymal cells found in developing fetus)
Type V	Present in most tissues but never as a major component; prominent in fetal membrane, cornea, heart valve; minor component of skin; synovial membranes
Type VI	Prevalent in most connective tissues
Type VII	May be involved in matrix and bone disorders, anchoring filaments of lymphatic vessels
Type VIII	Secreted by rapidly proliferating cells; found in basement membranes; may provide a molecular bridge between different types of matrix molecules
Type IX	Minor component in hyaline cartilage; vitreous humor (fluid of the eye)
Type X	Only formed in the epiphyseal growth plate cartilage; may have a role in angiogenesis; may be involved in matrix and bone disorders
Type XI	Hyaline cartilage
Type XII	Embryonic skin and tendon, periodontal ligament
Type XIII	Endothelial cells
Type XIV	Fetal skin and tendons; similar to Type I

cies,[6] whereas the presence of free radical scavengers inhibits the rate of collagen formation.[48] When either collagen or elastin becomes resorbed, elements are released into blood and concentrate in urine. Determining the presence of these components in tissues and body fluids provide important markers in the clinical investigation of various diseases.[60] Methods to quantify the number of collagen cross-links in tissue are also being further developed at this time.[59]

Special Implications for the Therapist 5-3

COLLAGEN

Much debate has been directed toward the role of the therapist in using myofascial techniques or soft tissue mobilization techniques (including friction massage) to change collagen structures and improve mobility, increase joint range or motion, or alter scar tissue. Whether these techniques can break the collagen cross-links and allow slippage to lengthen or realign the collagen fibers remains unproved at this time. Clinical research and determination of evidence-based intervention in this area is needed.

It has been found that regular mobility of affected tissues helps maintain lubrication and critical fiber distance.[1,28,70] Immobilization is associated with excessive deposition of connective tissue in associated areas with concomitant loss of water with subsequent dehydration and increase in intermolecular cross-linking, further restricting normal connective tissue flexibility and extensibility. The use of ultrasound to increase collagen tissue extensibility, increase enzymatic activity at the site of wound healing, absorb joint adhesions, and reduce fibrous tissue volume and density in scar tissue has been widely accepted, although some of these effects remain to be definitively proven. Ultrasound has been shown to facilitate the development of stronger and better-aligned scar tissue[10] and the first study to examine the ability of ultrasound to heat human tendon has been published.[11]

In the physiologic response of injury or wound healing, the key to growth or replacement tissue at sites of injury is stimulation of protein synthesis in fibroblasts. Exposure of injured tissue to ultrasound at clinically practical doses seems to provide this stimulation.[46] Continuous ultrasound during the first week of wound healing may hinder repair, but pulsed ultrasound at the lower ranges of intensity may be used during the acute phase to stimulate the release of vasodilator amine histamine from mast cells.[29] Other research has shown that 0.1 w/cm^2 continuous ultrasound provides the same total amount of ultrasound as 0.5 w/cm^2 pulsed, but the pulsed ultrasound was more effective in its nonthermal wound healing effects.[22]

It is thought that the nonthermal effects of ultrasound increase cellular diffusion, membrane permeability, and fibroblastic activities such as protein synthesis, which speeds up tissue regeneration during the proliferative phase.[11,55] After 3 weeks, collagen synthesis continues to occur for remodeling during the subacute stage of healing and ultrasound can be used as an adjunct to other interventions to promote this collagen synthesis and to minimize adhesions. Reducing adhesions occurs by raising the tissue temperature to increase viscoelastic properties during the proliferation to remodeling stage.[24,25] Combining ultrasound with other interventions such as electrical stimulation or laser photo stimulation may not be as effective as ultrasound alone.[33]

Ultrasound aids in reabsorption of joint adhesions by depolymerization of mucopolysaccharides, mucoproteins, or glycoproteins and may reduce the viscosity of hyaluronic acid in joints, thereby reducing joint adhesions. Slow, static stretching after ultrasound is important in increasing viscoelastic properties and maintaining length of the structure.[32,56] Tight capsular tissue, tendon, and mature scar tissue can also obtain increased extensibility with ultrasound when properly applied and followed immediately by slow, static stretching. This increased extensibility occurs as the mechanical effects of ultrasound disrupt the glucoside bonds forming scar tissue and the thermal effects increase the viscoelastic properties of the connective tissue. Again, ultrasound must be accompanied or immediately followed by a slow, controlled stretching and then active motion through the full available range of motion to assist in restoring mobility in tissue and between the tissue interfaces.[11,34] The stretch must be held until the collagen reaches a deformation phase. Without these follow-up techniques, the bond will reform in its original position.[32,41]

The therapist is advised to make careful assessment of the phase of injury and clinical results in the use of ultrasound and discontinue its use if there are increases in pain or edema or decreases in range of motion or function. Continuous ultrasound at low intensities may be used for nonthermal or thermal effects during the subacute and proliferative phase (fibroblastic infiltration and collagen formation) and early into the remodeling phase. ■

◆ Proliferation and Migration of Cells

Parenchymal Cells

Within a few hours after lethal injury to skin epithelial cells, the viable cells that surround the necrotic tissue detach from their extracellular matrix anchorage sites and separate from the other epithelial cells. The remaining epithelial cells flatten out to cover the area left bare by the necrotic cells. The remaining epithelial cells also divide and migrate into the tissue using the extracellular matrix support provided by the proteins secreted by the fibroblasts. This process of replacement of dead parenchymal cells by new cells is called *regeneration*. Regeneration is a very desirable healing process because it restores normal tissue structure and function.

Regeneration can only occur if the parenchymal cells can undergo mitosis. Cells are classified as permanent, stable, and labile based on their ability to divide. Permanent cells such as cardiac myocytes or central or peripheral neurons cannot divide; they are long-lived and irreplaceable. Very recent literature has revealed some capability of neurons to regenerate (neurogenesis) only in certain areas of the brain.[5] Stable cells such as hepatocytes, skeletal muscle fibers, and kidney cells normally do not divide but can be induced to undergo mitosis by an appropriate stimulus. For example, if a portion of the liver is removed by surgery or if liver cells are killed by a viral infection (hepatitis), the remaining hepatocytes divide and sometimes can fully replace the missing liver tissue. Labile cells, on the other hand, divide continuously. Examples include epithelial cells of the skin and gastrointestinal (GI) system. After each cell division, one daughter cell (stem cell) retains the ability to divide again. The second daughter cell becomes specialized (differentiates) and carries on its specific functions until it dies. Another example of labile cells is found in the bone marrow. Here, hematopoietic (blood cell forming) stem cells continuously divide giving rise to specialized cells such as erythrocytes and neutrophils with finite life spans (see Fig. 20-5). Another example of labile cells is found in epithelia such as skin, which contains basally located stem cells. The stem cells divide and produce daughter cells that progressively move to the surface of the epithelium and ultimately die, detach, and form a leading source of dust in the world.

Endothelial Cells

Within 2 days after a skin wound or injury, endothelial cells from viable blood vessels near the edge of the necrotic tissue begin to proliferate. The purpose of the endothelial cell proliferation is to establish a vascular network that can transport oxygen and nutrients and support the metabolism of the healing tissue. The endothelial cells bud out from the vessels and form new capillary channels that merge with each other as they develop and grow toward the tissue defect caused by the injury. This process of formation of new blood vessels is called *neovascularization* or *angiogenesis*.

The rich network of developing blood vessels with its connective tissue matrix can be seen with the naked eye in healing wounds. As described previously, the appearance of a reddish granular layer of tissue and was therefore given the name "granulation tissue." Histologically the main cellular components of granulation tissue are the endothelial cells and the fibroblasts although some inflammatory cells are also commonly present. Initially the newly formed vessels are leaky and this leak contributes to the edematous appearance of tissue undergoing repair. As tissue healing is completed, blood flow to the newly formed vasculature shuts down, and the nonfunctional vessels are degraded, leaving few blood vessels in mature scar tissue.

◆ Tissue Contraction and Contracture

As the healing process proceeds, the newly formed extracellular matrix draws together, causing a shrinkage (contraction) of the healing tissue. In this manner the size of the tissue defect caused by the injury is diminished. Some fibroblasts within the healing tissue differentiate and acquire some of the morphologic and functional characteristics of smooth muscle cells (myocytes). These specialized fibroblasts are called *myofibroblasts*. Myofibroblasts contain abundant contractile proteins and apparently contract and contribute to the shrinkage of the healing tissue. Tissue contraction is a normal process that contributes to tissue repair by approximating the margins of the healing tissue and speeding up the closure of wounds. In some cases, excessive shrinkage of the healing tissue occurs. This condition is called *contracture*. Contracture is an undesirable outcome of healing because it can be disfiguring and can impair movement or organ function. For example, people with severe burns often develop skin contractures due to the process of "hypertrophic scarring" that can result in significant movement impairments and subsequent disability.

◆ Tissue Regeneration

In some instances tissue healing occurs almost exclusively by the progress of regeneration (regrowth of original tissue). Regeneration can only occur in labile or stable tissues and currently does not occur in permanent tissues. This is the case if the inflammatory reaction that follows injury is short-lived and affects labile or stable parenchymal cells without disrupting their basement membranes and other extracellular components and vascular structures. Under these conditions the regenerating parenchymal cells can use the existing connective tissue scaffolding to reconstitute the normal structure and function of the organ. This type of tissue healing can be seen after superficial mechanical injury to epithelia. An example is a superficial abrasion of the skin that causes only necrosis of the epidermis. In this case, regeneration occurs with little or no scarring. In most cases, however, healing of tissue is achieved by both cell regeneration and replacement by connective tissue (scarring) called *repair*. In the case of skin, for example, this type of healing occurs after wounds that involve both the epidermis and dermis.

◆ Tissue Repair (Formation of Scar Tissue)

Tissue repair, the formation of a connective tissue scar, occurs with necrosis of permanent cells or excessive necrosis of tissues with removal of the connective tissue matrix. Without this matrix, labile cells do not regenerate or regenerate in an incomplete fashion. Therefore the structural integrity of the parenchymal tissue depends on the formation of this connective tissue scar (dense, irregular laying down of collagen). In many cases, however, healing of tissue is achieved by both cell regeneration and replacement by connective tissue (scarring). In the case of skin, for example, both types of healing occur in wounds that involve both the epidermis and dermis.

It is possible to minimize scarring by surgical obliteration of the tissue defect caused by injury and cell necrosis. For example, treatment of skin wounds begins with careful cleansing of the wound to remove foreign materials and bacterial contamination, which interfere with healing. This is followed by debridement to remove nonviable tissue that normally would be broken down by the inflammatory reaction. Careful attention to hemostasis minimizes the deposition of blood into the wound. During closure the wound margins are closely apposed under the right amount of tension by surgical sutures. A clean, closed wound is free of infectious and other foreign material, fibrin, and necrotic debris. As a result, the duration and intensity of the inflammatory reaction is minimized. Little granulation tissue forms and the epithelial cell surface is readily reconstituted.

The healing that occurs in the type of wound described above is called primary union or healing by first intention and results in a small scar (Fig. 5-18). In the presence of large tissue defects or infections, and in other conditions where surgical closure is not possible or desirable, healing occurs by secondary union. In this situation the time required for healing is longer and the amount of scarring is greater.

Minimizing tissue scarring is important not only for cosmetic reasons, as is the case in skin, but also because excessive scarring can interfere with organ function. Very large tissue defects may require the use of grafts or flaps of tissue to achieve optimal healing.

Even after healing is complete, degradation and resynthesis of collagen continues. This is, at least in part, a response to shifts in the stress forces to which the tissue is subjected. Cross-linking of collagen fibers continues for a period of several weeks, providing progressive strengthening of scar tissue. However, even under optimal conditions, the repaired tissue never fully regains its original stability. In the case of skin, a fully mature fibrous scar requires 12 to 18 months and is about 20% to 30% weaker than normal skin. In some people, an inherited tendency to produce excessive amounts of collagen during the healing process causes large amounts of collagen arranged in thick bundles

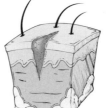

Incision with blood clot

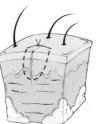

Edges approximated with suture

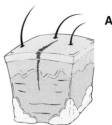

Fine scar

A

FIGURE   **5-18**   **A,** Healing by primary intention is the initial union of the edges of a wound, progressing to complete healing without granulation. **B,** Healing by secondary intention is wound closure in which the edges are separated, granulation tissue develops to fill the gap, and epithelium grows in over the granulations, producing a scar. **C,** Healing by *tertiary intention* is wound closure in which granulation tissue fills the gap between the edges of the wound, with epithelium growing over the granulation at a slower rate and producing a larger scar than results from healing from second intention. Suppuration is also usually found in tertiary wound closure. (Anderson KN, Anderson LE, Glanze WD: *Mosby's medical, nursing and allied health dictionary,* ed 5, St Louis, 1998, Mosby.)

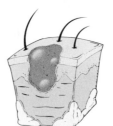

Irregular, large wound with blood clot

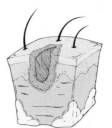

Granulation tissue fills in wound

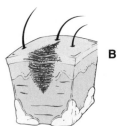

Large scar

B

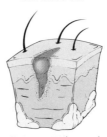

Contaminated wound

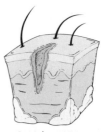

Granulation tissue

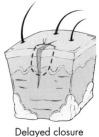

Delayed closure with suture

C

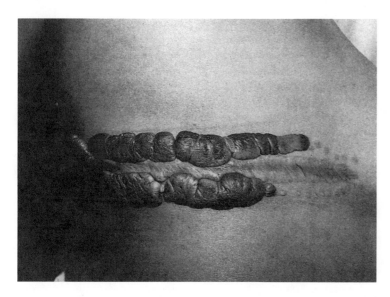

FIGURE 5-19 Keloid (hypertrophic) scar composed predominantly of type III collagen, rather than type I collagen. Keloids result from defective remodeling of scar tissue and the persistence of type III collagen, which is typical of immature scar. Epidermis is elevated by excess scar tissue, which may continue to increase long after healing occurs. Looks smooth, rubbery, "clawlike." Young women, black people, and people of Mediterranean descent are particularly susceptible to keloid formation. (Habif TP: *Clinical dermatology: a color guide to diagnosis and therapy*, ed 3, St Louis, 1996, Mosby.)

to accumulate in the tissue. These collagenous masses are called *keloids* and can be seen protruding from the skin surface (Fig. 5-19). Types of treatment include solid carbon dioxide, liquid nitrogen, intralesional corticosteroid injections, radiation, silicon gel, and surgery. However, treatment may worsen the condition. The treatment of keloids remains an area in which more effective intervention is warranted, but research in this area remains limited.

Necrosis of heart tissue (myocardial infarct) results in a fibrous scar because cardiac myocytes do not replicate to any great extent. Outcomes that can result from tissue repair in various tissue and conditions are summarized in Fig. 5-16. The CNS differs in its healing process because neurons are permanent cells and do not replicate. After tissue necrosis neither regeneration, nor tissue scarring occurs. No fibroblasts are present in the brain parenchyma, and no collagen is produced. After a brain infarct (stroke) the inflammatory cells arrive from the blood circulation and clear away the necrotic tissue, leaving behind an empty cavity (cyst). Specialized CNS cells called *astrocytes (glial cells)* proliferate, forming dense aggregates around the necrotic area called *glial scars* or *gliosis*.

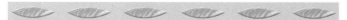

Special Implications for the Therapist 5-4

SCAR TISSUE

The clinical implications of tissue repair can be seen in the example presented earlier in this chapter (see the Special Implications for the Therapist: Collagen and Cell Injury in this chapter). In this example, after a transmural myocardial infarction, a symptom-limited stress test will usually be given after Phase II of cardiac rehabilitation, around 8 to 12 weeks post–myocardial infarction. With understanding of the material presented in this chapter, one can see the logical explanation. Heart healing, which occurs primarily through the process of tissue repair, requires 8 to 12 weeks for the formation of a dense connective tissue scar. This dense scar allows for structural integrity and force transduction of the viable myocardium, leading to a complete heart contraction. Since the connective tissue scar is not contractile, this area of the heart will never return to full function. Of great importance is the fact that after a myocardial infarction (heart attack), a person's aerobic fitness can improve (or exceed) to the level before his or her premorbid state with proper exercise. ■

◆ Factors That Affect Tissue Healing

Many variables regulate or affect the healing process and either facilitate, inhibit, or delay wound healing (Box 5-4). Since local blood supply is vital to the delivery of the materials necessary for wound healing, factors that impede local circulation or depletion of the necessary materials could delay rehabilitation. Certain tissues (e.g., tendons) have a decreased blood supply, and thus the healing process may require additional time.

Growth Factors

The cells involved in the tissue repair response produce proteins called *growth factors* that regulate a number of cellular reactions involved in healing. Growth factors regulate cell proliferation, differentiation, and migration; biosynthesis and degradation of proteins; and angiogenesis. Through all of these varying functions, growth factors integrate the inflammatory events with the reparative processes. When these complex mechanisms are disturbed, the result can be delayed healing and an inferior scar (hypotrophic) or elevated levels of growth factor, resulting in hypertrophic scarring such as occurs after a burn injury or in the formation of keloids.[53,67]

Growth factors act by binding to receptors on the plasma membranes of specific cells and have a stimulatory or inhibitory effect on these cells. This binding initiates a process of transmembrane signaling that results in the phosphorylation of proteins (the process of attaching a phosphate group to the protein). These steps lead to the activation of gene ex-

Factors Influencing Healing

Physiologic variables (e.g., age, growth factors, vascular sufficiency)

General health of the individual; immunocompetency; psychologic/emotional/spiritual well-being

Presence of comorbidities (examples):

- Diabetes mellitus
- Decreased oxygen perfusion (e.g., COPD, CHF, CAD, pneumonia)
- Hematologic disorders (e.g., neutropenia)
- Cancer (local and systemic effects)
- Incontinence
- Alzheimer's disease
- Neurologic impairment
- Immobility

Tobacco, alcohol, caffeine, other substance use/abuse

Nutrition (especially presence of protein, vitamins, and heavy metals depletion)

Local or systemic infection; presence of foreign bodies

Type of tissue

Medical treatment (e.g., prednisone, chemotherapy, radiation therapy)

COPD, chronic obstructive pulmonary disease; *CHF*, chronic heart failure; *CAD*, coronary artery disease.

pression and DNA synthesis in the cell. The signals that turn on proliferation of normal cells and cause tissue healing are also responsible for turning on proliferation of cancer cells. With continued growth of a neoplastic cells, a neoplasm or tumor may occur. The significant difference between the healing process and cancer is that the growth of the cancer cells goes on unchecked. These analogies have led to the designation of cancers as wounds that do not heal.

Platelets, endothelial cells, fibroblasts, macrophages, and cytokines are important sources of growth factors. Two important growth factors are platelet-derived growth factor (PDGF), which activates fibroblasts and macrophages, and fibroblast growth factor (FGF), which stimulates endothelial cells to form new blood vessels. An example of a growth factor that inhibits cell growth and inactivates macrophages is transforming growth factor–beta (TGF–β). Several growth factors are being tested clinically to establish if these can boost the healing process in people who have deficiencies in wound healing (e.g., diabetic lower extremity ulcers).[23] Wound dressings of the future may include several growth factors, each with a specific function. The application of topically active growth factors to chronic ulcers remains in the experimental phase.[20,69] Finally, it should be mentioned that cytokines such as IL-1, IL-2, IL-15, and TNF can also regulate some aspects of the healing response. Some ILs have been identified as T-cell growth factors with proinflammatory properties or the transforming growth factor associated with hypertrophic scarring. Further studies are necessary to clarify the mechanism of cytokine release in normal postoperative wounds before therapeutic use can be developed.[36]

Nutrition

Nutrition is an important factor to influence healing.* Adequate nutritional intake is necessary to support the active metabolism of cells involved in repair. Trauma, including surgery, or infections often increase the systemic rate of protein catabolism. This has adverse effects on the synthesis of proteins required for healing. Inadequate intake of specific nutritional factors can specifically affect collagen production and remodeling. Examples are vitamin C deficiency, which causes defective collagen molecules to form, and deficiency of zinc. Zinc is essential for the activity of enzymes that degrade collagen and of enzymes that are responsible ultimately for the induction of protein synthesis. Zinc deficiency therefore impairs healing. People with cancer often manifest delayed healing because of poor nutritional status often associated with the cancer process itself or the medical treatment (e.g., chemotherapy); particularly notable is the poor healing in tissues that have been subjected to radiation therapy.

Other Factors

Other factors that influence healing include vascular supply, presence of infection, immune reaction, client's age, and the presence of other medical conditions. An adequate vascular supply is critical to provide oxygen and nutrients to support healing. Vascular insufficiency, particularly in the lower limbs, is an important cause of slow- or nonhealing wounds. Infection interferes with healing by inciting a severe and prolonged inflammatory reaction that can increase tissue damage. Certain microorganisms can also release toxins that directly cause tissue necrosis and lysis. Foreign bodies may retard healing by inducing a chronic inflammatory reaction, by interfering with closure of a tissue defect and by providing a site protected from leukocytes and antibiotics where bacteria can multiply. Healing is often adversely affected in people who smoke, who are immunosuppressed, or who have other compromising medical conditions referred to as *co-morbidities*. For example, the presence of an immunocompromised state (e.g., acquired immunodeficiency syndrome [AIDS], the prolonged use of corticosteroids, or undergoing chemotherapy or radiation treatment), incontinence, peripheral vascular disease, confusion associated with dementia or Alzheimer's disease, or other neurologic impairment can contribute to delayed wound healing. Diseases associated with decreased oxygen perfusion (e.g., anemia, congestive heart failure, chronic obstructive pulmonary disease [COPD], or DM) can also delay healing. DM is associated with poor healing; one of the causes appears to be impaired function of phagocytic cells, another is a defect in granulation tissue formation.[17]

---

* For an excellent source of information related to nutrition and healing in the therapist's practice, see Nutrition Applied to Injury Rehabilitation and Sports Medicine.[8]

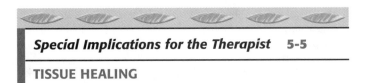

Special Implications for the Therapist 5-5

TISSUE HEALING

Understanding the interaction of the wound, wound microorganisms, and the immune response is central to developing successful therapeutic interventions for wound care and management. This chapter has carefully explained how wounding of normal skin initiates an inflammatory response that ordinarily contributes to the healing process that is orchestrated by specific and nonspecific immune responses. Inflammatory cells provide growth factors and stimulate the deposition of matrix proteins and phagocytose debris. However, the maturation and resolution of a wound may be complicated by the presence of microorganisms. The effects of microorganisms on oxygen consumption and pH or toxin production may interrupt the natural course of wound healing. The wound may not progress from the acute phase but may become a non-healing chronic or recalcitrant wound as long as the antigens from microorganisms or underlying pathology remain, leading to wound infection. Even so, most chronic wounds progress toward healing, depending on the wound care strategy employed.[66] For example, a venous leg ulcer will heal once the proper compression and support have been provided to counteract the underlying venous hypertension and appropriate wound care has been provided. Similarly, diabetic neuropathic foot ulcers do not heal until the disordered glucose metabolism is controlled, adequacy of the vascular supply is ensured, and causative pressure on the foot is offloaded.

Successful healing of chronic wounds involves intervention to address the underlying causes along with clinical wound management that provides an environment to tip the balance in favor of healing. The therapist is more likely to select appropriate intervention measures if the evaluation and assessment process takes into consideration the physiology of tissue repair along with the many factors that can affect wound healing. Investigating the status of these other factors (e.g., nutritional status; mobility status; turning schedule for the immobile; continence status; use of substances such as tobacco, alcohol, or caffeine; medication schedule) requires collaboration with other health care specialists and with the family.[64] Laboratory values such as albumin levels indicating nutritional status (see Table 39-15) and glucose levels, hemoglobin, and hematocrit (see Table 39-6) to monitor wound healing provide the therapist with necessary information when setting up and carrying out an appropriate intervention plan.

Specific techniques for wound management are beyond the scope of this text. The reader is referred to other texts with this information (see Chapter 9). ■

SPECIFIC TISSUE OR ORGAN REPAIR

Throughout this chapter, examples of cell types and healing processes within various organs and systems of the body have been discussed. Some organs are composed of cells that cannot regenerate (e.g., heart, central or peripheral nervous system cells), whereas other organs such as the liver and epithelial cells of the integumentary and GI systems can replace missing tissue through cell division (mitosis). Some cells such as skeletal muscle cells and renal cells do not divide but can be induced to undergo mitosis.

The extent to which cells can regenerate depends on the type of cell (e.g., permanent, stable, labile); the cell's ability to divide; the type of damage incurred (e.g., lethal, sublethal); and other factors discussed (e.g., nutrition, age, immunocompetency, vascular supply, presence of microorganisms leading to infection). The proliferation and migration of cells, including parenchymal cells is discussed; regeneration can only occur if the parenchymal cells can undergo mitosis. When regeneration of parenchymal cells is not possible, the inflammatory reaction can become chronic. Using an example of a person with traumatic brain injury, who also experiences a myocardial infarction (see Special Implications: Cell Injury: Multiple Cell Injuries), healing of brain and myocardial tissue is discussed. Only those tissues not specifically included in the main body of this chapter are presented further here.

◆ Lung

After lethal injury to alveolar cells (type I and II pneumocytes) with persistence of the basement membrane, regeneration can occur. After the phagocytic removal of the necrotic cells, adjacent living epithelial cells migrate onto the remaining basement membrane and differentiate into type II pneumocytes (cells that primarily produce surfactant). Eventually some of these cells differentiate into type I pneumocytes (cells that permit gas exchange) and full lung function is restored. This regeneration process occurs after a bout of pneumonia. If the damage to the lung disrupts the basement membrane, incomplete and inadequate regeneration occurs and healing must be achieved by repair. Also, certain injurious agents induce lung healing by the formation of scar tissue leading to restrictive lung disease. An example of this would include inhalation of asbestos.

◆ Peripheral Nerves

When a nerve is cut, the peripheral portion rapidly undergoes a myelin degeneration and axonal fragmentation. The lipid debris is removed by macrophages mobilized from the surrounding tissues in a process referred to as *Wallerian degeneration*. However, within 24 hours of section, new axonal sprouts from the central stump are observed with proliferation of Schwann cells from both the central and peripheral stumps. Careful microsurgical approximation of the nerve may result in reinnervation. The most important factor in achieving successful nerve regeneration after repair is the maintenance of the neurotubules (basement membrane and connective tissue endoneurium), along which the new axonal sprouts can pass.[9]

◆ Skeletal Muscle

Contrary to widespread belief, muscle tissue regenerates well, but the restoration of normal structure and function is strongly dependent on the type of injury sustained. In severe infections, the muscle fibers may be extensively destroyed. However, the sarcolemmal sheaths (basement membrane and connective tissue endomysium) usually remain intact, and rapid regeneration of muscle cells within the sheaths occurs so that the function of the muscle may be completely restored. After transection of a muscle, muscle fibers may regenerate either by growth from undamaged stumps or by growth of new, independent fibers.[9] This type of regeneration after lethal cell injury to skeletal muscle fibers regeneration is possible through mitotic division of "satellite cells" when the basement membrane remains intact. Satellite cells play an integral role in normal development of skeletal muscle and are essential to the repair of injured muscle by serving as a source of myoblasts for fiber regeneration.[4]

With death of the muscle cell and ensuing necrosis, chemotactic agents attract macrophages within the basement membrane confines to engulf the remnants of the dead cell.

Macrophages release growth factors stimulating the division of the satellite cells. These cells migrate to the central region and begin to differentiate into expressing the usual characteristics of a skeletal muscle fiber. This can occur with muscular dystrophy after lethal cell injury when the connective tissue matrix (primarily basement membrane) is disrupted and regeneration is attempted, but disruption of basement membrane leaves the satellite cells no direction where to set up and multiply. The end result is the muscle tissue heals by forming a connective tissue scar (i.e., repair). This at least maintains the structural integrity of the tissue but not the complete functional capability. This type of healing of muscle could occur after the trauma of a motor vehicle accident or a knife wound.

◆ Bone

A variety of conditions can affect bone and require a reparative process, including fracture; infection; inflammation (e.g., tuberculosis, sarcoidosis); metabolic disturbances (e.g., Paget's disease, osteoporosis, osteogenesis imperfecta); tumors; response to implanted prostheses; bone infarction; and as other systemic diseases that have skeletal manifestations (e.g., sickle cell disease, amyloidosis, hemochromatosis). For a discussion of these specific conditions and their impact on bone, the reader is referred to each individual chapter including those diseases. Only the bone response to injury and the reparative process (specifically fracture) will be discussed in this chapter.

Fracture repair is a healing process by regeneration and remodeling (i.e., without a scar) and with the potential for a return of optimal function in many cases. After an uncomplicated fracture, bone heals in several overlapping phases (Fig. 5-20). The first phase, the inflammatory phase, usually lasting several days, is clinically evidenced by pain, swelling, and heat. At the moment of fracture, tiny blood vessels through the haversian systems are torn at the fracture site. A brief period of local internal bleeding occurs, resulting in a fracture hematoma. Inflammatory cells arrive at the injured site accompanied by the vascular response and cellular proliferation. Clotting factors from the blood initiate the formation of a fibrin meshwork. This meshwork is the scaffolding for the ingrowth of fibroblasts and capillary buds around and between the bony ends. By the end of the first week, phagocytic cells have removed a majority of the hematoma, and neovascularization and initial fibrosis are occurring.

The second phase, the reparative phase, begins during the next few weeks and includes the formation of the soft callus, which is eventually replaced by a hard callus. During this phase, osteoclasts (bone macrophages) clear away the necrotic bone while the periosteum and endosteum regenerate and begin to differentiate into formation of hyaline cartilage (soft callus) and primary bony spicules (hard callus). Bone growth factors, including bone morphogenetic proteins, TGF-ß, platelet-derived growth factor, insulin-like growth factors I and II, and acid and basic fibroblasts growth factors are powerful components of the fracture healing (reparative) phase.[42] Once the callus is sufficient to immobilize the fracture site, repair occurs between the fractured cortical and medullary bones when the fibrocartilaginous union (soft callus) is replaced by a fibroosseous union (hard callus). Delayed union and nonunion result from errors in this phase of bone healing. The completion of the reparative phase (usually occurring between 6 and 12 weeks) is indicated by fracture stability. Radiographically, the fracture line begins to disappear.[37]

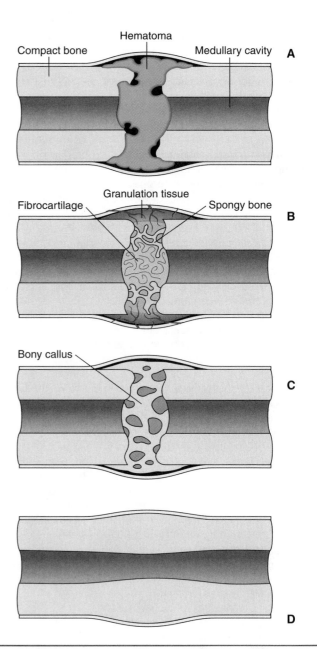

FIGURE 5-20 Fracture healing occurs in overlapping stages or phases. **A,** Immediate vascular response with hematoma formation and inflammatory response. **B,** Granulation tissue and fibrocartilage formation during early reparative phase. **C,** Fibrocartilaginous union (soft callus) is replaced by a fibroosseous union (bony callus). **D,** Remodeling phase with complete restoration of the medullary canal. (Damjanov I: *Pathology for the health-related professions*, ed 2, Philadelphia, 2000, WB Saunders.)

The third phase, the remodeling phase, begins with clinical and roentgenographic union (no movement occurs at the fracture site) and persists until the bone is returned to normal, including restoration of the medullary canal. During this phase, which may take months to years, the immature, disorganized woven bone is replaced with a mature organized lamellar bone that adds further stability to the fracture site. The excessive bony callus is resorbed, and the bone remodels in response to the mechanical stresses placed upon it.

The time for overall bone healing varies depending on the bone involved; the fracture site and type; treatment required (e.g., immobilization versus surgical repair, the need for bone grafting or use of bone graft substitutes); degree of soft tissue injury; treatment complications; and other factors mentioned previously (e.g., age, vascular supply, nutritional status, immunocompetency). Specific types of fractures, their treatment, and special implications for the therapist are discussed in greater detail in Chapter 26.

◆ Tendons and Ligaments

Tendons and ligaments are dense bands of fibrous connective tissue composed of 78% water, 20% collagen, and 2% glycosaminoglycans. This composition allows them to sustain high, unidirectional tensile loads, transfer forces, provide strong flexible support, and help the tissue respond to normal loads while resisting excessive mechanical or shearing forces and deformation. The viscoelastic characteristics of these tissues makes them capable of undergoing deformation under tensile or compressive force, yet still capable of returning to their original state after removal of the force.

Tendons attach muscles to their osseous origins and insertions, whereas ligaments provide support to joints through bone-to-bone attachments. Both are made up of parallel fibers of type I collagen produced by fibroblasts/cytes, glycosaminoglycans/proteoglycans, small vascular supply, and sensory innervation. The mechanical properties of tendons and ligaments are dependent not only on the architecture and properties of the collagen fibers but also on the proportion of elastin that these structures contain (e.g., minimal elastin in tendons and ligaments of the extremities, substantial elastin in the *ligamentum flava*).

Sprains and tears of the tendinous or ligamentous structures around a joint can be caused by abnormal or excessive joint motion. These injuries can be classified as first, second, or third degree, depending on the changes in structural or biomechanical integrity (ranging from injury of a few fibers without loss of integrity to a complete tear). Common sites for this type of injury include the ankle, knee, and fingers with clinical manifestations of local pain, edema, increased local tissue temperature, ecchymosis, hypermobility or instability, and loss of motion and/or function. If, after injury, the therapist notes quick onset of joint effusion, and the joint feels hot to the touch with extremely painful and limited movement, the joint needs to be examined by a physician to rule out hemarthrosis.

Tendons may heal either as a result of proliferation of the tenoblasts from the cut ends of the tendon or more likely as a result of vascular ingrowth and proliferation of fibroblasts derived from the surrounding tissues that were injured at the time of the tendon injury. Because the surrounding tissues contribute so much to the healing of a tendon, adhesions are very common. With rupture of the Achilles' tendon or cruciate ligament(s), functional restoration requires surgical repair to appose and suture the cut ends.[9]

After injury and/or surgical intervention, the inflammatory process begins, and the debris in the area is cleared away by macrophages. Granulation tissue is formed by the migration and proliferation of fibroblasts and vascular buds from the surrounding connective tissue. Capillary sprouts grow out of blood vessels around the edges of the wound-forming loops by joining with each other or with capillaries already carrying blood. Although this is occurring, the fibroblasts are secreting soluble collagen molecules, which form fibrils. Approximately 2 weeks into the healing process, the collagen fibrils are ori-

ented and rearranged into thick bundles, providing the tissue with greater strength. During this period, the affected area is immobilized to relieve stress from the healing tissue and prevent rupture from recurring. The lack of stress causes the newly forming collagen to be deposited in random alignment.

Once the healing tissue has achieved adequate integrity, motion is once again permitted. The remodeling collagen then aligns to the lines of stress produced by the motion, thereby permitting the healed tendons and ligaments to provide support in line with the stress. Realignment of collagen to its usual parallel arrangement also permits the restoration of full, normal range of motion after repair. Human tendons and ligaments regain normal strength in 40 to 50 weeks postoperatively; this means that even as long as a year after injury, the tendon or ligament still will not have achieved premorbid tensile strength.

Although the process of healing is by repair (formation of a connective tissue scar), this constitutes regeneration since tendons and ligaments are originally composed of connective tissue. However, the scar tissue is weaker and larger, and has compromised biomechanical integrity with an increased amount of minor collagens (types III, V, and VI); decreased collagen cross-links; and an increased amount of glycosaminoglycans.[35] These changes lead to impaired function, increased risk of reinjury, and increased risk of osteoarthritis. Research on ligament healing includes studies on low-load and failure-load properties, alterations in the expression of matrix molecules, cytokine modulation of healing, and gene therapy as a method to alter matrix protein and cytokine production.[45,49]

◆ Cartilage

Several forms of cartilage are recognized, including articular cartilage found at the ends of the bones; fibrocartilage found in the menisci of the knee, at the annulus fibrosis, at the insertions of the ligaments and tendons into the bone, and on the inner side of tendons as they angle around pulleys (e.g., at the malleoli); and elastic cartilage found in the *ligamentum flavum*, external ear, and epiglottis. Articular cartilage composed of hyaline cartilage (comprised of chondrocytes, type II collagen, and glycosaminoglycans/proteoglycans) is aneural, avascular, and does not appear to regenerate after adolescence most likely because of its avascularity and low cell-to-matrix ratio. In adults, the healing of articular cartilage occurs by fibrous scar tissue or fails to heal at all. This replacement tissue does not function as well as the original, and the adjacent joint surface can be affected. Fibrous scarring of the articular cartilage leads to local degenerative arthritis.

Animal studies of the biologic effects on articular cartilage of postoperative immobilization, intermittent active motion, and continuous passive motion suggest that postoperative immobilization results in degenerative arthritis (90% compared with only 20% in joints managed by continuous passive motion [CPM]).[57]

Current research is examining the effects of replacing damaged cartilage with cartilage harvested from the individual, grown in culture, and reinjected into the area of damaged cartilage to avoid this postoperative or post injury sequelae. This technology may allow the individual to regenerate a smooth, weight-bearing surface and avoid the rough, degenerative fibrocartilage formation that leads to osteoarthritis.

Advances in the fields of biotechnology and biomaterials are providing new techniques for regeneration or repair of tis-

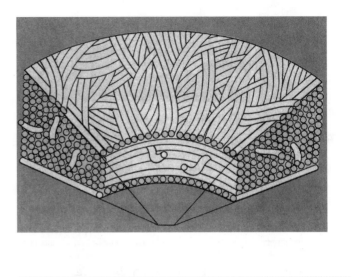

FIGURE 5-21 Diagrammatic representation of the distribution of collagen fibers in the meniscus of a knee. Collagen is oriented throughout the connective tissues in such a way as to maximally resist the forces placed upon these tissues. The majority of the fibers in the meniscus are circumferentially arranged with a few fibers on or near the tibial surface placed in a radial pattern. This structural arrangement enables the meniscus to resist the lateral spread that occurs during high loads generated during weight bearing. Longitudinally arranged collagen fibers facilitate shock absorption and sustain the tension generated between the anterior and posterior attachments. (Bullough PG: *Orthopaedic pathology*, ed 3, Baltimore, 1997, Mosby.)

sue lost to injury, disease, or aging. Bioengineered tissue including skin, bone, articular cartilage, ligaments, and tendons are under investigation for clinical use (see the section on Tissue Engineering in Chapter 20).[39,40]

◆ Menisci (Knee)

The menisci are composed mainly of collagen, although some proteoglycan is also present. The amount of proteoglycan increases dramatically in the injured, degenerate meniscus. The principal orientation of collagen fibers in the menisci is circumferential, designed to withstand the circumferential tension within the meniscus during normal loading (Fig. 5-21). A few small, radially oriented fibers present on the tibial surface, probably acting as ties to resist lateral splitting of the menisci from undue compression. In the young individual, the menisci are usually white, translucent, and supple on palpation. In the older individual, the menisci lose their translucency, become more opaque and yellow in color, and become less supple. Injury and degeneration leading to laceration are the two most common causes of symptoms that require surgical intervention.[9]

◆ Synovial Membrane

The synovial membrane lines the inner surface of the joint capsule and all other intraarticular structures (e.g., subcutaneous and subtendinous bursae sacs, tendon sheaths) with the exception of articular cartilage and the meniscus. Synovial membrane consists of two components: the intimal (cellular layer or synoviocytes) layer next to the joint space and the subintimal or supportive layer formed of fibrous and adipose tissue. The synovial membrane has three principal functions: secretion of synovial fluid hyaluronate, phagocytosis of waste material, and regulation of the movement of solutes, electrolytes, and proteins from the capillaries into the synovial fluid. This latter function provides a regulatory mechanism for maintenance of the matrix through various chemical mediators such as ILs. Injury to any of the joint structures affects the synovium and results in hemorrhage, hypertrophy and hyperplasia of the synovial lining cells, and mild chronic inflammation.[9] In the case of prolonged, chronic synovitis such as occurs in hemophilia, abnormal synovial fluid, joint immobilization, and fibrous adhesions a progressive destructive condition in the joint can result.

Special Implications for the Therapist **5-6**

SPECIFIC TISSUE OR ORGAN REPAIR

Therapists have an important role in the rehabilitation of acute injuries. Certain components of the inflammatory process must be controlled quickly for recovery to proceed. For example, if edema is a component of a joint injury, it must be controlled as quickly as possible. Studies have demonstrated that joint edema can inhibit or hinder local muscle activity, which could result in altered joint mechanics and further irritation.[19,61] The anticipated goals are to facilitate wound healing and maintain the normal function of noninjured tissue and body regions. The overall goal of the rehabilitation program is to return the person to normal activity as soon as possible, yet not so fast that irritation and further inflammation of the injured area occur. A fine line exists between maximizing activity and overdoing the activity to the point of injury aggravation.

Client education is essential regarding the injured individual's role in facilitating wound healing. Adherence to weight-bearing guidelines, avoiding prolonged sitting or flexion of the trunk, applying ice appropriately, and performing the prescribed exercises are key to the recovery process. Careful monitoring of the presenting symptoms and signs guides the therapist in deciding when and how to progress intervention and activity level. This monitoring can also be taught so the client understands the limits of his or her condition. This process is somewhat more difficult with acute back or neck injuries than with peripheral injuries. Owing to the depth of the tissues of the spine, increased temperature and erythema are not always present. The therapist must rely more on muscle tone and the degree of pain with movement changes in deciding when the program can be progressed.

A significant percentage of those coming to outpatient therapy clinics are taking salicylates or NSAIDs.[7] These medications can play a key role in recovery from an acute injury, facilitating the therapist's role and clinical decision making. Individuals respond very differently to NSAIDs so what works for one person may not work for another who presents with similar manifestations. If an acute injury is not responding to therapy intervention by 2 weeks, communicating with a physician regarding possibly trying a different antiinflammatory medication is warranted. This is based on the assumption that no other factors exist that could delay recovery.

Considering the widespread use of salicylates and NSAIDs, therapists must also be aware of potential side effects that would warrant communication with a physician (see Chapter 4). Irritation of the GI system is the most common potential side effect. The risk of developing peptic ulcer disease increases significantly if someone is taking more than one of these types of drugs. This pattern of drug use exists in the therapy population, in which significant numbers of subjects are taking one or more OTC antiinflammatory agents along with a prescribed NSAID.[7] See Chapter 15 for a description of peptic ulcer disease.

Besides ineffective medications, numerous other factors may delay or inhibit wound healing. Box 5-4 lists factors that could delay recovery from an injury. Since local blood supply is vital to the delivery of the materials necessary for wound healing, factors that impede local circulation or a depletion of the necessary materials could delay rehabilitation. Certain tissues (e.g., tendons) have a decreased blood supply, and thus the healing process may require additional time. Therapists should screen a client's medical history for the presence of conditions such as diabetes; chemical dependency (alcoholism); cigarette smoking; and so on to identify factors that could delay recovery. Lastly, local infection delays healing. If an abscess is present, the expected fever, chills, and sweats associated with infection may not be present in someone who is taking steroid medications. A sudden worsening of symptoms, the presence of a hot, acutely inflamed joint, or the onset of fever should warn the therapist that something more serious may exist. In general, the more compromised the host, the greater the chance of a slow or incomplete recovery.

Tissue Response to Immobilization

In addition to having an important role in the rehabilitation of acute injuries, therapists often deal with clinical problems secondary to the effects of immobilization. Although not traumatic in the classic sense, immobilization of a limb or joint can result in significant impairment and functional limitations. Immobilization takes a variety of forms, including bed rest, casting or splinting of a body part, or non–weight-bearing status of a lower extremity. On a tissue level, significant changes can occur with immobilization (Table 5-7). Besides the inert joint structures, changes also occur in muscle, particularly a loss of strength. Such changes can occur without injury, which magnifies the importance of maintaining function in noninjured tissue and body areas. A rehabilitation program should be designed to address the needs of each of the tissues.

While initiating rehabilitation after immobilization, the therapist must remain vigilant for the possible presence of deep vein thrombosis (DVT). A potential complication of DVT is pulmonary embolus, which represents one of the leading causes of morbidity and mortality after orthopedic surgical procedures.[27] Although a large percentage of clients with DVT are asymptomatic, severe local pain and edema, fever, chills, and malaise are all possible manifestations. The types of immobilization that carry the risk of DVT include bed rest, a limb being placed in a cast or splint, and non–weight-bearing status following a lower extremity injury, surgical procedure, or a long car or plane ride. (See Chapter 11 for more information about DVT.) ■

TABLE	5-7

Effects of Prolonged Immobilization

TISSUE	RESULTS OF IMMOBILIZATION
Muscle	Atrophy, decreased strength, contracture, reduced capillary to muscle fiber ratio, reduced mitochondrial density, reduced endurance
Bone	Generalized osteopenia of cancellous and cortical bone
Tendons and ligaments	Disorganization of parallel arrays of fibrils and cells; increased deformation with a standard load or compressive force
Ligament insertion site	Destruction of ligament fibers attaching to bone, reduced load to failure
Cartilage	Adherence of fibrofatty connective tissue to cartilage surfaces; loss of cartilage thickness; pressure necrosis at points of contact where compression has been applied
Synovium	Proliferation of fibrofatty connective tissue into joint space
Menisci	Adhesions of synovium villi; decreased synovial intima length; decreased synovial fluid hyaluronan concentrations; decreased synovial intima macrophages
Joint	*0-12 weeks:* Impaired range of motion; increased intraarticular pressure during movements; decreased filling volume of joint cavity *After 12 weeks:* Force required for the first flexion-extension cycle is increased more than 12-fold
Heart	Reduced strength of contraction (SV), reduced maximal cardiac output, reduced endurance, increased work of the heart for a submaximal load
Lung	Reduced airway clearance of mucous, increased likelihood of pneumonia, reduced maximal ventilatory volume
Blood	Reduced hematocrit and plasma volume, reduced endurance and temperature regulation

REFERENCES

1. Akeson WH et al: Effects of immobilization on joints, *Clin Orthop* 219:28-37, 1987.
2. Befus AD, Mathison R, Davison J: Integration of neuro-endocrine immune responses in defense of mucosal surfaces, *Am J Trop Med Hyg* 60(Suppl 4):26-34, 1999.
3. Berin MC, McKay DM, Perdue MH: Immune-epithelial interactions in host defense, *Am J Trop Med Hyg* 60(Suppl 4):16-25, 1999.
4. Best TM, Hunter KD: Muscle injury and repair, *Phys Med Rehabil Clin N Am* 11(2):251-266, 2000.
5. Biebl M et al: Analysis of neurogenesis and programmed cell death reveals a self-renewing capacity in the adult rat brain, *Neurosci Lett* 291(1):17-20, 2000.
6. Bode MK et al: Type I and III collagens in human colon cancer and diverticulosis, *Scand J Gastroenterol* 35(7):747-752, 2000.
7. Boissonnault WG, Koopmeiners MB: Medical history profile: Orthopaedic physical therapy outpatients, *J Orthop Sports Phys Ther* 20:2–10, 1994.
8. Bucci LR: *Nutrition applied to injury rehabilitation and sports medicine*, Boca Raton, Fla, 1995, CRC Press.

9. Bullough PG: *Bullough and Vigorita's orthopaedic pathology*, ed 3, St Louis, 1997, Mosby.

10. Cameron MH: *Physical agents in rehabilitation*, Philadelphia, 1999, WB Saunders.

11. Chan AK et al: Temperature changes in human patellar tendon in response to therapeutic ultrasound, *J Athletic Training* 33(2):130-135, 1998.

12. Christiansen DL, Huang EK, Silver FH: Assembly of type I collagen: fusion of fibril subunits and the influence of fibril diameter on mechanical properties, *Matrix Biol* 19(5):409-420, 2000.

13. Ciccone CD: Free-radical toxicity and antioxidant medications in Parkinson's disease, *Phys Ther* 78(3):313-319, 1998.

14. Culav EM, Clark CH, Merrilees MJ: Connective tissues: matrix composition and its relevance to physical therapy, *Phys Ther* 79(3):308-19, 1999.

15. Cyriax J: *Textbook of orthopaedic medicine: diagnosis of soft tissue lesions*, ed 8, vol 1, London, 1982, Bailliere-Tindall.

16. Damjanov, I: *Pathology for the health-related professions*, ed 2, Philadelphia, 2000, WB Saunders.

17. Darby IA et al: Apoptosis is increased in a model of diabetes-impaired wound healing in genetically diabetic mice, *Int J Biochem Cell Biol* 29(1):191-200, 1997.

18. Davies I: Cellular mechanisms of aging. In Tallis R, Fillit H, Brocklehurst JC, editors: *Brocklehurst's textbook of geriatric medicine and gerontology*, ed 5, London, 1998, Churchill Livingstone.

19. deAndrade JR, Grant C, Dixon AS: Joint distention and reflex muscle inhibition in the knee, *J Bone Joint Surg [Am]* 47:313–322, 1965.

20. Debus ES et al: The role of growth factors in wound healing, *Zentralbl Chir* 125(Suppl 1):49-55, 2000.

21. Dhaene K, Van Marck E, Parwaresch R: Telomeres, telomerase, and cancer: an update, *Virchows Arch* 437(1):1-16, 2000.

22. Dyson M, Suckling J: Stimulation of tissue repair by ultrasound: a survey of mechanisms involved, *Physiotherapy* 64:105-108, 1978.

23. Embil JM et al: Recombinant human platelet-derived growth factor-BB (becaplermin) for healing chronic lower extremity diabetic ulcers: an open-label clinical evaluation of efficacy, *Wound Repair Regen* 8(3):162-168, 2000.

24. Enwemeka CS: Inflammation, cellularity, and fibrillogenesis in regenerating tendon: implications for tendon rehabilitation, *Phys Ther* 69:816-825, 1989.

25. Enwemeka CS: The biomechanical effects of low-intensity ultrasound on healing tendons, *Ultrasound Med Biol* 16(8): 801-807, 1990.

26. Evans WJ: Vitamin E, vitamin C, and exercise, *Am J Clin Nutr* 72(Suppl 2):647S-52S, 2000.

27. Ferree BA et al: Deep venous thrombosis after spinal surgery, *Spine* 18(3):315-319, 1993.

28. Frank C, Akeson WH, Woo SL-Y: Physiology and therapeutic value of passive joint motion, *Clin Orthop* 185:113-125, 1984.

29. Fry F, Kosoff G, Eggleton RC: Threshold ultrasound dosage for structural changes in mammalian brain, *J Acoust Soc Am* 48:1413-1417, 1970.

30. Giovannucci E: Nutritional factors in human cancers, *Adv Exp Med Biol* 472:29-42, 1999.

31. Giovannucci E: Response: re: tomatoes, tomato-based products, lycopene, and prostate cancer: review of the epidemiologic literature, *J Natl Cancer Inst* 91(15):1331A-1331, 1999.

32. Griffin JE, Karselis TC: *Physical agents for physical therapists*, ed 2, Springfield Ill, 1982, Charles C Thomas.

33. Gum L et al: Combined ultrasound, electrical stimulation, and laser promote collagen synthesis with moderate changes in tendon biomechanics, *Am J Phys Med Rehabil* 76(4):288-296, 1997.

34. Hertling D, Kessler RM: *Management of common musculoskeletal disorders*, ed 3, Philadelphia, 1996, JB Lippincott.

35. Hildebrand KA, Frank CB: Scar formation and ligament healing, *Can J Surg* 41(6):425-429, 1998.

36. Holzheimer RG, Stenmeitz W: Local and systemic concentrations of pro- and anti-inflammatory cytokines in human wounds, *Eur J Med Res* 5(8):347-355, 2000.

37. Hoppenfeld S, Murthy VL: *Treatment and rehabilitation of fractures*, Philadelphia, 2000, Lippincott Williams and Wilkins.

38. Ishikawa F: Aging clock: the watchmaker's masterpiece, *Cell Mol Life Sci* 57(5):698-704, 2000.

39. Isogai N et al: Formation of phalanges and small joints by tissue-engineering, *J Bone Joint Surg Am* 81(3):306-316, 1999.

40. Jackson DW, Simon TM: Tissue engineering principles in orthopaedic surgery, *Clin Orthop* 367(Suppl):S31-S45, 1999.

41. Kahn J: *Principles and practice of electrotherapy*, New York, 1987, Churchill Livingstone, 1987.

42. Khan SN, Bostrom MP, Lane JM: Bone growth factors, *Orthop Clin North Am* 31(3):375-388, 2000.

43. Kletsas D et al: Fibroblast responses to exogenous and autocrine growth factors relevant to tissue repair: the effect of aging, *Ann NY Acad Sci* 908:155-166, 2000.

44. Kristal AR, Cohen JH: Invited commentary: tomatoes, lycopene, and prostate cancer, How strong is the evidence? *Am J Epidemiol* 151(2):109-118, 2000.

45. Majima T et al: Compressive compared with tensile loading of medial collateral ligament scar in vitro uniquely influences mRNA levels for aggrecan, collagen type II, and collagenase, *J Orthop Res* 18(4):524-531, 2000.

46. McDiarmid R, Ziskin MC, Michlovitz SL: Therapeutic ultrasound. In Michlovitz SL: *Thermal agents in rehabilitation*, ed 3, Philadelphia, 1996, FA Davis.

47. McDonald DM, Thurston G, Baluk P: Endothelial gaps as sites for plasma leakage in inflammation, *Microcirculation* 6(1):7-22, 1999.

48. Miles CA et al: Identification of an intermediate state in the helix-coil degradation of collagen by ultraviolet light, *J Biol Chem* 275(42):33014-33020, 2000.

49. Nakamura N et al: Decorin antisense gene therapy improves functional healing of early rabbit ligament scar with enhanced collagen fibrillogenesis in vivo, *J Orthop Res* 18(4):517-523, 2000.

50. Nerlich AG: Collagen types in the middle ear mucosa, *Eur Arch Otorhinolaryngol* 252(7):443-449, 1995.

51. Pedersen BK, Hoffman-Goetz L: Exercise and the immune system: regulation, integration, and adaptation, *Physiol Rev* 80(3):1055-1081, 2000.

52. Polidori MC et al: Physical activity and oxidative stress during aging, *Int J Sports Med* 21(3):154-157, 2000.

53. Polo M et al: Effect of TGF-beta2 on proliferative scar fibroblast cell kinetics, *Ann Plast Surg* 43(2):185-190, 1999.

54. Poulsen HE, Weimann A, Loft S: Methods to detect DNA damage by free radicals: relation to exercise, *Proc Nutr Soc* 58(4):1007-1014, 1999.

55. Ramirez A et al: The effect of ultrasound on collagen synthesis and fibroblast proliferation in vitro, *Med Sci Sports Exerc* 29(3):326-332, 1997.

56. Roberts M, Rutherford JH, Harris D: The effect of ultrasound on flexor tendon repairs in the rabbit, *Hand* 14:17-20, 1982.

57. Salter RB: *Textbook of disorders and injuries of the musculoskeletal system*, ed 3, Baltimore, 1999, Williams and Wilkins.

58. Sheldon H: *Boyd's introduction to the study of disease*, Philadelphia, 1992, Lea and Febiger, 1992.

59. Sims TJ, Avery NC, Bailey AJ: Quantitative determination of collagen cross-links, *Methods Mol Biol* 139:11-26, 2000.

60. Spacek P, Adam M: Enzymatic and nonenzymatic linking elements, their development and significance in physiologic, pathologic and gerontologic changes in the body, *Cas Lek Cesk* 139(4):102-110, 2000.

61. Spencer JD, Hayes KC, Alexander IJ: Knee joint effusion and quadriceps reflex inhibition in man, *Arch Phys Med Rehabil* 65:171-177, 1984.

62. Stanimirovic D, Satoh K: Inflammatory mediators of cerebral endothelium: a role in ischemic brain inflammation, *Brain Pathol* 1:113-26, 2000.

63. Sung KL et al: Signal pathways and ligament cell adhesiveness, *J Orthop Res* 14(5):729-735, 1996.

64. Sussman C, Bates-Jensen B, editors: *Wound care: a collaborative practice manual for physical therapists and nurses*, Gaithersburg, Md, 1998, Aspen.

65. Tepper SH, Mergner WJ: Role of the lymphatics in aiding regression of hypokalemic lesions in rat cardiac muscle, *Lymphology* 22:42-50, 1989.

66. Thomson PD: Immunology, microbiology, and the recalcitrant wound, *Ostomy Wound Manage* 46(Suppl 1A):77S-82S, 2000.

67. Tredgett EE et al: Transforming growth factor-beta mRNA and protein in hypertrophic scar tissues and fibroblasts: antagonism by IFN-alpha and IFN-gamma in vitro and in vivo, *J Interferon Cytokine Res* 20(2):143-151, 2000.

68. Uriquidi V, Tarin D, Goodison S: Role of telomerase in cell senescence and oncogenesis, *Annu Rev Med* 51:65-79, 2000.

69. Vogt PM et al: Clinical application of growth factors and cytokines in wound healing. *Zentralbl Chir* 125(Suppl 1):65-68, 2000.

70. Woo SL-Y et al: Connective tissue response to immobility, *Arthritis Rheum* 18:257-264, 1975.

71. Yang L, Tsai CM, Hsieh AH: Adhesion strength differential of human ligament fibroblasts to collagen types I and III, *J Orthop Res* 17(5):755-762, 1999.

72. Zhang S et al: A prospective study of folate intake and the risk of breast cancer, *JAMA* 281(17):1632-1637, 1999.

CHAPTER 6

THE IMMUNE SYSTEM

CATHERINE C. GOODMAN

*I*mmunology is the study of the physiologic mechanisms that allow the body to recognize materials as foreign and to neutralize or eliminate them. When the immune system is working properly, it protects the organism from infection and disease; when it is not, the failure of the immune system can result in localized or systemic infection or disease. In fact, the significance of a healthy immune system is apparent in states or diseases characterized by immunodeficiency, as occurs in human immunodeficiency virus (HIV) infection or in people on immunosuppressive medication.

Without an effective immune system, an individual is at risk for the development of overwhelming infection, malignant disease, or both. Not all immune system responses are helpful, as in the case of organ or tissue transplant rejection. Additionally, excessive or inappropriate activity of the immune system can result in hypersensitivity states, immune complex disease, or autoimmune disease. For a complete understanding of the immune system as it relates to injury, inflammation, and healing, the reader is encouraged to read this chapter along with Chapter 5.

TYPES OF IMMUNITY

◆ Innate and Acquired Immunity

Two types of immunity are recognized: innate (natural or native immunity) and acquired immunity (adaptive or specific immunity). *Innate immunity* acts as the body's first line of defense to prevent the entry of pathogens. Two nonspecific, nonadaptive* lines of defense are involved in innate immunity. The first is the skin and its mucosal barriers, and the second is a nonspecific inflammatory response to all forms of cellular injury or death. Innate responses occur to the same extent; however, many times the infectious agent is encountered.

Acquired immunity is characterized by specificity and memory. The primary role of the immune system as a more specific line of defense (acquired immunity) is to recognize and destroy foreign substances such as bacteria, viruses, fungi, and parasites and to prevent the proliferation of mutant cells such as those involved in malignant transformation.

*Nonspecific refers to the fact that this part of the immune system does not distinguish between different types of invaders (e.g., bacteria, fungus, virus, etc.) and is nonadaptive, i.e., does not remember the encounter with specific invaders for future encounters. Each time that potential pathogen is introduced, the innate immune system reacts in the same predictable manner.

This type of immunity results when a pathogen gains entry to the body, and the body produces a specific response to the invader. Acquired immunity has a memory so that when the same organism is encountered again, the body can respond even more rapidly to it and with a stronger reaction. The two components to acquired immunity (humoral immunity and cell-mediated immunity) are discussed in greater detail later in this section.

◆ Acquired Immunity: Active or Passive Immunity

Acquired immune responses can occur as a result of active or passive immunity. Active immunity includes natural immunity and artificial immunity, which is intended or deliberate (Table 6-1). Active acquired immunity refers to protection acquired by introduction (either naturally from environmental exposure or artificially by vaccination) of an antigen (microscopic component of pathogen that causes an immune response) into a responsive host. The concept of vaccination is based on the fact that deliberate exposure to a harmless version of a pathogen generates memory cells but not the pathologic sequelae of the infectious agent itself. In this way, the immune system is primed to mount a secondary immune response with strong and immediate protection should the pathogenic version of the microorganism be encountered in the future.[38] This type of immunity is expected to last a lifetime, but there are occasional exceptions.

Researchers are developing a new generation of vaccines to fight a variety of diseases. One of the most promising is the deoxyribonucleic acid (DNA) vaccine that allows DNA from a pathogen to be injected into the body where cells accept the added DNA instructions and make antigens that the body can recognize and fight. Genetic manipulation allows researchers to overcome the greatest deterrent to vaccination—the ability of common pathogens such as influenza and pneumococcal bacteria to mutate too rapidly for a vaccine to match the latest version. Some of the most promising new techniques are being investigated against malaria; cancer; ear infections; acquired immune deficiency syndrome (AIDS); sexually transmitted diseases; asthma; influenza; strep throat; diabetes; and hepatitis C. Improved administration of the vaccine using mucosal sprays, skin patches, time-released pills, and genetically engineered foods to replace needle injections is also under development.

Passive acquired immunity occurs when antibodies or sensitized lymphocytes produced by one person are transferred to another. Preformed antibodies made in a laboratory or made by someone else is another form of passive immunity. For example, the transplacental transfer of antibodies from mother to fetus,

---

TABLE	6-1

Types of Acquired Immunity

TYPE OF ACQUIRED IMMUNITY*	METHOD ACQUIRED	LENGTH OF RESISTANCE
Active		
Natural	Natural contact and infection with the antigen (environmental exposure)	Usually permanent but may be temporary
Artificial	Inoculation of antigen (vaccination)	Usually permanent but may be temporary (occasional exceptions)
Passive		
Natural	Natural contact with antibody transplacentally (mother to fetus) or through colostrum and breast milk	Temporary
Artificial	Inoculation of antibody or antitoxin; immune serum globulin	Temporary

*Active immunity occurs when a person produces his or her own antibodies to the infecting organism; passive immunity occurs when the antibody is formed in another host and transferred to an individual.

TABLE	6-2

The Immune System and Its Response

INNATE IMMUNITY	ACQUIRED IMMUNITY	
	HUMORAL	CELL-MEDIATED
Nonspecific interaction with different antigens; lacks immunologic memory	Specific interaction with different antigens	Specific interaction with different antigens
Exterior defenses: Skin, mucosa, secretions, nasal hair, ear wax	Mediated by antibody, present as serum globulins	Mediated by T lymphocytes
Phagocytes (leukocytes): Neutrophils (PMNs) Monocytes/macrophages Eosinophils Basophils	Antibodies are produced by plasma cells (differentiated form of B lymphocytes)	Production of helper T cells (CD4+) and cytotoxic T cells (CD8+)
Mast cells and platelets (inflammation)	Globulins having antibody activity (immunoglobulins) are produced	Secretion of lymphokines; Suppressor T cells may be activated
Soluble mediators: Complement and interferons; see Table 5-4 Natural killer (NK) cells or large granular lymphocytes	Primary and secondary (memory) antibody response	Primary and secondary (memory) T cell response

Courtesy Zoher F. Kapasi, PhD, PT Emory University School of Medicine, Department of Rehabilitation, Division of Physical Therapy, Atlanta, 2000.

---

the transfer of antibodies to an infant through breast milk or receiving immune serum globulin (γ-globulin) provides immediate protection but does not result in the formation of memory cells and therefore provides only temporary immunity. This type of immunity (passive acquired) lasts only until the antibodies are degraded, which may be only a few weeks to months.

THE IMMUNE RESPONSE

See Table 6-2.

◆ Antigens

Any foreign substance in the body that does not have the characteristic cell surface markers of that individual and is capable of eliciting an immune response is referred to as an *antigen* (from antibody generator). Bacteria, viruses, parasites, foreign tissue cells, and even large protein molecules are recognized as antigens or called *antigenic*. On encountering an antigen, the immune system recognizes it as nonself, and the appropriate immune response is mounted against the antigen. A single bacterium contains hundreds of antigenic sites, and therefore has multiple sites capable of stimulating an immune response.

The subunits of an antigen that elicit an immune response are called *epitopes*. These molecules protrude from the surface of an antigen and actually combine with an antibody (Fig. 6-1). Each antigen may display hundreds of epitopes. The more epitopes that are present, the greater is the antigenicity of a substance and the greater the immune response.

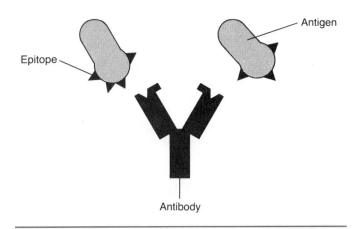

Epitope

Antigen

Antibody

FIGURE   **6-1** An antigen is recognized on the basis of shape. Epitopes protrude from the surface of an antigen and combine with the appropriate receptor of an antibody, much as a key fits a lock. For small antigens, the binding site on the antibody may be a pocket or cleft but in most cases it more closely resembles an undulating surface.[151] (From Black JM, Matassarin-Jacobs E, editors: *Medical-surgical nursing: clinical management for continuity of care*, ed 5, Philadelphia, WB Saunders, 1997, p 599.)

Antibodies produced in response to an antigen are protein molecules structured in such a way that they only interact with the antigen that induced their synthesis, much as a key is made to fit a lock.

◆ The Major Histocompatibility Complex

Since the basis of immunity depends on the immune cells' ability to distinguish self from nonself, all cells of the body contain specific cell surface markers or molecules that are as unique to that person as a fingerprint. The immune system recognizes these cell markers and tolerates them as self, in other words, produces self-tolerance. These cell markers are present on the surface of all body cells and are known as the major histocompatibility complex (MHC) proteins. They were originally discovered on leukocytes and are commonly called *human leukocytic antigens (HLAs)*. The six specific HLAs within the MHC markers are HLA-A, HLA-B, HLA-C, referred to as *class I antigens*, and HLA-DP, HLA-DQ, and HLA-DR, referred to as *class II antigens*.[83] The cell markers are essential for immune function. They not only determine which antigens an individual responds to and how strongly, but they also allow immune system cells to recognize and communicate with one another.

HLA antigens are inherited and can predispose or increase an individual's susceptibility to certain diseases (usually autoimmune) (see Table 39-17). Such diseases encompass many that affect the joints, endocrine glands, and skin, including rheumatoid arthritis, Graves' disease, psoriasis, and many others. Not all people with a certain HLA pattern develop the disease, but they have a greater probability for its development than the general population.

◆ Innate Immunity[74]

The innate immune system consists of all the immune defenses that lack immunologic memory. A characteristic of innate responses is that they remain unchanged however often the antigen is encountered. Innate immune responses use phagocytic cells (neutrophils, monocytes, and macrophages); cells that release inflammatory mediators (basophils, mast cells, and eosinophils); and natural killer (NK) cells. The molecular components of innate responses include complement, acute-phase proteins, and cytokines such as the interferons.[38]

The strategy of the innate immune response may not be to recognize every possible antigen but rather to focus on a few structures present in large groups of microorganisms. These structures are referred to as pathogen-recognition receptors.[106] A key cellular component of innate immunity and one of the most intensely studied components in the last decade is the interdigitating dendritic cell. Cells of this type (e.g., Langerhans' cells in skin) constantly but quietly endocytose extracellular antigens. Pattern-recognition receptors on these dendritic cells are a part of the innate immune response to differentiate between potentially harmful microorganisms and self-constituents.[38] These types of receptors are specific for structures found exclusively in microbial pathogens (pathogen-associated molecular pattern). This differs from the adaptive immune system, which has a tremendous capacity to recognize almost any antigenic structure but because antigen receptors are generated at random, they bind to antigens regardless of their origin—bacterial, environmental, or self.[106]

Exterior Defenses

As a covering for the entire body (with the exception of any openings), the skin offers the first and best line of protection, which is clearly demonstrated in cases of significant burns when infection becomes a major problem. The body openings also offer their own unique protection such as lysozyme in tears that can kill bacteria, waxy secretions in the ear canal to prevent bacteria from advancing inside, nasal hair, stomach acid for ingested organisms, protective low pH vaginal secretions, acidic urine, and so on.

When organisms enter the body by penetrating the epithelial surface of the respiratory, gastrointestinal (GI), or genitourinary tract, biochemical defenses offer additional protection such as acid secretions producing unfavorable pH, lysosomes that destroy cell walls of bacteria, phagocytes that engulf and destroy foreign particles, and NK cells that attack and destroy virus-infected cells and tumor cells.

Phagocytes.   Phagocytes are involved in nonspecific or innate immunity. These cells readily eat (ingest) microorganisms like bacteria or fungi and kill them as a means of protecting the body against infection. The two principal phagocytes are neutrophils and monocytes, but five types of phagocytic leukocytes are recognized: neutrophils, eosinophils, basophils,* monocytes, and lymphocyte. Phagocytes emigrate out of the blood and into the tissues in which an infection has developed, and each of these cell types has a specific phagocytic function in the immune system (see the section on Disorders of Leukocytes in Chapter 13). Neutrophils, eosinophils, basophils, and monocytes are classified as phagocytic leukocytes that function in nonspecific or innate immunity. A severe decrease in the blood level of these cells

---

*Class I antigens are found on nucleated cells and platelets; class II antigens are found on monocytes, macrophages, B cells, activated T cells, vascular endothelial cells, Langerhans' (skin) cells, and dendritic (nerve) cells. There is a third class of antigens (class III) including certain complement proteins (C2, C4, and factor B).

*Because of their granular appearance, neutrophils, eosinophils, and basophils are collectively referred to as *granulocytes*. Granulocytes are short-lived (2 to 3 days) compared with monocytes and macrophages, which may live for months or years.

is the principal cause of susceptibility to infection in people treated with intensive radio- or chemotherapy. These treatments suppress blood cell production in the marrow, resulting in deficiencies of these phagocytic cells.

Neutrophils, also referred to as polymorphonuclear cells (PMNs), the most numerous of these white blood cells (WBCs), derive from bone marrow and increase dramatically in number in response to infection and inflammation. Neutrophils can directly kill invading organisms but may also damage host tissues. In the process of phagocytosis (see Fig. 5-15), bacteria or debris is engulfed, and then digested by enzymes contained within the neutrophils. Neutrophils die after phagocytosis; the accumulation of dead neutrophils and phagocytosed bacteria contributes to the formation of pus.

Monocytes circulate in the blood but when they migrate to tissues, they mature into *macrophages,* which means large eaters. The engulfment of a pathogen by a macrophage is an essential first step leading to a specific immune response. After neutrophils kill the invading organism and the process of phagocytosis has begun, macrophages appear to clear up the debris produced by the neutrophils and to kill any damaged but not dead bacteria or bacteria that are too large for neutrophils. Neutrophils and macrophages both have receptors for antibodies and complement so that the coating of microorganisms with antibodies, complement, or both enhances phagocytosis.[1]

After phagocytes digest the pathogens, antigenic material appears on their surface to identify them more specifically as foreign invaders. In this process, phagocytes (primarily macrophages) serve as antigen-presenting cells (APCs) to introduce the pathogen to lymphocytes. The macrophage or APC processes the pathogen and presents a small part of it, the epitope (see Fig. 6-1), to a specific cell of the immune system known as the *helper/inducer lymphocyte,* or T4 lymphocyte (also referred to as *CD4 lymphocyte**). To prompt the T4 lymphocyte to recognize the processed pathogen, the macrophage releases interleukin-1 (IL-1),† a chemical messenger with many roles. In this way, the macrophage processes the antigen and then signals the lymphocytes to stimulate the specific immune response. Macrophages also participate in the defense against tumor cells and secrete numerous molecules called *monokines* that assist in the immune and inflammatory response. Stimulation of macrophages can boost the immune response.

Eosinophils are the next group of phagocytic leukocytes that participate in the innate immunity process. Eosinophils are derived from bone marrow and multiply in both allergic disorders and parasitic infestations. When organisms are too large for neutrophils and macrophages, eosinophils get within close proximity of the invading organisms and release the contents of their granules to kill them.

Basophils are WBCs (leukocytes) that circulate in peripheral blood and function similarly to mast cells in allergic disorders. Basophils and mast cells are located close to blood vessels throughout the body and have similar functional characteristics; *mast cells* contain histamine that dilates blood vessels when released. Mast cells are derived from stem cells and travel in the blood in such small numbers they are not recognized as blood cells. Arriving basophils and mast cells cause an increase in blood supply in the area where the bacteria or viral antigen is located. This increase in circulation also helps bring more phagocytes to the area thus counteracting bacteria indirectly. The increased circulation is accompanied by the feeling of congestion during an allergic reaction; antihistamines work by neutralizing the histamines and reducing the excessive immune (allergic) response.

The role of erythrocytes and *platelets* in immune responses is sometimes overlooked, but because they have complement receptors, they play an important part in the clearance of immune complexes consisting of antigen, antibody, and components of the complement system.[38]

Soluble (Inflammatory) Mediators

The complement system and interferons act as soluble inflammatory mediators along with phagocytes to destroy organisms that breech the first line of defense. The complement system consists of 20 serum proteins, which are key components in the acute inflammatory response designed to enhance immune function. When activated, these proteins interact in a cascadelike process to assist immune cells by coating microorganisms so they can be more easily phagocytosed and to participate in bacterial lysis. In some cases the invading organisms are eliminated from the body. Sometimes the inflammation produced by the complement cascade (immune response) walls off the microorganism by forming, for example, a cyst or tubercle that protects the rest of the body from infection. (See the section on The Complement System, in Chapter 5; see also Table 5-4.)

The second group of soluble mediators is the cytokines, especially interferons sometimes referred to as *biologic response modifiers (BRMs).* They act as messengers both within the immune system and between the immune system and other systems of the body, forming an integrated network that is highly involved in the regulation of immune responses.[108] In addition to acting as messengers, some cytokines have a direct role in defense such as the interferons. Interferons are produced by virally infected cells early in infection to limit the spread of the infection by protecting surrounding (noninfected) cells (interferons also inhibit tumor growth). Once a cell becomes infected by a virus, certain genes are turned on in the cell that will produce these interferons that coat the surrounding cells and make them viral resistant.

Natural Killer Cells

NK cells are also called *cytotoxic T cells,* or CD8, and are actually large granular lymphocytes that do not mature in the thymus but rather are always available and ready in the thymus. NK cells recognize virally infected cells where a bacteria or virus (or tumor cell) is hiding and directly attack and kill target invader cells with which they come into contact. The

---

*Microscopically, T lymphocytes appear identical, but they can be distinguished by means of distinctive molecules called *cluster designations* (CDs) located on their cell surface. For example, all mature T cells carry markers known as T2, T3, T5, and T7 (or CD2, CD3, CD5, and CD7). T4 (CD4) are the helper T cells, and T8 (CD8) are cytotoxic T cells. Another group of T lymphocytes are identified as natural killer (NK) cells for their ability to kill certain tumor cells and virus-infected cells without prior sensitization or activation.

†Interleukins are one type of cytokine, a protein released by macrophages to trigger the immune response. See Cytokines, later in this section. Some of the multiple functions of IL-1 include increasing the temperature set-point in the hypothalamus; increasing serotonin in the brainstem and duodenum causing sleep and nausea, respectively; stimulating the production of prostaglandins, leading to a decrease in the pain threshold, resulting in myalgias and arthralgias; increasing the synthesis of collagenases, resulting in the destruction of cartilage; and most important, kicking the T4 cells into action.

mechanism for how NK cells can recognize these invaders remains unknown, and sometimes NK cells kill the body's normal cells. A full-scale immune system response is not necessary when killer cells are available. These cells are used as an early marker of immune system function.

◆ Acquired Immunity

To establish an infection, the pathogen must first overcome numerous surface barriers and the innate immune responses. In these cases, acquired immunity is tailored to recognize each different type of organism and kill it. The two types of acquired immune responses that occur are *humoral immunity* (also called immunoglobulin-related immunity) and *cell-mediated immunity* (also referred to as T-cell immunity). Although these two responses are often discussed separately, they are two arms of the immune system and work together; failure in one can alter the effectiveness of the other. These two types of responses overlap and interact considerably but the distinction is useful in understanding how the immune system is activated.

The complexity of the cellular interactions that occur during acquired immune responses requires specialized microenvironments in which the relevant cells can collaborate efficiently. Because only a few lymphocytes are specific for any given antigen, T cells and B cells need to migrate throughout the body to increase the probability that they will encounter that particular antigen. In their travels, lymphocytes spend only about 30 minutes in the blood during each trip around the body.[117] More specific information about T-cell function and migration is available.[162]

Acquired responses involve the proliferation of antigen-specific B and T cells, which occurs when the surface receptors of these cells bind to antigen and initiate the immune response involving immunoglobulins, antibodies, suppressor T cells, and cytokines. The acquired immune system generates a highly diverse group of antigen receptors that allows the adaptive immune system to recognize virtually any antigen. However, the price for this diversity is the inability to distinguish foreign antigens from self-antigens.[106]

Humoral Immunity

The humoral immune response is mediated by antibodies present in different "humors" (body fluids or secretions) such as saliva, blood, or vaginal secretions. Antibodies produced by B lymphocytes are very effective against organisms that are free floating in the body that can be easily reached and neutralized. *B lymphocytes*, or B cells, are called such because they originate in the bone marrow and then circulate throughout the extracellular fluid.

The surface of B lymphocytes is coated with immunoglobulin, and each B cell has a receptor (an antibody) that can recognize a specific foreign substance or antigen. When this happens, B cells change into protein-synthesizing cells known as *plasma cells* and *memory B cells* (Fig. 6-2). The plasma cell

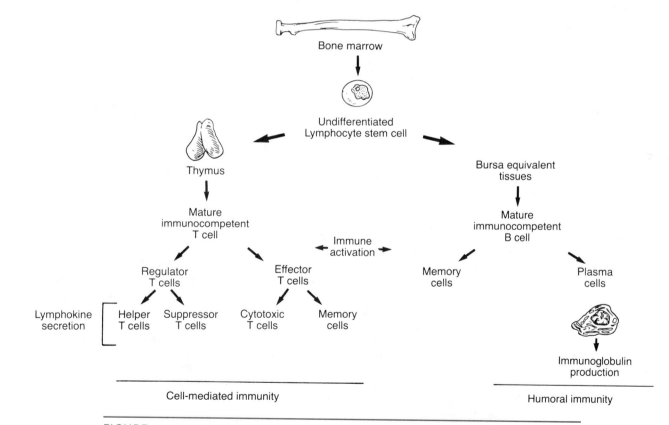

FIGURE 6-2 The pathway of lymphocyte maturation. Undifferentiated lymphocyte stem cells are derived from the bone marrow. B cells reach maturity within the bone marrow but T cells must travel to the thymus to complete their development. Activation of either T or B cells by antigens leads to proliferation of immune cells that mediate either cell-mediated immunity or humoral immunity, respectively. (From Black JM, Matassarin-Jacobs E, editor: *Medical-surgical nursing: clinical management for continuity of care*, ed 5, Philadelphia, 1997, WB Saunders, p 597.)

Major Functions of Immunoglobulins*

Immunoglobulins directly attack antigens, destroying or neutralizing them through the processes of agglutination, precipitating the toxins out of solution, neutralizing antigenic substances, and lysing the organism's cell wall.
Immunoglobulins activate the complement system.
Immunoglobulins activate anaphylaxis by releasing histamine in tissue and blood.
Immunoglobulins stimulate antibody-mediated hypersensitivity.

*Globulins with antibody activity are referred to as *immunoglobulins*.
From Thompson JM, McFarland GK, Hirsch JE, Tucker SM: *Mosby's clinical nursing*, ed 3, St Louis, 1993, Mosby.

produces and secretes into body fluids a specific antibody to that antigen. Memory cells produced in connection with humoral immunity circulate between the blood, lymphoid system, and tissues for about 1 year or even longer. They are responsible for the more rapid and sustained (stronger) immune response that occurs with repeated exposure to the same antigen. This humoral response is particularly useful in fighting bacterial infections.

The B lymphocyte/plasma cell interaction is capable of producing five types of antibodies, or immunoglobulins (Ig), in response to specific antigens. Because of these antibodies the humoral immune response may be referred to as the *antibody immune response*. The five types of antibodies are IgG, IgM, IgA, IgD, and IgE; major functions of immunoglobulins are listed in Box 6-1.

IgM predominates in the primary or initial immune response and is the largest immunoglobulin; because of its size, it is found almost exclusively in the intravascular compartment. IgG is the major antibacterial and antiviral antibody and is the predominant immunoglobulin in blood; it is responsible for the protection of the newborn during the first 6 months of life and is the only immunoglobulin to cross the placenta. It is the major immunoglobulin synthesized during the secondary immune response (after IgM initially responds to foreign pathogens), conferring long-term or permanent immunity. *IgA* defends external body surfaces, is the predominant immunoglobulin on mucous membrane surfaces, and is found in secretions such as saliva, breast milk (colostrum); urine; seminal fluid; tears; nasal fluids; and respiratory, GI, and genitourinary secretions. *IgD* is the predominant antibody found on the surface of B lymphocytes, serves mainly as an antigen receptor, and may function in controlling lymphocyte activation or suppression. *IgE* is a primary factor in eliminating parasitic infections such as roundworms and is therefore significant in the immune responses of people in developing countries where adequate nutrition, hygiene, and primary medical care are lacking. IgE also functions during allergic reactions by lysing the mast cells and releasing histamine in association with allergies, anaphylaxis, extrinsic asthma, and urticaria (hives). This response of IgE is a normal reaction but becomes excessive in people with allergies.

The type of antibody produced depends on genetic variability, the specific antigenic stimulus, and whether it is a first

or subsequent exposure to that antigen. The humoral immune response is more rapid than the cell-mediated response and is more often a factor in resistance to acute bacterial infections. Humoral immunity can be transmitted to another person, either by inoculation or by maternal transfer via placenta or breast milk. This transfer is called *passive immunity* (see Table 6-1).

Cell-Mediated Immunity

Some organisms (all viruses and some bacteria) actually hide inside the cells where the antibodies cannot reach them. A second arm of the immune system (cell-mediated immunity or cellular immunity) with more specific cells (T lymphocytes) can recognize these hidden organisms, search them out, and destroy them on a cell-to-cell basis. Lymphocytes originate from stem cells in the bone marrow and differentiate or mature into either B or T cells (see Figs. 6-2 and 20-5). The B cell (humoral immunity) is thought to mature and become immunocompetent in the bone marrow. *T lymphocytes*, or T cells (cell-mediated immunity), are called such because the precursors of these cells start from the bone marrow but then mature in the thymus located right behind the sternum where it learns to discriminate self from nonself (Fig. 6-3). Both T and B lymphocytes continuously recirculate between blood, lymph, and lymph nodes.

After interaction with a specific antigen, the activated lymphocyte will produce numerous additional lymphocytes called *sensitized T cells*. This T-cell subpopulation has three primary functions. The most numerous of the T cells, *helper T cells*, constituting 75% of all T cells, assist the B cells to mature and produce antibody by secreting protein mediators called *lymphokines*.* Some of their functions include (1) helping B cells augment the production of antibodies, (2) activating macrophages and helping them destroy large bacteria, (3) helping other T lymphocytes recognize and destroy virally infected cells, and (4) helping NK cells kill infected cells. HIV destroys or inactivates these helper T cells and leaves the body at risk for infectious agents such as cytomegalovirus (CMV).

T lymphocytes contribute to the immune response in two major ways. They are capable of turning the entire immune system on and just as capable of turning the entire immune system off through the actions of the helper/inducer T4 lymphocytes (the "on" cells) and the cytotoxic T8 lymphocytes (the "off" cells).† *Suppressor T cells*, the "peacemakers" downregulate and disarm the immune system by suppressing both helper and cytotoxic T-cell functions. These actions reduce the immune response, an important function in slowing down the immune response, especially when the body's immune system attacks its own normal tissue. This recognition and response is known as *immune tolerance*. The loss of immune tolerance can result in autoimmune disease in young and old. This production and activation of T cells is the component of the immune response called *cell-mediated immunity* and is primarily responsible for fighting invading pathogens such as viruses, fungi, bacteria, and so on.

*Many different lymphokines have been identified, including but not limited to, chemotactic factor, macrophage-activating factor, IL-1 and -2, interferon, T-cell replacement factor, and transfer factor.
†Autoimmune diseases are possible examples wherein suppressor T8 cells (CD8) are not functioning properly and do not get turned off.

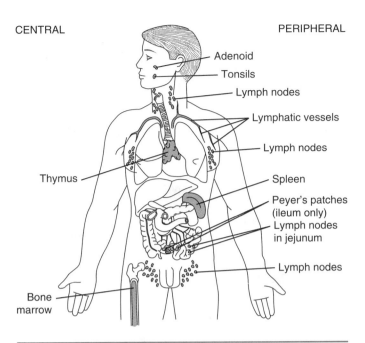

CENTRAL   PERIPHERAL

Adenoid
Tonsils
Lymph nodes
Lymphatic vessels
Lymph nodes
Thymus
Spleen
Peyer's patches (ileum only)
Lymph nodes in jejunum
Lymph nodes
Bone marrow

FIGURE   6-3   Organs of the immune system referred to as *lymphoid tissues*. The bone marrow and thymus are referred to as primary lymphoid organs since these organs are the central sites of all cells of the immune system and B- and T-cell differentiation, respectively. Immature lymphocytes migrate through the central lymphoid tissues and later reside as mature lymphocytes in the peripheral or secondary lymphoid tissues (e.g., lymph nodes, Peyer's patches, tonsils, spleen, mucosal associated lymphoid tissue or MALT from the mouth to the rectum).

Cell-mediated immunity is responsible for the rejection of transplanted tissue; delayed hypersensitivity reactions (e.g., contact dermatitis); and some autoimmune diseases. Cell-mediated immunity is the basis for many skin tests (e.g., tuberculin test, allergy testing). Cellular immunity cannot be transferred passively to another person.

Clinical conditions that compromise the cell-mediated T-lymphocyte function include HIV infection and AIDS, with a progressive reduction in T4 lymphocytes over the duration of the illness. Other conditions known to affect T-cell number or responsiveness include stress, malignancy, general anesthesia, thermal injury, surgery, diabetes, and immunosuppressive drugs (including corticosteroids). Older adults (65 years and older) show reduced numbers of circulating lymphocytes, and malnourished people show defects in most tests of T-cell function.

◆ Summary of the Immune Response
Immune responses are initiated according to the type of antigen presented. Adaptive immune responses are generated in the lymph nodes, spleen, and mucosa-associated tissue, referred to as the *secondary lymphoid tissues*. For example, blood-borne antigens usually initiate responses in the spleen, whereas responses to microorganisms are generated in local lymph nodes. Most pathogens are encountered after they are inhaled or ingested. Antigens entering the body through mucosal surfaces activate cells in the mucosa-associated lymphoid tissues (MALTs), including the tonsils, adenoids, and Peyer's patches (see Fig. 6-3).[39]

Keeping in mind that innate immunity and acquired immunity function in tandem together and that within the acquired immune system, humoral immunity and cellular immunity are also working simultaneously, a variety of immune responses can occur when an extracellular pathogen approaches the body. If the pathogenic organism gets past the first line of defense (innate immunity) and is presented to the body, the following can happen: (1) a B lymphocyte recognizes it as a bacteria and produces antibodies that bind to it and neutralize it (humoral response); (2) a T lymphocyte recognizes it as a bacteria and produce cytokines to help the macrophages lyse and phagocytose the bacteria (cell-mediated response); (3) in the case of a virus, a cytotoxic T lymphocyte can recognize the cell and destroy it (cell-mediated response); and (4) the complement system can recognize the invading organism and destroy it (innate immunity).

In some instances, innate and acquired immunity interact with each other, such as when bacteria enters the body and the B lymphocyte recognizes it and produces specific antibodies (acquired immunity). Examples of this interaction include (1) antibodies (acquired immunity) bind to the bacteria coating it and making it available for phagocytosis by the phagocytes of the innate immune system; (2) again, bacteria is recognized by the B lymphocyte (acquired immunity) and coated with the antibody produced by the lymphocyte; the complement (innate immunity) then recognizes it more clearly and destroy it; (3) activation of cytotoxic T lymphocytes (acquired immunity) and NK cells (innate immunity) result in a direct attack on cells that have been transformed by a virus or a malignant process; (4) the foreign invader is recognized by a T lymphocyte (from the acquired immune system) and the T lymphocyte then produces hormones (lymphokines) that help the macrophage (from the innate immune system) to destroy it.[74]

Dysfunction of the immune system can contribute to diseases. For example, two general types of genetic alterations could lead to immunologic abnormalities: mutations that inactivate the receptors or signaling molecules involved in innate immune recognition and mutations that render them active all the time. The first type of mutation would be expected to result in various types of immunodeficiencies. The second type of mutation would trigger antiinflammatory reactions and thereby contribute to a variety of conditions with an inflammatory component (e.g., asthma, allergy, arthritis, autoimmune diseases).[106]

AGING AND THE IMMUNE SYSTEM

Aging is accompanied by immune dysregulation as immune function declines with increasing age; this is described as the *Oxidative (Free Radical) Theory of Aging* (see the section Cellular Aging in Chapter 5). Changes are observed in both the innate and acquired immunity defenses; the end result is reduced resistance to pathogens and increased incidence of tumors and autoimmune disorders.

◆ Changes in Innate Immunity[74]
Exterior defenses are affected by thinning of the skin, making older adults more prone to pressure ulcers and increasing openings for bacteria to enter the body. Decreased acidity of the GI tract, shallower breathing with decreased air exchange, less acidic urine, and a less elastic bladder that retains more

urine are all examples of ways our exterior defenses are affected by aging, thus contributing to reduced effectiveness of the innate immune system.

Phagocytes (neutrophils and monocytes/macrophages) show decreased function with aging. *Eosinophils* accumulate in fewer numbers at sites of infection with age, perhaps predisposing us to parasitic infections as we age. *Basophils* are characterized by reduced degranulation with aging, although *mast cells* show no change in numbers or histamine release with aging. *Platelet aggregation* increases with aging, perhaps contributing to increased clot formation and decreased peripheral circulation.

Soluble mediators are characterized by increased serum levels of complement produced by the liver perhaps a compensatory mechanism but this remains unproved. A decreased production of interferons occurs by monocyte with increasing age.

NK cells (large granular lymphocytes) may experience a decrease in cell function, but this remains controversial and is not fully determined at this time.

◆ Changes in Acquired Immunity

With aging comes involution (shriveling) of the thymus, the central lymphoid organ for T-cell development that is responsible for training T cells to coordinate the body's immune system. The gradual degeneration of the thymus produces most of the effects of age on the immune system. By age 45 to 50 years, thymus size is only 5% to 15% of its maximum size, which is reached at sexual maturity. Thymic involution is hastened in young people after injuries, chemotherapy, and other forms of stress.[14]

As a result of thymic atrophy, the level of thymic hormone production and the capacity of the thymus to mediate T-cell differentiation decrease. No thymic hormone is detected by age 60. These changes in the thymus and T-cell responses result in much of the decrease in immunoresponsiveness that is seen in aging populations, especially including increased susceptibility to infection and cancer.

Numbers of circulating T cells decrease with age and those that remain are not as responsive. In addition to diminished T-cell function, specific antibody responses to antigenic challenge diminish by 50% to 80%, and increased antibody production against self-antigens (autoantibodies) occurs. The overall effect is an increased susceptibility to infection with advancing years (e.g., pneumonia, urinary tract infections, endocarditis, skin and soft tissue infections, diverticulitis) and the need for reimmunization with age.*

Aging, especially poor nutrition that often accompanies advancing age, is associated with the accumulation of mutations in regulatory genes, leading to the loss of coordinated control of cell growth and function. Mutations in regulatory genes interfere with specific hormones such as IL-1 and -2; tumor necrosis factor (TNF); and interferon, all of which control proliferation and differentiation in lymphocytes in response to antigenic exposure. New research has also shown that every cell has a preprogrammed defense that specifies if a cell cannot defend itself against a mutation, the cell will self-destruct (apoptosis). This apoptosis function also declines with age.

Cell-mediated immunity is similarly impaired, apparently by the same mechanisms, as fewer cells are available to mediate the reaction. The diminished cell-mediated immunity can result in the reactivation of dormant infections such as herpes zoster and tuberculosis. Age-related increase in autoimmune activity is both a cellular and a humoral phenomenon and limited studies suggest that reduced humoral and cellular immunocompetence, reduced suppressor cell activity, and increased autoantibody activity are all associated with reduced survival.

FACTORS AFFECTING IMMUNITY

In addition to the effects of aging, other factors can affect the immune system. These factors may include nutrition; environmental pollution and exposure to chemicals that influence the host defense; prior or ongoing trauma or illnesses; medications; splenectomy (removal of the spleen); influences of the enteric, endocrine, and neurochemical systems; stress; and psychosocial-spiritual well-being and socioeconomic status. These factors, as well as clinical conditions that contribute to an immunocompromised state, are listed in Table 6-3. Sleep deprivation has also been shown to have important effects similar to stress on the immune system by reducing cellular immunity.[10, 132] Some factors such as the iatrogenically introduced interventions listed and sexual practices do not alter the immune system directly but increase a person's exposure to pathogens.

New information is being discovered about the sensory functions of the intestine and how neural, hormonal, and immune signals interact. Representatives of all the major categories of immune cells are found in the gut or can be rapidly recruited from the circulation in response to an inflammatory stimulus. The gut immune system has 70% to 80% of the

TABLE	6-3

Factors Affecting Immunity

Factors That Alter the Immune System

Aging	Splenectomy
Sex and hormonal influences	Stress, psychospiritual well-being, socioeconomic status
Nutrition/malnutrition	
Environmental pollution	
Exposure to toxic chemicals	*Factors That Increase Exposure to Pathogens*
Trauma	Iatrogenic
Burns	• Urinary catheters
Sleep disturbance	• Nasogastric tubes
Presence of concurrent illnesses and diseases:	• Endotracheal tubes
• Malignancy	• Chest tubes
• Diabetes mellitus	• Intracranial pressure monitor
• Chronic renal failure	• External fixation devices
• HIV infection	• Implanted prostheses
Medications, immunosuppressive drugs	Sexual practices
Hospitalization, surgery, general anesthesia	

---

*Thirty-five percent of adults age 65 and older fail to respond to the influenza vaccine as a result of a failure of T lymphocytes to provide adequate help to B cells to form protective antibodies.[74]

body's immune cells and the protective blocking action of the secretory response in the gut is crucial to the integrity of the GI tract immune function and host defense.[13] Studies suggest that the development and expression of the regional immune system of the GI tract is independent of systemic immunity, but this remains an area of debate and investigation.

Nutritional status can have a profound effect on immune function. Nutrients have fundamental and regulatory influences on the immune response of the GI tract and therefore, on host defense. Reduction of normal bacteria in the gut after antibiotic treatment or in the presence of infection may interfere with the nutrients available for immune function in the GI tract. Severe deficits in calorie or protein intake or vitamins such as vitamin A or vitamin E can lead to deficiencies in T cell function and numbers. Deficient zinc intake can profoundly depress both T- and B-cell function. Zinc is required as a cofactor for at least 70 different enzymes, some of which are found in lymphocytes and are necessary for their function. Secondary zinc deficiencies may be associated with malabsorption syndrome, chronic renal disease, chronic diarrhea, or burns or severe psoriasis (loss of zinc through the skin). Dietary changes may alter aspects of immunity, although research in this area is ongoing. Additionally, morbid obesity may alter the immune system by creating a vulnerability to certain diseases, including cancer.

Some *medications* (e.g., cancer chemotherapeutic agents) profoundly suppress blood cell formation in the bone marrow. Other drugs (e.g., analgesics, antithyroid medications, anticonvulsants, antihistamines, antimicrobial agents, and tranquilizers) induce immunologic responses that destroy mature granulocytes. Many drugs also affect B- and T-cell function, especially against antigens that require the interaction of helper T cells and B cells for antibody production. These complications have been observed since the advent of potent immunosuppressive (e.g., corticosteroids) and chemotherapeutic drugs as treatment of people with autoimmune diseases, transplants, or cancer. Depression of B- and T-cell formation is manifested as a progressive increase in infections with opportunistic microorganisms (e.g., *P. carinii*, cytomegalovirus, and *Candida albicans* and other fungi).

Surgery and *anesthesia* can also suppress both T- and B-cell function for up to 1 month postoperatively.[99] Because of the invasive nature of any surgical procedure and because defects in immunity have been described in most major illnesses, it is logical to assume that the majority of hospitalized surgical clients are immunocompromised to some degree. Surgery to remove the spleen results in a depressed humoral response against encapsulated bacteria, especially *Streptococcus pneumoniae*, *Haemophilus influenzae*, *Staphylococcus aureus*, the group A streptococci, and *Neisseria meningitidis* (see Chapter 7).

Burns cause increased susceptibility to severe bacterial infections as a result of decreased external defenses (intact skin); neutrophil function; decreased complement levels; decreased cell-mediated immunity; and decreased primary humoral responses. Blood serum from clients with burns also contains nonspecific immunosuppressive factors that will suppress all immune responses, regardless of the antigen involved.

The relationship between *stress, psychosocial-spiritual well-being,* and *socioeconomic status* and susceptibility to disease through depressed immune function has become an area of intense research interest. In the past, there were anecdotal reports of increased incidence of infection, diseases, and malignancy associated with periods of both intense and relatively minor stress (see Box 2-9). In the new and expanding world of psychoneuroimmunology, almost any stress seems capable of altering immune function. The role of stress in the development of pathology is discussed in Chapter 2. Likewise, the role of environmental pollution and exposure to chemicals on susceptibility to immune system dysfunction and development of disease is discussed in Chapter 3.

INTERACTIONS BETWEEN THE IMMUNE AND CENTRAL NERVOUS SYSTEMS

The role of the nervous and endocrine systems in homeostasis has now been shown to include interaction with the immune system.* Two pathways link the brain and the immune system: the autonomic nervous system (ANS) and neuroendocrine outflow via the pituitary. Immune responses alter neural and endocrine functions, and in turn, neural and endocrine activity modifies immunologic function.

Many regulatory peptides and their receptors previously thought to be limited to the brain or to the immune system are now known to be expressed by both. It is now known that communication between the central nervous system (CNS) and the immune system is bidirectional,† that endocrine factors can alter immune function, and that immune responses can alter both endocrine and CNS responses.[9] Findings that link immune and neuroendocrine function may help explain how emotional state or response to stress can modify a person's capacity to cope with infection or cancer and influence the course of autoimmune disease. Whether emotional factors can influence the course of autoimmune disease, cancer, and infection in humans is a subject of intense research, but studies so far have shown reduced lymphocyte sensitivity with chronic distress.[8]

The CNS can be involved in immune reactions arising from within the brain or in response to peripheral immune stimuli. Activated immunocompetent cells such as monocytes, lymphocytes, and macrophages can cross the blood-brain barrier and take up residence in the brain, where they secrete their full repertoire of cytokines and other inflammatory mediators such as leukotrienes and prostaglandins. All aspects of immune and complement cascades can occur in the brain because of these nerve-macrophage communications. The CNS modulates immune cells by direct synaptic-like contacts in the brain and at peripheral sites, such as the lymphoid organs[159] (see Fig. 6-3).

A number of cytokines called *neurocytokines* (e.g., IL-1, -2, -4, and -6, neuroleukin, and TNF-α) are formed by glia, the supporting structure of nervous tissue. The activation of cytokines in the CNS occurs in response to local tissue injury and can lead to profound changes in neural functions, ranging from mild behavioral disturbances to anorexia, drowsiness,

---

*The study of immune responses involving the CNS has been called *neuroimmunology.* Newer terms include neuroimmunomodulation, psychoneuroimmunology, and neuroimmunoendocrinology (see Chapter 1).

†The immune system has the capacity not only to sense the presence of foreign molecules, but also to communicate this to the brain and neuroendocrine system. This interaction is termed *bidirectional communication* between the immune and neuroendocrine systems.

sleep disturbances, coma, dementia, and the destruction of neurons. The activation of cytokines in neural tissue by injury or toxins has a positive benefit as well, by stimulating the production of nerve growth factor.

Based on studies using animal models, researchers suggest that the brain can regulate immunocompetence. Much of this neuroimmunomodulation takes place through the hypothalamic-pituitary system and sympathetic nervous system, with the latter by the release of catecholamines at autonomic nerve endings and from the adrenal medulla. The principal immunoregulatory organs (lymph nodes, thymus, spleen, and intestinal Peyer's patches) are abundantly supplied by autonomic nerve fibers. Sensory neurons contain a variety of neurotransmitters and neuropeptides that can influence lymphocyte function.

EXERCISE IMMUNOLOGY

The effect of physical activity and exercise (aerobic, endurance, and resistance) on the immune and neuroimmune systems has been an area of research interest. A brief summary of the results is presented here, but a more detailed accounting of exercise and the immune system and future direction for studies is available.[116,119]

Depending on the intensity, activity or exercise can enhance or suppress immune function. In essence, the immune system is enhanced during moderate exercise. Moreover, regular, moderate physical activity can prevent the neuroendocrine and detrimental immunologic effects of stress.[49] In contrast to the beneficial effects of moderate exercise on the immune system, strenuous/intense exercise or long-duration exercise such as marathon running is followed by impairment of the immune system. Intense exercise can suppress the concentration of lymphocytes, suppress natural killer cell activity, and leave the host open to microbial agents, especially viruses that can invade during this open window of opportunity, and may lead to infections. Extreme and long-duration strenuous exercise appears to lead to deleterious oxidation of cellular macromolecules. The oxidation of DNA is important because the oxidative modifications of DNA bases are mutagenic and have been implicated in a variety of diseases including aging and cancer.[125]

◆ Effect on Neutrophils and Macrophages

Exercise triggers a rise in blood levels of neutrophils (PMNs) and stimulates phagocytic activity of neutrophils and macrophages. The exercise-evoked increase in the PMN count is greater if the exercise has an eccentric component, such as downhill running. If the exercise goes beyond 30 minutes, a second, or delayed, rise in PMNs occurs over the next 2 to 4 hours while the exerciser is at rest. This delayed rise in PMNs is probably the result of cortisol, which spurs release of PMNs from the bone marrow and hinders the exit of PMNs from the bloodstream.[104] After brief, gentle exercise, the PMN count soon returns to baseline, but after prolonged, strenuous exercise, this return to normal may take 24 hours or longer.[45] In many instances, exercise enhances macrophage function and can increase antitumor activity in mice, but many questions still remain regarding the mechanism(s) by which acute or chronic exercise affect macrophage function.[171]

◆ Effect on Natural Killer Cells

Most researchers agree that the number of NK cells and the function or activity of these cells in the blood increases during and immediately after exercise of various types, durations, and intensities.[119] This phenomenon, referred to as *NK enhancement*, is temporary and seems to be the result of a surge in epinephrine levels and from cytokines released during exercise. NK enhancement by exercise occurs in everyone regardless of sex, age, or level of fitness training; however, once a person is accustomed to a given exercise level, the NK enhancement falls off, suggesting it is a response not to exercise, per se, but to physiologic stress.

After intense exercise of long duration the concentration of NK cells and NK cytolytic activity declines below preexercise values. Maximal reduction in NK cell concentrations and lower NK cell activity occurs 2 to 4 hours after exercise.[119] Although this depression in NK cell count seems too brief to have major practical importance for health, there may be a cumulative adverse effect in athletes who induce these changes several times per week. Further study is warranted before specific exercise guidelines are determined.[150]

◆ Effect on Lymphocytes

Brisk exercise (even brief, heavy exertion such as maximal bicycle ergometry for 30 or 60 seconds) increases the WBC count in proportion to the effort.[62,114] This exercise-induced increase in WBCs (including lymphocytes and NK cells) is largely the result of the mechanical effects of an increased cardiac output and the physiologic effects of a surge in serum epinephrine concentration. Lymphocytes may be recruited to the circulation from other tissue pools during exercise (e.g., from the spleen, lymph nodes, GI tract). The number of cells that enter the circulation is determined by the intensity of the stimulus.[119]

The number of lymphocytes in circulation increases during exercise but decreases below the normal levels for several hours after intense exercise. Decreased numbers of lymphocytes are associated with decreased lymphocyte responsiveness and antibody response to several antigens after intense exercise.[77]

The effects of intense exercise on secondary antibody response in older adults remain unknown. In one study with older mice, no adverse effect(s) of multiple bouts of intense exercise on antibody levels occurred.[77] In contrast to intense exercise, moderate exercise training enhances secondary antibody response in young animals and is mediated in part by endogenous opioids.[76,77] Primary antibody response is not influenced by exercise training.

◆ Effect on Cytokines

Strenuous exercise* can suppress immune function and damage enough tissue to evoke the *acute phase response* in humans.[118] This complex cascade of reactions can modulate immune defense by activating complement and spurring the release of TNF, interferons, interleukins, and other cytokines. More research is needed to understand the clinical applications of this exercise-induced acute phase response. Strenuous exercise is accompanied by an increase in circulating proinflammatory and inflammation-responsive cytokines similar to the response to infection and trauma.[111] Eccentric exercise is

---

*Intense or strenuous exercise has been defined as exercising at a minimum of 80% of maximum oxygen consumption (VO_{2max}).

associated with an increase in serum interleukin (IL-6) concentration, whereas no changes are found after concentric exercise. The rise in IL-6 with eccentric exercise is accompanied by a corresponding increase in creatine kinase in the following days as a result of exercise-induced muscle damage.[120]

◆ Exercise and Apoptosis

The role of apoptosis, or programmed cell death, in exercise is the focus of much research in the area of exercise science. Apoptotic cell death differs morphologically and biochemically from necrotic cell death, although both appear to occur after exercise. Accelerated apoptosis has been documented to occur in a variety of disease states, such as AIDS and Alzheimer's disease, and in the aging heart. In striking contrast, failure to activate this genetically regulated cell death may result in cancer and certain viral infections. It is surmised that exercise-induced apoptosis is a normal regulatory process that serves to remove certain damaged cells without a pronounced inflammatory response, thereby insuring optimal body function.[123]

◆ Exercise and Infection[75]

From experimental studies, it is clear that effects of exercise stress on disease lethality varies with the type and time the exercise is performed. In general, exercise or training before infection has either no effect or decreases morbidity and mortality. Exercise during the incubation period of the infection appears either to have no effect or to increase the severity of infection. Several epidemiologic studies on exercise and upper respiratory tract infection (URTI) report an increased number of URTI symptoms (based on self-report rather than clinical verification) in the days after strenuous exercise (e.g., a marathon race), whereas moderate training has been claimed to reduce the number of symptoms. However, in neither strenuous nor moderate exercise have these symptoms been causally linked to exercise-induced changes in immune function.[119]

Special Implications for the Therapist   6-1

EXERCISE IMMUNOLOGY

Physical therapists employ exercise in treatment of all ages with a variety of clinical problems, thereby influencing immune function. Exercise as a means of preventing illness and attaining a healthy lifestyle and as an intervention tool in immunodeficiency states is becoming a larger part of preventive services. Research in the area of exercise immunology is in its infancy, with many results based on studies in animals. Keeping abreast of research results is the first step to examining the clinical implications in this area.

Aged adults constitute a growing and important consumer group of therapy services. Since immune function declines with advancing age, it is important that we understand the effects of exercise on immune function. Very few absolute guidelines have been developed; it seems intense or strenuous exercise may be detrimental to the immune system, whereas a lifetime of moderate exercise and physical activity enhances immune function. Further research is needed to clarify or modify this guideline.

It takes 6 to 24 hours for the immune system to recover from the acute effects of severe exercise. Each individual client must be evaluated after exercise to determine the perceived intensity of the exercise or intervention session. For example, in the deconditioned older adult with compromised cardiopulmonary function, reduced oxygen transport, and impaired mobility, ambulating from the bed to the bathroom may be perceived by their body as strenuous exercise.[74]

Intense exercise during an infectious episode should be avoided. For anyone, especially competitive athletes, who is wondering whether to exercise in the presence of an acute viral or bacterial infection (e.g., when manifesting constitutional symptoms), a neck check should be conducted. If the symptoms are located above the neck, such as a stuffy or runny nose, sneezing, or a scratchy throat, exercise should be performed cautiously through the scheduled workout at half speed. If, after 10 minutes, the symptoms are alleviated, the workout can be finished with the usual amount of frequency, intensity, and duration. If instead the symptoms are worse and the head is pounding or throbbing with every footstep, the exercise program should be stopped and the person should rest. If a fever or symptoms below the neck is evident, such as aching muscles, a hacking cough, diarrhea, or vomiting, exercise should not be initiated.[45] (See the specific exercise guidelines for the person with HIV in this chapter.) ∎

IMMUNODEFICIENCY DISEASES

In immunodeficiency, the immune response is absent or depressed as a result of a primary or secondary disorder. Primary immunodeficiency reflects a defect involving T cells, B cells, or lymphoid tissues. Secondary immunodeficiency results from an underlying disease or factor that depresses or blocks the immune response.

◆ Primary Immunodeficiency

The recognition of impaired immunity in children 50 years ago has resulted in tremendous increase in knowledge of the functions of the immune system. More than 95 inherited immunodeficiency disorders have now been identified. Genetically determined immunodeficiency can cause increased susceptibility to infection, autoimmunity, and increased risk of cancer. The defects may affect one or more components of the immune system, including T cells, B cells, NK cells, phagocytic cells, and complement proteins. No further discussion of these conditions is included in this book because the therapist rarely encounters these congenital conditions. A review of the pathophysiology of primary immunodeficiency is available.[19]

◆ Secondary Immunodeficiency

Secondary immunodeficiency disorders such as leukemia or Hodgkin's disease follow and result from an earlier disease or event. Multiple, diverse, and nonspecific defects in the immune defenses occur in viral and other infections, and also in malnutrition, alcoholism, aging, autoimmune disease, diabetes mellitus, cancer, chronic disease, steroid therapy, cancer chemotherapy, and radiation. More specific causes such as AIDS also contribute to secondary immunodeficiency.

Iatrogenic Immunodeficiency

Immunodeficiency induced by immunosuppressive drugs, radiation therapy, or splenectomy is referred to as *iatrogenic immunodeficiency*. Immunosuppressive drugs fall into several categories, including cytotoxic drugs, corticosteroids, cyclosporine, and antilymphocyte serum or antithymocyte globulin (ATG).

Cytotoxic drugs kill immunocompetent cells while they are replicating, but since most cytotoxic drugs are not selective, all rapidly dividing cells are affected. Not only are lymphocytes and phagocytes eliminated, but these drugs also interfere with lymphocyte synthesis and release of immunoglobulins and lymphokines. Other effects of this nonselectivity of cytotoxic drugs are discussed in Chapter 4 and may include bone marrow suppression with neutropenia, anemia, and cytopenia; gonadal suppression with sterility; alopecia; hemorrhagic cystitis; and vomiting, nausea, and stomatitis. The risk of lymphoproliferative malignancy is also increased (see Tables 4-10 and 8-8).

Corticosteroids are used to treat immune-mediated disorders because of their potent antiinflammatory and immunosuppressive effects. Corticosteroids stabilize the vascular membrane, blocking tissue infiltration by neutrophils and monocytes, thus inhibiting inflammation. They also kidnap T cells in the bone marrow, causing lymphopenia. Corticosteroids also appear to inhibit immunoglobulin synthesis and interfere with the binding of the immunoglobulin to antigen.

Cyclosporine (immunosuppressive drug) selectively suppresses the proliferation and development of helper T cells, resulting in depressed cell-mediated immunity. This drug is used primarily to prevent rejection of organ transplants but is also being investigated for use in several other disorders. *Antilymphocyte serum* or *antithymocyte globulin* is an anti–T-cell antibody that reduces T-cell number and function, thereby suppressing cell-mediated immunity. It has been used effectively to prevent cell-mediated rejection of tissue grafts or transplants. See the section on Immunosuppressants under Adverse Drug Reactions in Chapter 4.

Radiation therapy is cytotoxic to most lymphocytes, inducing profound lymphopenia, which results in immunosuppression. Irradiation of all major lymph node areas, a procedure known as *total nodal irradiation (TNI)*, is used to treat disorders such as Hodgkin's lymphoma. It is being investigated for its effectiveness in severe rheumatoid arthritis, lupus nephritis, and prevention of kidney transplant rejection. *Splenectomy* increases a person's susceptibility to infection, especially with pyogenic bacteria such as *Streptococcus pneumoniae*. This risk of infection is even greater when the person is very young or has an underlying reticuloendothelial disorder. These people should be observed carefully for any signs of infection (see Table 7-1).

◆ Consequences of Immunodeficiency

People who are immunocompromised from any of the immunodeficiency disorders are at increased risk of developing infection because their impaired immune system does not provide adequate protection against invading microorganisms. Normal mechanical defense mechanisms may be affected (respiratory, GI systems). Body flora that are normally harmless, such as *Candida*, may become pathogenic and a source of infection.

Additional risk factors for people who are already immunocompromised include poor physiologic and psychologic health status; old age; coexistence of other diseases or conditions, invasive procedures (e.g., surgery, invasive lines); and

treatments (e.g., chemotherapy, radiation therapy, bone marrow transplantation). The weakened immune system can cause the person to become susceptible to common everyday infectious agents, such as influenza viruses and *S. aureus*, as well as the more exotic organisms, such as *Histoplasma capsulatum* and *Toxoplasma gondii*.

Special Implications for the Therapist **6-2**

INFECTION CONTROL IN IMMUNODEFICIENCY DISORDERS

Although infection control strategies such as handwashing, standard precautions, and disinfection are important for all people treated in the health care system, they are especially critical for individuals whose immune systems are altered by primary immunodeficiency disorders, secondary immunodeficiency disorders, and HIV infection.

It is important that health care providers stop and think about altered defense mechanisms, infectious agents, reservoirs, modes of transmission, and infection control strategies to prevent infection in this population (Fig. 6-4). Pulmonary complications are common among the immunocompromised accompanied by poor cough reflexes, an inability to cough effectively, and susceptibility to pulmonary and other opportunistic infections. Additionally, these individuals are often debilitated and easily fatigued. Frequent mobilization and body positioning enhance gas exchange and promote comfort while maintaining strength.[36] ■

◆ Acquired Immune Deficiency Syndrome

Overview and Definition.   HIV can be considered an infection of the immune system, resulting in progressive and ultimately profound immune suppression. Currently one of the most widely publicized diseases, AIDS was first recognized in homosexual men in 1981 (the earliest sample of HIV-infected blood dates back to 1959,[68] but computer analysis suggests an emergence date of 1930[85]). The virus thought to be responsible for the transmission of AIDS was identified as HIV in July 1986. As new discoveries were made the classification scheme later included two subtypes as HIV-1 and HIV-2 with several strains of HIV-1 further identified.[147] This text deals primarily with HIV-1 (the cause of most of the AIDS cases in the United States), hereafter referred to as HIV.

AIDS is characterized by progressive destruction of cell-mediated (T-cell) immunity and changes in humoral immunity and even elements of autoimmunity because of the central role of the CD4+ T lymphocyte in immune reactions (see the section on Monocytes and Macrophages earlier in this chapter for a discussion of CD4+ cells). The resultant immunodeficiency leaves the affected person susceptible to opportunistic infections, including unusual cancers, and other abnormalities that characterize this syndrome. Additionally, up to 40% of Americans with HIV are believed to be infected with the hepatitis C virus (HCV), primarily among injection drug users and those with hemophilia as a result of blood products used to treat the hemophilia.

The Centers for Disease Control and Prevention (CDC) revised the definition of AIDS in 1992 to include those who

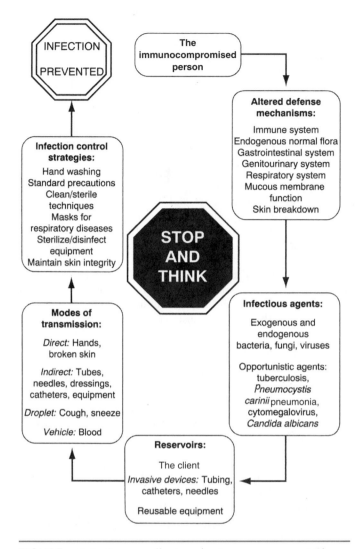

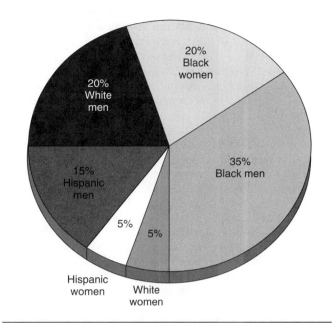

FIGURE   6-5   Estimates of new infections occurring by sex and ethnic group (1999). Although this illustration does not reflect it, there are a reported 5 to 10 million children infected with HIV-1 (worldwide) and this figure is expected to continue to increase in African countries. Centers for Disease Control and Prevention (CDC) media kit, 2000.

FIGURE   6-4   Factors affecting the immunocompromised person, leading to the selection of the correct infection control strategies to prevent infectious complications. (From Schaffer SD, Garzon LS, Heroux DL et al: *Pocket guide to infection prevention and safe practice,* St Louis, 1996, Mosby, p 222.)

have HIV-1 and a CD4 count below 200/mL (the normal CD4 lymphocyte count is 600 to 1200/mL) or 14% of the total lymphocyte count, even if the person has no other signs or symptoms of infection. The AIDS definition was further expanded in 1993 to include diseases affecting women (e.g., cervical cancer) and people with tuberculosis or depressed immune systems.

The term *HIV infection* includes the entire spectrum of illness from initial diagnosis to full-blown expression of AIDS. Three distinct points identify this continuum: (1) asymptomatic HIV seropositive, (2) early symptomatic HIV, and (3) HIV advanced disease (AIDS). Not everyone who is exposed to HIV becomes infected, and not everyone who is infected develops AIDS. The explanation for this phenomenon remains unknown, but researchers have shown that infection with HIV and progression to AIDS are controlled by both host genetic factors and viral factors. The human leukocyte antigen (HLA) region in humans controls immune response functions and influences susceptibility to infectious diseases, including HIV. There are HLA alleles* associated with sus-

ceptibility to and protection from HIV infection, and these differ among ethnic groups.[135] A single amino acid change in HLA molecules has a substantial effect on the rate of progression to AIDS.[59]

Incidence.   Since the first AIDS cases were reported in the United States in 1981, the number of cases and deaths among people with AIDS increased rapidly during the 1980s, followed by substantial declines in new cases and deaths in the late 1990s.† The greatest impact of the epidemic is among men who have sex with men (MSM) and among racial/ethnic minorities, with increases in the number of cases among women and those attributed to heterosexual transmission. The number of people living with AIDS has increased as deaths have declined.[112] New infections in the United States has declined to an estimated 40,000 per year since 1992 (down from a peak of 150,000 per year in the mid-1980s), and the number of people living with AIDS is the highest ever reported.

Half of all new cases are caused by injection drug use, and almost an equal amount (41%) are infected through MSM. Black women are four times as likely as white women to get HIV infection through the use of shared injection drug needles and sex with infected men (Fig. 6-5). Most people diagnosed with AIDS in the United States are age 20 to 49; however, the number of adolescents with HIV in the United States doubles every year. Teens account for one quarter of new sexually transmitted diseases reported each year, and AIDS in older adults accounts for 11% of all AIDS cases.[112]

---

* Alleles are situated at one or more sites on chromosomes and carry genetic information that determines a specific genetic characteristic or trait.

†AIDS remains an epidemic of vast proportions in other countries (e.g., one in four adults is infected in South Africa); soon, the number of deaths from AIDS is likely to exceed the estimated 25 million caused by the Black Death in the fourteenth century.[158]

Etiologic Factors, Transmission, and Risk Factors. The primary cause of AIDS is the type 1 retrovirus (HIV). Transmission of HIV occurs by exchange of body fluids (notably blood and semen) and is associated with high-risk behaviors. High-risk behaviors include unprotected anal and oral sex, including having six or more sexual partners in the past year; sexual activity with someone known to carry HIV; exchanging sex for money or drugs; or injecting drugs. HIV is not transmitted by fomites (e.g., coffee cups, drinking fountains, or telephone receivers) or casual household or social contact.

MSM has been the most common mode of exposure among people reported with AIDS (46%), followed by injection drug use (25%) and heterosexual contact (11%). The chief determinant of whether HIV is transmitted during heterosexual intercourse is the viral load* in the infected partner's bloodstream; transmission does not occur when serum HIV-1 ribonucelic [RNA] levels are less than 1500 copies/mL (i.e., low viral load).[128] Uncircumcised men have a greater risk of contracting HIV through sexual contact than do circumcised men. The thinner epithelial lining of the glans penis may be susceptible to increased trauma during sexual activity, increasing the likelihood of viral transmission.[92]

Nearly all transmission of HIV through transfusion of blood or blood products occurred before testing of the blood supply for HIV antibody and self-deferral programs were initiated in 1985. People with hemophilia were especially vulnerable and susceptible to transmission. In 1991, approximately 70% of people with hemophilia had seroconverted to being positive for HIV; however, since 1986, no further HIV transmission has occurred in that way. The number of people reported with AIDS who were exposed through blood transfusions was 284 in 2000, down from a peak of 1098 in 1993. The number of perinatally acquired AIDS cases peaked in 1992, followed by a sharp decline since then.[112]

Ethnicity is not directly related to increased AIDS risk, but it is associated with other determinants of health status such as poverty, illegal drug use, access to health care, and living in communities with a high prevalence of AIDS. Adolescents are one of the groups at greatest risk for HIV infection, particularly minority inner-city youth. Runaway and homeless youth are especially likely to engage in high-risk sexual activity. The use of amphetamines, ecstasy, and amyl nitrate is associated with increased frequency of unprotected anal sex, especially among homosexual and bisexual individuals under age 23.[44]

Pathogenesis. The rapid convergence of information from diverse areas of AIDS research makes it impossible to present the most up-to-date information. Scientists are reporting new discoveries daily about the pathogenesis of HIV disease. The natural history of AIDS begins with infection by the HIV retrovirus† detectable only by laboratory tests. This retrovirus predominantly infects human T4

(helper) lymphocytes, the major regulators of the immune response, and destroys or inactivates them. Macrophages and B cells are also infected. HIV is unique in that despite the body's immune responses after initial infection, some HIV invariably escapes. Large amounts of HIV have been discovered hiding in the immune cells lining the surface of adenoids.[50] This information alters the formally held view that HIV is a slow or covert process, when in fact the virus's growth continues in the period between infection and the onset of AIDS. It is theorized that the use of a preventive vaccine could stop hidden viral production.

Once HIV enters the body, cells containing the CD4 antigen, including macrophages and T4 cells, serve as receptors for the HIV retrovirus, allowing direct passage of the infection into target cells previously identified (e.g., GI tract, uterine cervical cells, and neuroglial cells). After invading a cell, a virus particle called a *virion* injects the core proteins and the two strands of viral RNA into the cell. As a retrovirus, HIV contains reverse transcriptase, an enzyme required for successful infection by the virus. Before viral replication can occur in the host cell, this enzyme must copy all the genetic information of the virus from viral RNA to viral DNA. Once the viral genome is transcribed, it can be integrated into the host's DNA and duplicated many times (Fig. 6-6).

Replication of the HIV virus can cause cell death, although the person remains asymptomatic. Seroconversion (becoming positive for HIV) usually takes place during the first 3 to 6 weeks of this replication process but can take longer. After a few months, very little virus is found in the blood; only HIV antibodies remain in the serum. During the asymptomatic period (also called the *early stage*), the virus migrates from the serum into the tissues to infect CD4 cells in lymph tissue. The virus continues to kill the CD4 cells in the lymph nodes, although the CD4 count remains above 500 cells/mm³ (average CD4 cell count is 1000 cells/mm³).*

Once all these cells are depleted, the virus once again enters the blood to infect any remaining lymphocytes and clinically apparent disease occurs. By the time this happens, the immune system has been compromised and is ineffective and unable to mount a specific immune response to these virions. The immune system dysfunction is even more exaggerated if the host has become further immunocompromised by opportunistic diseases.

HIV infection leads to profound pathology, either directly by destruction of CD4+ cells, other immune cells, or neuroglial cells or indirectly, through the secondary effects of CD4+ T-cell dysfunction and resultant immunosuppression. The decline in CD4 cells results in progressive loss of immune system function and the development of a wide variety of clinical signs and symptoms (see Table 6-4). This describes the middle stage or symptomatic phase of AIDS when CD4 count ranges between 200 and 500 cells/mm³. A decrease in the CD4 count to less than 200 and an elevated viral load occurs during the late-stage or advanced disease associated with the development of opportunistic infections.

---

*Viral load refers to the number of viral RNA particles present in the blood and correlates strongly with the stage of disease. Viral load tests measure the amount of HIV-specific RNA and is highest at the time of seroconversion when antibodies appear in the serum and the person is considered positive for HIV. This is a useful measurement for determining the effectiveness of drug treatment and also directly correlates with the risk of perinatal transmission in pregnant women with HIV.

†All human cells contain DNA and RNA, known collectively as *nucleic acids*. The DNA is located in the cell nucleus, and the RNA is located in the cytoplasm of the cell. Viruses contain only one of the nucleic acids and are categorized as belonging to the DNA group (e.g., herpes and mononucleosis) or the RNA group (e.g., measles and mumps). HIV is classified as a lentivirus, a subclass of retroviruses that contain RNA. When the RNA virus intitiates replication in the living host cell, it must convert its RNA genetic information into a DNA template to replicate.

---

*The regulation of HIV expression by modules secreted by immune cells is even more complex than previously realized. The initially expanded clones that can kill HIV-infected cells are found in the bloodstream rather than in the lymph nodes, where the virus is replicating. The gene, *vpr*, within HIV that stops production of the CD4 T lymphocytes has now been identified. Current research focuses on understanding how the *vpr* gene prevents these disease-fighting cells from dividing. New drugs to block the gene's actions and allow immune cells to continue multiplying and fighting HIV would be the next step.

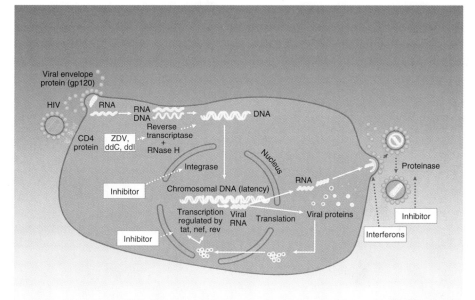

FIGURE **6-6** Stages of HIV replication cycle. (1) Attachment of the virus to the host cell, (2) Uncoating followed by reverse transcription, (3) Integration of newly synthesized DNA into the host cell DNA, with transcription and translation of the viral genetic message into viral protein; HIV possesses genes that code for proteins with important regulatory functions for the virus such as *tat* (transactivator), *nef* (negative factor), and *rev* (regulator of expression of virion proteins) (4) assembly with release of the virus out of the host cell. (Courtesy Patricia D. Salvato, MD, Houston, Texas, 2000.)

This infectious process may take one of three forms: (1) immunodeficiency with opportunistic infections and unusual malignancies; (2) autoimmunity such as rheumatoid arthritis, lymphoid interstitial pneumonitis, hypergammaglobulinemia, and production of autoimmune antibodies; and (3) neurologic dysfunction, including AIDS dementia complex, HIV encephalopathy, and peripheral neuropathies.

HIV has an extremely high mutation rate even within a single individual, producing competing strains of the same virus that fight for survival against the weapons produced by the immune system. Researchers are studying how different strains of HIV use recently discovered cell surface molecules, in addition to the well-known CD4 molecule, to bind to and enter target cells. Another consideration is how different strains of HIV have a preference for certain cells; strains that infect macrophages and T cells are the main ones found early in the disease. Later, strains appear that replicate efficiently in T cells but not in macrophages. Finally, mutations in the human genes for HIV co-receptors may help explain why some people do not become infected despite repeated exposure and why some who are infected may have different rates of disease progression.

Clinical Manifestations.   HIV infection manifests itself in many different ways (Table 6-4) and differs between adult and pediatric populations. The focus of this text is primarily adult populations; more specific discussion of pediatric HIV is available.[144,160] Great variation exists among individuals as to the amount of time that passes between acute HIV infection, the appearance of symptoms, the diagnosis of AIDS, and death.

Asymptomatic Stage [CD4 >500 cells/mm³].   During the early stage, the person demonstrates laboratory evidence of seroconversion (positive for HIV) but remains asymptomatic. Some individuals develop an acute, self-limiting infectious mononucleosis-like illness or a subtle, viral-like syndrome, followed by a period of clinical latency that may last a decade or more. During the asymptomatic period, the infected person is clinically healthy and capable of normal daily activities, normal work habits, and unrestricted level and duration of exercise.

Early Symptomatic Stage [CD4 = 200-500 cells/mm³]. As the infection progresses and the immune system becomes increasingly more compromised, a variety of symptoms may develop, including persistent generalized adenopathy; nonspecific symptoms such as weight loss, fatigue, night sweats, and fevers; neurologic symptoms resulting from HIV encephalopathy; or an opportunistic infection (e.g., *Pneumocystis carinii* pneumonia [PCP], cytomegalovirus [CMV], toxoplasmosis) or malignancy.

CMV can cause peripheral neuropathy and HIV retinitis (with possible blindness); PCP produces pulmonary symptoms such as dyspnea on exertion, nonproductive cough, and weight loss, and toxoplasmosis is a parasitic disease that affects the CNS. In addition to the symptoms that may occur with opportunistic diseases, treatment with multiple medications can cause adverse side effects, sometimes creating a confusing clinical picture.

HIV Advanced Disease (AIDS) [CD4 < 200 cells/mm³]. The neurologic manifestations of more advanced HIV disease are numerous and can involve the central, peripheral, and autonomic nervous systems. The CNS appears to be more commonly attacked by HIV than the peripheral nervous system. *HIV* or *AIDS encephalopathy,* also referred to as *HIV-associated dementia* (HAD), formerly AIDS dementia complex, is a primary infection of the brain by HIV. Symptoms can vary and are listed in Table 6-4. In the most advanced stages of the disease, severe dementia, mutism, incontinence, and paraplegia may occur. A detailed summary of nervous system disorders associated with HIV, including treatment, is available.[56,144,160]

Peripheral neuropathy, disease- or drug-induced myopathy, and musculoskeletal pain syndromes occur most often in advanced stages of HIV disease but can occur at any stage of HIV infection and may be the presenting manifestation. Peripheral neuropathies are usually distal, symmetric, and predominantly sensory, but other parts of the body may be affected such as the face or trunk. The pain of peripheral neuropathy is characterized by burning, tingling, contact hypersensitivity, proprioceptive losses, and in severe cases, secondary motor deficits. In the individual with HIV and newly acquired neuropathy with a strong major motor component, vasculitis may be the underlying cause (see the section on Vasculitis in Chapter 11). Involvement of the upper

Clinical Manifestations of HIV Disease

TABLE 6-4

Musculoskeletal	Neurologic/Neuromuscular	Cardiopulmonary	Integumentary	Other
Myalgia/arthralgia Rheumatologic manifestations: • Inflammatory joint disorders (e.g., Reiter's syndrome (e.g., Reiter's syndrome, reactive arthritis, psoriatic arthritis) • Myositis/pyomyositis • Connective tissue disease Avascular necrosis (osteonecrosis) Musculoskeletal pain syndrome/HIV wasting syndrome Myopathy (disease or drug-induced) Pelvic pain (e.g., pelvic inflammatory disease [PID]) Extrapulmonary tuberculosis	HIV encephalitis: • Gait disturbance • Intention tremor • Delayed release of reflexes HIV-associated dementia: • *Behavioral:* Apathy, lethargy, social withdrawal, irritability, depression • *Cognitive:* Memory impairment, confusion, disorientation • *Motor:* Ataxia, leg weakness with gait disturbances, loss of fine motor coordination, incontinence, paraplegia (advanced stage) Guillain Barré syndrome Headache, seizures (toxoplasmosis) HIV myelitis (osteomyelitis) Radiculopathy Peripheral neuropathy: • Pain (burning, tingling, hypersensitivity) • Sensory loss • Secondary motor deficits, gait disturbances Brachial neuropathy Vacuolar spinal myelopathy	Dyspnea, especially on exertion Nonproductive cough Hypoxia Sympotms associated with opportunistic infections of the pulmonary system Pericardial effusion Cardiomyopathy Endocarditis Vasculitis	Alopecia (hair loss) Basal cell carcinoma Kaposi's sarcoma Mucocutaneous ulcers Rash Urticaria (diffuse skin reaction, wheals)	Constitutional symptoms: • Flulike symptoms • Fever, sore throat • Generalized adenopathy • Weight loss • Lethargy, fatigue • Night sweats, fevers Opportunistic infections: • Cytomegalovirus • Bacterial pneumonia • Tuberculosis • Toxoplasmosis • *Pneumocystis carinii* pneumonia • Sinusitis • Vaginal infection Malignancy (most common forms): • Non-Hodgkin's lymphoma • Kaposi's sarcoma • Cervical cancer GI disturbance, including wasting syndrome Lymphedema Lipodystrophy Renal (kidney) failure Hepatic (liver) failure Oral thrush Gingivitis Visual disturbance (CMV) HIV-related psychiatric disorders

extremities can occur, but this is less common and usually later in the disease progression.

AIDS is associated with *neuromusculoskeletal diseases* such as osteomyelitis, bacterial myositis, non-Hodgkin's lymphoma, and infectious (reactive) arthritis. Avascular necrosis (osteonecrosis) of the femoral head(s) has been reported with the use of antiretroviral therapy containing protease inhibitors.[52]* Injection drug use (IDU) and hemophilia appear to be additional risk factors for development of musculoskeletal infections in people with HIV infection. The hip joint (hemophilia) and the sternocleidomastoid joint (IDU) are affected most often.

Musculoskeletal pain syndromes are associated with the wasting process in AIDS referred to as *HIV wasting syndrome*. HIV wasting is characterized by a disproportionate loss of metabolically active tissue, specifically body cell mass (i.e., tissue involved with glucose oxidation, protein synthesis, and immune system function). These conditions occur secondary to weight loss, chronic diarrhea, unexplained weakness, fever, and malnutrition (e.g., mineral and vitamin deficiencies, especially vitamin B deficiency).† As the HIV epidemic affects more women, increasing cases of pelvic inflammatory disease (PID) are being reported.[70] Pain is a common symptom in all these conditions.

Rheumatologic manifestations are transient or subtle and appear more often as HIV disease progresses. The arthritis can be severe and does not necessarily respond to conventional medications. Polymyositis involves bilaterally symmetrical proximal muscle weakness and arthritis may precede or accompany seroconversion. More detailed information regarding rheumatic disorders in HIV disease is available.[148]

HIV-associated myopathy presents with a progressive painless weakness in the proximal limb muscles. The weakness is symmetrical and often involves the muscles of the face and neck. This type of myopathy may occur in individuals with HIV at every stage of illness. Muscle biopsies have shown necrosis of muscle fibers with and without inflammatory infiltrates. No evidence has been found of direct HIV infection of the muscle, and the underlying cause has not been determined. The fact that these clients improve on corticosteroids or plasmapheresis may point to an underlying autoimmune defect. Drug-induced myopathy is discussed in Chapter 4.

Medical Management

Prevention. Two simple but effective interventions have been shown to limit the horizontal spread of HIV: (1) sex education and the practice of abstinence (or less effectively, the use of condoms) and (2) reducing/eliminating risky drug-abuse behavior including the provision of clean needles.[147]‡ Controlling the AIDS epidemic requires sustained prevention programs in all affected communities, particularly programs targeting MSM, sexually active women, and injection drug users.

Continued prevention education is important with sexually active individuals undergoing treatment. Even though potent antiviral treatment can eradicate HIV from the blood, these drugs cannot completely eliminate the virus from the body, especially the semen. Although antiretroviral therapy reduces shedding of HIV in semen thereby reducing HIV transmissibility, a substantial portion of people with HIV may still be infectious and may have drug-resistant strains of the virus.[7] Safe sex practices should continue to be reinforced in all people with HIV.

Healthy People 2010 has established three primary goals related to reducing the number of AIDS cases: (1) reduce AIDS among adolescents and adults to one new case per 100,000 people (from the current 19.5 cases in people age 13 years and older); (2) 25% improvement in the number of new AIDS cases among adolescent and adult men who have sex with them (*baseline:* 17,847 new cases of AIDS in 1998 among males age 13 years and older and *target:* 13,385 new cases); and (3) 25% improvement in the number of new AIDS cases among men and women who inject drugs (*baseline:* 12,099 new cases among injection drug users age 13 and older and *target:* 9075 new cases).[64]

A new generation of MSM has replaced those who benefited from early prevention strategies. Behavior intervention, the primary prevention tool, includes school-based programs, peer-to-peer interventions, strategies that limit needle sharing, parent-to-child communication, client-centered counseling, and personalized risk-reduction strategies (Box 6-2). The introduction of routine counseling, voluntary testing for women with HIV, and providing zidovudine (commonly known as *AZT*) to infected women and their infants has dramatically reduced mother-to-child transmission rates.[112]

Mycobacterium tuberculosis associated with AIDS is communicable, preventable, and treatable. Tuberculin (TB) skin testing should be available and routinely offered to individuals at HIV testing sites. Highest risk individuals for concomitant HIV and TB infections include the homeless, injection drug users, and incarcerated people[56] (see Chapter 14). Guidelines for the prevention of other opportunistic infections in people with HIV are also now available.[24]

Socioeconomic factors (e.g., high rates of poverty and unemployment, lack of access to health care) are associated with high rates of HIV risk behaviors among minority MSM and are barriers to accessing HIV testing, diagnosis, and treatment. Reaching minority MSM who may not identify themselves as homosexual or bisexual with prevention messages remains a challenge. The development of an HIV vaccine is important to control the global epidemic. Efforts to develop a microbicide that is safe and effective in reducing HIV transmission through sexual intercourse may be key to controlling the epidemic among women.[112]

Diagnosis. Early diagnosis is important so that early and preventive therapies may be initiated and sex partners can be notified of their risk of HIV and the subsequent need for HIV testing. To establish uniformity in reporting AIDS cases, the CDC has established diagnostic criteria for the confirmation of AIDS. The most commonly performed test is the enzyme-linked immunosorbent assay (ELISA) test, an antibody test to indicate HIV infection indirectly by revealing HIV antibodies (indicating exposure to the virus). However, antibody testing is not always reliable because the body takes a variable

---

*The increased incidence of osteonecrosis in HIV/AIDS may be due to the use of protease inhibitors or possibly as a result of an increased frequency of risk factors previously associated with osteonecrosis such as hyperlipidemia, corticosteroid use, alcohol abuse, and hypercoagulability.[145]

†Studies have shown a clear relationship between vitamin B$_{12}$ deficiency and dysfunction of the central and peripheral nervous systems. Some of the clinical abnormalities of the nervous system seen in people with HIV are similar to those that have been described in those with vitamin B$_{12}$ deficiency.

‡ While many studies and the NIH support the use of needle exchange in reducing transmission of HIV there is currently a ban on the use of Federal funds to support this program. Most states have a law in place (Model Drug Paraphernalia Act) prohibiting the acquisition of drug paraphernalia including needles. Needle exchange programs are available under limited circumstances in some states but this is not universally available.

BOX 6-2

Risk Reduction Behaviors for the Prevention of HIV Transmission

Obtain testing for HIV* if any of the following is true:
- You received blood or blood products before 1985.
- You have (or have had) multiple sex partners.
- You inject drugs and share needles.
- You have sexual intercourse (vaginal, anal, or oral) with someone else who injects drugs and shares needles.
- You have sex without a condom ("rubber") with someone who has HIV.
- You share used needles for tattooing or body piercing.

Protect yourself during sexual activities as follows:
- Abstinence or a monogamous relationship (sex with only one partner; both partners must be HIV free) is the only known prevention for the transmission of HIV.
- Use latex glove when inserting finger(s) into vagina or rectum.
- Use a new condom each time you have oral, anal, or vaginal sex.
  - Latex or polyurethane is best because HIV can pass through lambskin or natural condoms
- Do not use outdated condoms (check expiration date).
- Use the new condom with each sexual act from beginning to end (i.e., put on the condom before genital contact with partner and when the penis is erect; hold the condom firmly against base of penis during withdrawal; withdraw penis while still erect).
- Use water-based lubricants (e.g., KY jelly), NOT oils, lotions, or vaseline that can cause a condom to tear or break.
- Ensure that no air is trapped in tip of condom.

Protect yourself as follows if you use drugs:
- Never share drug needles or "works."
- Participate in clinic needle exchange programs or clean drug needles with 100% bleach, leave 30 seconds, repeat three times and then rinse three times with water between uses.
- Mixing sex, drugs, and alcohol increases your risk. If you are drunk or high, it is harder to make good decisions about sexual practices.

Protect yourself as follows if you are pregnant:
- You can pass on HIV to your unborn child during pregnancy, birth, or breastfeeding. If you are pregnant and you have engaged in HIV risk–behaviors, obtain HIV testing and appropriate treatment if you test positive for HIV.
- Medications taken during pregnancy can reduce your risk of HIV transmission to the fetus during pregnancy.

*A simple blood test (some centers offer a saliva test) can determine HIV infection 6 months after exposure. This test can be obtained anonymously (without giving out your name) and is free or low cost in most states. Contact your local Health Department.

From Montana Department of Health and Environmental Sciences, Doc No 20858 MT 4-98, Helena, Mont, 1998.

amount of time to produce a detectable level of antibodies. Consequently, a person with HIV could test negative for HIV antibodies. Antibody tests are also unreliable in neonates because transferred maternal antibodies persist for 6 to 10 months. The Western blot test is a more expensive test that may be used when there is a concern about false-positive tests because it is more specific—that is, in identifying individuals with negative test results.

The current CDC AIDS surveillance definition requires direct testing, including antigen tests (p24 antigen); HIV cultures; nucleic acid probes of peripheral blood lymphocytes; and the polymerase chain reaction (PCR). Additional laboratory confirmation of HIV infection is required; HIV RNA viral load testing as measured by the plasma HIV RNA assay and a CD4+ T lymphocyte count of less than 200 cells/mm³ is also considered diagnostic.* T-lymphocyte counts monitor the progression of HIV and should be viewed from a broad perspective rather than on a day-to-day basis; the overall trend is more important than single values.

A rapid noninvasive test that uses saliva to detect HIV antibodies is under investigation and primarily in use at testing clinics where it is more cost effective. This test is rapid, reliable, and easy to perform and interpret,[121,169] but concern exists that rapid tests will distract from risk reduction. Although some individuals may be reassured that they are negative for HIV, this does not necessarily translate into reduced risk without continued education. If the test is positive, then subsequent blood tests are ordered.

Treatment. No cure has been found for AIDS, but advances in treatment have successfully changed AIDS into a manageable chronic condition. The national HIV Vaccine Trials Network has been established to develop and test possible vaccine compounds but an effective vaccine is not imminent. Until a vaccine is available, the goal of intervention is to stop HIV from replicating.

Medical management centers on the CD4 cell count and viral load. When CD4 cell counts drop below 500 cells/mm³ highly active antiretroviral therapy (HAART) is initiated. HAART, a protease inhibitor plus two nucleoside-analog reverse transcriptase inhibitors, acts on reverse transcriptase, the enzyme necessary for transcribing HIV RNA to DNA, to achieve sustained suppression of HIV replication reducing the amount of virus in the blood to very low and even nondetectable levels. These drugs do not completely eliminate the virus and lifelong therapy is required until viral eradication is developed. In the United States, more than a dozen agents have been approved in three classes of drugs: (1) nucleoside analog reverse-transcriptase inhibitors, (2) nonnucleoside reverse-transcriptase inhibitors, and (3) protease inhibitors.[147]

Current efforts are focused on (1) simplifying the drug regimens to improve adherence, (2) developing alternatives for those in whom the current medications have failed, (3) preventing viral rebound (return of high levels of the virus when drugs are discontinued), and (4) managing the wide range of pharmacologic side effects. A highly controversial (investigational) approach to HIV infection is the structured treatment interruption or supervised treatment interruption (STI) designed to obtain immune control of the virus by boosting immunity to HIV. This approach is based on the hypothesis that limited reexposure to one's own virus may lead to augmented effective immunity.[163]

---

*T-cell measurement and viral load are both important indicators of HIV status. To use a train crash analogy, T-cell values represent the distance to the crash whereas viral load counts represent the speed of the train, i.e., how fast the person is declining.[143]

Development of drug resistance is the inevitable consequence of incomplete suppression of virus plasma levels in individuals with HIV treated with HAART. Several assays are available for testing HIV for resistance to antiretroviral agents. Genotypic and phenotypic testing has been implemented and should be carried out to establish an exact correlation between the genotype (individual's genetic makeup as determined by the specific combination and location of the genes on the chromosomes) and the clinical management, especially before the HAART regimen is discontinued.[22]

Potential toxicities from drug treatment include metabolic disorders (e.g., lipodystrophy, a syndrome of defective fat metabolism, dyslipidemia, and insulin resistance); avascular necrosis of the femoral head(s); and lactic acidosis. Lipodystrophy is characterized by a redistribution of fat with central obesity; dorsal fat pad, or "buffalo hump" (see Fig. 10-6); loss of fat in the extremities and face; and breast enlargement. Dyslipidemia may be associated with accelerated atherosclerosis and insulin resistance contributing to increased cardiovascular morbidity and mortality in the population with HIV.[60,86]

The lactic acidosis occurs as a result of injured cell mitochondria, giving off lactic acid in response to the effects of nucleoside reverse transcriptase inhibitors. AZT myopathy, a toxic mitochondrial myopathy is much less often seen today and is limited to people taking high doses of AZT. Both of these conditions are reversible with cessation of the drug therapy.[148]

The optimal time at which to initiate intervention remains controversial. When protease inhibitors were first introduced, the strategy was to "hit early, hit hard" because early intervention and the associated reduction of acute viral load might have positive effects on the subsequent course of the disease.[163] However, the development of resistance and the toxic side effects that occur have brought that philosophy into question. The complete eradication of the infection remains the focus of research today,[147] and the proper treatment of people with both HIV and HCV is still in its early stages.

Dosage adjustments are important considerations due to established gender-based response to antiretroviral side effects observed in women. Several antiretrovirals are now known to interact with oral contraceptives (e.g., nevirapine [Viraimune]; ritonavir [Navir]; nelfinavir [Viracept]). With HAART treatment, women are more likely to develop lipodystrophies, experience nausea, vomiting, fatigue, itching, abdominal pain, skin rashes, and perioral numbness while men experience more diarrhea.[65]

If, as suspected, multiple variants of HIV are in a single host and the virus is capable of mutating easily, treatment approaches geared toward enhancing host resistance and restoring or building the immune system will be more successful than trying to kill the virus.* Previous trials using interferon-α resulted in significant toxicity and its use has been limited. Other researchers are investigating the use of gene therapy and immune reconstitution or restoration in relation to AIDS.

Other pharmacologic intervention may be used to treat various clinical manifestations of HIV disease (e.g., antibiotics, nonsteroidal antiinflammatory drugs [NSAIDs]; corticosteroids; immunosuppressives; interferon therapy).

Nonpharmacologic intervention includes nutritional therapy, exercise, mental health support, and alternative or complementary methods. AIDS-associated weight loss, nutritional deficiencies, loss of muscle mass (wasting syndrome), and other effects contribute to immune dysfunction, faster disease progression in some people, and a variety of complications that can be ameliorated with proper nutrition. The use of alternative and complementary intervention techniques remains an area of controversy and investigation but may follow the same principles outlined elsewhere.[4,5,35]

Prognosis. The development of combination therapies is extending the lives of AIDS clients, keeping many healthy enough to avoid hospitalization and/or return to their baseline after illness, extending survival, and even resulting in return to work status for some people. People with AIDS are living longer with lower CD4 levels because prophylaxis and treatment of PCP saves many who would have died sooner in the earlier days of the AIDS epidemic.

Highly active antiretroviral therapy is improving survival but at the price of a variety of metabolic (and other) side effects. Patterns of morbidity and mortality are changing: the leading cause of death is now kidney or liver failure (instead of opportunistic infections) as a result of medical treatment (e.g., protease inhibitors are metabolized by the liver) and HCV.[20] For those people long infected with HIV or have both HIV and HCV, or who are manifesting the wasting syndrome, the prognosis remains poor.

A considerable body of evidence suggests that psychosocial factors play an important role in the progression of HIV infection, its morbidity and mortality. Psychosocial influences relating to faster disease progression include life-event stress, sustained depression, denial/avoidance coping, concealment of gay identity, and negative outlook. Conversely protective psychosocial factors include active coping, collaborative relationship with health care professionals, and stress management. Biologic factors such as genetics, age of the host, viral strain and virulence, medication, and immune response are also major determinants of disease progression and also impact on outcome. Scientists are continuing to investigate psychoneuroimmunologic pathways by which immune and neuroendocrine mechanisms might link psychosocial factors with health and survival.[6]

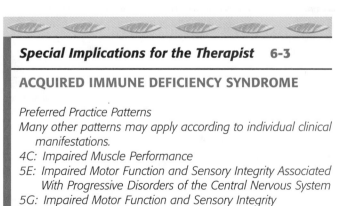

Special Implications for the Therapist   6-3

ACQUIRED IMMUNE DEFICIENCY SYNDROME

Preferred Practice Patterns
Many other patterns may apply according to individual clinical manifestations.
4C: *Impaired Muscle Performance*
5E: *Impaired Motor Function and Sensory Integrity Associated With Progressive Disorders of the Central Nervous System*
5G: *Impaired Motor Function and Sensory Integrity Associated With Acute or Chronic Polyneuropathies*
6B: *Impaired Aerobic Capacity/Endurance Associated With Deconditioning*

Continued

---

*This same principle of using drugs to boost the immune system, called biotherapy (immunotherapy), immunodilating, or immunologic therapy, is also being applied in the use of genetically engineered IL-2 to treat cancer.

6C: Impaired Ventilation, Respiration/Gas Exchange and Aerobic Capacity/Endurance Associated With Airway Clearance Dysfunction

With advances in treatment, improved care, and longer survival, therapists can expect to see increasing numbers of people in their practices who may have HIV. Maximal effectiveness from physical therapy requires a therapist who is knowledgeable about HIV disease and the unique rehabilitation issues surrounding individuals with HIV/AIDS.[142]

It is possible for individuals with HIV infection or AIDS to come to a therapy practice undiagnosed or unwilling to provide this information. Women who have been attacked or the victim of domestic violence have an increased risk of HIV transmission and do not always report this information. It is important to include questions in the history that consider the possibility of violence and HIV-related disease and correlate this information with objective evaluation results. For example, anyone presenting with musculoskeletal or neuromuscular symptoms of unknown origin, with or without constitutional symptoms, should be interviewed more specifically about the presence of past or current HIV risk behaviors. This may potentially lead to early medical referral, early diagnosis, and early, appropriate therapy. This is essential as early treatment choices will also determine future therapies because of viral resistance and other factors.

Prevention of Transmission

Health care workers (HCWs) may be concerned about potential contact in the workplace with clients who have AIDS; however, the risk of transmission of the virus from client to health care worker is exceedingly small.* Health care workers at potential risk of contact with HIV-containing body fluids include blood bank technologists, dialysis technicians, emergency department personnel, morticians, dentists, medical technicians, surgeons, and laboratory workers. Therapists are not considered at risk unless working in one of these capacities or performing wound care or débridement with a client with the virus.

The reported cases of occupational HIV transmission have been helpful in developing a definition of what constitutes exposure that could result in HIV transmission. Exposure routes implicated in occupational HIV transmission include (1) percutaneous injury (e.g., needle puncture or cut caused by a needle or other sharp object); (2) mucous membrane contamination with blood; and (3) nonintact skin (e.g., chapped, abraded, or afflicted with dermatitis) contamination. Contact of intact skin when the duration of contact is prolonged (i.e., several minutes or more) has not been associated with HIV transmission but is considered a potential exposure, in part because the skin may have unrecognized areas of disruption that could serve as portals of entry.[100]

Sources of HIV that may pose a risk of transmission through these routes include blood, visibly bloody fluids, tissues, and other body fluids including semen; vaginal secretions; and cerebrospinal, synovial, pleural, peritoneal, pericardial, and amniotic fluids. In addition, any direct cutaneous or mucosal contact, without barrier protection, to concentrated HIV in a research laboratory or production facility is considered to be an exposure.[100]

Although one nonoccupational episode of HIV transmission has been attributed to contact with blood-contaminated saliva, this incident was not analogous to the contact with saliva that occurs during dental or medical care. In the absence of visible blood in the saliva, exposure to saliva from a person with HIV is not thought to pose a risk for HIV transmission. Exposure to tears, sweat, or nonbloody urine or feces from individuals with the virus does not constitute exposure to HIV. Occupational exposure to breast milk does not constitute an exposure unless ingested directly.[100]

Health care considerations are primarily directed at preventing the transmission of the virus when caring for someone with AIDS by avoiding occupational blood exposure. Recommendations for preventing the spread of the virus consist of the use of standard precautions (e.g., using barriers for working with any liquid that comes from another person, excluding sweat [see Appendix A]). Specific recommendations for health care professionals working with AIDS and HIV-positive clients are included in Box 6-3. Everyone with AIDS is immunodeficient, and every precaution must be taken to prevent infection for that person.

An individual with HIV does not need a private room unless he or she has a communicable disease that requires respiratory isolation (e.g., tuberculosis) (see specific recommendations made in Chapter 14). Hepatitis would require standard precautions but not isolation. The virus is not transmitted through casual nonintimate contact or social encounters such as eating in restaurants or using public transportation or public bathroom facilities because the virus does not live long or replicate outside the body.

Few studies have evaluated the risk of transmission of blood-borne pathogens during sports or athletic activity. However, both the National Football League and the National Collegiate Athletic Association have evaluated the risk of transmission of HIV. Both groups conservatively estimate that the risk of HIV transmission on the playing field is well below one per 1 million games.[17,42]

BOX **6-3**

Standard AIDS/HIV Precautions for Health Care Workers

Use protective barriers (gloves, eye shields, gowns) when handling blood, body fluids, and infectious fluids.

Wash hands, skin, and mucous membranes immediately and thoroughly if contaminated by blood or other body fluids.

Prevent needle or scalpel sticks.

Ventilation devices are available for resuscitation.

Any health care worker (HCW) with open wounds or skin lesions should not treat clients or handle equipment until the lesion(s) heals.

Pregnant health care workers should take extra precautions. See Appendix A for additional information.

Occupational exposure to HIV should be followed immediately by evaluation of exposure source and postexposure prophylaxis.

---

* The health care worker is at far greater risk for the transmission of the hepatitis B virus (HBV) and should consider prophylactic vaccination for HBV or become familiar with postexposure prophylaxis (PEP) for HBV (see Chapter 16).

U.S. Public Health Service: Updated guidelines for the prevention of HIV and hepatitis virus transmission and the management of occupational exposures to HIV, BHV, and HCV, *MMWR* 50(RR-11):1-67, 2001.

Postexposure Prophylaxis

HIV postexposure prophylaxis (PEP) is a form of secondary HIV prevention that may reduce the incidence of HIV infections. The two types of PEP are occupational and nonoccupational. Occupational exposure should be considered an urgent medical concern requiring timely postexposure management.[24] Occupational HIV PEP is an accepted form of therapy for health care workers exposed to HIV through their jobs.[26] Well-established U.S. national guidelines for occupational HIV PEP exist. No national guidelines are available for nonoccupational HIV PEP; recommended use for after nonconsensual sexual intercourse (sexual abuse and assault); injected drug use; and needle-stick and sharp injuries (i.e., in non–health care individuals) has not been investigated.[107]

The presumed mechanism for HIV PEP comes from animal and human work suggesting that shortly after an exposure to HIV, a window period exists during which the viral load is small enough to be controlled by the body's immune system. Antiretroviral medications given during this period may help to diminish or end viral replication, thereby reducing the viral inoculum to a more potentially manageable target for the host's defenses. HIV PEP is accepted practice in the perinatal setting and for health care workers with occupational injuries. Determining level of risk and appropriateness of drug selection should be conducted as soon as possible after an exposure has occurred. HIV PEP should be administered within 1 hour of exposure. Other guidelines for HIV PEP are available.[24,107]

Guidelines for Health Care Workers with HIV

Any health care worker with HIV and/or HBV or HCV should not perform exposure-prone procedures in which blood contact might occur. Permission and guidance from special review committees is required before an infected health care worker can perform such procedures. For the therapist, this would primarily exclude internal pelvic floor examination and wound care, including débridement and dressing changes. According to guidelines drafted by the CDC, at a minimum the potential client must be informed of the worker's HIV, HBV, or HCV status if the therapist is to engage in high-risk activity such as vaginal examination of the pelvic floor muscles, debridement, or other wound care.[25]

HIV and Rehabilitative Therapy

From a rehabilitation point of view, HIV is considered a chronic illness on a continuum (i.e., from being asymptomatic to exhibiting mild to severe symptoms) rather than as a terminal illness. The individual with HIV disease may demonstrate clinical manifestations of overlapping pathologic processes and HIV-related physical disabilities that need appropriate rehabilitation intervention. For example, lesions of the CNS can be the site of more than one opportunistic disease process simultaneously[56] or the individual may experience a stroke in addition to an already existing peripheral neuropathy or other neuromusculoskeletal manifestations. The therapist may be involved in wound intervention when integumentary impairment is caused by HIV opportunistic infections while also providing intervention to relieve problems associated with rheumatologic dysfunctions.[142]

In addition to physical fitness and strength training, therapists must look at quality of life (QOL) issues; work simplification; and activities of daily living (ADLs), including community management skills such as access to transportation, socialization opportunities, shopping, banking, ability to negotiate health care,

and insurance systems[56]; and participation in church, synagogue, or other spiritual network. Home programs must be simple and easily incorporated into ADLs. Often individuals with AIDS are overwhelmed by the disease process, the complicated treatment, the multiple health care appointments, and scheduling to manage all of these tasks. Adding an exercise program may result in frustration and noncompliance unless the person can see a clear benefit and way to manage yet another aspect of the treatment program.

For the client with neurologic involvement rehabilitative therapy can help the person regain lost function and recover some skills. These clients seem to respond well to an eclectic blend of rehabilitation strategies such as for stroke or head-injured treatment programs. Proprioceptive neuromuscular facilitation (PNF) and Bobath techniques may be more beneficial for the lower-level functioning clients.[81] The therapist must be prepared for seizures, which may occur as a result of nervous system involvement, sometimes for the first time during a therapy session. Cognitive deficits in attention, concentration, and memory require consistency, structure, and environmental cures to minimize confusion.[56]

Quickly progressive peripheral neuropathy is one of the most common types of pain experienced by people with HIV, sometimes as a result of drugs used to treat HIV or possibly related to HIV-induced immune complexes.[57] The use of conventional transcutaneous electrical nerve stimulation (TENS) tends to exacerbate peripheral pain in HIV-related peripheral neuropathies. The alternate use of electroacupuncture has been reported to reduce pain, improve functional status, and increase perceived strength. Discussion of the possible mechanisms for these effects is available.[57]

The presence of peripheral neuropathies may also signal nutritional deficiencies requiring nutritional counseling. This is especially true for the client who has the wasting syndrome that often accompanies HIV infection and AIDS. The body may begin to draw from its own stores of fat, affecting the myelin sheaths of nerves, which are protected by fat. Without proper nutrition, therapy involving balance training, extremity strengthening and stretching, and motor skills, although extremely important, may be limited in benefit. Other guidelines for management of the lower extremity complications, balance, and postural derangements associated with distal symmetrical polyneuropathy (DSP) are available.[58,146]

For individuals with painful myopathy in the large muscle groups, progressive resistance training with weights or elastic band/tubing to strengthen specific muscles may be beneficial. Muscle spasms accompanying myopathy may respond well to gentle but consistent stretching exercises. Postexercise soreness is common in the AIDS group experiencing muscle pain. A longer rest period between exercises may be necessary.

Improper body mechanics, poor postural alignment, and biomechanical changes may occur in the person who has developed muscle weakness and fatigue following progression of the disease process, malnutrition, or the wasting syndrome. Again, postural awareness, stretching and strengthening of specific muscles, and attention to nutrition may be part of the treatment plan.

Cardiopulmonary complications (see Table 6-4) in advanced stages of AIDS contribute to morbidity and mortality. Oxygen transport mechanisms can be adversely affected. Muscle and joint mobilization techniques and breathing exercises are essential for the person who has been immobilized for any length of time as a result of respiratory or other disease involvement.

Continued

The rib cage is one area where normal respiratory and accessory movements are essential for adequate lung ventilation, energy conservation, correct posture, and balance reactions.

For the client with malignancy, guidelines for the management/treatment intervention of the oncologic client are discussed in Chapter 8 (see also the section on Kaposi's Sarcoma in Chapter 9).

Exercise and HIV/AIDS

Unlike other infections, HIV directly affects the immune system. Since exercise has clinically significant effects on immune responsiveness (see the section on Exercise Immunology in this chapter), a potential exists to alter the natural history of HIV infection in a beneficial manner through the use of exercise. A growing number of studies are now addressing the issue of the relationship between exercise and HIV infection. The results are summarized here.

Exercise is considered safe for people with HIV and an important way to increase the CD4 cells at earlier stages of the disease, possibly delaying symptoms while increasing muscle strength and size. During stage I (asymptomatic HIV) metabolic parameters are within normal limits with no limitations placed on the individual. During stages II and III, functional capacity is reduced, requiring more individualized exercise prescription and lower intensities.[93]

Exercise may provide pain relief; improve appetite, reduction of muscle atrophy, and regular bowel activity; and improve function; it can also enhance immune function by increasing T helper/inducer (CD4) cells and the inducer subset, which activate suppressor/cytotoxic (CD8) cells. Exercise can improve overall pulmonary function to help prevent pneumonia and other respiratory infections. Given the psychosocial influences on disease progression and the known effect of exercise on mood, QOL, and the immune system, exercise can benefit the psychoneuroimmunology interactions by reducing stress (see the section on Stress, Coping, and Adaptation in Chapter 2 and Theory of Psychoneuroimmunology in Chapter 1).

Exercise training at 70% to 80% of maximal heart rate is recommended to achieve the benefits listed. Higher intensities increase strength and aerobic fitness but have not been shown to change total lymphocyte cell counts or ratios.[134] A rate of perceived exertion (RPE) no greater than 14 is recommended[93] (see Table 11-13); other recommendations established by the American College of Sports Medicine (ACSM) are available for all three stages of HIV disease.

Monitoring vital signs (see Appendix B) and laboratory values (see Chapter 39) is an important part of determining exercise intensities especially in the presence of co-morbidities such as anemia, vitamin deficiency, wasting syndrome, or opportunistic infections. Proper caloric intake is also important in setting the standard for each type of exercise to meet energy expenditure required for the activity. Seeking the advice of a nutritionist is recommended.[56]

The effects of exercise demands on a high-level athlete with HIV in competition on levels of psychologic stress and immune function remain unclear. Potential adverse effects of the stresses of competition include increased upper respiratory infections in marathon runners.[115] Exercise recommendations for athletes with HIV are summarized in Box 6-4.

Exercise programs to increase strength and body mass are particularly relevant to HIV because wasting is one of the most devastating aspects of this infection. In contrast to people experiencing simple starvation who lose adipose tissue but initially retain lean body mass, people with HIV infection lose lean body mass too. Exercise training, including strength training, may have the potential to (possibly only temporarily) arrest and/or reverse the wasting effects. In the nonacute stage, improved muscle function and increased body dimensions and mass can occur following progressive resistive exercises three times per week for 6 weeks.[46,155]

The role of exercise in the treatment of lipodystrophy syndrome is important[15] and has been shown to have potential in normalizing insulin resistance, which is under investigation; to be effective in managing metabolic abnormalities without causing further side effects[33]; and to reduce trunk fat mass with fat redistribution.[138] Likewise, exercise has beneficial effects for those with the AIDS-related wasting syndrome. In either condition, the goal is to exercise enough to gain muscle and build lean body mass without causing degeneration with acidosis. Progressive resistive exercise can increase lean body mass significantly without increasing circulating HIV RNA concentrations.[136,137] ∎

BOX 6-4

Exercise Recommendations for Athletes with Human Immunodeficiency Virus* Disease

Before initiating any exercise program, the athlete must have a complete physical examination.

A graded exercise test may be a necessary part of the evaluation to determine how much exercise the person can tolerate and what baseline of exercise should be established to start.

Exercise is a safe and beneficial activity for the HIV-infected person.

For healthy individuals who are asymptomatic of HIV, unrestricted exercise activity and competition are acceptable; overtraining should be avoided.

For people with more advanced HIV infection, who are experiencing mild to moderate symptoms, athletic competition is not considered advisable given the stress of competition and its effect on the immune system; training may continue without competition.

Symptomatic people should avoid exhaustive exercise but may be able to continue exercise training under close supervision.

Exercise training programs may need to be modified to include mild exercise and energy conservation techniques for anyone during the acute stage of an opportunistic infection.

For the noncompetitive person, exercise should begin while healthy with strategies to help maintain an exercise program throughout the course of the illness.

People with HIV, through the use of exercise, can play an important role in the management of their illness while improving quality of life.

Exercise has the potential to offer subtle and effective behavioral therapeutic benefits regardless of ethnicity, exposure category, or gender.

*General principles included here apply to all individuals with HIV, including those who are not athletes or competitive in athletics or sports.
Modified from Calabrese LH, LaPerrierre A: Human immunodeficiency virus infection, exercise, and athletics, *Sports Med* 15:6, 1993.

◆ Chronic Fatigue and Immune Dysfunction Syndrome

Overview.   Chronic fatigue and immune dysfunction syndrome (CFIDS); chronic fatigue syndrome (CFS); chronic Epstein-Barr virus (CEBV); myalgic encephalomyelitis; neuromyasthenia; and the "yuppie-flu" all denote a highly publicized but not new illness. The name *chronic fatigue syndrome* indicates that this illness is not a single disease but the result of a combination of factors and is actually a subset of *chronic fatigue*, a broader category defined as unexplained fatigue of greater than or equal to 6 months' duration. This distinction is made to facilitate epidemiologic studies of populations with prolonged fatigue and chronic fatigue.

Incidence and Risk Factors.   From 1989 to 1993, the CDC used a physician-based surveillance team in four cities to determine the prevalence, incidence, course, and impact of this illness, but the resulting estimates were considered underestimates and could not be generalized to the U.S. population since the study did not randomly select its sites. Since that time, other studies have determined that the incidence among the general population appears to be approximately 200 per 100,000; this is considerably higher than the previously estimated 8 to 10 cases per 100,000. It is estimated that as many as a half million people in the United States have a CFS-like condition.[23]

Previously, it was thought that most people with CFS were middle-class, white women with an average age onset of 30 years, but the data only included people who were under a physician's care. Evidence exists now that CFS affects all ethnic groups and both genders fairly equally. Distribution by age has not been determined, but all age groups can be affected, perhaps with some symptom pattern variation in younger age groups.[23]

Etiologic Factors and Pathogenesis.   The etiologic factors and pathogenesis of CFS are still largely unresolved, although it is likely the interaction of multicausal variables, including biologic, social, behavioral, and psychologic factors. Considerable evidence exists of an underlying biologic process in most people who meet the CDC case definition of CFS.[84]

Although at this time the CDC reports no evidence to support the view that CFS is an infectious (contagious) disease[23] researchers continue to hypothesize the presence of a chronic infection that leads to increased immune activity over a long period with the production of various cytokines as the cause of the symptoms.[84] Research findings of immunologic dysfunction and neuroendocrine changes suggest the possible dysregulation of interactions between the nervous system and the immune system. It is clear that certain components of the immune system behave abnormally. IL-2 and interferon-γ produced in the presence of infectious processes or malignancy may not be made in normal amounts in people with CFS.

Other current hypotheses include oxidative stress and lipid peroxidation,[101] chronic immune activation in the brain,[84] overtraining in athletes,[149] and altered glucocorticoid regulation of the immune response secondary to hypothalamic-pituitary-adrenal (HPA)-axis dysfunction[161] to name just a few.

Clinical Manifestations.   At illness onset, the most commonly reported CFS symptoms are sore throat, fever, muscle pain, and muscle weakness. As the illness progresses, muscle pain and forgetfulness increase along with prolonged (lasting more than 6 months), often overwhelming fatigue that is exacerbated by minimal physical activity.

To aid the identification of this disease, the CDC has developed a working case definition with two criteria to distinguish CFS from other forms of fatigue (Box 6-5). The symptoms must have persisted or recurred during 6 or more consecutive months of illness and must not have predated the fatigue. Additionally, conditions that exclude a diagnosis of CFS and those that do not exclude a diagnosis of CFS are available.[23]

The degree of severity varies greatly; some people experience moderate symptoms, whereas others are completely bedridden. The pattern of symptoms (frequency and duration) varies from individual to individual. Some people are ill all the time, whereas others are well, except for a single fatigue episode every several weeks. Accurately predicting exacerbations and remissions is not possible, and the actual number of people who recover is unknown.

Neurally mediated hypotension (NMH) caused by disturbances in the autonomic regulation of blood pressure and pulse is common in people with CFS. This condition is characterized by lowered blood pressure and heart rate accompanied by lightheadedness, visual dimming, or slow response to verbal stimuli. Many people with NMH experience lightheadedness or worsening fatigue as they stand for prolonged periods or when in warm places (e.g., hot shower, sauna, indoor pool environment).

Medical Management

Diagnosis.   No single test confirms the presence of CFS; physicians must rely on the client's history and the CDC criteria (see Box 6-5). The presence of antibodies to Epstein-Barr virus (EBV), another herpes virus, does not necessarily mean the person has CFS, although some people with CFS do,

---

BOX	6-5

CDC Revised Case Definition: Chronic Fatigue Syndrome

1. Clinically evaluated, unexplained persistent or relapsing chronic fatigue that is any of the following:
   - New or definite onset (i.e., not lifelong)
   - Not the result of ongoing exertion
   - Not substantially alleviated by rest
   - Results in substantial reduction in previous levels of occupational, educational, social, or personal activities
2. The concurrent occurrence of four or more of the following symptoms:
   - Substantial impairment in short-term memory or concentration
   - Sore throat
   - Tender lymph nodes
   - Muscle pain
   - Multiple arthralgias without swelling or redness
   - Headaches of a new type, pattern, or severity
   - Unrefreshing sleep
   - Postexertional malaise lasting more than 24 hours

Centers for Disease Control and Prevention: Chronic fatigue syndrome: the revised case definition, 2001. Available at http://www.cdc.gov.

in fact, have high levels of EBV antibodies. Rising levels of antibodies to EBV were once thought to cause CFS but is now considered a result of this disease. Others with the syndrome have normal or no antibodies to the virus.

A new biologic marker, 37 kDa 2-5A (a binding protein), found in extracts of peripheral blood mononuclear cells has been discovered in people with CFS and is not evident in people with other fatiguing conditions such as fibromyalgia or depression. Whether this marker is present in all people with CFS remains to be determined.[40]

Treatment. Likewise, no treatment is known to cure CFS. A large variety of prescription medications may be used in the pharmacologic therapy directed toward the relief of specific symptoms experienced by each individual. Experimental drugs include ampligen, a synthetic nucleic acid product that stimulates the production of interferons; dehydroepiandrosterone (DHEA) to improve symptoms; gamma globulin (antibody molecules against common infectious agents); and dietary supplements and herbal preparation. In some people, avoidance of environmental irritants and certain foods may help relieve symptoms.

Prognosis. The outcome of this illness varies from person to person but approximately one third of all adults affected improve significantly within 5 years and nearly half improve within 10 years. However, "recovered" individuals may continue to have intermittent symptoms, although only a small proportion of people affected remain debilitated for more than 5 years.

Special Implications for the Therapist 6-4

CHRONIC FATIGUE SYNDROME

Preferred Practice Patterns
4B: Impaired Posture (fatigue-related)
4D: Impaired Joint Mobility, Motor Function, Muscle Performance, and Range of Motion Associated With Connective Tissue Dysfunction
5A: Primary Prevention/Risk Reduction for Loss of Balance and Falling (neurogenic hypotension)
6B: Impaired Aerobic Capacity/Endurance Associated With Deconditioning

The client with CFS is treated following guidelines and protocols for autoimmune disorders such as fibromyalgia (see the section on Fibromyalgia in this chapter). Pacing; energy conservation (see Box 8-2); physiologic quieting; stress management; and balancing life activities are extremely helpful in preventing worsening of fatigue and maintaining an even flow of energy from day to day. Support groups may be beneficial in providing emotional and psychologic support and in helping the individual keep up with latest research results and progress in medical intervention.

Exercise and Chronic Fatigue Syndrome
Carefully controlled and graded exercise is the center of effective intervention for CFS.[54,55,126] Many affected individuals fear a relapse and avoid physical activity and exercise but decondi-

tioning and muscle atrophy increases fatigue and makes other symptoms even worse. The physical therapist can be very instrumental in providing a prescriptive program of regular, moderate exercise to avoid deconditioning while advising against overexertion during periods of remission. During the acute onset or during flareups people with CFS are unable to sustain physical activity or exercise. Beginning with low-level, intermittent physical activity throughout the day to accumulate 30 minutes of exercise has been shown to be effective without exacerbating symptoms.[30]

Always assess for conditioning before initiating even a simple exercise program with anyone who has had CFS longer than 6 months. Although abnormal lung function or low concentration of oxygen with accompanying dyspnea or shortness of breath is not a clinical feature of this disease, anyone who is severely deconditioned and then tries to do even light exercise may experience dyspnea. People with CFS may also have a significantly reduced exercise capacity. Reaching age-predicted target heart rates may be limited by autonomic disturbances.[37] It may be better to begin a strengthening program before challenging the cardiovascular system.

The therapist must evaluate for altered breathing patterns, components of poor posture, and inefficient or biomechanically faulty movement patterns contributing to pain. Addressing these areas is an important part of the rehabilitation process. Stretching, strengthening, and cardiovascular training are essential aspects of therapy. Like people with fibromyalgia, those diagnosed with CFS must progress slowly and avoid overexertion since they often do not have the internal mechanism to alert them to stop an activity.

Soft tissue and joint mobilization combined with stretching are important components of intervention, especially in the presence of postural components or faulty mechanics. Prolonged inactivity, rest in poorly supported positions for long periods, and assuming postures dictated by pain can contribute to muscles shortening (see the sections on Modalities and Fibromyalgia in this chapter).

Over time, some individuals can be progressed to graded aerobic exercise therapy (some can begin at this level depending on the individual clinical presentation). Continuous exercise must be started at a short duration appropriate to the client's baseline ability. A more specific description of how to deliver a graded exercise therapy program to people with CFS is available.[53] This has been shown to be significantly more effective than just stretching and relaxation exercises.[54,168]

Monitoring Vital Signs
Assessment of vital signs in adults with CFS may demonstrate very large fluctuations in pulse rate and blood pressure, which are not consistent with the person's position or movement. Whereas the blood pressure and pulse rate normally show a slight increase as a physiologic response to a change in position from sitting to standing, orthostatic hypotension is marked in the CFS population. Vital signs may stay the same or even decrease, resulting in dizziness, lightheadedness, or loss of balance. The symptoms may result in decreased self-confidence in the ability to pursue activities.

During the initiation of an exercise program, it is advised to monitor blood pressure; RPE (see Table 11-13); heart rate; and respiratory rate for any signs of physiologic distress. Although the RPE may not change during the exercise session, the individual may perceive fatigue as worse after initiating exercise.

> However, if this increase in fatigue does not exceed 1 unit on a scale from 1 to 5 from the baseline level established before exercise, symptom exacerbation following exercise can potentially be avoided.[30] ■

HYPERSENSITIVITY DISORDERS

An exaggerated or inappropriate immune response may lead to various hypersensitivity disorders. Such disorders are classified as types I, II, III, or IV, although some overlap exists (Table 6-5). Overreaction to a substance, or hypersensitivity, is often referred to as an *allergic response* and although the term *allergy* is widely used, the term *hypersensitivity* is more appropriate. Hypersensitivity designates an increased immune response to the presence of an antigen (referred to as an *allergen*) that results in tissue destruction. The damage and suffering come predominantly from the immune response itself, rather than from the substances that provoke it.

The several types of hypersensitivity reactions include immediate, late-phase, and delayed, based on the rapidity of the immune response. *Immediate hypersensitivity reactions* usually occur within minutes of exposure to an allergen. If the skin is affected, blood vessels dilate and fluid accumulates, causing redness and swelling. In the eyes and nose, increased fluid and mucous secretions cause tearing and a runny nose. *Late phase* inflammation and symptoms persist for hours to day after the allergens are removed and can cause cumulative damage (e.g., progressive lung disease) if they persist. *Delayed hypersensitivity reaction* occurs after sensitization to certain drugs or chemicals (e.g., penicillin, poison ivy). These reactions often take several days to cause symptoms.

◆ Type I Hypersensitivity (Immediate Hypersensitivity, Allergic Disorders, Anaphylaxis)

Type I hypersensitivity reactions include hay fever, allergic rhinitis, urticaria, extrinsic asthma, and anaphylactic shock. In this type of immediate hypersensitivity response, IgE, instead of IgG, is produced in response to a pathogen (allergen). The term *atopy* is often used to describe IgE-mediated diseases. People with atopy have a hereditary predisposition to produce IgE antibodies against common environmental allergens* and have one or more atopic diseases.

IgE resides on mast cells in connective tissue, especially the upper respiratory tract, GI tract, and dermis. When IgE meets the pathogen again, an immediate response occurs with histamine release, along with other inflammatory mediators (e.g., chemotactic factors, prostaglandins, and leukotrienes) that enhance and prolong the response initiated by histamine.

If this response becomes systemic, widespread release of histamine (rather than just local tissue response) results in systemic vasodilation, bronchospasm, and increased mucous secretion, and edema referred to as *anaphylaxis*. Classic associated signs and symptoms are wheezing, hypotension, swelling, urticaria, and rhinorrhea (clear, runny nose often accompanied by sneezing). Anaphylaxis is a life-threatening emergency and requires immediate intervention with injected epinephrine to restore blood pressure, strengthen the heartbeat, and open the airways. Bee stings remain the number one cause of anaphylaxis; other triggers include penicillin, foods, animal dander, children, semen, and latex.

Marked increase in the prevalence of atopic disease has occurred in the United States during the last two decades, indicating the importance of environmental influences. The mechanisms for this action are outlined in greater detail elsewhere.[80]

◆ Type II Hypersensitivity (Cytotoxic Reactions to Self-Antigens)

When the body's own tissue is recognized as foreign or nonself, activation of complement occurs with subsequent agglutination (clumping together) and phagocytosis of the identified pathogens. This means the cellular membrane of normal tissues (e.g., red blood cells [RBCs], leukocytes, and platelets) is disrupted and ultimately destroyed. Self-antigen disorders include blood transfusion reactions, hemolytic disease of the newborn, autoimmune hemolytic anemia, and myasthenia gravis.

A second type of hypersensitivity response occurs when a cross-reaction from exogenous pathogens with endogenous body tissues as occurs in rheumatic fever. For example, group A hemolytic streptococci (the exogenous pathogen) are attacked by the immune system but the body also misinterprets the mitral valve (endogenous body tissue) as a foreign microorganism (i.e., as streptococcus) and attacks normal, healthy tissue in the same way it attempts to destroy the true pathogenic microorganisms. Another example of this type of cross-reaction is an exogenous virus causing the immune system to attack the peripheral nervous system as nonself, as occurs in Guillain-Barré acute syndrome.

◆ Type III Hypersensitivity (Immune Complex Disease)

Normally, excessive circulating antigen-antibody complexes called *immune complexes* are effectively cleared by the reticuloendothelial system. When circulating immune complexes (antigen-antibody complexes) successfully deposit in tissues around small blood vessels, they activate the complement cascade and cause acute inflammation and local tissue injury. The subsequent vasculitis most commonly affects the skin, causing urticaria (wheals); joints, causing synovitis, as in rheumatoid arthritis; kidneys, causing nephritis; pleura, causing pleuritis; and pericardium, causing pericarditis.

Systemic lupus erythematosus (SLE) is the classic picture of vasculitis, occurring in various organ systems. The antigen is the individual's own nucleus of cells; antinuclear antibodies (ANAs) are made, which in turn form a complex with the antigen and are deposited in the skin, joints, and kidneys, causing acute immune injury. Other examples of this hypersensitivity reaction occur in association with infections such as hepatitis B and bacterial endocarditis, malignancies, or after drug or serum therapy.

◆ Type IV Hypersensitivity (Cell-Mediated Immunity)

Type IV is a delayed hypersensitivity response such as the reaction that occurs in contact dermatitis after sensitization to an allergen (commonly a cosmetic, adhesive, topical medication, or plant toxin such as poison ivy); latex sensitivity; or

---

*Allergens are a special class of antigens that cause an allergic response. These normally harmless substances are inhaled (e.g., mold spores, animal dander, dust mites, grasses, weeds); eaten (e.g., nuts, fruits, shellfish, eggs); or injected (e.g., venom from fire ants, wasps, bees, hornets), or they come in contact with the skin or mucous membranes (e.g., plants, cosmetics, metals, drugs, dyes, latex).

| TABLE | 6-5 |

Clinical Manifestations of Hypersensitivity Disorders

TYPE I	TYPE II	TYPE III	TYPE IV
Varies according to the allergies present	*General:* malaise, weakness	Headache	Fever
Classic symptoms	*Dermal:* hives, erythema	Back (flank) pain	Arthralgias
• Wheezing	*Respiratory:* sneezing, rhinorrhea, dyspnea	Chest pain similar to angina	Lymphadenopathy
• Hypotension	*Upper airway:* hoarseness, stridor; tongue and pharyngeal edema	Nausea and vomiting	Urticaria
• Swelling	*Lower airway:* dyspnea, bronchospasm, asthma (air trapping), chest tightness, wheezing	Tachycardia	Anemia
• Urticaria	*Gastrointestinal:* increased peristalsis, vomiting, dysphagia, nausea, abdominal cramps, diarrhea	Hypotension	
• Rhinorrhea	*Cardiovascular:* tachycardia, palpitations, hypotension, cardiac arrest	Hematuria	
Anaphylaxis	*Central nervous system:* anxiety, seizures	Urticaria	

the response to a tuberculin skin test present 48 to 72 hours after the skin test. In this type of reaction, the antigen is processed by macrophages and presented to T cells. The sensitized T cells then release lymphokines, which recruit other lymphocytes, monocytes, macrophages, and PMNs. Graft-versus-host disease (GVHD) and transplant rejection are also examples of type IV reactions (see Chapter 20).

Special Implications for the Therapist   6-5

HYPERSENSITIVITY DISORDERS

Preferred Practice Pattern
7A: Primary Prevention/Risk Reduction for Integumentary Disorders

Immediate action is required for any client experiencing a type I hypersensitivity reaction or anaphylaxis. When a severe reaction occurs, the health care professional must call for emergency assistance.

Type IV reactions may occur in response to lanolin added to lotions, ultrasound gels, or other preparations used in massage or soft tissue mobilization, requiring careful observation of all people for delayed skin reactions to any of these substances. With the first exposure, no reaction necessarily occurs, but antigens are formed and on subsequent exposures, hypersensitivity reactions are triggered. Anyone with known hypersensitivity should have a small area of skin tested before use of large amounts of topical agents in the therapy setting. Careful observation throughout treatment is recommended. ∎

AUTOIMMUNE DISEASES

Definition and Overview.   Autoimmune diseases fall into a category of conditions in which the cause involves immune mechanisms directed against self-antigens. More specifically, the body fails to distinguish self from nonself, causing the im-

mune system to direct immune responses against normal (self) tissue and become self-destructive. More than 56 autoimmune diseases have been identified, affecting everything from skin and joints to vital organs. Autoimmune diseases can be viewed as a spectrum of disorders, some of which are systemic and others of which involve a single organ. A portion of the known diseases most likely to be seen in a rehabilitation setting is listed in Table 6-6.

At one end of the continuum are organ-specific diseases, in which localized tissue damage occurs, resulting from the presence of specific autoantibodies. An example is Hashimoto's disease of the thyroid, characterized by a specific lesion in the thyroid gland with production of antibodies with absolute specificity for certain thyroid constituents.

In the middle of the continuum are disorders in which the lesion tends to be localized in one organ, but the antibodies are not organ specific. An example is primary biliary cirrhosis, in which inflammatory cell infiltration of the small bile ductule occurs, but the serum antibodies are not specific to liver cells.

At the other end of the spectrum are non–organ-specific diseases, in which lesions and antibodies are widespread throughout the body and not limited to one target organ. SLE is an example of this type of autoimmune disease. Identification of ANAs that attack the nucleic acids (DNA and RNA) and other components of the body's own tissues established SLE as an autoimmune disease.

In this book, with the few exceptions included in this chapter (e.g., fibromyalgia, CFS, SLE), autoimmune disorders are discussed individually in the most appropriate chapter. For example, Reiter's syndrome, rheumatoid arthritis, and Sjögren's syndrome are discussed in Chapter 26. Polymyositis, dermatomyositis, and progressive systemic sclerosis are discussed in Chapter 9. Giant cell arteritis is discussed in Chapter 11, sarcoidosis in Chapter 14, and so on. More information is available on autoimmune-related diseases.[3]

Etiologic and Risk Factors.   Although the autoimmune disorders are regarded as acquired diseases, their causes often cannot be determined. Autoimmunity is believed to result from a combination of factors, including genetic; hormonal

TABLE	6-6

Autoimmune Disorders

ORGAN-SPECIFIC	SYSTEMIC
Addison's disease	Amyloidosis
Crohn's disease	Ankylosing spondylitis
Chronic active hepatitis	Mixed connective tissue disease
Diabetes mellitus	Multiple sclerosis
Giant cell arteritis	Myasthenia gravis
Hemolytic anemia	Polymyalgia rheumatica
Idiopathic thrombocytopenic purpura	Progressive systemic sclerosis (scleroderma)
Polymyositis/dermatomyositis	Psoriasis (psoriatic arthritis)
Postviral encephalomyelitis	Reiter's syndrome
Primary biliary cirrhosis	Rheumatoid arthritis
Thyroiditis	Sarcoidosis
Graves' disease	Sjögren's syndrome
Hashimoto's disease	Systemic lupus erythematosus
Ulcerative colitis	

(women are affected more often than men by autoimmune diseases); and environmental influences (e.g., exposure to chemicals, other toxins, or sunlight and drugs that may destroy suppressor T cells).

Although no single gene has been identified as responsible for autoimmune diseases, clusters of genes seem to increase susceptibility. In most autoimmune disorders, a known or suspected genetic susceptibility is evident, and certain HLA types show increased risk, such as ankylosing spondylitis with HLA-B27 (see Table 39-17). The influence or hormonal factors is confusing since some autoimmune diseases occur among women in their 20s and 30s when estrogen is high, and others develop after menopause or before puberty when estrogen levels are low. During pregnancy, many women with rheumatoid arthritis or multiple sclerosis (MS) experience complete remission, whereas pregnant women with SLE often experience exacerbations.

Other factors implicated in the development of immunologic abnormalities resulting in autoimmune disorders include viruses, stress, cross-reactive antibodies, and various autoimmune diseases occurring in women who have had silicone gel breast implants. This organ-specific autoimmune disease has been associated with musculoskeletal problems (see Chapter 7).

Pathogenesis.   Autoimmune disorders involve disruption of the immunoregulatory mechanism, causing normal cell-mediated and humoral immune responses to turn self-destructive, resulting in tissue damage. The exact pathologic mechanisms for this process remain unknown. The importance of the innate immune system in determining whether T cells become activated and functional in autoimmune disorders has been shown.[106] Researchers suspect that more than one part of the immune system must be involved for autoimmune disease to develop. Some autoimmune diseases affect a single organ (e.g., pancreas in type 1 diabetes), whereas others affect a large system or more than one system (e.g., MS). In some cases the autoimmune process overstimulates organ function, as in Graves' disease, in which excess thyroid hormone is produced.

Gene-mapping studies have demonstrated that allergy and autoimmunity must involve not only the recognition of antigen by T cells, but also the very important immunoregulatory effects of cytokines, inhibitory receptors, and survival factors. Linkage analysis of the human genome has revealed candidate loci for susceptibility to MS, type 1 diabetes, SLE, and Crohn's disease. Continued genetic analysis is ongoing to identify the specific genetic link in hopes of finding a more specific treatment.[78]

Although antibodies and T-cell receptors can accurately distinguish between closely related antigens, they sometimes cross-react with apparently unrelated antigens, either because the two antigens happen to share an identical epitope (see Fig. 6-1) or because two different epitopes have similar shapes and charges. Such cross-reactions may be the underlying pathogenesis of some autoimmune diseases.[39]

Many autoimmune diseases are associated with characteristic autoantibodies. In other words, the body begins to manufacture antibodies directed against the body's own cellular components or specific organs. These antibodies are known as *autoantibodies*, in this case, producing autoimmune diseases. For example, SLE is associated with anti-DNA and anti–splicesosomal (Sm) antigen; Sjögren's syndrome is associated with antiribonucleoproteins (SS-A and SS-B); progressive systemic sclerosis is associated with anticentromere and anti–Scl-70 (DNA topoisomerase); psoriasis and psoriatic arthritis are associated with HLA-B13; and mixed connective tissue disease is associated with antiribonucleoprotein without anti-DNA.

Antibodies specific to hormone receptors on the surface of cells have been found and determined to be partially responsible for some conditions. Examples include myasthenia gravis, in which antiacetylcholine receptor antibodies are involved; Graves' disease, in which antibodies against components of thyroid cell membranes, including the receptors for thyroid-stimulating hormone (TSH), are responsible; and certain cases of insulin-resistant diabetes mellitus, in which the antibodies affect insulin receptors on cells. Other diseases involving autoimmune mechanisms include rheumatic fever, rheumatoid arthritis, autoimmune hemolytic anemia, idiopathic thrombocytopenic purpura, and postviral encephalomyelitis.

Clinical Manifestations.   Autoimmune disorders share certain clinical features and differentiation among them is often difficult because of this. Common findings include synovitis, pleuritis, myocarditis, endocarditis, pericarditis, peritonitis, vasculitis, myositis, skin rash, alterations of connective tissues, and nephritis. Constitutional symptoms such as fatigue, malaise, myalgias, and arthralgias are also common.

Medical Management

Diagnosis.   Diagnosis can be difficult because autoimmune diseases are poorly understood, mimic one another, and often consist of vague symptoms like lethargy or migratory joint pain. Laboratory tests may reveal thrombocytopenia, leukopenia, immunoglobulin excesses or deficiencies, ANAs, rheumatoid factor, cryoglobulins, false-positive serologic tests, elevated muscle enzymes, and alterations in serum complement. Coombs' test will be positive when hemolytic anemia is present. Some of the laboratory alterations that occur in autoimmune diseases (e.g., false-positive serologic tests, rheumatoid factor) occur in asymptomatic people. These changes may also be demonstrated in certain asymptomatic relatives of people with connective tissue diseases, in older individuals, those taking certain medications, and people with chronic infectious diseases.

Treatment. Treatment of autoimmune diseases varies with the specific disease. Treatment must maintain a delicate balance between adequate suppression of the autoimmune reaction to avoid continued damage to the body tissues, and maintenance of sufficient functioning of the immune mechanism to protect the person against foreign invaders. In general, autoimmune diseases are treated by the administration of corticosteroids to produce an antiinflammatory effect and salicylates to provide symptomatic relief.

The wealth of new information gleaned from research in the last decade has been used to improve immunization strategies and hopefully will lead to new approaches to the reinduction of immune tolerance. The development of an effective vaccine is under close scrutiny,[78] as is the use of intense immunosuppression (immunoablation), followed by stem cell transplantation for the treatment of autoimmune diseases.

Since autoimmune disease is the result of genetic dysregulation, gene therapy may become a viable alternative in the future. Scientists have been involved in developing new drugs aimed at the mechanism of autoimmunity rather than treating its effects. Based on new information about the function of *Fc* receptors, which bind antibodies that are instructing the immune system in the destructive inflammation characteristic of autoimmune diseases, scientists are looking for blocking compounds to prevent this interaction.

◆ Systemic Lupus Erythematosus

Definition and Overview. Lupus erythematosus, sometimes referred to as *lupus*, is a chronic inflammatory autoimmune disorder that appears in several forms, including *discoid lupus erythematosus (DLE)*, which affects only the skin (usually face, neck, scalp) (see Chapter 9), and *systemic lupus erythematosus (SLE)*, which can affect any organ or system of the body.

The clinical picture of SLE presents on a continuum with different combinations of organ system involvement. The most common of these presentations are latent lupus, drug-induced lupus, antiphospholipid antibody syndrome, and late-stage lupus. *Latent lupus* describes a constellation of features suggestive of SLE but does not qualify as classic SLE (Box 6-6). Many people with latent lupus persist with their clinical presentation of signs and symptoms over many years without ever developing classic SLE.

Drug-induced lupus may be diagnosed in people without prior history suggestive of SLE in whom the clinical and serologic manifestations of SLE develop while the person is taking a drug (most often hydralazine used to treat hypertension or procainamide used to treat arrhythmia). The symptoms cease when the drug is stopped, with gradual resolution of serologic abnormalities.

Antiphospholipid antibody syndrome describes the association between arterial and venous thrombosis, recurrent fetal loss, and immune thrombocytopenia with a variety of antibodies directed against cellular phospholipid (lipids in cell membranes containing phosphorus) components. This syndrome may be part of the clinical manifestations seen in SLE, or it may occur as a primary form without other clinical features of lupus.

BOX 6-6

American Rheumatism Association Diagnostic Criteria for Systemic Lupus Erythematosus

A person is considered to have SLE if four or more of the following 11 criteria are present, serially or simultaneously, during any interval of observation:

1. Abnormal titer of antinuclear antibodies (ANA)
2. Butterfly (malar) rash
3. Discoid rash
4. Hemolytic anemia, leukopenia, lymphopenia, or thrombocytopenia
5. Neurologic disorder: seizures or psychosis
6. Nonerosive arthritis of two or more peripheral joints characterized by tenderness, swelling, or effusion
7. Oral or nasopharyngeal ulcerations
8. Photosensitivity
9. Pleuritis or pericarditis
10. Positive lupus erythematosus cell preparation, anti-DNA, or anti-Sm test or chronic false-positive serologic test for syphilis
11. Renal disorder: profuse proteinuria (>0.5 g/day) or excessive cellular casts in urine

---

Late-state lupus is defined as chronic disease duration of greater than 5 years. In such cases, morbidity and mortality are affected by long-term complications of SLE that result either from the disease itself or as a consequence of its therapy. These late complications may include end-stage renal disease, atherosclerosis, pulmonary emboli, and avascular necrosis. In late-stage lupus, when no evidence of active disease exists and the client is on low-dose or no corticosteroids, cognitive disabilities are a common manifestation.

Incidence. SLE is primarily a disease of young women; it is rarely found in older people. Disease onset may occur from infancy to advanced age, but its peak incidence occurs between the ages of 15 and 40; women are affected 10 to 15 times more often than men. The female-to-male ratio is less dramatic (2:1) in SLE with onset in childhood or older age. The dramatic age and gender relationship in SLE has led researchers to investigate the importance of the hormonal influence in the pathogenesis. SLE occurs worldwide but is most prevalent among blacks and some Asian and Native American groups; at least 1.4 million Americans have been diagnosed with SLE.

Etiologic and Risk Factors. The cause of SLE remains unknown, but evidence points to interrelated immunologic, environmental, hormonal, and genetic factors. Whether SLE represents a single pathologic entity with variable expression or a group of related conditions remains unknown. Immune dysregulation in the form of autoimmunity is thought to be the prime causative mechanism. SLE shows a strong familial link with a much higher frequency among first-degree relatives. Evidence for genetic susceptibility is present and linkage studies in conjunction with genome scans may delineate this more specifically in the future.[172]

Genetically determined immune abnormalities may be triggered by both exogenous and endogenous factors. Although the predisposition to disease is hereditary, it is likely to involve different sets of genes in different individuals. As the human genome becomes more extensively mapped, a susceptibility gene may be found, although it remains possible that the differences in disease course among ethnic groups relates solely to their environment and other social factors.

Other factors predisposing to SLE may include physical or mental stress, which can provoke neuroendocrine changes affecting immune cell function; streptococcal or viral infections; exposure to sunlight or ultraviolet light, which can cause inflammation and tissue damage; immunization; pregnancy*; and abnormal estrogen metabolism.† The role of EBV as a possible risk factor for SLE remains under investigation with conflicting results.[71,79] SLE may also be triggered or aggravated by treatment with certain drugs (e.g., hydralazine, anticonvulsants, penicillins, sulfa drugs, and oral contraceptives), which could modify both cellular responsiveness and immunogenicity of self-antigens.

Pathogenesis.   The central immunologic disturbance in SLE is autoantibody production. The body produces antibodies (e.g., ANAs) against its own cells. Deposition of the formed antigen-antibody complexes at various tissue sites can suppress the body's normal immunity and damage tissues. In fact, one significant feature of SLE is the ability to produce antibodies against many different tissue components such as RBCs, neutrophils, platelets, lymphocytes, or almost any organ or tissue in the body. This wide range of antigenic targets has resulted in SLE being classified as a disease of generalized autoimmunity. Given the clinical diversity of SLE, the disease may be mediated by more than one autoantibody system and several immunopathogenic mechanisms..

Specific pathologic findings are organ-dependent; for example, repeat biopsies of the kidney show inflammation, cellular proliferation, basement membrane abnormalities, and immune complex deposition comprised of IgM, IgG, and IgA. Skin lesions demonstrate inflammation and degeneration at the dermal-epidermal junction with the basal layer being the primary site of injury. Other organ systems affected by SLE are usually studied only at autopsy. Although these tissues may show nonspecific inflammation or vessel abnormalities, pathologic findings are sometimes minimal, suggesting a mechanism other than inflammation as the cause of organ damage or dysfunction.

Clinical Manifestations.   Generally, SLE is more severe than discoid lupus, and no two people with systemic lupus will have identical symptoms. For some people, only the skin and joints will be involved. For others, joints, lungs, kidneys, blood, or other organs, and/or tissues may be affected.

Musculoskeletal.   Arthralgias and arthritis constitute the most common presenting manifestations of SLE, but the onset of SLE may be acute or insidious and may produce no characteristic clinical pattern. Other early symptoms may include fever, weight loss, malaise, and fatigue. Acute arthritis can involve any joint but typically affects the small joints of the hands, wrists, and knees. It may be migratory or chronic; most cases are symmetrical, but asymmetrical polyarthritis is not uncommon. Unlike rheumatoid arthritis, the arthritis of SLE is not usually erosive or destructive of bone, and symptoms are not usually severe enough to cause joint deformities, but pain can cause temporary functional impairment. When deformities do occur, ulnar deviation, swan-neck deformity, or fixed subluxations of the fingers often occur as well. Tenosynovitis and tendon ruptures may occur.

Cutaneous and Membranous Lesions.   The skin rash occurs most commonly in areas exposed to sunlight (ultraviolet rays) and may be exacerbated by the use of cosmetic products containing alpha hydroxy acids. The classic butterfly rash over the nose and cheeks is common (see Fig. 9-17). Discoid lesions associated with DLE are raised, red, scaling plaques with follicular plugging and central atrophy (see Fig. 9-16). This raised edging and sunken center gives them a coin-like appearance (see Chapter 9).

Vasculitis (inflammation of cutaneous blood vessels) involving small- and medium-size vessels may cause other skin lesions, including infarctive lesions of the digits (see Fig. 26-12), splinter hemorrhages, necrotic leg ulcers, or digital gangrene. Raynaud's phenomenon occurs in about 20% of people. Diffuse or patchy alopecia (hair loss) may be temporary with hair regrowth once the disease is under control. However, permanent hair loss can occur from the extensive scarring of discoid lesions. Painless ulcers of the mucous membranes are common involving the mouth, vagina, and nasal septum.

Cardiopulmonary System.   Signs of cardiopulmonary abnormalities may develop such as pleuritis, pericarditis, and dyspnea. Myocarditis, endocarditis, tachycardia, and pneumonitis (acute or chronic) may also occur. Pulmonary hypertension and congestive heart failure are less common and usually secondary to a combination of factors. Anyone with SLE with the antiphospholipid antibody syndrome is at a high risk of thrombosis. (See the section on Collagen-Vascular Disease in Chapter 11.)

Central Nervous System.   A significant number of people with SLE will have CNS involvement at some point in their illness, sometimes referred to as *neuropsychiatric manifestations*. Clinical manifestations may be related to specific autoantibodies that react with nervous system antigens and/ or cytokine-mediated brain inflammation and include headaches, irritability, and depression (most commonly). Emotional instability, psychosis, seizures, cerebrovascular accidents, cranial neuropathy, peripheral neuropathy, and organic brain syndrome can also occur. Return to the previous level of intellectual function may follow remission of the neuropsychiatric flare, or permanent cognitive impairment may occur.

The pattern of cognitive dysfunction is diverse, intensity can vary within the same person, and can be affected by mood.[41] The person may have difficulties with verbal memory,

---

*Whether pregnancy induces lupus flareups has not been established; existing data suggest both that it does and does not. More studies are needed to further determine the effects of pregnancy on this condition.

†A higher incidence of SLE exacerbation occurs among women taking even low-dose estrogen contraceptives. Since an increased risk of thrombosis is possible in young women with SLE, estrogen-containing contraceptives are avoided or used at the lowest effective dose. No evidence exists that postmenopausal estrogen replacement therapy is associated with SLE flareups and since women in this age range are at increased risk for coronary artery disease and osteoporosis, estrogen replacement therapy can be taken. For all women with SLE who have been treated with cyclophosphamide, an increased risk of gynecologic malignancy is evident.[122]

attention, language skills (verbal fluency, productivity), and psychomotor speed. Progressive cognitive impairment, sometimes subtle and sometimes obvious, may develop even in the absence of clinically diagnosed episodes of neuropsychiatric disease. People with SLE may or may not have other signs of lupus when they experience neurologic symptoms.

Other Systems. Pathologic changes may also occur in the kidneys where the glomerulus is the usual site of destruction; other renal effects may include hematuria and proteinuria, progressing to kidney failure. Antiphospholipid antibodies are a significant cause of morbidity and mortality in cases of renal involvement as a result of thrombosis and the development of thrombotic microangiopathy.[72]

Anemia from decreased erythrocytes is a common finding with associated amenorrhea (cessation of menstrual flow) among women. Sometimes the spleen and cervical, axillary, and inguinal nodes are enlarged; hepatitis may also develop. Nausea, vomiting, diarrhea, and abdominal pain may occur with GI involvement. All symptoms mentioned in this section can occur at the onset or at any time during the course of lupus. Nearly all people with SLE experience fluctuations in disease activity with exacerbations and remissions.

Medical Management

Diagnosis. Diagnosis of SLE is difficult because SLE often mimics other diseases and the symptoms are often vague, varying greatly from individual to individual. The American Rheumatism Association has issued a list of criteria for classifying SLE to be used primarily for consistency in epidemiologic surveys. Usually, four or more of these signs are present at some time during the course of the disease (see Box 6-6).

In addition to the routine history and physical examination, laboratory findings are an important part of the diagnosis of SLE and subsequent monitoring of clinical disease activity. Specific test procedures and their significance are available.[89] ANA is present in all cases of SLE, but its presence does not make a definitive diagnosis. However, if ANA is absent, SLE is probably not present. Lupus anticoagulant testing and immunologic anti-phospholipid (aPL) establish the presence of antiphospholipid syndrome.

Magnetic resonance imaging (MRI) scans of the head are usually ordered for all people experiencing new episodes of focal neurologic deficits, seizures, altered consciousness, or psychosis. Neuropsychologic assessment may be helpful for identifying subtle, clinically latent sequelae of CNS events such as stroke and in monitoring the response to drug treatment.[41]

Prevention. Preventive measures can reduce the risk of flareups. For photosensitive people, avoidance of (excessive) sun exposure and/or the regular application of sunscreen usually prevents rashes. Regular exercise helps prevent muscle weakness and fatigue. Immunization protects against specific infections. Support groups, counseling, and talking to family members, friends, and health care professionals can help alleviate the effects of stress. Lifestyle choices and personal behavior are very important for people with SLE. These include smoking, excessive consumption of alcohol, too much or too little of prescribed medication, or postponing regular medical checkups.[90]

Treatment. The objectives of medical intervention are to reverse the autoimmune and inflammatory processes and prevent exacerbations and complications. At the present time, pharmacologic interventions are the primary means of accomplishing these goals. Mild symptoms can be managed with NSAIDs to relieve muscle and joint pain while reducing tissue inflammation. Corticosteroid-sparing agents (e.g., methotrexate) used earlier preserve bone and offer protection from premature cardiovascular disease. Anticoagulants for individuals who have antiphospholipid antibody syndrome and coagulopathies will ensure a more favorable outcome.

Antimalarial agents (e.g., chloroquine [Aralen], hydroxychloroquine [Plaquenil]) are useful against the dermatologic, arthritic, and renal symptoms of this disease. Immunomodulating drugs (e.g., azathioprine [Imuran], cyclophosphamide [Cytoxan]) are immunosuppressive drugs used to suppress inflammation and subsequently, the immune system. These are used only with active disease, especially with severe kidney involvement. Corticosteroids and cytotoxic drugs are given in more severe disease that has not responded to these other types of drug therapy.

Treatment in the future may be more specific as knowledge of genes that participate in the predisposition, pathogenesis, pharmacogenetics of, and protection against this disease come to light. Better understanding of the role of sex hormones has allowed trials of weak androgens or prolactin inhibitors. New immunomodulators or immunosuppressants, immune ablation with subsequent stem cell transplantation, and more precise immunoregulation (e.g., tolerance-induction strategies, intervention at the level of T cell co-stimulation) may become standard intervention tools.[16]

Prognosis. The prognosis improves with early detection and intervention that prevents organ damage and improves life expectancy. The overall reduction in the use of large doses of corticosteroids over the past two decades has significantly reduced morbidity and mortality. People with SLE have an increased prevalence of valvular and atherosclerotic heart disease, apparently because of factors related to the disease itself and to drug therapy necessary in severe cases. Symptomatic large vessel occlusive disease in SLE, occurring several years after the diagnosis of the disease, is associated with a relatively poor short-term outcome.

Prognosis is less favorable for those who develop cardiovascular, renal, or neurologic complications, or severe bacterial infections. High-stress, poor social support, and psychologic distress are modifiable factors associated with health outcomes for people with SLE.[43,165]

Special Implications for the Therapist **6-6**

SYSTEMIC LUPUS ERYTHEMATOSUS

Preferred Practice Patterns
Other patterns may apply depending on individual clinical
manifestation and presentation.
4A: Primary Prevention/Risk Reduction for Skeletal
Demineralization (osteoporosis as a side effect of some
medications; prolonged bedrest)

4B: Impaired Posture (fatigue related)

4D: Impaired Joint Mobility, Motor Function, Muscle Performance, and Range of Motion Associated With Connective Tissue Dysfunction

6B: Impaired Aerobic Capacity/Endurance Associated With Deconditioning

7A: Primary Prevention/Risk Reduction for Integumentary Disorders (vasculitis)

7E: Impaired Integumentary Associated With Skin Involvement Extending Into Fascia, Muscle, or Bone and Scar Formation

Like fibromyalgia, physical and occupational therapy intervention can be important components of the overall treatment plan. Recurrence of disease can be managed with carefully controlled and sometimes restricted activities. After an exacerbation, gradual resumption of activities must be balanced by maximum rest periods, usually 8 to 10 hours of sleep a night and several rest periods during the day. Most of the principles and reference materials outlined in the following section, Fibromyalgia, also apply to SLE. Management of joint involvement follows protocols for rheumatoid arthritis (see Special Implications for the Therapist: Rheumatoid Arthritis, 26-6). Clients with skin lesions should be examined thoroughly at each visit. The therapist can be instrumental in teaching and assisting with skin care and prevention of skin breakdown.

Functional limitations among people with SLE vary according to the type and degree of the disease. Generalized fatigue defined as "the inclination to rest, even though pain and weakness are not limiting factors," is a common problem and can be very debilitating, especially for those individuals with both SLE and fibromyalgia.[2] The therapist can be very instrumental in teaching clients how to pace activities and conserve energy (see Box 8-2), follow a prescriptive exercise plan, avoid excessive bed rest, and protect joints. Excessive bedrest can worsen fatigue, promote muscle disuse and atrophy, and promote osteoporosis. Prescriptive exercise should strengthen the muscles and improve endurance while avoiding undue stress on inflamed joints.

Septic arthritis or osteonecrosis may develop as a complication of SLE or its treatment. Septic arthritis is uncommon in SLE, but it should be suspected when one joint is inflamed out of proportion to the others. People with SLE may develop a drug-related myopathy secondary to corticosteroids or as a complication of antimalarials (see the section on Corticosteroid Myopathy in Chapter 4). Anyone taking corticosteroids or immunosuppressants must be monitored carefully for signs of infection, especially people at heightened risk of infection such as those with renal failure, cardiac valvular abnormalities, or ulcerative skin lesions. (See specific side effects and Special Implications for the Therapist: Corticosteroids in Chapter 4.) The client should contact the physician if a fever or any other new symptoms develop. The therapist can provide osteoporosis prevention and intervention management.

High-dose oral corticosteroid treatment remains the major predisposing cause of avascular necrosis in SLE and other autoimmune disorders. The most common site is the femoral head of the hip; less commonly, the femoral condyle of the knee is affected. Although the condition may be bilateral, it most often presents with an insidious onset of unilateral hip or knee pain that is worse with ambulating but often present at rest. Symptoms are progressive over weeks to months.

Observe carefully for any sign of renal involvement such as weight gain, edema, or hypertension. Take seizure precautions if there are signs of neurologic involvement. The therapist may recognize signs of cognitive dysfunction or decline, either directly observed in the client or by family report. These manifestations should be reported to the physician for consideration in evaluating medications. If Raynaud's phenomenon is present, teach the client to warm and protect the hands and feet. (See Special Implications for the Therapist: Peripheral Vascular Disease/Raynaud's Phenomenon, 11-23.)

A discussion of pregnancy and SLE is beyond the scope of this text but may be of importance to the therapist involved in women's health issues. More detailed information is available elsewhere.[109,130,131] ∎

◆ Fibromyalgia

Definition and Overview.   Fibromyalgia or fibromyalgia syndrome (FMS), formerly mislabeled or misdiagnosed as fibrocytis, fibromyositis, myofascial pain, CFS, or SLE, is a chronic muscle pain syndrome. It is considered a syndrome and not a disease and has now been defined by the American College of Rheumatology as pain that is widespread in at least 11 of 18 tender points (see Clinical Manifestations and Diagnosis in this section).

FMS currently falls under the auspices of rheumatology, having originally been determined to have no known organic basis. However, with the recent advances in understanding of FMS with documented objective biochemical, endocrine, and physiologic abnormalities, it may be best characterized as a biologic (organic) disorder associated with neurohormonal dysfunction of the ANS. It is commonly associated with many other conditions (e.g., hypothyroidism, rheumatoid arthritis, connective tissue disease, systemic lupus erythematosus, chronic fatigue syndrome); the link between these disorders is under investigation.

Fibromyalgia has been differentiated from myofascial pain (see the section on Myofascial Pain Syndrome in Chapter 26) in that fibromyalgia is considered a systemic problem with widespread multiple tender points as one of the key symptoms. Myofascial pain is a localized condition specific to a muscle and may involve as few as one or as many as several areas with characteristic trigger points that are painful and refer pain to other areas when pressure is applied. The person with FMS may have both tender points and trigger points requiring specific treatment interventions for each. The person with myofascial pain syndrome does not exhibit other associated constitutional or systemic signs or symptoms unless palpation elicits a painful enough response to elicit an ANS response with nausea and/or vomiting, increased blood pressure, and increased pulse.

It has been proposed that fibromyalgia and CFS are two names for the same syndrome with CFS being an early form of FMS, but at present, CFS is thought to differ by the greater degree of fatigue. However, people with fibromyalgia tend to experience more pain. In contrast to CFS, fibromyalgia is associated with a variety of initiating or perpetuating factors such as psychological distressing events, primary sleep disorders, inflammatory rheumatic arthritis, and acute febrile illness. Fibromyalgia and CFS have similar disordered sleep physiology and evidence suggests a reciprocal relationship of the immune and sleep-wake systems. Interference with either system has effects on the other and will be accompanied by the symptoms of CFS.[110] A significant number of people with FMS meet the criteria for CFS and vice versa.

Incidence.   Fibromyalgia occurs in 5% to 8% of the U.S. population, affecting at least 6 million Americans and possibly as many as 10 to 12 million. It has now surpassed rheumatoid arthritis as the most common musculoskeletal disorder in the United States. Women are affected more often than men (75% to 80% are women), generally between the ages of 14 and 68 years, although it has been reported in children as young as 6 and adults as old as 85 years.

Risk Factors.   Risk factors or triggering events for the onset of fibromyalgia may include prolonged anxiety and emotional stress, trauma (e.g., motor vehicle accident, work injury, surgery), rapid steroid withdrawal, hypothyroidism, and viral and nonviral infections. Fibromyalgia may also develop with no obvious precipitating events or illnesses. It is more prevalent in minimally to moderately physically fit persons and is not usually found in highly trained athletes; a strong correlation exists between fibromyalgia and anxiety or depression (it remains unclear whether these factors are contributory or a result of this condition). Women with extracapsular silicone (silicone gel outside of the fibrous scar that forms around breast implants) as a result of rupture are more likely to report having fibromyalgia, but more data is needed to confirm this association.[18]

Etiologic Factors.   Research is now ongoing to determine the cause of fibromyalgia; most likely the initiation of this condition is multifactorial (Fig. 6-7). Debate continues over whether fibromyalgia is even an organic disease and if so, whether it is caused by abnormal biochemical, metabolic, or immunologic pathology. Possible etiologic theories include diet; viral origin; sleep disorder; occupational, seasonal, or environmental influences; psychologic distress; adverse childhood experiences, including sexual abuse[47,102]; and a familial or hereditary link.

The basis of most viral theories (i.e., FMS as a postinfectious disorder or syndrome) was the discovery that people with cancer temporarily develop fibromyalgia (or CFS) while they receive treatment with IL-2 and interferon-α. These two cytokines are produced by the immune system when the body is fighting an infection. Overproduction of interleukins (the IL-1β inhibitory theory) has been documented to cause musculoskeletal pain, fatigue, memory problems, and other symptoms of fibromyalgia and CFS that may explain the cause and pathology of both these conditions.[164]

Pathogenesis.   Both central and peripheral mechanisms may operate in the pathophysiology of impaired muscle function and pain in fibromyalgia. A disturbance in four regulatory systems of the body has been identified in people with FMS: (1) the hypothalamic-pituitary-adrenal axis (HPA); (2) the ANS; (3) the reproductive hormone axis (RHA); and (4) the immune system. Although these systems function independently, each system influences the other, and each helps regulate cellular function. Disruption of one system can influence the other systems, disrupting cellular function.[69]

Hypothalamic-Pituitary-Adrenal Axis.   The HPA axis is considered the stress system of the body, affecting the body's ability to cope with stress, both psychoemotional and bio-

logic, including dysfunction in metabolic and physiologic processes controlling blood pressure, blood sugar levels, infection control, and so on. The hypothalamus, pituitary, and adrenal glands produce chemical messengers that modulate pain, sleep, mood, sex drive, appetite, energy, and circulation. Many of the HPA axis hormones are found to be at abnormal levels in FMS (see Fig. 6-7).[69]

Substance P, a neurotransmitter for pain, may play a role in the transmission of nociceptive information. The inhibitory system acts to lessen or filter out some of the painful signals transmitted to the brain. These pain stimuli are usually transmitted by substance P. Increased activity of substance P may explain an abnormally decreased pain threshold in fibromyalgia.[173] Elevated levels of substance P have been found in the cerebrospinal fluid of fibromyalgia clients, resulting in an exaggerated response to normal stimuli and an amplified effect on pain. People with FMS are not just sensitive to pain, they also find loud noises, odors, and bright lights aversive.

The role of other pain-inhibiting neurotransmitters, such as serotonin, gamma-aminobutyric acid (GABA), enkephalins, epinephrine, and norepinephrine has been studied.[61] Although substance P is elevated, decreased levels of all of these neurotransmitters in the cerebrospinal fluid have been observed. Serotonin, a CNS neurotransmitter that is made from tryptophan (an essential amino acid obtained from diet), is necessary for restorative sleep and appears to play a role in pain control, immune system function, vascular constriction and dilation, and even emotions that may contribute to such feelings as depression or anxiety. Earlier studies found the concentration of serotonin end products (metabolites) to be lower than normal in clients with fibromyalgia, supporting a hypothesis of aberrant pain perception resulting from a deficiency of serotonin.[139,140,141]

However, clinical trials showed that conventional FMS interventions such as tricyclic antidepressants used to increase the amount of serotonin at synapses were no more effective than placebos in improving or alleviating FMS symptoms.[21] This suggests that it is unlikely FMS results primarily from a serotonin deficiency but perhaps another mechanism that causes serotonin deficiency and the other features of this condition.

Available new evidence suggests that impaired metabolism caused by inadequate thyroid hormone regulation at the cellular level may be the underlying pathogenesis. The inadequate regulation of cell function may result from a thyroid hormone deficiency or from cellular resistance to normal levels of thyroid hormone.[96,98] Whether this inadequate thyroid hormone regulation is triggered by genetic mutations[133] and/or can be attributed to environmental contaminants[105] remains unproved.

Abnormalities in the function of the HPA-kidney-bladder axis may account for the irritable bladder syndrome and the female urethral syndrome characterized by urinary frequency and urgency. Low blood pressure and blood volume (ANS dysfunction) may also contribute to this condition. Studies in this area are very limited at this time.

Autonomic Nervous System.   The activity of the skeletal muscles, heart, stomach, intestines, blood vessels, and sweat glands during daily stress tends to be excessive in fibromyalgia. These organs overactivate, resulting in the heart beating faster, the stomach secreting excessive digestive

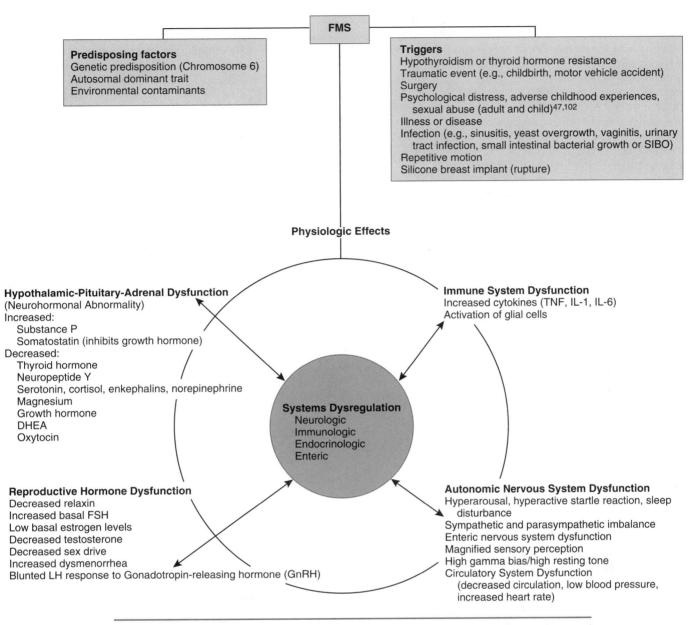

FIGURE   **6-7**   Multifactorial Causes of Fibromyalgia Syndrome. There are many hypotheses and models of how multiple factors contribute to the development of fibromyalgia syndrome (FMS). This model represents data thus far to support FMS as a biologic (organic) disorder caused by neurohormonal dysfunction of the ANS. The physiologic effects of four primary systems dysfunction are listed.

juices and contracting erratically, the smooth muscles of the intestines and bowel contracting abnormally, breathing becoming rapid and shallow, and blood vessels constricting, which decreases blood flow to body parts. These and other ANS responses may occur in response to a relatively mild life stressor and linger even after cognitive memory of the event is gone.

People who do not have fibromyalgia experience these changes, but the autonomic responses occur in smaller amplitude and for a shorter period before returning to normal levels. In fibromyalgia, the nervous system's ability to modulate and return to normal is fragile and lacks the subtle ability to respond quickly; responses are more exaggerated and the return to normal takes more time.[69,173]

The enteric system (autonomic nervous control of the digestive system) is often significantly disrupted in fibromyalgia. Digestion is often compromised, and the absorption of nutrients into the bloodstream where it can be used by the body for cell function is often inadequate for healthy daily function. The enteric system's interaction with other systems (e.g., brain, immune system) links effects of nutritional deficits to other functions as well.[69]

Sleep disturbances may contribute to fibromyalgia symptoms; researchers are investigating alterations of the neuroimmunoendocrine systems that accompany disordered sleep physiology, resulting in the nonrestorative sleep, pain, fatigue, and cognitive and mood symptoms that people with fibromyalgia (and CFS) experience. People affected do not enter restorative sleep (phase IV sleep), or rapid eye movement (REM) sleep. Deficiency of non-REM sleep also contributes to sleep disturbance by reducing the amount of time the muscles enter a state of resting muscle tone. Eighty percent of the body's growth hormone is secreted by the pituitary gland (under hypothalamic control) during deep sleep, and it is crucial for normal muscle metabolism and tissue repair. Substantial nighttime decreases in growth hormone have been reported in FMS.[91] These types of sleep disturbances are not unique to fibromyalgia but have been observed in many people with rheumatoid arthritis, osteoarthritis, and other painful rheumatic diseases.

The Reproductive Hormone Axis.

Reproductive hormones help regulate the HPA axis in a bidirectional feedback loop (see Fig. 10-2). During chronic stress, a decrease in function in both the HPA and the RHA with diminished reproductive capability, fatigue, sleep disruption, and illness or exacerbation of FMS. Female reproductive hormones, especially estrogen and progesterone, exert influence over menstrual cycle, bowel and bladder function, blood pressure, sleep cycles, endorphins, serotonin levels, thyroid function, digestive activity, sex drive, sense of well-being, and much more.

The onset or exacerbations of fibromyalgia often occur around or during the time of sex hormone–related events (e.g., menses, pregnancy, childbirth, peri-menopause, menopause) but few studies exist to study the relationship between these cycles and fibromyalgia. The possibility of inadequate thyroid hormone regulation of the hypothalamic-pituitary-gonadal axis for men and women has been suggested.[96]

Immune System.

Finally, a new model (Watkins Pain Model) for pathologic pain syndromes such as FMS and CFS has been formulated based on pain facilitory effects produced by the immune system. Immune cells, activated in response to infection, inflammation, or trauma release proinflammatory cytokines that signal the CNS to release glia within the brain and spinal cord. Pain has been classically viewed as being mediated solely by neurons, but the discovery that spinal cord glia (microglial and astrocytes) amplify pain has changed this view.

When glial cells become activated by sensory signals arriving from the periphery, they can release a variety of substances known to be involved in chronic pain (e.g., nerve growth factor, excitatory amino acids, nitric oxide), and they can also control the release of neurotransmitters (e.g., substance P).

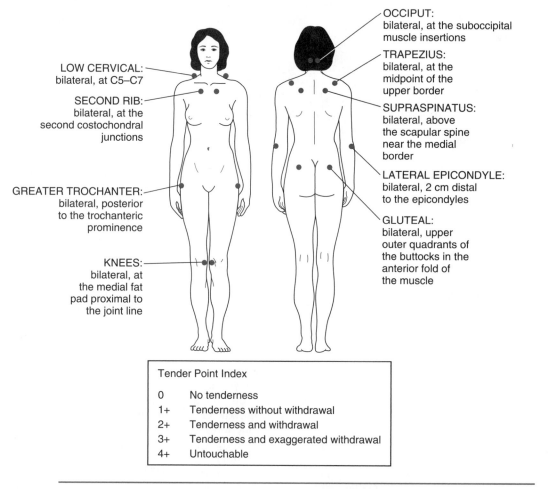

LOW CERVICAL: bilateral, at C5–C7

SECOND RIB: bilateral, at the second costochondral junctions

GREATER TROCHANTER: bilateral, posterior to the trochanteric prominence

KNEES: bilateral, at the medial fat pad proximal to the joint line

OCCIPUT: bilateral, at the suboccipital muscle insertions

TRAPEZIUS: bilateral, at the midpoint of the upper border

SUPRASPINATUS: bilateral, above the scapular spine near the medial border

LATERAL EPICONDYLE: bilateral, 2 cm distal to the epicondyles

GLUTEAL: bilateral, upper outer quadrants of the buttocks in the anterior fold of the muscle

Tender Point Index

0	No tenderness
1+	Tenderness without withdrawal
2+	Tenderness and withdrawal
3+	Tenderness and exaggerated withdrawal
4+	Untouchable

FIGURE   6-8   Anatomic locations of tender points associated with fibromyalgia, according to the American College of Rheumatology 1990 classification of fibromyalgia. Digital palpation should be performed using the thumb or the first two fingers. Apply a steady, uniform pressure with an approximate force of 4 kg/cm² (approximately the pressure needed to indent a tennis ball; enough to blanch the examiner's thumbnail). Using the Tender Point Index, a composite score can be assessed by adding up the individual scores for each of the 18 fibromyalgia tender point sites.

Once activated, such as when viruses and bacteria enter the CNS, glial cells cause prolonged release of proinflammatory cytokines (e.g., TNF, IL-1 and -6), creating an exaggerated pain state. Glia may be the key driving force for the pain created by tissue inflammation and nerve injury because they can increase the release of pain transmitters and cytokines from the neurons in the surrounding area and they are connected to large networks that allow activation of glia at distant sites. This pain model emphasizes again the need for anyone with FMS to minimize pain-generating aggravants such as infectious agents, trauma, and inflammation or other triggers (see Fig. 6-7).[166,167]

Clinical Manifestations.   Fibromyalgia is characterized by muscle pain as the major symptom, often described as aching or burning, a "migraine headache of the muscles." Diffuse pain or tender points is present on both sides of the body in many muscle groups, including the neck, back, arms, legs, jaw, feet, and hands (Fig. 6-8). Sleep disturbances result in fatigue and exhaustion, even after a night's sleep. Men with fibromyalgia typically have fewer symptoms and milder tender points (less "hurt-all-over" reports), less fatigue, and fewer incidences of irritable bowel syndrome compared with women who have FMS.[174]

Other symptoms or associated problems occur with a high frequency (Table 6-7) sometimes more incapacitating than the pain and tender points. Symptoms are often exacerbated by stress; overloading physical activity, including overstretching; damp or chilly weather; heat exposure or humidity; sudden change in barometric pressure; trauma; or another illness. Those people with fibromyalgia who are aerobically fit manifest fewer symptoms than those who remain physically deconditioned and aerobically unfit. Biofeedback specialists have shown that blood circulation to the affected areas is often significantly decreased while at rest and a noticeable decrease in circulation occurs with changes in barometric pressure. During exercise, when circulation should normally increase to muscles and brain, in fibromyalgia, just the opposite happens, and circulation is decreased significantly.[69]

The diaphragm is significantly affected in fibromyalgia to the point that it ceases to function as the major breathing muscle and accessory muscles of the neck and upper chest take over. This overwork results in tender points or tightness of the neck and chest muscles. In general, the level of muscular activity in fibromyalgia is high, even when the body is sitting or reclining. During daily activities such as cleaning, cooking, typing, and even socializing, the muscles used for these activities are at a higher level of activity than the muscles of a normal person doing the same tasks. When the activity is over and the person with fibromyalgia is resting, those same muscles continue to repeat the activity over and over at a lower intensity so that no outward movement is apparent.

TABLE	6-7

Clinical Manifestations of Fibromyalgia

Sign/Symptom	Incidence (%)*	Sign/Symptom	Incidence (%)*
Muscle pain (myalgia), tender points	99†	Pelvic pain	43
Visual problems (e.g., blurring, double vision, bouncing images)	95	Irritable bladder syndrome, female urethral syndrome	40
Mental and physical fatigue	85	Hypotension (low blood pressure, elevated heart rate); neurally mediated hypotension or vasopressor syncope	40
Sleep disturbance/morning fatigue	80		
Morning stiffness (persists >30 min)	75		
Mitral valve prolapse	75	Raynaud's phenomenon	38
Global anxiety	72	Sicca syndrome (dry eyes/mouth)	33
Cognitive (memory) problems (e.g., decreased attention span, impaired short-term memory, decreased concentration, increased distractibility)	71	Respiratory dysfunction (e.g., dyspnea, erratic breathing patterns during exertion)	33
Irritable bowel syndrome	70	Restless leg syndrome, nocturnal myoclonus, periodic leg movement disorder (PLMD)	30-60
Inflammatory bowel disease (Crohn's disease, ulcerative colitis)	50-60	Auditory problems	31
Headaches	70	Temporomandibular dysfunction	25
Hypersensitivity to noise, odors, heat, or cold (cold intolerance)	50-60	Depression	20
		Allergies	Unknown
Paresthesias	50	Lack of libido	Unknown
Swollen feeling (joint or soft tissues)	50	Skin discoloration	Unknown
Muscle spasms or nodules	50	Sciatica	Unknown
Reactive hypoglycemia (e.g., weakness, irritability, disorientation)	45-50		

*These figures were compiled from a variety of sources but represent a fairly accurate clinical perspective.
†Although the American College of Rheumatology requires the identification of at least 11 out of 18 tender points to qualify for a diagnosis of FMS, some clinicians report isolated individuals without pain but characterized by the physiologic effects and manifestations of FMS.
Modified from Hulme J: *Fibromyalgia: a handbook for self-care and treatment,* ed 3, Missoula, Mont, 2000, Phoenix.

Medical Management

Diagnosis. No definitive test is currently available to determine the presence of fibromyalgia, and usually the organs involved are not the cause but merely the messenger of a problem originating elsewhere in the body. According to the American College of Rheumatology two criteria must be met before a medical diagnosis of FMS can be made: (1) widespread (four-quadrants) pain both above and below the waist present for at least 3 months and (2) subjective report of pain when pressure is applied to 11 of the 18 common FMS tender points on the body (see Fig. 6-8). Subjective assessment of tender points can be elicited by the use of an instrument called a *dolorimeter*, which distributes pressure equally over a discrete point. With a dolorimeter, the pressure required to produce pain in a given area can be recorded.

Often, the diagnosis is determined as a process of elimination by ruling out other conditions based on clinical presentation and past medical history (Box 6-7). In addition to the presence of tender points, skin fold tenderness, increased reactive skin hyperemia, and low tissue compliance (in the trapezius and paraspinal regions) provide further diagnostic information.

Laboratory tests and radiologic studies give essentially normal results with the exception of substance P, a chemical involved in pain transmission (higher levels in FMS) and decreased serotonin levels. Altered brain waves during deep sleep also suggest abnormal growth hormone production necessary for restoring muscles and other soft tissues. The antipolymer antibody (APA) assay detects antipolymer antibodies in the blood of many, but not all, people with FMS. This is an indication that the body is mounting an immunologic response associated with the symptoms present. This is the first objective laboratory marker to correlate with severity of symptoms in this population.[170]

Treatment. Until recently, no single intervention (allopathic or alternative) has been found effective in changing the status of clients with FMS (either altering pain levels or affecting functional impairment).[21,48] Rather, normalizing the ANS, metabolism, and hormones in combination with lifestyle management, nutritional support, and coping strategies seems to be the most successful. Recent evidence supporting metabolic insufficiency of thyroid hormone has shown that administration of supraphysiologic dosages of triiodothyronine (T_3) is the first to demonstrate long-term effectiveness of an FMS treatment. This treatment is referred to as *metabolic rehabilitation*.[98]

Even with this new information, approaches to helping clients with fibromyalgia must be holistic and multidisciplinary, including education and support; stress management; nutrition and lifestyle training (e.g., coping strategies, applying work simplification and ergonomic principles, and psychotherapy); medications; local modalities and techniques for muscle pain (e.g., relaxation techniques, biofeedback, physiologic quieting, or soft tissue techniques); and conditioning and aerobic exercise. Cognitive behavioral therapy aimed at altering sensory, affective, cognitive, and behavioral aspects of chronic pain (e.g., pain severity, emotional distress, depression, anxiety, pain behavior) have been shown to be effective over a long period, even when the disease process cannot be controlled and symptoms worsen.

Alternative and complementary intervention (e.g., acupuncture, herbal or vitamin supplements, chiropractic,

---

BOX 6-7

Differential Diagnosis of Fibromyalgia

Endocrine Disorders	Infection/Inflammation
Hypothyroidism	Subacute bacterial endo-
Hypopituitary	carditis
	Lyme disease
Illness	AIDS
	Chronic syphilis
Rheumatoid arthritis	Tuberculosis
Systemic lupus erythematosus	
Sjögren's syndrome	**Other**
Polymyositis/dermatomyositis	
Polymyalgia rheumatica/	Temporomandibular joint
giant cell arteritis	dysfunction
Metabolic myopathy (e.g.,	Disk disease
alcohol)	Myofascial pain syndrome
Metastatic cancer	Silicone breast implant
Chronic fatigue syndrome	Neurosis (depression/
	anxiety)

---

hypnotherapy, and others) is available and often provides palliative relief from symptoms for periods. Like most interventions (medical or nonconventional), no single intervention is effective all the time, and the person with FMS may cycle through various modalities over time.

Prognosis. Many people with mild symptoms are managed without a specialist and have an expected good long-term outcome, but most people experience persistent symptoms of fibromyalgia for many years or a lifetime. Symptoms usually remain unchanged or increase with concomitant decrease in function, but new hope abounds with the advent of metabolic rehabilitation combined with a team approach for those individuals with a thyroid component.

Special Implications for the Therapist 6-7

FIBROMYALGIA

Preferred Practice Patterns
4A: *Primary Prevention/Risk Reduction for Skeletal Demineralization (osteoporosis as a side effect of some medications)*
4B: *Impaired Posture (metabolic-based fatigue)*[96]
4D: *Impaired Joint Mobility, Motor Function, Muscle Performance, and Range of Motion Associated With Connective Tissue Dysfunction*
5A: *Primary Prevention/Risk Reduction for Loss of Balance and Falling (neurogenic hypotension)*
6B: *Impaired Aerobic Capacity/Endurance Associated With Deconditioning*

Therapists are often the first to recognize the history and clinical manifestations suggestive of fibromyalgia and then request medical diagnosis and intervention. Efforts to assess the accuracy of thumb nailbed blanching as a means of determining the presence of tender points suggest that the therapist can quickly learn to use the 4 kg/cm^2 of force required to administer a tender point examination (Manual Tender Point Survey or MTPS).[154] Accurate assessment allows the therapist to establish a baseline sensitivity to aid in determining progress and direct intervention.[29] Specific procedures for identifying and palpating each site are available.[87,157] A complete compendium of blank assessment forms and information on how to obtain assessment instruments for FMS is also available.[69,96]

Rehabilitative therapy is an important component in managing fibromyalgia. Many people with FMS have undergone unnecessary exploratory or corrective surgery and have residual functional limitations. Chronic musculoskeletal conditions that are sources of noxious neural input to the CNS often involve the shoulder(s) and spine. Therapy is helpful first in directing individuals to reach goals of lessening pain and fatigue, and eliminating sleep disturbance. Outcomes can be measured in a variety of ways, not only by reduction in tender points but also by global scores of pain, fatigue, sleep, reduction of other distressing symptoms, improved quality of life, reduced visits to the physician, reducing or eliminating medications, increased sexual activity, improved work performance, and so on.

Many people with FMS have been told they must "learn to live with it." A more positive approach is to suggest working together to learn how to move forward with FMS, respecting limitations but not being controlled by them. The therapist can be very instrumental in guiding that person to understand how to manage this condition. Prevention programs for osteoporosis and falls related to low blood pressure are additional services the therapist can provide.

Strategies for work modification and applying ergonomic techniques to increase efficiency and decrease pain are important interventions. A chronic pain program may be appropriate (see the section on Chronic Pain in Chapter 2). The reader is referred to more specific literature for treatment regimens, self-stabilizing techniques, and therapy protocols for this condition.[28,69,129]

Monitoring Vital Signs

Monitoring tests provide an indication of the present physiologic status but cannot predict future status so regular monitoring is necessary. Depending on the current status, the individual may have to self-monitor every 2 hours, whereas others are able to maintain a balance by monitoring twice daily or less often. For most people with FMS, the sensory system and the ANS are overactive. Monitoring tests are a helpful tool in developing techniques to quiet these hypersensitivities and achieve a state of physiologic quiet.[69]

Blood pressure and heart rate are indicators of cardiac and circulatory system function and should be monitored. Most people with FMS have low blood pressure and usually an elevated pulse rate even at rest (some individuals have a slow pulse). Hypotension in people with FMS is now referred to as *neurogenic hypotension* (see Chapter 11). It has been suggested that thyroid hormone regulation will normalize the heart rate and contractility and often normalizes the blood pressure.[98]

For some individuals with a hypoglycemic component, blood glucose assessment may be necessary. Hand temperature is one indicator of ANS function and can be easily assessed using a handheld biofeedback device (e.g., Thermister®)[124] designed to measure hand temperature. This tool provides a mean of modulating the ANS, improving circulation, and reducing pain levels. The therapist can monitor medical and physical therapy intervention outcomes by assessing vital signs and documenting results..

Modalities and Fibromyalgia

Very little research is available to determine the outcomes of modality use (i.e., physical therapy intervention with thermal or mechanical properties such as physical agents, cryotherapy, moist heat, massage, manual therapy, soft tissue treatment) with FMS. Investigation into the use of cranial electrotherapy stimulation (sending minicurrents of electricity through the brain) is under investigation. Limited study shows that this treatment intervention provided a significant improvement in tender point scores and in self-rated scores of general pain level, along with dramatic gains in six stress-related psychologic test measures.[82,94]

Ultrasound can be an effective therapeutic modality for its thermal effects and for the treatment of myofascial trigger points often present in people with FMS when combined with the complete trigger point (TrP) protocol. Continuous ultrasound is preferable to pulsed ultrasound, and the intensity must be reduced from standard settings to accommodate hypersensitivity in most people with FMS. Specific positions, tissue effects, intervention techniques, and treatment parameters are available.[66,67] Again, additional steps must be taught to sustain pain relief (e.g., using biofeedback or physiologic quieting to avoid contracting the involved muscle, gentle stretching combined with moist heat several times each day, appropriate changes in work style, patterns of movement, postures, and over-the-counter analgesics such as ibuprofen or naproxen when approved by the physician).[67]

Soft tissue techniques may correct the neurocirculatory abnormality and thereby reduce or eliminate the nociceptive signal transmission from the muscle. The result should be to relieve pain and improve Tender Point Index scores or other FMS pain scores assessed. Given the proposed mechanism of muscle pain (hyperresponsive myofascial mechanoreceptors/impaired CNS pain-inhibiting system), soft tissue techniques must be applied gently and slowly to increase circulation while avoiding an increase in nociceptive signal transmission. With the typical FMS client, posttreatment discomfort can be avoided by keeping the discomfort level during treatment between 1 and 5 on a self-assessment scale from 1 to 10. Cross-friction massage is not advised.[97]

Exercise and Fibromyalgia

The primary nonpharmacologic modality in the management of FMS is prescriptive exercise. Improvement in both subjective pain and objective measurement has been demonstrated with cardiovascular fitness training or simple flexibility training.[103] Increases in β-endorphin; adrenocorticotropic hormone (ACTH); and cortisol levels in response to exercise at aerobic levels (i.e., 60% of maximal oxygen consumption) have also been shown in this population.[113] Aerobic exercise also contributes by increasing the metabolic rate of the lean tissues for those individuals with a thyroid component.[152] Resistance exercise contributes to the increase in metabolism by increasing

Continued

lean tissue mass, which has a higher metabolic rate than fat tissue.[127] Well-managed prescriptive exercise regimens improve sleep and result in a decrease in pain and fatigue.[32] Only general concepts are included in this text; other texts are available for specific exercise regimens.[11,69]

Combining self-care and management strategies with an exercise program helps the individual reach the goals of optimal function and fitness while maintaining decreased pain and fatigue and increasing endurance for daily activities. A number of excellent self-care books are available for consumers.[27,34,51,156] Gentle stretching exercises performed routinely throughout the day may reduce fatigue. A cardiopulmonary fitness component should be included at whatever level the individual presents with at the time of assessment.

Sometimes the person's condition is so acute that exercise is not tolerated immediately. This is often the reason for using modalities in the early stage of therapy. Exercising too soon and commiting to too much can set the person back considerably, but at the same time the therapist must keep in mind the long-term goal to increase strength and improve aerobic fitness. Aquatic therapy* is an ideal way to begin conditioning, especially for those individuals with FMS who have injuries, are overweight, or are sensitive to axial load. Aquatic therapy provides low-level progressive exercises, gradually increasing strength and endurance while improving overall cardiovascular fitness.

As with all exercise programs with this population (whether aquatic or other therapy), people with fibromyalgia fatigue quickly and may have a low tolerance for exertion. The key is to avoid activating the peripheral sensory mechanisms in order to avoid increasing pain postexercise. The person with FMS will respond to stimuli that would not ordinarily be perceived as painful (referred to as *allodynia*). This requires short exercise sessions, according to individual tolerance using the rate of perceived exertion (see Chapter 11), that are possibly even only 3 to 5 minutes at first. The client is encouraged to increase exercise duration in small daily increments, sometimes only by seconds or minutes. Reaching a goal of 30 minutes of daily exercise may take weeks to months; some individuals are only able to tolerate one to three daily exercise cycles, each lasting only 5 to 10 minutes, but this will produce beneficial effects.

The individual with FMS must be taught to set aside the philosophy of "no pain, no gain" and to avoid "pushing through the pain." In the normal individual, growth hormone is increased with exercise, but this does not happen in the person with FMS. Rather, as a result of ANS dysfunction, reduced microcirculation (capillary flow and other small vessels that supply muscles) causes microtrauma in muscles with vigorous, strenuous, or excessive exercise. The resulting postexertional muscle pain or discomfort aggravates the abnormal pain filter experienced by this population. All causes of increased pain should be minimized, reduced, or eliminated.[12]

Poor compliance is common when the use of muscle relaxants, sedatives, or other medications reduce desire or drive to exercise. Symptoms of pain and fatigue increase during exercise, resulting in limited compliance and limited long-term benefits. The therapist can explain that pain may result in part from muscle spasm and reduced blood flow to muscles, both of which can be aided by persistence in managing exercise. Using training intensity as a measure of improvement may be helpful. Before performing the physical activity or exercise, compute the maximum heart rate (MHR = 220 − age). During the activity/exercise, take the pulse and record this for later calculations. Once the activity/exercise is completed, compute the intensity of work: I_w = Pulse/MHR. Multiply I_w by the number of minutes exercised to determine the Training Index (TI) [TI = I_w × number of minutes]. Keep track of the TI for each activity/exercise session and total them up for 1 week. Track this value over time to assess improved outcomes.[31]

People with fibromyalgia are also more vulnerable to overuse syndromes than people with normal muscle histology, requiring a slower, longer rehabilitation process. This may not be activity-induced as once thought, but rather may occur as a result of sarcolemmal abnormality.[73] At present, until more is known and understood about this phenomenon, whenever possible, an aerobic exercise routine should become a part of the client's life before individual muscle group strengthening is started.

Additionally, TrPs, a separate entity from tender points, must be detected and eliminated before initiating exercise using those muscles. Specific assessment and intervention for TrP therapy is available,[28,63,153] but it should be noted that TrPs are treatment resistant in some individuals with inadequate thyroid hormone at the cellular level. For these individuals, treatment of the underlying hypothyroidism and/or thyroid resistance is essential first.[95]

Other resources include the Fibromyalgia Network Newsletter; P.O. Box 31750; Tucson, AZ 85751 (http://www.fmnetnews.com) and the American Fibromyalgia Syndrome Association; P.O. Box 9699; Bakersfield, CA 93389 (http://www.afsafund.org). ■

ISOIMMUNE DISEASE

◆ Organ and Tissue Transplantation

With recent advances in technology and immunology, organ and tissue transplantation is becoming commonplace. In fact, transplantation of almost any tissue is feasible, but the clinical use of transplantation to remedy disease is still limited for many organ systems because of the rejection reaction. Transplant rejection, an isoimmune phenomenon, occurs in response to transplantation because the body usually recognizes the donor tissue as nonself and attempts to destroy the tissue shortly after transplantation.

In all cases of graft rejection, the cause is incompatibility of cell surface antigens. The rejection of foreign or transplanted tissue occurs because the recipient's immune system recognizes that the surface HLA proteins of the donor's tissue are different from the recipient's. For this reason, HLA matching of donor and recipient greatly enhances the probability of graft acceptance. Certain antigens are more important than others for a successful transplant, including ABO and Rh antigens present on RBCs and histocompatibility antigens, most importantly the HLA. As expected, a better chance of graft acceptance is evident with syngeneic or autologous transplants because the cell surface antigens are identical.

For a complete discussion of histocompatibility, graft rejection (acute versus chronic), GVHD, and immunosuppression, see Chapter 20.

---

*Ideal pool temperature is between 84° F and 90° F (compared with 82° F to 84° F for the general population and 90° F to 94° F for people with arthritic conditions).[88]

REFERENCES

1. Aderem A, Underhill DM: Mechanisms of phagocytosis in macrophages, *Annu Rev Immunol* 17:593-623, 1999.

2. Albano SA, Wallace DJ: Managing fatigue in patients with SLE, *J Musculoskel Med* 18(3):149-152, 2001.

3. American Autoimmune Related Diseases Association, Detroit, Mich, 2001. Available at http://www.aarda.org or by calling (800) 598-4668.

4. American Cancer Society: *Guide to complementary and alternative cancer methods*, New York, 2000, The Society.

5. Anastasi JK: Alternative and complementary therapies. In Ungvarski PJ, Flaskerud JH: *HIV/AIDS: a guide to primary care management*, ed 4, Philadelphia, 1999, WB Saunders.

6. Balbin EG, Ironson GH, Solomon GF: Stress and coping: the psychoneuroimmunology of HIV/AIDS, *Baillieres Best Pract Res Clin Endocrinol Metabol* 13(4):615-633, 1999.

7. Barroso PF et al: Effect of antiretroviral therapy on HIV shedding in semen, *Ann Intern Med* 133(4):280-284, 2000.

8. Bauer ME et al: Chronic stress in caregivers of dementia patients is associated with reduced lymphocyte sensitivity to glucocorticoids, *J Neuroimmunol* 103(1):84-92, 2000.

9. Befus AD, Mathison R, Davison J: Integration of neuro-endocrine immune responses in defense of mucosal surfaces, *Am J Trop Med Hyg* 60(4):26-34, 1999.

10. Benca RM, Quintas J: Sleep and host defenses: a review, *Sleep* 20(11):1027-1037, 1997.

11. Bennett K: Exercise in fibromyalgia and chronic fatigue syndrome. In Hall CM, Brody LT: *Therapeutic exercise*, Philadelphia, 1998, Lippincott-Raven.

12. Bennett R: A balanced view on exercise, *Fibromyalgia Net*, p. 5, 1997.

13. Berin MC, McKay DM, Perdue MH: Immune-epithelial interactions in host defense, *Am J Trop Med Hyg* 60(4):16-25, 1999.

14. Berthiaume F et al: Age- and disease-related decline in immune function: an opportunity for "thymus–boosting" therapies, *Tissue Eng* 5(6):499-514, 1999.

15. Borderi M et al: Metabolic complications of HIV-1 antiretroviral therapy: the lipodystrophy syndrome, *New Microbiol* 24(3):303-315, 2001.

16. Brodsky RA, Petri M, Jones RJ: Hematopoietic stem cell transplantation for systemic lupus erythematosus, *Rheum Dis Clin North Am* 26(2):377-387, 2000.

17. Brown L, Drotman P: *What is the risk of HIV infection in athletic competition?* Presented at Ninth International Conference on AIDS, Berlin, June 6-11, 1993.

18. Brown SL et al: Silicone gel breast implant rupture, extracapsular silicone, and health status in a population of women, *J Rheumatol* 28:996-1003, 2001.

19. Buckley RH: Primary immunodeficiency diseases due to defects in lymphocytes, *N Engl J Med* 343(18):1313-1324, 2000.

20. Calabrese LH: Changing patterns of morbidity and mortality in HIV disease, *Cleve Clin J Med* 68(2):105, 109-110, 2001.

21. Carette S: What have clinical trials taught us about the treatment of fibromyalgia? *J Musculo Pain* 3:133-140, 1995.

22. Caride E et al: Drug-resistant reverse transcriptase genotyping and phenotyping of B and non-B subtypes (F and A) of human immunodeficiency virus type I found in Brazilian patients failing HAART, *Virology* 275(1):107-115, 2000.

23. Centers for Disease Control and Prevention: *Chronic fatigue syndrome: the revised case definition*, 2001. Available at http://www.cdc.gov.

24. Centers for Disease Control and Prevention: Draft of guidelines for the prevention of opportunistic infections (OIs) in people infected with human immunodeficiency virus, *MMWR* 50(32):687, 2001. Available at http://www.hivatis.org.

25. Centers for Disease Control and Prevention: Guidelines for prevention of HIV and hepatitis B virus transmission to health care and public safety workers, *MMWR* 38:S1-6, 1989.

26. Centers for Disease Control and Prevention: Public Health Service guidelines for the management of health care worker exposures to HIV and recommendations for postexposure prophylaxis, *MMWR* 47(RR-7):1-33, 1998.

27. Chaitow L: *Fibromyalgia & muscle pain*, ed 2, Thorson Health Series, 1999. Available by calling (800) 367-7393.

28. Chaitow L: *Fibromyalgia syndrome: a practitioner's guide to treatment*, Philadelphia, 2000, Churchill Livingstone.

29. Chinnock L et al: Is thumb nailbed blanching consistent with 4 kg of pressure when performing the Manual Tender Point Survey? *Phys Ther* (abstr) 81(5):A25, 2001.

30. Clapp LL et al: Acute effects of thirty minutes of light-intensity, intermittent exercise on patients with chronic fatigue syndrome, *Phys Ther* 79(8):749-756, 1999.

31. Clark S: Health care professionals teaming up, *Fibromyalgia Net*, 1999. Available at http://www.fmnetnews.com.

32. Clark SR et al: Exercise and patient outcome in fibromyalgia, *Arthritis Rheum* 34:S190, 1991.

33. Currier JS: How to manage metabolic complications of HIV therapy: what to do while we wait for answers, *AIDS Read* 10(3):162-169, 2000.

34. Davies C: *The trigger point therapy workbook: your self-treatment guide for pain relief*, Oakland, Calif, 2001, New Harbinger Publishers.

35. Davis CM, editor: *Complementary therapies in rehabilitation: holistic approaches for prevention and wellness*, Thorofare, NJ, 1997, Slack, Inc.

36. Dean E: Oxygen transport deficits in systemic disease and implications for physical therapy, *Phys Ther* 77(2):187-202, 1997.

37. De Becker P et al: Exercise capacity in chronic fatigue syndrome, *Arch Intern Med* 160(21):3270-3277, 2000.

38. Delves PJ, Roitt IM: The immune system (I), *N Engl J Med* 343(1):37-49, 2000.

39. Delves PJ, Roitt IM: The immune system (II), *N Engl J Med* 343(2):108-117, 2000.

40. De Meirleir K et al: A 37kDa 2-5A binding protein as a potential marker for chronic fatigue syndrome, *Am J Med* 108:99-105, 2000.

41. Denburg SD, Carbotte RM, Denburg JA: Identifying cognitive deficits in systemic lupus erythematosus, *J Musculoskel Med* 16(6):356-363, 1999.

42. Dick R, Worthman F: Frequency of bleeding and risk of HIV transmission in intercollegiate athletics, *Med Sci Sports Exer* 5(Suppl):S13, 1994.

43. Dobkin PL et al: Psychosocial contributors to mental and physical health in patients with systemic lupus erythematosus, *Arthritis Care Res* 11(1):23-31, 1998.

44. Donenberg GR et al: Understanding AIDS-risk behavior among adolescents in psychiatric care: links to psychopathology and peer relationships, *J Am Acad Child Adolesc Psychiatry* 40(6);642-653, 2001.

45. Eichner ER: Infection, immunity, and exercise: what to tell patients? *Physician Sportsmed* 21(1):125-135, 1993.

46. Evans WJ, Roubenoff R, Shevitz A: Exercise and the treatment of wasting: aging and human immunodeficiency virus infection, *Semin Oncol* 25(2 Suppl 6):112-122, 1998.

47. Finestone HM et al: Chronic pain and health care utilization in women with a history of childhood sexual abuse, *Child Abuse Negl* 24(4):547-556, 2000.

48. Fitzcharles MA, Esdaile JM: Nonphysician practitioner treatments and fibromyalgia syndrome, *J Rheumatol* 24(5):937-940, 1997.

49. Fleshner M: Exercise and neuroendocrine regulation of antibody production: protective effect of physical activity on stress-induced suppression of the specific antibody response, *Int J Sports Med* 21(Suppl 1):S14-19, 2000.

50. Frankel SS et al: Replication of HIV-1 in dendritic cell-derived syncytia at the mucosal surface of the adenoid, *Science* 272:115-117, 1996.

51. Fransen J, Russell IJ: The fibromyalgia help book: practical guide to living better with fibromyalgia, Smith House, 1997. Available by calling (800) 367-7393.

52. Franzen C, Salzberger B, Fatkenheuer G: Avascular necrosis of both femoral heads in an HIV-infected patient receiving protease inhibitors, *Eur J Med Res* 6(2):83-4, 2001.

53. Fulcher KY, White PD: Chronic fatigue syndrome: a description of graded exercise treatment, *Physiotherapy* 84:223-226, 1998.

54. Fulcher KY, White PD: Randomised control led trial of graded exercise in patients with the chronic fatigue syndrome, *BMJ* 314(7095):1647-1652, 1997.

55. Fulcher KY, White PD: Strength and physiological response to exercise in patients with chronic fatigue syndrome, *J Neurol Neurosurg Psychiatry* 69(3):302-307, 2000.

56. Galantino ML: Human immunodeficiency virus (HIV) infection: living with a chronic illness. In Humphred D, editor: *Neurological rehabilitation*, ed 4, St Louis, 2001, Mosby.

57. Galantino ML et al: Use of noninvasive electroacupuncture for the treatment of HIV-related peripheral neuropathy: a pilot study, *J Alt Complem Med* 5(2):135-142, 1999.

58. Galantino ML et al: Physical therapy management for the patient with HIV. Lower extremity challenges, *Clin Podiatr Med Surg* 15(2):329-346, 1998.

59. Gao X et al: Effect of a single amino acid change in MHC class I molecules on the rate of progression to AIDS, *N Engl J Med* 344(22):1668-1675, 2001.

60. Garg A: Lipodystrophies, *Am J Med* 108:143-152, 2000.

61. Goldstein JA: What important brain neurotransmitters does TRH alter? *Fibromyalgia Net*, April 1999. Available at http://www.fmnetnews.com or by contacting Fibromyalgia Network; P.O. Box 31750; Tuscon, AZ 85751 (800) 853-2929.

62. Gray AB et al: Anaerobic exercise causes transient changes in leukocyte subsets and IL-2R expression, *Med Sci Sports Exerc* 24:1332, 1992.

63. Headley B: *When movement hurts: a self-help manual for treating trigger points*, Longmont, Colo, 1997, Innovative Systems.

64. Healthy People 2010: Ojectives: AIDS, 2001. Available at http://www.health.gov/healthypeople/.

65. Hirschhorn L: Women, HIV, and HAART: closing the gender gap, *Internal Med* 20(1):32-39, 1999.

66. Honeyman-Lowe G: *Ultrasound treatment of the fibromyalgia patient.* Presented at the conference of the French Fibromyalgia Association conference, May 6, 2000, Grenoble, France. Available by contacting the Fibromyalgia Research Foundation; P.O. Box 396; Tulsa OK 74101 (DrGHL@drlowe.com)

67. Honeyman-Lowe G: Ultrasound treatment of trigger points: differences in techniques for myofascial pain syndrome and fibromyalgia patients, *Myalgia '99* (2):12-15, 1999. Available by contacting the Fibromyalgia Research Foundation; P.O. Box 396; Tulsa OK 74101 (DrGHL@drlowe.com).

68. Hooper E, Hamilton WD: *The river: a journey to the source of HIV and AIDS*, Boston, 2000, Back Bay Press.

69. Hulme J: *Fibromyalgia: a handbook for self-care and treatment*, ed 3, Missoula, Mont, 2000, Phoenix.

70. Irwin KL et al: Potential for bias in studies of the influence of human immunodeficiency virus infection on the recognition, incidence, clinical course, and microbiology of pelvic inflammatory disease, *Obstet Gynecol* 84:463-469, 1994.

71. James JA et al: Systemic lupus erythematosus in adults is associated with previous Epstein-Barr virus exposure, *Arthritis Rheum* 44(5):1122-1126, 2001.

72. Joseph RE, Radhakrishnan J, Appel GB: Antiphospholipid antibody syndrome and renal disease, *Curr Opin Nephrol Hypertens* 10(2):175-181, 2001.

73. Jubrias SA, Bennett RM, Klug GA: Increased incidence of a resonance in the phosphodiester region of 31P nuclear magnetic resonance spectra in the skeletal muscle of fibromyalgia patients, *Arthritis Rheum* 37:801-807, 1994.

74. Kapasi ZF: *Exercise and the aging immune system.* Presented at the Combined Sections Meeting, New Orleans, La, February 12-14, 2000.

75. Kapasi ZF: Personal communication, 2001.

76. Kapasi ZF et al: The role of endogenous opioids in exercise-induced enhancement of the secondary antibody response in mice, *Phys Therap* 81(11): 1801-1809, 2001.

77. Kapasi ZF et al: The effects of intense physical exercise on secondary antibody response in young and old mice, *Phys Therap* 80(11):1076-1086, 2000.

78. Kamradt T, Mitchison NA: Tolerance and autoimmunity, *N Engl J Med* 344(9):655-664, 2001.

79. Katz BZ et al: Epstein-Barr virus burden in adolescents with systemic lupus erythematosus, *Pediatr Infect Dis J* 20(2):148-153, 2001.

80. Kay AB: Allergy and allergic disease, *N Engl J Med* 344(1):30-37, 2001.

81. Keller P: Physical therapy management of patients with HIV-positive/AIDS, *Adv Phys Therapists* 5:6-7, 17, 1994.

82. Kirsch DL, Smith RB: The use of cranial electrotherapy stimulation in management of chronic pain: a review, *NeuroRehabil* 14(2):85-94, 2000.

83. Klein J, Sato A: The HLA system (I), *N Engl J Med* 343(10): 702-709, 2000.

84. Komaroff AL: The biology of chronic fatigue syndrome, *Am J Med* 108(2):169-171, 2000.

85. Korber B et al: Timing the ancestor of the HIV-1 pandemic strains, *Science* 288(5472):1789-1796, 2000.

86. Krishnaswamy G et al: The cardiovascular and metabolic complications of HIV infection, *Cardiol Rev* 8(5):260-268, 2000.

87. Krsnich-Shriwise S: Fibromyalgia syndrome: an overview, *Phys Therap* 77(1):68-75, 1997.

88. Kuhne L: *Improving functional mobility for fibromyalgia patients with aquatic exercise.* Presented at the Aquatic Therapy Rehabilitation Institute Conference, Las Vegas, August 1995.

89. Lahita RG: *Laboratory tests used in the diagnosis of lupus*, Lupus Foundation of America, 2001. Available at http://www.lupus.org/.

90. Lahita RG: Treatment of lupus, Lupus Foundation of America, 2001. Available at http://www.lupus.org/.

91. Landis CA et al: Decreased nocturnal levels of prolactin and growth hormone in women with fibromyalgia, *J Clin Endocrinol Metab* 86(4):1672-1678, 2001.

92. Lavreys L: Effect of circumcision on incidence of human immunodeficiency virus type 1 and other sexually transmitted diseases, *J Infect Dis* 180(2):330-336, 1999.

93. Leuthotlz BC, Ripoll I: Exercise and disease management, Baco Raton, Fla, 1999, CRC Press.

94. Lichtbroun AS, Raicer MMC, Smith RB: The treatment of fibromyalgia with cranial electrotherapy stimulation, *J Clin Rheum* 7(2):72-78, 2001.

95. Lowe JC: Revised edition of the trigger point manual, vol 1 (book report): fibromyalgia, *J Bodywork Move Ther* 4(3):197-201, 2000.

96. Lowe JC: *The metabolic treatment of fibromyalgia*, Boulder, Colo, McDowell, 2000.

97. Lowe JC, Honeyman-Lowe G: Facilitating the decrease in fibromyalgic pain during metabolic rehabilitation: an essential role for soft tissue therapies, *J Bodywork Move Ther* 2(4):208-217, 1998.

98. Lowe JC, Honeyman-Lowe G: The metabolic rehabilitation of fibromyalgia patients. In Chaitow L, editor: *Fibromyalgia syndrome: a practitioner's guide to treatment*, Philadelphia, 2000, Churchill Livingstone.

99. Lynch FA, Kirov SM: Changes in blood lymphocyte populations following surgery, *J Clin Lab Immunol* 20:75, 1986.

100. Mandell GL: *Principles and practice of infectious diseases*, ed 5, Philadelphia, 2000, Churchill Livingstone.

101. Manuel y Keenoy B et al: Antioxidant status and lipoprotein peroxidation in chronic fatigue syndrome, *Life Sci* 68(17):2037-2049, 2001.

102. McBeth J et al: The association between tender points, psychologic distress, and adverse childhood experiences: a community-based study, *Arthritis Rheum* 42(7):1397-1404, 1999.

103. McCain GA et al: A controlled study of the effects of a supervised cardiovascular fitness training program on the manifestations of primary fibromyalgia, *Arthritis Rheum* 31:1135-1141, 1988.

104. McCarthy DA, Dale MM: The leukocytosis of exercise: a review and model, *Sports Med* 6:333-363, 1988.

105. McKinney JD, Pedersen LG: Do residue levels of polychlorinated biphenyls (PCBs) in human blood produce mild hypothyroidism? *J Theoret Biol* 129:231-241, 1987.

106. Medzhitov R, Janeway C: Innate immunity, *N Engl J Med* 343(5):338-344, 2000.

107. Merchant RC, Keshavarz R: Human immunodeficiency virus postexposure prophylaxis for adolescents and children, *Pediatrics* 108(2):E38, 2001.

108. Mire-Sluis AR, Thorpe R, editors: *Cytokines*, San Diego, 1998, Academic Press.

109. Mok CC, Wong RW: Pregnancy in systemic lupus erythematosus, *Postgrad Med J* 77(905):157-165, 2001.

110. Moldofsky H: Fibromyalgia, sleep disorder and chronic fatigue syndrome, *Ciba Found Symp* 173:262-271, 1993.

111. Moldoveanu AI, Shephard RJ, Shek PN: The cytokine response to physical activity and training, *Sports Med* 31(2):115-144, 2001.

112. MMWR: HIV and AIDS: United States, 1981-2000, *MMWR* 50(21):430-434, 2001.

113. Nichols DS, Glenn TM: Effects of aerobic exercise on pain perception, affect, and level of disability in individuals with fibromyalgia, *Phys Ther* 74:327-332, 1994.

114. Nieman DC et al: Effects of brief, heavy exertion on circulating lymphocyte subpopulations and proliferative response, *Med Sci Sports Exerc* 24:1339, 1992.

115. Nieman DC et al: Infectious episodes in runners before and after the Los Angeles Marathon, *J Sports Med Phys Fitness* 30:316, 1990.

116. Nieman DC, Pedersen BK: *Nutrition and exercise immunology*, Boca Raton, Fla, 2000, CRC Press.

117. Pabst R, Westerman J, Binns RM: Lymphocytic trafficking. In Delves PJ, Roitt JM, editors: *Encyclopedia of immunology*, vol 3, ed 2, London, 1998, Academic Press.

118. Pedersen BK et al: Cytokines in aging and exercise, *Int J Sports Med* 21(Suppl 1) 4:S4-9, 2000.

119. Pedersen BK, Hoffman-Goetz L: Exercise and the immune system: regulation, integration, and adaptation, *Physiol Rev* 80(3):1055-1081, 2000.

120. Pedersen BK, Ostrowski K, Rohde T: The cytokine response to strenuous exercise, *Can J Physiol Pharmacol* 76(5):505-511, 1998.

121. Peralta L et al: Evaluation of youth preferences for rapid and innovative human immunodeficiency virus antibody tests, *Arch Pediatr Adolesc Med* 155(7):838-843, 2001.

122. Petri M: Is estrogen therapy safe in women with lupus? *J Musculoskel Med* 11(12):11, 1994.

123. Phaneuf S, Leeuwenburgh C: Apoptosis and exercise, *Med Sci Sports Exerc* 33(3):393-396, 2001.

124. Phoenix, Inc: Thermister product available at http://www.phoenix-pub.com. This is not a product endorsement; the authors receive no compensation for the sale of any products mentioned.

125. Poulsen HE, Weimann A, Loft S: Methods to detect DNA damage by free radicals: relation to exercise, *Proc Nutr Soc* 58(4):1007-1114, 1999.

126. Powell P et al: Randomised controlled trial of patient education to encourage graded exercise in chronic fatigue syndrome, *BMJ* 322(7283):387-390, 2001.

127. Pratley R et al: Strength training increases resting metabolic rate and norepinephrine levels in healthy 50 to 65 year old men, *J Appl Physiol* 76(1):133-137, 1994.

128. Quinn TC et al: Viral load and heterosexual transmission of human immunodeficiency virus type 1, *N Engl J Med* 342(13):921-929, 2000.

129. Rachlin ES, editor: Diagnosis and comprehensive management of myofascial pain, St Louis, 1994, Mosby.

130. Ramsey-Goldman R: Assessing disease activity in SLE patients during pregnancy, *Lupus* 8(8):677-684, 1999.

131. Ramsey-Goldman R, Schilling E: Immunosuppressive drug use during pregnancy, *Rheum Dis Clin North Am* 23(2):149-167, 1997.

132. Redwine L et al: Effects of sleep deprivation on interleukin-6, growth hormone, cortisol, and melatonin levels in humans, *J Clin Endocrinol Metab* 85(10):3597-3603, 2000.

133. Refetoff S, Weiss RE, Usala SJ: The syndromes of resistance to thyroid hormone, *Endocrine Rev* 14:348-399, 1993.

134. Rigsby LW: Effects of exercise training on men seropositive for HIV-1, *Med Sci Sports Exer* 24(1):6-12, 1992.

135. Roe DL, Lewis RE, Cruse JM: Association of HLA-DQ and -DR alleles with protection from or infection with HIV-1, *Exp Mol Pathol* 68(1):21-28, 2000.

136. Roubenoff R: Acquired immunodeficiency syndrome wasting, functional performance, and quality of life, *Am J Manage Care* 6(9):1003-1016, 2000.

137. Roubenoff R, Abad LW, Lundgren N: Effect of acquired immune deficiency syndrome wasting on the protein metabolic response to acute exercise, *Metabolism* 50(3):288-292, 2001.

138. Roubenoff R et al: A pilot study of exercise training to reduce trunk fat in adults with HIV-associated fat distribution, *AIDS* 12(11):1373-1375, 1999.

139. Russell IJ: Neurohormonal aspects of fibromyalgia syndrome, *Rheum Dis North Am* 15:149-168, 1989.

140. Russell IJ et al: Platelet 3H-imipramine uptake receptor density and serum serotonin levels in patients with fibromyalgia/fibrositis syndrome, *J Rheumatol* 19:104-109, 1992.

141. Russell IJ, Vaeroy H: Cerebrospinal fluid (CSF) biogenic amines in fibromyalgia syndrome, *ACR Sci Abstracts* S55, 1990.

142. Sacky K, Shankle D, Hobbs J: Just sweat it out: physical therapy's role in the HIV pandemic, *Res Initiat Treat Action* 4(4):8-10, 1998.

143. Salvato PD: *HIV update: treatment therapies for the millennium.* Presented at the Combined Sections Meeting, New Orleans, February 4, 2000.

144. Sande MA, Volberding PA: The medical management of AIDS, ed 6, Philadelphia, 1999, WB Saunders.

145. Scribner AN et al: Osteonecrosis in HIV: a case control study, *J Acquir Immune Defic Syndr* 25(1):19-25, 2000.

146. Senneff JA: Numb toes and aching soles: coping with peripheral neuropathy, San Antonio, Tex, 1999, Medpress. Available at http://www.medpress.com or by calling (888) 633-9898.

147. Sepkowitz KA: AIDS: the first 20 years, *N Engl J Med* 344(23):1764-1772, 2001.

148. Serhal D, Calabrese LH: Diagnosing and managing rheumatic disorders in HIV-infected persons, *J Musculo Med* 17(10):606-620, 2000.

149. Shephard RJ: Chronic fatigue syndrome: an update, *Sports Med* 31(3):167-194, 2001.

150. Shephard RJ, Shek PN: Effects of exercise and training on natural killer cell counts and cytolytic activity: a meta-analysis, *Sports Med* 28(3):177-195, 1999.

151. Sheriff S: Antibody-antigen complexes, three-dimensional structures. In Delves PJ, Roitt IM, editors: Encyclopedia of immunology, vol 1, ed 2, London, 1998, Academic Press.

152. Shinkai S et al: Effects of 12 weeks of aerobic exercise plus dietary restriction on body composition, resting energy expenditure, and aerobic fitness in mildly obese middle-aged women, *Euro J Applied Physio Occup Physio* 68:258-265, 1994.

153. Simons DG, Travell JG, Simons LS: Travell and Simons' myofascial pain and dysfunction, the trigger point manual, vol 1 and 2, Baltimore, 1999, Williams and Wilkins.

154. Smythe H: Examination for tenderness: learning to use 4 kg force, *J Rheumatol* 25(1):149-151, 1998.

155. Spence DW et al: Progressive resistance exercise: effect on muscle function and anthropometry of a select AIDS population, *Arch Phys Med Rehabil* 71(9):644-648, 1990.

156. Starlanyl DJ, Copeland M: *Fibromyalgia and chronic pain syndrome: a survival manual*, ed 2, Oakland, Calif, 2001, New Harbinger.

157. Starz TW et al: Putting the finger on fibromyalgia: the manual tender point survey, *J Musculoskel Med* 14(1):61-67, 1997.

158. Steinbrook R, Drazen JM: AIDS: Will the next 20 years be different? (editorial), *N Engl J Med* 344(23):1781-1782, 2001.

159. Straub RH et al: Neuropeptide Y cotransmission with norepinephrine in the sympathetic nerve-macrophage interplay, *J Neurochem* 75(6):2464-2471, 2000.

160. Ungvarski PJ, Flaskerud JH: *HIV/AIDS: a guide to primary care management*, ed 4, Philadelphia, 1999, WB Saunders.

161. Visser JT, De Kloet ER, Nagelkerken L: Altered glucocorticoid regulation of the immune response in chronic fatigue syndrome, *Ann NY Acad Sci* 917:868-875, 2000.

162. von Andrian UH, MacKay CR: T-cell function and migration, *N Engl J Med* 343(14):1020-1034, 2000.

163. Walker BD: Immunopathogenesis of HIV infection, *Medscape HIV/AIDS: Annual Update*, 2001, Medscape. Available at http://www.medscape.com/Medscape/HIV/Annual Update/2001.

164. Wallace D: Cytokine and immune regulation in FMS, *Arthritis Rheum* 32:1334-1335, 1989.

165. Ward MM et al: Psychosocial correlates of morbidity in women with systemic lupus erythematosus, *J Rheumatol* 26(10):2153-2158, 1999.

166. Watkins LR, Maier SF: The pain of being sick: implications of immune-to-brain communication for understanding pain, *Annu Rev Psychol* 51:29-57, 2000.

167. Watkins LR, Milligan Ed, Maier SF: Glial activation: a driving force for pathological pain, *Trends Neurosci* 24(8):450-455, 2001.

168. Wearden AJ et al: Randomised double-blind, placebo-controlled treatment trial of fluoxetine and graded exercise for chronic fatigue syndrome, *Br J Psychiatry* 172:485-490, 1998.

169. Webber LM et al: Evaluation of a rapid test for HIV antibodies in saliva and blood, *S Afr Med J* 90(10):1004-1007, 2000.

170. Wilson RB et al: Antipolymer antibody reactivity in a subset of patients with fibromyalgia correlates with severity, *J Rheumatol* 26(2):402-407, 1999.

171. Woods JA: Exercise and neuroendocrine modulation of macrophage function, *Int J Sports Med* 21(Suppl 1):S24-S30, 2000.

172. Yim YS, Wakeland EK: The genetics of lupus, *Curr Opin Nephrol Hypertens* 10(3):437-443, 2001.

173. Yunus MB: Towards a model of pathophysiology of fibromyalgia: aberrant central pain mechanisms with peripheral modulation, *J Rheumatol* 19:846-850, 1992.

174. Yunus MB et al: Plasma tryptophan and other amino acids in primary fibromyalgia: a controlled study, *J Rheumatol* 19:90-94, 1992.

175. Yunus MB et al: Fibromyalgia in men: comparison of clinical features with women, *J Rheumatol* 27(2):485-490, 2000.

CHAPTER 7

INFECTIOUS DISEASE

CATHERINE C. GOODMAN AND TERESA E. KELLY SNYDER

Although humans are continually exposed to a vast array of microorganisms in the environment, only a small proportion of those microbes are capable of interacting with the human host in such a way that infection and disease result. With the steady advances being made in medicine, people are living longer, but infection is still a frequent cause of hospital admission and remains an important cause of death, especially in the aging population.

From 1950 until 1980 the management of communicable infectious diseases was well under control; morbidity and mortality from infectious diseases such as yellow fever, cholera, typhus, malaria, typhoid fever, and plague were no longer serious threats in the United States. The widespread availability and use of sulfa drugs and antibiotics successfully treated tuberculosis, syphilis, gonorrhea, bacterial meningitis, scarlet fever, rheumatic fever, and nosocomial (hospital- or nursing home–acquired) infections. Organized efforts to immunize all children lowered the incidence of vaccine-preventable diseases such as measles, mumps, rubella, diphtheria, tetanus, and poliomyelitis. Research was then directed toward preventing and managing chronic disease.

Unfortunately, this period of reduced morbidity and mortality secondary to infectious disease did not last, and in the 1970s and 1980s, new infectious agents appeared. *Legionella*, human immunodeficiency virus (HIV), antibiotic-resistant organisms, and a resurgence of tuberculosis are examples of infectious processes that have returned the focus to the prevention and treatment of infectious diseases. Infectious diseases are spreading more rapidly throughout the world than in the past, facilitated by a combination of environmental disruption and increasing human mobility.

At the same time, infectious agents are now suspected in the origins of chronic diseases such as sarcoidosis, various forms of inflammatory bowel disease, scleroderma, rheumatoid arthritis, systemic lupus erythematosus (SLE), diabetes mellitus, primary biliary cirrhosis, Kawasaki disease and many forms of heart disease, Alzheimer's disease, multiple sclerosis, Hashimoto's thyroiditis, cerebral palsy, and many forms of cancer.[21,87]

In addition, an area of major public health concern is the continued emergence of antibiotic-resistant microorganisms that appear in hospitals and communities. The most common of these resistant bacteria are methicillin-resistant *Staphylococcus aureus* (MRSA); vancomycin-resistant *enterococci* (VRE), and multiple-drug–resistant *Mycobacterium tuberculosis* (MDR-TB). Additionally, a strain of *S. aureus* is developing a resistance to vancomycin, which will make treatment of this organism extremely difficult.

The cause of antibiotic resistance is primarily associated with the misuse and overuse of antibiotics in treatment of infections or potential infections. Other variables include large numbers of children in day care facilities; a sicker population base when hospitalized (therefore more susceptible to infection); and modern agriculture relying on antibiotics to boost growth and limit disease among cattle, chickens, and other animals leading to the spread of more dangerous microbes. The resistant organisms spread quickly and easily when inadequate precautions are taken to prevent transmission (e.g., poor use of handwashing and contact precautions).[1]

Although a number of new infectious diseases have appeared in recent years, a worldwide resurgence of long-standing diseases once thought to be well controlled has occurred. Epidemics of destructive organisms have accelerated; one third of the world's population now carries *Mycobacterium tuberculosis*. Organisms travel on the shoes of tourists, in the ballast of cargo ships, within the confines of jetliners, and in the blood of humans. When natural systems are weakened or altered by ecologic stresses (e.g., pollution, habitat destruction, weather disasters, climate change, famine), they become more vulnerable to damage or destruction by invading organisms, which can result in the spread of infection. Opportunistic organisms take advantage of the weakened defenses.

All health care professionals must maintain a vigilant attitude to preventing infectious disease. This requires an understanding of the infectious process, the chain of transmission, and selected aspects of control. In this chapter, a basic understanding of these concepts is provided along with a discussion of a few infectious diseases. Other pertinent infectious diseases are presented in appropriate chapters according to the primary clinical pathology (such as pneumonia in Chapter 14, bacterial meningitis in Chapter 28, and Sjögren's syndrome in Chapter 26).

SIGNS AND SYMPTOMS OF INFECTIOUS DISEASES

Clinical manifestations of infectious disease are many and varied depending on the etiologic agent (e.g., viruses, bacteria) (see the section on Types of Organisms in this chapter) and the system affected (e.g., respiratory, central nervous system [CNS], gastrointestinal [GI], genitourinary). Systemic symptoms of infectious disease can include fever and chills, sweating, malaise, and nausea and vomiting. Changes in blood composition may occur, such as an increased number of leukocytes or a change in the types of leukocytes. Older adults may experience a change in mentation (e.g., confusion, memory loss, difficulty concentrating). When observing any person for early signs of infection, the therapist will most likely see one or only a few symptoms listed (Table 7-1).

A change in body temperature is a characteristic systemic symptom of infectious disease but fever may accompany noninfectious causes such as inflammatory, neoplastic, and immunologically mediated diseases (Box 7-1). *Fever*, a sustained temperature above normal, can be caused by abnormalities of the hypothalamus, brain tumors, dehydration, or toxic substances affecting the temperature-regulating center of the hypothalamus. Certain protein substances and toxins can cause the set-point of the hypothalamic thermostat to rise. This re-

sults in activation of the hypothalamus to conserve heat and increase heat production. Substances that cause these effects are called *pyrogens*.

In infectious disease the endotoxins of some bacteria and the extracts of normal leukocytes (cytokines) are pyrogenic. They act to raise the thermostat in the hypothalamus, thus raising the body temperature. Fever patterns may differ depending on the specific infectious disease present and occur clinically on a continuum from fever associated with an acute illness lasting 7 to 10 days, to sepsis and ongoing infection lasting longer than 10 days, to fever of unknown origin (FUO) associated with a possible infectious origin lasting at least 3 weeks. Other causes of FUO include neoplasm (lymphoma and leukemia are the most common); autoimmune disorders such as Still's disease, SLE, and polyarteritis nodosa; and miscellaneous diseases, including temporal arteritis, sarcoidosis, alcoholic hepatitis, and drug-induced fever, among others.[45]

A general rule, the 102° F rule, divides conditions into two groups: those that do not cause temperature elevations exceeding 102° F (39° C) and those that regularly exceed 102° F. Table 7-2 reflects hospital data, whereas the outpatient population is more likely to experience fever accompanied by generalized arthralgias and myalgias associated with a self-limiting illness or fever with localized symptom(s) such as a sore throat, cough, or right lower quadrant pain, as occurs with bacterial infection. Temperature elevation to 104° F (40° C) may cause delirium and convulsions, particularly in children. An extremely high fever may damage cells irreversibly. Some people with serious infection do not initially develop fever but instead become *tachypneic, confused*, or develop *hypotension*. Most often, this situation occurs in older adults, hospitalized client with a nosocomial infection or in the immunocompromised person.

Inflammation and its *exudates* may remain localized, permeate the tissue, or spread throughout the body via the blood or lymph. Infection can develop, as is the case with an *abscess*, a localized infection and inflammation with purulent exudate. Leukocytes form a wall around the organisms. The abscess deepens as more leukocytes are drawn into the area, more organisms are killed, and more necrotic tissue is dissolved. The exudate may eventually be autolyzed and resorbed by the body, in which case the inflammation and infection are resolved. Rupture of the abscess and drainage into other tissues can spread the infection to other areas of the body.

For example, infectious abdominal disorders (e.g., Crohn's disease, diverticulitis, appendicitis); tuberculosis of the spine; pelvic inflammatory disease (PID); vertebral osteomyelitis; septic arthritis of the sacroiliac joint; and tumor of the thigh can result in abscess formation in the space between the posterior peritoneum and the psoas and iliac fascia.[30,61] A psoas

---

TABLE	7-1

Signs and Symptoms of Infectious Disease

Fever, chills, malaise (most common early symptoms)
Englarged lymph nodes

Integument	Purulent drainage from abscess, open wound, or skin lesion
	Skin rash, red streaks
	Bleeding from gums or into joints; joint effusion or erythema
Cardiovascular	Petechial lesions
	Tachycardia (see the sections on Aneurysm and Thrombophlebitis in Chapter 11)
	Hypotension
	Change in pulse rate (may increase or decrease depending on the type of infection)
Central nervous system	Altered level of consciousness, confusion, convulsions
	Headache
	Photophobia
	Memory loss
	Stiff neck, myalgia
Gastrointestinal	Nausea
	Vomiting
	Diarrhea
Genitourinary	Dysuria or flank pain
	Hematuria
	Oliguria
	Urgency, frequency
Upper respiratory	Tachypnea
	Cough
	Dyspnea
	Hoarseness
	Sore throat
	Nasal drainage
	Sputum production
	Oxygen desaturation
	Decreased exercise tolerance
	Prolonged ventilatory support

BOX	7-1

Common Causes of Fever in the Hospitalized Person

Atelectasis	Urinary tract infection
Pneumonia	Drugs
Catheter-related infection	Pulmonary emboli
Surgical wound infection	Infected pressure ulcers

TABLE 7-2

Most Common Causes of Prolonged Fever*

Conditions in Which Fever Generally Does Not Exceed 102° F	Conditions in Which Fever Regularly Exceeds 102° F
Catheter-associated bacteriuria	Malignant hyperthermia (secondary to anesthesia)
Atelectasis	Transfusion reactions
Phlebitis	Urosepsis
Pulmonary emboli	Intravenous (IV) line sepsis
Dehydration	Prosthetic valve endocarditis
Pancreatitis	Intraabdominal or pelvic peritonitis or abscess
Myocardial infarction	*Clostridium difficile* colitis
Uncomplicated wound infections	Procedure-related bacteremia
Any malignancy	Nosocomial pneumonia
Cytomegalovirus	Drug fever
Hepatitis	HIV infection
Infectious mononucleosis (Epstein-Barr virus)	Heat stroke
Subacute bacterial endocarditis	Acute bacterial endocarditis
Tuberculosis	Tuberculosis (usually disseminated or extrapulmonary)
	Lymphoma
	Metastasizing carcinoma to liver or central nervous system

*The evaluation of fever magnitude with the 102° F rule is most often done in the acute care setting. This is a general guideline that must be taken into consideration with other presenting factors.

abscess is usually confined within the psoas fascia, but occasionally, because of anatomic relations, infection extends to the buttock, hip, or upper thigh. Such an abscess causes true musculoskeletal symptoms of back pain, or pain referred to the hip or knee, and limited range of hip motion from an underlying systemic cause. Flexion contracture of the hip (positive Thomas test) may develop from reflex spasm, and extension of the thigh is very painful; hip abduction and adduction evoke minimal discomfort. An unexplained limp may be the initial symptom, and this will be an important clinical clue when taking a history (see Figs. 15-10 and 15-11). Only days to weeks later does lower abdominal pain develop, and the person becomes acutely ill with a high fever.

Rash with fever can result from a local infectious process caused by any microbe that has successfully penetrated the stratum corneum (see Fig. 9-1) and multiplied locally. Skin rashes may also occur with infection elsewhere in the body unrelated to local skin disease (e.g., scarlet fever caused by streptococci, also called *scarlatina*). The most common types of localized skin lesions associated with infectious disease are maculopapular eruptions (e.g., classic childhood viral illnesses such as measles, rubella, roseola, fifth disease); nodular lesions (e.g., streptococcus, *Pseudomonas*); diffuse erythema (e.g., scarlet fever, toxic shock syndrome); vesiculobullous eruptions (e.g., varicella, herpes zoster); and petechial purpuric eruptions (e.g., Epstein-Barr virus [EBV] and cytomegalovirus [CMV]). Specific types of skin lesions are discussed in Chapter 9.

Red streaks radiating from an infection site, known as *blood poisoning,* in the direction of a regional lymph node may be associated with lymphangitis secondary to an infection such as cellulitis. Lymphangitis, an acute inflammation of the subcutaneous lymphatic channels, usually occurs as a result of hemolytic streptococci or staphylococci (or both) entering the lymphatic channels from an abrasion or local trauma, wound, or infection (see Chapters 9 and 12). The red streak may be obvious, or it may be faint and easily overlooked, especially in dark-skinned people. The nodes most often affected are the submandibular, cervical, inguinal, and axillary nodes, in that order. Involved nodes are usually tender and enlarged (greater than 3 cm).

Inflamed lymph nodes can be associated with other infectious diseases and may be palpated by the therapist, especially in cervical, axillary, or inguinal areas when presenting musculoskeletal symptoms are evident in those areas. For example, intraoral infection may cause an inflamed cervical node leading to spasm of the sternocleidomastoid muscle causing neck pain. Palpation may appear to aggravate a primary spasm as if originating in the muscle, when in fact a lymph node under the muscle is the source of the symptom. In acute infections, nodes are tender asymmetrically, enlarged, and matted together. The overlying skin may be erythematous (red) and warm. Unilaterally warm, tender, enlarged, and fluctuant lymph nodes sometimes associated with elevated body temperature may be caused by pyogenic infections and requires medical referral.

Supraclavicular and inguinal nodes are also common metastatic sites for cancer. Nodes involved with metastatic cancer are usually hard and fixed to the underlying tissue. Any suspicious lymph node (e.g., changes in size: greater than 1 cm; changes in shape: matted together; or changes in consistency: rubbery) or the presence of painless, enlarged lymph nodes must be evaluated by a physician. See the section on lymph nodes in Special Implications for the Therapist: Anatomy of the Lymphatic System, 12-1.

Joint effusion, usually of one joint (monarticular), associated with infectious arthritis can occur as a result of bacterial, mycobacterial, fungal, or viral etiologic agents. Streptococcal bacteremia from any cause can result in suppurative arthritis (inflammatory with pus formation). Bone and joint infections are discussed more completely in Chapter 24.

AGING AND INFECTIOUS DISEASES

Aging is a state of immune dysregulation. Not only does involution (shriveling) of the thymus and altered T-cell–mediated immunity occur, but increased antibody production to self-antigens also takes place. Diminished cell-mediated immunity results in the reactivation of dormant infections such as herpes zoster and tuberculosis. Influenza deaths after age 65 are increased, and the antibody response to influenza vaccine is decreased.[13]

The aging process at the tissue and cellular level may lead to increased susceptibility to infection because of atrophic skin; achlorhydria (absence of hydrochloric acid in gastric juice); decreased cough and gag reflexes; and decreased bronchiolar elasticity and mucociliary activity.[13] The most important determining factors of how well aging people can handle infections are related to their underlying mental and physical disability, nutritional status, and the presence of chronic disease such as renal and cardiac impairment or peripheral vascular insufficiency. Environmental factors also play a role in preventing infections.

In many aging people, physical or psychologic impairment and decline may result in indifference to personal hygiene and loss of manual dexterity, body mobility, or vision. Denture-associated infections may occur in up to 60% of older adult denture-wearing clients. Predisposing factors include flaccid, sagging cheeks, deepened labial angles constantly moistened by saliva, and ill-fitting dentures, often worn for a considerable time without replacement or repair.[25]

Many types of infections are seen in the aging adult, but early recognition of infection in the older adult is difficult because people underreport symptoms, the presentation is often vague or atypical, and symptoms are difficult to assess. The older adult may be unable to describe the present illness or past history or list the medications being taken. A complete physical examination may be difficult because of the person's uncooperativeness, cognitive impairment, neurologic deficits, or contracted limbs. Pain may be poorly localized or absent, as in appendicitis, or it may be confused with preexisting conditions, as in septic arthritis or degenerative joint disease (DJD).

The aging person can have more serious infections with little or no fever because of an impaired thermoregulatory system* or secondary to the masking effects of drugs such as aspirin, other antiinflammatory drugs, and corticosteroids. If the febrile response is absent in an older adult with a serious infection, it is a grave sign. Acute infections in the aging may cause confusion even in the absence of fever. A change in mental state with confusion or lethargy may be the earliest sign of acute infection. Chronic infections of the lungs, bone, skin, kidneys, and CNS may also present as dementia.[77]

Aging spouse caregivers of aging people are significantly more likely to have communicable upper respiratory tract infections than are others. Many aging adults are in acute or extended care settings and are therefore more likely to be exposed to nosocomial pathogens such as aerobic gram-negative bacilli and *S. aureus* and VRE.[13]

INFECTIOUS DISEASES

◆ Definition and Overview

Infection is a process in which an organism establishes a parasitic relationship with its host. This invasion and multiplication of microorganisms produces an immune response and subsequent signs and symptoms. Such reproduction injures the host by causing cellular damage from microorganism-producing toxins or intracellular multiplication or by competing with the host's metabolism. The host's immune response may compound the tissue damage; such damage may be localized (e.g., as in infected pressure ulcers) or systemic. However, in some instances, microorganisms may be present in the tissues of the host and yet not cause symptomatic disease. This process is called *colonization of organisms*. The person with colonization may be a carrier and

transmit the organisms to others but does not have detectable symptoms of infection.

The development of an infection begins with transmission of an infectious organism (agent, pathogen, pathogenic agent) and depends on a complex interaction of the pathogen, an environment conducive to transmission of the organism, and the susceptibility of the human host. Even after successful transmission of a pathogen, the host may experience more than one possible outcome. The pathogen may merely contaminate the body surface and be destroyed by first-line defenses such as intact skin or mucous membranes that prevent further invasion or a subclinical infection may occur in which no apparent symptoms are evident other than an identifiable immune response of the host. A rise in the titer of antibody directed against the infecting agent is often the only detectable response. Antibiotic treatment is not necessary, although infection control procedures remain in force to prevent spreading the bacteria to others. A third possible outcome is the development of a clinically apparent infection in which the host-parasite interaction causes obvious injury and is accompanied by one or more clinical symptoms. This outcome is called *infectious disease* and ranges in severity from mild to fatal depending on the organism and the response and underlying health of the host.[44]

The period between the pathogen entering the host and the appearance of clinical symptoms is called the *incubation period*. This period may last from a few days to several months, depending on the causative organism and type of disease. Disease symptoms herald the end of the incubation period. A *latent* infection occurs after a microorganism has replicated but remains dormant or inactive in the host, sometimes for years (e.g., tuberculosis, herpes zoster). The host may harbor a pathogen in sufficient quantities to be shed at any time after latency and toward the end of the incubation period. This time period when an organism can be shed is called the *period of communicability*.

From this concept of communicability, communicable diseases can be defined as any disease whereby the causative agent may pass or be carried from one person to another directly or indirectly. It usually precedes symptoms and continues through part or all of clinical disease, sometimes extending to convalescence, but it is important to note that an asymptomatic host can still transmit a pathogen. The communicable period, like the incubation period and mode of transmission, varies with different pathogens and different diseases.[84]

◆ Types of Organisms

A great variety of microorganisms are responsible for infectious diseases, including viruses; mycoplasmas; bacteria; rickettsiae; chlamydiae; protozoa; fungi (yeasts and molds); helminths (e.g., tapeworms); mycobacteria; and prions. All microorganisms can be distinguished by certain intrinsic properties such as shape, size, structure, chemical composition, antigenic makeup, growth requirements, ability to produce toxins, and ability to remain alive (viability) under adverse conditions such as drying, sunlight, or heat. These properties provide the basis for identification and classification of the organisms. Knowledge of the properties permits diagnosis of a specific pathogen in specimens of body fluids, secretions, or exudates. All these properties are important to consider when looking for ways to interfere with the mechanisms of transmission.

---

*Fever in older people may not be high enough to cause concern because the basal body temperature is low. Temperatures should be taken in the evening and a lower threshold for infection should be used (e.g., oral temperature of 99° F or 100° F with a change in function).

Viruses are subcellular organisms made up only of a ribonucleic acid (RNA) or a deoxyribonucleic acid (DNA) nucleus covered with proteins. They are the smallest known organisms, visible only through an electron microscope. Viruses are completely dependent on host cells and cannot replicate unless they invade a host cell and stimulate it to participate in the formation of additional virus particles. The estimated 400 viruses that infect humans are classified according to their size; shape (spherical, rod-shaped, or cubic); or means of transmission (respiratory, fecal, oral, or sexual). Viruses are not susceptible to antibiotics and cannot be destroyed by pharmacologic means. However, antiviral medications can mitigate (moderate) the course of the viral illness. For example, acyclovir, an antiviral medication used for herpesvirus interferes with DNA synthesis, causing decreased viral replication and decreasing the time of lesional healing.

Mycoplasmas are unusual, self-replicating bacteria that have no cell wall components and very small genomes. For this reason, antibiotics that are active against bacterial cell walls have no effect on mycoplasmas. At present, mycoplasmas remain sensitive to some antibiotics. They require a strict dependence on the host for nutrition and sustenance and are able to pass through many bacteria-retaining filters or barriers because they are very small.[6]

Bacteria are single-celled microorganisms with well-defined cell walls that can grow independently on artificial media without the need for other cells. Bacteria can be classified according to shape. Spherical bacterial cells are called *cocci*; rod-shaped bacteria, *bacilli*; and spiral-shaped bacteria, *spirilla* or *spirochetes*. Bacteria can also be classified according to their response to staining (gram-positive, gram-negative, or acid-fast); motility (motile or nonmotile); tendency toward capsulation (encapsulated or nonencapsulated); and capacity to form spores (sporulating or nonsporulating).

Bacteria can also be classified according to whether oxygen is needed to replicate and develop (aerobic) or whether they can sustain life in an oxygen poor (anaerobic) environment. Anaerobic bacteria are organisms that require reduced oxygen tension for growth. Normal human flora is primarily anaerobic, and disease can be produced when these normal organisms are displaced from their usual tissue sites (e.g., mouth, skin, large bowel, female genital tract) into other tissues or closed body spaces.[18] Other common anaerobic organisms include the spore-forming bacilli such as *Clostridium* (*botulinum* or *tetani*) that thrive in a strictly anaerobic environment.

Rickettsiae are primarily animal pathogens that generally produce disease in humans through the bite of an insect vector such as a tick, flea, louse, or mite. They are small, gram-negative, obligate intracellular organisms that often cause life-threatening infections. Like viruses, these microorganisms require a host for replication. Three categories of the family Rickettsiaceae are *Rickettsia*, *Coxiella*, and *Bartonella*.[10] Chlamydiae are smaller than rickettsiae and bacteria but larger than viruses. They too depend on host cells for replication, but unlike viruses, they always contain both DNA and RNA and are susceptible to antibiotics.

Protozoa have a single cell unit or a group of nondifferentiated cells, loosely held together and not forming tissues. They have cell membranes rather than cell walls, and their nuclei are surrounded by nuclear membranes. Larger parasites include roundworms and flatworms. *Fungi* are unicellular to filamentous organisms possessing hyphae (filamentous outgrowths) surrounded by cell walls and containing nuclei (eukaryocyte). Fungi show relatively little cellular specialization and occur as yeast (single-cell, oval-shaped organisms) or molds (organisms with branching filaments). Depending on the environment, some fungi may occur in both forms. Fungal diseases in humans are called *mycoses*.

Prions are newly discovered proteinaceous, infectious particles consisting of proteins but without nucleic acids. These particles are transmitted from animals to humans and are characterized by a long, latent interval in the host. When reactivated, they cause a rapidly progressive deteriorating state in the host (e.g., Creutzfeldt-Jakob disease, bovine spongiform encephalopathy or "mad cow disease").[26]

◆ The Chain of Transmission

Infection begins with transmission of a pathogen to the host. Successful transmission depends on a pathogenic agent, a reservoir, a portal of exit from the reservoir, a mode (mechanism) of transmission, a portal of entry into the host, and a susceptible host. This sequence of events is called the *chain of transmission* (Table 7-3).

Pathogens

Humans coexist with many microorganisms in complex, mutually beneficial relationships. Even so, many organisms are parasitic, maintaining themselves at the expense of their host. Some parasites arouse a pathologic response in the host and

TABLE 7-3

Chain of Transmission of Infectious Disease

TRANSMISSION CHAIN	FACTORS
Pathogen or agent	Viruses, mycoplasmas, bacteria, rickettsiae, chlamydiae, protozoa, fungi, prions
Reservoir	Humans (clinical cases, subclinical cases, and carriers)
	Animal, arthropod, plant, soil, food, organic substance
Portal of exit	Genitourinary tract, gastrointestinal tract, respiratory tract, oral cavity, open lesion, blood, vaginal secretions, semen, tears, excretions (urine, feces)
Transmission	Contact (direct or indirect)
	Airborne (float on air currents and remain suspended for hours; small particles)
	Droplet (fall out within 3 feet of source; large particles)
	Vehicle (through a common source such as water or food)
	Vectorborne (carried by insects or animals)
Modes of entry	Ingestion, inhalation, percutaneous injection, transplacental entry, mucous membranes
Susceptible host	Specific immune reactions
	Nonspecific body defenses
	Host characteristics: age, sex, ethnic group, heredity, behaviors
	Environmental and general health status

are called *pathogens* or *pathogenic agents*. A *pathogen* is defined as any microorganism that has the capacity to cause disease.[76] As such, pathogens are ineffective parasites because they stimulate a disease response, which may harm the host and eventually kill the pathogen.

The ability of a pathogen to stimulate an immune response in the host (antigenicity) varies greatly among organisms, depending on the site of invasion, the number of pathogenic organisms, and the dissemination of organisms in the body. The immune status of a person plays the largest role in determining the risk for infection and the ability of the host to combat organisms that have gained entry.

The mode of action of a pathogen refers to how the organism produces a pathologic process. Great variation exists among the various pathogens. Some intracellular pathogens, like viruses, invade cells and interfere with cellular metabolism, growth, and replication, whereas others invade and cause hyperplasia and cell death. Yet other organisms, such as the influenza virus, have the potential to alter their antigenic characteristics. This virus is capable of extensive gene rearrangements, resulting in significant changes in surface antigen structure. This ability allows new strains to evade host antibody responses directed at earlier strains.

Some viruses (e.g., all members of the herpesvirus group) cause a persistent latent infection that can be reactivated in certain circumstances. HIV causes immunosuppression by destroying helper T lymphocytes. Some pathogens such as the tetanus bacillus, produce a toxin that interferes with intercellular responses. Some bacteria, such as diphtheria and tetanus, secrete water-soluble antigenic exotoxins that are quickly disseminated in the blood, causing potentially severe systemic and neurologic manifestations. Larger parasites such as roundworms cause anemia and interfere with the function of the GI system.

The characteristics of the organism and the susceptibility of the host influence the likelihood of a pathogen producing infectious disease and the type of disease produced. Not all pathogens have an equal probability of inducing disease in the same host population. *Principle* pathogens are those pathogens that regularly cause disease in people with apparently intact defense systems. *Opportunist* pathogens are those pathogens that do not cause disease in people with intact host defense systems but can clearly cause devastating disease in many hospitalized and immunocompromised clients.[76] Organisms that may be harmless members of normal flora in healthy people may act as virulent invaders in people with severe defects in host defense mechanisms.[60]

Pathogenicity, the ability of the organism to induce disease, depends on the organism's speed of reproduction in the host, the extent of damage it causes to tissues, and the strength of any toxin released by the pathogen. *Virulence* refers to the potency of the pathogen in producing severe disease and is measured by the case-fatality rate (i.e., the number of people who die of the disease divided by the number of people who have the disease). Virulence provides a quantitative measure of pathogenicity. The amount and destructive potential of released toxin is closely related to virulence.

Reservoir

A reservoir is an environment in which an organism can live and multiply such as an animal, plant, soil, food, or other organic substance or combination of substances. The reservoir provides the essentials for survival of the organism at specific stages in its life cycle. Some parasites have more than one reservoir such as the yellow fever virus, which can maintain life in humans and other animals. Some parasites require more than one reservoir at different growth stages and still others such as most sexually transmitted organisms require only a human reservoir.

Human and animal reservoirs can be symptomatic or asymptomatic carriers of the pathogen. A carrier maintains an environment that promotes growth, multiplication, and shedding of the parasite without exhibiting signs of disease. Hepatitis is a common example of this carrier state in humans.

Portal of Exit

The portal of exit is the place from which the parasite leaves the reservoir. Generally, this is the site of growth of the organism and corresponds to the system of entry into the next host. For example, the portal of exit for GI parasites is usually the feces, and the portal of entry into a new host is the mouth. Exceptions to the case include hookworm eggs, which are shed in the feces but enter through the skin of a person walking barefoot in soil containing hatched eggs.

Common portals of exit include secretions and fluids (e.g., respiratory secretions, blood, vaginal secretions, semen, tears); excretions such as urine and feces; open lesions; and exudates such as pus from an open wound or ulcer. Some organisms such as HIV have more than one portal of exit. Knowledge of the portal of exit is essential for preventing transmission of a pathogen.

Mode of Transmission

For infection to be transmitted, the invading organism must be transported from the infected source to a susceptible host. Microorganisms are transmitted by several possible routes, and the same microorganism can travel by more than one route. The five main routes of transmission are contact, airborne, droplet, vehicle, and vector borne. *Contact transmission* occurs directly or indirectly. Direct contact is the direct transfer of microorganisms that come into physical contact either by skin-to-skin or mucous membrane-to-mucous membrane (e.g., sexual contact, biting, touching, kissing). Indirect contact involves transfer of microorganisms from a source to a host by passive transfer from an inanimate, intermediate object,* called a *fomite*. An example of indirect transmission is transfer of human immunodeficiency virus from a contaminated source to a host through a needlestick. Another example of indirect contact includes oral-fecal transmission by the ingestion of enteric pathogens from a food prepared by a person who does not wash his or her hands.[44]

Airborne transmission occurs when disease-causing organisms are so small (under 5 microns) that they are capable of floating on air currents within a room and remain suspended in the air for several hours. They are often propelled from the respiratory tract through coughing or sneezing. A host then inhales the particles directly into the respiratory tract (e.g. tuberculosis, chickenpox, rubeola measles).[34]

---

*Inanimate objects can include items such as the telephone, sphygmomanometer, bedside rails, tray tables, countertops, and other items that come into direct contact with the infected person, thus emphasizing the need for thorough handwashing at all times.

Droplet transmission is different from airborne transmission because droplets are larger particles (greater than 5 microns) than airborne particles and they do not remain suspended in air but fall out within 3 feet of the source. They are produced when a person coughs or sneezes and then travel only a short distance. A common example of droplet-spread infection is influenza. Those people who are in closest proximity to the infected source have the highest risk for infection.[44]

Vehicle transmission occurs when infectious organisms (e.g., Salmonellosis) are transmitted through a common source (e.g., contaminated food, water, and intravenous [IV] fluid) to many potential susceptible hosts. *Vectorborne* transmission of infectious organisms involves insects and/or animals that act as intermediaries between two or more hosts. Lyme disease, Rocky Mountain spotted fever, and Creutzfeldt-Jakob disease are examples of vectorborne diseases. Nosocomial infections are infections acquired during hospitalization. In the United States, about 5% of people who enter the hospital without infection acquire a nosocomial infection.

Nosocomial infections result in prolongation of hospital stays, increase in cost of care, significant morbidity, and a mortality rate of about 5%.[45] The most common infections are urinary tract infections (usually associated with Foley catheters or urologic procedures) or bloodstream infections. Bloodstream infections can occur as a result of indwelling IV catheters but also from surgical wound infections; abscesses; pneumonia; especially in intubated individuals or those with altered levels of consciousness; and GI and genitourinary infections.

In general, increases in nosocomial infections can be related to more frequent use of invasive devices for monitoring or therapy; more colonization and infection by multiple-drug–resistant organisms (both viral and bacterial); and greater debilitation and severity of illness of hospitalized clients who acquire these infections. Additionally, nosocomial infections are more virulent and more resistant to treatment. The increased use of invasive and surgical procedures, immunosuppressants, antibiotics, and the lack of handwashing predispose people to such infections and superinfections. At the same time, the growing number of personnel that come into contact with the client makes the risk of exposure greater.

Prevention is of critical importance in controlling nosocomial infections. The concept of standard precautions emphasizes that all clients must be treated as though each one has a potential bloodborne, transmissible disease and thus all body secretions are handled with care to prevent disease. Handwashing has been cited as the easiest and most effective means of preventing nosocomial infection and must be done routinely even when gloves are used (Box 7-2).[45]

Portal of Entry

A pathogen may enter a new host by ingestion, inhalation, or bites or through contact with mucous membranes, percutaneously or transplacentally. Infectious diseases vary as to the number of organisms and the duration of exposure required to start the infectious process in a new host.

Host Susceptibility

Each person has his or her own susceptibility to infectious disease, and this susceptibility can vary throughout time. A susceptible host has personal characteristics and behaviors that

---

BOX **7-2**

Effective Handwashing Technique

Use plain soap and water scrubbing at least take as long as it takes to sing "Happy Birthday" or "Twinkle, Twinkle Little Star" twice.

Both sides of both hands must be scrubbed along with wrists, web between the fingers, and under the nails.

Use a paper towel to turn off the faucet and if leaving the room; use the paper towel to open the door before discarding the towel.

Hands must also be washed after taking gloves off and before touching anything.

Wash hands before and after each and every client (before to protect the client and after to protect yourself and others).

Do not touch a chart with gloved hands.

When dealing with antimicrobial-resistant gram-positive cocci (e.g., methicillin resistant *Staphylococcus aureus*, vancomycin-resistant *Enterococci*) an antimicrobial soap is recommended.

---

increase the probability of an infectious disease developing. Biologic and personal characteristics such as age, sex, ethnicity, and heredity influence this probability. General health and nutritional status, hormonal balance, and the presence of concurrent disease also play a role. Likewise, living conditions and personal behaviors such as drug use, diet, hygiene, and sexual practices influence the risk of exposure to pathogens and resistance once exposed.

Older adults in hospitals and long-term care facilities are already susceptible hosts, especially if poorly nourished. Immunosuppressive agents and corticosteroids decrease the body's ability to resist infection. Inadequate or absent handwashing or other breaches of aseptic technique result in spread of microorganisms from health care workers (HCWs) to clients and between individuals receiving health care. Surfaces of equipment can become contaminated and then transmit microorganisms that cause infection. Incorrect isolation procedures such as leaving doors open to rooms in which airborne precautions are in effect or not using masks increase the risk of transmitting organisms that cause nosocomial infections.

The presence of underlying medical disorders (e.g., malignancy, diabetes, renal failure, acquired immune deficiency syndrome [AIDS], and cirrhosis) decrease T cell– and B-cell–mediated immune function. Breaches of body integrity such as nasogastric and chest tubes, intubation, urinary catheters, and IV devices impair the body's defense mechanisms, decreasing the ability of the integumentary, GI, genitourinary, and respiratory systems to resist invasion by microorganisms.[98]

Lines of Defense

Susceptibility is also influenced by the presence of anatomic and physiologic defenses, sometimes called *lines of defense*. The *first-line defenses* are external such as intact skin and mucous membranes, oil and perspiration on skin, cilia in respiratory passages, gag and coughing reflexes, peristalsis in the GI tract, and the flushing action of tears, saliva, and mucus.

These first-line defenses act to inhibit invasion of pathogens and remove them before they have an opportunity to multiply. The chemical composition of body secretions such as tears and sweat, together with the pH of saliva, vaginal secretions, urine, and digestive juices, further prevents or inhibits growth of organisms. Compromise in any of these natural defenses increases host susceptibility to pathogen invasion.

Another important first-line defense is the normal flora of microorganisms that inhabit the skin and mucous membranes in the oral cavity, GI tract, and vagina. These organisms occur naturally and usually coexist with their host in a mutually beneficial relationship. Through a mechanism called *microbial antagonism* they control the replication of potential pathogens. The importance of this mechanism is evident when it is disturbed, as happens when extensive antibiotic therapy destroys normal flora in the oral or vaginal cavity, resulting in *Candida albicans,* an overgrowth of yeast. Some normal flora can become pathogenic under specific conditions such as immunosuppression or displacement of the pathogen to another area of the body. Displacement of normal flora is a common cause of nosocomial infections. This can occur when *Escherichia coli,* ordinarily normal flora in the GI tract, invade the urinary tract. Invasive procedures increase the risk of displacing these organisms.

The *second-line defense,* the inflammatory process, and the *third-line defense,* the immune response, share several physiologic components. These include the lymphatic system, leukocytes, and a multitude of chemicals, proteins, and enzymes that facilitate the internal defenses. Once a microorganism penetrates the first line of defense, the inflammatory response is initiated. Inflammation is a local reaction to cell injury of any type whether from physical, chemical, or thermal damage, or microbial invasion. As a response to microbial injury, inflammation is aimed at preventing further invasion by walling off, destroying, or neutralizing the invading organism.

The early inflammatory response is protective, but it can continue for sustained periods in some infections, leading to granuloma formation. The production of new leukocytes may be stimulated for weeks or months and is reflected in an elevated WBC count. However, sustained inflammation can become chronic and result in destruction of healthy tissues. Extensive necrosis from persistent inflammation can increase tissue susceptibility to the infectious agent or provide an ideal setting for invasion by other pathogens.

The first- and second-line defenses are nonspecific—that is, they operate against all infectious agents in the same way. In contrast, the immune system responds in a specific manner to individual pathogens, as long as the organism has antigenic characteristics. Generally, antigens are proteins, large polysaccharides, or large lipoprotein complexes that stimulate an immune response. Not all microorganisms are antigenic, but some are bound by complement or other host-produced substances to form an antigen that elicits an immune response. An immune response is triggered after foreign materials have been cleared from an area of inflammation. For specific details regarding cell-mediated versus humoral immune responses, see Chapter 6.

◆ Control of Transmission
Much can be done to prevent transmission of infectious diseases, including the use of barriers and isolation; comprehensive immunizations, including the required immunization of travelers to or emigrants from endemic areas; drug prophylaxis; improved nutrition, living conditions, and sanitation; and correction of environmental factors. Breaking the transmission chain at any of these links can help control transmission of infectious diseases. The link most amenable to control varies with the characteristics of the organism, its reservoirs, the type of pathologic response it produces, and the available technology for control. The general goal is to break the chain at the most cost-effective point or points—that is, the point at which the greatest number of people can be protected with available technology and the least amount of resources.

Isolation and barriers can be used to prevent the transmission of microorganisms from infected or colonized people to other nonaffected people. In hospital or institutional settings, the purpose of isolating individuals or residents is to prevent the transmission of colonized or infectious microorganisms among clients, visitors, and HCWs. In 1996 the Centers for Disease Control and Prevention (CDC) and the Hospital Infection Control Practices Advisory Committee (HICPAC) issued a revision of the isolation guidelines. The new guidelines outline a two-tiered approach with standard precautions that apply to all clients and transmission-based precautions that apply to anyone with documented or suspected infection or colonization with specific microorganisms.

These *transmission-based precautions* are defined according to the major modes of transmission of infectious agents (contact, airborne, and droplet) in the health care setting (Table 7-4). Standard precautions have replaced universal precautions. Barrier precautions stipulate that gloves should be worn to touch any of the following: blood; all body fluids; secretions and excretions except sweat, regardless of whether these are visibly bloody; nonintact skin; and mucous membranes. *Infectious waste* is defined as free-flowing blood/body fluids present in sufficient quantity to drip, splash, or flake from dressings or containers (Box 7-3).

Hands must be washed immediately after gloves are removed and between clients. For procedures that are likely to generate splashes or sprays of body fluid, a mask with eye protection or a face shield and gown should be worn. Gowns should be of a material that prevents penetration by microorganisms and subsequent contamination of the skin or clothing.[7,34] Needles should not be recapped, bent or broken, but should be disposed of in a puncture-resistant container.[28]

Immunization, by decreasing host susceptibility, can now control many diseases, including diphtheria, tetanus, pertussis, measles, mumps, rubella, some forms of meningitis, poliomyelitis, hepatitis A and B, pneumococcal pneumonia, influenza (certain strains),* and rabies. Vaccines, which contain live but attenuated (weakened) or killed microbes, induce active immunity against bacterial and viral diseases by stimulating antibody formation.† These molecules lock onto specific proteins made by a virus or bacterium, which are often those proteins lodged in the microbe's outer coat. Once antibodies attach to an invading microbe, other immune defenses are

---

*Each year the CDC issues updated information on the vaccine and antiviral agents available for controlling influenza during the current influenza season.
†Side effects to immunization can occur, but the incidence of significant adverse effects of immunization among humans remains very small.[2,3,4] The potential increase in susceptibility to influenza and death from respiratory illness in high-risk people (e.g., those with rheumatoid arthritis, the aging adult, and chronically ill or immunosuppressed individual) suggests that the influenza and pneumococcal vaccines should include these groups in standard immunization programs.[3]

TABLE	7-4

Type of Transmission-Based Precautions and Prevention Guidelines

TYPE OF PRECAUTION	TYPE OF MICROORGANISM	MEASURES TAKEN
Standard precautions	Bloodborne pathogens; applies to all clients	See Appendix A
Airborne precautions	Microorganisms transmitted by small particle residue; can suspend in the air and be dispersed by air currents (i.e., coughing, sneezing, talking) EXAMPLES: • Measles (rubeola) • *M. tuberculosis* (MDRT) • Varicella (chickenpox) • Zoster (disseminated shingles)	• Private room with monitored negative airflow • ROOM DOOR CLOSED and client in room • Respiratory protection when entering room (specialized, approved filter masks in suspected or known tuberculosis) • Restrict entry of certain susceptible people (immunosuppressed, pregnant women) when rubella or varicella is suspected or known • Limit transport of client from room (only when essential); place surgical mask on restricted individual transported
Droplet precautions	Microorganisms transmitted by large particle droplets about 3 feet from the source; generated by sneezing, coughing, talking, or during procedures EXAMPLES: • Invasive *Haemophilus influenza B* including meningitis, pneumonia, epiglottitis, sepsis • Invasive *Neisseria meningitidis* • Diptheria, pertussis • Mycoplasma pneumonia • Pneumonia plaque • Streptococcal pharyngitis, pneumonia, or scarlet fever in infants and young children • Adenovirus • Influenza, RSV • Mumps, rubella • Parvovirus B19	• Private room or house with others with same infection • Door may remain open • Wear mask when working within 3 feet of affected person • Limit client transport to only when necessary; place surgical mask on person when transported
Contact precautions	Microorganisms that can be transmitted by *direct contact* with the client (hand/skin to skin contact); or *indirect contact* (touching environmental surfaces or client/care items) EXAMPLES: • Gastrointestinal, respiratory, skin or wound infections • Multiple-drug–resistent bacteria (MRSA, VRE) • Enteric infections (low infectious dose or prolonged environmental survival) *(Clostridium difficile)* • Diapered or incontinent clients: *(Enterohemorrhagic E. coli; Shigella; Hepatitis A; Rotavirus)* • In infants and young children: • RSV • Parainfluenza virus • Enteroviral infections • Highly contagious skin infections or those that may occur on dry skin: *Diphtheria; herpes simplex virus; impetigo; noncontained abscesses, cellulitis or decubiti; pediculosis; scabies; herpes zoster (disseminated)* • Viral/hemorrhagic conjunctivitis • Viral hemorrhagic infections (e.g., *Ebola*)	• Private room • Glove when entering room • Change gloves after having contact with infective material that may contain high concentrations of microorganisms (e.g., fecal material; wound drainage) • Remove gloves before leaving the client environment and wash hands immediately with antimicrobial soap or waterless antiseptic • After removing gloves and washing hands, DO NOT TOUCH potentially contaminated surfaces or materials • Wear a clean gown when entering the room if you anticipate substantial contact with the contaminated materials or surfaces *(particularly if the person is incontinent, has diarrhea, ileostomy, colostomy, or noncontained draining wound)* • Remove gown before leaving; do not touch contaminated areas • Limit transport of person from room • Dedicate use of non-critical client care items to only this person *(e.g., stethoscope)* • Disinfect equipment with approved disinfectant if to be used with other people

MDRT, Multiple drug resistant tuberculosis; *RSV*; respiratory syncytial virus; *MRSA*, methicillin resistant *staphylococcus aureus*; *VRE*, vancomycin resistant enterococci.
Modified from Centers for Disease Control and Prevention: Guidelines for infection control in health care personnel, *AJIC* 26(3):289-343, 1998.

BOX 7-3

Infectious and Safe Waste

Infectious Waste	Safe Waste
Blood and components	Cotton balls, bandaids
All disposable sharps (used or unused)	Latex gloves, masks, or other personal protective devices
Urine, stool, or emesis if visibly contaminated with blood	Nasal secretions
Vaginal secretions	Sputum
Semen	Feces
Cerebrospinal fluid (CSF)	Urine
Synovial fluid	Vomitus
Pericardial fluid (mediastinal tubes)	Tears
Amniotic fluid	Sweat

evoked to destroy it. Immune globulins contain previously formed antibodies from hyperimmunized donors or pooled plasma and provide temporary passive immunity. Passive immunization is generally used when active immunization is life-threatening or when complete protection requires both active and passive immunization (e.g., immunoglobulins used for hepatitis B or for tetanus) (see Table 6-1).

Prophylactic antibiotic therapy may prevent certain diseases and is usually reserved for people at high risk of exposure to dangerous infections (e.g., pneumocystis carinii pneumonia in clients with HIV/AIDS; postexposure of HCWs to percutaneous contamination from individuals with HIV; preoperatively before joint replacement surgery).[50] Antibiotic-resistant bacteria are on the rise in part because antibiotics have been misused and overused.* Crowded conditions (e.g., day care centers, hospitals, military barracks, and prisons) and prior antibiotic therapy are the principal factors predisposing to colonization and disease.

Some bacteria, such as enterococci, which cause wound and blood infections, have developed mutant strains that do not respond to any antibiotic therapy. Enterococcal infections are primarily limited to hospitals. At present, certain strains of pneumococcus are resistant to only one antibiotic so that other antibiotics remain effective against these pneumococci. If those strains become resistant to other (currently effective) antibiotics, there may be no treatment available. Before 1980, only a few cases of pneumococcus were resistant to penicillin but within a year, strains resistant to penicillin were reported everywhere and are now common throughout the world.

Because resistance to many mainline antibiotics has developed, including resistance to vancomycin, an aggressive search is under way for newer and more effective antimicrobial agents. Cellular enzymes such as synthetases that are universal and essential for cellular via-

bility are being studied as one of the targets for new antibiotics.[79,93] New fluoroquinolones such as gatifloxacin have shown promise against some gram-positive cocci such as *Streptococcus pneumoniae* but less promise against resistant strains of staphylococcus.[29,71]

In April 2000 the Food and Drug Administration (FDA) approved linezolid for the treatment of individuals with infections caused by gram-positive bacteria. Linezolid comes from the first completely new class of antibiotics to reach hospitals in 35 years, the oxazolidinones. Linezolid is indicated for adults in the treatment of numerous gram-positive organisms *S. aureus*, including methicillin resistant *S. aureus*, and has shown efficacy in experimental treatment for resistant otitis and *M. tuberculosis*, including strains resistant to the usual antituberculosis agents.[27,74] Current research is focused on the epidemiology of resistant bacteria, including investigation about the receptors and mechanisms of cellular action and resistance. The study and potential use of inhibitors of resistance mechanisms is an area that might prove useful as a new direction in drug development.[105]

Improved nutrition, living conditions, and *sanitation* through the use of disinfection, sterilization, and antiinfective drugs can inactivate pathogens such as *S. aureus.** This is important because drug-resistant strains of *S. aureus* have developed. Transmission to a new portal of entry can be prevented by environmental disinfection; use of barrier precautions (gloves, masks, condoms); proper handling of food; and protection from vectors. Decreasing host susceptibility can be achieved through personal hygiene and avoidance of high-risk behaviors (unsafe sex practices, injection drug use, recapping needles); and effective handwashing. Maintaining the first-line defense is an important consideration for the client whose health status has already been compromised by disease or diagnostic and treatment procedures. Some ways to accomplish this include preoperative and postprocedure assistance to encourage deep breathing; coughing; ambulation; skin care; and maintaining adequate hydration, fluid and electrolyte balance, and proper nutrition to strengthen resistance.

Correction of environmental factors, particularly water treatment, food and milk safety programs, and control of animals, vectors, rodents, sewage, and solid wastes, can best eradicate nonhuman environments (reservoirs) and thus control pathogens. Other prevention methods in this category include proper handling and disposal of secretions, excretions, and exudates; isolation of infected clients (doors must remain closed, especially in negative-pressure rooms); and quarantine of contacts. The CDC has recommended specific transmission precautions, based on knowledge of the transmission chain for individual infections. The precautions were designed to prevent transmission of pathogens among hospitalized people, health care personnel, and visitors (see Table 7-4). Specific recommendations have been made for individual diseases.

---

*This is only a small part of the total picture regarding this issue. Other components of this problem include the extensive use of antibiotics in animals later consumed or whose products are consumed (e.g., milk products).

---

*This is important since one strain of staphylococcus, MRSA, is resistant to most antibiotics. Over the past 10 years, MRSA and other resistant strains of *S. aureus* have become the most common causes of hospital and community-acquired infections. MRSA usually develops when multiple antibiotics are used in the treatment of infection and in older adults who are debilitated, having surgery or multiple invasive procedures, or being treated in critical are units.

TABLE	7-5

The 1996 CDC Recommendations for Immunization of Health Care Workers (HCWs)

DISEASE	SCHEDULE	INDICATIONS
Hepatitis B	Recombinant vaccine (three-dose series)	Health care worker (HCW) at risk of exposure to blood and body fluids
Influenza	Annual vaccination with current vaccine; inactivated whole-virus and split virus vaccines	HCWs who have contact with clients at high risk for influenza or its complications; who work in chronic care facilities; who work with high-risk medical conditions; or who are ≥ 65 years
Measles, Mumps, Rubella (MMR)	Live virus vaccine, 2 doses needed ≥ 4 weeks apart	*All* HCWs who work in health care should be immune to measles, mumps, and rubella; CONTRAINDICATED IN PREGNANCY *Measles:* HCWs born during or after 1957 who do not have documentation of having received two doses of live vaccine, a history of physician diagnosed measles, or serologic evidence of immunity *Mumps:* HCWs believed to be susceptible; adults born before 1957 can be considered immune *Rubella:* HCWs (men and women) who do not have documentation of receiving live vaccine on or after their first birthday or serologic evidence of immunity; adults born before 1957 can be considered immune *except women who can become pregnant*
Varicella zoster	Live vaccine; two doses 4-8 weeks apart If ≥13 years of age	HCWs who do not have either a reliable history of varicella or serologic evidence of immunity; CONTRAINDICATED IN PREGNANCY
Bacille Calmette Guérin BCG (BBC for tuberculosis)	BCG vaccination, one dose Not used in the United States	HCWs only in areas where multiple drug–resistant TB (MDRTB) is prevalent; a strong likelihood of infection exists and where comprehensive infection-control precautions have not worked to protect HCWs; CONTRAINDICATED IN PREGNANCY

Immunizing Agents Available in Special Circumstances

DISEASE	SCHEDULE	INDICATIONS
Hepatitis B (HBV)	Hepatitis B immune globulin (HBIG)	Postexposure prophylaxis for persons exposed to blood or body fluids containing HbsAg and who are not immune to HBV; also given to infants of hepatitis B positive mother
Varicella zoster	Varicella zoster immune globulin (VZIG)	HCWs know or likely to be susceptible (particularly pregnant women or immunocompromised clients) who have close and prolonged exposure to a contact case or to an infectious hospital staff member or client
Hepatitis A (HAV)	Hepatitis A vaccine, two doses 6-12 months apart	Not routinely indicated for HCWs in the United States. Used for people who work with HAV-infected primates or with HAV in a laboratory setting; safety of vaccine not evaluated in pregnancy, probably low risk
Meningococcal disease (vaccine is available)	Rifampin (2 days) or ceftriazone (one dose) or Ciprofloxacin (one dose)	HCWs with direct contact with respiratory secretions from infected persons without the use of proper precautions (e.g., mouth-to-mouth resuscitation; endotracheal intubation or management)
Typhoid	Vaccine administered intramuscularly—one dose with booster every 3 years; two doses ≥ 4 weeks apart; booster every 3 years; or four oral doses on alternate days	Workers in microbiology laboratories who often work with *Salmonella typhi*
Smallpox	Vaccine no longer available for routine use	–
Polio	Inactivated polio vaccine (IPV), two doses subcutaneously 4-8 weeks apart followed by a third dose 6-12 months; after second booster, doses may be IPV or oral polio vaccine (OPV)	HCWs in close contact with persons who may be excreting wild virus and laboratory personnel handling specimens that may contain wild poliovirus; also if traveling to polio-endemic areas; SAFETY IN PREGNANCY NOT EVALUATED, CONTRAINDICATED

TABLE	7-5—cont'd

The 1996 CDC Recommendations for Immunization of Health Care Workers (HCWs)

DISEASE	SCHEDULE	INDICATIONS
Pertussis	Erythromycin or trimethoprim sulfamethoxazole for 14 days	Personnel with direct contact with respiratory secretions or large aerosol droplets from infected people
Rabies	Two types of vaccine available: pre- and post exposure; sequence of injections (deltoid): days 0, 3, 7, 14, 28; one booster	Personnel who work with rabies virus or infected animals in research laboratories
Tetanus and diphtheria (Td)	Two doses intramuscular injection 4 weeks apart; third dose 6-12 months after second dose; booster every 10 years	All adults; tetanus prophylaxis in wound management; used after needle-stick injury; pregnant women should receive Td to decrease risk of neonatal tetanus

Modified from Centers for Disease Control and Prevention. Immunization of health-care workers: recommendations of the advisory committee on immunization practices (ACIP) and the hospital infection control practices advisory committee (HICPAC), *MMWR* 46 (RR-18), 1-42, December 26, 1997.

Special Implications for the Therapist 7-1

CONTROL OF TRANSMISSION

The CDC has set up guidelines for the care of all clients regarding precautions against the transmission of infectious disease (see Appendix A). These should be used with all clients regardless of their disease status. All blood and body fluids are potentially infectious and should be handled as such (see Box 7-3).

All clients receiving therapy (and thus in contact with HCWs) may be asymptomatic hosts during the period of communicability. The careful use of precautionary measures severely limits the transmission of any disease. In addition, each hospital has transmission-based precautions organized according to categories of transmission routes to prevent the spread of infectious disease to others. Every HCW must be familiar with these procedures and follow them carefully. Transmission prevention guidelines and accompanying basic isolation procedures are provided in Table 7-4.

HCWs should be concerned about improving their resistance and decreasing their susceptibility to infectious diseases. Maintaining an adequate immunization status is one approach. Every HCW should be adequately immunized against hepatitis B, measles, mumps, rubella, polio, tetanus, diphtheria, and varicella. The most recent CDC recommendations for immunization of HCWs are given in Table 7-5.

Second to immunization, handwashing is the most effective disease-preventing measure anyone can practice. A single hand can carry 200 million organisms, including bacteria, viruses, and fungi. It takes a full 5 minutes of handwashing to cleanse 99% of the bacteria from fingernails, thumbs, palm creases, and backs of the hands. The average wash-and-rinse in the hospital setting is less than 10 seconds, and the dominant hand is often underwashed.[101]

However, many HCWs suffer severe hand irritation with cracking and bleeding as a consequence of frequent handwashing and glove use. Integumentary breakdown has major implications for nosocomial infection control and promotes the spread of blood-borne viruses. An adjunct to handwashing is an alcohol gel fortified with a skin-protecting emollient (e.g., glycerin) or an alcohol-based towelette. These sanitizers are to be used only when there is no visible soiling of the hands and only when a source of soap and water for washing is unavailable. Alcohol hand rinses may increase compliance with hand disinfection, but used without the added skin protection, alcohol has a significant drying effect leading to the same skin problems associated with frequent washing.[65]

Nosocomial Infections

Therapists can help prevent transmission of nosocomial infections from themselves to others (Table 7-6), from client to client, and from client to self by following standard precautions (see Appendix A) and guidelines as follows:

- Follow strict infection-control procedures. Make sure to identify each client's individual transmission precautions and procedures. When in doubt, ask the nursing staff regarding the status of the person in question.
- Strictly follow necessary isolation techniques. Doors must remain closed, especially in negative pressure rooms.
- Observe *all* clients for signs of infection (see Table 7-1), especially those people at high risk. Notify nursing or medical staff of these observations.
- Always follow proper handwashing technique or use an alcohol-based hand antiseptic, and encourage other staff members to do so as well. Take time to wash or disinfect hands before and after each and every client.
- Stay away from susceptible, high-risk clients when you have an obvious infection. Make arrangements for some other therapist to treat that client until the contagious period has passed. If in doubt, consult a physician.
- Take special precautions with vulnerable clients—that is, those with Foley catheters, mechanical ventilators, or IV lines and those recuperating from surgery. Specific tips for preventing infection in these situations are listed in Box 7-4.
- Avoid the use of acrylic nails that harbor pathogens[64]

Continued on p. 208

TABLE 7-6

Summary of Important Recommendations and Work Restrictions for Personnel with Infectious Diseases

DISEASE/PROBLEM	WORK RESTRICTION	DURATION
Conjunctivitis	Restrict from client contact and contact with the client's environment	Until discharge ceases
Cytomegalovirus infections	No restriction	
Diarrheal Diseases		
Acute stage (diarrhea with other symptoms)	Restrict from client contact, contact with the client's environment, or food handling	Until symptoms resolve
Convalescent stage, *Salmonella* species	Restrict from care of high-risk clients	Until symptoms resolve; consult with local and state health authorities regarding need for negative stool cultures
Diphtheria	Exclude from duty	Until antimicrobial therapy completed and 2 cultures obtained ≥ 24 hours apart are negative
Enteroviral infections	Restrict from care of infants, neonates, and immunocompromised persons and their environments	Until symptoms resolve
Hepatitis A	Restrict from client contact, contact with client's environment, and food handling	Until 7 days after onset of jaundice
Hepatitis B		
Personnel with acute or chronic hepatitis B surface antigemia who do not perform exposure-prone procedures	No restriction*; refer to state regulations; standard precautions should always be observed	
Personnel with acute or chronic hepatitis B e antigenemia who perform exposure-prone procedures	Do not perform exposure-prone invasive procedures until counsel from an expert review panel has been sought; panel should review and recommend procedures the worker can perform, taking into account specific procedure and skill and technique of worker; refer to state regulations	Until hepatitis B e antigen (a marker of a high titer of virus) is negative
Hepatitis C	No recommendation	
Herpes Simplex		
Genital	No restriction	
Hands (herpetic whitlow)	Restrict from client contact and contact with client's environment	Until lesions heal
Orofacial	Evaluate for need to restrict from care of high-risk clients	
Human immunodeficiency virus	Do not perform exposure-prone invasive procedures until counsel from an expert review panel has been sought; panel should review and recommend procedures the worker can perform, taking into account specific procedure and skill and technique of the worker; standard precautions should always be observed; refer to state regulations	
Measles		
Active	Exclude from duty	Until 7 days after the rash appears
Postexposure (susceptible)	Exclude from duty	From 5th day after first exposure through 21st day after last exposure and/or 4 days after rash appears
Meningococcal infections	Exclude from duty	Until 24 hours after start of effective therapy

TABLE	7-6—cont'd

Summary of Important Recommendations and Work Restrictions for Personnel with Infectious Diseases

DISEASE/PROBLEM	WORK RESTRICTION	DURATION
Mumps		
Active	Exclude from duty	Until 9 days after onset of parotitis
Postexposure (susceptible personnel)	Exclude from duty	From 12th day after first exposure through 26th day after last exposure or until 9 days after onset of parotitis
Pediculosis	Restrict from client contact	Until treated and observed to be free of adult and immature lice
Pertussis		
Active	Exclude from duty	From beginning of catarrhal stage through 3rd week after onset of paroxysms or until 5 days after start of effective antimicrobial therapy
Postexposure (asymptomatic personnel)	No restriction, prophylaxis recommended	
Postexposure (symptomatic personnel)	Exclude from duty	Until 5 days after start of effective antimicrobial therapy
Rubella		
Active	Exclude from duty	Until 5 days after rash appears
Postexposure (susceptible personnel)	Exclude from duty	From 7th day after first exposure through 21st day after last exposure
Scabies	Restrict from client contact	Until cleared by medical evaluation
Staphylococcus aureus infection		
Active, draining skin lesions	Restrict from contact with client and client's environment or food handling	Until lesions have resolved
Carrier state	No restriction, unless personnel are epidemiologically linked to transmission of the organism	
Streptococcal infection, group A	Restrict from client care, contact with client's environment or food handling	Until 24 hours after adequate treatment started
Tuberculosis		
Active disease	Exclude from duty	Until proved noninfectious
PPD converter	No restriction if not an active case and if cleared medically	
Varicella		
Active	Exclude from duty	Until all lesions dry and crust
Postexposure (susceptible personnel)	Exclude from duty	From 10th day after first exposure through 21st day (28th day if VZIG given) after last exposure
Zoster		
Localized, in healthy person	Cover lesions; restrict from care of high-risk clients†	Until all lesions dry and crust
Generalized or localized in immunosuppressed person	Restrict from client contact	Until all lesions dry and crust
Postexposure (susceptible personnel)	Restrict from client contact	From 10th day after first exposure through 21st day (28th day if VZIG given) after last exposure or, if varicella occurs, until all lesions dry and crust
Viral respiratory infections, acute febrile	Consider excluding from the care of high risk clients‡ or contact with their environment during community outbreak of RSV and influenza	Until acute symptoms resolve

*Unless epidemiologically linked to transmission of infection.
†Those susceptible to varicella and who are at increased risk of complications of varicella, such as neonates and immunocompromised persons of any age.
‡High-risk patients as defined by the Advisory Committee of Immunization Practices for complications of influenza.
VZIG, varicella zoster immunoglobulin; *RSV*, respiratory syncytial virus; *PPD*, purified protein derivative.
Modified from: Centers for Disease Control and Prevention: Guidelines for infection control in health care personnel, 1998, *AJIC* 26(3):289-343, 1998.

Hydrotherapy and Therapeutic Pool Protocol

In the past, routine cultures of hydrotherapy and pool equipment were performed to identify and supposedly eliminate colonization of infectious bacteria. In this way, the spread of infection was prevented from equipment to client and from client to client, especially in the acute care setting. Now, under the outcomes-based management philosophy, infection control is cost-driven so that the outcome is managed, as long as the outcome is what was predicted and intended or improving. For example, in the case of preventing the spread of infection through hydrotherapy or therapeutic pool equipment, good disinfection and cleaning procedures are practiced and monitored closely. This plan is both cost effective and is accompanied by a high degree of safety. Routine environmental cultures are not cost effective and therefore are not performed. Many organisms are present normally, and if present and no one is infected, these pathogens are not considered a functional problem. Under outcomes-based management, when an infectious problem develops, the cause is traced back to the source and eliminated at that point.

When using hydrotherapy (e.g., pulsatile lavage with suction; whirlpool) for wound care, clients should be treated in a private treatment room with all walls and doors closed. Proper personal protective equipment (PPE) such as masks, gloves, and eyewear must be worn by the therapist when treating the individual and cleaning hydrotherapy equipment. Whirlpool equipment should be cleaned before and after treatment.[57]

Home Health Care

Preventing spread of an infectious disease to the family, the home health therapist, and perhaps the community is a primary concern when preparing the client for return home. The therapist should work closely with the home health nurse and seek guidance if unsure how to handle a specific situation. A list of helpful hints for home health care includes the following[84]:

- Handwashing is the best protection against transmission of infectious diseases, and it is essential after providing direct care and when gloves are removed before touching anything.

BOX 7-4

Tips for Preventing Infection

Chest Tube

Prevent chest tube from kinking by carefully coiling the tubing on top of the bed and securing it to the bed linen, leaving room for the person to turn.

Tracheostomy

Contact with secretions occurs with a tracheostomy; follow standard precautions. When direct contact is made and potential splash secondary to expelled secretions occurs, gown, mask, protective facewear, and gloves are needed.

Urinary Catheter

Follow standard precautions for handwashing techniques.
Do not allow the drainage bag spigot to come in contact with a contaminated surface.
When the drainage tubing becomes disconnected, do not touch the ends of the tubing or catheter. Contact the nursing staff for reconnecting.
Before turning, moving, or transferring a catheterized person, locate the proximal end of the tubing and either clamp it to the person's gown or hold it to allow necessary slack during movement. This will help prevent the catheter from accidentally and traumatically being pulled out.
Whenever possible, avoid raising the drainage bag above the level of the person's bladder.
If it becomes necessary to raise the bag during transfers, clamp the tubing but avoid prolonged clamping or kinking of the tubing (except during bladder conditioning).
Avoid allowing large loops of tubing to dangle from the bedside, wheelchair, or walker.
Drain all urine from tubing into the bag before the person exercises or ambulates.

Intravenous Devices

If you have exudative lesions or weeping dermatitis, refrain from all direct contact with intravenous (IV) or invasive equipment until the condition resolves.
Notify the nursing staff of any suspicious observations such as if the IV device is not dripping at a steady rate (either none at all or flowing very fast); if the IV bag is empty; or if blood is flowing from insertion of the IV catheter tip into the person's body out into the IV line.

Nasogastric and Feeding Tubes

Care must be taken to avoid excessive movement or pulling and tugging of these tubes.
Wash your hands before and after touching the entry point of the tube into the body.

Hydrotherapy

Hydrotherapy for wound care (pulsatile lavage with suction, whirlpool) should be performed in a private treatment room with all walls and doors closed.
Proper personal protective equipment (PPE) must be worn when treating the client and/or cleaning hydrotherapy equipment.
Whirlpool equipment should be cleaned before and after treatment.

- Staff should leave extraneous clothing and equipment outside the client's area and take in only items that are needed.
- Equipment needed on a regular basis, such as the blood pressure cuff and stethoscope,* should be in the room at the beginning of home health care. When it is no longer needed, equipment should be bagged or covered and taken to the appropriate area for decontamination and reprocessing. Disposable equipment should be contained, labeled, and discarded.
- The therapist should be adequately supplied with gloves, masks, gowns, and disposable plastic aprons. Some plastic bags of different sizes should be carried for the therapist's own use and to demonstrate to the client's family how to handle soiled linens and trash.
- Paper towels are useful when working in the client's area. Use them as a clean surface during care and to wipe your hands.
- Before going into the client's area, plan what to do and gather the items needed.
- It is important to remember that isolation or precautions can have a negative effect on the family. Help the family feel comfortable with the techniques needed for isolation. Encourage them to visit with the client and not just be with him or her during care.
- Should the client have a fecesborne infectious disease such as hepatitis A or salmonellosis, it is important to show the family how to bag and launder soiled linens. It is equally important to demonstrate how to bag and dispose of soiled paper products such as linen savers, which cannot be flushed down the toilet. Remind the family to wash their hands afterward, and the therapist should do so as well.
- If the client has hepatitis A or salmonellosis, the family and the client should be reminded not to handle raw food served to others, such as lettuce or tomatoes, until the physician determines the client is past the infectious stage.
- In treating clients with bloodborne illnesses, if the client accidentally sustains a cut, any spilled blood on inanimate objects or surfaces should be cleaned off with household bleach and water. Razors and toothbrushes should not be shared.
- The therapist should practice self-protection at all times. Use good handwashing technique and when in doubt, ask for assistance from other, more knowledgeable health care staff. ■

◆ Diagnosis of Infectious Diseases

Five basic laboratory techniques can be used in the diagnosis of infectious diseases: (1) direct visualization of the organism; (2) detection of microbial antigen; (3) a search for clues produced by the host immune response to specific microorganisms; (4) detection of specific microbial nucleotide sequences; and (5) isolation of the organism in culture. Each technique has its use and each has associated advantages and disadvantages.

In many infectious diseases, pathogenic organisms can be directly visualized by microscopic examination of readily available tissue fluids, such as sputum, urine, pus, and pleural, peritoneal, or cerebrospinal fluid (CSF). Detection of specific antigens establishes the presence of some diseases such as meningitis, hepatitis B, and some respiratory and genitourinary tract infections. Histopathologic examination of biopsied or excised tissue often reveals patterns of the host inflammatory response that can provide clues to narrow down the diagnostic possibilities. Some viral infections, such as skin or respiratory infections caused by herpesviruses, or pneumonia due to cytomegalovirus produce characteristic changes in host cells visible on cytologic examination. Recent techniques to amplify microbial DNA or RNA sequences for detection have been used to diagnose some infections and are expected to be developed enough to diagnose numerous other infectious diseases. Finally, isolation of a single microbe from an infected site is generally considered evidence that the infection is caused by this organism.

SPECIFIC INFECTIOUS DISEASES

Most infections are confined to specific organ systems. In this book, many of the important infectious disease entities are discussed in the specific chapter dealing with the affected anatomic area. Only the most commonly encountered infectious problems not covered elsewhere are included in this chapter.

◆ Bacterial Infections
Staphylococcal Infections
Overview and Incidence.   *Staphylococcus aureus* is one of the most common bacterial pathogens normally residing on the skin and is easily inoculated into deeper tissues where it causes suppurative (pus formation) infections. Staphylococci bacteria are the leading cause of nosocomial and community acquired infections accounting for about 13% of all hospital infections each year. This figure translates into approximately 2 million hospital infections annually, resulting in 60,000 to 80,000 deaths each year. It is the most common cause of suppurative infections affecting all ages and involving the heart, lung, soft tissue, joints, and bones. It is a leading cause of infective endocarditis.

Risk Factors.   *S. aureus* spreads by direct contact with colonized surfaces or people. Most people (both children and adults) are intermittently colonized with S. aureus, carrying the organism on the skin, in the nares, or on clothing. The organism also survives on inanimate surfaces but the role of contaminated surfaces in transmission of S. aureus has not been well-documented and remains controversial. Heavy contamination of fomites may facilitate transmission to clients by the hands of personnel.[7] Predisposing factors are multiple and varied depending on the type of disease outcome (Table 7-7). The principal factor associated with the reemergence of these pathogens is the frequent use of intravascular devices such as Hickman catheters, central lines, and peripheral IV catheters, both in hospitals and outpatient settings.

Burns and surgical wounds often become infected with S. aureus from the person's own nasal passages or from contact with medical personnel. Newborns and older adults and malnourished, diabetic, and obese individuals all have increased susceptibility. S. aureus is the causative organism in half of all cases of septic arthritis, mostly in people ages 50 to 70.

---

*Stethoscopes are often contaminated with staphylococci and therefore a potential vector of infection. Such contamination poses a risk to people with open wounds such as burns. This contamination is greatly reduced by frequent cleaning with alcohol or nonionic detergent; cleaning with antiseptic soap is only 75% effective in reducing the bacterial count.[49]

TABLE	7-7

Staphylococcal Infections

Type	Predisposing Factors	Type	Predisposing Factors
Bacteremia	Infected surgical wounds	Enterocolitis	Broad-spectrum antibiotics as prophylaxis for bowel surgery or treatment of hepatic coma
	Abscesses		Elderly; newborn infants (associated with staphylococcal skin lesions)
	Infected intravenous or intra-arterial catheter sites; catheter tips	Osteomyelitis	Hematogenous organisms (blood-borne)
	Infected vascular grafts or prostheses		Skin trauma
	Infected pressure ulcers		Infection spreading from adjacent joint or other infected tissues
	Osteomyelitis		*Staphylococcus aureus* bacteremia
	Injection drug abuse		Orthopedic surgery or trauma
	Source unknown (primary bacteremia)		Cardiothoracic surgery
	Cellulitis		Usually occurs in growing bones, especially femur and tibia of children <12 yr
	Burns		Male sex
	Immunosuppression	Food poisoning	Contaminated food
	Debilitating diseases (e.g., diabetes, renal failure)		
	Infective endocarditis	Skin infections	Decreased resistance
	Cancer (leukemia) or neutropenia after chemotherapy or radiation		Burns or pressure ulcers
Pneumonia	Immunodeficiency (especially elderly and children [2 yr])		Decreased blood flow
	Chronic lung disease and cystic fibrosis		Skin contamination from nasal discharge
	Malignancy		Foreign bodies
	Antibiotics that kill normal respiratory flora but spare *Staphylococcus aureus*		Underlying skin diseases, such as eczema and acne
	Viral respiratory infections, especially influenza		Common in persons with poor hygiene living in crowded quarters
	Blood-borne bacteria spread to the lungs from primary sites of infections (e.g., heart valves, abscesses, pulmonary emboli)		
	Recent bronchial or endotracheal suctioning or intubation		

Rheumatoid arthritis and corticosteroid therapy are common predisposing conditions.

Pathogenesis.　　S. *aureus* cannot invade through intact skin or mucous membranes; infection usually begins with traumatic inoculation of the organism. Once inside the body, the organism is a virulent pathogen, secreting at least five different membrane-damaging enzymes and toxins that harm host tissues and are capable of destroying erythrocytes, leukocytes, platelets, fibrinoblasts, and other cells.

Many S. *aureus* infections begin as localized infections of the skin and skin appendages and then invade beyond the initial site, spreading by the bloodstream or lymphatic system to almost any location in the body. The bones, joints, and heart valves are the most common sites of metastatic S. aureus infections.

Clinical Manifestations.　　When S. *aureus* is inoculated into a previously sterile site, infection usually produces suppuration and abscess formation. The abscesses range in size from microscopic to lesions several centimeters in diameter, and they are filled with pus and bacteria. The clinical manifestations vary enormously according to the site and type of infection and may include furuncles (boils); paronychia (staphylococcal infection of the nail bed); felons (staphylococcal infections on the palmar side of the fingertips); carbuncles (clusters of infected boils); os-

teomyelitis, infections of burns or surgical wounds; respiratory tract infections; bacterial arthritis; septicemia; bacterial endocarditis; toxic shock syndrome; and food poisoning. Fever, chills, and symptoms associated with the affected area may accompany staphylococcal infection of any body part.

Acute staphylococcus *osteomyelitis*, usually in the bones of the legs, most commonly affects boys between ages 3 and 10, most of whom have a history of infection or trauma. Osteomyelitis presenting in the vertebrae affects adults older than age 50, often following staphylococcal infections of the skin or urinary tract or prostatic surgery or after pinning of a fracture. Clinical manifestations include abrupt onset of fever, usually 101° F (38.3° C) or lower, shaking chills, pain and swelling over the infected area, restlessness, and headache (see the section on Osteomyelitis in Chapter 24).

Staphylococcus-associated *skin infections* include cellulitis (see the section on Cellulitis in Chapter 9); boil-like lesions (furuncles and carbuncles); and small macules or skin blebs that may develop into pus-filled vesicles. Associated symptoms may include mild or spiking fever and malaise.

Medical Management
Diagnosis, Treatment, and Prognosis.　　Culture of the organism from pus or drainage is usually diagnostic; antibiotic

sensitivity testing is important. Isolation of the organism in blood cultures confirms endocarditis in the presence of a new murmur or positive echocardiogram. Treatment may include drainage of any abscesses, administration of antibiotics, and supportive therapy for the specific type and site.

Prognosis is good with treatment, although antibiotic resistance is increasingly associated with morbidity and mortality. Methicillin-resistant *Staphylococcus aureus* is resistant to available antimicrobials except vancomycin. Reports of reduced susceptibility to vancomycin among strains of *S aureus* are on the rise.[14] Untreated skin infections can become systemic and cause infective endocarditis and visceral abscesses or osteomyelitis; staphylococcal sepsis is potentially lethal. Studies are under way to develop an effective vaccine to prevent *S. aureus*. Although it may be several years before vaccines against *S. aureus* are available for humans, immunization may represent an important step toward solving the problem of antimicrobial resistance.[69]

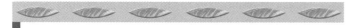

Special Implications for the Therapist 7-2

STAPHYLOCOCCAL INFECTIONS

Preferred Practice Patterns
7A: Prevention/Risk Reduction for Integumentary Disorder
7B: Impaired Integumentary Integrity Associated With Superficial Skin Involvement
7E: Impaired Integumentary Associated With Skin Involvement Extending into Fascia, Muscle, or Bone, and Scar Formation (osteomyelitis, lymphangitis)

Some organisms such as *S. aureus* (and streptococci) are considered resident organisms because they are not easily removed by scrubbing and often can be cultured from the HCW's skin. Many HCWs carry *S. aureus* without sequelae but are able to shed organisms into nonintact skin areas of susceptible hosts, causing infections.

For the most part, good handwashing with plain soap is adequate in the therapy or home setting, but therapists need to consistently educate family members and caregivers about infection control through handwashing and environmental management. Antimicrobial soaps that contain chemicals to kill transient and some resident organisms may be recommended. The choice of using an antimicrobial soap or plain soap is usually based on the need to reduce and maintain minimal counts of resident organisms and to mechanically remove transient organisms such as *Pseudomonas, E. coli, Salmonella,* or *Shigella.* When working with people who are infected with drug-resistant, gram-positive cocci such as MRSA or VRE, antimicrobial soap is recommended since some studies have shown that these organisms persist on hands until an antimicrobial product is used.[37]

Some questions have been raised regarding isolation procedures for methicillin- or vancomycin-resistant clients who have been discharged from an isolation setting as an inpatient but are now returning to therapy as an outpatient. Is a separate area required? Are special precautions necessary? Anyone with an active, resistant infection should not be discharged from an inpatient setting. However, if such a case is encountered, the therapist must remember that these organisms are spread by contact. Therefore the same germicidal cleaning measures used in a hospital or institutional setting are required. All equipment that comes in direct contact with a draining area needs to be cleaned with an approved germicidal before and after use. Isolation (e.g., private room or separate area of the gym or clinic) is not required. American Physical Therapy Association (APTA) infection control guidelines for hydrotherapy and physical therapy aquatic programs recommend that clients with MRSA may attend therapy programs, provided the area of colonization can be contained. If it is in a wound, the drainage must be contained within the dressing without evidence of breakthrough. ■

Streptococcal Infections
Group A Streptococci

Streptococcus pyogenes, the prototype of group A streptococci (GAS), is one of the most common bacterial pathogens of humans of any age. It causes many diseases of diverse organ systems ranging from skin infections, to acute self-limited pharyngitis, to major illnesses such as rheumatic fever (Table 7-8).

The diseases caused by *S. pyogenes* may be considered in two categories: suppurative (formation of pus) and nonsuppurative. Suppurative diseases occur at sites where the bacteria invade and cause tissue necrosis, usually inciting an acute inflammatory response. By contrast, nonsuppurative diseases (see Table 7-8) occur at sites remote from the site of bacterial invasion.

TABLE	7-8

Streptococcal Infections

Streptococcus pyogenes (group A streptococci)	
Suppurative	Streptococcal pharyngitis
	Scarlet fever (scarlatina)
	Impetigo (streptococcal pyoderma)
	Streptococcal gangrene (necrotizing fasciitis)
	Streptococcal cellulitis
	Streptococcal myositis
	Puerperal sepsis (following vaginal delivery or abortion)
	Toxic shock syndrome (TSS)
	Pneumonia (rare)
Nonsuppurative	Rheumatic fever
	Acute poststreptococcal glomerulonephritis

Streptococcus agalactiae (group B streptococci)
Neonatal streptococcal infections
Adult group B streptococcal infection

Streptococcus pneumoniae
Pneumococcal pneumonia
Otitis media
Meningitis
Endocarditis

Group A streptococcus (GAS) has been transmitted from infected clients to HCWs after contact with infected secretions. The infected personnel have subsequently acquired a variety of GAS-related illnesses (e.g., toxic shock–like syndrome, cellulitis, and pharyngitis). HCWs who are GAS carriers have infrequently been linked to sporadic outbreaks of surgical site, postpartum, or burn wound infection and to foodborne transmission of GAS causing pharyngitis. Contact is the major mode of GAS transmission in health care settings, but some airborne transmission has been suggested during severe outbreaks. Adherence to standard precautions or other transmission-based precautions can prevent nosocomial transmission of GAS to personnel. Restriction from client care activities and food handling is indicated for personnel with GAS (see Table 7-6).

Signs and symptoms of GAS depend on the location but typically include fever, chills, sore throat, and enlarged lymph nodes with pharyngitis; red honey-crusted lesions with impetigo; diffuse inflammation of the skin and subcutaneous tissues with swelling and redness with erysipelas (skin strep), a type of skin cellulitis; and new onset of heart murmur with endocarditis.

Streptococcal Pharyngitis. Streptococcal pharyngitis, commonly known as *strep throat*, accounts for 95% of all cases of bacterial pharyngitis. Occurring most commonly from October to April in children age 5 to 10 years, a recent increase has occurred among adults age 30 to 50 years. This organism often colonizes in throats of people with no symptoms; up to 20% of schoolchildren may be carriers (pets may also be carriers).

After a 1- to 5-day incubation period, a temperature of 101° F to 104° F (38.3° C to 40° C); sore throat with severe pain on swallowing; beefy red pharynx; tonsillar exudate; edematous tonsils and uvula; swollen glands along the jaw line; generalized malaise and weakness; anorexia; and occasional abdominal discomfort may develop. Up to 40% of affected children may have symptoms too mild for diagnosis.

Complications may include otitis media or sinusitis; rarely, bacteremic spread may cause arthritis, endocarditis, meningitis, osteomyelitis, or liver abscess; and poststreptococcal sequelae include acute rheumatic fever or acute glomerulonephritis. Diagnosis is usually by throat culture and treatment is pharmacologic with supportive measures for symptoms.

Scarlet Fever. Scarlet fever usually follows untreated streptococcal pharyngitis, but may also occur after wound infections or puerperal sepsis. It is caused by a streptococcal strain that releases an erythrogenic toxin and is most common in children 2 to 10 years old. It is spread by inhalation or direct contact and presents as a streptococcal sore throat; fever; strawberry tongue (white-coated tongue with prominent red papillae); and fine erythematous rash that blanches on pressure and resembles sunburn with goose bumps. The rash first appears on the upper chest and then spreads to the neck, abdomen, legs, and arms, sparing the soles and palms. The cheeks may be flushed, with pallor around the mouth. Rarely, complications may include high fever, arthritis, and jaundice.

Impetigo. Impetigo, or streptococcal pyoderma, occurs most commonly in children age 2 to 5 years, especially in hot, humid weather. Predisposing factors include close contact in schools, overcrowded living quarters, poor skin hygiene, and minor skin trauma. Small macules appear and rapidly develop into vesicles that become pustular and encrusted, causing pain, surrounding erythema, and itching. Scratching spreads infection and may develop into adenitis (glandular inflammation) or cellulitis. Lesions often affect the face, heal slowly, and leave depigmented areas (see Chapter 9).

Streptococcal Gangrene. Group A β-hemolytic streptococcal infections have shown remarkable virulence in recent years, resulting in severe local tissue destruction as occurs in streptococcal gangrene. This is a rare form of gangrene, due to group A (or C or G) streptococci,* which usually develops at a site of trauma on an extremity or from an intraoral abscess or dental source affecting the face, head, and neck. It may also occur in the absence of an obvious portal of entry. Predisposing factors include surgery, wounds, skin ulcers, intramuscular administration of drugs such as nonsteroidal antiinflammatory agents (NSAIDs), diabetes mellitus, chronic alcoholism, and peripheral vascular disease.

This condition mimics gas gangrene because it develops within 72 hours of onset with the affected person showing a red-streaked, painful skin lesion with dusky red surrounding tissue. Bullae containing yellowish to red-black fluid develop and rupture; the lesion evolves into a sharply demarcated area covered by a necrotic eschar and surrounded by an erythematous border. The involved area resembles a third-degree burn. Extensive necrotic sloughs can result because of deep penetration of the infection along fascial planes.[52]

Other symptoms may include fever, tachycardia, lethargy, prostration, disorientation, hypotension, jaundice, hypovolemia, and severe pain followed by anesthesia due to nerve destruction. Complications may include bacteremia (bacteria in the blood), metastatic abscesses, and death; and secondary thrombophlebitis when the lower extremities are involved.

Streptococci can usually be cultured from the early bullous lesions and often from the blood. Treatment is immediate, with wide, deep surgical debridement of all necrotic tissue accompanied by high-dose IV antibiotics.[81] If surgical therapy is not an option, the prevention of secondary complications such as infection becomes the goal of treatment until the necrotic process stops and healing begins. In such situations, a moist environment is a recommended choice for topical therapy.

Necrotizing Fasciitis. Necrotizing fasciitis, an invasive infection of fascia, is predominantly an adult disorder of polymicrobial bacterial origin. In children, it is relatively rare and has a high mortality rate. In the pediatric population, varicella (chickenpox)† is an important risk factor for necrotizing fasciitis (varicella gangrenosa) caused by more virulent strains of group A β-hemolytic streptococci.[91,102] In the newborn, necrotizing fasciitis can be a serious complication of omphalitis (inflammation of the umbilical cord).

Other predisposing risk factors include trauma (laceration, abrasion, burn, insect bite); ischemia; surgery (e.g., hemorrhoidectomy, vasectomy); anatomic sites regularly exposed to fecal or oral contamination, such as wounds associated with intestinal surgery; pressure and diabetic ulcers; human bites; infected pilonidal (containing hair) cysts; alcoholism; and injection drug abuse.[18]

---

*Other pathogens for this disease include *S. aureus*,[41] *Staphylococcus epidermidis*,[54] a case where a nonvirulent organism becomes pathogenic as a result of age alone, and *Streptococcus pneumoniae*.[20]

†Isolated cases of this condition caused by chickenpox in adults have been reported.[39]

This condition is characterized by infectious thrombosis of vessels passing between the skin and deep circulation, producing skin necrosis superficially resembling ischemic vascular or clostridial gangrene. The affected area is initially erythematous, swollen, without sharp margins, hot, shiny, exquisitely tender, and painful. The process progresses rapidly over several days, with sequential skin color changes from red-purple to patches of blue-gray. Within 3 to 5 days of onset, skin breakdown with bullae containing thick pink or purple fluid and cutaneous gangrene resembling a thermal burn occurs. By this time, the involved area is no longer tender but has become anesthetic secondary to the thrombosis of small blood vessels and destruction of superficial nerves located in the necrotic subcutaneous tissues.

Necrotizing fasciitis can affect any part of the body but is most common on the extremities, particularly the legs. Necrotizing fasciitis from intestinal sources may extend along the psoas muscle to affect the lower extremities, groin, or abdominal wall. Although the superficial and/or deep fascia is predominantly involved, the overlying skin and subcutaneous fat may also be affected.

Aggressive surgery beyond the necrotic tissue is mandatory and usually requires multiple procedures, as the demarcation line is difficult to differentiate. Pulsatile lavage with suction (PLWS) has been an excellent intervention in decreasing bacteria, irrigating and débriding and in allowing for increased ease of sharp debridement with hydration of necrotic tissue.[56]

Streptococcal Cellulitis. Streptococcal cellulitis, an acute spreading inflammation of the skin and subcutaneous tissues, usually results from infection of burns or wounds. Recurrent episodes of cellulitis may occur in extremities in which lymphatic drainage has been impaired (e.g., postaxillary node dissection). Lymphangitis may accompany cellulitis or may occur after clinically minor or unapparent skin infection. Lymphangitis is readily recognized by the presence of red, tender, linear streaks directed toward enlarged, tender regional lymph nodes. It is accompanied by systemic symptoms such as chills, fever, malaise, and headache (see the sections on Cellulitis in Chapter 9 and Lymphangitis in Chapter 12).

Streptococcal Myositis. Streptococcal myositis* is a rare but potentially life-threatening entity characterized by severe pain and inflammation in the affected muscle. This condition can also be caused by bacteria, mycobacteria, fungi, viruses, and protozoan forms. Gas gangrene, discussed in the following section, is a type of myositis, as is psoas abscess associated with enteric infection and pyomyositis, an accumulation of pus in the skeletal muscles, usually caused by *S. aureus*. Therapy includes aggressive surgical debridement and IV penicillin. Mortality in reported cases has been high.[92] (See the section on Myositis in Chapter 24 and Streptococcal Gangrene in this chapter.)

Puerperal Sepsis. Puerperal sepsis follows abortion or normal delivery when streptococci colonizing the woman or transmitted from medical personnel invade the endometrium and surrounding structures, lymphatics, and bloodstream. The resulting endometritis and septicemia may be complicated by pelvic cellulitis, septic pelvic thrombophlebitis, peritonitis, or pelvic abscess. Before the antibiotic era and the benefits of handwashing between clients was known, this disease was associated with high mortality.

Group B Streptococci. Group B streptococcal infection (*Streptococcus agalactiae*) is the leading cause of neonatal pneumonia, meningitis, and sepsis. The organism is also an infrequent cause of pyogenic infections in adults. Several thousand neonatal infections with group B streptococci occur in the United States each year, and about 10% of the infants with the infection die. Group B streptococci are part of the normal vaginal flora and are found in 30% of women. Most newborns born to colonized women acquire the organism as they pass through the birth canal, but less than 1% of these infants develop group B streptococcal infections.

Symptoms of infection in the newborn are not specific, but group B streptococcal infection typically presents as lethargy, poor feeding, and respiratory distress. In the first few days of life, fever may not be present, but if infection occurs several weeks after birth, fever is prominent.

Streptococcus pneumoniae
Etiologic and Risk Factors. Pneumonia and other infections, such as sepsis, otitis media, and meningitis, can be caused by *Streptococcus pneumoniae* (pneumococcal pneumonia or pneumococcus). This is the most common cause of community-acquired pneumonia, accounting for 70% of all cases of bacterial pneumonia. *S. pneumoniae* is the most common cause of meningitis in adults and the second most common cause in children over age 6. Head trauma, CSF leaks, and sinusitis may precede pneumococcal meningitis.[13] Pneumococcal pneumonia often follows influenza or viral respiratory infection and is often seen in clients with chronic diseases, during immunosuppression, and in alcohol abusers. Other risk factors are included in Box 7-5.

Clinical Manifestations. Clinical manifestations include acute onset of fever, chills, pleuritis with pleuritic chest pain, and dyspnea with productive cough or purulent sputum that may be blood-tinged. Other complications may include empyema, bacteremia, sepsis, meningitis, pericarditis, endocarditis primarily involving the aortic valve, and septic arthritis. Septic arthritis can occur in a natural or prosthetic joint.[94] or as a complication of rheumatoid arthritis; underlying chronic joint disease may delay diagnosis. Pneumococcal (septic) arthritis secondary to this pathogen is relatively uncommon and occurs principally in the older adult and in individuals with HIV. The clinical symptoms are similar to other forms of hematogenous pyogenic joint infections. Adjacent osteomyelitis involving the vertebral bones may be detected on radiologic examination.

Diagnosis of *S. pneumoniae* is made by recognition of abrupt onset of symptoms typical of pneumonia, defining chest film, and laboratory examination of sputum (culture). Currently, immunization for pneumococcal pneumonia is available and is recommended in specific circumstances of susceptibility as defined by the CDC[11,66] (see Table 7-5). Adults age 65 and older should receive one dose of the vaccine. Individuals ages 2 to 64, with defined conditions such as im-

---

*This condition can also be caused by bacteria, mycobacteria, fungi, viruses, and protozoan forms. Gas gangrene, discussed in the following section, is a type of myositis, as is psoas abscess associated with enteric infection and pyomyositis, and accumulation of pus in the skeletal muscles, usually caused by *S. aureus*.

BOX **7-5**

Risk Factors for Pneumococcal Disease

65 years of age or older
Recent episode of influenza or viral respiratory infection
Chronic illness (e.g., diabetes, heart disease, pulmonary disease, renal disease)
Immunosuppression
Human immunodifeciency virus/acquired immune-deficiency syndrome
Cancer or Hodgkin's disease
History of alcoholism
Liver disease (e.g., cirrhosis)
Asplenia (absent, removed, or nonfunctioning spleen)
Neurologic impairment
Aspiration of oral contents
Cigarette smoking
Resident of a long-term facility

munocompromise, asplenia, chronic liver or renal dysfunction, and diabetes mellitus, should be vaccinated and then revaccinated in 3 to 5 years based on CDC guidelines.[17]

Vaccination is also recommended in certain Native American populations (e.g., Native Alaskans); children under age 2; older children with CDC-specified problems; economically disadvantaged children; and children in group day care who have frequent or complicated otitis media. The Otitis Media Working Group of the CDC has recommended specific treatment guidelines for otitis media since resistant *S. pneumoniae* has increased significantly in incidence.[11,66]

Medical Management

Diagnosis, Treatment, and Prognosis. Clinical diagnosis of streptococcal infections is based on recognition of spreading skin infections and other defining clinical presentation. Laboratory diagnosis isolates the organism from the infected region (or blood as in endocarditis). Treatment is with antibiotic therapy (usually penicillin) and prevents long-term sequelae in heart and kidneys. Prognosis is usually good with therapy even though drug resistance has developed in certain situations; toxic shock syndrome associated with streptococcus has a high mortality. Infection of any joint is considered an orthopedic emergency, and if left untreated, it can destroy a joint within 24 hours.

Special Implications for the Therapist 7-3

STREPTOCOCCAL INFECTIONS

Health care personnel can transmit and acquire streptococcal infections. Guidelines for preventing transmission must be followed at all times (see Boxes 7-2 and 7-4 and Table 7-4).

Preferred Practice Patterns
7A: *Prevention/Risk Reduction for Integumentary Disorder*
7B: *Impaired Integumentary Integrity Associated With Superficial Skin Involvement*
7E: *Impaired Integumentary Integrity Associated With Skin Involvement Extending into Fascia, Muscle, or Bone*

Gas Gangrene (Clostridial Myonecrosis)

Definition and Overview. *Gangrene* is the death of body tissue usually associated with loss of vascular (nutritive, arterial circulation) supply and followed by bacterial invasion and putrefaction. The three major types of gangrene are dry, moist, and gas gangrene. Dry and moist gangrene result from loss of blood circulation due to various causes; gas gangrene occurs in wounds infected by anaerobic bacteria, leading to gas production and tissue breakdown. This is a rare but severe and painful condition that usually follows trauma or surgery in which muscles and subcutaneous tissues become filled with gas and exudate. The disease spreads rapidly to adjacent tissues and can be fatal within hours of onset.

Pathogenesis. Fortunately, the anaerobic conditions necessary to foster clostridial growth are uncommon in human tissues and produced only in the presence of extensive devitalized tissue, as occurs with severe trauma, wartime injuries, and septic abortions. Contributing factors include hypoxia from injury to blood vessels near the wound site, pressure dressings, tourniquets, local injection of vasoconstrictors, foreign bodies, damaged tissues from earlier injury, and concurrent microbial infections. Gas gangrene is most often found in deep wounds, especially those in which tissue necrosis further reduces oxygen supply. Such necrosis releases both carbon dioxide and hydrogen subcutaneously, producing interstitial gas bubbles. Gas gangrene (clostridial myonecrosis) is rare when wounds are promptly and thoroughly cleaned and debrided of traumatized tissue.

Clinical Manifestations. The incubation period for gas gangrene is usually 2 to 4 days after injury. Sudden, severe pain occurring at the site of the wound, which is tender and edematous, are early signs and symptoms of gas gangrene. The skin darkens because of hemorrhage and cutaneous necrosis. The lesion develops a thick discharge, which has a foul odor and may contain gas bubbles. Crepitation may be felt on palpation of the skin from the gas bubbles in muscles and subcutaneous tissue. True gas gangrene produces myositis and anaerobic cellulitis, affecting only soft tissue. The skin over the wound may rupture, revealing dark-red or black necrotic muscle tissue, accompanied by a foul-smelling watery or frothy discharge. Associated symptoms may include sweating, low-grade fever, and disproportionate tachycardia followed by hemolytic anemia, hypotension, and renal failure.

Medical Management

Diagnosis, Treatment, and Prognosis. Prevention is the key to avoiding gas gangrene before treatment is required. To prevent gangrene in an open wound, the wound should be kept as clean as possible. Special wound care is particularly important in people with diabetes mellitus, malnutrition, and immunodeficiency.

Diagnosis based on history and clinical presentation is confirmed by anaerobic cultures of wound drainage and radiographs showing gas in the tissues. Once diagnosed, treatment involves opening the wound widely to admit air and permit drainage. Large, multiple incisions are made through the skin and fascia, sutures and any gangrenous material are removed, and the wound is irrigated. Antiinfective agents are administered but if massive gangrene develops, amputation may be necessary. With prompt treatment, 80% of people with gas gangrene of the extremities survive; prognosis is poorer for gas gangrene in other sites such as the abdominal wall, uterus, or bowel.

Special Implications for the Therapist   7-4

GAS GANGRENE

Preferred Practice Patterns
7A: Prevention/Risk Reduction for Integumentary Disorders
7B: Impaired Integumentary Integrity Associated With
*   Superficial Skin Involvement*
7E: Impaired Integumentary Integrity Associated With Skin
*   Involvement Extending into Fascia, Muscle, or Bone and*
*   Scar Formation*

Careful observation may result in early diagnosis. With any postoperative or posttraumatic injury, look for signs of ischemia such as cool skin, pallor or cyanosis, sudden, severe pain, sudden edema, and loss of pulses in the involved limb. Record carefully and immediately report these findings to the medical staff. Throughout this illness, adequate fluid replacement is essential; assess pulmonary and cardiac functions often.

Special care to prevent skin breakdown is important, and meticulous wound care following surgery is imperative. To prevent gas gangrene, routinely take precautions to render all wound sites unsuitable for growth of clostridia by attempting to keep granulation tissue viable; adequate debridement is imperative to reduce anaerobic growth conditions. Notify the physician immediately of any devitalized tissue. Position the client to facilitate drainage.

Psychologic support is critical, as these clients can remain alert until death, knowing that death is imminent and unavoidable. The therapist must be prepared for the foul odor from the wound and prepare the client emotionally for the large wound after surgical excision. Wound care requires sterile procedures to prevent spread of bacteria; dispose of drainage material and dressings in double plastic bags for incineration. No special cleaning measures are required after the client is discharged. ■

Pseudomonas

Overview.   *Pseudomonas aeruginosa* is a major opportunistic pathogen and one of the most common hospital- or nursing home-acquired (nosocomial) pathogens. The organism infrequently colonizes humans, but it can cause disease, particularly in the hospital environment, where it is associated with pneumonia, wound infections, urinary tract disease, and sepsis in debilitated people. Burns, urinary catheterization, cystic fibrosis, chronic lung diseases, neutropenia associated with chemotherapy, and diabetes all predispose to infections with P. aeruginosa. This bacterium produces the pigments that give the color to the green pus seen in some suppurative infections. It thrives on moist environmental surfaces, making swimming pools, Hubbard tanks, whirlpool tubs, respiratory therapy equipment, and liquid soap dispensers prime targets for growth. This organism is among the most antibiotic-resistant bacteria.

Discrete (i.e., isolated incidences, nonepidemic) hospital outbreaks of P. aeruginosa have been traced to specific reservoirs such as respiratory equipment, endoscopes, transvenous pacemakers, contaminated antistatic mattresses, antiseptics, orthopedic plaster, operating room suction apparatus, contaminated nursery formula and hydrotherapy tanks and pools.

Pathogenesis.   *P. aeruginosa* consists of an array of proteins, which allow it to attach to, invade, and destroy host tissues, while avoiding host inflammatory and immune defenses. Injury to epithelial cells uncovers surface molecules that serve as binding sites for P. aeruginosa. Many strains of this pathogen produce a proteoglycan that surrounds the bacteria, protecting them from mucociliary action, complement, and phagocytes. The organism releases extracellular enzymes, which facilitate tissue invasion and are partially responsible for the necrotizing lesions associated with pseudomonas infections. This pathogen can also invade blood vessel walls and produce systemic pathologic effects through endotoxin and several systemically active exotoxins.

Clinical Manifestations.   Signs and symptoms of pseudomonas infection vary with the site of infection and the state of host defenses.[75] If the host has the capacity to respond to the invading bacteria with neutrophils, an acute inflammatory response results. The pseudomonas organism often invades small arteries and veins, producing vascular thrombosis and hemorrhagic necrosis, particularly in the lungs and skin. Blood vessel invasion predisposes to bacteremia; dissemination (spread); and sepsis (toxins in the blood). Vascular invasion often leads to the rapid development of multiple metastatic nodular lesions in the lungs. Disseminated infections are marked by the development of typical skin lesions called *ecthyma gangrenosum*. These bullous or pustular eruptions represent sites where the organism has disseminated to the skin, invaded blood vessels, and produced localized hemorrhagic infarctions.

This bacterium can cause infective endocarditis on native heart valves in injection drug users and on prosthetic heart valves in the general population; pneumonia in people with chronic lung disease, congestive heart failure, and malignancies, especially those involving the hematopoietic system and in those who are neutropenic as a result of chemotherapy; CNS infections such as meningitis and brain abscess; and infections of the ear, eye, urinary tract, GI tract, skin and soft tissues, and bone and joints.

Central Nervous System Infections.   Pseudomonas infections of the CNS result from extension from a contiguous structure such as ear, mastoid, or paranasal sinus; direct inoculation into the subarachnoid space or brain by means of head trauma, surgery, or invasive diagnostic procedures (e.g., lumbar punctures, spinal anesthesia, intraventricular shunts); and bacteremic spread from a distant site of infection such as the urinary tract, lung, or endocardium.

The clinical manifestations of pseudomonas meningitis are like those of other forms of bacterial meningitis (see Chapter 28) and include fever, headache, and confusion. The onset of disease may be acute and occur suddenly or may be more gradual and insidious in the absence of systemic signs and symptoms, as in those whose meningitis is related to neurosurgery or extension from a contiguous site of chronic infection or in people who are immunosuppressed or have cancer.

Skin and Soft Tissue Infections.   Pseudomonas disease of the skin and mucous membranes can result from primary or metastatic foci of infections. Primary skin and soft tissue infections may be either localized or diffuse. Common predisposing factors are a breakdown in the integument, especially resulting from burns, trauma, pressure ulcers, whirlpool use, and chemotherapy-induced neutropenia. Wound infections may have a characteristic fruity odor (sweet, grapelike odor) with a blue-green exudate that forms a crust on wounds. Pseudomonas bacteria may produce distinctive skin lesions known as *ecthyma gangrenosum*, characterized by hemorrhage, necrosis, and surrounding erythema. Associated symptoms may include headache, dizziness, earache, sore throat, swollen breasts, sore eyes, sore nose, and abdominal cramps. Fever is uncommon and remains low grade when it occurs.

Pseudomonas burn wound sepsis is a dreaded complication of extensive thermal injuries and is characterized by multifocal black or dark-brown discoloration of the burn eschar; degeneration of the underlying granulation tissue with rapid eschar separation and hemorrhage into subcutaneous tissue; edema or hemorrhagic necrosis of previously healthy tissue adjacent to infected burn sites; and erythematous nodular lesions in unburned skin. Systemic manifestations may include fever or hypothermia, disorientation, hypotension, oliguria, ileus, and leukopenia.

Bone and Joint Infections.   Pseudomonas infections of the bones and joints result from hematogenous spread from other primary sites or extension from other sites of infection. Contiguous infections are usually related to penetrating trauma, surgery, or overlying soft tissue infections. *Pseudomonas osteochondritis* can follow puncture wounds of the foot; the sternoclavicular and sacroiliac joints, vertebrae, and symphysis pubis are affected in injection drug users; osteomyelitis occurs in conjunction with vascular insufficiency of the lower extremities in people with diabetes mellitus; diseased large synovial joints are infected in people with underlying rheumatoid disease; and infections of the long bones follow open fractures and internal fixation procedures.

P. osteochondritis following a puncture wound involves the cartilage of the small joints and the bones of the foot. Typically, the person experiences early improvement in pain and swelling following a puncture wound only to have the symptoms recur or worsen several days later. The average duration of symptoms before diagnosis is several weeks, and fever and other systemic signs are usually absent. An area of superficial cellulitis is evident on the plantar surface of the foot, or there may merely be tenderness to deep palpation.

Bloodborne pseudomonas appears to have a predilection for the fibrocartilaginous joints of the axial skeleton involving joint space, cartilage, synovium, and contiguous bone. Vertebral osteomyelitis caused by *P. aeruginosa* is occasionally associated with complicated urinary tract infections and genitourinary surgery or instrumentation. This disease occurs most often in older adults and involves the lumbosacral spine. Physical signs include local tenderness and decreased range of motion in the spine; fever and other systemic symp-

toms are relatively uncommon. Mild neurologic deficits may be present.

Medical Management

Diagnosis, Treatment, and Prognosis.   Diagnosis requires isolation of the pseudomonas organism in blood, spinal fluid, urine, exudate, or sputum culture. Antibiotic therapy is initiated immediately; local pseudomonas infections or septicemia secondary to wound infection requires acetic acid irrigations, topical drug therapy, and debridement or drainage of the infected wound.

P. aeruginosa infections are among the most aggressive human bacterial infections, often progressing rapidly to sepsis, especially in people with poor immunologic resistance (e.g., premature infants; aging adults; and those with debilitating disease, burns, or wounds). In local pseudomonas infections, treatment is usually successful and complications are rare. Immediate medical intervention is necessary; septicemic pseudomonas infections are associated with a high mortality. Medical management is directed according to the site of infection and may include antibiotics, surgery, pulmonary therapy, respiratory assistance if necessary, and other supportive measures dictated by the presence of septic shock and other complications.

Special Implications for the Therapist   7-5

PSEUDOMONAS INFECTIONS

Preferred Practice Patterns
7A: Primary Prevention/Risk Reduction for Integumentary Disorders
7B: Impaired Integumentary Integrity Associated With Superficial Skin Involvement
7E: Impaired Integumentary Integrity Associated With Skin Involvement Extending Into Fascia, Muscle, or Bone and Scar Formation
4E: Impaired Joint Mobility, Motor Function, Muscle Performance, and Range of Motion Associated with Localized Inflammation (arthropathy associated with infection)
5C: Impaired Motor Function and Sensory Integrity Associated with Nonprogressive Disorders of the Central Nervous System: Congenital Origin or Acquired in Infancy or Childhood (meningitis)
5D: Impaired Motor Function and Sensory Integrity Associated With Nonprogressive Disorders of the Central Nervous System: Acquired in Adolescence or Adulthood
6D: Impaired Aerobic Capacity/Endurance Associated With Cardiovascular Pump Dysfunction or Failure (endocarditis)

Pseudomonas is a transient organism that is able to survive less than 24 hours on the skin and is easily removed by washing or scrubbing. These organisms use the hands as a short-lived mode of transmission while looking for a susceptible host or reservoir where they can survive. Such transient organisms readily cause infection once they enter a susceptible host. For this reason, person-to-person transmission of Pseudomonas via the hands of hospital staff is often assumed but difficult to track.[75] These types of organisms can be removed by mechanical friction and soap-and-water washing and become the focus of handwashing to prevent further spread.[78] Proper cleaning of any equipment in contact with mucous membranes or a moist environment is absolutely critical.[67]

Anyone who is immunocompromised should be protected from exposure to this infection. Wound care requires strict sterile technique. ■

VIRAL INFECTIONS

◆ Bloodborne Viral Pathogens

The bloodborne viruses that most endanger HCWs are the bloodborne pathogens hepatitis B virus (HBV); hepatitis C virus (HCV); and HIV. In 1991 the U.S. Congress passed the Bloodborne Pathogens Standard prepared by the Occupational Safety and Health Administration (OSHA) and written to help eliminate or minimize occupational exposure to hepatitis B, hepatitis C, HIV, and other bloodborne pathogens.[7] The guidelines are based on the use of standard precautions, including appropriate handwashing and barrier precautions to reduce contact with body fluids potentially contaminated by these viruses. The use of safety devices and techniques to reduce the handling of sharp instruments can help in reduction of significant contact with body fluids, particularly blood or blood-containing fluids.[100]

Special Implications for the Therapist   7-6

BLOODBORNE VIRAL PATHOGENS

Preferred Practice Patterns
See individual disease discussion.

Hepatitis B

NOTE: See discussion on hepatitis B in Chapter 16. Nosocomial transmission of HBV is a serious risk for HCWs. The risk of acquiring HBV infection from occupational exposure is dependent on the nature and frequency of exposure to blood or body fluids containing blood. An approximate 30% chance exists of acquiring HBV after percutaneous (needle-stick) contact with a surface antigen seropositive source.[7] HBV is transmitted by percutaneous or mucosal exposure to blood and serum-derived body fluids from people who have either the acute or chronic form of HBV infection. The incubation period is 45 to 180 days (average 60 to 90 days).

Hepatitis B vaccination of HCWs who are at risk (e.g., those that work in an area likely to have contact with blood and body fluids) can prevent transmission of HBV and is strongly recommended[15] (see Table 7-5). The need for postexposure prophylaxis with hepatitis B immune globulin (HBIG) vaccination or both depends on the surface antigen status of the source person and the immunization status of the HCW who was exposed. The OSHA bloodborne pathogen standard mandates that hepatitis B vaccine be made available, at the employer's expense, to all HCWs with potential occupational exposure. In addition to

the vaccine, strict adherence to handwashing and standard precautions (see Appendix A) are critical in prevention of the transmission of hepatitis-contaminated body fluids. Transmission is also prevented by use of barriers during sexual activity and by not sharing personal or other items that may have blood on them.

For the HCW who is positive for HIV, HBV, or HCV, the CDC guidelines are based on the assumption that the risk of transmission to others is greatest during invasive procedures that include (for the therapist) sharp debridement or digital palpation of needle tip (or other sharp instrument) in a poorly visualized or highly confined anatomic site. Any therapist performing such procedures should determine his or her own HIV, hepatitis B e antigen, and hepatitis C antigen status. Those who are infected should not perform the procedures unless they have obtained guidance from an expert panel about when and how they may safely do so. Although the CDC does not mandate restricted practice, the requirement that clients of an infected HCW be notified of the provider's infection status before undergoing these procedures is a restriction on practice.[36]

Some experts consider these practice guidelines and the idea of mandatory testing of all clinicians performing invasive procedures cost-prohibitive and unnecessary, given the fact that HCWs are far more likely than their clients to contract bloodborne pathogens from exposure to infected blood. Viewed in this context, extraordinary measures to protect clients undergoing these interventions may not be warranted, and the current CDC recommendations are considered overly conservative.[36]

Hepatitis C

NOTE: See the section on Heptatis C in Chapter 16.

Hepatitis C is the most common etiologic agent in cases of non-A, non-B hepatitis in the United States. Seroprevalence studies among HCWs have shown a significant association between acquisition of disease and health care employment, specifically client care or laboratory work. Accidental percutaneous injuries (needle sticks or cuts with sharp instruments) are the highest risk vehicle for transmission to HCWs from people with acute or chronic hepatitis C. The incubation period for hepatitis C is 6 to 7 weeks, and nearly all individuals with acute infection will have chronic (more than 3 to 6 months' duration) HCV infection with persistent viremia and the potential for transmission to others over an extended period. Serologic assays to detect HCV antibodies (not protective antibodies) are available and are used to determine source and HCW status after exposure. More than 80% of all people with hepatitis C develop chronic hepatitis, and cirrhosis may develop in up to 30% of those with chronic hepatitis C. A risk of developing hepatocellular carcinoma (approximately 3% to 5% per year) exists, and a small percentage of people with hepatitis C may progress to fulminant liver failure.[31]

Currently no vaccine against hepatitis C is available, and no postexposure prophylaxis can be recommended. Postexposure prophylaxis with immune globulin, used with hepatitis B, does not appear to be effective in preventing HCV infection. No current information is available regarding the use of antiviral interferon alpha (used in some cases of chronic hepatitis C) in the post exposure setting, and such prophylaxis is not recommended by the CDC.[7] Strict adherence to handwashing and standard precautions (see Appendix A) are critical in prevention of transmission of hepatitis-contaminated body fluids.

Continued

Transmission is also prevented by use of barriers during sexual activity and by not sharing personal or other items that may have blood on them.

Human Immunodeficiency Virus

NOTE: See the section on HIV in Chapter 6.

Nosocomial transmission of HIV from clients to HCWs may occur after percutaneous or, infrequently, mucocutaneous exposure to blood and body fluids containing blood. According to recent prospective studies done by the CDC, the average risk for HIV infection has been estimated to be about 0.3% for HCWs.[7] HIV seroconversion among HCWs after percutaneous exposure to blood containing HIV is associated with the following factors: (1) presence of visible blood on the device prior to injury, (2) a procedure that involved needle placement into a person's vein or artery, or (3) deep injury with the contaminated device. Transmission of HIV infection was also associated with injuries in which the source was terminally ill with AIDS, thus exposing the HCW to high titers of active virus. The findings of these studies suggested that postexposure treatment of HCWs with zidovudine and lamivudine may be protective for them.

In 1998 the CDC updated previously published provisional recommendations for postexposure chemoprophylaxis and use of antiretroviral therapies. HCWs who sustain needle-stick or other high-risk exposures should be counseled and offered HIV baseline and follow-up blood testing as soon as possible and should then be treated with antiretroviral therapy per CDC protocol. Postexposure, the involved area of contact should be immediately washed thoroughly (not scrubbed) with antiseptic soap and then rinsed with water. Therapy with antiretrovirals should be initiated immediately in high-risk situations and should be continued for 4 weeks.[50] Prevention of transmission includes the use of meticulous handwashing, standard precautions, and the same precautions described above for the bloodborne hepatitis viruses. ■

◆ Herpesviruses

Overview and Definition.   The term *herpes* is derived from the Greek word *herpein*, which means *to creep*. The word refers to the tendency for this type of viral infection to become chronic, latent, and recurrent. The known herpesviruses (HHVs) are divided by genomic and biologic behavior into eight types (Box 7-6). All herpesviruses are morphologically similar but the biologic and epidemiologic features of each are distinct. Subclinical primary infection with the herpesviruses is more common than clinically symptomatic illness and each type then persists in a latent state for the rest of the life of the host. With the herpes simplex virus (HSV) and varicella-zoster virus (VZV), the virus remains latent in sensory ganglia and upon reactivation, lesions appear in the distal sensory nerve distribution. Virus reactivation in immunocompromised hosts may lead to widespread lesions in affected organs such as the viscera or the CNS. Severe or fatal illness may occur in infants and the immunocompromised. Association with malignancies includes EBV with Burkett's lymphoma and nasopharyngeal carcinoma and HHV-8 with Kaposi's sarcoma and body cavity lymphoma.[8,22]

Herpes Simplex Viruses Types 1 and 2
See Table 7-9.

BOX **7-6**

Types of Herpesviruses

Herpes simplex virus (HSV)	Type 1
Herpes simplex virus (HSV)	Type 2
Varicella-zoster virus (VZV)	Type 3
Epstein-Barr infectious mononucleosis virus (EBV)	Type 4
Cytomegalovirus (CMV)	Type 5
Roseola (exanthema subitum) human herpes virus (HHV)	Type 6
Herpes virus serologically associated with roseola, human herpes virus (HHV)	Type 7
Human herpes virus associated with Kaposi's sarcoma (HHV)	Type 8

Incidence, Etiologic Factors, and Risk Factors.   Four out of five Americans harbor HSV-1, which is usually responsible for cold sores; one in five over the age of 12 has HSV-2, the principal cause of genital herpes. Both strains can infect any part of the body and HSV-1 can be transmitted to the genital area during oral sex. Due to the universal distribution of these viruses most individuals have been inoculated by the ages of 1 to 2 years.

Asymptomatic shedding is common and appears to be responsible for transmission, usually during the period immediately preceding appearance of sores. Sexual contact during asymptomatic periods is less likely to result in transmission of the virus than when sores are present. However, since people with genital herpes are more likely to engage in sexual contact when they are free of sores, the rate of asymptomatic transmission is still significant.

Infants born to women with genital herpes can be infected with HSV when they pass through an infected birth canal. The virus can also be passed to other regions of the body by hand contact, particularly in people who are immunosuppressed (e.g., older adults, transplant recipients, people with cancer undergoing chemotherapy, anyone with AIDS or other conditions that weaken the immune system).

Pathogenesis.   Even though HSV-1 and 2 are the two most closely related herpesviruses and share antigenic cross-reactivity, these two agents are genetically and serologically distinct and produce different clinical symptoms. HSV-1 and 2 primarily affect the oral mucocutaneous (cold sores and mouth sores) and genital areas (genital herpes), respectively. Seroprevalence for both agents increases with age and with sexual activity for HSV-2. Primary infection occurs through a break in the mucous membranes of the mouth, throat, eye or genitals, or via minor abrasions in the skin. Initial infection is often asymptomatic, although minor localized vesicular lesions may be evident.

Local multiplication occurs, followed by viremia and systemic infection with a subsequent lifelong latent infection and periodic reactivation of the virus. During primary infection, the virus enters peripheral sensory nerves and migrates along axons to sensory nerve ganglia in the CNS, allowing the virus to escape immune detection and response. During latent infection of nerve cells, viral DNA is maintained and not integrated into surrounding cellular structures, thus maintaining true latency. Various disturbances such as physical or psychologic stress can disrupt the delicate balance of latency, and reactivation of the latent virus occurs. The virus travels back down sensory nerves to the surface of the body and replicates, forming new lesions. Although painful, most recurrent infections resolve spontaneously, recurring at a later time. More serious infections are herpetic keratitis (ulceration of the cornea due to repeated infection) that can lead to blindness and encephalitis, which is very rare but often fatal. Incidence of genital herpes has increased sharply during the last 20 years. Currently HSV-1 is under active development as a vector for gene therapy.[95]

Clinical Manifestations.

Mucocutaneous disease usually involves HSV-1 and affects the mouth and oral cavity (cold sores, mouth sores) but also includes whitlows (herpetic infection of the fingers) and a minority of urogenital infections. Vesicles typically form moist ulcers after several days and if untreated, epithelialize over 2 to 3 weeks. Primary infection may be asymptomatic. Recurrences are usually milder, involve fewer lesions, and heal faster. They are most commonly induced by stress, fever, sunlight, infection, or undetermined factors.[8]

HSV-2 primarily involves the genital tract with latent virus present in the presacral ganglia. Lesions are usually painful, small, grouped, and vesicular with possible burning and itching. The blisterlike lesions break and weep after a few days, leaving ulcerlike sores that usually crust over and heal in 1 to 3 weeks. Genital ulcers may occur on the genital area, buttocks, urethra, or bladder. Aseptic meningitis may be a manifestation of primary infection in women.[22]

Ocular problems such as keratitis, blepharitis, and conjunctivitis can be caused by HSV. Symptoms are usually unilateral and visual acuity may be impaired from adjacent corneal involvement. Both HSV-1 and 2 can infect the fetus and can cause congenital malformations. Neonatal herpes may also occur from unknown shedding in the mother's genital tract at the time of delivery.

Encephalitis and *recurrent meningitis* can also be caused by HSV. Encephalitis usually presents with a flulike prodrome, followed by headache, fever, behavioral and speech disturbances, and seizures. A masslike lesion can appear on scan with HSV encephalitism, and HSV can be identified in CSF. Untreated disease with coma has a very high mortality rate. HSV-2 has been associated as a major cause of lymphocytic meningitis. HSV can also appear as disseminated infection and serious esophagitis in immunocompromised people. An association between HSV-1 and Bell's palsy has also been established.

Medical Management

Diagnosis, Treatment, and Prognosis. Diagnosis is usually made with clinical symptoms, but viral cultures of vesicular fluid or direct fluorescent antibody staining of scraped lesions can confirm the diagnosis. An HSV vaccine that showed promise in animals ultimately failed human testing. Although no immunization against HSV infection is available, new antiviral drugs can minimize recurrences. Drugs commonly used that inhibit replication of HSV-1 and 2 include oral and topical acyclovir, foscarnet, and ophthalmic drops (acyclovir, trifluridine). Acyclovir, however, does not change the clinical course of Bell's palsy. Infections

are recurrent but treatable in most cases.[8] Herpes in a child less than 4 months of age can cause serious illness and can be fatal in some circumstances.

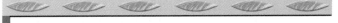

Special Implications for the Therapist   7-7

HERPES SIMPLEX VIRUS

Preferred Practice Pattern
7B: Impaired Integumentary Integrity Associated With
Superficial Skin Involvement
5C, 5D: Acquired Neuromuscular Involvement (meningitis)

Recurrent disease is best treated with acyclovir, and recurrent genital disease requires barrier precautions during sexual activity in addition to medication. Although herpes simplex is contagious, nosocomial transmission is rare. However, it has been reported in some high-risk areas such as nurseries, intensive care units, burn units, and other areas where immunocompromised individuals might be placed. Nosocomial transmission of HSV occurs primarily through contact with lesions or with virus-containing secretions such as saliva, vaginal secretions, or amniotic fluid. Exposed areas of skin, particularly when minor cuts, abrasions, or other skin lesions are present are the most likely sites of viral entry. The incubation period of HSV is 2 to 14 days. HCWs may acquire a herpetic infection of the fingers (herpetic whitlow or paronychia) from exposure to contaminated oral secretions. Such exposures are a distinct risk for HCWs who have direct contact with either oral or respiratory secretions from clients.

HCWs can protect themselves from acquiring HSV by adhering to standard precautions and handwashing before all client care and by the use of appropriate barriers such as a mask, gloves, or gauze dressing to prevent hand contact with the lesion. Some work restrictions may be appropriate for affected HCWs when active lesions are present (e.g., herpetic whitlow) (see Table 7-6). No reports are evident that HCWs with genital HSV infections have transmitted HSV to clients, so no work restriction for people with HSV-2 are indicated.[7]

During the prodromal stage of herpes simplex, the levator scapulae becomes vulnerable to activation of its trigger points by mechanical stresses that are usually well within its tolerance. However, a stiff neck syndrome can develop a day or two before the fully developed symptoms of herpes simplex.[86] Careful questioning regarding previous history of herpes, presence of prodromal symptoms, and observing for the development of a new outbreak of sores during the episode of care will be helpful in making an accurate physical therapy diagnosis. ■

Varicella-Zoster Virus (herpes virus type 3)

Incidence. VZV is human herpes virus type 3 and is known as *chickenpox* or *shingles* (see the section on Viral Infections: Herpes Zoster in Chapter 9). In its primary form (first infection), VZV accounts for about 3.5 million cases of chickenpox per year in the United States. Approximately 10% to 20% of the population develops the secondary or reactivation form of VZV, resulting in herpes zoster or shingles.

TABLE	7-9

Most Common Sexually Transmitted Infections*

INFECTION	INCIDENCE[†]	TRANSMISSION
Human papilloma virus (HPV) (genital warts)	5.5 million new cases/year; incidence is rapidly escalating	Unprotected sexual contact; condoms do not provide 100% protection since the virus can be spread by contact with an infected part of the genitals not covered by a condom; vertical transmission from mother to newborn with vaginal delivery
Chlamydia	3 million new cases/year	Unprotected vaginal or anal intercourse; infection of fetus in pregnant women
Herpes simplex virus 2 (Genital herpes)	1 million new cases/year 45 million carriers	Oral, genital, or anal sex; kissing or touching an infected area when there is a break in the skin; can be spread by asymptomatic person; transmission from mother to child during vaginal birth
Gonorrhea (the "clap")	650,000 new cases/year	Unprotected oral, vaginal, or anal sex; infection of fetus in pregnant women
Hepatitis B	77,000 new cases/year	Infected blood; sexual contact; fecal-oral route
Syphilis (primary)	70,000 new cases/year (primary and secondary combined); overall incidence is declining	Unprotected sexual contact; contact with exudates of skin and mucous membranes of infected person; transplacental infection of fetus if mother is infected; can transmit though blood transfusion§
Syphilis (secondary)		
Syphilis (latent)		
Syphilis (late; can occur up to 20 years after second stage)		
HIV/AIDS	45,000 new cases/year; half caused by sexual contact	Exposure to blood/blood products; exposure to body fluids (blood, semen, vaginal secretions, breast milk); sexual contact; shared needles in injection drug users; transmission from mother to child during vaginal delivery or breast feeding

*Listed in descending order by incidence.
†Statistics provided by Kaiser Family Foundation and American Social Health Association, Menlo Park, Calif, 1998.
‡All sexually transmitted diseases can be prevented by sexual abstinence and mutually monogamous sex between two uninfected partners. The Centers for Disease Control and Prevention has come under criticism by the medical community for not stressing this point in their prevention programs for young people.
§Centers for Disease Control and Prevention: *Control of communicable diseases manual*, CDC, ed 17, Atlanta, 2000, The Centers.

Approximately 300,000 to 600,000 cases of shingles occur in the United States every year, although these numbers for both primary and secondary infection are expected to decline with the increased use of the varicella virus vaccine (Varivax).

Pathogenesis. Like other herpes viruses, VZV has the capacity to persist in the body (in sensory nerve ganglia) as a latent infection after the primary (first) infection. Transmission is via face-to-face airborne droplets, although the disease can also spread through virus-contaminated ventilation in institutions. VZV enters the host through the respiratory tract and conjunctiva and has a short survival time outside the infected host. The virus is believed to multiply at the site of entry in the nasopharynx and in regional lymph nodes. A primary viremia occurs 4 to 6 days after infection and then disseminates to other organs such as the liver, spleen, and sensory ganglia. Further replication occurs in the viscera, followed by a secondary viremia with viral infection of the skin and mucosa,

CLINICAL MANIFESTATIONS	TREATMENT‡
Warts on the genitals, anal region, vagina, cervix, mouth, or throat: 1-6 months after sexual contact with infected person; *in women*; abnormal pap smear, HPV can cause cervical cancer	Can be removed using chemical, ablative, or surgical therapies. Recurrence is not uncommon.
In men: none or urethritis *In women:* none or vaginal discharge with pus or mucus; pain; burning during urination; genital reddening can cause pelvic inflammatory disease (PID) and infertility if untreated; eye infections in newborn	Can be cured with antibiotics. Partner must be treated as well. PID may require additional treatment.
None or vesicular (blister-like) lesions on the genitals, vagina, cervix, anal region, mouth, or throat; can cause serious complications if untreated	Cannot be cured but healing can be accelerated and recurrence of outbreaks can be reduced with antivirals; partner must be informed.
In men: urethritis with discharge, frequent urge to urinate and pain during urination *In women:* none or slight vaginal discharge and difficulty or pain during urination; pelvic pain; abnormal menstrual cycle *Both:* Cardiac valvular disease, arthritis (if untreated)	Can be cured with antibiotics, although some strains are drug resistant.
Jaundice, arthralgias, rash, dark urine, anorexia, nausea, painful abdominal bloating, clay-colored stools, fever	Can be prevented with hepatitis B vaccine. In unvaccinated people, hepatitis B immune globulin (HIBG) and antiviral agents are used but relapse on cessation of treatment is common.
Painless sore at site of infection (genitals, mouth) occurring 3-8 weeks after infection	Can be cured with antibiotics in primary, secondary, and latent stages. Late-stage disease may cause irreversible damage.
Flulike symptoms and rash occurring 6-12 weeks to 1 to 2 years after infection None Cardiovascular and central nervous system damage	
Widespread illness due to immune system decline; may not develop symptoms for 10 years or more after infection	Cannot be cured but combined antiviral therapy can prolong life for many people.

producing vesicles filled with high titers of infectious virus, which then shed more virus. The incubation period is from 14 to 16 days from exposure with a range of 10 to 21 days. This may be prolonged in immunocompromised people and those who have received varicella zoster immune globulin (VZIG).[5]

The exact mechanism for the reactivation of VZV remains unknown, although shingles occurs more often in immunocompromised adults such as the older adult; those with hematologic malignancies, especially leukemia and lymphoma; and people with HIV.

Clinical Manifestations. Disease manifestations are either chickenpox (varicella) or shingles (herpes zoster).

(See Chapter 9 for discussion of clinical manifestations of herpes zoster.) Primary VZV is virtually always symptomatic and second episodes of chickenpox are uncommon unless the child is under the age 1. A mild prodrome consisting of fever and malaise may precede the onset of the rash. Adults may have 1 to 2 days of fever and malaise, but in children, the rash is often the first sign of disease. The rash is an itchy rash that is generalized and rapidly progresses from macules to papules to vesicular lesions before crusting. It usually appears first on the scalp and moves to the trunk and then the extremities with the highest concentration of lesions on the trunk. Lesions also can appear on mucous membranes of the oropharynx, respiratory tract, vagina, conjunctiva and the cornea. The vesicles contain clear fluid on an erythematous base that may rupture or become pustular before they dry and crust. Successive crops appear over several days, with lesions present in several stages of evolution at any one time. The crusts slough in 7 to 14 days.[5] Some varicella infections are subclinical and in immunocompromised people, VZV can occur with no visible skin lesions but can be present viscerally. The generalized pattern of eruption without specific dermatome distribution distinguishes varicella from herpes zoster (see Fig. 9-6).

Complications of varicella include secondary bacterial infections, which are the most common; interstitial pneumonia, which can result in adult respiratory distress syndrome (ARDS); and rarely, meningitis, encephalitis, and Reye's syndrome.[99] When contracted during the first or second trimesters of pregnancy, varicella carries a small risk of congenital malformations. If a mother develops varicella within 5 days after delivery, the newborn is at risk of serious disseminated disease and should receive VZIG.

Medical Management

Diagnosis, Treatment, and Prognosis. Diagnosis is usually made based on clinical symptoms. Lowered white blood cell count (leukopenia) is common and VZV may be isolated in tissue culture. The most common source of isolation is vesicular fluid. Stained smears from vesicular scrapings may reveal multinucleated giant cells consistent with VZV infection. A reliable history of chickenpox has been found to be a valid measure of immunity to varicella because the rash is distinctive and subclinical cases are unusual. Serologic testing is not routinely used but may be useful in adult vaccination programs.

Bedrest is important until the fever has gone down, and the person's skin should be kept clean to avoid secondary bacterial contamination. Itching can be relieved with oral antihistamines, topical calamine lotion, and other skin soothing lotions and baths. Antiviral therapy is necessary in some situations but is not usually used in uncomplicated, low-risk situations. In immunocompromised individuals and pregnant women (during the third trimester), antiviral therapy with high-dose acyclovir is recommended. Antiviral therapy is also used for pneumonitis; corneal infection (herpes zoster); or trigeminal infection in immunocompetent adults. Topical acyclovir and steroids are also used for eye involvement. Secondary bacterial infections of lesions are treated with antibacterial ointment or oral antibiotics if severe. Postherpetic neuralgia, persistent nerve pain following shingles, may be treated palliatively with a skin patch that delivers an analgesic drug.

The total duration of varicella from onset to resolution of crusts is usually less than 2 weeks. Fatalities are rare but may occur in cases of neonatal chickenpox or among immunocompromised people. Recovery from varicella infection usually results in lifetime immunity. Herpes zoster resolves in 2 to 6 weeks. Antibodies persist longer and at higher levels with zoster than with primary varicella. Varicella vaccine is recommended for all children at 12 to 18 months of age and for all children by the thirteenth birthday if they have not had chickenpox. It is recommended for all susceptible adolescents and adults (see Table 7-5).[5]

Special Implications for the Therapist 7-8

VARICELLA-ZOSTER VIRUS

NOTE: See Special Implications for the Therapist: Herpes Zoster in Chapters 9 and 38.

Preferred Practice Pattern
7B: Impaired Integumentary Integrity Associated with Superficial Skin Involvement

Varicella is highly contagious. The period of communicability extends from 1 to 2 days before the onset of the rash through the first 4 to 5 days or until all lesions have formed crusts. Immunocompromised individuals with progressive varicella are probably contagious during the entire period new lesions are appearing.

Nosocomial transmission of VZV is well known. Sources for nosocomial exposures include clients or residents, HCWs, and visitors, including children or HCWs, with either varicella or zoster. It is generally advisable to allow only workers who are immune to varicella to take care of clients with VZV. Because of the possibility of transmission to and development of severe illness in high-risk clients, HCWs with localized zoster should not take care of such clients until all lesions are dry and crusted. However, they may take care of others if they cover their lesions (see the section on Herpes Zoster in Chapter 9).

To prevent transmission of VZV affected individuals should be isolated until crusts have dried. HCWs who do take care of VZV clients should use standard precautions including careful use of barriers such as gloves, gowns, and masks whenever in contact with active lesions. If serologic immunity of the HCW cannot be verified, varicella vaccine is recommended (see Table 7-5). When unvaccinated susceptible HCWs are exposed to varicella, they are potentially infectious 10 to 21 days after exposure and exclusion from duty is indicated from day 10 through day 21 after the last exposure or until all lesions are dry and crusted. When vaccinated HCWs are exposed to varicella, serotesting for antibodies may be done, and exclusion from duty can occur if they are seronegative or develop varicella symptoms. VZIG and acyclovir are not routinely recommended postexposure for healthy HCWs (exceptions may be made for pregnant or immunocompromised HCWs).[5,7] ∎

Infectious Mononucleosis (Herpesvirus Type 4)

Overview. Infectious mononucleosis (herpesvirus type 4) is an acute infectious disease caused by EBV, a member of the herpesvirus group. Although it may be seen at any age, it primarily affects young adults and children. In children, it is usually so mild that its presence often goes unnoticed.

Incidence, Etiologic Factors, and Risk Factors.

Infection with EBV is fairly common in the United States and both genders are affected equally. Incidence varies seasonally among college students but not among the general population. The reservoir of EBV is limited to humans and probably spreads by the oral-pharyngeal route (most likely in saliva), since about 80% of people carry EBV in the throat during the acute infection and for an indefinite period afterward. For this reason, it is sometimes called the *kissing disease*. It can also be transmitted by blood transfusion and has been reported after cardiac surgery as the postpump perfusion syndrome.

Pathogenesis and Clinical Manifestations. EBV causes lymphoid proliferation in the blood, lymph nodes, and spleen. Characteristically, the virus produces fever, sore throat, headache, painful cervical lymphadenopathy, hepatic dysfunction, and increased lymphocytes and monocytes. The incubation period is about 10 days in children and from 30 to 50 days in adults.

Temperature fluctuations occur throughout the day, peaking in the evening (101° F to 102° F [38.3° C to 38.9° C.]). A maculopapular rash closely resembling the rash of rubella occurs in 10% to 15% of those affected. Hepatomegaly may develop and the spleen may enlarge to two to three times its normal size, causing left upper quadrant pain with possible referral to the left shoulder and left upper trapezius region. Both the peripheral and central nervous systems can be involved.

Overall, major complications are rare but may include splenic rupture, aseptic meningitis, encephalitis, hemolytic anemia, idiopathic thrombocytopenia, and Guillain-Barré syndrome. Symptoms subside about 6 to 10 days after onset of the disease but may persist for weeks. A recent study supports an association between a history of infectious mononucleosis and the subsequent development of multiple sclerosis within the following 12 months. A history of infectious mononucleosis (IM) was associated with a greater than five times risk of multiple sclerosis.[63]

Medical Management

Diagnosis, Treatment, and Prognosis. The symptoms of EBV infection mimic those of other infectious diseases such as hepatitis, rubella, and toxoplasmosis. Diagnosis is based on three criteria: physical assessment, laboratory tests, and a positive heterophil* (Monospot) test. Rising levels of antibodies to EBV were once thought to be the cause of chronic fatigue syndrome (CFS) but are now considered a result of CFS (see the section on Chronic Fatigue and Immune Dysfunction Syndrome in Chapter 6). EBV is also associated with several other diseases or syndromes including Burkett's lymphoma, Hodgkin's lymphoma, nasopharyngeal carcinoma, oral hairy leukoplakia, and other lymphoproliferative syndromes.[8,80]

The prognosis is excellent with rest and supportive care, but no lifetime immunity exists against this virus; the virus can live indefinitely in B lymphocytes. No other specific intervention alters or shortens the disease process.

---

*Heterophil antibodies (agglutinins for sheep red blood cells) in serum drawn during the acute illness and at 3- to 4-week intervals rise to four times normal.

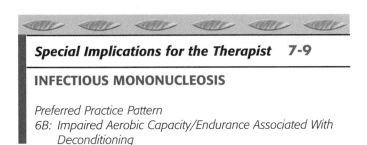

Special Implications for the Therapist 7-9

INFECTIOUS MONONUCLEOSIS

Preferred Practice Pattern
6B: Impaired Aerobic Capacity/Endurance Associated With Deconditioning

Infectious mononucleosis is probably contagious before symptoms develop until the fever subsides and the oral and pharyngeal lesions disappear. Although infectious mononucleosis appears to be only mildly contagious, adherence to standard precautions, especially good handwashing and avoiding shared dishware or food items with other people, is essential in preventing the HCW from contracting this condition.

The person with infectious mononucleosis should be cautioned against engaging in excessive activity, especially contact sports, which could result in splenic rupture or lowered resistance to infection. Usually this guideline is appropriate for a period of at least 1 month. Any sign of splenic rupture (e.g., abdominal or upper quadrant pain; Kehr's sign, or sudden left shoulder pain; or shock) requires immediate medical evaluation. Any soft tissue mobilization or myofascial techniques necessary in the left upper quadrant, especially up and under the rib cage, must take into consideration the enlarged liver and/or spleen; indirect techniques away from the spleen are indicated. ∎

Cytomegalovirus (Herpesvirus Type 5)

Overview and Incidence. Cytomegalovirus (herpesvirus type 5) or cytomegalic inclusion disease (CID) is a commonly occurring DNA herpes virus group. CMV may occur congenitally, peri- or postnatally, or disseminated in immunocompromised people; it increases in frequency with age. One percent of newborns have it, and four out of five adults over age 35 have CMV (usually contracted during childhood or early adulthood) and are seropositive. Multiple sites may be affected, including the brain (in utero infection); salivary glands; kidneys; liver; lung; pancreas; thyroid; adrenals; and GI tract.

Etiologic and Risk Factors. CMV is transmitted by human contact such as through the placenta, urine, breast milk, feces, blood, and semen, vaginal, and cervical secretions and through blood transfusions and transplanted organs (organ recipients have the greatest risk). CMV is extremely common with AIDS.

Pathogenesis and Clinical Manifestations. CMV probably spreads through the body via lymphocytes or mononuclear cells to the lungs (CMV pneumonitis); liver (CMV hepatitis); GI tract (CMV gastroenteritis); eyes (CMV retinitis); and CNS, where it produces inflammatory reactions. Lesions include diffuse interstitial pneumonitis leading to respiratory distress syndrome; hepatitis, adrenalitis, and intestinal ulcerations; and calcifications around ventricles in neonatal CNS infections.

In normal adults, the infection is usually asymptomatic and runs a self-limiting course. In immunosuppressed people, transplant recipients, or neonates, fever, splenomegaly, hepatitis, pneumonitis or other pulmonary involvement or multisystem involvement is evident. In people with AIDS, infection with CMV can cause the various clinical illnesses listed, but the most common manifestation is chorioretinitis. Early symptoms include mild visual impairment and deficits of peripheral vision; blindness can occur. CMV commonly causes peripheral neuropathies and distal sensory axonal neuropathies occurring in the later phases of HIV infection.

Medical Management

Diagnosis, Treatment, and Prognosis. Diagnosis is made by isolating the virus in cultures of urine, saliva, the throat, or cervix; serum antibody titers may indicate prior infection that has been reactivated. Treatment is toward relief of symptoms and preventing complications. In the immunosuppressed person, pharmacologic treatment with ganciclovir, foscarnet, or cidofovir has been proven effective (acyclovir is ineffective). Transplant recipients are most at risk the first 100 days following transplantation (see Chapter 20). The prognosis for people with transplanted organs or who are immunocompromised is poor, as they may have fatal disseminated infections with respiratory failure.

Special Implications for the Therapist 7-10

CYTOMEGALOVIRUS

Practice Patterns
6B: Impaired Aerobic Capacity/Endurance Associated with
Deconditioning
Other practice patterns depend on organ systems involved
and clinical presentation.

The two principle reservoirs of CMV in health care institutions are (1) infants and young children and (2) immunocompromised individuals. However, HCWs who provide care to these high-risk populations have a rate of primary CMV that is no higher than among personnel without such client contact. CMV transmission appears to occur directly, either through close, intimate contact with contaminated secretions or through excretions, especially saliva or urine.[23] Transmission by the hands of HCWs or individuals with the virus has also been suggested. The incubation period for person-to-person is not known, and although CMV can survive on environmental surfaces or objects for a very short time, no evidence of fomite transmission exists.[7]

Pregnant women and immunosuppressed people should avoid exposure to confirmed or suspected CMV infection. Pregnant women or women of childbearing age need to be counseled regarding the risks and prevention of transmission of CMV, but no data show that HCWs can be protected from infection by transfer to areas with less contact with individuals who have been diagnosed with CMV. Work restrictions for HCWs who contract CMV are not necessary since the risk of transmission of CMV can be reduced by careful adherence to handwashing and standard precautions.[7]

Clients with CMV infection should be encouraged to wash their hands thoroughly and frequently to prevent spreading it. It is especially important to impress this on young children. As difficult as it may be, the child should not be allowed to kiss others, and parents and others should also avoid kissing the affected child. ∎

Herpesviruses Types 6, 7, and 8

Human herpesvirus 6 (HHV-6) is a B-cell lymphotropic virus that is the principle cause of exanthema subitum (roseola infantum or Sixth disease). Primary HHV-6 is common in children under age 2, but its occurrence in adults is more complicated and associated with immunocompromised states such as AIDS and lymphoma. It has been associated with graft rejection and bone marrow suppression in transplant recipients and has recently been mentioned as a factor in the cause of multiple sclerosis.[8]

Human herpesvirus 7 (HHV-7) is a T-cell lymphotropic virus that has also been serologically associated with roseola. HHV-8 is associated with Kaposi's sarcoma in AIDS and other immune-related diseases (e.g., body cavity lymphoma)[40,58] (see the section on Kaposi's Sarcoma in Chapter 9).

◆ Viral Respiratory Infections

Viral respiratory infections (influenza, respiratory syncytial virus) are common problems in health care settings. Many viral pathogens can cause nosocomial respiratory infections but influenza and respiratory syncytial virus (RSV) are associated with significant morbidity and mortality in health care situations.

Influenza

Nosocomial transmission of influenza has been reported in acute and long-term health care facilities and has occurred from clients to HCWs, from HCWs to clients, and among HCWs. The mode of transmission from person to person is believed to be by direct deposition of virus-laden large droplets onto the mucosal surfaces of the upper respiratory tract of an individual during close contact with a person with the virus rather than by fomites or large particle aerosols. The incubation period is usually 1 to 5 days after illness onset. Although sporadic cases occur, epidemics usually appear at varying intervals, usually in the fall or winter. The three types of influenza are designated by A, B, and C. Antigenic types A and B influenza produce clinically very similar infections, whereas type C is usually a minor illness. Only types A and B can cause human influenza epidemics and are included in the vaccine.

Influenza resembles many other mild fever-causing illnesses but is almost always accompanied by a nonproductive cough. The onset is usually abrupt, with fever, chills, malaise, muscular aching, substernal soreness, headache, nasal stuffiness, sore throat, and occasionally nausea. The fever lasts about 1 to 7 days (usually 3 to 5). The virus may be isolated from throat washings and cultured, and leukopenia (low white blood cell count) and occasional proteinuria (protein in the urine) are common.[8]

Genetic mutations in the influenza virus create hundreds of variations within the three main types; being immune to one variant does not ensure immunity to another. Trivalent influenza virus vaccine provides partial immunity (about 85% efficacy) for a few months to 1 year. The CDC updates the vaccine annually to include the most current influenza A and B virus strains. Vaccination is recommended before the beginning of each influenza season for people over age 50,* children and teenagers receiving chronic aspirin therapy, nursing home residents, those with chronic lung or heart disease or other debilitating illnesses, and HCWs, including pregnant women (see Table 7-5). During institutional outbreaks of in-

---

*In April 2000 the Advisory Committee on Immunization Practices (ACIP) lowered the age by 15 years from 65 and older to 50 and older. This policy changed because under the old guidelines, many people at risk for complications from influenza were being missed. About 25% of people between the ages of 50 and 64 have chronic medical conditions that place them at risk for influenza-related hospitalizations and possible death. The new plan recognizes that mass immunization programs based on age have been more successful than those targeting people with chronic diseases.

fluenza, prophylactic influenza antiviral agents (e.g., amantadine, rimantadine, zanamivir, and oseltavir) may be used in conjunction with vaccine.[103] Many people with influenza prefer to rest in bed; analgesics and a cough medicine mixture are often used. The antiviral agents used to treat influenza are given in the same doses as are those used for prophylaxis.

These help decrease the duration and severity of signs and symptoms. Droplet precautions (see Table 7-4) are imperative for all diagnosed and suspected cases of influenza. Ribavirin delivered as an aerosol with oxygen has helped severely ill individuals with influenza A or B. Newer agents such as nasally applied zanamivir are under development. Antibacterial antibiotics are used only for treatment of bacterial complications.

The duration of the uncomplicated illness is 1 to 7 days, and the prognosis is usually very good in previously healthy people. Frequent complications of influenza, particularly in older adults and a chronically ill person, are acute sinusitis, otitis media, purulent bronchitis, and pneumonia. Pericarditis, myocarditis, and thrombophlebitis sometimes occur; Reye's syndrome is a rare (almost eradicated) and severe complication of influenza and other viral diseases, especially in young children (acetaminophen should be used for fever instead of aspirin in children). Most fatalities related to influenza are due to bacterial pneumonia. The mortality rate is low except in debilitated individuals. People at greatest risk for influenza-related complications are (1) individuals older than 65 years, (2) residents of chronic health care facilities such as nursing homes, (3) people with chronic pulmonary or cardiovascular disease, and (4) people with diabetes mellitus.[7]

Respiratory Syncytial Virus. Respiratory syncytial virus (RSV) causes annual outbreaks of pneumonia, bronchiolitis, and tracheobronchitis in infants and very young children. In adults and older children, reinfection is common and manifests itself as mild upper respiratory tract infection and tracheobronchitis. Serious pulmonary RSV infections have been described in older adults and immunocompromised individuals with a high mortality rate in bone marrow transplant and pediatric liver transplant recipients.[33,59] In addition, infants with congenital heart disease, intensive care unit clients, and older adults are at high risk for serious and complicated RSV. Annual epidemics occur in winter and spring. The average incubation period is 5 days. Inoculation may occur through the eyes or nose.

Nosocomial transmission of RSV occurs among clients, visitors, and HCWs. RSV is present in large numbers in the respiratory secretions of people with symptomatic RSV infections. It can be transmitted through large droplets during close contact with such individuals or indirectly by hands or fomites that are contaminated with RSV. Hands can become contaminated through touching or handling of fomites or respiratory secretions and can transmit RSV by touching the nose or eyes. Usually, people shed the virus for 3 to 8 days, but young infants may shed the virus for as long as 3 to 4 weeks. Signs include low-grade fever, tachypnea, and wheezing. Hyperinflated lungs, decreased gas exchange, and increased work of breathing are also often present, and otitis media is a common complication.

Rapid diagnosis of RSV may be made by viral antigen identification of nasal washings using an enzyme-linked immunosorbent assay (ELISA) or immunofluorescent assay. Culture of nasopharyngeal secretions remains the standard of diagnosis. Treatment consists of hydration, humidification of inspired air, and ventilatory support as needed. In infants, aerosolized ribavirin (an antiviral agent used in chronic hepatitis C therapy) given with oxygen may be beneficial; pregnant women should avoid ribavirin exposure, since it is associated with fetal malformation or fetal death. Respiratory syncytial virus immune globulin (human) (RSV-IGIV) has been shown to be safe and effective prophylaxis against lower respiratory tract infection in infants and young children who are at high risk of serious RSV, but the vaccine is expensive and must be administered intravenously. A vaccine given to pregnant women may provide passive protection against respiratory syncytial virus in neonates. A significant number of people have recurrent episodes of bronchiolitis and wheezing and may develop asthma later in life. Avoidance of exposure to tobacco smoke, cold air, and air pollutants is also beneficial to long-term recovery from RSV bronchiolitis. A number of vaccines to prevent this infection are currently being studied.[51,58]

Special Implications for the Therapist 7-11

VIRAL RESPIRATORY INFECTIONS

Influenza

HCWs must follow the guidelines in Tables 7-4 and 7-5 regarding prevention of transmission of influenza, both for themselves and their clients. Recommendations for immunization must be reviewed and acted on individually. Since the immunization for influenza does not provide immunity for the entire year or for all strains of influenza, common sense must prevail in the case of a HCW who suspects he or she has early signs and symptoms of influenza. An early diagnosis can result in the use of antivirals to minimize intensity and duration of the symptoms. HCWs must be aware of their responsibility to avoid transmission of infectious diseases such as influenza and either use personal protective equipment or practice self-isolation by staying home. This is especially important for the therapist in a setting with aged, immunocompromised, or chronically ill individuals.

Respiratory Syncytial Virus

Nosocomial RSV infections disseminate quickly, requiring rapid diagnosis; droplet and contact precautions (see Table 7-4); handwashing; and sometimes, passive immunization to achieve prevention in hospitals. Because viral respiratory infections are so common during the winter and spring months, it is difficult for health care facilities to restrict workers with the virus from all client care duties. However, restricting HCWs with acute viral respiratory infections from care of high-risk clients may be necessary during community outbreaks of RSV and influenza. ∎

MISCELLANEOUS INFECTIOUS DISEASES

◆ Infections with Prostheses and Implants

Overview. Over the past decades joint replacement surgery has become commonplace, which is largely attributed to the success of these procedures in restoring function to people with disabling arthritis. People receiving total joint replacements number in the hundreds of thousands each year worldwide, and virtually millions of people have indwelling prosthetic joints. Likewise, during the past 30 years, many new instrumentation systems for internal fixation of the spine have been developed.[9]

Other types of prostheses or implants susceptible to infection include breast implants, dental implants, cardiac implants, other orthopedic devices and hardware, shunts, and even contact lenses (external to epithelial surfaces that can give rise to serious sight-threatening infections).

Incidence. The successful development of synthetic materials and the introduction of artificial devices into nearly all body systems has been accompanied by the adaptation of microorganisms to the opportunities these devices provide for eluding defenses and invading the host. With improvements in surgical procedures and prophylactic antibiotics, the incidence of infection has been reduced to less than 1.5%. The incidence of infection does increase with longer procedures and revisions.[73] However, as the number of people undergoing replacements has grown, reoperations have become increasingly common. Bioprostheses, implanted in large numbers in the 1970s and early 1980s, have now gone into the second decade of life since implantation, a time when biodegradation becomes more common. Multiple reoperations carry a higher risk of infection. Likewise, as the population ages, an increasing number of total hip, knee, shoulder, elbow, wrist, and finger arthroplasties are coming up for revision.

Infection of a prosthetic joint causes loosening of the prosthesis and sepsis with significant mortality and morbidity. Two thirds of prosthetic joint infections occur within 1 year of surgery and are due to intraoperative inoculations of bacteria into the new joint or postoperative bacteremias. Early infections have been substantially reduced due to preoperative use of antibiotics, the use of cleaner air systems in operating rooms, and improved surgical technique.[68,73]

Risk Factors. Certain groups have been identified as predisposed toward infection of their prosthetic joints, including those with prior surgery at the site of the prosthesis, rheumatoid arthritis, corticosteroid therapy, diabetes mellitus, poor nutritional status, low albumin, obesity, and extremely advanced age.[9] One case of skin breakdown with sequential infection of silicone metacarpophalangeal joint arthroplasty was attributed to excessive and improper use of the hand.[38] Risk factors for infection of spinal instrumentation may include IV drug use, paraplegia with neurogenic bladder, and pyelonephritis secondary to renal calculi.

Certain factors or events can enhance the ability of bacteria to multiply rapidly and increase the risk of infection. For example, wound hematomas, seromas, and hemarthroses; fresh operative wounds; ischemic wounds; and tissues in diabetic and steroid-treated people. In the early postimplantation period the fascial layers have not yet healed, and the deep, periprosthesis tissue is not protected by the usual physical barriers. Any superficial infection that develops, such as ischemic necrosis, an infected wound hematoma, wound infection, or suture abscess, can become a preceding event for joint replacement sepsis.

Joint replacement has been shown to be responsible for reactivation of quiescent infections that occurred earlier in a person's life. Knowledge of a previous history of osteomyelitis, tuberculosis, HIV, or other bacteria with latent capabilities is extremely important before joint replacement surgery.[24]

Etiologic Factors and Pathogenesis. The four major pathologic processes that may arise in response to any biomedical implant are infection, inflammation, thrombosis, and neoplasia. Only infection is discussed in this section. Prosthetic joints and other implants become infected by two different pathogenic routes: the hematogenous route and the locally introduced route. Any bacterium can induce infection of a total joint replacement by the hematogenous route, which accounts for 20% to 40% of prosthetic joint infections. Hematogenous spread may occur from dentogingival infections, pyogenic skin processes, and genitourinary or GI tract infections or procedures.

Locally introduced forms of infection account for 60% of all prosthetic joint infections and occurs as a result of wound sepsis next to the prosthesis or operative contamination. This can occur as a result of direct implantation (seeding) at the time of the operation by the operating team, from environmental sources, or from contaminated implant materials. Generally, these infections are caused by a single pathogen, but polymicrobial sepsis can occur.

Staphylococci (coagulase-negative staphylococci and S. aureus) are the principal causative agents in a locally introduced infection; aerobic streptococci and gram-negative bacilli are each responsible for 20% to 25% of cases; and anaerobes are involved in about 10% of these infections.[9] Locally introduced forms of infection can be the result of wound sepsis in the near vicinity of the prosthesis or operative contamination. Any factor that delays or impairs wound healing increases the risk of infection. Rarely, latent foci of chronic, nonactive osteomyelitis are reactivated by the disruption of tissue associated with prosthetic surgery. Previous S. aureus and M. tuberculosis infections can recur postoperatively.[9]

Prostheses that are cemented into place with polymethyl methacrylate develop infection at the bone-cement interface, whereas cementless prostheses may develop sepsis in the bone contiguous with the metallic alloy. As foreign bodies, these prostheses contribute to local sepsis by decreasing the quantity of bacteria necessary to establish infection and by permitting pathogens to persist on their avascular surface, sequestered from circulating immunologic defenses (leukocytes, antibodies, and complement) and from systemic antibiotics.[9] Before the development of cementless prostheses, the cement used appeared to predispose toward infection by inhibiting phagocytic, lymphocytic, and complement function. Today, these devices have textured surfaces to provide fixation by the growth of adjacent bone into the porous interface of the prosthesis. The performance and durability of this new form of arthroplasty remain uncertain.[9]

In the presence of prosthetic or implantable devices, many bacteria form a fibrous material called *glycocalyx*. Organisms can reproduce within this matrix and form a thick biofilm that is protected in part from host defense mechanisms. Biofilms are an important issue for surgery involving prosthetic or implantable devices. For example, only 32% of infections caused by slime-producing staphylococci resolved with antibiotics compared with 100% recovery in non–slime-producing strains. The implant and its adherent biofilm must be removed for the infection to resolve since recurrent, acute infections or disseminated, persistent infection may develop if these reservoirs are allowed to continue. Meticulous protocols for sterilization of implants should be followed since biofilms may be identified as an important mechanism of bacterial resistance to disinfectants and germicides in the hospital.[106]

Clinical Manifestations.

The pattern and clinical presentation is determined largely by three factors: the virulence of the infecting pathogen, the nature of the host tissue in which the microorganism grows, and the route of infection. *S. aureus* and β-hemolytic streptococci are particularly virulent pathogens in this situation and usually produce a fulminant (occurring suddenly with great intensity) infection, occasionally with septic shock. Coagulase-negative staphylococci are avirulent but tenacious pathogens consistently associated with a more indolent (slow) course of events.

Prosthetic joint sepsis produces the cardinal symptoms of inflammation with a wide variability of severity. Most people present with a long course, characterized by a progressive increase in joint pain and occasionally the formation of cutaneous draining sinuses, but without fever, soft tissue swelling, or systemic toxicity. Others present with an acute illness with high fever, severe joint pain, local swelling, and erythema. When a bloodborne infection arises in a prosthetic joint several months or years after implantation surgery, the fully healed connective tissue often is capable of restricting the septic process to a relatively small focus at the bone-cement interface. Joint pain is the principal symptom of deep tissue infection irrespective of mode of presentation and suggests either acute inflammation of the periarticular tissue or loosening of the prosthesis due to subacute erosion of bone at the bone-cement interface.

Medical Management

Diagnosis.

Clinical manifestations of joint pain, swelling, erythema, and warmth all reflect an underlying inflammatory process in the surrounding tissues but are not specific for infection. When a painful prosthesis is accompanied by fever or purulent drainage from overlying cutaneous sinuses, infection is investigated further. The physician must differentiate infection from aseptic and mechanical problems (e.g., hemarthrosis, gout, mechanical loosening, or dislocation), which are more common causes of inflammatory and painful symptoms in this population. Constant joint pain is suggestive of infection, whereas mechanical loosening commonly causes pain only with motion or with weight bearing.

The specific diagnosis of joint replacement infection is dependent on isolation of the pathogen by aspiration of joint fluid or by culture of tissue obtained at arthrotomy. Elevated serum leukocyte counts; elevated erythrocyte sedimentation rates (ESRs); and creatinine protein levels are suggestive but not diagnostic of joint sepsis. Ultrasound-guided (ultrasonography) aspiration in suspected sepsis of arthroplasty has been developed to facilitate this process. Arthrocentesis (joint aspiration) is effective in demonstrating the involved pathogen in 85% to 90% of cases.

Radiologic abnormalities may be helpful but generally require 3 to 6 months to demonstrate changes. When both the distal and proximal components of a prosthetic joint demonstrate pathology on radiography, sepsis is more likely than simple mechanical loosening. However, such radiographic changes are not specific for infection and may also be seen with aseptic processes. Radioisotope scans demonstrate increased uptake in areas of bone with enhanced blood supply or increased metabolic activity (a normal finding during the first 6 months post implantation). Positive scans after 6 months following implantation are abnormal but do not differentiate among inflammation, possible loosening, and infection.

Treatment.

Prosthesis removal accompanied by extensive and meticulous surgical debridement of surrounding tissue and effective antimicrobial therapy are usually necessary to treat deep infections, especially infections involving the interface between prosthesis and bone. Simple surgical drainage (with retention of the prosthesis), followed by a course of antibiotics or treatment with antibiotics without prosthesis removal has had limited success. For more predictably effective treatment of prosthetic joint replacement sepsis, complete removal of all foreign materials (metallic prosthesis, cement, and any accompanying biofilm) is essential. This can be done in a one-stage or two-stage exchange. The most successful protocol incorporates standardized antimicrobial therapy with a two-stage surgical procedure: (1) removal of prosthesis and cement and placement of an antibiotic impregnated cement spacer, followed by a 6-week course of bactericidal antibiotic therapy; and (2) reimplantation of a new prosthesis using cement impregnated with an antibiotic at the conclusion of the 6-week antibiotic course.[19,72]

Sometimes surgical intervention is not possible, owing to a medical or surgical condition or refusal on the part of the affected client. In such cases, lifelong oral antibiotic treatment may be required to suppress the infection and retain function of the joint. Serial radiographs are needed to monitor progressive bone resorption at the bone-cement interface. In such cases, the localized septic process may still extend into adjacent tissue compartments or become a systemic infection, or the person may develop side effects of chronic antibiotic administration.

Prognosis.

Infection associated with prostheses and implants can produce significant morbidity and occasionally death. Early recognition and prompt therapy for infection in any location is critical to reducing the risk of seeding the joint implant hematogenously. Situations likely to cause bacteremia should be avoided.[9]

The American Dental Association and the American Academy of Orthopedic Surgeons have jointly advised that a single dose of prophylactic antibiotic be given to selected individuals undergoing dental procedures associated with significant bleeding and potential hematogenic bacterial contamination (e.g., pyogenic dentogingival pathology, obstructive uropathy, dermatologic conditions). The selected populations include people with inflammatory arthropathies, immunosuppression, diabetes mellitus, malnutrition, hemophilia, or previous prosthetic joint infection and anyone undergoing these procedures within 2 years after joint replacement.

Perioperative antibiotic prophylaxis has been shown to reduce deep wound infection effectively in total joint replacement surgery. Cephalosporins continue to be the antibiotic of choice for orthopedic surgeons because of the broad spectrum of activity against the most common pathogens. The antibiotic is given a half hour before the incision is made, and if the procedure is long, another dose is administered during surgery. The medication is then continued for about 24 to 48 hours after surgery.[35]

Special Implications for the Therapist   7-12

INFECTIONS WITH PROTHESES AND IMPLANTS

Preferred Practice Patterns
4B: Impaired Posture
4C: Impaired Muscle Performance
4E: Impaired Joint Mobility, Motor Function, Muscle
*   Performance, and Range of Motion Associated With*
*   Localized Inflammation*
4H: Impaired Joint Mobility, Motor Function, Muscle
*   Performance, and Range of Motion Associated With Joint*
*   Arthroplasty*

Many cases of infection after instrumentation or prosthetic implantation occur months to years after the surgery. In most cases, a distant cause of infection can be identified, but usually no preceding breakdown of the overlying skin occurs to help identify the presence of underlying infection. The therapist may not be aware of existing hardware and must include questions in the interview to elicit this information. A recent history of infection from dental caries, pulmonary or upper respiratory tract, gastrointestinal tract, or genitourinary tract in such a person requires medical evaluation. Any spontaneous drainage from previous scars or sites of surgery may be a sign of infection and must also be evaluated by a physician.

Anyone with implants of any kind with onset of increasing musculoskeletal symptoms (especially in the area of the surgery) must be screened for the possibility of infection. Normal radiographs and negative needle aspirates can delay medical diagnosis of infection. Knowing the risk factors for developing an antibiotic-resistant infection (e.g., multiple surgical procedures, previous *S. aureus* infection, multiple antibiotics) and recognizing red flag symptoms of infection can help the therapist in recognizing the need for persistence in obtaining follow-up medical care.

Breast Implantation

Silicone breast implants (SBIs) are medical devices implanted subcutaneously or subpectorally for cosmetic breast augmentation or reconstruction. Most women with silicone gel-filled breast implants do not experience serious problems, but some women have reported symptoms otherwise associated with connective tissue and immune-related disorders. Such symptoms may include joint pain and swelling; skin tightness, redness, or swelling; swollen glands or lymph nodes; unusual and unexplained fatigue; swollen hands and feet; and unusual hair loss. The term *human adjuvant disease* is sometimes used to describe the musculoskeletal symptoms accompanying breast

implantation. Evidence to support an autoimmune response to silicone breast implants has not been conclusively proven, and to date, the largest studies have found no association between the implants and connective tissue diseases or signs and symptoms of these diseases.[47,70,90]

The consensus is that the reported cases of connective tissue diseases or immune-related disorders in women with breast implants do not exceed the number of cases normally expected in women. In the meantime, silicone breast implant litigation escalated in the early 1990s so that despite the FDA's statement that no medical evidence supports that silicone causes autoimmune disease, silicone gel implants were removed from the market in 1992.* In addition, other studies have demonstrated that human immune system activation and response to implantation of silicone-based medical devices occurs in both adults and children born to mothers with mammary implants placed before pregnancy.[82,83,88] However, after at least two large studies, no epidemiologic evidence exists showing any clear association between breast implants and connective tissue disorders or breast cancer.[90]

Women who have implants for reconstruction following mastectomy for breast cancer are nearly three times more likely to have complications than those who receive implants for cosmetic reasons only. The most common complication of SBIs is capsule contracture or contracture of the fibrous tissue surrounding the prosthesis, leading to a firmness and distortion of the breast that can be painful. Other complications may include gel bleed, implant rupture, calcifications around the implant, and possibly interference with mammography in the diagnosis of breast cancer. Some recent studies have shown that silicone devices can prolong wound healing and formation of granulation tissue.[82]

Other tissue problems related to cancer therapy affect surrounding tissue and contribute greatly to the overall complication rate in this group.[32] Any woman (with or without breast implants) experiencing breast pain or discomfort, changes in size or shape of the breast, color changes in the breast area, discharge from or unusual sensation around the nipple, or unexplained symptoms possibly related to breast tissue should see a medical doctor. ■

◆ Lyme Disease

Definition and Overview.   Lyme disease is an infectious multisystemic disorder caused by a spiral-shaped form of bacteria, *Borrelia burgdorferi*. It is carried by a deer tick† and was first recognized (but did not originate) in 1975 when a group of children in Lyme, Conn. developed an unusual type of arthritis and also had a history of a tick bite and an unusual bull's-eye rash. Ticks carrying *B. burgdorferi* can transmit it to the mammals and birds on which they feed. In the United States, the disease is only transmitted to humans by certain ticks of the Ixodes species: *Ixodes scapularis* (formerly called

---

*Silicone implants are still used in FDA clinical trials for women needing reconstructive surgery, but no date has been set for when silicone gel implants will again be approved for general use. To report a problem with an implant, write to The Problem Reporting Program; 12601 Twinbrook Parkway; Rockville, MD 20852. For other information on breast implants, write the FDA, Breast Implant Information, HFE-88; 5600 Fishers Lane; Rockville, MD 20857 or call (301) 443-3170.

†In addition to deer, these ticks are found on birds and rodents; they are about the size of the period at the end of a sentence. Not all of these ticks carry the bacteria.

I. dammini), known as the deer, bear, or black-legged tick in the Northeast (from Massachusetts to Maryland) and North Central United States (Wisconsin and Minnesota); and *I. pacificus*, the Western black-legged tick found on the western Coast of northern California and Oregon.[97] The ticks are about the size of the period at the end of this sentence. Several more genospecies of Borrelia are known to cause the disease in Europe, Asia and Australia.[46]

Incidence. Lyme disease has become the most prevalent vectorborne infectious disease in the United States in the last decade and is being reported with increasing frequency although, over-reporting has been cited as a problem.[43,46] Most cases (more than 90%) have been reported from the mid-Atlantic, Northeastern, and North Central regions of the country. It has been reported in 49 states and the District of Columbia with nearly 17,000 new cases recorded in 1998.[97] In the United States, Lyme disease is often seen in the late spring and summer months.

Pathogenesis. Lyme disease occurs when the tick bites the host and ingests the host's blood. The tick becomes engorged with the blood and turns a grayish color. After at least 48 hours, the bacteria from an infected tick are passed into the host when a tick injects spirochete-laden saliva into the bloodstream of the host. Most commonly, however, the tick falls off or is removed before the bacteria are injected into the host's bloodstream. Between 70% and 90% of bites are caused by nymphs, the immature tick, most active between May and September.[48]

After incubating for 3 to 32 days, the spirochetes migrate out to the skin, causing characteristic skin lesions (see Clinical Manifestations below). Then the bacteria disseminate to other skin sites or organs via the bloodstream or lymphatic system.[89] The spirochetes' life cycle is not completely understood; it remains unclear whether they survive for years in areas that receive minimal blood supply (e.g., tendons or the synovium in joints) or perhaps just trigger an inflammatory response in the host and then die.

Clinical Manifestations. Lyme disease is often described as the "Great Imitator," since its signs and symptoms mimic those of many other diseases. Symptoms vary widely and may not develop for as long as a month after a bite and in some cases, symptoms do not develop at all. Within 7 to 14 days following a tick bite, about 80% of affected individuals will have a red, slowly expanding bull's-eye rash called *erythema migrans (EM)* (Fig. 7-1). Not all people with the disease develop the telltale rash, and because early symptoms are often mild, some people may remain undiagnosed and untreated in *stage 1, the early, localized state.* EM resolves spontaneously without treatment within an average of 4 weeks. Use of antibiotics speeds up the process of rash resolution.[97] Flulike symptoms such as chills, fever, headache, lethargy, muscle pain, or a stiff neck may also develop early in the course of the infection.*

In *stage 2, early-disseminated infection*, the spirochete may spread in the blood or lymph to cause a wide variety of signs and symptoms. Stage 2 is marked by generalized fatigue, loss of appetite, and vomiting. These symptoms may occur weeks

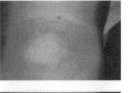
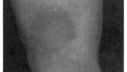
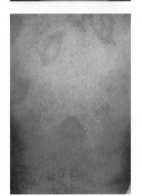

FIGURE 7-1 Examples of erythema migrans associated with Lyme disease. Other types of rashes can also occur. (From National Institutes of Health [NIH]: *Lyme disease: the facts, the challenge*, NIH Publ No 92-3193, Bethesda, Md, 1992, US Department of Health and Human Services, p 6.)

BOX 7-7

Neurologic Manifestations of Lyme Disease

Facial nerve palsy (Bell's palsy)
Cognitive impairment (e.g., forgetfulness, decreased concentration, personality changes)
Inflammation of the brain, spinal cord, or nerves
- Cranial neuritis
- Encephalitis
- Encephalomyelitis
- Encephalopathy
- Meningitis
- Radiculoneuropathies

to months after a tick bite. Neurologic symptoms may be the first to arise (Box 7-7) and occur in 10% to 20% of all cases, most commonly manifested as aseptic meningitis with mild headache and stiff neck.*

About half of those diagnosed may go on to develop painful Lyme arthritis characterized by unilateral inflammation and swelling in the large joints, especially the knees. Migratory musculoskeletal pain in joints, bursae, tendons, muscle, or bone may occur in one or a few locations at a time, often lasting only hours or days in a given location. Weeks to months later, after the development of a marked cellular and humoral response to the spirochete, untreated people often have intermittent or chronic monarticular (one joint) or oligoarticular (affecting only a few joints) arthritis.

---

*Large joints, particulary the knees, are most commonly affected.

*Recent studies indicate that the bacteria may invade the brain and spinal cord early in the disease.

Skin lesions or benign skin tumors and liver abnormalities such as hepatitis can appear.[97] Some people (4% to 10%) experience cardiac signs and symptoms including myocarditis and varying types of heart block and dysrhythmias, which can result in irregular, rapid, or slowed pulses; dizziness; fainting; and shortness of breath. Involvement of the eye can include optic nerve inflammation, conjunctivitis, diplopia, and retinal detachment.

Stage 3, late disseminated disease may not become apparent until months to years after the initial infection. It occurs in more than half of people with the disease who have not received early treatment. Stage 3 is primarily characterized by rheumatoid arthritis with marked swelling, especially in the large joints (Fig. 7-2); profound fatigue; fibromyalgia; or chronic neurologic manifestations such as encephalopathy, polyneuropathy, or leukoencephalitis. In addition, demyelinating-like symptoms similar to multiple sclerosis, severe headache, and cognitive changes such as memory loss, mood changes, and sleep disturbances can also occur in this stage.[89] Recurrent acute joint flareups may precede the development of chronic arthritis with severe cartilage and bone erosion; chronic arthritis occurs in about 10% to 20% of untreated people.

Medical Management

Diagnosis. Because of the wide range of symptoms possible with Lyme disease, it is easily misdiagnosed as rheumatoid arthritis, fibromyalgia, chronic fatigue syndrome, meningitis, or multiple sclerosis. On the other hand, the fatigue, mood changes and neurologic problems associated with Lyme disease are often mistaken for mental illness or chronic fatigue syndrome. In the early, localized stage 1, diagnosis of Lyme disease is based on both clinical symptoms and laboratory findings. Infection may be present without the signs used by the CDC as indicative of Lyme disease. CDC criteria for diagnosis include (1) exposure to tick habitat 30 days before developing EM, (2) EM diagnosed, (3) at least one late manifestation of the disease, or (4) laboratory confirmation of the disease (detection of specific antibodies to *B. burgdorferi*).[16]

Laboratory tests for Lyme disease are often used inappropriately to screen for the condition after a tick bite. The tests now available are unreliable and should be used only to support a diagnosis. A positive laboratory test result should not be used to diagnose Lyme disease in the absence of clinical findings.[96] Immunofluorescent antibody (IFA) test and ELISA are indirect tests that measure the immune system's response to the bacterium. Since it takes 4 to 6 weeks for the immune system to mount a response, many people in the early stages have little or no detectable antibody in their serum and those who receive antibiotics may never seroconvert. Positive IFA or ELISA is further tested using the Western blot analysis.

A newer test called *polymerase chain reaction* (PCR) uses gene slicing techniques to detect the DNA of the bacterium itself, enabling earlier diagnosis than the previously used antibody tests. PCR has detected bacterium DNA in synovial fluid, CSF, skin, blood, and urine. The PCR has its limitations, as it remains unknown whether persisting PCR positivity means ongoing infection or merely persistence of dead organisms.[96] Synovial fluid may be tested to distinguish Lyme arthritis from acute septic arthritis.

Treatment. Lyme disease is treated with oral antibiotics; severe cases may require IV antibiotics for several months or longer. Supportive measures are essential for the associated constitutional symptoms (e.g., rest for fatigue and for swollen, inflamed joints; analgesics for pain). Treatment of long-term complications varies according to the affected organs. Arthroscopic surgery may be required for joints damaged by the disease.

Prognosis. Early treatment is vital for the prevention of long-term complications, but even so, complications involving the heart, joints, and nervous system occur in about 15% of people who do undergo early treatment. For most people, Lyme disease is curable with standard antibiotic therapy and the effects of Lyme disease resolve completely within a few weeks or months of treatment. Unfortunately, no natural immunity develops from exposure to Lyme disease, and anyone can be reinfected. Although Lyme disease is rarely fatal, heart complications may cause life-threatening cardiac arrhythmias.

Great concern came about in the past regarding potential fetal infection and teratogenicity from Lyme disease contracted during pregnancy. However, in recent prospective studies, no cases of congenital infection have been linked to the Lyme disease spirochete. Although it is possible that *B. burgdorferi* may cause an adverse fetal outcome in humans, it has not been conclusively documented in humans or animals.[62,85,104]

Prevention. Prevention is the key to avoiding Lyme disease. Lyme disease is most common during the late spring and summer months in the United States when nymphal ticks are most active and human populations are frequently outdoors and most exposed. People who live or work in residential areas surrounded by woods or overgrown brush infested by ticks or favored by white-tailed deer and live in the endemic geographic areas are at risk. In addition, people who participate in outdoor recreational activities in tick habitat are also at risk for Lyme disease (Box 7-8).

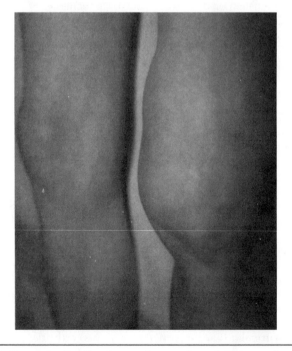

FIGURE 7-2 Swollen knee of a youth with Lyme arthritis. (From National Institutes of Health [NIH]: *Lyme disease: the facts, the challenge*, NIH Publ No 92-3193, Bethesda, Md, 1992, US Department of Health and Human Services, p 12.)

BOX | **7-8**

Prevention of Lyme Disease

These precautions are provided for people living in tick-infested areas:

Avoid tick-infested areas, especially in May, June, and July (check with local health departments or park services for the seasonal and geographic distribution in your area).

Walk along cleared or paved surfaces rather than through tall grass or wooded areas.

Wear long-sleeved shirts, long pants tucked into socks, and closed shoes (no part of foot exposed).

Wear light-colored clothing to make it easy to detect ticks.

Shower as soon as possible after being outdoors. Ticks take several hours to attach themselves to the skin and can be washed away first.

Wash clothing worn outdoors immediately and use a dryer (heat kills the ticks). If no access to laundry facilities is available, the clothing should not be stored in the bedroom, or if camping, the clothing should not be stored in the same area where people are sleeping.

If bitten by a tick, remove the tick immediately by grasping it as close to the skin as possible with tweezers and tugging gently. Do not twist or turn the tweezers; pull straight away from the skin. A cotton ball soaked in rubbing alcohol or fingernail polish remover and rubbed against the head while tugging gently may help loosen the tick more readily.

To lessen the chance of contact with the bacterium, do not crush the tick's body or handle the tick with bare hands. Clean the bite area thoroughly with soap and water, then swab the area with an antiseptic to prevent bacterial infection.

Whenever possible, save the tick in a glass jar for identification should symptoms develop.

If living in an area in which deer ticks are common, keep the weeds and grass around the house mowed.

Use flea and tick collars on pets; brush and examine them carefully after they have been outdoors. People can use insecticides such as permethrin or insect repellents containing diethyltoluamide (DEET).*

*The use of such chemicals may be objectionable to some people because they may cause neurotoxicity in children. Alternative methods are available.

In December 1998 the FDA licensed the vaccine LYMErix to aid in the prevention of Lyme disease in people ages 15 to 70 that engage in activities that put them at risk. The vaccine is given by injection in three doses and is about 76% effective after the third dose. Regular boosters may be necessary to maintain protection. The decision to be vaccinated depends primarily on risk of exposure status, and even after vaccination, tick precaution measures are very important. The long-term safety and effectiveness of the vaccine are not known, and presence of the vaccine in the serum of the recipients can confuse antibody findings when a diagnosis is being made.[48] The vaccine has not been studied in the United States in people over 70 years or in pregnant or breastfeeding women. Studies of children under age 15 have shown promising results for effectiveness of the vaccine in that age group.[97]

Special Implications for the Therapist   **7-13**

LYME DISEASE

Preferred Practice Patterns
Stage 1
   7B: Impaired Integumentary Integrity Associated With Superficial Skin Involvement
Stages 2 and 3
   4D: Musculoskeletal Impairment Associated With Connective Tissue Disorder (rheumatoid arthritis)
5C, 5D: Impaired Neuromuscular Function With Acquired Nonprogressive Disorder of the CNS
   6D: Impaired Aerobic Capacity/Endurance Associated With Cardiovascular Pump Dysfunction (cardiac arrhythmias)

Chronic arthritis is the most widely recognized result of untreated Lyme disease in the United States. Unlike other forms of rheumatoid arthritis, Lyme arthritis does not affect the joints bilaterally, though both sides may be affected alternately. The condition has been called chronic because episodes can last months, occurring intermittently over a period of 1 to 3 years.[89] Permanent joint damage and cartilage destruction can occur if excessive use occurs during the inflammatory period. Range-of-motion and strengthening exercises are important but must be carried out carefully and without overexertion.

Nervous system abnormalities can develop weeks, months, or even years following an untreated infection. These symptoms often last for weeks or months and may recur. The therapist may treat such a client at any time during the course of symptomatic presentation. For anyone with known Lyme disease, frequent assessment of the person's neurologic function and level of consciousness is important. Any signs of cardiac abnormality or increased intracranial pressure and cranial nerve involvement (e.g., ptosis, strabismus, diplopia) must be reported to the physician immediately. Both upper- and lower-extremity peripheral nerve problems can occur and are managed as any neuropathy from other causes.

It has been hypothesized that people who present with symptoms of multiple sclerosis but respond to antibiotics may have been bitten by ticks years ago. However, in theory, if the person had true multiple sclerosis, antibiotics would not have altered the symptoms present as they do with Lyme disease. Along the same lines, the question has been raised whether Lyme disease triggers fibromyalgia or does Lyme disease just manifest clinically as indistinguishable from fibromyalgia? It is possible that fibromyalgia-like symptoms develop as a result of sleep disturbances during the dissemination stage of Lyme disease. Since the cause of fibromyalgia (independent of Lyme disease) is unknown, linking its development to Lyme disease is even more difficult.

Continued

For the present, therapists are encouraged to treat adults with long-term manifestations of Lyme disease using the treatment philosophy adopted for autoimmune disorders (see the sections on Fibromyalgia and Systemic Lupus Erythematosus in Chapter 6). Conversely, anyone diagnosed as having fibromyalgia should be screened for Lyme disease. The therapist can start this screening process by asking about a history of exposure (i.e., frequency and location of outdoor activities) if the physician has not already posed these questions. ■

◆ Sexually Transmitted Diseases

Overview and Incidence. Each year 15 million Americans become contract a sexually transmitted disease (STD), and it is estimated that at least one out of every four sexually active people (56 million Americans) are carrying an infection other than HIV. Although the incidences of syphilis and gonorrhea have reached all-time lows in the United States, chlamydia and human papillomavirus (HPV) remain problems of epidemic proportions. Chlamydia is the fastest-spreading STD in the United States affecting more than 3 million men and women each year. Among college-age women, HPV, which causes genital warts and can lead to cervical cancer, is more common than all other STDs combined. Additionally, 45 million people have chronic genital herpes, and one million new cases occur every year. There are 77,000 new cases of hepatitis B every year caused by sexual transmission, despite the availability of a preventive vaccine, and an estimated 900,000 Americans currently have the HIV/AIDS virus with an additional 45,000 cases reported every year, half of which occurred through sexual contact.

STDs are spread primarily through sexual contact but also by sharing infected needles and some by transmission from mother to child during vaginal childbirth. Many STDs are easily treated and cured, but others remain chronic. Although more than 50 different STDs are evident, only the most common ones are included here (Table 7-9).

Etiologic and Risk Factors.
All groups of people are potentially at risk for STDs but women, teens, and they have disproportionately affected minorities. Young people under the age of 18 years are considered at greatest risk for getting a sexually transmitted disease but in fact, the over-50 population is also at risk. Although 25% of all STDs occur in people under the age of 25, numerous surveys of healthy adults have verified that older people are sexually active and less likely to practice safe sex. Risk factors vary but most often include multiple sex partners, a partner with a known risk factor, or a history of a blood transfusion between 1977 and 1984, failure to use a condom (or use it properly) during sexual intercourse, or sharing needles during illicit drug use. The presence of STDs is a risk factor itself for facilitating the transmission of HIV.

Pathogenesis and Clinical Manifestations.
STDs are caused by bacteria, viruses, or occasionally, parasites and may have a considerable latency period when the infectious organism lies dormant before triggering symptomatic presentation. Clinical manifestations vary according to the STD present (see Table 7-9). STDs may be completely asymptomatic

and are less likely to produce symptoms in women and therefore are less likely to be diagnosed until serious problems develop. Complications of STDs are more severe and more frequent among women than men. Once infected, women are more susceptible to reproductive cancers, infertility, and contracting other STDs.

Medical Management

Prevention. Prevention is the most important key to managing STDs. The only prevention that is 100% effective is abstinence and/or a mutually monogamous sexual relationship (single partner) between two uninfected people. For those who are sexually active, protection with proper use of high quality latex condoms combined with the use of a spermicidal foam or jelly containing nonoxynol-9 is only effective for vaginal and anal intercourse; some STDs can be transmitted by kissing, touching, and oral sex.

Every pregnant woman should have blood tests for syphilis and hepatitis B. A vaccine is available to protect anyone, especially women of childbearing age against hepatitis B (see Table 7-5). Pregnant women should also be tested for gonorrhea, HPV, and HIV. Those with recurrent genital herpes and open sores may benefit from cesarean section delivery to protect the child. Anyone with a STD or known possibility of infection must inform a physician and all partners to obtain appropriate treatment and prevent spreading the disease to others.

Other prevention measures include to never, under any circumstance, use injection equipment (e.g., needles, syringes, and "works") that has been used by another person. Contact any sexual partners of an infected person and recommend an examination even if the person is asymptomatic.

Diagnosis, Treatment, and Prognosis.
STDs can often be identified by the clinical manifestations, but various screening tests are also available for different STDs. Experts recommend that sexually active adolescents and women (early 20s or younger) be screened for chlamydia every 6 months regardless of symptoms.[12] Older women with multiple partners should be screened once a year. Since HPV can lie dormant for years before triggering cell changes that can lead to cervical cancer, a woman with HPV (like any woman) should have yearly Pap smears to detect any abnormal cells.

Antibiotics can cure some STDs (see Table 7-9), although some may be drug resistant. Practicing abstinence and safe sex until all sores have healed is recommended. Intercourse during an active infection transmits the virus and dramatically increases the risk of contracting HIV and other STDs. Frequent handwashing and avoiding self-injection by avoiding touching the affected areas during an outbreak are essential practices. Researchers are working on topical microbicides that could be applied like spermicides to protect women from a range of STDs.[42,53] A vaccine is now available for hepatitis B, and vaccines against HPV, HIV, and herpes are under investigation.

The prognosis varies with each STD but with treatment, symptoms can be minimized and complications prevented. Without treatment, serious complications can occur such as infertility, chronic pelvic pain, ectopic pregnancy and miscarriage, cardiovascular disease, central nervous system impairment, blindness, cervical cancer, and even death.

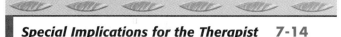

Special Implications for the Therapist   7-14

SEXUALLY TRANSMITTED DISEASES

Preferred Practice Patterns
NOTE: *These are variable depending on specific disease entity and clinical presentation.*

Any therapist treating men or women with clinical presentation of pelvic, buttock, hip, or groin pain of apparent unknown cause must be prepared to ask the client about past history of STDs; sexual activity; changes in sexual function; and presence of urogenital signs or symptoms (e.g., discharge from penis or vagina, painful urination, difficulty initiating or continuing a stream of urine). Any suspicion that the clinical manifestations may be correlated to an STD must be further evaluated by a medical doctor. ■

Special Implications for the Therapist   7-15

INFECTIONS IN DRUG ADDICTS

NOTE: *See Special Implications for the Therapist: Substance Abuse, 2-2.*

Being aware of the signs of substance abuse or drug addiction and the patterns of infection associated with drug addiction may assist the therapist in recognizing early signs of infection requiring medical evaluation and treatment. Any therapist involved in wound care management, needle electromyography, or other high-risk practice techniques who has not already been immunized against hepatitis B should undergo this series of vaccinations. ■

◆ Infections in Drug Addicts[45]

The abuse of parenterally administered narcotic drugs has increased enormously in recent years. An estimated 300,000 or more narcotic addicts are in the United States, mostly in or near large urban centers. Consequently, HCWs in urban and suburban populations may encounter many problems related to drug abuse, including infections.

Common infections that occur with greater frequency in drug users include (1) skin infections associated with poor hygiene and multiple needle punctures, commonly caused by *S. aureus*; myositis and necrotizing fasciitis are uncommon but life-threatening; (2) hepatitis, which is nearly universal among habitual injection drug users and is transmissible both by the parenteral route (B, C, D) and the fecal-oral route (A); (3) aspiration pneumonia and its complications (lung abscess, empyema, brain abscess) resulting from altered consciousness associated with drug abuse; (4) pulmonary septic emboli originating from venous thrombi or endocarditis; (5) sexually transmitted diseases, which are not directly related to drug abuse but occur with greater frequency in population groups that are also involved in drug abuse; (6) higher incidence of AIDS among injection drug abusers and their sexual contacts as well as the offspring of infected women; (7) tuberculosis, which has spread much more rapidly in HIV infected drug users; and (8) infective endocarditis. Coinfection with HIV and infective endocarditis has a very poor outcome.

Osteomyelitis involving vertebral bodies, sternoclavicular joints, and other sites are found in drug abusers usually from hematogenous distribution of injected organisms or septic venous thrombi. Intravenous drug abuse is increasingly related to infection of joints. About one third of septic arthritis cases are associated with drug users and many of these cases are HIV positive. The majority of joint infections occur in the joints and bones of the axial skeleton (sternoclavicular, costochondral, hip, shoulder, vertebrae, symphysis pubis, sacroiliac) but can also occur in peripheral joints. The most commonly associated organism is *S. aureus*, but others include gram-negative organisms such as *Enterobacter*, *P. aeruginosa*, and *Serratia marcescens*. Gram-negative infections are harder to diagnose and more difficult to treat.[68] Pain and fever precede radiographic changes by several weeks.

REFERENCES

1. Advisory Committee on Immunization Practices: APIC (Association for Professionals in Infection Control and Epidemiology) brochure, 2000. Available at http://www.apic.org.
2. Advisory Committee on Immunization Practices: Prevention and control of influenza, *MMWR* 45(5):1-24, 1996a.
3. Advisory Committee on Immunization Practices (ACIP): Update, vaccine side effects, adverse reactions, contraindications and precautions, *MMWR* 45(12):1-35, 1996b.
4. Agha R: Complications of immunizations, *Pediatr Rev* 18(2):66-67, 1997.
5. Atkinson W et al, editors: *Epidemiology and prevention of vaccine preventable diseases*, ed 6, Centers for Disease Control and Prevention (Department of Health and Human Services), 2000.
6. Baseman J, Tully J: Mycoplasmas, sophisticated, reemerging and burdened by their notoriety, *Emerg Infect Dis* 3(1):21-32, 1997.
7. Bolyard E et al and the Hospital Infection Control Practices Advisory Committee: Guidelines for infection control in health care personnel, 1998, *AJIC* 26(3):289-343, 1998.
8. Bouckenooghe A, Shandera W: Infectious diseases: viral and rickettsial. In Tierney L, McPhee S, Papadakis M, editors: *Current medical diagnosis and treatment*, ed 39, New York, 2000, Lange Medical Books/McGraw-Hill.
9. Brause B: Infections with prostheses in bones and joints. In Mandell G, Bennett J, Dolin R, editors: *Principles and practice of infectious diseases*, ed 5, Philadelphia, 2000, Churchill Livingstone.
10. Brouqui P: Chronic *Bartonella quintana* bacteremia in homeless patients, *N Eng J Med*, 340:21-32, 1999.
11. Brueggmann A, Doern G, Wingert E: Antimicrobial resistance with streptoccocus pneumoniae in the United States, 1997/1998, *Emerg Infect Dis*, 5(6):757-765, 1999.
12. Burstein GR et al: Screening for gonorrhea and chlamydia by DNA amplification in adolescents attending middle school health centers. Opportunity for early intervention, *Sex Transm Dis* 25(8):395-402, 1998.
13. Cantrell M, Norman D: Infections. In Duthrie E, Katz P, editors: *Practice of geriatrics*, ed 3, Philadelphia, 1998, WB Saunders.
14. Centers for Disease Control and Prevention: *Staphylococcus aureus* with reduced susceptibility to vancomycin—United States, 1997, *MMWR* 46:813-815, 1997a.
15. Centers for Disease Control and Prevention: Immunization of healthcare workers recommendations of the Advisory Committee on Immunization Practices (APIC) and the Hospital Infection Control Practices Advisory Committee (HICPAC), *MMWR* 46(RR-18):1-41, 1997b.

16. Centers for Disease Control and Prevention: Lyme disease—United States, 1994, *MMWR* 44:459-462, 1995.

17. Centers for Disease Control and Prevention: National Immunization Program, Summary of adolescent/adult immunization recommendations, 1998. Available at http://www.cdc.gov.

18. Chambers H: Infectious diseases: bacterial and chlamydial. In Tierney L, McPhee S, Papadakis M, editors: *Current medical diagnosis and treatment*, ed 39, New York, 2000, Lange Medical Books/McGraw-Hill.

19. Chohfi M et al: Pharmacokinetics, uses, and limitations of vancomycin-loaded bone cement, *Int Orthop* 22(3):171-177, 1998.

20. Choudhri SH et al: A case of necrotizing fasciitis due to *Streptococcus pneumoniae*, *Br J Dermatol* 133:128-131, 1995.

21. Cochran GM, Ewald PW, Cochran KD: Infectious causation of disease: an evolutionary perspective, *Perspect Biol Med* 43(3):406-408, 2000.

22. Corey L: Herpes simplex virus. In Mandell G, Bennett J, Dolin R, editors: *Principles and practice of infectious diseases*, ed 5, Philadelphia, 2000, Churchill Livingstone.

23. Crumpacker C: Cytomegalovirus. In Mandell G, Bennett J, Dolin R, editors: *Principles and practice of infectious diseases*, ed 5, Philadelphia, 2000, Churchill Livingstone.

24. DeBraun BJ: Prevention of infection in the orthopedic surgery patient, *Nurs Clin North Am* 33(4):671-684, 1998.

25. Devlin H, Ferguson MW: Aging and the orofacial tissues. In Tallis RC, Fillit HM, Brocklehurst JC, editors: *Brocklehurst's textbook of geriatric medicine and gerontology*, ed 5, New York, 1998, Churchill Livingstone.

26. Dobos K, Quinn F, Ashford D, Horsburgh C, King C: Emergence of a unique group of necrotizing mycobacterial diseases, *Emerg Infect Dis* 5(3):367-378, 1999. Available at http://www.cdc.gov.

27. Donowitz G: Oxazolidones. In Mandell G, Bennett J, Dolin R, editors: *Principles and practice of infectious diseases*, ed 5, Philadelphia, 2000, Churchill Livingstone.

28. Edmond M, Wenzel R: Isolation. In Mandell G, Bennett J, Dolin R, editors: *Principles and practice of infectious diseases*, ed 5, Philadelphia, 2000, Churchill Livingstone.

29. Entenza J: Y-688, new quinolone active against quinolone-resistant *Staphylococcus aureus*: Lack of in vivo efficacy in experimental endocarditis, *Antimicrob Agents Chemother* 42(18): 1889-1894.

30. Feldman M, Scharschmidt BF, Sleisenger MH, editors: *Sleisenger & Fordtran's gastrointestinal and liver disease*, ed 6, Philadelphia, 1998, WB Saunders.

31. Freidman L: Liver, biliary tract and pancreas. In Tierney L, McPhee S, Papadakis M, editors: *Current medical diagnosis and treatment*, ed 39, New York, 2000, Lange Medical Books/McGraw-Hill.

32. Gabriel S et al: Complications leading to surgery after breast implant, *N Engl J Med* 336(10): 677-682, 1997.

33. Garcia R et al: Nosocomial RSV infections: Prevention and control in bone marrow transplant patients, *Infect Control Hosp Epidemiol* June 18(6):412-416, 1997.

34. Garner J: Guidelines for isolation precaution in hospitals, *Infect Control Hosp Epidemiol* 17:54-80, 1996.

35. Garvin K, McKillip T: Preventing and managing infection following joint replacement, *J Musculoskel Med* 14(6):9-18, 1997.

36. Gerberding JL: The infected health care provider, *N Engl J Med* 334(9):594-595, 1996.

37. Goldman D, Weinstein R, Wensel R: Strategies to prevent and control the emergence and spread of antimicrobial-resistant micro-organisms in hospitals: a challenge to hospital leadership, *JAMA* 275:234-240, 1996.

38. Golz R, Kuschner SH, Gellman H: Sequential infection of silicone metacarpophalangeal joint arthroplasties resulting from skin breakdown, *J Hand Surg* 17:150-152, 1992.

39. Gonzales-Ruiz GL et al: Varicella gangrenosa with toxic shock-like syndrome due to group A streptococcus in an adult: case report, *Clin Infect Dis* 20:1058-1060, 1995.

40. Hall C: Human herpesviruses at sixes, sevens, and more, *Ann Intern Med* 125(6):481-483, 1997.

41. Henrich DE, Smith TL, Shockley WW: Fatal craniocervical necrotizing fasciitis in an immunocompetent patient: A case report and literature review, *Head Neck* 17:351-357, 1995.

42. Howett MK et al: A broad-spectrum microbicide with virucidal activity against sexually transmitted viruses, *Antimicrob Agents Chemother* 43(2):314-321, 1999.

43. Hunder G, Kaye R, Lane NE: Osteoporosis, fibromyalgia, Lyme disease, polymyalgia, lupus, and gout, *J Musculoskel Med* 16(1):12-32, 1999.

44. Ignativicius D, Workman M, Mishler M: *Medical-surgical nursing across the health care continuum*, ed 3, Philadelphia, 1999, WB Saunders.

45. Jacobs R: Infectious diseases: Spirochetal. In Tierney L, McPhee S, Papadakis M, editors: *Current medical diagnosis and treatment*, ed 39, New York, 2000a, Lange Medical Books/McGraw Hill.

46. Jacobs R: General problems in infectious diseases. In Tierney L, McPhee S, Papadakis M, editors: *Current medical diagnosis and treatment*, ed 39, New York, 2000b, Lange Medical Books/McGraw-Hill.

47. Janowsky E, Kupper L, Hulka B: Meta-analyses of the relation between silicone breast implants and the risk of connective tissue diseases, *N Engl J Med* 342(11):781-790, 2000.

48. Johns Hopkins University: Lyme disease: is vaccination right for you? *Med Letter* 12(2):3, 2000.

49. Jones JS, Hoerle D, Riekse R: Stethoscopes: a potential vector of infection? *Ann Emerg Med* 26:296-299, 1995.

50. Katz M, Hollander H: HIV infection. In Tierney L, McPhee S, Papadakis M, editors): *Current medical diagnosis and treatment*, ed 39, New York, 2000, Lange Medical Books/McGraw-Hill.

51. Kneyber MC, Moll HA, de Groot R: Treatment and prevention of respiratory syncytial virus protection, *Eur J Pediatr* 159(6):399-411, 2000.

52. Ko T, Adal K, Tomecki K: Infectious diseases, *Med Clin North Am* 82(5): 1001-1031, 1998.

53. Krebs FC, Miller SR, Catalone BJ: Sodium dodecyl sulfate and C31G as microbicidal alternatives to nonoxynol 9: comparative sensitivity of primary human vaginal keratinocytes, *Antimicrob Agents Chemother* 44(7):1954-1960, 2000.

54. Leibowitz MR, Ramakrishnan KK: Necrotizing fasciitis: the role of *Staphylococcus epidermidis*, immune status, and intravascular coagulation, *Austr J Dermatol* 36:29-31, 1995.

55. Levy J: Three new human herpesviruses (HHV-6, 7 and 8), *Lancet* 349(9051):558-563, 1997.

56. Loehne H: Personal communication, Winston-Salem, NC, 2000.

57. Loehne H et al: *Aerosolization of microorganisms during pulsatile lavage with suction*. Presented at the international conference of Association for Professionals in Infection Control and Epidemiology (APIC), Washington, DC, 1999.

58. Loveys DA, Kulkarnia S, Atreya PL: Role of type I IFNs in the in vitro attenuation of live, temperature-sensitive vaccine strains of human respiratory syncytial virus, *Virology* 271(2):390-400, 2000.

59. Malhotra A, Krilov LR: Influenza and respiratory syncytial virus. Update on infection, management, and prevention, *Pediatr Clin North Am* 47(2):353-372, 2000.

60. Mandell G: Intro to microbial disease. In Goldman L, Bennett J, editors: *Cecil textbook of medicine*, ed 21, Philadelphia, 2000, WB Saunders.

61. Mandell GL, Bennett JE, Dolin R, editors: *Principles and practice of infectious diseases*, ed 5, New York, 2000, Churchill Livingstone.

62. Maraspin V et al: erythema migrans in pregnancy, *Wien Clin Wochenschr* 111(22-23):933-940, 1999.

63. Marrie RA et al: Multiple sclerosis and antecedent infections: a case-control study, *Neurology* 54(12):2307-2310, 2000.

64. Mathias JM: Acrylic nails harbor pathogens, *OR Manager* 16(1):10, 2000.

65. Maury E et al: Availability of an alcohol solution can improve hand disnfection complaiance in an intensive care unit, *Am J Respir Crit Care Med* 162(1): 324-327, 2000.

66. Musher D: Streptococcus pneumoniae. In Mandell G, Bennett J, Dolin R, editors: *Principles and practice of infectious diseases*, ed 5, Philadelphia, 2000, Churchill Livingstone.

67. Nafziger D: Infection control in ambulatory care, *Infect Dis Clin North Am* 11(2):279-296, 1997.

68. Naides S: Infectious disorders: Septic arthritis. In Klippel J, editor: *Primer on the rheumatic diseases*, Atlanta, 1997, Arthritis Foundation.

69. Nilsson IM: Protection against *Staphylococcus aureus* sepsis by vaccination with recombinant staphylococcal enterotoxin A devoid of superantigenicity, *J Infect Dis* 180(4):1370-1373, 1999.

70. Nyren O et al: Risk of connective tissue disease and related disorders among women with breast implants: a nationwide retrospective cohort study in Sweden, *BMJ* 316(7129):417-422, 1998.

71. Odland B et al: Antimicrobial activity of gatifloxacin and four other fluroquinolones tested against 2,284 recent clinical strains of Streptococcus pneumoniae from Europe, Latin America, Canada and the United States: The SENTRY Antimicrobial Surveillance Group (Americas and Europe), *Diagn Microbiol Infect Dis* 34(4):315-320, 1999.

72. Pagnano M et al: Blood management in two-stage revision knee arthroplasty for deep prosthetic infection, *Clin Orthop* 367:238-242, 1999.

73. Palmer L: Management of the patient with a total joint replacement: the primary care practitioner's role, *Lippincott's Primary Care Practice* 3(4):419-427, 1999.

74. Pelton S, Figueria M, Albut R et al: Efficacy of linezolid in experimental otitis media, *Antimicrob Agents Chemther* 44(3):654-657, 2000.

75. Pollack M: *Pseudomonas aeruginosa*. In Mandell G, Bennett J, Dolin R, editors: *Principles and practice of infectious diseases*, ed 5, Philadelphia, 2000, Churchill Livingstone.

76. Relman D, Falkow S: A molecular perspective of microbial pathogenicity. In Mandell G, Bennett J, Dolin R, editors: *Principles and practice of infectious diseases*, ed 5, Philadelphia, 2000, Churchill Livingstone.

77. Resnick N: Geriatric medicine. In Tierney L, McPhee S, Papadakis M, editors: *Current medical diagnosis and treatment*, ed 39, New York, 2000, Lange Medical Books/McGraw-Hill.

78. Schaffer SD et al: *Infection prevention and safe practice*, St Louis, 1996, Mosby.

79. Schimmel P, Tao J, Hill J: Aminoacyl tRNA synthetases as targets for new anti-infectives, *FASEB J* 12(15): 1599-1609, 1998.

80. Schooley R: Epstein-Barr virus (*Infectious mononucleosis*). In Mandell G, Bennett J, Dolin R, editors: *Principles and practice of infectious diseases*, ed 5, Philadelphia, 2000, Churchill Livingstone.

81. Schurr M, Englehardt S, Helgerson R: Limb salvage for streptococcal gangrene of the extremity, *Am J Surg* 175(3):213-217, 1998.

82. Shanklin D, Smalley D: Dynamics of wound healing after silicone device and implantation, *Exp Mol Pathology* 67(1):26-39, 1999.

83. Shanklin D, Smalley D: The immunopathology of siliconosis; history, clinical presentation and relation to silicosis and the chemistry of silicon and silicone, *Immunol Res* 18(3):125-173, 1998.

84. Sharkey C: Infectious disorders. In Black JM, Matassarin-Jacobs E, editors: *Medical-surgical nursing, clinical management for continuity of care*, ed 5, Philadelphia, 1997, WB Saunders.

85. Silver H: Lyme disease during pregnancy, *Infec Dis Clin North Am* 11(1): 93-97, 1997.

86. Simons DG, Travell JG, Simons LS: *Travell & Simons' myofascial pain and dysfunction. The trigger point manual, vol 1: upper half of body*, ed 2, Baltimore, 1999, Williams and Wilkins.

87. Siscovick D et al: Collaborative multidisciplinary workshop report: the role of epidemiology studies in determining a possible relationship between chlamydia pneumoniae infection and atherothrombotic diseases, *J Infect Dis* 181(Suppl 3):S430-S431, 2000.

88. Smalley D et al: Lymphocyte response to silica among offspring of silicone breast implant recipients, *Immunobiology* 196(5):567-574, 1996-1997.

89. Steere A: *Borrelia burgdorferi* (Lyme disease, Lyme borreliosis). In Mandell G, Bennett J, Dolin R, editors: *Principles and practice of infectious diseases*, ed 5, Philadelphia, 2000, Churchill Livingstone.

90. Stein Z: Silicone breast implants: Epidemiological evidence of sequelae, *Am J Public Health* 89(4):484-487, 1999.

91. Swartz M: Cellulitis and subcutaneous tissue infections. In Mandell G, Bennett J, Dolin R, editors: *Principles and practice of infectious diseases*, ed 5, Philadelphia, 2000a, Churchill Livingstone.

92. Swartz M: Myositis. In Mandell G, Bennett J, Dolin R, editors: *Principles and practice of infectious diseases*, ed 5, Philadelphia, 2000b, Churchill Livingstone.

93. Trauger JW, Walsh CT: Heterologous expression in *Escherichia coli* of the first module of the nonribosomal peptide synthetase for chloroeremomycin, a vancomycin-type glycopeptide antibiotic, *Proc Natl Acad Sci USA* 97(7):3112-3117, 2000.

94. Trivalle C, Cremieux A, Carbon C: Pneumococcal septic arthritis in HIV infection, *Presse Med* 24(33):1566-1568, 1995.

95. Varenne O et al: Percutaneous gene therapy using recombinant adenoviruses encoding human herpes simplex virus thymidine kinase, human PAI-1, and human NOS3 in balloon-injured porcine coronary arteries, *Hum Gene Ther* 11(9):1329-1339, 2000.

96. Verdon M, Sigal L: Recognition and management of Lyme disease, *Am Fam Physician* 56(2):427-436, 1997.

97. Wade C: Keeping Lyme disease at bay: an integrated approach to prevention, *Am J Nurs* 100(7):27-32, 2000.

98. Weinstein R: Nosocomial infection update, *Emerg Infect Dis* 4(3): 416-420, 1998.

99. Whitley R: Varicella-zoster virus. In Mandell G, Bennett J, Dolin R, editors: *Principles and practice of infectious diseases*, ed 5, Philadelphia, 2000, Churchill Livingstone.

100. Wilburn S: Preventing needlestick injuries in your facility, *Am J Nurs* 100(2):96, 2000.

101. Williams G: The biology of handwashing, *Discover Mag* 36-38, 1999.

102. Wilson GJ et al: Group A streptococcal necrotizing fasciitis following varicella in children: case reports and review, *Clin Infect Dis* 20:1333-1338, May 1995.

103. Winquist A et al: Neuraminidase inhibitors for treatment of influenza A and B infections, *MMWR* 48(14): 1-9, 1999.

104. Woodrum JE, Oliver JH: Investigation of venereal, transplacental, and contact transmission of the lyme disease spirochete, *Borrelia burgdorferi*, in Syrian hamsters, *J Parasitol* 85(3):426-430, 1999.

105. Wright G: Resisting resistance; new chemical strategies for battling superbugs, *Chem Bio* 7(6):127-132, 2000.

106. Zaidi M, Wenzel R: Disinfection, sterilization and control of hospital waste. In Mandell G, Bennett J, Dolin R, editors: *Principles and practice of infectious diseases*, ed 5, Philadelphia, 2000, Churchill Livingstone.

CHAPTER 8

ONCOLOGY

CATHERINE C. GOODMAN AND TERESA E. KELLY SNYDER

Cancer is a term that refers to a large group of diseases characterized by uncontrolled cell proliferation and spread of abnormal cells. Other terms used interchangeably for cancer are malignant neoplasm, tumor, malignancy, and carcinoma. According to the American Cancer Society (ACS) about 5% of cancer is genetic whereas 95% is related to other factors. About one third of cancers are due to cigarette smoking, one third are related to diet and nutrition, and one third are caused by numerous other factors including genetics.[40] Only oncologic concepts are presented in this chapter; individual cancers are discussed in the chapters devoted to the affected system. See also Chapter 4.

DEFINITIONS

◆ Differentiation

Normal tissue contains cells of uniform size, shape, maturity, and nuclear structure. Differentiation is the process by which normal cells undergo physical and structural changes as they develop to form different tissues of the body. Differentiated cells specialize in different physiologic functions. In malignant cells, differentiation is altered and may be lost completely so that the malignant cell may not be recognizable in relationship to its parent cell. When a tumor has completely lost identity with the parent tissue, it is considered to be undifferentiated (anaplastic; anaplasia). In this case, it may become difficult or impossible to identify the malignant cell's tissue of origin. In general, the less differentiated a tumor becomes, the faster the metastasis (spread) and the worse the prognosis.

◆ Dysplasia

A variety of other tissue changes can occur in the body. Some of these changes are benign, whereas others denote a malignant or premalignant state. Dysplasia is a general category that indicates a disorganization of cells in which an adult cell varies from its normal size, shape, or organization. This is often caused by chronic irritation, such as is seen with changes in cervical (uterine) epithelium as a result of long-standing irritation of the cervix. Dysplasia may reverse itself or may progress to cancer.

◆ Metaplasia

Metaplasia is the first level of dysplasia (early dysplasia). It is a reversible and benign but abnormal change in which one adult cell changes from one type to another. For example, the most common type of epithelial metaplasia is the change of columnar epithelium of the respiratory tract to squamous epithelium. Another example of metaplasia is Barrett's esophagus (also called Barrett's epithelium), in which squamous epithelium of the esophagus is replaced by the glandular epithelium of the stomach. Although metaplasia usually gives rise to an orderly arrangement of cells, it may sometimes produce disorderly cellular patterns (i.e., cells varying in size, shape, and orientation to one another).

Anaplasia (loss of cellular differentiation) is the most advanced form of metaplasia and is a characteristic of malignant cells only.

◆ Hyperplasia

Hyperplasia refers to an increase in the number of cells in tissue, resulting in increased tissue mass. This type of change can be a normal consequence of physiologic alterations (physiologic hyperplasia), such as increased breast mass during pregnancy, wound healing, or bone callous formation. Neoplastic hyperplasia, however, is the increase in cell mass because of tumor formation and is an abnormal process. Atypical "hyperplasia" of the breast can develop into a "proliferative" hyperplasia (both are premalignant conditions) and then later into breast carcinoma. The presence of these types of hyperplastic breast tissue increases the risk of later development of breast cancer.[63]

◆ Tumors

Tumors, or neoplasms, are defined as abnormal growths of new tissue that serve no useful purpose and may harm the host organism by competing for vital blood supply and nutrients. These new growths may be benign or malignant (see the following discussion) and primary or secondary. A primary tumor arises from cells that are normally local to the given structure, whereas a secondary tumor arises from cells that have metastasized from another part of the body. For example, a primary neoplasm of bone arises from within the bone structure itself, whereas a secondary neoplasm occurs in bone as a result of metastasized cancer cells from another (primary) site.

Carcinoma in situ refers to preinvasive epithelial tumors of glandular or squamous cell origin. These tumors have not broken through basement membranes of the squamous cells and occur in the cervix, skin, oral cavity, esophagus, bronchus, and breast. Carcinoma in situ affecting glandular epithelium occurs most commonly in the cervix, breast, stomach, endometrium, large bowel, and prostate gland (prostate intraepithelial neoplasia [PIN]). How long the characteristic cell disorganization and atypical changes last before becoming invasive remains unknown.

CLASSIFICATIONS OF NEOPLASM

A neoplasm can be classified on the basis of cell type, tissue of origin, degree of differentiation, anatomic site, or whether it is benign or malignant. A benign growth is usually considered harmless and does not spread or invade other tissue. Certain benign growths, recognized clinically as tumors, are not truly neoplastic but rather represent overgrowth of normal tissue elements (e.g., vocal cord polyps, skin tags, hyperplastic polyps of the colon). However, benign growths can become large enough to distend, compress, or obstruct normal tissues and to impair normal body functions, as in the case of benign central nervous system (CNS) tumors. These tumors can cause disability and even death.

When tumors (benign or malignant) are classified by cell type, they are named according to the tissue from which they arise (Table 8-1). The five major classifications of normal body tissue are epithelial, connective and muscle, nerve, lymphoid, and hematopoietic tissue. Not all tissue types fit into one of these five categories, requiring a miscellaneous category (not included in Table 8-1) for other tissues, such as the tissues of the reproductive glands, placenta, and thymus. Malignant tumors usually carry the same name as the benign tumor except the suffix *carcinoma* is applied to epithelial cancers and *sarcoma* refers to those of mesenchymal origin.

Epithelium covers all external body surfaces and lines all internal spaces and cavities. The skin, mucous membranes, gastrointestinal tract, and lining of the bladder are examples of epithelial tissue. The functions of epithelial tissues are to protect, excrete, and absorb. Cancer originating in any of these epithelial tissues is called a *carcinoma*. Tumors derived from glandular tissues are called *adenocarcinomas*.

Connective tissue consists of elastic, fibrous, and collagenous tissues, such as bone, cartilage, and fat. Cancers originating in connective tissue and muscle are called *sarcomas*. Nerve tissue includes the brain, spinal cord, and nerves and consists of neurons, nerve fibers, dendrites, and a supporting tissue composed of glial cells. Tumors arising in *nerve tissue* are named for the type of cell involved. For example, tumors arising from astrocytes, a type of glial cell thought to form the blood-brain barrier, are called *astrocytomas*. Tumors arising in nerve tissue are often benign, but because of their critical location they are more likely to be harmful than benign tumors in other sites.

Malignancies originating in *lymphoid tissues* are called *lymphomas*. Lymphomas can arise in many parts of the body, wherever lymphoid tissue is present. The most common sites to find lymphoid malignancies are the lymph nodes and spleen. However, lymphomas can appear in other parts of the body such as the skin, central nervous system, stomach, small bowel, bone, and tonsils.[19] *Hematopoietic* malignancies include leukemias, multiple myeloma, myelodysplasia, and the myeloproliferative syndromes.

TABLE	8-1

Classification of Neoplasms by Cell Type of Origin

TISSUE OF ORIGIN	BENIGN	MALIGNANT
Epithelial tissue		
Surface epithelium (skin) and mucous membrane	Papilloma	Squamous cell, basal cell, and transitional cell carcinoma
Epithelial lining of glands or ducts	Adenoma	Adenocarcinoma
Pigmented cells (melanocytes of basal layer)	Nevus (mole)	Malignant melanoma
Connective tissue and muscle		
Fibrous tissue	Fibroma	Fibrosarcoma
Adipose	Lipoma	Liposarcoma
Cartilage	Chondroma	Chondrosarcoma
Bone	Osteoma	Osteosarcoma
Blood vessels	Hemangioma	Hemangiosarcoma
Smooth muscle	Leiomyoma	Leiomyosarcoma
Striated muscle	Rhabdomyoma	Rhabdomyosarcoma
Nerve tissue		
Nerve cells	Neuroma	
Glia		Glioma or neuroglioma
Ganglion cells	Ganglioneuroma	Neuroblastoma
Nerve sheaths	Neurilemoma	Neurilemic sarcoma
Meninges	Meningioma	Meningeal sarcoma
Retina		Retinoblastoma
Lymphoid tissue		Lymphoma
Lymph nodes		
Spleen		
Intestinal lining		
Hematopoietic tissue		
Bone marrow		Leukemias, myelodysplasia, and myeloproliferative syndromes
Plasma cells		Multiple myeloma

TABLE	8-2

TNM Staging System

T: *Primary Tumor*

TX	Primary tumor cannot be assessed
T_0	No evidence of primary tumor
T_{IS}	Carcinoma in situ (confined to site of origin)
T_1, T_2, T_3, T_4	Progressive increase in tumor size and involvement locally

N: *Regional Lymph Nodes*

N_x	Nodes cannot be assessed
N_0	No metastasis to regional lymph nodes
N_1, N_2, N_3	Increasing degrees of involvement of regional lymph nodes

M: *Distant Metastasis*

M_x	Presence of distant metastasis cannot be assessed
M_0	No distant metastasis
M_1	Distant metastasis

Note: Extension of primary tumor directly into lymph nodes is considered metastasis to lymph nodes. Metastasis to a lymph node beyond the regional ones is considered distant metastasis.

◆ Staging and Grading

Staging is the process of describing the extent of disease at the time of diagnosis in order to aid treatment planning, predict clinical outcome (prognosis), and compare different treatment approaches. The stage of disease at the time of diagnosis reflects the rate of growth and the extent of the neoplasm.

In the TNM classification scheme, developed by the American Joint Committee on Cancer (AJCC), tumors are staged according to three basic components (Table 8-2): (1) primary tumor (T), (2) regional lymph nodes (N), and (3) metastasis (M). Numbers are used with each component to denote extent of involvement; for example, T0 indicates undetectable, and T1, T2, T3, and T4 indicate a progressive increase in size or involvement.[70]

Grading, another way to define a tumor, classifies the degree of malignancy and differentiation of malignant cells. For example, a low-grade tumor typically has cells more closely resembling normal cells and tends to remain localized, whereas a high-grade tumor has poorly differentiated cells that tend to metastasize early.

CANCER AND AGING

Advancing age is a significant risk factor for the development of cancer. The association of cancer and aging is becoming more common because of the aging of the general population.[10] Data on cancer that emphasize the impact of this disease on older persons have been described using population-based statistics on incidence and mortality. Sixty percent of all cancers and 70% of all cancer mortality occur in people older than 65 years.[102] The risk of multiple diseases (co-morbidity) also increases with age, creating limitations in the life expectancy of individual aging adults and enhancing the likelihood of treatment complications.

Older people may be more susceptible to cancer simply because they have been exposed to carcinogens longer than younger people. The effects of age on immune function and host defense are being studied to determine what the association is between cancer and age (see the section on Aging and the Immune System in Chapter 6). Studies on mutations in cancer-causing structures such as telomeres, DNA repair aberrations, and dysregulation of important hormonal and immune modulators, such as cytokines, are all being reported as potential reasons for the increasing incidence of cancer in older adults.[11,29]

Clues about the life span of a cell and about aging in general are emerging from recent research on telomeres, which are chromosomal structures located at the end of each chromosome. In normal cells, the telomere shortens each time a cell divides. The cell dies when the telomere becomes so short that it can no longer divide. An important enzyme, telomerase, helps keep normally dividing cells healthy by rebuilding the telomeres; it normally shuts down when cells are mature, but in cancer, the enzyme enables cancer cells to grow with unlimited cell divisions. Telomerase is active in up to 95% of all human cancers.[16,17] See also the section on Cellular Aging in Chapter 5.

This understanding has led to discoveries regarding the life span of human cells, their relationship to aging, and the development of many illnesses associated with aging, such as cancer. It has been reported that normal cells do not divide indefinitely during the life span of a human because of a stopping process called *cellular senescence*. The acquisition of one or more short telomeres attached to cellular chromosomes appears to influence the development of cellular senescence and the stopping or modulating of cell division. It is theorized that dysfunctional senescence, caused by years of mutation, may lead to an increasing chance for developing cancer as people age.[15,95] Creating telomerase inhibitors could produce a means of supporting anticancer activity.

People age 65 years and older have a risk of cancer development 11 times greater than younger persons. All the highest-incidence cancers affect older adults in larger numbers. In both men and women over 65 years, cancers of the colon/rectum, stomach, pancreas, and bladder accounted for two thirds to three fourths of the total number of these malignancies. More than 65% of lung cancers and 50% of non-Hodgkin's lymphomas occur in older men and women. Seventy-seven percent of the cases of prostate cancer occurred in men older than 65 years; and 48% of breast and 46% of ovarian cancer occurred in women over 65 years. Malignancies of the lung, colon/rectum, breast, and prostate account for the highest number of cancer deaths in the United States, with malignancies of the pancreas, stomach, ovary, and bladder and non-Hodgkin's lymphomas also a major cause of cancer deaths. For each of these cancers, more than one half of the cancer deaths occur in persons older than 65 years.[102]

INCIDENCE

The American Cancer Society (ACS) publishes annual cancer statistics and estimates cancer trends (Fig. 8-1). Each year

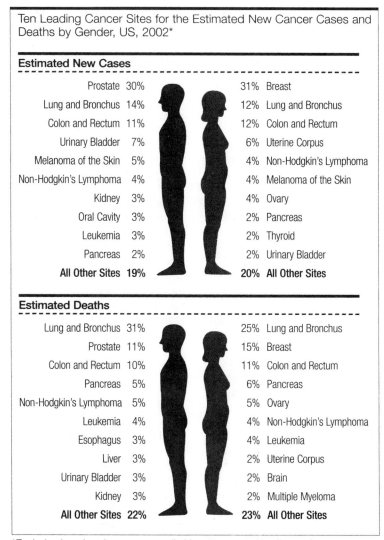

Ten Leading Cancer Sites for the Estimated New Cancer Cases and Deaths by Gender, US, 2002*

Estimated New Cases

Prostate	30%		31%	Breast
Lung and Bronchus	14%		12%	Lung and Bronchus
Colon and Rectum	11%		12%	Colon and Rectum
Urinary Bladder	7%		6%	Uterine Corpus
Melanoma of the Skin	5%		4%	Non-Hodgkin's Lymphoma
Non-Hodgkin's Lymphoma	4%		4%	Melanoma of the Skin
Kidney	3%		4%	Ovary
Oral Cavity	3%		2%	Pancreas
Leukemia	3%		2%	Thyroid
Pancreas	2%		2%	Urinary Bladder
All Other Sites	**19%**		**20%**	**All Other Sites**

Estimated Deaths

Lung and Bronchus	31%		25%	Lung and Bronchus
Prostate	11%		15%	Breast
Colon and Rectum	10%		11%	Colon and Rectum
Pancreas	5%		6%	Pancreas
Non-Hodgkin's Lymphoma	5%		5%	Ovary
Leukemia	4%		4%	Non-Hodgkin's Lymphoma
Esophagus	3%		4%	Leukemia
Liver	3%		2%	Uterine Corpus
Urinary Bladder	3%		2%	Brain
Kidney	3%		2%	Multiple Myeloma
All Other Sites	**22%**		**23%**	**All Other Sites**

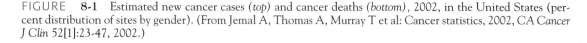

*Excludes basal and squamous cell skin cancers and in situ carcinomas except urinary bladder.
Percentages may not total 100% due to rounding.

FIGURE   **8-1**   Estimated new cancer cases *(top)* and cancer deaths *(bottom)*, 2002, in the United States (percent distribution of sites by gender). (From Jemal A, Thomas A, Murray T et al: Cancer statistics, 2002, CA *Cancer J Clin* 52[1]:23-47, 2002.)

the ACS calculates estimates of the number of new cancer cases and expected cancer deaths in the United States and compiles the most recent data on cancer incidence, mortality, and survival.[35] The National Cancer Institute (NCI) established the surveillance, epidemiology, and end results (SEER) program in 1973 as a way to report population-based data of site-specific incidences and outcomes of cancer. Because the United States does not have a nationwide cancer registry, the precise number of new cases of cancer diagnosed each year in the United States is not fully known. As a result of this, the number of new cancer cases occurring annually is estimated using complex statistical measures.

Overall incidence of cancer has declined in the last decade by an average of 1.1% annually with a 1.4% decline in cancer death rates. The largest decreases in deaths oc-

curred among men, especially among black men, who bear the heaviest cancer burden. Officials have attributed the steady downward trends to improved vigilance among Americans, who are benefiting from early screening and advances in treatment, as well as smoking less, improving their diets, and exercising more. About a dozen cancers continue to rise in incidence or mortality, including breast and female lung cancer, melanoma, non-Hodgkin's lymphoma, thyroid, and esophageal cancer.[45]

Based on statistical estimates, in the year 2002, the ACS is predicting about 1.3 million new cases of invasive cancer in the United States and approximately 555,500 cancer-related deaths. This figure does not include most skin cancers, and new cases of skin cancer are expected to exceed 1 million people per year.[39] Among men, the most common cancers are predicted to be cancers of the prostate, lung and bronchus, and colon/rectum. Among women, the three most commonly diagnosed cancers are expected to be cancers of the breast, lung and bronchus, and colon/rectum. Although death rates from breast cancer continue to decline, the incidence of the disease climbed 1.2% annually between 1992 and 2000. Breast cancer alone is expected to account for 203,500 new cancer cases in women.[35,45]

It is estimated that at least one in three people will be diagnosed with some form of invasive cancer in their lifetime and three of five people will be cured and/or survive 5 years after cancer treatment. However, cancer is still the second leading cause of death in the United States, exceeded only by heart disease. Poor health and nutrition habits, continued smoking, ozone destruction, and a long-term lack of exercise among many people continue to be discussed as contributors to the overall rise of this disease.[80]

ETIOLOGY

The cause of cancer varies, and causative agents are generally subdivided into two categories: those of endogenous (genetic) origin and those of exogenous (environmental or external) origin. It is likely that most cancers develop as a result of multiple environmental, viral, and genetic agents working together to disrupt the immune system and failure of an aging immune system to recognize and scavenge cells that have become less differentiated. Certain cancers show a familial pattern, giving people a hereditary predisposition to cancer. The most common cancers showing a familial pattern include prostate, breast, ovarian, and colon cancers. Research efforts have been directed at finding genes associated with various cancers that could identify high-risk individuals for screening and early detection.

The ACS estimates that 50% of all cancers are caused by one or more of nearly 500 different cancer-causing agents (e.g., tobacco use, viruses, chemical agents, physical agents, drugs, alcohol, hormones).[80] Etiologic agents capable of initiating the malignant transformation of a cell (i.e., carcinogenesis) are called *carcinogens*. The study of *viruses* as carcinogens is one of the most rapidly advancing areas in cancer research today. Researchers now have evidence that viruses play a role in the pathogenesis of cervical carcinomas, some hepatomas, Burkitt's lymphomas, nasopharyngeal carcinomas, adult T-cell leukemias, and indirectly, many Kaposi's sarcomas.[40] Viruses, such as the human immunodeficiency virus (HIV), the causative agent of acquired immunodeficiency syndrome (AIDS), weaken cell-mediated immunity, resulting in malignancies.

Chemical agents (e.g., tar, soot, asphalt, dyes, hydrocarbons, oils, nickel, arsenics) and *physical agents* (e.g., radiation, asbestos) may cause cancer after close and prolonged contact. Most people affected by chemical agents are industrial workers. Radiation exposure is usually from natural sources,* especially ultraviolet radiation from the sun, which can cause changes in deoxyribonucleic acid (DNA) structure that lead to malignant transformation. Basal and squamous cell carcinomas and malignant melanoma are all linked to ultraviolet exposure. See further discussion of chemical and physical agents in Chapter 3.

Some *drugs*, such as cancer chemotherapeutic agents, are in themselves carcinogenic. Cytotoxic drugs, including steroids, decrease antibody production and destroy circulating lymphocytes. Cancer clients treated with chemotherapy are at risk for future development of leukemia and other cancers. Cancer itself is immunosuppressive; advanced cancer exhausts the immune response.

Hormones have been linked to tumor development and growth, such as estrogen stimulating the growth of the endometrial lining, which over time becomes anaplastic. Other types of cancer occurring in target or hormone-responsive tissues include ovary and prostate cancers.

Excessive *alcohol* consumption is associated with cancer of the mouth, pharynx, larynx, esophagus, and pancreas. It can also indirectly contribute to liver cancer (i.e., alcohol causes liver cirrhosis, which is associated with cancer). The possible association between alcohol and breast cancer is under investigation. The pathophysiologic link remains unclear, but researchers postulate that alcohol influences the metabolism of estrogen, and increased estrogen exposure is a known risk factor for breast cancer (see the section on Breast Cancer in Chapter 19).

RISK FACTORS

As discussed previously (see Cancer and Aging, this chapter), *advancing age* is one of the most significant risk factors for cancer. In addition to age and the carcinogens described earlier under Etiologic Factors, predisposing factors also influence the host's susceptibility to various etiologic agents (Box 8-1). Experimental and epidemiologic evidence has established an association between at least eight viruses and various cancer sites. At least 10% of cancer worldwide is caused by viruses, tobacco, and diet. Some risk factors are interactive and become exponential rather than additive (e.g., alcohol and smoking for oral pharyngeal cancers).

BOX **8-1**

Cancer Risk Factors

Advancing age	Geographic location and
Lifestyle or personal behaviors	environmental variables
Tobacco use	(see Chapter 3)
Diet and nutrition	Gender
Alcohol use	Ethnicity
Sexual and reproductive	Socioeconomic status
behavior	(see Chapter 2)
Exposure to viruses	Occupation (see Chapter 3)
Human papillomavirus (HPV)	Heredity
Hepatitis B virus (HBV)	Presence of precancerous
Hepatitis C virus (HCV)	lesions
Helicobacter pylori	Stress
Herpesvirus 8	

---

*Notable exceptions include past history of radiation treatment for acne, thymus, or thyroid conditions.

◆ Lifestyle

Lifestyle or personal behaviors, such as tobacco use, diet and nutrition, alcohol use, and sexual and reproductive behavior, are cited as risk factors for the development of cancer. Both epidemiologic and experimental data support the conclusion that *tobacco* (including smokeless tobacco) is carcinogenic and remains the most important cause of cancer. Lung cancer is now the leading cancer-causing death in both genders. Cigarette smoking is related to nearly 90% of all lung cancers, and accumulating evidence suggests that cigarette smoking increases the incidence of cancer of the bladder, pancreas, and, to a lesser extent, the kidney, larynx, oral cavity, and esophagus.

The major role of *diet and nutrition* in affecting cancer risk is well established.[4,5,14] Consumption of a poor diet may blunt the immune system's natural defense mechanisms against genetic damage caused by long-term exposure to an environmental carcinogen. Diet and nutrition can directly influence various hormonal factors affecting growth and differentiation in the carcinogenic process. A healthful diet is thought to act, at least in part, to detoxify carcinogens and to inhibit certain processes in carcinogenesis, particularly at the stage of growth and spread. Diet and nutrition can influence these processes (positively or negatively) by providing bioactive compounds to specific tissues via the circulatory system or by modulating hormone levels.

Differences in certain dietary patterns among populations explain a proportion of cancers. These dietary patterns in combination with physical inactivity contribute to obesity and metabolic consequences, such as increased levels of growth factor, insulin, estrogen, and possibly testosterone. These hormones tend to promote cellular growth.[34]

It is estimated that approximately one third of cancer mortality in developing countries may result from dietary causes.[6,96] The intake of cured, pickled, smoked, salted, and preserved food has been conclusively linked to stomach cancer, and it is suspected that there is a correlation between the amount of fat in the diet and the incidence of colorectal cancer in the United States. There is a similar correlation between excessive red meat consumption and colon cancer. Epidemiologic data also suggest links between fat intake and prostate and ovarian cancers although not all findings are consistent.[40]

The role of fruits and vegetables and their antioxidant qualities in reducing cancer of various sites has been proved. Reduction of cancer risks for most epithelial tumors, especially colorectal cancer, has been demonstrated repeatedly in the presence of increased dietary intake of fresh fruits and vegetables and fiber. High cruciferous vegetable consumption may reduce bladder cancer risk and the risk of non-Hodgkin's lymphoma.[57,104]

Alcohol consumption has been linked to increased rates of cancer of the mouth, pharynx, larynx, esophagus, and liver (closely controlled for tobacco use). With tobacco use, alcohol interacts with smoke synergistically, increasing the risk of malignant tumors by acting as a solvent for the carcinogenic smoke products and thus increasing the absorption of carcinogens. Evidence is suggestive (but not yet convincing) in associating alcohol consumption and cancers of the colon, pancreas, breast, bladder, and head and neck.[40]

Sexual and reproductive behaviors are linked to the risk of developing various cancers. For example, the risk of developing cervical cancer is related to age of first sexual intercourse (increased incidence with earlier intercourse), to the number and type of sexually transmitted diseases, and to the number of sexual partners (increased incidence with increasing number of sexual partners). Pregnancy and childbearing seem to be protective against cancers of the endometrium, ovary, and breast. Prolonged lactation may also have a significant impact in the reduction of breast cancer risk by reducing the cumulative exposure of breast tissue to estrogen.[40] Other risk factors for breast cancer are discussed in Chapter 19.

◆ Geographic Location and Environmental Variables

The incidence of different types of cancer varies geographically. Colon cancer is more prevalent in urban than in rural areas, but in rural areas, especially among farmers, skin cancer is more common. People living in rural areas are less likely to use preventive screening services or to exercise regularly. Availability of specialty care is also a contributing issue for this group of people.[39] The greater susceptibility of certain geographic areas within the United States is probably related to exposure to different carcinogens.[20] The increased incidence of cancer found in urban areas may be related to the increased pool of minorities, increased poverty represented in this group, local smoking ordinances, and diet (e.g., cost and availability of fresh fruits and vegetables).[67]

Researchers are investigating the possible causal relationship between environmental exposure and the increased incidence of childhood cancers. The U.S. Environmental Protection Agency (EPA) has identified the carcinogenic effects from hazardous exposures. Heritable genetic and chromosomal mutations caused by environmental or occupational exposures to agents (e.g., chemicals, radiation) can be passed on to the next generation. For further discussion, see Chapter 3.

◆ Ethnicity

Black Americans are diagnosed with cancer and die from it more often than any other racial group in the United States. At present this increased incidence is attributed to preventable risk factors, such as the absence of early screening, delayed diagnosis, and smoking and diet. The number of black American men who smoke is decreasing, but the incidence of lung cancer and other smoking-related diseases remains high, possibly because black men tend to smoke cigarettes with a higher tar and nicotine content. The incidence rates of prostate cancer among black men are at least 50% higher than rates for men of other ethnic groups.[35]

Lung cancer is the leading cause of cancer death among black American women. The number of black American women (aged 45 to 54 years) who have died from lung cancer has increased 30% over the last two decades. The number of black American women of all ages who have died from breast cancer has risen nearly 20% over the last 25 years. Breast cancer is the second leading cause of death for black American women. Colorectal cancer has increased in both black American men and women; black women are twice as likely to develop cervical cancer and nearly three times as likely to die from it as other women; black American men have the world's highest rate of prostate cancer.[98]

Some specific forms of cancer affect other ethnic groups at rates higher than the national average (e.g., stomach and liver cancers among Asian American populations and colorectal [CRC] cancer among Alaska Natives). Certain racial and ethnic groups have lower survival rates than whites for most cancers.

Differences among ethnic groups represent both a challenge to understand the reasons and an opportunity to reduce illness and death and to improve survival rates. The Hispanic cancer experience also differs from that of the non-Hispanic white population, with Hispanics having higher rates of cervical, esophageal, gallbladder, and stomach cancers. New cases of female breast and lung cancers are increasing among Hispanics, who are diagnosed at later stages and have lower survival rates than whites.[39]

◆ Precancerous Lesions

Precancerous and some benign tumors may undergo transformation later into cancerous lesions and tumors. Common precancerous lesions include pigmented moles, burn scars, senile keratosis, leukoplakia, and benign adenomas or polyps of the colon or stomach. All such lesions need to be examined periodically for signs of changes.

◆ Stress

Recent research suggests a strong link between stress and cancer. Chronic physical or emotional stress can cause hormonal or immunologic changes or both, which in turn can facilitate the growth and proliferation of cancer cells. There is substantial evidence from both healthy populations and people with cancer linking psychologic stress with immune down regulation. Distress and depression are associated with two important processes for carcinogenesis: poorer repair of damaged DNA and alterations in apoptosis. Conversely, the possibility that psychologic interventions and social support may enhance immune function and survival is under further investigation.[48] See the section on Psychoneuroimmunology Theory in Chapter 1; see also the section on Stress in Chapter 2.

PATHOGENESIS

Early in the study of cancer the concept that neoplasia originates in a single cell by acquired genetic change was proposed and remains today the view of cancer pathogenesis most supported by experimental evidence. This hypothesis, called the *somatic mutation theory*, was first substantiated when investigations of tumors confirmed that tumor cells are characterized by chromosomal abnormalities, numerical as well as structural.* The discovery that chromosomal aberration is one of the basic mechanisms of tumor cell proliferation laid the foundation of modern cancer cytogenetics (study of chromosomes in cancer).

At first the question arose: are acquired chromosomal abnormalities the cause of the neoplastic changes in cells or merely the result of the neoplastic state? Chromosomal banding techniques developed in the 1970s have allowed precise

identification of chromosomal changes. This information, along with molecular genetic techniques developed during the 1980s, has enabled researchers to investigate this question by examining tumor cells at the level of individual genes.

From these studies two functionally different classes of cancer-relevant genes have been detected: (1) the dominant oncogenes and (2) the recessive tumor suppressor genes. Both gene classes have been detected at just those chromosomal sites that are visibly involved in cancer-associated rearrangements. To date, over 100 genes have been found to be structurally or functionally altered following neoplasia-associated chromosomal abnormalities.

Exactly how these chromosomal changes contribute to the malignant process remains unclear. Chromosomal rearrangements may lead to oncogene activation, either by a regulatory change causing increased production of normal oncogene-encoded peptides or by creating a deranged oncogene template that codes for an abnormal protein product. Another proposed mechanism suggests that chromosomal changes inactivate a tumor suppressor gene through chromosomal deletion. Loss of tumor suppressor genes is suspected because chromosomal regions found to be consistently missing in tumor cells have been observed in carcinomas of the lung, breast, bladder, and kidney.

An important tumor suppressor gene currently under study is p53. The p53 gene appears to trigger programmed cell death (apoptosis) as a way of regulating uncontrolled cellular proliferation. Mutations in the p53 gene result in loss of the ability of the gene protein to bind with DNA and act as a suppressor for the division of that cell.[62] Another genetic suppressor of cell growth and division also plays a part in the aging process. As cells divide and grow older, there is continuous progressive shortening of the end portions of the chromosomes or telomeres of those cells. Studies of human fibroblasts and other human tissues have shown a very close association between the development of cancer and the overproduction of an enzyme called *telomerase*. This enzyme, when present, prevents the telomeres from shortening, thus lengthening the life span of the cell indefinitely. Telomerase has been found to be present in about 85% of malignant tumors but is absent in most normal human tissues.[76,94]

Although much remains to be learned about the cascade of genetic changes for every kind of cancer, continued increasing understanding may suggest a means for interrupting the genetic events leading to cancer and for diagnosing the early stages of tumorigenesis.

◆ Current Theory of Oncogenesis

The study of viruses in tumors has led researchers to discover small segments of genetic DNA called *oncogenes*. Oncogenes, also called cancer-causing genes or *protooncogenes*, have the ability to transform normal cells into malignant cells, independently or incorporated with a virus. Oncogenes are thought to be the abnormal counterparts of protooncogenes, which aid in regulating biologic functions, such as cell division, in normal cells. Oncogenes may be activated by carcinogens, at which point they alter the regulation of growth in the cell. Oncogenes force a cell to grow even when its surroundings contain none of the cues that normally provoke growth. Oncogenes are hyperactivated versions of normal cellular growth-promoting genes. By releasing strong, unrelenting growth-stimulating signals into a cell, oncogenes can drive cell growth ceaselessly.

---

*Chromosomal changes can include addition or deletion of entire chromosomes (numerical changes) or translocations, deletions, inversions, and insertions of parts of chromosomes (structural changes). Translocations occur when two or more chromosomes exchange material and are common in leukemias and sarcomas. Deletions or losses of chromosomal material are common in epithelial adenocarcinomas of the large bowel, lung, breast, and prostate. Chromosomal deletions may lead to neoplastic development when a tumor suppressor gene is lost. Chromosomal inversions and insertions are less common but still cause abnormal juxtaposition (side-by-side placement) of genetic material.[75]

Researchers have also discovered a group of regulatory genes, called *antioncogenes* and now called *tumor suppressor genes,* that have the opposite effect of oncogenes. When activated, tumor suppressor genes can regulate growth and inhibit carcinogenesis. Tumor suppressor genes are the "brakes" to the "stuck accelerator" of the activated oncogene (e.g., p53, telomeres). When defects in the oncogene occur simultaneously with inactivation of growth-suppressing genes, aggressive cell proliferation takes place with the creation of certain types of tumor cells.

Tumor Biochemistry and Pathogenesis

Carcinogenesis is the process by which a normal cell undergoes malignant transformation. Usually it is a multistep process, involving progressive changes following genetic damage to or alteration of cellular DNA through the development of hyperplasia, metaplasia, dysplasia, carcinoma in situ, invasive carcinoma, and metastatic carcinoma in that order.[59] These discrete stages in tumor development suggest that a single altered gene only suffices to push a cell part of the way down the path to actual malignancy. The process is completed when multiple, successive changes occur in distinct cellular genes, including activation or overexpression of oncogenes and loss or mutation of tumor suppressor genes.

The number of genetic events required for conversion of normal cells to malignant cells is still debated, but at least in the case of many solid tumors (e.g., colon carcinomas), this number may be as great as seven or eight. This high number of genetic events may imply that genetic instability occurs during cancer progression.[59] This requirement for multiple changes creates an important protective mechanism against cancer. If a small number of genetic changes sufficed to transform a normal cell into a malignant one, multiple tumors would develop easily. These multiple barriers, along with the normal circuitry inside cells, ensure that only the rare cell will sustain the requisite number of changes for making a cancer cell.

INVASION AND METASTASES

Malignant tumors differ from benign tumors in their ability to metastasize or spread from the primary site to other locations in the body. Metastasis occurs when cells break away from the primary tumor, travel through the body via the blood or lymphatic system, and become trapped in the capillaries of organs. From there, they infiltrate the organ tissue and grow into new tumor deposits. Cancer can also spread to adjacent structures and penetrate body cavities by direct extension. For example, ovarian tumors frequently shed cells into the peritoneal cavity, where they grow to cover the surface of abdominal organs.

Patterns of metastasis differ from cancer to cancer. Although there is no clear explanation of the exact mechanism of metastasis, certain cancers tend to spread to specific organs or sites in the body in a predictable manner. The five most common sites of metastasis are the lymph nodes, liver, lung, bone, and brain.

The spread of cancer may be negatively influenced by a variety of host factors, such as the aging or dysfunctional immune system, increasing age, hormonal environment, pregnancy, and stress. Factors that may slow the spread of metastasis include radiation, chemotherapy, anticoagulants, steroids, and other antiinflammatory agents.

Incidence of Metastasis

Approximately 30% of clients with newly diagnosed cancers have clinically detectable metastases. At least 30% to 40% of the remaining clients who are clinically free of metastases harbor occult (hidden) metastases. Unfortunately, most people have multiple sites of metastatic disease, not all of which present at any one time. The formation of metastatic colonies is a continuous process, commencing early in the growth of the primary tumor and increasing with time.

Even metastases have the potential to metastasize; the presence of large, identifiable metastases in a given organ can be accompanied by a greater number of micrometastases that have been disseminated more recently from the primary tumor or the metastasis. The size variation in metastases and the dispersed anatomic location of metastases can make complete surgical removal of disease impossible, limiting the effective concentration of anticancer drugs that can only be delivered to tumor cells in metastatic colonies.

Mechanism of Metastasis

A complicated series of tumor-host interactions resulting in a metastatic colony is called the *metastatic cascade* and is similar for all tumor cells. Once a primary tumor is initiated and starts to move by local invasion, blood vessels from surrounding tissue grow into the solid tumor, a process called *tumor angiogenesis.*

The ability of a tumor to grow beyond a very small mass (1 to 2 mm) depends on its ability to gain access to an adequate supply of blood and in some cases (e.g., breast, prostate) the presence of hormonal factors. The supply of blood allows the tumor to obtain essential nutrients, such as oxygen, and to eliminate metabolic waste products, such as carbon dioxide and acids. The blood supply to tumors is provided by growth of new capillaries and larger vessels into the tumor mass from the blood supply of adjacent normal tissues. Tumor-derived proteins called *angiogenesis factors* facilitate the use of nearby blood vessels from normal tissues and promote the growth of new blood vessels into the malignant tissue.[75]

The actual factors involved in tumor angiogenesis are very complex, but two cytokines have been identified as primary stimulators of vascular proliferation. Both vascular endothelial growth factor (VEGF) and fibroblast growth factor stimulate proliferation of vascular cells and even allow the newly formed blood vessels to be easily invaded by the cancer cells that are closely adjacent to them.[28] Increased tumor contact with the circulatory system provides tumors with a mechanism to enter the general circulation and colonize at distant sites. Antiangiogenic therapy shows promise as a strategy for cancer treatment (see the section on Treatment in this chapter).

For rapidly growing tumors, millions of tumor cells can invade the vascular system each day. Only a very small percentage of circulating tumor cells initiate metastatic colonies because most cells that have invaded the bloodstream are quickly eliminated. The greater the number of invasive tumor cells in the bloodstream, the greater the probability that some cells will survive to form metastases.

Tumors generally lack a well-formed lymphatic network, so communication of tumor cells with lymphatic channels occurs only at the tumor periphery and not within the tumor mass. Lymphatic dissemination and hematogenous dissemination occur in parallel. Where lymph nodes drain into veins (e.g., lymphatic intersection with the subclavian vein), cancer cells can enter the bloodstream.

◆ Clinical Manifestations of Metastasis

Metastatic spread usually occurs within 3 to 5 years after initial diagnosis and treatment of malignancy, although some low-grade lesions can reappear as much as 15 to 20 years later. It is therefore very important to conduct a thorough past medical history as part of any client interview. Metastases occur most commonly to areas of the body that provide an environment rich in nutrition to the colonized tumor cells, such as the lung, brain, liver, and bone. However, metastases can also be found in the lymph nodes, skin, ovaries, and adrenal glands.

Pulmonary System (Lungs). Pulmonary metastases are the most common of all metastatic tumors because venous drainage of most areas of the body is through the superior and inferior venae cavae into the heart, making the lungs the first organ to filter malignant cells. Parenchymal metastases are asymptomatic until tumor cells have obstructed bronchi resulting in pulmonary symptoms or until tumor cells have expanded and reached the parietal pleura where pain fibers are stimulated.

Most initial pulmonary metastases are asymptomatic. A dry, persistent cough is often the first symptom of pulmonary metastases. Pleural pain can indicate pleural invasion, and shortness of breath (dyspnea) usually occurs in the presence of a malignant pleural effusion. If hemoptysis occurs, there is usually bronchial tissue invasion either by a primary lung malignancy or metastatic disease.[92]

Tumor cells traveling from the lung via the pulmonary veins and carotid artery can result in metastases to the CNS. Lung cancer is the most common primary tumor to metastasize to the brain. Any neurologic sign may be the presentation of a silent lung tumor.[36]

Hepatic System (Liver). Liver metastases are among the most ominous signs of advanced cancer. The liver filters blood coming in from the gastrointestinal tract, making it a primary metastatic site for tumors of the stomach, colorectum, and pancreas. Symptoms include abdominal and/or right upper quadrant pain, general malaise and fatigue, anorexia, early satiety and weight loss, and sometimes low-grade fevers.

Skeletal System (Bone). Primary bone tumors, such as osteogenic sarcoma, metastasize initially to the lungs, whereas a large proportion of cancer cases metastasize first to the bone, often with a poor prognosis (see also Chapter 25). Bone is one of the three most favored sites of solid tumor metastasis, indicating that the bone microenvironment provides fertile ground for the growth of many tumors. Although lung, breast, and prostate are the three primary sites responsible for most metastatic bone disease, tumors of the thyroid and kidney, lymphoma, and melanoma can also metastasize to the skeletal system.

In any person with metastasized cancer, bone metastases may be the osteolytic type, marked by areas of decreased bone density, or osteoblastic, appearing as areas of dense scarring and increased bone density. Osteolytic metastases predominate in lung, kidney, and thyroid cancer, whereas osteoblastic metastases occur in breast and prostate cancer. The axial

skeleton is most commonly involved with spread to the spine, pelvis, ribs, proximal femora, proximal humeri, and skull.

The primary symptom associated with bone metastases (osteolytic or osteoblastic) is pain. Pain is usually deep and worsened by activity, especially weight bearing. Disabling pathologic fractures, especially of the vertebral bodies and proximal ends of the long bones, may occur in up to one half of people with osteolytic metastases and are sometimes one of the first signs of a malignant process.[36]

Hypercalcemia (abnormally high concentration of blood calcium) is a frequent complication of neoplastic disease and is associated with bony metastases, particularly osteolytic lesions as a result of increased bone resorption. Although more than 80% of people with hypercalcemia have bony metastasis, the severity of the hypercalcemia does not correlate with the extent of the bony disease. Hydration and administration of bisphosphonates (e.g., pamidronate [Aredia], clodronate) are the mainstays of current treatment and have contributed to the decrease in the frequency of hypercalcemia and to minimizing or preventing bone loss. Bisphosphonates prevent thinning of the bone by preventing cells that dissolve osteoclasts from doing so. There is no life-prolonging benefit with bisphosphonates but a substantial reduction of morbidity associated with bone metastases.[23,43]

Central Nervous System

Brain. Many primary tumors may lead to CNS metastases. Lung carcinomas account for approximately one-half of all metastatic brain lesions. Breast carcinoma and malignant melanoma also commonly metastasize to the brain. Metastatic disease in the brain is life-threatening and emotionally debilitating. Metastatic brain tumors can increase intracranial pressure, obstruct the normal flow of cerebrospinal fluid, change mentation and contribute to cognitive impairment, and reduce sensory and motor function. The management of cognitive impairments is important, and the therapist can use the same strategies known for people with traumatic brain injuries (see Chapter 32).

Clinical manifestations of brain metastases depend on the location, either in the brain or outside the brain in the bony cranium exerting compression externally. The therapist can look at computed tomography (CT) scan results, see the location of pathologic conditions, and correlate these to signs and symptoms observed clinically (see Table 29-2).

Primary tumors of the CNS rarely develop metastases outside the CNS despite the highly invasive capacity of these tumors. Microscopically, some CNS (brain) tumor cells (astrocytomas) may spread widely within the CNS but rarely metastasize outside it.

Spinal Cord. Metastatic involvement of the vertebrae may result in epidural spinal (usually anterior) cord compression because severe, destructive osteolytic lesions lead to fracture and fragility of one or more vertebral bodies. In such cases, compression of the cord occurs as a result of the subsequent deformity.[60] Spinal cord and nerve root compression cause either insidious or rapid loss of neurologic function. This compression phenomenon occurs in approximately 5% of people with systemic cancer, most often caused by carcinoma of the lung, breast, prostate, or kidney. Lymphoma and multiple myeloma may also result in spinal cord and nerve root compression.

The earliest neurologic symptoms include gradual onset of distal weakness and sensory changes, including numbness, paresthesias, and coldness. The incidence of permanent motor dysfunction has markedly decreased in the past two decades because of earlier diagnosis and treatment.[23] The client who presents with spinal cord symptoms caused by metastatic epidural disease and resultant compression may have only transient symptoms with proper medical treatment. More than 95% of people with spinal cord compression complain of progressive central or radicular back pain often aggravated by recumbency, weight bearing, sneezing, coughing, or Valsalva's maneuver. Sitting often relieves it.

Lymphatic System.   Cancer-related surgery or radiation treatment affecting the lymph nodes may result in dysfunction of the lymphatic system presenting as lymphedema. It has a wide range of onset from weeks to years from the initial insult to the lymphatic system. The therapist may be the first health care professional to assess for abnormalities or changes in the extremities. See further discussion in Chapter 12.

◆ Diagnosis of Metastasis

Metastases usually reproduce the cellular structure of the primary growth well enough to enable a pathologist to determine the site of the primary tumor. For example, bone metastases from a carcinoma of the thyroid not only exhibit a microscopic structure similar to the original tumor but also may produce thyroid hormone. Sometimes, symptoms of a cancer will present in the metastatic site rather than the site of origin (primary site). If the metastatic sites are difficult to identify regarding origin, the malignant tissue is called *carcinoma of unknown primary*. Special histologic stains can be done on the unknown tissue and compared to slides of a previous malignancy to determine similarity.

◆ Cancer Recurrence

Disease-free survival describes the time between diagnosis and recurrence or relapse. Recurrences may be local, regional, disseminated, or a combination of these. The most important predictors of recurrent cancer are stage at the time of initial therapy and histologic findings. Recurrence of cancer may be first recognized by the return of systemic symptoms associated with paraneoplastic phenomena. The metabolic or toxic effects of the syndrome (e.g., hypercalcemia, hyponatremia) may constitute a more urgent hazard to life than the underlying cancer.

CLINICAL MANIFESTATIONS

◆ Local and Systemic Effects

Most cancers in their earliest stages are asymptomatic but treatable if found. Most primary site cancers cause certain symptoms that are recognizable causes for suspicion or concern. For example, endometrial cancer causes abnormal bleeding so often that it is usually detected in its early stages. Laryngeal cancer causes hoarseness, which is also an early sign. However, lung cancer is usually quite extensive before it causes enough symptoms to warrant investigation, as is true with breast cancer if it is a deeply buried tumor that is difficult to palpate. Most cancer is detected early and can be cured or successfully treated.

Nausea, vomiting, and retching (NVR) accompanied by anorexia and subsequent weight loss is common in people with advanced cancer as a result of the malignant process and its treatment. NVR is especially prevalent in association with lung carcinoma, hypernephroma, and pancreatic carcinoma. Anorexia has been attributed to tumor production of a protein (a cytokine) called *tumor necrosis factor (TNF)** or *cachectin*. Cancer-related anorexia/cachexia (CAC) is a complex phenomenon in which metabolic abnormalities, proinflammatory cytokines produced by the host immune system, circulating tumor-derived catabolic factors, decreased food intake, and possibly other unknown factors all contribute. Profound muscle loss is prominent in CAC syndrome as a result of decreased protein synthesis and abnormal muscle proteolysis.

Later, the rapid growth of the tumor encroaches on healthy tissue, causing destruction, necrosis, ulceration, and hemorrhage and producing many local and systemic effects. Pain may or may not occur depending on how close tumor cells, swelling, or hemorrhage occurs to the nerve cells. Systemically with advanced or stage IV cancer, the host presents with muscular weakness, anemia, and coagulation disorders (granulocyte and platelet abnormalities; see the section on Disorders of Hemostasis and Thrombocytopenia in Chapter 13).

Fever may be seen with cancer in the absence of infection and is produced either by white blood cells inducing a pyrogen (an agent that causes fever) or by direct tumor production of a pyrogen. Continued spread of the cancer may lead to gastrointestinal, pulmonary, or vascular obstruction. Secondary infections frequently occur as a result of the host's decreased immunity and can lead to death.

Other vital organs may be affected, such as the brain, where increased intracranial pressure by tumor cells can cause stroke-like symptoms. In addition to the local effects of tumor growth, cancer can produce systemic signs and symptoms that are not direct effects of either the tumor or its metastases, for example, paraneoplastic syndromes such as proximal leg weakness in small cell lung cancers (Eaton-Lambert syndrome) or fever with renal cancer. Pain may occur as a late symptom caused by infiltration, compression, or destruction of nerves.

◆ Cancer Pain

One of the most common symptoms of cancer is pain, affecting between 50% and 70% of clients in its early stages and 60% to 90% of clients in its late stages. It is estimated that 1.1 million Americans experience cancer-related pain annually.[18] Depression and anxiety may increase the person's perception of pain or may be the result of the cancer pain. Symptoms often go unreported or underreported because clients are reluctant to take the pain medication prescribed.†

The cause of cancer pain is multifaceted, and the characteristics of the pain depend on the tissue structure as well as on the mechanisms involved (Table 8-3). Some pain is caused

---

*Tumor necrosis factors are believed to play an important role in mediating inflammation and cytotoxic reactions (along with interleukins). TNFs produce necrosis of tumor cells by eliminating the blood supply to these growths. Small amounts of TNF are beneficial in promoting wound healing and preventing tumors, but uncontrolled production is accompanied by symptoms of fever, weight loss, and tissue damage that can cause more problems than the benefits provided.

†An unfounded fear of tolerance, addiction, or adverse effects from pain medication may result in underreporting of painful symptoms with subsequent inadequate cancer pain control and unnecessary pain-induced loss of function. Likewise, physicians may hesitate to provide adequate pain medications based on this misconception of client addiction.

TABLE	8-3

Common Patterns of Pain Referral

Pain Mechanism	Site of Lesion	Referral Site
Visceral	Diaphragmatic irritation	Shoulder
	Urothelial tract	Inguinal region and genitalia
Somatic	C7, T1 vertebrae	Interscapular
	L1, L2 vertebrae	Sacroiliac joint and hip
	Hip joint	Knee
	Pharynx	Ipsilateral ear
Neuropathic	Nerve or plexus	Anywhere in the distribution of a peripheral nerve
	Nerve root	Anywhere in the corresponding dermatome
	Central nervous system	Brain
		Spinal cord
		Anywhere in the region of the body innervated by the damaged structure

Modified from Cherny NI, Portenoy RK: The management of cancer pain, CA *Cancer J Clin* 44:271, 1994.

by pressure on nerves or by the displacement of nerves. Microscopic infiltration of nerves by tumor cells can result in continuous, sharp, stabbing pain generally following the pattern of nerve distribution. Ischemic pain (throbbing) may also result from interference with blood supply or from blockage within hollow organs.

A common cause of cancer pain is metastasis of cancer to bone. Lung, breast, prostate, thyroid, and the lymphatics are the primary sites responsible for most metastatic bone disease. Bone metastasis results in increased release of prostaglandins and cytokines and subsequent bone destruction caused by breakdown and resorption. Bone pain may be mild to intense. Movement, weight bearing, and ambulation exacerbate painful symptoms from bone destruction. Pathologic fractures with resultant muscle spasms can develop; in the case of vertebral involvement, nerve pain may also occur.

Signs and symptoms accompanying mild to moderate superficial pain may include hypertension, tachycardia, and tachypnea (rapid, shallow breathing) as a result of a sympathetic nervous system response. In severe or visceral pain, a parasympathetic nervous system response is more characteristic, with hypotension, bradycardia, nausea, vomiting, tachypnea, weakness, or fainting.

Spinal cord compression from metastases may present as radicular back pain, leg weakness, and unilateral loss of bowel or bladder control. Back pain may precede the development of neurologic signs and symptoms. The presence of jaundice in association with an atypical presentation of back pain may in-

dicate hepatobiliary obstruction and/or liver metastasis. Signs of nerve root compression may be the first indication of a cancer, in particular of lymphoma, multiple myeloma, or cancer of the lung, breast, prostate, or kidney. Other neurologic or musculoskeletal manifestations of neoplasm are discussed under Paraneoplastic Syndromes below.

Pain may also result from iatrogenic causes, such as surgery, radiation therapy, or chemotherapy (e.g., mucositis, stomatitis, esophageal inflammation, localized skin burns). Immobility and inflammation can lead to pain. Inflammation with its accompanying symptoms of redness, edema, pain, heat, and loss of function may progress to infection, necrosis, and sloughing of tissue. If the inflammatory process alone is present, the pain is characterized by tenderness. Pain may be excruciating in the presence of tissue necrosis and sloughing.

◆ Cancer-Related Fatigue

Fatigue, or more specifically, cancer-related fatigue syndrome is a syndrome with multiple characteristics and problems. Fatigue affects up to 70% of all people during chemotherapy and radiotherapy; reduced physical performance and fatigue are universal after bone marrow transplantation. Up to 30% of cancer survivors report a loss of energy for years after cessation of treatment. For many people with cancer, fatigue is severe and imposes limitations on normal daily activities.[25]

◆ Paraneoplastic Syndromes
Overview and Definition.   In addition to the local effects of tumor growth, cancer can produce systemic signs and symptoms that are not direct effects of either the tumor or its metastases. When tumors produce signs and symptoms at a site distant from the tumor or its metastasized sites, these remote effects of malignancy are collectively referred to as paraneoplastic syndromes.

Although malignant cells frequently lose the function, appearance, and properties associated with the normal cells of the tissue of origin, in some cases they can acquire new cellular functions uncharacteristic of the originating tissue. Many of these syndromes involve ectopic hormone production by tumor cells or the secretion of biochemically active substances that cause metabolic abnormalities. For example, tumors in nonendocrine tissues sometimes acquire the ability to produce and secrete hormones that are distributed by the circulation and act on target organs at a site other than the location of the tumor. The most common cancer associated with paraneoplastic syndromes is small cell cancer of the lung, which can produce adrenocorticotropic hormone (ACTH) in amounts sufficient to cause Cushing's syndrome.

Malignancy is often associated with a wide variety of musculoskeletal disorders, which may be the presenting symptoms of an occult tumor. Although musculoskeletal symptoms often result from direct invasion by the malignancy or its metastases into bone, joints, or soft tissue, they may also occur without invasion as a result of the paraneoplastic disorders, including well-recognized syndromes as well as less well-defined disorders referred to as *cancer arthritis*.[89]

Neurologic complications are common in cancer. The most frequent neurologic problems are caused directly by three phenomena: (1) tumor metastases to the brain; (2) endocrine, fluid, and electrolyte abnormalities; and (3) paraneoplastic syndromes. The focus in this chapter is on the musculoskeletal and neurologic manifestations of malignancy caused by paraneoplastic syndromes. See Chapter 4 for a discussion of fluid and electrolyte imbalances and Chapter 29 for a discussion of CNS neoplasms.

Incidence and Etiology. Previously, these syndromes occurred in 10% to 20% of all cancer clients. Paraneoplastic nervous system syndromes are now being identified with increasing frequency because of greater physician awareness and the availability of serodiagnostic tests for some syndromes.

The causes of these syndromes are not well understood, but four groups of mechanisms have been identified: (1) effects initiated by a variety of vasoactive tumor products, such as serotonin, histamine, catecholamines, prostaglandins, and vasoactive peptides, which usually occur in the small bowel and less commonly in the lung or stomach; (2) effects caused by the destruction of normal tissues by tumor, such as occurs when osteolytic skeletal metastases cause hypercalcemia; (3) effects caused by unknown mechanisms, such as unidentified tumor products or circulating immune complexes stimulated by the tumor (e.g., osteoarthropathy as a result of bronchogenic carcinoma); and (4) effects caused by autoantibodies (antibodies directed against the host's tissue).

The neurologic syndromes are generally produced by cancer stimulation of antibody production. Cancer cells produce antibodies that impair presynaptic calcium channel activity hindering the release of the neurotransmitter acetylcholine, resulting in muscle weakness.

Clinical Manifestations. The paraneoplastic syndromes are of considerable clinical importance because they may accompany relatively limited neoplastic growth and provide an early clue to the presence of certain types of cancer. Nonspecific symptoms, such as neurologic changes, anorexia, malaise, diarrhea, weight loss, and fever, may be the first clinical manifestations of a paraneoplastic syndrome. Even these types of nonspecific symptoms occur as a result of the production of specific biochemical products by the tumor itself.

Paraneoplastic syndromes with musculoskeletal manifestations are listed in Table 8-4. Gradual, progressive muscle weakness may develop over a period of weeks to months. The proximal muscles (especially of the pelvic girdle) are most likely to be involved; the weakness does stabilize. Reflexes of the involved extremities are present but diminished. Proximal leg weakness (Eaton-Lambert myasthenic syndrome) is associated with small cell carcinoma of the lung.

Muscular and cutaneous disorders associated with malignancy are presented in Table 8-5. Myositis may precede, follow, or arise concurrently with the malignancy and tends to occur most often in older people. Cutaneous paraneoplastic syndromes are a large group of dermatoses that may be associated with an internal malignancy.

There may be rheumatologic symptoms referred to as *carcinoma polyarthritis*. This condition can be differentiated from rheumatoid arthritis by the presence of asymmetric joint involvement, involvement of primarily the lower extremity (although symmetric involvement of the hands has been reported),[89] explosive onset, late age of onset, and the presence of malignancy and arthritis together.

Neurologic paraneoplastic syndromes are of unknown cause and include subacute cerebellar degeneration, amyotrophic lateral sclerosis, sensory or sensorimotor peripheral neuropathy, Guillain-Barré syndrome, dermatomyositis, polymyositis, myasthenia gravis, and the Lambert-Eaton myasthenic syndrome (LEMS).

Medical Management
Diagnosis, Treatment, and Prognosis. Serodiagnostic tests are available for some paraneoplastic syndromes, and characteristic abnormalities in magnetic resonance imaging (MRI) have been identified in association with neurologic paraneoplastic syndromes. Biochemical markers in urine provide specific monitoring of the response of bone metastases to treatment. This early diagnosis of paraneoplastic syndromes provides for prevention of tumor progression and subsequent problems, such as bone pain, fracture, and hypercalcemia. In the case of cancer polyarthritis, the absence of rheumatoid nodules, absence of rheumatoid factor, and absence of family history of rheumatoid disease help in the diagnostic process.

Interestingly, paraneoplastic syndromes do not necessarily parallel the course of the disease but can be more related to

---

TABLE 8-4

Paraneoplastic Syndromes: Rheumatologic Associations and Clinical Features

MALIGNANCY	RHEUMATOLOGIC ASSOCIATIONS	CLINICAL FEATURES
Lung cancer	Myasthenic syndrome	Proximal leg weakness
Lymphoproliferative disease (leukemia)	Vasculitis	Necrotizing vasculitis
Plasma cell dyscrasia	Cryoglobulinemia	Vasculitis, Raynaud's disease, arthralgia, neurologic symptoms
Hodgkin's disease	Immune complex disease	Nephrotic syndrome
Ovarian cancer	Complex regional pain syndrome	Palmar fasciitis and polyarthritis
Carcinoid syndrome	Scleroderma	Scleroderma-like changes: anterior tibia
Colon cancer	Pyogenic arthritis	Enteric bacteria cultured from joint
Mesenchymal tumors	Osteogenic osteomalacia	Bone pain, stress fractures
Renal cell cancer (and other tumors)	Severe Raynaud's phenomenon	Digital necrosis
Pancreatic cancer	Panniculitis	Subcutaneous nodules, especially males
Lung cancer, small cell		Eaton-Lambert syndrome

TABLE	8-5

Muscular and Cutaneous Disorders Associated with Malignancy

MUSCULAR	CUTANEOUS
Amyloidosis	Acanthosis (diffuse thickening)
Amyotrophic lateral sclerosis	Dermatomyositis
Polymyositis	Extramammary Paget's disease
Lambert-Eaton myasthenic syndrome (LEMS)	Nigricans (blackish discoloration; changes in skin pigmentation)
Myasthenia gravis	Pemphigus vulgaris (water blisters)
Metabolic myopathies	Pruritus (itching)
Primary neuropathic diseases	Pyoderma gangrenosum (eruption of skin ulcers)
Type II muscle atrophy	Reactive erythemas (skin redness)

Data from Gilkeson GS, Caldwell DS: Rheumatologic associations with malignancy, *J Musculoskel Med* 7(1):70, 1990; Cohen PR: Cutaneous paraneoplastic syndromes, *Am Fam Physician* 50:1273-1282, 1994.

the amount of antibody present rather than the amount of tumor volume. Some of the cutaneous paraneoplastic syndromes will respond to specific measures, such as systemic corticosteroid therapy, but for the most part, successful resolution requires eradication of the underlying malignancy.

MEDICAL MANAGEMENT OF CANCER

◆ Prevention

The goal of *Healthy People 2010* is to reduce the number of new cancer cases as well as the illness, disability, and death caused by cancer. Evidence suggests that several types of cancer can be prevented and that the prospects for surviving cancer continue to improve. The ability to reduce cancer death rates depends, in part, on the existence and application of various types of resources. First, the means to provide culturally and linguistically appropriate information on prevention, early detection, and treatment to the public and to health care professionals are essential. Second, mechanisms or systems must exist for providing people with access to state-of-the-art preventive services and treatment. Third, a mechanism for maintaining continued research progress and for fostering new research is essential. Genetic information that can be used to improve disease prevention strategies is emerging for many cancers and may provide the foundation for improved effectiveness in clinical and preventive medicine services.[39]

Primary Prevention.   Prevention is the first key to the management of cancer. Primary prevention may include *screening* to identify high-risk people and subsequent *reduction or elimination of modifiable risk factors* (e.g., tobacco use, diet high in unsaturated fats and low in fiber). Physical activity and weight control also can contribute to cancer prevention.

Chemoprevention, the use of agents to inhibit and reverse cancer, has focused on diet-derived agents. More than 40 promising agents and agent combinations (e.g., green and black tea phenols, lycopene, soy isoflavones, vitamins D and E, selenium, calcium) are being evaluated clinically as chemopreventive agents for major cancer targets, including breast, prostate, colon, and lung cancer.[47] In addition, low-dose aspirin intake and nonsteroidal antiinflammatory drug (NSAID) intake have shown promising results in the prevention of gastrointestinal cancers.

Research focusing on a *cancer vaccine* to stimulate an immune response against cancer cells is being investigated in clinical studies although currently no known specific immunization prevents cancer in general. The most promising vaccines are for malignant melanoma and prostate cancer; vaccines for cancer viruses (human papillomavirus [HPV] associated with cervical cancer and hepatitis B virus [HBV] associated with liver cancer) are already in use.[30] The person's own tumor cells can be obtained during surgery, radiated to inactivate them, and then reinfused. This stimulates the immune system to react and make antibodies against these specific cells. The vaccine specifically evokes the activity of killer T cells to directly target and destroy tumors in all vaccine recipients. A vaccine given on an outpatient basis would be less dangerous than surgery and less toxic than other cancer treatments, such as chemotherapy and radiation therapy.

Secondary Prevention.   Secondary prevention aimed at preventing morbidity and mortality uses early detection[85] and prompt treatment (Table 8-6). Some drugs, such as tamoxifen (Nolvadex), are used in both primary and secondary prevention of breast cancer. Tamoxifen has been approved by the FDA as a preventive agent in women who have a high risk for possible development of breast cancer.[97] The preliminary results of a randomized trial comparing tamoxifen to a placebo in women considered at high risk for breast cancer suggested that the risk of breast cancer in this group of high-risk women could be decreased by approximately 50% with the administration of tamoxifen.[63] Multifactor risk reduction is an important part of secondary prevention for people diagnosed with cancer at risk for recurrence. This is especially true because the adverse effect of several risk factors is cumulative and many risk factors are interrelated.

Tertiary Prevention.   Tertiary prevention focuses on managing symptoms, limiting complications, and preventing disability associated with cancer or its treatment.

◆ Diagnosis

Medical history and physical examination are usually followed by more specific diagnostic procedures. Useful tests for the early detection and staging of tumors include radiography, endoscopy, isotope scan, CT scan, mammography, MRI, and

TABLE   8-6

Early Detection of Cancer

These are guidelines for the early detection of cancer in people without symptoms. Some people have a higher risk for certain cancers and may need to have tests more often, start tests at a younger age, or have additional tests.

Cancer-related checkups are recommended every 3 yr for people ages 20-39 yr and every year for people 40 yr and older. This examination should include health counseling (e.g., smoking cessation, diet and nutrition) and examinations for cancers of the thyroid, mouth, skin, and lymph nodes in both men and women. An examination of the testicles for men and of the ovaries and uterus for women is recommended.

For Women

Breast

Women age 40 yr and older should have an annual mammogram and an annual clinical breast exam by their health care professional and should do monthly breast self-examination. Ideally the clinical breast exam should be scheduled near to the time of and before the mammogram. Women ages 20-39 yr should have a clinical breast exam every 3 years and should do monthly self-breast examination.

Uterus

Cervix

All women who are or have been sexually active or are 18 yr or older should have an annual Pap test and pelvic exam. After three tests in a row with normal results, the Pap test may be done less often.

Endometrium

Women with or at high risk for hereditary nonpolyposis colon cancer (a genetic condition leading to an increased risk of colon cancer and endometrial cancer) should be offered an endometrial biopsy annually, starting at age 35 yr.

For Men

Prostate

Starting at age 50 yr, men should have the prostate antigen (PSA) blood test and a digital rectal exam. Those men at higher risk for prostate cancer (African-American or father/brother diagnosed with prostate cancer at a young age) should begin having these tests at age 45 yr.

Women and Men

Colon and Rectum

Men and women who are age 50 yr and older may have one of the exams listed below (depending on their health professional's advice):

- Fecal occult blood test (FOBT) every year and flexible sigmoidoscopy every 5 yr (the ACS prefers this option to having either FOBT or flexible sigmoidoscopy alone), or
- Flexible sigmoidoscopy every 5 yr, or
- Fecal occult blood test every year, or
- Colonoscopy every 10 yr, or
- Double-contrast barium enema every 5 yr

The complete ACS guidelines for early detection of cancer are available.[85] The cancers that can be found by these tests and exams account for about half of all cancer cases in the U.S. The overall 5-yr survival rate for people with these cancers is about 81% but is much worse for those individuals whose cancer is diagnosed after symptoms develop. If all these cancers were diagnosed at a localized stage through the use of early detection tests according to ACS guidelines, the 5-yr survival rate would improve to about 96%.

From American Cancer Society (ACS), Atlanta, 2001. This table can be copied and given to the public per ACS guidelines.

---

biopsy. Advances in nuclear medicine have made it possible to examine images of organs, structures, and physiologic or pathologic processes and detect the distribution of radiopharmaceuticals according to their uptake and metabolism.

Biopsy of tissue samples is the single most important diagnostic method for the study of tumors. Tissue for biopsy may be taken by curettage (Papanicolaou [Pap] smear), fluid aspiration (pleural effusion, lumbar puncture or spinal tap), needle aspiration (breast, thyroid), dermal punch (skin or mouth), endoscopy (rectal polyps), or surgical excision (visceral tumors and nodes).

Sentinel node biopsy has become a standard diagnostic procedure to assess lymph node status of various tumors (e.g., breast, melanoma, endometrial, valvular, head and neck) and to assess staging. A blue dye is injected around the cancerous tumor (or the biopsy site if the tumor has been removed). The dye flows through the ducts, and the first node or nodes it reaches is identified as the sentinel or sentinels. An incision is made over the nodes and the blue-stained sentinel node or

nodes are removed and analyzed. Information on the lymphatic drainage from the cancer can have a direct impact on surgery. Sentinel node biopsy has reduced the number of unnecessary axillary dissections in breast cancer. The status of axillary nodes is the most important prognostic factor in breast cancer and in determining the medical management.

Tumor markers, substances produced and secreted by tumor cells, may be found in the blood serum. The level of tumor marker seems to correlate with the extent of disease. A tumor marker is not diagnostic itself but can signal malignancies. Carcinoembryonic antigen (CEA) is one tumor marker that may indicate malignancy of the large bowel, stomach, pancreas, lungs, and breasts. CEA and other serum titers, such as CA-125 (ovarian), CA-27-29 (breast), and PSA (prostate), may be valuable during chemotherapy to evaluate the extent of response and detect tumor recurrence.

Other tumor markers found in the blood (no more specific than CEA) include alpha-fetoprotein (AFP), a fetal antigen uncommon in adults and suggestive of testicular cancer. The beta-2 (β_2) microglobin is used in the monitoring of lymphomas, and lactic dehydrogenase (LDH) is particularly elevated in fast-growing malignancies. Human chorionic gonadotropin (b subunit) may indicate testicular cancer or choriocarcinoma. Prostate-specific antigen (PSA) helps evaluate prostatic cancer. Because of the lack of specificity of the markers individually (except PSA), test panels are used more frequently rather than just individual tumor marker evaluations.[70]

Several research institutes have developed a monoclonal antibody that identifies breast cancer and other cancer cells. The monoclonal antibody is used to devise a simple blood test for use in diagnosis and monitoring treatment of breast and ovarian cancers and will be used in the future to diagnose colon cancer. Combining the breast cancer antibody with nuclear medicine scanning techniques will provide a noninvasive means of determining lymphatic spread and guide surgeons in determining the extent of surgery required.[8]

◆ Treatment

Changes in the health care system have shifted much of cancer care to the ambulatory and home settings. The medical management of cancer may be curative (i.e., with the intent to cure) or palliative (i.e., provides symptomatic relief but does not cure). Major therapies that are the focus of curative cancer treatment at this time include surgery, radiation, chemotherapy, biotherapy (also called immunotherapy or molecularly based therapy), angiogenesis therapy, and hormonal therapy. Complementary and alternative methods in the cure and palliation of cancer (sometimes designed for use with conventional medicine, sometimes used in place of standard medical therapy) have received consumer attention and concern on the part of those who provide conventional or standard medical therapy. The ACS has published a guide to help consumers make these kinds of treatment decisions.[3] Major research institutions and universities are beginning to investigate the effectiveness of these types of interventions for cancer.

Palliative treatment may include radiation, chemotherapy, physical therapy (e.g., physical agents, exercise, positioning, relaxation techniques, biofeedback, manual therapy), medications, acupuncture, chiropractic care, alternative medicine (e.g., homeopathic and naturopathic treatment), and hospice care. The palliative treatment of nausea, vomiting, and retching (NVR) may incorporate both pharmacologic and nonpharmacologic approaches with the overall goal of improving and/or maintaining the person's quality of life.[74] In the case of hospice care, attempts are made to help the person achieve as full a life as possible, with minimal pain, discomfort, and restriction. Many medications, especially morphine, are used for pain control. Emphasis of hospice care is toward emotional and psychologic support for the client and the family, focusing on death as a natural end to life.

Major Treatment Modalities.   Each of the five curative therapies mentioned earlier may be used alone or in combination, depending on the type, stage, localization, and responsiveness of the tumor and on limitations imposed by the person's clinical status. *Surgery,* once a mainstay of cancer treatment, is now used most often in combination with other therapies. Surgery may be used curatively, for tumor biopsy and tumor removal, or palliatively to relieve pain, correct obstruction, or alleviate pressure. Surgery can be curative in persons with localized cancer, but 70% of clients have evidence of micrometastases at the time of diagnosis, requiring surgery in combination with other treatment modalities to achieve better response rates. Adjuvant therapy used following surgery eradicates any residual cells.

Radiation therapy is used to destroy the dividing cancer cells by destroying hydrogen bonds between DNA strands within the cancer cells, while damaging resting normal cells as little as possible. Radiation consists of two types: ionizing radiation and particle radiation. Both types have the cellular DNA as their target; however, particle radiation produces less skin damage. Radiation treatment approaches include external beam radiation and intracavitary and interstitial implants. Radiation may be used preoperatively to shrink a tumor, making it operable while preventing further spread of the disease during surgery. After the surgical wound heals, postoperative doses prevent residual cancer cells from multiplying or metastasizing.

Radiation therapy may be delivered externally or internally depending on the type and extent of the tumor by (1) external beam (teletherapy), (2) sealed source (brachytherapy), and (3) unsealed source (systemic therapy). When the distance between the radiation source and the target is short, the term *brachytherapy* is used. Brachytherapy allows for a rapid falloff in dose away from the target volume. When the radiation source is at a distance from the target, the term *teletherapy* is used. Teletherapy allows for a more uniform dose across the target volume.

X-rays, radioactive elements, and radioactive isotopes are most often used. Isotopes implanted in the tumor or a body cavity by external beam sources are delivered in the form of electromagnetic waves (e.g., x-rays or gamma rays) or as streams of particles (e.g., electrons). X-rays generated by linear accelerators and gamma rays generated by radioactive isotopes (e.g., cobalt-60, radium-226, cesium-137) are referred to as sealed source radiation therapies or brachytherapy. This form of radiation is used for the treatment of visceral tumors, because they penetrate to great depths before reaching full intensity and thereby spare the skin from toxic effects. Strontium and yttrium aluminum garnet (YAG) lasers have been administered for the palliation of bone pain related to metastatic bone disease in both prostate and breast cancer.[49,88] Electron beam irradiation is most useful in the treatment of superficial tumors, since energy is deposited at the skin and quickly dissipates, sparing the deeper tissues from toxic effects.

Normal and malignant cells respond to radiation differently, depending on blood supply, oxygen saturation, previous irradiation, and immune status. Generally, normal cells recover from radiation faster than malignant cells. The success of the treatment and damage to normal tissue also vary with the intensity of the radiation. Although a large single dose of radiation has greater cellular effects than fractions of the same amount delivered sequentially, a protracted schedule allows time for normal tissue to recover in the intervals between individual sublethal doses.

Chemotherapy includes a wide array of chemical agents to destroy cancer cells. It is particularly useful in the treatment of widespread or metastatic disease, whereas radiation is more useful for treatment of localized lesions. Chemotherapy is used in eradicating residual disease as well as inducing long remissions and cures, especially in children with childhood leukemia and adults with Hodgkin's disease or testicular cancer. Several major chemotherapeutic agents are listed in Table 8-7.

TABLE   8-7

Major Chemotherapeutic Agents

AGENT	ACTION
Alkylating agents (e.g., Cytoxan)	Inhibit cell growth and division by reacting with DNA
Nitrosourea (e.g., BCNU)	Inhibits cell growth and division by reacting with DNA
Antimetabolites (e.g., methotrexate)	Prevent cell growth by competing with metabolites in production of nucleic acid
Antitumor antibiotics (e.g., Adriamycin)	Inhibit cell growth by binding with DNA and interfering with DNA-dependent RNA synthesis
Plant alkaloids (e.g., vincristine)	Prevent cellular reproduction by disrupting cell mitosis
Steroid hormones (e.g., tamoxifen)	Block the growth of hormone-susceptible tumors by changing their chemical environment

Chemotherapeutic drugs can be given orally, subcutaneously, intramuscularly (IM), intravenously (IV), intracavitarily (into a body cavity such as the thoracic, abdominal, or pelvic cavity), intrathecally (through the sheath of a structure, such as through the sheath of the spinal cord into the subarachnoid space), and by arterial infusion, depending on the drug and its pharmacologic action and on tumor location. Administration in any form is usually intermittent to allow for bone marrow recovery between doses.

Biotherapy, formerly called immunotherapy, relies on biologic response modifiers (BRMs) to change or modify the relationship between the tumor and host by strengthening the host's biologic response to tumor cells. Much of the work related to BRMs is still experimental so the availability of this type of treatment varies regionally within the United States. The most widely used agents include interferons,* which have a direct antitumor effect, and interleukin-2, one type of cytokine, a protein released by macrophages to trigger the immune response (see Chapter 5).[41]

Other forms of biotherapy include bone marrow or stem cell transplantation, monoclonal antibodies, colony-stimulating factors, and hormonal therapy. Bone marrow transplantation (BMT) or peripheral stem cell transplantation (PSCT) is used for cancers that are responsive to high doses of chemotherapy or radiation. These high doses kill cancer cells but are also toxic to bone marrow; BMT provides a method for rescuing people from bone marrow destruction while allowing higher doses of chemotherapy for a better antitumor result.

BMT was a technique developed to restore the marrow to people who had lethal injury to that site because of bone marrow failure, destruction of bone marrow by disease, or intensive chemical or radiation exposure. At first, the source of the transplant was the marrow cells of a healthy donor who had the same tissue type (human leukocyte antigen [HLA]; mark-

ers on the white blood cells) as the recipient (usually a sibling or close family relative). Now donor programs have been established to identify unrelated donors who have a matching HLA. The transplant product is a very small fraction of the marrow cells called *stem cells.* These cells occur in the bone marrow and also circulate in the blood and can be harvested from the blood of a donor by treating the donor with an agent or agents (e.g., granulocyte colony-stimulating factor [G-CSF]) that cause a release of larger numbers of stem cells into the blood and collecting them by hemapheresis. Since blood (peripheral site) as well as marrow is a good source of cells for transplantation, the term *stem cell transplantation* has replaced the general term for these procedures (see the section on Bone Marrow Transplantation in Chapter 20).

Monoclonal antibodies (MAbs) are laboratory-engineered copies of proteins produced from a single clone (monoclonal) of B-lymphocytes that can stimulate the immune system to attack cancer cells. These antibodies can be used alone to produce a massive amount of one specific antibody or bound with radioisotopes and injected into the body to detect cancer by attaching to tumor cells.

Research is under way to find a way to use these antibodies as a means of destroying specific cancer cells without disturbing healthy cells. Rituximab (Rituxan) and trastuzumab (Herceptin) are monoclonal antibodies currently in use for cancer treatment. Rituximab is used primarily in the treatment of non-Hodgkin's lymphoma. Rituximab binds to lymphoid cells in the thymus, spleen, lymph nodes, and peripheral blood in order to lyse and destroy specific immune target cells. Trastuzumab is used in the treatment of metastatic breast cancer in women who have overexpression of the human epidermal growth factor receptor 2 (HER-2) protein. It binds with this protein and both inhibits proliferation of cells with this protein and also mediates an antibody-mediated destruction of the cancer cells that have the HER-2 receptor overexpression.[31] Both agents are usually used in combination with or in addition to other chemotherapeutic agents for treatment.

Colony-stimulating factors (CSFs) may be used to support the person with low blood counts related to chemotherapy. CSFs function primarily as hematopoietic growth factors, guiding the division and differentiation of bone marrow stem cells. They also influence the functioning of mature lymphocytes, monocytes, macrophages, and neutrophils. Currently, erythropoietin (EPO), human granulocyte colony-stimulating factor (G-CSF), granulocyte macrophage colony-stimulating factor (GM-CSF), and thrombopoietin (opreleukin) and various interleukins* are being used for chemotherapy-induced pancytopenia (deficiency of all cellular components of blood). EPO is used to treat anemia by stimulating bone marrow production of red blood cells. Both G-CSF and GM-CSF are very useful in protecting individuals from prolonged neutrophil nadirs (lowest points after neutrophil count has been depressed by chemotherapy). Thrombopoietin (opreleukin) has been recently identified and has shown promise in promoting elevation in platelet counts.[77] In addition, GM-CSF has shown significant antitumor effects that prolong survival and disease-free survival in adults with stage

---

*In addition to their desired immune effects, interferons cause a number of significant toxicities, including constitutional, hematologic, hepatic, and prominent effects on the nervous system, especially depression.

Interleukins are a large group of cytokines sometimes called *lymphokines* when produced by the T-lymphocytes or *monokines* when produced by mononuclear phagocytes. Interleukins have a variety of effects, but most interleukins direct other cells to divide and differentiate.

III and IV melanoma who are at high risk for recurrence after surgical resection.[87]

Antiangiogenic therapy shows promise as a strategy for cancer treatment. Thalidomide, a drug that has been used in the past as a sedative, has strong antiangiogenic properties. Although its mechanism of action is still unclear, thalidomide has been used successfully as a treatment for some people with multiple myeloma, and it continues to be carefully studied regarding its role in the suppression of blood supply formation in other types of cancers.[73,90] A very active area of experimental cancer therapy involves the study of other antiangiogenesis factors, such as angiostatin and endostatin. These substances have shown dramatic inhibition of primary tumor growth in animals. Treatment with antiangiogenesis factors focuses on blocking the general process of tumor growth rather than on the destruction of an already formed cancerous mass.[75]

Hormonal therapy is used for certain types of cancer that have been shown to be affected by specific hormones. For example, the luteinizing-releasing hormone leuprolide is now used to treat prostate cancer. With long-term use, this hormone inhibits testosterone release and tumor growth. Goserelin acetate (Zoladex) is a newer hormone used in prostate cancer that is a synthetic form of leuteinizing hormone-releasing hormone. Goserelin acetate inhibits pituitary gonadotropic secretion, thus decreasing serum testosterone levels.[97] Tamoxifen, an antiestrogen hormonal agent, is used in breast cancer to block estrogen receptors in breast tumor cells that require estrogen to thrive.

Pain Control.   Pain management and control may depend on the cause of the pain syndrome (see the section on Cancer Pain in this chapter). Treatment approaches may include narcotic* and nonnarcotic analgesics; chemotherapy or radiation therapy or both; surgery; nerve blocks; or other more invasive pain control measures, such as intraspinal opioids, rhizotomy, or cordotomy. Newer drugs, such as the bisphosphonates (e.g., pamidronate), have been useful in the treatment of refractory bone pain.[18]

In 1994 the U.S. Department of Health and Human Services released a clinical practice guideline for clinicians advising medical professionals on the treatment of cancer pain.[2] The National Comprehensive Cancer Network (NCCN) has also published the Cancer Pain Treatment Guideline, which outlines the process of screening, evaluation, and intervention.[61] Whereas severe cancer pain is treated pharmaceutically, mild to moderate joint and muscle pain can be addressed by the rehabilitation professional. Pain elimination through the use of medication may not be possible without accompanying severe loss of function, an undesirable outcome. Noninvasive physical agents, such as cryotherapy, thermotherapy, electrical stimulation, immobilization, exercise, massage, biofeedback, and relaxation techniques, may be effective in pain management.

People with cancer may also experience pain because of nerve damage. This damage can be caused directly by tumor invasion or indirectly as a side effect of cytotoxic drug therapy. The treatment of neuropathic pain remains a dilemma since conventional analgesic drugs do not always provide relief. Recommended treatment for this type of pain includes antidepressant drugs (e.g., amitriptyline); antiepileptics (e.g., carbamazepine, gabapentin); and steroids (e.g., methylprednisolone, dexamethasone). Pain relief is usually not immediate, and the drugs used must be taken continuously so side effects, such as sedation and bone marrow depression, can be additional problems.[18,42]

Management of pain in people with cancer who live in long-term care facilities remains an ongoing concern. Consistent, daily pain is prevalent among nursing home residents with cancer and is frequently untreated, particularly among older and minority clients.[13]

◆ Prognosis

Prognosis is influenced by the type of cancer, the stage and grade of disease at diagnosis, the availability of effective treatment, and the response to treatment. Cancer cells that develop resistance to anticancer drugs can regrow with fatal consequences. Researchers are close to understanding the mechanisms underlying chemotherapeutic failure and developing new strategies to circumvent drug resistance. Generally, the earlier cancers are found, the simpler treatment may be and the greater likelihood of a cure.

Cancer survival statistics are usually reported as 5-year survival rates. When adjusted for normal life expectancy (accounting for factors such as diabetes, heart disease, injuries, dying of old age) a relative 5-year survival rate of 60% is seen for cancer. This means that the chance of a person recently diagnosed with cancer being alive in 5 years is 60% of the chance of someone not diagnosed with cancer. The person who is alive and without evidence of disease for at least 5 years after diagnosis is considered cured.* Even without complete remission, cancer can be controlled to provide longer survival time and improved quality of life, but these factors are not reflected in survival rates. Cancer statistics reported usually include a lag time so that rates may not reflect the most recent treatment advances.

Survival rates for many cancers have increased from 1960 to the present, but not all cancers have been characterized by this increase. For example, while survival rates for Hodgkin's disease and prostate, testicular, and bladder cancers have increased by at least 25%, the survival rates for cancers of the oral cavity and pharynx, liver, pancreas, esophagus, and colon have decreased or increased less than 5% during the same period.

A significantly lower survival rate in black American men for most cancer classifications has been noted. This difference may be due to a variety of factors, including limited access to health care, little or no insurance, lack of a primary health care provider, limited knowledge of the benefits of early diagnosis and treatment, and greater exposure to carcinogens. Central to these social forces is access to health care, including prevention, information, early detection, and quality treatment.[98]

In terminally ill individuals, rates of change are more important indicators of survival than absolute measures. Using a modified Barthel index comprised of 10 activities of daily living, each with five levels of dependency (maximum score =

---

*A method of pain relief called *patient-controlled analgesia* (PCA) is now being used in many cancer care centers. This system permits the person to self-administer a premeasured dose of analgesic by pressing a button that activates a pump syringe containing the analgesic. Small intermittent doses of the analgesic administered IV maintain blood levels that ensure comfort and minimize the risk of oversedation. Clinical studies report that people using PCA effectively maintain comfort without oversedation and use less drug than the amount normally given by IM injection.

---

*The terms *survival* and *cure* do not always portray the functional status of a cancer survivor. Many people considered cured are left with physical limitations and movement dysfunctions that interfere with their daily lives.

100 points), can provide important predictions about length of time until death. Half of those individuals with advanced cancer who lose 10 or more points per week die within 2 weeks, and three-fourths are dead at 3 weeks. In contrast, 50% of all cases without declines in score survive for 2 months or more. This may be a useful tool for planning and end-of-life issues in a hospice setting.[12]

Special Implications for the Therapist   8-1

ONCOLOGY/CANCER

Preferred Practice Patterns
See individual cancer as discussed in each chapter. Practice patterns are determined by site-specific clinical manifestations and resulting level of disability and presence of functional limitations. Side effects of treatment may also determine appropriate practice patterns.

Cancer treatment and therapy have improved over the past 20 years, but cancer treatment often results in functional deficits caused by the removal of a diseased organ or segmental bone, joint, or limb amputation. Treatment can cause severe disfigurement and is the major cause of amputation in children. Site-specific cancer issues (e.g., cognitive impairment with brain tumors); postsurgical problems (e.g., limited motion, soreness, disuse, pain, fatigue, sensory loss, weakness, deep venous thrombosis and emboli, lymphedema, sleep disturbance); and side effects of radiotherapy, chemotherapy, and bone marrow or stem cell transplantation often require physical therapy intervention and education.[65,69]

Psychosocial-spiritual issues (e.g., loss, grief, anger) and client diversity (e.g., life span, socioeconomic class, ethnicity) require consideration in planning an effective therapeutic approach.[69] The psychosocial-spiritual status can be a driving factor in successful outcomes. Engaging the individual in honest discussion, listening to concerns or feelings, and sharing rehabilitation needs to set mutually achievable goals will enhance outcomes.[9]

Side Effects of Cancer Treatment
Table 8-8 compares the potential side effects associated with the major treatment modalities discussed in this section. See Chapter 4 for discussion of the effects of chemotherapy agents, radiation sickness, CNS effects of immunosuppression, and steroid-induced myopathy.

The risk of falling is one of the more serious sequelae of both the local effects of cancer and the systemic consequences of cancer treatment. (See the section on Adverse Drug Reactions: Radiation Injuries and Chemotherapy in Chapter 4.) Weakness, pain, fatigue, orthostatic hypotension, peripheral neuropathy, decreased bone density (osteoporosis), and diminished flexibility, in various combinations, may result in falls. Anyone with metastasized cancer to the spine or long bones may fracture these bones in a fall (or fall because of pathologic fractures), resulting in serious, long-term disability.

Fall prevention and education are important aspects of the rehabilitation or exercise program. In addition, the therapist must evaluate each client individually, possibly selecting an assistive device in appropriate cases. A walker with auto-stop wheels in the front may be a safer choice for some people than a standard walker that must be repeatedly lifted during ambulation. A wheelchair may be necessary for someone who experiences dizziness, weakness, fatigue, or signs of disorientation.

Recommended rehabilitation during medical intervention with consideration for the specific cancer treatment is available for physical therapists.[33,103]

Precautions
The therapist must practice Standard Precautions carefully (especially proper hand washing and infection control principles) to help the individual undergoing cancer treatment avoid infection. Closely monitoring blood counts (and other laboratory values) and vital signs and observing for signs of infection, bleeding, or arrhythmias are important. Radiated tissue must be treated with care to avoid local trauma, extreme temperatures must be avoided, management of lymphedema may be required, and specific guidelines for the use of physical agents must be followed.[69]

Many people are using complementary and alternative medications that can have an adverse effect when combined with radiation or chemotherapy. If the client perceives disapproval, this information may not be relayed to the appropriate health care professional. By being open and nonjudgmental and inviting more discussion about the use of these techniques, the therapist may be able to bring to light potential risks involved. The client should be advised that most herbal or natural supplements and complementary interventions are designed to support not replace traditional medical interventions that have been proven effective.

Physical Agents
Various forms of electric, electromagnetic, and other biophysical energy sources have been investigated in light of their potential to relieve some of the symptoms and side effects of cancer, as well as to slow, halt, or destroy tumors. The physical modalities have the capacity to break down cell membrane barriers and stimulate changes in transmembrane potentials, which can trigger growth and development of abnormal tissue.[22]

The use of physical agents in people who have cancer is summarized in Table 8-9. The reader is encouraged to consult the bibliography for references and more specific information about the use of thermal and mechanical agents with this population.[68] Heat modalities should not be used in people undergoing radiation because the thermal effect may enhance the effect of the radiation. Risk for modality use based on stage of medical management is listed in Table 8-10.

The application of therapeutic ultrasound over tumors is contraindicated (especially continuous ultrasound), presumably because it is believed that there is an increased risk of metastasis.[91] Studies conducted on mice have shown that a tumor given large doses of ultrasound will spread because of increasing blood supply to the area.[44,51,84] The concern that electrical and thermal modalities increase blood flow and possibly increase micrometastases in humans has not yet been proved in clinical studies.*

The clinical behavior of the majority of musculoskeletal tumors is such that the symptoms are shared with a wide range of nontumorous orthopedic disorders. Pain, swelling, and local heat accompanying musculoskeletal tumors are also common to inflammatory conditions. In addition, the most likely sites of musculoskeletal tumors are regions frequently involved in

Continued

---

*For a detailed explanation of the possible physiologic effects of therapeutic ultrasound on tumor angiogenesis, see reference 56. For further discussion of the electrical field around cells and how percutaneous application of biophysical modalities can change the electrical potential of tissues for cell division and growth, see reference 22.

sports injuries.[53] Occasionally the client does recall some sort of injury at the site of a previously unsuspected tumor, and this information further confuses the relationship between trauma and malignancy.[56]

As a general guideline, some therapists caution that people with cancer should not be treated with electrical or deep-heating thermal physical agents (ultrasound in particular), even at a site distant from the neoplasm, because the effect of ultrasound on micrometastases is not known. There may come a time in the client's situation (especially in the case of advanced-stage cancer or limited life expectancy) when palliation (e.g., especially pain control) is more important than the risks of metastasis with the use of some modalities. However, this must still be determined based on clinical presentation, potential risks, and benefits. For example, if a tumor is impinging or even wrapped around a nerve, ultrasound over the site may increase tumor growth, causing further nerve compression. Short-term pain relief using this modality may result in more pain even in the short term and would not be advised.[68]

Sexual Issues

Sexual dysfunction is a frequent side effect of cancer treatment, especially for those adults with cancer of the reproductive organs (e.g., breast, prostate, testicle, ovary, uterus) and after Hodgkin's disease. The most common problems include loss of desire for sexual activity, erectile dysfunction in men, and dyspareunia in women. Unlike many other physiologic side effects, sexual problems do not tend to resolve within the first year or two of disease-free survival but remain constant.[79]

Physical therapists are often in a unique position to assist people with sexual concerns because of their repeated close contact with the affected individual. Sexual function is an important aspect of quality of life and requires a brief assessment. In oncology settings, it is often helpful to designate and train a member of the team as the expert on sexuality issues.[79]

The therapist who is comfortable and knowledgeable in discussing sexual issues may be able to provide more focused assistance to the individual who is trying to adjust to changes in sexual style and practices as a result of the illness. Understanding the range of values and sexual history that clients bring to the clinical situation and respecting appropriate provider-client boundaries are important.[71] More specific information on this topic is readily available.[7,46,64,81]

Hospice Care

Physical therapy can enhance the quality of life of dying individuals receiving hospice care and the family and friends who care for them. Intervention is aimed at achieving symptom control, maximizing remaining functional abilities, providing caregiver education, and contributing to interdisciplinary team communication.[54]

Radiation Hazard for the Health Care Worker

Implant radiation therapy requires personal radiation protection for all staff members who come in contact with the client (see the section on Radiation Hazard for Health Care Professionals in Chapter 4). ■

Text continues on page 258

TABLE 8-8

Side Effects of Cancer Treatment

Surgery	Radiation (See Table 4-9)	Chemotherapy	Biotherapy	Hormonal Therapy
Fatigue	Fatigue	Fatigue	Fever	Hypertension
Disfigurement	Radiation sickness	Gastrointestinal effects	Chills	Steroid-induced
Loss of	Immunosuppression	Anorexia	Nausea	diabetes
function	Decreased platelets	Nausea	Vomiting	Myopathy
Infection	Decreased white blood	Vomiting	Anorexia	(steroid-
Increased pain	cells	Diarrhea	Fatigue	induced)
Deformity	Infection	Constipation	Fluid retention	Weight gain
Bleeding	Fatigue	Fluid/electrolyte imbalance from GI effects	CNS effects	Hot flashes
Scar tissue	Fibrosis	Hepatotoxicity	Slowed thinking	Impotence
Fibrosis	Burns	Hemorrhage	Memory	Decreased libido
	Mucositis	Bone marrow suppression	problems	Vaginal dryness
	Diarrhea	Anemia	Inflammatory	
	Edema	Leukopenia (infection)	reactions at	
	Hair loss	Thrombocytopenia	injection sites	
	Ulceration, delayed wound	Decreased bone density with ovarian failure[82]	Anemia	
	healing	Muscle weakness	Leukopenia	
	CNS/PNS effects	Skin rashes	Altered taste	
	Malignancy	Neuropathies	sensation	
		Hair loss		
		Sterilization		
		Stomatitis, mucositis (oral, rectal, vaginal)		
		Sexual dysfunction		

CNS, central nervous system; GI, gastrointestinal; PNS, peripheral nervous system.

TABLE 8-9

Common Physiologic Effects and Uses of Physical Agents and Modalities in People with Cancer

Superficial Heating Agents: Hot packs, paraffin baths, infrared lamps, fluidotherapy, local immersion

POTENTIAL BENEFITS	CONTRAINDICATIONS (DO NOT USE)	EFFECTIVENESS*
Increases blood flow to affected area Increases metabolism Reduces pain, muscle spasm, chronic inflammation Increases relaxation, increases ROM Provides mild heat (≤40° C) to trunk; vigorous heat (≥40° C) to extremities	Over dysvascular tissue (after radiation therapy) and with people who are insensate to temperature or pain in application area Over areas of bleeding or hemorrhage (i.e., if there has been long-term corticosteroid therapy or chemotherapy) Over an acute injury or inflammation Presence of thrombophlebitis Directly over a tumor Over open wounds (except whirlpool at warm temperature)	Heat and stretch may decrease pain and muscle spasm in abnormal tissue; modulates pain and facilitates relaxation (gating effect) Not effective with deep cancer pain or bone pain (NSAIDs used)

Deep Heating Agents: Diathermy, ultrasound, full-body immersion hydrotherapy

POTENTIAL BENEFITS	CONTRAINDICATIONS (DO NOT USE)	EFFECTIVENESS*
Increases extensibility of collagen tissue (scar tissue, tendons) (ultrasound) Reduces pain and muscle spasm Increases range of motion Alters threshold of nerve conduction Provides mild heat (≤40° C) to trunk; vigorous heat (≥40° C) to extremities Increases metabolism	Over growing epiphyses Over areas of acute hemorrhage (long-term use of corticosteroids or NSAIDs) Over acute injury of inflammation Over insensitive skin; dysvascular or irradiated skin Over tumors (unless trained in hyperthermia) Over implants (devices such as pacemakers or defibrillators, insulin pumps, morphine pumps, breast implants, plastic components, joint prosthetics—ultrasound over joint) Over reproductive organs; lumbosacral, pelvic, and lumbar regions if pregnant	Acute stage—there is a cancer treatment used for tumor hyperthermia to kill tumor tissue, administered at greater than therapeutic doses Advanced cancer/terminal stage—not indicated over tumor: this will increase tumor growth, often increasing the severity of symptoms such as pain

Cryotherapy: Cold packs, ice massage, cold hydrotherapy or baths, vapocoolant spray, cold compression

POTENTIAL BENEFITS FOR ACUTE MUSCULOSKELETAL TRAUMA	CONTRAINDICATIONS (DO NOT USE)	EFFECTIVENESS*
Reduces acute inflammation or inhibits edema, muscle spasm, spasticity (transient decrease of spasticity) Alters threshold of nerve conduction Decreases metabolism Decreases blood flow with later increase in blood flow	Over dysvascular tissue (after radiation therapy) and with people who are insensate to temperature or pain in application area When transient increase of blood pressure might be dangerous (monitor anyone with hypertension) When wound healing is delayed If nerve injury has occurred (applies especially to irradiation- or chemotherapy-induced nerve injury) If Raynaud's disease or peripheral vascular disease is present (exacerbated by chemotherapy)	Acute stage or advanced cancer—tumor treatment: supercooled at below therapeutic temperatures for local, superficial tumor destruction (e.g., liquid nitrogen for precancerous skin lesions) Immediate postchemotherapy cancer treatment—cold packs (cold cap) to head are suggested to reduce hair loss Chronic stage and cured or in remission—used for usual indications for cold therapy Occasionally selected by clients for pain relief; must be monitored by health or personal caregiver Treatment of pain in advanced cancer—not as acceptable to some for comfort care

Continued

TABLE	8-9—cont'd

Common Physiologic Effects and Uses of Physical Agents and Modalities in People with Cancer

Mechanical Agents

Traction (sustained or intermittent, mechanical or manual, spinal or peripheral)

POTENTIAL BENEFITS	CONTRAINDICATIONS (DO NOT USE)	EFFECTIVENESS*
Improves motion and mobility in clients with degenerative joint disease, joint hypomobility, or herniated disks	Structural disease (tumor, infection) Acute injury Positive vertebral artery test Positive alar ligament test	Effective when there has not been previous spinal surgery or previous radiation therapy to spine

External Compression (Mechanical or manual—Jobst pump, Lymphopress, Wright linear pump, garments, bandages)

POTENTIAL BENEFITS	CONTRAINDICATIONS (DO NOT USE)	EFFECTIVENESS*
Reduces edema or lymphedema and pain secondary to edema or lymphedema; improves ROM problems related to edema	Difficulty tolerating treatment (impaired circulation) Phlebitis, DVT, thrombosis in area to be compressed Compression setting should not be greater than 45 mm Hg (see Chapter 12)	Acute stage—may not be indicated. Immediate postcancer treatment, advanced or terminal stage, chronic stage or cured—not indicated for lymphedema management unless cleared of cancer metastasis or recurrence or new cancer in region(s) to be treated

Hydrotherapy with Agitation (Agitation and local immersion hydrotherapy)

POTENTIAL BENEFITS	CONTRAINDICATIONS (DO NOT USE)	EFFECTIVENESS*
Depending on temperature, same as for superficial heat and/or cold in region to be immersed Wound healing—stimulates circulation to promote healing; removes exudates and necrotic tissue Facilitates exercise Relaxation; pain control	Depending on water temperature, same as for superficial heat and/or cold in region to be immersed Agitation should be minimized with painful open lesions, severely traumatized tissue, or recent skin grafts Risk of cross infection must be controlled, especially for immunocompromised clients	Same as for superficial heat in region to be immersed

Electrical Stimulation

Neuromuscular electrical nerve stimulation (and FES)

POTENTIAL BENEFITS	CONTRAINDICATIONS (DO NOT USE)	EFFECTIVENESS*
Reduces or eliminates muscle spasm Minimizes disuse atrophy Strengthens weak but innervated muscle Increases circulation secondary to muscle pump Functions as a substitute orthotic	If there is a potential for pathologic fracture in the area Any type of implanted devices (see above list) Severe cardiopulmonary insufficiency Active phlebitis, DVT, thrombosis in area to be treated	Would healing—high-volt pulsed current (HVPC) low-intensity direct (LIDC) (microcurrent) Strengthening Increased endurance

TABLE	8-9—cont'd

Common Physiologic Effects and Uses of Physical Agents and Modalities in People with Cancer

TENS and Electrical Stimulation at Acupuncture Points

POTENTIAL BENEFITS	CONTRAINDICATIONS (DO NOT USE)	EFFECTIVENESS*

Partial or complete alleviation of pain
  Acute pain
  Postoperative incisional pain
  Chronic pain
  Phantom pain
  Peripheral neuropathy pain
  Post-herpetic neuralgia
  Advanced malignancy (but not
    over tumor)
	Any type of implanted electronic device (pacemaker, insulin
	  pump, morphine pump, defibrillator)
	Not useful in control of generalized pain or deep bone pain
	Occasional allergic reactions to gel or adhesive
	Decreased effectiveness over time
		Advantages over narcotic anal-
		  gesics—few side effects, rela-
		  tively inexpensive and easy
		  to use
		Allows interpersonal interaction
		  and is controlled by the client
		During treatment (chemother-
		  apy)—effective as an
		  antiemetic for nausea and
		  vomiting
		Immediately after treatment—
		  postoperative pain and chronic
		  pain control for 2-4 mo

Courtesy Lucinda Pfalzer, P.T., Ph.D., University of Michigan, 2001. Used with permission.
ROM, Range of motion; *NSAID,* nonsteroidal antiinflammatory drug; *DVT,* deep vein thrombosis; *FES,* functional electrical stimulatin; *TENS,* transcutaneous electrical nerve stimulation.
*Safe if cleared for possible cancer recurrence, metastasis, or new cancer in area or areas to be treated and if the sensation and circulation in the area or areas to be treated are not impaired.

TABLE	8-10

Risks for Modality Use Based on Stage of Medical Management

Acute Stage
Medical diagnosis and treatment for new or newly recurrent cancer
Potential for disseminated cancer until the medical diagnostic
  process is completed (except cases of local cancer)
Stage I cancer: local disease, usually receives a local treatment
  (e.g., surgery and/or radiation therapy)
Stage II cancer: option of local treatment (surgery and radiation
  therapy) without systemic therapy (e.g., chemotherapy); higher
  risk of metastases or recurrence
Stage III cancer: systemic therapy, often chemotherapy; the process
  of micrometastases is unlikely in someone responding to
  chemotherapy
Risk: high risk; thermal agents should not be used during or in
  close time proximity to radiation or chemotherapy; general con-
  traindications/precaustions apply (e.g., insensate or dysvascular
  tissue with decreased sensation or decreased blood flow)

Subacute Stage
Immediately after cancer treatment; may extend 6-12 mo depending on treatment intervention (e.g., surgery, chemotherapy,
  radiation); hormone therapy (e.g., tamoxifen for breast cancer)
  continues for 5 yr
Acute side effects or toxicities from treatment (e.g., radiation or
  chemotherapy) begin to subside
Risk: high risk; thermal agents should not be used during or in
  close time proximity to radiation or chemotherapy; general
  contraindicatins/precautions apply (e.g., insensate or dysvascular tissue with decreased sensation or decreased blood flow)

Continued

TABLE   8-10—cont'd

Risks for Modality Use Based on Stage of Medical Management—cont'd

Chronic Stage

Remission or recurrence may occur from 6-12 mo up to 5 yr after cancer treatment

Risk of recurrence decreases over time so that the likelihood of recurrence diminishes the farther the client is from the time of diagnosis and treatment

Risk: Stage I*—no restrictions on use of physical agents or modalities in the absence of clinical signs or symptoms of potential recurrence or new cancer; client has had recent medical checkup including testing for cancer (e.g., bone scan, serum markers) that is negative; general contraindications/precautions apply (e.g., insensate or dysvascular tissue with decreased sensation or decreased blood flow)

Stage II*—moderate-to-low-risk group; same restrictions as stage I

Stage III*—moderate risk group; same restrictions as stage I

Stage IV* (advanced)—high-risk group; caution should be taken over any painful area or mass; thermal agents should not be used during or in close proximity to radiation or chemotherapy; general contraindications/precautions apply

Statistically Cured Stage

Remission more than 5 yr after cancer treatment

Statistical risk of recurrence is minimal

Return to lifetime risk of cancer as an individual statistical measure

Risk: low-risk group; no restrictions on use of physical agents or modalities in the absence of clinical signs or symptoms of potential recurrence or new cancer; general contraindications/precautions apply

Courtesy Lucinda Pfalzer, P.T., Ph.D., University of Michigan, 2001. Used with permission.
*At the time of diagnosis.

CANCER, PHYSICAL ACTIVITY, AND EXERCISE TRAINING

◆ Exercise as a Cancer Prevention Strategy

Physical activity is defined as body movement caused by skeletal muscle contraction that results in quantifiable energy expenditure. Both epidemiologic and laboratory data indicate that the level of physical activity in which an individual engages may affect cancer risk. Exercise is distinguished from other types of physical activity by the fact that the intensity, duration, and frequency of the activity are specifically designed to improve physical fitness.

Based on available data, a role for exercise in specifically reducing cancer risk has been conjectured and is referred to as the exercise-cancer hypothesis. Despite the problems of interpreting epidemiologic studies and the difficulty in developing appropriate animal models, there is growing evidence that moderate habitual physical activity can protect against certain types of neoplasm, particularly tumors of the colon and the female reproductive tract.[83]

Exercise programs also appear to have a beneficial influence on the clinical course, at least in the early stages of the disease. At the present time, cytokine modulation with exercise is getting most of the research attention. Recent demonstration of exercise-induced changes in the activity of macrophages, natural killer cells, lymphokine-activated killer cells, neutrophils, and regulating cytokines suggests that immunomodulation may contribute to the protective value of exercise (see also the section on Exercise, Physical Activity, and the Immune System in Chapter 6).[58,101]

◆ Exercise for the Person with Cancer

With almost 8 million Americans alive today who have been through the cancer experience, it is important to develop interventions to enhance immune function, prevent or minimize muscle wasting thus counteracting the detrimental physiologic effects of cancer and chemotherapy, and maintain

quality of life (QOL) following cancer diagnosis. Physical activity and exercise training are interventions that address a broad range of QOL issues, including physical (e.g., muscular strength, body composition, nausea, fatigue), functional (e.g., functional capacity), psychologic (e.g., coping, mood changes), spiritual, emotional, and social well-being.[21]

Screening and Assessment.   Medical screening should be conducted with all clients before their participation in an exercise program.[1] This type of screening is especially important for people with cancer who receive various levels of treatment that can affect the physiologic response to exercise. For example, fatigue is a common symptom of nearly every form of cancer treatment. The therapist will need to take a detailed history of treatment administered to date, examine laboratory results, and distinguish between fatigue from deconditioning and fatigue from medical interventions in order to determine the most effective and efficient approach to rehabilitation.

A detailed medical history is essential and should include conditions not related to cancer, such as hypertension, diabetes, coronary artery disease, and preexisting orthopedic conditions. The person's current physical condition, condition before disease onset, and age are also important variables.[100] A self-reporting survey instrument called the Cancer Rehabilitation Evaluation System (CARES; formerly called the Cancer Inventory of Problem Situations [CIPS]) is a useful tool for evaluating rehabilitation needs and interventions.[32,78]

The therapist must understand the stages of the disease and know the type and timing of the medical intervention, especially for radiation and chemotherapy. The body's physiologic response to these agents may affect tolerance for exercise and alter the normal training response.

Monitoring Vital Signs.   Monitoring physiologic responses to exercise is important in the immunosuppressed population. Exercise intensity determined by training heart rate may be difficult to use since some people have inappropriate heart responses to exercise and large physiologic changes on a day-to-day basis from disease and treatment (e.g., changes in medications). Exercise intensity can be guided by heart rate ranges based on oxygen consumption or metabolic equivalent (MET) levels (see the section on Myocardial Infarction: Monitoring Vital Signs in Chapter 11).

The therapist (or client) should always monitor oxygen saturation with pulse oximetry and monitor heart rate (for arrhythmia), pulse rate, breathing frequency, and blood pressure throughout the treatment session. Borg's ratings of perceived exertion scale (see Table 11-13) or other scales can be used to determine level of symptom distress or severity. Watch closely for early signs (dyspnea, pallor, sweating, fatigue) of cardiopulmonary complications of cancer treatment. The activity level of someone with anemia also may require adjustment. This client may have elevated pulse and respiratory rates because of hypoxia, with increased cardiac output resulting from the body's effort to maintain an adequate oxygen supply.

Exercise During and After Chemotherapy.

Bone marrow suppression is a common and serious side effect of many chemotherapeutic agents and can be a side effect of radiation therapy in some instances. Therefore it is extremely important to monitor the hematologic values in clients receiving these treatment modalities. The therapist must review these values before any type of vigorous exercise or activity is initiated. Current guidelines recommend that individuals undergoing chemotherapy or radiation therapy should not exercise within 2 hours of the treatment because increases in circulation may attenuate (increase) the effects of the treatment.[33]

Fatigue is a frequent and severe problem during and after treatment. People in cancer treatment are often advised to rest after chemotherapy, but aerobic exercise and physical activity have been shown to help improve energy level and stamina, reduce fatigue, reduce nausea, increase muscle mass, and increase daily activities without increasing fatigue. Physical activity can also improve mood and reduce anxiety and mental stress for people undergoing chemotherapy. Independence and quality of life improve as functional ability improves.[24,26,72]

A helpful guideline to indicate when aerobic exercise is contraindicated (or when reevaluation of the exercise program is indicated) in chemotherapy clients is given in Table 8-11. See also exercise guidelines provided in Tables 39-6 and 39-7, keeping in mind that most oncology settings have their own guidelines that are more liberal. For example, in some oncology settings, exercise is contraindicated when white blood cell count drops below 500/mm³ (compared to 5000/mm³ listed in Table 39-6) and when platelets drop below 5000/mm³ (compared to 20,000/mm³ listed in Table 39-7).

The American College of Sports Medicine (ACSM) guidelines for termination of testing or training may also be consulted.[1] People with cancer are advised to contact their physician if any of the following abnormal responses develop: fever; extreme or unusual tiredness; unusual muscular weakness; irregular heart beat, palpitations, or chest pain; leg pain or cramps, unusual joint pain, unusual bruising, or nosebleeds; sudden onset of nausea during exercise; rapid weight loss, severe diarrhea, or vomiting; disorientation, confusion, dizziness or light-headedness, or blurred vision; pallor or gray-colored appearance; night pain or pain not associated with an injury.[27]

Prescriptive Exercise.

Types of prescriptive exercise intervention in the treatment of cancer, especially cancer pain, limitations, and precautions, are being studied.[93] Peak exercise capacity is normally between 3 and 5 METs. The exercise intensity should be prescribed at 40% to 65% of the peak heart rate, the heart rate reserve, $VO_{2\,max}$, or just below the anaerobic threshold depending on the person's ability to exercise. Non-weight-bearing activities may be recommended in the presence of muscle wasting and increased risk of fracture.

A perceived exertion of no greater than 12 may be used as a guide when exercise testing is not possible (see Table 11-13). The frequency and duration of exercise are determined by the clinical status of the person. If weight training is prescribed, high-repetition, low-weight circuit programs are recommended that do not exceed a rate of perceived exertion (RPE) of 14.[52] Other clinical tools for monitoring and more specific guidelines for exercise are available.[25,27,65]

Generalized weakness associated with cancer treatment can be more debilitating than the disease itself. Whenever possible, exercise, including strength training and cardiovascular training, is an essential component for many people with cancer. Improving strength and endurance aids in countering the effects of the disease and the effects of medical interventions. Not all people with cancer are able to participate in aerobic exercise. People who ambulate less than 50% of the time or who are confined to bed and those who fatigue with mild exertion may not be candidates for aerobic exercise.[99] Range of motion and gentle resistive work until tolerance for activity improves are still important.

Some people may become easily fatigued with minimal exertion. Energy-conservation techniques and work simplification (Box 8-2) may be necessary for the person with chronic fatigue and for those whose functional status is declining. Therapeutic exercise should be scheduled during periods when the person has the highest level of energy.

Interval exercise or a bedside exercise program may be preferred at first. Interval exercise may be the only treatment possible in this circumstance. This is performed during frequent but short sessions throughout the day with work-rest intervals beginning at the person's level of tolerance. See also the section on Special Implications for the Therapist: Anemia in Chapter 13. This may be no more than 1 minute of exercise activity followed by 1 minute of rest, then 1

TABLE	8-11

Winningham Precautions to Aerobic Exercise in Chemotherapy Clients

Platelet count	<50,000/ml
Hemoglobin	<10 g/ml
White blood cell count	<3000/ml
Absolute granulocytes	<500/ml

Modified from Winningham ML, MacVicar MG, Burke CA: Exercise for cancer patients; guidelines and precautions, *Physician Sportsmed* 14:125-134, 1986.

BOX **8-2**

Tips for Energy Conservation

Energy conservation is an organized procedure for finding ways to reduce the amount of effort and energy needed to accomplish a given task. By reducing the amount of energy needed to accomplish a task, more energy is available.

Applying principles of energy conservation requires self-examination and assessment of habits and priorities. Making these types of changes requires patience but can result in continued activity over a longer period of time:

Schedule the most strenuous activities during periods of highest energy.

Before starting any activity, analyze the task and answer the following questions:
Is the task necessary?
Can it be eliminated or combined?
Am I doing this out of habit?
Can it be simplified by combining or eliminating steps?
Can a larger job be divided into smaller tasks?
Are there any assistive devices or tools that could make the task easier?
Can this be done by someone else?

Alternate more strenuous tasks with easier ones.

Plan frequent rest periods, sit down, or take naps as needed.

Cluster activities so that it is not necessary to make frequent trips or walk long distances at home, school, or work.

Avoid or keep to a minimum the climbing of stairs.

Keep certain tasks, such as housekeeping, to a minimum.

Sit down to perform activities of daily living (e.g., tooth brushing, hair combing) or household tasks, including meal preparation.

Avoid sitting on low or soft furniture that requires more energy expenditure to get up again.

Modified from Hamburgh RR: Principles of cancer treatment, *Clin Manage* 12:37–41, 1992.

minute of exercise, and so on. As the person's endurance level increases, the duration of work may be increased and the interval of rest decreased.

Compromised skeletal integrity may prevent weight-bearing activities. Non–weight-bearing aerobic activities that may be used for people with bone and joint disease include cycling, rowing, and swimming (aquatics for those who are not immunosuppressed). People with severe muscle weakness may tolerate cycling better than walking.[66]

Exercise and Lymphedema. In the past, therapists were cautioned to carefully design a program that did not cause or exacerbate cancer-related complications, such as edema. It was advised that repetitive or strenuous exercise would increase the production of lymph fluid and lymphedema would be the result because lymph nodes were removed during surgery, damaged by radiation therapy, or invaded by the tumor, leaving scar tissue that prevented normal lymph drainage. In fact, it is now known that exercise activates muscle groups and joints in the affected

extremity and does not induce lymphedema.[37,38] Combining a specific exercise program for each individual with the use of sufficient compression will facilitate the process of decongestion by using the natural pumping effect of the muscles to increase lymph flow while preventing limb refilling. Most clinicians experienced in lymphedema treatment agree on basic guidelines for exercise. See further discussion in Chapter 12.

CHILDHOOD CANCER

◆ Incidence and Overview

Each year approximately 8400 children in the United States are diagnosed with cancer. With recent advances in treatment, 65% of these children will survive 5 years or more, an increase of almost 40% since the early 1960s. Cancer is the second leading cause of death among children between 1 and 14 years of age.[35,55] Treatment-related deaths have declined as a result of advances in clinical supportive care (e.g., antibiotic therapy, indwelling venous access lines, blood products, enteral and parenteral nutrition) that maximize the benefits and minimize the side effects of cancer therapy.

The types of cancers that occur in children vary greatly from those seen in adults. Leukemias (particularly acute lymphoblastic leukemia [ALL]) and lymphomas (almost half of all childhood cancers involve the blood or blood-forming organs), brain tumors, embryonal tumors, and sarcomas are the most common pediatric malignancies, whereas adenocarcinomas (e.g., lung, breast, colorectal) are more common in adults.[50,55]

Other differences that must be taken into account when treating the child with cancer include the stage of growth and development, stage of psychosocial and cognitive development, and emotional response to the illness and its treatment. The immaturity of the child's organ systems often has important treatment implications.

◆ Types of Childhood Cancers

The most common pediatric malignancies are acute leukemia, non-Hodgkin's lymphoma, Hodgkin's disease, and primary CNS tumors. Neuroblastoma, Wilms' tumor, rhabdomyosarcoma, and retinoblastomas are the types of solid tumors occurring most frequently in children.[55]

Acute lymphoblastic leukemia (ALL), the most common childhood malignancy, accounts for almost one-third of all pediatric cancers. White males are affected most often, and although the exact cause is unknown, radiation, chromosomal abnormalities, viruses, and congenital immunodeficiencies have all been associated with an increased incidence of leukemia. See also the section on The Leukemias in Chapter 13.

Wilms' tumor, a malignancy that may affect one or both kidneys, occurs in children under the age of 14 years and is slightly more prevalent in females than males. Epidemiologic research suggests an increased incidence in children of men exposed to lead or hydrocarbons. Recently, an association between Wilms' tumor and chromosomal abnormalities has been established, specifically deletion of a suppressor gene located on the short arm of chromosome 11. This chromosomal anomaly is an autosomal dominant trait requiring evaluation of other family members.

Neuroblastoma is the most common extracranial solid tumor in children and the most commonly diagnosed neoplasm during the first year of life. Approximately 500 new cases are diagnosed annually in the United States, and the incidence is higher among whites than nonwhites. Neuroblastoma can originate anywhere along the sympathetic nervous system, but more than half the tumors occur in the retroperitoneal area and present as an abdominal mass. Other common sites include the posterior mediastinum, pelvis, and neck. If the bone marrow is involved, bone pain may occur. See the section on Neuroblastoma in Chapter 29.

Rhabdomyosarcoma is the most common soft tissue sarcoma and the seventh leading cause of cancer in children. This tumor, which is more prevalent in males than females, originates from the same embryonic cells that give rise to striated muscle. The peak incidence is between the age of 2 and 5 years with a second peak occurring between 15 and 19 years. The most common tumor sites include the head and neck, genitourinary tract, and extremities. Head and neck tumors can lead to CNS involvement including cranial nerve palsies, meningeal symptoms, and respiratory paralysis. Ninety percent of children with lesions extending into the CNS die.

Other common cancers seen in children are bone cancers, both osteogenic and Ewing's sarcomas (see Chapter 25), and brain tumors (see Chapter 29).

◆ Late Effects and Prognosis

As advances in cancer therapy improve, the prognosis of children with malignancies continues to improve. Over the past 25 years there have been significant improvements in the 5-year survival rate for many childhood cancers, especially acute lymphocytic and myeloid leukemias, non-Hodgkin's lymphoma, and Wilms' tumor. Between 1974 and 1996, 5-year survival rates among children for all cancer sites combined improved from 56% to 75%.[35] With increasing survival rates, there is a growing concern about the late effects of disease and treatment.

The term *late effects* refers to the damaging effects of surgery, radiation, and chemotherapy on nonmalignant tissues, as well as to the social, emotional, and economic consequences of survival. These effects can appear months to years after treatment and can range in severity from subclinical, to clinical, to life-threatening. Fortunately, not all children experience such effects, but those that do often end up in the rehabilitation setting.

Late effects have been identified in almost every organ system. Treatment involving the CNS can cause deficits in intelligence, hearing, and vision. Treatment involving the CNS, head and neck, or gonads can cause endocrine abnormalities, such as short stature, hypothyroidism, or delayed secondary sexual development. Children treated with anthracyclines (e.g., doxorubicin [Adriamycin]) are at risk for development of cardiomyopathies, especially with increasing cumulative doses.[86]

Surgery and radiation involving the musculoskeletal system have been associated with defects such as kyphosis, scoliosis, and spinal shortening. Finally, the child who has received radiation or chemotherapy has a tenfold greater chance of developing a second malignancy than a child who has never had cancer.

REFERENCES

1. ACSM (American College of Sports Medicine): *Guidelines for exercise testing and prescription*, ed 6, Philadelphia, 2000, Lippincott.
2. AHCPR (Agency for Health Care Policy and Research): *Management of cancer pain for adults/Management of cancer pain for children and adolescents*. Guideline no. 9, 1994. Available by calling the National Cancer Institute, (800) 4-CANCER; or write Cancer Pain Guideline, AHCPR Publications Clearinghouse, P.O. Box 8547, Silver Spring, MD 20907.
3. American Cancer Society: *Guide to complementary and alternative cancer methods*, New York, 2000, The Society.
4. American Cancer Society: Nutrition and cancer prevention, *CA Cancer J Clin* 46(6):323-341, 1996.
5. American Cancer Society: Nutrition and cancer: strategy 2000, *CA Cancer J Clin* 49(6):331-361, 1999.
6. American Institute for Cancer Research: *Food, nutrition and the prevention of cancer: a global perspective*, Washington, DC, 1997, The Institute.
7. Anllo LM: Sexual life after breast cancer, *J Sex Marital Ther* 26(3):241-248, 2000.
8. Austin Research Institute: *ARI achievements* (on-line), 2000: www.ari.unimelb.edu.au/achieve
9. Bach EC: Cancer rehabilitation in the home care setting, *Rehabilitation Oncology* 18(1):32-33, 2000.
10. Balducci L, Extermann M: Cancer and aging, an evolving panorama, *Hematol Oncol Clin North Am* 14:1-16, 2000.
11. Baraldi-Jenkins C, Beck A, Rothstein G: Hematopoeisis and cytokines: relevance to cancer and aging, *Hematol Oncol Clin North Am* 14:45-62, 2000.
12. Bennett M, Ryall N: Using the modified Barthel index to estimate survival in cancer patients in hospice: observational study, *BMJ* 321:1381-1382, 2000.
13. Bernabei R, Gambassi M, Lapane K et al: Management of pain in elderly patients with cancer, *JAMA* 279:1877-1882, 1998.
14. Brown J, Byers T, Thompson K et al: Nutrition during and after cancer treatment: a guide for informed choices by cancer survivors, *CA Cancer J Clin* 51(3):153-187, 2001.
15. Campisi J: Cancer, aging and cellular senescence, *In Vivo* 14:183-188, 2000.
16. Cech T: Life at the end of the chromosome: telomeres and telomerase, *Angew Chem Int Ed Engl* 39(1):34-43, 2000.
17. Cech TR, Egan LW, Doyle C et al: The biomedical research bottleneck, *Science* 293(5530):573, 2001.
18. Cherny N: The management of cancer pain, *CA Cancer J Clin* 50:70-120, 2000.
19. Cheson B: Hodgkin's disease and the non-Hodgkin's lymphomas. In Lenhard R, Osteen R, Gansler T, editors: *The American Cancer Society's clinical oncology*, Atlanta, 2002, American Cancer Society, pp 497-516.
20. Costanza M, Li F, Finn L, et al: Cancer prevention: strategies for practice. In Lenhard R, Osteen R, Gansler T, editors: *The American Cancer Society's clinical oncology*, Atlanta, 2001, American Cancer Society, pp 55-74.
21. Courneya KS, Friedenreich CM: Physical exercise and quality of life following cancer diagnosis: a literature review, *Ann Behav Med* 21(2):171-179, 1999.
22. Dalzell MA: *Biophysical modalities in oncology: guidelines for the use of electrical stimulation, laser and ultrasound*. Proceedings from Cancer rehabilitation: the multidisciplinary integration of traditional and "whole person" care, Montreal, L'Espirit Rehabilitation Centers, Jan 21-23, 2000.
23. DeMichele A, Glick J: Cancer-related emergencies. In Lenhard R, Osteen R, Gansler T, editors: Cancer-related emergencies. In Lenhard R, Osteen R, Gansler T, editors: *The American Cancer Society's clinical oncology*, Atlanta, 2001, American Cancer Society, pp 733-764.
24. Dimeo F: Exercise programs for cancer patients during chemo- and radiotherapy, *Rehabilitation Oncology* 18(3):5, 2000.
25. Dimeo F: Strategies in managing cancer fatigue, *Rehabilitation Oncology* 17(3):27-28, 1999.
26. Dimeo F, Rumberger BG, Keul J: Aerobic exercise as therapy for cancer fatigue, *Med Sci Sports Exerc* 30:475-478, 1998.
27. Drouin J, Pfalzer LA: Aerobic exercise guidelines for the person with cancer, *Acute Care Perspectives* 10(1&2):18-24, 2001.
28. Eatock AM, Scatzlein A, Kayes L: Tumour vasculature as a target for anticancer therapy, *Cancer Treat Rev* 26:191-204, 2000.

29. Fernendez-Pol J, Douglas M: Molecular interactions of cancer and age, *Hematol Oncol Clin North Am* 14:25-44, 2000.

30. Franceschi S: Strategies to reduce the risk of virus-related cancers, *Ann Oncol* 11(9):1091-1096, 2000.

31. Gahart B, Nazareno A: *2001 Intravenous medications,* ed 16, St Louis, 2001, Mosby.

32. Ganz PA: Quality of life and cancer rehabilitation, *Rehabil Oncol* 17(3):9-11, 1999.

33. Gerber L, Augustine E: Rehabilitation management: restoring fitness and return to functional activity. In Harris J, Lippman M, Morrow M, et al, editors: *Diseases of the breast*, Philadelphia, 2000, Lippincott, pp 1001-1007.

34. Giovannucci E: Nutritional factors in human cancers, *Adv Exp Med Biol* 472:29-42, 1999.

35. Jemal A, Thomas A, Murray T: Cancer statistics, 2001, *CA Cancer J Clin* 51:15-36, 2001.

36. Gudas S: The physical therapy challenge in disseminated cancer, *APTA Newsletter* 5:3, 1987.

37. Harris SR: Challenging myths in physical therapy, *Physical Therapy* 81(6):1180-1183, 2001.

38. Harris SR, Niesen-Veertommen SL: Challenging the myth of exercise-induced lymphedema following breast cancer: a series of case reports, *J Surg Oncol* 74(2):95-98, 2000.

39. *Healthy people 2001: objectives* (on-line), 2001: http://health.gov/healthypeople/

40. Heath C, Fontham E: Cancer etiology. In Lenhard R, Osteen R, Gansler T, editors: *The American Cancer's Society clinical oncology*, Atlanta, 2001, American Cancer Society, pp 37-54.

41. Herberman R: Basis for current major therapies for cancer, section E. In Lenhard R, Osteen R, Gansler T, editors: *The American Cancer Society's clinical oncology*, Atlanta, 2001, American Cancer Society, pp 215-229.

42. Hill C, Cleeland C, Gustein H: Effective pain treatment in cancer patients. In Lenhard R, Osteen R, Gansler T, editors: *The American Cancer Society's clinical oncology*, Atlanta, 2001, American Cancer Society, pp 765-809.

43. Hillner BE, Ingle JN, Berenson JR, et al: American Society of Clinical Oncology guideline on the role of bisphosphonates in breast cancer, *J Clin Oncol* 18(6):1378-1391, 2000.

44. Hogan RD, Burke KM, Franklin TD: The effect of ultrasound on microvascular haemodynamics in skeletal muscle: effects during ischaemia, *Microvasc Res* 23:370-379, 1982.

45. Howe HL, Wingo PA, Thun MJ, et al: Annual report to the nation on the status of cancer (1973 through 1998), featuring cancers with recent increasing trends, *J Natl Cancer Inst* 93(11):824-842, 2001.

46. Hughes MK: Sexuality and the cancer survivor: a silent coexistence, *Cancer Nurs* 23(6):477-482, 2000.

47. Kelloff GJ, Crowell JA, Steele VE, et al: Progress in cancer chemoprevention: development of diet-derived chemopreventive agents, *J Nutr* 130(2S, suppl):467S-471S, 2000.

48. Kiecolt-Glaser JK, Glaser R: Psychoneuroimmunology and cancer: fact or fiction? *Eur J Cancer* 35(11):1603-1607, 1999.

49. Kraeber-Bodere F, Champion L, Rousseau C, et al: Treatment of bone metastases of prostate cancer with strontium-89 chloride: efficacy in relation to the degree of bone involvement, *Eur J Nucl Med* 27(10):1487-1493, 2000.

50. Landier W: Childhood acute lymphoblastic leukemia: current perspectives, *Oncol Nurs Forum* 28:823-833, 2001.

51. Lejbkowicz F, Zwiran M, Salzberg S: The response of normal and malignant cells to ultrasound in vitro, *Ultrasound Med Biol* 19:75-82, 1993.

52. Leutholtz BC, Ripoll I: *Exercise and disease management*, Boca Raton, Fla, 1999, CRC Press.

53. Lewis MM, Reilly JF: Sports tumors, *Am J Sports Med* 15:362-365, 1987.

54. Mackey KM, Sparling JW: Experiences of older women with cancer receiving hospice care: significance for physical therapy, *Phys Ther* 80(5):459-468, 2000.

55. Marcus K: Pediatric solid tumors. In Lenhard R, Osteen R, Gansler T, editors: *The American Cancer Society's clinical oncology*, Atlanta, 2001, American Cancer Society, pp 577-609.

56. Maxwell L: Therapeutic ultrasound and tumor metastasis, *Physiotherapy* 81:272-275, 1995.

57. Michaud D, Spiegelman D, Clinton S, et al: Fruit and vegetable intake and incidence of bladder cancer in a male prospective cohort, *J Natl Cancer Inst* 91:605-613, 1999.

58. Moldoveanu AI, Shepard RJ, Shek PN: The cytokine response to physical activity and training, *Sports Med* 31(2):115-144, 2001.

59. Monier R: Fundamental aspects, mechanisms of carcinogenesis and dose-effect relationships, *CR Acad Sci III* 323:603-610, 2000.

60. Mundy GR: Mechanisms of bone metastasis, *Cancer Supplement* 80(8):1546-1553, 1997.

61. National Comprehensive Cancer Network (NCCN): *Cancer pain treatment guideline* (on-line), 2000: www.nccn.org

62. Olumi A: A critical analysis of the use of p53 as a marker for management of bladder cancer, *Urol Clin North Am* 27:75-82, 2000.

63. Osteen R: Breast cancer. In Lenhard R, Osteen R, Gansler T, editors: *The American Cancer Society's clinical oncology*, Atlanta, 2001, American Cancer Society, pp 251-268.

64. Penson RT, Gallagher J, Gioiella, ME et al: Sexuality and cancer: conversation comfort zone, *Oncologist* 5(4):336-344, 2000.

65. Pfalzer L: *Clinical monitoring tools and guidelines for exercise.* Proceedings from Cancer rehabilitation: the multidisciplinary integration of traditional and "whole person" care, Montreal, L'Espirit Rehabilitation Centers, Jan 21-23, 2000.

66. Pfalzer L: Exercise for patients with disseminated cancer, *APTA Newsletter* 5:5-7, 1987.

67. Pfalzer L: Personal communication, 2000.

68. Pfalzer L: Physical agents/modalities for survivors of cancer, *Rehabilitation Oncology* 19(2):12-24, 2001.

69. Pfalzer L: *Research models and tools for physical therapy in cancer rehabilitation.* Proceedings from Cancer rehabilitation: the multidisciplinary integration of traditional and "whole person" care, Montreal, L'Espirit Rehabilitation Centers, Jan 21-23, 2000.

70. Pfeifer J, Wick M: Pathologic evaluation of neoplastic diseases. In Lenhard R, Osteen R, Gansler T, editors: *The American Cancer Society's clinical oncology*, Atlanta, 2001, American Cancer Society, pp 123-145.

71. Plaut SM, Rutter MA: Addressing sexual issues in patients with cancer, *Acute Care Perspectives* 10(1&2):41-44, 2001.

72. Porock D, Kristjanson LJ, Tinnelly K, et al: An exercise intervention for advanced cancer patients experiencing fatigue: a pilot study, *J Palliative Care* 16(3):27, 30-36, 2000.

73. Rajkumar S: A review of angiogenesis and antiangiogenic therapy with thalidomide in multiple myeloma, *Cancer Treat Rev* 26:351-362, 2000.

74. Rhodes VA, McDaniel RW: Nausea, vomiting, and retching: complex problems in palliative care, *CA Cancer J Clin* 51(4):232-248, 2001.

75. Ringer D, Schnipper L: Principles of cancer biology. In Lenhard R, Osteen R, Gansler T, editors: *The American Cancer Society's clinical oncology*, Atlanta, 2001, American Cancer Society, pp 21-35.

76. Romanov S, Kozakiewicz B, Holst C, et al: Normal human mammary epithelial cells spontaneously escape senescence and acquire genomic changes, *Nature* 409:633-637, 2001.

77. Rosenthal P: Complications of cancer and cancer treatment. In Lenhard R, Osteen R, Gansler T, editors: *The American Cancer Society's clinical oncology*, Atlanta, 2001, American Cancer Society, pp 231-249.

78. Schag CAC, Heinrich RL: Development of a comprehensive quality of life measurement tool: the CARES, *Oncology* 4(5):135-138, 1990.

79. Schover LR, McKee AL: Sexuality rehabilitation, *Rehabilitation Oncology* 18(1):16-18, 2000.

80. Seffrin J: An endgame for cancer, *CA Cancer J Clin* 50:4-5, 2000.

81. Sexual Information and Education Council (provides annotated bibliographies about sexuality with illness and disability), 2001: www.siecus.org

82. Shapiro CL, Manola J, Leboff M: Ovarian failure after adjuvant chemotherapy is associated with rapid bone loss in women with early-stage breast cancer, *J Clin Oncol* 19(14):3306-3311, 2001.

83. Shepard RJ, Shek PN: Cancer, immune function, and physical activity, *Can J Appl Physiol* 20(1):1-25, 1995.

84. Sicard-Rosenbaum L, Danoff JV, Guthrie JA, et al: Effects of energy-matched pulsed and continuous ultrasound on tumor growth in mice, *Phys Ther* 78(3):271-277, 1998.

85. Smith RA, von Eschenbach AC, Wender R, et al: American Cancer Society guidelines for the early detection of cancer, *CA Cancer J Clin* 51(1):38-75, 2001.

86. Sorensen K, Levitt G, Bull C et al: Anthracycline dose in childhood acute lymphoblastic leukemia: issues of early survival versus late cardiotoxicity, *J Clin Oncol* 15:61-68, 1997.

87. Spitler L, Grossbard M, Ernstoff M et al: Adjuvant therapy of stage III and IV malignant melanoma using granulocyte-macrophage colony stimulating factor, *J Clin Oncol* 18:1614-1621, 2000.

88. Strohl P: Radiation therapy. In Miaskowski C, Buchsel P, editors: *Oncology nursing: assessment and clinical care*, St Louis, 1999, Mosby, pp 59-81.

89. Stummvoll GH, Aringer M, Machold KP, et al: Cancer polyarthritis resembling rheumatoid arthritis as a first sign of hidden neoplasms, *Scand J Rheumatol* 30:40-44, 2001.

90. Takayama K: Suppression of tumor angiogenesis and growth by gene transfer of a soluble form of vascular endothelial growth factor receptor into a remote organ, *Cancer Res* 60:2169-2177, 2000.

91. ter Haar G, Dyson M, Oakley S: Ultrasound in physiotherapy in the United Kingdom: results of a questionnaire, *Physiother Pract* 4:69-772, 1988.

92. Thomas C, Williams T, Cobos E: Lung cancer. In Lenhard R, Osteen R, Gansler T, editors: *The American Cancer Society's clinical oncology*, Atlanta, 2001, American Cancer Society, pp 269-295.

93. University of Northern Colorado Rocky Mountain Cancer Rehabilitation Institute, Greeley, Colorado (on-line), 2000: www.univnorthco.edu

94. Urquidi V, Tarin D, Goodison S: Role of telomerase in cell senescence and oncogenesis, *Annu Rev Med* 51:65-79, 2000.

95. Vasiri H, Benchimol S: Alternative pathways for the extension of cellular life span, inactivation of p53/pRb and expression of telomerase, *Oncogene* 18:7676-7680, 1999.

96. Willett W: Goals for nutrition in the year 2000, CA *Cancer J Clin* 49:331-352, 1999.

97. Wilson B, Shannon M, Stang C: *Nursing drug guide 2001*, Upper Saddle River, NJ, 2001, Prentice-Hall Health.

98. Wingo P, Parkin D, Eyre H: Measuring the occurrence of cancer, impact and statistics. In Lenhard R, Osteen R, Gansler T, editors: *The American Cancer Society's clinical oncology*, Atlanta, 2001, American Cancer Society, pp 1-19.

99. Winningham ML: Walking program for people with cancer, *Cancer Nurs* 14:270-276, 1991.

100. Winningham ML, MacVicar MG, Burke CA: Exercise for cancer patients: guidelines and precautions, *Physician Sportsmed* 14:121-134, 1986.

101. Woods J, Lu Q, Ceddia MA, et al: Special feature for the Olympics: effects of exercise on the immune system: exercise-induced modulation of macrophage function, *Immunol Cell Biol* 78(5):545-553, 2000.

102. Yancik R, Ries L: Aging and cancer in America: demographic and epidemiologic perspectives, *Hematol Oncol Clin North Am* 14:17-24, 2000.

103. Yarbro C, Frogge MH, Goodman M, editors: *Cancer symptom management*, Sudbury, Mass, 1999, Jones & Bartlett.

104. Zhang SM, Hunter DJ, Rosner BA, et al: Intakes of fruits, vegetables, and related nutrients and the risk of non-Hodgkin's lymphoma among women, *Cancer Epidemiol Biomarkers Prev* 9(5):477-485, 2000.

CHAPTER 9

THE INTEGUMENTARY SYSTEM

PAMELA UNGER AND CATHERINE C. GOODMAN

Skin is the largest body organ, constituting 15% to 20% of the body weight and consisting of three primary layers (Fig. 9-1). The dermis is more distinctly divided into two separate layers referred to as the papillary dermis and reticular dermis. The structures included in each layer are listed in Table 9-1. The skin differs anatomically and physiologically in different areas of the body, but the overall primary function of the skin is to protect underlying structures from external injury and harmful substances. The skin is primarily an insulator, not an organ of exchange. It has many other different functions, including holding the organs together, sensory perception, contributing to fluid balance, controlling temperature, absorbing ultraviolet (UV) radiation, metabolizing vitamin D, and synthesizing epidermal lipids.

SKIN LESIONS

Approximately one in every four people who consult a physician has a skin disorder. Skin lesions can occur as a result of a wide variety of etiologic factors (Box 9-1). Lesions of the skin or systemic disorders with skin manifestations can be classified as *primary* or *secondary* lesions. The primary lesion is the first lesion to appear on the skin and has a visually recognizable structure (e.g., macule, papule, plaque, nodule, tumor, wheal, vesicle, pustule). When changes occur in the primary lesion, it becomes a secondary lesion (e.g., scale, crust, thickening, erosion, ulcer, scar, excoriation, fissure, atrophy). These changes may result from many factors, including scratching, rubbing, medication, natural disease progression, or processes of healing.

Birthmarks, commonly caused by a nevus (pl., nevi), may involve an overgrowth of one or more of any of the normal components of skin, such as pigment cells, blood vessels, and lymph vessels. Birthmarks may be classified as pigment cell (e.g., mongolian spot, café au lait spot); vascular (e.g., portwine stain, strawberry hemangioma); epidermal (e.g., epidermal nevus, nevus sebaceus), or connective tissue (e.g., juvenile elastoma, collagenoma) birthmarks.

Most birthmarks do not require treatment. Vascular birthmarks may be removed with laser therapy for cosmetic reasons. The presence of six or more café au lait spots over 5 cm in length requires medical investigation because these may be diagnostic of neurofibromatosis or Albright's syndrome. Mongolian spots (blue-black macules) are found over the lumbosacral area in 90% of Native American, black, and Asian infants and can easily be mistaken for a large bruise by uninformed individuals.

SIGNS AND SYMPTOMS OF SKIN DISEASE

Pruritus (itching) is one of the most common manifestations of dermatologic disease and a symptom of underlying systemic disease in up to 50% of people with generalized itching, especially among the chronically ill and older populations.[104] It can lead to damage if scratching injures the skin's protective barrier, possibly resulting in increased inflammation, infection, and scarring. Many systemic disorders may cause pruritus, most commonly diabetes mellitus, drug hypersensitivity, and hyperthyroidism (Box 9-2).

Urticaria, more commonly known as hives, is a vascular reaction of the skin marked by the appearance of smooth, slightly elevated patches (wheals). These are redder or paler than the surrounding skin and are often accompanied by severe itching. These eruptions are usually an allergic response to drugs or infection and rarely last longer than 2 days but may exist in a chronic form, lasting more than 3 weeks and, rarely, months to years. There is approximately a 50% reduction in numbers of mast cells responsible for urticaria in intrinsically aged skin. This explains the relative rarity of urticaria in the older adult population.

Rash is a generalized term for an eruption on the skin, most often on the face, trunk, axilla, and groin, and is often accompanied by itching. As such, a rash can present as a continuum anywhere from erythema, to macular lesions, to a raised papular appearance. Rashes typically occur as a secondary response to some primary agent, such as exposure to the sun, allergens, irritants, or medications or in association with systemic disease. The most common rashes are diaper rash, drug rash, heat rash, and butterfly rash (a cutaneous reaction across the nose and adjacent areas of the cheeks in the pattern of a butterfly, most often encountered in systemic lupus erythematosus; see Fig. 9-17). Rash appearing on the breast, especially a rash on the areola or nipple with or without accompanying symptoms of itching, soreness, or burning, may be a sign of Paget's disease of the nipple, a rare form of breast cancer.

Blisters (vesicle or bulla) are fluid-containing elevated lesions of the skin with clear watery or bloody contents; they can occur as a manifestation of a wide variety of diseases. Blisters may be primarily associated with diseases of a genetic or autoimmune origin or secondary to viral or bacterial infections of the skin (e.g., herpes simplex, impetigo), local injury to the skin (e.g., burns, ischemia, dermatitis), or drug-induced (e.g., penicillamine, captopril).[29] Blisters associated with underlying neoplasm called paraneoplastic pemphigus may be the first sign of underlying malignancy.

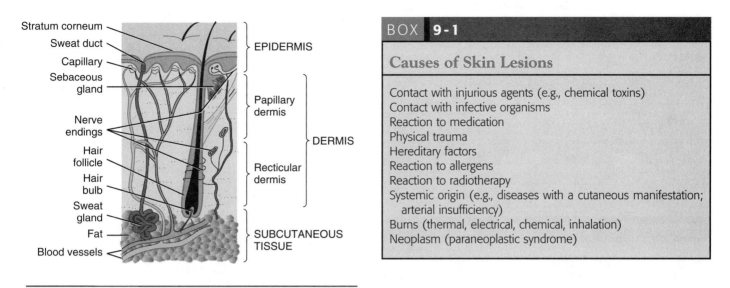

FIGURE **9-1** Overall skin structure.

BOX **9-1**

Causes of Skin Lesions

Contact with injurious agents (e.g., chemical toxins)
Contact with infective organisms
Reaction to medication
Physical trauma
Hereditary factors
Reaction to allergens
Reaction to radiotherapy
Systemic origin (e.g., diseases with a cutaneous manifestation; arterial insufficiency)
Burns (thermal, electrical, chemical, inhalation)
Neoplasm (paraneoplastic syndrome)

TABLE **9-1**

Skin Structure

LAYER	STRUCTURE*	FUNCTION
Epidermis	Stratum corneum	Protection (from trauma, microbes); barrier (prevents fluid, electrolyte, and chemical loss)
	Keratinocytes (squamous cells)	Synthesis of keratin (skin protein)
	Melanocytes	Melanosome production; synthesis of melanin, a pigment to protect against sunburn, ultraviolet carcinogenesis; determines skin color
	Langerhans' cells	Antigen presentation; immune response
	Basal cells	Epidermal reproduction
Dermis	Collagen, reticulum, elastin	Skin proteins; skin texture
	Fibroblasts	Collagen synthesis for skin strength and wound healing
	Macrophages	Phagocytosis of foreign substances; initiates inflammation and repair
	Mast cells	Provide histamine for vasodilation and chemotactic factors for inflammatory responses
	Lymphatic glands	Removal of microbes and excess interstitial fluids; provide lymphatic drainage
	Blood vessels	Provide metabolic skin requirements; thermoregulation
	Nerve fibers	Perception of heat and cold, pain, itching
Epidermal appendages	Eccrine unit	Thermoregulation by perspiration
	Apocrine unit	Production of apocrine sweat; no known significance
	Hair follicles	Protection; cavity enclosing hair
	Nails	Protection; mechanical assistance
	Sebaceous glands	Produce sebum (oil to lubricate skin)
Subcutaneous tissue	Adipose (fat)	Energy storage and balance; trauma absorption

Modified from Nicol NH: Structure and function: assessment of clients with integumentary disorders. In Black JM, Matassarin-Jacobs E, editors: *Medical-surgical nursing*, ed 5, Philadelphia, 1997, Saunders, p 2176.
*Understanding the structure of the integument is important in wound management. Knowing why a wound closes the way it does is an essential assessment tool.

Xeroderma is a mild form of ichthyosis or excessive dryness of the skin characterized by dry, rough, discolored skin with the formation of scaly desquamation (shedding of the epithelium in small sheets). This problem is accentuated by the use of drying skin cleansers, soaps, disinfectants, solvents, and dry climates.

Other symptoms, such as unusual spots, moles, cysts, fibromas, nodules, swelling, or changes in nail beds, may be observed frequently since more than half of all people have some basic skin problem at some point in their lives (Box 9-3). Any unusual spot that has appeared recently or changed since its

BOX **9-2**

Systemic Causes of Pruritus

Diabetes mellitus	Leukemia
Drug hypersensitivity	Liver disease
Hyperthyroidism	Lymphomas
Intestinal parasites	Polycythemia rubra vera
Iron deficiency anemia	Renal disease
Kidney disease	Solid tumor malignancies

BOX **9-3**

Signs and Symptoms of Skin Disorders

Pruritus
Urticaria
Rash
Blisters
Xeroderma (dry skin)
Unusual spots, moles, nodules, cysts
Edema or swelling
Changes in appearance of nails
Changes in skin pigmentation, turgor, texture

initial appearance should be documented and brought to the physician's attention. On the legs, varicosities and stasis changes from poor venous return may be signaled by changes in skin pigmentation, skin turgor (see Fig. 4-1), and skin texture. Edema of the legs can be a sign of multiple systemic illnesses, such as heart, kidney, or liver disease.

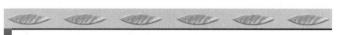

Special Implications for the Therapist **9-1**

SKIN LESIONS

Preferred Practice Patterns
4D: Impaired Joint Mobility, Motor Function, Muscle Performance, and Range of Motion Associated With Connective Tissue Dysfunction
7A: Primary Prevention/Risk Reduction for Integumentary Disorders
7B: Impaired Integumentary Integrity Associated With Superficial Skin Involvement
7C: Impaired Integumentary Integrity Associated With Partial-Thickness Skin Involvement and Scar Formation
7D: Impaired Integumentary Integrity Associated With Full-Thickness Skin Involvement and Scar Formation

Any time a client reports signs or symptoms of skin lesions, further evaluation is necessary; and documentation and possible medical referral may be required. The therapist must remain alert to any skin changes that may indicate the onset or progression of a systemic condition. Any rash on the breast, whether or not symptomatic or accompanied by other symptoms, raises the suspicion of Paget's disease and must be examined by a medical doctor. Blisters of unknown cause may be the first sign of underlying malignancy requiring immediate medical evaluation.

Certain skin lesions—for example, actinic keratosis, slightly raised, red, scaly papules; sebaceous cysts, enclosed cysts in the dermis; skin tears as a result of aging—should be examined by a physician because of their premalignant status and infectious potential, respectively. Seborrheic keratosis can be moved with friction and may bleed, causing alarm, but this is not a malignancy; the therapist must avoid contact with the skin in that area. In the case of pruritus, regardless of the cause, the therapist can offer some practical suggestions to help soothe skin, ease the itching, and prevent skin damage (Box 9-4). Bullous skin lesions, including blisters, are associated with risk of exposure to human immunodeficiency virus (HIV) at least comparable to that from blood. Standard Precautions while treating anyone with skin lesions or burns are required.[27]

When examining and documenting the presence of a skin disorder, note the location, size, and any irregularities in skin color, temperature, moisture, ulceration, texture, thickness, mobility, edema, turgor, odor, and tenderness (Box 9-5). If more than one lesion is present, note the pattern of distribution: localized or isolated; regional; general; or universal (total), involving the entire skin, hair, and nails. Note whether the lesions are unilateral or bilateral, note whether they are symmetric or asymmetric, and note the arrangement of the lesions (clustered or linear configuration), especially if these occur as a result of contact with clothing, jewelry, or another external object.

Blisters may be associated with a variety of skin conditions, such as frostbite, dermatitis, burns, or malignancy, or possibly as a side effect of medications. All blisters should be opened and debrided. Although an intact blister is theoretically sterile, few blisters are substantial enough to remain intact for long. Blister fluid will "set" into a gelatinous film if debridement is delayed. In a burn, this film is the beginning of eschar and is an ideal culture medium for bacteria. Blister fluid impairs normal function of neutrophils and lymphocytes, which reduces the effectiveness of local immunity. Blister fluid also contains arachidonic acid metabolites that increase the inflammatory response and retard the fibrolytic process. All these effects delay healing of the wound.[99]

Special care must always be taken when working with the older adult. Avoiding shear and friction forces during treatment and particularly during repositioning is essential. Extreme caution is also necessary whenever using electrical or thermal modalities (heat or cold) with older people. Decreased circulation, reduced subcutaneous adipose, and altered metabolism create a situation where initial skin resistance to electricity or poor dissipation of heat or cold can lead to tissue damage. Extra toweling and close supervision are necessary to prevent complications. Utilize protective dressings and appropriate moisturizers for treatment intervention, and avoid using adhesives.

Laboratory Values
Many factors affect the progression of a skin lesion to wound status and subsequent ability to heal, including use of to-

BOX 9-4

Skin Care Strategies

Reduce Pruritus

Gently rub the skin, and avoid scratching.

Keep fingernails trimmed short to prevent damage in case of unconscious or nighttime scratching.

Bathe with nondrying, nonfragranced or unscented soap or other agent when indicated. Use soothing bath products, such as Aveeno oatmeal, mineral oil, cottonseed oil, or cornstarch (make a paste with 2 cups cornstarch and 4 cups warm water) added to warm not hot bath water.

Scleroderma: Apply cooling agents, such as menthol or camphor (e.g., contained in Sarna lotion), to the affected areas.

Psoriasis: Try skin preparations such as creams containing capsaicin,[68,98] chaparral, or aloe (some advocate the use of pure aloe). Do not apply hot-pepper creams on broken skin.

Discuss with your physician the possible use of an alpha-hydroxy acid (AHA) product or other prescription cream containing urea to dissolve the outer layer of skin and get rid of the dead scales.

Second rinse all clothing and bedding to remove residual laundry soap; avoid the use of fabric softeners.

Wear open weave, loose-fitting, cotton blend fabrics to allow air to circulate and minimize perspiration, thereby reducing the risk of pruritus; avoid rough, wool, or tightly woven fabrics.

Avoid temperature extremes that can trigger itching secondary to vasodilation and increased cutaneous blood flow. Avoid hot water (baths or hot tubs) for this same reason.

Take antihistamines to reduce itching according to physician recommendation.

Take a shower or bath immediately after swimming; wash with mild soap to remove any residual chlorine or chemicals from the skin.

Reduce Inflammation

Apply topical steroids (available as lotion, solution, gel, cream, or ointment) to affected areas twice daily or as directed. Topical steroids are used to reduce skin inflammation, relieve itching, and control flare-ups of dermatitis and psoriasis. The proper preparation depends on the location and severity of the lesions and should not be applied to normal skin.

Apply tar preparations (available as lotion, solution, gel, cream, ointment, or shampoo) to affected skin as directed. (Some tar preparations can be added to bath water). The antiinflammatory properties of tars are not as fast-acting as topical steroids, but the effect is longer lasting with fewer side effects.

Tar preparations should not be used on acutely inflamed skin because this may cause burning or irritation.

Maintain Skin Hydration

Bathing has been discouraged because of its alleged drying effect, but some skin care professionals advocate the use of long soaks in a warm (not hot) bath for 15 to 20 minutes, suggesting that soaking for 15 to 20 minutes allows the stratum corneum to become saturated with water. Others recommend only showers or brief baths. Both groups agree that drying of the skin is the result of failure to immediately apply the appropriate occlusive moisture, thereby allowing evaporation to occur. Avoid vigorous or brisk towel drying since this removes more water from the skin and increases vasodilation; gently and quickly pat dry. Immediately (within 2 to 4 minutes of leaving the bath) apply an appropriate emollient or prescribed topical agent.

Avoid Sun (Light) Exposure

Wear sun protective clothing with tightly woven material covering as much of the body as possible (e.g., long sleeves, long pants, neckline with a collar, hat with broad brim, UVA/UVB protective sunglasses).

Avoiding sitting near a window at work or for prolonged periods of time.

Avoid outdoor activities during peak sunlight hours (10:00 AM to 4:00 PM in most time zones but may vary geographically). Limit sun exposure during nonpeak hours.

Avoid fluorescent lighting or reflected sunlight.

Wear sunscreen daily and year round, even if driving inside an automobile or on cloudy days.

Apply sunscreen 30 to 60 minutes before sun exposure to assure maximum absorption. Sunscreen preparations must provide a minimum ultraviolet B sun protective factor (SPF) of 30 plus an ultraviolet A sunscreen for anyone with a current skin condition or who is at risk for skin cancer. A sunscreen of SPF 15 is considered adequate for anyone else who does not meet this criterion.

Reapply every 2 hours if you are in the water or perspiring. Sunscreens are not recommended for infants under 6 months of age.

Do not increase sun exposure because you are wearing a sunscreen. High SPF has been shown to lead to increased time spent in the sun by 25%. Sunscreen is most effective against squamous cell carcinoma.[42]

---

bacco, psychosocial status (e.g., comatose, homeless), and nutritional status. Laboratory values, such as albumin levels indicating nutritional status and glucose levels, hemoglobin, and hematocrit to monitor wound healing provide the therapist with necessary information when setting up and carrying out an appropriate intervention plan. ■

AGING AND THE INTEGUMENTARY SYSTEM

The skin undergoes numerous changes that can be seen and felt throughout the life span. The most obvious changes occur first during puberty and again during older adulthood. Hormone changes during puberty stimulate the maturation of

BOX 9-5

Documentation of Skin Lesions

Characteristics

Size (measure all dimensions)
Shape or configuration
Color; temperature
Tenderness, pain, or pruritus
Texture
Mobility; skin turgor
  (see Fig. 4-1)
Elevation or depression
Pedunculation
  (stemlike connections)

Exudates

Color
Odor
Amount
Consistency

Pattern of Arrangement

Annular (rings)
Grouped
Linear
Arciform (bow-shaped)
Diffuse

Location and Distribution

Generalized, localized, or
  universal
Region of the body; unilateral
  or bilateral; symmetric or
  asymmetric
Patterns (dermatomal, flexor
  or extensor, random,
  related to clothing lines)
Discrete or confluent
  (running together)

Modified from Hill MJ: *Skin disorders*, St Louis, 1994, Mosby, p 18.

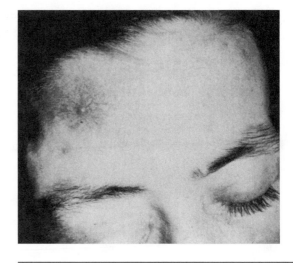

FIGURE 9-2 Spider angioma (arterial spider, spider telangiectasia, vascular spider) is so called because it consists of a central arteriole, radiating from which are numerous small vessels resembling a spider's legs (ranging from pinhead size to 0.5 cm in diameter). Common sites are the necklace area, face, forearms, and dorsum of the hand; may be associated with rosacea, basal cell carcinoma, scleroderma, pregnancy, liver disease, or estrogen therapy or may occur by itself. (From Callen JP, Jorizzo J: *Dermatological signs of internal disease*, ed 2, Philadelphia, 1995, Saunders, p 234.)

hair follicles, sebaceous glands, and apocrine and eccrine units in certain body areas. Mild acne, perspiration and body odor, freckles (promoted by sun exposure), and pigmented nevi (moles) are common occurrences.

During adolescence and adulthood, the use of birth control pills or pregnancy may result in temporary changes in hair growth patterns or hyperpigmentation of the cheeks and forehead known as *melasma* or *pregnancy mask*. Other hormonal abnormalities may result in excessive facial and body hair in women (androgen-related). Hormonal and genetic changes also produce male baldness (alopecia). Smoking is an independent causative factor of facial wrinkles.[33]

The skin exhibits changes that denote the onset of senescence (the process or condition of growing old). These changes may be due to the aging process itself (intrinsic aging), to the cumulative effects of exposure to sunlight (photoaging), or to environmental factors (extrinsic aging). As aging occurs both structural and functional changes occur in the skin (Table 9-2), resulting clinically in diminished pain perception, increased vulnerability to injury, decreased vascularity, and a weakened inflammatory response.

Visible indications of skin changes associated with aging include gray hair, balding and loss of secondary sexual hair, increased facial hair,* lax skin, vascular changes (e.g., decreased elasticity of blood vessel walls; angiomas) (Fig. 9-2), dermal or epidermal degenerative changes, and wrinkling. Wrinkling signifies loss of elastin fibers, weakened collagen, and decreased subcutaneous fat and is accelerated by smoking and excessive sun exposure.

Blood vessels within the reticular dermis are reduced in number, and the walls are thinned. This compromises blood flow and appears physiologically as pale skin and an impaired capacity to thermoregulate, a possible contributing factor to the increased susceptibility in older individuals to hypothermia and hyperthermia. Many other benign changes may occur, including seborrheic keratoses (raised brown or black wartlike growths), lentigines (liver spots, unrelated to the liver but rather secondary to sun exposure), and skin tags (small flesh-colored papules).

A primary factor in the loss of protective functions of the skin is the diminished barrier function of the stratum corneum (outermost layer of the epidermis; see Fig. 9-1). As this layer becomes thinner, the skin becomes translucent and paper-thin, reacting more readily to minor changes in humidity, temperature, and other irritants. There are fewer melanocytes, with decreased protection against UV radiation. A significant decrease in the number of Langerhans' cells occurs so that by the time a person reaches 70 years old there is only half the number of Langerhans' cells compared to the number in early adulthood. A reduction in Langerhans' cell number represents a loss of immune surveillance and an increased risk of skin cancer.[44] The epidermis is also one of the body's principal suppliers of vitamin D, which is produced when a hormone, 7-dehydrocholesterol, is exposed to sunlight. At 65 years of age, the levels of that hormone are only about 25% of what they were in youth, contributing to vitamin D deficiency and, because vitamin D plays a vital role in building bone, to osteoporosis as well.

It is generally agreed that one of the major and important contributions to skin aging, skin disorders, and skin diseases is the oxidative damage that occurs to the skin as a result of environmental exposures and endogenous (within the skin

---

*For women, excessive facial hair may occur along the upper lip and around the chin. Women may also experience balding after menopause. Men frequently develop increased facial hair in the nares, eyebrows, and helix of the ear.

TABLE 9-2	

Effects of Aging on the Skin

STRUCTURAL	FUNCTIONAL
Epidermis	
Flattening of the dermal-epidermal junction	Altered skin permeability
Changes in basal cells	Decreased inflammatory responsiveness
Decreased number of Langerhans' cells	Decreased immunologic responsiveness; increased risk of skin
Decreased number of melanocytes	cancer; increased sensitivity to allergens
	Impaired wound healing; loss of photoprotection with increased
	risk of skin cancer
Dermis	
Decreased dermal thickness; degeneration of elastin fibers	Decreased elasticity; increased wrinkling, slow wound healing, less
	scar tissue (cosmetic benefit)
Decreased vascularization	Decreased vitamin D production
Appendages	
Decreased number and distorted structure of sweat glands	Decreased eccrine sweating; altered skin thermoregulation
Decreased number and distorted structure of specialized	Impaired sensory perception; increased pain threshold
nerve endings	
Decreased hair bulb melanocytes and decreased number	Change in hair color (gray, white); hair loss
of hair follicles	

itself) factors. The skin is rich in lipids, proteins, and deoxyribonucleic acid (DNA), all of which are extremely sensitive to the oxidation process. Scientists are striving to understand the mechanisms involved in skin oxidation and the skin defense systems in order to understand skin aging and the mechanisms involved in various pathologic processes of the skin.[65]

Special Implications for the Therapist   9-2

AGING AND THE INTEGUMENTARY SYSTEM

Preferred Practice Patterns
4D: Impaired Joint Mobility, Motor Function, Muscle
Performance, and Range of Motion Associated With
Connective Tissue Dysfunction
7A: Primary Prevention/Risk Reduction for Integumentary
Disorders
7B: Impaired Integumentary Integrity Associated With
Superficial Skin Involvement

The therapist must remain alert to all skin changes because age-associated blunting of vascular and immune responses may make skin findings more subtle in older adults compared to younger clients with similar disorders. Vascular changes affecting thermoregulation and wound healing require careful consideration when planning therapy intervention. Likewise, loss of collagen increases susceptibility to shearing force trauma, increasing the risk for pressure ulcers. Wound healing is impaired in intrinsically aged as compared to young skin in that the rate of healing is appreciably slower, but paradoxically the resultant scar is usually more cosmetically acceptable.[44]

Skin diseases and symptoms caused by skin disorders are exceedingly common among the older population. Although these disorders are not usually life-threatening they provoke anxiety and psychologic distress. Often, the client has not brought these concerns to the attention of a physician and the therapist is the first health care professional to observe the skin lesion.

It is important to ask about physical findings in other parts of the body (e.g., the client may not mention genital lesions or may be unaware of the significance of other symptoms). All dermatologic lesions must be examined by a physician, and anyone with evidence of sun damage, particularly those with actinic keratoses (see discussion), should have a full skin examination annually. ■

COMMON SKIN DISORDERS

◆ Atopic Dermatitis
Definition and Incidence.   Atopic dermatitis (AD) is a chronic inflammatory skin disease. It is the most common type of eczema, frequently already present during the first year of life and affecting more than 10% of children. AD is considered an early manifestation of atopy* that appears before the development of allergic rhinitis or asthma. There is usually a personal or family history of allergic disorders present, and AD is often associated with food allergies as well.

Etiologic and Risk Factors and Pathogenesis.   The exact cause of atopic dermatitis is unknown although recent studies have demonstrated the complex interrelationship of genetic, physical environment, skin barrier, pharmacologic,

---

*The word *atopic* (from atopy) refers to a group of three associated allergic disorders: asthma, allergic rhinitis (hay fever), and atopic dermatitis.

psychological, and immunologic etiologic factors that contribute to the development and severity of AD.[70] The pathomechanisms associated with AD are also unknown but most likely include both immediate and cellular immune responses. Two possibilities include the release of inflammatory mediators by autoallergens or the release of proinflammatory cytokines by autoreactive T cells in response to autoallergens mediated by IgE.[121] AD is often associated with increased levels of serum immunoglobulin E (IgE) and with sensitization to food allergens. Some foods may be responsible for exacerbations of skin inflammation, but their pathogenic role must be clinically assessed before an avoidance diet is recommended.[57] Xerosis (abnormal dryness) associated with AD is usually worse during periods of low humidity and over the winter months in northern latitudes.

The underlying biochemical abnormality in xerosis is unknown, and the pathologic findings may be a result of the dry skin rather than the cause of the drying effects of this condition. Compared with normal skin, the dry skin of AD has a reduced water-binding capacity, a higher transepidermal water loss, and a decreased water content. Rubbing and scratching of itchy skin are responsible for many of the clinical changes seen in the skin. Hands frequently in and out of water make the condition worse.

Clinical Manifestations. Atopic dermatitis begins in many people during infancy in the form of a red, oozing, crusting rash classified as acute dermatitis (Fig. 9-3). As the child grows, the chronic form of dermatitis results in skin that is dry, thickened, and brownish-gray in color. The rash tends to become localized to the large folds of the extremities as the person becomes older. It is found mainly on flexor surfaces such as the elbows and knees, neck, sides of the face, eyelids, and the backs of hands and feet. Hand and foot dermatitis can become a significant problem for some people.

Xerosis and pruritus are the major symptoms of AD and cause the greatest morbidity with severely excoriated lesions, infection, and scarring. Viral, bacterial, and fungal secondary skin infections may cause further changes in the skin. *Staphylococcus aureus* is the most common bacterial infection, resulting in extensive crusting with serous weeping, folliculitis (inflammation of hair follicles), pyoderma (pus), and furunculosis (boils).

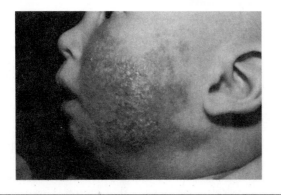

FIGURE 9-3 Infantile atopic dermatitis with oozing and crusting lesions. (From Weston WL, Lane AT: *Color textbook of pediatric dermatology*, St Louis, 1991, Mosby.)

Medical Management

Diagnosis, Treatment, and Prognosis. Although no cure exists, atopic dermatitis often resolves spontaneously, and more than 90% of cases of AD can be effectively controlled through proper management. The goal of medical therapy is to break the inflammatory cycle that causes excess drying, cracking, itching, and scratching. Personal hygiene, moisturizing the skin, avoidance of irritants, topical pharmacology, and systemic medications (e.g., antibiotics, antihistamines, and rarely, systemic corticosteroids) are treatment techniques currently available. *Staphylococcus aureus*, known to colonize the skin of people with AD, may exacerbate skin lesions and need to be treated with antibiotics. Advancing knowledge in understanding the immunologic basis of this disease will continue to result in effective new local and systemic treatments in the decade to come.[84,110]

Special Implications for the Therapist 9-3

ATOPIC DERMATITIS

Preferred Practice Patterns
7A: *Primary Prevention/Risk Reduction for Integumentary Disorders*
7B: *Impaired Integumentary Integrity Associated With Superficial Skin Involvement*

The therapist may be instrumental in providing client education that results in avoiding factors that precipitate or exacerbate inflammation and then teaching proper management techniques for flare-ups. Daily care (hydration and lubrication) of the skin is important, and applications (two or three times daily) of emollients that occlude the skin to prevent evaporation and retain moisture should be recommended. Creams or ointments containing petrolatum or lanolin may be used unless the person is sensitized to lanolin (see the section on Contact Dermatitis), and those that contain urea or lactic acid improve the binding of water in the skin and prevent evaporation. In the case of skin redness, the skin lesion must be identified first because of possible fungal origin requiring an antifungal preparation.

Understanding the individual disease pattern and identifying exacerbating factors are crucial to effective management of this disorder. It is important to identify and eliminate triggers that cause the atopic dermatitis to flare. Older clients should be encouraged to bathe with tepid water using a nondrying, nonfragranced or unscented soap or other agent when indicated. Emollients must be applied to the body within 5 minutes after showering or bathing, especially in dry, winter weather, to prevent further skin drying.

Dermatitis must be considered a precaution, if not contraindication, to some treatment modalities used by therapists. The use of water, alcohol, or any topical agents containing alcohol should be avoided. Topical agents, such as ultrasound gel and mobilization creams, must be used carefully, observing for any skin reaction. A nonreactive response does not guarantee the client will not react when such agents are subsequently applied in future interventions. Caution and careful observation are encouraged. ■

◆ Contact Dermatitis

Etiologic Factors, Incidence, and Pathogenesis. Contact dermatitis can be an acute or chronic skin inflammation caused by exposure to a chemical, mechanical, physical, or biologic agent. It is one of the most common environmental skin diseases occurring at any age. As people age, they may develop delayed cell-mediated hypersensitivity to a variety of substances that come in contact with the skin.

Common sensitizers include nickel (found in jewelry and many common foods), chromates (used in tanning leathers), wool fats (particularly lanolin found in moisturizers and skin creams), rubber additives (see the section on Latex Rubber Allergy in Chapter 3), topical antibiotics (typically neomycin), and topical anesthetics, such as benzocaine or lidocaine.[46] Dermatitis of unknown cause is more commonly diagnosed in the older population.

A small percentage of the population is allergic to silicone. The therapist is most likely to see this reaction in a sensitized person with an amputation using a silicone type of interface in a prosthetic device (designed to reduce shear, decrease repetitive stress, and absorb shock). Silicone sheets used for scar reduction in the postburn population may also result in an episode of contact dermatitis.

Clinical Manifestations. Intense pruritus (itching), erythema (redness), and edema of the skin occur 1 to 2 days after exposure in previously sensitized persons. Clinical manifestations begin at the site of exposure but then extend to more distant sites. These conditions may progress to vesiculation, oozing (watery discharges), crusting, and scaling (Fig. 9-4). If these symptoms persist the skin becomes thickened with prominent skin markings and pigmentation changes. Older people have a less pronounced inflammatory response to standard irritants than do younger persons.

Medical Management

Diagnosis, Treatment, and Prognosis. If contact dermatitis is suspected, the client should be referred to a physician. A detailed history and careful examination are frequently all that are needed to make the diagnosis. It may be necessary to perform patch testing to identify the causative agent.

Primary treatment is removal of the offending agent; treatment of the skin is secondary. The client should be instructed to avoid contact with strong soaps, detergents, solvents, bleaches, and other strong chemicals. The involved skin should be lubricated frequently with emollients. Topical anesthetics or steroids (topical or sometimes systemic) or both may be prescribed. For those people unable to avoid known allergens, immunosuppressant therapies (including phototherapy) can be helpful.[7]

Acute lesions usually resolve in 3 weeks; chronic lesions persist until the causative agent has been removed.

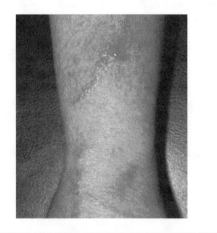

FIGURE **9-4** Primary contact dermatitis, a local inflammatory reaction, can occur in response to an irritant in the environment or an allergy. Characteristic location of lesions often gives a clue to the cause. Erythema occurs first, followed by swelling, wheals or urticaria, or maculopapular vesicles accompanied by intense pruritus. The example shown here is a result of contact with poison ivy. (From Hurwitz S: *Clinical pediatric dermatology: a textbook of skin disorders of childhood and adolescence,* Philadelphia, 1981, Saunders, p 381.)

Special Implications for the Therapist   9-4

CONTACT DERMATITIS

Preferred Practice Patterns
7A: Primary Prevention/Risk Reduction for Integumentary Disorders
7B: Impaired Integumentary Integrity Associated With Superficial Skin Involvement

The therapy professional should always consider the client's reactions to external substances. This is of particular importance when applying any cream, topical agent, or solution. Various modalities used within the profession may involve causative substances (e.g., whirlpool additives, ultrasound gels, self-sticking electrode pads). The client's skin must always be examined before and after intervention for the appearance of any adverse reactions. The client should be instructed to report any discomfort or unusual findings during or after treatment to the therapist.

The person with contact dermatitis associated with the use of a silicone sleeve or interface with a prosthetic device should be cautioned about the use of soaps that do not include a rinsing agent. Many antibacterial and antiperspirant soaps leave particles on the surface of the skin that act as a barrier on the skin's surface against bacterial invasion. A rash or blister may occur in patchy areas corresponding to pressure points when the friction of the interface drives the soap particles back into the skin.[19]

The therapist may suggest one of several care plans for this type of contact dermatitis. The use of alcohol-based lubricants or soaps, antifungal or antibacterial soaps without a rinsing agent, and lanolin should be avoided. Soap-free cleansing agents or a soft soap should be used for daily cleansing, and a petroleum-based ointment can be applied to the limb before putting on the liner. Water-based ointments should be avoided when using urethane liners because these can cause the normally tacky urethane to adhere to the skin so that when the liner is removed, bits of skin may be pulled off as well. Alcohol-based lubricants or soaps should also be avoided with urethane products because these components act as a solvent on urethane, increasing the stickiness of the urethane.[19] ■

◆ Eczema and Dermatitis

Definition and Overview. *Eczema* and *dermatitis* are terms that are often used interchangeably to describe a group of disorders with a characteristic appearance. Eczema or dermatitis is a superficial inflammation of the skin caused by irritant exposure, allergic sensitization (delayed hypersensitivity), or genetically determined idiopathic factors. Many types of dermatitis are represented according to these major etiologic categories (e.g., allergic dermatitis, irritant dermatitis, seborrheic dermatitis, nummular eczema, atopic dermatitis, stasis dermatitis).

Eczema or dermatitis has three primary stages; this condition can manifest in any one of the three stages, or the three stages may coexist. *Acute dermatitis* is characterized by extensive erosions with serous exudate or by intensely pruritic, erythematous papules and vesicles on a background of erythema. *Subacute dermatitis* is characterized by erythematous, excoriated (scratched or abraded), scaling papules or plaques that are either grouped or scattered over erythematous skin. Often the scaling is so fine and diffuse the skin acquires a silvery sheen. *Chronic dermatitis* is characterized by thickened skin and increased skin marking (called *lichenification*) secondary to rubbing and scratching; excoriated papules, fibrotic papules, and nodules (prurigo nodularis); and postinflammatory hyperpigmentation and hypopigmentation.

Incidence and Etiologic Factors. Dermatitis is a common skin disorder in older people. It may be caused by hypoproteinemia, venous insufficiency, allergens, irritants, or underlying malignancy, such as leukemia or lymphoma. Because older people often take multiple medications, dermatitis from drug-drug interaction can occur. The normal aging process with the flattened epidermal-dermal junction and loss of dermis results in skin fragility that contributes to the development of skin tears and dermatitis.

Stasis Dermatitis

Stasis dermatitis is the development of areas of very dry, thin skin and sometimes shallow ulcers of the lower legs primarily as a result of venous insufficiency. The client commonly has a history of varicose veins or deep vein thrombosis (see also the section on Venous Diseases in Chapter 11). The process of stasis dermatitis begins with edema of the leg as a result of slowed venous return. As the venous insufficiency continues, the tissue becomes hypoxic from inadequate blood supply. This poorly nourished tissue begins to necrose. The clinical manifestations include itching, a feeling of heaviness in the legs, brown-stained skin, and open shallow lesions (Fig. 9-5). The lesions are very slow to heal because of a lack of oxygenated blood. Gait training is an important part of compression in the treatment of stasis dermatitis. Support hose works well in the recumbent position, but ambulation with the muscular contract-relax cycle pushes the venous return within the compressive field.

Environmental Dermatoses

It is well documented that exposure to various environmental chemicals and to physical stimuli (Box 9-6) is capable of inducing adverse cutaneous responses. Common environmental skin diseases seen in a therapy practice may include irritant and allergic dermatitis, acne lesions, pigmentary changes (hyperpigmentation, hypopigmentation, absence of pigment), photosensitivity reactions, scleroderma, infectious disorders, and cutaneous malignancy. Each of these environmentally in-

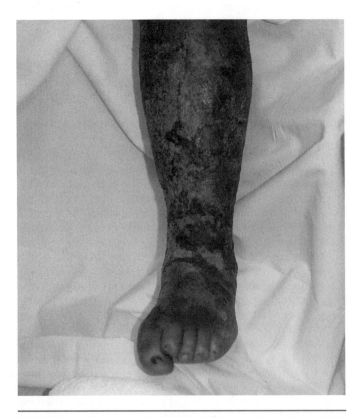

FIGURE **9-5** Stasis dermatitis. (Courtesy Pam Unger, P.T., Community General Hospital, Center for Wound Management, Reading, Pa, 1995.)

BOX **9-6**

Environmental Factors That Induce Skin Disease

Mechanical Factors	**Chemical Agents**
Superficial	Primary irritants
Friction	Sensitizers
Pressure	Photoirritants
Vibration	Photosensitizers
Cuts	
Internal: shearing (skin is forced in opposite direction)	**Biologic Agents**
	Insect and animal parasites
Physical Factors	Bacteria
	Rickettsiae
Heat	Fungi
Cold	Viruses
Humidity	Irritant and sensitizing plants
Water	and woods
Sunlight	
Ultraviolet light	
Ionizing radiation	

From Brooks SM, Gochfeld M, Herzstein J et al: *Environmental medicine*, St Louis, 1995, Mosby.

duced skin conditions is discussed separately in this chapter (see also Chapter 3).

◆ Rosacea

Rosacea* is a chronic facial disorder of middle-aged and older people. Although it is a form of acne, it is differentiated by age, the presence of a large vascular component (erythema, telangiectasis), and usually the absence of comedones. An acneiform rosacea can occur with papules, pustules, and oily skin. No known cause or factor has been identified to explain the pathogenesis of this disorder. A statistically significant incidence of migraine headaches accompanying rosacea has been reported.

Rosacea has often been linked with gastrointestinal (GI) disturbances, and a causal relationship between *Helicobacter pylori* (a bacterium that causes gastritis) and rosacea was reported in the early 1990s. Many studies linking rosacea to *H. pylori* infection were uncontrolled and were performed in areas where the endemic rates of both *H. pylori* infection and rosacea are high.[116] Continued investigation of this issue is required before a causal relationship can be confirmed.

Clinically, the cheeks, nose, and chin (sometimes the entire face) may have a rosy appearance marked by reddened skin. This benign but obvious condition is most common in people with fair skin who flush easily. Sun, hot weather, and humidity can all trigger flare-ups; the condition is worse in the summer. The affected person reports burning or stinging with episodes of flushing that come and go, but the condition may worsen over time, causing lasting redness, pimples, red lines, or nasal bumps. Inflammatory papules are prominent, and there may be pustules. It is not uncommon to have associated ophthalmic disease, including blepharitis and keratitis.

Medical management aimed at the inflammatory papules, pustules, and surrounding erythema may include topical or systemic therapy. Rosacea tends to be a persistent condition that can be controlled with drugs. Rosacea associated with *H. pylori*–induced gastritis can be effectively treated by addressing the underlying problem. Although therapists do not treat this condition, clients with other diagnoses often present with this condition also. Clients with this condition should see a physician for adequate medical treatment.

SKIN INFECTIONS

Many bacterial, viral, fungal, and other parasitic skin infections encountered by the therapist are not the primary focus of intervention but rather occur in clients who are hospitalized or being treated for some other condition. Many of these skin disorders are contagious (Table 9-3) and require careful handling by all health care professionals to avoid spreading the infection and becoming contaminated themselves. Sources of infection differ depending on the disease and mode of transmission (see also Chapter 7). Predisposing factors to skin infections include decreased resistance, dehydrated skin, burns or pressure ulcers, decreased blood flow, contamination from nasal discharge, poor hygiene, and crowded living conditions. Only the most common skin infections encountered in the therapy or rehabilitation setting are discussed further in this section.

*For further information contact the National Rosacea Society, Barrington, Illinois, (847) 382-8971 or www.rosacea.com.

TABLE 9-3

Infections of the Skin

TYPE OF INFECTION	TRANSMISSION
Bacterial	
Impetigo contagiosa	Contagious
Pyoderma	Contagious
Folliculitis (pimple, boil)	Contagious; minimal chance of spread
Cellulitis	Contagious*
Viral	
Verrucae (warts)	Contagious; autoinoculable†
Verruca plantaris (plantar wart)	Contagious; autoinoculable
Herpes simplex	
Type 1: cold sore, fever blister	Contagious
Type 2: genital lesion	Contagious
Varicella-zoster virus (herpes zoster; shingles)	Contagious; chickenpox can occur in anyone not previously exposed
Fungal	
Tinea corporis (ringworm)	Person-to-person Animal-to-person Inanimate object–to–person
Tinea capitis (affects scalp)	Person-to-person Animal-to-person
Tinea cruris (jock itch)	Person-to-person
Tinea pedis (athlete's foot)	Transmission to other people rare despite general opinion to the contrary
Candidiasis	Person-to-person; sexually transmitted during birth from colonized vagina to neonatal oropharynx
Other	
Scabies	Person-to-person; sexually transmitted Inanimate object–to–person
Lice	Same as scabies

*Technically, cellulitis is contagious, but from a practical point of view the chances of this spreading are very low and would require a susceptible host, for example, an open cut on the therapist's hand coming in contact with blood or pus from the client's open wound.
†Capable of spreading infection from one's own body by scratching.

◆ Bacterial Infections

Normally the skin harbors a variety of bacterial flora, including the major pathogenic varieties of staphylococci and streptococci. The degree of their pathogenicity depends on the invasiveness and toxigenicity of the specific organisms, the integrity of the skin, the barrier of the host, and the immune and cellular defenses of the host. Organisms usually enter the skin through abrasions or puncture wounds of the hands. In the therapist's practice, periwound care requires cleaning away from the wound opening to avoid introducing bacteria from the surrounding skin into the wound. Clinical infection develops 3 to 7 days after inoculation. Septicemia can develop if treatment is not provided or if the person is immunocompromised.

People at risk for the development of bacterial infections include children and adults who are immunocompromised, such as occurs with acquired or inherited immunodeficiency; anyone in a debilitated physical condition; those receiving immunosuppressive therapy; and those with a generalized malignancy, such as leukemia or lymphoma. All these factors emphasize the importance of careful hand washing and cleanliness to prevent spread of infection before and after caring for infected people and their lesions.

Some conditions (e.g., impetigo) are easily spread by self-inoculation; therefore the affected person must be cautioned to avoid touching the involved area. Follicular lesions should not be squeezed because this will not hasten the resolution of the infection and may increase the risk of making the lesion worse or spreading the infection.

Impetigo

Definition and Overview. Impetigo is a superficial skin infection commonly caused by staphylococci or streptococci. It is most commonly found in infants, young children 2 to 5 years of age, and older people. Predisposing factors include close contact in schools, overcrowded living quarters, poor skin hygiene, anemia, malnutrition, and minor skin trauma. It can be spread by direct contact, environmental contamination, or an arthropod vector. Impetigo often occurs as a secondary infection in conditions characterized by a cutaneous barrier broken to microbes, such as eczema or herpes zoster excoriations.

Clinical Manifestations. Small macules (flat spots) rapidly develop into vesicles (small blisters) that become pustular (pus-filled). When the vesicle breaks, a thick yellow crust forms from the exudate, causing pain, surrounding erythema, regional adenitis (inflammation of gland), cellulitis (inflammation of tissue), and itching. Scratching spreads infection, a process called *autoinoculation*. Lesions frequently affect the face, heal slowly, and leave depigmented areas. If the infection is extensive, malaise, fever, and lymphadenopathy may also be present.

Medical Management. Single small lesions can often be managed by soaking them for 10 minutes with drying agents (Burow's solution). Oral antibiotics may be required. Rarely, extensive lesions require systemic antibiotics to reduce the risk of glomerulonephritis and to prevent this contagious condition from spreading. A skin swab may be necessary to determine the contaminating organism.

Cellulitis

Cellulitis is a suppurative inflammation of the dermis and subcutaneous tissues that spreads widely through tissue spaces. *Streptococcus pyogenes* or *Staphylococcus* are the usual cause of this infection although other pathogens may be responsible. Clients at increased risk for cellulitis include older adults and people with lowered resistance from diabetes, malnutrition, steroid therapy, and the presence of wounds or ulcers. Other predisposing factors include the presence of edema or other cutaneous inflammation or wounds (e.g., tinea, eczema, burns, trauma). There is a tendency for recurrence, especially at sites of lymphatic obstruction. See also the sections on Streptococcal Cellulitis in Chapter 7 and Lymphangitis in Chapter 12.

Cellulitis of the breast can occur following breast conservation therapy for breast cancer. Although only a minority of women who undergo this therapy will develop breast cellulitis, the therapist may be the first to observe signs of this disorder. A definitive pathogen has not been identified, and recurrent breast cellulitis is possible months to years after the procedure is completed. Local breast findings include the skin changes typical of cellulitis with or without fever.[4]

Cellulitis usually occurs in the loose tissue beneath the skin, but it may also occur in tissues beneath mucous membranes or around muscle bundles. The skin is erythematous, edematous, tender, and sometimes nodular. Erysipelas, a surface cellulitis of the skin, is characterized by patches of skin that are red with sharply defined borders and that feel hot to the touch. Red streaks extending from the patch indicate that the lymph vessels have been infected. Facial cellulitis involves the face, especially the cheek or periorbital or orbital tissues; the neck may also be affected. Pelvic cellulitis involves the tissues surrounding the uterus and is called *parametritis*.

Intravenous antibiotic infusion is the primary treatment; extensive cellulitis requires surgical debridement of the necrotic tissue. Lymphangitis may occur if cellulitis is untreated; and gangrene, metastatic abscesses, and sepsis can result.

◆ Viral Infections

Viruses are intracellular parasites that produce their effect by using the intracellular substances of the host cells. Viruses are composed only of DNA or ribonucleic acid (RNA), not both, usually enclosed in a protein shell, and are unable to provide for their own metabolic needs or to reproduce themselves. After a virus penetrates a cell of the host organism, it sheds the outer shell and disappears within the cell, where the nucleic acid core stimulates the host cell to form more virus material from its own intracellular substance. In a viral infection the epidermal cells react with inflammation and vesiculation (as in herpes zoster) or by proliferating to form growths (warts).

Herpes Zoster

Definition, Incidence, and Risk Factors. Herpes zoster, or shingles, is a local disease brought about by the reactivation of the same virus that causes a systemic disease called *varicella-zoster virus* (VZV; chickenpox). The initial infection with varicella is common during childhood. Shingles may occur and recur at any age, although peak incidence occurs between ages 50 and 70 years. An estimated 300,000 episodes of zoster occur annually. Of these episodes 95% are first occurrences and 5% are recurrences. By age 80 years, almost 15% of persons will have experienced at least one episode of zoster.[3] The disease is usually brought on by an immunocompromised state, such as occurs with advancing age, underlying malignancy, organ transplantation, or acquired immunodeficiency syndrome (AIDS).

Pathogenesis. Herpes zoster results from reactivation of varicella virus that has been dormant in the cerebral ganglia (extramedullary ganglia of the cranial nerves) or the ganglia of posterior nerve roots from a previous episode of chickenpox. The immunologic mechanism that controls latency of VZV is not well understood. One explanation is that the virus multiplies as it is reactivated and that it is neutralized by antibodies remaining from the initial infection. If effective antibodies are not present, the virus continues to multiply in the ganglia, destroying the host neuron and spreading down the sensory nerves to the skin. Factors associated with recurrent disease include aging, immunosuppression, intrauterine exposure to VZV, and varicella at a young age (<18 months).[3]

Clinical Manifestations.   The vesicular eruption of zoster generally occurs unilaterally in the distribution of a dermatome supplied by a dorsal root or extramedullary cranial nerve sensory ganglion. Most often, this involves the trunk or the area of the fifth cranial nerve. Two to four days before the eruption the affected person may have some warning (prodromal symptoms) that the virus has become reactivated, especially in repeat incidences. Early symptoms of pain and tingling along the affected spinal or cranial nerve dermatome are usually accompanied by fever, chills, malaise, and GI disturbances. One to three days later red papules are seen along a dermatome (Fig. 9-6). The lesions most commonly spread unilaterally around the thorax or vertically over the arms or legs.

Herpes papules rapidly develop into vesicles that vary in size and may be filled with clear fluid or pus. The vesicles are confined to the distribution of the infected nerve root and begin to dry 5 days after eruption with gradual, progressive healing over the next 2 to 4 weeks.

Postherpetic neuralgia, or pain in the area of the recurrence that persists after the lesions have resolved, is a distressing complication of zoster with no adequate therapy currently available. Incidence of postherpetic neuralgia increases sharply in people over the age of 60 years and may last as long as 1 year after the episode of zoster. Children are unaffected by postherpetic pain. In the adult, severe neuralgic pain can occur in peripheral areas innervated by the nerves arising in the inflamed root ganglia. The pain may be constant or intermittent and vary from light burning to a deep visceral sensation. The cause of postherpetic neuralgia is not fully understood. Scarring and degenerative changes involving the nerve trunks, ganglia, and skin may be important factors. The incidence of scarring and hyperpigmentation is much higher in older adults.

Occasionally herpes zoster involves the cranial nerves, especially the trigeminal and geniculate ganglia or the oculomotor nerve. Geniculate zoster may cause vesicle formation in the external auditory canal, ipsilateral facial palsy, hearing loss, dizziness, and loss of taste. Trigeminal ganglion involvement causes eye pain and possibly corneal and scleral damage with loss of vision.

In rare cases, herpes zoster leads to generalized central nervous system (CNS) infection, muscle atrophy, motor paralysis (usually transient), acute transverse myelitis, and ascending myelitis. More often, generalized infection causes acute retention of urine and unilateral paralysis of the diaphragm.

Medical Management

Diagnosis.   Diagnosis is usually based on clinical examination and recognition of the skin lesions with accompanying systemic signs of infection. Laboratory diagnosis may include culture and histologic examination of skin biopsy. Differentiation of herpes zoster from localized herpes simplex requires staining antibodies from vesicular fluid and identification using a fluorescent monoclonal antibody test that is very sensitive and specific. For those individuals who are uncertain whether they have had childhood varicella, a variety of serologic tests for the varicella antibody are available.

Treatment.   There is no curative agent for shingles, but supportive treatment to relieve itching and neuralgic pain is provided. The use of systemic corticosteroids within the first week of eruption may abort the attack and appears to reduce both the acute symptoms and the risk of postherpetic neuralgia in older persons. Acyclovir (Zovirax) seems to stop the progression of the rash and prevents visceral complications. Famciclovir, an oral drug, is comparable to acyclovir in effectiveness but has a longer duration of action and requires less frequent dosage. Hospitalized clients with varicella-zoster should be placed in isolation rooms, and personnel entering the room should wear gowns, gloves, and masks. Eye involvement in zoster requires ophthalmologic evaluation and treatment.

A live varicella vaccine (Varivax) is available for use in persons 12 months of age or older who have not had varicella.* The Advisory Committee on Immunization Practices (ACIP) also recommends the vaccine for use in susceptible persons following exposure to varicella. Data from the United States and Japan in a variety of settings indicate that varicella vaccine is effective in preventing illness or modifying the severity of illness if used within 3 days, and possibly up to 5 days, of exposure.[3]

Prognosis.   Overall prognosis is good unless the infection spreads to the brain (rare). Most people recover com-

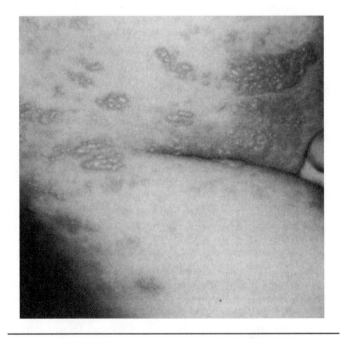

FIGURE   **9-6** Herpes zoster of the groin. (From Black JM, Matassarin-Jacobs E, editors: *Luckmann and Sorensen's medical-surgical nursing,* ed 4, Philadelphia, 1993, Saunders, p 1975.)

*Immunity appears to be long-lasting and is probably permanent in the majority of vaccines, but the actual duration of protection from the vaccine remains unknown and the need for booster doses has not been determined. Studies are ongoing to evaluate the need and timing for booster vaccination. Because seroconversion does not take place until 4 to 6 weeks after vaccination VZIG remains the only immediate treatment for some people. Women should not get pregnant for 3 months after getting the chickenpox vaccine.

pletely, with the possible exception of scarring and, with corneal damage, visual impairment. Occasionally, intractable pain associated with neuralgia may persist for months or years. Those persons who develop postherpetic neuralgia may require further medical intervention.

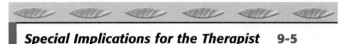

Special Implications for the Therapist   9-5

HERPES ZOSTER (see the discussion on herpesviruses in Chapter 7; also see the discussion on herpes zoster in Chapter 38)

Preferred Practice Patterns
7A: *Primary Prevention/Risk Reduction for Integumentary Disorders*
7B: *Impaired Integumentary Integrity Associated With Superficial Skin Involvement*

Adults with shingles are infectious to persons who have not had chickenpox, and the person with shingles can develop shingles more than one time. For this reason, therapists who have never had chickenpox should receive the vaccination; complications and morbidity associated with adult onset of varicella warrant this precaution. Any female therapist who is pregnant or planning a pregnancy should be tested for immune status if unsure about her previous history of varicella. This is especially important because transmissibility of the virus occurs 2 to 3 days before symptoms develop; immunocompromised clients with shingles are probably contagious during the entire period new lesions are appearing until all lesions are crusted over. This means anyone receiving intervention by a therapist may be an asymptomatic host during the period of communicability; exposure to self and further transmission to others can occur without the therapist's awareness.

Susceptible health care workers with significant exposure to varicella should be relieved from direct client contact from day 10 to day 21 after exposure. If workers develop chickenpox, varicella lesions must be crusted before they return to direct client contact.

The Centers for Disease Control and Prevention (CDC) has set up guidelines for the care of all clients regarding precautions for the transmission of infectious skin diseases (see Tables 9-3 and 7-6). These Standard Precautions (see Appendix A) should be used with all clients regardless of their disease status. All skin lesions are considered potentially infectious and should be handled as such. The careful use of these precautionary measures severely limits the transmission of any disease. In addition, each hospital has isolation precautions organized according to categories of disease to prevent the spread of infectious disease to others. Every health care professional must be familiar with these procedures and follow them carefully. See also the section on Isolation Procedures in Chapter 7 and Table 7-4.

Neither heat nor ultrasound should be used on a person with shingles because these modalities can increase the severity of the person's symptoms. For the person with severe herpetic pain, relaxation techniques may be useful. In the case of unresolved postherpetic neuralgia, the individual may benefit from a program of chronic pain management. ■

Warts (Verrucae)

Warts are common, benign viral infections of the skin and adjacent mucous membranes caused by human papillomaviruses (HPVs). There are more than 50 different varieties of these viruses depending on their location on the skin. The incidence of warts is highest in children and young adults, but warts can occur at any age. Transmission is probably through direct contact, but autoinoculation is possible.

Warts may appear singly or as multiple lesions with thick white surfaces containing many pointed projections. Clinical manifestations depend on the type of wart and its location. The most common wart (verruca vulgaris) is referred to as such and appears as a rough, elevated, round surface most frequently on the extremities, especially the hands and fingers. Plantar warts are slightly elevated or flat, occurring singly or in large clusters referred to as mosaic warts, primarily at pressure points of the feet.

Medical Management

Diagnosis.   Diagnosis is usually made on the basis of visual examination. Plantar warts can be differentiated from corns and calluses by certain distinguishing features. Plantar warts obliterate natural lines of the skin, may contain red or black capillary dots that are easily discernible if the surface of the wart is shaved down with a scalpel, and are painful on application of pressure. Both plantar warts and corns have a soft, pulpy core surrounded by a thick callous ring; plantar warts and calluses are flush with the skin surface.

Treatment.   Some warts respond to simple treatment, and some disappear spontaneously. Warts can be chronic or recurrent. Many treatment regimens are available. The specific choice of treatment method is influenced by the location of the wart or warts, the size and number of warts, presence of secondary infection, amount of tenderness present on palpation, age and gender of the client, history of previous treatment, and individual compliance with treatment. Over-the-counter salicylic acid preparations (e.g., Duofilm, Wart-off, Clear Away, or other wart-removing compounds) applied topically may be used to induce peeling of the skin.

Cryotherapy is performed with either liquid nitrogen or solid carbon dioxide. This procedure is widely used as the cosmetically preferred treatment choice, but it is painful. The procedure causes epidermal necrosis; the area dries and peels off together with the wart. *Acids* in liquid form or as a paste (salicylic acid, lactic acid) can be painted on warts daily, removed after 24 hours, and reapplied. This treatment choice is not recommended for areas where perspiration is heavy, for areas likely to get wet, or for exposed body parts where patches are cosmetically undesirable. Acid therapy requires a commitment from the client or family to perform it on a daily basis. Electrodesiccation and *curettage* of warts are widely used for common warts and occasionally for plantar warts. High-frequency electric current destroys the wart and is followed by surgical removal of dead tissue at the base with application of an antibiotic ointment and bandage for 48 hours. Atrophic scarring may occur, and the recurrence rate is 20% to 40%. The use of mechanical (nonthermal) ultrasound has been advocated by some in the treatment of plantar warts, but this has not been widely accepted by the medical community.

◆ Fungal Infections (Dermatophytoses)

Fungal infections such as ringworm are caused by a group of fungi that invade the stratum corneum, hair, and nails.[46] These are superficial infections that live on, not in, the skin and are confined to the dead keratin layers, unable to survive in the deeper layers. Since the keratin is being shed (desquamated) constantly, the fungus must multiply at a rate that equals the rate of keratin production to maintain itself; otherwise the infection would be shed with the discarded skin cells.

Fungal infections will proliferate without treatment; antifungal creams are available over the counter, but diagnosis is required to identify the skin lesion.

Ringworm (tinea corporis)

Dermatophytoses, or fungal infections of the hair, skin, or nails, are designated by the Latin word *tinea*, with further designation related to the affected area of the body (see Table 9-3). Tinea corporis, or ringworm, has no association with worms but rather is marked by the formation of ring-shaped pigmented patches covered with vesicles or scales that often become itchy (Fig. 9-7). Transmission can occur directly through contact with infected lesions or indirectly through contact with contaminated objects, such as shoes, towels, or shower stalls.

Diagnosis can be made through laboratory examination of the affected skin. Treatment for any type of ringworm requires maintaining clean, dry skin and the application of antifungal powder or topical agent as prescribed. Treatment with the drug griseofulvin may take weeks to months to complete and should be continued throughout the prescribed dosage schedule even if symptoms subside. Possible side effects of this agent include headache, GI upset, fatigue, insomnia, and photosensitivity. Prolonged use of this drug requires monitoring of liver function.

Occasionally an obese client with tinea corporis is referred to therapy for wound care secondary to skin breakdown. Open wet dressings may be applied two or three times daily to areas of moist, denuded skin to help decrease inflammation.

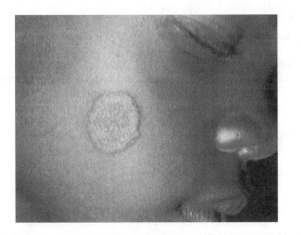

FIGURE **9-7** Scales forming multiple circular lesions with clear centers are characteristic of tinea corporis (ringworm). These lesions are hyperpigmented in whites, are depigmented in dark-skinned people, and occur most often on the face, chest, abdomen, and back of arms. (From Hurwitz S: *Clinical pediatric dermatology: a textbook of skin disorders of childhood and adolescence*, Philadelphia, 1981, Saunders, p 381.)

Athlete's Foot (tinea pedis)

Tinea pedis, or athlete's foot, causes erythema, skin peeling, and pruritus between the toes that may spread from the interdigital spaces to the sole. Severe infection may result in inflammation, with severe itching and pain on walking. Clean, dry socks and adequate footwear (well-ventilated, properly fitting) are important. After washing the feet and drying thoroughly between the toes, antifungal cream or powder (the latter to absorb perspiration and prevent excoriation) can be applied.

Special Implications for the Therapist **9-6**

FUNGAL INFECTIONS

Preferred Practice Patterns
7A: *Primary Prevention/Risk Reduction for Integumentary Disorders*
7B: *Impaired Integumentary Integrity Associated With Superficial Skin Involvement*

The infectious nature of fungal infections requires specific hygienic measures common to all infectious conditions. Affected persons should not share hair care products (e.g., combs, brushes, headgear), clothes, or other articles that have been in proximity to the infected area. Affected persons must use their own towels and linens.

Since fungal infections are superficial (living on the skin), the therapist is advised to avoid shaving body hair for the application of electrodes or other adhesives. Cutting the hair closely will avoid providing microscopic nicks that can give entrance for the transmission of surface pathogens.

Ringworm
Since ringworm can be acquired by animal-to-human transmission (see Table 9-3), all household pets must be examined for the presence of ringworm as well. Other sources of infection include seats with headrest (e.g., theater seats, seats on public transportation, or other public seats that can be shared).

Athlete's Foot
Athlete's foot, often observed by the therapist (see previous description), should be discussed with the client. Although the client may consider this condition a nuisance or a minimal problem that does not require medical attention, it can be an entry point for bacterial infections, especially in older adults. Keeping athlete's foot under control is an important way to prevent cellulitis, a bacterial infection in the legs, and is especially important in the presence of diabetes.[48] ∎

◆ Other Parasitic Infections

Some parasitic infections of the skin are caused by insect and animal contacts. Contact with insects that puncture the skin for the purpose of sucking blood, injecting venom, or laying their eggs is relatively common. Substances deposited by insects are considered foreign to the host and may create an allergic sensitivity in that individual and produce pruritus, urticaria, or systemic reactions of a greater or lesser degree, depending on the individual's sensitivity.

Scabies

Definition. Scabies (mites) is a highly contagious skin eruption caused by a mite, *Sarcoptes scabiei*. It is a common public health problem with an estimated prevalence of 300 million worldwide. The female mite burrows into the skin and deposits eggs that hatch into larvae in a few days. Scabies are easily transmitted by skin-to-skin contact or from contact with contaminated objects, such as linens or shared inanimate objects. Infections with human T-cell leukemia/lymphoma virus I (HTLV-I) and HIV are associated with scabies.[24] Mites can spread rapidly between members of the same household, nursing home, or institution, but the inflammatory response and itching do not occur until approximately 30 to 60 days after initial contact.

Clinical Manifestations. The symptoms include intense pruritus (worse at night), usually excoriated skin, and the burrow, which is a linear ridge with a vesicle at one end. The mite is usually found in the burrow, commonly in the interdigital web spaces, flexor aspects of the wrist (volar surface), axillae, waistline, nipples in females, genitalia in males, and the umbilicus. Intense scratching can lead to severe excoriation and secondary bacterial infection. Itching can become generalized secondary to sensitization.

Medical Management

Diagnosis and Treatment. The mite can be excavated from one end of a burrow with a needle or a scalpel blade and examined under a microscope. In long-standing cases, a mite may not be found. At that point treatment is based on a presumptive diagnosis. Treatment has traditionally been with a scabicide, usually a lotion or cream containing permethrin or lindane, applied to the entire body from the neck down. Single oral-dose therapy of ivermectin (Stromectol) is a new treatment for this infestation. Permethrin is generally the treatment of choice for head lice and scabies because of its residual effect and because toxicity and absorption are minimal. Ivermectin may be reserved for cases where permethrin fails[31]; further research is advocated regarding the safety and effectiveness of ivermectin.

Special Implications for the Therapist   9-7

SCABIES

Preferred Practice Patterns
7A: *Primary Prevention/Risk Reduction for Integumentary Disorders*
7B: *Impaired Integumentary Integrity Associated With Superficial Skin Involvement*

If a hospitalized person has scabies, prevent transmission to self and others by practicing good hand-washing technique and by wearing gloves when touching the affected person and a gown when in close contact. Observe wound and skin precautions for 24 hours after treatment of scabies. Gas-autoclave blood pressure cuffs or other equipment used with the affected person before using them on other people. All linens and toweling used must be isolated after use until the person is noninfec-

---

tious. If treated anywhere outside the hospital room (e.g., on a plinth or treatment mat), the area must be thoroughly disinfected after each session.

In using a scabicide, the individual must understand that NO area can be missed. After 24 hours, the affected person should bathe. All bed linens and clothes must be laundered in hot water or dry-cleaned. Other household members and those in close contact with the affected person should be treated. A second application of the cream or lotion is applied 7 days later. The same procedure is followed. Itching may persist for 1 to 2 weeks after treatment until the stratum corneum is replaced, but lesions on the forearms or legs can be occluded with Unna's boots to eliminate the scratch-itch cycle (Fig. 9-8). Widespread bacterial infections require additional treatment with systemic antibiotics. ∎

Pediculosis (Lousiness)

Pediculosis is an infestation by *Pediculus humanus*, a very common parasite infecting the head, body, and genital area. Transmission is from one person to another, usually on shared personal items, such as combs, lockers, clothes, or furniture. Lice are not carried or transmitted by pets. School-age children are easily infected as are people who live in overcrowded surroundings and those older adults who have poor personal hygiene, depend on others for care, or live in a nursing home.

Pediculus humanus var. *capitis*, the head louse, is transmitted through personal contact or through shared hairbrushes or shared head wear. Severe itching accompanied by secondary eczematous changes develops, and small grayish or white nits (eggs) are usually seen attached to the base of the hair shafts.

Pediculus corporis, the body or clothes louse, produces intense itching, which in turn results in severe excoriations from scratching and possible secondary bacterial infections. The lice or nits are generally found in the seams of the affected individual's clothing.

Pediculus pubis (*Phthirus pubi*), the pubic or crab louse, is usually transmitted by sexual contact but can be transferred on clothing or towels. The lice and nits are usually found at the base of the pubic hairs. Sometimes dark brown particles (louse excreta) may be seen on underclothes.

Medical Management. Traditional treatment has been with the appropriate cleaning solution (e.g., shampoo or soap containing permethrin) specific to the type of louse present. As with scabies, single oral-dose therapy of ivermectin (Stromectol) is a new treatment for this infestation (see previous section on Scabies).

Special Implications for the Therapist   9-8

PEDICULOSIS

Preferred Practice Patterns
7A: *Primary Prevention/Risk Reduction for Integumentary Disorders*
7B: *Impaired Integumentary Integrity Associated With Superficial Skin Involvement*

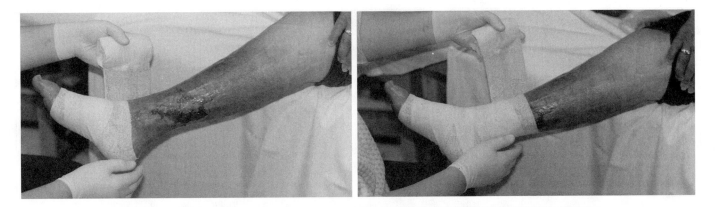

FIGURE **9-8** Although most often used in cases of venous insufficiency, the application of Unna's boot to the forearms or legs can be used with a variety of skin lesions to eliminate the scratch-itch cycle. Unna's boot is a dressing made of gauze impregnated with gelatin, zinc oxide, calamine, and glycerin. The bandage is applied in a spiral fashion and allowed to dry, forming a rigid dressing. This dressing can be allowed to stay intact for 7 days. (Courtesy Pam Unger, P.T., Community General Hospital, Center for Wound Management, Reading, Pa, 1995.)

The therapist must always be conscious of the personal hygiene of all clients. Anyone can get pediculosis regardless of age, socioeconomic status, or status of personal cleanliness. Wear gloves while carefully inspecting the head of any adult or child who scratches excessively. Look for bite marks, redness, and nits or movement that indicates a louse. If exposure to lice occurs, treatment for the client as well as the therapist may be required depending on the exposure level. Use the same precautions outlined earlier in the section on Scabies.

All combs and brushes should be soaked in the cleaning agent, and clothing must be boiled, dry-cleaned, or washed in a machine (hot cycle). The seams of the clothing should be pressed with a hot iron. Carpets, car seats, pillows, stuffed animals, rugs, mattresses, upholstered furniture, and similar objects that come in contact with the affected person must be vacuumed or cleaned thoroughly with hot water and the cleaning agent. Any item that cannot be cleaned can be stored in a sealed plastic bag for 2 to 3 weeks until all lice have been killed. ■

SKIN CANCER

The American Cancer Society (ACS) estimates that skin cancers are the most prevalent form of cancer, eventually affecting nearly all white people older than 65 years of age. Skin cancer is the most rapidly increasing cancer in the United States with over 1 million new cases of nonmelanoma (i.e., basal and squamous cell) skin cancer diagnosed annually in the United States. There is no evidence that this epidemic has peaked.[43] Solar radiation (exposure to midrange-wavelength ultraviolet B [UVB] radiation) causes most skin cancers, and protection from the sun during the first 2 decades of life significantly reduces the risk of skin cancer (Box 9-7). The melanoma rate is rising most rapidly in persons younger than 40 years of age and is now the most common cancer in women between the ages of 25 and 29 years and second only to breast cancer in the age-group from 30 to 34 years.

In this chapter, skin cancer is discussed in three broad categories: benign, premalignant, and malignant (Table 9-4). Malignant lesions of the skin are considered as either melanoma or nonmelanoma. Kaposi's sarcoma, which occurs in the skin, is not included in these categories and is discussed separately in this chapter.

Benign skin lesions, such as seborrheic keratosis, keratoacanthoma, or nevi (moles), do not usually undergo transition to malignant melanoma* and do not usually require treatment. Precancerous lesions, such as actinic keratosis or Bowen's disease, may progress to malignancy and must be carefully evaluated. The most common types of (nonmelanoma) malignant skin cancer are basal call carcinoma and squamous cell carcinoma. These carcinomas occur twice as often in white men as in white women, and the incidence increases steadily with age. A third type of malignant skin cancer (also affecting white men more than white women), malignant melanoma, is the most serious skin cancer, resulting in early metastasis and possible death.

◆ Benign Tumors
Seborrheic Keratosis
Seborrheic keratosis is a benign proliferation of basal cells occurring most frequently after middle age and presenting as multiple lesions on the chest, back, and face. The lesions often appear following hormonal therapy or inflammatory dermatoses. The areas are waxy, smooth, or raised lesions that vary in color from yellow to flesh tones to dark brown or black. Their size varies from barely palpable to large verrucous (wartlike) plaques. These tumors are usually left untreated unless they itch or cause pain. Otherwise, cryotherapy with liquid nitrogen is an effective treatment.

Nevi (Moles)
Nevi are pigmented or nonpigmented lesions that form from aggregations of melanocytes beginning early in life. Most

*Although most moles remain benign skin lesions, when malignant melanoma does occur, it often arises from a preexisting mole, derived from pigment cells (melanocytes) of the skin.

BOX 9-7

Important Trends in Skin Cancer

Incidence

More than 1 million cases per year with the majority being the highly curable basal or squamous cell cancers; not as common is the most serious skin cancer (malignant melanoma) with an estimated 53,600 new cases per year.

Mortality

Total estimated deaths in 2002 were 9600: 7400 from malignant melanoma and 2200 from other skin cancers.

Risk Factors

Excessive exposure to ultraviolet radiation from the sun; fair complexion; occupational exposure to coal tar, pitch, creosote, arsenic compounds, and radium; chronic immunosuppression; skin cancer is negligible in blacks because of heavy skin pigmentation.

Warning Signals

Any unusual skin condition, especially a change in the size or color of a mole or other darkly pigmented growth or spot.

Prevention and Early Detection

Avoidance of sun when ultraviolet light is strongest (e.g., between 10 AM and 4 PM); use sunscreen preparations; basal and squamous cell skin cancers often form a pale, waxlike, pearly nodule or a red, sharply outlined patch; melanomas are usually dark brown or black; they start as small molelike growths that increase in size, change color, become ulcerated, and bleed easily from a slight injury.

Treatment

There are four methods of treatment: surgery, electrodesiccation (tissue destruction by heat), radiation therapy, and cryosurgery (tissue destruction by freezing); for malignant melanomas, wide and often deep excisions and removal of nearby lymph nodes are required.

Survival

For basal cell and squamous cell cancers, cure is virtually ensured with early detection and treatment; malignant melanoma, however, metastasizes quickly; this accounts for a lower 5-year survival rate for white people with this disease.

TABLE 9-4

Types of Skin Cancer

BENIGN	PREMALIGNANT	NONMELANOMA	MELANOMA
Seborrheic keratosis	Actinic keratosis	Basal cell carcinoma	Superficial spreading melanoma
Nevi (moles)	Bowen's disease	Squamous cell carcinoma	Nodular melanoma
			Lentigo maligna melanoma
			Acral lentiginous melanoma

moles are either brown, black, or flesh-colored and may appear on any part of the skin. They vary in size and thickness, occurring in groups or singly. Nevi seldom undergo transition to malignant melanoma, but as previously mentioned, when malignant melanoma does occur, it often arises from a preexisting mole; the chances of cancerous transformation are increased as a result of constant irritation. Any change in size, color, or texture of a mole; bleeding; or any excessive itching should be reported to a physician.

◆ Precancerous Conditions

There are two common premalignant skin lesions: actinic keratosis and Bowen's disease.

Actinic Keratosis

Actinic keratosis (also known as solar keratosis) is a skin disease resulting from many years of exposure to the sun's UV rays. The damage caused by overexposure to sunlight results in abnormal cell growth, causing a well-defined, crusty, or sandpaper-like patch or bump that appears on chronically sun-exposed areas of the body (e.g., face, ears, lower lip, bald scalp, dorsa of hands and forearms). The base may be light or dark, tan, pink, red, or a combination of these, or it may be the same color as the skin. The scale or crust is horny, dry, and rough; it is often recognized by touch rather than sight. Occasionally it itches or produces a pricking or tender sensation. The skin abnormality or lesion develops slowly to reach a size that is most often 3 to 6 mm. It may disappear only to reappear later. Often there are several actinic keratoses present at one time.

Actinic keratosis affects nearly 100% of the older white population. It is most common in fair-complexioned, blue- or green-eyed, middle-aged men with a history of sun exposure (solar radiation). The number of lesions that develop is directly related to heredity and lifetime exposure to the sun. There is a known risk of malignant degeneration and subsequent metastatic potential in neglected lesions. Almost half of the estimated 5 million current cases of skin cancer began as actinic keratosis lesions. It is important that this condition be diagnosed properly because it is often difficult to distinguish a large or hypertrophic actinic keratosis from a squamous cell carcinoma. A biopsy may be indicated.

Not all keratoses need to be removed. The decision about treatment protocol is based on the nature of the lesion and the age and health of the affected person. Treatment may be with 5-fluorouracil (5-FU, Efudex), a topical antimetabolite that inhibits cell division, or masoprocol cream; cryosurgery using liquid nitrogen; or curettage by electrodesiccation (superficial tissue destruction through the use of bursts of electrical current). These clients should be advised to avoid sun exposure and use a high-potency (sun protection factor [SPF] 15+)* sunscreen 30 to 60 minutes before going outside. Some conditions call for more invasive treatments, such as laser resurfacing (outer layers of the skin are vaporized) or chemical peels (outer layers are burned off via chemical solution). In June 2000 the U.S. Food and Drug Administration (FDA) approved the use of photodynamic treatment of actinic keratosis of the face and scalp using a topical application (Levulan Kerastick) followed by exposure to a nonlaser blue light source.

Bowen's Disease

Bowen's disease can occur anywhere on the skin (exposed and unexposed areas) or mucous membranes (especially the glans penis in uncircumcised males). It presents as a persistent, brown to reddish brown, scaly plaque with well-defined margins. Often the person has a history of arsenic exposure in youth. Multiple lesions have been associated with an increased number of internal malignancies and therefore require close follow-up. Treatment is with surgical excision and topical 5-FU.

◆ Malignant Neoplasms
Basal Cell Carcinoma
Definition and Overview.   Basal cell carcinoma is a slow-growing surface epithelial skin tumor originating from undifferentiated basal cells contained in the epidermis. This type of carcinoma rarely metastasizes beyond the skin and does not invade blood or lymph vessels but can cause significant local destruction. Until recently, this tumor rarely appeared before age 40 years and was more prevalent in blond, fair-skinned males. In the age-group under 30 years, more women than men develop skin cancer associated with the use of indoor tanning booths with concentrated doses of UV radiation.† It is the most common malignant tumor affecting whites, with a reported 100,000 new cases each year; blacks and Asians are rarely affected.

Etiologic and Risk Factors.   Prolonged sun exposure and intermittent sun exposure are the most common causes of basal cell carcinoma; but arsenic ingestion (in drinking water, insecticides), UV radiation exposure, burns, immunosuppres-

sion (e.g., organ transplant recipients, individuals who are HIV-positive),* genetic predisposition, and rarely, the site of vaccinations are other possible causes. These lesions are seen most frequently in geographic regions with intense sunlight in people with outdoor occupations and on those areas most exposed, the face and neck. Dark-skinned people are rarely affected because their basal cells contain the pigment melanin, a protective factor against sun exposure. Anyone who has had one basal cell carcinoma is at increased risk of developing others. Recurrences of previously treated lesions are possible, usually within the first 2 years after initial treatment.

Pathogenesis.   The pathogenesis of basal cell tumors remains uncertain, and basal cell carcinoma is considered biologically unusual. It is a stable growth characterized by monotonous structure (the same in small as well as large tumors), the absence of progression to metastasis, and the small amount of chromosomal damage (as compared with moderate chromosomal damage associated with squamous cell carcinoma). To the dismay of investigators seeking to design experiments, basal cell carcinomas are very seldom seen in animals and not found in laboratory rodents at all. Whereas squamous cell carcinoma is often preceded by a precursor (actinic keratosis), there are no known precursors to basal cell carcinoma. This fact suggests that basal cell carcinoma tumors need only a few mutations to induce malignant transformation.[91]

One theory suggests that these tumors arise as a result of a defect that prevents the cells from being shed by the normal keratinization process. The process of epidermal cell maturation is called *keratinization* because the cells synthesize a fibrous protein called *keratin*. Basal cells that lack the normal keratin proteins form basal cell tumors. Another hypothesis is that undifferentiated basal cells become carcinomatous instead of differentiating into sweat glands, sebum, and hair. See also the section on Squamous Cell Carcinoma: Pathogenesis.

Clinical Manifestations.   Basal cell carcinoma (Fig. 9-9) typically has a pearly or ivory appearance, has rolled edges, and is slightly elevated above the skin surface, with small blood vessels on the surface (telangiectasia) (see Fig. 9-2). The nodule is usually painless and slowly increases in size and may ulcerate centrally. More than 65% of basal cell carcinomas are found on the head and neck. Other locations are the trunk, especially the upper back and chest. If these lesions are not detected and treated early, they may invade deep tissues and ulcerate (see Prognosis).

Medical Management

Diagnosis and Treatment.   Diagnosis by clinical examination of appearance must be confirmed via biopsy and histologic study. Treatment depends on the size, location, and depth of the lesion and may include curettage and electrodesiccation, chemotherapy, surgical excision, Mohs' chemosurgery (serial application and removal of pathologic tissue using a fixative paste such as zinc chloride), and irradiation. Irradiation is used if the tumor location requires it and in older or debilitated people who cannot tolerate surgery. Radiation

---

*SPF 30+ is recommended for people of fair complexion. Sunscreens are not recommended for infants under 6 months of age. Infants should be kept out of the sun or shaded from it. Fabric with a tight weave, such as cotton, is suggested.

†About 80% of indoor tanning patrons are women, with an average age of 26 years.

---

*Immunosuppressed organ transplant recipients are more likely to develop squamous cell carcinoma, whereas HIV-infected adults are far more likely to have basal cell carcinoma.

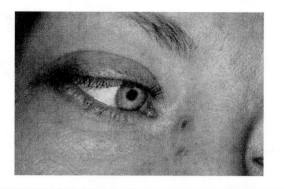

FIGURE   **9-9**   Basal cell carcinoma can appear as a red patch; a shiny, pearly, or translucent pink, red, or white bump; a crusty, open sore that will not heal; or a scarlike area. There may be a rolled border with an indented center. (From Skin Cancer Foundation: *What you need to know about skin cancer*, New York, 1993, The Foundation.)

therapy is generally contraindicated in persons less than 50 years of age because of the risk of recurrence and the development of secondary radiation-induced tumors of the skin.*

If the tumor is identified and treated early, local excision or even nonexcisional destruction is usually curative. Skin grafting may be required in cases where large areas of tissue have been removed. A new experimental treatment called *photodynamic therapy (PDT)* is being investigated in the treatment of superficial nonmelanoma skin cancers. This technique requires the administration of a drug that induces photosensitivity, followed in 48 to 72 hours by exposure to light that helps outline the tumor. The tumor cells concentrate this drug so as to allow selective destruction of the cancer cells when exposed to a laser light of 630 nanometers (nm).[63,117] Clinical trials are under way investigating the use of chemopreventive agents, such as vitamin A analogs called *retinoids*. These topical agents may potentially complement sunscreens and result in decreased incidence, morbidity, and mortality of skin cancer.[112] Investigation continues in the use of immunotherapy with interferon in skin cancer management.

Prognosis.   If left untreated, basal cell lesions slowly invade surrounding tissues over months and years, destroying local tissues such as bone and cartilage, especially around the eyes, ears, and nose.

Squamous Cell Carcinoma
Definition and Overview.   Squamous cell carcinomas are the second most common skin cancer in whites, usually arising in sun-damaged skin, such as the rim of the ear, the face, the lips and mouth, and the dorsa of the hands (Fig. 9-10). It is a tumor of the epidermal keratinocytes and rarely occurs in dark-skinned people.

Squamous cell tumors may be one of two types: in situ (confined to the site of origin) and invasive (infiltrate surrounding tissue). *In situ* squamous cell carcinoma is usually confined to the epidermis but may extend into the dermis.

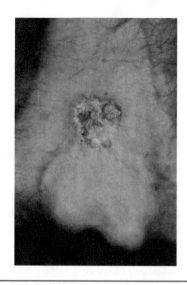

FIGURE   **9-10**   Squamous cell carcinoma can take the form of a persistently scaly, red patch that sometimes crusts or bleeds; an open sore that does not heal; or a raised or wartlike growth that may bleed. (From Skin Cancer Foundation: *What you need to know about skin cancer*, New York, 1993, The Foundation.)

Common premalignant skin lesions associated with in situ carcinomas are actinic keratosis and Bowen's disease (see earlier section). *Invasive* squamous cell carcinoma can arise from premalignant lesions of the skin, including sun-damaged skin, actinic dermatitis, scars, whitish discolored areas (leukoplakia), radiation-induced keratosis, tar and oil keratosis, and chronic ulcers and sinuses.

Incidence.   As with basal cell carcinoma, fair-skinned people have a higher incidence of squamous cell carcinoma. This particular type of tumor has a peak incidence at 60 years of age and affects men more than women.

Etiologic and Risk Factors.   Predisposing factors associated with squamous cell carcinoma include cumulative overexposure to UV radiation (e.g., outdoor employment or residence in a warm, sunny climate), presence of premalignant lesions such as actinic keratosis or Bowen's disease, radiation therapy, ingestion of herbicides containing arsenic, chronic skin irritation and inflammation, exposure to local carcinogens (tar, oil), and hereditary disease such as xeroderma pigmentosum and albinism. Organ transplant recipients who are chronically immunosuppressed are at risk for the development of recurring squamous cell carcinoma. Rarely, squamous cell carcinoma may develop on the site of a smallpox vaccination, psoriasis, or chronic discoid lupus erythematosus.

Pathogenesis.   UV radiation continues to be one of the most important causes of skin cancer because the sun's UV rays damage the DNA inside the nuclei of the epidermal cells, triggering enzymes to repair the damage. We differ in our ability to produce repair enzymes, which may explain our differences in tanning ability as well as susceptibility to skin cancer. Not all DNA lesions are properly repaired, increasing the risk of skin cancer. Newer studies show that when DNA damage occurs, a cell surface molecule (Fas ligand; FasL) belonging to the tumor necrosis factor family binds to its receptor Fas and

---

*Radiotherapy can be followed by chronic skin ulcers that are difficult to close, much less heal. Some radiation-induced ulcers open on and off for years, and some just develop 10 to 20 years after the radiation therapy.[107]

attaches to the damaged cells, inducing them to die by apoptosis (i.e., programmed cell death).

These suicidal cells known as keratinocytes take themselves out of action, and the less damaged ones repair themselves. After many years of cumulative sun exposure keratinocytes can become malignant. But even then, the cancers (either basal or squamous cell) grow slowly and do not spread easily. On the other hand, melanocytes, the cells that give rise to melanomas, seem highly resistant to self-destruction. After a person gets badly sunburned, damaged melanocytes continue to replicate, increasing the chance that some will turn malignant. These studies suggest that Fas ligand is a critical defense against the accumulation of mutations caused by sunlight exposure. Its absence or inactivation may be key to the development of skin cancer.[54,89]

Clinical Manifestations.
Squamous cell lesions are more difficult to characterize than basal cell tumors. The squamous cell tumor has poorly defined margins since the edge blends into the surrounding sun-damaged skin. This type of carcinoma can present as an ulcer, a flat red area, a cutaneous horn, an indurated plaque, or a nodule. It may be red to flesh-colored and surrounded by scaly tissue. More than 80% of squamous cell carcinomas occur in the head and neck region.

Usually lesions on unexposed skin tend to be more invasive and more likely to metastasize with the exception of lesions on the lower lip and ears. These sites tend to metastasize early, beginning with the process of induration and inflammation of the lesion. Metastasis can occur to the regional lymph nodes, producing characteristic systemic symptoms of pain, malaise, fatigue, weakness, and anorexia.

Medical Management

Diagnosis, Treatment, and Prognosis. An excisional biopsy provides definitive diagnosis and staging (Table 9-5) of squamous cell carcinoma. Other laboratory tests may be appropriate depending on the presence of systemic symptoms. The size, shape, location, and invasiveness of a squamous cell tumor and the condition of the underlying tissue determine the treatment method selected (see the section on Basal Cell Carcinoma; see also Box 9-7). A deeply invasive tumor may require a combination of techniques. As with all benign, premalignant, or malignant skin lesions, sun protection is vitally important (see Box 9-4).

All the major treatment methods have excellent rates of cure; generally, the prognosis is better with a well-differentiated lesion in an unusual location.

Malignant Melanoma
Definition and Overview. Malignant melanoma is a neoplasm of the skin originating from melanocytes or cells that synthesize the pigment melanin. The melanomas occur most frequently in the skin but can also be found in the oral cavity, esophagus, anal canal, vagina, or meninges or within the eye. The clinical varieties of cutaneous melanoma are classified into four types (Fig. 9-11):

1. *Superficial spreading melanoma* (SSM) is the most common type of melanoma and accounts for 75% of cutaneous melanomas.* SSM can occur on any part of the

---

*Percentages of each of the four classifications in this section were obtained from reference 13.

TABLE 9-5

Staging of Squamous Cell Carcinoma

*Primary Tumor (T)**

TX	Primary tumor cannot be assessed
T0	No evidence of primary tumor
Tis	Carcinoma in situ
T1	Tumor ≤ 2 cm in greatest dimension
T2	Tumor >2 cm but not >5 cm in greatest dimension
T3	Tumor >5 cm in greatest dimension
T4	Tumor invades deep extradermal structures (i.e., cartilage, skeletal muscle, bone)

Regional Lymph Nodes (N)

NX	Regional lymph nodes cannot be assessed
N0	No regional lymph node metastasis
N1	Regional lymph node metastasis

Distant Metastasis (M)

MX	Presence of distant metastasis cannot be assessed
M0	No distant metastasis
M1	Distant metastasis

Used with permission of the American Joint Committee on Cancer (AJCC), Chicago. The original source for this material is the *AJCC handbook for staging of cancer,* ed 5, Philadelphia, 1998, Lippincott-Raven.
*In the case of multiple simultaneous tumors, the tumor with the highest T category will be classified and the number of separate tumors will be indicated in parentheses, for example, T2 (5).

---

body, especially in areas of chronic irritation, the legs of females between the knees and ankles, or the upper back in both genders. SSM is usually diagnosed in people between 20 and 60 years of age. It usually arises in a preexisting mole and presents as a brown or black, raised patch with an irregular border and variable pigmentation (red, white, and blue; brown-black; black-blue). It is usually asymptomatic. With advanced lesions, itching and bleeding may occur.

2. *Nodular melanoma* can be found on any part of the body with no specific site preference. Men between 20 and 60 years of age are affected more often than women. It is often described as a small, suddenly appearing but quickly enlarging, uniformly and darkly pigmented papule (may be grayish) accounting for approximately 12% of cutaneous melanomas. This type invades the dermis and metastasizes early.

3. *Lentigo maligna melanoma (LMM)* is a less common type of lesion occurring predominantly on sun-exposed areas, especially the head, neck, and dorsa of hands or under the fingernails, in the 50- to 80-year-old age-group, accounting for 6% to 10% of cutaneous melanomas. This lesion looks like a large (3 to 6 cm), flat freckle with an irregular border containing varied pigmentation of brown, black, blue-black, red, and white found in a single lesion. These lesions enlarge and become progressively irregularly pigmented over time. Approximately one-third develop into malignant melanoma and therefore bear careful watching.

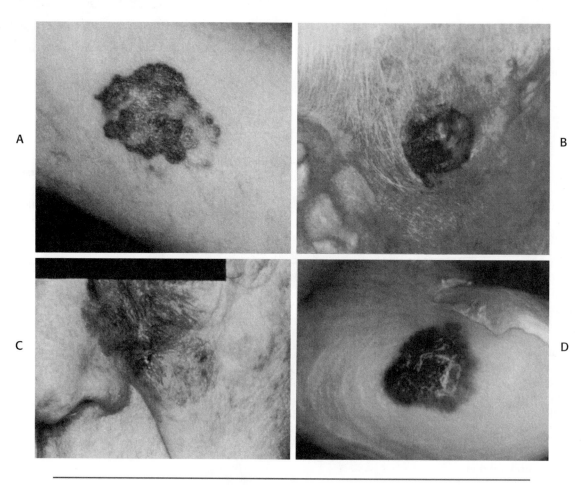

FIGURE **9-11** **A,** Superficial spreading melanoma: an irregular margin with multiple colors of black, blue, pale red, and white may be seen. **B,** Nodular lesion of melanoma. **C,** Lentigo maligna: if left alone, progression to lentigo maligna melanoma occurs. **D,** Acral lentiginous melanoma. (Courtesy Dr. Neil A. Fenske, Tampa. From Callen JP, Jorizzo J, editors: *Dermatological signs of internal disease*, ed 2, Philadelphia, 1995, Saunders, pp 173-174.)

4. *Acral lentiginous melanoma (ALM)* is a relatively uncommon form of melanoma accounting for 5% of all cutaneous melanomas. It is the most common form of melanoma in dark-skinned people (e.g., Africans, Asians). These lesions usually have flat, dark brown portions with raised bumpy areas that are predominantly brown-black or blue-black. Most common areas include low-pigment sites where hair is absent, such as the palms of the hands, soles of the feet, nail beds of fingers and toes, and mucous membranes.

Incidence. Malignant melanoma accounts for up to 5% of all cancers, currently affecting 1 in 75 people in the course of a lifetime.* Epidemiologists, who report that the incidence of melanoma is doubling every 10 to 20 years, call this a melanoma epidemic. The ACS estimates 53,600 new cases of malignant melanoma in 2002,[43] accounting for 7400 deaths, more than from any other skin disorder. The peak incidence is between 40 and 60 years, affecting women more than men but with a greater mortality rate among men. The incidence is rising in younger age groups but remains rare in children before adolescence.

Etiologic and Risk Factors. Most people who develop melanoma have blond or red hair, fair skin, and blue eyes; are prone to sunburn; and are of Celtic or Scandinavian ancestry (Box 9-8). These risk factors are believed to be linked to variations in a gene called *MC1R* that assists in producing melanin pigment to help protect the skin against UV rays.*[50,97] Melanomas appear to be more prevalent among whites of high socioeconomic status who work indoors and tend to take short vacations with intense sun exposure than in people who are at risk of chronic sun exposure. This correlation appears to be related to education not income.[49]

Melanoma occurs more often within families and among people who have dysplastic nevus syndrome, also known as the atypical mole syndrome. This is a familial disorder that results in a large number of irregular moles that have an almost 50% chance of developing melanoma during the person's lifetime. Puberty and pregnancy may enhance growth. Previous

*This has increased dramatically from a 1 in 1500 risk of developing melanoma in the 1930s.

*Not all UVB radiation (280 to 320 nm) but UVA (320 to 400 nm) radiation, the type produced by sun lamps, may promote skin cancer. For these reasons, tanning parlors should also be considered a significant risk factor for the development of skin cancer..

BOX 9-8

Risk Factors for the Development of Malignant Melanoma

Family history of malignant melanoma
Presence of blond or red hair
Presence of marked freckling on the upper back
History of three or more blistering sunburns before age 20 years
History of 3 or more years of an outdoor summer job during adolescence
Presence of actinic keratosis (sharply outlined horny growth)

Modified from Friedman RJ, Rigel DS, Silverman MK et al: Malignant melanoma in the 1990s, CA *Cancer J Clin* 41:201-225, 1991.

history of melanoma places the individual at greater risk of developing a second melanoma.

Other risk factors include excessive exposure to UV radiation through sunlight or tanning booths, especially intense intermittent exposure, and immune suppression from chemotherapy. There is some controversy over reports that commercial airline pilots have high rates of malignant melanoma.* Although the evidence is clear that this occupation has the highest incidence ratio of skin cancer, whether this is a result of excessive exposure to cosmic and UV radiation (which can easily penetrate the cockpit), from flying over multiple time zones (disturbance of circadian rhythm), or from factors related to lifestyle (excessive sunbathing) rather than work conditions remains inconclusive.[47,95] Supportive research shows that an 8% to 10% increase in UVB radiation occurs for every 1000 feet of elevation, suggesting a higher incidence of skin cancer at higher elevations.[101]

Pathogenesis. See the section on Squamous Cell Carcinoma: Pathogenesis.

The majority of malignant melanomas appear to be associated with the intensity rather than the duration of sunlight exposure; that is, most people who develop melanoma work indoors and have intense but limited exposure to the sun on weekends or vacations. This accounts for the location of most melanomas most commonly on skin that is covered most of the year.

Clinical Manifestations. Melanoma can appear anywhere on the body, not just on sun-exposed areas. Common sites are the head and neck in men, the legs in women, and the backs of people exposed to excessive UV radiation. Up to 70% arise from a preexisting nevus. Any change in a skin lesion or nevus (increased size or elevation; bleeding; soreness or inflammation; changes in color, pigmentation, or texture) must be examined for melanoma.

Medical Management

Diagnosis. Early recognition of cutaneous melanomas can have a major impact on the surgical cure of this disease.

The ACS suggests a monthly self-examination. A skin biopsy with histologic examination can distinguish malignant melanoma from other lesions, determine tumor thickness, and provide staging. There are several techniques for staging skin cancer. The Breslow method measures the thickness of the melanoma; the thinner the melanoma, the better the prognosis. Generally, melanomas less than 1 mm in depth have a very small chance of spreading. A second system used to determine the appropriate stage is to evaluate the layers of skin that are invaded by the melanoma (Fig. 9-12). A third method of staging, TNM, combines both previously described methods (Table 9-6). Depending on the depth of the tumor invasion and metastatic spread, other testing procedures may include baseline laboratory studies, a bone scan for metastasis, or computed tomography (CT) scan for metastasis to the chest, abdomen, CNS, and brain.

Diagnostic accuracy will continue to improve as digitalized images of lesions can be analyzed enabling the physician to determine whether a biopsy is needed. Computer-aided microscopic examination of biopsy slides may lead to better diagnosis, and teledermatology will add additional assistance in melanoma diagnosis. This technology makes it possible to compress digital images of suspicious lesions and transmit them electronically anywhere in the world, making consultation easier.[100]

Scientists are continuing to seek complementary ways of predicting metastatic potential so that preventive therapies can be initiated earlier. Tests that can detect submicroscopic melanoma cells circulating in the blood vessels and lymphatics could prove invaluable since melanoma generally metastasizes via these systems. The recently developed reverse transcriptase polymerase chain reaction (RT-PCR) assay designed to detect genetic markers or indicators of potential metastatic melanoma in the blood has been seriously hampered by false-negative reports. Additional assays that make use of multiple melanoma markers are being investigated.[28,40]

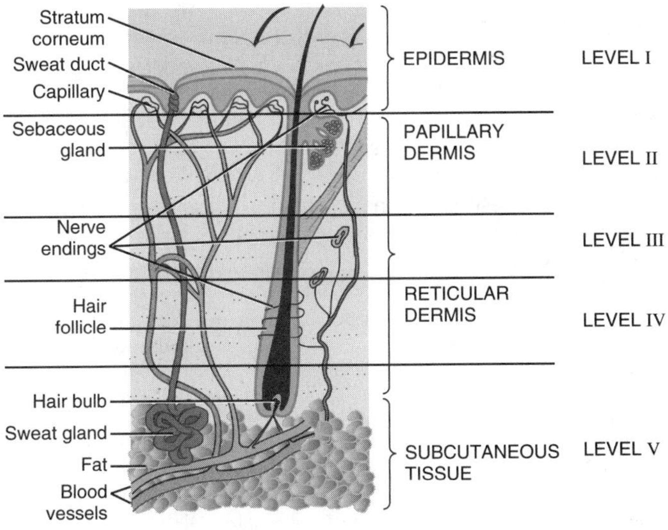

FIGURE 9-12 Clark's levels, a system of classifying tumor progression according to skin layer penetration. Level I involves only the epidermis, level II has spread to the dermis, level III involves most of the upper dermis, level IV has spread to the lower dermis, and level V indicates the cancer has spread to the subcutis. The higher the level, the greater the chance that metastasis has occurred.

---

*Increased cancer risk among all flight personnel has been previously noted, including breast cancer among flight attendants and acute myeloid leukemia among pilots. Further studies are needed to identify specific and potentially preventable risk factors.[6]

TABLE 9-6

Staging of Malignant Melanoma*

Primary Tumor (pT)

pTX	Primary tumor cannot be assessed
pT0	No evidence of primary tumor
pTis	Melanoma in situ (atypical melanocytic hyperplasia, severe melanocytic dysplasia, not an invasive lesion; Clark's level I)
pT1	Tumor ≤0.75 mm in thickness and invades the papillary dermis (Clark's level II)
pT2	Tumor >0.75 mm but not >1.5 mm in thickness or invades to papillary-reticular dermal interface (Clark's level III)
pT3	Tumor >1.5 mm but not >4 mm in thickness or invades reticular dermis (Clark's level IV)
pT3a	Tumor >1.5 mm but not >3 mm in thickness
pT3b	Tumor >3 mm but not >4 mm in thickness
pT4	Tumor >4 mm in thickness or invades subcutaneous tissue (Clark's level V) and/or satellite(s) within 2 cm of primary tumor
pT4a	Tumor >4 mm in thickness or invades subcutaneous tissue
pT4b	Satellite(s) within 2 cm of primary tumor

Regional Lymph Nodes (N)

NX	Regional lymph nodes cannot be assessed
N0	No regional lymph node metastasis
N1	Metastasis ≤3 cm in greatest dimension in any regional lymph node(s)
N2	Metastasis >3 cm in greatest dimension in any regional lymph node(s) or in-transit metastasis
N2a	Metastasis >3 cm in greatest dimension in any regional lymph node(s)
N2b	In-transit metastasis†
N2c	Both (N2a and N2b)

Distant Metastasis (M)

MX	Presence of distant metastasis cannot be assessed
M0	No distant metastasis
M1	Distant metastasis
M1a	Metastasis in skin or subcutaneous tissue or lymph node(s) beyond regional lymph nodes
M1b	Visceral metastasis

Used with permission of the American Joint Committee on Cancer (AJCC), Chicago. The original source for this material is the *AJCC handbook for staging of cancer*, ed 5, Philadelphia, 1998, Lippincott-Raven.
*Several systems exist for staging malignant melanoma, including the TNM (tumor, node, metastasis) system, developed by the American Joint Committee on Cancer, and Clark's system, which classifies tumor progression according to skin layer penetration (see Fig. 9-12).
†In-transit metastasis involves skin or subcutaneous tissue more than 2 cm from the tumor but not beyond the regional lymph nodes.

Treatment.   Neither cryosurgery with liquid nitrogen nor electrodesiccation is used to treat melanoma, although they are among the acceptable procedures for squamous cell and basal cell tumors. The treatment of choice for melanoma without evidence of distant metastatic spread is surgical exci-

sion. Surgery is combined with postoperative adjuvant radiation therapy and/or chemotherapy when there is evidence of regional spread. Surgery is not usually recommended in tumors that have metastasized to distant sites.[81] Previously, surgical excision of the primary lesion site may have been accompanied by removal of regional lymph nodes (regional lymphadenectomy), but sentinel node biopsy (see Chapter 8) has been shown to be a reliable diagnostic tool for selecting individuals to be submitted to lymph node dissection, thereby reducing the extent of surgery for those who do not need this procedure.*[18, 82]

Surgeons are now able to use aggressive surgical approaches on a more selective basis and therefore decrease treatment-related complications and disfigurement without compromising surgical goals. This change in treatment approach came as a result of the knowledge that the recurrence rate for people with melanoma clinically localized to the skin correlates directly with tumor thickness or depth of invasion, whereas the prognosis for people whose disease has spread to the regional lymph nodes depends primarily on the number of nodes that have tumors.[102]

Deep primary lesions may warrant adjuvant chemotherapy and biotherapy to eliminate or reduce the number of tumor cells, but there is no role at present for chemotherapy or radiation therapy as the initial treatment. Radiation therapy is used for metastatic disease to reduce tumor size and provide palliative relief from painful symptoms; it does not prolong survival time.

Ongoing research to develop immunomodulation therapy remains a large area of study. In addition to immunotherapy to stimulate the immune system, research to treat people with a vaccine made from their own cancer cells is under way. This antimelanoma immunization is currently undergoing multiple clinical trials and has shown evidence of clinical effectiveness with minimal side effects.[14,119] Long-term effectiveness remains unknown. Other more investigational techniques may include incorporating Fas ligands (a protein found to provide defense against the accumulation of mutations caused by sun exposure) into short-acting drugs or mixing them into sunscreens to boost people's natural resistance to skin cancer.

Prognosis.   Malignant melanoma is a more serious problem than other skin cancers because it can spread quickly and insidiously, becoming life-threatening at an earlier stage of development. However, it is essentially 100% curable if detected early. The prognosis for all types of melanoma depends primarily on the tumor's thickness and depth of invasion, not on the histologic type; that is, the more superficial or thin the tumor, the better the prognosis. For example, melanoma lesions less than 0.76 mm deep have an excellent prognosis (5-year survival rate is 90%), whereas deeper lesions (more than 0.76 mm) are at risk for metastasis (5-year survival rate with local metastasis is 65%; 30% to 35% when distant metastases are present). Metastases, usually to the brain, lungs, bones, liver, skin, and CNS, are universally fatal, usually within 1 year.

---

*There is considerable debate about the use of sentinel node biopsy in staging melanoma at this time. Some studies report that this type of biopsy is highly reliable in experienced hands but a low-yield procedure in most thin melanomas,[22] whereas others argue against its use except in clinical trials[118] and claim that there is not enough evidence to support the current combined use of sentinel node biopsy and systemic interferon for melanoma.[88]

Prognosis is better for a tumor on an extremity that is drained by one lymphatic network than for one on the head, neck, or trunk drained by several lymphatic networks. Tumors can recur more than 5 years after primary surgery, requiring close long-term medical follow-up. Local recurrence without metastases may not represent a poor prognosis if the recurrence is simply an outgrowth of residual undetected microscopic cells from the previously excised primary tumor.[15,129] Education on the effects of UVB exposure can dramatically reduce the incidence and recurrence of skin cancer.

Special Implications for the Therapist   9-9

MALIGNANT MELANOMA

Preferred Practice Patterns
For potential treatment intervention for nonhealing skin graft
*   following excision:*
7D: *Impaired Integumentary Integrity Associated With Full-*
*   Thickness Skin Involvement and Scar Formation*
7E: *Impaired Integumentary Integrity Associated With Skin*
*   Involvement Extending Into Fascia, Muscle, or Bone and*
*   Scar Formation*

During observation and inspection of any client, the therapist should be alert to the potential signs of skin cancer. Therapists should not become overly concerned about small pink spots on the client's skin, since other common skin conditions, such as eczema, psoriasis, and seborrheic dermatitis, are prevalent in more than half of all people at some time in their lives. Therapists should look for abnormal spots, especially in sun-exposed areas, that are rough in texture, are persistently present, and bleed on minimal contact or with minimal friction.*

As discussed in the text, *any* change in a wart or mole (color, size, shape, texture, ulceration, bleeding, itching) should be inspected by a physician. The Skin Cancer Foundation advocates the use of the ABCD method of early detection of melanoma and dysplastic (abnormal in size or shape) moles (Box 9-9). Other signs and symptoms that may be important include irritation and itching; tenderness, soreness, or new moles developing around the mole in question; or a sore that keeps crusting and does not heal within 6 weeks. For any client with a previous history of skin cancer, emphasize the need for continued close follow-up to detect recurrence early. Education on the effects of UV radiation and taking precautions (Box 9-10) can dramatically reduce the incidence of skin cancer.

If surgery included lymphadenectomy, the therapist may be involved in minimizing lymphedema or treating residual lymphedema (see the section on Lymphedema in Chapter 12). Wound care may involve care of a skin graft and the associated donor site; the graft may be as painful as the tumor excision site and just as much at risk for infection. Standard Precautions (see Appendix A) are essential for the postoperative as well as immunosuppressed client.

---

*Keep in mind that seborrheic keratosis commonly bleeds; once diagnosed, this bleeding should not cause undue alarm.

BOX 9-9

ABCD Method of Early Melanoma Detection

A: Asymmetry: uneven edges, lopsided in shape, one half unlike the other
B: Border: irregularity, irregular edges scalloped or poorly defined edges
C: Color: black, shades of brown, red, white, pink, occasionally blue
D: Diameter: Larger than a pencil eraser

BOX 9-10

Guidelines for Prevention of Skin Cancer

1. Avoid peak hours of sunlight.
2. Wear close-woven protective clothing.
3. Use a sunscreen of SPF 15 or higher.
4. Teach children sun protection.
5. Do not work on getting a tan.
6. Do not patronize tanning salons.
7. Examine your skin regularly.
8. If you notice any changes, see your physician promptly.

For the dying client, hospice care may include pain control and management. It is important that pain relief not be delayed until after pain occurs but rather that a schedule of analgesia to prevent pain or to prevent an increase in pain levels is instituted. ■

◆ Kaposi's Sarcoma

Definition and Overview.   Kaposi's sarcoma (KS) is a malignancy of vascular tissue that presents as a skin disorder. Until recently, this tumor was most commonly seen in older men of Mediterranean or Eastern European origin, especially men of Jewish or Italian ancestry (now referred to as *classic KS*). The sudden emergence of this malignancy in the Western world is directly related to AIDS-associated immunodeficiency, and the incidence has risen dramatically along with the incidence of AIDS (*epidemic KS*). KS may also occur in kidney transplant recipients taking immunosuppressive drugs.

Etiologic Factors and Incidence.   Research in the mid-1990s confirmed that KS is caused by a herpesvirus infection. The human herpesvirus 8 (HHV-8) or Kaposi's sarcoma–associated herpesvirus (KSHV) is present in all AIDS-related KS and has been linked to all forms of KS.*

---

*Human herpesvirus 8 is found in tissues from all four forms of KS (classic, iatrogenic, endemic [African], HIV-associated); however, only iatrogenic KS and HIV-associated KS have been shown to be linked to impairment of the host immune response. This universal detection of KSHV/HHV-8 suggests a central role for the virus in the development of KS and a common etiologic factors for all KS types.[58] Genetic or hereditary predisposition may be a factor in the classic form.

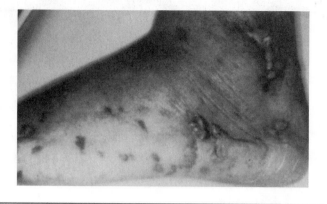

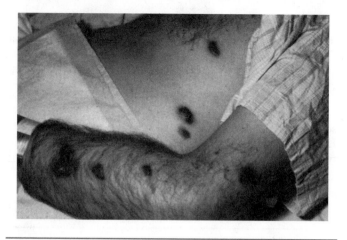

FIGURE **9-13** Classic Kaposi's sarcoma is present as typical nodular lesions on this ankle and foot. (From Callen JP, Jorizzo J, editors: *Dermatological signs of internal disease*, ed 2, Philadelphia, 1995, Saunders, p 161.)

FIGURE **9-14** Epidemic Kaposi's sarcoma in the plaque stage. Evolving lesions develop into raised papules or thickened plaques that are oval in shape and vary in color from red to brown. (From Swartz MH: *Textbook of physical diagnosis*, Philadelphia, 1989, Saunders, plate IV.)

Epidemiologic surveys indicate that the seroprevalence for HHV-8 parallels the risk of developing KS—5% to 10% in the general population of the Western world but ranging up to 20% to 70% in homosexual HIV-infected clients. Among the people who develop AIDS, KS is seen almost exclusively among homosexual or bisexual men and among homosexual men, with the probability of HHV-8 seropositivity directly proportional to the number of previous male sex partners. If a person contracts AIDS as a result of IV drug use or from a transfusion, the chance of developing KS is less than 2%. Rates are lower (10%) among HIV-infected women, people with hemophilia, and injection drug users. Overall incidence has been reduced among adults with AIDS associated with the use of antiretroviral therapy to control HIV replication and limit the associated immunodeficiency.[22,41]

Pathogenesis. Although HHV-8 is detectable in saliva and semen, the exact mechanism of transmission is not known and the details of the pathogenesis remain unknown. KS is an angioproliferative tumor. It is suspected that endogenous substances produced by HIV-infected cells and/or a viral-induced tumorigenesis may promote angiogenesis and the growth of KS.[1,80] Recent experimental studies have demonstrated the role of vascular endothelial growth factor (VEGF) and its receptors in the pathogenesis of KS.[2]

Clinical Manifestations. This neoplasm involves the skin and mucous membranes as well as other organs and can lead to tumor-associated edema and ulcerations. Classic KS occurs commonly on the lower extremities, and the affected areas are red, purple, or dark blue macules (Fig. 9-13) that slowly enlarge to become nodules or ulcers. Itching and pain in the lesions that impinge on nerves or organs may occur; and as the sarcoma progresses causing lymphatic obstruction, the legs become edematous. The lesions may spread by metastasis through the upper body to the face and oral mucosa.

Unlike classic forms of the disease, AIDS-associated KS is a multicentric entity that appears on the upper body (including face, chest, and neck) but can occur on the legs. It frequently involves lymph nodes, lung, and the GI tract; it may be the first

manifestation of AIDS (Fig. 9-14). Early lesions are faint pink and can easily be mistaken for bruises or nevi and be ignored. Systemic involvement may present with one or more signs and symptoms, including weight loss (10% of body weight), fever of unknown origin that exceeds 100° F (37.8° C) for more than 2 weeks, chills, night sweats, lethargy, anorexia, and diarrhea. Pulmonary involvement may be characterized by dyspnea, cough, chest pain, and hemoptysis (in order of prevalence).

Medical Management

Diagnosis, Treatment, and Prognosis. Diagnosis is by skin biopsy using a highly sensitive and specific test for this neoplasm. A CT scan may be performed to detect and evaluate possible metastasis. Dermatologic manifestations of KS can be alarming, but it is visceral involvement associated with AIDS KS that is most life-threatening. However, new antiretroviral therapies, in particular the protease inhibitors, appear to be changing the clinical course of KS. It is now possible to see a complete resolution and control of KS with the use of these new agents. As researchers continue to unravel the pathogenesis of KS, new treatment modalities will target its pathogenic pathways. Chemotherapy remains an integral part of treatment, and new agents are becoming available. Experimental therapies being evaluated in ongoing clinical trials include angiogenesis inhibitors, hormonal therapies, retinoic acid derivatives, and immune modulators, such as interleukin-12.[37] See discussion of AIDS in Chapter 6.

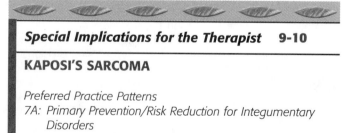

Special Implications for the Therapist **9-10**

KAPOSI'S SARCOMA

Preferred Practice Patterns
7A: *Primary Prevention/Risk Reduction for Integumentary Disorders*
7B: *Impaired Integumentary Integrity Associated With Superficial Skin Involvement*

7C: Impaired Integumentary Integrity Associated With Partial-Thickness Skin Involvement and Scar Formation

7D: Impaired Itegumentary Integrity Associated With Full-Thickness Skin Involvement and Scar Formation

7E (Skin and soft tissue): Impaired Integumentary Integrity Associated With Skin Involvement Extending Into Fascia, Muscle, or Bone and Scar Formation

6H (Lymph nodes): Impaired Circulation and Anthropometric Dimensions Associated With Lymphatic System Disorders

The KS skin lesions in the AIDS client are not contagious, and the health care provider need have no fear of transmission of KS or HIV through daily contact with the client. Standard Precautions must be followed whenever providing care for clients with KS to prevent the spread of infection to the client. Prevention of skin breakdown and wound care is the usual focus of intervention. Clients receiving radiation therapy must keep the irradiated skin dry to avoid possible breakdown and subsequent infection (see the section on Radiation Injuries: Special Implications for the Therapist in Chapter 4). ■

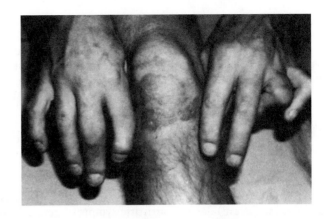

FIGURE   9-15   Deforming asymmetric oligoarticular (affecting only a few areas) arthritis of the hands in a person with plaque psoriasis of the knee. (From Callen JP, Jorizzo J, editors: *Dermatological signs of internal disease*, ed 2, Philadelphia, 1995, Saunders, p 44.)

SKIN DISORDERS ASSOCIATED WITH IMMUNE DYSFUNCTION

◆ Psoriasis

Definition and Incidence.   Psoriasis is a chronic, inherited, recurrent inflammatory but noninfectious dermatosis characterized by well-defined erythematous plaques covered with a silvery scale (Fig. 9-15). There are several types of psoriasis, including plaque, guttate, erythrodermic, and pustular psoriasis.

Psoriasis occurs equally in both genders and most commonly in young adults (mean age of onset is 27 years of age) but can occur at any point in a person's life and once present, becomes a chronic condition that may go in and out of remission. Although psoriasis can occur in infancy, it is uncommon in children under the age of 6 years. It is uncommon among blacks but affects 1% to 2% of the white population; more than 6 million Americans are affected, with more than 100,000 classified as severe cases.

Etiologic and Risk Factors.   The cause of psoriasis is unknown, but it appears to be hereditary; that is, the tendency to develop psoriasis is genetically determined. Researchers have discovered a significantly higher than normal incidence of certain human leukocyte antigens (HLAs) in families with psoriasis, suggesting a possible immune disorder. In the search for a psoriasis gene, researchers have discovered that, although there may be a primary "gatekeeper" gene, multiple genes seem to be involved. If one parent has psoriasis, a child has a 10% to 15% chance of developing the disease; if both parents have psoriasis, the chances increase to 50%.

Although psoriasis is believed to be genetically linked, it may be triggered by mechanical, ultraviolet, and chemical injury; various infections (especially beta-hemolytic streptococci); prescription drug use; psychologic stress; smoking; and pregnancy and other endocrine changes.[90] Cold weather and severe anxiety or emotional stress tend to aggravate psoriasis. Flare-ups are often related to specific systemic and environmental factors but may be unpredictable. New epidemiologic studies present evidence that both smoking and drinking have an influence on psoriasis, suggesting that simple modifications in lifestyle may reduce both the prevalence and the severity of psoriasis.[53]

Pathogenesis.   The underlying abnormality in psoriasis has not been definitively identified. It is a disorder of the keratinocytes, which form in the lower epidermis, flatten with age, and move toward the surface as new cells are generated below. Normally, the life cycle of a skin cell is 26 to 28 days: 14 days to move from the basal layer to the stratum corneum and 14 days of normal wear and tear before the cell is sloughed off. In contrast, the turnover time of psoriatic skin is 3 to 4 days. This shortened cycle does not allow time for the cell to mature; thus cells stick and build up on the skin, resulting in a thick and flaky stratum corneum, which in turn produces the cardinal manifestations of psoriasis.

A second component in the pathogenesis of psoriasis is the immune system reaction since T cells appear at the sites of heightened keratinocyte activity, much as they would at the site of an infection or tumor. The accelerated activity also triggers capillary growth supplying blood and nutrients to the tissue at that site. It remains uncertain whether the accelerating keratinocyte turnover initiates the immune system reaction. One theory is that psoriasis is an autoimmune condition in which T-cell attack is provoked by a protein present in the skin, yet other animal studies suggest the pathogenesis begins in the T lymphocytes and initiates the disease process.[87]

Clinical Manifestations.   Psoriasis appears as erythematous papules and plaques covered with silvery scales. The lesions in ordinary cases have a predilection for the scalp, chest, nails, elbows, knees, groin, skinfolds, lower back, and buttocks. The occurrence may vary from a solitary lesion to countless patches covering large areas of the body in a symmetric pattern. Two clearly distinguishing features are the tendency for this condition to recur and to persist. Lesions that develop at the site of a previous injury are known as

Koebner's phenomenon. Flare-ups are more common in the winter as a result of dry skin and lack of sunlight, and, as is true for many skin ailments, the severity of psoriasis varies over time, and its exacerbations and remissions often correlate with stress levels and mental outlook.

The most common subjective complaint is itching and, occasionally, pain from dry, cracked, encrusted lesions. In approximately 30% of cases, psoriasis spreads to the fingernails, producing small indentations and yellow or brown discoloration. In severe cases, the accumulation of thick, crumbly debris under the nail causes it to separate from the nail bed (nail dystrophy).

Approximately 10% of people with psoriasis (usually moderate to severe) develop arthritic symptoms referred to as psoriatic arthritis (see Chapter 26). Psoriatic arthritis usually affects one or more joints of the fingers or toes, or sometimes the sacroiliac joints, and may progress to spondylitis. These clients report morning stiffness that lasts more than 30 minutes. Joint symptoms show no consistent linkage to the course of the cutaneous manifestations of psoriasis but rather demonstrate remissions and exacerbations similar to those of rheumatoid arthritis. No other systemic effects of psoriasis have been reported, but hyperuricemia (gout) is fairly common in clients, precipitated by treatment with methotrexate and as a result of nucleic acid turnover caused by cellular breakdown in lesions of psoriasis.[126]

Medical Management

Diagnosis.   Diagnosis depends on the previous history, clinical presentation, and, if needed, skin biopsy to identify psoriatic changes in skin or rule out other causes for the lesions. Typically, the serum uric acid level is elevated because of accelerated nucleic acid degradation but without the corresponding gout usually associated with increased uric acid levels. Psoriasis must be distinguished from eczema, seborrheic dermatitis, and lichenlike papules.

Treatment.   In the absence of a cure, the goal of treatment is to maximize remission and lessen outbreaks. Psoriasis therapy is highly individualized and often determined by trial and error because different people respond to different treatments. Psoriasis does not spread, and early treatment does not prevent the condition from progressing.

New options exist that adequately suppress the disease process and help provide better control of the psoriasis through the use of a combination of therapies. Various forms of local or systemic treatment routinely offered fall into five general categories: (1) topical preparations, (2) phototherapy, (3) antimetabolites, (4) oral retinoid therapy, and (4) immunosuppressants. Topical treatment of psoriasis is usually the first line of therapy, and therapeutic agents include corticosteroids; synthetic vitamin D_3; vitamin A analogs (retinoids); occlusive ointments (e.g., petroleum jelly, salicylic acid preparations, urea-containing topical ointments); oatmeal baths, emollients, and open wet dressings to relieve pruritus; and occasionally tar preparations.

Corticosteroids are the most commonly prescribed therapy for psoriasis but should be used sparingly because of the incidence of side effects that have increased with the use of the superpotent fluorinated preparations. Only weak preparations, such as 0.5% or 1.0% hydrocortisone, should be used on the face, perineum, or other sensitive areas (e.g., the flexor surfaces of the arms, abdomen).*

Crude coal tar, one of the oldest remedies for psoriasis, is assumed to work by an antimitotic effect (helps retard rapid cell production). This treatment consists of the daily application of 2% to 5% crude coal tar combined with a tar bath and UV light.† Exposure to UV light (phototherapy), such as UVB or natural sunlight, also helps retard rapid cell production. Widespread involvement may improve with whole-body irradiation with UV light. PUVA refers to the combination of an orally administered photosensitizing drug plus exposure to 1 to 1½ hours of UVA radiation. It is more effective for the thick plaque type of psoriasis, pustular psoriasis, and generalized erythroderma.‡

Methotrexate, originally an anticancer drug, affects DNA synthesis and inhibits reproduction in rapidly growing cells, such as the prolific keratinocytes in psoriasis. Methotrexate also has an immunosuppressant effect, tempering the inflammatory response. Cyclosporine (Neoral), an immunosuppressant most often used to prevent organ transplantation rejection, has also been approved as a psoriasis treatment. These pharmaceuticals have potentially serious side effects and must be monitored closely.

A new treatment strategy called *sequential therapy* involving a deliberate sequence to optimize therapeutic outcome is being explored for those who require systemic therapy without methotrexate. The rationale for this strategy in psoriasis is that it is a chronic disease requiring long-term maintenance therapy as well as quick relief of symptoms and that some medical interventions are better suited for rapid clearance whereas others are more appropriate for long-term care. In sequential therapy, an acute exacerbation of psoriasis is brought under control promptly with the use of cyclosporine followed by phototherapy and then acitretin administered in a maintenance phase.[66,67]

Prognosis.   Psoriasis usually recurs at intervals and lasts for increasingly longer periods, but treatment advances bring relief during flare-ups in approximately 85% to 90% of cases. Spontaneous cure is uncommon, and the risk of infection is high because of the greater than normal amounts of staphylococci present on psoriatic plaques. People with psoriasis who are HIV-positive are at high risk of infection from self-inoculation. As many as 20% of clients who develop psoriatic arthritis may sustain early and severe joint damage with accompanying deformity and disability. Finally, psoriasis treatment involving PUVA has been shown to contribute to an increased risk of skin cancer decades after the treatment has stopped.[111] New research shows that it may be possible to reduce the risk of skin cancer from PUVA with meditation and stress reduction techniques that reduced healing time to half, thus reducing UV exposure.[61]

---

*The major concerns with all corticosteroid preparations are dermal atrophy, skin fragility, fast relapse times, and in rare cases, adrenal suppression resulting from systemic absorption. See also the section on Corticosteroids in Chapter 4.

†The disadvantages of this treatment are the extended time commitments required by the client and the associated mess. More recently, the use of liquid carbonis detergens (LCD) has replaced the use of crude coal tar.

‡PUVA also has its disadvantages as a treatment option, including premature skin aging, nonmelanoma skin and other cancers, and premature cataract formation. This type of therapy is contraindicated in pregnancy and for anyone with abnormal moles or otherwise at risk for skin cancer.

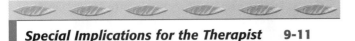

Special Implications for the Therapist 9-11

PSORIASIS

Preferred Practice Patterns
7A: Primary Prevention/Risk Reduction for Integumentary Disorders
7B: Impaired Integumentary Integrity Associated With Superficial Skin Involvement

Physical therapy and occupational therapy are key components in the treatment of moderate to severe psoriasis with desired outcomes based on minimizing functional limitations.* Client instruction and direct intervention to provide skin care should emphasize the following: (1) steroid cream application must be in a thin film, rubbed gently into the skin until all the cream disappears; (2) all topical medications, especially those containing anthralin and tar, should be applied with a downward motion to avoid rubbing them into the hair follicles causing inflammation (folliculitis); (3) medication should be applied only to the affected lesions, avoiding contact with normal surrounding skin; and (4) gloves must be worn when applying the cream since anthralin stains and injures the skin. After application, the client must dust himself or herself with powder to prevent anthralin from rubbing off on the clothes. Mineral oil followed by soap and water can be used to remove the anthralin; the skin should never be rubbed vigorously, but a soft brush can be used to remove the scales.

Any side effects, especially allergic reactions to anthralin, atrophy and acne from steroids, and burning, itching, and nausea, must be reported to the physician immediately. Squamous cell epithelioma may develop from PUVA. Cytotoxins from methotrexate therapy may cause hepatic or bone marrow toxicity; methotrexate may be teratogenic (harmful to fetal development) and should not be prescribed for women who are pregnant, trying to become pregnant, or breast feeding. Other immunosuppressants when used over a long period have an accumulative effect and therefore the potential to cause serious side effects, such as poor wound healing, high blood pressure, kidney damage, and many other complications (see the section on Immunosuppressants in Chapter 4).

Teaching relaxation techniques and stress management are valuable tools that should be encouraged on a daily basis but especially during periods of exacerbation.

Psoriatic Arthritis

Clinically, psoriatic arthritis differs from rheumatoid arthritis in the more frequent involvement of the distal interphalangeal joints, asymmetric distribution of affected joints, presence of spondyloarthropathy (including the presence of both sacroiliitis and spondylitis), and characteristic extraarticular features (e.g., psoriatic skin lesions, iritis, mouth ulcers, urethritis, colitis, aortic valve disease). Joints are less tender in psoriatic arthritis, which may lead to underestimation of the degree of inflammation. Pain and stiffness of inflamed joints are usually increased by prolonged immobility and alleviated by physical activity.

Evidence of inflammation is pain on stressing the joint, tenderness at the joint line, and the presence of effusions.

The increasing use of nuclear magnetic resonance imaging (MRI) techniques, with their ability to delineate cartilage and ligamentous structures and to identify edema, is providing a radical improvement in ascertainment of musculoskeletal abnormalities associated with this disease. It is expected that in the decade to come new information about this aspect of the disease will offer greater information and improved treatment regimens.[125]

Psychologic Considerations

Psoriasis can result in psychologic problems because the skin lesions may cause the person to feel contagious and untouchable. In addition, ongoing treatment may not work and the smell of some topical preparations and the stain may add to the psychological reaction. Assure the client that psoriasis is not contagious. Flare-ups can be controlled with treatment, and stress control can help prevent recurrences. Relaxation techniques, group counseling, stress management, and medications to treat depression or anxiety may be suggested. ∎

◆ Lupus Erythematosus

Definition. Lupus erythematosus is a chronic inflammatory disorder of the connective tissues. It appears in several forms, including cutaneous lupus erythematosus primarily affecting the skin and systemic lupus erythematosus (SLE), which affects multiple organ systems (including the skin) with considerably more morbidity and associated mortality (see complete discussion in Chapter 6). *Lupus* is the Latin word for wolf, referring to the belief in the 1800s that the skin erosion of this disease was caused by a wolf bite. The characteristic rash of lupus is red, hence the term *erythematosus*.

Cutaneous Lupus Erythematosus

Overview and Incidence. The subsets of lupus erythematosus (LE) involving the skin include chronic cutaneous LE, acute cutaneous LE, and subacute cutaneous LE.* Chronic cutaneous LE, formerly known as discoid lupus, is marked by chronic skin eruptions on sun-exposed skin that can lead to scarring and permanent disfigurement if left untreated. Usually a systemic disorder does not develop, but in 5% to 10% of cases SLE does develop later; conversely, discoid lesions occur in 20% of people with SLE.[105] It is estimated that approximately 60% of persons with chronic cutaneous LE are women in their late 20s or older. The disease is rare in children.

Acute cutaneous LE occurs in 30% to 50% of clients who have SLE and includes malar erythema, widespread erythema, and bullous lesions. Association with systemic disease is highest in acute cutaneous LE, with virtually all clients meeting the American College of Rheumatology criteria for SLE (see Chapter 6).

Etiologic and Risk Factors and Pathogenesis. The exact cause of cutaneous LE is unknown, but evidence suggests an autoimmune defect. There appear to be interrelated

---

*For an interesting and comprehensive article on establishing a practical and effective psoriasis treatment center including phototherapy, debridement, and whirlpool, see reference 5.

*Only the skin-related components of LE are discussed in this chapter. See also the section on Systemic Lupus Erythematosus in Chapter 6.

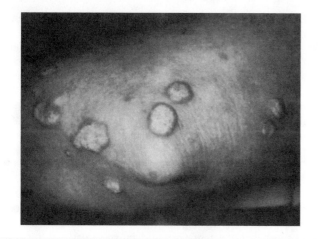

FIGURE **9-16** Wartlike lesions referred to as hypertrophic lupus erythematosus present in a person with typical discoid lupus erythematosus. They simulate warts, keratoacanthoma (benign, craterlike papular lesion), or squamous cell carcinoma. (From Callen JP, Jorizzo J, editors: *Dermatological signs of internal disease*, ed 2, Philadelphia, 1995, Saunders, p 5.)

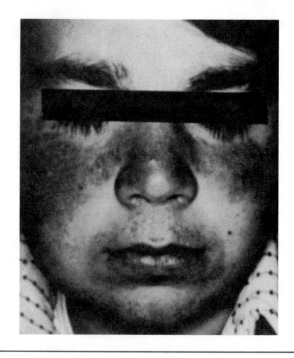

FIGURE **9-17** Butterfly rash of systemic lupus erythematosus across the bridge of the nose and the cheeks. (From Callen JP, Jorizzo J, editors: *Dermatological signs of internal disease*, ed 2, Philadelphia, 1995, Saunders, p 9.)

immunologic, environmental, hormonal, and genetic factors involved. Smoking is considered a risk factor for the development of the discoid lesions associated with chronic cutaneous LE and for resistance to treatment with antimalarial agents in this subgroup.[35,59]

Just how the sun causes skin rash flare-ups remains unknown. One theory is that the DNA of people with lupus, when exposed to sunlight, becomes more antigenic (able to induce a specific immune response). This antigenicity causes accelerated antigen-antibody reactions and thus more deposition of immune complexes in the skin at the dermal-epidermal junction. The photosensitivity is most commonly associated with LE and not other rheumatologic diseases.

Clinical Manifestations. Discoid lesions (*chronic cutaneous LE*) can develop from the rash typically seen in lupus and become raised, red, scaling plaques with follicular plugging and central atrophy. The raised edges and sunken centers give them a coinlike appearance (Fig. 9-16). Although these lesions can appear anywhere on the body, they usually erupt on the face, scalp, ears, neck, and arms or any part of the body that is exposed to sunlight. Hair tends to become brittle, and scalp lesions can cause localized alopecia (bald patches). Facial plaques sometimes assume the classic butterfly pattern with lesions appearing on the cheeks and the bridge of the nose. The rash may vary in severity from a sunburned appearance to discoid (plaquelike) lesions. These lesions can occur in the absence of other lupus-related symptoms and tend to leave hypopigmented and hyperpigmented scars that can become a cosmetic concern.

The most recognized skin manifestation of SLE (*acute cutaneous LE*) is the classic butterfly rash over the nose, cheeks, and forehead (Fig. 9-17) commonly precipitated by exposure to sunlight (UV rays). This classic rash over the nose and cheeks occurs in a large percentage of affected people, but rash can occur on the scalp, neck, upper chest, shoulders, extensor surface of the arms, and dorsum of the hands. These rashes begin abruptly and last from hours to days. They may be precip-

itated by sun exposure and often coincide with a flare of systemic disease.[105] Other skin manifestations may point to the presence of vasculitis (inflammation of cutaneous blood vessels) leading to infarctive lesions in the digits (see Fig. 26-12), necrotic leg ulcers, or digital gangrene.

Acute cutaneous LE is usually accompanied by other symptoms of SLE, commonly including malaise, overwhelming fatigue, arthralgia, fever, arthritis, anemia, hair loss, Raynaud's phenomenon, and urologic symptoms associated with kidney involvement.

Medical Management

Diagnosis and Treatment. The client history and appearance of the rash itself are diagnostic. Skin biopsy of the discoid lesions may be performed. The client must report any changes in the lesions to the attending physician. Drug treatment consists of topical, intralesional, or systemic medication. Potential side effects of systemic therapy (antimalarial agents) for chronic cutaneous LE include diarrhea, nausea, myopathy, cardiomyopathy, and anemia. The lesions resolve spontaneously in 20% to 40% of affected individuals or may cause hypopigmentation or hyperpigmentation, atrophy, and scarring. Discoid lesions are not life-threatening (unless accompanied by complications of SLE) but are associated with psychologic distress and altered quality of life.

Skin lesions require topical treatment, maintaining an optimal wound environment (moist enough to allow tissue healing but not swamplike) while preventing further deterioration or infection. Most often, topical corticosteroid creams are used. The disease process can cause loss of skin integrity and subsequent loss of function.

Clients with any form of cutaneous lupus should avoid prolonged exposure to the sun, fluorescent lighting, or reflected sunlight. They are encouraged to wear protective clothing, use sun-screening agents, and avoid engaging in outdoor activities during periods of intense sunlight (see Box 9-4).

Prognosis. The survival rate has improved dramatically in recent years although death can occur from renal failure when there is kidney involvement causing progressive changes in the glomeruli; cardiac involvement with deposition of immune complexes in the coronary vessels, myocardium, and pericardium; or cerebral infarct.

Special Implications for the Therapist 9-12

LUPUS ERYTHEMATOSUS

Preferred Practice Patterns
4A: Primary Prevention/Risk Reduction for Skeletal
Demineralization
4B: Impaired Posture
6B: Impaired Aerobic Capacity/Endurance Associated With
Deconditioning
7A: Primary Prevention/Risk Reduction for Integumentary
Disorders

Clients with lupus erythema with skin involvement require careful assessment, supportive measures, and emotional support. Skin lesions should be checked thoroughly at each visit. The client should be urged to get plenty of rest, follow energy conservation guidelines, and practice good nutrition. The therapist can be instrumental in teaching and assisting with skin care and prevention of skin breakdown, range-of-motion (ROM) exer-

cises, prevention of orthopedic deformities, ergonomic and postural training, and relief of joint pain associated with SLE. Persons with lupus erythematosus exposed to the long-term effects of corticosteroids should be followed carefully. See specific side effects and the section on Corticosteroids: Special Implications for the Therapist in Chapter 4. See also the section on SLE: Special Implications for the Therapist in Chapter 6. ∎

◆ Systemic Sclerosis
Definition and Overview. Systemic sclerosis (SSc, progressive systemic sclerosis [PSS], scleroderma*) is a diffuse connective tissue disease that causes fibrosis of the skin, joints, blood vessels, and internal organs. SSc is a chronic disease, lasting for months, years, or a lifetime, and is classified according to the degree and extent of skin thickening. There are two distinct subtypes: systemic scleroderma and localized scleroderma (Table 9-7). *Systemic scleroderma* can take one of three forms: limited (lSSc), diffuse (dSSc), and an overlap form with either diffuse or limited skin thickening.

Limited cutaneous SSc is also known as the CREST syndrome from its manifestations (calcinosis, Raynaud's phenomenon, esophageal dysmotility, sclerodactyly, telangiectasia [see Fig. 9-2]). Persons with this form of SSc have a much lower incidence of serious internal organ involvement, although pulmonary hypertension and esophageal disease are not uncommon. Skin tightness is limited to the hands and face (excluding the trunk).

---

*The presence of a distinctive, widespread vascular lesion characterized by endothelial abnormalities as well as by proliferative reaction of the vascular intima was a significant factor in changing terminology from scleroderma to systemic sclerosis (SSc). General clinical vernacular still refers to this condition as scleroderma although that term simply refers to thickening or hardening of the skin.

TABLE 9-7

Classification of Scleroderma

SYSTEMIC SCLEROSIS	LOCALIZED
Limited (75%-80%)	Morphea
• Symmetric skin thickening	• Single or multiple plaques of skin fibrosis without systemic disease
• Restricted to distal extremities and face	Linear
• Slow progression of skin changes	• Single or multiple fibrotic bands involving skin and deeper tissues
• Late development of visceral involvement	
• CREST syndrome	
• Relatively good prognosis (≥70% survival at 10 yr)	
Diffuse (15%-20%)	
• Symmetric skin thickening	
• Widespread, affecting distal and proximal extremities, face, trunk	
• Rapid progression of skin changes	
• Early appearance of visceral involvement (GI tract, lungs, heart, kidneys)	
• Overall poor prognosis (40%-60% survival at 10 yr)	
Overlap (5%-10%)	
• Either diffuse or limited skin thickening	
• Associated with one or more connective tissue diseases (e.g., systemic lupus erythematosus, polymositis, dermatomyositis)	

CREST, Calcinosis, Raynaud's phenomenon, esophageal dysmobility, sclerodactyly, telangiectasia; *GI,* gastrointestinal.

Although the diffuse form is less common than the limited form, it is by far the more debilitating because of the more frequent renal and pulmonary involvement. Some measurable degree of heart, lung, or kidney involvement, or any combination of these, can be found in the majority of people with SSc. Diffuse scleroderma is characterized by involvement of all body parts, including the skin. In most people, this involvement tends to progress slowly, if at all, but if involvement is to become severe, it tends to do so early, within the first 5 years. The severity of the disease depends on the number of organs affected and the extent of the effect.

Localized scleroderma affects primarily the skin in one or many different areas without visceral organ involvement and is therefore a benign form of this disease. Localized scleroderma should not be confused with limited cutaneous scleroderma. The latter is a form of systemic rather than localized disease. There is further differentiation of localized scleroderma: *morphea* is characterized by hard, oval-shaped patches on the skin, generally on the trunk. These patches are usually white with a purple ring around them. *Linear* refers to the bandlike lesions that occur in the areas of the arms, legs, and forehead. The bones and muscles beneath these areas may also be affected. Ultimately, ROM and a child's growth are greatly affected. Linear scleroderma often occurs in childhood.

Other forms include *chemically induced localized scleroderma, eosinophilic myalgia syndrome* (previously associated with ingestion of L-tryptophan), toxic oil syndrome (associated with ingestion of contaminated rapeseed oil), and *graft-versus-host disease*.

Incidence.

The annual incidence of SSc based on epidemiologic studies of hospital records and death certificates is 10 to 20 cases per 1 million, affecting approximately 400,000 Americans. Until the 1980s, SSc was considered a rare disease, but studies at that time reported a prevalence as much as five times greater than the highest prevalence rate previously reported. Some evidence suggests continued rising incidence rates among adults as well as children, but whether this reflects worldwide incidence or merely regional differences remains unknown.[12,32]

SSc affects women two to three times more often than men, with the female/male ratio peaking at 15:1 during the childbearing years. Preliminary studies show that fetal cells persist in maternal blood for as long as 27 years postpartum even if the pregnancy does not go to full term. This phenomenon, referred to as *fetomaternal cell trafficking,* may provide an explanation for the increased prevalence of autoimmune disorders such as SSc in adult women following childbearing.[11]

Etiologic and Risk Factors.

The cause of scleroderma is reportedly unknown. However, several groups suggest that scientific evidence accumulated over the last 50 years strongly points to SSc as an acquired disease triggered by bacteria (mycoplasma).[20,71] It has also been suggested that an autoimmune mechanism is the underlying cause because specific autoantibodies occur in the sera of these clients. Other possible triggers suggested include cytomegalovirus (CMV; increased levels of anti-CMV antibodies present in scleroderma) or immune reactions to viral or environmental factors.[62]

The potential role of placental transfer of fetal cells in the pathogenesis of autoimmune diseases has been mentioned

(see Incidence). In childbearing women with scleroderma, fetal cell–derived DNA is detected more frequently in the peripheral blood than in controls. This finding of a limited number of fetal cells in maternal tissues leading to microchimerism (see explanation of chimerism in Chapter 20) has been proposed to have a role in the induction of scleroderma.[115]

The occasional onset after trauma suggests the possibility of trophoneurosis (a trophic disorder consequent to disease or injury to nerves). The onset of scleroderma immediately following a severe emotional shock is in some cases a manifestation and result of a psychosomatic disturbance that causes vascular spasm.

Chemicals, especially from occupational exposure to silica, vinyl chloride, or various organic solvents (whether through direct contact or by inhalation), may also induce scleroderma-like changes. Exposure to organic solvents such as benzene and trichloroethane, chemicals common in paint thinners, stains, epoxy resins, and degreasers associated with recreational hobby or occupation causes the body to produce an antibody called *Scl-70* associated with scleroderma-like illnesses.[85,86] The toxic oil syndrome and eosinophilia-myalgia syndrome are best-known examples of chemically induced localized forms of scleroderma.[26]

Pathogenesis.

Widespread small-vessel vasculopathy and fibrosis set systemic sclerosis apart from other connective tissue diseases. The relentless deposition of extracellular matrix (collagen) in the intima of blood vessels, the pericapillary space, and the interstitium of the skin is distinctive for SSc and distinguishes it from other autoimmune disorders. Endothelial injury, obliterative microvascular lesions, and increased vascular wall thickness preferentially affecting small arteries, arterioles, and capillaries are present in all involved organs. Autonomic nerve dysfunction (parasympathetic impairment and marked sympathetic overactivity) seems to be linked to the development of microvascular, cardiac, and GI alterations.[38]

The vascular pathologic condition is characterized by altered vascular function with increased vasospasm, reduced vasodilatory capacity, and increased adhesiveness of the blood vessels to platelets and lymphocytes. The connection between the vascular pathologic condition and development of tissue fibrosis remains unknown, but it is hypothesized that SSc modifies the activity of both the endothelium and the peripheral nervous system, eventually leading to the clinical manifestations of this condition.[39] The extent of injury and dysfunction is reflected by changes in the circulating levels of vascular markers.[62]

Clinical Manifestations.

The three stages in the clinical development of scleroderma are the *edematous stage*, the *sclerotic stage,* and the *atrophic stage.* In the edematous stage, bilateral nonpitting edema is present in the fingers and hands and, rarely, in the feet. The edema can progress to the forearms, arms, upper chest, abdomen, back, and face. After a few weeks to several months, edema is replaced by thick, hard skin.

The replacement of edema takes place in the sclerotic stage, when the skin becomes tight, smooth, and waxy and seems bound down to underlying structures. Accompanying changes include a loss of normal skinfolds, decreased flexibility, and skin hyperpigmentation and hypopigmentation.

The skin changes may stabilize for periods (years) and may then either progress to the third stage or soften and return to normal. Actual atrophy of skin may occur, particularly over joints at sites of flexion contractures, such as the proximal interphalangeal joints and the elbows. Such thinning of the skin contributes to the development of ulcerations at these sites. Softening and return to normal of the skin may occur to some extent. Improvement typically begins centrally, so that the last areas to become classically involved are the first to show regression.

Not all people pass through all the stages. Subcutaneous calcification (calcinosis) is a late-developing complication that is considerably more frequent in lSSc. Sites of trauma are often affected, such as the fingers, forearms, elbows, and knees. These calcifications vary in size from tiny deposits to large masses ulcerating the overlying skin.

Raynaud's Phenomenon.
Scleroderma affects everyone in a different fashion. Each previously mentioned form affects the body in different ways (Table 9-8). Raynaud's phenomenon is very often the first manifestation of SSc preceding the onset of all the other signs and symptoms of the disease by months or years.[39] It appears almost universally in lSSc and in approximately 75% of cases of dSSc.

Raynaud's phenomenon is characterized by sudden blanching, cyanosis, and erythema of the fingers and toes as the walls of the blood vessels that supply the hands and feet become narrowed, making it difficult for the blood to pass through. Closure of the muscular digital arteries, precapillary arterioles, and arteriovenous shunts of the skin causes the hands or feet to become white and numb and then bluish in color as blood flow remains blocked. As the spasm eases and blood flow returns (approximately 10 to 15 minutes after the triggering stimulus has ended), rewarming occurs and the fingers or toes become red and painful. This cycle is initiated in response to stress or exposure to cold. Progressive phalangeal resorption may shorten the fingers, and compromised circulation resulting from abnormal thickening of the arterial intima may cause slowly healing ulcerations on the tips of the fingers or toes that may lead to gangrene.[124]

Skin.
Other symptoms include pain, stiffness, and swelling of the fingers and joints. Skin thickening produces taut, shiny skin over the entire hand and forearm. As tightening progresses, contractures may develop. Flexion contractures are especially severe in people with dSSc (Fig. 9-18). Facial skin may also become tight and inelastic, and the face takes on a stretched and masklike appearance, with thin lips and a pinched nose. Peripheral nervous system involvement affects nerve terminals, reducing sensory fibers in SSc skin. Neuropeptides released by sensory nerve endings are reduced, resulting in vasoconstriction in the skin.

Neuromusculoskeletal System.
Most persons with dSSc have disuse atrophy of muscle because of limited joint motion secondary to skin, joint, or tendon involvement. A small percentage of people may have overlap syndromes and demonstrate marked weakness and inflammatory myopathy indistinguishable from polymyositis or dermatomyositis. Some individuals develop myositis or erosive arthropathy that complicates the joint retraction induced by skin fibrosis. SSc also targets the peripheral nervous system with distal mononeuropathy of the median nerve as a frequent and early feature.[38] Neuropathy from carpal tunnel syndrome is also common.

Polyarthralgias affect both small and large joints and are especially frequent early in dSSc; polyarthritis is unusual.

TABLE 9-8

Characteristics Likely to Be Seen in Clients with Systemic Sclerosis Early and Late in the Disease Course

	LIMITED DISEASE	DIFFUSE DISEASE

Early (≤5 yr)	Rapidly progressive
	  Renal crisis (5%)
	  Interstitial lung disease (severe in 10%-15%)
	Slowly progressive
	  Raynaud's phenomenon
	  Cutaneous ulceration
	  Esophageal dysmotility
		Rapidly progressive
		  Skin thickening
		  Heart involvement (severe in 10%-15%)
		  Interstitial lung disease (severe in 15%)
		Renal crisis (15%-20%)
		  Contractures, joint pain
		  Cutaneous ulcerations
		  Esophageal dysmotility
		  Gastrointestinal complications

Late (>5 yr)	Slowly progressive
	  Raynaud's phenomenon
	  Cutaneous ulcerations
	  Esophageal dysmotility
	  Gastrointestinal complications
	Very late
	  Pulmonary artery hypertension
	  Biliary cirrhosis
		Improvement
		  Skin thickening
		  Musculoskeletal pain
		Slowly progressive
		  Heart, lung, kidney involvement
		  Raynaud's phenomenon
		  Cutaneous ulceration
		  Esophageal dysmotility
		  Gastrointestinal complications

Modified from Clements PJ: Systemic sclerosis: natural history and management strategies, *J Musculoskel Med* 11(11):43-50, 1994.

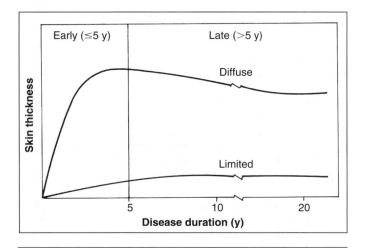

FIGURE   9-18 The progression of skin thickening in systemic sclerosis is greatest in the early period (first 5 years), especially in those with diffuse disease. (From Clements PJ: Systemic sclerosis: natural history and management strategies, *J Musculoskel Med* 11[11]:43-50, 1994.)

Tenosynovial involvement with inflammation and fibrosis of the tendon sheath or adjacent tissues is characterized by the presence of carpal tunnel syndrome and by coarse, leathery friction rubs palpated during motion over the extensor and flexor tendons of the fingers, distal forearms, knees, ankles, and other sites. These friction rubs are found almost exclusively in persons with dSSc, and their presence signifies a poorer overall clinical outcome.[124]

Viscera.   GI motility dysfunction affects the esophagus and anorectal regions causing frequent reflux, heartburn, dysphagia, and bloating after meals. Other effects include abdominal distention, diarrhea, constipation, and malodorous, floating stools. In advanced disease, cardiac and pulmonary fibrosis develops. Cardiac involvement can be manifested as myocardial disease, pericardial disease, conduction system disease, or arrhythmias. Pulmonary involvement is characterized by impaired diffusing capacity for carbon monoxide. Kidney involvement and scleroderma renal crisis are now considered rare because of the introduction of angiotensin-converting enzyme (ACE) inhibitors.[38]

Other.   Nearly 50% of adults with scleroderma report other symptoms, such as major depression, sexual dysfunction, trigeminal neuralgia, hypothyroidism, dental involvement, and corneal tears.

Medical Management

Diagnosis.   Early diagnosis and accurate staging of visceral involvement are fundamental for appropriate management and therapeutic approach to this disease. However, diagnosis can be delayed because there is no single laboratory test diagnostic for SSc. A thorough physical examination and history are the first steps to a definitive diagnosis. Laboratory tests (skin biopsy, urinalysis, blood studies, including erythrocyte sedimentation rate [ESR], presence of rheumatoid factor [found to be positive in 30% of SSc cases], presence of anti-

nuclear antibodies*) are used to determine the extent of involvement and rule out other disease processes. Other tests may include chest films and pulmonary function studies, GI series, and electroencephalogram (ECG).

Treatment.   Presently there is no cure for SSc. A global vision of SSc is necessary for this multisystem disease, and each treatment program is individualized to manage the specific disease process. Treatment ranges from merely symptomatic for a person with only limited skin involvement after 5 years to aggressive treatment for a person with early, diffuse skin involvement. When organ involvement occurs, it most often develops early in the disease course, and in the acute phase it requires aggressive management. The program may include medications (e.g., immunosuppressants, penicillamine,† antiinflammatory drugs), exercises, joint protection techniques, skin protection techniques, and stress management. See also the section on Raynaud's Phenomenon in Chapter 11.

Treatment of the pulmonary complications (pulmonary hypertension, interstitial lung disease) remains difficult. Home blood pressure monitoring can screen for acute hypertension signaling a renal crisis; treatment with ACE inhibitors (see Chapter 11)may be life-saving.

Research remains ongoing to investigate various treatment regimens for scleroderma, including the use of recombinant human relaxin to reduce skin thickening, improve mobility, and improve function in people with moderate to severe diffuse scleroderma[108] and the use of antibiotics such as minocycline‡ without the use of any disease-modifying drugs or steroids.[69]

Prognosis.   The prognosis in SSc principally depends on early diagnosis; the intensity and rapidity of involvement of the lungs, heart, gut, and kidneys; and appropriate medical management. A model to predict mortality based on a combination of three factors (proteinuria, elevated ESR, low carbon monoxide diffusing capacity) has been reported to have an accuracy of more than 80% in predicting mortality. The absence of these three factors is associated with 93% survival.[17]

Spontaneous recovery is common in children, but approximately 30% of clients with SSc die within 5 years of onset. Persons with dSSc who have lived beyond the 5-year mark with no significant visceral involvement are unlikely to experience such organ involvement. Those in whom significant visceral disease developed early can expect a slowing in its progression or at least a stabilization of its course. This 5-year mark is also a time when skin softening begins and musculoskeletal aches and pains begin to ease. Treatment with ACE inhibitors, started early, now prevents previously fatal complications (acute hypertension, renal failure) Aggressive treatment of early interstitial lung disease may further survival.[45] Localized scleroderma may reach an end point beyond which the disease does not progress.

***

*Distinctive serum autoantibodies are found in more than 90% of cases.[79]

†Penicillamine, a disease-modifying drug, is a penicillin-derivative immunomodulating agent that has been shown to improve the skin by interfering with cross linking of collagen and prolonging survival in people with early, rapidly progressive SSc.

‡Oral tetracyclines have been found to be the most effective and have the fewest side effects, with minocycline or doxycycline being the antibiotic of choice. Brand names (Minocin, Vibramycin) are preferred because some generics are ineffective.[120]

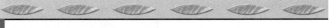

Special Implications for the Therapist 9-13

SYSTEMIC SCLEROSIS

Skin (Pruritus and Ulcers)
Integumentary Practice Patterns
7A: Primary Prevention/Risk Reduction for Integumentary Disorders
7B: Impaired Integumentary Integrity Associated With Superficial Skin Involvement
7C: Impaired Integumentary Integrity Associated With Partial-Thickness Skin Involvement and Scar Formation

Itching can be a major problem in this condition, and excoriation from scratching can cause open wounds susceptible to infection. The therapist can offer some simple suggestions to soothe skin, ease the itching, and prevent skin damage (see Box 9-4).

Local management of digital tip ulcers may include an occlusive dressing to promote wound healing and protect against trauma and infection. Commercial occlusive dressings are particularly helpful with larger noninfected ulcers. Infected ulcers are treated with a trial of oral antistaphylococcal antibiotics and may require surgical debridement of necrotic tissue. Local skin care requires avoidance of excessive bathing or using moisturizing creams containing glycerin. (See also the sections on Peripheral Vascular Disease: Special Implications for the Therapist, and Raynaud's Phenomenon in Chapter 11).

Muscle
Integumentary Practice Pattern
7E: Impaired Integumentary Integrity Associated With Skin Involvement Extending Into Fascia, Muscle, or Bone and Scar Formation
Musculoskeletal Practice Patterns
4B: Impaired Posture
4C: Impaired Joint Mobility, Motor Function, Muscle Performance, and Range of Motion Associated With Connective Tissue Disorders

Myositis (muscle inflammation) is treated with corticosteroids and sometimes requires the addition of immunosuppressive drugs, whereas fibrotic myopathy (fibrotic tissue laid down within the muscle) is best managed with strengthening and ROM exercises. The efficacy of using soft tissue mobilization or similar techniques has not been investigated. Caution must be used when attempting such treatment because the skin of these people is usually very sclerosed and sensitive to pressure. Aquatic therapy is an excellent choice for clients with this condition.

Joints and Tendons
Integumentary Practice Pattern
7E: Impaired Integumentary Integrity Associated With Skin Involvement Extending Into Fascia, Muscle, or Bone and Scar Formation
Musculoskeletal Practice Pattern
4E: Impaired Joint Mobility, Motor Function, Muscle Performance, and Range of Motion Associated With Localized Inflammation

Joint and tendon sheath involvement is common and may be treated successfully with nonsteroidal antiinflammatory drugs (NSAIDs). In early dSSc, tenosynovitis can be very painful, limiting joint movement. In addition to NSAIDs, early aggressive therapy is important in preventing or minimizing contractures. For clients with scleroderma, regular exercise will assist with keeping the skin and joints flexible, maintaining better blood flow, and preventing contractures. Active and passive stretching exercises are necessary but difficult in the presence of extreme pain. Analgesia is required to optimize participation in an exercise program. Protecting swollen and painful joints from stresses and strains is also an important factor. This may require teaching activities of daily living (ADLs) without causing strain on the joint or joints. Lightweight splints may be necessary to provide joint protection. Dynamic splinting has not been found effective in preventing flexion contractures. Carpal tunnel syndrome, which often occurs before the diagnosis of scleroderma, usually responds well to conservative treatment without requiring surgery.

Exercise
Cardiovascular/Pulmonary Practice Patterns
6B: Impaired Aerobic Capacity/Endurance Associated With Deconditioning
6D: Impaired Aerobic Capacity/Endurance Associated With Cardiovascular Pump Dysfunction or Failure

Practice patterns in this area will vary depending on the form of cardiovascular or pulmonary involvement manifested. When cardiopulmonary involvement occurs, intervention must take into consideration effects of this disease on the individual's activity and lifestyle. The client's primary diagnosis and primary intervention may be integument- or orthopedic-related, but functional limitations may be present secondary to systemic involvement (e.g., decreased aerobic capacity, endurance, and overall general physical condition secondary to cardiovascular and/or pulmonary involvement).

Psychologic Considerations
Persons with early dSSc with or without organ involvement are often anxious because their bodies are changing rapidly and in unexpected ways. They may not understand the grave nature of the disease. Since persons with dSSc are at greatest risk for early visceral disease and early mortality, education about the disease is important as is identifying where they are in the natural history of SSc. They should be encouraged to take their blood pressure at home at least three times per week, since this is the best method of screening for acute hypertension. The therapist may screen blood pressure as well. ■

◆ Polymyositis and Dermatomyositis
Definition and Overview. Polymyositis and dermatomyositis are the two most common idiopathic inflammatory diseases of muscle (Box 9-11). Other types of inflammatory muscle disease have been distinguished, but no satisfactory classification of the idiopathic inflammatory myopathies exists; however, histologic analysis allows differentiation among the types of dermatomyositis.[15] They are diffuse, inflammatory myopathies that produce symmetric weakness of striated muscle, primarily the proximal muscles of the shoulder and pelvic girdles, neck, and pharynx. These related illnesses belong to the family of rheumatic diseases. These diseases often progress slowly, with frequent exacerbations and remissions.

Types of Inflammatory Myopathies*

Primary idiopathic polymyositis
Primary idiopathic dermatomyositis
Dermatomyositis or polymyositis associated with malignancy (lung, breast, ovarian, gastric, colon)
Juvenile polymyositis or dermatomyositis
Polymyositis associated with other connective tissue diseases (overlap):
Sjögren's syndrome
Mixed connective tissue disease
Rheumatoid arthritis
Systemic lupus erythematosus
Scleroderma

*Listed in descending order of frequency. Primary idiopathic polymyositis and dermatomyositis account for nearly three-fourths of all cases.

Incidence.   Polymyositis and dermatomyositis are not very common in the United States, affecting approximately 5 to 10 persons per 1 million; the incidence appears to be increasing. Myositis can affect people of any age, but mostly adults between 45 and 65 years and children between 5 and 15 years are affected. Twice as many women as men are affected with the exception of dermatomyositis associated with malignancy, which is most common in men over age 40 years.

Etiologic Factors.   The cause of these conditions remains unknown, although there appears to be some autoimmune mechanism whereby the T cells inappropriately recognize muscle fiber antigens as foreign and attack muscle tissue. Autoantibodies are present in most cases. Polymyositis and dermatomyositis may be drug-induced; possibly triggered by a virus; or associated with other disorders as listed in Box 9-11. The association of dermatomyositis with malignancy, particularly ovarian, gastric, and colonic malignancies, may suggest that the neoplasm may stimulate the dermatomyositis.[15]

Pathogenesis.   If these conditions are caused by an autoimmune reaction, diffuse or focal muscle fiber degeneration is followed by regeneration of new muscle cells, producing remission. Muscle biopsy reveals focal or diffuse inflammatory infiltrates consisting primarily of lymphocytes and macrophages surrounding muscle fibers and small blood vessels. Muscle cells show evidence of degeneration and regeneration, and fiber atrophy is often most severe at the periphery of the muscle bundle. Extensive interstitial fibrosis and fatty replacement are common in long-standing cases.

Clinical Manifestations.   Symmetric proximal muscle weakness is the dominant feature of these diseases, although it is variable in its onset, progression, and severity. In some people, symptoms appear suddenly, progress rapidly, and quickly result in a bedridden state, sometimes requiring ventilatory assistance and tube feeding. More typically, malaise and weight loss develop insidiously over months or even years, with some people either unable to identify the onset of the disease or unaware of the gradual disability developing. Fatigue, rather than weakness, is a commonly reported symptom, but close questioning usually reveals functional losses indicating weakness as well. Pain is not a key feature of these diseases in the adult population, although aching muscles are not uncommon. Muscle wasting is observed in long-standing or severe cases.

Cardiac involvement is not uncommon and contributes significantly to mortality. Nearly half of all people with polymyositis or dermatomyositis have arrhythmias, congestive heart failure, conduction defects, ventricular hypertrophy, or pericarditis. Pulmonary disease (progressive pulmonary fibrosis) can result from weakness of the respiratory muscles, intrinsic lung pathologic conditions, or aspiration. Swallowing difficulties, nasal regurgitation, and esophageal dysphagia and reflux are common, especially in severe cases.

Polymyositis.   Polymyositis begins acutely or insidiously with muscle weakness, tenderness, and discomfort. The proximal muscles of the shoulder and pelvic girdle are affected more often than the distal muscles, usually in a symmetric pattern, but asymmetry is common. The legs are affected more often than the arms, and the anterior thigh is more frequently involved than the posterior thigh. Initially, the muscles may be slightly swollen, but as the disease progresses muscular atrophy and induration become more noticeable, reflecting the deposition of fibrous tissue. Some persons have a mild peripheral neuropathy with loss of deep tendon reflexes.

Early signs of muscle weakness may include impaired functional status, such as difficulty climbing stairs, getting up from a chair, reaching into an overhead cupboard, combing the hair, or lifting the head from a pillow; difficulty with balance; or a tendency to fall, often resulting in a fracture. Other muscular effects may include decreased deep tendon reflexes, contractures, arthralgias, arthritis, an inability to move against resistance (e.g., pushing open a heavy door, opening a car door), proximal dysphagia (difficulty swallowing), and dysphonia (difficulty speaking).

Dermatomyositis.   When a rash is associated with polymyositis, it is referred to as dermatomyositis. A characteristic purplish rash appears on the eyelids (heliotrope erythema), accompanied by periorbital edema (puffy eyelids). The rash may progress to the anterior neck, upper chest and back, shoulders, and arms and may appear around the nail beds. Gottron's papules (red or violet, smooth or scaly patches) may appear on the knuckles, elbows, knees, or medial malleoli (Fig. 9-19). Although the disease usually begins with erythema and swelling of the face and eyelids, cutaneous manifestations can develop concomitantly with muscle involvement or even afterward. The cutaneous lesions of dermatomyositis are nearly always present by the time proximal muscle weakness manifests itself. In some persons, muscle involvement is minimal, whereas in others it may progress to wasting and contractures associated with extreme disability.[126]

Medical Management

Diagnosis.   The diagnosis of myositis is often difficult because it resembles closely several other diseases and the pathologic manifestation can be localized, sometimes resulting in

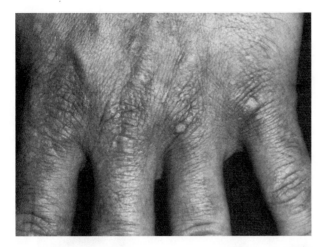

FIGURE   **9-19** Gottron's papules or Gottron's sign. Typical lesions over bony prominences on the extensor surfaces of the hand. (From Callen JP, Jorizzo JL, editors: *Dermatological signs of internal disease*, Philadelphia, 1988, Saunders, p 15.)

nondiagnostic biopsies. The physician must rule out internal malignancy first, requiring appropriate medical testing. Laboratory studies to evaluate muscle enzymes,* biopsy to assess muscle fibers, and electromyography (EMG) to measure the electrical activity of the muscles are all necessary to properly diagnose myositis. MRI can reveal muscle inflammation and may help to select the site on which to do a biopsy in difficult cases.

Treatment.   The treatment must be individualized; the components include medication, exercise, and rest. High-dose daily oral systemic corticosteroid therapy is the usual initial pharmacologic treatment for polymyositis or dermatomyositis. Steroids reduce the inflammation, shorten the time to normalization of muscle enzymes, and reduce morbidity. Persons who do not respond well to steroids or who are unable to tolerate the high dosages required may be treated with immunosuppressive drugs.

Prognosis.   The adult prognosis varies depending on age and progression of the disease process, but overall prognosis has improved with the introduction of systemic glucocorticoid therapy. At present, 85% of people with dermatomyositis can be expected to survive. Approximately 50% are left with residual weakness and have persistently elevated serum creatinase (CK) levels or experience a relapse when corticosteroids are reduced, and 20% are substantially disabled. Generally, the prognosis is worse with visceral organ involvement and death occurs from associated malignancy, respiratory disease, or heart failure. Side effects of therapy (corticosteroids, immunosuppressants) contribute to long-term morbidity. The prognosis for children is guarded if left untreated; it progresses rapidly to disabling contractures and muscular atrophy.

---

*Most people with these diseases have an elevated creatine kinase (CK) level at presentation. The CK represents striated muscle involvement, although in people with chronic disease CK may be of the cardiac MB isotype (see Table 35-13).

Special Implications for the Therapist   9-14

POLYMYOSITIS AND DERMATOMYOSITIS

The abrupt onset of any of the cutaneous lesions associated with polymyositis or dermatomyositis could also be a sign of underlying malignancy, particularly genitourinary or gastrointestinal. The differential diagnosis requires medical evaluation before proceeding with therapy intervention.

Preferred Practice Patterns
4D: *Impaired Joint Mobility, Motor Function, Muscle Performance, and Range of Motion Associated With Connective Tissue Dysfunction*
7E: *Impaired Integumentary Integrity Associated With Skin Involvement Extending Into Fascia, Muscle, or Bone and Scar Formation*

The therapist plays a pivotal role in the management of myositis. Manual muscle testing and tests of functional abilities are useful tools in following disease progression and therapeutic response over a long period. The individualized exercise program can help improve muscle strength and function.[51] Aerobic exercise testing may be a useful functional assessment tool in some cases.[123]

It is suggested that the medication regimen be well established before beginning exercise. In the early stages of treating myositis, the muscle fibers are fragile and could be damaged further, causing rhabdomyolysis (disintegration of muscle fibers) from exercises and other forms of therapy. The therapist treating a client with myositis should keep in close contact with the physician, who will be using physical examination and laboratory tests to determine the most opportune time for initiating a graded exercise program (i.e., when muscle enzyme levels fall to acceptable levels indicating effective medical intervention). Often heat, whirlpools, and massages are very effective adjunctive treatments. Pool therapy may be initiated sooner than other forms of exercise.

If the person is confined to bed, protection from footdrop and contractures and prevention of pressure ulcers are essential. If the client has a skin rash, the therapist should caution about the possibility of infection from scratching. If antipruritic medications do not relieve severe itching, tepid sponges or compresses can be applied (see also Box 9-4). If the client is receiving corticosteroids, observe for side effects (weight gain, acne, edema, hypertension, purplish stretch marks [striae], easy bruising). Long-term use of steroids lowers resistance to infection, may induce diabetes, causes myopathy and/or neuropathy, and is associated with loss of potassium in the urine and gastric irritation (see Table 4-7 and the section on Corticosteroids in Chapter 4). If side effects are marked, advise against abruptly discontinuing corticosteroids until the client consults the physician first. A low-sodium diet will help prevent fluid retention.

Progressive pulmonary fibrosis complicates dermatomyositis and polymyositis in 10% of adults. During the acute phase of illness, clients must be closely monitored for signs of respiratory weakness that requires ventilatory assistance and for overwhelming infection that can lead to circulatory collapse.[15] ∎

THERMAL INJURIES

◆ Cold Injuries

Cold injuries result from overexposure to cold air or water and occur in two major forms: localized injuries (e.g., frostbite) and systemic injuries (e.g., hypothermia). Untreated or improperly treated frostbite can lead to gangrene and may necessitate amputation requiring therapy and rehabilitation. Hypothermia is a medical emergency and is not discussed in detail here.

Incidence and Etiologic and Risk Factors. Cold injuries, once almost exclusively a military problem, are becoming more prevalent among the general population, especially in athletes using localized cryotherapy or participating in outdoor sports. Frostbite results from prolonged exposure to dry temperatures far below freezing. The risk of serious cold injuries is increased by lack of insulating body fat, old age, homelessness, drug or alcohol use, cardiac disease, psychiatric illness, motor vehicle problems, or smoking when combined with unplanned circumstances leading to cold exposure without adequate protective clothing.[113]

Research is ongoing to reduce the risk of hypothermia and frostbite through the use of nuclear, biologic, and chemical (NBC) protective clothing combined with the Extreme Cold Weather Clothing System (ECWCS) for those individuals engaging in cold weather outdoor activities. It is undetermined yet whether wearing protective clothing may increase the risk of hypothermia during periods of strenuous activity followed by subsequent periods of inactivity accompanied by sweat accumulation in clothing, which may compromise insulation.[127]

Pathogenesis and Clinical Manifestations. Cold-induced injuries can be local or systemic. Severe cold affects all organ systems and especially the central nervous and cardiovascular systems. Many biologic reactions and pathways become distorted or slowed at low body core temperatures. Low body shell temperature can interfere with athletic ability by weakening and slowing muscle contractions, by delaying nerve conduction time, and by facilitating injury.[106]

Typically, an initial vasoconstriction in the skin will protect body parts from a drop in core temperature, but when tissue temperature drops to $-2°$ C, ice crystals form in the tissues and expand extracellular spaces resulting in localized cold injuries. With compression of cells, cell membranes rupture, interrupting enzymatic and metabolic activities. Additional injury occurs with thawing when increased capillary permeability accompanies the release of histamine, resulting in aggregation of red blood cells and microvascular occlusion. Research into the pathophysiology of cold injuries has revealed marked similarities in inflammatory processes to those seen in thermal burns and ischemia/reperfusion injury.[83]

Frostbite may be deep or superficial. Superficial frostbite affects the skin and subcutaneous tissue, especially of the face, ears, extremities, and other exposed body areas. Although it may go unnoticed at first, on returning to a warm place, frostbite produces burning, tingling, numbness, swelling, and a mottled, blue-gray skin color. When the affected area begins to rewarm, the person will feel pain and numbness followed by hypoesthesia. Deep frostbite extends beyond subcutaneous tissue and usually affects the hands or feet. The skin becomes white until it has thawed and then turns purplish blue. Deep frostbite produces pain, blisters, tissue necrosis, and gangrene (Fig. 9-20).

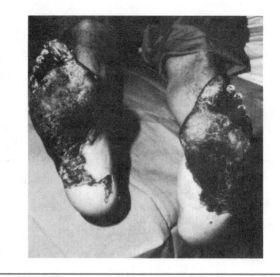

FIGURE 9-20 Frostbite of the feet. Blackened areas in the photo show tissue necrosis and gangrene, the result of deep frostbite that extends beyond the subcutaneous tissue. (From Norris J, McMahon E, Fandek N et al, editors: *Professional guide to diseases*, ed 5, Springhouse, Pa, 1995, Springhouse, p 298.)

Medical Management
Diagnosis and Treatment. Diagnosis is usually made based on the history and presenting symptoms; measures to prevent and treat general hypothermia are taken before managing the local frostbite injuries. Evidence of the role of thromboxanes and prostaglandins in cold injuries has resulted in more active approaches in the medical treatment of frostbite wounds, including the use of vasodilators, thrombolysis, and hyperbaric oxygen.[83] Triple-phase bone scans can be used to distinguish between tissue that is irreversibly destined for necrosis and tissue that is at risk for necrosis but potentially salvageable. These improvements in radiologic assessment have led to earlier surgical intervention to provide at-risk tissue with a new blood supply and preserve both function and length in an extremity.[113]

In a localized cold injury, treatment consists of rewarming the injured part without rubbing or massaging the area to avoid further tissue damage, and supportive measures (e.g., analgesics for pain [200 mg of ibuprofen every 6 hours][96] and proper positioning to avoid weight bearing with gauze between the toes to prevent maceration). More severe and deeper injuries should not be thawed until medical treatment can be given in a hospital.

The management of blisters was at one time controversial, but current practice indicates that all blisters should be opened and debrided (see the section on Skin Lesions: Special Implications for the Therapist, 9-1). Milky blisters may be treated with alcohol-free aloe vera products.[96] Bulky dressings may be applied to permit drainage and provide protection. A bed cradle may be needed to keep the weight of bed covers off the affected part or parts.

In the case of a developing compartment syndrome a fasciotomy may be performed to increase circulation by lowering edematous tissue pressure. If gangrene occurs, amputation may be necessary. Smoking causes vasoconstriction and slows healing; the client should be advised to quit smoking, at least during the recovery period.

Prognosis. The prognosis depends on the extent of localized cold injury and development of any complications, such as compartment syndrome, necrosis, or gangrene. Rapid triage and treatment of frostbite can lead to dramatic improvements in outcome and prognosis.[96] Long-term effects may include increased sensitivity to cold, burning and tingling on reexposure to cold, and increased sweating of the affected area.

Future cold injuries may be prevented through the use of wind-proof, water-resistant, many-layered clothing; moisture-wicking socks; a head covering; mittens instead of gloves; and heat-generating devices in pockets or battery-operated socks.

Special Implications for the Therapist 9-15

COLD INJURIES

Preferred Practice Patterns
4J: *Impaired Motor Function, Muscle Performance, Range of Motion, Gait, Locomotion, and Balance Associated With Amputation*
7D: *Impaired Integumentary Integrity Associated With Full-Thickness Skin Involvement and Scar Formation*
7E: *Impaired Integumentary Integrity Associated With Full-Thickness Skin Involvement Extending Into Fascia, Muscle, or Bone and Scar Formation*

Local cold injury subsequent to prolonged exposure may not be seen in a therapy practice until complications such as necrosis and gangrene result in amputation. Whirlpool with gentle agitation directed away from the affected area may be prescribed as part of the rewarming procedure. Water temperature is based on tissue temperature and should be determined in conjunction with the medical staff.

Use of cryotherapy as a modality among the general population can result in localized tissue damage requiring documentation (e.g., filing an accident report) and possible medical evaluation and treatment. Massage may cause further tissue damage and should not be carried out until local tissue has healed. ∎

◆ Burns

Definition and Overview. Injuries that result from direct contact or exposure to any thermal, chemical, electrical, or radiation source are termed *burns*. Burn injuries occur when energy from a heat source is transferred to the tissues of the body. The depth of injury is a function of temperature or source of energy (e.g., radiation) and duration of exposure.

The severity of burn injury is assessed with respect to the risk of infection, mortality, and cosmetic or functional disability.[94] Factors that influence injury severity include burn depth, burn size (percentage of total body surface area [TBSA]), burn location, age, general health, and mechanism of injury. Burn depth can be divided into categories based on the elements of the skin that are damaged (Fig. 9-21). Most burn wounds that require medical intervention are a combination of partial- and full-thickness burns.

Burn size is determined by one of two techniques: the rule of nines (Fig. 9-22) and the Lund-Browder method (Figs. 9-23 and 9-24). The rule of nines is based on the division of the body into anatomic sections, each of which represents 9% or a multiple of 9% of the TBSA. This is an easy method to quickly assess the percentage of TBSA injured and is most commonly used in emergency departments where the initial evaluation takes place. The Lund-Browder method modifies the percentages for body segments and provides a more accurate estimate of burn size according to age. For the most accurate estimate of burn size, the burn diagram should be confirmed following the initial wound debridement.[74]

Incidence. In the United States, approximately 1.4 to 2 million burn injuries occur each year; 70,000 people are hospitalized with severe injuries; and 7500 are fatalities. Extensive autografts are required in over 1500 third-degree burns every year and 40,000 second-degree burns. Burn injuries are the third leading cause of accidental death in all age-groups. Males tend to be injured more frequently than females, except for the older population (older than 70 years).[93] The incidence of burn injuries is expected to increase as an aging society characterized by a striving for independence becomes more apparent.[77]

Etiologic Factors. Burn injuries are categorized according to their mechanism of injury: thermal, chemical, electrical, or radiation. *Thermal* burns are caused by exposure to or contact with sources such as flames, hot liquids, steam, semisolids (tar), or hot objects. *Chemical* burns are caused by tissue contact, ingestion, inhalation, or injection with strong acids, alkalis, or organic compounds. Chemical burns can result from contact with certain household cleaning agents and various chemicals used in industry, agriculture, and the military. *Electrical* burns are caused by heat that is generated by the electrical energy as it passes through the body. Electrical burns can result from contact with exposed or faulty electrical wiring, high-voltage power lines, or lightning. *Radiation* burns are the least common burn injury and are caused by exposure to a radioactive source. These types of injuries have been associated with the use of ionizing radiation in industry or from therapeutic radiation sources in medicine. A sunburn from prolonged exposure to UV rays is also considered a type of radiation burn.

Risk Factors. Data collected from the National Burn Information Exchange indicate that 75% of all burn injuries result from the actions of the injured person, occurring most often in the home. Children under 3 years and adults over 70 years are at the highest risk for burn injury. Risk factors include inadequate adult supervision (in the case of children), psychomotor disorders (e.g., impaired judgment, impaired mobility, drug or alcohol use), rural location, mobile home residence, occupation, lack of smoke detectors, fireworks, and misuse of cigarettes.[23,77,78]

New data demonstrate a change in the epidemiology of burns from previous studies. These data point out the relationship between epileptic seizures and domestic scald injuries. Scald injuries are now the major cause of burns in people with epilepsy and account for approximately 2% of all burn admissions.[60]

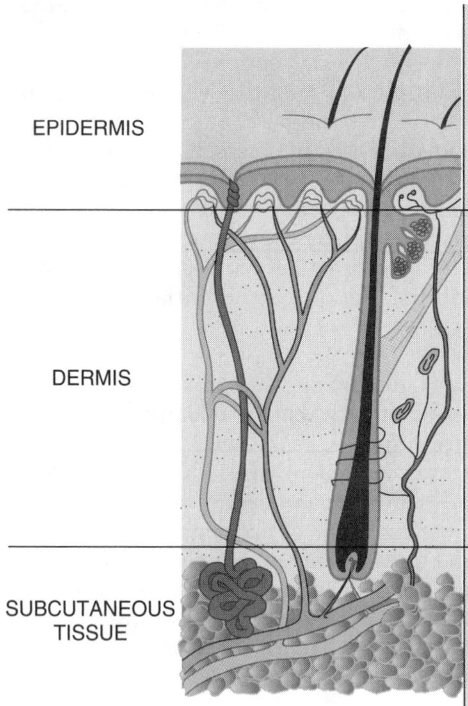

		CAUSE	APPEARANCE	SENSATION	COURSE
EPIDERMIS	SUPERFICIAL BURN First-degree burn	Sunburn Ultraviolet exposure Brief exposure to flash, flame, or hot liquids	Mild to severe erythema; skin blanches with pressure; dry, no blisters; edema variable amount	Painful Hyperesthetic Tingling Pain eased by cooling	Discomfort lasts about 48 hours Desquamation in 3–7 days
DERMIS	PARTIAL-THICKNESS BURN Second-degree burn	Superficial: Scalding liquids, semi liquids (oil, tar), or solids Deep: Immersion scald, flame	Large thick-walled blisters covering extensive area (vesication) Edema; mottled red base; broken epidermis; wet, shiny, weeping surface	Painful Sensitive to cold air	Superficial partial-thickness burn heals in 14–21 days Deep partial-thickness burn requires 21–28 days for healing Healing rate varies with burn depth and presence or absence of infection
SUBCUTANEOUS TISSUE	FULL-THICKNESS BURN Third-degree or fourth-degree burn	Prolonged exposure to: Chemical, electrical, flame, scalding liquids, steam	Variable, e.g., deep red, black, white, brown Dry surface Edema Fat exposed Tissue disrupted	Little or no pain Insensate	Full-thickness dead skin suppurates and liquefies after 2–3 weeks Spontaneous healing may be impossible but small areas may be left alone to form scarring without grafting (called secondary intent) Requires removal of eschar and subsequent split- or full-thickness skin grafting Hypertrophic scarring and wound contractures likely to develop without preventive measures

FIGURE **9-21** Burn injury classification according to depth of injury. This information is important to review because it will help determine the practice pattern to use when making a physical therapy diagnosis. A *partial-thickness* burn involves loss of epidermis and/or a portion of the dermis. Because part of the dermis is intact and that is where the regenerating elements are, a partial-thickness wound has the ability to heal via epithelialization. A *full-thickness* burn involves total destruction of the epidermis and dermis and cannot heal independently without contraction, therefore requiring a flap or skin graft procedure.[30]

Pathogenesis

Cutaneous Burn.   The pathophysiologic changes that occur immediately following a cutaneous burn injury depend on the extent or size of the burn. For smaller burns, the body's response to injury is localized to the injured area. With more extensive burns (25% or more of the TBSA), the response is systemic, potentially affecting all major systems of the body. The systems more obviously affected include the cardiovascular, renal, gastrointestinal, immune, and respiratory systems.

Cardiovascular changes occur immediately following a burn injury as vasoactive substances (catecholamines, histamine, serotonin, leukotrienes, prostaglandins) are released from the injured tissue causing an increase in capillary permeability. Extensive burns result in generalized body edema in both burned and nonburned tissues and a decrease in circulating intravascular blood volume. Heart rate increases in response to catecholamine release and to the hypovolemia, but overall cardiac output falls. If the intravascular space is not replenished with IV fluids, hypovolemic (burn) shock and death may result. Within 18 to 36 hours after the burn, capillary permeability decreases and continues to return to normal for several weeks following the injury. Cardiac output returns to normal and then increases approximately 24 hours after the injury to meet the hypermetabolic needs of the body. The body begins to reabsorb the edema fluid and excretes the excess fluid over the ensuing days and weeks. See also the section on Common Causes of Fluid and Electrolyte Imbalances in Chapter 4.

The *renal* and *gastrointestinal systems* are affected as the body responds initially by shunting blood from the kidneys and intestines leading to oliguria (decreased urine output) and intestinal dysfunction, respectively, in clients with burns greater than 25% of TBSA. *Immune system function* is depressed, increasing the risk of infection and life-threatening sepsis. The *respiratory system* may respond with pulmonary artery hypertension and decreased lung compliance, even when there has been no inhalation injury.

Smoke Inhalation.   Smoke inhalation may result in injury secondary to inhalation of carbon monoxide, smoke poisoning from the inhalation of byproducts of combustion, or direct ther-

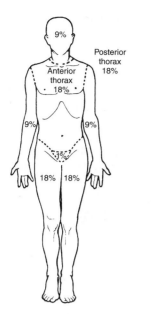

Posterior
thorax
18%

Anterior
thorax
18%

9%

9%

9%

9%

18% 18%

FIGURE   9-22   The rule of nines provides a quick method for estimating the extent of a burn injury.

mal burns to the pulmonary airways. See the section on Noxious Gases, Fumes, and Smoke Inhalation in Chapter 14.

Electrical and Chemical Burns.

In electrical burns, heat is generated as the electricity travels through the body, resulting in internal tissue damage. However, entrance and exit wounds may be significant, distracting medical personnel from internal injuries. Cutaneous burn injuries associated with electrical burns may be negligible, but soft tissue and muscle damage may be extensive, particularly in high-voltage electrical injuries. However, it is possible for electrical burns to ignite the person's clothes, causing thermal burns as well. The voltage, type of current (direct or alternating), contact site, and duration of contact are important factors in the amount and type of damage sustained. Alternating current is more dangerous than direct and is often associated with cardiopulmonary arrest, ventricular fibrillation, and tetanic muscle contractions. Other significant injuries, such as long-bone or vertebral compression fractures, spinal cord injury, or traumatic brain injury, can occur if the victim falls on electrical contact. Chemical burns are associated with systemic toxicity from cutaneous absorption. See also Chapter 3.

Clinical Manifestations.

Appearance, sensation, and course of injury of superficial, partial-thickness, and full-thickness burns are outlined in Fig. 9-21. Burn location influences injury severity in that burns of certain areas of the body are commonly associated with specific complications. For example, burns of the head, neck, and chest frequently have associated pulmonary complications. Burns involving the face may have associated corneal abrasions. Burns of the hands and joints can result in permanent physical and vocational disability requiring extensive therapy and rehabilitation. Circumferential burns of extremities may produce a tourniquet-like effect and lead to total occlusion of circulation.

Theoretically, with a full-thickness burn the nerve endings have been destroyed and no pain should be associated with this type of injury. However, most full-thickness burns occur with superficial and partial-thickness burns in which nerve endings are intact and exposed. Excised eschar (dead tissue produced by a burn) and donor sites expose nerve fibers as well. As peripheral nerves regenerate, painful sensation returns. Consequently, people with burn injuries often experience severe pain that is related to the size and depth of the burn.

The clinical course of the (major) burn client can be divided into three phases: the emergent and resuscitation phase, the acute phase, and the rehabilitation phase. The *emergent period* begins at the time of injury and concludes with the restoration of capillary permeability, usually 48 to 72 hours following injury. The *resuscitation period* begins with initiation of fluid resuscitation measures and ends when capillary integrity returns to near-normal levels and the large fluid shifts have decreased. The *acute phase* of recovery begins when the person is hemodynamically stable, capillary permeability is restored, and diuresis has begun, usually 48 to 72 hours after the initial injury occurred. The acute phase continues until wound closure is achieved. The *rehabilitation phase* represents the final phase of burn care, often overlaps the acute care phase, and lasts well beyond the period of hospitalization. This phase focuses on gaining independence through achievement of maximal functional recovery.

Infection is the most common and life-threatening complication of burn injuries. Burn wound infections can be classified on the basis of the causative organism, the depth of invasion, and the tissue response. Individuals with extensive burns and in whom wound closure is difficult to achieve are at greatest risk for infection and other complications. Inhalation injury with major burns and added staphylococcal septicemia are often fatal.[36] The multiple organ system response that occurs following a burn injury may result in the multiple organ dysfunction syndrome and death (see Chapter 4).

Hypertrophic scarring is a second complication that although not life-threatening is associated with considerable morbidity and potential lifelong disfigurement. Children and blacks are at greatest risk for hypertrophic scarring presumably because of the abundance of collagen in these groups. Aging white adults with wrinkled, loose skin have little to no hypertrophic scarring because of the absence of collagen.

Medical Management

Treatment.

The emergency department therapist may be involved in wound care for minor burns consisting of cleansing; removal of any damaging agents (chemicals, tar, etc.); debridement of loose, nonviable tissue; and application of topical antimicrobial creams or ointment and a sterile dressing. Blister management usually includes debridement of the blister (see the section on Skin Lesions: Special Implications for the Therapist, 9-1). Although the blister fluid is theoretically sterile most blisters break and the fluid is an ideal medium for bacteria.[103] Instructions for home care include observation for clinical manifestations of infection and active ROM exercises to maintain normal joint function, decrease edema formation, and decrease possible scar formation.

Treatment of major burns includes life-saving measures (ABCs: *airway*, *breathing*, *circulation*) immediately after the

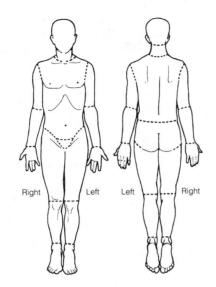

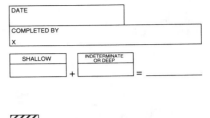

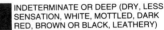

SHALLOW (PINK, PAINFUL, MOIST)

INDETERMINATE OR DEEP (DRY, LESS SENSATION, WHITE, MOTTLED, DARK RED, BROWN OR BLACK, LEATHERY)

Per cent surface area burned
(Berkow formula)

AREA	1 YEAR	1 to 4 YEARS	5 to 9 YEARS	10 to 14 YEARS	Y 15 YEARS	ADULT	SHALLOW	INDETER-MINATE OR DEEP
Head	19	17	13	11	9	7		
Neck	2	2	2	2	2	2		
Ant. Trunk	13	13	13	13	13	13		
Post.Trunk	13	13	13	13	13	13		
R. Buttock	2½	2½	2½	2½	2½	2½		
L. Buttock	2½	2½	2½	2½	2½	2½		
Genitalia	1	1	1	1	1	1		
R. U. Arm	4	4	4	4	4	4		
L. U. Arm	4	4	4	4	4	4		
R. L. Arm	3	3	3	3	3	3		
L. L. Arm	3	3	3	3	3	3		
R. Hand	2½	2½	2½	2½	2½	2½		
L. Hand	2½	2½	2½	2½	2¼	2½		
R. Thigh	5½	6½	8	8½	9	9½		
L. Thigh	5½	6½	8	8½	9	9½		
R. Leg	5	5	5½	6	6½	7		
L. Leg	5	5	5½	6	6½	7		
R. Foot	3½	3½	3½	3½	3½	3½		
L. Foot	3½	3½	3½	3½	3½	3½		
TOTAL								

FIGURE   9-23   A sample chart for recording the extent and depth of a burn injury using the Lund-Browder formula.

injury followed by restorative care (e.g., infection control, wound care, skin grafts, pain management) during the acute phase until wound closure is achieved. Therapists are closely involved early in the acute phase of recovery to maximize functional recovery and cosmetic outcome. Therapeutic interventions include wound care, positioning and immobilization following skin grafting to prevent unwanted movement and shearing of grafts, scar and contracture prevention and management, exercise, ambulation, and ADL. Elasticized garments help reduce scar hypertrophy and may be worn for months to 2 years after hospitalization.

Bioengineered temporary biologic dressings may be used to minimize fluid and protein loss from the burn surface, prevent infection, and reduce pain. Types of temporary grafts include *allografts* (homografts), which are usually cadaver skin; *xenografts* (heterografts), which are typically pigskin; and *biosynthetic grafts*, which are a combination of collagen and synthetics. To treat a full-thickness burn, an *autograft* (the person's own skin) may be required.

The transplanted skin graft will be used intact over areas where appearance or joint movement is important but the graft may be meshed (fenestrated) to cover up to three times its original size. Several new permanent skin substitutes are being utilized to aid in replacing dermal thickness and to assist in coverage of large surface area injuries.[92] Cultured skin is usually used in conjunction with allograft dermis. See the section on Skin Transplantation in Chapter 20.

Prognosis.   Burn care has improved in recent decades, resulting in a lower mortality rate for victims of burn injuries. Current techniques of burn wound care, such as effective topical antimicrobial chemotherapy and early burn wound excision, have significantly reduced the overall occurrence of invasive burn wound infections.[94]

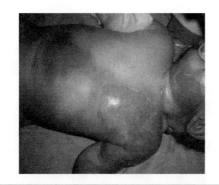

A

B

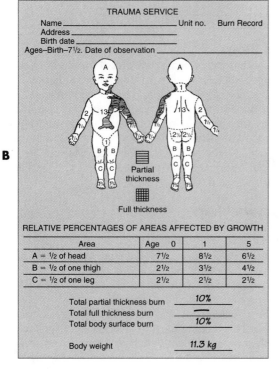

TRAUMA SERVICE

Name_____ Unit no.   Burn Record
Address_____
Birth date_____
Ages–Birth–7½. Date of observation _____

Partial
thickness

Full thickness

RELATIVE PERCENTAGES OF AREAS AFFECTED BY GROWTH

Area	Age 0	1	5
A = ½ of head	7½	8½	6½
B = ½ of one thigh	2½	3½	4½
C = ½ of one leg	2½	2½	2½

Total partial thickness burn	10%
Total full thickness burn	—
Total body surface burn	10%
Body weight	11.3 kg

FIGURE   **9-24   A,** Pediatric scald burn. **B,** Corresponding Lund-Browder chart. (Courtesy Katherine S. Biggs, P.T., Yale New Haven Hospital, New Haven, Conn.)

The client's age affects the severity and outcome of the burn. Mortality rates are higher for children less than 4 years of age and for clients over 65 years although survival rates after burns have improved significantly for children. At present most children, even children with large burns, should survive.[109] Survival rate for older clients is 70% with at least 60% of those individuals becoming fully functional 6 months after hospital discharge.[77]

Factors such as obesity, alcoholism, and cardiac disorders affecting general health, especially disorders that impair peripheral circulation, such as peripheral vascular disease, increase the complication and mortality rates for adults with burns. Delay in amputation results in prolonged hospital stay, delayed rehabilitation, and a higher mortality rate. Early amputation is associated with a 14% mortality rate compared with a 50% mortality rate for cases of delayed amputation. Earlier identification of nonsalvageable limbs may decrease infectious complications and improve chances of survival.[128]

Special Implications for the Therapist   9-16

BURNS

Preferred Practice Patterns
6C: Impaired Ventilation, Respiration/Gas Exchange, and Aerobic Capacity/Endurance Associated With Airway Clearance Dysfunction
6E: Impaired Ventilation and Respiration/Gas Exchange Associated With Ventilatory Pump Dysfunction or Failure
7B: Impaired Integumentary Integrity Associated With Superficial Skin Involvement
7C: Impaired Integumentary Integrity Associated With Partial-Thickness Skin Involvement and Scar Formation
7D: Impaired Integumentary Integrity Associated With Full-Thickness Skin Involvement and Scar Formation
7E: Impaired Integumentary Integrity Associated With Skin Involvement Extending Into Fascia, Muscle, or Bone and Scar Formation

In light of statistics showing that the population over 70 years old is at highest risk of burn injury, prevention of burn accidents, especially in this population, is an important part of client education.* Reviewing simple cooking precautions may be helpful; for example, do not leave burners in use unattended, do not use high heat, do not wear clothing with loose sleeves or belts (especially bathrobes), use front burners whenever possible, and avoid leaning over front burners when using back burners.

Unless employed in an emergency department, most therapists do not begin to treat the burn client until the acute phase (as soon as the person is physiologically stable), continuing intervention through much of the rehabilitation phase. However, initiating bedside intervention before the person is medically stable is ideal in reducing morbidity and functional loss. The therapist will direct treatment intervention to encourage deep breathing and facilitate lung expansion; promote wound healing; reduce dependent edema formation and promote venous return; prevent or minimize deformities and hypertrophic scarring; increase ROM, strength, and function; increase independence in daily activities and self-care; and encourage emotional and psychologic well-being. Specific compression, lymphatic movement, debridement, and wound care procedures are beyond the scope of this book; the reader is referred to other texts for more detailed information.[21,52,76,99,114]

Throughout the acute and rehabilitation phases of burn care, the therapist must remain alert to the development of medical complications, such as ileus, gastric ulcers, respiratory distress, infection, and impaired circulation. Monitor vital signs (e.g., heart rate, blood pressure, oxygen saturation levels) to ensure the person can tolerate therapy. Notify the nursing staff of any new or unusual findings observed during assessment and intervention (Table 9-9). Daily inspection of the wound must be made; any change in wound appearance must be reported.

The amount of body surface area exposed during wound care must be minimized to prevent hypothermia because heat is lost in open wounds and after hydrotherapy by evap-

Continued

---

*Additional resources for the therapist are available.[21,99]

TABLE	9-9

Assessing Medical Complications in the Burn-Injured Adult

SYSTEM	COMPLICATIONS
Urinary	Visible red or dark brown urine (catheter)
Respiratory	Signs of respiratory distress
	Restlessness
	Confusion
	Labored breathing
	Tachypnea (>24 respirations/min)
	Dyspnea
	PaO_2 <90 mm Hg; O_2 <95%
Peripheral vascular	Pulses absent on palpation
	Capillary refill (unburned area) >2 sec
	Numbness or tingling
	Increased pain with active range-of-motion exercises
	Increased edema, changes in skin color
Infection	Discoloration of wounds or drainage, odor, delayed healing
	Headache, chills, anorexia, nausea
	Increased pain
	Change in vital signs
	Paralytic ileus, confusion, restlessness, hallucinations
Gastrointestinal	Paralytic ileus (painful, distended abdomen)
	Stress-induced gastric ulcer (epigastric pain, abdominal distention, loss of appetite, nausea)

oration. Hydrotherapy treatment must be limited to 30 minutes or less with water temperature in the 98° to 102° F range. External heat shields or radiant heat lamps can provide a source of external heat. Clients excluded from hydrotherapy are generally those who are hemodynamically unstable and those with new grafts. In recent years, hydrotherapy has been challenged and alternative methods are being advocated (e.g., shower versus tub, smaller tub versus tank).*[114]

People with burns are at high risk of infection because of the significant loss of skin barrier and impaired immune response. Infection control techniques must be practiced carefully at all times (see Appendix A). Skin donor sites require the same care and precautions as other partial-thickness wounds in order to promote healing and prevent infection.

Arrange any therapy likely to elicit a painful response to coincide with medications (allow 45 minutes for oral, 30 minutes for intramuscular [IM], 5 to 10 minutes for IV administration). Combining relaxation techniques, music therapy, distraction, and other techniques for pain modulation may be helpful. Burned areas must be maintained in positions of physiologic function within the limits imposed by associated injuries, grafting, and other therapeutic devices (see Table 9-10 for positioning recommendations).

Burned areas are prone to develop contractures requiring close assessment of ROM and muscle strength. Encourage active ROM exercises at least every 2 hours while the person is awake unless this is contraindicated by a recent grafting procedure. Prolonged stretching is sometimes combined with splinting or orthoses to maintain motion. Provide honest, positive reinforcement throughout intervention, being aware that each individual will progress through stages of denial, grief, and acceptance of injury and recovery. During the rehabilitation phase, chronic pain protocols may be helpful (see Box 2-13). ■

MISCELLANEOUS SKIN DISORDERS

◆ Skin Ulcers

Skin ulcers can be caused by a variety of underlying disorders, including diabetes, arterial insufficiency, radiation damage, systemic sclerosis, vasculitis, and prolonged pressure. In keeping with the focus of this text of recognizing the underlying pathology for various conditions, skin ulcers are discussed in individual sections according to the pathogenesis (e.g., diabetic ulcer, see the section on Diabetes Mellitus in Chapter 10; arterial insufficiency ulcers, see the section on Peripheral Vascular Disease in Chapter 11).

◆ Pressure Ulcers

Definition and Overview. A pressure ulcer (formerly called bed sore, decubitus ulcer) is a lesion caused by unrelieved pressure resulting in damage to underlying tissue. Pressure ulcers usually occur over bony prominences, such as the elbows, scapula, sacrum, heels, ischial tuberosities, and greater trochanters, and are graded or staged to classify the degree of tissue damage observed (Table 9-11).* It should be noted that this staging classification is only for pressure ulcers. Other types of ulcers, such as arterial, venous, or neuropathic ulcers† (see Table 11-21), are staged using Wagner's classifications (Table 9-12).

Incidence. Consistent data concerning incidence of pressure ulcers in the United States are difficult to find. Studies differ in a number of significant ways, and methodologies vary considerably.[9,10] Given these limitations it is estimated that 1.5 million people develop pressure ulcers each year, including 500,000 people in nursing homes and another 400,000 people with diabetic foot ulcers. Pressure ulcers are viewed as high-volume, high-risk problems in most health care settings. In long-term care facilities, regulatory agencies have designated the development of pressure ulcers as an indicator of quality of care provided to clients.[34] *Healthy People 2010* has set as an objective to reduce the proportion of nursing home residents

---

*Clinicians working with this client population are encouraged to review this resource for more specific details.

*In 1975 a landmark paper was published describing a method of classifying pressure ulcers, defined by the anatomic depth of soft tissue damage. Since that time the original staging system has been modified and developed into the current staging system adopted by the Agency for Health Care Policy and Research (AHCPR) Pressure Ulcer Guideline Panels and published in both sets of Pressure Ulcer Clinical Practice Guidelines (1992, 1994).[8,56] The revised stage I definition adopted by the NPUAP in 1998 that is more inclusive of the range of skin pigmentation is included in Table 9-11.

†The term *neuropathic ulcer* is used interchangeably with *diabetic ulcer*, but a diabetic ulcer is really a neuropathic ulcer in someone with diabetes. Neuropathic ulcers can occur in anyone with loss of sensation (e.g., alcoholic neuropathy, peripheral neuropathy).

TABLE	9-10

Therapeutic Positioning for the Burn-Injured Client

BURNED AREA	THERAPEUTIC POSITION	POSITIONING TECHNIQUES
Neck		
Anterior	Extension	No pillow; small towel roll beneath cervical spine to promote neck extension
Circumferential	Neutral toward extension	No pillow
Posterior or asymmetric	Neutral	No pillow
Shoulder, axilla	Arm abduction to 90-110 degrees	Splinting; arms positioned away from body and supported on arm troughs; elbow splint
Elbow	Arm extension	Elbow splint; elbow(s) positioned in extension with slight bend at elbow (≤10 degrees of elbow flexion)
		Arms supported on arm troughs with the forearm in slight pronation
Hand		
Wrist	Wrist extension	Hand splint
Metacarpophalangeal (MCP) joints	MCP flexion at 90 degrees	Hand splint
Proximal or distal interphalangeal (PIP/DIP) joints	PIP/DIP extension	Hand splint
Thumb	Thumb abduction	Hand splint with thumb abduction
Web spaces	Finger abduction	Web spacers of gauze, foam, or thermoplastics to decrease webbing formation
Hip	Hip extension	Supine with the head of bed flat and legs extended
		Trochanter roll to maintain neutral rotation (toes pointing toward ceiling)
		Prone positioning
Knee	Knee extension	Supine with knees extended and toes pointing toward ceiling
		Prone with feet extended over end of mattress
		Sitting with legs extended and elevated
		Knee splint
Ankle	Neutral	Padded footboard
		Ankle positioning devices (avoid position of ankle inversion or eversion)
		Portect heels to prevent pressure ulcer

Modified from Carrougher GJ: Nursing care of clients with burns. In Black JM, Matassarin-Jacobs E, editors: *Medical-surgical nursing*, ed 5, Philadelphia, 1997, Saunders, p 2260.

with current diagnosis of pressure ulcers from 16/1000 residents to no more than 9/1000 residents.*

Etiologic and Risk Factors. Pressure ulcers are caused by unrelieved pressure that results in damaged skin, muscle, and underlying tissue, usually over bony prominences. The primary causative factors for the development of pressure ulcers are (1) interface pressure (externally); (2) friction (rubbing of the skin against another surface); (3) shearing forces (two layers sliding against each other in opposite directions causing damage to the underlying tissues); (4) maceration (softening caused by excessive moisture); and (5) decreased skin resilience (e.g., dehydration).

*The target setting method used by *Healthy People 2010* in conjunction with the National Pressure Ulcer Advisory Panel is based on a 50% reduction in prevalence and improvement over the baseline. Incidence refers to the rate at which new cases occur in a population over a given period of time, whereas prevalence refers to the number of both new and old cases at any one time in the population.

Pressure contributes to other types of ulcers (e.g., arterial, venous, neuropathic), and likewise, the underlying cause of the other types of ulcers can contribute to the development of pressure ulcers (see Table 11-21). However, pressure ulcers are a separate entity from these other types of ulcers. A systemic risk assessment evaluating both sensation and physiologic risk of pressure ulcers can be made using a validated risk assessment tool, such as the Braden Scale (Table 9-13) or the Norton Scale (Table 9-14). Intrinsic factors most commonly associated with pressure ulcer development include impaired mobility of activity levels, incontinence, nutritional status, and altered levels of consciousness. Extrinsic factors include pressure, shear, friction, and moisture.

Bed- and chair-bound clients and those with impaired ability to reposition themselves should be assessed for additional factors that increase the risk of developing pressure ulcers. These factors include decreased mobility or immobility; hip or femoral fractures; contractures; increased muscle tone; loss of

TABLE **9-11**

Stages of Pressure Ulcers

Stage I*
An observable pressure-related alteration of intact skin whose indicators as compared to an adjacent or opposite area on the body may include changes in one or more of the following:
- Skin temperature (warmth or coolness)
- Tissue consistency (firm or boggy feel)
- Sensation (pain, itching)

The ulcer appears as a defined area of persistent redness in lightly pigmented skin, whereas in darker skin tones, the ulcer may appear with persistent red, blue, or purple hues.
NOTE: Reactive hyperemia can normally be expected to be present for one half to three fourths as long as the pressure-occluded blood flow to the area; it should not be confused with a stage I pressure ulcer.

Stage II
Partial-thickness skin loss involving epidermis or dermis or both. The ulcer is superficial and presents clinically as an abrasion, blister, or shallow crater.

Stage III
Full-thickness skin loss involving damage or necrosis of subcutaneous tissue that may extend down to, but not through, underlying fascia. The ulcer presents clinically as a deep crater with or without undermining of adjacent tissue.

Stage IV
Full-thickness skin loss with extensive destruction, tissue necrosis, or damage to muscle, bone, or supporting structures (e.g., tendon or joint capsule).
NOTE: Undermining and sinus tracts may also be associated with stage IV pressure ulcers.

Modified from U.S. Department of Health and Human Services: *Pressure ulcers in adults: prediction and prevention.* Clinical practice guideline no. 3. AHCPR publication no. 92-0047, Rockville, Md, 1992, The Department.
*Revised 1998 Stage I pressure ulcer definition; the NPUAP has not changed the definitions of Stages II-IV pressure ulcers.

---

sensation; incontinence; obesity; nutritional factors*; chronic disease accompanied by anemia, edema, renal failure, or sepsis; and altered level of consciousness.

Pathogenesis. Pressure is the external factor causing ischemia and tissue necrosis. Continuous pressure on soft tissues between bony prominences and hard or unyielding surfaces compresses capillaries and occludes blood flow. Normal capillary blood pressure at the arterial end of the vascular bed averages 32 mm Hg. When tissues are externally compressed, that pressure may be exceeded, reducing blood supply to, and lymphatic drainage of, the affected area.[55,56] Shearing (when

---

*Nutritional factors may include malnutrition or inadequate nutrition leading to weight loss and subsequent reduction of subcutaneous tissue and muscle bulk. The Agency for Health Care Policy and Research (AHCPR) guidelines for clinically significant malnutrition impairing wound healing include serum albumin less than 3.5 mg/dl and total lymphocyte count less than 1800/mm³ (see Tables 39-4 and 39-15).

TABLE **9-12**

Wagner's Ulcer Grade Classification

GRADE	CHARACTERISTICS
0	Preulcerative lesions; healed ulcers; presence of bony deformity
1	Superficial ulcer without subcutaneous tissue involvement
2	Penetration through the subcutaneous tissue; may expose bone, tendon, ligament, or joint capsule
3	Osteitis, abscess, or osteomyelitis
4	Gangrene of digit
5	Gangrene of foot requiring disarticulation

This classification scheme for ulceration is used for arterial, venous, or neuropathic ulcers and does not represent pressure ulcers. It is included here for comparison with the stages of pressure ulcers (see Table 9-11).

From Wagner REW: The dysvascular foot: a system for diagnosis and treatment, *Foot Ankle* 2:64-122, 1981.

---

the skin layers move in opposite directions) is the intrinsic factor that contributes to ripping or tearing of blood vessels, further damaging the integument.

If the pressure is relieved, a brief period of rebound capillary dilation (called *reactive hyperemia*) occurs and no tissue damage develops. If the pressure is not relieved, the endothelial cells lining the capillaries become disrupted by platelet aggregation, forming microthrombi that occlude blood flow and cause anoxic necrosis of surrounding tissues. Necrotic tissue predisposes to bacterial invasion and subsequent infection, preventing healthy granulation of scar tissue (Fig. 9-25). Muscle and tendon tissue can tolerate less pressure loading than skin before ischemic damage.[75]

In the case of neuropathic ulcers associated with diabetes, the primary pathogenesis is the absence of protective sensation combined with high pressure. The absence of protective sensation indicates a high risk for pressure ulcers on the feet; diabetic ulcers are typically present on the soles of the feet (see the section on Diabetes Mellitus: Ulceration in Chapter 10).

Clinical Manifestations. Pressure ulcers usually occur over bony prominences and often in a circular pattern shaped like an inverted volcano with the greatest tissue ischemia at the apex next to the bone, or they may assume the shape of objects causing the pressure, such as tubing. Irregular patterns indicate additional shearing forces or other contributing factors. Sacral ulcers are often deep to the bone and large since the tissue mass over the sacrum is thin and erodes easily to the deep tissues. Pressure ulcers are manifested at the surface as the deeper tissues die so that a stage I ulcer can become a stage III or IV quickly without further injury.

The wounds (Fig. 9-26) can be described, measured, and categorized with respect to surface area, exudates, and type of wound tissue.* When present, infection can be localized and

---

*Therapists may want to utilize the PUSH Tool to assess and document pressure ulcers. This tool is available from the National Pressure Ulcer Advisory Panel (NPUAP): www.npuap.org.

TABLE 9-13

The Braden Scale for Predicting Ulcer Risk

Category	1	2	3	4
Sensory Perception (ability to respond to discomfort)	1. Completely limited: Unresponsive to painful stimuli, either because of state of unconsciousness or severe sensory impairment, which limits ability to feel pain over most of body surface.	2. Very limited: Responds only to painful stimuli (but not verbal commands) by opening eyes or flexing extremities. Cannot communicate discomfort verbally OR has a sensory impairment that limits the ability to feel pain or discomfort over 1/2 body surface.	3. Slightly limited: Responds to verbal commands by opening eyes and obeying some commands but cannot always communicate discomfort or needs OR has some sensory impairment that limits ability to feel pain or discomfort in one or two extremities.	4. No impairment: Responds to verbal commands by obeying. Can communicate needs accurately. Has no sensory deficit that would limit ability to feel pain or discomfort.
Moisture (degree to which skin is exposed to moisture)	1. Very moist: Skin is kept moist almost constantly by perspiration and urine. Dampness is detected every time patient is moved or turned. Linen must be changed more than one time each shift.	2. Occasionally moist: Skin is frequently, but not always, kept moist; linen must be changed 2 or 3 times every 24 hr.	3. Rarely moist: Skin is rarely moist more than 3 or 4 times per week, but linen does require changing at that time.	4. Never moist: Perspiration and incontinence are never a problem; linen changed at routine intervals only.
Activity (degree of physical activity)	1. Bed-fast: Confined to bed.	2. Chair-fast: Ability to walk severely impaired or nonexistent and must be assisted into chair or wheelchair. Is confined to chair or wheelchair when not in bed.	3. Walks occasionally: Walks occasionally during day but for very short distances, with or without assistance. Spends majority of each shift in bed or chair.	4. Walks frequently: Walks a moderate distance at least once every 1-2 hr during waking hours.
Mobility (ability to change and control body position)	1. Completely immobile: Unable to make even slight changes in position without assistance.	2. Very limited: Makes occasional slight changes in position without help but unable to make frequent or significant changes in position independently.	3. Slightly limited: Makes frequent although slight changes in position without assistance but unable to make or maintain major changes in position independently.	4. No limitations: Makes major and frequent changes in position without assistance.
Nutrition (usual food intake pattern)	1. Very poor: Never eats a complete meal. Rarely eats more than 1/3 of any food offered. Intake of protein is negligible. Takes even fluids poorly. Does not take a liquid dietary supplement OR is NPO or maintained on clear liquids or IV feeding for more than 5 days.	2. Probably inadequate: Rarely eats a complete meal and generally eats only about 1/2 of any food offered. Protein intake is poor. Occasionally will take a liquid dietary supplement OR receiving less than optimum amount of liquid diet or tube feeding.	3. Adequate: Eats over 1/2 of most meals. Eats moderate amount of protein source 1 or 2 times daily. Occasionally will refuse a meal. Will usually take a dietary supplement if offered OR is on tube feeding or TPN, which probably meets most nutritional needs.	4. Excellent: Eats most of every meal. Never refuses a meal. Frequently eats between meals. Does not require a dietary supplement.
Friction and Shear	1. Problem: Requires moderate to maximum assistance in moving. Complete lifting without sliding against sheets is impossible. Frequently slides down in bed or chair, requiring frequent repositioning with maximum assistance. Either spasticity, contractures, or agitation leads to almost constant friction.	2. Potential problem: Moves feebly independently or requires minimum assistance. Skin probably slides against bedsheets or chair to some extent when movement occurs. Maintains relatively good position in chair or bed most of the time but occasionally slides down.	3. No apparent problem: Moves in bed and in chair independently and has sufficient muscle strength to lift up completely during move. Maintains good position in bed or chair at all times.	

TABLE 9-14

Norton Scale

PHYSICAL CONDITION		MENTAL CONDITION		ACTIVITY		MOBILITY		INCONTINENT		TOTAL SCORE
Good	4	Alert	4	Ambulant	4	Full	4	Not	4	
Fair	3	Apathetic	3	Walk/help	3	Slightly limited	3	Occasional	3	
Poor	2	Confused	2	Chairbound	2	Very limited	2	Usually/urine	2	
Very bad	1	Stupor	1	Bed	1	Immobile	1	Doubly	1	
Name		Date								

From Norton D, McLaren R, Exton-Smith AN: *An investigation of geriatric nursing problems in the hospital,* London 1962, National Corporation for the Care of Old People (now the Centre for Policy on Ageing).

self-limiting or can progress to sepsis. Proteolytic enzymes from bacteria and macrophages dissolve necrotic tissues and cause a foul-smelling discharge that appears like, but is not, pus.

Necrosis associated with pressure ulcers is not painful, but the surrounding tissue is often painful in individuals who do not have loss of sensation from spinal cord trauma or neuropathy. Trauma to the tissues produces an acute inflammatory response with hyperemia, fever, and increased white blood cell count.

However, many individuals never initiate a significant acute inflammatory response because of the heavy bioburden from large amounts of necrotic tissue but rather develop an unresolved chronic inflammation. Individuals who are immunosuppressed or who have diabetes mellitus are often unable to mount a sufficient inflammatory response to start the healing cascade and thus are at greater risk for infection.

Medical Management

Diagnosis. Prevention is the key to this condition (Table 9-15), starting with assessment of people at high risk for the development of pressure ulcers. In fact, risk prediction should be an ongoing assessment carried out by all health care professionals. In addition to the Braden Scale (see Table 9-13) or Norton Scale (see Table 9-14), laboratory data on hemoglobin, hematocrit, albumin, total protein, and lymphocytes should be assessed by all health care professionals involved.

The diagnosis is reached by looking at the location of the wound and the type of tissue response. The pressure ulcer is then staged (see Tables 9-11 and 9-12). If there is evidence of infection, the wound is cleaned with isotonic saline and debrided if necrosis is present, and then viable tissue is cultured (not a swab culture of the exudates or necrotic tissue).* Sensitivity testing to identify infecting organisms and to help determine appropriate topical or systemic antibiotics* may be needed. Topical antibiotics (e.g., Polysporin, Neosporin, Bacitracin, Bactroban, Metrogel) can be effective on local infections without systemic involvement to control bacterial concentration. Antiseptics are not recommended because these are cytotoxic.

TISSUE LOAD
MANAGEMENT

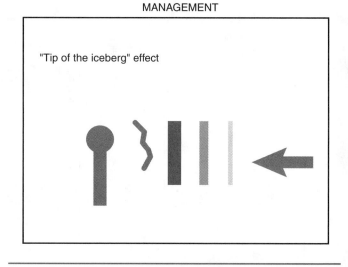

"Tip of the iceberg" effect

FIGURE 9-25 Evolving stages of a stage IV pressure ulcer. This diagram represents a trochanter partially surrounded by tendon, with subcutaneous, dermis, and epidermis layers (*vertical lines left to right*). As pressure occurs from the outside (*arrow*), the tendon becomes ischemic first, and then the subcutaneous layer is affected because it is less vascular than the dermis. The last tissue to become ischemic is the epidermis. The observer would initially identify the epidermal tissue change as a stage I pressure ulcer. Initially, the ischemic inner tissue layers would not be known. Only as the necrosis moves superficially will the full impact of tissue damage become observable, identifying the area as a stage IV pressure ulcer with extensive damage to the bone. (Courtesy Karen Kendall, P.T., C.W.S., Medical Center for Continuing Education, Gulf Breeze, Fla., 2000.)

Treatment. Prevention and removing the causative factor are the first step in the treatment intervention of pressure ulcers. Preventing shear and friction forces requires education of the client and primary caretakers. The pressure ulcer is cleaned thoroughly; spontaneous healing will occur more quickly when the ulcer is kept moist.† The use of antiseptics

---

*The definition of infection is invasion into viable tissue. Cultures of the organisms that have invaded the tissue causing the infection must be determined following these procedures. Clinical practice of wound cultures must be careful to avoid culturing wound exudate contaminants, of which there are usually a minimum of three per wound.[64]

*The AHCPR (no. 15) recommends blood cultures for ulcer-related sepsis to determine appropriate systemic antibiotics.

†Many plastic surgeons continue to advocate the initial use of wet-to-dry dressing (application of open wet dressing, allowing it to dry on the ulcer, and mechanically debriding exudate by removal of the dressing) for debridement. Because there is a risk of removing viable tissue, as well as bleeding, with this procedure, it no longer has universal approval.[8, 75]

TABLE	9-15

Guidelines for Prevention of Pressure Ulcers in Adults

- All clients at risk should have a systematic skin inspection at least once each day, paying particular attention to the bony prominences. Results of skin inspection should be documented (see Box 9-5).
- Clean skin at the time of soiling and at routine intervals. Individualize the frequency of skin cleaning according to need and client preference. Avoid hot water, and use a mild cleaning agent that minimizes irritation and dryness of the skin. During the cleaning or wound care process, minimize the force and friction applied to the skin.
- Minimize environmental factors leading to skin drying, such as low humidity (< 40%) and exposure to cold. Treat dry skin with moisturizers.
- Do NOT perform massage over bony prominences in the population at risk. Perform indirect soft tissue mobilization techniques or massaging the tissue around and toward the area with caution.
- Minimize skin injury caused by friction and shear forces through proper positioning, transferring, and turning techniques. Reduce friction injuries by the use of lubricants such as cornstarch and creams, protective films such as transparent film dressings and skin sealants, protective dressings such as hydrocolloids, and protective padding.
- Maintain current activity level, mobility, and range of motion. Evaluate the potential for improving the person's mobility and activity status, and institute rehabilitation efforts.
- Monitor and document interventions and outcomes.
- Reposition any person in bed who is assessed to be at risk of developing pressure ulcers at least every 2 hr if consistent with overall treatment goals.
- For persons in bed, use positioning devices such as pillows or foam wedges to keep bony prominences (e.g., knees, ankles) from direct contact with one another.
- Provide persons in bed who are completely immobile with devices that completely relieve pressure on the heels. Do not use doughnut-type devices.
- When side-lying position is used in bed, avoid positioning directly on the greater trochanter.
- Maintain the head of the bed at the lowest degree of elevation (30-degree lateral incline; see Fig. 9-28) consistent with medical conditions and other restrictions. Limit the amount of time the head of the bed is elevated.
- Use lifting devices, such as a trapeze, hydraulic lift, slide board, or linen, to move (rather than drag) persons in bed who cannot assist during transfers and position changes.
- Place any person assessed to be at risk of developing pressure ulcers, when lying in bed, on a pressure-reducing surface, such as foam, static air, alternating air, gel, or water mattresses.
- Avoid uninterrupted sitting in any chair or wheelchair for any person at risk of developing a pressure ulcer. Reposition the person, shifting the points under pressure at least every hour, or put him or her back to bed if consistent with overall management goals. Persons who are able should be taught to shift weight every 15 min.
- For chair-bound persons, use a pressure-reducing device. Do not use doughnut-type devices.

Modified from Panel on the Prediction and Prevention of Pressure Ulcers in Adults: *Pressure ulcers in adults: prediction and prevention*. Clinical practice guidelines. CPR publication no. 92-0050, Rockville, Md, 1992, Agency for Health Care Policy and Research, Public Health Service, U.S.

such as hydrogen peroxide or iodine is not recommended because these are cytotoxic and can be damaging to marginal granulation tissue.

Successful healing requires continued adequate relief of pressure (e.g., turning, positioning, support surfaces) and absence of infection. The presence of necrotic tissue in a wound may provide an optimal environment for bacteria to grow, hence the importance of removing necrotic material from a wound as rapidly as possible. Therapeutic intervention may include hydrotherapy (e.g., pulsatile lavage with suction), electrical stimulation, ultrasound, debridement (autolytic, enzymatic, mechanical, sharp), or any combination of these. An appropriate wound covering is then applied to provide an optimal wound environment.

Large deep pressure ulcers may require chemical debridement using proteolytic enzyme agents or surgical debridement of necrotic tissue and opening of deep pockets for drainage. A variety of skin-grafting techniques may be used if the wound is closed. In stage III ulcers, undamaged tissue near the wound is rotated to cover the ulcer. In stage IV ulcers, musculoskeletal flaps (a single unit of skin with its underlying muscle and vasculature), as well as a variety of other skin-grafting techniques, may be used effectively to close the wound. Bioactive human dermal tissue capable of interacting with the wound bed is now available commer-

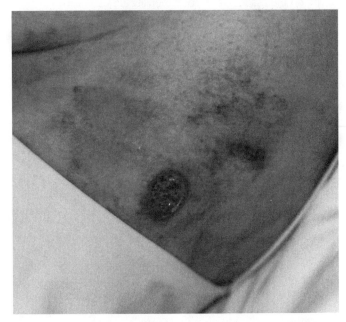

FIGURE   9-26 Pressure ulcer. (Courtesy Pam Unger, P.T., Community General Hospital, Center for Wound Management, Reading, Pa., 1995.)

cially for use in pressure and neuropathic ulcer wound management.*

Prognosis. Most clients have multiple complicating medical factors that contribute to the poor wound closure. Each client responds differently to a course of therapy. Provided there is no infection, there is a good blood supply, the pressure has been eliminated, and the client has no medical complications, the wound should heal successfully. The presence of any of these factors alters the prognosis negatively.

---

*These skin substitutes derived from living human tissue (human fibroblasts) represent an important advance in the treatment of burns and skin ulcers, including neuropathic foot ulcers, venous ulcers, and pressure ulcers. See the extensive section on Skin Transplantation in Chapter 20.

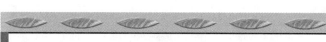

Special Implications for the Therapist 9-17

PRESSURE ULCERS

Preferred Practice Patterns
7B: Impaired Integumentary Integrity Associated With Superficial Skin Involvement
7C: Impaired Integumentary Integrity Associated With Partial-Thickness Skin Involvement and Scar Formation
7D: Impaired Integumentary Integrity Associated With Full-Thickness Skin Involvement and Scar Formation
7E: Impaired Integumentary Integrity Associated With Skin Involvement Extending Into Fascia, Muscle, or Bone and Scar Formation

The therapist plays a pivotal role in the prevention and management of pressure ulcers. Not only is the therapist an expert in the delivery of therapeutic modalities, but also appropriate positioning, management of tissue load (mechanical factors acting on the tissues), and good mobility are essential to the success of the intervention.

High-risk clients should be identified, possibly using the Braden Scale or Norton Scale (see Tables 9-13 and 9-14), but all people in the health care delivery system should be evaluated for risk levels and reassessed every 3 months for changes in status (or when there is a change in medical status). Anyone with a history of previous pressure ulcer is considered high risk requiring a prevention protocol immediately.

The high-risk client will need frequent position changes (at least every 2 hours). Utilizing all turning surfaces, position the client at a 45-degree oblique angle when side-lying (Fig. 9-27). Elevate the head of the bed no greater than 30 degrees when the client is supine (Fig. 9-28); if the head of the bed is elevated beyond 30 degrees (e.g., for eating, watching television, nursing care, or therapy intervention) the duration of this position needs to be limited to minimize both pressure and shear forces. A trapeze bar, turning sheet, or transfer board can be used to prevent shearing injury to the skin during movement or position change. Frequent shifting of body weight prevents ischemia by redistributing the weight and allowing blood to recirculate. Static or dynamic pressure-reducing devices using air, gel or water, foam, or other substances are commercially available, but the therapist must be aware that the material covering these devices can also create heat and friction contributing to pres-

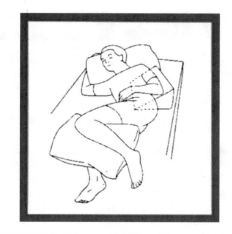

FIGURE 9-27 Following the "rule of 30s" (head position at 30 degrees; see Fig. 9-28) and bed positioning should include side-lying at oblique angles, usually described as a 30- to 45-degree side-lying position to either side. (Courtesy National Pressure Ulcer Advisory Panel, 2000.)

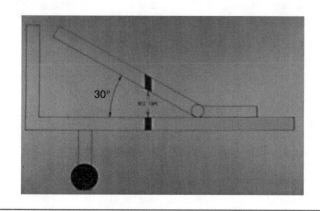

FIGURE 9-28 Head of bed at 30 degrees. Using a goniometer to determine a 30-degree angle, the therapist can mark the bed frame and raised headboard with colored tape to signify maximum inclination for pressure ulcer prevention. Client, family, and staff education and cooperation are vitally important and remain key intervention strategies. (Courtesy Anthony Stabler, Byron Health Center, Fort Wayne, Ind. National Pressure Ulcer Advisory Panel, 2000.)

sure. Electric or battery-operated alternating pressure pads (vinyl- or plastic-covered) are also available that compensate for lack of response to pain and pressure. These devices work by pumping air alternately into different chambers, thereby distributing pressure and simulating the normal changes in pressure over time. Reducing pressure on the skin must be accompanied by adequate fluid and nutrition intake (see also Table 9-15). Donut cushions are to be avoided because they can cause tissue ischemia.

The person who is incontinent presents an additional challenge to keeping the skin clean and dry. Stool or urine becomes an irritant and places the person at additional risk for skin breakdown. Contamination of an already existing wound by wound drainage, perspiration, urine, or feces is also a concern for the incontinent and immobile population. Fecal containment products are available for use in the case of acute diarrhea or fecal incontinence when these conditions contribute to the development of ulcers.*

Cleaning should be carried out using a mild agent that minimizes irritation and dryness of the skin. Avoid harsh alkali soaps, alcohol-based products that can cause vasoconstriction, tincture of benzoin (may cause painful erosions), and hexachlorophene (may irritate the CNS). During cleaning or wound care, the force and friction applied to the skin should be minimized.

Anyone performing pulsatile lavage with suction (PLWS) must beware of the potential for aerosolization of microorganisms from a wound during this intervention. Therapists and others in the room during PLWS should wear appropriate personal protective equipment to limit contact with infectious agents. To prevent possible exposure of other clients, PLWS should be performed in a private room or in a treatment room.[72] Concerns that high-pressure (output pressure of 70 psi) lavage may disseminate contaminants to surrounding tissues have not been substantiated. Until further research establishes safe levels of irrigation pressure in wound cleansing, therapists are advised to use the AHCPR guideline of irrigation pressures between 4 and 15 psi.[73] ■

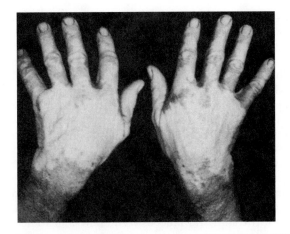

FIGURE   **9-29** Vitiligo. (From Callen JP, Jorizzo J, editors: *Dermatological signs of internal disease*, ed 2, Philadelphia, 1995, Saunders, p 191.)

◆ Pigmentary Disorders

Definition and Overview.   Skin color or pigmentation is determined by the deposition of melanin, a dark polymer found in the skin, as well as in the hair, ciliary body, choroid of the eye, pigment layer of the retina, and certain nerve cells. Melanin is formed in the melanocytes in the basal layer of the epidermis and is regulated (dispersion and aggregation) through the release of melatonin, a pineal hormone. *Hyperpigmentation* is the abnormally increased pigmentation resulting from increased melanin production. *Hypopigmentation* is the abnormally decreased pigmentation resulting from decreased melanin production.

Pigmentary disorders (either hyperpigmentation or hypopigmentation) may be primary or secondary. Secondary pigmentary changes occur as a result of damage to the skin, such as irritation, allergy, infection, excoriation, burns, or dermatologic therapy, such as curettage, dermabrasion, chemical peels, or freezing with liquid nitrogen.

Etiologic and Risk Factors.   The formation and deposition of melanin can be affected by external influences such as exposure to heat, trauma, solar or ionizing radiation, heavy metals, and changes in oxygen potential. These influences can result in hyperpigmentation, hypopigmentation, or both. Local trauma may destroy melanocytes temporarily or permanently, causing hypopigmentation, sometimes with hyperpigmentation in surrounding skin.

Other pigmentary disorders may occur from exposure to exogenous pigments, such as carotene, certain metals, and tattooing inks. Carotenemia occurs as a result of excessive carotene in the blood, usually from ingesting certain foods (e.g., carrots, yellow fruit, egg yolk). It may also occur in dia-

betes mellitus and in hypothyroidism. Exposure to metals such as silver can cause argyria, a poisoning marked by a permanent ashen-gray discoloration of the skin, conjunctivae, and internal organs. Gold, when given long term for rheumatoid arthritis, can also cause pigmentary changes.

Clinical Manifestations

Hyperpigmentation.   Primary disorders in this category include pigmented nevi, mongolian spots, juvenile freckles (ephelides), lentigines (also called *liver spots*) from sun exposure, café au lait spots associated with neurofibromatosis, and hypermelanosis caused by increased melanocyte-stimulating hormone (e.g., Addison's disease).

Secondary hyperpigmentation most commonly occurs after another dermatologic condition, such as acne (e.g., postinflammatory hyperpigmentation seen in dark-skinned people). *Melasma*, a patterned hyperpigmentation of the face, can occur as a result of steroid hormones, estrogens, and progesterones, such as occurs during pregnancy and in 30% to 50% of women taking oral contraceptives. Secondary hyperpigmentation may also develop as a phototoxic reaction to medications, oils in perfumes, and chemicals in the rinds of limes, citrus fruits, and celery.

Hypopigmentation and Depigmentation.   The disorder most commonly seen by a therapist in this category is vitiligo. In *vitiligo*, pigment cells (melanocytes) are destroyed resulting in small or large circumscribed areas of depigmentation often having hyperpigmented borders and enlarging slowly (Fig. 9-29). This condition may be associated with hyperthyroidism, hypothyroidism, pernicious anemia, diabetes mellitus, Addison's disease, and carcinoma of the stomach.

Hypopigmentation can also occur on black skin from the use of liquid nitrogen. Intraarticular injections of high concentrations of corticosteroids may also cause localized temporary hypopigmentation.

◆ Blistering Diseases

Definition, Incidence, and Etiologic Factors.   On occasion, blistering diseases may be seen in a therapy practice when severe enough to warrant localized treatment interven-

---

*New products for urinary or fecal incontinence are available to help prevent skin maceration from back flow of urine or feces. The thin, tapered skin barrier provides comfort for the wearer and allows an extended wear time (see www.hollister.com). Mention of these products does not indicate endorsement.

tion (usually similar to wound care, ulcer care, or burn care). Blisters occur on skin and mucous membranes in a condition called *pemphigus*, which is an uncommon intraepidermal blistering disease in which the epidermal cells separate from one another. This disease occurs almost exclusively in middle-aged or older adults of all races and ethnic groups.

The exact cause of blistering diseases is unknown, but they may occur as a secondary event associated with viral or bacterial infections of the skin (e.g., herpes simplex, impetigo) or local injury of the skin (e.g., burns, ischemia, dermatitis), or they may be drug-induced (e.g., penicillamine, captopril). In other diseases, blistering of the skin occurs as a primary autoimmune event characterized by the presence of autoantibodies directed against specific adhesion molecules of the skin and mucous membranes.[29] Paraneoplastic pemphigus, an autoantibody-mediated mucocutaneous disease associated with underlying neoplasm, is a syndrome that has a distinct clinical and histologic presentation. This form of pemphigus has a poor prognosis because of the underlying malignancy.

Clinical Manifestations. Blistering diseases are characterized by the formation of bullae, or blisters. These bullae appear spontaneously, often on the oral mucous membranes or scalp, and are relatively asymptomatic. Erosions and crusts may develop over the blisters, causing toxemia and a mousy odor. The lesions become extensive, and the complications of the disease, especially infection, can lead to great toxicity and debility. Disturbances of electrolyte balance are also common because of fluid losses through the involved skin in severe cases. See the section on Fluid and Electrolyte Balance in Chapter 4.

Medical Management. Medical management may include hospitalization (bed rest, IV antibiotics and feedings) when the disease is severe. For others, treatment may be with corticosteroids (e.g., prednisone) and local measures. The course of this disorder tends to be chronic in most people, and high-dose corticosteroids can mask the signs and symptoms of infection. If untreated, this condition is usually fatal within 2 months to 5 years as a result of infection. In the case of paraneoplastic pemphigus, early diagnosis and treatment of the underlying neoplasm are imperative.

◆ Cutaneous Sarcoidosis

Sarcoidosis is a multisystemic disorder characterized by the formation of granulomas, inflammatory lesions containing mononuclear phagocytes usually surrounded by a rim of lymphocytes. These granulomas may develop in the lungs, liver, bones, or eyes (see Table 14-15) and may be accompanied by skin lesions (see Fig. 14-18). Subcutaneous nodules around the knee and elbow joints may occur in association with pulmonary or cardiac involvement and resolve in response to systemic corticosteroids. In the United States, sarcoidosis occurs predominantly among blacks, affecting twice as many women as men. Acute sarcoidosis usually resolves within 2 years. Chronic, progressive sarcoidosis, which is uncommon, is associated with pulmonary fibrosis and progressive pulmonary disability. See Chapter 14 for a complete discussion of this condition.

REFERENCES

1. Aboulafia DM: The epidemiologic, pathologic, and clinical features of AIDS-associated pulmonary Kaposi's sarcoma, *Chest* 117(4):1128-1145, 2000.
2. Arasteh K, Hannah A: The role of vascular endothelial growth factor (VEGF) in AIDS-related Kaposi's sarcoma, *Oncologist* 5(suppl 1):28-31, 2000.
3. Atkinson W, Wolfe, C, Humiston S, et al: *Epidemiology and prevention of vaccine-preventable diseases,* Bethesda, Md, 2000, Centers for Disease Control and Prevention, Department of Health and Human Services.
4. Baddour LM: Breast cellulitis complicating breast conservation therapy, *J Intern Med* 245(1):5-9, 1999.
5. Bagel J: Establishing a practical and effective psoriasis treatment center, *Dermatol Clin* 18(2):349-357, 2000.
6. Ballard T, Lagorio S, De Angelis G, et al: Cancer incidence and mortality among flight personnel: a meta-analysis, *Aviat Space Environ Med* 71(3):216-224, 2000.
7. Belsito DV: The diagnostic evaluation, treatment, and prevention of allergic contact dermatitis in the new millennium, *J Allergy Clin Immunol* 105(3):409-420, 2000.
8. Bergstrom N: *Treatment of pressure ulcers: clinical practice guideline no. 15,* Bethesda, Md, 1994, Health and Human Services Department, Public Health Service, Agency for Health Care Policy and Research (AHCPR).
9. Bergstrom N, Braden B, Kemp M, et al: Multi-site study of incidence of pressure ulcers and the relationship between risk level, demographic characteristics, diagnoses, and prescription of preventive interventions, *J Am Geriatr Soc* 44(1):22-30, 1996.
10. Berlowitz DR, Anderson JJ, Ash AS, et al: Reducing random variation in reported rates of pressure ulcer development, *Med Care* 36(6):818-825, 1998.
11. Bianchi DW: Fetomaternal cell trafficking: a new cause of disease? *Am J Med Genet* 91(1):22-28, 2000.
12. Bodemer C, Belon M, Hamel-Teillac D, et al: Scleroderma in children: a retrospective study of 70 cases, *Ann Dermatol Venereol* 126(10):691-694, 1999.
13. Bouffard D, Wong TY, Hernandez M, Mihm MO: Suspicion of early desmoplastic melanoma, *Melanoma Lett* 11(3):1, 1993.
14. Brinckerhoff LH, Thompson LW, Slingluff CL: Melanoma vaccines, *Curr Opin Oncol* 12(2):163-173, 2000.
15. Brown CD, Zitelli JA: The prognosis and treatment of true local cutaneous recurrent malignant melanoma, *Dermatol Surg* 21(4):285-290, 1995.
16. Brown CW, Marschall SF: Connective tissue update: focus on dermatomyositis, *Consultant* 39(10):2867-2875, 1999.
17. Bryan C, Knight C, Black CM: Prediction of five-year survival following presentation with scleroderma: development of a simple model using three disease factors at first visit, *Arthritis Rheum* 42(12):2660-2665, 1999.
18. Cafiero F, Peressini A, Percivale PL, et al: Selective lymph node dissection in patients with intermediate thickness melanoma: our experience, *Anticancer Res* 20(1B):497-500, 2000.
19. Callaghan S: Skin considerations with silicone–type interfaces, *Adv Phys Ther* 7:22-23, 1996.
20. Cantwell A: Infection with bacteria as the cause of scleroderma, *The Physician's Page* 5(1):5-8, 2000 (www.roadback.org).
21. Carrougher GJ: *Burn care and therapy,* St Louis, 1998, Mosby.
22. Cathomas G: Human herpes virus 8: a new virus discloses its face, *Virchows Arch* 436(3):195-206, 2000.
23. Cerovac S, Roberts AH: Burns sustained by hot bath and shower water, *Burns* 26(3):251-259, 2000.
24. Chosidow O: Scabies and pediculosis, *Lancet* 355(9206):819-826, 2000.
25. Clements PJ, Furst DE, Wong WK, et al: High-dose versus low-dose D-penicillamine in early diffuse systemic sclerosis: analysis of a two-year, double-blind, randomized, controlled clinical trial, *Arthritis Rheum* 42(6):1194-1203, 1999.
26. D'Cruz D: Autoimmune diseases associated with drugs, chemicals and environmental factors, *Toxicol Lett* 112-113:421-432, 2000.
27. Descamps V: HIV-1 infected patients with toxic epidermal necrolysis: an occupational risk for healthcare workers, *Lancet* 353(9167):1855-1856, 1999.

28. deVries TJ, Fourkour A, Punt CJ, et al: Melanoma-inhibiting activity (MIA) mRNA is not exclusively transcribed in melanoma cells: low levels of MIA mRNA are present in various cell types and in peripheral blood, *Br J Cancer* 81(6):1066-1170, 1999.

29. Diaz LA, Giudice GJ: End of the century overview of skin blisters, *Arch Dermatol* 136(1):106-112, 2000.

30. Driscoll J: Integumentary management of the patient with multiple traumatic injuries, *Acute Care Perspectives* 7(3):1, 3-4, 16-18, 1999.

31. Elgart ML: Current treatments for scabies and pediculosis, *Skin Therapy Lett* 5(1):1-3, 2000.

32. Englert H, Small-McMahon J, Davis K, et al: Systemic sclerosis prevalence and mortality in Sydney 1974-1988, *Aust NZ J Med* 29(1):42-50, 1999.

33. Frances C: Smoker's wrinkles: epidemiological and pathologic considerations, *Clin Dermatol* 16(5):565-570, 1998.

34. Frantz RA: Measuring prevalence and incidence of pressure ulcers, *Adv Wound Care* 10(1):21-24, 1997.

35. Gallego H, Crutchfield CE, Lewis EJ, et al: Report of an association between discoid lupus erythematosus and smoking, *Cutis* 63(4):231-234, 1999.

36. Gang RK, Sanyal SC, Bang RL, et al: Staphylococcal septicaemia in burns, *Burns* 26(4):359-366, 2000.

37. Gascon P, Schwartz RA: Kaposi's sarcoma: new treatment modalities, *Dermatol Clin* 18(1):169-175, 2000.

38. Generini S, Fiori G, Moggi PA, et al: Systemic sclerosis: a clinical overview, *Adv Exp Med Biol* 455:73-83, 1999.

39. Generini S, Matucci CM: Raynaud's phenomenon and vascular disease in systemic sclerosis, *Adv Exp Med Biol* 455:93-100, 1999.

40. Ghossein RA, Carusone L, Bhattacharya S: Review: polymerase chain reaction detection of micrometastases and circulating tumor cells: application to melanoma, prostate, and thyroid carcinomas, *Diagn Mol Pathol* 8(4):165-175, 1999.

41. Gnann JW, Pellett PE, Jaffe HW: Human herpesvirus 8 and Kaposi's sarcoma in persons infected with human immunodeficiency virus, *Clin Infect Dis* 30(suppl 1):S72-S76, 2000.

42. Green A: Daily sunscreen application and beta-carotene supplementation in prevention of basal-cell and squamous-cell carcinomas of the skin: a randomized controlled trial, *Lancet* 354(9180):723-729, 1999.

43. Jemal A, Thomas A, Murray T, et al: Cancer statistics 2002, *CA Cancer J Clin* 52(1):23-47.

44. Griffiths CEM: Aging of the skin. In Tallis RC, Fillit HM, Brocklehurst JC: *Brocklehurst's textbook of geriatric medicine and gerontology*, ed 5, New York, 1998, Churchill Livingstone, pp 1293-1298.

45. Gulin J, Korn JH: Systemic sclerosis: challenges in diagnosis and management, *J Musculoskel Med* 16:288-300, 1999.

46. Habif TP: *Skin disease: diagnosis and treatment*, St Louis, 2000, Mosby.

47. Haldorsen R, Reitan JB, Tveten U: Cancer incidence among Norwegian airline pilots, *Scand J Work Environ Health* 26(2):106-111, 2000.

48. Halpern A: *P.T.s can help patients by recognizing signs of skin disorders.* Presented at the Hospital of the University of Pennsylvania (HUP), 1993.

49. Harrison RA, Haque AU, Roseman JM, et al: Socioeconomic characteristics and melanoma incidence, *Ann Epidemiol* 8(5):327-333, 1998.

50. Healy E, Flannagan N, Ray A, et al: Melanocortin-1-receptor gene and sun sensitivity in individuals without red hair, *Lancet* 355(9209):1072-1073, 2000.

51. Henry KD: Effect of physical therapy on a patient with dermatomyositis, *Phys Ther Case Reports* 2(4):157-161, 1999.

52. Hess CT, Salcido R: *Wound care: clinical guide*, Springhouse, Pa, 1999, Springhouse Publishing.

53. Higgins E: Alcohol, smoking, and psoriasis, *Clin Exp Dermatol* 25(2):107-110, 2000.

54. Hill LL, Ouhtit A, Loughlin SM, et al: Fas ligand: a sensor for DNA damage critical in skin cancer etiology, *Science* 285(5429):898-900, 1999.

55. HHS (U.S. Department of Health and Human Services): *Pressure ulcer treatment.* AHCPR publication no. 95-0652, Rockville, Md, 1995, The Department.

56. HHS (U.S. Department of Health and Human Services): *Pressure ulcers in adults: predilection and prevention.* AHCPR publication no. 92-0047, Rockville, Md, 1992, The Department.

57. Hofer MF: Atopic dermatitis: the first allergic step in children, *Rev Med Suisse Romande* 120(3):263-267, 2000.

58. Iscovich J, Boffetta P, Franceschi S, et al: Classic Kaposi sarcoma: epidemiology and risk factors, *Cancer* 88(3):500-517, 2000.

59. Jewell ML, McCauliffe DP: Patients with cutaneous lupus erythematosus who smoke are less responsive to antimalarial treatment, *J Am Acad Dermatol* 42(6):983-987, 2000.

60. Josty IC, Narayanan V, Dickson WA: Burns in patients with epilepsy: changes in epidemiology and implications for burn treatment and prevention, *Epilepsia* 41(4):453-456, 2000.

61. Kabat-Zinn J, Wheeler E, Light T, et al: Influence of a mindfulness mediation-based stress reduction intervention on rates of skin clearing in patients with moderate to severe psoriasis, *Psychosom Med* 60(5):625-632, 1998.

62. Kahaleh MB, LeRoy EC: Autoimmunity and vascular involvement in systemic sclerosis (SSc), *Autoimmunity* 31(3):195-214, 1999.

63. Kalka K, Merk H, Mukhtar H: Photodynamic therapy in dermatology, *J Am Acad Dermatol* 42(3):389-413, 2000.

64. Kendall, K: Personal communication, Gulf Breeze, Fla, 2000, Medical Center for Continuing Education.

65. Kohen R: Skin antioxidants: their role in aging and in oxidative stress—new approaches for their evaluation, *Biomed Pharmacother* 53(4):181-192, 1999.

66. Koo J: Systemic sequential therapy of psoriasis: a new paradigm for improved therapeutic results, *J Am Acad Dermatol* 41(3, pt 2):S25-S28, 1999.

67. Koo J, Liao W: Update on psoriasis therapy: a perspective from the USA, *Keio J Med* 49(1):20-25, 2000.

68. Krogstad AL, Lonnroth P, Larson G, et al: Capsaicin treatment induces histamine release and perfusion changes in psoriatic skin, *Br J Dermatol* 141(1):87-93, 1999.

69. Le C, Morales, A, Trentham DE: Minocycline in early diffuse scleroderma, *Lancet* 352(9142):1755-1756, 1998.

70. Leung DY: Atopic dermatitis: new insights and opportunities for therapeutic intervention, *J Allergy Clin Immunol* 105(5):860-876, 2000.

71. Livingston Wuerthele-Caspe V, Brodkin E, Mermod C: Etiology of scleroderma: preliminary clinical report, *J Med Soc NJ* 44:256-259, 1947.

72. Loehne H, Streed SA, Gaither B, et al: Aerosolization of microorganisms during pulsatile lavage with suction, 1999.

73. Luedtke-Hoffmann KA, Schafer DS: Pulsed lavage in wound cleansing, *Phys Ther* 80(3):292-300, 2000.

74. Lund CC, Browder NC: The estimation of areas of burn, *Surg Gynecol Obstet* 79:352-358, 1994.

75. Maklebust J, Sieggreen M: *Pressure ulcers guidelines for prevention and nursing management,* ed 2, Springhouse, Pa, 1996, Springhouse Publishing.

76. McColloch JM, Kloth L, editors: *Wound healing: alternatives in management (contemporary perspectives in rehabilitation),* Philadelphia, 1994, FA Davis.

77. McGill V, Kowal-Vern A, Gamelli RL: Outcome for older burn patients, *Arch Surg* 135(3):320-325, 2000.

78. McGwin G, Chapman V, Rousculp M: The epidemiology of fire-related deaths in Alabama, 1992-1997, *J Burn Care Rehabil* 21(1, pt 1):75-83, 2000.

79. Medsger TA: Systemic sclerosis (scleroderma). In Stein JH, editor: *Internal medicine,* ed 4, St Louis, 1994, Mosby, pp 2443-2449.

80. Mitsuyasu RT: Update on the pathogenesis and treatment of Kaposi's sarcoma, *Curr Opin Oncol* 12(2):174-180, 2000.

81. Morton DL, Ollila MD, Eddy C, et al: Cytoreductive surgery and adjuvant immunotherapy: a new management paradigm for metastatic melanoma, *CA Cancer J Clin* 49:101-116, 1999.

82. Muller MG, Borgstein PJ, Pijpers R, et al: Reliability of the sentinel node procedure in melanoma patients: analysis of failures after long-term follow-up, *Ann Surg Oncol* 7(6):461-468, 2000.

83. Murphy JC, Banwell PE, Roberts AH, et al: Frostbite: pathogenesis and treatment, *J Trauma* 48(1):171-178, 2000.

84. Nicol NH: Managing atopic dermatitis in children and adults, *Nurse Pract* 25(4):58-70, 2000.

85. Nietert PJ, Sutherland SE, Silver RM, et al: Is occupational organic solvent exposure a risk factor for scleroderma? *Arthritis Rheum* 41(6):1111-1118, 1998.

86. Nietert PJ, Sutherland SE, Silver RM, et al: Solvent oriented hobbies and the risk of systemic sclerosis, *J Rheumatol* 26(11):2369-2372, 1999.

87. Ortonne JP: Recent developments in the understanding of the pathogenesis of psoriasis, *Br J Dermatol* 140(suppl 54):1-7, 1999.

88. Otley CC, Zitelli JA: Review of sentinel lymph node biopsy and systemic interferon for melanoma: promising but investigational modalities, *Dermatol Surg* 26(3):177-180, 2000.

89. Owen-Schaub L, Chan H, Cusack JC, et al: Fas and fas ligand interactions in malignant disease, *Int J Oncol* 17(1):5-12, 2000.

90. Peters BP, Weissman FG, Gill MA: Pathophysiology and treatment of psoriasis, *Am J Health Syst Pharm* 57(7):645-659, 2000.

91. Ponten J: How do skin cancers get their start? *Skin Cancer Foundation J* 17:34-35, 94, 1999.

92. Pruitt BA: The evolutionary development of biologic dressings and skin substitutes, *J Burn Care Rehabil* 18:S2-S5, 1997.

93. Pruitt BA, Mason AD, Goodwin CW: Epidemiology of burn injury and demography of burn care facilities, *Problems in General Surgery* 7(2): 235-251, 1990.

94. Pruitt BA, McManus AT, Kim SH, et al: Burn wound infections: current status, *World J Surg* 22(2):135-145, 1998.

95. Rafnsson V, Hrafnkelsson J, Tulinius H: Incidence of cancer among commercial airline pilots, *Occup Environ Med* 57(3):175-179, 2000.

96. Reamy BV: Frostbite: review and current concepts, *J Am Board Fam Pract* 11(1):34-40, 1998.

97. Rees JL, Birch-Machin M, Flanagan N, et al: Genetic studies of the human melanocortin-1 receptor, *Ann NY Acad Sci* 885:134-142, 1999.

98. Reimann S, Luger R, Metze D: Topical administration of capsaicin in dermatology for treatment of itching and pain, *Hautarzt* 51(3):164-172, 2000.

99. Richard R, Staley M, editors: *Burn care and rehabilitation: principles and practice*, Philadelphia, 1994, FA Davis.

100. Rigel DS: Recent advances in diagnostic techniques, *Skin Cancer Foundation J* 16:36-37, 1998.

101. Rigel DS, Rigel EG, Rigel AC: Effects of altitude and latitude on ambient UVB radiation, *J Am Acad Dermatol* 40(1):114-116, 1999.

102. Rivers J, editor: Surgery, *Worldwide Melanoma Update* 1:11, 1997.

103. Rockwell WB, Ehrlich HP: Fibrinolysis inhibition in human burn blister fluid, *J Burn Care Rehabil* 11:1-6, 1990.

104. Rupp JF, Kaplan DL: Pruritus: causes—cures, part 1, *Consultant* 39(11):3157-3160, 1999.

105. Sabir AM, Werth VP: Cutaneous manifestations of lupus erythematosus, *J Musculoskel Med* 16:482-491, 1999.

106. Sallis R, Chassay CM: Recognizing and treating common cold-induced injury in outdoor sports, *Med Sci Sports Exerc* 31(10):1367-1373, 1999.

107. Schindl A, Schindl M, Pernerstorfer-Schon H, et al: Low intensity laser irradiation in the treatment of recalcitrant radiation ulcers in patients with breast cancer, *Photodermatol Photoimmunol Photomed* 16(1):34-37, 2000.

108. Seibold JR, Korn JH, Simms R, et al: Recombinant human relaxin in the treatment of scleroderma: a randomized, double-blind, placebo-controlled trial, *Ann Intern Med* 132(11):871-879, 2000.

109. Sheridan RL, Remensnyder JP, Schnitzer JJ, et al: Current expectations for survival in pediatric burns, *Arch Pediatr Adolesc Med* 154(3): 245-249, 2000.

110. Sidbury R, Hanifin JM: Old, new, and emerging therapies for atopic dermatitis, *Dermatol Clin* 18(1):1-11, 2000.

111. Stern RS, Liebman EJ, Vakeva L: Oral psoralen and ultraviolet-A light (PUVA) treatment of psoriasis and persistent risk of nonmelanoma skin cancer: PUVA follow-up study, *J Natl Cancer Inst* 90(17):1278-1284, 1998.

112. Stratton SP, Dorr RT, Alberts DS: The state-of-the-art in chemoprevention of skin cancer, *Eur J Cancer* 36(10):1292-1297, 2000.

113. Su CW, Lohman R, Gottlieb LJ: Frostbite of the upper extremity, *Hand Clin* 16(2):235-247, 2000.

114. Sussman C, Bates-Jensen BM, editors: *Wound care: a collaborative practice manual for physical therapists and nurses*, Gaithersburg, Md, 1998, Aspen Publishers.

115. Tanaka A, Lindor K, Ansari A, et al: Fetal microchimerisms in the mother: immunologic implications, *Liver Transpl* 6(2):138-143, 2000.

116. Thiboutot DM: Acne and rosacea, *Dermatol Clin* 18(1):63-71, 2000.

117. Thissen MR, Schroeter CA, Neumann HA: Photodynamic therapy with delta-aminolaevulinic acid for nodular basal cell carcinomas using a prior bulking technique, *Br J Dermatol* 142(2):338-339, 2000.

118. Thomas JM, Patocskai EJ: The argument against sentinel node biopsy for malignant melanoma: its use should be confined to patients in clinical trials, *BMJ* 321(7252):3-4, 2000.

119. Trefzer U, Weingart G, Chen Y, et al: Hybrid cell vaccination for cancer immune therapy: first clinical trial with metastatic melanoma, *Int J Cancer* 85(5):618-626, 2000.

120. Trentham DE: Minocycline in early diffuse scleroderma SSc—the next step, *The Physician's Page* 3(2):3, 2000 (www.roadback.org).

121. Valenta R, Seiberler S, Natter S, et al: Autoallergy: a pathogenetic factor in atopic dermatitis? *J Allergy Clin Immunol* 105(3):432-437, 2000.

122. Wagner JD, Corbett, L, Park HM, et al: Sentinel lymph node biopsy for melanoma: experience with 234 consecutive procedures, *Plast Reconstr Surg* 105(6):1956-1966, 2000.

123. Weisinger GF, Quittan M, Nuhr M, et al: Aerobic capacity in adult dermatomyositis/polymyositis patients and healthy controls, *Arch Phys Med Rehabil* 81(1):1-5, 2000.

124. Wigley FM: Systemic sclerosis and related syndromes. B. Clinical features. In Klippel JH, editor: *Primer on the rheumatic diseases*, ed 11, Atlanta, 1997, Arthritis Foundation, pp 267-272.

125. Winchester R: Psoriatic arthritis and the spectrum of syndromes related to the SAPHO (synovitis, acne, pustulosis, hyperostosis, and osteitis) syndrome, *Curr Opin Rheumatol* 11(4):251-256, 1999.

126. Wooldridge WE: Psoriasis, joint swelling, and draining plaques, *J Musculoskel Med* 13(7):61-62, 1996.

127. Young AJ, O'Brien C, Sawka MN, et al: Physiological problems associated with wearing NBC protective clothing during cold weather, *Aviat Space Environ Med* 71(2):184-189, 2000.

128. Yowler CJ, Mozingo DW, Ryan JB, et al: Factors contributing to delayed extremity amputation in burn patients, *J Trauma* 45(3):522-526, 1998.

129. Zitelli JA, Brown CD, Hanusa BH: Surgical margins for excision of primary cutaneous melanoma, *J Am Acad Dermatol* 37(3, pt 1):422-429, 1997.

CHAPTER 10

THE ENDOCRINE AND METABOLIC SYSTEMS

CATHERINE C. GOODMAN AND TERESA E. KELLY SNYDER

ENDOCRINE SYSTEM

The endocrine system is composed of various glands located throughout the body (Fig. 10-1). These glands are capable of synthesis and release of special chemical messengers called *hormones,* which are transported by the bloodstream to the cells and organs on which they have a specific regulatory effect (Table 10-1). The endocrine system and the nervous system control and integrate body function to maintain homeostasis. Whereas the nervous system sends its messages along nerve fibers, eliciting swift and selective neural responses, the endocrine system sends its messages in the form of hormones via the bloodstream. Hormonal effects have a slower onset than neural effects, but they maintain a longer duration of action. The actions of the endocrine system may be localized to one area or generalized to all the cells of the body.[62]

The endocrine system has five general functions: (1) differentiation of the reproductive and central nervous system of the developing fetus; (2) stimulation of sequential growth and development during childhood and adolescence; (3) coordination of the male and female reproductive systems; (4) maintenance of optimal internal environment throughout the lifespan; and (5) initiation of corrective and adaptive responses when emergency demands occur.[63]

The endocrine system meets the nervous system at the hypothalamic-pituitary interface. The hypothalamus, the main integrative center for the endocrine and autonomic nervous systems, controls the function of endocrine organs by neural and hormonal pathways. Although the communicative and integrative roles of the endocrine and nervous systems are similar, the precise ways in which each system functions differ.

◆ Hypothalamic Control

Neural pathways connect the hypothalamus to the posterior pituitary (or neurohypophysis), providing the hypothalamus direct control over both the anterior and posterior portions of the pituitary gland (Fig. 10-2). Disorders of the hypothalamic-pituitary axis are manifested clinically usually either by syndromes of hormone excess or deficiency or by visual impairment from optic nerve compression because of the location of the hypothalamus and pituitary.

Neural stimulation to the posterior pituitary provokes the secretion of two effector hormones: antidiuretic hormone (ADH) and oxytocin. The hypothalamus also exerts hormonal control at the anterior pituitary through releasing and inhibiting factors. Hypothalamic hormones stimulate the pituitary to release tropic (stimulating) hormones, such as adrenocorticotropic hormone (ACTH), thyroid-stimulating hormone (TSH), luteinizing hormone (LH), and follicle-stimulating hormone (FSH) (see Fig. 10-2). At the same time, effector hormones such as growth hormone and prolactin are released or inhibited, affecting the adrenal cortex, thyroid, and gonads. Endocrine pathology develops as a result of dysfunction of releasing, tropic, or effector hormones or when defects occur in the target tissue.

In addition to hormonal and neural controls, a negative feedback system regulates the endocrine system. The mechanism may be simple or complex. Simple feedback occurs when the level of one substance regulates the secretion of a hormone. For example, low serum calcium levels stimulate parathyroid hormone (PTH) secretion; high serum calcium levels inhibit it. Complex feedback occurs through the hypothalamic-pituitary-target organ axis. For example, after an injury or major stress, secretion of the hypothalamic corticotropin-releasing hormone (CRH) releases pituitary ACTH, which in turn stimulates adrenal cortisol secretion. Subsequently, a rise in serum cortisol inhibits ACTH by decreasing CRH secretion (see Fig. 10-2). Steroid therapy disrupts the hypothalamic-pituitary-adrenal (HPA) axis by suppressing hypothalamic-pituitary secretion. Abrupt withdrawal of exogenous steroid can induce life-threatening adrenal insufficiency because the HPA axis does not have enough time to recover sufficiently to stimulate cortisol secretion.

◆ Hormonal Effects

In response to the hypothalamus, the *posterior pituitary* secretes oxytocin and ADH. Oxytocin stimulates contraction of the uterus and is responsible for the milk letdown reflex in lactating women. ADH controls the concentration of body fluids by alteration of the permeability of the kidney's distal convoluted tubules and collecting ducts to conserve water. The secretion of ADH depends on plasma volume and osmolality as monitored by hypothalamic neurons. Circulatory shock and severe hemorrhage are the most powerful stimulators of ADH; other stimulators include pain, emotional stress, trauma, morphine, tranquilizers, certain anesthetics, and positive-pressure breathing.

The *anterior pituitary* secretes prolactin, which stimulates milk production, and human growth hormone (HGH), which affects most body tissues. HGH stimulates growth by increasing protein synthesis and fat mobilization and by decreasing carbohydrate utilization. Hyposecretion of HGH results in dwarfism; hypersecretion causes gigantism in children and acromegaly in adults.

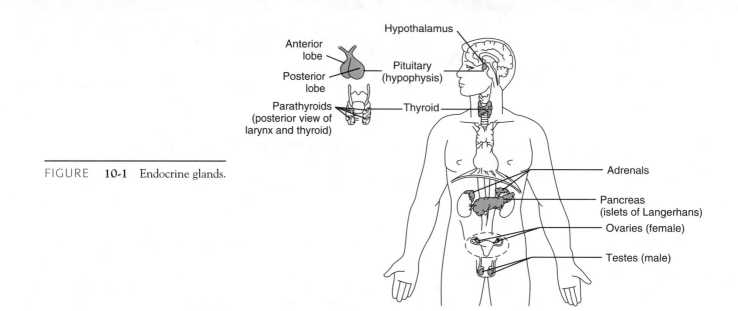

Hypothalamus

Anterior lobe

Pituitary (hypophysis)

Posterior lobe

Parathyroids (posterior view of larynx and thyroid)

Thyroid

Adrenals

Pancreas (islets of Langerhans)

Ovaries (female)

Testes (male)

FIGURE **10-1** Endocrine glands.

The *thyroid gland* secretes the iodinated thyroid hormones thyroxine (T_4) and triiodothyronine (T_3).* Thyroid hormones, necessary for normal growth and development, act on many tissues to regulate our basal metabolism (i.e., the rate at which we convert food and oxygen into energy) and to increase metabolic activity and protein synthesis. Deficiency of thyroid hormone causes varying degrees of hypothyroidism, from a mild, clinically insignificant form to the life-threatening extreme, myxedema coma. Congenital hypothyroidism causes a condition in children previously referred to as *cretinism* (now considered an undesirable term). Hypersecretion of thyroid hormone causes hyperthyroidism and, in extreme cases, thyrotoxic crisis. Excessive secretion of TSH from the pituitary gland causes thyroid gland hyperplasia, resulting in goiter in chronic iodine deficiency states. Other causes of goiter are discussed in this chapter (see the section on Thyroid Gland in this chapter).

The *parathyroid glands* secrete PTH, which regulates calcium and phosphate metabolism. PTH elevates serum calcium levels by stimulating resorption of calcium and phosphate from bone, reabsorption of calcium and excretion of phosphate by the kidneys, and, by combined action with vitamin D, absorption of calcium and phosphate from the gastrointestinal (GI) tract. Hyperparathyroidism results in hypercalcemia; hypoparathyroidism causes hypocalcemia. Altered calcium levels also may result from nonendocrine causes, such as metastatic bone disease. Pathologic changes in calcium affecting bone bring these conditions to the therapist's attention.

The *endocrine pancreas* produces glucagon from the alpha-cells and insulin from the beta-cells. Glucagon, the hormone of the fasting state, releases stored glucose to raise the blood glucose level. Insulin, the hormone of the nourished state, facilitates glucose transport, promotes glucose storage, stimulates protein synthesis, and enhances free fatty acid uptake and storage. Insulin deficiency causes diabetes mellitus; insulin excess can be exogenous (i.e., a person with diabetes may receive more insulin than is required) or insulin excess

may result from a tumor of the beta-cells called *insulinoma*. Whatever the cause of excess insulin, hypoglycemia (abnormally low level of glucose in the blood) is the result.

The *adrenal cortex* secretes mineralocorticoids, glucocorticoids, and sex steroids. Aldosterone, a mineralocorticoid, regulates the reabsorption of sodium and the excretion of potassium by the kidneys and is involved intimately in the regulation of blood pressure. An excess of aldosterone (aldosteronism) can result primarily from hyperplasia or from adrenal adenoma or secondarily from many conditions, such as congestive heart failure or cirrhosis. The *adrenal medulla* is an aggregate of nervous tissue that produces the catecholamines epinephrine and norepinephrine, which are involved in the fight-or-flight response. (See the section on Neuroendocrine Response to Stress in this chapter.)

The *testes* and *ovaries* are also endocrine glands responsible for synthesizing and secreting hormones (see Chapters 18 and 19).

◆ Endocrine Pathology

Dysfunctions of the endocrine system are classified as hypofunction and hyperfunction. The source of hypofunction and hyperfunction may be inflammation or tumor originating in the hypothalamus, the pituitary gland, or in other endocrine glands. Inflammation may be acute or subacute but is usually chronic, which results in glandular hypofunction. Chronic endocrine abnormalities (e.g., deficiencies of cortisol, thyroid hormone, or insulin) are common health problems requiring life-long hormone replacement for survival. Rarely, some endocrine gland tumors result in ectopic hormone production and may affect the musculoskeletal system.

Ectopic hormone production is the production and secretion of hormone or hormone-like substances from a source other than the normal source of the hormone. For example, some endocrine gland tumors can metastasize and produce excess hormone from those new tumor sites (e.g., some types of thyroid, parathyroid, and adrenal cancers). Some nonendocrine cancers, particularly certain lung cancers, can secrete ACTH and growth hormone. (See Chapter 8 for a discussion of paraneoplastic syndromes associated with this phenomenon.)

---

*For reference values of thyroid hormone levels mentioned throughout this chapter see Table 39-16.

TABLE	10-1

Endocrine Glands: Secretion, Target, and Actions

When reading a client's chart, it is important to know basic hormone functions or effects that may have an impact on therapy treatment. At least 30 different hormones have been identified, but only those most common to therapy clients are included here.

GLAND	HORMONE	TARGET	BASIC ACTION
Pituitary			
Anterior lobe	Somatotropin (growth hormone [GH])	Bones, muscles, organs	Retention of nitrogen to promote protein anabolism
	Thyroid stimulating hormone (TSH)	Thyroid	Promotes secretory activity
	Follicle stimulating hormone (FSH)	Ovaries, seminiferous tubules	Promotes development of ovarian follicle, secretion of estrogen, and maturation of sperm
	Luteinizing hormone	Follicle, interstitial cell	Promotes ovulation and formation of corpus luteum, secretion of progesterone, and secretion of testosterone
	Prolactin (luteotropic hormone)	Corpus luteum, breast	Maintains corpus luteum and progesterone secretion; stimulates milk secretion
	Adrenocorticotropic hormone (ACTH)	Adrenal cortex	Stimulates secretory activity
Posterior lobe	Antidiuretic hormone (ADH)	Distal tubules of kidney	Reabsorption of water
	Oxytocin	Uterus	Stimulates contraction
Thyroid	Thyroxine (T$_4$) and triiodothyronine (T$_3$)	Widespread	Regulate oxidation rate of body cells and growth and metabolism; influence gluconeogenesis, mobilization of fats, and exchange of water, electrolytes, and protein
	Calcitonin	Skeleton	Calcium and phosphorus metabolism
Parathyroids	Parathyroid hormone (PTH)	Bone, kidney, intestinal tract	Essential for calcium and phosphorus metabolism and calcification of bone
Adrenal			
Cortex	Mineralocorticoid (aldosterone)	Widespread, primarily kidney	Maintains fluid/electrolyte balance; reabsorbs sodium chloride; excretes potassium
	Glucocorticoids (cortisol)	Widespread	Concerned with food metabolism and body response to stress; preserves carbohydrates and mobilizes amino acids; promotes gluconeogenesis; suppresses inflammation
	Sex hormones (testosterone, estrogen, progesterone)	Gonads	Ability to influence secondary sex characteristics
Medulla	Epinephrine	Widespread	Cardiac: Myocardial stimulation, tachycardia, dysrhythmias; vasoconstriction with increased blood pressure; increased blood glucose via glycolysis; stimulates ACTH production
	Norepinephrine	Widespread	Vasoconstriction
Pancreas	Insulin	Widespread	Increased utilization of carbohydrate, decreased lipolysis, and protein catabolism; decreased blood glucose
	Glucagon	Widespread	Hyperglycemic factor; increases blood glucose via glycogenolysis
Gonads			
Ovaries	Estrogen	Widespread	Secondary sex characteristics; maturation and sexual function
	Progesterone	Uterus, breast	Preparation for and maintenance of pregnancy; development of mammary gland secretory tissue
Testes	Testosterone	Widespread	Secondary sex characteristics; maturation and normal sex function

From Goodman CC, Snyder TE: *Differential diagnosis in physical therapy,* ed 2, Philadelphia, 1995, WB Saunders, pp 327-328.

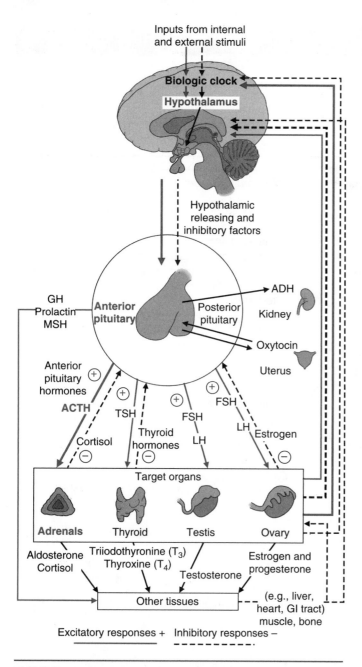

Excitatory responses + **Inhibitory responses −**

FIGURE 10-2 Control of the endocrine system by the nervous system. One example of the complex feedback loops described in the text is highlighted here. The hypothalamus controls the pituitary gland through releasing and inhibiting factors. The anterior lobe of the pituitary gland then releases tropic (stimulating) hormones that act on target glands (thyroid, adrenals, gonads). Endocrine pathology occurs when dysfunction occurs in releasing, tropic, or effector hormones, or when defects occur in the target tissue.

◆ Neuroendocrine Response to Stress*

The concept that stress of any kind (emotional, physical, psychological, spiritual) may influence immunity and resistance to disease has been the subject of investigation for many years. The endocrine system, together with the immune sys-

tem and the nervous system, mounts an integrated response to stressors. Evidence to support a psychoneuroimmunologic basis for disease is discussed elsewhere in this text (see Chapters 2 and 6).[70]

Hormones of the neuroendocrine system affect components of the immune system,[18] and mediators produced by immune components regulate the neuroendocrine response. The sympathetic nervous system is aroused during the stress response and causes the medulla of the adrenal gland to release catecholamines, such as epinephrine, norepinephrine, and dopamine, into the bloodstream. Simultaneously, the pituitary gland releases a variety of hormones, including antidiuretic hormone (from the posterior pituitary gland), prolactin, growth hormone, and adrenocorticotropic hormone (ACTH) from the anterior pituitary gland.

Catecholamines. Catecholamines are organic compounds that play an important role in the body's physiologic response to stress. Their release at sympathetic nerve endings increases the rate and force of muscular contraction of the heart, thereby increasing cardiac output; constricts peripheral blood vessels, resulting in elevated blood pressure; elevates blood glucose levels by hepatic and skeletal glycogenolysis*; and promotes an increase in blood lipids by increasing the catabolism (breakdown) of fats. These well-known metabolic effects of adrenal catecholamines prepare the body to take physical action in the fight-or-flight phenomenon. Stressors commonly associated with catecholamine release include exercise, thermal changes, and acute emotional states.

Cortisol. Cortisol is the principal glucocorticoid hormone released from the adrenal cortex, also known as *hydrocortisone* when synthesized pharmaceutically. Cortisol has multiple functions (Table 10-2), but it primarily regulates the metabolism of proteins, carbohydrates, and lipids to cause an elevation in blood glucose level. These effects on glucose level and fat metabolism result in increased blood glucose and plasma lipid levels and promote the formation of ketone bodies when insulin secretion is insufficient. For this reason, glucocorticoids (including cortisol) are referred to as *anti-insulin diabetogenic hormones*.[6]

Cortisol is essential to norepinephrine-induced vasoconstriction and other physiologic phenomena necessary for survival under stress. The production of glucose promoted by cortisol provides a source of energy for body tissues (nerve cells in particular), and the pooling of amino acids from catabolized proteins may ensure amino acid availability for protein synthesis at sites where replacement is critical, such as muscle or cells of damaged tissue.

Another effect of cortisol is that of dampening the body's inflammatory response to invasion by foreign agents. This antiinflammatory protective mechanism helps preserve the integrity of body cells at the site of the inflammatory response and provides the basis for the major therapeutic use of this steroid. Cortisol also inhibits fibroblast proliferation and function at the site of an inflammatory response and accounts for the poor wound healing, increased susceptibility to infection, and decreased inflammatory response often

---

*Only a brief review of the neuroendocrine response to stress contributing to disease is presented in this section. The reader is referred to a more specific text for detailed description of the endocrine system.

*Glycogenesis is the splitting of glycogen, a starch stored primarily in the liver but also in the muscles, yielding glucose.

TABLE	10-2

Physiologic Effects of Cortisol

FUNCTIONS AFFECTED	PHYSIOLOGIC EFFECTS
Protein metabolism	Increases protein synthesis in the liver and depresses protein synthesis in muscle, lymphoid tissue, adipose tissue, skin, and bone; increases plasma level of amino acids
Carbohydrate and lipid metabolism	Diminishes peripheral uptake and utilization of glucose; increases output of glucose from the liver; enhances the elevation of blood glucose promoted by other hormones
Lipid metabolism	Breakdown of fat in the extremities (lipolysis) and production of fat in the face and trunk (lipogenesis)
Inflammatory effects	Decreases circulating eosinophils, lymphocytes, and monocytes; increases release of polymorphonuclear leukocytes from the bone marrow; decreases accumulation of leukocytes at the site of inflammation; delays healing; essential for vasoconstrictive action of norepinephrine
Digestive function	Promotes gastric secretion
Urinary function	Enhances urinary excretion
Connective tissue function	Decreases proliferation of fibroblasts in connective tissue (and thus delays healing)
Muscle function	Maintains normal contractility and maximal work output for skeletal and cardiac muscle
Bone function	Decreases bone formation
Vascular system and myocardial function	Maintains normal blood pressure; permits increased responsiveness of arterioles to the constrictive action of adrenergic stimulation; optimizes myocardial performance
Central nervous system function	Modulates perceptual and emotional functioning (mechanism unknown); essential for normal arousal and initiation of activity

Modified from Bucher L, Melander S, editors: *Critical care nursing,* ed 1, Philadelphia, 1999, WB Saunders, p 609.

seen in individuals with chronic glucocorticoid excess. Whether cortisol-induced effects are adaptive or destructive depends on the subsequent concentration and length of cortisol exposure.

Other Hormones.   Other hormones such as endorphins, growth hormone, prolactin, and testosterone may be released as part of the response to stressful stimuli. *Endorphins,* a term derived from *endogenous* and *morphine,* are a group of opiate-like peptides produced naturally by the body at neural synapses in the central nervous system. These hormones serve to modulate the transmission of pain perceptions by raising the pain threshold and producing sedation and euphoria.

As its name implies, *growth hormone* stimulates and controls the rate of skeletal and visceral growth by directly influencing protein, carbohydrate, and lipid metabolism. GH levels increase in the blood after a variety of physically or psychologically stressful stimuli, such as surgery, fever, physical exercise, or the anticipation of exhausting exercise, cardiac catheterization, electroshock therapy, or gastroscopy.[4]

Prolactin stimulates the growth of breast tissue and sustains milk production in postpartum mammals. Prolactin levels in plasma increase with a variety of stressful stimuli, including such procedures as gastroscopy, proctoscopy, pelvic examination, and surgery, but they show little change after exercise. *Testosterone,* a hormone that regulates male secondary sex characteristics and sex drive (libido), decreases after stressful stimuli such as anesthesia, surgery, marathon running, and acute illness (e.g., respiratory failure, burns, congestive heart failure). Decreased testosterone during these circumstances restrains growth and reproduction to preserve energy for protective responses.[4]

◆ Aging and the Endocrine System[19,48]

The exact effects of aging on the endocrine system are not clear. In particular, the question of whether changes in endocrine function are a cause of aging or a natural consequence of aging remains unresolved. The endocrine system has never been implicated as the direct cause of aging. Coexisting age-related variables such as acute and chronic nonendocrine disease, use of medications, alterations in diet, changes in body composition and weight, and changes in sleep-wake cycle affecting the endocrine system confuse the picture. New analytical tools to evaluate the neuroregulation of the endocrine axes are predicted to yield important information in the next decade.

Age-associated declines in physiologic performance of the endocrine system are well documented and it is accepted that the basis of this decline is a *failure of homeostasis.* The conventional view is that "normal" aging changes predispose to age-related disease and contribute to the poor recovery of aging adults after illness or severe stresses such as surgery. Equilibrium concentrations of the principal hormones necessary to maintain homeostasis are not necessarily altered with age, but what may differ as we get older is the way we achieve equilibrium hormone levels, which points to changes in regulatory control.

Collectively, available clinical data suggest a general model of early neuroendocrine aging in the human (both males and females) with variable but predictable disruption in the time-delayed feedback and feedforward interconnections among neuroendocrine glands.[90] Thus with advancing age, significant alterations in hormone production, metabolism, and action are found. The continuum of the age-related changes is highly variable and sex-dependent. Whereas only subtle changes occur in the pituitary, adrenal, and thyroid function,* changes in glucose homeostasis, reproductive function, and calcium metabolism are more apparent.

Aging is associated with a higher incidence of disorders or diseases of the endocrine system, including type 2 diabetes mellitus, hypothyroidism, and an increased incidence of atypical endocrine diseases during later life. Cellular damage associated with aging, genetically programmed cell change, and chronic wear and tear may contribute to endocrine gland dysfunction or alterations in responsiveness of target organs (as a result of changes with aging and disease, the target organs may lose their ability to respond to hormones).

Other endocrine changes that may be associated with aging and especially contribute to the age-associated failure in homeostasis include the *neuroendocrine theory of aging*. This theory attempts to explain the altered biologic activity of hormones, altered circulating levels of hormones, altered secretory responses of endocrine glands, altered metabolism of hormones, and loss of circadian control of hormone release. These changes are postulated to occur as a result of a genetic program encoded in the brain and then controlled and relayed to peripheral tissues through hormonal and neural agents.[63] This theory suggests that cells are programmed to function only for a given time. Menopause as a result of programmed changes in the reproductive system is an example of this theory.

The relationship between aging and the structure and function of the endocrine system cannot be separated from the changes in the immune system and the central nervous system. Evidence is increasing in support of an immune–neuroendocrine homeostatic network in humans with the thymus gland playing a key role in the immunoregulation of the nervous and endocrine systems. The early onset of thymus involution may act as a triggering event that initiates the gradual decline in endocrine homeostasis resulting in the aging process.[38]

Additionally, as the nervous system ages, a progressive reduction takes place in the body's capacity to maintain homeostasis in the face of environmental stress. The overall effect of the changes in aging in the neuroendocrine system is a progressive resistance to the inhibitory feedback of the end-organ hormonal secretion (see Fig. 10-2). Thus, although the initial response to a stressful stimulus may be appropriate, as the body ages, the response is more likely to be persistent and ultimately inappropriate or even harmful.[25]

Anatomic Changes with Aging.   The *pituitary gland* undergoes both anatomic and histologic changes associated with aging. By age 80 years, the weight of the anterior pituitary lobe (adenohypophysis) is reduced approximately 75% from its peak during young adulthood. The blood supply is reduced, and a higher incidence of adenomas and cysts is described during later life.

The *thyroid gland* becomes relatively smaller and fibrotic, and its position becomes lower-lying and retrosternal with age. As with the pituitary gland, blood supply to the thyroid gland is decreased. Secretion of thyroid hormones may diminish with age. The *parathyroid gland* demonstrates tissue changes with ad-

vancing age, but no major change is apparent in parathyroid hormone (PTH) levels. Hyperparathyroidism occurs primarily in persons older than 50 years and most commonly results from a single adenoma. It occasionally occurs with multiple adenomas or hyperplasia of two or more parathyroid glands. It is rarely caused by parathyroid carcinoma.

The *adrenal glands* have more fibrous tissue with aging, but because of compensatory feedback mechanisms, no relative alteration is apparent in functional cortisol levels. The most common cause of hypercortisolism occurs with the use of corticosteroids for medical conditions. As previously mentioned, because steroid use can suppress the pituitary-adrenal axis, adrenal insufficiency can occur after discontinuation of steroid therapy.

Changes in the *reproductive glands* have been shown clearly to have physiologic effects, most notably on the cardiovascular system and the skeleton (ovary) and muscle mass and libido (testis).[72] These effects are discussed elsewhere (see Chapters 18, 19, and 23).

Hormonal Changes with Aging.   Much of the available data regarding changes in hormonal levels and function are contradictory. The female reproductive system undergoes changes as part of the normal aging process. Menopause leads to changes in the genitourinary tract and accelerates the loss of minerals from bone and leads to an alteration in the lipid composition in the mature woman. Male hormones have been linked to preservation of bone and muscle mass and to an increased tendency toward developing certain diseases (e.g., benign prostatic hypertrophy, liver disease) during later life.

Loss of body hair, changes in the skin's collagen content and thickness, an increase in the percentage of body fat, a decrease in lean body mass, a decrease in bone mass, and a decrease in protein synthesis are signs of endocrinopathy that may be associated with decreased growth hormone levels.[48] With the decline of growth hormone secretion, sleep cycles are disrupted, and the potential for sequelae associated with sleep deprivation (e.g., depression, fibromyalgia) is now recognized.[89]

As mentioned, interactions between the endocrine and immune systems also influence the aging process. Declining hormonal levels are accompanied by increased activity of tumor-suppressor genes in the aging population unless these genes have been mutated so that suppressor function is lost. In fact, the most common somatic mutation of human cancers is the loss of tumor-suppressor genes as a result of exposures to a lifetime of mutagens. In the presence of decreased hormonal levels, loss of tumor-suppressor genes accounts for the increased probability of tumors with advancing age, again demonstrating the link between the endocrine and immune systems.[48]

◆ Signs and Symptoms of Endocrine Disease

Signs and symptoms of endocrine pathology vary depending on the gland affected and whether the pathology is as a result of an excess (hyperfunction) or insufficiency (hypofunction) of hormonal secretions.[37] In a therapy setting, the most common signs and symptoms associated with endocrine pathology are observed in the musculoskeletal system.

Growth and development of connective tissue structures are influenced strongly, and sometimes controlled, by various hormones and metabolic processes. When these processes are altered, structural and functional changes can occur in various connective tissues, producing musculoskeletal signs and symp-

---

*The role of the thyroid gland in the metabolism of the healthy older person remains unclear. No major defects are apparent in healthy individuals; however, during episodes of ill health, the thyroid's ability to maintain homeostasis is often limited.[19]

toms in addition to other systemic signs and symptoms of endocrine dysfunction (Table 10-3).

The therapist must be aware that clients with an underlying but undiagnosed endocrine disorder may present initially with a musculoskeletal problem and that clients with established endocrine disorders are not cured by hormonal replacement or suppression. Rather, they may develop progression of musculoskeletal impairment in response to hormone fluctuations.

Musculoskeletal System. *Rheumatoid arthritis* can be an indicator of an underlying endocrine disease. Early rheumatic symptoms such as myalgias and arthralgias are seen commonly with a number of endocrine diseases. Diabetes mellitus is associated with a variety of rheumatic syndromes, such as the stiff-hand syndrome and limited joint motion syndrome. Although rheumatic symptoms can appear suddenly in people with an endocrine disorder, an insidious onset is much more common.

Muscle weakness, atrophy, myalgia, and *fatigue* that persist despite rest may be early manifestations of thyroid or parathyroid disease, acromegaly, diabetes, Cushing's syndrome, or osteomalacia. In endocrine disease, most proximal muscle weakness is usually painless and may be unrelated to either the severity or the duration of the underlying disease. However, when true demonstrative weakness occurs (particularly in hyperthyroidism and hyperparathyroid disease), proximal muscle weakness is related to the severity and duration of the underlying endocrine problem. Any compromise of muscle energy metabolism aggravates and perpetuates trigger points such as are associated with myofascial pain syndrome (see Chapter 26) or tender points in muscle associated with fibromyalgia syndrome (see Chapter 6).

Carpal tunnel syndrome (CTS)* (see discussion, Chapter 38) resulting from median nerve compression at the wrist is a common finding in people with certain endocrine and metabolic disorders such as acromegaly and hypothyroidism (see Table 38-6). Any increase in the volume of contents of the carpal tunnel impinges on the median nerve (e.g., neoplasm, calcium, gouty tophi deposits, edema, tenosynovitis). Tenosynovitis (inflammation of the tendon sheaths) occurs with some infectious processes and many musculoskeletal conditions. Fluid infiltrating the tunnel may soften the transverse carpal ligament, which can make the bony arch flatten and compress the nerve.[36] Thickening of the transverse carpal ligament also may occur with systemic disorders such as acromegaly or myxedema.

Carpal tunnel syndrome in persons with diabetes represents one form of diabetic neuropathy caused by ischemia-related microvascular damage of the median nerve. This ischemia then causes increased sensitivity to even minor pressure exerted in the carpal tunnel area.[46] Vitamin B$_6$ deficiency may also be a factor in the development of CTS for the person with diabetes.[26]

CTS occurring during pregnancy may be caused by extra fluid and/or fat, diabetes (gestational or previously diagnosed), vitamin deficiencies, or other causes unrelated to the pregnancy itself (e.g., rheumatoid arthritis, job-related biomechanical stress). The fact that many women develop CTS at or near menopause may suggest that the soft tissues about the wrist may be affected in some way by hormones.[23]

---

*In endocrine disorders, CTS is frequently bilateral, which is one characteristic that may distinguish it from overuse syndromes and other causes of CTS. Unreported tarsal tunnel syndrome may also occur, another distinguishing characteristic of an underlying systemic origin of symptoms when present along with carpal tunnel syndrome.

TABLE	10-3

Signs and Symptoms of Endocrine Dysfunction

Neuromusculoskeletal	Systemic
Rheumatic-like signs and symptoms	Excessive or delayed growth
Muscle weakness	Polydipsia
Muscle atrophy	Polyuria
Myalgia	Mental changes (nervousness, confusion, depression)
Fatigue	Changes in hair (quality and distribution)
Carpal tunnel syndrome	Changes in skin pigmentation
Synovial fluid changes	Changes in distribution of body fat
Periarthritis	Changes in vital signs (elevated body temperature, pulse rate, increased blood pressure)
Adhesive capsulitis (diabetes mellitus)	Heart palpitations
Chondrocalcinosis	Increased perspiration
Spondyloarthropathy	Kussmaul's respirations (deep, rapid breathing)
Diffuse idiopathic skeletal hyperostosis (DISH)	Dehydration or excessive retention of body water
Osteoarthritis	
Osteoporosis	
Osteonecrosis	
Hand stiffness	
Arthralgia	
Pseudogout	

Periarthritis (inflammation of periarticular structures including the tendons, ligaments, and joint capsule) and *calcific tendinitis* occur most often in the shoulders of people who have endocrine disease. *Chondrocalcinosis* is the deposition of calcium salts in the joint cartilage; when accompanied by attacks of goutlike symptoms, it is called *pseudogout*. In 5% to 10% of people with chondrocalcinosis, an associated underlying endocrine or metabolic disease occurs, such as hypothyroidism, hyperparathyroidism, or acromegaly.[32] People diagnosed with fibromyalgia also may have altered thyroid function[57] and present with shoulder impingement secondary to chondrocalcinosis (see the section on Fibromyalgia in Chapter 6).

Spondoarthropathy (disease of joints of the spine) and *osteoarthritis* occur in individuals with various endocrine or metabolic diseases, including hemochromatosis (disorder of iron metabolism with excess deposition in the tissues; also known as *bronze diabetes* and *iron storage disease*), ochronosis (metabolic disorder caused by alkali deposits, resulting in discoloration of body tissues), acromegaly, and diabetes mellitus.

Hand stiffness, hand pain, and arthralgias of the small joints of the hand may occur with endocrine and metabolic diseases. Flexor tenosynovitis with stiffness is a common finding in persons with hypothyroidism. This condition often accompanies CTS.[59]

Other clinical presentations of musculoskeletal symptoms, such as CTS, rheumatoid arthritis, or adhesive capsulitis, may be referred to the therapist without accurate diagnosis of the underlying endocrine pathology. The therapist always must remain alert to the client's report of systemic signs and symptoms (usually a constellation of symptoms, rather than an isolated few) preceding, accompanying, or developing with the current musculoskeletal problems.

Additionally, the lack of progress in therapy should signal to the therapist the possibility of a systemic origin of musculoskeletal symptoms. Failure to recognize a metabolic cause of symptoms may result in prolonged, ineffective therapy; visits to a variety of therapists; and, occasionally, one or more unsuccessful surgical procedures.

Any client who is taking diuretics must be monitored for signs or symptoms of potassium depletion or fluid dehydration (see Chapter 4) before initiating exercise and then throughout the duration of exercise. Cortisol suppresses the body's inflammatory response, masking early signs of infection. Any unexplained fever without other symptoms in the immunocompromised client must be reported to the physician. ■

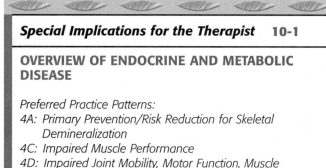

Special Implications for the Therapist 10-1

OVERVIEW OF ENDOCRINE AND METABOLIC DISEASE

Preferred Practice Patterns:
4A: Primary Prevention/Risk Reduction for Skeletal Demineralization
4C: Impaired Muscle Performance
4D: Impaired Joint Mobility, Motor Function, Muscle Performance, and Range of Motion Associated with Connective Tissue Dysfunction
4E: Impaired Joint Mobility, Motor Function, Muscle Performance, and Range of Motion Associated with Localized Inflammation
6B: Impaired Aerobic Capacity/Endurance Associated with Deconditioning

Disorders of the endocrine and metabolic systems may present with recognizable clinical signs and symptoms (see Table 10-3). Clients with a variety of endocrine and metabolic disorders report symptoms of fatigue, muscle weakness, and, occasionally, muscle or bone pain. Painless muscle weakness associated with endocrine and metabolic disorders usually involves proximal muscle groups. This muscle weakness and other symptoms, such as periarthritis and calcific tendinitis, may respond to treatment of the underlying endocrine pathology.

In most cases, the person who has received a diagnosis of an endocrine or metabolic disorder has undergone a combination of clinical and laboratory tests. This person may be in the care of a therapist for some other unrelated musculoskeletal problem that can be affected by symptoms associated with hormone imbalances.

SPECIFIC ENDOCRINE DISORDERS

◆ Pituitary Gland

The pituitary gland, or hypophysis, is a small (1 cm in diameter), oval gland located at the base of the skull in an indentation of the sphenoid bone directly posterior to the sphenoid sinus (see Figs. 10-1 and 10-2). It is often referred to as the *master gland* because of its role in regulating other endocrine glands. It is joined to the hypothalamus by the pituitary stalk (neurohypophyseal tract) and is influenced by the hypothalamus through releasing and inhibiting factors. The pituitary consists of two parts: the anterior pituitary (adenohypophysis) and the posterior pituitary (neurohypophysis) lobes. The anterior pituitary secretes six different hormones (ACTH, TSH, LH, FSH, human growth hormone, and prolactin) (see Fig. 10-2).

The posterior pituitary is a downward offshoot of the hypothalamus and contains many nerve fibers; it produces no hormones of its own. The hormones ADH (also called *vasopressin*) and oxytocin are produced in the hypothalamus and then stored and released by the posterior pituitary. These hormones pass down nerve fibers from the hypothalamus through the pituitary stalk to nerve endings in the posterior pituitary; they accumulate in the posterior pituitary during less active periods of the body. Transmitter substances, such as acetylcholine and norepinephrine, are thought to activate release of these substances by the posterior pituitary gland when they are stimulated by nerve impulses from the hypothalamus.[4]

Anterior Lobe Disorders. Disorders of the pituitary gland occur most frequently in the anterior lobe, most often caused by tumors, pituitary infarction, genetic disorders, and trauma. The three principal pathologic consequences of pituitary disorders are hyperpituitarism, hypopituitarism, and local compression of brain tissue by expanding tumor masses.[5] (See also Chapter 29.)

Hyperpituitarism

Overview. Hyperpituitarism is an oversecretion of one or more of the hormones secreted by the pituitary gland, especially growth hormone, resulting in acromegaly or gigantism. It is caused primarily by a hormone-secreting pituitary tumor, typically a benign adenoma. Other syndromes associated with hyperpituitarism include Cushing's disease,* amenorrhea, and hyperthyroidism.

Pituitary tumors produce both systemic effects and local manifestations. Systemic effects include (1) excessive or abnormal growth patterns resulting from overproduction of growth hormone; (2) hyperprolactinemia (increased prolactin secretion) resulting in amenorrhea, galactorrhea (spontaneous milk flow in women without nursing), and gynecomastia and impotence in men; and (3) overstimulation of one or more of the target glands, resulting in the release of excessive adrenocortical, thyroid, or sex hormones. Local pituitary tumors produce symptoms as the growing mass expands within the bony cranium. Local manifestations may include visual field abnormalities (pressure on the optic chiasma where the optic nerve crosses over), headaches, and somnolence (sleepiness).

Gigantism and Acromegaly. Gigantism, an overgrowth of the long bones, and acromegaly, increased bone thickness and hypertrophy of the soft tissues, result from growth hormone-secreting adenomas of the anterior pituitary gland. Although growth hormone–producing tumors that cause these conditions are rare, they are the second most common type of hyperpituitarism. Gigantism develops in children before the age when the epiphyses of the bones close; people who develop gigantism may grow to a height of 9 feet. Acromegaly is a disease of adults and develops after closure of the epiphyses of the long bones, so the bones most affected are those of the face, jaw, hands, and feet. In adults, acromegaly occurs equally among men and women and usually between ages 30 and 50 years.[5]

Gigantism develops abruptly, whereas acromegaly develops slowly. Both conditions are characterized by the same skeletal abnormalities because hypersecretion of growth hormone produces cartilaginous and connective tissue overgrowth, resulting in coarsened facial features; protrusion of the jaw (prognathism); thickened ears, nose, and tongue; and broad hands, with spadelike fingers (Fig. 10-3). In gigantism, as the tumor enlarges and invades normal tissue, target organ functions are impaired by the loss of other tropic (stimulating) hormones, such as TSH, LH, FSH, and ACTH. Clients with acromegaly may experience local manifestations such as headache, diplopia, blindness, and lethargy as the tumor compresses brain tissue.

Medical Management. Pituitary tumors are treated usually by surgical removal, drug therapy, and/or external beam radiation therapy. Drugs are now available that effectively reduce levels of growth hormone and prolactin and decrease pituitary tumor size. Drug therapy has replaced surgery in most cases of prolactin-secreting adenomas, but surgery is still the treatment of choice for pituitary adenomas that cause acromegaly. Some drug or radiation therapy may be required if levels of growth hormone remain high after surgery. Radiation therapy is also

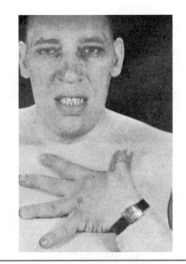

FIGURE 10-3 Acromegaly (hyperpituitarism). Acromegaly occurs as a result of excessive secretion of growth hormone after normal completion of body growth. The resulting overgrowth of bone in the face, head, and hands are pictured here. (From Jarvis C: *Physical examination and health assessment*, Philadelphia, 1992, WB Saunders, p 219.)

useful when surgery is not curative. Frequently, after pituitary surgery, pituitary function is lost and at that time, treatment with thyroid, cortisone, and hormone replacement may be necessary. Growth hormone therapy also is added in many cases.[86]

Special Implications for the Therapist 10-2

HYPERPITUITARISM

Preferred Practice Patterns:
4D: *Impaired Joint Mobility, Motor Function, Muscle Performance, and Range of Motion Associated with Connective Tissue Dysfunction*
4E: *Impaired Joint Mobility, Motor Function, Muscle Performance, and Range of Motion Associated with Localized Inflammation*
4F: *Impaired Joint Mobility, Motor Function, Muscle Performance, Range of Motion, and Reflex Integrity Associated with Spinal Disorders*
5F: *Impaired Peripheral Nerve Integrity and Muscle Performance Associated with Peripheral Nerve Injury*

Postoperative Care

Ambulation and exercise are encouraged within the first 24 hours after surgery. Coughing, sneezing, and blowing the nose are contraindicated after surgery, but deep breathing exercises are encouraged. Postoperatively, vital signs and neurologic status must be closely monitored. Any alteration in level of consciousness or visual acuity, falling pulse rate, or rising blood pressure may signal an increase in intracranial pressure resulting from intracranial bleeding or cerebral edema and must be reported immediately. Observe for signs of meningitis (e.g., severe headache, irritability, nuchal [back of the neck] rigidity), a potential complication of surgery.

Continued

---

*Cushing's disease is one form of Cushing's syndrome and results from oversecretion of ACTH by a pituitary tumor, which in turn, results in oversecretion of adrenocortical hormones (see section on Cushing's Syndrome in this chapter).

The nursing staff members monitor blood glucose levels often, because growth hormone levels fall rapidly after surgery, removing an insulin-antagonist effect in many people and possibly precipitating hypoglycemia (low blood glucose level). The therapist is advised to consult with nursing staff to determine the possible need for blood glucose monitoring during or after exercise. The therapist should be familiar with signs and symptoms and special implications of hypoglycemia (see the section on Hypoglycemia in this chapter).

Tumors causing visual changes may require the therapist to consciously remain within the client's visual field. Unexpected mood changes can occur, requiring patience and understanding on the part of health care workers. Although surgical removal of the tumor and/or pituitary gland prevents permanent soft-tissue deformities, bone changes already present do not change.

Orthopedic Considerations

Skeletal manifestations, such as arthritis of the hands and osteoarthritis of the spine, may develop with these conditions. Osteophyte formation and widening of the joint space owing to increased cartilage thickening may be seen on x-rays. In late-stage disease, joint spaces become narrowed, and chondrocalcinosis occasionally may be present. CTS is seen in up to 50% of people with acromegaly and is thought to be caused by intrinsic and extrinsic factors (e.g., compression of the median nerve at the wrist from soft tissue hypertrophy, bony overgrowth, and hypertrophy of the median nerve).[64]

About half of individuals with acromegaly have thoracic and/or lumbar back pain. X-ray studies demonstrate increased intervertebral disk spaces and large osteophytes along the anterior longitudinal ligament (ALL).

The therapist may be called on to provide a program that promotes maximum joint mobility, muscle strength, and functional skills. Assistance with activities of daily living (ADL) may be an important aspect of intervention. Home health staff should assess the home to remove any obstacles and recommend necessary adaptive equipment or assistive devices. ■

Hypopituitarism

Hypopituitarism (also *panhypopituitarism* and *dwarfism*) results from decreased or absent hormonal secretion by the anterior pituitary gland. Panhypopituitarism refers to a generalized condition caused by partial or total failure of all six of the anterior pituitary's vital hormones (ACTH, TSH, LH, FSH, human growth hormone, and prolactin).[86]

Hypopituitarism and panhypopituitarism are rare disorders that occur as a result of (1) hypophysectomy (removal or destruction of the pituitary by surgery, irradiation, or chemical agents); (2) nonsecreting pituitary tumors; (3) postpartum hemorrhage (the fall in blood pressure and subsequent hypoxia after delivery causes necrosis of the gland); and (4) reversible functional disorders (such as starvation, anorexia-nervosa, severe anemia, and GI tract disorders).

Clinical manifestations are dependent on the age at onset and the hormones affected (Table 10-4). More than 75% of the pituitary must be obliterated by tumors or thromboses before symptoms develop. Specific disorders resulting from pituitary hyposecretion include *growth hormone deficiency*, with subsequent short stature, delayed growth, and delayed puberty; *secondary adrenocortical insufficiency* from diminished

---

TABLE	10-4

Clinical Manifestations of Hypopituitarism

Growth hormone deficiency	Gonadal failure
Short stature	Secondary amenorrhea
Delayed growth	Impotence
Delayed puberty	Infertility
Adrenocortical insufficiency	Decreased libido
Hypoglycemia	Absent secondary sex
Anorexia	characteristics (children)
Nausea	Neurologic signs (produced
Abdominal pain	by tumors)
Orthostatic hypotension	Headache
Hypothyroidism (see also	Bilateral temporal hemianopia
Table 10-7)	Loss of visual acuity
Tiredness	Blindness
Lethargy	
Sensitivity to cold	
Menstrual disturbances	

---

synthesis of ACTH by the pituitary gland, which in turn causes diminished secretion of adrenocortical hormones by the adrenal cortex; *hypothyroidism* (thyroid hormone is dependent on TSH secreted by the pituitary); and *sexual and reproductive disorders* from deficiencies of the gonadotropins (LH and FSH). Treatment for hypopituitarism involves removal (if possible) of the causative factor, such as tumors, and lifetime replacement of the missing hormones.

Special Implications for the Therapist **10-3**

HYPOPITUITARISM

Although rarely encountered in a therapy setting, the client with hypopituitarism may report symptoms associated with hormonal deficiencies until hormone replacement therapy is complete. The therapist may observe weakness, fatigue, lethargy, apathy, and orthostatic hypotension (see Special Implications for the Therapist: Orthostatic Hypotension, Chapter 11). Nailbeds and skin may demonstrate pallor associated with anemia (see Special Implications for the Therapist: Anemia, Chapter 13).

Infection prevention requires meticulous skin care following the guidelines outlined in Table 11-22. Impaired peripheral vision associated with bilateral hemianopia (blindness in half of the visual field) requires special consideration. The therapist must be certain to stand where the affected individual can see others and to move slowly in and out of the client's visual field. ■

Posterior Lobe Disorders

Diabetes Insipidus. Diabetes insipidus, a rare disorder, involves a physiologic imbalance of water secondary to ADH deficiency. Injury or loss of function of the hypothalamus, the neurohypophyseal tract, or the posterior pituitary gland can result in diabetes insipidus (Box 10-1).

BOX 10-1

Causes of Diabetes Insipidus

Intracranial or pituitary neoplasm
Metastatic lesions (e.g., breast or lung cancer)
Surgical hypophysectomy or other neurosurgery
Skull fracture or head trauma (damages the neurohypophyseal structures)
Infection (e.g., meningitis, encephalitis)
Granulomatous disease
Vascular lesions (e.g., aneurysm)
Idiopathic
Autoimmune; heredity
Drugs or medications (e.g., phenytoin; alcohol)
Nephrogenic diabetes insipidus (congenital; drug induced)

BOX 10-2

Causes of Syndrome of Inappropriate Antidiuretic Hormone Secretion (SIADH)*

Oat cell carcinoma (accounts for 80% of cases)
Pulmonary disorders
    Pneumonia
    Tuberculosis
    Lung abscess
    Mechanical ventilation (e.g., positive pressure)
Central nervous system disorders
    Brain tumor or abscess
    Cerebrovascular accident
    Head injury
    Guillain-Barré syndrome
    Systemic lupus erythematosus
Other neoplasms (e.g., pancreatic or prostatic cancer, Hodgkin's disease, thymoma)
Infection
Stress (e.g., surgery) or trauma
Medications (e.g., chlorpropamide, antineoplastic drugs, morphine, thiazides)
Myxedema
Psychosis
Porphyria

*Listed in descending order.

Because the major functions of ADH are to promote water resorption by the kidney and to control the osmotic pressure of the extracellular fluid, when ADH production decreases, the kidney tubules fail to resorb water. The end result is excretion of large amounts of dilute urine. Unlike urine in diabetes mellitus, which contains large amounts of glucose, urine in diabetes insipidus is dilute and contains no glucose. Other clinical manifestations include polydipsia (excessive thirst), nocturia (excessive urination at night), and dehydration (e.g., poor tissue turgor, dry mucous membranes, constipation, muscle weakness, dizziness, and hypotension) (see Box 4-6). Fatigue and irritability may develop secondary to sleep disruption and in association with nocturia.

If a person is conscious and able to respond appropriately to the thirst mechanism, hydration can be maintained. However, if a person is unconscious or confused and unable to take in necessary fluids to compensate for fluid loss, rapid dehydration, shock, and death can occur. Treatment is usually exogenous replacement of ADH with vasopressin or a synthetic derivative, such as Pitressin, along with administration of diuretics. When this condition is caused by tumor, resection of the tumor can affect a cure.

Special Implications for the Therapist   10-4

DIABETES INSIPIDUS

The therapist must be alert for possible serious side effects of any type of ADH administration. ADH stimulates smooth muscle contraction of the vascular system (causing increased blood pressure), the GI tract (causing diarrhea), and the coronary arteries (causing angina or myocardial infarction).[46] Increases in blood pressure can cause additional serious problems in some people, particularly those with hypertension or coronary artery disease (CAD) and cerebrovascular disease (CVD). Additionally, after receiving vasopressin, clients must be assessed for signs and symptoms of water intoxication, which can lead to fluid overload, cerebral edema, and seizures. See also Special Implications for the Therapist: Fluid and Electrolyte Imbalances, Chapter 4. ■

Syndrome of Inappropriate Antidiuretic Hormone Secretion (SIADH).

SIADH is a disorder associated with excessive release of ADH, which disturbs fluid and electrolyte balance, resulting in a water imbalance. SIADH has a wide variety of causes, including pituitary damage resulting from infection, trauma, or neoplasm; the stress of surgery or many systemic disorders; and response to certain medications (Box 10-2).

SIADH is the opposite of diabetes insipidus, so treatment of diabetes insipidus with vasopressin can lead to SIADH if excessive amounts are administered. In SIADH, instead of large fluid losses, water intoxication occurs as a result of fluid retention. Under normal circumstances, ADH regulates serum osmolality.* When serum osmolality falls, a feedback mechanism causes inhibition of ADH, which promotes increased water excretion by the kidneys to raise serum osmolality to normal. When this feedback mechanism fails and ADH levels are sustained, fluid retention results. Ultimately, serum sodium levels fall, resulting in hyponatremia (sodium depletion) and water intoxication.[46]

Although fluid retention is the primary symptom, edema is rare unless water overload exceeds 4 L; much of the free water excess is within cellular boundaries. Neurologic and neuro-

*Serum osmolality is a measure of the number of dissolved particles per unit of water in serum. In a solution, the fewer the particles of solute in proportion to the number of units of water (solvent), the less concentrated the solution. A low serum osmolality indicates a higher-than-usual amount of water in relation to the amount of particles dissolved in it. In other words, serum osmolality provides a measure of hydration of cells. For example, a low serum osmolality accompanies overhydration (i.e., edema); an increased serum osmolality is present in a state of fluid volume deficit. Osmolality is proportional with dilutional or depletional states (true for water and sodium). The normal value for serum osmolality is 280 to 300 mOsm/kg of water.[14]

muscular signs and symptoms predominate and are directly related to the swelling of brain tissue and to sodium changes within neuromuscular tissues. Central nervous system dysfunction, characterized by alterations in level of consciousness, seizures, and coma, can occur when serum sodium falls to 120 mEq/L or less. Hyponatremia can result in diminished GI function; this problem is complicated further by the need for fluid restriction.

Correction of life-threatening sodium imbalance is the first aim of treatment followed by correction of the underlying cause. If SIADH is caused by malignancy, success in alleviating water retention may be obtained by surgical resection, irradiation, or chemotherapy. Otherwise, treatment for SIADH is symptomatic and includes restriction of water intake, careful replacement of sodium chloride, and administration of diuretics. Other pharmaceuticals (e.g., demeclocycline and tetracycline or lithium) also may be used to block the renal response to ADH.

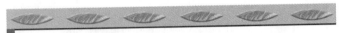

Special Implications for the Therapist 10-5

SYNDROME OF INAPPROPRIATE ANTIDIURETIC HORMONE SECRETION (SIADH)

Anyone at risk for SIADH (see conditions listed in Box 10-2) should be monitored for sudden weight gain or fluid retention and changes in urination and fluid intake. Observe for headache, lethargy, muscle cramps, restlessness, irritability, convulsions, or weight gain without visible edema (2 lb or more a day). Throughout therapy, the client's cardiovascular status should be assessed regularly so that any unusual alterations can be noted immediately. (See also Special Implications for the Therapist: Fluid Imbalances, Chapter 4.)

Continued need for sodium and fluid restrictions may be necessary for the person discharged to home or who is in a facility other than the acute care setting (hospital). People with unresolved SIADH should avoid the use of aspirin or nonsteroidal antiinflammatory agents without a physician's approval, because these drugs can increase hyponatremia. ∎

◆ **Thyroid Gland**

The thyroid gland is located in the anterior portion of the lower neck, below the larynx, on both sides of and anterior to the trachea (see Fig. 10-1). The primary hormones produced by the thyroid are thyroxine (T_4), triiodothyronine (T_3), and calcitonin. Both T_3 and T_4 regulate the metabolic rate of the body and increase protein synthesis. Calcitonin has a weak physiologic effect on calcium and phosphorus balance in the body. Thyroid function is regulated by the hypothalamus and pituitary feedback controls and by an intrinsic regulator mechanism within the gland.[39]

Disorders of the thyroid gland may be functional abnormalities leading to hyperfunction or hypofunction of the gland or anatomic abnormalities such as thyroiditis, goiter, and tumor. Enlargement of the thyroid gland or neoplasm may or may not be associated with abnormalities of hormone secretion.

Susceptibility to thyroid disease is largely determined by the interaction of genetic makeup, age, and sex. Women, particularly those with a family history of thyroid disease, are much more likely to have thyroid pathology than are men. Although most thyroid conditions cannot be prevented, they respond well to treatment.

Thyroid hormone acts on nearly all body tissues, so excessive or deficient secretion affects various body systems. Alterations in thyroid function produce changes in nails, hair, skin, eyes, GI tract, respiratory tract, heart and blood vessels, nervous tissue, bone, and muscle.[39] Both hyperthyroidism and hypothyroidism can adversely affect cardiac function. Sustained tachycardia in hyperthyroidism and sustained bradycardia with cardiac enlargement in hypothyroidism can result in cardiac failure. Both conditions affect the general rate of metabolism, the muscular system, the nervous system, the gastrointestinal system, and, as mentioned, the cardiovascular system.

Hyperthyroidism
Definition and Overview. Hyperthyroidism is an excessive secretion of thyroid hormone, sometimes referred to as *thyrotoxicosis*, a term used to describe the clinical manifestations that occur when the body tissues are stimulated by increased thyroid hormone. Excessive thyroid hormone creates a generalized elevation of body metabolism, the effects of which are manifested in almost every system.

The most common form of hyperthyroidism is Graves' disease, which increases T_4 production and accounts for 85% of cases of hyperthyroidism. Like most thyroid conditions, hyperthyroidism affects women more than men (4:1), especially women between ages 20 and 40 years.

Rarely, a person with inadequately treated hyperthyroidism may experience what is called a *thyroid storm*. This potentially fatal condition is an acute episode of thyroid overactivity characterized by high fever, severe tachycardia, delirium, dehydration, and extreme irritability or agitation. Stress occurring in the presence of undiagnosed or untreated hyperthyroidism may precipitate such an event. Stressors may include surgery, infection, toxemia of pregnancy, labor and delivery, diabetic ketoacidosis, myocardial infarction, pulmonary embolus, and medication overdose.

Etiologic and Risk Factors. Hyperthyroidism may result from both immunologic and genetic factors. Graves' disease, the most common form of hyperthyroidism, is most likely autoimmune in development, and although it is more common in women with family histories of thyroid abnormalities, major risk factors have not been identified. In addition, autoimmune hyperthyroid disease is present in people with other immune-related disorders such as Sjögren's syndrome,[52] rheumatoid arthritis, and psoriatic arthritis.[61] Hyperthyroidism also may be due to the overfunction of the entire gland such as in Graves' disease, or less commonly, to hyperfunctioning of a single adenoma or multiple toxic nodules. Rarely, overtreatment of myxedema associated with hypothyroidism (see next section) may result in hyperthyroidism. And more rarely, thyroid cancer can cause glandular hyperfunction.

Pathogenesis. About 95% of people with Graves' disease have circulating autoantibodies called thyroid-stimulating immunoglobulins (TSI) that react against thyroglobulin (precursor for thyroid hormones). These autoantibodies may be due to a defect in suppressor T-lymphocyte function that allows formation of TSIs. Evidently, the presence of TSIs in the serum of hyperthyroid Graves' clients are autoantibodies that react against a component of the thyroid cell membranes, stimulating enlargement of the thyroid gland and secretion of excess thyroid hormone.

Because the action of thyroid hormone on the body is stimulatory, hypermetabolism results with increased sympathetic nervous system activity. The excessive amounts of thyroid hormone stimulate the cardiac system and increase the number of beta-adrenergic receptors throughout the body. This excess thyroid hormone secretion, coupled with the increased secretion of catecholamines, leads to tachycardia, increased stroke volume, and increased peripheral blood flow. The increased metabolism also leads to a negative nitrogen balance, lipid depletion, and a resultant state of nutritional deficiency.

Clinical Manifestations.

Because hyperthyroidism is caused by an excess secretion of thyroid hormone, the clinical picture of Graves' disease is in many ways the opposite of that of hypothyroidism. The classic symptoms of Graves' disease are mild symmetric enlargement of the thyroid (goiter), nervousness, heat intolerance, weight loss despite increased appetite, sweating, diarrhea, tremor, and palpitations. Hyperthyroidism may induce atrial fibrillation, precipitate congestive heart failure, and increase the risk of underlying coronary artery disease for myocardial infarction.

Exophthalmos (abnormal protrusion of the eyes) (Fig. 10-4) is considered most characteristic but is absent in many people with hyperthyroidism, and may exacerbate after adequate treatment of the hyperthyroid state. Changes such as swelling behind the eyes are mediated by autoimmune production of antibodies to soft tissues (particularly the fibroblasts). Highly specialized ophthalmic surgery (surgical decompression) may be effective for correcting the severe exophthalmus when vision is impaired and proctosis is severe. Retroorbital radiation has also been shown to be effective.[93] Many other symptoms are commonly present, because this condition affects many body systems (Table 10-5). Complications such as thyroid storm and heart disease can occur (see previous discussion, this section).

Emotions are adversely affected by the increased metabolic activity within the body. Moods may be cyclic, ranging from mild euphoria to extreme hyperactivity or delirium and, infrequently, depression, which may persist even after successful treatment of hyperthyroidism. Excessive hyperactivity may be associated with extreme fatigue.

Hyperthyroidism in older adults is notorious for presenting with atypical or minimal symptoms.[88] Signs and symptoms are not the usual ones and may be attributed to aging. Many older people actually appear apathetic instead of hyperactive. Cardiovascular abnormalities, as described above, are much more common in older adults.

Neuromuscular Manifestations.

Chronic periarthritis also is associated with hyperthyroidism. Inflammation that involves the periarticular structures, including the tendons, ligaments, and joint capsule, is termed *periarthritis*. This syndrome is characterized by pain and reduced range of motion. Calcification, whether periarticular or tendinous, may be seen on x-ray studies. Both periarthritis and calcific tendinitis can occur most often in the shoulder in clients

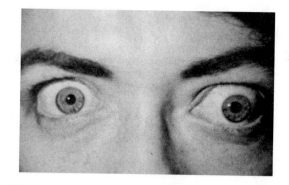

FIGURE   **10-4**   Exophthalmos, or protruding eyes. This is a forward displacement of the eyeballs associated with thyroid disease. Because the eyes are surrounded by unyielding bone, fluid accumulation in the fat pads and muscles behind the eyeballs causes protruding eyes and a fixed stare. Without treatment of the underlying cause, the client with severe exophthalmos may be unable to close the eyelids and may develop corneal ulceration or infection, eventually resulting in loss of vision. Note the lid lag; the upper eyelid rests well above the limbus (edge of the cornea where it joins the sclera), and white sclera is visible. This is evident when the person moves the eyes from up to down. (From Jarvis C: *Physical examination and health assessment,* ed 3, Philadelphia, 2000, WB Saunders, p 336.)

who have undiagnosed, untreated, or inadequately treated endocrine disease. The involvement can be unilateral or bilateral and can worsen progressively to become adhesive capsulitis, or frozen shoulder. Acute calcific tendinitis of the wrist also has been described in such clients. Although antiinflammatory agents may be needed for acute symptoms, chronic periarthritis usually responds to treatment of the underlying hyperthyroidism.*

Proximal muscle weakness (most marked in the pelvic girdle and thigh muscles) accompanied by muscle atrophy, known as *myopathy*, can occur in cases of undiagnosed, untreated, or inadequately treated hyperthyroidism. The therapist may first notice problems with coordination or balance or notice weakness of the legs causing a client difficulty in ambulating, rising from a chair, or climbing stairs.[28] Respiratory muscle weakness can present as dyspnea. The pathogenesis of the weakness is still a subject of controversy; muscle strength seems to return to normal in 6 to 8 weeks after medical treatment, with a slower resolution of muscle wasting. In severe cases, normal strength may not be restored for months.

The incidence of myasthenia gravis, which is also an antibody immune disease, is increased in clients with hyperthyroidism, which in turn can aggravate muscle weakness. If the hyperthyroidism is corrected, improvement of the myasthenia gravis usually follows.

Sudden, periodic paralysis while at rest characterized by recurrent episodes of motor weakness of variable intensity can occur in a selective population (more common among people of Asian origin). This phenomenon is precipitated by intracellular shifts of potassium triggered by thyroid overactivity and hyperinsulemia after ingestion of carbohydrates and increased physical activity. Administration of potassium is required to prevent life-threatening arrhythmias.[69,76]

---

*Physical therapy is not recommended in these cases until after the endocrine problem is resolved. Then therapeutic intervention with ultrasound, joint mobilization, stretching, and strengthening may be indicated to treat any residual dysfunction.

TABLE 10-5

Systemic Manifestations of Hyperthyroidism

CNS Effects	Cardiovascular and Pulmonary Effects	Musculo-skeletal Effects	Ingegumentary Effects	Ocular Effects	Gastrointestinal Effects	Genitourinary Effects
Tremors Hyperkinesis (abnormally increased motor function or activity) Nervousness Emotional lability Weakness and muscle atrophy Increased deep tendon reflexes	Increased pulse rate/ tachycardia/ palpitations Increased cardiac output Increased blood volume Dysrhythmias (especially atrial fibrillation) Weakness of respiratory muscles (breathlessness, hypoventilation) Increased respiratory rate	Muscle weakness and fatigue Muscle atrophy Chronic periarthritis Myasthenia gravis	Capillary dilation (warm, flushed, moist skin) Heat intolerance Onycholysis (separation of the fingernail distally from the nail bed) Easily broken hair and increased hair loss Hard, purple area over the anterior surface of the tibia with itching, erythema, and, occasionally, pain	Exophthalmos Weakness of the extra-ocular muscles (poor convergence, poor upward gaze) Sensitivity to light Visual loss Spasm and retraction of the upper eyelids, lid tremor	Hypermetabolism (increased appetite with weight loss) Diarrhea, nausea, and vomiting Dysphagia	Polyuria (frequent urination) Amenorrhea (absence of menses) Female infertility Increased risk of spontaneous miscarriage Gynecomastia (males)

Modified from Goodman CC, Snyder TE: *Differential diagnosis in physical therapy*, ed 3, Philadelphia, 2000, WB Saunders, p 300.

Medical Management

Diagnosis. Diagnosis is based on clinical history, physical presentation, examination findings, and laboratory test results. Hyperthyroidism is almost always associated with suppressed thyroid stimulating hormone (TSH). The very rare exception is that of a TSH-secreting pituitary adenoma. In very mild hyperthyroidism the thyroxine (T_4) would be normal but the measurement of triiodothyronine (T_3) usually would be elevated or at the upper range of normal. This is called T_3 *toxicosis* and almost always precedes Graves' disease. Diagnostic tests such as radioactive iodine uptake (RIU) can confirm the presence of hyperthyroidism and differentiate among causes of hyperthyroidism.[14]

Radioactive iodine uptake studies are elevated in Graves' disease and nodular thyrotoxicosis but are very low or negative in thyroiditis-caused hyperthyroidism. Thyroid stimulating immunoglobulin (TSI) is positive in almost all people with Graves' disease. It is essential to distinguish hyperthyroidism caused by Graves' disease and nodular thyrotoxicosis from thyroiditis because the treatment for each is different.[97]

Treatment. The three major forms of therapy are antithyroid medication, radioactive iodine, and surgery. Most endocrine specialists would now recommend radioactive iodine as first line therapy in anyone older than 18 years of age who is not pregnant. Some physicians treat down to the age of 12 because long-term studies have shown no increased incidence of thyroid cancer or leukemia in people receiving such treatment.[99] Iodine 131 therapy takes several months before it is effective, so adrenergic blocking agents are sometimes given in the interim to control the activity of the sympathetic nervous system. Typically everyone who receives radioactive iodine becomes hypothyroid and requires thyroid hormone replacement for the rest of their lives. Almost everyone treated with radioactive iodine is hypothyroid during the first year of therapy but eventually normalizes with replacement therapy.

Use of antithyroid drugs (propylthiouracil and methimazole) is also effective and is the usual choice of therapy during pregnancy and for children under the age of 12. Side effects from drug treatment include rheumatoid-like arthritis and agranulocytosis (serious and potentially fatal) and usually resolve after 10 days of discontinuing the drug. About half of the people treated with antithyroid drugs have a later recurrence of hyperthyroid activity. Again, adrenergic blocking agents may be used with these drugs.[93]

Partial or subtotal thyroidectomy is an effective way to treat hyperthyroidism caused by Graves' disease and single or multinodular thyrotoxicosis. The ideal surgical treatment leaves a small portion of the functioning thyroid gland to avoid permanent hormone replacement. Surgical treatment is effective in most cases although surgical complications can develop such as vocal cord paralysis (resulting from laryngeal nerve damage) or hypoparathyroidism leading to hypocalcemia (resulting from inadvertent removal of parathyroid gland tissue).[5]

Prognosis. Antithyroid drugs may be tapered and discontinued if remission is possible. Remission rates are higher in people with mild degrees of hyperthyroidism, small goiters, and for those who are diagnosed early. Even with remission, lifelong follow-up is recommended because many remissions are not permanent. Relapses are most likely to occur in the postpartum period.[97]

After radioiodine treatment, regular life-long medical supervision is required. Frequently, hypothyroidism develops even as long as 1 to 3 years after treatment. Exophthalmos may not be reversed by intervention. In severe cases, the person may be unable to close the eyelids and must have the lids taped shut to protect the eyes. Without intervention, severe exophthalmos can progress to corneal ulceration or infection and loss of vision.

Special Implications for the Therapist   10-6

HYPERTHYROIDISM

Preferred Practice Patterns:
4C: Impaired Muscle Performance
4D: Impaired Joint Mobility, Motor Function, Muscle
       Performance, and Range of Motion Associated with
       Connective Tissue Dysfunction
4E: Impaired Joint Mobility, Motor Function, Muscle
       Performance, and Range of Motion Associated with
       Localized Inflammation
6B: Impaired Aerobic Capacity/Endurance Associated with
       Deconditioning

Any time a therapist examines a client's neck and finds unusual swelling, enlargement, with or without symptoms of pain, tenderness, hoarseness, or dysphagia (difficulty swallowing), a medical referral is required. For the client requiring life-long thyroid hormone replacement therapy, nervousness and palpitations may develop with overdosage. A small number of people experience fever, rash, and arthralgias as side effects of antithyroid drugs. The physician should be notified of these or any other unusual symptoms, because it may be possible to use an alternative drug.

Monitoring Vital Signs
Monitoring vital signs is important to assess cardiac function if the involved person is an older adult[88], has coronary artery disease, or presents with symptoms of dyspnea, fatigue, tachycardia, and/or arrhythmia. If the heart rate is more than 100 beats/minute, check the blood pressure and pulse rate and rhythm frequently. The person with dyspnea is most comfortable sitting upright or in a high Fowler's position (head of the bed raised 18 to 20 inches above a level position with the knees elevated).

Because clients with Graves' disease may suffer from heat intolerance, they should avoid exercise in a hot aquatic or pool physical therapy setting. Exercise in a warm pool would be safe and would not be contraindicated as long as the person's temperature is monitored. True heat intolerance usually is associated with severe hyperthyroid states such as thyroid storm and probably would not occur in a nonhospitalized individual.

Postoperative Care
Postoperatively, observe for signs of hypoparathyroidism (muscular twitching, tetany, numbness and tingling around the mouth, fingertips, or toes), a complication that results from the accidental removal of the parathyroid glands during surgery. Symptoms can develop 1 to 7 days after surgery.

Any health care worker in contact with clients who have undergone radioiodine therapy must follow necessary precautions (see Chapter 4). Saliva is radioactive for 24 hours after ^{131}I therapy; health care professionals in contact with clients while they are coughing or expectorating must take precautions.

Side Effects of Radioiodine Therapy
Radioiodine therapy has few immediate side effects. Rarely, anterior neck tenderness may develop 7 to 10 days after therapy, consistent with radiation-induced thyroiditis.[78] The potential exists for worsening hyperthyroidism soon after radioiodine therapy, secondary to inflammation and release of stored thyroid in the bloodstream. Older adults and anyone with cardiac disease usually are pretreated with antithyroid agents before receiving radioiodine to prevent this occurrence.

The major adverse reaction from radioiodine is iatrogenic hypothyroidism. This development is so characteristic that it is considered an inevitable consequence of therapy rather than a side effect. Hypothyroidism develops in at least 50% of all cases treated with radioiodine therapy within the first year after therapy, with a gradual increased incidence thereafter. This complication necessitates life-long follow-up with close monitoring of thyroid function.

For further discussion of radiation side effects and precautions for health care workers coming in contact with a person who has been irradiated, see Chapter 4.

Hyperthyroidism and Exercise
Hyperthyroidism is associated with exercise intolerance and reduced exercise capacity although the exact relationship is unknown. Cardiac output is either normal or enhanced (e.g., increased heart rate) during exercise in the hyperthyroid state and blood flow to muscles is augmented during submaximal exercise. However, proximal muscle weakness with accompanying myopathy is characteristic in individuals with Graves' disease and may affect exercise capability.

Impaired cardiopulmonary function (more noticeable in older people with hyperthyroidism) also may affect exercise capacity. Thyrotoxicosis can aggravate preexisting heart disease and can lead to atrial fibrillation, congestive heart failure, worsening angina pectoris, and increase the risk for myocardial infarction. These factors must be considered in the overall discussion and planning of any exercise program for clients who are hyperthyroid.

Fatigue as a result of the hypermetabolic state and rapid depletion of nutrients may affect exercise capacity.[27] Using perceived exertion or exercise tolerance as a guide, exercise parameters (frequency, intensity, duration) remain the same for the person treated for hyperthyroidism as for anyone who does not have this condition. However, the therapist must remain alert for signs of subclinical hyperthyroidism (especially reduced VO_{2max} and other signs of impaired exercise performance) in the person receiving long term TSH—suppressive therapy. These manifestations improve or disappear after careful tailoring of the medications.[65] ■

Hypothyroidism
Definition and Etiologic Factors.   Hypothyroidism (hypofunction) refers to a deficiency of thyroid hormone in the adult that results in a generalized slowed body metabolism; it is the most common disorder of thyroid function in the United States and Canada. More than 50% of cases occur in families in which thyroid disease is present.

TABLE 10-6

Causes of Hypothyroidism

PRIMARY	SECONDARY
Congenital defects	Pituitary tumor
Loss of thyroid tissue	Pituitary insufficiency
Radioiodine treatment of hyperthyroidism	Postpartum necrosis of the pituitary (Sheehan's syndrome)
Surgical removal	
Radiation treatment for Hodgkin's disease or throat cancer	
Defective hormone synthesis	
Chronic autoimmune thyroiditis (Hashimoto's disease)	
Iodine deficiency	
Antithyroid drugs	

The condition may be classified as either primary or secondary. *Primary hypothyroidism* results from reduced functional thyroid tissue mass or impaired hormonal synthesis or release. *Secondary hypothyroidism* accounts for a small percentage of all cases of hypothyroidism and occurs as a result of inadequate stimulation of the gland because of pituitary or hypothalamic disease (failure to produce TSH and TRH, respectively) (Table 10-6). (See section on Hashimoto's Thyroiditis in this chapter.)

In the United States and Canada, this disease commonly is due to congenital autoimmune thyroiditis, thyroid ablation via surgery or radioactive iodine therapy, or medication with thiouracil or lithium; rarely it is a result of subacute thyroiditis, iodine deficiency, dietary factors, congenital abnormalities in iodination, or pituitary failure.[96]

Incidence.   Hypothyroidism is about four times more prevalent in women than in men. Although hypothyroidism may be congenital and therefore present at birth, the highest incidence is between ages 30 and 60 years. More than 95% of all people with hypothyroidism have the primary form of the disease.[46]

Pathogenesis.   In primary hypothyroidism, the loss of thyroid tissue leads to decreased secretion of thyroid hormone. In response to a decrease in thyroid hormone, TSH secretion is increased from the anterior pituitary gland as the body attempts to stimulate increased production of thyroid hormone. Secondary hypothyroidism is most commonly the result of failure of the pituitary gland to synthesize and release adequate amounts of TSH.

Decreased levels of thyroid hormone lead to an overall slowing of the basal metabolic rate. This slowing of all body processes leads to bradycardia, decreased GI tract motility, slowed neurologic functioning, a decrease in body heat production, and achlorhydria (absence of hydrochloric acid from gastric juice). Lipid metabolism also is altered by hypothyroidism with a resultant increase in serum cholesterol and triglyceride levels and a concomitant increase in arteriosclerosis and coronary heart disease. Thyroid hormones also play a role in the production of red blood cells with the potential for the development of anemia.

Clinical Manifestations.   As with all disorders affecting the thyroid and parathyroid glands, clinical signs and symptoms associated with hypothyroidism affect many systems of the body (Table 10-7). Typically, the early clinical features of hypothyroidism are vague and ordinary, so they escape detection (e.g., fatigue, mild sensitivity to cold, mild weight gain resulting from fluid retention [10 to 15 lb], forgetfulness, depression, and dry skin or hair).

As the disorder progresses, myxedema and its associated signs and symptoms appear. Myxedema is a result of an alteration in the composition of the dermis and other tissues, causing connective tissues to be separated by increased amounts of mucopolysaccharides and proteins. This mucopolysaccharide-protein complex binds with water, causing a nonpitting, boggy edema, especially around the eyes, hands, feet, and in the supraclavicular fossae. Thickening of the tongue, laryngeal and pharyngeal structures, hoarseness, and slurred speech occur as a result of myxedema.[96]

Other clinical manifestations associated with hypothyroidism may include decreasing mental stability; dry, flaky, inelastic skin; dry, sparse hair; hoarseness; upper eyelid droop; and thick, brittle nails. Cardiovascular involvement leads to decreased cardiac output, slow pulse rate, and signs of poor peripheral circulation. Other possible effects of hypothyroid function are anorexia, abdominal distention, menorrhagia, decreased libido, infertility, ataxia, intention tremor, and nystagmus.

Neuromuscular symptoms are among the most frequent manifestations of hypothyroidism seen in a therapy practice. Flexor tenosynovitis with stiffness can accompany CTS in persons with hypothyroidism. CTS arising from myxedematous tissue in the carpal tunnel area can develop before other signs of hypothyroidism become evident. Most people with CTS associated with hypothyroidism do not require surgical treatment because symptoms of median nerve compression respond to thyroid replacement.

A wide spectrum of rheumatic symptoms occurs in people with hypothyroidism. A fibromyalgia-like symptom complex with muscle aches and tender points may be seen early; replacement therapy with thyroid hormone eliminates the symptoms and distinguishes it from classic fibromyalgia. An inflammatory arthritis indistinguishable from rheumatoid arthritis may be seen. The arthritis predominantly involves the small joints of the hands and apparently differs from the viscous noninflammatory effusions observed in large joints of individuals with hypothyroidism. In general, the arthritis resolves with normalization of the thyroid hormone levels.[64]

Proximal muscle weakness can occur in persons with hypothyroidism; sometimes accompanied by pain. Trigger points are frequently detected on examination, and diffuse muscle tenderness may be the major finding. Muscle weakness is not always related to either the severity or the duration of hypothyroidism; it can be present several months before a medical diagnosis of hypothyroidism is made. Deep tendon reflexes show delayed relaxation time (i.e., prolonged reflexes), especially in the Achilles tendon.[28]

Medical Management

Diagnosis.   A substantial delay in diagnosis resulting from the vague onset of symptoms is not uncommon. Specific testing of TSH levels is the most sensitive indicator of primary hypothyroidism. TSH levels are always elevated in primary hypothyroidism. T_3 (triiodothyronine) levels do not change dra-

TABLE   **10-7**

Systemic Manifestations of Hypothyroidism

CNS Effects	Musculoskeletal Effects	Cardiovascular Effects	Hematologic Effects	Respiratory Effects	Integumentary Effects	Gastrointestinal Effects
Slowed speech and hoarseness	Proximal muscle weakness	Bradycardia	Anemia	Dyspnea	Myxedema (periorbital and peripheral)	Anorexia
Slow mental function (loss of interest in daily activities, poor short-term memory)	Myalgias	Congestive heart failure	Easy bruising	Respiratory muscle weakness	Thickened, cool, and dry skin	Constipation
	Trigger points	Poor peripheral circulation (pallor, cold skin, intolerance to cold, hypertension)	Menorrhagia		Scaly skin (especially elbows and knees)	Weight gain disproportionate to caloric intake
Fatigue and increased sleep	Stiffness				Carotenosis (yellowing of the skin)	Decreased absorption of nutrients
Headache	Carpal tunnel syndrome	Severe atherosclerosis			Coarse, thinning hair	Decreased protein metabolism (retarded skeletal and soft-tissue growth)
Cerebellar ataxia	Prolonged deep tendon reflexes (especially Achilles)	Angina			Intolerance to cold	
Depression	Subjective report of paresthesias without supportive objective findings				Nonpitting edema of hands and feet	Delayed glucose uptake
Psychiatric changes	Muscular and joint edema				Poor wound healing	Decreased glucose absorption
	Back pain				Thin, brittle nails	
	Increased bone density					
	Decreased bone formation and resorption					

Modified from Goodman CC, Snyder TE: *Differential diagnosis in physical therapy*, ed 3, Philadelphia, 2000, WB Saunders, p 301.

matically, even in severe hypothyroidism. T_4 (thyroxine) levels, however, decrease gradually until they are well below normal in advanced hypothyroidism. Serum cholesterol, alkaline phosphatase, and triglyceride levels also can be significantly elevated in the presence of hypothyroidism. In addition, the presence of antithyroid antibodies documents the existence of autoimmune thyroiditis resulting in progressive destruction of thyroid tissue by circulating antithyroid antibodies.[97]

Treatment.   The goals of treatment for hypothyroidism are to correct thyroid hormone deficiency, reverse symptoms, and prevent further cardiac and arterial damage. If treatment with (life-long) administration of synthetic thyroid hormone preparations is begun soon after symptoms appear, recovery may be complete. Older people with underlying heart disease (particularly underlying coronary artery disease) can be started on very low doses of thyroxine and be gradually increased in dosage to ultimately return the TSH to within the normal range. Cardiac complications can occur, including angina severe enough that intervention may be required. Only small doses should be initiated in anyone with preexisting heart problems.

Prognosis.   Severely hypothyroid conditions accompanied by pronounced atherosclerosis (resulting from abnormal lipid metabolism) may cause angina and other symptoms of coronary artery disease. Treatment of hypothyroidism-induced angina can be difficult because thyroid hormone replacement increases the heart's need for oxygen by increasing body metabolism. This increase in metabolism then precipitates

angina and aggravates the anginal condition. In severe hypothyroidism, psychiatric abnormalities can occur and are described as "myxedema madness" in the older literature.

Rarely, severe or prolonged hypothyroidism may progress to myxedema coma when aggravated by stress such as surgery, infection, or noncompliance with thyroid treatment. Myxedema coma can be fatal because of the extreme decrease in the metabolic rate, hypoventilation leading to respiratory acidosis, hypothermia, and hypotension.

Special Implications for the Therapist   10-7

HYPOTHYROIDISM

Preferred Practice Patterns:
4C: Impaired Muscle Performance
4D: Impaired Joint Mobility, Motor Function, Muscle Performance, and Range of Motion Associated with Connective Tissue Dysfunction
4E: Impaired Joint Mobility, Motor Function, Muscle Performance, and Range of Motion Associated with Localized Inflammation
4F: Impaired Joint Mobility, Motor Function, Muscle Performance, Range of Motion, and Reflex Integrity Associated with Spinal Disorders

Continued

6B: Impaired Aerobic Capacity/Endurance Associated with Deconditioning

7A: Primary Prevention/Risk Reduction for Integumentary Disorders

In the case of myxedematous hypothyroidism, distinctive changes in the synovium can occur, resulting in a viscous non-inflammatory joint effusion. Often the fluid contains calcium pyrophosphate dihydrate (CPPD) crystal deposits that may be associated with chondrocalcinosis (i.e., calcium salts in the synovium). When these hypothyroid clients have been treated with thyroid replacement, some have experienced attacks of acute pseudogout caused by the crystals in the periarticular joint structures (found in both the hyaline cartilage and fibrocartilage). Without medical treatment, this condition can lead to permanent joint damage.

CPPD disease (pseudogout) usually affects larger joints, but symptomatic involvement of the spine with deposition of crystals in the ligamentum flavum and atlantooccipital ligament can result in spinal stenosis and subsequent neurologic syndromes.[77] Effective treatment of pseudogout may include joint aspiration to relieve fluid pressure, steroid injection, and nonsteroidal antiinflammatories.*[86] The role of the therapist is similar to the treatment of rheumatoid arthritis (see Chapter 26).

Muscular complaints (aches, pain, and stiffness) associated with hypothyroidism are likely to develop into persistent myofascial trigger points. Clinically, any compromise of the energy metabolism of muscle aggravates and perpetuates trigger points. These do not resolve just with specific intervention by a therapist (e.g., trigger point therapy, myofascial release); they also require thyroid replacement.[82]

Hypothyroidism and Fibromyalgia

The correlation between hypothyroidism and fibromyalgia syndrome (FMS) continues to be investigated.†[58] Studies have shown an association between hypothyroidism and fibromyalgia. Persons with FMS may have a blunted response to a hypothalamic-releasing hormone (thyrotropin) that stimulates the anterior pituitary to secrete TSH, or, in some cases, a possible tissue-specific resistance may exist to thyroid hormone.[58] Reduced high-energy phosphate in muscle, related to impairment of carbohydrate metabolism (glycolysis abnormalities), may explain the chronic fatigue that can approach lethargy; it is noticeable on arising in the morning and is usually worse during midafternoon. These clients are particularly weather conscious and have muscular pain that increases with the onset of cold, rainy weather.[86]

Acute Care Setting

Dry, edematous tissues associated with hypothyroidism are more prone to skin tears and breakdown. Prevention of pressure ulcers requires careful monitoring of the usual pressure points (e.g., sacrum, coccyx, scapulae, elbows, greater trochanter, heels, malleoli).

Hypothyroidism and Medication

Clients with cardiac complications are started on small doses of thyroid hormone because large doses can precipitate heart failure or myocardial infarction by increasing body metabolism, myocardial oxygen requirements, and, consequently, the workload of the heart. Carefully observe for any signs of aggravated cardiovascular disease, such as chest pain and tachycardia. Report any signs of hypertension or congestive heart failure in the older adult.

After thyroid replacement therapy begins, watch for symptoms of hyperthyroidism (e.g., restlessness, tremor, sweating, dyspnea, excessive weight gain; see also Table 10-5).

Hypothyroidism and Exercise

Activity intolerance, weakness, and apathy secondary to decreased metabolic rate may require developing increased tolerance to activity and exercise once thyroid replacement has been initiated. Increased activity and exercise are especially helpful for the client who is constipated secondary to slowed metabolic rate and decreased peristalsis. Exercise-induced myalgia leading to rhabdomyolysis (disintegration of striated or skeletal muscle fibers with acute edema and excretion of myoglobin in the urine) has been reported in untreated or undiagnosed hypothyroidism. Rhabdomyolysis also could occur possibly as a result of poor drug compliance in combination with other aggravating factors, such as exercise.[56,80] Although they occur infrequently, the therapist should remain alert to any signs or symptoms of rhabdomyolysis (e.g., unexplained muscle pain and weakness) in exercising clients with hypothyroidism. Rhabdomyolysis can progress to renal failure.

Reduction in stroke volume and heart rate associated with hypothyroidism causes lowered cardiac output, increased peripheral vascular resistance to maintain systolic blood pressure, and a variety of ECG changes (e.g., sinus bradycardia, prolonged PR interval, depressed P waves). In animal models, exercise can affect skeletal and cardiac muscle systems independent of thyroid hormone replacement, which supports the role of exercise in improving muscle and cardiovascular function for the person with hypothyroidism.[22,49]

Because changes in lipid and lipoprotein levels occur with exercise, an exercise program can improve the lipid profile. This is especially important for the person with altered lipid metabolism and associated cardiovascular complications (see preceding section on Clinical Manifestations). However, if the client is hypothyroid with lipid abnormalities, the thyroid deficit should be corrected first and if, after treatment, any lipid abnormality remains, exercise should be instituted to treat it. ■

Goiter.   Goiter, an enlargement of the thyroid gland, may be a result of lack of iodine, inflammation, or tumors (benign or malignant). Enlargement also may appear in hyperthyroidism, especially Graves' disease. Goiter occurs most often in areas of the world in which iodine, which is necessary for the production of thyroid hormone, is deficient in the diet. Factors that inhibit normal thyroid hormone production result in a negative feedback loop, with hypersecretion of thyroid-stimulating hormone (TSH). The TSH increase results in the production and secretion of huge amounts of thyroglobulin (colloid) into the glandular follicles and the gland grows in size. Thyroglobulin is the large glycoprotein molecule in which thyroid hormones (T3 and T4) are produced in the presence of io-

---

*Although the synovium contains noninflammatory joint effusion, crystals may loosen, resulting in crystal shedding into the joint fluid, thereby causing an inflammatory response.

†Despite the correlation between hypothyroidism and FMS, thyroid dysfunction is seen at least three times more often in women with rheumatoid arthritis (RA) than in women with similar demographic features with noninflammatory rheumatic diseases, such as osteoarthritis and fibromyalgia.[61]

dine. When iodine is absent, only the thyroglobulin is made by the gland in response to repeated TSH stimulation. Because the thyroglobulin molecule is large, its increased production causes rapid glandular growth and a marked increase in overall glandular mass occurs called a *colloid goiter*.[39]

With the use of iodized salt, and iodine-containing binders in commercial foods, this problem almost has been eliminated in the United States and Canada. Although the younger population in the United States may be goiter-free, aging adults may have developed goiter during their childhood or adolescent years and may still have clinical manifestations of this disorder. Increased neck size may be observed, and when the thyroid increases to a certain point, pressure on the trachea and esophagus may cause difficulty breathing, dysphagia (difficulty swallowing), and hoarseness. Compression of the upper airway can be a fatal complication. Surgical intervention is essential when the trachea is compromised.

Thyroiditis.   Thyroiditis, inflammation of the thyroid, may be classified as *acute suppurative* (pus forming and very rare), *subacute granulomatous* (uncommon) and *lymphocytic*, or *chronic* (Hashimoto's disease). Acute and subacute thyroiditis are uncommon conditions caused by bacterial (*Streptococcus pyogenes*, *Staphylococcus aureus*, and *Pneumococcus pneumoniae*) and viral agents, respectively. Infected glands are painful and associated with systemic symptoms of fever and hyperthyroidism. Several varieties of related autoimmune causes of thyroiditis exist, such as Hashimoto's (lymphocytic) thyroiditis and postpartum thyroiditis. These types of thyroiditis are generally painless with only a rare case of Hashimoto's causing pain. Only the most common form of Hashimoto's thyroiditis is discussed further.

Hashimoto's (chronic) thyroiditis affects women more frequently than it does men (10:1) and is most often seen in the 30- to 50-year age group. The disorder has an autoimmune basis, and genetic predisposition appears to play a role in the etiology. It is associated with HLA-DR3, which is also present in other autoimmune conditions (e.g., Graves' disease, systemic lupus erythematosus, type 1 diabetes mellitus, pernicious anemia, myasthenia gravis, rheumatoid arthritis).[61]

Hashimoto's thyroiditis causes destruction of the thyroid gland because of the infiltration of the gland by lymphocytes and antithyroid antibodies. This infiltration results in decreased serum levels of T_3 and T_4, thus stimulating the pituitary gland to increase the production of TSH. The increased TSH causes hyperfunction of the tissue and goiter formation (enlargement of the gland) results. In some cases, this increase in function helps maintain a normal hormonal level, but eventually, when enough of the gland is destroyed, hypothyroidism develops. Hashimoto's thyroiditis is one of the most common causes of hypothyroidism in women older than 50 years.

Signs of chronic thyroiditis usually include painless symmetric or asymmetric enlargement of the gland and an irregular surface, which occasionally causes pressure on the surrounding structures. This pressure may subsequently cause dysphagia and respiratory distress. Most clients are euthyroid (have a normally functioning thyroid), about 20% are hypothyroid, and fewer than 5% are hyperthyroid with these people having combined Hashimoto's and Graves' disease caused by a genetic component.[46] The course of Hashimoto's thyroiditis varies. Most people see a decrease in the size of the goiter and remain stable for years with treatment. Treatment is directed toward suppressing the TSH to the lower end of the normal range to decrease TSH

stimulation of the gland, and to correct hypothyroidism if present. Tablets containing thyroxine (T_4) can help regulate and maintain adequate levels of circulating hormones. Generally, long-term or permanent therapy is advised.

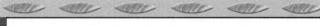

Special Implications for the Therapist   10-8

THYROIDITIS

Because the symptoms of thyroiditis are related to glandular function, and because the condition may be associated with hypothyroidism or hyperthyroidism, the therapist is referred to the sections relevant to client presentation (see Special Implications for the Therapist: Hypothyroidism or Hyperthyroidism in this chapter). ■

Thyroid Cancer.   Malignant tumors of the thyroid are rare; they affect women more than men (2:1 ratio), mainly between the ages of 40 and 60 years. A past medical history of radiation to the head, neck, or chest (e.g., for an enlarged thymus or tonsils, acne, or Hodgkin's disease) is the most obvious risk factor.

The usual presentation of thyroid cancer is the appearance of a hard, painless nodule on the thyroid gland or a gland that is multinodular. Most palpable nodules of the thyroid are benign adenomas and rarely become malignant or grow to a significant size to cause pressure against the trachea. About 5% of palpable nodules are malignant. Of the malignant nodules, most are a variety that seldom metastasizes beyond regional lymph nodes of the neck, resulting in a good prognosis for most people. A very small percentage of thyroid cancers, most often in aging adults, are anaplastic and can be fatal.[78]

Women have more thyroid nodules and more thyroid cancer than men. However, the presence of a thyroid nodule in a man is regarded with greater suspicion for cancer. Thyroid cancer is diagnosed by fine-needle aspiration and biopsy or open biopsy. Treatment usually involves removal of all or part of the thyroid. Neck resection of involved lymph nodes may be done for metastases to the neck. Radioactive ablation of remaining thyroid tissue is standard practice for most thyroid cancers. External radiation may be used in some situations. Major postoperative complications may involve damage to the laryngeal nerve, hemorrhage, and hypoparathyroidism.[71] Most thyroid cancers are treatable and the person can expect a normal life expectancy.

Special Implications for the Therapist   10-9

THYROID CANCER

A thyroid neoplasm can be the incidental finding in persons being treated for a musculoskeletal condition involving the head and neck. Most thyroid nodules are benign, but as mentioned previously, any time a therapist examines a client's neck and finds an asymptomatic nodule or unusual swelling or enlargement (with or without symptoms of pain), hoarseness, dyspnea, or dysphagia (difficulty swallowing), a medical referral is required. ■

◆ Parathyroid Glands

Two parathyroid glands are located on the posterior surface of each lobe of the thyroid gland. These glands secrete parathyroid hormone (PTH), which regulates calcium and phosphorus metabolism. PTH exerts its effect by (1) increasing the release of calcium and phosphate from the bone (bone demineralization); (2) increasing the absorption of calcium and excretion of phosphate by the kidneys; and (3) promoting calcium absorption in the GI tract.[46]

Disorders of the parathyroid glands may come to the therapist's attention because these conditions can cause periarthritis and tendinitis. Both types of inflammation may be crystal-induced, with formation of periarticular or tendinous calcification. Rarely, ruptured tendons resulting from bone resorption at the insertions occur in cases of primary hyperparathyroidism. These complications and problems are seen infrequently because most cases are diagnosed earlier with the advent of blood screening for identification of asymptomatic hypercalcemia.

Hyperparathyroidism

Definition and Incidence. Hyperparathyroidism is a disorder caused by overactivity of one or more of the four parathyroid glands that disrupts calcium, phosphate, and bone metabolism. Women are affected more than men (2:1), usually after age 60 years.

Hyperparathyroidism frequently is overlooked in the over-60 population. Symptoms in the early stages for this group are subtle and easily attributed to the aging process, depression, or anxiety. Eventually the symptoms intensify as the level of serum calcium rises, but this situation is accompanied by increased bone damage and other complications.

Etiologic and Risk Factors. Hyperparathyroidism is classified as primary, secondary, or tertiary. *Primary hyperparathyroidism* develops when the normal regulatory relationship between serum calcium levels and PTH secretion is interrupted. This occurs when one or more of the parathyroid glands enlarge, increasing PTH secretion and elevating serum calcium levels. The most common cause is a single adenoma of the parathyroid gland. Hyperplasia of the gland without an identifying injury and multiple adenomas are less common causes.

Secondary hyperparathyroidism occurs when the glands are hyperplastic from malfunction of another organ system. A hypocalcemia-producing abnormality outside the parathyroid gland results in a compensatory response of the parathyroid glands to chronic hypocalcemia. This is usually the result of renal failure (decreased renal activation of vitamin D), but it also may occur with osteogenesis imperfecta, Paget's disease, multiple myeloma, carcinoma with bone metastasis, laxative abuse, and vitamin D deficiency. *Tertiary hyperparathyroidism* is seen almost exclusively in dialysis clients who have long-standing secondary hyperparathyroidism. Hyperplasia occurs and the parathyroid glands ultimately become autonomous in function and unresponsive to serum calcium levels. Parathyroidectomy is required even after successful renal transplantation has resolved the cause of the secondary hyperparathyroidism.[29]

Pathogenesis and Clinical Manifestations. The primary function of parathyroid hormone (PTH) is to maintain a proper balance of calcium and phosphorus ions within the blood. PTH is not regulated by the pituitary or the hypothalamus and maintains normal blood calcium levels by increasing bone resorption and GI absorption of calcium. It also maintains an inverse relationship between serum calcium and phosphate levels by inhibiting phosphate reabsorption in the renal tubules. Abnormal PTH production disrupts this balance; symptoms of hyperparathyroidism are related to this release of bone calcium into the bloodstream. Excessive circulating PTH leads to bone damage, hypercalcemia, and kidney damage (Table 10-8).

Bone Damage. Oversecretion of PTH causes excessive osteoclast growth and activity within the bones. Osteoclasts are active in promoting resorption of bone, which then releases calcium into the blood, causing hypercalcemia. This calcium loss leads to bone demineralization, and in time, the bones may become so fragile that pathologic fractures, deformity (e.g., kyphosis of the thoracic spine), and compression fractures of the vertebral bodies occur. If uncontrolled, osteoclast proliferation may cause lytic bone lesions (bone disintegrates, leaving holes). Surgical treatment of hyperparathyroidism (parathyroidectomy) can be expected to result in biochemical cure and increased bone mineral density of the lumbar spine and femoral neck, (areas rich in cancellous bone), in both symptomatic and asymptomatic clients. Cortical bone loss, however, is not as readily reversible in either group.[81] Early surgical treatment of hyperparathyroidism may assist in the prevention of spine and hip fractures in this population.

Hypercalcemia. As excessive parathyroid hormone secretion results in bone resorption and hypercalcemia as just described, hypercalciuria (excessive calcium in the urine) eventually develops because the excessive filtration of calcium overwhelms this renal mechanism. High serum calcium levels also stimulate hypergastrinemia (excess gastrin, a hormone that stimulates secretion of gastric acid and pepsin in the blood), abdominal pain, peptic ulcer disease, and pancreatitis.

Kidney Damage. As serum calcium levels rise in response to excessive PTH levels, large amounts of phosphorus and calcium are excreted and lost from the body. Excretion of these compounds occurs through the renal system, leaving deposits of calcium phosphate within the renal tubules. This produces a kidney condition called *nephrocalcinosis*. Because calcium salts are insoluble in urine, kidney stones composed of calcium phosphate develop. Serious renal damage may not be reversible with parathyroidectomy.

Some people with hyperparathyroidism may be completely asymptomatic, but even asymptomatic clients with elevated serum and PTH levels have been found to have paresthesias, muscle cramps, and loss of pain and vibratory sensation in a stocking-glove distribution. Others suffer from a wide range of symptoms as a result of skeletal disease, renal involvement, GI tract disorders, and neurologic abnormalities.

Medical Management

Diagnosis. The diagnosis of hyperparathyroidism depends on measurement of parathyroid hormone (PTH) levels in persons found to be hypercalcemic. Serum calcium and PTH levels are elevated, serum phosphorus may be low normal or depressed, and urine calcium can range from low to

TABLE   10-8

Systemic Manifestations of Hyperparathyroidism

Early CNS Symptoms	Musculoskeletal Effects	Gastrointestinal Effects	Genitourinary Effects
Lethargy, drowsiness, paresthesias	Mild-to-severe proximal muscle weakness of the extremities	Peptic ulcers	Renal colic associated with kidney stones
Slow mentation, poor memory	Muscle atrophy	Pancreatitis	Hypercalcemia (polyuria, poly-
Depression, personality changes	Bone decalcification (bone pain, es-	Nausea, vomiting,	dipsia, constipation)
Easily fatigued	pecially spine; pathologic frac-	anorexia	Kidney infections
Hyperactive deep tendon reflexes	tures; bone cysts)	Constipation	Renal hypertension
Occasionally glove-and-stocking distribution sensory loss	Gout and pseudogout	Abdominal pain	
	Arthralgias involving the hands		
	Myalgia and sensation of heaviness in the lower extremities		
	Joint hypermobility		

Modified from Goodman CC, Snyder TE: *Differential diagnosis in physical therapy*, ed 3, Philadelphia, 2000, WB Saunders, p 304.

high. Radiographic evidence of skeletal damage is important to measure in asymptomatic clients with mild hyperparathyroidism. Skeletal damage can be seen on x-ray as diffuse demineralization of bones, bone cysts, subperiosteal bone resorption, and loss of the laminae durae surrounding the teeth.

Treatment and Prognosis.   Treatment for primary hyperparathyroidism is surgical removal (parathyroidectomy). The prognosis is good if the condition is identified and treated early. Emergency medical management of severe hypercalcemia includes use of drugs to lower serum calcium such as hydration and loop diuretics, which promote calcium loss through the kidneys; and antiresorption agents, which inhibit calcium release from bone. Long-term medical management of hypercalcemia with drugs is not as effective as parathyroid surgery but if needed for short-term treatment, drugs such as phosphonate, estrogen, and calcitonin can prevent progressive bone demineralization.[86]

Special Implications for the Therapist   10-10

HYPERPARATHYROIDISM

Preferred Practice Patterns:
4A: *Primary Prevention/Risk Reduction for Skeletal Demineralization*
4D: *Impaired Joint Mobility, Motor Function, Muscle Performance, and Range of Motion Associated with Connective Tissue Dysfunction*
4E: *Impaired Joint Mobility, Motor Function, Muscle Performance, and Range of Motion Associated with Localized Inflammation*
4G: *Impaired Joint Mobility, Muscle Performance, and Range of Motion Associated with Fracture*
6B: *Impaired Aerobic Capacity/Endurance Associated with Deconditioning*

The therapist is likely to see skeletal, articular, and neuromuscular manifestations associated with hyperparathyroidism. Chronic low back pain and easy fracturing resulting from bone demineralization may be compounded by marked muscle weakness and atrophy, especially in the legs.[46]

Inflammatory erosive polyarthritis may be associated with chondrocalcinosis and calcium pyrophosphate dihydrate (CPPD) crystal deposits in the synovial fluid in some cases of hyperparathyroidism. This erosion, described as *osteogenic synovitis,* occurs as part of the bone destruction that can occur with hyperparathyroidism. When this complication develops, the Achilles, triceps, and obturator tendons are most commonly affected; other affected areas may include hands and wrists (CTS), shoulders, knees, clavicle, and axial skeleton. Because of better and earlier diagnosis, inflammatory erosive polyarthritis and chondrocalcinosis are much less common today than they were several decades ago. However, some older adults still experience these complications and may present with these problems. Concurrent illness and surgery (e.g., parathyroidectomy) are recognized inducers of acute arthritic episodes.

The therapist may be involved in treating the arthritis associated with this (or any other endocrine) condition, but unless the underlying cause is treated first, intervention for the arthritis will be frustrating and poorly effective. After medical treatment, the therapist's treatment of the residual arthritis is the same as for arthritis, regardless of the cause.

Acute Care

In the acute care setting, auscultate for lung sounds and listen for signs of pulmonary edema in the person receiving large amounts of saline solution IV, especially in the presence of pulmonary or cardiac disease. Monitor the person on digitalis carefully for any toxic effects produced by elevated calcium levels because clients with hypercalcemia are hypersensitive to digitalis and may quickly develop toxic symptoms (e.g., arrhythmias, nausea, fatigue, visual changes) (see Table 11-4).

Clients with osteopenia are predisposed to pathologic fractures and must be treated with caution to minimize the risk of injury. Take every safety precaution, assisting carefully with walk-

Continued

ing, keeping the bed at its lowest position, raising the side rails, and lifting the immobilized person carefully to minimize bone stress. Schedule care to allow the person with muscle weakness recovery time and rest between all activities.

Postoperative Care

Postoperatively, after parathyroidectomy, the person should use a semi-Fowler's position with support for the head and neck to decrease edema, which can cause pressure on the trachea. Observe for any signs of mild tetany, such as reports of tingling in the hands and around the mouth. These symptoms should subside quickly but may be prodromal signs of tetany resulting from hypocalcemia. Watch for increased neuromuscular irritability and other signs of severe tetany and report them immediately. Acute postoperative arthritis may occur secondary to gout or pseudogout.

Early ambulation (although uncomfortable) is essential, because weight bearing and pressure on bones speed up recalcification. The use of light ankle weights or light weight-resistive elastic for the lower extremities provides tension at the musculotendinous/bone interface, accomplishing the same response. The physician first must approve the same type of exercise program for the upper extremities because care must be taken not to disturb the surgical site.

Home Health Care

For the person at home, fluids are important, and the use of cranberry or prune juice to increase urine acidity and help prevent stone formation may be recommended. Evaluate the living environment for any potential safety hazards that may predispose the client to injury, such as throw rugs, tub or shower stall without a rubber mat or decals to prevent slipping, missing hand and guard rails wherever necessary, and improper lighting. Encourage the use of a night-light in dark areas at all times. ■

Hypoparathyroidism

Definition. Hyposecretion, hypofunction, or insufficient secretion of parathyroid hormone (PTH) are ways to describe hypoparathyroidism.[5] Because the parathyroid glands primarily regulate calcium balance, hypoparathyroidism causes hypocalcemia and produces a syndrome opposite that of hyperparathyroidism with abnormally low serum calcium levels, high serum phosphate levels, and possible neuromuscular irritability (tetany) (Table 10-9).

Etiologic Factors and Incidence.

Hypoparathyroidism is either iatrogenic, which is most common, or idiopathic. *Iatrogenic* (acquired) causes include accidental removal of the parathyroid glands during thyroidectomy or anterior neck surgery,* infarction of the parathyroid glands resulting from an inadequate blood supply to the glands during surgery, strangulation of one or more of the glands by postoperative scar tissue, and, rarely, massive thyroid irradiation. Other secondary causes of hypoparathyroidism may include

---

*Variations in location and color in addition to the minute size of parathyroid glands make identification difficult and may result in glandular damage or accidental removal during thyroid removal or anterior neck surgery.

TABLE	10-9

Characteristics of Hyperparathyroidism and Hypoparathyroidism

HYPERPARATHYROIDISM	HYPOPARATHYROIDISM
Increased bone resorption	Decreased bone resorption
Elevated serum calcium levels	Depressed serum calcium levels
Depressed serum phosphate levels	Elevated serum phosphate levels
Hypercalciuria and hyperphosphaturia	Hypocalciuria and hypophosphaturia
Decreased neuromuscular irritability	Increased neuromuscular activity, which may progress to tetany

From Black JM, Matassarin-Jacobs E, editors: *Medical surgical nursing*, ed 5, Philadelphia, 1997, WB Saunders, p 2031.

hemochromatosis, sarcoidosis, amyloidosis, tuberculosis, neoplasms, or trauma.

Idiopathic causes affect children nine times as often as adults and affect twice as many women as men. Like Graves' disease and Hashimoto's thyroiditis, idiopathic hypoparathyroidism may be an autoimmune disorder with a genetic basis.

Pathogenesis. See the section on Pathogenesis of Hyperparathyroidism in this chapter for a description of the regulation of calcium and phosphate by PTH and the parathyroid glands. PTH normally functions to increase bone resorption to maintain a proper balance between serum calcium and phosphate. When parathyroid secretion of PTH is reduced, bone resorption and GI tract absorption slow, serum calcium levels fall, and severe neuromuscular irritability develops. Calcifications may form in various organs, such as the eyes and basal ganglia. Serum phosphate levels rise without sufficient PTH because fewer phosphorus ions are secreted by the distal tubules of the kidneys with decreased renal excretion of phosphorus.

Clinical Manifestations. Mild hypoparathyroidism may be asymptomatic, but it usually produces hypocalcemia and high serum phosphate levels that affect the CNS and other body systems (Table 10-10). The most significant clinical consequence of hypocalcemia associated with hypoparathyroidism is neuromuscular irritability. In people with chronic hypoparathyroidism, this neuromuscular irritability may result in tetany. Hypocalcemia resistant to PTH, called *pseudohypoparathyroidism*, is determined genetically and is associated with shortened metacarpals and metatarsals.[51]

Acute (overt) tetany begins with a tingling in the fingertips, around the mouth, and, occasionally, the feet. This tingling spreads and becomes more severe, producing painful muscle tension, spasms, grimacing, laryngospasm, and arrhythmias. Trousseau's sign (carpal spasm) and Chvostek's sign (hyperirritability of the facial nerve, producing a characteristic spasm when tapped) are apparent on examination (see Figs. 4-4 and 4-5). In severe cases, a tracheostomy may be required to correct acute respiratory obstruction secondary to laryngospasm.

TABLE	10-10			

Systemic Manifestations of Hypoparathyroidism

CNS EFFECTS	MUSCULOSKELETAL EFFECTS*	CARDIOVASCULAR EFFECTS*	INTEGUMENTARY EFFECTS	GASTROINTESTINAL EFFECTS
Personality changes (irritability, agitation, anxiety, depression) Convulsions	Hypocalcemia (neuromuscular excitability and muscular tetany, especially involving flexion of the upper extremity) Spasm of intercostal muscles and diaphragm compromising breathing Positive Chvostek's sign	Cardiac arrhythmias Eventual heart failure	Dry, scaly, coarse, pigmented skin Tendency to have skin infections Thinning of hair, including eyebrows and eyelashes Fingernails and toenails become brittle and form ridges	Nausea and vomiting Constipation or diarrhea Neuromuscular stimulation of the intestine (abdominal pain)

*The therapist should be aware of musculoskeletal and cardiovascular effects, which are the most common and important.
Modified from Goodman CC, Snyder TE: *Differential diagnosis in physical therapy,* ed 3, Philadelphia, 2000, WB Saunders, p 305.

Medical Management

Diagnosis. Diagnosis of this condition is based on history, clinical presentation, examination, and laboratory values (low serum calcium, high serum phosphate, low or absent urinary calcium). Radioimmunoassay for parathyroid hormone demonstrates decreased PTH concentration.

Treatment. Acute hypoparathyroidism, with its major manifestation of acute tetany, is a life-threatening disorder. Treatment is directed toward elevation of serum calcium levels as rapidly as possible, with intravenous calcium, prevention or treatment of convulsions, and control of laryngeal spasm and subsequent respiratory obstruction. Treatment of chronic hypoparathyroidism with pharmacologic management is accomplished more gradually than treatment for an acute situation. Surgical intervention is not appropriate and, in fact, is often the cause of this condition (see the section on Etiologic Factors).

Prognosis. Full recovery from the effects of hypoparathyroidism is possible when the condition is diagnosed early, before the development of serious complications. Unfortunately, once formed, cataracts and brain (basal ganglion) calcifications are irreversible. Death can occur from respiratory obstruction secondary to tetany and laryngospasms if treatment is not initiated early in acute hypoparathyroidism.

Special Implications for the Therapist   10-11

HYPOPARATHYROIDISM

Anyone experiencing acute tetany will be receiving acute medical care and will not be a likely candidate for therapy until the condition has resolved with treatment.

Chronic Hypoparathyroidism

For the person with chronic hypoparathyroidism, observe carefully for any minor muscle twitching or signs of laryngospasm because these may signal the onset of acute tetany. Chronic tetany is less severe, usually affects one side only, and may cause difficulty with gait and balance. Gait training and prevention of falls are key components of a therapy program. Hyperventilation may worsen tetany; focus on breathing during exercise is important.

Chronic hypoparathyroidism can lead to cardiac complications (e.g., arrhythmia, heart block, decreasing cardiac output) that necessitate careful monitoring. Calcium in vitamin D preparations prescribed for this condition may result in hypercalcemia, which potentiates* the effect of digitalis, thus requiring close monitoring for signs of digitalis toxicity and mild hypercalcemia (see Table 11-4).

Home Health Care

Life-long medication, dietary modifications, and medical care are required for the person with chronic hypoparathyroidism. Serum calcium levels must be checked by a physician at least three times a year to maintain normal serum calcium levels. If hypophosphatemia persists, cheese and milk should be omitted from the diet because they have a high calcium content. Other foods high in calcium but low in phosphorus are encouraged. ■

◆ Adrenal Glands.

The adrenals are two small glands located on the upper part of each kidney (see Fig. 10-1). Each adrenal gland consists of two relatively discrete parts: an outer cortex and an inner medulla. The outer cortex is responsible for the secretion of mineralocorticoids (steroid hormones that regulate fluid and mineral balance), glucocorticoids (steroid hormones responsible for controlling the metabolism of glucose), and androgens (sex hormones).

The centrally located adrenal medulla is derived from neural tissue and secretes epinephrine and norepinephrine, which exert widespread effects on vascular tone, the heart, and the nervous system, and affect glucose metabolism.

*When one agent potentiates the effects of another agent, the enhancement is such that the combined effect is greater than the sum of the effects of the individual agents.

Together, the adrenal cortex and medulla are major factors in the body's response to stress.

Glandular hypofunction and hyperfunction characterize the major disorders of the adrenal cortex. Underactivity of the adrenal cortex results in a deficiency of glucocorticoids, mineralocorticoids, and adrenal androgens. Overactivity results in excessive production of these same hormones.

Adrenal Insufficiency.
Hypofunction of the adrenal cortex can originate from a disorder within the adrenal gland itself (primary adrenal insufficiency) or it may be due to hypofunction of the pituitary-hypothalamic unit (secondary adrenal insufficiency).[86] Adrenocortical insufficiency, whether primary or secondary, can be either acute or chronic.

Primary Adrenal Insufficiency (Addison's Disease)

Definition and Overview. Addison's disease is a condition that occurs as a result of a disorder within the adrenal gland itself, named for the physician who first studied and described the associated symptoms. Adrenal insufficiency affects both sexes equally across the lifespan. Primary forms of adrenal insufficiency are uncommon; the therapist is most likely to see secondary adrenal insufficiency as a result of suppression of ACTH by steroid therapy.

Etiologic Factors. At one time, most causes of Addison's disease occurred as a complication of tuberculosis, but now most cases are considered idiopathic or autoimmune. Because more than half of all people with idiopathic Addison's disease have circulating autoantibodies that react specifically against adrenal tissue, this condition is considered to have an autoimmune basis. Less frequent causes of primary insufficiency include bilateral adrenalectomy, adrenal hemorrhage or infarction, radiation to the adrenal glands, malignant adrenal neoplasm, infections (e.g., histoplasmosis, cytomegalovirus), and rarely, destruction of the adrenal glands by chemical agents.[71]

Risk Factors. Surgery (including dental procedures); pregnancy (especially with postpartum hemorrhage); accident, injury, or trauma; infection; salt loss resulting from profuse diaphoresis (hot weather or with strenuous physical exertion); or failure to take steroid therapy in persons who have chronic adrenal insufficiency can cause acute adrenal insufficiency. In anyone who has previously been diagnosed with Addison's disease, it is called *Addisonian crisis*.

Pathogenesis and Clinical Manifestations. This adrenal gland disorder results in decreased production of cortisol (a glucocorticoid) and aldosterone (a mineralocorticoid), two of the primary adrenocortical hormones. Glucocorticoid deficiency causes widespread metabolic disturbances. Glucocorticoids promote gluconeogenesis* and have an antiinsulin effect. Consequently, when glucocorticoids become deficient, gluconeogenesis decreases, with resultant hypoglycemia and liver glycogen deficiency. The person grows weak, exhausted, hypotensive, and suffers from anorexia, weight loss, nausea, and vomiting. Emotional disturbances can develop,

ranging from mild neurotic symptoms to severe depression. Glucocorticoid deficiency also diminishes resistance to stress.

Cortisol deficiency results in a failure to inhibit anterior pituitary secretion of adrenocorticotropic hormone (ACTH). The result is a simultaneous increase in ACTH secretion and melanocyte-stimulating hormone (MSH) (see Fig. 10-2); excessive MSH increases skin and mucous membrane pigmentation. Persons with Addison's disease may have a bronzed or tanned appearance, which is the most striking physical finding with primary adrenal insufficiency (not present in all people with this disorder).

This change in pigmentation may vary in the white population from a slight tan or a few black freckles to an intense generalized pigmentation. The change in pigmentation is most commonly observed over extensor surfaces, such as the backs of the hands (metacarpophalangeal joints), elbows, knees, creases of the hands, lips, and mouth. Increased pigmentation of scars formed after the onset of the disease is common. Members of darker-skinned races may develop a slate-gray color that is obvious only to family members.

Aldosterone deficiency causes numerous fluid and electrolyte imbalances. Aldosterone normally promotes conservation of sodium and therefore conserves water and excretion of potassium. A deficiency of aldosterone causes increased sodium excretion, dehydration (see symptoms listed in Box 4-6), hypotension (low blood pressure causing orthostatic symptoms, see Chapter 11), and decreased cardiac output affecting heart size (decrease in size). Eventually, hypotension becomes severe and cardiovascular activity weakens, leading to circulatory collapse, shock, and death. Excess potassium retention (greater than 7 mEq/L) can result in arrhythmias and possible cardiac arrest.

Other clinical effects include decreased tolerance for even minor stress, poor coordination, fasting hypoglycemia (resulting from decreased gluconeogenesis), and a craving for salty food. Addison's disease may also retard axillary and pubic hair growth in females, decrease the libido (from decreased androgen production), and, in severe cases, cause amenorrhea (absence of menstruation).[95]

Medical Management
Diagnosis, Treatment, and Prognosis. Diagnosis of Addison's disease depends primarily on blood and urine hormonal assays and cortisol response to synthetic ACTH administration. Medical management is primarily pharmacologic, consisting of life-long administration of synthetically manufactured corticosteroids and mineralocorticoids (fludrocortisone). If untreated, Addison's disease is ultimately fatal. Adrenal crisis requires immediate hospitalization and treatment.

Special Implications for the Therapist **10-12**

PRIMARY ADRENAL INSUFFICIENCY (ADDISON'S DISEASE)

Preferred Practice Patterns:
4A: Primary Prevention/Risk Reduction for Skeletal Demineralization
6B: Impaired Aerobic Capacity/Endurance Associated with Deconditioning

---

*Gluconeogenesis (formerly called *glyconeogenesis*) is the synthesis of glucose from noncarbohydrate sources, such as amino acids; it occurs primarily in the liver and kidneys whenever the supply of carbohydrates is insufficient to meet the body's energy needs.

With pharmacologic therapy, listlessness and exhaustion should gradually lessen and disappear, making exercise possible. Stress should be minimized and infectious illnesses monitored by a physician. Any signs of infection, such as sore throat or burning on urination (see Table 7-1), should be reported to the physician. The client may be directed by the physician to increase medication dosage during times of stress and self-limiting illnesses (e.g., colds and flu). The therapist may need to advise the person to check with the physician if illness or any of the listed risk factors develop at home or during outpatient care.

Clients with Addison's disease should be assessed carefully for signs or hypercortisolism, which can result from excessive long-term cortisol therapy (see Tables 4-7 and 4-8). Assess for signs of sodium and potassium imbalance as well. If steroid replacement therapy is inadequate or too high, changes in amounts of sodium and water are observed (see Table 4-14). Persons receiving glucocorticoid alone may need mineralocorticoid therapy if signs of orthostatic hypotension or electrolyte abnormalities develop.

Older adults may be more sensitive to the side effects of steroid therapy, such as osteoporosis, hypertension, and diabetes, when these conditions already exist. The therapist must not overlook the presence of these other conditions when providing treatment intervention.

Anyone with identified Addison's disease should wear an identification bracelet and carry an emergency kit containing dexamethasone or hydrocortisone. Steroids administered in the late afternoon or evening may cause stimulation of the CNS and insomnia in some people. Anyone reporting sleep disturbances should be encouraged to discuss this with the physician. ■

Secondary Adrenal Insufficiency.   Secondary adrenal insufficiency is caused by other conditions outside the adrenals, such as hypothalamic or pituitary tumors, removal of the pituitary, or other causes of hypopituitarism, or rapid withdrawal of corticosteroid drugs. Long-term exogenous corticosteroid stimulation suppresses pituitary ACTH secretion and results in adrenal gland atrophy. Untimely discontinuation of adrenocorticosteroid therapy results in acute adrenal insufficiency and can become a life-threatening emergency. Anyone receiving adrenocorticosteroid therapy should be identified through the use of a bracelet or necklace. Steroid therapy must be discontinued gradually so that pituitary and adrenal function can normalize.

Clinical manifestations of secondary disease are somewhat different from symptoms of primary adrenal insufficiency. Whereas most symptoms of primary adrenal insufficiency arise from cortisol and aldosterone deficiency, symptoms of secondary disease are related to cortisol deficiency only. Because the gland is still intact, aldosterone is secreted normally, but the lack of stimulation from ACTH results in deficient cortisol secretion. Arthralgias, myalgias, and tendon calcification can occur, which resolve with treatment of the underlying condition.

Hyperpigmentation is not part of the clinical presentation because ACTH and MSH levels are low. Additionally, because aldosterone secretion may continue at fairly normal levels in secondary adrenal hypofunction this condition does not necessarily cause accompanying hypotension and electrolyte abnormalities.[4]

As with primary adrenal insufficiency, treatment involves replacement of ACTH and monitoring for fluid and electrolyte imbalances. Too much cortisol replacement can result in the development of Cushing's syndrome (see next section).

Adrenocortical Hyperfunction.   Hyperfunction of the adrenal cortex can result in excessive production of glucocorticoids, mineralocorticoids, and androgens. The three major conditions of adrenocortical hyperfunction are Cushing's syndrome (glucocorticoid excess), Conn's syndrome or aldosteronism (aldosterone excess), and adrenal hyperplasia (adrenogenital syndrome). This last condition, rare and congenital, is not discussed further in this text.

Cushing's Syndrome

Definition and Overview.   *Hypercortisolism* is a general term for an excess of cortisol in the body. This condition can occur as a result of hyperfunction of the adrenal gland (usually benign or malignant adenomas), an excess of corticosteroid medication, or an excess of ACTH stimulation from the pituitary gland (or other sites). Hypercortisolism resulting from adrenal gland oversecretion or from hyperphysiologic doses of corticosteroid medications is called *Cushing's syndrome*. When the hypercortisolism results from oversecretion of ACTH from the pituitary, the condition is called *Cushing's disease*. The clinical presentation is the same for both conditions.[63]

Etiologic Factors and Incidence.   The primary causes of Cushing's syndrome are hyperphysiologic doses of adrenocorticosteroids and adrenocortical tumors. Cushing's disease results from pituitary adenomas, which secrete an excess of ACTH causing overstimulation of a normal adrenal gland. A similar condition can occur as a result of ectopic production of ACTH by lung cancer and more rarely, by carcinoid tumors. Therapists are more likely to treat people who have developed medication-induced Cushing's syndrome. This condition occurs after these individuals have received large doses of cortisol (also known as hydrocortisone) or cortisol derivatives. Exogenous steroids are administered for a number of inflammatory and other disorders (see Box 4-5). Noniatrogenic Cushing's syndrome occurs mainly in women, with an average age at onset of 20 to 40 years, although it can be seen in people up to age 60 years.

Pathogenesis and Clinical Manifestations.   When the normal function of the glucocorticoids becomes exaggerated, multiple physiologic responses occur (Table 10-11; see also Table 4-7). Overproduction of cortisol causes liberation of amino acids from muscle tissue with resultant weakening of protein structures (specifically muscle and elastic tissue). The end result may include a protuberant abdomen (Fig. 10-5) with purple striae (stretch marks), poor wound healing, thinning of the skin, generalized muscle weakness, and marked osteoporosis that is made worse by an excessive loss of calcium in the urine. In severe cases of prolonged Cushing's syndrome, muscle weakness and demineralization of bone may lead to pathologic fractures and wedging of the vertebrae, kyphosis (Fig. 10-6), osteonecrosis (especially of the femoral head), bone pain, and back pain.

The effect of increased circulating levels of cortisol on the muscles varies from slight to marked. Muscle wasting can be so extensive that the condition simulates muscular dystrophy. Marked weakness of the quadriceps muscle often prevents affected people from rising out of a chair unassisted. Cortisone-induced myopathies are discussed in Chapter 4.

TABLE	10-11

Pathophysiology of Cushing's Syndrome

PHYSIOLOGIC EFFECT	CLINICAL RESULT
Persistent hyperglycemia	"Steroid diabetes"
Protein tissue wasting	Weakness as a result of muscle wasting; capillary fragility resulting in ecchymoses; osteoporosis as a result of bone matrix wasting
Potassium depletion	Hypokalemia (Table 4-14), cardiac arrhythmias, muscle weakness, renal disorders
Sodium and water retention	Edema and hypertension
Hypertension	Predisposes to left ventricular hypertrophy, congestive heart failure, cerebrovascular accidents
Abnormal fat distribution	Moon-shaped face; dorsocervical fat pad; truncal obesity, slender limbs, thinning of the skin with striae on the breasts, axillary areas, abdomen, and legs
Increased susceptibility to infection; lowered resistance to stress	Absence of signs of infection; poor wound healing
Increased production of androgens	Virilism in women (e.g., acne, thinning of scalp hair, hirsutism or abnormal growth and distribution of hair)
Mental changes	Memory loss, poor concentration and thought processes, euphoria, depression ("steroid psychosis," see Chapter 4)

Data from Black JM, Matassarin-Jacobs E, editors: *Medical surgical nursing*, ed 5, Philadelphia, 1997, WB Saunders, p 2051

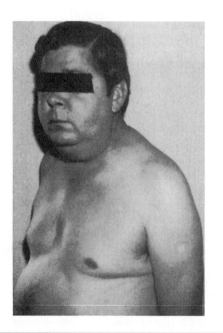

FIGURE 10-5 Central obesity of Cushing's syndrome. (From Callen JP, Jorizzo J, editors: *Dermatological signs of internal disease*, ed 2, Philadelphia, 1995, WB Saunders, p 204.)

Whenever corticosteroids are administered, the increase in serum cortisol levels triggers a negative feedback signal to the anterior pituitary gland to stop its secretion of ACTH. This decrease in ACTH stimulation of the adrenal cortex results in adrenocortical atrophy during the period of exogenous corticosteroid administration. If these medications are stopped suddenly rather than reduced gradually, the atrophied adrenal gland will not be able to provide the cortisol necessary for physiologic needs. A life-threatening situation known as *acute adrenal insufficiency* can develop, requiring emergency cortisol replacement (see the section on Addisonian Crisis in this chapter).[86]

Medical Management
Diagnosis, Treatment, and Prognosis. Although there is a classic cushingoid appearance in persons with hypercortisolism (Fig. 10-7), diagnostic laboratory studies including measurement of urine and serum cortisol are used to confirm the diagnosis. Treatment to restore hormone balance and reverse Cushing's syndrome or disease may require radiation, drug therapy, or surgery, depending on the underlying cause (e.g., resection of pituitary tumors). Prognosis depends on the underlying cause and the ability to control the cortisol excess.

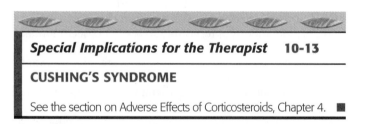

Special Implications for the Therapist **10-13**

CUSHING'S SYNDROME

See the section on Adverse Effects of Corticosteroids, Chapter 4. ∎

Conn's Syndrome
Definition and Overview. Conn's syndrome, or primary aldosteronism, occurs when an adrenal lesion results in hypersecretion of aldosterone, the most powerful of the mineralocorticoids. Its primary role is to conserve sodium, and it also promotes potassium excretion. The major cause of primary aldosteronism (an uncommon condition present most often in women aged 30 to 50 years) is a benign, aldosterone-secreting tumor called *aldosteronoma*.[33] Rarely, Conn's syndrome develops as a consequence of adrenocortical carcinoma.

Secondary hyperaldosteronism also can occur as a consequence of pathologic lesions that stimulate the adrenal gland to increase production of aldosterone. For example, conditions that reduce renal blood flow (e.g., renal artery stenosis), induce renal hypertension (e.g., nephrotic syndrome, ingestion of oral contraceptives), and edematous disorders (e.g., cardiac failure, cirrhosis of the liver with ascites) can cause secondary hyperaldosteronism.

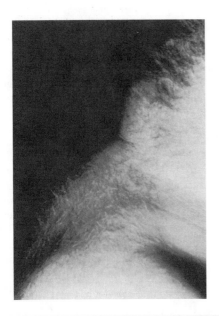

FIGURE   10-6   Buffalo hump and hypertrichosis (excessive hairiness; hirsutism) in a male with Cushing's syndrome. This hump is a painless accumulation of fat that also may occur idiopathically in (usually) women. A familial pattern may exist (i.e., affected women report a similar anatomic change in their mothers). In the case of steroid-induced changes, this condition resolves when the individual stops taking the medication; in such cases, therapeutic intervention by the therapist has no permanent effect. Idiopathic fat deposits and underlying postural changes can be altered with postural correction and soft tissue and joint mobilization techniques. No studies have substantiated whether these changes are long term. (From Callen JP, Jorizzo J, editors: *Dermatological signs of internal disease*, ed 2, Philadelphia, 1995, WB Saunders, p 204.)

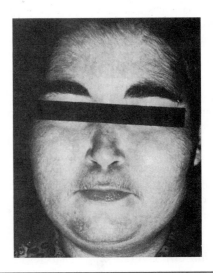

FIGURE   10-7   Round facies in a woman with Cushing's disease. This condition is sometimes referred to as moon face. Other characteristics include telangiectasia and hirsutism. (From Callen JP, Jorizzo J, editors: *Dermatological signs of internal disease*, ed 2, Philadelphia, 1995, WB Saunders, p 204.)

Pathogenesis and Clinical Manifestations.   Aldosterone affects the tubular reabsorption of sodium and water and the excretion of potassium and hydrogen ions in the renal tubular epithelial cells; an excess of aldosterone enhances sodium reabsorption by the kidneys. This leads to the development of hypernatremia (excess sodium in blood, indicating water loss exceeding sodium loss), hypervolemia (fluid volume excess, increase in the volume of circulating fluid or plasma in the body), hypokalemia (low blood levels of potassium), and metabolic alkalosis (see Chapter 4). With the hypervolemia and hypernatremia, the blood pressure increases, often to very high levels, and renin production is suppressed. This hypertension can lead to cerebral infarctions and renal damage.

Without intervention, complications of chronic hypertension develop in the presence of hypertension, hypernatremia, and hypokalemia, heart failure, renal damage, and cerebrovascular accident. Hypokalemia results from excessive urinary excretion of potassium causing muscle weakness; intermittent, flaccid paralysis; paresthesias; or cardiac arrhythmias (see Table 4-14).

This excessive urinary excretion of potassium (hypokalemia) leads to polyuria and resulting polydipsia (excessive thirst). Diabetes mellitus is common because hypokalemia interferes with normal insulin transport. Finally, hypokalemia leads to metabolic alkalosis, which can cause a decrease in ionized calcium levels, resulting in tetany and respiratory suppression. However, low serum potassium and alkalosis are not always present at the time of diagnosis.

Medical Management

Diagnosis, Treatment, and Prognosis.   Diagnosis of primary hyperaldosteronism is based on elevations in serum and urine aldosterone studies, and CT scanning of the abdomen for evidence of unilateral and sometimes bilateral adenomas of the adrenal gland.[33] Radiographic studies can reveal cardiac hypertrophy resulting from chronic hypertension. Radionuclide scanning techniques using radiolabeled substances allow visualization of any tumors present.

The goals of treatment are to reverse hypertension, correct hypokalemia, and prevent kidney damage. Usually, surgical removal of the aldosterone-secreting tumor (may require adrenalectomy) completely resolves the hypertension within 1 to 3 months. However, without early diagnosis and treatment, renal complications from long-term hypertension may be progressive. Pharmacologic treatment to increase sodium excretion and treat the hypertension and hypokalemia is a nonsurgical alternative.

Special Implications for the Therapist   **10-14**

CONN'S SYNDROME

The therapist treating someone with hyperaldosteronism, primary or secondary, may observe signs of tetany (muscle twitching, Chvostek's sign; see Fig. 4-3) and hypokalemia-induced cardiac dysrhythmias, paresthesias, or muscle weakness. If these are encountered in an acute care setting, the medical team is usually well aware of such symptoms and is working to establish a fluid-electrolyte balance. When such signs and symptoms are observed in the outpatient setting, the client must seek medical attention. ■

◆ Pancreas (Islets of Langerhans)

The pancreas lies behind the stomach, with the head and neck of the pancreas located in the curve of the duodenum and the body extending horizontally across the posterior abdominal wall (see Figs. 10-1 and 15-1). It has two functions, acting as both an endocrine gland (secreting the hormones insulin and glucagon) and an exocrine gland (producing digestive enzymes). The cells of the pancreas that function in the endocrine capacity are the islets of Langerhans.

The islets of Langerhans have three major functioning cells: (1) the alpha-cells produce glucagon, which increases the blood glucose levels by stimulating the liver and other cells to release stored glucose (glycogenolysis); (2) the beta-cells produce insulin, which lowers blood glucose levels by facilitating the entrance of glucose into the cells for metabolism; and (3) the delta-cells produce somatostatin, which is believed to regulate the release of insulin and glucagon (Table 10-12).[46]

Diabetes Mellitus

Definition and Overview.   Diabetes mellitus (DM) is a chronic, systemic disorder characterized by hyperglycemia (excess glucose in the blood) and disruption of the metabolism of carbohydrates, fats, and proteins. Insulin, produced in the pancreas, normally maintains a balanced blood glucose level. Diabetes mellitus is characterized as a group of metabolic diseases resulting from defects in the secretion of insulin, action of insulin, or both. The chronic hyperglycemia of diabetes mellitus is associated with long-term damage and dysfunction and failure of tissues and organs, especially the eyes, kidneys, nerves, heart, and blood vessels.

The majority of cases of diabetes mellitus (DM) fall into two large categories, type 1 DM and type 2 DM, related to differences in etiology and pathogenesis of the disease. In type 1 DM (previously called insulin-dependent diabetes mellitus [IDDM] or juvenile onset DM), the cause of hyperglycemia is an absolute deficiency of insulin production and secretion. Most individuals with type 1 DM can be identified by serologic evidence showing an autoimmune process occurring in the islet cells of the pancreas along with specific genetic markers.* People with type 1 diabetes are prone to ketoacidosis and specific metabolic derangements associated with hyperglycemia; they require exogenous insulin to maintain life.

Type 2 DM (previously called *non–insulin-dependent diabetes mellitus [NIDDM]* or *adult-onset DM*), is a much more prevalent form of diabetes and the cause is a combination of cellular resistance to insulin action and an inadequate compensatory insulin secretory response. These individuals are not as likely to exhibit the metabolic derangements common to the person with type 1 DM and usually can be controlled with diet, exercise, and oral hypoglycemic agents. In some cases, however, people with type 2 DM do require insulin replacement.[23] A comparison of the primary differences between the two types of diabetes is shown in Table 10-13.

Other Types and Categories of Diabetes Mellitus.   In addition to the main categories of type 1 and type 2 DM, other rare specific types of DM exist, which are associated with a variety of etiologies, including the following:

- Genetic beta-cell defects
- Genetic defects in insulin action
- Disorders of the exocrine pancreas such as injury, neoplasm, or infection
- Other endocrinopathies that antagonize insulin action (e.g., increased growth hormone, cortisol, glucagons, or epinephrine)

---

*A certain number of people with very rare cases of type 1 DM have no clear etiology for their disease and are defined as idiopathic.

TABLE	10-12

Regulation of Glucose Metabolism

GLAND	REGULATING FUNCTION
Pancreas	
α cells (islets of Langerhans)	Secrete glucagon; increase blood glucose level
β cells (islets of Langerhans)	Secrete insulin (glucose-regulating hormone); decrease blood glucose level
δ cells (islets of Langerhans)	Secrete somatostatin; regulate the release of insulin and glucagon
Adrenal Gland	
Medulla: Epinephrine	Responds to stress; epinephrine stimulates liver and muscle glycogenolysis to increase the blood glucose level
Cortex: Glucocorticoids	Increase blood glucose levels by promoting the flow of amino acids to the liver, where they are synthesized into glucose
Anterior Pituitary	
Adrenocorticotropic hormone (ACTH)	Increases blood glucose levels
Human growth hormone (GH)	Limits storage of fat; favors fat catabolism; inhibits carbohydrate catabolism, raising blood glucose levels
Thyroid	
T_3 and T_4	May raise or lower blood glucose levels

- Drug or chemically induced DM (e.g., glucocorticoids, thiazides, thyroid hormone)
- Uncommon forms of immune or genetically associated syndromes (e.g., stiff-man syndrome, Down syndrome, Klinefelter's syndrome, Turner's syndrome, and Wolfram's syndrome)
- Infections (certain viruses, including rubella, coxsackievirus B, cytomegalovirus, adenovirus, and mumps, have been associated with beta-cell destruction in people with existing genetic markers).

According to the American Diabetes Association,[23] two categories of hyperglycemia classifications fall between normal and a true diagnosis of diabetes. *Impaired glucose tolerance (IGT)* and *impaired fasting glucose (IFG)* refer to intermediate metabolic stages that fall between normal glucose metabolism and diabetes. Individuals with IGT (impaired glucose tolerance) often manifest hyperglycemia only when challenged with the oral glucose load used in the oral glucose tolerance test (OGTT). IFG includes people whose fasting blood glucose levels are equal to or greater than 110 mg/dL but less than 126 mg/dL. (Normal blood glucose as defined by the ADA is less than 110 mg/dL.)

The final category of diabetes classification is gestational diabetes mellitus (GDM). This category is defined as any degree of glucose intolerance recognized with the onset of pregnancy. Approximately 6 weeks or more after pregnancy ends, the woman should be reclassified into one of the other categories depending on whether or not her glucose tolerance resolves. She could be reclassified as normal if no glucose intolerance remains after the pregnancy is completed. Most women who have GDM return to normal glucose metabolism after pregnancy.[23]

Incidence.   According to the American Diabetes Association, more than 16 million Americans have been diagnosed with diabetes, and approximately 5 million more people have undiagnosed cases. Diabetes, with its severe complications of heart disease, stroke, kidney disease, blindness, and loss of limbs, is the most common endocrine disorder, ranked as the third cause of death from disease in the United States (mostly because of increased rates of coronary artery disease). It is the leading cause of blindness and renal failure in adults.[86]

Black, Native, Hispanic, and Asian Americans are three times more likely to develop DM than are white Americans, with increasing incidence associated with advancing age. Nearly one third of all Americans with DM are older than 60 years; males and females are affected equally. Approximately 90% of all cases of DM are type 2. Type 1 DM and secondary causes (e.g., medications, genetic disease, hormonal changes) account for the remaining 10%. Since the mid-1970s, the incidence of diabetes has steadily increased as a result of prolonged life expectancy; increased incidence of obesity; and reduced mortality resulting in increased live births to people with type 1 DM, whose children are predisposed to future development of type 1.

Etiologic and Risk Factors
See Box 10-3.

Type 1 Diabetes Mellitus.   Type 1 DM results from cell-mediated autoimmune destruction of the beta-cells of the pancreas and is a condition of absolute insulin deficiency. This autoimmune process is detectable because markers of cellular destruction called *autoantibodies* are specific to pancreatic beta cells. One, and sometimes more, of these autoantibodies are present and detectable in 85% to 90% of individuals with type 1 DM when the disease initially is detected.

In type 1 DM diabetes, the rate of beta-cell destruction is rapid in some people (mainly infants and children), and slow in others. Even though immune-mediated diabetes commonly occurs in childhood and adolescence, it can occur at any age, even late in life. Both genetic and environmental factors are associated with autoimmune destruction of the beta-cell, although the environmental relationship is still poorly defined.[23] Certain HLA antigens (HLA-DR3 and HLA-DR4) on specific chromosomes appear to predispose persons to the development of type 1 DM. Experimental research is underway in the development of a vaccine that may help stop the immune system attack of the insulin-producing beta-cells of the pancreas.[17] People with autoimmune destruction of beta-

TABLE 10-13		

Differences Between Types of Diabetes Mellitus

FEATURES	TYPE I (KETOSIS-PRONE)	TYPE 2 (NOT KETOSIS-PRONE)
Age at onset	Usually <20 yr	Usually >40 yr
Proportion of all cases	<10%	>90%
Type of onset	Abrupt (acute or subacute)	Gradual
Etiologic factors	Possible viral/autoimmune, resulting in destruction of islet cells	Obesity-associated insulin receptor resistance
HLA association	Yes	No
Insulin antibodies	Yes	No
Body weight at onset	Normal or thin, obesity uncommon	Majority are obese (80%)
Endogenous insulin production	Decreased (little or none)	Variable (above or below normal)
Ketoacidosis	May occur	Rare
Treatment	Insulin, diet, and exercise	Diet, oral hypoglycemic agents, exercise, insulin, and weight control

Modified from Goodman CC, Snyder TE: *Differential diagnosis in physical therapy,* ed 3, Philadelphia, 2000, WB Saunders, p 307.

Risk Factors for Type 1 and Type 2 Diabetes Mellitus

Type 1 DM Risk Factors

Presence of type 1 diabetes in a first degree relative (sibling or parent)

Type 2 DM Risk Factors

Positive family history
Ethnic origin: Black, Native American, Hispanic, Asian American, Pacific Islander
Obesity
Increasing age ($\geq$45 yr)
Previous history of gestational diabetes (GDM) or delivery of babies weighing more than 9 lb
Previously identified impaired fasting glucose (IFG) or impaired glucose tolerance (IGT)
Hypertension ($\geq$140/90 mmHg in adults)
HDL cholesterol level <35 mg/dL and/or triglyceride level $\geq$250 mg/dL

---

cells are also prone to other autoimmune disorders such as Graves' disease, Hashimoto's thyroiditis, Addison's disease, vitiligo, and pernicious anemia.

In about 10% of cases of type 1 DM, no definable etiology exists. Some individuals in this category (usually of African or Asian origin) have permanent hypoinsulinemia and are prone to ketoacidosis but have no evidence of autoimmunity. Their need for insulin replacement is usually inconsistent.

Type 2 Diabetes Mellitus. Type 2 DM is a form of diabetes in which individuals have endogenous insulin production but have difficulty with effective insulin action at the cellular level. People with type 2 DM may not need insulin treatment to survive but need other forms of therapy to prevent hyperglycemia and its resulting complications. Although the specific etiologies of type 2 diabetes are not clear, autoimmune destruction of beta-cells does not occur. Recently, however, the first genetic defect linked to insulin resistance in humans has been identified on chromosomes 12 and 20.[3,74]

People with this form of diabetes may have normal or elevated insulin levels, but the insulin produced is ineffective and resistant to cellular attachment and action. Insulin secretion also is impaired and the beta-cells are unable to secrete increased amounts of insulin when it is needed. The person with type 2 diabetes frequently goes undiagnosed for many years because onset of type 2 DM is often gradual enough that the classic signs of hyperglycemia are not noticed. Most people with type 2 DM are obese and obesity causes some degree of insulin resistance. At least 80% of all persons with type 2 DM are obese and the remaining 20%, who are not obese by traditional weight criteria, may have an increased percentage of body fat distribution, particularly in the abdominal area.[23] Ketoacidosis seldom occurs in this type of diabetes but people with type 2 DM are at increased risk for developing macrovascular and microvascular complications. The risk of developing this form of diabetes increases with age, obesity, low cardiorespiratory fitness, and lack of exercise.[94] Type 2 DM occurs more frequently in women with prior gestational DM and in individuals with hypertension or dyslipidemia. Its frequency varies in different racial/ethnic groups (see Box 10-3). Type 2 DM is associated with a stronger genetic predisposition than type 1 DM but the genetics of this form of diabetes are complex and not easily described.[23]

Pathogenesis. Insulin is a hormone secreted by the beta-cells of the pancreas that transports glucose into the cell for use as energy and storage as glycogen: it turns food into energy. It also stimulates protein synthesis and free fatty acid storage in the fat deposits. In DM, insulin is either insufficient in amount (type 1) or ineffective in action (type 2). Insulin deficiency compromises the body tissues' access to essential nutrients for fuel and storage.[86] When glucose levels are elevated normally (e.g., after eating a meal), beta-cells increase secretion of insulin to transport and dispose of the glucose into peripheral tissues, thereby lowering blood glucose levels and reestablishing blood glucose homeostasis. Defects in the pancreas, liver, or skeletal muscle, singularly or collectively, can contribute to abnormal glucose homeostasis.

Normally, after a meal, the blood glucose level rises. The liver takes up a large amount of this glucose for storage or for use by other tissues, such as skeletal muscle and fat. When insulin is deficient or its function is impaired, the glucose in the general circulation is not taken up or removed by these tissues; thus it continues to accumulate in the blood. Because new glucose has not been deposited in the liver, the liver synthesizes more glucose and releases it into the general circulation, which increases the already elevated blood glucose level.[86]

When a true deficiency of insulin exists, such as that which occurs in type 1 DM diabetes, three major metabolic problems exist: (1) decreased utilization of glucose (as described above), (2) increased fat mobilization, and (3) impaired protein utilization. Cells that require insulin as a carrier for glucose, such as skeletal and cardiac muscle and adipose tissue, are affected most, whereas nerve tissue, erythrocytes, and the cells of the intestines, liver, and kidney tubules, which do not require insulin for glucose transport, are affected the least. In an attempt to restore balance and normal levels of glucose, the kidney excretes the excess glucose resulting in glucosuria (sugar in the urine). Glucose excreted in the urine acts as an osmotic diuretic and causes excretion of increased amounts of water. This process results in fluid volume deficit (FVD) (see Chapter 4). The conscious person becomes extremely thirsty and drinks large amounts of water (polydipsia).

Increased fat mobilization occurs because the body can rely on fat stores for energy when glucose is not available. The process of fat metabolism leads to the formation of breakdown products called *ketones*, which accumulate in the blood and are excreted through the kidneys and lungs. Ketones can be measured in the blood and the urine to indicate the presence of diabetes. Ketones interfere with acid-base balance by producing hydrogen ions. The pH can fall, and the affected person can develop metabolic acidosis (see Chapter 4). After the renal threshold for ketones is exceeded, the ketones appear in the urine as acetone (ketonuria). When large amounts of glucose and ketones are excreted, osmotic diuresis becomes more severe and fluid and electrolyte loss through the kidneys increases. Sodium, potassium, and other critical electrolytes are lost in the urine, resulting in severe dehydration electrolyte deficiency and worsening acidosis. When fats are used for a primary source of energy, the body lipid level can rise to five times the normal amount. This elevated level can lead to atherosclerosis and its subsequent cardiovascular complications (see Chapter 11).

Impaired protein utilization occurs because the transport of amino acids (the chief constituent of proteins) into cells requires insulin. Normally, proteins are constantly being broken down and rebuilt. Without insulin to transport amino acids, thereby contributing to protein synthesis, the balance is altered and protein catabolism increases. Catabolism of body proteins and resultant protein loss hamper the inflammatory process and diminish the tissue's ability to repair itself. Because the person with type 2 DM continues to produce and use some amount of endogenous insulin, the metabolic problems associated with inappropriate use of fat and protein for energy do not occur as severely. People with type 2 DM are not prone to ketoacidosis and the metabolic derangements associated with type 1 DM. They are, however, still at great risk for hyperglycemic osmotic diuresis, dehydration, shock, and loss of electrolytes.[86]

Clinical Manifestations

Cardinal Signs and Symptoms.   In type 1 diabetes, symptoms of marked hyperglycemia include polyuria, polydipsia, weight loss with polyphagia, and blurred vision (Table 10-14). These symptoms occur as a result of the inability of the body to use glucose appropriately and the resulting osmotic diuresis, dehydration, and starvation of body tissues. In type 1 DM, the utilization of fats and proteins for energy causes severe hunger, fatigue, and weight loss. The person with this type of diabetes may present initially in diabetic ketoacidosis (DKA).

People with type 2 diabetes also may have some of these cardinal signs and symptoms, but the aging population may not recognize the abnormal thirst or frequent urination as abnormal for their age. More commonly, they may experience visual blurring, neuropathic complications (e.g., foot pain), infections, and significant blood lipid abnormalities. Type 2 DM is commonly diagnosed while the client is hospitalized or receiving medical care for another problem. Frequently, the person presents with one of the long-term complications of DM such as neuropathy, retinopathy, or nephropathy.

Long-term effects of DM affect the large blood vessels (macrovascular), small blood vessels (microvascular), and nerves throughout the body. The chronic hyperglycemia of diabetes is associated with long-term damage to blood vessels and eventual dysfunction or failure of various organs, particularly the eyes (retinopathy), the kidneys (nephropathy), the nerves (neuropathy) and the coronary, cerebral, and peripheral arteries. The blood vessel changes caused by lipid accumulation and thickening of vessel walls result in decreased vessel lumen size, compromised blood flow, and ischemia to adjacent tissues.[46]

Neuropathy in diabetes is presumably related to the accumulation in the nerve cells of sorbitol, a byproduct of improper glucose metabolism. This accumulation then results in abnormal fluid and electrolyte shifts and nerve-cell dysfunction.[46] The combination of this metabolic derangement and the diminished vascular perfusion to nerve tissues contributes to the severe problem of diabetic neuropathy. (See the section on Diabetic Neuropathy in Chapter 38.)

Atherosclerosis.   Because of the hyperglycemia and increased fat metabolism associated with type 1 DM, atherosclerosis begins earlier and is more extensive among people with diabetes than in the general population. Atherosclerosis and the accompanying large-vessel changes result in cardiovascular and cerebrovascular changes, skin and nail changes, poor tissue perfusion, decreased or absent pedal pulses, and impaired wound healing. Atherosclerosis combined with peripheral neuropathy and the subsequent foot deformities increases the risk for ulceration of skin and underlying tissues.

Individuals with undiagnosed type 2 DM are at significantly higher risk for coronary artery disease, stroke, and peripheral vascular disease than the population without diabetes. Screening of the type 2 at-risk population is essential in

---

TABLE	10-14

Cardinal Signs of Diabetes at Diagnosis

CLINICAL MANIFESTATIONS	PATHOPHYSIOLOGIC BASES
Polyuria (excessive urination, types 1 and 2)	Water is not reabsorbed from renal tubules because of osmotic activity of glucose in the tubules
Polydipsia (excessive thirst, types 1 and 2)	Polyuria causes dehydration, which causes thirst
Polyphagia (excessive hunger, type 1)	Starvation secondary to tissue breakdown causes hunger
Weight loss (type 1)	Glucose is not available to the cells; body breaks down fat and protein stores for energy; dehydration
Recurrent blurred vision (types 1 and 2)	Chronic exposure of the lenses and retina to hyperosmolar fluids causes blurring of vision
Ketonuria (type 1)	Fatty acids are broken down so ketones are present in urine
Weakness, fatigue and dizziness (types 1 and 2)	Dehydration leads to postural hypotension; energy deficiency and protein catabolism contribute to fatigue and weakness
Often asymptomatic (type 2)	Physical adaptation often occurs because rise in blood glucose is gradual

the prevention and treatment of diabetes-related complications. In addition, all individuals with diabetes should be aware of the strong and consistent data regarding the risks of smoking and the exacerbation of atherosclerosis-related diabetic complications. Clients and families should be consistently and continuously counseled and encouraged in smoking cessation. The combination of smoking and diabetes dramatically increases the risks related to atherosclerotic vessel disease, impaired wound healing, and the associated morbidity and mortality rates.[40]

Infection. Chronic, poorly controlled diabetes mellitus, can lead to a variety of blood vessel and tissue changes that result in impaired wound healing and markedly increased risk for infections. Impaired vision and peripheral neuropathy contribute to the decreased ability of the person with diabetes to feel or see breaks in skin integrity and developing wounds. Vascular disease contributes to tissue hypoxia, which further decreases healing ability. In addition, once pathogens are inside the body, they multiply rapidly because the increased glucose content in body fluids and tissues fosters bacterial growth. Because the blood supply to tissues is already compromised, white blood cells are not mobilized to the affected areas efficiently or adequately. Diabetes results in higher incidences of skin, urinary tract, vaginal, and other types of tissue infections.[46]

Retinopathy and Nephropathy. Diabetic retinopathy is a highly specific vascular complication in persons with both type 1 and type 2 DM and its prevalence is correlated closely with duration and control of high blood glucose levels. After 20 years with diabetes mellitus, nearly all individuals with type 1 DM and more than 60% of type 2 DM have some degree of retinopathy. Diabetic retinopathy poses a serious threat to vision. Underlying microvascular occlusion of the retina resulting in progressive areas of retinal ischemia and tissue death causes diabetic retinopathy. Recent studies have established that intensive management of blood glucose level control to consistent near-normal levels can prevent and delay the progression of diabetic retinopathy.[21]

Diabetes also has become the most common single cause or end-stage renal disease (ESRD) in the United States and Europe. Hardening and thickening of the glomerular basement membrane, which result in eventual destruction of critical renal filtration structures, cause diabetic nephropathy. The presence of small amounts of albumin in the urine is the earliest clinical evidence of nephropathy. The eventual destruction of the filtering ability of the kidney causes chronic renal failure and the need for permanent dialysis or renal transplantation. Renal destruction, as with retinopathy, can be slowed significantly with early detection and monitoring, tight glucose control, early treatment of hypertension (particularly with ACE inhibitors),* careful monitoring of dietary protein, and strong encouragement of cessation of smoking.[24,43]

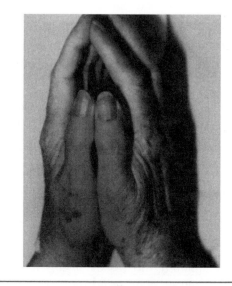

FIGURE **10-8** The prayer sign. The individual is unable to press the palms flat against each other, a diagnostic sign for the syndrome of limited joint mobility in diabetic persons. Other conditions also may result in loss of extension with a positive prayer sign. (From Kaye T: Watching for and managing musculoskeletal problems in diabetes, *J Musculoskel Med* 11:25-37, 1994.)

Musculoskeletal Problems. Musculoskeletal complications are common, often involving the hands, shoulders, spine, and feet. Carpal tunnel syndrome, Dupuytren's contracture, trigger finger, and adhesive capsulitis occur more frequently in people with diabetes compared with those who do not have diabetes.[9] Although these disorders are not life threatening, they can add significant functional impairment to a person's life. See also discussion of orthopedic problems that can develop secondary to sensory and motor neuropathy (see the section on Sensory, Motor, and Autonomic Neuropathy in this chapter).

Upper Extremity. In the hand, the *syndrome of limited joint mobility* (SLJM or LJM) and the stiff hand syndrome are unique to diabetes. SLJM is characterized by painless stiffness and limitation of the finger joints (Fig. 10-8). Flexion contractures typically progress to result in loss of dexterity and grip strength. The SLJM is an underdiagnosed complication of diabetes, largely because this type of loss of hand range of motion is considered a common normal sign of aging.[87] The severity of this syndrome in diabetes is correlated with the duration of disease, duration and quantity of insulin therapy, and smoking. Joint contractures also may develop in larger joints, such as the elbows, shoulders, knees, and spine.

The *stiff hand syndrome* often is confused with or included in SLJM, but it has a distinct pathogenesis and clinical presentation. The stiff hand syndrome occurs uniquely with diabetes and is seen more frequently with type 1 DM and poor blood glucose control. Paresthesias, which eventually become painful, are accompanied by subcutaneous tissue changes such as stiffness and hardness. Vascular insufficiency may be the underlying cause or may be secondary to neuropathy, nodular tenosynovitis, and osteoarthritis.

Dupuytren's contracture is characterized by the formation of a flexion contracture and thickening band of palmar fascia (Fig. 10-9), usually involving the third and fourth digits in the

---

*Hypertension is managed with ACE inhibitors initially and if blood pressure is not less than 130/85, a beta blocker may be added. However, combining a beta blocker with a diuretic can blunt awareness and symptoms of low glucose, so this combination usually is not recommended.

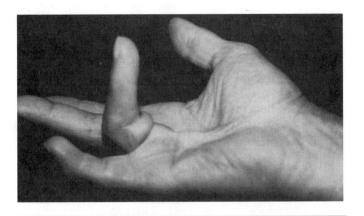

FIGURE 10-9 Dupuytren's contracture. Painless nodules develop in the distal palmar crease, often in line with the ring finger, that slowly mature into a longitudinal cord that is readily distinguishable from a tendon. The skin overlying the nodules is usually puckered. The contracture may be symptomatic (painful), but with or without pain it results in impaired hand function. (From Kaye T: Watching for and managing musculoskeletal problems in diabetes, *J Musculoskel Med* 11:25-37, 1994.)

population with diabetes (rather than the fourth and fifth digits in the population without diabetes). Pain and decreased range of motion are the primary presentation. Painless nodules develop in the distal palmar crease, often in line with the ring finger, which slowly mature into a longitudinal cord that is readily distinguishable from a tendon. The skin overlying the nodules is usually puckered.

Flexor tenosynovitis (also called *chronic stenosing tenosynovitis*) is another rheumatologic condition seen more commonly in persons with diabetes. Tenosynovitis is caused by accumulation of fibrous tissue in the tendon sheath and can cause aching, nodularity along the flexor tendons, and contracture. Locking of the digit, called *trigger finger,* can occur in flexion or extension and may be associated with crepitus or pain. In the population with diabetes, tenosynovitis is found predominantly in women and affects the thumb, middle, and ring fingers most often.

Diabetes is the systemic disease most often seen in connection with *peripheral neuropathy of the hand,* including CTS. The clinical presentation of CTS is the same for the person with diabetes as for the person without diabetes, although in diabetes CTS is more likely to be a neuropathic process than an entrapment problem. Both neuropathy and compression within the carpal tunnel may exist together.

Adhesive capsulitis (also known as *periarthritis* or *frozen shoulder*) is characterized by diffuse shoulder pain and loss of motion in all directions, often with a positive painful arc test and limited joint accessory motions. The pattern is slightly different from that of typical adhesive capsulitis, in which regional tightness in the anteroinferior joint capsule primarily compromises external rotation, followed by loss of abduction and, less often, internal rotation and flexion. The pattern in diabetes is one of significant global tightness with external and internal rotation equally limited in the dominant shoulder, followed by limitations in abduction and hyperextension. External rotation and hyperextension are most limited in the nondominant shoulder, followed by internal rotation and abduction. The pathogenesis of the capsular thickening and ad-

herence to the humeral head remains unknown. The long head of the biceps tendon may become glued down in its tendon sheath on the anterior humeral head.[87]

Adhesive capsulitis may be accompanied by vasomotor instability of the hand previously referred to as reflex sympathetic dystrophy (RSD) but now classified as the complex regional pain syndrome (CRPS). This condition is characterized by severe pain, swelling, and trophic skin changes of the hand* (e.g., thinning and shininess of the skin with loss of wrinkling, sometimes with increased hair growth). Skin and subcutaneous tissue atrophy and tendon flexion contractures develop. The natural history of this condition ranges from spontaneous remission to permanent loss of function. (See the section on Complex Regional Pain Syndrome in Chapter 38.)

Spine. Diffuse idiopathic skeletal hyperostosis (DISH; also known as *ankylosing hyperostosis*) is a condition of the spine seen most often in people with type 2 DM, although it can occur in a person who does not have diabetes. In DISH, osteophytes develop into bony spurs, typically right-sided syndesmophytes that may join to form bridges (Fig. 10-10). The thoracic spine most commonly is involved. In contrast to ankylosing spondylitis, the sacroiliac joints are spared, and vertebral body osteoporosis is absent. Calcaneal and olecranon spurs may develop, and new bone may form around hips, knees, and wrists.

People with DISH may be asymptomatic or they may experience back pain and stiffness without limitations in range of motion. Dysphagia may develop if extensive cervical spine involvement occurs. The pathogenesis of DISH is unknown and apparently no correlation exists between the degree of diabetic control and the extent of hyperostosis.

Osteoporosis. Generalized osteoporosis usually develops within the first 5 years after the onset of diabetes mellitus and is more severe in persons with type 1 DM. It is hypothesized that bone matrix formation may be inadequate in the absence of normal circulating insulin levels. Results of bone density studies in persons with type 2 DM are conflicting, with some studies demonstrating decreased bone density and others indicating increased bone density. People with type 2 DM have decreased circulating insulin levels because of beta-cell exhaustion, and others are hyperinsulinemic because of insulin resistance.

As in any case of osteoporosis, regardless of the underlying cause, this condition places the person at greater risk for fractures. With the additional loss of sensation associated with diabetes, minor trauma easily produces injury. Microfractures can occur in already weakened bone and cartilage and may remain unrecognized because of the lack of pain appreciation. A vicious circle is started, leading to further damage.

Sensory, Motor, and Autonomic Neuropathy. Sensory, motor, and autonomic neuropathy is a common phenomenon. Neuropathy may affect the central nervous system, peripheral nervous system, or autonomic nervous system. The

---

*Skin changes in diabetic hand arthopathy, in addition to changes because of RSD, may occur in association with adhesive capsulitis. Other skin changes associated with diabetes include scleroderma diabeticorum, an asymptomatic thickening of the skin that may lead to a peau d'orange appearance, which usually involves the posterior neck, upper back, and shoulders.[8]

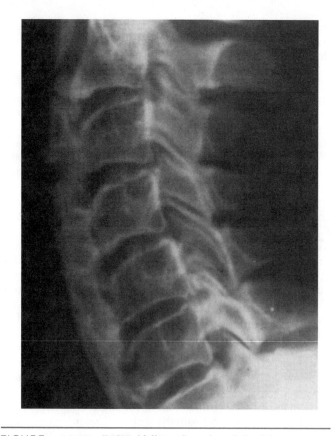

FIGURE 10-10 DISH (diffuse idiopathic skeletal hyperostosis; ankylosing hyperostosis) associated with type 2 diabetes mellitus. DISH can occur with other conditions such as ankylosing spondylitis. Although the dense anterior bony bridging of the cervical vertebrae is pictured on this lateral roentgenogram, the thoracic spine most commonly is involved in diabetes. This type of DISH can be distinguished from ankylosing spondylitis by the preservation of sacroiliac joints, a site of typical involvement in ankylosing spondylitis. (From Kaye T: Watching for and managing musculoskeletal problems in diabetes, *J Musculoskel Med* 11:25-37, 1994.)

most common form of diabetic neuropathy is a *sensory polyneuropathy*, usually affecting the hands and feet and causing symptoms that range from mild tingling, burning, or numbness to a complete loss of sensation (usually feet).

The loss of sensation in diabetic neuropathy predisposes joints to repeated trauma and progressive joint destruction. Chronic progressive degeneration of the stress-bearing portion of a joint associated with loss of proprioceptive sensation in the joint produces a condition called *Charcot's disease, Charcot's arthropathy,* or *neuropathic arthropathy.* Diabetes is the most common cause of neuropathic joints.*

Subluxation of the tarsal and metatarsal joints commonly result in a rocker-bottom foot deformity with progressive development of ulceration. A neuropathic joint is swollen, warm, and edematous, but pain is minimal because of the underlying altered sensation. Left untreated, neuropathic changes progress to complete destruction of the joint.

---

*The health care team must assess the presence of macrovascular or peripheral vascular disease, which may be present in diabetes and diabetic foot disease, caused by neuropathy, a microvascular problem. Improving circulation may be a goal with macrovascular or peripheral vascular disease (see Chapter 11), whereas foot care and orthoses are more appropriate treatments for microvascular-caused neuropathy.

Joints with less movement transmit abnormal forces through the foot to injure already damaged joints. This is especially true during walking, when large forces are placed on the midtarsal and tarsometatarsal joints. Obesity further increases these forces and in the presence of any preexisting gait abnormalities or deformities both create additional stress that compounds the condition. The underlying neurologic disorder should be treated but this has no effect on the existing arthropathy. Reduction of weight bearing, joint immobilization, and joint protection are important conservative treatment tools. Surgical fusion can be performed if all else fails but joint replacement is contraindicated in this condition.[12]

Motor neuropathy produces weakness (bilateral but asymmetric proximal muscle weakness, called *diabetic amyotrophy*) and deformity (e.g., claw toes, severe flatfoot with valgus of the midfoot, collapse of the longitudinal arch) that contribute to biomechanical changes in foot function resulting in abnormal patterns of loading. Pain and erythema of the forefoot may constitute forefoot osteolysis, sometimes considered another form of neuropathy distinguished from cellulites or osteomyelitis by laboratory values (leukocyte count) and roentgenographic appearance.

Autonomic neuropathy may manifest itself in several ways, including loss of normal regulation of sweating (skin becomes dry and cracked with buildup of callus), temperature control, and blood flow in the limbs. Skin changes such as these can create more openings for bacteria to enter. The combination of all three types of neuropathy can ultimately lead to gangrene and possible amputation, largely preventable with proper care (see Special Implications for the Therapist: Diabetes and Foot Care in this section). Other forms of neuropathy include gastroparesis (decreased gastrointestinal motility accompanied by diarrhea and fecal incontinence) and dysregulation of the heart with increased heart rate and postural hypotension.

Ulceration. Neuropathy occurring as a result of improper glucose metabolism and diminished vascular perfusion to nerve tissues places the diabetic person at risk for the development of ulcers. Diabetic foot ulcers are caused primarily by repetitive stress on the insensitive skin with increased pressure and/or horizontal (shear) stress. Body weight and activity level increase the force that the foot must transmit, and this also may increase pressure and shear force, especially in the presence of an underlying bony prominence or foot imbalance. In addition, previously healed ulcers leave scars that transmit force to underlying tissues in a more concentrated manner and hold the fat pad locally so that it cannot function physiologically. As a result, it cannot transmit shear forces, and it becomes damaged easily.

The normal response to damaged areas is to spare them from pressure because they are painful. However, in the insensitive foot of a person with diabetes, this normal alteration of weight-bearing surface, pressure, and duration does not take place, resulting in repetitive stress and injury with subcutaneous and cutaneous necrosis and skin breakdown. The loss of autonomic nerve function eliminates the production of sweat, leaving the skin dry and inelastic. Changes in pressure and gait, fat atrophy, and muscle weakness are mechanical factors that, along with sensory neuropathy, influence the development of plantar skin abnormalities, especially ulceration.[7,85]

The skin is likely to contribute to ulceration because the collagen and keratin* may be glycosylated (saturated with glucose) with increased cross-linking, which makes the skin stiff. Keratin builds up in response to the increased pressure, covering the openings of unhealed ulcers, and cannot be removed as readily as normal keratin. The areas most commonly affected by foot ulcers are the plantar areas of the metatarsal heads, the toes, and the plantar area of the hallux (Fig. 10-11). In the Charcot foot, the incidence of ulceration beneath the talus and navicular bones becomes more common because of the rigid rocker-bottom deformity.

Medical Management

Diagnosis.   Diagnostic assessment may include a variety of testing procedures such as blood glucose, blood glucose finger-stick, fasting blood sugar, glucose tolerance test, glycosylated hemoglobin, and urine ketone levels, to name just a few (see Table 39-10). A diagnosis of diabetes is confirmed by symptoms of hyperglycemia and blood and urine glucose and ketone abnormalities. Current defined criteria for definitive diagnosis of diabetes mellitus are the following[23]:

Classic symptoms of diabetes plus a casual plasma glucose concentration of ≥200 mg/dL (*Casual* is defined as any time of day without regard to time since last meal.)

or

Fasting plasma glucose (FPG) ≥126 mg/dL after no caloric intake for at least 8 hours (If the FPG is repeated and continues to be ≥126 mg/dL on a subsequent day, a glucose tolerance test does not need to be done to confirm diagnosis.)

or

2-hour postload glucose ≥200 mg/dL during an oral glucose tolerance test.

Frequent self-monitoring by performing a direct blood sampling (fingerstick or laser technique) is an important management tool in the long-term treatment of this disease. Early screening and assessment of people at risk for diabetes is critical so that prevention and treatment of complications can be initiated before the onset of significant blood vessel and tissue damage. The American Diabetes Association recommends universal screening at age 45 (earlier for high-risk groups such as non-Caucasians, obese individuals, and those with a family history of type 2 DM in a first-degree relative). In response to the statistic that one fourth of all new cases of DM under age 20 are diagnosed as type 2 DM, the Centers for Disease Control and Prevention now recommends diabetes testing begin at age 25 years.

Treatment.   No known cure exists for diabetes. The goal of overall care for persons with diabetes is control or regulation of blood glucose. Researchers continue to investigate drugs that would prevent the formation of fat cells, thereby reducing the problem of obesity before type 2 DM can develop. Studies of the use of gene therapy as a treatment for both types of diabetes is ongoing utilizing a variety of approaches such as direct delivery of the insulin gene to non–beta-cells, improving insulin secretion from existing beta-cells, and implanting genetically modified cells.[30,35]

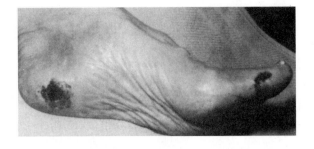

FIGURE   **10-11** Neurotrophic ulcers associated with diabetic neuropathy.   (From Callen JP, Jorizzo JL, editors: *Dermatological signs of internal disease*, Philadelphia, 1995, WB Saunders, p 187.)

Type 1 DM requires exogenous insulin administration and dietary management to achieve tight (near normal) blood glucose control. Although exercise has not been proven to provide increased glycemic control for the person with type 1 DM, it should be taken into account as part of the total picture. The insulin dosage schedule varies depending on the individual's age, level of compliance, and severity of diabetes (sometimes referred to as how brittle the diabetes is) (Tables 10-15 and 10-16). Poorly controlled diabetes is ideally treated with more frequent administration of insulin (e.g., four times per day), whereas other individuals may receive insulin once or twice daily, sometimes mixing different types of insulin (e.g., rapid-acting [human analog; Humalog]; short-acting [regular] with intermediate-acting [NPH] insulin).* From a therapist's point of view, the client receiving more frequent dosages is less likely to develop hypoglycemia, especially when beginning an exercise program.

An insulin pump is now available to deliver fixed amounts of regular insulin continuously, thereby more closely imitating the release of the hormone by the islet cells. This lightweight device is worn conveniently on a belt or a shoulder holster (Fig. 10-12); a waterproof design makes swimming (especially competitive swimming) possible. Although this type of insulin administration provides better control, it has some disadvantages. It cannot be removed for more than 1 hour, reactions to the needle are common, and like any other mechanical device, it is subject to malfunction. New, implantable pump options are being tested and can dispense insulin in constant, steady pulses throughout the day. This type of pump would eliminate the need for an open needle site in the skin. Penlike injection cartridges also are in use, and possible oral or inhaled forms of insulin and an artificial pancreas are being researched.[55]

Type 2 DM most often is treated with diet and exercise, sometimes in conjunction with oral hypoglycemic drugs (OHDs); insulin occasionally is required. Exercise is a recognized therapy for the prevention of complications in type 2 DM. Several long-term studies have shown a consistent positive effect of regular exercise training on carbohydrate metabolism and insulin sensitivity. Some of the beneficial effects include prevention of cardiovascular disease and obesity, management of hypertension, and reduction in VLDL cholesterol.[23]

---

*A protein that is the principal constituent of epidermis, hair, and nails.

* Humalog (Lispro) is a new type of insulin that has rapid action. It works faster than short-acting insulin and must be taken with a meal to prevent hypoglycemia.[47]

TABLE   10-15

Insulin Dosage Schedule

Insulin Type	Insulin Preparation	Onset	Peak (Hr)	Duration (Hr)
Rapid-acting	Human analog (humalog)	10-30 min	0.5-2	3-4
Short-acting	Insulin injection (regular)	30-60 min	2-4	4-12
	Prompt insulin zinc suspension (semilente)	1-3 hr	2-8	12-16
Intermediate-acting	Isophane insulin suspension and regular insulin	30 min	4-12	24
	NPH, isophane insulin suspension	3-4 hr	6-12	24-48
	Insulin zinc suspension (lente)	1-3 hr	8-12	24-48
Long-acting	Extended insulin zinc suspension (ultralente)	4-6 hr	18-24	36

TABLE   10-16

Therapeutic Regimens for Insulin

Insulin Schedule	Indications
Single daily injections	Primarily for older adult clients
	Long-term complications less likely
	Usually use intermediate- or long-acting insulin
	May be combined with short-acting insulin to maximize control
Twice-daily injections	Used in people with reasonably stable activity and diet
	Combined short- and intermediate-acting insulin
Multiple injections	Used in younger people (more flexible to fit their lifestyle)
	Frequently use one-time long-acting dose to establish baseline effect
Infusion pump	Used to maintain tighter control
	Short-acting insulin
Intraperitoneal	Used in people with peritoneal dialysis for renal failure
	Insulin added to dialysis fluid

Courtesy Michael B. Koopmeiners, MD, Associate Professor, Institute of Physical Therapy, St. Augustine, Florida, 1996.

Several types of OHDs are available, including those used to stimulate islet cells to increase endogenous insulin secretion and enhance insulin receptor binding (sulfonylureas), those that act by slowing the digestion of sugars in the intestine (acarbose), those referred to as *insulin-resistance reducers* (thiazolidinediones such as pioglitazone and rosiglitazone, which do not cause liver problems as seen with troglitazone [Rezulin] which was removed from the market in March 2000); and those* used to improve hepatic and peripheral tissue sensitivity to insulin (metformin [Glucophage]), thereby increasing the effectiveness of insulin found in the body.

*The advantage of this OHD is that it does not stimulate activity with concomitant weight gain. However, diarrhea develops for 2 to 3 weeks in approximately one third of people using this drug. One potentially serious side effect (rare) is lactic acidosis, a life-threatening buildup of lactic acid in the blood. This condition can be fatal in people with kidney or liver disease or alcoholism. The main clinical feature of lactic acidosis is hyperventilation.

Medical treatment of long-term diabetic complications may include dialysis or kidney transplantation for renal failure and vascular surgery for large-vessel disease. Currently the American Diabetes Association advises that people with diabetes take low-dose aspirin (81 to 325 mg) daily to help minimize risks such as heart attacks and strokes. Prophylactic aspirin therapy is recommended in both men and women with diabetes who are 50 years and older, although some diabetologists suggest that aspirin prophylaxis should begin at age 35.[23]

The therapist often is involved in prevention and wound care for diabetic ulcers, which sometimes necessitate amputation. Topical application of growth factors on wounds without infection and with at least a minimal level of vascularization was introduced in the early 1990s and has progressed to include new techniques in skin transplantation (see the section on Skin Transplantation in Chapter 20). Also on the horizon in wound prevention and glucose monitoring is the development of an experimental device that monitors glucose levels without the use of fingersticks. The device, worn like a watch, uses electrical currents to obtain interval measurements of glucose levels in the skin. This type of monitoring device would prevent the invasive and often painful skin punctures by needle or laser, now in use for blood glucose monitoring.[34]

Some people with type 1 DM are now receiving pancreas transplants, but life-long immunosuppression and its complications make this treatment option less than ideal. Research is being conducted on the use of transplanted pancreatic islet cells rather than the entire pancreas (see the section on Pancreas Transplantation in Chapter 20). Some recent research advances have been made in this area and in the use of genetically altered human liver cells as possible producers of human insulin. See the section on Pancreas Transplantation in Chapter 20.

Prognosis.   Diabetes control depends on the proper interaction between three factors: (1) food, (2) insulin or oral medication to lower blood glucose, and (3) activity (e.g., sedentary or exertional) or exercise. When diabetes is regulated successfully, complications of hyperglycemia and hypoglycemia can be avoided with minimal disruption to a normal lifestyle. However, diabetes can be fatal even with medical treatment, or it can cause major permanent disabilities and seriously impair functional abilities. In fact, about 50% of myocardial infarctions and 75% of strokes are attributable to diabetes, and it is the leading cause of new blindness and is a contributory cause to renal failure and peripheral vascular disease.

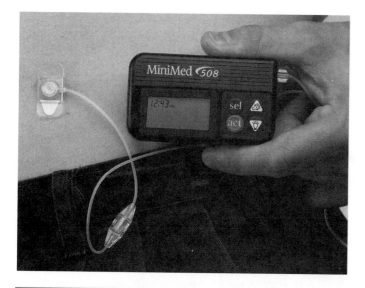

FIGURE 10-12 The programmable insulin pump. Compact and worn like a pager, the programmable insulin pump delivers fixed amounts of insulin continuously, based on blood glucose levels determined by regular fingerstick glucose monitoring. (Courtesy Mini-Med, Sylmar, California, 2000.)

TABLE   10-17

Clinical Signs and Symptoms of Hypoglycemia

SYMPATHETIC ACTIVITY (INCREASED EPINEPHRINE)	CNS ACTIVITY (DECREASED GLUCOSE TO BRAIN)
Pallor	Headache
Perspiration*	Blurred vision
Piloerection (erection of the hair)	Thickened speech
Increased heart rate (tachycardia)	Numbness of the lips and tongue
Heart palpitation	Confusion
Nervousness* and irritability	Emotional lability
Weakness*	Convulsion*
Shakiness/trembling	Coma
Hunger	

*Signs most often reported by clients.
From Black JM, Matassarin-Jacobs E, editors: *Medical-surgical nursing*, ed 5, Philadelphia, 1997, WB Saunders, p 1988.

Regardless of the modality of treatment used for the person with type 1 or type 2 DM, recent studies have shown clearly that tight glucose control (plasma glucose levels consistently within normal limits, approximately 110 mg/dL) delays onset and progression of diabetic complications. The only apparent danger in maintenance of tight control is the greater possibility of hypoglycemia, particularly in those people with type 1 DM who receive frequent exogenous insulin administration.[23]

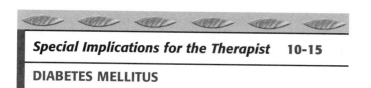

Special Implications for the Therapist   10-15

DIABETES MELLITUS

Preferred Practice Patterns:
4C: Impaired Muscle Performance
4J: Impaired Motor Function, Muscle Performance, Range of Motion, Gait, Locomotion, and Balance Associated with Amputation
5G: Impaired Motor Function and Sensory Integrity Associated with Acute or Chronic Polyneuropathies
6A: Primary Prevention/Risk Reduction for Cardiovascular/Pulmonary Disorders
6B: Impaired Aerobic Capacity/Endurance Associated with Deconditioning
7A: Primary Prevention/Risk Reduction for Integumentary Disorders
7B: Impaired Integumentary Integrity Associated with Superficial Skin Involvement

Client education is the key to therapeutic, nonsurgical treatment of the neuromusculoskeletal complications associated with diabetes. Extensive self-management is the focus of the educa-

tional program.* Exercise is a key component of the overall intervention plan.[23] The client must be taught the importance of assessing glucose levels before and after exercise and to judge what carbohydrate and insulin requirements are suitable for the activity or workout (see the section on Diabetes and Exercise in this chapter).

People with diabetes and peripheral neuropathy have a high incidence of injuries (e.g., falls, fractures, sprains, cuts, bruises) during walking or standing and a low level of perceived safety. Suggested strategies for appropriate clinical intervention to reduce these complications are available.[16]

Complications of Insulin Therapy

Hypoglycemia.   Insulin therapy can result in hypoglycemia (low blood glucose, also called an insulin reaction); tissue hypertrophy, atrophy, or both, at the site of injection; insulin allergy; erratic insulin action; and insulin resistance. Symptoms of hypoglycemia are related to two body responses; increased sympathetic activity and deprivation of CNS glucose supply (Table 10-17). The clinical picture may be varied from a report of headache and weakness to irritability and lack of muscular coordination (much like drunkenness) to apprehension, inability to respond to verbal commands, and psychosis.

Symptoms can occur when the blood glucose level drops to 70 mg/dL or less, although this value varies among those with diabetes and can be lower than 70 mg/dL before symptoms are elicited. In diabetes, an overdose of insulin, late or skipped meals, or overexertion in exercise may cause hypoglycemic reactions. Immediately provide carbohydrates in some form (e.g., fruit juice, honey, hard candy, commercially available glucose tablets or gel); a blood glucose test should be performed as soon as the symptoms are recognized. The
Continued

Diabetes Self-Management magazine is an invaluable asset for anyone with diabetes: available by title at P.O. Box 51125, Boulder, CO 80321-1125.

unconscious person needs immediate medical attention; to prevent aspiration, fluids should not be forced. Hospitalization is recommended when

- The blood glucose is less than 50 mg/dL and/or the treatment of hypoglycemia has not resulted in prompt recovery of altered mental status
- Seizures or unconsciousness are present
- A responsible adult cannot be with the person for the next 12 hr
- A sulfonaurea drug causes the hypoglycemia. This type of drug reduces liver conversion of glycogen to glucose and prolongs the period of hypoglycemia.

It is important to note that clients can exhibit signs and symptoms of hypoglycemia when their elevated blood glucose level drops rapidly to a level that is still elevated (e.g., 400 to 200 mg/dL). The rapidity of the drop is the stimulus for sympathetic activity-based symptoms; even though a blood glucose level appears elevated, affected individuals may still have symptoms of hypoglycemia.

When a person with diabetes mentions the presence of nightmares, unexplained sweating, and/or headache causing sleep disturbances, this may be an indication of hypoglycemia during nighttime sleep (most often related to the use of intermediate and long-acting insulins given more than once a day). These symptoms should be reported to the physician.

Erratic insulin action (i.e., low blood glucose followed by high blood glucose) can occur as a result of a variety of factors such as overeating, irregular meals, irregular exercise, irregular rest periods, chronic overdosage of insulin (Somogyi effect),* emotional or psychologic stress, failure to administer insulin, or intermittent use of hyperglycemic or hypoglycemic drugs (e.g., aspirin, phenylbutazone, steroids, birth control pills, alcohol). The therapist may be a helpful source of education to help clients remember the many factors affecting their condition.

Lipogenic Effect of Insulin.   Frequent injections of insulin at the same site can cause thickening of the subcutaneous tissues (hypertrophy or lipohypertrophy) and a loss of subcutaneous fat (atrophy or lipoatrophy) resulting in a dimpling of the skin that is lumpy and hard or spongy and soft. These abnormal tissue changes may cause decreased absorption of the injected insulin and poor glucose control.

The client usually is instructed to choose an injection site that is easily accessible (e.g., thighs, upper arms, abdomen, lower back) and relatively insensitive to pain (away from the midline of the body). Sites of injection should be rotated, and rotation within each area is recommended. An individual can rotate within an area using 1 inch of the surrounding tissue at a time. The client who is going to exercise should avoid injecting sites or muscles that will be exercised heavily that day, because exercise increases the rate of absorption. Following a definite injection plan can help avoid tissue damage.

Diabetic Ketoacidosis.   The therapist must always be alert for signs of ketoacidosis (e.g., acetone breath, dehydration, weak and rapid pulse, Kussmaul's respirations) progressing to hyperosmolar coma (polyuria, thirst, neurologic abnormalities, stupor).

Immediate medical care is essential. If it is not clear whether the symptoms are the result of hypoglycemia or hyperglycemia (Table 10-18), the health care worker is advised to administer fruit juice or honey. This procedure does not harm the hyperglycemic person but could potentially save the hypoglycemic person. (See discussion in next section.) Everyone with diabetes should be wearing a medical alert identification tag.

Diabetes and Exercise

An overwhelming body of evidence now exists that acute muscle contractile activity and chronic exercise improve skeletal muscle glucose transport and whole-body glucose homeostasis in the person with type 2 DM (Table 10-19). Therapists must recognize, understand, and use the role of skeletal muscle in glucose homeostasis because of the high prevalence of people with underlying skeletal muscle insulin resistance or impaired skeletal muscle glucose disposal such as occurs with inactivity, bedrest, limb immobilization, or denervation.*

A program of planned exercise including all the elements of fitness (flexibility, muscle strength, cardiovascular endurance) can benefit greatly persons with diabetes, especially those with type 2 DM. Exercise increases carbohydrate metabolism (which lowers the blood glucose level); aids in maintaining optimal body weight; increases high-density lipoproteins (HDLs); and decreases triglycerides, blood pressure, and stress and tension (Table 10-20).

Many people with diabetes may not be able to exercise intensely to a calculated heart rate because of preexisting heart conditions, deconditioning, age, neuropathies, arthritis, or other joint problems. Some people with autonomic neuropathy may have silent myocardial infarctions without angina. The first symptom may be shortness of breath resulting from congestive heart failure. Decrease in nerve innervation to the heart associated with this type of neuropathy may prevent a normal increase in heart rate with stress or exercise, requiring careful observation and monitoring of vital signs during exercise. Before beginning any exercise program, the person with diabetes should undergo a detailed medical evaluation with appropriate diagnostic studies. Screening should be done for the presence of macro and microvascular complications that may be worsened by the exercise program. A careful history and physical examination should be done by the physician and should focus on the signs and symptoms of disease affecting the heart, blood vessels, eyes, kidneys, and nervous system.[23]

Exercise in Type 1 DM.   The person with type 1 DM tends to be thin, may be poorly nourished, and, because of the islet cell deficiency, always needs exogenous insulin for adequate control of blood glucose. Exercise can increase strength and facilitate maintenance of weight and provide other important benefits (see Table 10-20), but unfortunately exercise has not been proven to provide increased glycemic control for the person with type 1 DM. During exercise in individuals without diabetes, blood glucose levels remain normal largely as a result of hormonal mediation with an increase in glucagon and catecholamines, which supply the necessary glucose for use by muscles and other body tissues. In a person with type 1 DM,

---

*The Somogyi effect occurs when the blood glucose level decreases to the point at which stress hormones (epinephrine, growth hormone, and corticosteroids) are released, causing a rebound hyperglycemia. Treatment consists of increasing the amount of food eaten and/or decreasing the insulin.

* See Sinacore and Gulve (1993) for an excellent, detailed review of the pathways for glucose transport into skeletal muscle and the pathophysiology of insulin action in skeletal muscle as it contributes to disturbances of whole-body glucose metabolism.[84]

TABLE	10-18

Comparison of Manifestations of Hypoglycemia and Hyperglycemia

VARIABLE	HYPOGLYCEMIA	HYPERGLYCEMIA
Onset	Rapid (minutes)	Gradual (days)
Mood	Labile, irritable, nervous, weepy	Lethargic
Mental status	Difficulty concentrating, speaking, focusing, coordinating	Dulled sensorium, confused
Inward feeling	Shaky, hungry, headache, dizziness	Thirst, weakness, nausea/vomiting, abdominal pain
Skin	Pallor, sweating	Flushed, signs of dehydration (see Box 4-9)
Mucous membranes	Normal	Dry, crusty
Respirations	Shallow	Deep, rapid (Kussmaul's respirations)
Pulse	Tachycardia	Less rapid, weak
Breath odor	Normal	Fruity, acetone
Neurologic	Tremors; late: dilated pupils, convulsion	Diminished reflexes, paresthesias
Blood Values		
Glucose	Low: <50 mg/dL	High: ≥250 mg/dL
Ketones	Negative	High/large
pH	Normal	Low: ≤7.25
Hematocrit	Normal	High
Urine Values		
Output	Normal	Polyuria (early) to oliguria (late)
Glucose	Negative	High
Ketones	Negative/trace	High

From Ignativicius D, Workman M, Mishler M et al: *Medical-surgical nursing across the health care continuum*, ed 3, WB Saunders, 1999, Philadelphia, p 1675.

these hormonal adaptations are lost and, as a consequence, when too little insulin is available, the cells are sensing starvation so an excessive release of glucagon and catecholamines occurs. These hormones further increase glucose mobilization into the bloodstream and significantly increase an already high level of glucose and ketones. If the hyperglycemia and ketosis is high enough and/or if the person is dehydrated, diabetic ketoacidosis can be precipitated.[23]

The person with well-controlled type 1 DM may commonly work out for approximately 30 to 45 minutes of sustained intense aerobic exercise without problems. Lack of adequate glycogen stores (i.e., decreased glycogen stores in the liver and, to a lesser extent, in skeletal muscle) leads to impaired aerobic exercise endurance when compared with the nondiabetic person.

Hypoglycemia is a common occurrence in persons with type 1 DM who are exercising. In those who do not have diabetes, plasma insulin levels decrease during exercise and insulin counter regulatory hormones (glucagon and epinephrine) promote increased hepatic glucose production, which matches the amount of glucose used during exercise. For the person with type 1 DM, who is not insulin deficient, plasma insulin concentrations may not fall during exercise and may even increase if exercise occurs within 1 hour of insulin injection. These sustained insulin levels during exercise enhance peripheral glucose uptake and stimulate glucose oxidation by exercising muscle. For this reason, insulin should not be injected into muscles or at sites close to areas involved in exercise within 1 hour of exercise.

Moderate periods of exercise provide beneficial effects, but longer periods may result in hypoglycemia. The greatest risk of severe hypoglycemia occurs 6 to 14 hours after strenuous exercise. Muscle and hepatic glycogen must be restored during periods of rest. Insulin and caloric intake must be adjusted after strenuous exercise to avoid severe nocturnal hypoglycemia.

Exercise in Type 2 DM. In contrast, people with type 2 DM are often obese and exercise is a major contributor in controlling hyperglycemia. Exercise can improve short-term insulin sensitivity and reduce insulin resistance, making it possible to prevent type 2 DM in those persons at risk and to improve glycemic control in those with diabetes.[15] These effects disappear a few days after exercise is discontinued.

Hypoglycemia is not as common a problem for the person with type 2 DM because endogenous insulin levels usually can be maintained. Control of blood glucose levels by lowering the medication dose or increasing carbohydrate intake (or both) before exercise can prevent hypoglycemia. However, individuals with type 2 diabetes who receive insulin or sulfonylureas may have a risk for hypoglycemia similar to that of people with type 1 DM.[23]

General Exercise Considerations. For anyone with diabetes, type 1 or type 2, the exercise prescription must take into account any of the complications present, especially cardiovascular changes, autonomic and sensory neuropathy, and retinopathy. Generally, individuals with autonomic neuropathy have a poor ability to perform aerobic exercise owing to decreased maximal heart rate and increased resting heart rate. Persons with a generalized form of autonomic neuropathy may have hypotensive episodes after exercising, especially those who are deconditioned. They also demonstrate a predisposition toward dehydration in the heat and poor exercise tolerance in cold environments. Silent myocardial infarction during exercise and postexercise hypotension are likely prob-

Continued

TABLE	10-19

Diabetes Mellitus: Key Points to Remember

General Guidelines

Although "safe" blood glucose levels are between 100 and 250 mg/dL (i.e., the person is not likely to experience diabetic ketoacidosis), the goal of therapy may be toward tighter control (e.g., in a young person with type 1 DM, 80 to 120 mg/dL) or moderate control (e.g., in an adult with type 2 DM, up to 150 mg/dL). A measurement more than 120 mg/dL should still be monitored closely in any age group

If the blood glucose level is ≤100 mg/dL, a carbohydrate snack should be given and the glucose retested in 15 minutes to ensure an appropriate level. Food eaten in response to blood glucose levels between 70 and 100 mg/dL is symptom dependent (i.e., if a person's blood glucose is 80 mg/dL but no signs or symptoms of hypoglycemia are present, no snack is necessary)

Observe carefully for signs or symptoms of diabetic ketoacidosis: acetone breath, dehydration, weak and rapid pulse, Kussmaul's respirations

Avoid exercise if blood glucose >250 mg/dL with evidence of ketosis

Administer fruit juice or honey to anyone with diabetes who is in a hypoglycemic state. If uncertain whether the person is hypoglycemic or hyperglycemic, provide juice or honey anyway

Exercise must be carefully planned in conjunction with food intake and administration of insulin or oral hyperglycemic agents

Do *not* exercise during peak insulin times. The peak activity of insulin occurs at different times depending on the type, dose, and time of the insulin injection (see explanation in text)

When under stress, the person with diabetes has increased insulin requirements and may become symptomatic even though the disease is usually well-controlled in normal circumstances

Avoid exercising late at night if this has not been gradually and consistently incorporated into the overall lifestyle. Delayed hypoglycemic reactions can occur during sleep hours after heavy, unaccustomed exercise late in the evening

Before Exercise

Take at least 17 ounces of fluid before exercise (approx. two 8 oz. glasses)

Glucose levels must be monitored immediately before exercise

Do not exercise when blood glucose levels are at or near 300 mg/dL with or without urinary ketones; or at or near 250 mg/dL with urinary ketones

Do *not* exercise without eating at least 2 hr before exercise (exercise about 1 hr *after* a meal is best, but individual variations must be determined)

Before Exercise—cont'd

Do *not* inject short-acting insulin in muscles or sites close to areas involved in exercise within 1 hr of exercise because insulin is absorbed much more quickly in an active extremity

Clients with type 1 DM may have to reduce the insulin dose or increase food intake when initiating an exercise program

Ketosis can be checked by means of a urine test before exercise (e.g., if the blood glucose is close to 250 mg/dL). If the test is positive (i.e., showing large numbers of ketones in the urine), exercise should be delayed until the urine test shows negative or low numbers of ketones. The person should administer added insulin. Delay exercise until glucose and ketones are under control

Do not use drugs that may contribute to exercise-induced hypoglycemia (e.g., beta blockers, alcoholic beverages, diuretics, estrogens, phenytoin)

Menstruating women need to increase their insulin during menses, especially those who are inactive or who do not exercise on a regular basis

During Exercise

It is best to exercise regularly (5 times/wk or at least every other day) and consistently at the same time each day

Duration of exercise is optimal at 40 to 60 min, although as little as 20 to 30 min of continuous aerobic exercise is beneficial in improving glucose homeostasis

During prolonged activities, a readily absorbable carbohydrate snack (e.g., fruit) is recommended for each 30 minutes of activity. After exercise, a more slowly absorbed carbohydrate snack (e.g., bread, pasta, crackers) helps prevent delayed-onset hypoglycemia. Activities should be stopped with the development of any symptoms of hypoglycemia, and blood glucose tested

Replace fluid losses adequately

Monitor blood glucose every 30 min during prolonged exercise

Anyone with diabetes should not exercise alone. Health care workers, partners, teammates, and coaches must understand the possibility of hypoglycemia and how to manage it

After Exercise

Glucose levels must be monitored 15 min after exercise, especially if exercise is not consistent

Increase caloric intake for 12 to 24 hr after activity, according to intensity and duration of exercise

Reduce insulin, which peaks in the evening or night, according to intensity and duration of exercise

---

lems. Exercise, unless specifically approved by a physician, is contraindicated in anyone with a severe form of autonomic neuropathy (Box 10-4), including anyone with vasomotor instability, angina, and a history of myocardial infarction.[23]

Muscle damage, with accompanying insulin resistance and impaired glucose uptake and disposal, can occur when untrained individuals begin to exercise.[84] For this reason, clients with diabetes must start any new activity at a well-tolerated intensity level and duration, gradually increasing over a period of

weeks or even months.[15] Unplanned exercise can be dangerous for people taking insulin or oral hypoglycemic agents. During periods of exercise, muscles are stimulated to take up glucose to supply the fuel to the working muscles, causing blood glucose levels to fall abruptly. However, anyone with blood glucose levels at or near 300 mg/dL should *NOT* exercise, because vigorous activity also can raise the blood glucose level by releasing stored glycogen. Exercise or therapy sessions should be scheduled to avoid peak insulin times (see Table

TABLE	10-20

Benefits and Potential Risks of Exercise in People with Diabetes Mellitus

BENEFITS	POTENTIAL RISKS*
Improves cardiovascular function	Hypoglycemia in people taking oral hypoglycemics or insulin
Improves maximum oxygen uptake	Worsening of hyperglycemia
Improves insulin binding and sensitivity	Cardiovascular disease, such as myocardial infarction, arrhythmias, excessive increases in blood pressure during exercise, postexercise orthostatic hypotension, or sudden death
Lowers insulin requirements (type 2 DM)	
Improves sense of well-being and quality of life	
Promotes other healthy lifestyle activities	Microvascular disease, such as retinal hemorrhage or increased proteinuria
Increases carbohydrate metabolism	Degenerative joint disease
Improves blood glucose control†	Orthopedic injury related to neuropathy
Reduces hypertension	
May help with weight reduction	
Improves lipid profile	
Reduces stress	

*These are potential risks over the long term. In general, the benefits of regular exercise outweigh the risks.
†Not confirmed for insulin-dependent diabetes mellitus (type 1 DM).

10-15) and to avoid periods of fasting (e.g., missed meal, just before the next meal).

Exercise in the morning is recommended to avoid hypoglycemia resulting from fluctuations in insulin sensitivity caused by factors such as diurnal variations in growth hormone. Growth hormone levels remain low in the afternoon, and less gluconeogenesis occurs. Too-vigorous exercise late in the day or evening could lead to delayed hypoglycemia during sleep, which is dangerous.

Some thought should be given to the specific type of exercise selected. The young individual, in good metabolic control, can safely participate in most activities. The middle-aged and older person with diabetes should be encouraged to be physically active, but because the aging process leads to degeneration of musculoskeletal structures, exercise can exacerbate these problems.[23] However, even for the person with type 1 DM in good control, sports in which hypoglycemia may be life-threatening (e.g., scuba diving, rock climbing, parachuting) should be discouraged.

Walking necessitates care toward proper footwear for the person who does not already have evidence of peripheral neuropathy. Swimming may be a good choice, once again taking care to provide meticulous foot care (see the section on Diabetes and Physical Agents in this chapter). Wearing boat shoes (specially designed shoes for water wear available in many local stores) can help prevent scraping the feet along the sides or bottom of the pool. Care must be taken to gently dry the feet, especially between the toes, after swimming; to prevent infection. Anyone with abrasions or open sores should not enter a swimming pool environment.

Intermittent, high-intensity activities (e.g., racquetball, baseball)* or contact sports (e.g., basketball or soccer) should be avoided to prevent trauma (especially to the feet or eyes). High resistance strength-training programs should be limited to the young diabetic with no diabetic complications. Low-resistance strength training programs should be encouraged unless retinopathy is present (weightlifting is contraindicated in anyone with proliferative retinopathy; see Box 10-4). Exercise involving jarring or rapid head motion may precipitate hemorrhage or retinal detachment. Outdoor activities must be evaluated carefully, taking into consideration the weather extremes (hot or cold) and the person's ability to maintain distal circulation. Stationary indoor equipment (many types are now available) may be the best overall choice.

Balancing Insulin, Food, and Exercise. As mentioned, insulin should be injected in sites away from the part of the body involved in exercising. Because glucose can enter the cells without insulin during exercise, food should be eaten if the person is exercising more than usual. Conversely, when exercising less often, a lighter diet or more insulin is required.

Glucose levels should be monitored before and after exercise (or therapy activities), remembering that the effect of exer-

Continued

BOX	10-4

Contraindications to Exercise in Diabetes Mellitus

Poor control of blood glucose levels
Unevaluated or poorly controlled associated conditions:
   Retinopathy
   Hypertension
   Neuropathy (autonomic or peripheral)
   Nephropathy
Recent photocoagulation or surgery for retinopathy
Dehydration
Extreme environmental temperatures (hot or cold)

*More specific recommendations for the long-distance runner and other athletes are available (see Hough, 1994[45]; Landry, 1994[54]; Campaigne, 1998[10]).

cise can be felt up to 12 to 24 hours later. Those clients taking insulin should have their own glucose monitoring devices (fingerstick or laser punctures). After exercise, available glucose is important for the replenishment of muscle glycogen stores. Bouts of hypoglycemia can be delayed until hours after completion of exercise. The insulin-dependent person must regulate activity so that the rate of energy expenditure balances the amount and type of insulin and food intake (Table 10-21). Women who are menstruating need to increase their insulin during menses.

Glucose monitoring is not as crucial for a person who has an established pattern of activities and/or exercise. When a new activity is introduced, such as occurs in an exercise or rehabilitation program, monitoring blood glucose levels is recommended until the individual's response to the change is known and predictable in maintaining stable blood glucose levels.

Diabetes and Musculoskeletal Complications

The treatment of musculoskeletal problems outlined in Clinical Manifestations (previous discussion, this section) does not differ from treatment for these same conditions in the nondiabetic population. Early aggressive therapy for the adhesive capsulitis usually results in restoration of functional motion, even though full range of motion may not be achieved. Hand function can be maintained and disease progression delayed with hand therapy, especially for the stiff hand syndrome. SLJM does not always benefit from therapy, but treatment intervention should be tried. For either of these conditions, the client must understand the importance of a self-directed exercise program established by the therapist to prevent recurrence of symptoms and to maintain functional outcomes.

Intervention for CTS must take into account the neuropathic and the entrapment components in the person with diabetes; surgical decompression may not be beneficial because of the neuropathic component. Nonsurgical efforts should be the focus of treatment. In conditions such as adhesive capsulitis and CRPS, a successful outcome is more likely with early medical and therapeutic intervention.

Diabetes and Foot Care

Disorders of the feet constitute a source of increasing morbidity associated with diabetes. Foot problems are a leading cause of hospital admission in people with diabetes, and diabetes is the most common reason for lower limb amputation. Half of those cases are preventable with proper foot care.[85] Treatment of the underlying diabetes has little effect on any joint disease already present. The most beneficial intervention includes stabilizing the joint, minimizing trauma, maintaining muscular strength, and performing daily foot care.

Assess for signs of diabetic neuropathy (e.g., numbness or pain in hands or feet, footdrop*; see Table 11-21) and teach each person with diabetes proper foot and skin care (see Table 11-22).

---

*For a description of an easy and reliable method to test for protective sensation using the Semmes-Weinstein monofilaments, see the reference section.[68] This test is an easily used clinical indicator for identifying people who are at risk for developing foot ulcers and requiring subsequent amputations. The results of this test provide a definitive idea of who can benefit most from preventive care, education, and prescription of appropriate therapeutic footwear.[68]

TABLE   10-21

Making Food Adjustments for Exercise: General Guidelines

Type of Exercise and Examples	If Blood Glucose is*:	Increase Food Intake By:	Suggestions of Food to Use
Exercise of short duration and low to moderate intensity (walking a half mile or leisurely bicycling for <30 min)	<100 mg/dL	10-15 g of carbohydrate per hour of exercise	1 fruit or 1 starch/bread exchange
	≥100 mg/dL	Not necessary to increase food	
Exercise of moderate intensity (1 hr of tennis, swimming, jogging, leisurely bicycling, golfing)	<100 mg/dL	25-50 g of carbohydrate before exercise, then 10-15 g per hour of exercise	½ meat sandwich with a milk or fruit exchange
	100-180 mg/dL	10-15 g of carbohydrate	1 fruit or 1 starch/bread exchange
	180-300 mg/dL	Not necessary to increase food	
	≥300 mg/dL	Do not begin exercise until blood glucose is under better control	
Strenuous activity or exercise (about 1 to 2 hr of football, hockey, racquetball, or basketball games; strenuous bicycling or swimming; shoveling heavy snow)	<100 mg/dL	50 g carbohydrate; monitor blood glucose carefully	1 meat sandwich (2 slices of bread) with a milk and fruit exchange
	100-180 mg/dL	25-50 g carbohydrate, depending on intensity and duration	½ meat sandwich with a milk or fruit exchange
	180-300 mg/dL	10-15 g carbohydrate	1 fruit or starch/bread exchange
	≥300 mg/dL	Do not begin exercise until blood glucose is under better control	

*100 mg/dL = 100 mg/100 mL. The 100 mg/dL is a general guideline. Wide individual variations occur in this area. The timing of food intake may be symptom-dependent. Some individuals may experience symptoms of hypoglycemia when the blood glucose is 150 mg/dL, others not until the level is below 80 mg/dL, and so on.

Decreased sensation in the feet associated with diabetic neuropathy requires retraining of the somatosensory and vestibular systems to help compensate for the somatosensory deficit.[42]

Note the location of any foot ulcerations for possible causes that can be corrected. For example, ill-fitting shoes may cause ulcers on the medial or lateral borders of the feet, whereas ulcers on top of the foot may be caused by deformities such as hammer (claw) toes. The pressure exerted during standing and other weight-bearing activities may cause ulcers appearing on the bottom of the foot. The presence of corns or calluses is an indication that footwear fits poorly and should be carefully evaluated by the therapist. Additionally, cartilage requires insulin for glucose uptake, metabolism of carbon dioxide, and collagen synthesis. Lacking an adequate supply, the articular cartilage in the person with diabetes does not tolerate repetitive trauma, compression, and motion, making proper footwear all the more important.[75]

Although the management of the diabetic foot (Charcot joint) sometimes requires surgery, most people can be treated nonsurgically with appropriate cast, shoe, and orthotic techniques. When a neuropathic joint is detected early, complete avoidance of weight bearing for 8 weeks may prevent progression of disease. Because wound healing (surgical and nonsurgical) is impaired in the diabetic foot, surgery can be accompanied by increased risks of poor healing and infection. Sympathectomy, arthrodesis, and joint immobilization have not been proved helpful. This underscores the importance of therapists providing nonsurgical alternatives such as appropriate shoes, insoles, and orthoses for these problems.* The presence of a previous history of plantar ulceration may alert the therapist to the need to teach the client how to control activity levels to lessen shear forces on scars from previous ulcers.[8]

Total contact casting (TCC) is now recognized as an effective intervention for neuropathic plantar ulcers. Healing of foot ulcers may be delayed in those who are selectively immunosuppressed after organ transplantation.[83] Monitoring of foot problems through the use of skin temperature changes using dermal thermography may provide valuable information to the clinician in the detection, treatment, and prevention of neuropathic foot problems.[2] The prevention of foot problems before they begin, however, is always the most effective method in offsetting the development of foot ulceration and infection and their potentially devastating effects. The use of proper footwear, proper cleaning and lubrication of the feet, safe removal of corns or calluses, and the removal of mechanical sources of foot pressure are critical components in the prevention of foot problems. Client education is a key component in the monitoring and detection of potential difficulties.[75]

The detrimental effects of cigarette smoking on wound healing and peripheral circulation are well documented (see the section on Substance Abuse in Chapter 2). Substance abuse of any kind can impair or slow the rehabilitation process, especially delaying wound healing. Client education in this area is an important aspect of treatment.

Diabetes and Physical Agents

Numerous studies from the 1980s and continued ongoing research have documented the large inter- and intra-individual variability in subcutaneous insulin absorption, a major contributing factor in the variability of blood glucose. The therapist must be aware of these factors and plan intervention accordingly. Specifically, insulin absorption is impaired or altered by smoking, injection site, thickness of skin fold (adipose tissue), exercise, subcutaneous edema, local subcutaneous blood flow, ambient and skin temperature, and local massage.[1,44]

The application of heat causes local vasodilation and hyperemia (excess blood to an area) necessitating burn precautions in this population. In a therapy practice, heat application may take the form of hot packs, paraffin, hydrotherapy, fluidotherapy, infrared radiation, ultrasound, or aquatic (pool) physical therapy. Heat from the use of hot baths, whirlpools, saunas, or sun beds have been shown to accelerate the absorption of subcutaneous injections of insulin, by increasing skin blood flow. To reduce the risk of hypoglycemia, local application of heat to the site of a recent insulin injection should be avoided. The use of cryotherapy (cold) with its effects of vasoconstriction and decreased skin blood flow would be expected to slow or delay insulin absorption from the injection site.

Diabetes and Aquatic Physical Therapy*[13]

See Appendix B: Guidelines for Aquatic Physical Therapy.

A rise in ambient (surrounding) temperature such as a client might experience in an indoor, warm, and humid pool setting also causes an increase in insulin absorption from subcutaneous injection sites. The insulin disappearance rate may be as much as 50% to 60% greater with an increase of 15° in ambient temperature.[53] Additionally, the ease of movement in the water allows increased activity without the same perceived intensity of exertion for the same amount of work performed outside the water. The combination of increased temperatures and increased activity can result in hypoglycemia. The therapist and client must work closely together to maintain a balance of activity, food intake, and insulin dosage.

When a client with diabetes begins aquatic physical therapy, both the time in the water and the intensity of exercise should be systematically progressed and monitored, with one of the parameters being increased with each session according to the client's tolerance. Before pool therapy, the client must not miss any meals or snacks and must measure blood glucose levels. A snack or beverage such as orange juice should be readily available throughout the therapy session for anyone developing symptoms of hypoglycemia. Glucose testing should be performed after completion of the pool program. Exercise can have a positive effect in reducing blood glucose levels in persons with type 2 DM, but sudden drops in blood glucose levels after exercise should be avoided.

With careful management, the individual should be able to adjust food intake and exercise tolerance to avoid having to increase insulin dosage. Throughout the pool program, the therapist must closely monitor each individual with diabetes for any signs of hypoglycemia (see Table 10-17). The affected individuals must be cautioned to carry out self-monitoring and to respond to the earliest perceived symptoms. ■

---

*For an excellent discussion of how to provide a good fit in shoes, including proper shoe lacing patterns to match foot type, and a review of the Diabetic Shoe Bill, see Bottomley JM: "Diabetic Shoe Bill" provides assistance in Medicare part B, *The ADVANCE Magazine for Physical Therapists,* Dec 12, 1994, pp 20, 23.

---

*The Aquatics Section of the American Physical Therapy Association (APTA) has an annotated bibliography with relevant articles related to pool therapy including the use of aquatics with medical conditions such as diabetes mellitus. This document is available through the section by calling (334) 990-5713.

Insulin Resistance Syndrome.   A syndrome of insulin resistance has been proposed to explain the frequent association of hypertension, carbohydrate intolerance, abdominal obesity, dyslipidemia, and accelerated atherosclerosis associated with type 2 DM. Although a primary insufficiency of insulin secretion is the pathology in the development of type 2 DM, obesity is a major risk factor for the development of this type of DM, owing in part to the associated insulin resistance. Insulin resistance refers to the phenomenon of having high levels of both circulating insulin and glucose in the bloodstream, but the insulin molecules cannot bind properly to the insulin receptor sites on the surface of the cell to allow glucose to enter the cells and be used for energy.

This condition occurs primarily in women but also can develop in men when weight gain is accompanied by alterations in the fat cells. With increased fat storage, these cells become distorted in shape and the receptor site for insulin becomes "warped" or out of proper alignment, so the insulin molecule "key" no longer fits in the receptor. Insulin resistance makes it more difficult to lose weight because the cells are not getting enough fuel and the individual perceives hunger when adequate amounts of circulating glucose exist. The affected individual may develop elevated blood pressure and problems with reactive hypoglycemia when the excess insulin is suddenly used, glucose rushes into the cells and the blood glucose drops suddenly. This sequence creates intense sweet cravings and the cycle repeats itself with increasing insulin resistance.[91]

In offspring of people with type 2 DM, insulin resistance appears inherited and may be the best predictor of future diabetic state. *Syndrome X* is sometimes referred to as the *insulin resistance syndrome*; but these are two separate entities (see the section on Syndrome X in Chapter 11).

Hyperglycemia   Two primary life-threatening metabolic conditions can develop if uncontrolled or untreated DM progresses to a state of severe hyperglycemia (greater than 300 mg/dL: diabetic ketoacidosis (DKA) and hyperglycemic, hyperosmolar, nonketotic coma (HHNK). Between diabetic ketoacidosis and hyperosmolar nonketotic coma is a continuum of metabolic abnormalities.

Diabetic Ketoacidosis

Definition and Overview.   Diabetic ketoacidosis (DKA) is most commonly seen in type 1 diabetes when complications develop from severe insulin deficiency. About one half of the people who require hospitalization for DKA develop this hyperglycemic emergency secondary to an acute infection or failure to follow their prescribed dietary or insulin therapy.[92] Most episodes of DKA occur in persons with previously diagnosed type 1 DM. However, the condition may occur in new cases of type 1 and in persons with type 2 DM (under stressful conditions in the latter, such as during a myocardial infarction). It is characterized by the triad of hyperglycemia, acidosis, and ketosis.[86]

Etiologic Factors.   Any condition that increases the insulin deficit in a person with diabetes can precipitate DKA. Causes of DKA commonly include taking too little insulin; omitting doses of insulin; failing to meet an increased need for insulin because of surgery, trauma, preg-

nancy, stress, puberty, or infection; and development of insulin resistance caused by insulin antibodies. Other precipitating causes are listed in Box 10-5.

The most common precipitating factor is infection, which occurs in up to half of all cases and may seem like a trivial condition, such as mild cellulitis or upper respiratory tract infection. Omission of insulin, either because of noncompliance or because people mistakenly believe that insulin is not required on sick days when they are not eating well, is another important and preventable cause of DKA. In approximately 15% to 30% of cases, no identifiable cause can be determined.[86]

Pathogenesis.   The initiating metabolic defect in diabetic ketoacidosis is an insufficient or absent level of circulating insulin. Insulin may be present, but not in a sufficient amount for the increase in glucose resulting from the stressor (see Box 10-5).

Inadequate insulin creates a biologic state of starvation, which triggers the excess secretion of counter regulatory hormones, particularly glucagon in an attempt to get more glucose to the cells and tissues. The abnormal insulin-to-glucagon ratio, along with excess circulating catecholamine, cortisol, and growth hormone levels, initiates a host of complex metabolic reactions, leading to hyperglycemia, acidosis, and ketosis.

When the body lacks insulin and cannot use carbohydrates for energy, it resorts to fats and proteins. The process of catabolizing fats for fuel gives rise to incomplete lipid metabolism, dehydration, metabolic acidosis, and electrolyte and acid-base imbalances. (See more complete discussion in the section on Pathogenesis of Diabetes Mellitus in this chapter.)

BOX 10-5

Precipitating Causes of Diabetic Ketoacidosis*

Inadequate insulin under stressful conditions
Infection
Missed insulin doses
Trauma
Medications
    Beta blockers
    Calcium-channel blockers
    Pentamidine (NebuPent, Pentam)
    Steroids
    Thiazides (diuretics)
Alcohol abuse (inability to manage insulin because of mentation change; alcoholic ketoacidosis)
Hypokalemia
Myocardial ischemia
Surgery
Pregnancy
Renal failure
Stroke

*Listed in descending order.

TABLE	10-22

Clinical Symptoms of Life-Threatening Glycemic States

HYPERGLYCEMIA		HYPOGLYCEMIA
Diabetic Ketoacidosis (DKA)	*Hyperglycemic, Hyperosmolar, Nonketotic Coma (HHNK)*	*Insulin Shock*
Gradual onset*	Gradual onset	Sudden onset
Headache	Thirst	Pallor
Thirst	Polyuria leading quickly to decreased urine output	Perspiration
Hyperventilation	Volume loss from polyuria leading quickly to renal	Piloerection
Fruity odor to breath	insufficiency	Increased heart rate
Lethargy/confusion/coma	Severe dehydration	Palpitations
Abdominal pain and distention	Lethargy/confusion	Irritability/nervousness
Dehydration	Seizures	Weakness
Polyuria	Coma	Hunger
Flushed face	Abdominal pain and distention	Shakiness
Elevated temperature	Blood glucose level	Headache
Blood glucose level	>300 mg/dL	Double/blurred vision
>300 mg/dL		Slurred speech
Serum pH <7.30		Fatigue
		Numbness of lips/tongue
		Confusion
		Convulsion/coma
		Blood glucose level <70 mg/dL

*Less gradual than HHNK.
From Goodman CC, Snyder TE: *Differential diagnosis in physical therapy,* ed 3, Philadelphia, 2000, WB Saunders, p 311.

Clinical Manifestations. The signs and symptoms of DKA vary, ranging from mild nausea to frank coma (Table 10-22). Common symptoms are thirst, polyuria, nausea, and weakness that have progressed over several days. This condition also may develop quickly, with symptoms progressing to coma over the course of only a few hours.

Other symptoms may include dry mouth; hot, dry skin; fruity (acetone) odor to the breath, indicating the presence of ketones; overall weakness, possible paralysis; confusion, lethargy, or coma; and deep, rapid respirations (Kussmaul's respirations). Fever is seldom present even though infection is common. Severe abdominal pain, possibly accompanied by nausea and vomiting, easily mimics an acute abdominal disorder.

Medical Management
Diagnosis, Treatment, and Prognosis. Prevention of DKA through client education is the key to avoiding this serious condition. Once DKA is suspected, the diagnosis must be established quickly, with immediate treatment after diagnostic confirmation (blood glucose level >250 mg/dL, pH <7.3, bicarbonate level <18 mEq/L, serum ketones).

Treatment includes fluid administration, insulin therapy, and correction of metabolic abnormalities, in addition to correction of any underlying illnesses (e.g., infection). Before the discovery of insulin in the 1920s, DKA was almost universally fatal. This complication is still potentially lethal with an average mortality rate between 5% and 10%.

Special Implications for the Therapist   10-16

DIABETIC KETOACIDOSIS (DKA)

Preferred Practice Patterns:
5E: Impaired Motor Function and Sensory Integrity Associated with Progressive Disorders of the Central Nervous System
5I: Impaired Arousal, Range of Motion, and Motor Control Associated with Coma, Near Coma, or Vegetative State

The therapist will be an active member of the health care team, emphasizing to anyone with type 1 DM the need for regular, daily self-monitoring of blood glucose, adherence to the diabetes management program, and early recognition of and intervention for mild ketosis. The therapist also must be able to recognize early signs and symptoms of DKA in addition to signs of infection, a major cause of DKA (see Table 7-1). The first sign of an infection in a foot or leg or an upper respiratory, urinary tract, or vaginal infection should be reported immediately to the physician.

DKA can cause major potassium shifts accompanied by muscular weakness that can progress to flaccid quadriparesis. The weakness is initially most prominent in the legs, especially the quadriceps, and then extends to the arms with involvement of the respiratory muscles. (See Chapter 4 for further discussion of hypokalemia in addition to a discussion of the other conditions associated with DKA, such as dehydration, metabolic acidosis, and electrolyte and acid-base imbalances.) ■

Hyperglycemic, Hyperosmolar, Nonketotic Coma

Overview. Hyperglycemic, hyperosmolar, nonketotic coma (HHNK) is another acute complication of diabetes, a variation of diabetic ketoacidosis. HHNK is characterized by extreme hyperglycemia (800 to 2000 mg/dL), mild or undetectable ketonuria, and the absence of acidosis. It is seen most commonly in older adults with type 2 DM.[46]

The precipitating factors of HHNK may be similar to those for DKA, such as infections, inadequate fluid intake, medications (see Box 10-5), or stress. HHNK may be the first indication of undiagnosed diabetes and it may occur in the case of someone who is receiving total parenteral nutrition (hyperalimentation) or who is on renal dialysis and is receiving solutions containing large amounts of glucose.

The major difference between HHNK and DKA is the lack of ketosis with HHNK. Because some residual ability exists to secrete insulin in NIDDM, the mobilization of fats for energy is avoided. When adequate insulin is lacking, blood becomes concentrated with glucose. Because glucose molecules are too large to pass into cells, osmosis of water occurs from the interstitial spaces and cells to dilute the glucose in the blood. Osmotic diuresis occurs, and eventually the cells become dehydrated. If not treated promptly, the severe dehydration leads to vascular collapse and death.

Clinical manifestations of HHNK are polyphagia, polydipsia, polyuria, glucosuria, dehydration, abdominal discomfort, changes in sensorium, coma, hypotension, and shock (see Table 10-22). Lactic acidosis also can develop if tissue perfusion is compromised. Treatment is with short-acting insulin, electrolyte replacement, and careful fluid replacement, to avoid congestive heart failure and intercerebral swelling in older adults, who often have other cardiovascular or renal disorders.

Special Implications for the Therapist 10-17

HYPERGLYCEMIC, HYPEROSMOLAR, NONKETOTIC COMA

The therapist should be alert to any signs of HHNK in the aging adult who may have a previous diagnosis of type 2 DM. Early recognition and treatment to restore fluid and electrolyte balance are important for a good prognosis in this condition. (See also Special Implications for the Therapist: Diabetes Mellitus, 10-15.) ∎

METABOLIC SYSTEM

As noted earlier, the endocrine system works with the nervous system to regulate and integrate the body's metabolic activities. Metabolism is the physical and chemical (physiologic) processes that allow cells to utilize food to continually rebuild body cells and transform food into energy. Metabolism is broken down into two phases: the anabolic (tissue-building) and catabolic (energy-producing) phases. The *anabolic phase* converts simple compounds derived from nutrients into substances the body cells can use, whereas the *catabolic phase* is a consumptive phase when these organized substances are reconverted into simple compounds with the release of energy necessary for the proper functioning of body cells.[39]

The body gets most of its energy by metabolizing carbohydrates, especially glucose. A complex interplay of hormonal and neural controls regulates the homeostasis of glucose metabolism. Hormone secretions of five endocrine glands dominate this regulatory function (see Table 10-12). The rate of metabolism can be increased by exercise, elevated body temperature (e.g., high fever, prolonged exertional exercise), hormonal activity (e.g., thyroxine, insulin, epinephrine), and increased digestive action after the ingestion of food.

◆ Fluid and Electrolyte Balance

Fluid and electrolyte balance is a key component of cellular metabolism. Homeostasis, maintaining the body's chemical and physical balance, involves the proper functioning of body fluids to preserve osmotic pressure, acid-base balance, and anion-cation balance. The goal of metabolism and homeostasis is to maintain the complex environment of body fluid that nourishes and supports every cell.

Body fluids, classified as intracellular and extracellular, contain two kinds of dissolved substances: those that dissociate (separate) in solution (electrolytes) and those that do not. For example, when dissolved in water, glucose does not break down into smaller particles, but sodium chloride dissociates into sodium cations (positively charged) and chloride anions (negatively charged). The composition of these electrolytes in body fluids is electrically balanced, so the positively charged cations (sodium, potassium, calcium, and magnesium) equal the negatively charged anions (chloride, bicarbonate, sulfate, phosphate, carbonic acid). Although these particles are present in relatively low concentrations, any deviation from their normal levels can have profound physiologic effects.

Because many situations in the body cause both normal and abnormal fluid shifts, it is important to have a clear understanding of fluid compartments. The recognition of pathologic conditions such as edema, dehydration, ketoacidosis, and various types of shock can depend on the understanding of these concepts. In the healthy body, fluids and electrolytes are constantly lost or exchanged between compartments. This balance must be maintained for the body to function properly. The amount used in these functions depends on such factors as humidity; body and environmental temperature; physical activity; metabolic rate; and fluid loss from the GI tract, skin, respiratory tract, and renal system. Normal balance is achieved through fluid intake and dietary consumption. Alterations in fluid and electrolyte balance are discussed more completely in Chapter 4.

◆ Acid-Base Balance

The proper balance of acids and bases in the body is essential to life. The body maintains the pH of extracellular fluid (fluid found outside cells) between 7.35 and 7.45 through a complex chemical regulation of carbonic acid by the lungs and base bicarbonate by the kidneys. The pH is essentially a measure of hydrogen ion concentration in body fluid. Nutritional deficiency or excess, disease, injury, or metabolic disturbance may interfere with normal homeostatic mechanisms and cause a lowering of pH called *acidosis* or a rise in pH called *alkalosis*.

Various bodily functions operate to keep the pH at a relatively constant level. Acid-base regulatory mechanisms include chemical buffer systems, the respiratory system, and the renal system. These systems interact to maintain a normal acid-base ratio of 20:1 bicarbonate to carbonic acid. The consequences of an acid-base metabolism disorder can result in many signs and symptoms encountered by the therapist. These conditions are discussed more completely in Chapter 4.

◆ Aging and the Metabolic System

Aging as measured by loss of physiologic function has not yet been defined precisely, so the distinction between usual, normal, and ideal metabolic changes remains undetermined. Studies of the aging population have shown that several physiologic parameters such as body weight, basal metabolism, renal clearance, and cardiovascular function decline with age. Protein-calorie nutritional status has pervasive effects on metabolic regulatory systems; nutritional status often declines with age, which contributes to metabolic dysfunction.[48]

Because the respiratory and renal systems are largely responsible for maintaining acid-base balance, changes in these systems associated with aging also have an impact on metabolic function. A common measure for metabolic loss in tissues is the decline in VO_{2max}, the maximum oxygen extraction capacity of the lungs. (See also Chapters 14 and 17.) Loss of muscle mass associated with aging can affect stroke volume capacity and oxidative metabolism.[73] The low level metabolic acidosis that appears to occur in many people with advancing age may play a role in age-associated bone loss, a factor that has received little attention from those who study bone loss and aging.[60]

Oxidative stress has been implicated in the pathogenesis of a number of diseases and has been labeled the free radical theory of aging; studies indicate that protection from the consequences of excess metabolic activity result in a slowing of the aging process, particularly in the postreproductive period of life.[11,31] Links between oxidative stress and aging focus on mitochondria in a theory called the *mitochondrial theory of aging*.

Mitochondria, the principal site of adenosine triphosphate (ATP) synthesis (also containing DNA and RNA) is the cellular site of energy production from oxygen and the principal site of free radical damage.[20] Free radical derivatives of oxygen are generated as a result of normal metabolic activity, producing destructive oxidation of membranes, proteins, and DNA. These free radicals (unstable oxygen molecules robbed of electrons) attempt to replace their missing electrons by scavenging the body and taking electrons from healthy cells, causing a chain reaction called *oxidation* (see Fig. 5-2).

The formation of free radicals can be triggered by many exogenous (outside) factors such as cigarette smoke, air pollution, anticancer drugs, ultraviolet lights, pesticides and other chemicals, uncontrolled diabetes, radiation, and emotional stress. The major defenses against these destructive byproducts of normal metabolism are the protective enzymes, which remove the free radicals and remove, repair, and replace cell constituents. Impairment of cellular function and metabolism occurs as proteins and DNA (which turn over slowly or not at all) are damaged over time.[25] The use of antioxidants found naturally in fruits and vegetables or ingested as a nutritional supplement to counteract this process is believed to increase longevity but remains under scientific investigation.[66,67]

◆ Signs and Symptoms of Metabolic Disease

Clinical manifestations of metabolic disorders vary depending on the specific pathology present. Fluid and electrolyte disorders, disorders of acid-base metabolism leading to metabolic (nonrespiratory) alkalosis or acidosis, and their associated signs and symptoms are discussed in Chapter 4.

SPECIFIC METABOLIC DISORDERS

Metabolic bone disease is discussed in Chapter 23, and *disorders of purine and pyrimidine metabolism* resulting in gout and pseudogout are discussed in Chapter 26.

◆ Metabolic Bone Disease

Metabolic disorders involving the connective tissue may result in pathologic loss of bone mineral density such as occurs in osteomalacia or osteoporosis or acceleration of both deposition and resorption of bone as seen in Paget's disease. These disorders differ in pathogenesis and treatment and are discussed in Chapter 23.

◆ Metabolic Neuronal Diseases

Metabolic neuronal diseases are rare and are not likely seen in a therapy practice. Phenylketonuria (PKU), Wilson's disease, and porphyrias are the three most often encountered and are briefly discussed in this section.

Phenylketonuria.   PKU is an autosomal recessive disease resulting from a genetic defect in the metabolism of the amino acid phenylalanine. This condition is transmitted recessively through apparently healthy parents, who show signs of the disease only on testing. The lack of an enzyme (phenylalanine hydroxylase) necessary for the conversion of the amino acid phenylalanine into tyrosine results in an accumulation of phenylalanine (Phe) in the blood with excretion of phenylpyruvic acid in the urine. If untreated, the condition results in mental retardation and other manifestations such as tremors, poor muscular coordination, excessive perspiration, mousy odor (resulting from skin and urinary excretion of phenylpyruvic acid), and seizures.

Although PKU cannot be cured, a simple screening test for PKU can be administered to newborns and is required by law in most states in the United States and in all provinces in Canada. Currently, between 160 and 400 of the 4 million babies born in the United States each year are affected. The practice of discharging newborns in 24 hours is resulting in an increase in the number of babies at risk of PKU.

Treatment is primarily through Phe restriction of the infant's diet to control the effects of PKU and is prescribed on an individual basis with the additional administration of a dietary protein substitute. The start of newborn screening for PKU during the early 1970s has given rise to an increasing number of women who have been identified and successfully treated for the disease in childhood and initiation of nutritional therapy before conception for a successful pregnancy outcome.[50] A need remains for maternal screening before pregnancy to identify undiagnosed maternal phenylketonuria and subsequent prophylactic treatment to prevent maternal PKU syndrome.[41]

The prognosis for people with PKU has improved greatly with early institution of treatment after birth. However, hyperphenylalaninemia can cause white matter abnormalities, psychiatric illness, and decreased performance on neuropsychologic tests for people with PKU compared with subjects without PKU. It has been shown that the diet necessary to reduce phenylalanine levels cannot be terminated after adolescence without elevation of plasma levels resulting in poor neuropsychologic performance.[21]

Wilson's Disease.   Wilson's disease, also known as *hepatolenticular degeneration*, is a progressive disease inherited as an autosomal recessive trait (both parents must carry the abnormal gene). This condition produces a defect in the metabolism of copper, with accumulation of copper in the liver, brain, kidney, cornea, and other tissues. Although the pathogenesis of Wilson's disease is still uncertain, it seems likely that defective biliary excretion of copper is involved.

The disease is characterized by the presence of Kayser-Fleischer rings around the iris of the eye (from copper deposits), cirrhosis of the liver (see Chapter 16), and degenerative changes in the brain, particularly the basal ganglia. Liver disease is the most likely manifestation in the pediatric population and neurologic disease is most common in young adults. Cerebellar intoxication from deposition of copper in the brain results in athetoid movements and an unsteady gait. Other CNS symptoms may include pill-rolling tremors in the hands, facial and muscular rigidity, dysarthria, and emotional and behavioral changes. Musculoskeletal effects occur in severe disease and may include muscle atrophy and wasting, contractures, deformities, osteomalacia, and pathologic fractures.[86]

Treatment is pharmacologic (e.g., lifetime administration of vitamin B_6 and D-penicillamine) and is aimed at reducing the amount of copper in the tissues by promoting its urinary excretion. Managing hepatic disease is also important; if left untreated, Wilson's disease progresses to fatal hepatic failure.

Special Implications for the Therapist   10-18

WILSON'S DISEASE

Preferred Practice Patterns:
4C: Impaired Muscle Performance
4D: Impaired Joint Mobility, Motor Function, Muscle Performance, and Range of Motion Associated with Connective Tissue Dysfunction
4G: Impaired Joint Mobility, Muscle Performance, and Range of Motion Associated with Fracture
5E: Impaired Motor Function and Sensory Integrity Associated with Progressive Disorders of the Central Nervous System

For the person with Wilson's disease, physical or vocational rehabilitation may be required. In the advanced stage of this disease, self-care is promoted to prevent further mental and physical deterioration. An exercise schedule is essential to encourage consistent focus on rehabilitation. Sensory deprivation or overload should be avoided and prevention of injuries that could occur as a result of neurologic deficits is important (see Table 11-22). ■

Porphyrias.   Porphyrias are a group of hereditary and sometimes acquired diseases characterized by enzymatic abnormalities in biosynthesis of the heme molecule. Normally, porphyrins and their precursors are necessary for the synthesis of the heme molecule. In porphyrias, because of enzyme deficiencies, an accumulation of excessive amounts of porphyrins and their precursors occurs. This accumulation results in generalized clinical symptoms. Neurologic abnormalities, acute abdominal pain, skin fragility, and photosensitivity and psychiatric problems are symptoms that characterize the porphyrias. Various drugs and chemicals can cause porphyria (e.g., large amounts of alcohol, hemodialysis, other chemical toxins) or can trigger acute, potentially life-threatening attacks in susceptible individuals. Diagnosis is suspected when clinical symptoms are combined with substantial increases in porphyrins or porphyrin-precursors in the blood and urine.[14]

REFERENCES

1. Ariza-Andraca CR, Altamirano-Bustamante E, Frati-Munari AC et al: Delayed insulin absorption due to subcutaneous edema, *Arch Invest Med* 22(2):229-33, 1991.
2. Armstrong D, Lavery L, Liswood P et al: Infrared dermal thermometry for the high riskdiabetic foot, *Physical Therapy* 77:169-75, 1997.
3. Bektas A, Suprenant ME, Wogan LT et al: Evidence of a novel type 2 diabetes locus 50 cM centromeric to NIDDM2 on chromosome 12q, *Diabetes* 48(11):2246-51, 1999.
4. Berne RM, Levy MN: *Principles of physiology*, ed 3, St Louis, 1999, Mosby.
5. Birch C: Nursing care of clients with adrenal, pituitary and gonadal disorders. In Black JM, Matassarin-Jacobs E, editors: *Medical-surgical nursing, clinical management for continuity of care*, ed 5, Philadelphia, 1997, WB Saunders, pp 2041-70.
6. Birch C, Greear K: Nursing care of clients with endocrine disease of the pancreas. In Black JM, Matassarin-Jacobs E, editors: *Medical-surgical nursing, clinical management for continuity of care*, ed 5, Philadelphia, 1997, WB Saunders, pp 1955-2004.
7. Birke JA, Patout CA, Foto JG: Factors associated with ulceration and amputation in the neuropathic foot, *J Orthop Sports Phys Ther* 30(2):91-97, 2000.
8. Bruen J, Blair K, Haynie S: Addressing risk factors and functional mobility in diabetic wound care, *Phys Ther Case Rep* 1(5): 227-37, 1998.
9. Bunker TD, Anthony PP: The pathology of frozen shoulder, a Dupuytren-like disease, *T Bone Joint Surg (Br)* 77-B:677-83, 1995.
10. Campaigne BN: Exercise and diabetes mellitus. In ACSM's *Resource Manual for Guidelines for exercise testing and prescription*, ed 3, Philadelphia, 1998, Lippincott, Williams & Wilkins, pp 267- 74.
11. Carlson JC, Riley JC: A consideration of some notable aging theories, *Exp Gerontol* 33(1-2):127-34, 1998.
12. Chan A, Meyer C: Right ankle pain and foot swelling, *J Musculoskel Med* 16(7):416-417, 1999.
13. Charness A: Personal communication (Past President, Aquatics Section, American Physical Therapy Association; faculty, Medical College of Pennsylvania, Philadelphia), 2000.
14. Chernecky C, Berger B: *Laboratory tests and diagnostic procedures*, ed 2, Philadelphia, 1997, WB Saunders.
15. Clinical Update in Musculoskeletal Medicine: Question remains: How to motivate patients? To reduce the risk of diabetes, exercise must pass threshold, *J Musculoskel Med* 14(2): 76-7, 1997.
16. Colan B: Taking control of diabetes with exercise, *ADVANCE for the Physical Therapist*, Feb 23, 1998; pp 11-3.
17. Coon B: DNA immunization to prevent autoimmune diabetes, *J Clin Invest* 104:189-99, 1999.
18. Cutolo M: Macrophages as effectors of the immunoendocrinologic interactions in autoimmune rheumatic diseases, *Ann N Y Acad Sci* 22: 32-41, 1999.
19. Davies J: Aging and the endocrine system. In Tallis R, Fillit H, Brocklehurst JC, editors: *Brocklehurst's textbook of geriatric medicine and gerontology*, ed 5, London, 1998, Churchill Livingstone, pp 1003-11.

20. de Grey AD: The reductive hotspot hypothesis: an update, *Arch Biochem Biophys* 373(1):295-301, 2000.

21. de Valk HW, de Sonneville LM, Duran M et al: Phenylketonuria: a children's disease in adulthood, *Ned Tijdschr Geneeskd (German)* 144(1):11-5, 2000.

22. Delp MD, McAllister RM, Laughlin MH: Exercise training alters aortic vascular reactivity in hypothyroid rats, *Am J Physiol* 268(4 pt 2): H1428-35, 1995.

23. Diabetes Care, Supplement 1: Clinical Practice Recommendations 2000. American Diabetes Association, *J Clin Appl Res Educ* 23:S1-S116, Jan. 2000.

24. Eberhard R, Orth S: Nephropathy in patients with type 2 diabetes mellitus, *N Engl J Med* 341 (15):1127-33, 1999.

25. Ebersole P, Hess P: *Toward healthy aging: human needs and nursing response*, ed 5, St Louis, 1998, Mosby.

26. Ellis JM, Folkers K, Minadea M et al: A deficiency of vitamin B_6 is a plausible molecular basis of the retinopathy of patients with diabetes mellitus, *Biochem Biophys Res Commun* 179:615-9, 1991.

27. Erkintalo M, Bendahan D, Mattei JP et al: Reduced metabolic efficiency of skeletal muscle energetics in hyperthyroid patients evidenced quantitatively by in vivo phosphorus-31 magnetic resonance spectroscopy, *Metabolism* 47(7):769-76, 1998.

28. Everts ME: Effects of thyroid hormones on contractility and cation transport in skeletal muscle, *Acta Physiologic Scandinavia Mar* 156(3):325-33, 1996.

29. Fletcher S, Kanagasundaram NS, Rayner HC et al: Assessment of ultrasound guided percutaneous ethanol injection and parathyroidectomy in patients with tertiary hyperparathyroidism, *Nephrol Dialysis Transplant* 12:3111-7, 1998.

30. Freeman DJ, Leclerc I, Rutter GA: Present and potential future use of gene therapy for the treatment of noninsulin dependent diabetes mellitus, *Int J Mol Med* 4(6):585-92, 1999.

31. Fukagawa NK: Aging: is oxidative stress a marker or is it causal? *Proc Soc Exp Biol Med* 222(3):293-98, 1999.

32. Fye KH, Weinstein PR, Donald F: Compressive cervical myelopathy due to calcium pyrophosphate dihydrate deposition disease, *Arch Intern Med* (2):189-93, 1999.

33. Ganguly A: Primary aldosteronism, *N Engl J Med* 339(25):1828-34, 1998.

34. Garg S: Correlaton of fingerstick blood glucose measurements with GlucoWatch biographer glucose results in young subjects with type 1 diabetes, *Diabetes Care* 22:1708, 1999.

35. Giannoukakis N, Rudert WA, Robbins PD et al: Targeting autoimmune diabetes with gene therapy, *Diabetes* 48(11):2107-21, 1999.

36. Gleeson PB, Pauls J: Carpal tunnel syndrome during pregnancy and lactation, *PT Magazine* 9:52-4, 1993.

37. Goodman CC, Snyder TE: *Differential diagnosis in physical therapy*, ed 3, Philadelphia, 2000, WB Saunders.

38. Goya RG, Bolognani F: Homeostasis, thymic hormones, and aging, *Gerontology* 45(3):174-8, 1999.

39. Guyton A: *Human physiology and mechanisms of disease*, ed 6, Philadelphia, 1996, WB Saunders.

40. Haire-Joshu D, Glasgow RE, Tibbs TL: Smoking and diabetes, *Diabetes Care* 22 (11):1887-98, 1999.

41. Hanley WB, Platt LD, Bachman RP et al: Undiagnosed maternal phenylketonuria: the need for prenatal selective screening or case finding, *Am J Obstet Gynecol* 180(4):986-94, 1999.

42. Herdman, SJ, editor: *Vestibular rehabilitation: contemporary perspectives in rehabilitation*, ed 2, Philadelphia, 1999, FA Davis, 1999.

43. Hernendez D: Hospitalization can exacerbate complications of type II diabetes, including retinopathy, neuropathy and nephropathy, *AJN* 98 (6):27-32, 1998.

44. Hildebrandt P: Subcutaneou absorption of insulin in insulin-dependent diabetic patients. Influence of species, physico-chemical properties of insulin and physiological factors, *Dan Med Bull* 38(4):337-46, 1991.

45. Hough DO: Diabetes mellitus in sports, *Sports Med* 78:423-37, 1994.

46. Ignativicius D, Workman M, Mishler M: *Medical-surgical nursing across the health care continuum*, ed 3, Philadelphia, 1999, WB Saunders.

47. Joslin Diabetes Center: Humalog Insulin (Lispro); http://www.joslin.harvard.edu/education/library/humalog.html, Boston 2000.

48. Kane R, Ouslander J, Abrass I: *Essentials of clinical geriatrics*, ed 4, New York, 1999, McGraw-Hill.

49. Katzeff HL, Ojamaa KM, Klein I: Effects of exercise on protein synthesis and myosin heavy chain gene expression in hypothyroid rats, *Am J Physiol* 267:E63-7, 1994.

50. Kirby RB: Maternal phenylketonuria: a new cause for concern, *J Obstet Gynecol Neonatal Nurs* 28(3):227-34, 1999.

51. Klippel JH, editor: *Primer on the rheumatic diseases*, ed 11, Atlanta, 1997, Arthritis Foundation, 1997.

52. Kohriyama D, Katayama Y, Tsurusakoy T: Relationship between primary Sjögrens syndrome and autoimmune thyroid disease, *Nippon Rinsho* 57(8):1878-81, 1999.

53. Koivisto VA, Fortney S, Hendler R et al: A rise in ambient temperature augments insulin absorption in diabetic patients, *Metabolism* 30:402-4, 1981.

54. Landry GL, Allen DB: Diabetes mellitus and exercise, *Clin Sports Med* 11:403-18, 1994.

55. Leslie C: New insulin replacement technologies: overcoming barriers to tight glycemic control, *Cleve Clin J Med* 66(5):293-302, 1999.

56. Lochmuller H, Reimers CD, Fischer P et al: Exercise-induced myalgia in hypothyroidism, *Clin Invest* 71:999-1001, 1993.

57. Lowe J, Honeyman-Lowe G: Facilitating the decrease in fibromyalgia pain during metabolic rehabilitation: an essential role for soft tissue therapies, *J Body Work Movement Ther* 2(4): 208-17, 1998.

58. Lowe J, Reichman A, Yellin J: A case-control study of metabolic therapy for fibromyalgia; long-term follow-up comparison of treated and untreated patients, *Clin Bull Myofascial Ther* 3(1):65-79, 1998.

59. Louthrenoo W, Schumacher HR: Musculoskeletal clues to endocrine or metabolic disease, *J Musculoskel Med* 7:33-56, 1990.

60. Masoro EJ: Physiology of Aging. In Tallis R, Fillit H, Brocklehurst JC, editors: *Brocklehurst's textbook of geriatric medicine and gerontology*, ed 5, London, 1998, Churchill Livingstone, pp 85-95.

61. MasukoHongo K, Kato T: The association between autoimmune thyroid diseases and rheumatic diseases: a review, *Nippon Rinsho* 57(8):1873-7, 1999.

62. Matassarin-Jacobs E: Structure and function of the endocrine system. In Black J, Matassarin-Jacobs JE, editors: *Medical-surgical nursing, clinical management for continuity of care*, ed 5, Philadelphia, 1997, WB Saunders, pp 1937-41.

63. McCance E, Huether S, Parkinson C: *Pathophysiology: the biologic basis for disease in adults and children*, ed 3, St Louis, 1999, Mosby.

64. McQuire JL, Van Vollenhoven, RF: Arthropathies associated with endocrine disease. In Klippel JH, editor: *Primer on the rheumatic diseases*, ed 11, Atlanta, 1997, Arthritis Foundation, pp 351-3.

65. Mercuro G, Panzuto MG, Bina A et al: Cardiac function, physical exercise capacity, and quality of life during long-term thyrotropin-suppressive therapy with levothyroxine: effect of individual dose tailoring, *J Clin Endocrinol Metab* 85(1):159-64, 2000.

66. Meydani M: Dietary antioxidants modulation of aging and immune-endothelial cell interaction, *Mech Ageing Dev* 111(2-3):123-32, 1999.

67. Meydani M, Lipman RD, Han SN et al: The effect of long-term dietary supplementation with antioxidants, *Ann NY Acad Sci* 854:352-60, 1998.

68. Mueller MJ: Identifying patients with diabetes mellitus who are at risk for lower-extremity complications: use of Semmes-Weinstein monofilaments, *Phys Ther* 76:68-71, 1996.

69. Navarro V, Fournier E, Girard S et al: Periodic hypokalemic paralysis as the manifestation of Graves' disease: clinical and electrophysiological study, *Rev Neurol* (Paris) 156(1):59-61, 2000.

70. Neidhart M, Gay RE, Gay S: Prolactin and Prolactin-like polypeptides in rheumatoid arthritis, *Biomed Pharmacotherap* 53:218-222, 1999.

71. Painter J: Thyroid and parathyroid cancer. In Miaskowski C, Buchsel P, editors: *Oncology nursing assessment and clinical care*, St Louis, 1999, Mosby, pp 1203-21.

72. Parker CR, Slayden SM, Azziz R et al: Effects of aging on adrenal function in the human, *J Clin Endocrinol Metab* 85(1):48-54, 2000.

73. Patterson DH, Cunningham DA: The gas transporting systems: limits and modifications with age and training, *Can J Appl Physiol* 24(1):28-40, 1999.

74. Pizzuti A: A polymorphism (K121Q) of the human glycoprotein PC-1 Gene coding region is strongly associated with insulin resistance, *Diabetes* 48:1881-8, 1999.

75. Postellec M: PTs help patients with diabetes put their best feet forward, *ADVANCE for Physical Therapists and PT Assistants*, July 13, 1998; pp 11-2, 32.

76. Ramirez R, Flores AD: Sudden periodic paralysis: rare manifestations of thyrotoxicosis, *Bol Asoc Med P R* 90(4-6):88-90, 1998.

77. Ryan LM: Calcium pyrophosphate dihydrate crystal deposition. In Klippel JH, editor: *Primer on the rheumatic diseases*, ed 11, Atlanta, 1997, Arthritis Foundation, pp 226-9.

78. Schlumberger M: Papillary and follicular thyroid carcinoma; *N Engl J Med* 338(5):297-306, 1998.

79. Schlumberger M, Vathaire F: 131 iodine: Medical use. Carcinogenic and genetic effects, *Ann Endocrinol* (Paris) 57(3):166-76, 1996.

80. Sekine N, Yamamoto M, Michikawa M, et al: Rhabdomyolysis and acute renal failure in a patient with hypothyroidism, *Intern Med* 32:269-71, 1993.

81. Silverberg S, Shane E, Jacobs T et al: A 10-year prospective study of primary hyperparathyroidism with or without parathyroid surgery, *N Engl J Med* 341(17):1249-56, 1999.

82. Simons DG, Travell JG, Simons LS: *Travell & Simons' myofascial pain and dysfunction: the trigger point manual*, vol 1, Williams and Wilkins, Baltimore, 1999.

83. Sinacore DR: Healing times of pedal ulcers in diabetic immunosuppressed patients after transplantation, *Arch Phys Med Rehabil* 80(8):935-40, 1999.

84. Sinacore DR, Gulve EA: The role of skeletal muscle in glucose transport, glucose homeostasis, and insulin resistance: implications for physical therapy, *Phys Ther* 73:878-91, 1993.

85. Slovenkai M: Getting and keeping—a leg up on diabetes-related foot problems, *J Musculoskel Med* 15(12):46-54, 1998.

86. Smeltzer S, Bare B: *Brunner and Suddarth's textbook of medical-surgical nursing*, ed 9, Philadelphia, 2000, Lippincott.

87. Swedler WI, Baak S, Lazarevic MB et al: Rheumatic changes in diabetes: shoulder, arm, and hand, *J Musculoskel Med* 12:45-52, 1995.

88. Trivalle C, Doucet J, Chassagne P et al: Differences in the signs and symptoms of hyperthyroidism in older and younger patients, *J Am Geriatr Soc* 44(1):50-3, 1996.

89. Van Cauter E, Plat L, Leproult R et al: Alterations of circadian rhythmicity and sleep in aging: endocrine consequences, *Horm Res* 49(3-4):147-52, 1998.

90. Veldhuis JD: Nature of altered pulsatile hormone release and neuroendocrine network signaling in human aging: clinical studies of the somatotropic, gonadotropic, corticotropic and insulin axes, *Novartis Found Symp* 227:163-85, 2000.

91. Vliet EL: *Screaming to be heard: hormonal connections women suspect ... and doctors ignore*, New York, 1995, M Evans and Co.

92. Wagner KD: Altered glucose metabolism. In Kidd P, Wagner KD, editors: *High acuity nursing*, ed 2, Stamford, Conn, 1997, Appleton and Lange, pp 565-90.

93. Wartofsky L: Diseases of the thyroid. In Fauci A, Brunwold E, Isselbacher K et al, editors: *Harrison's principles of internal medicine*, ed 14, New York, 1998, McGraw-Hill, pp 2018-30.

94. Wei M, Gibbons L, Mitchell T, Kampert J et al: The association between cardiorespiratory fitness and fasting glucose and type 2 DM in men, *Ann Intern Med* (130):89-96, 1999.

95. Williams G, Dluhy R: Diseases of the adrenal cortex. In Fauci A, Brunwold E, Isselbacher K et al, editors: *Harrison's principles of internal medicine*, ed 14, New York, 1998, McGraw-Hill.

96. Wilson J: Endocrinology and metabolism. In Fauci A, Brunwold E, Isselbacher K et al, editors: *Harrison's principles of internal medicine*, ed 14, New York, 1998, McGraw-Hill, pp 1965-98.

97. Wilson JD, Foster DW: *Williams' textbook of endocrinology*, ed 9, Philadelphia, 1998, WB Saunders.

CHAPTER 11

THE CARDIOVASCULAR SYSTEM

CATHERINE C. GOODMAN

The cardiovascular system functions in coordination with the pulmonary system to circulate oxygenated blood through the arterial system to all cells. The deoxygenated blood is then collected from the venous system and delivered to the lungs for reoxygenation (Fig. 11-1). Pathologic conditions of the cardiovascular system are varied, multiple, and complex. This chapter presents cardiovascular structure and function according to how diseases affect each individual part, including diseases of the heart muscle, cardiac nervous system, heart valves, pericardium, and blood vessels. Other factors, such as surgery, pregnancy, and complications from other pathologic conditions (e.g., collagen vascular diseases,* acquired immunodeficiency syndrome [AIDS], cancer treatment, metabolic diseases) can also adversely affect the normal function of the cardiovascular system. Discussion of these additional factors is limited in this chapter (see specific chapters for each subject).

A section reporting gender differences as these relate to the cardiovascular system and diseases has been added. Whenever possible, ethnicity as it relates to cardiovascular diseases is included in each section. Ethnic differences are an area just coming under closer review, and the knowledge available is limited at this time.

SIGNS AND SYMPTOMS OF CARDIOVASCULAR DISEASE

Cardinal symptoms of cardiac disease usually include chest, neck, or arm pain or discomfort; palpitations; dyspnea; syncope (fainting); fatigue; cough; and cyanosis. Edema and leg pain (claudication) are the most common symptoms of the vascular component of cardiovascular pathologic conditions. Symptoms of cardiovascular involvement should be reviewed by system as well (Table 11-1).

Chest pain or discomfort is a common presenting symptom of cardiovascular disease and must be evaluated carefully. Chest pain of systemic origin may be cardiac or noncardiac and may radiate to the neck, jaw, upper trapezius, upper back, shoulder, or arms (most commonly the left arm). Radiating pain down the arm is in the pattern of ulnar nerve distribution. Noncardiac chest pain can be caused by an extensive list of disorders and is not covered in this text. Cardiac-related chest pain may arise secondary to ischemia, myocardial infarction

(MI), pericarditis, endocarditis, mitral valve prolapse, or aortic dissection with or without aneurysm. Location and description (frequency, intensity, duration) vary according to the underlying pathologic condition (see each individual condition). Chest pain is often accompanied by associated signs and symptoms, such as nausea, vomiting, diaphoresis, dyspnea, fatigue, pallor, or syncope. Cardiac chest pain or discomfort can also occur when coronary circulation is normal, as in the case of anemia causing lack of oxygenation of the myocardium (heart muscle) during physical exertion although this situation is uncommon.

Palpitations, the presence of an irregular heartbeat, may also be referred to as arrhythmias or dysrhythmias, which may be caused by a relatively benign condition (e.g., mitral valve prolapse, athlete's heart, caffeine, anxiety, exercise) or a severe condition (e.g., coronary artery disease [CAD], cardiomyopathy, complete heart block, ventricular aneurysm, atrioventricular valve disease, mitral or aortic stenosis). Palpitations may occur as a response to the bursts of adrenaline in the brain that occur with drops in estrogen levels, as a response to excess or erratic production of adrenaline-type compounds associated with panic disorder, or as a result of hyperthyroidism through other mechanisms. Palpitations have been described as a bump, pound, jump, flop, flutter, or racing sensation of the heart. Associated symptoms may include light-headedness or syncope. Palpated pulse may feel rapid or irregular, as if the heart has skipped a beat. Some people report fluttering sensations in the neck rather than in the chest or thoracic area.

Dyspnea, also referred to as breathlessness or shortness of breath, can be cardiovascular in origin, but it may also occur secondary to pulmonary pathologic conditions (see also Chapter 14), trauma, fever, certain medications, or obesity. Early onset of dyspnea may be described as a sensation of having to breathe too much or as an uncomfortable feeling during breathing after exercise or exertion. Shortness of breath with mild exertion (dyspnea on exertion [DOE]) can be caused by an impaired left ventricle that is unable to contract completely. The result is an abnormal accumulation of blood in the pulmonary vasculature. Pulmonary congestion and shortness of breath then ensue. With severe compromise of the cardiovascular or pulmonary systems, dyspnea may occur at rest.

The severity of dyspnea is determined by the extent of disease; the more severe the heart disease, the more readily episodes of dyspnea occur. More extreme dyspnea includes paroxysmal nocturnal dyspnea (PND) and orthopnea. PND, which is sudden, unexplained episodes of shortness of breath,

---

*Collagen vascular disorders are now more commonly referred to as *diffuse connective tissue diseases*. See Box 11-11 for a specific listing of these diseases.

TABLE	11-1

Cardiovascular Signs and Symptoms by System

SYSTEM	SYMPTOM
General	Weakness
	Fatigue
	Weight change
	Poor exercise tolerance
Integumentary	Pressure ulcers
	Loss of body hair
	Cyanosis (lips, nail beds)
Central nervous system	Headaches
	Impaired vision
	Dizziness or syncope
Respiratory	Labored breathing, dyspnea
	Productive cough
Cardiovascular	Chest, shoulder, neck, jaw, or arm pain or discomfort
	Palpitations
	Peripheral edema
	Intermittent claudication
Genitourinary	Urinary frequency
	Nocturia
	Concentrated urine
	Decreased urinary output
Musculoskeletal	Muscular fatigue
	Myalgias
	Chest, shoulder, neck, jaw, or arm pain or discomfort
	Peripheral edema
	Intermittent claudication
Gastrointestinal	Nausea and vomiting
	Ascites (abdominal distention)

awakens a person sleeping in a supine position, because the amount of blood returning to the heart and lungs from the lower extremities increases in this position. This type of dyspnea frequently accompanies congestive heart failure (CHF). During the day, the effects of gravity in the upright position and the shunting of excessive fluid to the lower extremities permit more effective ventilation and perfusion of the lungs, keeping the lungs relatively fluid-free, depending on the degree of CHF. Orthopnea is the term used to describe breathlessness that is relieved by sitting upright, using pillows to prop the head and trunk. Orthopnea can occur anytime during the day or night.

Cardiac syncope (fainting or, in a milder form, light-headedness) can be caused by reduced oxygen to the brain. Cardiovascular conditions resulting in syncope include arrhythmias, orthostatic hypotension, aortic dissection, hypertrophic cardiomyopathy, CAD, and vertebral artery insufficiency. Predictors of syncope include a history of stroke or transient ischemic attacks, use of cardiac medication, and high blood pressure. Marginally associated risk factors also include lower body mass index, increased alcohol intake, and diabetes or elevated glucose level.

Light-headedness as a result of orthostatic hypotension (sudden drop in blood pressure) may occur with any quick change in a prolonged position (e.g., going from a supine position to an upright posture or standing up from a sitting position) or with physical exertion involving increased intraabdominal pressure (e.g., straining with a bowel movement, lifting). Any client with aortic stenosis is more likely to experience light-headedness as a result of these activities. During the period of initiation and regulation of cardiac medications (e.g., vasodilators), side effects such as orthostatic hypotension may occur. Implantable loop recorders are available to assess falls associated with syncope of unknown cause. Implantable recorders allow for continuous electrocardiograph (ECG) monitoring for recurrent but infrequent syncope.

Noncardiac conditions, such as anxiety and emotional stress, migraine headaches, seizures, or psychiatric conditions, can cause hyperventilation and subsequent light-headedness.

Fatigue provoked by minimal exertion indicates a lack of energy that may be cardiac in origin (e.g., CAD, aortic valve dysfunction, cardiomyopathy, myocarditis), or it may occur secondary to neurologic, muscular, metabolic, or pulmonary pathologic conditions. Often fatigue of a cardiac nature is accompanied by associated symptoms, such as dyspnea, chest pain, palpitations, or headache.

Cough (see also Chapter 14) is usually associated with pulmonary conditions but may occur as a pulmonary complication of a cardiovascular pathologic condition. Left ventricular dysfunction, including mitral valve dysfunction as with resulting pulmonary edema, may result in a cough when aggravated by exercise, metabolic stress, supine position, or PND. The cough is often hacking and may be productive of large amounts of frothy, blood-tinged sputum. In the case of CHF, cough develops because a large amount of fluid is trapped in the pulmonary tree, irritating the lung mucosa. A persistent, dry cough can develop as a side effect of some cardiovascular medications (see Table 11-4).

Cyanosis is a bluish discoloration of the lips and nail beds of the fingers and toes that accompanies inadequate blood oxygen levels (reduced amounts of oxygenated hemoglobin). Although cyanosis can accompany cardiac, pulmonary, hematologic, or central nervous system (CNS) disorders, visible cyanosis most often accompanies cardiac and pulmonary problems.

Peripheral edema is the hallmark of right ventricular failure; it is usually bilateral and dependent and may be accompanied by jugular venous distention (JVD; see Fig. 11-13), cyanosis (lips, appendages), and abdominal distention from ascites (see Fig. 16-4). Right upper quadrant pain, described as constant, aching, or sharp, may occur secondary to an enlarged liver with this condition. Right-sided heart failure and subsequent edema can also occur as a result of cardiac surgery, venous valve incompetence or obstruction, cardiac valve stenosis, CAD, or mitral valve dysfunction. Noncardiac causes of edema may include pulmonary hypertension resulting in right-sided heart failure, kidney dysfunction, cirrhosis, burns, infection, lymphatic obstruction, or allergic reaction.

Claudication, sometimes described as cramping or leg pain, is brought on with a consistent amount of exercise or activity. It develops as a result of peripheral vascular disease (PVD) (arterial or venous), often occurring simultaneously with CAD. Claudication can be more functionally debilitating than other associated symptoms, such as angina or dyspnea, and may occur in addition to these other symptoms. The presence of pitting edema along with leg pain is usually associated

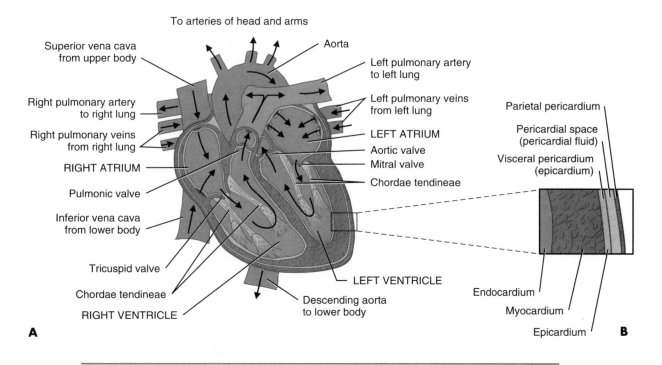

To arteries of head and arms

Superior vena cava
from upper body

Aorta

Left pulmonary artery
to left lung

Right pulmonary artery
to right lung

Left pulmonary veins
from left lung

Right pulmonary veins
from right lung

LEFT ATRIUM

Aortic valve

RIGHT ATRIUM

Mitral valve

Chordae tendineae

Pulmonic valve

Inferior vena cava
from lower body

Tricuspid valve

LEFT VENTRICLE

Chordae tendineae

Descending aorta
to lower body

RIGHT VENTRICLE

A

Parietal pericardium

Pericardial space
(pericardial fluid)

Visceral pericardium
(epicardium)

Endocardium

Myocardium

Epicardium

B

FIGURE   **11-1   A,** Structure and circulation of the heart. Blood flows from the superior and inferior venae cavae into the right atrium through the tricuspid valve to the right ventricle. The right ventricle ejects the blood through the pulmonic valve into the pulmonary artery during ventricular systole. Blood enters the pulmonary capillary system where it exchanges the carbon dioxide for oxygen. The oxygenated blood then leaves the lungs via the pulmonary veins and returns to the left atrium. From the left atrium, blood flows through the mitral valve into the left ventricle. The left ventricle pumps blood into the systemic circulation through the aorta to supply all the tissues of the body. From the systemic circulation, blood returns to the heart through the superior and inferior venae cavae to begin the cycle again. **B,** Sagittal view of the layers of the heart.

with venous disease. Other noncardiac causes of leg pain (e.g., sciatica, pseudoclaudication,* anterior compartment syndrome, gout, peripheral neuropathy) must be differentiated from pain associated with PVD.

---

*Low back pain associated with *pseudoclaudication* often indicates spinal stenosis. The typical person affected is approximately 60 years old and bothered less by back pain than by a discomfort occurring in the buttock, thigh, or leg that (like true claudication) is brought on by walking but (unlike true claudication) can also be elicited by prolonged standing. The discomfort associated with pseudoclaudication is frequently bilateral and improves with rest or with flexion of the lumbar spine.

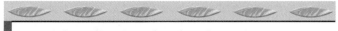

Special Implications for the Therapist   **11-1**

SIGNS AND SYMPTOMS OF CARDIOVASCULAR DISEASE

As part of the evaluation, the physical therapist will assess cardiac signs and symptoms, assess the degree of risk of an adverse cardiac event, assess the type and degree of impairment (dysfunction at the level of the tissue, organ or organ system, and circulation), assess the level of disability (difficulty performing activities of daily life), and assess functional limitations (restrictions in the ability to perform specific actions).[59]

In some cases, monitoring individuals closely and minimizing risk of an adverse event are a priority (e.g., the person with oxygen transport impairment with or without symptoms). If the individual is symptomatic, recommendations are given to minimize life-threatening risks; interventions are directed at the underlying impairments whenever possible. As a general guideline, the therapist monitors the unstable cardiac client (whether or not an initial ECG readout is available) during initial exercise to keep intensity lower than the threshold at which cardiac symptoms appear. In other cases, when the degree of risk is low, the need for monitoring may be reduced accordingly and treatment can be less conservative.[59]

The evaluation and intervention strategies for clients with cardiac symptoms described go beyond the scope of this text, and the clinician is referred to any of the specific cardiopulmonary texts available. Special implications included in this chapter should be supplemented by other such materials. An excellent review of physiologic measures in a cardiopulmonary setting in relation to the Preferred Practice Patterns listed in the Guide is also available.[59]

Signs and Symptoms

Cervical disk disease and arthritic changes can mimic atypical *chest pain* requiring screening for medical disease. Pain of cardiac origin can be experienced in the shoulder because the heart (and diaphragm) are supplied by the C5-6 spinal seg-

Continued

ment, which refers visceral pain to the corresponding somatic area. Chest pain attributed to trigger points and other noncardiac causes is discussed in detail elsewhere.[91]

Palpitations lasting for hours or occurring in association with pain, shortness of breath, fainting, or severe light-headedness or dizziness require medical evaluation. Palpitations in any person with a personal history of cardiac disease or a family history of unexplained sudden death require medical referral. Clients describing palpitations or similar phenomena may not be experiencing symptoms of heart disease. Palpitations can be considered physiologic (i.e., fewer than six occur per minute may be considered within the normal function of the heart), or they may occur as a result of an overactive thyroid, secondary to caffeine sensitivity, as a side effect of some medications, during menopause when estrogen levels decline, and through the use of drugs, such as cocaine. Encourage the client to report any such symptoms to the physician if this has not already been brought to the physician's attention. ECG monitoring of the heart's electrical impulses along with a diary of symptoms while wearing the monitor is most often used to identify the underlying condition. See also the section on Arrhythmias: Disturbances of Rate or Rhythm in this chapter.

Before referring the client to the physician, the therapist can help the client characterize the symptom or symptoms by asking a series of questions: Is the sensation long-lasting or transient? Palpitations that begin and end abruptly are more often true sustained arrhythmias. Episodes that gradually appear and disappear tend to be normal alterations in heart rhythm. Does anything precipitate the symptom or symptoms? Eliminating possible triggers (e.g., caffeine) one at a time may reduce or eliminate palpitations. Is there an association between hormonal status and palpitations (e.g., onset or change in frequency associated with ovulation or start or stop of menstruation)? If exercise brings on the palpitations, ventricular tachycardia may be the underlying cause. On the other hand, sometimes starting an exercise program reduces the frequency of palpitations. Some people find that deep breathing, coughing, or relaxation can stop the symptom when it begins. If fainting occurs with the palpitations and there is a family history of sudden death, there may be an inherited cardiomyopathy or primary arrhythmia. For the experienced clinician, auscultation may provide additional useful information. Gathering this type of information for the physician's consideration can be very helpful in making the medical diagnosis.

Dyspnea may be a sign of poor physical conditioning, obesity, or asthma or allergies. Anyone who cannot climb a single flight of stairs without feeling moderately to severely winded or who awakens at night or experiences shortness of breath when lying down should be evaluated by a physician. Anyone with known cardiac involvement in whom progressively worse dyspnea develops must also notify the physician of these findings. Dyspnea relieved by specific breathing patterns (e.g., pursed-lip breathing) or by specific body positions (e.g., leaning forward on arms to lock the shoulder girdle) is more likely to be pulmonary than cardiac in origin. Because breathlessness can be a terrifying experience, any activity that provokes the sensation is avoided, which quickly reduces functional activities. Pulmonary rehabilitation can favorably influence both exertional and clinically assessed dyspnea. The therapist is key in preventing this vicious circle and in delaying decline of function in the cardiopulmonary population.

Syncope without any warning period of light-headedness, dizziness, or nausea may be a sign of heart valve or arrhythmia problems but rarely occurs as a result of myocardial ischemia. Sudden death can occur; therefore medical referral is recommended for any unexplained syncope, especially in the presence of heart or circulatory problems or if the client has any risk factors for heart attack or stroke.

Physical therapy orthopedic examination of the cervical spine may include vertebral artery tests for compression of the vertebral arteries that can contribute to the development of syncope. Specific test procedures are available.[14,147,192] Traditionally, if signs of eye nystagmus, changes in pupil size, or report of visual disturbances and symptoms of dizziness or light-headedness occurred, this was considered an indication of vertebral artery compromise requiring special care with any subsequent intervention. However, the effect of these tests (known as the vertebral basal artery test, vertebral artery compression test, Wallenberg test, or the de Kleyn hanging head test) on blood flow velocity has come under question. For example, the extension-rotation test as a valid clinical screening procedure to detect decreased blood flow in the vertebral artery has been reviewed with variable results. Although one study found it to be a useful test of the adequacy of collateral circulation[193] it has been suggested that other factors, such as individual sensitivity to extreme head positions, age, and vestibular responsiveness, could affect the results of this test for vertebral artery compression.[54,230] Larger studies are needed to determine whether subjects testing positive significantly differ from those testing negative.

Athletes may experience neurocardiogenic syncope (neurally mediated hypotension; also known as vasodepressor syncope, vasovagal attack), a benign noncardiac cause of fainting in athletes. This disorder of autonomic cardiovascular regulation (i.e., blood pressure control system) is precipitated by prolonged standing after exertion, a warm environment, or stress, or it may occur during or after exercise and is not life-threatening. Fainting during exertion should always be evaluated by medical personnel.

Fatigue beyond expectations during or after exercise, especially in a client with a known cardiac condition, must be closely monitored. It should be remembered that beta-blockers prescribed for cardiac problems can also cause unusual fatigue symptoms. For the client experiencing fatigue without a prior diagnosis of heart disease, monitoring vital signs may indicate a failure of the blood pressure to rise with increasing workloads. Such a situation may indicate inadequate cardiac output* to meet the demands of exercise. However, poor exercise tolerance is often the result of deconditioning, especially in the older adult population. Further testing (e.g., exercise treadmill test) may be helpful in determining whether fatigue is related to cardiac problems.

Peripheral edema in the form of a 3-lb or greater weight gain or gradual, continuous gain over several days with swelling of the ankles, abdomen, and hands, and shortness of breath, fatigue, and dizziness may be a red flag symptom of CHF. When such symptoms persist despite rest, medical referral is required. Edema of a cardiac origin may require ECG monitoring during exercise or activity (the physician may not want the client stressed when extensive ECG changes are present), whereas

---

*Cardiac output is the amount of blood that the heart is able to pump per minute and is directly affected by stroke volume (the amount the ventricle pumps out with each heartbeat) and the heart rate (the number of heartbeats per minute).

edema of peripheral origin requires medical treatment of the underlying cause.

Claudication may occur in the absence of physical findings, but it is usually accompanied by skin discoloration and trophic changes (e.g., thin, dry, hairless skin) in the presence of vascular disease. Core temperature, peripheral pulses, and skin temperature should be assessed. Cool skin is more indicative of vascular obstruction; warm to hot skin may indicate inflammation or infection. Abrupt onset of ischemic rest pain or sudden worsening of intermittent claudication may be due to thromboembolism and must be reported to the physician immediately. If persons with intermittent claudication have normal-appearing skin at rest, exercising the extremity to the point of claudication usually produces marked pallor of the skin over the distal one third of the extremity. This postexercise cutaneous ischemia occurs in both upper and lower extremities and is due to selective shunting of the available blood to the exercised muscle and away from the more distal parts of the extremity. ■

AGING AND THE CARDIOVASCULAR SYSTEM

Cardiovascular disease, especially coronary atherosclerosis, is the most common cause of hospitalization and death in the older population in the United States. With the aging of America, by the year 2030, nearly 50% of all Americans will be 45 years old or older. By that time the number of people 65 years and older will more than double and the population 85 years and older is expected to triple.[168] With this increase in the number of older persons, cardiovascular disease is likely to be even more of a major health problem in the future.

Aging of the heart is associated with a number of typical morphologic, histologic, and biochemical changes although not all observed changes with age are associated with deterioration in function. The high prevalence of hypertension and ischemic heart disease makes distinction between normal aging changes and the effects of underlying cardiovascular disease processes difficult. Disease-independent changes in the aging heart associated with a reduction in function include (1) reduction in the number of myocytes and cells within the conduction tissue, (2) the development of cardiac fibrosis, (3) a reduction in calcium transport across membranes, (4) lower capillary density, (5) decreases in the intracellular response to beta-adrenergic stimulation (sometimes referred to as blunted beta-adrenoceptor responsiveness), and (6) impaired autonomic reflex control of heart rate.[194]

Other characteristic changes, such as epicardial fat deposition and "brown atrophy" caused by intracellular lipofuscin deposits, appear to be signs of the aging process but without any obvious effects on function. The hearts of older subjects, even fit, healthy, and active subjects, pump less blood to the skin and require the heart of the older person to work much harder under the same circumstances (e.g., exercise in warm environments) as a younger person. None of these changes have clinical relevance at rest but may have considerable consequences during cardiovascular stress, such as occurs with increased flow demand (e.g., exercise, postoperative), demand for acute autonomic reflex control (e.g., change in posture), or severe disease (e.g., uncontrolled hypertension, tachyarrhythmias, myocardial ischemia). Physiologic aging is accompanied by a progressive decline in resting organ function. Con-

sequently, the reserve capacity to compensate for impaired organ function, heat, drug metabolism, and added physiologic demands is impaired and functional disability will occur more quickly and take longer to resolve.[187]

The heart itself undergoes some changes associated with advancing age, such as moderate thickening of the left ventricular wall (exaggerated in hypertensive clients) and increased left atrial size. Thickening of the cardiac tissue occurs as a result of myocyte enlargement or replacement by fibrous tissue, but overall enlarging or atrophy of the aging heart is not representative of normative aging. Decreased ventricular filling compensated by increased systolic blood pressure occurs as a result of the changes in the ventricular wall. Left ventricular functioning is compromised in the presence of stress such as vigorous exercise or disease. Arrhythmia or hypertension may occur as a result. The vasculature changes with aging as the arterial walls stiffen with age and the aorta becomes dilated and elongated. The incidence and severity of atherosclerosis do increase with aging, and this contributes to changes in vasculature function. Calcium deposition and changes in the amount and loss of elasticity in elastin and collagen most often affect the larger and medium-sized vessels. The unpredictable interaction between age-related and disease-associated changes in all organ functions (including the heart) and the altered neurohormonal response to various forms of stress in the aging older adult may result in atypical clinical presentations of disease delaying diagnosis and medical intervention.[143, 187]

Resting cardiac function (e.g., cardiac output, heart rate) shows minimal age-related changes; a small increase in stroke volume may occur. Changes in functional capacity are more apparent during exercise than at rest. The maximal heart rate or the highest heart rate during exercise does decline with age, possibly because of a decreased cardiovascular response to catecholamines. This decline in maximal heart rate is reflected in the target zone heart rates for exercising senior citizens. See Appendix B for calculation of target heart rates for sedentary and physically fit older adults. The effect of the Frank-Starling mechanism* is unaltered with age and is used effectively during exercise to maintain cardiac output through a higher stroke volume.

It is commonly accepted that a decline in maximal oxygen uptake, heart rate, and reduced maximal cardiac output with aging occurs during exercise, even in older athletes. These cardiovascular alterations parallel changes that occur with deconditioning or disuse, including the decrease in maximal oxygen intake and maximal cardiac output. These functions normalize with increased activity, and exercise can reverse some of the age-associated changes in the heart at least partially,[194] supporting the hypothesis that age-related cardiovascular changes are simply the result of inactivity. In older people, aerobic exercise training lowers heart rate at rest, reduces heart rate and levels of plasma catecholamine at the same absolute submaximal workload, improves heat tolerance,[231] and, at least in men, improves left ventricular perfor-

---

*The Frank-Starling law states that the greater the myocardial fiber length (or stretch), the greater will be its force of contraction. The more the left ventricle fills with blood, the greater will be the quantity of blood ejected into the aorta. This is like a rubber band: The more it is stretched, the stronger it recoils or snaps back. Thus a direct relationship exists between the volume of blood in the heart at the end of diastole (the length of the muscle fibers) and the force of contraction during the next systole.

mance during peak exercise.[202] It may be that the effect of training is relatively greater in older subjects.

Although the specific organ changes associated with aging are discussed here, disease and lifestyle may have a greater impact on cardiovascular function than aging. Research now shows that even children need to control their modifiable risk factors for heart disease. Heart studies of adolescents and young adults who have died from accidental causes demonstrate that heart disease begins earlier than formerly expected. Cholesterol deposits and blood vessel changes have been demonstrated in early adolescence with substantial changes observed by age 30 years in some people. As the arteries age, increased collagen and calcium content and progressive deterioration of the arterial media combined with atherosclerotic plaque formation result in stiff arterial walls, increased systolic blood pressure, and increased fatigue of arterial walls, all of which accelerate arterial damage, producing a self-perpetuating cycle.

Finally, although the benefits of physical activity and exercise among older persons are becoming increasingly clear, the role of exercise stress testing and safety monitoring for older people who want to start an exercise program is unclear. Current guidelines regarding exercise stress testing may not be applicable to the majority of adults aged 75 years or older who are interested in restoring or enhancing their physical function through a program of physical activity and exercise. Recommendations and precautions to minimize the risk of adverse cardiac events among previously sedentary older adults who do not have symptomatic cardiovascular disease and are interested in starting an exercise program are available.[86] The therapist is very instrumental in conducting an examination and performing exercise testing to identify the specific level of pathology, impairment, or functional limitations. An individual exercise prescription is made (mode, intensity, duration, frequency) based on the results of the examination and testing.

GENDER DIFFERENCES AND THE CARDIOVASCULAR SYSTEM

Interest in gender differences in all of medicine but especially the cardiovascular system has come to the forefront in the new millennium. Only a small, representative portion of the new information now available can be presented here; the reader is referred to other more complete sources.[140,141] Female hearts not only are smaller than male hearts but also are constructed differently and respond to age and hypertrophic stimuli differently. Structural differences in the mitral valve may explain why women are more prone to mitral valve prolapse than men. At puberty, a young woman's QT interval* lengthens, and the woman with an extra long QT interval is at greater risk for a serious form of ventricular arrhythmia (known as *torsades de pointes*) and sudden cardiac death, especially when taking drugs that prolong the QT interval.[20]

Left ventricular mass increases with age in healthy women but remains constant in men. Under increased cardiac loading

conditions (e.g., hypertension, aortic stenosis) this disparity between genders is even more obvious, especially in adults older than 50 years.[104] Women also have a three times greater risk of potentially fatal arrhythmias from some cardiac and psychotropic medications.*[200] Complications from antiarrhythmic drug use are most common during the first 3 days or after a dosage increase. Women also tend to have a decreased therapeutic response to anticoagulants and from thrombolytic agents (see Table 11-4) but paradoxically, a higher incidence of bleeding episodes.

◆ Coronary Artery Disease in Women

It was long believed that CAD was a more benign process in females, but this has been soundly disproved. A woman presenting with angina postmenopausally has the exact same mortality as a man presenting with angina in his 60s. CAD is the single leading cause of death and a significant cause of morbidity among women in the United States. Certain characteristics and clinical conditions may place women at higher risk of CAD development or progression, such as depression, being black, menopausal status, age, type 2 diabetes mellitus, and thyroid function. In addition, female gender may adversely influence the relative benefits of some risk modification interventions in older adults (e.g., cholesterol lowering, sedentary behavior, smoking cessation).[119]

Many studies have suggested that women with acute MI receive less aggressive therapy than men and have a poorer outcome when treatment is received. Until recently, women in all age-groups have been less likely to undergo diagnostic catheterization than men, and this difference was especially pronounced among older women (>85 years). Women have been less likely than men to receive preventive care (drug treatment for lipid management; risk factor management through exercise, nutrition, and weight reduction), invasive treatments (revascularization procedures), and thrombolytic therapy within 60 minutes.[81,247] Women delay longer than men before seeking help for symptoms of acute MI, referred to as *decision delay*, further compromising effective treatment and improved outcomes.[195] This is especially true given the evidence that first heart attacks in women may be more severe and that women are more likely to die in the first weeks and months after a heart attack.

For many years, women and minorities were underrepresented in studies conducted on heart disease and stroke, but this has changed over the last decade along with concomitant expansion of prevention and educational outreach programs for heart attack, stroke, and other cardiovascular diseases in women. The use of noninvasive testing in women was controversial because of a perception of diminished accuracy, limited female representation, and technical limitations. Large observational studies now report marked improvements in the accuracy of results for women undergoing exercise treadmill, echocardiography, and nuclear testing as a result of expanding risk parameters in the test interpretations and improved diagnostic accuracy of such tests.[208] Because of technologic advances, improved surgical techniques, greater awareness of

---

*The QT interval is a measure of the duration of ventricular depolarization and repolarization. A prolonged period of time for depolarization prolongs the suprathreshold period of an action potential and upsets the critical influx and efflux of electrolytes during action potential activity that may predispose a person to ventricular tachycardia.

*The risk for drugs other than cardiac and psychotropic ones in causing prolongation of the QT interval has recently been recognized. It is anticipated that the list of drugs known to produce such effects will grow.[200]

gender differences in heart disease, and increased funding for gender-based research, these trends are improving and women now seem to do as well as men after surgical (revascularization) procedures to restore blood flow to the heart.

Although the American Heart Association reports a decline in death rates in women for coronary heart disease (CHD) and stroke, women are still twice as likely as men to die within 1 year of having a heart attack and women are at greater risk for second heart attacks and for disability because of heart failure. The death rate for stroke among black women is 33.7% higher than for white women and 69% higher for heart disease.[8,12] Many women die of CHD without any warning signs and by age 65 years one in four women has heart disease (the same proportion as in men). CHD claims the lives of nearly 250,000 women annually in the United States, compared with 40,200 from breast cancer and 63,000 from lung cancer. Despite these statistics, misperceptions still exist that cardiovascular disease is not a real problem for women and that, despite the fact that some risk factors for CHD can be prevented, CHD is not curable. For these reasons, education and prevention are vitally important to reduce risk of heart disease.

◆ Coronary Artery Surgery and Women

The number of women undergoing coronary artery bypass surgery (CABG, pronounced "cabbage") has continued to increase (from 146,000 in 1995 to 237,000 in 2001).[12] Women may experience more chest wall discomfort as a common side effect of CABG than men, most often reported in those women who had an internal mammary artery graft (IMA). Following angioplasty (or bypass surgery), the rates of complication and mortality among women are similar to men with a slightly higher mortality in women within the first 30 days. This difference in outcome is attributed to older age and greater co-morbidity of women rather than a difference in the use of therapeutic modalities, including thrombolysis and invasive coronary procedures.[95]

◆ Hormonal Status

Influence of Hormones on Coronary Artery Disease.
Estrogen has been considered a cardioprotective benefit for women via a variety of mechanisms. It stimulates the formation of high-density lipoprotein (HDL), the good cholesterol, which carries plaque away from the artery wall and back to the liver to be broken down and excreted while also stimulating low-density lipoprotein (LDL) receptors in the liver and possibly the walls of arterial blood vessels. These receptors bind the LDL, which removes LDL from the circulation and from its damaging effects in plaque formation. Estradiol acts as a calcium-channel blocker to relax artery walls, which helps dilate the arteries, improves blood flow throughout the brain and body, and helps to reduce blood pressure. Estrogen maintains the normal balance of prostacyclin and thromboxane, two chemicals that regulate clot formation. Estrogen increases artery production of prostacyclin, which improves blood flow and reduces platelet aggregation. Estrogen receptors have located molecules that attract and bind to estrogen in the cells of the smooth muscle layer of blood vessels. Atherosclerosis may develop because blood vessel cells cannot extract needed estrogen from the blood without the necessary receptors. Another possible mechanism by which estrogen protects against heart disease before menopause is the release of endothelium-derived relaxing factor (EDRF, thought to be nitric oxide), a chemical stimulated by estrogen and responsible for dilating blood vessels to maintain normal pressure and flow.* As women lose the biologically active estradiol, gender differences become gender similarities and the incidence of cardiovascular disease (CVD) increases dramatically, matching the incidence among men within 10 years of menopause without hormone replacement therapy.

Myocardial ischemia may be more easily induced when estrogen concentrations are low, a finding that may be important for timing the assessment and evaluating treatment in women with CHD. Early follicular phase, when estradiol and progesterone concentrations are low, may be associated with poor exercise performance as measured by onset to myocardial ischemia. These findings are preliminary and have not been reproduced or confirmed.

Hormone Replacement for Postmenopausal Women.
The use of hormones for cardioprotection has been under investigation for many years. Because heart attacks tend to occur 10 years later in women than in men, it was assumed that the protective effect of estrogen was responsible. Exogenous (externally administered) estrogen has been reported to improve plasma lipid profiles, carbohydrate metabolism, and vascular reactivity, but surprisingly, hormonal therapy does not alter the progression of CAD or protect against MI or coronary death. The Heart and Estrogen/Progestin Replacement Study (HERS) failed to demonstrate cardioprotection and even showed an early adverse outcome in women with documented CHD who received daily hormone replacement therapy. Several large randomized clinical trials for primary and secondary prevention are under way.[100,113]

Fifty percent of all women who have had a hysterectomy (without removal of the ovaries) and all women who have an oophorectomy (ovary removal) become endocrinologically menopausal by 3 years after surgery, regardless of age. Their heart disease risk increases when they become menopausal regardless of their age or the means by which menopause occurs.

Oral Contraceptives.   Studies show that women smokers over 35 years who use oral contraceptives are much more likely to have a heart attack or stroke than nonsmokers who use birth control pills. In the last 20 years, cardiovascular complications in all women taking oral contraceptives have become less common because current contraceptives contain the lowest dose of estrogen possible without breakthrough bleeding.[12] At this dose, the risk of thromboembolic disease is reduced to about 40 events per 100,000 women per year, approximately the same risk as in the general population.[36] However, much debate continues about the use of so-called third-generation (newest) oral contaceptives containing low doses of estrogen and a type of progestin known as *desogestrel*. Women taking this contraceptive are twice as likely to develop superficial venous blood clots compared to women taking second-generation oral contraceptives containing progestins, such as levonorgestrel and norethindrone. It is

---

*Endothelium-derived nitrous oxide (NO) is an important mediator of exercise-induced changes in skeletal muscle blood flow. Given the recently documented effects of estrogens on NO synthase, it was hypothesized that oral contraceptives containing estrogen would increase NO production at rest and after endurance exercise. These proposed findings have not been substantiated.

estimated that 425 ischemic strokes are attributed to oral contraceptives each year in the United States even with the newer low-estrogen preparations.[87]

◆ Hypertension in Women

More women than men eventually develop hypertension in the United States because of their higher numbers and longer longevity. White coat hypertension (rise in blood pressure when being evaluated by a physician or other health care worker) and hypertension among blacks are more prevalent among women. Alcohol,* obesity, and oral contraceptives are important causes of rise in blood pressure among women. Women with left ventricular hypertrophy are at greater risk of death than men. Angiotensin-converting enzyme (ACE) inhibitors and angiotensin receptor blockers are contraindicated in pregnancy and should be avoided in women with childbearing potential.[189]

◆ Cholesterol Concerns for Women

The National Heart, Lung, and Blood Institute estimates that more than half of all women over age 55 years need to lower their blood cholesterol. In the past, women with high blood cholesterol were less likely to receive appropriate cholesterol-lowering therapy than men and when they did receive drug therapy, dosages were often inadequate. Women have better outcomes from treatment for hyperlipidemia than men— sometimes lowering their risk of heart attack by twice as much.

Reference guides for cholesterol testing and recommendations based on lipid levels have not been standardized for women. Whether the current established guidelines (based on data derived from studies of men) are most appropriate for women remains unknown. After menopause, women have higher concentrations of total cholesterol than men do, but the significance of this finding remains unknown. Research results at this time suggest that women need higher levels of the good cholesterol (HDL)† for protection against heart disease and that other blood markers, such as serum triglycerides and homocysteine, may play more meaningful roles in defining women's heart disease risk. Low levels of HDL cholesterol are predictive of CHD in women and appear to be a stronger risk factor for women older than 65 years than for men of the same age.[164]

DISEASES AFFECTING THE HEART MUSCLE

◆ Ischemic Heart Disease

Coronary arteries carry oxygen to the myocardium. When these arteries become narrowed or blocked, the areas of the heart muscle supplied by that artery become ischemic and injured, and infarction may result. Major disorders of the myocardium owing to insufficient blood supply are collectively

known as ischemic heart disease, coronary heart disease (CHD), or coronary artery disease (CAD).

Despite improved clinical care, heightened public awareness, and widespread use of health innovations, atherosclerotic diseases and their thrombotic complications remain the number one cause of mortality and morbidity in the United States (see Table 2-1). An estimated 12 million persons in the United States have CHD. Of the 1.1 million who are expected to have a CHD event during 2001, approximately 650,000 will be first events and 450,000 will be recurrences. Each year approximately 220,000 fatal CHD events occur suddenly among unhospitalized people. Eleven million Americans who are alive today have a history of angina pectoris, MI, or both, and an estimated 2 million middle-aged and older adults (>75 years) have silent myocardial ischemia.[163] Although CHD death rates in the United States have decreased since reaching a peak during the late 1960s (146.2 cases per 100,000 in 1948 with a peak of 220.3 in 1963 to 87 cases per 100,000 in 1996), a decline in the incidence of coronary disease has not been achieved. In 1940, the rate of cardiovascular disease was 26.4 per 100,000 people compared to 173.5 in 2000.[11] The declining mortality rate does not apply to those adults with diabetes and has been attributed to improvements in lifestyle (e.g., reduced smoking in men, improved treatment for lipid lowering, improved coronary care) whereas the increased incidence may be related to the increasing number of people who are surviving past age 65 years.

Nonatherosclerotic causes of coronary artery obstruction and subsequent ischemic heart disease (Box 11-1) are uncommon; each of these conditions is discussed more completely elsewhere in this chapter. Mediastinal radiotherapy for left-sided breast cancer, Hodgkin's disease, or non-Hodgkin's disease may be an independent risk factor in the development of ischemic heart disease. Radiotherapy causes cardiac perfusion defects 6 months after treatment in most people, but it remains unknown if these changes are transient or permanent. Improvements in radiation technique have reduced complications, especially late cardiac deaths. At the present time, the benefit of treatment for operable breast cancer for individuals who may be cured of the disease appears to outweigh the risks

---

*Alcohol is known to have specific toxic effects on heart muscle fibers, and excessive alcohol consumption is increasing in women; yet women are less likely than men to be identified as alcohol abusers at early stages of the illness and are less often referred for alcohol treatment until later stages of abuse, when cardiac and other severe complications have occurred.[241]

†Total cholesterol is broken into HDL, or good cholesterol, which carries cholesterol away from the cells, and LDL, or bad cholesterol, which carries cholesterol to the cells. A helpful way to remember the function of these is to think of HDL as "Healthy" or beneficial cholesterol and LDL as "Lousy" or detrimental cholesterol. Lipoproteins are complexes that help dissolve, transport, and utilize the cholesterol molecule. For normal reference values see Table 39-12. For target measurement, see Table 11-3.

BOX **11-1**

Nonatherosclerotic Causes of Coronary Artery Obstruction

Kawasaki disease	Arteritis
Coronary embolism	Syphilis
Infective endocarditis	Polyarteritis nodosa
Prosthetic valves	Lupus erythematosus
Cardiac myxomas	Rheumatoid arthritis
Cardiopulmonary bypass	Connective tissue diseases
Coronary arteriography	Radiotherapy
Syndrome X	
Insulin resistance syndrome	
(hyperinsulinemia)	
Trauma to coronary arteries	
Penetrating	
Nonpenetrating	

TABLE	11-3

Heart Disease Prevention Target Measurements*

RISK FACTORS	TARGETS
Body Measurements	
• Body mass index (BMI): multiply your weight in pounds by 700, then divide that number by the square of your height in inches	18.5-24.9 (see also Table 2-5)†
• Waist/hip ratio (WHR): divide your waist measurement in inches by your hip measurement in inches	≤0.8
Lipids, Lipoproteins	
• Total cholesterol	<200 mg/dL
• HDL cholesterol	≥40 mg/dL (men)‡
	≥50 mg/dL (women)‡
• LDL cholesterol	≤130 mg/dL (optimal: 100 mg/dL)‡
• Triglycerides	≤200 mg/dL (<150 mg/dL)‡
• Total cholesterol/HDL ratio	<4.5
Blood Pressure	<140/90 mm Hg and lower if tolerated (optimal: 120/80 mm Hg); some sources suggest the following:
	130/85 mm Hg = normal
	139/89 mm Hg = high normal
	140/90 mm Hg = high risk

*These target measures are for healthy adults without evidence of heart disease.
†Federal guideline standards as represented here may be overly restrictive when applied to adults >74 yr. Studies do not support overweight (as opposed to obesity) as conferring an excess mortality risk.[106]
‡The current standard for all adults is set at ≥35 mg/dL. Proposed targets of ≥40 mg/dL for men and ≥50 mg/dL for women are the new guidelines from the National Heart, Lung, and Blood Institute.[171] Some experts recommend 55 mg/dL or higher for women, but this remains unproven and is under investigation.

greater effect on reducing the incidence of ischemic heart disease than the modification of the other three risk factors. Regular aerobic exercise lowers resting pulse rate and blood pressure, improves the ratio of good to bad cholesterol, and helps prevent and control diabetes and osteoporosis. The risk of heart attack and death from heart disease declines steadily as the frequency of vigorous exercise increases. Occasional exercise (one or two times per week) reduces the risk of heart attack by 36%, moderate exercise (three or four times per week) reduces it by 38%, and regular, vigorous exercise (five or more times per week) reduces it by 46%. The benefit of habitual exercise toward reducing heart attack was greatest among those who worked out for 11 to 24 minutes and did not change or increase further after 24 minutes of exercise.[3]

Impaired glucose metabolism (e.g., insulin resistance, hyperinsulinemia, glucose intolerance) is reported to be atherogenic. Diabetes mellitus (DM), impaired glucose tolerance, and high-normal levels of glycosylated hemoglobin in the Framingham study are powerful contributors to atherosclerotic cardiovascular events.[252] The association is complex, and the pathways by which elevated insulin adversely affects both CAD risk factors and the risk of developing CAD remain unknown. The risk for CHD in participants younger than 65 years was double in men and triple in women with diabetes compared with nondiabetic counterparts. Individuals with type 2 DM have a risk of myocardial infarction equivalent to that of someone without diabetes who has had a previous MI.

Kidney disease accompanied by hypertension is a serious complication affecting the cardiovascular system among people with diabetes. More than 80% of persons who have diabetes die of some form of cardiovascular disease. Bypass surgery provides significantly better survival than angioplasty for individuals with diabetes. This may be attributed to the more extensive CAD among people with diabetes and the greater tendency for their arteries to restenose after angioplasty.

Low levels of HDL cholesterol (and high levels of triglycerides) produce twice as many cases of CAD as any other lipid abnormality; this effect is exaggerated in women (see Table 11-3). Increasing HDL cholesterol has a more cardioprotective effect in the female than in the male population. The total cholesterol/HDL cholesterol ratio is also more predictive of CAD in women than in men.

Hormonal status in the menopausal or postmenopausal woman is now known to be a likely contributing risk factor in the development of CAD. The mechanism through which a protective effect is mediated by estrogen has not been explained completely (see previous discussion in this chapter).

Modification of Risk Factors That Might Reduce Incidence of CAD. *Psychologic factors and emotional stress* (e.g., depression, anxiety, personality factors and character traits, social isolation, chronic life stress) contribute significantly to the pathogenesis and expression of CAD. People who are negative, insecure, and distressed (type D personality) are three times more likely to experience a second heart attack than non-D types.[62] Other personality traits likely to affect the heart are free-floating hostility associated with anger and a sense of time urgency (two major components of the type A personality). The long-held belief that anger can increase the risk of acute MI and can be an immediate trigger of heart attacks has been verified.[249] The relationship between these entities and CAD can be divided into behavioral mechanisms, whereby psychosocial conditions contribute to a higher frequency of adverse health behaviors such as poor diet and smoking, and direct stress-induced pathophysiologic mechanisms, which contribute to neuroendocrine activation, hemodynamic and catecholamine responses, and platelet activation.[219] Personality traits are more difficult to change than other psychologic risk factors, such as depression or anxiety.[62]

Improved technologies and research demonstrate that acute mental or emotional stress triggers myocardial ischemia, promotes arrhythmogenesis, stimulates platelet function, and increases blood viscosity through hemoconcentration. Moderate to severe depression is associated with altered cardiac autonomic modulation, including elevated heart rate, elevated norepinephrine, and reduced heart rate variability, known risk factors for cardiac morbidity and mortality.

In the presence of atherosclerosis in people with CAD, acute stress also causes coronary vasoconstriction. Hypersensitivity of the sympathetic nervous system to perceived adversity (manifested by exaggerated heart rate and blood pressure responses to psychologic stimuli) is an intrinsic characteristic among these individuals; in addition, the calming response of the parasympathetic nervous system is diminished in persons who are hostile and the parasympathetic counterbalance does not stop the effects of adrenaline on the heart. These emotions trigger the stress response, increasing blood pressure and heart rate and altering platelet function. Increasing evidence suggests that cognitive behavioral therapy and anger management may benefit cardiac clients by improving medical outcome. (See also the section on Stress: Special Implications for the Therapist in Chapter 2.)

Discriminatory medicine, the idea that women (and minorities) are treated less aggressively than men for heart problems, has been strongly debated. On the one hand, it has been suggested that a woman's symptoms are more likely to be misinterpreted, overlooked, or dismissed as psychosomatic and that women are less likely to undergo diagnostic procedures. On the other hand, lower rates of cardiac catheterization among women may be related to women's lower rate of positive exercise test results and older age at the time of symptomatic presentation rather than bias based on gender. As mentioned in this chapter, there is evidence to suggest that this trend is changing toward improved gender equity. Research to understand ethnic differences remains limited.

Oxidative stress, or the oxidation of LDL particles as part of the atherosclerotic formation, is under active investigation. Much of the research has originated from observational studies where greater intake of antioxidant nutrients, particularly vitamin E and beta-carotene, has been associated with reduced risk for CAD. See further discussion of the oxidation process in Chapter 5; see also the section on Myocardial Infarction: Pathogenesis in this chapter.

Moderate alcohol consumption decreases the risk of heart disease in some people because of an associated elevated level of an enzyme called *tissue-type plasminogen activator (t-PA)* that helps to keep blood flowing smoothly by dissolving clots (fibri-

nolysis). The highest levels of endogenous t-PA antigen have been found among daily consumers of red wine, and the lowest levels were found among subjects who never (or rarely) consumed alcohol.*[1] The cardioprotective benefits appear to be effective only in men over age 45 years and women over age 55 years when limited to one or two drinks per day.[110] Greater concentrations of alcohol cause direct coronary artery constriction, which may explain the relationship between ethanol and sudden coronary ischemia that is seen clinically. In addition, the depressive effect of excessive alcohol on the function of myocardial cells decreases myocardial contractility and can be very disabling. Chronic abuse of alcohol is also related to a higher incidence of hypertension, which places greater stress on a heart already compromised by CAD. Chemical dependency is also associated with increased stress on the diseased heart.

In addition, several epidemiologic studies have suggested that *sleep-disordered breathing* is a risk factor for cardiovascular disease, particularly hypertension, stroke, and ischemic heart disease.

Nonmodifiable Risk Factors.   The risk of CVD or CAD increases with *increasing age*, and the person older than 40 years is more likely to become symptomatic. *Gender* as a nonmodifiable risk factor is reflected in the fact that heart disease is more prevalent among men; women generally experience heart attacks 10 years later than men, possibly because of the biologic protection factor provided premenopausally by estrogen. By age 45 years, heart disease affects one woman in nine. By age 65 years, this ratio becomes one in three, more closely approximating rates among men. These statistics represent the outcome when no hormone replacement therapy is initiated, but as previously mentioned, the effectiveness of hormone replacement therapy in reducing morbidity and mortality associated with CAD is still under investigation.

A *family history* (i.e., one or more members of the immediate family) of cardiovascular disease is associated with increased incidence of heart disease. It is proposed that a mix of environmental and genetic factors leads to atherosclerosis of the coronary arteries in a complex, unpredictable, and unknown series of interactions. For selected individuals, genetic predisposition, especially abnormalities in lipoprotein metabolism, can play a very important role in their risk of developing atherosclerosis. Current research is exploring the possibility of "candidate genes"† that may be associated with an increased risk of CHD. For example, *apo E-4*, one of three forms of a gene involved in clearing cholesterol from the body, is associated with an increase in LDL and total cholesterol. Another candidate gene (*DSCAM*) present in individuals with Down syndrome and CHD has been identified, and a

---

*Although a small amount of daily alcohol taken with meals may elevate levels of HDL cholesterol and the bioflavonoids in red wine reduce atherosclerosis, most researchers oppose recommending drinking as a public health measure to fight heart disease and stress that no one, particularly people with a personal or family history of alcohol abuse, should drink alcohol to improve cholesterol. It should always be remembered that heavy alcohol consumption and binge drinking increase risk of blood clot formation, cardiac arrhythmia, elevated blood pressure, and cardiovascular disease. Dietary supplements containing flavonoids and antioxidants are now available without the sugar in grape juice or the alcohol in wine.

†Previously, genetic studies were often labor-intensive and lengthy unless a focus was placed on biologic candidate genes. Current technology and information from the Genome Project now allow linkage in family studies to be supplemented with accurate localization of a disease-causing or susceptibility (candidate) gene.

mutation in the *ABC-1* (ATP-binding cassette transporter 1) protein involved in lipoprotein metabolism can disrupt normal transport and processing of cholesterol. In the future, inherited markers in combination with traditional risk factor assessment will be used first to prevent and then to manage vascular disease through better utilization of diagnostic testing and individualized pharmacologic intervention.

Ethnicity is a risk factor, and certain ethnic groups have a higher rate of heart disease. The risk of heart disease is highest among blacks, who are three times more likely to have extremely high blood pressure, a major risk factor for CAD, and who have a higher prevalence of other risk factors, such as diabetes mellitus, obesity, and cigarette smoking. Native Americans have an unusually high rate of diabetes and obesity, although lower total and LDL cholesterol levels appear to offset the difference. Conflicting comparisons of CHD mortality between Mexican Americans and non-Hispanic whites have been reported. Despite their adverse cardiovascular risk profiles, especially a greater prevalence of diabetes, Mexican-Americans are reported to have lower mortality rates from CHD. However, when death certificates are more carefully examined and coded, Mexican Americans have rates equal to or higher than those of non-Hispanic whites.[179] Hispanics are less likely than whites to receive catheterization and angioplasty procedures.[73]

Infections (bacterial and viral) as a cause of atherosclerosis and thereby CAD in some people have been supported by experimental and clinical data. This discovery came about as researchers identified the presence of a common virus (cytomegalovirus) in arterial plaque as a contributing factor to angioplasty failure. Atherosclerosis is very similar to an inflammatory process, and injury to the inner layer of the artery may be triggered by acute or chronic infection, particularly in more susceptible disease states such as diabetes. Epidemiologic studies have suggested a link between chronic *Helicobacter pylori* infection or prior infection with *Chlamydia pneumoniae* and ischemic heart disease, but this has not yet been proven conclusively and the underlying mechanism remains unknown. See also the section on Germ Theory in Chapter 1.

New Predictors. Investigators may have identified markers for heart disease present in apparently healthy people, that is, components of blood or other factors that can help identify risk of CHD before symptoms develop (see Table 11-2). Serum cholesterol has been used for a long time, but many more potential predictors of risk are being examined. *Homocysteine* (Hcy), an amino acid that is generated as the body metabolizes another amino acid, methionine (found in animal-derived foods), occurs naturally in blood and tissues and is more common in people with CHD. Elevated levels of homocysteine may be as much of a risk factor as high cholesterol or smoking.

C-reactive protein (CRP), produced by the liver in response to trauma, tissue inflammation, and infection, seems to predict heart attacks and strokes before they occur. People with even slightly elevated blood levels of CRP appear to be at increased risk for CHD and its complications regardless of age, gender, general health, or the presence of other CHD risk factors. Cigarette smokers have elevated levels of CRP, and individuals experiencing a heart attack who have high levels of CRP have a slower than normal response to antithrombotic medication. Preliminary data suggest that the relative effectiveness of secondary preventive therapies, such as cholesterol-lowering drugs and aspirin, may depend on an individual's baseline CRP level.[4]

Fibrinogen, a blood protein essential for proper clotting, may predict first heart attacks (and strokes) in people with unstable CHD and is a risk factor for future cardiovascular problems in those who have not yet developed CHD. *Lipoprotein (a)*, an LDL cholesterol particle with an additional protein attached, slows the breakdown of blood clots. People with high levels of Lp(a) are at greater risk for myocardial infarction than those with lower levels of Lp(a). *Troponin T*, a component of the actin-myosin contractile portion of muscle, is quite specific for myocardial ischemia and necrosis. It remains elevated 5 to 7 days after an MI and is a predictor of cardiovascular mortality.

Dermatologic indicators of coronary risk, such as baldness, graying of the hair, thoracic hairiness, and diagonal earlobe crease are additional risk indicators of MI in men under age 60 years, independent of age and other established coronary risk factors.

Erectile dysfunction (impotence) is a hemodynamic event that can warn of ischemic heart disease in some men. Researchers may eventually call impotence a "penile stress test" that can be as predictive as a treadmill exercise stress test.[176]

Pathogenesis. The exact mechanism by which the development of CVD/CAD can be explained has yet to be determined. The recent implication of infectious agents initiating the inflammatory cascade may help explain the pathogenesis in some (but not all) cases.[198] Clinical and laboratory studies have shown that inflammation plays a major role in the initiation, progression, and destabilization of atheromas. C-reactive protein (CRP), an acute-phase reactant that reflects low-grade systemic inflammation, has been found in a variety of cardiovascular diseases. However, whether CRP is a contributing cause or an aftereffect remains undetermined. Many new studies emphasize the fact that cholesterol deposits are only one of many mechanisms through which acute CAD develops. New information points to the endothelium as a modulating factor in the pathogenesis of CAD through the production of nitric oxide* and angiotensin II, which maintain the homeostatic environment influencing the progression of CAD. This imbalance tends to promote CAD in individuals who have multiple risk factors.

In the normal artery, the endothelial lining is tightly packed with cells that allow the smooth passage of blood and act as a protective covering against harmful substances circulating in the bloodstream. The normal endothelium presents a nonreactive surface to blood, but injury triggers the thrombotic process. In the earliest stage of atherosclerosis, damage to arteries arises from a combination of factors. In some cases, the initial damage comes from LDL cholesterol that has been modified by free radicals (see Fig. 5-2). Free radicals are abundant in people who smoke and who have high blood pressure or diabetes. In other cases, high levels of homocysteine or bacteria may contribute to early damage of arterial linings.

---

*This molecule composed of one nitrogen atom and one oxygen atom is responsible for the natural dilation of blood vessels. Nitric oxide (NO) is an antilipid that provides a nonstick coating to the lining of blood vessels, much like Teflon. These two effects have helped explain how NO might prevent heart attacks and strokes and why nitroglycerin works—nitroglycerin is converted to NO inside vascular tissue, where it relaxes smooth muscle in arteries and causes blood vessels to dilate.

In general, most current theories include the following major events in the development of an atherosclerotic plaque (Fig. 11-2): arterial wall damage occurs either from injury caused by harmful substances in the blood or by physical wear and tear as a result of high blood pressure. This injury to the blood vessel wall permits the infiltration of macromolecules (especially cholesterol) from blood through the damaged endothelium to the underlying smooth muscle cells. Naked collagen acts like flypaper for platelets, causing them to aggregate at the site of injury and plug up the wound. The core of a coronary thrombus is composed of platelets, forming a so-called white thrombus. Early-stage plaque formations known as fatty streaks consist of foam cells (white blood cells coated with LDL particles, smooth muscle cells that move in from deeper layers of the artery wall, and platelets).

Although platelet activation is a normal response to injury, in atherosclerosis, once the platelets adhere, they also release chemicals that alter the structure of the blood vessel wall, so that what starts out as a small erosion in the wall can end up a swollen mound of platelets, muscle cells, and fibrous clots, a process called *proliferation* that obstructs the flow of blood through the vessel. After a thrombus forms and causes static or reduced blood flow in the vessel, the clot stabilizes with fibrin. This is commonly referred to as a *red thrombus* because of the presence of entrapped red blood cells. Within the thrombus is thrombin, which remains active and can activate

platelets. Platelets also release plasminogen activator inhibitor-1, a potent natural inhibitor of fibrinolysis, and vasoactive amines that can lead to vessel spasm, further platelet aggregation, and thrombus formation or reocclusion. This cycle of injury, platelet activation, and lipid deposition can lead to complete blockage of a vessel and result in ischemia and necrosis of tissue supplied by the obstructed blood vessel.

Clinical Manifestations.   Atherosclerosis by itself does not necessarily produce symptoms. For manifestations to develop, there must be a critical deficit in blood supply to the heart or other structures supplied by affected blood vessels. For example, symptoms of CAD may not appear until the lumen of the coronary artery narrows by 75%. Then, pain and dysfunction referable to the region supplied by an occluded artery may occur. When atherosclerosis develops slowly, collateral circulation develops to meet the heart's needs. Complications from atherosclerosis occur because it is a progressive disorder that results in more severe cardiac disease if it is not prevented or untreated. Common sequelae of atherosclerosis affecting coronary arteries include angina pectoris, MI or heart attack, or sudden death.

Men experience angina as the first symptom of CHD in one third of all cases and heart attack or sudden death in the majority of cases, whereas one half of all women experience angina and remain asymptomatic or present with atypical symptoms in the remaining cases. Atypical symptoms of angina in women include breathlessness, pain in the left chest, upper abdominal pain, and back or arm pain (especially isolated pain in the right biceps muscle) in the absence of substernal chest pain. The pain may be more diffuse and is described as sharp or fleeting, unrelated to exercise, unrelieved by rest or nitroglycerin but relieved by antacids, and characterized by palpitations without chest pain. The pain may be repeated and prolonged. Chest pain in women with chronic stable angina is more likely to occur during rest, sleep, or periods of mental stress.

Medical Management

Diagnosis.   Advances in technology are rapidly changing the diagnostic tools available to physicians for diagnosing and evaluating CAD. Coronary angiography (angiogram or arteriography; x-ray examination of the arteries with dye injection) has been the most widely used anatomic test to assess the degree of obstructive coronary disease and left ventricular contractility. Angiograms are limited by their inability to detect which plaques represent vulnerable sites for rupture, and all forms of chest pain in women are associated with a lower prevalence of positive findings on angiography making the diagnosis challenging. Tests using traditional contrast agents are less reliable in women because signals are blocked by breast tissue.

Noninvasive echocardiography has begun to substitute for cardiac catheterization and is now providing more accurate diagnostic and prognostic assessment of CAD. Echocardiography is a group of interrelated applications of ultrasound imaging (including Doppler, contrast, stress, and real-time three-dimensional [RT-3D] echocardiography). Advances in echocardiography have expanded its use in assessment of regional myocardial function, analysis of diastolic function, and quantification of regional myocardial function in different pathologic conditions, including ischemic heart disease. Echocardiography has the potential to image myocardial per-

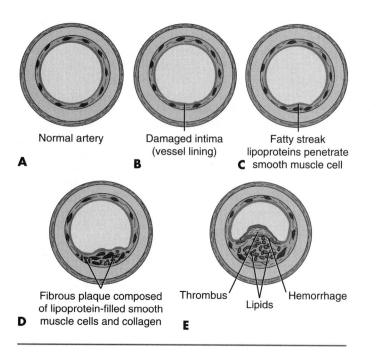

Normal artery

A

Damaged intima
(vessel lining)

B

Fatty streak
lipoproteins penetrate
C smooth muscle cell

Fibrous plaque composed
of lipoprotein-filled smooth
D muscle cells and collagen

Thrombus   Hemorrhage
Lipids
E

FIGURE   **11-2   A,** Cross section of a normal artery. **B,** Atherosclerosis begins with an injury to the endothelial lining of the artery (intimal layer) that makes the vessel permeable to circulating lipoproteins. **C,** Circulating immune cells (monocytes) rush to the site of injury causing inflammation. Arterial cells proliferate in an effort to heal the lesion, and penetration of lipoproteins into the smooth muscle cells of the intima causes plaque to form on the vessel lining producing fatty streaks. **D,** A fibrous plaque large enough to decrease blood flow through the artery develops. **E,** Calcification with rupture or hemorrhage of the fibrous plaque is the final advanced stage. Thrombosis may occur, further occluding the lumen of the blood vessel.

fusion along with wall motion and wall thickening. Stress echocardiography showing responses of the heart to changes in the environment can be performed during or after a number of different physical and even mental stressors. This is important because responses of the heart to stressors are probably even more important than how the heart functions at rest.

Until this technology is available everywhere exercise treadmill testing to record symptoms and the electrical activity of the heart under stress continues to offer a means of assessing risk of future cardiac events in most groups (obese, sedentary, middle-aged or older men and women; studies among ethnic groups are under way).[92] Heart rate recovery after submaximal exercise has been confirmed as a predictor of mortality. This measurement is routinely obtained during exercise testing; it is determined by subtracting the heart rate 2 minutes after exercise from the heart rate at the end of exercise. Abnormal heart rate recovery is defined as a reduction of 12 beats/min or less from the heart rate at peak exercise as compared to the heart rate measured 2 minutes after exercise cessation. People with an abnormal heart rate recovery are four times as likely to die as those with a normal heart rate recovery. This screening tool can be used with healthy adults as well as with those who have known heart disease.[50, 51] A delay in decline of systolic blood pressure after graded exercise is another independent correlate of CAD.

Other diagnostic test procedures available include ultrafast computed tomography (fast CT; "heart scan") that allows for a computer image accommodating for the heart's pumping cycle, and magnetic resonance angiography (MRA), the use of a powerful cylinder-shaped magnet able to vibrate in distinctive ways, creating a signal that is translated into a picture. This technique is also synchronized to the heart cycle, able to detect plaques and determine which ones are most likely to rupture. Thermography using probes to check the temperature of arteries may also reveal vulnerable plaques that are at risk for rupture since these will be inflamed with elevated temperatures. The routine measurement of newer predictors, such as Lp(a), CRP, or Hcy, is not recommended at this time for prognostic use and will be delayed until the clinical benefits of altering these concentrations are made available.

Prevention.   Overwhelming evidence indicates that CVD and CAD are largely preventable; therefore whenever possible, prevention of CVD and CAD is the goal for persons with a high-risk profile. *Healthy People 2010* has identified the following goals for heart disease and stroke: improvement of cardiovascular health and quality of life through the prevention, detection, and treatment of risk factors; early identification and treatment of heart attacks and strokes; and prevention of recurrent cardiovascular events. An excellent guide to evidence-based primary prevention of cardiovascular disease and similar recommendations for prevention of cerebrovascular disease (i.e., stroke) are available.[93,98,107,181,182]

Health perceptions, health care–seeking behavior, and willingness to participate in long-term preventive therapies are significantly influenced by age, cultural, and socioeconomic factors. Many physicians underestimate the life expectancy in older adults. For example, the average 65-year-old can expect to live an additional 15 to 20 years and function independently for more than 70% of this time. Adults older than 80 years can expect to live 7 to 10 more years and function independently for one half of that time. Older individuals are less likely to be referred to cardiac rehabilitation and exercise-training programs and less likely to attend than younger adults. Preventive cardiology including primary and secondary preventive efforts directed at the older adult is important.[139]

Primary and secondary prevention programs are needed that are modified for the language, cultural, and medical needs of all age-groups and ethnic backgrounds but especially for older ethnic minorities who are at increased risk for CVD.[221] Ethnic comparisons of health behaviors and prevalence of risk factors among teenagers support the need for health promotion intervention among urban, ethnic teenagers.[70] Women are less likely than men to receive health care advice on risk reduction while they are still healthy (i.e., before a significant cardiac event) even though they are more likely to die with the first heart attack. For this reason, new guidelines for prevention of heart disease in women were published in 1999.[164]

Modifying risk factors whenever possible can decrease the risk of CVD/CAD, especially prevention or cessation of cigarette smoking, managing diabetes and hypertension, and modifying diet. For example, folate deficiency is believed to be a major determinant of the increased risk of cardiovascular disease related to elevated total homocysteine (tHcy) because these nutritional components benefit both the vascular wall structure and the blood coagulation system.[67] Folate, riboflavin, vitamin B_6, and vitamin B_{12} are essential in homocysteine metabolism. Changing dietary habits by increasing intake of these nutrients may substantially influence the plasma tHcy concentration in the general population. Reduction of fat intake can result in regression and disappearance of fatty streaks consisting of lipid-laden macrophages, T-lymphocytes, and smooth muscle cells before these progress to form a fibrous plaque.

Dietary changes are recommended for everyone, including children and adults, since it is now recognized that blood vessel changes associated with heart disease begin as early as 15 years old and the progression of the lesions is strongly influenced by the same risk factors that predict risk of clinically manifest coronary disease in middle-aged adults.[220,257] In addition, at least 25% of all Americans under age 19 years are overweight or obese. There is a need for early and aggressive control of all risk factors in young persons for long-range prevention of CHD and related diseases. The Unified Dietary Guidelines have been published as nutritional guidelines by experts from the American Heart Association, American Cancer Society, American Dietetic Association, American Academy of Pediatrics, and National Institutes of Health.[60] In addition, an excellent guide to risk reduction outlining goals, screening, and recommendations for lifestyle factors and pharmacologic interventions is available.[164] The National Heart, Lung, and Blood Institute also has a validated health risk appraisal instrument (ATP III scale) that is easy to use.[171]

Exercise and physical activity according to recommendations from the Centers for Disease Control and Prevention (CDC) (i.e., moderate-intensity exercise for at least 30 minutes on most days of the week)* have been shown to reduce the risk for coronary events, ischemic stroke,[111] insulin resis-

---

*In recent years the view that physical activity has to be vigorous to achieve a reduction in risk of CHD has been under question. Substantial evidence supports the benefit of continued regular physical activity that does not need to be strenuous or prolonged and includes daily leisure activities, such as walking or gardening. Taking up regular light or moderate physical activity in middle or older age confers significant benefit for CVD.[242]

tance, and diabetes mellitus for men and women.[150,242] The American College of Sports Medicine's position on the quantity and quality of exercise for developing and maintaining cardiorespiratory and muscular fitness and flexibility in healthy adults recommends aerobic endurance training at least 2 days per week at 50% or higher VO$_2$* and for at least 10 minutes. The National Runners' Health Study reports that substantial health benefits occur (in men) at exercise levels that exceed the CDC guidelines, suggesting that intense exercise offers one set of benefits whereas lengthy exercise provides another.[250] Other studies report the benefits of shorter periods of physical activity in decreasing the risk of CHD as being equal to one longer, continuous session of exercise, as long as the total caloric expenditure is equivalent.[94]

The effect of exercise on cholesterol has been documented, but it remains unclear which component of exercise is the underlying beneficial mechanism. Exercise frequency may be more important than intensity in improving HDL cholesterol and cholesterol ratios,[133] and resistive exercise training has been reported to raise HDL cholesterol levels, but studies in these areas have been limited.[90,184] Even so, many health benefits from physical activity can be achieved in shorter bouts at less intensity.[6] More studies are required to identify the ideal prescriptive exercise. Interestingly, endothelial damage has been reported after intense aerobic exercise, raising additional questions about exercise for athletes with cardiovascular risk factors.[21] It is likely that in the future, different exercise regimens for specific heart disease risk factors will be individually prescribed.

Exercise alone independent of weight loss or diet changes can have significant beneficial effects on cardiovascular risk factors in overweight people with elevated cholesterol levels.[34] Exercise is the one single intervention with the ability to influence the greatest number of risk factors (e.g., aids in smoking cessation, alters cholesterol levels, reduces blood pressure, helps control blood glucose levels, reverses the effects of a sedentary lifestyle, contributes to weight loss, helps in managing stress-induced increases in heart rate and blood pressure). In fact, researchers at the University of Texas using real-time 3D echocardiography to compare the effects of medications with the effects of exercise on coronary artery perfusion declare exercise to be "the most powerful drug available in preventing cardiac events."[47] Exercise can lessen depression, anger, and stress, which frequently interfere with recovery, and heart attack survivors who follow the CDC exercise guidelines reduce their risk of a fatal second episode by up to 25%.[120]

Chemoprevention is an established method in the primary and secondary prevention of cardiovascular (and cerebrovascular) disease. Clinical trials have proven conclusively that both fatal and nonfatal coronary events and strokes can be prevented.[236] Pharmacologic management is used to reduce the risk of clotting, to treat hypertension, and to decrease serum cholesterol level when it exceeds 200 mg/dl. Medications are now available (3-hydroxy-3-methylglutaryl coenzyme A [HMG-CoA] reductase inhibitors, better known as "statins") that have been proven effective not only in lowering LDL levels and raising HDL levels but also in reducing

cardiac events (primary and secondary prevention of MI). There is no known way to reduce Lp(a) levels; recommendations are for aggressive reduction or elimination of other modifiable risk factors to minimize overall CHD risk. Target measurements to reduce risk factors developed by the American College of Cardiology and the American Heart Association are listed in Table 11-3.

Researchers are actively examining the potential benefits of antioxidants in the prevention and treatment of blood vessel disease. Antioxidants such as garlic oil; vitamins A, C, and E; ginkgo biloba; black and green teas; and a variety of plant substances are under investigation. To date, results support the idea that antioxidants can prevent and even counteract the adverse effects of oxygen free radicals by preventing the formation of radicals, scavenging them, or promoting their decomposition.[32, 255]

Treatment. Medical management is directed toward the specific blood vessel occlusion and depends on complications, for example, occlusive disease of the peripheral vasculature, arterial disease in diabetic clients, occlusive cerebrovascular disease, or visceral artery insufficiency (intestinal ischemia) (see discussion of each individual complication). Surgical management of atherosclerosis of the coronary arteries may include percutaneous transluminal coronary angioplasty (PTCA) (Fig. 11-3), coronary artery bypass graft (Fig. 11-4), and coronary stents (Fig. 11-5). Angioplasty is performed 10 times more often than bypass surgery; angioplasty combined with a stent reduces the incidence of restenosis, especially for people with diabetes who have a high mortality rate when treated by standard balloon angioplasty.[237]

The use of a combined antiplatelet treatment with aspirin and glycoprotein IIb/IIIa receptor blockers (Table 11-4) is a standard pharmacologic regimen after coronary artery stenting for the prevention of thrombosis. For the person with significant coronary and carotid artery disease, the importance of treating symptomatic stenosis of the carotid artery as a means of stroke prevention is now widely accepted. Some centers are combining carotid endarterectomy (CEA) and coronary revascularization (CABG) for low-risk individuals for convenience and cost savings by avoiding a second hospitalization and operation. Carotid artery angioplasty and stenting constitute a procedure that is an alternative to CEA, especially for people considered at high risk for postoperative complications.

Blockages that are heavily calcified and that involve long stretches of coronary artery are difficult to treat successfully with angioplasty or stenting. In such cases, rotational atherectomy can be accomplished using a device called a *rotoblator* (catheter tipped with a tiny rotary blade). This procedure makes sharp cuts in plaque, shaving away the blockage and producing a relatively smooth luminal surface. Other surgical techniques such as mechanical thrombectomy using a device (AngioJet System) that removes blood clots in the coronary (or carotid) arteries before angioplasty or the use of laser-assisted balloon angioplasty (LABA, a laser beam at the tip of a catheter) are viable options in some cases but carry higher rates of major complications, especially for women. Intravascular ultrasound, a technology that combines echo with catheterization, may eventually allow diagnosis and therapy to be combined as the cardiologist uses a camera on the tip of a catheter to precisely target atherosclerotic blockage. In keep-

---

*VO$_2$ is a measure of oxygen uptake sometimes described as aerobic capacity, ventilatory uptake, or physical working capacity. Maximal oxygen consumption is referred to as VO$_2$ max. This measurement reflects the integration of three components of the delivery system that transports O$_2$ from the outside air to the working muscles: pulmonary ventilation, blood circulation, and muscle tissue.

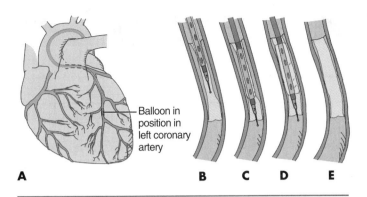

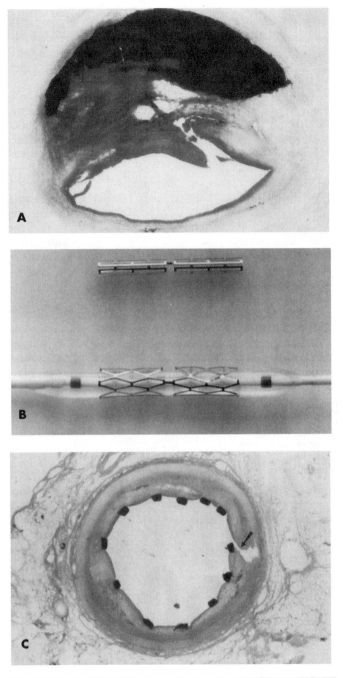

FIGURE   **11-3** Percutaneous transluminal coronary angioplasty (PTCA) can open an occluded coronary artery without opening the chest, an important advantage over bypass surgery. **A,** Once coronary angiography has been performed to determine the presence and location of an arterial occlusion, a guide catheter is threaded through the femoral artery into the left coronary artery. **B,** When the angiography shows the guide catheter positioned at the site of occlusion, the uninflated balloon is centered in the obstruction. **C,** A smaller double-lumen balloon catheter is inserted through the guide catheter. **D,** The balloon is inflated and deflated until the angiogram confirms arterial dilation with a reduced pressure gradient in the vessel. **E,** The balloon is removed, and the artery is left unoccluded.

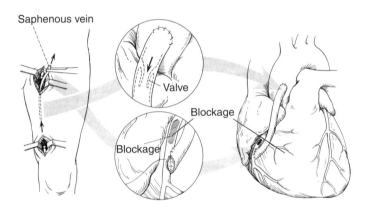

FIGURE   **11-4** Coronary bypass surgery (CABG). This procedure involves taking a portion of a vein or artery from the chest or leg and grafting it onto the coronary artery. In this illustration, a section of the saphenous vein is used as a graft to route blood around areas of blockage. Bypassing the clogged vessel provides an alternative route for blood to reach the heart muscle. The internal mammary artery can be used as an alternate vein site for grafting. CABG has been a major surgery requiring a sternotomy but is being refined to possibly become an off-pump bypass grafting through a partial sternotomy. It is considered most effective in individuals who have several severely blocked coronary arteries and a previously damaged heart muscle or when repeated revascularization has failed. (From Black JM, Matassarin-Jacobs E, editors: *Medical-surgical nursing,* ed 5, Philadelphia, 1997, Saunders, p 1250.)

FIGURE   **11-5** **A,** Cross section of a severely occluded coronary artery. **B,** Blocked coronary artery can be held open using a balloon-expandable device called a *coronary stent.* **C,** Stent shown here is in place to maintain opened vessel allowing blood to pass through freely. Biodegradable stents are under development to reduce or eliminate problems associated with metal stents.[233] Delivery of gene therapy to inhibit intimal hyperplasia and prevent postangioplasty restenosis is under investigation.[72] (Courtesy Thomas Jefferson University, Philadelphia.)

ing with the new data on the time of day that cardiac events occur (i.e., thrombus formation is more likely to occur in the morning hours), researchers are now investigating the possibility that postoperative complications are related to the time the procedure takes place.[228]

Although surgical intervention has been a mainstay for the treatment of CAD, researchers are questioning the necessity of heart surgery and studying the benefits of pharmacologic intervention combined with exercise and lifestyle changes. The role of exercise in the prevention of atherosclerosis has been

TABLE **11-4**

Common Cardiovascular Medications

MEDICATIONS: TRADE NAMES (GENERIC NAMES)	INDICATIONS AND SIDE EFFECTS*
Alpha-Adrenergic Blockers (-zosin) Cardura (doxazosin) Hytrin (terazosin HCl) Minipress (prazosin HCl) Cardura (doxazosin)	**Indication:** to lower blood pressure by dilating peripheral blood vessels reducing peripheral resistance **Side effects:** headache, palpitations, fatigue, nausea, weakness, drowsiness, palpitations,† dizziness,‡ fainting‡
Angiotensin-Converting Enzyme (ACE) Inhibitors (-pril) Capoten (captopril) Lotensin (benazepril) Vasotec (enalapril maleate) Prinivil, Zestral (lisinopril) Altace (ramipril) Accupril (quinapril)	**Indication:** to treat high blood pressure and heart failure; prevent constriction of blood vessels and retention of sodium and fluid; improve sympathetic heart rate response during exercise in the early phase of MI to prevent heart failure **Side effects:** persistent, dry cough, skin rash, loss of taste, weakness, headaches, palpitations,† swelling of feet or abdomen,† dizziness or fainting‡ (because of low blood pressure), numbness or tingling of the hands, feet, or lips, renal failure
Angiotensin II (ATII) Receptor Antagonists (-sartan) Atacand (candesartan) Avapro (irbesartan) Cozaar (losartan) CS-866 Diovan (valsartan) Micardis (telmisartan) Teveten (eprosartan) Verdia (tasosartan)	**Indication:** to vasoconstrict arterioles by blocking the effects of angiotensin II; enhance renal clearance of sodium and water **Side effects:** dizziness,‡ insomnia,† anxiety,† confusion,† stroke,‡ hypotension,‡ visual changes,‡ GI/GU effects,† cough,† upper respiratory infection,† myalgia; many other various but less common side effects
Antiarrhythmics Cardioquin (quinidine) Procan (procainamide HCl) Rythmol (propafenone HCl)	**Indication:** to alter conduction patterns in the heart **Side effects:** nausea, palpitations, vomiting, rash,† insomnia,† dizziness,‡ symptoms of CHF (shortness of breath, swollen ankles, coughing up blood)‡
Anticoagulants (Antithrombotic) Coumadin (warfarin sodium) Unfractionated heparin (Lovenox [enoxaparin]) Low–molecular weight heparin (Fragmin [dalteparin], Orgaran [danaparoid], Normiflo [ardeparin]) Hirudin (Refludan [lepirudin])	**Indication:** to prevent blood clot formation **Side effects:** easy bruising, joint or abdominal pain,‡ difficulty in breathing or swallowing,‡ paralysis,‡ unexplained swelling, unusual or uncontrolled bleeding,‡ rib and vertebral fractures (long-term use of anticoagulants)[41]
Beta-Blockers (-olol) Inderal (propranolol HCl) Lopressor (metoprolol tartrate) Tenormin (atenolol) Kerlone (betaxolol) Cartrol (carteolol) Corgard (nadolol) Coreg (carvedilol) Levatol (penbutolol) Blocadren (timolol) Not registered (clinical trial status): bucindolol	**Indications:** to relax the blood vessels of the heart muscle by blocking sympathetic conduction at beta-receptors on the SA node and myocardial cells, producing a decline in the force of contraction and a reduction in heart rate; decrease blood pressure, dysrhythmias, and angina; decrease myocardial oxygen demand **Side effects:** insomnia, nausea, fatigue, slow pulse, weakness, increased cholesterol and blood glucose levels, nightmares,† depression,† sexual dysfunction,† asthmatic attacks,‡ dizziness‡
Calcium-Channel Blockers (-pine) Procardial (nifedipine) Cardizem (diltiazem HCl)	**Indications:** to dilate coronary arteries to lower blood pressure and suppress some arrhythmias

TABLE	11-4—cont'd

Common Cardiovascular Medications

MEDICATIONS: TRADE NAMES (GENERIC NAMES)	INDICATIONS AND SIDE EFFECTS*
Calcium-Channel Blockers (-pine)—cont'd Calan, Verelan (verapamil) Norvasc (amlodipine) Plendil (felodipine) Cardene (nicardipine)	**Side effects:** fluid retention, palpitations, headache from vasodilation, flushes, rash,† dizziness‡
Central Antiadrenergic Agents Aldomet (methyldopa) Catapres (clonidine) Wytensin (guanabenz acetate) Tenex (guanfacine)	**Indication:** to lower high blood pressure by dilating the blood vessels **Side effects:** drowsiness, depression, sexual dysfunction, fatigue, dry mouth, stuffy nose, fever, upset stomach, change in bowel habits, weight gain, fluid retention, dizziness‡
Digitalis Compounds (Cardiac Glycosides) Lanoxin (digoxin) Crystodigin (digitoxin)	**Indications:** to strengthen the heart's pumping force to increase cardiac output and decrease electrical conduction through the AV node **Side effects:** fatigue, lethargy, weakness, headache,† visual disturbances (blurred vision, yellow-green halos, blind spots in visual field or scotamata, double vision),† cardiac disturbances (bradycardia, irregular heart rhythms),‡ hypotension,† anorexia, nausea, vomiting,† diarrhea,† CNS disturbance† (depression, irritability, confusion, restlessness, drowsiness, seizures‡), electrolyte disturbances (hypokalemia)†
Diuretics Thiazide diuretics (e.g., Hydrodiuril [hydrochlorothiazide]) Potassium-sparing diuretics (e.g., Aldactone [spironolactone]) Loop diuretics (e.g., Lasix [furosemide], Bumex [bumetanide], Demadex [torsemide])	**Indications:** to increase the excretion of sodium and water and control high pressure and fluid retention **Side effects:** drowsiness, dehydration, electrolyte imbalances, gout, nausea, pain, hearing loss, blood glucose abnormalities, elevated cholesterol and lipoprotein levels, muscle cramps,† dizziness,‡ light-headedness‡
Lipid-Lowering Drugs (statins); HMG-CoA reductase inhibitors) Lipitor (atorvastatin) Mevacor (lovastatin) Zocor (simvastatin) Loecol (fluvastatin) Baycol (cerivistatin) Pravachol (pravastatin) Lopid (gemfibrozil) Questran (cholestyramine) Nia-Bid, Niacor, Nicobid (niacin)	**Indication:** to interfere with the metabolism of blood fats in various ways by lowering cholesterol, low-density lipoproteins, and/or triglyceride levels in the blood; non–lipid lowering effects include improving endothelial function, antiproliferative actions on smooth muscle, and reducing platelet aggregation **Side effect:** nausea, vomiting,† diarrhea,† constipation,† flatulence, abdominal discomfort, myalgia, increased liver enzymes; more rarely, statins can cause myositis or rhabdomyolysis (a debilitating muscle-wasting condition resulting in acute renal failure), peripheral neuropathy, sleep disturbances (insomnia, bad or vivid dreams), or rash; statins may stimulate bone growth and reduce osteoporosis (under investigation)
Nitrates (vasodilators) Nitrostat, Nitro-Bid (nitroglycerin) Iso-Bid, Isordil (isosorbide dinitrate)	**Indication:** for dilation of coronary arteries **Side effects:** headache, dizziness,†, orthostatic hypotension,†, tachycardia†
Platelet Inhibitors (antiplatelet) Aspirin Ticlid (Ticlopidine) Plavix (Clopidogrel) Glycoprotein IIb/IIa receptor blockers ("super aspirin") ReoPro (Abciximab) Integrilin (Eptifibadtide) Aggrastat (Tirofiban)	**Indication:** to prevent platelet aggregation and subsequent clot formation **Side effects:** gastric irritation (aspirin),† bleeding or hemorrhage,‡ leg or pelvic pain,† rash, atrial fibrillation,‡ tachycardia,‡ dizziness,† confusion†

Continued

TABLE 11-4—cont'd	

Common Cardiovascular Medications

MEDICATIONS: TRADE NAMES (GENERIC NAMES)	INDICATIONS AND SIDE EFFECTS*
Thrombolytics Streptokinase Urokinase Tissue-type plasminogen activator (t-PA) (Activase [alteplase], Tenecteplase or TNKase [reteplase])	**Indication:** break down and dissolve already formed blood clots **Side effects:** bleeding (GI, GU, intracranial, surface),‡ headache,† fever,† nausea,† low back pain†
Vasodilators Nitroglycerin Isosorbide dinitrate (Isordil, Iso-Bid)	**Indication:** to dilate the peripheral blood vessels (used in combination with diuretics) **Side effects:** headache, drowsiness, nausea, vomiting, diarrhea, hair growth (minoxidil only), increased heart rate,† swollen ankles,† dizziness,‡ difficulty in breathing‡
Human B-type natriuretic peptide (vasodilator/diuretic; genetically engineered form of naturally occurring cardiac hormone; BNP) Nesiritide (Natrecor)	**Indication:** combination of effects including rapid dilation of arteries and veins; promotes diuresis; used in decompensated CHF and arrhythmias **Side effects:** dose-related hypotension†

HCl, Hydrochloride; *GI*, gastrointestinal; *GU*, genitourinary; *CHF*, congestive heart failure; *SA*, sinoatrial; *AV*, atrioventricular; *CNS*, central nervous system.

*The therapist is more likely to see potential side effects not otherwise present since these develop when the person is physically challenged. Any unusual signs or symptoms and potential side effects should be documented and reported to the prescribing physician but especially for any specialty marked.

†Document and call physician when possible.

‡Call physician immediately; document findings.

discussed, but the role of exercise as a treatment modality is equally important. Cardiac rehabilitation exercise training consistently improves objective measures of exercise tolerance, without significant cardiovascular complications or other adverse outcomes. Appropriately prescribed and conducted exercise training is recommended as an integral component of the treatment of atherosclerosis and CAD.[2] See further discussion in Special Implications for the Therapist, this section.

Results from the Stanford Coronary Risk Intervention Project (SCRIP) conducted over 4 years have demonstrated that intensive multifactor risk reduction favorably alters the rate of luminal narrowing in coronary arteries of men and women with CAD and decreases hospitalizations for clinical cardiac events. In cases of low-risk, stable CAD, aggressive lipid-lowering therapy is at least as effective as angioplasty in reducing the incidence of ischemic events.[35] The development of new fibrin-specific thrombolytic agents for establishing coronary patency in acute MI in combination with platelet inhibitors may replace angioplasty procedures.[232]

Numerous other trials (e.g., Leiden Intervention Trial, Heidelberg Diet and Exercise Study, St. Thomas's Atherosclerosis Regression Study, Cholesterol Lowering Atherosclerosis Study [CLAS]) have focused on the effect of diet-induced reductions in LDL cholesterol and the resultant changes in CAD. Restricting the intake of saturated fat and cholesterol has a favorable result in changing the course of coronary atherosclerosis. In addition, dietary and lifestyle interventions slowed CAD progression, decreased the incidence

and severity of angina, and reduced the number of cardiac events. The effect of exercise alone without a comprehensive cardiac rehabilitation intervention has not been evaluated, but exercise-based cardiac rehabilitation is effective in reducing cardiac deaths.[122]

Because pharmaceutical agents, surgery, and lifestyle changes including diet and exercise have been unable to maintain blood flow without restenosis in some people, new technologic approaches to intervention are being investigated. Emerging treatment of restenosis include antiproliferative-coated stents and photoangioplasty. Photoangioplasty uses a photosensitive drug that selectively accumulates in atheromatous plaque and remains inactive until exposed to an endovascularly delivered far-red light that reduces or destroys the deposits without damage to the normal vessel wall.[103] Gene therapy (i.e., gene transfer-based antirestenosis therapy) is one strategy with the potential to prevent some of the sequelae after arterial injury, induce growth of new vessels, or remodel preexisting vessels.[72] Several groups have injected a gene that makes a protein called *vascular endothelial growth factor (VEGF)*. When injected directly into the heart, this gene prompts the heart to sprout tiny new blood vessels to bypass the blocked vessels, a process referred to as *therapeutic angiogenesis* or *biologic revascularization*.[173,258] Alternately, endothelial stem cells derived from bone marrow and injected into the region bordering an infarction have been shown to regenerate new myocardium or new blood vessels in animal studies. The increase in oxygen and nutrients accompanying this new tissue formation has the potential of preventing death of my-

TABLE	11-5

Medical Management of Cardiovascular Conditions*

CORONARY ARTERY DISEASE/MYOCARDIAL INFARCTION	ANGINA PECTORIS	HYPERTENSION	CONGESTIVE HEART FAILURE	ARRHYTHMIAS
Lifestyle changes (see text)	Lifestyle changes	Lifestyle changes	Lifestyle changes	Cardioversion (electrical or pharmacologic)
Prescriptive exercise	Prescriptive exercise	Prescriptive exercise	Prescriptive exercise	
Medications	Medications	Medications (frequently combination therapy)	Medications	Medications
Antilipids (especially statins)	Organic nitrates (vasodilators)	Diuretics	Cardiac glycosides	Sodium channel blockers
Antiplatelets†	Beta-adrenergic blockers	Beta-adrenergic blockers	Diuretics	Beta-adrenergic blockers
Anticoagulants	Calcium-channel blockers	ACE inhibitors	ACE inhibitors	Calcium-channel blockers
Thrombolytics	Antiplatelets (platelet inhibitors)	Vasodilators	Vasodilators	Agents prolonging depolarization
Beta-adrenergic blockers	Anticoagulants	Calcium-channel blockers	Angiotensin II receptor antagonists	Human B-type natriuretic peptide (BNP)
Angiotensin-converting enzyme (ACE) inhibitors	Antithrombins	Alpha₁-blockers	Beta-adrenergic blockers	
		Angiotensin II receptor blockers (ARB; antagonists)	Human B-type natriuretic peptide (BNP)	
		Anticoagulants		
		Antiplatelets		
Surgery	Surgery	Surgery	Surgery	Surgery
Percutaneous transluminal coronary angioplasty (PTCA)	Revascularization procedures for unstable angina (see Coronary Artery Disease/Myocardial Infarction, this table)	Transplantation	Revascularization procedures (see Coronary Artery Disease/Myocardial Infarction, this table)	Maze procedure (surgical or catheter)
Coronary artery bypass graft (CABG)	Transmyocardial revascularization (TMR)		Intraaortic balloon pump (IABP)	Pacemaker
Coronary stent implantation			Left ventricular assistive device (see Chapter 20)	Implantable cardioverter-defibrillator (ICD)
Atherectomy			Cardiac resynchronization therapy (CRT)	Ventricular resynchronization therapy
Mechanical thrombectomy			Implantable cardioverter-defibrillator (ICD)	
Transmyocardial revascularization (TMR)			Transplantation	
Photoangioplasty				
Intraaortic balloon pump (IABP)				
Transplantation				
Gene therapy	External counterpulsation (EECP)		External counterpulsation (EECP)	
Stem cell therapy				

Modified with permission from Susan Queen, P. T., Ph.D., University of Kentucky, Lexington, 2001.

*The use of complementary or alternative therapies in the adjunctive treatment of each of these conditions is under investigation at this time (see text discussion, Atherosclerosis: Treatment). Research centered on pharmacologic and surgical approaches to these conditions is changing rapidly. This information represents a broad overview and my not include every option available.

†Antiplatelets, anticoagulants, and thrombolytics are used to treat overactive clotting but have distinct uses and mechanisms of action. Antiplatelets inhibit platelet aggregation and platelet-induced clotting, anticoagulants inhibit the synthesis of clotting factors, and thrombolytics facilitate clot breakdown after the formation of a clot.

ocardial cells, reducing myocardial remodeling and scarring, and improving heart function by levels of 30% to 40%.[80,177]

Finally, a review of alternative or complementary interventions, sometimes referred to as mind-body therapies, and their effects on heart disease, blood pressure, lipid levels, morbidity, and mortality is available.[145] These techniques remain under investigation and include prayer or mediation and/or religious attendance at church or services; yoga, Tai Chi, and other forms of martial arts; acupuncture; social support and/or support groups; cognitive-behavioral therapy; imagery; hypnosis; physiologic quieting; relaxation techniques; music therapy; and others (Table 11-5).

Prognosis.   The American Heart Association reports compelling scientific evidence that comprehensive risk factor interventions in people with cardiovascular heart disease extend overall survival, improve quality of life, decrease the need for interventional procedures, and reduce the incidence of subsequent MI. Even so, despite the well-documented benefit of preventive measures and cardiac rehabilitation, compliance with recommendations for reducing risk factors and utilization rates of rehabilitation programs remain low, especially among women.[164]

Prognosis depends on the site and extent of necrosis, but nearly 500,000 deaths each year in the United States are attributable to CAD/CHD. Fatality rates for CAD remain low before age 35 years, but these figures increase exponentially until age 75 years, with men generally experiencing mortality at approximately twice the rate of women until age 65 years. Total CAD mortality in women after age 65 years now exceeds that of men. Of the nearly 20,000 persons eligible for heart transplants, only 10% receive a new heart each year. Advanced atherosclerosis is usually fatal if vessels to the brain or heart are affected, but new technology and new surgical intervention may reduce mortality in the decade ahead. The newest, most predictive value of future cardiac events is the pulse pressure, a measure of arterial stiffness (systolic–diastolic blood pressure). Pulse pressure (>60 mm Hg) as an independent predictor of the incidence of CHD, CHF, and overall mortality among community-dwelling older adults has been verified.[235]

Surgical procedures are considered safe, and although complications can occur, the rates of complications (e.g., reintervention or repeat procedures, reexploration for bleeding) following CABG surgery have declined substantially in the last 10 years despite higher client risks. In the case of angioplasty, the risks of failure, reoperative procedures, and operative mortality are higher with advanced age, female gender, diabetes mellitus, elevated serum cardiac enzymes following the procedure, the presence of certain viruses,* and impaired left ventricular dysfunction.[217] Percutaneous transluminal coronary angioplasties (PTCAs) are associated with greater rates of restenosis especially among women, who are at greater risk for complications and have a higher mortality rate. Most studies attribute the higher mortality rate to the fact that women more often undergo the surgery during an emergency, they are usually older at the time of diagnosis than men, they are more likely to have other complicating conditions (e.g., hypertension, diabetes), and they may have smaller, more delicate coronary arteries, making surgery more difficult. The higher rates of morbidity and mortality associated with angioplasty have resulted in the use of the balloon-expandable stent, which is associated with a low restenosis rate and a favorable clinical outcome with event-free survival rate at 1 year. The need for repeat revascularization has also been significantly reduced.

---

*The presence of *cytomegalovirus* (CMV) as a causative agent in the calcification that occurs after angioplasty has been documented. Other infections may also be implicated, such as *Chlamydia pneumoniae* and *H. pylori*, but the strength of this association and the mechanism of entry into the arterial wall remain unclear; antiviral pharmacologic interventions to prevent restenosis in high-risk clients has not been proven effective yet.[58]

Special Implications for the Therapist   **11-2**

ATHEROSCLEROSIS (Cardiovascular Disease, Coronary Artery Disease)

Preferred Practice Pattern:
6A: Primary Prevention/Risk Reduction for Cardiovascular/Pulmonary Disorders

Other practice patterns may be necessary depending on the clinical manifestations and disease outcomes (see discussion of each specific disease). The therapist can be very instrumental in guiding individuals through a preoperative wellness program including client education, risk factor reduction, and exercise program. See also the section on Stroke in Chapter 31.

Postoperative Considerations
Cardiac rehabilitation (phases I to IV) is an important component of intervention for anyone treated medically for congestive heart failure, arrhythmias, unstable angina, coronary artery disease, myocardial infarction, valvular disease, and heart transplantation. This multidisciplinary program of education and exercise is designed to promote the development of and maintenance of a desirable level of physical, social, and psychologic function in those individuals with an acute cardiovascular illness. Specific goals of cardiac rehabilitation include risk stratification, improving emotional well-being and psychologic factors, reducing CHD risk factors, and decreasing symptoms. In addition, older adults often have reduced functional capacity and quality of life scores compared with younger CHD clients, making this an important goal for those individuals.[139] Implementation of phase I by physical therapists begins day 1 to 3 following CABG (or other) surgery or an MI. Primary emphasis is on postsurgical mobilization; client education is essential given the presence of co-morbidities and the need for individualized prescriptive exercise.

During this phase the therapist uses and teaches the client sternal precautions (Box 11-2; see also the section on The Cardiac Client and Surgery in this chapter) and adjusts the intensity of mobilization to optimize recovery from surgery and tissue injury, thereby minimizing length of stay without compromising the client.[116] In the past, chest physical therapy was recommended routinely for persons who had abdominal or cardiothoracic surgery, but the efficacy of chest physical therapy for reducing complications after coronary artery surgery has been repeatedly studied and never been proven. With advances in surgical techniques, smaller incisions, reduced postoperative pulmonary dysfunction, and earlier mobilization, techniques such as postural drainage and manual techniques now are limited to clients who are very acutely ill and cannot participate in early mobilization.[49]

Postoperative brachial plexus injury can occur following cardiac surgery that requires a sternotomy when prolonged sternal separation or asymmetric traction of the sternal halves causes nerve compression or overstretching. Uncomplicated cases are usually transient and do not require intervention by a therapist. In rare cases, peripheral neuropathy will persist resulting in impaired function and disability. As cardiac operative techniques continue to improve and move toward noninvasive methods, this type of injury will become obsolete.

BOX **11-2**

Sternal Precautions

It is important to know whether the chest has been closed; the skin may be sutured, but the underlying chest structures may not be closed.

To evaluate chest wall stability at rest, the therapist places his or her hands on the client's chest and asks the client to cough. Observe chest movement; any type of asynchronous movement between the two chest sides is a sign of an unstable chest requiring sternal precautions. These precautions vary from center to center and sometimes from surgeon to surgeon based on the surgical procedure performed but usually include the following:

- No pulling up in bed during acute care is allowed; client must roll into side-lying position and use the top arm to assist in pushing up while allowing the feet to drop off the side of the bed as a pendulum type of assist.
- Hand-held assistance during mobilization may be required initially in place of assistive devices, such as walkers or canes.
- No pushing, pulling, or lifting more than 10 lb (some precautions list 5 lb) for 6 weeks postoperatively is allowed; this includes vacuuming, lifting pets (or walking pets on a leash), furniture, bowling balls, doors, children, or anything that weighs more than 1 gallon of milk.

- No driving motorized vehicles (e.g., automobile, golf cart, or other similar large conveyance) for 4 weeks postoperatively (some centers require 6 to 8 weeks) is permitted; during this time, person should not sit in the front seat of any vehicle and especially vehicles equipped with airbags.
- Full neck, shoulder, and torso range of motion may be permitted as long as the sternum is stable but not if a sternectomy with skin or muscle flap is present; presence of a flap limits range of motion to 90 degrees (flexion or abduction) or until the point of movement at the chest wall or rib cage.
- Avoid shoulder horizontal abduction with extreme external rotation.
- Progression is based on client tolerance and signs of wound healing; once the incision is fully healed, scar mobilization is permissible. The usual precautions for scar mobilization apply, including mobilizing the tissue in the direction of the scar before using any cross-transverse techniques and mobilizing toward the scar rather than away from the scar to avoid overstretching the healing tissue.
- Use of the more conservative precautions is advised with anyone who has diabetes mellitus, severe osteoporosis, or other equally compromising co-morbidities.

Home monitoring of symptoms for the first weeks after surgery is essential following the guidelines in Table 11-6. The physician should be notified if the client experiences one or more of the signs and symptoms outlined. Transfusion is no longer a standard part of open-heart surgery so hematocrit levels are usually low (20% to 25%) following this procedure, requiring modification of exercise guidelines (see Table 39-6) unless directed otherwise by the physician. Carotid artery disease is a risk factor for CNS complications after CABG surgery requiring close monitoring for signs and symptoms of CNS involvement. Discharge instructions for the cardiovascular surgical population may vary according to physician and institution, but some general guidelines apply (Box 11-3). The therapist can be helpful in teaching about unexpected symptoms and ways to manage them. For example, women experiencing postoperative chest discomfort can be reassured that this is not uncommon, will subside over time, and may be minimized by wearing a snug all-cotton undershirt under loose clothing to decrease friction. Reassurance and education are extremely important for clients who are emotionally distressed. Although these people are successful in improving their functional status and physical capacity, they are more likely to experience angina during activities of daily living (ADLs) and during exercise and less successful in returning to work.

Prescriptive Exercise

The known benefits of regular physical activity and exercise in both primary and secondary prevention of cardiovascular disease have been thoroughly documented (and discussed in this section; see Prevention). Exercise training increases cardiovascular functional capacity and decreases myocardial oxygen demand at any level of physical activity in apparently

healthy people as well as in most people with cardiovascular disease. Regular dynamic exercise is considered adjunctive therapy for lipid management along with dietary management and reduction of excess weight but must be maintained in order to sustain the training effects. Both short- and long-term endurance exercise can contribute to an improvement in blood lipid abnormalities.[10]

Although exercise and physical training have been shown to improve exercise capacity and recovery of the autonomic nervous activity,[226] there is an increased risk that exercise may precipitate cardiovascular complications and silent symptoms of ischemia, arrhythmias, or abnormal blood pressure. Heart responses to exercise and fatigue necessitate special considerations for the formulation and execution of physical conditioning programs. Determining how heart rate and blood pressure respond to exercise (e.g., at what point symptoms of oxygen deprivation occur) forms the basis for an exercise prescription.

Frequent premature ventricular contractions (PVCs) are considered a contraindication to exercise unless approved by the physician (e.g., as in the case of automatic implantable cardioverter-defibrillators). Indications for stopping an exercise test can be used as precautions during therapy or exercise (Table 11-6; see also Box 11-6). Therapists in all settings are encouraged to read the complete American Heart Association Exercise Standards.[10] Risks associated with resistance exercise in older adults and recommended guidelines for resistance exercise prescription in this population of cardiac rehabilitation clients are also available.[26]

Postoperative Exercise

People recovering from cardiac surgery, despite an excellent hemodynamic result, may be disabled by persistent left ventricu-

Continued

BOX 11-3

Discharge Instructions After Cardiovascular Surgery

Showers: Permitted 2 days after surgery or hospitalization. Avoid tub baths or soaking in water until incisions are healed; avoid extremely hot water.

Incisions: The incision should be kept dry but can be gently washed with mild soap and warm water (directly over the tapes); lotions, creams, oils, or powders are not permitted until the wound is completely healed unless prescribed by the physician.

Care of surgical leg (for bypass graft involving the leg): Avoid crossing the legs, which impairs circulation; avoid sitting in one position or standing for prolonged periods. Elevate the involved leg when sitting or lying down. Swelling in the grafted leg is common until collateral circulation develops. Swelling should decrease after leg elevation but may recur when standing. Progressive edema must be reported to the physician.

Elastic stockings: Worn for at least 2 weeks after discharge during the daytime and removed at bedtime.

Rest: A balance of rest and exercise is an essential part of the recovery process. Resting between activities and short naps are encouraged. Resting may include sitting quietly or reading for 20 to 30 minutes; loss of appetite is common for the first 2 weeks and may contribute to fatigue.

Walking: Walking increases circulation throughout the body and to the heart muscle and is encouraged. Activity must be increased gradually, but frequent walks of short duration are recommended initially. Pacing of activities throughout the day, combined with energy conservation, is important.

Stairs: Climbing stairs is permitted unless the physician indicates otherwise.

Sexual relations: Sexual relations can be resumed when the client feels physically comfortable (usually 2 to 4 weeks after discharge; see also text discussion).

Sternal precautions: See Box 11-2.

Stop any activity immediately if dyspnea, palpitations, chest pain or discomfort, or dizziness or fainting develops. Notify the physician if symptoms do not subside with rest in 20 minutes.

---

lar hypertrophy and years of presurgical restricted activity and deconditioning. Exercise rehabilitation is an important part of the recovery process. Easy fatigability related to muscular weakness lessens with increased physical activity. Exercise-induced symptoms of angina and light-headedness or syncope disappear immediately after surgery with a successful result.

The exercise capacity of clients soon after MI and bypass surgery is determined by the same parameters as in healthy individuals or for other cardiac problems, including time since MI, age, physical training status, and amount of myocardial dysfunction that occurs with exercise. CNS dysfunction (see Table 11-6) is a common consequence of otherwise uncomplicated CABG surgery that may affect exercise capacity. The exact cause of this neurologic phenomenon remains unknown, but it may be the result of preoperative intracranial or extracranial carotid artery disease contributing to compromised hemodynamics and cerebral hypoperfusion.

A program to increase the strength and flexibility of the pectoral and leg muscles is usually recommended. During this time, elastic stockings are usually worn to prevent fluid accumulation at the site of the leg incisions. Special exercises are prescribed to improve chest wall function, facilitate breathing, and prevent adhesive capsulitis, a common finding 6 to 12 weeks after a CABG or other open-chest procedure. Data to support the need for early range of motion (ROM) to prevent loss associated with surgery are limited. One small study of the effect of shoulder ROM exercises after CABG surgery reported that ROM exercises do not ameliorate the early loss of ROM associated with surgery since the loss is a function of the surgical procedure and not lack of ROM challenge.[207] The delay in presentation of adhesive capsulitis suggests other variables may be present during the time when clients are enrolled in phase I (inpatient) and phase II (outpatient) cardiac rehabilitation programs to account for this development.

Monitoring During Exercise

More than one half of all ischemic episodes are not accompanied by angina. Ask any client with identified CAD risk factors or diagnosed CAD to report all unusual sensations, not just episodes of chest pain or discomfort. Exercise testing should be performed before beginning an exercise program, but if this has not been accomplished and baseline measurements are unavailable for use in planning exercise, use pulse oximetry; monitor the heart rate and rhythm, respiratory rate, and blood pressure; and note any accompanying symptoms before, during, and after exercise (see Appendix B). This type of monitoring can be modified for each individual and is recommended throughout therapy intervention. Documentation of vital signs can be an excellent way to demonstrate evidence-based outcomes of intervention.

Side effects of cardiovascular medications may not appear until the cardiovascular system is challenged, such as occurs during therapy intervention. Monitoring for drug-related problems is essential, and a basic understanding of how these medications work is helpful (see Table 11-4). Striking a balance between the benefits of cardiovascular medications and acceptable or tolerable side effects can be a challenge, and the therapist must keep in mind when documenting and reporting drug-related effects that these medications often produce physiologic responses that increase the effectiveness of physical therapy. A more comprehensive discussion of this topic is available.[48] Several drugs used in the treatment of CAD are known to alter the heart rate. For example, beta-adrenergic blocking agents used in the treatment of angina and hypertension cause a reduction in resting and exercise heart rate. Anyone taking these medications may not be able to achieve a target heart rate above 90 beats/min; therefore using symptoms (e.g., angina, diaphoresis, shortness of breath, dizziness, pallor, isolated [arm or leg] or overall fa-

TABLE	11-6

Indications for Discontinuing or Modifying Exercise*

Symptoms

New-onset or easily provoked anginal chest pain

Increasing episodes, intensity, or duration of angina (unstable angina)

Discomfort in the upper body, including chest, arm, neck, or jaw; chest pain unrelated to chest incision

Fainting, light-headedness, dizziness

Sudden, severe dyspnea

Severe fatigue or muscle pain

Nausea or vomiting

Back pain during exercise

Bone or joint pain or discomfort during or after exercise

Severe leg claudication

Clinical Signs

Pallor; peripheral cyanosis; cold, moist skin

Staggering gait, ataxia

Confusion or blank stare in response to inquiries

Resting heart rate >130 beats/min or <40 beats/min

>6 arrhythmias (irregular heartbeats; palpitations) per hour

Frequent premature ventricular contractions (PVCs)

Clinical Signs—cont'd

Uncontrolled diabetes mellitus (blood glucose >250 mg/dL)

Oxygen saturation <90% (98% is normal); some variability (individual and geographic)

Acute infection or fever >100° F

Persistent drainage or change in drainage from any incision

Increased swelling, tenderness, and redness around any incision site

Inability to converse during activity

Blood pressure (BP) abnormalities

  Fall in systolic BP with increase in workload; specifically, a decrease of 10 mm Hg or more below any previously recorded BP accompanied by other signs or symptoms

  Rise in systolic BP above 250 mm Hg or diastolic BP above 120 mm Hg

Signs of CNS involvement (e.g., confusion or delirium, cognitive decline, encephalopathy, seizure, stroke)

Other

Person indicates need or desire to stop

From Fletcher GF, Froelicher VG, Hartley H et al: AHA Medical/Scientific Statement. Exercise standards: a statement for health professionals from the American Heart Association, *Circulation* 82:2286, 1990.

*Not all signs and symptoms require immediate cessation of exercise or intervention. The therapist is advised to document any clinical signs or symptoms observed or reported along with any modifications made in the intervention and notify the physician accordingly.

tigue) and rating perceived exertion may be a more appropriate means of monitoring. Avoid increases of more than 20 beats/min over the resting rate for individuals taking these medications.

Conservative limits postoperatively include a maximal heart rate of 130 beats/min, 120 beats/min for medically managed cases, or an increase of 30 beats/min for surgical cases and 20 beats/min for medical cases. A safe rate of exercise will allow the heart rate to return to the resting level within 5 minutes after stopping exercise.

Almost all antihypertensive agents, including diuretics that may have a dual action of peripheral dilation and volume depletion, can have a profound effect on postexercise blood pressure. In some healthy people, when exercise is terminated abruptly, precipitous drops in systolic blood pressure can occur owing to venous pooling. Some people with CAD have higher levels of systolic blood pressure that exceed peak exercise values; a proper cool-down after vigorous exercise is important to prevent such an occurrence. More detailed information on the effects of various drugs on the exercise response during training in clients with CAD can be found in *Guidelines for Exercise Testing and Prescription* by the American College of Sports Medicine.[5] ■

Angina Pectoris

Definition and Incidence. As blood vessels become obstructed by the formation of atherosclerotic plaque, the blood supply to tissues supplied by these vessels becomes restricted. When the cardiac workload exceeds the oxygen supply to myocardial tissue, ischemia occurs, causing temporary chest pain or discomfort, called *angina pectoris*. The exact incidence of angina is unknown, although it is considered common, especially in people age 65 years and older; it occurs more often in men.

Overview. There are several types of anginal pain (Box 11-4). *Chronic stable angina*, classified as classic, exertional angina, occurs at predictable levels of physical or emotional stress and responds promptly to rest or to nitroglycerin. No pain occurs at rest; and the location, duration, intensity, and frequency of chest pain are consistent over time (60 days). *New-onset angina* describes angina that has developed for the first time within the last 60 days and is also considered unstable. *Nocturnal angina* may awaken a person from sleep with the same sensation experienced during exertion usually caused by

BOX	11-4

Types of Angina Pectoris

Chronic (stable) angina; classic exertional angina

New-onset (unstable) angina

Nocturnal angina

Postinfarction angina

Preinfarction angina (unstable); progressive, crescendo angina

Prinzmetal's (variant) angina; vasospastic

Resting angina (decubitus)

Syndrome X; microvascular angina

increased heart rate associated with dreams or in response to underlying CHF.

Postinfarction angina occurs after MI when residual ischemia triggers an episode of angina. *Preinfarction angina* or *unstable angina*, also known as progressive angina or crescendo angina, is unpredictable and is characterized by an abrupt change (increase) in the intensity and frequency of symptoms or decreased threshold of stimulus. This angina lasts longer than 15 minutes and is a symptom of worsening cardiac ischemia.

Prinzmetal's, vasospastic, or *variant angina* produces symptoms similar to those of typical angina, but it is caused by coronary artery spasm. These spasms periodically squeeze arteries shut and keep the blood from reaching the heart. In this type of angina, coronary arteries are usually clear of plaque or free of physiologic changes that cause obstruction of the vessels. The pattern of Prinzmetal's angina is characterized by early morning occurrence, frequently at the same time each day, and it occurs at rest (i.e., it is unrelated to exertion). Prinzmetal's angina is more common in women younger than 50 years; it is often associated with various types of arrhythmias or conduction effects.

Decubitus or *resting angina* is considered atypical; it occurs most often when at rest and frequently occurs at the same time every day. This type of anginal chest pain is atypical in that it is paroxysmal in nature, not brought on by exercise, and not relieved by rest, but it is reduced when the person sits or stands up.

Syndrome X is an unusual form of ischemic heart disease used to describe microvascular angina, exertional angina, or angina without obvious coronary atherosclerosis. This is seen as a positive response to exercise testing suggestive of ischemia but with normal coronary arteries on angiograph. It is more prevalent among women, particularly those who have undergone hysterectomy. Microvascular angina associated with syndrome X affects the microcirculatory system, a network of tiny blood vessels that branch from the large coronary vessels and that provide oxygen to each of the millions of myocardial cells. Why these vessels spasm and cause decreased blood flow remains undetermined; the cause may be a decrease in estrogen during menopause or a specific trigger from within the heart. Long-term survival rates are not reduced in women with this syndrome.

Syndrome X is sometimes referred to as the insulin resistance syndrome, characterized by a constellation of interrelated CHD risk factors, including dyslipidemia (improper lipids),* obesity, elevated systolic blood pressure, and hyperinsulinemia (excess insulin in the blood). There may be some overlap between syndrome X (microvascular angina) and insulin resistance syndrome (also called hyperinsulinemia syndrome), but they are two separate entities.

Etiologic and Risk Factors.

Any condition that alters the blood (oxygen) supply or demand of the myocardium can cause ischemia (Table 11-7). Increased oxygen needs of the heart, increased cardiac output, or reduced blood flow to the heart can cause angina. CAD accounts for 90% of all cases of

TABLE	11-7

Causes of Myocardial Ischemia

DECREASED OXYGEN SUPPLY	INCREASED OXYGEN DEMAND
Vessels	
Atherosclerotic narrowing	Hyperthyroidism
Inadequate collateral circulation	Arteriovenous fistula
Spasm caused by smoking, emotion, or cold	Thyrotoxicosis
Coronary arteritis	Exercise or exertion
Hypertension	Emotion or excitement
Hypertrophic cardiomyopathy	Digestion of large meal
Circulatory Factors	
Arrhythmias ($\downarrow$blood pressure)	
Aortic stenosis	
Hypotension	
Bleeding	
Blood Factors	
Anemia	
Hypoxemia	
Polycythemia	

From Goodman CC, Snyder TE: *Differential diagnosis in physical therapy,* ed 3, Philadelphia, 2000, Saunders, p 97.

angina, although other conditions affecting normal vessels can also cause angina. Disorders of circulation, such as relative hypotension secondary to spinal anesthesia, antihypertensive drugs, or blood loss, can also result in decreased blood return to the heart and subsequent ischemic pain.

Various known triggers are associated with plaque rupture and the subsequent onset of angina: physical exertion or exercise, especially involving thoracic or upper extremity muscles or walking rapidly uphill; increase in pulse rate or blood pressure (e.g., psychologic or emotional stress); or vasoconstriction. The threshold for angina is often lower in the morning or after strong emotion; the latter can provoke attacks in the absence of exertion. Angina may also occur less commonly during sexual activity, at rest, or at night during sleep.

Pathogenesis.

Angina is a symptom of ischemia usually brought on by an imbalance between cardiac workload and oxygen supply to myocardial tissue usually secondary to CAD (see previous discussion on pathogenesis of atherosclerosis). Disruption of a formed plaque with sudden total or near-total arterial occlusion may bring on unstable angina. Rupture leads to the activation, adhesion, and aggregation of platelets and the activation of the clotting cascade, resulting in the formation of an occlusive thrombus. If this process leads to complete occlusion of the artery, then myocardial infarction occurs. If the process leads to severe stenosis but the artery remains open, then unstable angina occurs. Metabolites within the ischemic segment of the myocardium (e.g., histamines, bradykinin, prostaglandins) and buildup of lactic acid or abnormal stretching of the myocardium irritate myocardial fibers resulting in myocardial pain. Afferent sympathetic fibers

---

*Dyslipidemias constitute elevations of LDL cholesterol (hypercholesterolemia) as well as abnormalities in the metabolism of triglyceride-rich lipoproteins (hypertriglyceridemia) and lipoprotein (hypoalphalipoproteinemia).

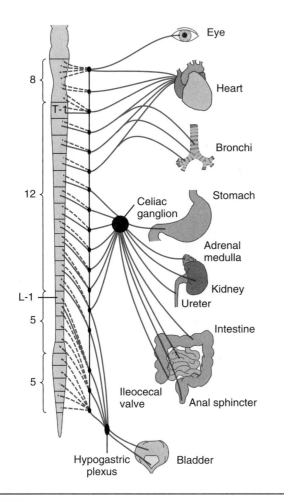

FIGURE   **11-6** Diagram of the autonomic nervous system. The visceral afferent fibers mediating cardiac pain travel with the sympathetic nerves and enter the spinal cord from multiple levels (C3 to T4). This multisegmental innervation results in a variety of pain patterns associated with myocardial ischemia and infarction.

enter the spinal cord from levels C3 to T4 (Fig. 11-6) accounting for the varied locations and radiation patterns of anginal pain. The effects of temporary ischemia are reversible; if blood flow is restored, no permanent damage or necrosis of the heart muscle occurs.

Clinical Manifestations.   Angina is characterized by temporary pain or, more often, discomfort that starts suddenly in the chest (substernal or retrosternal) and sometimes radiates to other parts of the body, most commonly to the left shoulder and down the ulnar border of the arm to the fingers. Pain or discomfort may also be referred to any dermatome from C3 to T4, presenting at the back of the neck, lower jaw, teeth, left upper back, interscapular area, abdomen occasionally, and possibly down the right arm (Fig. 11-7). The sensation described is often referred to as squeezing, burning, pressing, heartburn, indigestion, or choking. It is usually mild to moderate (rarely reported as severe); it usually lasts 1 to 3 minutes, sometimes 3 to 5 minutes, but can persist up to 15 to 20 minutes. Symptoms are usually relieved by rest or nitroglycerin; in women, symptoms may be relieved by taking an antacid.

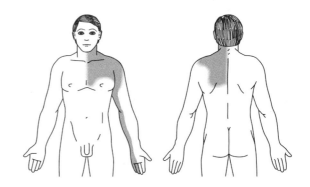

FIGURE   **11-7** Pain patterns associated with angina. *Left,* Area of substernal discomfort projected to the left shoulder and arm over the distribution of the ulnar nerve. Referred pain may be present only in the left shoulder or in the shoulder and along the arm only to the elbow. *Right,* Occasionally, anginal pain may be referred to the back in the area of the left scapula or the interscapular region. See Fig. 11-11 for pain pattern associated with myocardial ischemia or infarction experienced by some women (see text for complete description).

Recognizing symptoms of myocardial ischemia in women is more difficult, since the symptoms are less reliable and do not follow the classic pattern described. Many women describe the pain in ways consistent with unstable angina, suggesting that they first become aware of their chest discomfort or have it diagnosed only after it reaches more advanced stages. Some experience a sensation similar to that of inhaling cold air, rather than the more typical shortness of breath. Other women note only weakness and lethargy, and some have observed isolated pain in the midthoracic spine or throbbing and aching in the right biceps muscle.

Medical Management
Diagnosis.   The diagnosis of angina pectoris is strongly suspected by history and is supported if sublingual nitroglycerin shortens an attack and if prophylactic nitrates permit greater exertion or prevent angina entirely. Medical evaluation includes examination for signs of diseases that may produce angina or contribute to or accompany atherosclerotic disease (see the previous section on Clinical Manifestations). Early and accurate triage to assess risk (low, intermediate, high) can help identify those people for whom medical therapy will probably fail and lead to better outcomes through a more appropriate management strategy. ECG is normal in about 25% to 30% of people with angina, so the exercise tolerance test (ETT) is a more useful noninvasive procedure for evaluating the ischemic response to exercise in the client with angina. Diagnostic testing continues as for CAD (see the previous section on Atherosclerosis: Diagnosis and the next section on Myocardial Infarction: Diagnosis).

Prevention and Treatment.   Prevention of attacks is the first step after the acute attack subsides. Treatment of underlying disorders such as hypertension is essential. The client is also encouraged to avoid situations and stressors that precipitate angina. This usually requires modifying all possible risk factors through changes in lifestyle and modifications of lifelong habits.

Short-acting sublingual nitroglycerin is the drug of choice for the acute attack, usually relieving symptoms within 1 to 2 minutes. Nitroglycerin oral spray is also available in a metered delivery system, which is especially useful for anyone having difficulty handling or swallowing pills. The spray is also easy to use in the dark and is more rapid-acting. Pharmacologic therapy may include other vasodilators, such as long-acting nitrates (e.g., oral sustained-release nitroglycerin, transdermal nitroglycerin patches, nitroglycerin ointment), beta-blockers (i.e., beta-adrenergic receptor blockers), and calcium-channel blockers (see Table 11-4). Intravascular thrombosis is a key element in the pathophysiology of unstable angina and its progression to MI. Anticoagulation therapy using aspirin and/or heparin is an important part of treatment for unstable angina.* Second-line alternatives to aspirin (sometimes referred to as "clot busters" or "super aspirins"; e.g., ticlopidine, clopidogrel) are more effective than aspirin in preventing platelet aggregation and thereby reducing the combined risk of ischemic stroke, MI, or death from vascular disease and may be useful in preventing coronary-stent thrombosis.

Revascularization procedures are recommended for persons who do not become ischemia-free on medical therapy, especially the client with progressive unstable angina. Surgical intervention, such as PTCA, has been shown to relieve angina, but it does not halt the progress of atherosclerosis or prolong life. CABG can diminish the probability of ischemia leading to necrosis and lethal infarction. Enhanced external counterpulsation (EECP) is a noninvasive outpatient procedure to reduce chronic angina by improving perfusion of areas in the heart deprived of adequate blood supply. EECP uses a series of pneumatic compression cuffs enclosing the lower extremities (upper thigh, lower thigh, calf) to produce an acute hemodynamic effect with increased blood flow to the heart similar to the effects of an (invasive) intraaortic balloon pump (see Fig. 11-14). Rapid inflation and deflation create a pressure wave that raises diastolic aortic pressure, increases coronary perfusion pressure, and provides improved venous return with subsequent increase in cardiac output.[17] In addition to providing symptomatic relief, EECP also improves exercise tolerance[234] and provides psychosocial benefits (e.g., reduced depression, anxiety, and somatization).[215]

For people who are not good candidates for any of the proven procedures or whose angina persists despite angioplasty or bypass surgery, transmyocardial revascularization (TMR) may be recommended. In TMR, a computer-controlled laser drills tiny channels through the wall of the left ventricle while the chamber is filled with oxygenated blood. In theory, this allows blood to flow through the channels to the oxygen-deprived tissue, relieving angina. The openings on the heart's surface scar over quickly, but it is not known how long the channels stay open on the inside of the heart; long-term results remain unknown. TMR is still considered experimental and may not be available in all centers, but studies consistently report success relieving severe angina that has been refractory to medical and surgical intervention.[124] This procedure is performed through a 4-inch incision between the ribs and does not require a bypass machine; efforts to develop noninvasive techniques of TMR using fiberoptic catheters are under investigation.

Prognosis. Myocardial ischemia leaves the heart vulnerable to arrhythmias and MI, which can be fatal. About one-third of all people who experience angina pectoris die suddenly from MI or arrhythmias. Prognosis depends on type of angina, ability to prevent angina, and severity of underlying disease, such as hypertension or atherosclerosis.

Special Implications for the Therapist   11-3

ANGINA PECTORIS

Preferred Practice Patterns:
6B: Impaired Aerobic Capacity/Endurance Associated With Deconditioning
6D: Impaired Aerobic Capacity/Endurance Associated With Cardiovascular Pump Dysfunction or Failure
See also Special Implications for the Therapist: Atherosclerosis, 11-2.

Identifying Angina

Referred pain from the external oblique abdominal muscle and the pectoral major muscle can cause the sensation referred to as heartburn in the anterior chest wall, which mimics angina. When active trigger points are present in the left pectoralis major muscle, the referred pain is easily confused with that from coronary insufficiency. Physical therapy to eliminate the trigger points can aid in the diagnostic process.

Anterior chest wall syndrome with localized tenderness of intercostal muscles, Tietze's syndrome with inflammation of the chondrocostal junctions, intercostal neuritis, and cervical or thoracic spine disease involving the dorsal nerve roots can all produce chest pain that mimics angina. Evaluation of range of motion, palpation of soft tissue structures, and analysis of relieving or aggravating factors usually differentiate these conditions from true angina.[91] Likewise, heartburn from indigestion, hiatal hernia, peptic ulcer, esophageal spasm, and gallbladder disease can also cause angina-like symptoms that require a medical evaluation for an accurate medical diagnosis.

The development of unstable angina also requires immediate medical referral and may be reported as the onset of angina at rest, occurrence of typical angina at a significantly lower level of activity than usual, changes in the typical anginal pattern (e.g., symptoms occurring more frequently), or changes in blood pressure (decrease) or heart rate (increase) with levels of activity previously well tolerated. Educating the public about reducing delays and getting to an emergency department at the earliest signs of heart attack is essential. Reperfusion therapy within the first 60 to 70 minutes of a heart attack can make a significant difference in outcome.

Nitroglycerin

A person experiencing angina should reduce the pace or, if necessary, stop all activity and sit down for a few minutes until the symptoms disappear. Exercise can be reinitiated at a reduced intensity, and interval-type training may be required (i.e., slow activity alternating with activity requiring more effort). Nitroglycerin may be used prophylactically 5 minutes before activities likely to precipitate angina. This is especially true in the intervention or exercise setting of the person with chronic, stable, exertional

---

*Anticoagulants, such as aspirin and heparin, prevent clot formation, whereas antithrombotic agents (thrombolytics), such as urokinase and streptokinase, break down clots already formed. Aspirin blocks platelet cyclooxygenase, preventing the formation of thromboxane A2, thereby inhibiting platelet aggregation.

angina. The use of nitroglycerin must be by physician order and cannot be decided solely by the therapist and client.

Clients must be reminded that they are not to alter their prescribed drug schedule without consulting their health care provider and that nitrates should be taken as prescribed. For example, taking sublingual nitroglycerin orally markedly decreases its effectiveness. Clients should be seated when taking nitroglycerin to avoid syncope and falls. For anginal pain or discomfort that is not relieved by rest or relieved by up to three nitroglycerin doses in 10 to 15 minutes (i.e., the initial dose followed by a second dose 5 minutes later and a third dose 5 minutes after the second dose), the physician should be contacted. Until the angina is controlled and coronary blood flow reestablished, the client is at risk of myocardial damage from myocardial ischemia.

Nitroglycerin tablets are inactivated by light, heat, air, and moisture, and they should be stored in the refrigerator in a tight-fitting amber container. Nitroglycerin has a short shelf life and needs to be replaced about every 3 months. A potent nitroglycerin tablet should produce a burning sensation under the tongue when taken sublingually (if it does not, check the expiration date).

Orthostatic Hypotension

Orthostatic hypotension (see discussion later in this chapter) is one of the most common side effects of prophylactic medications for angina. Caution on the part of the therapist is required when exercising or ambulating clients who take these medications. If the person becomes hypotensive, have him or her assume a supine position with legs elevated to increase venous return and to ensure cerebral blood flow. Extra caution must be taken when placing anyone with orthostatic hypotension and CHF supine with legs elevated because this may overload an already stressed ventricle. Keeping the head elevated and monitoring carefully are required in this circumstance. Support hose may be recommended, and the person should be reminded to change positions slowly to minimize the effects of orthostatic hypotension. Headache, weakness, increasing pulse, or other unusual signs or symptoms should be reported to the physician. In a home health setting, the home should be evaluated for potentially hazardous conditions. All clients should be encouraged to avoid hazardous activities until their condition is stabilized by medication, especially in the presence of dizziness.

Monitoring Vital Signs

Exercise testing should be performed before a client begins an exercise program, but if this has not been accomplished and baseline measurements are unavailable for use in planning exercise, monitor the heart rate and blood pressure and note any accompanying symptoms during exercise (see Appendix B). Exercise and activity should be performed below the anginal threshold. The therapist must document heart rate and blood pressure when the ischemia began (as evidenced by symptoms of angina) to establish these parameters. Angina occurring after an MI is not considered normal and should be reported to the physician. Exercise testing is recommended before a client resumes an exercise program. ■

◆ Hypertensive Cardiovascular Disease

Hypertensive cardiovascular disease includes hypertensive vascular disease, hypertensive heart disease, pulmonary hypertension, and pulmonary heart disease. The latter two conditions affecting the heart are caused by an underlying pulmonary pathologic condition and are discussed in Chapter 14.

Hypertension (Hypertensive Vascular Disease)
Definition and Overview. Blood pressure is the force exerted against the walls of the arteries and arterioles; diastolic pressure (bottom number) is the pressure in these vessels when the heart is relaxed between beats, and systolic pressure (top number) is the pressure exerted in the arteries when the heart contracts. Between ages 55 and 60 years, diastolic blood pressure often begins to plateau and may even decline whereas systolic blood pressure often starts to rise. Hypertension, or high blood pressure, is defined by the World Health Organization (WHO) as a persistent elevation of diastolic blood pressure (>90 mm Hg), systolic blood pressure (>140 mm Hg), or both measured on at least two separate occasions at least 2 weeks apart (i.e., sustained elevation of blood pressure). Based on epidemiologic data from the Framingham Heart Study, the development of hypertension is neither inevitable nor beneficial; systolic pressure is more important than diastolic pressure as a determinant of cardiovascular sequelae.

Hypertension can be classified according to type (systolic or diastolic), cause, and degree of severity. Hypertension can also be classified based on risk according to the most recent guidelines (Table 11-8).[212] *Primary* (or *essential*) *hypertension* is also known as idiopathic hypertension and accounts for 90% to 95% of all cases of hypertension. *Secondary hypertension* accounts for only 5% to 10% of cases and results from an identifiable cause. Intermittent elevation of blood pressure interspersed with normal readings is called *labile hypertension* or borderline hypertension. *Malignant hypertension* is a syndrome of markedly elevated blood pressure (diastolic blood pressure >125 mm Hg) with target organ damage (e.g., retinal hemorrhages, papilledema, heart failure, encephalopathy, renal insufficiency). The elevation of systolic blood pressure independent of change in the diastolic blood pressure is now recognized as a medical condition referred to as *isolated systolic hypertension.*

Incidence. The incidence of hypertension varies considerably among different groups in the American population, but it is estimated that one in four adult Americans (50 million) have high blood pressure. Hypertension is twice as prevalent and more severe among blacks than whites. This phenomenon has been attributed to heredity, greater environmental stress, and greater salt intake or salt sensitivity (i.e., responsiveness to changes in sodium balance and extracellular fluid and volume status), although the actual cause is not clear; reduced access to health care increases the prevalence of untreated hypertension. Hypertension control rates are no longer improving and fell short of the U.S. *Healthy People 2000* goal of blood pressure control in 50% of all hypertensive adults. These goals are now modified for *Healthy People 2010* to include the following: (1) reduce the proportion of adults ages 20 years and older with high blood pressure from the current incidence (28%) to 16% and (2) increase the proportion of adults ages 18 years and older with high blood pressure whose blood pressure is under control from current rates of 18% to a target rate of 50%.[105]

Etiologic and Risk Factors. *Primary (essential) hypertension* has no established etiology but is probably related to genetics and other risk factors, such as smoking, obesity, high

TABLE	11-8

Classification of Blood Pressure and Recommended Treatment*

STAGES	BLOOD PRESSURE (SYSTOLIC/ DIASTOLIC, mm Hg)	RISK GROUP A†	RISK GROUP B‡	RISK GROUP C§
Optimal	<120/<80			
Normal	<130/<85			
High normal	130-139/85-89	Lifestyle changes	Lifestyle changes	Lifestyle changes; drug therapy
Hypertension				
Stage 1 (mild)	140-159/90-99	Lifestyle changes (up to 12 mo, followed by drug therapy if necessary)	Lifestyle changes (up to 6 mo, followed by drug therapy if necessary)	Lifestyle changes; drug therapy
Stage 2 (moderate)	160-179/100-109	Drug therapy; lifestyle changes	Drug therapy; lifestyle changes	Drug therapy; lifestyle changes
Stage 3 (severe)	≥180/≥110	Drug therapy; lifestyle changes	Drug therapy; lifestyle changes	Drug therapy; lifestyle changes

From the Sixth Report of the Joint National Committee on Detection, Evaluation, and Treatment of High Blood Pressure (JNCW), Arch Intern Med 157(21):2413-2446, 1997.

*For adults aged 18 yr and older not taking antihypertensive drugs and not acutely ill.

†High normal blood pressure; no associated cardiovascular disease risk factors; no target organ damage or cardiovascular disease.

‡Hypertension with ≥1 associated cardiovascular disease risk factor (excluding diabetes); no target organ damage or cardiovascular disease; no target organ damage or cardiovascular disease.

§Hypertension in the presence of diabetes or target organ damage or cardiovascular disease.

cholesterol levels, and being of black descent. In the past 10 years, hypertension research has shifted strongly in the direction of molecular genetics. A familial association with hypertension has been documented, possibly attributable to common genetic background, shared environment, or lifestyle habits. Using the candidate gene approach, allelic variants in the genes for angiotensinogen, beta$_2$-adrenergic receptor, mutation in the beta subunit of the epithelial sodium channel, and several others have been identified, but the mechanisms by which these contribute to hypertension have not been identified.[144]

Small arteries branching from the aorta, called arterioles, regulate blood pressure. Any condition that can narrow the opening of these arterioles can increase the blood pressure in the arteries. A variety of specific diseases or problems, such as chronic renal failure, renal artery stenosis, or endocrine disease, can cause *secondary hypertension* (Table 11-9). The risk for cardiovascular disease in adults with hypertension is determined not only by level of blood pressure but also by the presence or absence of target organ damage or factors such as smoking, dyslipidemia, and diabetes. *Isolated hypertension* has very distinct causes, often not directly vascular and often related to a specific organ or tissue, such as aortic diseases, heart malformations, or thyrotoxic crisis.

Risk factors for hypertension may be modifiable or non-modifiable (Box 11-5). The risk of hypertension increases with age as arteries lose elasticity and become less able to relax. Hypertension occurs slightly more often in men than in women and at an earlier age, but after age 50 years, hypertension begins to develop in more women than men. In all groups the incidence of hypertension increases with age, with a poorer prognosis for people whose hypertension begins at a young age. White coat hypertension increases the risk of heart disease because rise in blood pressure occurs in other anxiety-provoking situations as well. Personality traits such as hopelessness and hostility are important factors in cardiovascular disease including hypertension; research is under way to identify the neuroendocrine and CNS mechanisms underlying these associations and to identify other possible personality traits.[68] Hypertension itself represents a significant risk factor for the development of CHD, stroke, CHF, and renal failure, preceding heart failure in 90% of all cases and increasing in all other associated conditions.

The influence of nonsteroidal antiinflammatory drugs (NSAIDs) on blood pressure in normotensive and hypertensive persons remains in question. At the very least it has been determined that there is always the potential for NSAIDs to interact with antihypertensive agents, most notably diuretics, beta-receptor antagonists, and ACE inhibitors. Given the high prevalence of NSAID use by older adults, especially for conditions such as arthritis, gout, and similar problems, the association between this drug use and blood pressure must be observed carefully. Alcohol has been estimated to be responsible for as many as 10% of all cases of hypertension and may be the actual unknown cause of "essential" hypertension.[79]

Blood pressure is linked to salt intake and modulated by the "salt gene" (angiotensinogen) in some people. Those who are salt-sensitive (including those who do not yet have high blood pressure) may have an increased risk of death. Salt sensitivity is a measure of how blood pressure responds to sodium and is independent of other risk factors (including elevated blood pressure) for death from cardiovascular disease.

TABLE 11-9

Causes of Secondary Hypertension

Coarctation of the aorta
Pheochromocytoma
    (rare catecholamine-
    secreting tumor)
Alcohol abuse
Pregnancy induced
Thyrotoxicosis
Increased intracranial
    pressure from tumors or
    trauma
Collagen disease
Endocrine disease
    Acromegaly
    Cushing's disease
    Diabetes
    Hypothyroidism
    Hyperthyroidism
Renal disease (e.g., connective
    tissue diseases, diabetic
    nephropathy)
Effects of drugs (e.g., oral
    contraceptives, cyclosporine,
    cocaine)

Acute stress
    Surgery
    Psychogenic hyperventilation
    Alcohol withdrawal
    Burns
    Pancreatitis
    Sickle cell crisis
Neurologic disorders
    Brain tumor
    Respiratory acidosis
    Encephalitis
    Sleep apnea
    Guillain-Barré syndrome
    Quadriplegia
    Lead poisoning

Modified from Kaplan NM: Systemic hypertension: mechanisms and diagnosis. In Braunwald E: *Heart disease: a textbook of cardiovascular medicine*, ed 4, Philadelphia, 1992, Saunders, p 820.

BOX 11-5

Risk Factors of Primary (Essential) Hypertension

Modifiable

High sodium intake (causes water retention, increasing blood volume)
Obesity (associated with increased intravascular volume)
Diabetes mellitus
Hypercholesterolemia and increased serum triglyceride levels
Smoking (nicotine restricts blood vessels)
Long-term abuse of alcohol (increases plasma catecholamines)
Continuous emotional stress (stimulates sympathetic nervous system)
Personality traits (hostility, sense of hopelessness)
Sedentary lifestyle
White coat hypertension (see explanation in text)
Hormonal status (menopause, especially before age 40 years and without hormone replacement therapy; hysterectomy/oophorectomy)

Nonmodifiable

Positive family history of cardiovascular disease
Age (>55 years)
Gender (male <55 years; female >55 years)
Ethnicity (black,* Hispanic)

*From a pathogenetic point of view, recent research findings have suggested that beta-adrenergic receptor down regulation is characteristic of hypertension in whites, whereas heightened vascular alpha-receptor sensitivity or early vascular hypertrophy may be a feature of hypertension in blacks.[209]

Pathogenesis.   Blood pressure is regulated by two factors: blood flow and peripheral vascular resistance. Blood flow is determined by cardiac output (strength, rate, rhythm of heartbeat; blood volume). The resistance to flow is primarily determined by the diameter of blood vessels and, to a lesser degree, by the viscosity of blood.

Increased peripheral resistance as a result of the narrowing of the arterioles is the single most common characteristic of hypertension. Constriction of the peripheral arterioles may be controlled by two mechanisms, each with several components: (1) sympathetic nervous system activity (autonomic regulation) and (2) activation of the renin-angiotensin system. In the case of the sympathetic nervous system, norepinephrine is released in response to psychogenic stress or baroreceptor activity. The blood vessels constrict, which increases peripheral resistance. At the same time, epinephrine is secreted by the adrenal medulla, resulting in increased force of cardiac contraction, increased cardiac output, and vasoconstriction. With prolonged hypertension, the elastic tissue in the arterioles is replaced by fibrinous collagen tissue. The thickened arteriole wall becomes less distensible, offering even greater resistance to the flow of blood. This process leads to decreased tissue perfusion, especially in the target organs of high blood pressure (i.e., heart, kidneys, brain). Atherosclerosis is also accelerated in persons with high blood pressure.

Within the renin-angiotensin system, vasoconstriction results in decreased blood flow to the kidney. Whenever blood flow to the kidney diminishes, renin is secreted and an-

giotensin is formed, causing vasoconstriction within the renal system and increased total peripheral resistance. Angiotensin also stimulates the secretion of aldosterone, which promotes sodium and water retention by the kidney tubules, causing an increase in intravascular volume. All these factors increase blood pressure. Evidence from animal, clinical, and epidemiologic studies points to an association between high blood pressure and abnormal calcium metabolism, leading to increased calcium loss, secondary activation of the parathyroid gland, increased movement of calcium from bone, and increased risk of urinary tract stones and osteoporosis.[40]

Clinical Manifestations.   Hypertension is frequently asymptomatic (except for elevated blood pressure when measured) especially in the early stages; this creates a significant health care risk for affected people. When symptoms do occur, they may include headache (usually occipital and present in the morning, worse on waking, and slowly improving with activity), vertigo, flushed face, spontaneous epistaxis, blurred vision, and nocturnal frequency. Sleep-disordered breathing is also associated with systemic hypertension in middle-aged and older individuals of both genders and different ethnic backgrounds.[172] Progressive hypertension may be characterized by cardiovascular or cerebral symptoms, such as dyspnea, orthopnea, chest pain, and leg edema (cardiovascular) or nausea, vomiting, drowsiness, confusion, and fleeting numbness or tingling in the limbs (cerebral). Hypertensive encephalopathy, a neurologic syndrome that occurs as a result of a sudden sustained rise in blood pressure, may be accompanied by nonspecific neurologic symptoms, such as confusion, headache, nausea, and even coma. It is also well-recognized that end-stage renal disease (ESRD) is associated with accelerated and malignant hypertension; hypertension is associated with increased urinary calcium excretion and subsequent bone loss and osteoporosis especially at the femoral neck.[22]

Medical Management

Diagnosis. In the past, hypertension was diagnosed primarily on the basis of the diastolic measurement, which was considered a better representation of the overall condition of the circulatory system. The rise of systolic pressure with age was considered to be normal and therefore not a risk factor. Today, it is recognized that although diastolic hypertension (>90 mm Hg) is common and usually controllable, systolic hypertension (>140 mm Hg) is the most common in older adults and the most powerful risk factor for stroke and strongly linked with heart attack, heart failure, and kidney failure even when the diastolic blood pressure is within normal limits. Systolic pressure measures the maximal strain on the heart and blood vessels and is a more precise measure of future damage to the system.

Blood pressure varies over the course of any single day depending on exertion, emotional state, ingestion of food, medications, and the presence of risk factors described previously. Thus it is important that blood pressure be measured at several different times and under consistent circumstances before a diagnosis of hypertension is made. Twenty-four–hour blood pressure monitoring using a portable device that automatically takes blood pressure readings at regular intervals is available and especially helpful in mapping out labile hypertension. The individual maintains a log of activities and emotions corresponding to the times when readings are taken; this information is compared with the computer-generated map of blood pressures generated from the data collected by the measurement device. No other tests are specific for essential hypertension. Studies used in the routine evaluation of hypertension may include a complete blood count (CBC); urinalysis; serum potassium, cholesterol, and creatinine assays; fasting blood glucose level; ECG; and chest radiography. Other more specific tests may be needed for secondary hypertension or more complete cardiac assessment for selected individuals.

Prevention. The American Society of Hypertension recommends that everyone, regardless of age, should know his or her blood pressure (the actual numbers). An annual blood pressure check is important for everyone; more frequent blood pressure measurements should be taken in anyone with risk factors or known hypertension. Elevated blood pressure in a younger adult (<50 years) can cause long-term accumulated damage, irreversible by age 50 or 60 years; therefore any elevation in blood pressure at any age must be addressed. The most important prevention factor is physical activity and exercise; other key variables include weight control, limitations on salt and alcohol intake, and modification of other risk factors present (see Box 11-5). Combining a low-sodium diet with the DASH diet (Dietary Approaches to Stop Hypertension; high intake of fruits, vegetables, and low-fat dairy foods) helps reduce blood pressure more than diet alone, both for healthy people and for those with high blood pressure. Reducing salt intake also lowers the risk of osteoporosis and possible fracture since a high salt intake increases urinary calcium excretion and hypertension has been found to be associated with bone loss.

Treatment. Once diagnosed, hypertension requires ongoing management (see Table 11-5) despite the absence of symptoms. According to the Joint National Committee (JNC VI), the goal is to achieve and maintain the lowest safe arterial blood pressure (without side effects); the intended target goal is to reduce blood pressure to less than 140/90 mm Hg or 130/85 mm Hg in those at highest risk. The decision to treat and the method and intensity of intervention are based on the concept of total risk not just blood pressure measurements. This approach takes into account cardiovascular risk factors in people with hypertension (see Box 11-5) and the presence of target organ damage or clinical cardiovascular disease (e.g., prior coronary revascularization, MI, stroke, peripheral arterial disease, retinopathy). The World Health Organization has published guidelines for the management of hypertension that review the management of risk factors in detail and prognosis based on risk stratification.[254]

Management of hypertension may begin with a "stepped care" approach including smoking cessation and other nonpharmacologic interventions through lifestyle modification as initial therapy for primary hypertension (including those with blood pressure on the high side of normal or a family history of hypertension). This approach has been shown effective in lowering blood pressure and can reduce other cardiovascular risk factors. Even when lifestyle modifications alone are not adequate in controlling hypertension, they may reduce the dosage of medication needed to manage the condition.[212] This program may include weight reduction; smoking cessation; a regular program of aerobic exercise; moderation of alcohol, dietary fat, caffeine, and dietary sodium; administration of nutritional supplements (e.g., potassium, calcium, magnesium); and behavioral cognitive therapy for those with hypertension associated with certain personality traits. See the previous section on Atherosclerosis: Treatment.

If nonpharmacologic measures fail to produce the desired results or if the blood pressure is very high at the time of diagnosis, blood pressure–lowering medications are prescribed starting with the lowest effective dose (to avoid intolerable side effects) and modifying accordingly. Antihypertensive medications can be classified by mode of action as diuretics, adrenergic inhibitors, vasodilators, ACE inhibitors, and calcium antagonists (see Table 11-4). More than 50% of cases of mild hypertension can be controlled with one drug; a combination of medications may be required for others. Diuretics are often the first step in the pharmacologic management of hypertension. Although these drugs decrease plasma volume, potassium depletion and renal complications may require the use of beta-blockers, calcium-channel blockers, or ACE inhibitors. Black people are generally more responsive to calcium antagonists and diuretics than to beta-blockers or ACE inhibitors. Older adults with hypertension are generally equally responsive to all classes of antihypertensive medications, but they have an increased likelihood of side effects. Pharmacologic therapy is individualized, matching the individual's clinical presentation with medications available.

More aggressive early treatment of people with diabetes and elevated blood pressure is recommended. Hypertensive people who tend to be hostile may be told to take their medication at bedtime to avoid the sharp rises in blood pressure in the early morning hours associated with heart attacks. The use of home monitoring devices is an important part of the management program both to monitor the blood pressure and to evaluate the effect of antihypertensive medication. Home monitoring can also distinguish between sustained hypertension and white coat hypertension and improves program compliance. In individuals with hypertension, the blood pressure readings taken in a clinic setting tend to be 5 to 10 mm Hg higher than measurements taken at home. Recommended frequency of readings is twice daily (morning and evening) on work and nonwork days for anyone newly diagnosed or in whom antihypertensive medication has recently been initiated or changed. Anyone with stable hypertension can take blood pressure reading several days per week.

Obesity has long been associated with hypertension and is an independent risk factor for CVD and CAD as well. Regular exercise enhances weight loss and reduces blood pressure independent of weight loss. (For further discussion see Special Implications for the Therapist: Exercise in this section.) Older individuals, blacks, and hypertensive individuals are more sensitive to change in dietary sodium chloride than are other individuals. A reduction of sodium intake alone may be enough to control blood pressure in persons with mild hypertension and may reduce the medication requirements in those who require drug therapy. It is also recommended that individuals with high blood pressure limit their intake of alcohol to 2 oz of liquor, 10 oz of red wine, or 24 oz of beer. Women and lighter-weight men should limit ethanol intake to half of these amounts/day.[212]

Dietary potassium deficiency may have a role in increasing blood pressure; individuals may also become hypokalemic from increased urinary magnesium excretion during diuretic therapy and require additional potassium. Magnesium and calcium influence vascular tone because magnesium acts to relax blood vessels and calcium assists in blood vessel contraction. A proper balance of these two substances is essential, since they compete for entry into the cell. When magnesium is low, an abnormally large amount of calcium enters the cells so that blood vessels begin to lose their ability to relax. Progressive vasoconstriction and subsequent spasms result in elevated blood pressure and eventual ischemia. Muscle weakness with depressed tendon reflexes may accompany this condition. A fall in serum potassium level also enhances the effects of digitalis, increasing the risk of digoxin toxicity.

Prognosis.   Hypertension is a major risk factor for atherosclerosis, implicating hypertension as a common cause of death in the United States. Among black Americans, hypertension is also the most common fatal familial disease. More than one-half of persons with angina pectoris, sudden death, stroke, and thrombotic occlusion of the abdominal aorta or its branches have hypertension. Three fourths of people with congestive heart failure, dissecting aortic aneurysm, intracerebral hemorrhage, or rupture of the myocardial wall also have elevated blood pressure. If it is untreated, nearly 50% of people with hypertension die of heart disease, 33% die of stroke, and 10% to 15% die of renal failure.

When a person with hypertension achieves the target blood pressure, it must be emphasized that blood pressure control does not equal cure. Adherence to treatment and follow-up monitoring must be continued on an ongoing basis. Unfortunately, the cost of antihypertensives, side effects, and lack of symptoms sometimes lead to poor compliance with treatment. Treatment prolongs life, and antihypertensive medications have dramatically reduced the mortality rate associated with hypertension. See also the section on Atherosclerosis: Prognosis (especially regarding pulse pressure as the newest predictor of mortality).

Special Implications for the Therapist   11-4

HYPERTENSION (HYPERTENSIVE VASCULAR DISEASE)

Preferred Practice Patterns:
4A: Primary Prevention/Risk Reduction for Skeletal Demineralization (osteoporosis prevention)
5A: Primary Prevention/Risk Reduction for Loss of Balance and Falling (side effect of medication: dizziness)
6A: Primary Prevention/Risk Reduction for Cardiovascular/Pulmonary Disorders
6B: Impaired Aerobic Capacity/Endurance Associated With Deconditioning
See also Special Implications for the Therapist: Atherosclerosis, 11-2.

It is estimated that hypertension remains undiagnosed in nearly one half of the 60 million Americans who have it. It is possible that many people in a therapy practice will be hypertensive without knowing it. Cardiac pathology may be unknown, requiring the therapist to remain alert for risk factors that require medical screening. For anyone with identified risk factors, a baseline blood pressure measurement should be taken on two or three separate occasions, and any unusual findings should be reported to the physician. The role of the therapist in screening to identify conditions such as hypertension is important since an essential early component of intervention for this condition includes exercise.

The potential for osteoporosis and subsequent hip fractures in older adults (especially women) with hypertension points to the importance of osteoporosis screening and prevention in this population. The physical therapist has an important role in the primary prevention of impairments and functional limitations in people with hypertension. A sudden increase in blood pressure such as occurs with any increase in intraabdominal pressure (e.g., Valsalva's maneuver; see also Box 15-1) during exercise or stabilization exercises can be dangerous for already hypertensive persons. The therapist must alert individuals with hypertension to this effect and teach proper breathing techniques during all activities.

Medications

People with coronary artery disease taking NSAIDs may also be at slight risk for a myocardial event during times of increased myocardial oxygen demand (e.g., exercise, fever). In addition,

Continued

older adults taking NSAIDs and antihypertensive agents must be monitored carefully. Regardless of the NSAID chosen, it is important to check blood pressure within the first few weeks after therapy or exercise is initiated and periodically thereafter.

Whenever a health care provider knows that a client has been prescribed antihypertensive medications, appropriate follow-up questions as to whether the client is taking the medication and taking it as prescribed must be addressed. Many people take the medication only when symptoms are perceived and are at risk for the complications described previously (especially during an exercise program, when oxygen demands of the myocardium increase). Obtain as much information as possible about a client's medications so that potential side effects can be anticipated and intervention planned accordingly. Any side effects noted may indicate that a medication adjustment is needed and should be brought to the physician's attention (see Table 11-4).

The following brief description of the impact of various drug classes (all vasodilators) on exercise may assist the therapist in prescribing activities for those who require pharmacologic agents and provide insight into therapeutic decisions for active hypertensive individuals. Antihypertensive medications reduce resting blood pressure levels and may influence blood pressure changes during submaximal and maximal exertion, which affects exercise capacity. Vasodilators selectively inhibit an increase in heart rate. Clinically, this means that when the person increases his or her activity or exercise level, the normal physiologic response of increased heart rate is blunted. This requires a longer warm-up and cool-down period. Sudden changes in position (e.g., supine to standing) should be avoided to prevent dizziness and falls associated with the resulting orthostatic hypotension (see Special Implications for the Therapist: Orthostatic Hypotension, 11-8). Vasodilators such as *nitroglycerin* and other nitrates act as a prophylactic for angina by dilating the coronary arteries and improving collateral cardiac circulation, increasing oxygen to the heart muscle, and decreasing the blood pressure, thereby decreasing symptoms of angina.

β-adrenoreceptor antagonists (β-*blockers*) diminish catecholamine-induced elevations of heart rate, myocardial contractility, and blood pressure. These effects reduce myocardial oxygen requirements during exertion and stress, thereby preventing angina and allowing the person to exercise for longer periods before the onset of angina. The intended action of β-blockers may prevent normal blood pressure and heart rate responses to exercise; therefore using heart rate as an index for monitoring response to exercise is not recommended. Although β-blockers are effective antihypertensives, most of them adversely alter aerobic capacity so that exercise capacity is reduced. An exercise prescription should be based on exercise stress test results using recommended guidelines.[5] Side effects of β-blockers include bronchospasm, which causes difficulty breathing, or chest tightness, which mimics angina; orthostatic hypotension; syncope; headache; or fatigue and weakness.

Diuretics have been first-line antihypertensive agents for many years, but few studies have observed the effect of diuretic therapy on exercise performance. Existing evidence reveals that peak blood pressures induced by physical activity may not always be controlled with diuretics. Diuretic therapy can result in hypokalemia accompanied by muscular cramps and skeletal muscle fatigue (see also Chapter 4). Potassium-sparing diuretics may cause hyperkalemia, which can in turn cause ventricular arrhythmias. Exercise tolerance may be reduced with ar-

rhythmias because of a decrease in left ventricular filling time. Prolonged exercise in the heat is not recommended for people taking diuretics because of the cumulative effects of heat, exercise, and diuretics on blood volume and electrolytes. The length of time an individual who is taking a diuretic can safely exercise in the heat varies with the heat index and the physical condition of the person.

Calcium plays a role in the electrical excitation of cardiac cells and in the mechanical contraction of the myocardial and vascular smooth muscle cells. *Calcium-channel antagonists* inhibit calcium ion influx across the cell membrane during cardiac depolarization, relax coronary vascular smooth muscle, dilate coronary and peripheral arteries, and increase myocardial oxygen delivery in people with vasospastic angina. This class of vasodilators decreases peripheral vascular resistance at rest and during physical activity, thereby altering exercise tolerance by affecting heart rate and blood pressure during exercise. During exercise, calcium-channel antagonists have been observed to reduce systolic and diastolic pressure at submaximal loads, but higher systolic blood pressures measured during maximal exercise are not lowered. Side effects of calcium antagonists (e.g., drowsiness, dizziness, headache, peripheral edema, tachycardia or bradycardia) may interfere with a client's ability to participate in an exercise program.

ACE inhibitors reduce blood pressure by lowering peripheral vascular resistance. Despite the benefits of ACE inhibitors on the prognosis of individuals who are taking them, there is a lack of consistency in the results of trials investigating the effects of ACE inhibitors on exercise capacity. These inconsistencies cannot be readily explained by variations in effects on known neurohormonal or conventional hemodynamic factors. Investigators propose that the conflicting observations on the effects of inhibitors on exercise capacity suggest that there is an optimal dosage of ACE inhibitors that will most enhance exercise capacity, but further studies are required to verify this theory.[251] Use of calcium antagonists and ACE inhibitors in hypertension increased dramatically in the 1990s whereas the use of less expensive agents, such as diuretics and beta-blockers, declined. In the absence of convincing evidence that the more expensive medications reduced stroke and coronary disease and prevented heart disease in the hypertensive population, the use of less expensive but just as effective diuretics and beta-blockers has regained prominence.

Exercise and Blood Pressure

The benefits of resistive or dynamic exercise in people with and without cardiovascular disease are well-known and available for review.[186] A regular program of aerobic exercise, introduced gradually, facilitates cardiovascular conditioning, may assist in weight reduction, and may provide some benefit in reducing blood pressure. Exercising using primarily the lower extremities (e.g., cycling, walking) can also reduce blood pressure. Postexercise hypotension (lowered blood pressure in response to exercise) in mildly hypertensive individuals has been observed for up to 7 hours after exercise independent of other variables.[185] Diastolic blood pressure reduction seems to be related to the duration of the exercise program (i.e., the longer the program, the more likely the hypotensive effect). Blood pressure reduction has occurred after just several weeks to 6 months of regular training.[101] On the other hand, blood pressure will return to its previous elevated level if training is discontinued.

Heavy isometric exercises and heavy weightlifting may be harmful, since the blood pressure often rises because of vaso-vagal reflexes that occur. During fatiguing isometric exercise, the rate and rise of systolic blood pressure appear to be higher in hypertensive individuals, but studies in this area are limited. Generally, antihypertensive drugs have not been found to affect the blood pressure response to isometric exertion. However, the use of isometric exercise to lower blood pressure has not been studied in hypertensive individuals; a fall in resting blood pressure has been observed in normotensive individuals after repetitive isometric contractions equal to 30% of maximal capacity.[248]

Exercise Training Guidelines

The intensity of exercise required to produce health benefits and decrease blood pressure has been confused with the level of exercise necessary to improve physical fitness. Health benefits can be achieved without large gains in fitness. Encouraging people to increase their level of total energy expenditure is the key to increasing activity levels, rather than emphasizing physical fitness. The type, intensity, duration, and frequency of training, as well as progression, should be assessed regularly. A preexercise evaluation and exercise testing may be prescribed by the physician. This information is helpful in establishing submaximal and maximal blood pressure responses. Monitoring vital signs before, during, and after exercise or activity is essential. Any person with an exaggerated systolic blood pressure response (>250 mm Hg) or failure to reduce diastolic pressure (<90 mm Hg) should be referred to the physician for reevaluation.

Training intensity does not need to be high, and it appears that low-intensity activity (65% to 70% of maximal heart rate) three times per week is as effective as high-intensity activity in blood pressure reduction. Training intensity should be based on maximal heart rate using the calculated formulas (see Appendix B) or measured during a maximal exercise test. After 12 to 16 weeks, if the blood pressure is adequately controlled, the physician may reduce the antihypertensive medication slowly to determine the long-term effect of training on blood pressure. Several resources are available for determining the appropriate exercise program for the hypertensive client whether symptomatic or asymptomatic.[5,25]

Monitoring During Exercise

Therapists often treat people who are diagnosed with conditions that are highly correlated with hypertension, such as stroke, obesity, diabetes mellitus, alcoholism, CAD, and pregnancy (see Table 11-9). Monitoring tolerance to exercise by observing for unusual symptoms and measuring blood pressure before, during, and after therapy are important steps in identifying a potential cardiovascular event. Many factors can cause an increase in blood pressure (see Appendix B). ■

Hypertensive Heart Disease

Definition and Overview.   The term *hypertensive heart disease* is used when the heart is enlarged as a result of persistently elevated blood pressure (hypertension) (see previous discussion). Left ventricular hypertrophy (LVH) and diastolic dysfunction are found in 10% to 30% of the adult population with chronic hypertension, and it may present with many of the signs and symptoms of CHF. Both the prevalence and the severity of the disease are greater in blacks than in whites. In all adults, it increases progressively with age.

Medical Management

Diagnosis, Treatment, and Prognosis.   Cardiac enlargement viewed on x-ray and ECG changes of left ventricular hypertrophy are diagnostic of hypertensive heart disease. Treatment is as for hypertension unless heart failure develops, in which case treatment is as for heart failure (see each section for more discussion). The most common cause of death in hypertensive heart disease is CHF, accounting for 40% of all deaths from hypertension.

Special Implications for the Therapist   11-5

HYPERTENSIVE HEART DISEASE

Preferred Practice Patterns:
6B: Impaired Aerobic Capacity/Endurance Associated With Deconditioning
6D: Impaired Aerobic Capacity/Endurance Associated With Cardiovascular Pump Dysfunction or Failure
See Special Implications for the Therapist: Atherosclerosis, 11-2, Special Implications for the Therapist: Hypertension, 11-4 and Special Implications for the Therapist: Congestive Heart Failure, 11-7. ■

◆ Myocardial Infarction

Definition and Incidence.   MI, also known as a heart attack or coronary, is the development of ischemia with resultant necrosis of myocardial tissue. Any prolonged obstruction depriving the heart muscle of oxygen can cause an MI. Myocardial infarction occurs in $1\frac{1}{2}$ million persons each year and represents the leading cause of death (500,000 deaths annually) in the adult American population. See the previous section on Ischemic Heart Disease in this chapter.

Etiologic and Risk Factors.   Etiologic and risk factors are the same as for all forms of CVD, especially angina pectoris associated with CAD (see the previous section on Angina Pectoris). Eighty percent to ninety percent of MIs result from coronary thrombus at the site of a preexisting atherosclerotic stenosis. New cases of MI occur in many people with only a borderline risk profile or even lack of known risk factors suggesting other unidentified risk factors. Other causes may include cocaine use (causes vasoconstriction of the coronary arteries), vasculitis, aortic stenosis, or aortic root or coronary artery dissection. Smokers have more than twice as many heart attacks as nonsmokers, and sudden cardiac death occurs two to four times more frequently in smokers. After an infarction, smokers have a poorer chance of recovery than nonsmokers. Exertion-related MI, which may include weakness or shortness of breath while working with the arms extended overhead in habitually inactive people, has also been reported associated with single-vessel rather than triple-vessel disease.[88]

It is a well-established fact that heart attacks occur more frequently in the early morning hours. This peak incidence is attributed to an increase in catecholamines with the resultant

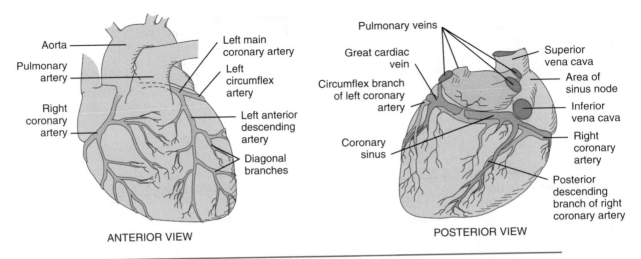

ANTERIOR VIEW   POSTERIOR VIEW

FIGURE 11-8 Areas of myocardium affected by arterial insufficiency of specific coronary arteries. The right and left coronary arteries branch off the aorta just above the aortic valve and normally supply the myocardium with oxygenated blood. The most commonly affected arteries and the area of myocardium supplied are listed in order of decreasing occurrence.

Coronary Artery Supply	Area of Myocardium Involved
Left coronary artery (LCA), left anterior descending (LAD) branch	Anterior
Right coronary artery (RCA)	Posterior
RCA	Inferior
LCA, LAD branch	Anteroseptal
Circumflex artery, marginal branch, or LCA, diagonal branch	High lateral
Usually LCA, left anterior branch, may be RCA, posterior descending branch	Apical

increased blood pressure, increased workload of the heart, as well as increased clotting factors in the early morning. Heart attacks also occur in a seasonal pattern with an increased incidence between Thanksgiving and New Year's Day across all ages, in both genders, and across geographic regions. Whether this is attributed to mood changes, weather, circadian rhythms, or some other mechanism remains unknown.

The association between periodontal disease and acute MI is under investigation. Researchers have found that bacteria in the mouth spill into the bloodstream and can be found in the walls of major arteries. Whether treating periodontal disease reduces the risk of heart attack or stroke has not been established. Acute respiratory tract infections, such as the common cold, flu, and bronchitis, may also increase the risk of heart attack occurring within 2 weeks of a first heart attack and may account for some cases of MI although researchers point out that early symptoms of heart attacks may be mistaken for acute upper respiratory infection.[158]

Silent ischemia is highly prevalent among people with diabetes; plasminogen activator inhibitor (PAI-1)* has been identified as a risk factor for MI in persons with diabetes as well as for postmenopausal women not receiving hormone replacement therapy. Research now shows that diabetic clients have higher PAI-1 activity than nondiabetic clients, both at hospital admission for acute MI and at follow-up 1 year later. Raised PAI-1 activity may predispose diabetic clients to MI and may also impair pharmacologic and spontaneous reperfusion after acute MI, contributing to the poor outcome in this population.[225]

Pathogenesis. The myocardium receives its blood supply from the two large coronary arteries and their branches (Fig. 11-8). One or more of these blood vessels may become occluded by a clot that forms suddenly when an atheromatous plaque ruptures through the sublayers of a blood vessel or when the narrow, roughened inner lining of a sclerosed artery becomes completely filled with thrombus. In most cases, infarcts result from an occlusive thrombus superimposed on an atherosclerotic plaque. Researchers have found that plaque most likely to rupture (vulnerable plaque) is comprised of the soft form of cholesterol (cholesteryl ester) and is vulnerable to mechanical forces such as occur with the increase in hormones early in the morning or even the vibration of the heartbeat. Rupturing plaque does not always result in an MI. It is likely that plaque breaks off frequently without triggering a heart attack and the large plaques visible on angiograms are often the healed over and more stable plaque. Although these plaques occlude the coronary vessels resulting in obstruction, ischemia, and angina, they are not as likely to cause rupture and sudden death as happens with the soft, smaller, and usually undetected plaques.

The most common site involved is the left ventricle, the chamber of the heart with the greatest workload. Thrombosis of the anterior descending branch of the left coronary artery is the most common location of infarction and affects the anterior left ventricle (Fig. 11-9). Occlusion

---

*PAI-1 is a naturally occurring substance that inhibits another natural substance, t-PA; t-PA is an enzyme released endogenously as part of the body's defense against thrombosis; it lyses fibrin and dissolves forming blood clots. The effect of PAI-1 on t-PA is to *prevent* clot destruction in the bloodstream.

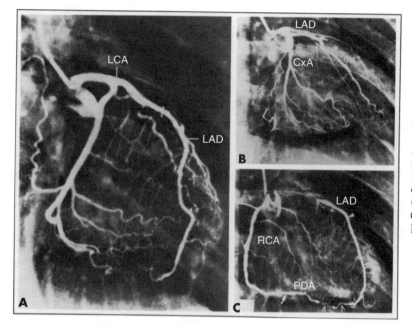

FIGURE   **11-9**   **A,** Angiogram of a normal coronary artery (LCA). **B,** Angiogram of a totally obstructed left anterior descending (LAD) coronary artery. **C,** Angiogram of the right coronary artery (RCA) and its major branch, the posterior descending artery (PDA) (same heart as in **B**). The LAD is seen because of collateral vessels connecting the LAD and the RCA system. (From Boucek R, Morales A, Romanelli R, et al: *Coronary artery disease: pathologic and clinical assessment,* Baltimore, 1984, Williams & Wilkins, pp 4, 9.)

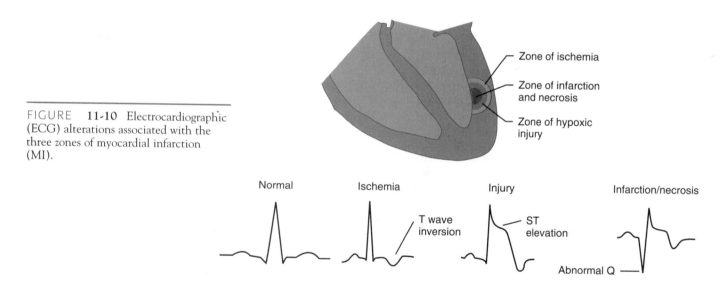

FIGURE   **11-10**   Electrocardiographic (ECG) alterations associated with the three zones of myocardial infarction (MI).

of the left circumflex artery produces anterolateral or posterolateral infarction. Right coronary artery thrombosis leads to infarction of the posteroinferior portion of the left ventricle and may involve the right ventricular myocardium and interventricular septum. The arteries supplying the atrioventricular node and the sinus node more commonly arise from the right coronary artery; thus atrioventricular block at the nodal level and sinus node dysfunction occur more frequently during inferior infarctions.

Myocardial ischemia/reperfusion injury is accompanied by an inflammatory response comprised of three major components: (1) molecular oxygen, (2) cellular blood elements (especially neutrophils), and (3) activated complement system. When the myocardium has been completely deprived of oxygen, cells die and the tissue becomes necrotic in an area called the *zone of infarction* (Fig. 11-10; see also Figs. 5-5 and 5-6). In response to this necrosis, leukocytes aid in removing the dead cells, and fibroblasts form a connective tissue scar within the area of infarction. The remaining heart muscle cells enlarge to compensate for the loss in heart pump function (see also the

section on Cell Injury in Chapter 5; a complete discussion of the role of oxidative stress and complement activation in heart disease is available[45,65]). Usually the formation of fibrous scar tissue is complete within 6 to 8 weeks (Table 11-10; see Fig. 5-6).

Immediately surrounding the area of infarction is a less seriously damaged area of injury called the *zone of hypoxic injury.* This zone is able to return to normal, but it may also become necrotic if blood flow is not restored. With adequate collateral circulation, this area may regain its function within 2 to 3 weeks. Adjacent to the zone of hypoxic injury is another reversible zone called the *zone of ischemia.* Ischemic and injured myocardial tissues cause characteristic ECG changes; as the myocardium heals, the ST segment and T waves gradually return to normal, but abnormal Q waves may persist.

Oxygen deprivation is accompanied by electrolyte disturbances, particularly cellular loss of potassium, calcium, and magnesium. Myocardial cells deprived of necessary oxygen and nutrients lose contractility, thereby diminishing the pumping ability of the heart. Normally the myocardium takes up varying quantities of catecholamines (epinephrine, no-

TABLE   11-10

Tissue Changes After Myocardial Infarction

TIME AFTER MI	TISSUE CHANGES
6-12 hr	No gross changes; healing process has not begun
18-24 hr	Inflammatory response; intercellular enzyme release
2-4 days	Visible necrosis; proteolytic enzymes remove debris; catecholamines, lipolysis, and glycogenolysis elevate plasma glucose and increase free fatty acids to assist depleted myocardium recovery from anaerobic state
4-10 days	Debris cleared; collagen matrix laid down
10-14 days	Weak, fibrotic scar tissue with beginning revascularization; area vulnerable to stress
6 wk	Scarring usually complete; tough, inelastic scar replaces necrotic myocardium; unable to contract and relax like healthy myocardial tissue

Modified from McCance KL, Huether SE: *Pathophysiology: the biologic basis for disease in adults and children,* ed 2, St Louis, 1994, Mosby, p 1028.

repinephrine), which are released when significant arterial occlusion occurs. Released catecholamines predispose the individual to serious imbalances of sympathetic and parasympathetic function, irregular heartbeats (arrhythmia), and heart failure.

Clinical Manifestations.   The most notable symptom of MI is a sudden sensation of pressure, often described as prolonged crushing chest pain, occasionally radiating to the arms, throat, neck (as high as the occipital area), and back (Fig. 11-11). The pain is constant, lasting 30 minutes up to hours, and may be accompanied by pallor, shortness of breath, and profuse perspiration. Catecholamine release resulting in sympathetic stimulation may produce diaphoresis and peripheral vasoconstriction that cause the skin to become cool and clammy. Angina pectoris pain can be similar, but it is less severe, does not last for hours, and is relieved by cessation of activity, rest, or nitrates.

Symptoms do not always follow the classic pattern, especially in women. Two major symptoms in women are shortness of breath, sometimes occurring in the middle of the night, and chronic, unexplained fatigue. Atypical presentation may include continuous pain in the midthoracic spine or interscapular area, neck and shoulder pain, stomach or abdominal pain, nausea, unexplained anxiety, or heartburn that is not altered by antacids. Silent attacks (painless infarction without acute symptoms) are more common among nonwhites, older adults (>75 years), all smokers, and adults (men and women) with diabetes, presumably because of reduced sensitivity to pain. Nausea and vomiting may occur because of reflex stimulation of vomiting centers by pain fibers. Fever may develop in the first 24 hours and persist for a week because of inflammatory activity within the myocardium.

Postinfarction complications include arrhythmias, congestive heart failure, cardiogenic shock, pericarditis, rupture of the heart, thromboembolism, recurrent infarction, and sudden death. Arrhythmias affecting more than 90% of individuals are the most common complication of acute MI and are caused by ischemia, hypoxia, autonomic nervous system imbalances, lactic acidosis, electrolyte imbalances, drug toxicity, or alterations of impulse conduction pathways or conduction defects.

Medical Management
Prevention.   See the sections on Atherosclerosis: Prevention and Angina Pectoris: Prevention.

Diagnosis.   Diagnosis of acute MI and determination of the site and extent of necrosis rely on the clinical history, interpretation of the electrocardiogram, and measurement of serum levels of cardiac enzymes. Diagnostic uncertainty frequently arises because of a variety of factors. Many people with acute MI have atypical symptoms, and one half of all cases with typical symptoms do not have acute MI. One half of the people with acute MI have nondiagnostic ECGs, and some people are unable to provide a history. Biochemical markers of cardiac injury are commonly relied on to diagnose or exclude acute MI. These laboratory tests dramatically reduce the cost of treating heart attacks by allowing physicians to quickly discharge people with noncardiac chest pain.

Newer biochemical markers of myocardial injury, such as cardiac troponin I (TnI) and cardiac troponin T (TnT) (regulatory proteins that help the heart muscle contract), are now being used instead of or along with the standard markers, isoenzyme of creatine kinase (CK-MB) and lactate dehydrogenase. Troponin I is a better cardiac marker than CK-MB for myocardial infarction because it is equally sensitive but more specific to myocardial injury, but troponin T is a better predictor of cardiovascular mortality (as well as all-cause mortality). Both TnI and TnT are useful markers for myocardial injury that help determine the prognosis in people who have unstable angina but no evidence of CK-MB elevation. (See also the section on Cardiac Enzymes and Markers in Chapter 39; see Tables 39-13 and 39-14).

Researchers are continuing to investigate other hemostatic markers based on the knowledge that coronary thrombosis involves both coagulation and fibrinolysis cascades. For example, increases of fibrinogen and D-dimer, a circulating marker of fibrin turnover, are significantly higher in people with acute ischemic events such as MI and unstable angina than in nonischemic individuals, but it has not been determined to what extent this is causal. Other tests may include nuclear scanning, coronary angiography, echocardiography, CT, cardiac magnetic resonance (CMR) stress test, and MRA. Serum cholesterol must be determined because of its importance as a modifiable risk factor. See the previous sections on Angina Pectoris: Diagnosis and Atherosclerosis: Diagnosis.

Other cardiac markers include homocysteine, Lp(a) (lipoprotein little a), and C-reactive protein (CRP). Although these have not become "standard" laboratory values they can be used as independent predictors of future coronary events in apparently healthy men and women. For example, elevated plasma total homocysteine (tHcy) is a risk factor for atherosclerosis and endothelial dysfunction and CRP may be used as a marker of subclinical atherosclerosis and cardiovascular risk specifically linked to MI and sudden death.

Infarcted tissue is electrically silent and does not contribute to the ECG. Most clients with acute infarction have ECG changes, although this test provides only a crude estimate of the

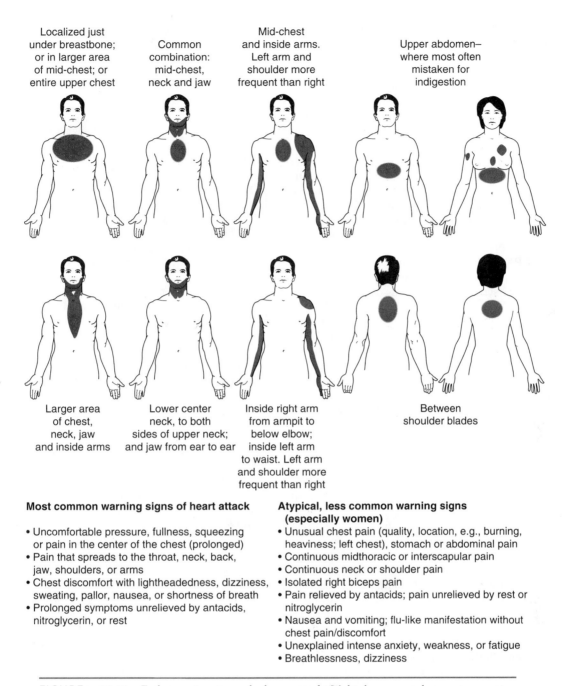

Localized just under breastbone; or in larger area of mid-chest; or entire upper chest

Common combination: mid-chest, neck and jaw

Mid-chest and inside arms. Left arm and shoulder more frequent than right

Upper abdomen— where most often mistaken for indigestion

Larger area of chest, neck, jaw and inside arms

Lower center neck, to both sides of upper neck; and jaw from ear to ear

Inside right arm from armpit to below elbow; inside left arm to waist. Left arm and shoulder more frequent than right

Between shoulder blades

Most common warning signs of heart attack

- Uncomfortable pressure, fullness, squeezing or pain in the center of the chest (prolonged)
- Pain that spreads to the throat, neck, back, jaw, shoulders, or arms
- Chest discomfort with lightheadedness, dizziness, sweating, pallor, nausea, or shortness of breath
- Prolonged symptoms unrelieved by antacids, nitroglycerin, or rest

Atypical, less common warning signs (especially women)

- Unusual chest pain (quality, location, e.g., burning, heaviness; left chest), stomach or abdominal pain
- Continuous midthoracic or interscapular pain
- Continuous neck or shoulder pain
- Isolated right biceps pain
- Pain relieved by antacids; pain unrelieved by rest or nitroglycerin
- Nausea and vomiting; flu-like manifestation without chest pain/discomfort
- Unexplained intense anxiety, weakness, or fatigue
- Breathlessness, dizziness

FIGURE 11-11 Early warning signs of a heart attack. Multiple segmental nerve innervation shown in Fig. 11-6 accounts for the varied pain patterns possible. A woman can experience any of the various patterns described but is more likely to develop atypical symptoms of pain as depicted here. (Modified from Goodman CC, Snyder TE: *Differential diagnosis in physical therapy,* ed 3, Philadelphia, 2000, Saunders, p 127.)

magnitude of infarction. When diagnosis by ECG and enzymes is not possible (e.g., when people seek medical attention after MI), scintigraphic studies (radionuclide imaging) can show areas of necrotic myocardium and diminished perfusion. These tests, which use radiotracers, do not distinguish old damage from recent infarction, and false-positive results can occur.

Other test procedures may include echocardiography, which is useful in assessing the ability of the heart walls to contract and relax, and transesophageal echocardiography (TEE), an ultrasonic technique that provides a clearer image of the heart, including the posterior wall, valvular anatomy, and thoracic aortic structure, providing identification of structural heart diseases. Newer technology, such as three-dimensional real-time imaging, has the potential to improve evaluation of heart function (especially ventricular) with TEE. Magnetic resonance imaging (MRI) to evaluate structural defects of the heart and positron emission tomography (PET) to evaluate cardiac physiology and metabolism and assess tissue perfusion have contributed significantly to the understanding of the pathophysiology of the ischemic heart.

Another new technique being investigated is the use of a contrast agent called EchoGen, used in conjunction with an ultrasound procedure. This agent infiltrates healthy heart muscle but not muscle that has been deprived of blood or oxygen. Existing contrast agents only image the heart chambers, which provides information about the flow of blood through the chamber but not about the structure of the heart muscle itself.

Treatment. The goal of treatment is reestablishing the flow of blood in blocked coronary arteries. Pharmacologic intervention is used to provide pain relief (essential since angina is evidence of ongoing ischemia), limit infarction size, reduce vasoconstriction, prevent thrombus formation, and augment repair. MI caused by intracoronary thrombi can be relieved by infusion of thrombolytic agents (e.g., streptokinase, urokinase, t-PA*) that dissolve clots, promote vasodilation, and reduce infarct size. This intervention initiated within 70 minutes of symptom onset is associated with improved outcome.[245] After a thrombolytic agent is administered, intravenous (IV) heparin therapy is usually administered with adjunctive drug therapy during and after MI because platelet inhibitor and other cardiovascular medication (see Table 11-4) administration is known to further reduce mortality when administered during the acute phase.

Right now, only 5% of heart attack victims receive reperfusion therapy within that crucial first hour after symptom onset primarily because people delay (sometimes by hours) coming to the emergency department. This points out the extreme importance of early intervention and education of the general population (and especially for those with known risk factors, such as hypertension, previous heart attack, diabetes, smoking, or hyperlipidemia) as to the importance of getting to an emergency department at the earliest sign of heart attack. Educating the public about the less common or atypical warning signs and symptoms is essential. Information about public education, reducing delays at home or at work, and the National Heart Attack Alert Program is available.[56,169]

Other treatment interventions, including identification and modification of risk factors, angioplasty, stenting, atherectomy, angiogenesis, tissue engineering, gene therapy, stem cell transplantation, and cardiac rehabilitation utilizing exercise programs, have been previously discussed in detail (see the sections on Atherosclerosis: Medical Management and Hypertension: Medical Management). Studies to determine whether early, rapid use of cholesterol-lowering therapy can reduce recurrent ischemic events in acute coronary syndromes is under way through the MIRACL (Myocardial Ischemia Reduction with Aggressive Cholesterol Lowering) program.

Exercise has been recommended as a means of increasing pain tolerance, increasing the stimulus required to induce angina, alleviating depression, reducing anxiety, and inducing collateral circulation. Increasing evidence suggests that combining a low-fat diet and intensive exercise training can improve myocardial perfusion by regression of coronary atherosclerosis. Exercise training may be contraindicated for some people (Box 11-6; see also Table 11-6). Medical clearance

---

BOX **11-6**

Contraindications to Exercise After Myocardial Infarction

Acute MI (<1 or 2 days after an MI without physician approval)
Unstable angina; easily provoked angina
New electrocardiogram (ECG) signs and symptoms of MI (e.g., nausea, dyspnea, light-headedness, chest pain)
PaO_2 <60 mm Hg
O_2 saturation <85%
Hemoglobin <8 g/dl; hematocrit <26%
Severe aortic outflow obstruction
Suspected or known dissecting aneurysm
Acute myocarditis or pericarditis
Uncontrolled complex arrhythmias
Active severe congestive heart failure (CHF); resting respiratory rate >45 breaths/min
Recent pulmonary embolism or thrombophlebitis
Untreated third-degree heart block
Severe systemic hypertension unresponsive to medication
Uncontrolled diabetes
Acute infections
Digoxin toxicity (see Table 11-4)

Modified from Kavanaugh T: Cardiac rehabilitation. In Goldberg L, Elliot DL: *Exercise for prevention and treatment of illness,* Philadelphia, 1994, Davis, p 55.

---

must be obtained for entry into an exercise-training program. Exercise testing is the most useful tool to establish guidelines for exercise training in apparently healthy adults and is mandatory for people with known or suspected cardiovascular disease. The majority of exercise testing can be done within 3 days of MI with a very low incidence of complications. Criteria for testing usually include clients who are off IV nitroglycerin with no angina at rest, uncontrolled cardiac failure, or arrhythmias. Early testing can lead to early triage and potential cost savings.

Prognosis. The size and anatomic location of the infarction, together with the amount of damage from previous infarctions, determine the acute clinical picture, the early complications, and the long-term prognosis. The first 24 hours after onset of symptoms is the time of highest risk for sudden death. The sooner someone reaches the hospital, the better the prognosis. Eighty percent of those experiencing an acute MI survive the initial attack when transported to a coronary care unit (CCU). Substantial reductions in post-MI death have occurred over the last four decades because of improved intervention.

Factors negatively affecting prognosis include age (clients older than 80 years have a 60% mortality); evidence of other cardiovascular diseases, respiratory diseases, or uncontrolled diabetes mellitus; anterior location of MI (30% mortality rate); and hypotension (clients whose systolic blood pressure is less than 55 mm Hg have a 60% mortality rate). The risk of reinfarction is increased in women, people with elevated blood pressure, and people with elevated serum cholesterol. As MI survivors with long-standing hypertension live longer,

---

*Tissue plasminogen activator (t-PA), a naturally occurring enzyme that acts directly on blood clots to dissolve them, is now a genetically engineered drug used in thrombolytic therapy. However, a single dose of recombinant t-PA (rt-PA) costs about $1000, whereas other drugs are less expensive (e.g., streptokinase costs about $300).

cardiac failure has become an increasingly important long-term sequela of MI.

Prognostic testing predictive of cardiac events includes standard exercise testing such as functional capacity and heart rate recovery and imaging using single-photon emission computed tomography (SPECT) with contrast agents (e.g., thallium 201, technetium Tc 99m sestamibi). In the imaging studies, a radioisotope is taken up by adequately perfused tissue detecting myocardial perfusion defects at rest and during exercise (areas of infarction appear as regions of diminished isotope activity or no activity referred to as *cold spots*). The prognostic value of treadmill exercise testing in older persons has shown that workload (measured in metabolic equivalents) is the only treadmill exercise testing predictive of death both in younger persons and in adults over 65 years of age.[92] An abnormal exercise test is a more powerful predictor of risk in those people with conventional risk factors compared to those without such risk factors.

Special Implications for the Therapist   11-6

MYOCARDIAL INFARCTION

Preferred Practice Patterns:
6A: Primary Prevention/Risk Reduction for
  Cardiovascular/Pulmonary Disorders
6B: Impaired Aerobic Capacity/Endurance Associated With
  Deconditioning
Other patterns may apply depending on postinfarction complications (e.g., arrhythmias, congestive heart failure, embolism, side effects of medications). See also Special Implications for the Therapist: Atherosclerosis.

Early Post-MI Considerations

Although the myocardium must rest, bed rest puts the client at risk for development of hypovolemia, hypoxemia, muscle atrophy, and pulmonary embolus (see also the section on The Cardiac Client and Surgery in this chapter). Developing a program of progressive physical activity with adequate pacing and rest periods begins within 24 hours for the acute care client in uncomplicated cases. Gentle movement exercises, deep breathing, and coughing are usually begun immediately as prophylactic measures. Incisional pain or discomfort from cardiac surgery may cause a person to exhibit rapid, shallow respirations in an attempt to ease the discomfort. If analgesics are prescribed to prevent severe discomfort, the drug can be administered before therapy to better enable the person to carry out breathing exercises. This problem is of limited duration and usually resolves when the incision heals. The therapist must be aware that analgesics also mask pain response, making it possible for the client to overexert.

Early therapeutic exercise helps prevent cardiopulmonary complications, venous stasis, joint stiffness, and muscle weakness. Relaxation is often promoted with low-intensity activity. Activities that increase intrathoracic or intraabdominal pressure, such as breath-holding and Valsalva's maneuvers (see Box 15-1), can precipitate bradycardia followed by increased venous return to the heart, causing possible cardiac overload. For this reason, these actions are contraindicated and should not be performed in any stage of the rehabilitation program.[59] During the first 6 weeks post-MI, the client is cautioned to avoid saunas, hot tubs, whirlpools, and excessively warm swimming pools. Early rehabilitation lasting 2 to 3 weeks is often followed by exercise testing, at which time water therapy may be permissible per physician approval (see Guidelines for Aquatic Therapy in Appendix B). Specific aspects of cardiac rehabilitation and postoperative care are beyond the scope of this text. Other more specific texts are available to guide the therapist in this area.[78,109,117] See also the Agency for Health Care Policy and Research's *Clinical Guidelines for Cardiac Rehabilitation.*[2]

Monitoring Vital Signs

The therapist must continually monitor for signs of impending infarction, including generalized or localized pain anywhere over the thorax, upper limbs, and neck; palpitations; dyspnea; lightheadedness; syncope; sensation of indigestion; hiccups; and nausea (see Fig. 11-11). Pain medications, such as morphine, used to minimize discomfort initially may also depress the respiratory drive. The CCU therapist must monitor corresponding vital signs. The home health therapist must monitor pulse and blood pressure measurements for hypotension because of the side effects precipitated by antihypertensive medications, vasodilators, and other antianginal agents. (See also Special Implications for the Therapist: Angina Pectoris, 11-3.) Initial ambulation and activities at home should be roughly equivalent to levels achieved at the hospital at the time of discharge, depending on the client's physiologic response to the transition from hospital to home.

The client must increase activities gradually to avoid overtaxing the heart as it pumps oxygenated blood to the muscles. The metabolic equivalent system provides one way of measuring the amount of oxygen needed to perform an activity: 1 metabolic equivalent of the task (MET) equals 3.5 ml of oxygen per kilogram of body weight per minute; 1 MET is approximately equivalent to the oxygen uptake a person requires when resting. Early mobilization activities after acute MI should not exceed 1 to 2 MET (e.g., brushing teeth, eating). By comparison, people who can exercise to 8 or more MET (oxygen uptake of 28 ml/kg/min or more) can perform most daily physical activities.

As activity level increases, the therapist must monitor heart rate, blood pressure, and fatigue, adjusting activity level accordingly. During phase I (acute hospital) care, the heart rate should not rise more than 25% above resting level, and blood pressure must not rise more than 25 mm Hg above resting level. When systolic blood pressure falls or fails to increase as the intensity of exercise increases, exercise intensity should be immediately reduced. A drop in systolic blood pressure during exercise below the rest value as measured in the standing position is associated with increased risk of lethal arrhythmia in clients with a prior MI or myocardial ischemia.

Supplemental oxygen may be used to supply the myocardium with oxygen when the demand exceeds supply, thereby reducing myocardial stress and eliminating dyspnea. Blood gas analysis is usually performed within 1 hour of initiating oxygen therapy to establish a baseline of arterial saturation. By monitoring blood gases, oxygen dose can be altered to regulate blood gases and acid-base balance. The therapist must monitor oxygen saturation levels during exercise or intervention because these activities may increase myocardial oxygen demand (see Table 39-21).

Continued

The client with chronic obstructive pulmonary disease (COPD) who receives oxygen therapy must be monitored very closely for symptoms of decreased ventilation, such as headache, giddiness, tinnitus (ringing in the ears), nausea, weakness, and vomiting. Frequently persons with COPD retain carbon dioxide (CO_2) making the use of oxygen a deadly drug. CO_2 levels are elevated in the COPD client, eliminating the drive to breathe normally that is initiated by rising levels of CO_2. The only drive to breathe in the COPD client is hypoxia (reduced oxygen levels). The administration of oxygen in a person with CO_2 retention can further depress the respiratory drive, resulting in death.

Exercise After Myocardial Infarction

As little as 10 years ago, exercise was avoided following a heart attack, but research has shown that a reasonable amount of regular exercise is the best way to strengthen the heart and control blood pressure, cholesterol, diabetes, and weight. Survivors who exercise usually require less medication, are less likely to need future invasive procedures (e.g., angioplasty, bypass graft), and are less likely to die of a second heart attack than those who remain sedentary. Traditionally, isometric exercises have been contraindicated, and resistance training or weightlifting has been excluded from the cardiac client's program. Although weight training is not an isometric (static) exercise, it is similar during maximal lifts.* Now, low-risk cardiac clients have undertaken supervised and prescribed weight-training programs without ill effects, especially if regimens incorporate moderate levels of resistance and high numbers of repetitions.[120,218] Thrombolytic agents reduce the client's blood-clotting ability, necessitating special care to avoid tissue trauma during therapy (e.g., resistive exercises, soft tissue or scar mobilization).

Heart attack survivors are often people who have never exercised before and need sound advice and careful supervision by a physical therapist. Exercise may induce cardiac arrhythmias during diuretic and digitalis therapy, and recent ingestion of caffeine may exacerbate arrhythmias. Exercise-induced arrhythmias are generated by enhanced sympathetic tone, increased myocardial oxygen demand, or both. The immediate postexercise period is particularly dangerous because of high catecholamine levels associated with a generalized vasodilation. Sudden termination of muscular activity is accompanied by diminished venous return and may lead to a reduction in coronary perfusion while heart rate is elevated. A careful cool-down period is required with continued monitoring of vital signs after exercise.

Sexual Activity

People with cardiac disease, both men and women, are prone to sexual dysfunction. Often their concerns are voiced to the therapist. Problems may be caused by medications, anxiety, depression, or limited physical capacity. Hypertensive medications are the most common drugs to cause sexual dysfunction (e.g., loss of sexual desire or ability to reach orgasm). Marijuana increases myocardial oxygen consumption and heart rate and results in decreased testosterone levels and decreased libido.

Cocaine can hinder erection, ejaculation, and orgasm; it may also cause coronary artery vasoconstriction and resulting chest pain and fatal MI. Fear of death during sexual intercourse, fear of another infarction caused by sexual activity, and diminished sexual ability caused by illness and aging may occur. The sexual partner may have many similar fears and may want to be included in any information provided about return to sexual function. The relative risk of triggering an MI by sexual activity is less than 1%.[167]

Sexual intercourse with orgasm is physiologically equivalent to activities such as a brisk walk or climbing a flight of stairs. It has been equated to 5 MET of work on an exercise stress test; preorgasmic and postorgasmic phases require about 3.7 METs. Advice to clients should be based on consultation with the physician. Some general guidelines include the following: (1) when the client can sustain a heart rate of 110 to 120 beats/min with no shortness of breath or anginal pain, he or she can resume sexual activity; (2) sexual activity should be resumed gradually and only after activities such as walking moderate distances (equivalent to 3 or 4 miles on a level treadmill) or climbing stairs comfortably have been accomplished; (3) sexual activity causes the least amount of stress when it occurs in familiar surroundings with the usual partner in a comfortable environment; (4) gradual foreplay helps the heart prepare for coitus; less strenuous sexual activities, such as cuddling, kissing, touching, and hugging, can be engaged in without sexual intercourse; (5) positions requiring isometric contractions should be avoided; (6) eating a large meal or drinking alcohol 1 to 3 hours before sexual activity should be avoided; (7) anal stimulation and anal intercourse should be avoided because this stimulates the vagus nerve and may cause chest pain and slows down the heart rate and rhythm, impulse conduction, and coronary blood flow[156]; and (8) the physician should be asked about whether the client should take prophylactic nitroglycerin before intercourse.[134] ■

◆ Congestive Heart Failure

Definition and Overview. CHF is a condition in which the heart is unable to pump sufficient blood to supply the body's needs. Backup of blood into the pulmonary veins and high pressure in the pulmonary capillaries lead to subsequent pulmonary congestion and pulmonary hypertension. Failure may occur on both sides of the heart or may predominantly affect the right or left side. Heart failure is not a disease but rather represents a group of clinical manifestations caused by inadequate pump performance from either the cardiac valves or the myocardium. It may be chronic over many years, requiring management by oral medications, or it may be acute and life-threatening, requiring more dramatic medical management to maintain an adequate cardiac output.

Four distinct types of CHF have been recognized: (1) systolic heart failure (caused by contractile failure of the myocardium), (2) diastolic failure (occurs when increased filling pressures are required to maintain adequate cardiac output despite normal contractile function), (3) left-sided heart failure (occurs when the left ventricle can no longer maintain a normal cardiac output), and (4) right-sided heart failure (right-sided ventricular dysfunction secondary to either left-sided heart failure or to pulmonary disease). Strictly classified, left ventricular failure is referred to as congestive

---

*A static muscle contraction that involves 70% or more of maximal effort results in a disproportionate increase in heart rate and blood pressure for the absolute level of oxygen uptake, which is potentially harmful for the ischemic heart.[129] For some people, use of a cane or walker is an isometric use of muscles that can increase heart rate; therefore, careful monitoring of vital signs and indications of perceived exertion is required.

heart failure; acute right ventricular failure, seen almost exclusively in association with massive pulmonary embolism, is labeled cor pulmonale. Cor pulmonale is heart disease, but it arises from an underlying pulmonary pathologic condition; therefore it is discussed in Chapter 14. Right-sided heart dysfunction secondary to left-sided heart failure, vascular dysfunction, or congenital heart disease is excluded in the definition of cor pulmonale (see the section on Cor Pulmonale in Chapter 14).

Incidence.   CHF is a common complication of ischemic and hypertensive heart disease, occurring most often in the older adult and in its chronic form, referred to as a cardiogeriatric syndrome. Because the heart muscle is damaged during a heart attack, many heart attack survivors develop CHF. In the United States, heart failure develops in an estimated 500,000 individuals annually: it is the most common cause for hospitalization in people older than 65 years with an estimated 5 million men and women living with CHF in the United States today. This condition is on the increase as the population ages and more people survive heart attacks.

Etiologic and Risk Factors.   Many cardiac conditions predispose individuals to CHF, but hypertension is one of the most prevalent (Table 11-11). People with preexisting heart disease are at greatest risk for the development of CHF because when the heart is stressed, compensatory mechanisms may be inadequate. For example, a faster redistribution of blood volume and increased demand for oxygen by the myocardium occur with increased activity, such as exercise, resulting in heart failure. Pulse pressure appears to be the best single measure of blood pressure in predicting mortality in older people and helps explain apparently discrepant results

for low diastolic blood pressure. Pulse pressure is more predictive than even systolic blood pressure alone. Each elevation of 10 mm Hg between systolic and diastolic blood pressure increases the risk of CHF by 14%.[44,89]

CHF occurring during middle age as distinguished from CHF at advanced age includes an increasing proportion of women, a shift from coronary heart disease to hypertension as the most common etiology, and intact left ventricular systolic function.[191] Women tend to have more risk factors and concurrent medical problems, such as hypertension, diabetes, or renal insufficiency. In addition, there may be other gender differences contributing to the development of CHF in women, such as differences in myocardial distensibility (the degree to which muscle fibers stretch) or hormonal differences as yet undetermined.

Paget's disease causes vascular proliferation in the bones. When the disease involves over one third of the skeleton, a high cardiac output state exists and may tax the compromised heart. Medications such as steroids or NSAIDs and drug toxicity are also risk factors. For the person with chronic, stable heart failure, acute exacerbations may occur caused by alterations in therapy, client noncompliance with therapy, excessive salt and fluid intake, arrhythmias, excessive activity, pulmonary emboli, infection, or progression of the underlying disease.

Pathogenesis and Clinical Manifestations.   Over the last 10 years, major advances have occurred in our understanding of heart failure, involving the complex interactions that take place among the adrenergic nervous system, the renin-angiotensin axis, the immune system, the peripheral circulation, and other vasoactive substances in response to impaired cardiac function. The pathophysiology involves structural changes such as loss of myofilaments, apoptosis (programmed cell death), disturbances in calcium homeostasis, and alteration in receptor density, signal transduction, and collagen synthesis. A neurohormonal hypothesis has replaced the hemodynamic model focusing on the neuroendocrine activation of a progressive disorder of left ventricular remodeling. This cascade of events occurs as a result of a cardiac event (e.g., myocardial infarction) that develops into a clinical syndrome characterized by impaired cardiac function and circulatory congestion.[76]

CHF is a complex event involving one or both ventricles. This discussion is based on left ventricular failure. See the section on Cor Pulmonale in Chapter 14 for a complete discussion of right-sided heart failure. When the heart fails to propel blood forward normally (such as occurs with left ventricular failure), the body utilizes three neurohormonal compensatory mechanisms; these are effective for a short time but eventually become insufficient to meet the oxygen needs of the body. First, the failing heart attempts to maintain a normal output of blood by enlarging its pumping chambers so that they can hold a greater volume of blood. This lengthening of the muscle fibers, called *ventricular dilation*, increases the amount of blood ejected from the heart. This compensatory mechanism has limits, because contractility of ventricular muscle fibers ceases to increase when they are stretched beyond a certain point.

During this *first compensatory phase*, the right ventricle continues to pump more blood into the lungs. Congestion occurs in the pulmonary circulation with accumulation of blood

TABLE	**11-11**

Etiologic and Risk Factors Associated with Congestive Heart Failure

ETIOLOGIC FACTORS	RISK FACTORS*
Hypertension	Emotional stress
Coronary artery disease	Physical inactivity
Myocardial infarction	Obesity
Valvular heart disease	Diabetes mellitus
Congenital heart disease	Nutritional deficiency (vitamin C,
Endocarditis	thiamin)
Pericarditis	Fever
Myocarditis	Infection
Cardiomyopathy	Anemia
Chronic alcoholism	Thyroid disorders
Atrioventricular	Pregnancy
malformation	Paget's disease
Thyrotoxicosis	Pulmonary disease
(arrhythmia)	Medications (e.g., steroids, NSAIDs)
Chronic anemia	Drug toxicity
	Renal disease

NSAIDs, Nonsteroidal antiinflammatory drugs.
*Risk factors for new onset or exacerbation of previous CHF.

in the lungs. The immediate result is shortness of breath (most common symptom), and if the process continues, actual flooding of the air spaces of the lungs occurs, with fluid seeping from the distended blood vessels; this is called *pulmonary congestion* or *pulmonary edema.* Congestion in the vascular system interferes with the movement of body fluids in and out of the various fluid compartments, resulting in fluid accumulation in the tissue spaces and progressive edema.

During the *second compensatory phase,* the sympathetic nervous system responds to increase the stimulation of the heart muscle, causing it to pump more often. In response to failing contractility of the myocardial cells, the sympathetic nervous system activates adaptive processes that increase the heart rate and increase its muscle mass to strengthen the force of its contractions. This results in ventricular hypertrophy and a need for more oxygen. Eventually, the coronary arteries cannot meet the oxygen demands of the enlarged myocardium, and the person may experience angina pectoris owing to ischemia. Secondary compensatory mechanisms activate the sympathetic nervous system and release endothelin from vascular linings, vasopressin (antidiuretic hormone [ADH]) from the pituitary gland, and atrial natriuretic hormone from the heart.

The *third compensatory phase* involves activation of the renin-angiotensin-aldosterone system. With less blood coming from the heart, less blood passes through the kidneys. The kidneys respond by retaining water and sodium in an effort to increase blood volume, which further exacerbates tissue edema. The expanded blood volume increases the load on an already compromised heart. These mechanisms are responsible for the symptoms of diaphoresis, cool skin, tachycardia, cardiac arrhythmias, and oliguria (reduced urine excretion).

When the combined efforts of these three compensatory mechanisms achieve a normal level of cardiac output, the client is said to have compensated CHF. Ultimately, however, the body's efforts to compensate may backfire and produce higher blood volume, higher blood pressure, and more stress on the already weakened heart. The heart's ongoing failure to supply the body with blood compels the body to keep compensating in ways that further burden the heart, and the cycle perpetuates itself. When these mechanisms are no longer effective and the disease progresses to the final stage of impaired heart function, the client has decompensated CHF.

This condition ranges from mild congestion with few symptoms to life-threatening fluid overload and total heart failure (Table 11-12). Symptoms usually develop very gradually so that many people do not recognize or report signals of serious disease. The older adult in particular may wrongly associate early symptoms with a lack of fitness or as a sign of aging. Confusion and impaired thinking can characterize heart failure in older adults.

Left-Sided Heart Failure.

Failure of the left ventricle (Fig. 11-12) prevents the heart from pumping enough blood through the arterial system to meet the body's metabolic needs and causes either pulmonary edema or a disturbance in the respiratory control mechanisms. The degree of respiratory distress varies with the client's position, activity, and level of emotional or physical stress, but any of the symptoms listed under Pulmonary Edema in Chapter 14 may occur.

Dyspnea is subjective and does not always correlate with the extent of heart failure; exertional dyspnea occurs in all clients to some degree. Time for dyspnea to subside is an indi-

---

TABLE	11-12

Clinical Manifestations of Heart Failure

LEFT VENTRICULAR FAILURE	RIGHT VENTRICULAR FAILURE
Progressive dyspnea (exertional first)	Progressive failure
Paroxysmal nocturnal dyspnea	Dependent edema (ankle or pretibial first)
Orthopnea	Jugular vein distention
Productive spasmodic cough	Abdominal pain and distention
Pulmonary edema	Weight gain
Extreme breathlessness	Right upper quadrant pain (liver congestion)
Anxiety	Cardiac cirrhosis
Frothy pink sputum	Ascites
Nasal flaring	Jaundice
Accessory muscle use	Anorexia, nausea
Rales	Cyanosis (nail beds)
Tachypnea	Psychologic disturbances
Diaphoresis	
Cerebral hypoxia	
Irritability	
Restlessness	
Confusion	
Impaired memory	
Sleep disturbances	
Fatigue, exercise intolerance	
Muscular weakness	
Renal changes	

---

cation of progress or deterioration in a client's status, and it can be measured for documentation. Paroxysmal nocturnal dyspnea resembles the frightening sensation of awakening with suffocation. Once the client is in the upright position, relief from the attack may not occur for 30 minutes or longer. The client often assumes a three-point position, sitting up with both hands on the knees and leaning forward. In severe heart failure, the client may resort to sleeping upright in a chair or recliner. Other sleep disturbances may occur from central sleep apnea present in approximately 40% of all adults with heart failure.

Fatigue and *muscular weakness* are often associated with left ventricular failure, since dyspnea develops along with weight gain and a faster resting heart rate, which decrease the person's ability to exercise. Inadequate cardiac output leads to decreased peripheral blood flow and blood flow to skeletal muscle. The resultant tissue hypoxia and slowed removal of metabolic wastes cause the person to tire easily. Disturbances in sleep and rest patterns may aggravate fatigue; muscle atrophy is common in advanced CHF.

Renal changes can occur in both right- and left-sided heart failure, but they are more evident with left-sided failure. During the day, the client is upright, decreased cardiac output reduces blood flow to the kidneys, and the formation of urine is reduced (oliguria). Sodium and water not excreted in the urine are retained in the vascular system, adding to the blood volume. Diminished blood supply to the renal system causes the kidney to secrete renin, stimulating angiotensin, which causes vasoconstriction, thereby causing an increase in peripheral vascular resistance, increasing blood pressure and cardiac work and resulting in worse heart failure. Renin secretion also indirectly stimulates the secretion of aldosterone from the adrenal gland. Aldosterone acts on the renal tubules, causing them to increase reabsorption of sodium and water, further increasing fluid volume. At night, urine formation increases with the recumbent position as blood flow to the kidney improves. *Nocturia* may interfere with effective sleep patterns, which contributes to fatigue as mentioned.

Right-Sided Heart Failure.

Failure of the right ventricle (see Fig. 11-12) to adequately pump blood to the lungs results in peripheral edema and venous congestion of the organs. Symptoms result from congestion in the heart's right side and throughout the venous system (see Table 11-12) (see also the section on Cor Pulmonale in Chapter 14). *Dependent edema* is one of the early signs of right ventricular failure, although significant CHF can be present in the absence of peripheral edema. In CHF, fluid is retained because the baroreceptors of the body sense a decreased volume of blood as a result of the heart's inability to pump an adequate amount of blood. The receptors subsequently relay a message to the kidneys to retain fluid so that a greater volume of blood can be ejected from the heart to the peripheral tissues. Unfortunately this compounds the problem and makes the heart work even harder, which further decreases its pumping ability causing a sense of weakness and fatigue.

The retained fluid commonly accumulates in the extracellular spaces of the periphery. The resultant edema is usually symmetric and occurs in the dependent parts of the body, where venous pressure is the highest. In ambulatory persons, edema begins in the feet and ankles and ascends up the lower legs (pretibial areas). It is most noticeable at the end of a day and often decreases after a night's rest. In the recumbent person, pitting edema may develop in the presacral area and, as it worsens, progress to the medial thighs and genital area.

Jugular venous distention also results from fluid overload. The jugular veins empty unoxygenated blood directly into the superior vena cava. Since no cardiac valve exists to separate the superior vena cava from the right atrium, the jugular veins give information about activity on the right side of the heart. As fluid is retained and the heart's ability to pump is further compromised, the retained fluid backs up into both the lungs and the venous system, and the jugular veins reveal this. Jugular venous pulsations are examined by inspecting the silhouette of the neck with the person reclining at a 45-degree angle (Fig. 11-13). The right internal jugular vein is recommended because the left internal jugular may be falsely elevated in some people.

As the liver becomes congested with venous blood it becomes enlarged, and *abdominal pain* occurs. If this occurs rapidly, stretching of the capsule surrounding the liver causes severe discomfort, and the person may notice either a constant aching or a sharp *right upper quadrant pain*. In chronic CHF, long-standing congestion of the liver with venous blood and anoxia can lead to ascites (see Fig. 16-4) and jaundice, which are symptoms of liver damage. Anorexia, nausea, and bloating develop secondary to venous congestion of the gastrointestinal (GI) tract. Anorexia and nausea may also result from digitalis toxicity, which is a common problem since digitalis is usually prescribed for CHF.

Cyanosis of the nail beds appears as venous congestion reduces peripheral blood flow. Clients with CHF often feel anxious, frightened, and depressed. Fears may be expressed as frightening nightmares, insomnia, acute anxiety states, depression, or withdrawal from reality.

Medical Management

Diagnosis. Diagnosis is based on the clinical picture and depends on where symptoms are on the continuum of mild to severe. Because the two sides of the heart serve different functions, distinguishing the symptoms of left-sided heart failure from those of right-sided heart failure is critical in both diagnosis and treatment. Equally important is consideration of systolic and diastolic dysfunction, both of which indicate a functional or structural defect in the ventricles. Echocardiogram is the main diagnostic tool; noninvasive cardiac tests such as ECG, chest radiography, and echocardiography are secondary tools that can determine left ventricular size and function well enough to confirm the diagnosis. Cardiac catheterization is not routinely performed, but it may be useful in certain cases (e.g., atherosclerotic heart disease, which is potentially correctable). Arterial blood gases are drawn to measure oxygen saturation. Liver enzymes (e.g., aspartate transaminase [AST], alkaline phosphatase) are often elevated (see Tables 39-15 and 39-21); liver involvement with hyperbilirubinemia commonly occurs, resulting in jaundice.

A new screening tool for individuals with suspected left ventricular dysfunction has been introduced. Measuring B-type natriuretic peptide (BNP), a protein secreted from the cardiac ventricles in response to wall tension and pressure overload, can reliably predict the presence or absence of heart failure, even helping to identify when dyspnea is associated with heart failure or some other underlying pathologic condition.[149]

Prevention and Treatment.

Managing heart failure begins with treatment of the underlying cause whenever possible. Nonpharmacologic interventions, such as diet, medications, and exercise, that alter interactions between the heart and the periphery are now accepted therapeutic approaches. Alterations in lifestyle reduce symptoms and the need for additional medication. There is an urgent need to develop more effective strategies for the prevention and treatment of this increasingly common disorder. Multiple co-morbidities in older clients require a multidisciplinary approach to management. Persons with CHF are placed on a sodium-restricted diet, sometimes with limited fluid intake. Emotional and physical rest during the initial phases of intervention is also important in diminishing the workload of the heart.

Traditionally, the diagnosis of CHF was a contraindication for participation in exercise training because of concerns that further decline in cardiac function would occur. It is now clear that activity restriction is no longer appropriate, since exercise programs have proved to quantitatively achieve similar results to those attained with most effective drug therapies. These findings have shifted attention away from treating the heart toward exercising the muscles. Whenever possible, physical activity and exercise are prescribed per client tolerance. Physical training for clients with CHF results in an increase in muscular strength and better adaptation to effort owing to the effect of training on peripheral muscles (e.g., decreased vascular resistance in the muscles, delay in the onset of anaerobic metabolism). Exercise training has also been shown to improve exercise capacity, reduce symptoms, improve psychosocial status, and improve functional capacity.[18,132]

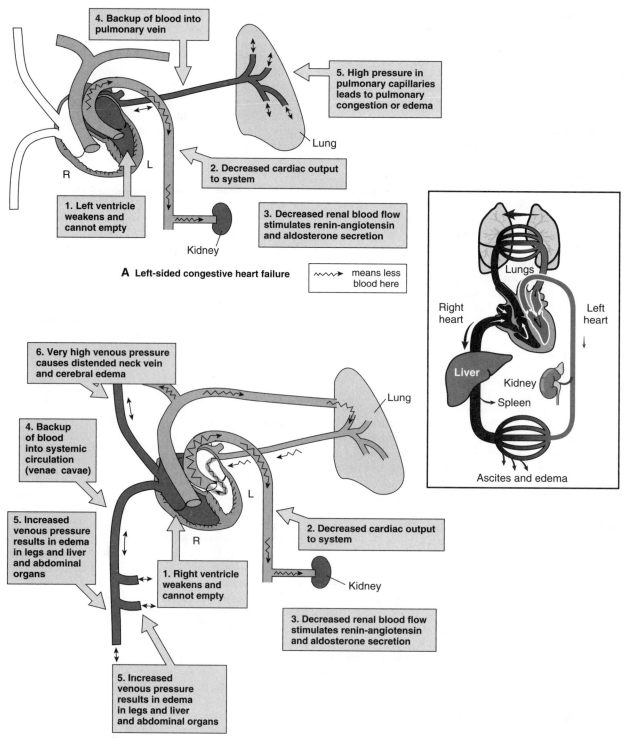

4. Backup of blood into pulmonary vein

5. High pressure in pulmonary capillaries leads to pulmonary congestion or edema

Lung

2. Decreased cardiac output to system

1. Left ventricle weakens and cannot empty

R

L

3. Decreased renal blood flow stimulates renin-angiotensin and aldosterone secretion

Kidney

A Left-sided congestive heart failure

∿∿∿➤   means less blood here

Lungs

Right heart

Left heart

Liver

Kidney

Spleen

Ascites and edema

6. Very high venous pressure causes distended neck vein and cerebral edema

4. Backup of blood into systemic circulation (venae cavae)

Lung

5. Increased venous pressure results in edema in legs and liver and abdominal organs

L

R

2. Decreased cardiac output to system

1. Right ventricle weakens and cannot empty

Kidney

3. Decreased renal blood flow stimulates renin-angiotensin and aldosterone secretion

5. Increased venous pressure results in edema in legs and liver and abdominal organs

B Right-sided congestive heart failure

FIGURE   **11-12**   Pathophysiologic mechanisms of congestive heart failure. **A,** Left-sided heart failure leads to pulmonary edema (see text description). **B,** Right ventricular failure causes peripheral edema that is most prominent in the lower extremities. *Inset,* Integration of the pulmonary and systemic circulation. When the heart contracts normally, it pumps blood simultaneously into both loops, but pump failure causes circulatory or pulmonary problems depending on the underlying pathologic mechanism. (**A** and **B** from Gould B: *Pathophysiology for the health-related professions,* Philadelphia, 1997, Saunders, p 192; inset from Damjanov I: *Pathology for the health-related professions,* ed 2, Philadelphia, 2000, Saunders, p 157.)

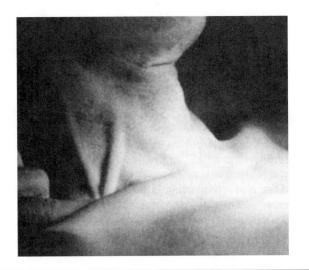

FIGURE 11-13 Jugular venous distention occurs bilaterally if there is a cardiac cause such as congestive heart failure; a unilateral distention indicates a localized problem. (From Daily EK, Schroeder JP: *Techniques in bedside hemodynamic monitoring*, ed 2, St Louis, 1981, Mosby.)

Pharmacologic therapy is now responsive to the updated understanding of CHF as a cascade of neurohormonal events centered on ventricular remodeling. Pharmacologic agents are used to reduce the heart's workload, increase muscle strength and contraction, and inhibit neuroendocrine responses to heart failure (see Tables 11-4 and 11-5). ACE inhibitors have become standard therapy for heart failure because of their ability to block the renin-angiotensin-aldosterone system, increasing renal blood flow and decreasing renal vascular resistance, thereby enhancing diuresis. ACE inhibitors reduce left ventricular filling pressure and moderately increase cardiac output. Vasodilator therapy in combination with ACE inhibitors prolongs life in persons with moderate to severe heart failure. Diuretics are used to control fluid buildup and prevent congestion, and digoxin may be added to stimulate the heart's pumping action if symptoms persist despite treatment with ACE inhibitors and diuretics. Angiotensin II receptor antagonists have been added to function as an antihypertensive and enhance the clearance of sodium and water. Beta-blockers, once rarely considered in the treatment of CHF, have been shown effective in reducing symptoms, improving clinical status, reducing hospitalizations, and reducing the risk of death. Combining beta-blockers with ACE inhibitors can produce additive effects on two neurohormonal systems (renin-angiotensin system and sympathetic nervous system). A new drug, nesiritide (human recombinant B-type natriuretic peptide [BNP]) has been introduced as a first-line medication for decompensated CHF that inhibits sympathetic activity and dilates arterial and venous vessels. Nesiritide binds to receptors in the vasculature, kidney, and other organs to mimic the vasodilatory and diuretic actions of endogenous natriuretic peptides.[53]

Surgical intervention may include CABG (see Fig. 11-4) for underlying myocardial ischemia and infarction reconstruction of incompetent heart valves; ventricular remodeling or heart reduction (e.g., Batista procedure, in which a piece of the heart tissue is removed and the heart muscle is sutured back together making a smaller, tauter heart with a stronger heartbeat); internal counterpulsation (Fig. 11-14) or external counterpulsation, which uses an external pump or balloon to adjust the aortic blood pressure; temporary ventricular assistive devices for people unable to come off bypass (see Chapter 20); and use of an artificial heart or cardiac transplantation. The implantation of skeletal muscle (removed from the individual's thigh and multiplied in the laboratory) injected into the postinfarction scar after infarction in the case of severe ischemic heart failure has been shown experimentally to improve heart function.[159] A review of surgical innovations for chronic heart failure in the context of cardiopulmonary rehabilitation for the therapist is available.[115] See also the sections on Atherosclerosis: Treatment in this chapter and Heart Transplantation in Chapter 20. Cardiac transplantation is now more common for treatment of heart failure. Transplantation is successful for selected individuals, usually those who are treated early in the course of heart failure, before advanced symptoms develop. Reform of the selection process is recommended to identify people who, although not critically ill, will not survive without early transplantation. See further discussion in Chapter 20.

A pacemaker-like device designed to deliver electrical stimulation to the ventricles (biventricular pacing) in an effort to improve the heart's overall cardiac efficiency by coordinating the heart's contractions (both ventricles pump at the same time making the heart pump more forceful) has been approved by the U.S. Food and Drug Administration (FDA). This technique, referred to as cardiac resynchronization therapy, is available on a limited basis for selected individuals with severe heart failure. The results are promising for people who because of age criteria or lack of donor hearts are not able to receive cardiac transplantation. Other similar devices are under continued investigation and development as well as the combined use of resynchronization therapy with pharmacologic therapy and/or cardioverter-defibrillator as adjunct treatment for CHF.

Prognosis.   Treatment of CHF remains difficult, and the prognosis is poor, even with recent advances in pharmacologic therapy. Annual mortality rates range from 10% in stable clients with mild symptoms to over 50% in people with advanced, progressive symptoms. About 40% to 50% of clients with heart failure die suddenly, probably owing to ventricular arrhythmias. To achieve the maximal benefit from drug therapy, symptoms must be recognized as early as possible and intervention initiated. Because this condition often develops gradually, intervention is delayed, full resolution is not usually possible, and CHF becomes a chronic disorder.

Exercise capacity was the most powerful predictor of survival in CHF, but a new test that measures swings in heart rate during the day has been developed that can identify individuals who are at the highest risk of dying from CHF. The test measures the amount by which the heart rate changes from slow rates to fast rates in one 24-hour period. The less the heart rate varies over 24 hours, the more likely a person is to die of CHF.[174] Other signs of poor prognosis include severe left ventricular dysfunction, severe symptoms and limitation of exercise capacity, secondary renal insufficiency, and elevated plasma catecholamine levels.

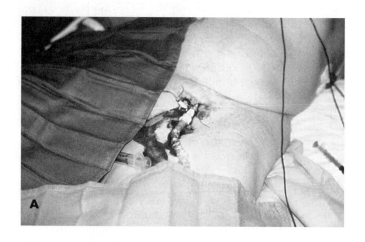

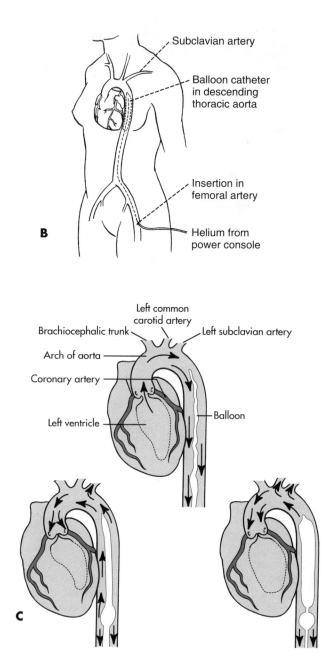

FIGURE 11-14 The intraaortic balloon pump (IABP) is a common type of cardiac assist device that is used to improve myocardial oxygen supply-demand for individuals with deteriorating hemodynamics or ongoing ischemia, as evidenced by rest pain or electrocardiographic changes in the region of the infarct. The primary functions of balloon counterpulsation are to reperfuse the coronary arteries at the end of systole and decrease the left ventricular afterload reduction (the amount of work the ventricle must do), thereby decreasing myocardial oxygen consumption and improving cardiac output. These intravascular catheter-mounted counterpulsation devices are traditionally used for cases of cardiogenic shock following cardiac surgery or an acute myocardial infarction as well as for people who have chronic end-stage heart failure and who are not candidates for long-term ventricular assistive device (VAD) support. The rationale for IABP counterpulsation in this latter situation is to maintain systemic perfusion and preserve end-organ function until cardiac transplantation occurs. **A,** The catheter is usually placed through the femoral artery, and the balloon is moved up the iliac artery to the descending aorta where it is then placed, **B,** above the renal arteries and below the subclavian artery. This position is critical in order to prevent ischemia to the upper extremities or kidneys. **C,** When the heart contracts (systole), the balloon is deflated, creating a decline in aortic pressure. After the heart contracts (during diastole), the balloon is filled with air, causing the blood to regurgitate back toward the root of the aorta, thereby perfusing the coronary arteries. When the left ventricle is ready to pump, the balloon is deflated (cardiac systole again), reducing ventricular afterload. (**A** courtesy Chris Wells, P.T., M.S., Ph.D, University of Pittsburgh Medical Center, 2001. **B** from Polaski AL, Tatro SE: *Luckmann's core principles and practice of medical-surgical nursing,* Philadelphia, 1996, Saunders. **C** from Lewis SM, Collier IC, Heitkemper MM: *Medical-surgical nursing: assessment and management of clinical problems,* ed 4, St Louis, 1996, Mosby.)

Special Implications for the Therapist **11-7**

CONGESTIVE HEART FAILURE

Preferred Practice Patterns:
6A: Primary Prevention/Risk Reduction for Cardiovascular/Pulmonary Disorders
6B: Impaired Aerobic Capacity/Endurance Associated With Deconditioning
6C, 6F may apply for complications associated with mechanical vascular devices or implants (see Chapter 20).
7A: Primary Prevention/Risk Reduction for Integumentary Disorders (prevent complications of bed rest)

Therapists have a unique role in the prevention, medical management, and rehabilitation of people with heart failure. Physical therapists can provide programs that profoundly improve the exercise tolerance and functional status of individuals with CHF. Medical intervention can be more objectively implemented by using information obtained during physical therapy assessments and interventions. Tests such as the 6-minute walk test may be helpful in predicting peak oxygen consumption and early survival as well as implementing a proper exercise conditioning program for people with advanced heart failure.[39] Education of physicians and other health care professionals about the role of the physical therapist in defining prescriptive exercise is important. Consideration for the complex pathologic conditions and co-morbidities of people in this population is an important contribution to cardiac rehabilitation from the physical therapist's training. Clients should be referred to rehabilitation before the VO_2 max drops below 14 ml/kg/min and when the wedge pressure is still greater than 16 mm Hg (i.e., before they progress in a downward spiral requiring transplantation). See further discussion in Chapter 20.

Early Considerations

Clients hospitalized with severe CHF require a therapy program to maintain pulmonary function and prevent complications of bed rest (e.g., skin breakdown, venous stasis, venous thrombus, pulmonary emboli). An important aspect of intervention includes functional assessment (Box 11-7) and physical exercise within the limitations set by the physician. See also established guidelines for exercise training in CHF.[38,39] Physical therapy assessment of cardiopulmonary status is beyond the scope of this text. The clinician is referred to any of the specific examination and assessment texts available.[78,109,117]

The therapist should be aware of psychosocial considerations in older adults with CHF. Neuropsychiatric conditions such as Alzheimer's dementia and complications such as delirium are common in older adults with CHF. Persistent alcohol abuse and cigarette smoking often contribute to the onset and progression of heart failure. Major depression, other depressive disorders, anxiety, and social isolation are common and have adverse effects on functional status, quality of life, and prognosis. Working as a team with psychologists and social workers can address these issues effectively.

Monitoring Vital Signs

Aerobic capacity is likely impaired and even more so if the client is deconditioned; adaptive responses to activity may be attenuated or inadequate; activity may exacerbate cardiovascular pump dysfunction; and signs of fatigue and shortness of breath are common. The downward cycle of disease, deconditioning, decreased activity, and disability necessitates the monitoring of vital signs.[33] Progressing activities from bed rest to transfers or ambulation requires vital sign assessment immediately after the major activity and 3 minutes later to assess for return to baseline. Oxygen may be administered by mask or cannula; team members should consult respiratory therapy staff to determine appropriate oxygen levels during exercise.

Monitor the client for signs of increasing peripheral edema by assessing jugular neck vein distention, peripheral edema in the legs or sacrum, and any report of right upper quadrant pain. In the outpatient or home health setting, the client is advised to call the nurse or physician if shoes, belt, or pants become too tight to fasten, usual activities of daily living or tasks become difficult, extra sleep is needed, or urination at night becomes more frequent. Monitoring blood pressure is essential to detect heart failure; observe for decreasing blood pressure and report any change in status to the nurse or physician immediately. Observe for flat or falling systolic blood pressure in response to activity indicative of inadequate pump function (should see a linear increase of systolic blood pressure with increased activity). Exaggerated increases in heart rate may be observed as the heart attempts to maintain adequate cardiac output. Observe for dyspnea at rest and/or with activity, and auscultate for changes from baseline during activity.[33] See also Appendix B.

Continuous supervision and frequent monitoring of blood pressure are necessary when starting an exercise program for someone with CHF. Rating of perceived exertion should range from 11 to 14 (light to somewhat hard; Table 11-13). Anginal symptoms should not exceed 2+ on the 0 to 4 angina scale (moderate to bothersome), and exertional dyspnea should not exceed a rating of mild, some difficulty with activity. Initially, full resuscitation equipment should be available.[24]

Positioning

Positioning is important, and the client is taught to use a high Fowler's position (head of the bed elevated at least 20 inches above the level) or chair to reduce pulmonary congestion, facilitate diaphragmatic expansion and ventilation, and ease dyspnea. The legs are maintained in a dependent position as much as possible to decrease venous return. Range of motion to decrease venous pooling and monitoring for the development of thrombophlebitis (e.g., unilateral swelling, calf pain, pallor) are required.

Exercise and CHF

The American College of Sports Medicine's guidelines[7] suggest that CHF clients entering an exercise program should start with moderate intensity exercise (40% to 60% VO_2 max) for a duration of 2 to 6 minutes, followed by 2 minutes of rest. Blood pressure and heart rhythm should be routinely monitored at rest, during peak exercise, and after cool down. The goal is to gradually increase the intensity and duration of exercise. Others advocate starting CHF clients at a low to moderate exercise intensity (less than 40% VO_2max) with a shorter duration of exercise initially and a shorter rest period less than 2 minutes). Recommendations for interval exercise training (following work phases of 30 seconds by recovery phases of 60 seconds) have also been reported.[160]

The best guideline is to customize initial exercise intensity for each individual, keeping in mind the individual's goals and expected outcomes (e.g., preparation for transplantation, improved functional daily living, perceived quality of life). Exercise

Continued

<table>
<tr><td colspan="3">TABLE 11-13</td></tr>
</table>

Borg Scale of Perceived Exertion*

NUMERICAL RATING		
15-GRADE SCALE	10-GRADE SCALE	VERBAL RATING
6	0	No exertion at all
8	0.5	Extremely light
9	1	Very light
11	2	Light
13	3	Moderate
14	4	Somewhat hard
15	5	Hard
16	6	
17	7	Very hard
18	8	
19	9	
20	10	Very, very hard
—	—	Maximal exertion

Modified from Borg GA: Psychosocial bases of perceived exertion, *Med Sci Sports Exerc* 472:194-381, 1982.

*Using a perceived exertion scale (6 to 20 scale or 0 to 10 scale) is a useful approach to activity prescription. The individual is asked to identify a desirable rating of perceived exertion and uses that level of intensity as a daily guideline for activity. A suggested rating of perceived exertion for most healthy individuals is 3 to 5 (moderate to heavy on the 10-grade scale); for the compromised person, a more moderate level of perceived exertion may be recommended by the physician.

should be avoided immediately after eating or after taking vasodilator medication. Using an interval training approach is helpful with those individuals who demonstrate marked exercise intolerance. Symptoms and general fatigue level serve as a guideline to determine frequency, and warm-up/cool-down periods should be longer than normal for observation of possible arrhythmias. Determination of appropriate exercise intensity of 40% to 60% VO$_2$ max is recommended (rather than based on heart rate peak) because the response to exercise is frequently abnormal in people with CHF. Alternately, the initial exercise intensity should be 10 beats below any significant symptoms, including angina, exertional hypotension, arrhythmias, and dyspnea. Rehabilitation personnel must observe for symptoms of cardiac decompensation during exercise, including cough or dyspnea, hypotension, light-headedness, cyanosis, angina, and arrhythmias. Exercise progression following these recommendations is available in detail[24]; see also Monitoring Vital Signs in this section. Endurance exercise training has been shown to modify neuroendocrine activation in heart failure and may have a long-term beneficial impact.[25]

The therapist should keep in mind that some older CHF clients are unable to increase their exercise intensity or duration despite starting very slowly. These people do not achieve the goal of increased endurance and often leave the program owing to increased symptoms and exercise intolerance. Maintaining or even improving functional activities and independence at home may be more appropriate goals for this group. An excellent review of exercise assessment, exercise training, and exercise training guidelines in heart failure for all clients is available.[37,38]

Medications

Diuretics can produce mild to severe electrolyte imbalance requiring special consideration (see Chapter 4). A small drop in the serum potassium level can precipitate digoxin poisoning (digitalis toxicity) and serious arrhythmias. This situation is a life-threatening condition that occurs in one of every five clients and may present with systemic or cardiac manifestations. Any sign or symptom of digitalis toxicity should be reported to the physician (see Table 11-4). Digitalis toxicity can cause a dip in the ST segment on ECG; whenever possible, the ECG should be monitored during exercise. Activity should not increase the magnitude of the altered ST segment. Side effects from digitalis can occur when digitalis levels are within the therapeutic range (<2.0 ng/ml), but the albumin level will be low (<3.5 g/dl; see Table 39-15) because digitalis binds to albumin in the serum. If the serum albumin level is low, digitalis may not be bound to the albumin-binding sites and would be circulating as "free" digoxin. Watch for a low, irregular pulse (<60 beats/min); the heart rate normally increases to compensate for congestive heart failure, but in the presence of digoxin, heart rate decreases.

NSAIDs, including over-the-counter drugs such as ibuprofen, increase fluid retention independently and significantly blunt the action of diuretics and other cardiovascular drugs (especially ACE inhibitors), exacerbating preexisting CHF and causing isolated lower extremity edema. The major consideration for exercise in clients taking ACE inhibitors is the possibility of hypotension and accompanying arrhythmias. These problems should be reported to the physician and can be addressed by maintaining proper hydration and by altering dosages and the simultaneous use of other medications. ∎

◆ Orthostatic (Postural) Hypotension

Definition and Overview. The term *orthostatic (postural) hypotension* signifies a decrease of 20 mm Hg or greater in systolic blood pressure or a drop of 10 mm Hg or more of both systolic and diastolic arterial blood pressure with a concomitant pulse increase of 15 beats/min or more on standing from a supine or sitting position.

Orthostatic hypotension may be acute and temporary or chronic. Orthostatic hypotension occurs frequently in older adults and occurs in more than one half of all frail, older adults, contributing significantly to morbidity from syncope, falls, vital organ ischemia (e.g., myocardial infarction, transient ischemic attacks), and mortality among older adults with diabetic hypertension. It is highly variable over time but most prevalent in the morning when supine blood pressure is highest and on first arising.

Etiologic Factors. Orthostatic hypotension is recognized in all groups as a cardinal feature of autonomic nervous dysfunction as well as other nonneurogenic etiologies (Box 11-8). In young adults, orthostatic intolerance and tachycardia may be associated with norepinephrine-transporter deficiency. A single gene that clears norepinephrine does not function in some individuals pointing to a genetic etiology.

Postural reflexes are slowed as part of the aging process for some, but not all, persons. Normal aging is associated with various changes that may lead to postural hypotension. Cardiac output falls with age; in the older adult with hyper-

BOX 11-8

Causes of Orthostatic Hypotension

Volume depletion (e.g., burns, diabetes mellitus, sodium or potassium depletion)

Venous pooling (e.g., pregnancy, varicosities of the legs)

Side effects of medication (e.g., antidepressants, antihypertensives; see Table 11-4)

Prolonged immobility

Starvation, malnutrition, eating disorders

Performing Valsalva's maneuver

Chronic: sluggish normal regulatory mechanisms (e.g., anatomic variation, altered body chemistry)

Chronic: autonomic nervous system dysregulation (e.g., diabetes mellitus, Parkinson's disease, aging, fibromyalgia syndrome, chronic renal failure)

tension, it is even lower. When older subjects (>65 years) are put under passive postural stress (60-degree upright tilt), their stroke volume falls even further. These normal changes obviously predispose the aging adult to postural hypotension from any process that further reduces fluid volume or vascular integrity. For example, pooling of blood after eating may lead to profound hypotension, called *postprandial hypotension*. In addition, as systolic pressure rises from atherosclerosis, baroreceptor sensitivity and vascular compliance are reduced further, increasing the likelihood of postural hypotension. In the older adult with hypertension and cardiovascular disease receiving vasoactive drugs, the circulatory adjustments to maintain blood pressure are disturbed, leaving the person vulnerable to postural hypotension.[131]

Drugs are a major cause of orthostatic hypotension in the aging adult. Many have effects on the autonomic nervous system, both centrally and peripherally, and on fluid balance. Diuretics, calcium-channel blockers, nitrates, and L-dopa have hypotensive effects. Antidepressants are a common, overlooked cause of orthostasis, even though this is a known side effect of these medications. A general result of treatment for hypertension may be hypotension. In addition, many older adults with systolic hypertension have postural hypotension that may require management before the hypertension is addressed.

Chronic orthostatic hypotension may occur secondary to a specific disease, such as endocrine disorders, metabolic disorders, nephropathy, or neurogenic disorders affecting the autonomic or central nervous systems. Alcohol and drugs such as vincristine used in the treatment of cancer can cause autonomic neuropathy.

Pathogenesis.   Orthostasis is a physiologic stress related to upright posture. When a normal individual stands up, the gravitational changes on the circulation are compensated for by several mechanisms, including the circulatory and autonomic nervous systems. On standing, the force of gravity in the vertical axis causes venous pooling in the lower limbs, a sharp decline in venous return, and reduction in filling pressure of the heart, which increase further on prolonged standing because of shifting of water to interstitial spaces and hemoconcentration.

These mechanical events can cause a marked reduction in cardiac output and consequent fall in arterial blood pressure. In normal people, cardiac output and blood pressure regulation are maintained by powerful compensatory mechanisms involving a rise in heart rate. Blood pressure is maintained by a rise in peripheral resistance. These compensatory mechanisms are initiated by the baroreceptors located in the aortic arch and carotid bifurcation. Orthostatic hypotension results from failure of the arterial baroreflex, most commonly because of disorders of the autonomic nervous system.[131]

In people with autonomic failure or dysreflexia (e.g., Parkinson's disease, aging, diabetes, fibromyalgia), orthostatic hypotension results from an impaired capacity to increase vascular resistance during standing. This dysfunction leads to increased downward pooling of venous blood and a consequent reduction in stroke volume and cardiac output that exaggerates the orthostatic fall in blood pressure. Approximately 80% of the blood pooled in the lower limb is contained in the upper leg (thighs, buttocks) with less pooling in the calf and foot. The location of the additional venous pooling has not been clearly identified, but present data suggest the abdominal compartment and perhaps leg skin vasculature. The pooled blood in the veins of the feet and calves is arterial in origin in that it arises as a result of decreased venous drainage of that region. In contrast, the blood pooled in the thighs, buttocks, pelvis, and abdomen arises primarily from venous reflux. The pooled blood is not actually stagnant; its mean circulatory time through the dependent region is merely increased by changes in the pressure gradient across the vascular bed and by increases in venous volume. The identification of venous pooling may offer insights for intervention techniques in the future.

Clinical Manifestations.   Orthostatic hypotension is often accompanied by dizziness, blurring or loss of vision, and syncope or fainting. There are three main modes of presentation in the older adult: (1) falls or mobility problems, (2) acute or chronic mental confusion, and (3) cardiac symptoms. A common clinical picture is the person whose legs give way when attempting to stand, usually after prolonged recumbency, after physical exertion, or in a warm environment. These episodes may be accompanied by confusion, pallor, tremor, and unsteadiness. Loss of consciousness may cause frequent falls and additional injuries that can be quite serious. Ischemic neck pain in the suboccipital and paracervical region is often reported by individuals with autonomic failure and orthostatic hypotension.[23] Other reported ischemic symptoms of orthostatic hypotension are nonspecific, such as lethargy, weakness, low backache, calf claudication, and angina. Some older adults may experience unexpected and unexplained falls associated with orthostatic hypotension. The cause of such falls may be circulatory impairment that causes a drop in blood pressure on standing upright quickly, an early sign of some other illness, or effects of medication.

Medical Management.   There are several general and specific approaches to the management of orthostatic hypotension but no curative intervention for orthostatic hypotension of unknown cause. Prevention is important, and whenever the underlying disorder causing hypotension is corrected, symptoms cease. Nonneurogenic causes, such as diminished intravascular volume, are treated specifically. In orthostatic hypotension caused by autonomic failure there are considerable difficulties in reestablishing sympathetic or parasympathetic efferent activity.

Tilt study or tilt-table test may be used to assess hypotension by monitoring blood pressure and pulse while tilting a person from horizontal supine to 60 degrees upright. This test has proved very valuable in determining the cause of dizziness or syncope and can reveal irregularities in the vascular regulating system. A combination of general measures and pharmacologic measures is needed in the management of neurogenic postural hypotension.[97]

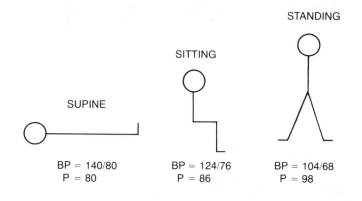

FIGURE   **11-15**   Assessing postural hypotension. After measuring the blood pressure (BP) and pulse in the supine position, leave the blood pressure cuff in place and assist the person to sit. Remeasure the blood pressure within 15 to 30 seconds. Assist the person to stand, and measure again. A drop of more than 20 mm Hg systolic and more than 10 mm diastolic accompanied by a 10% to 20% increase in heart rate (pulse) indicates postural hypotension. Sample measurements are given. (From Black JM, Matassarin-Jacobs E, editors: *Luckmann and Sorensen's medical-surgical nursing,* ed 4, Philadelphia, 1993, Saunders, p 1111.)

Special Implications for the Therapist   11-8

ORTHOSTATIC HYPOTENSION

Preferred Practice Patterns:

5A: Primary Prevention/Risk Reduction for Loss of Balance and Falling (side effects of medication)

6D: Impaired Aerobic Capacity/Endurance Associated With Cardiovascular Pump Dysfunction or Failure

Many medications used to treat hypertension can result in hypotension, especially when combined with interventions or exercise that results in vasodilation. Of particular concern are heat modalities, such as the whirlpool or Hubbard tank. In addition, moderate to vigorous exercise of large muscle groups can produce significant vasodilation and can result in hypotension. This is particularly true following exercise, when venous return diminishes as exercise abruptly ceases. A cool-down period is essential, and safety measures must be employed.[244] Aerobic conditioning is an important part of orthostatic hypotension resulting from autonomic insufficiency, perhaps best accomplished through aquatic exercise therapy.[97]

Stationary standing, as is performed in many activities of daily living, can produce hypotension, especially among those individuals with autonomic failure. With autonomic failure, symptoms of postural hypotension are increased on standing after exercise. The therapist can instruct the individual in protective measures that reduce excessive orthostatic blood pooling including avoidance of precipitating factors. Anyone with orthostatic hypotension, especially persons taking antihypertensive agents, should be instructed to rise slowly from the bed or chair after a long period of recumbency or sitting to avoid loss of balance and prevent falls. Dorsiflexing the feet (ankle pumps), raising the arms overhead with diaphragmatic breathing, and abdominal compression before standing often promote venous return to the heart, accelerate the pulse, and increase blood pressure. The use of abdominal binders and elastic stockings may also help with venous return. Stockings should not be taken off at night to avoid falls when getting up to go to the bathroom or when getting out of bed in the morning. Elevating the head of the bed 5 to 20 degrees prevents the nocturnal diuresis and supine hypertension caused by nocturnal shifts of interstitial fluid from the legs to the rest of the circulation. Eating small meals may help to avoid postprandial (after eating) hypotension. The person who becomes hypotensive should assume a supine position with legs elevated to increase

venous return and to ensure cerebral blood flow. As previously mentioned, this position must be monitored carefully for anyone with orthostatic hypotension and CHF, possibly requiring modifying the position to include slight head and upper body elevation. Crossing the legs, which involves contraction of the agonist and antagonist muscles, also has been shown to increase cardiac output, thereby increasing blood pressure.[214]

The physician should be notified if the person remains symptomatic after these measures have been taken. Anyone who is considered borderline hypotensive when tested in the supine position should have blood pressures measured and pulses counted in a sitting position with the legs dangling. If no change occurs when this is done, repeat the measurements with the person standing, if possible. A drop in systolic pressure of 10 to 20 mm Hg or more associated with an increase in pulse rate of more than 15 beats/min suggests depleted intravascular volume (Fig. 11-15). Some normovolemic persons with peripheral neuropathies or those taking antihypertensive medications may demonstrate an orthostatic fall in blood pressure but without an associated increase in pulse rate. ■

◆ Myocardial Disease

Myocarditis.   Myocarditis is a relatively uncommon inflammatory condition of the muscular walls of the heart (myocardium); it is most often a result of bacterial or viral infection, but it also includes those inflammatory processes related to infectious and noninfectious causes of ischemic heart disease. Other possible causes of myocarditis include chest radiation for treatment of malignancy, sarcoidosis, and drugs, such as lithium and cocaine.

The therapist is most likely to treat the person with systemic lupus erythematosus (SLE) (see Chapter 6) who may have a type of myocarditis called *lupus carditis* (see also the section on Collagen Vascular Diseases: Lupus Carditis in this chapter). SLE is a multisystem autoimmune disease characterized by a release of autoantibodies into the circulation, with a subsequent inflammatory process that can target the heart and vasculature.

Clinical evidence of cardiac involvement among people with SLE occurs in up to one half of all cases. Clinical manifestations may include mild continuous chest pain or soreness in the epigastric region or under the sternum, palpitations, fatigue, and dyspnea; and onset may follow a viral upper respiratory illness in the population at large as well as in persons with SLE. Complications include heart failure, arrhythmias, dilated (congestive) cardiomyopathy (see next section), and sudden death.

Myocarditis usually resolves with treatment of the underlying condition or cause; specific antimicrobial therapy is prescribed if an infectious agent can be identified. Management of myocarditis in SLE is usually with corticosteroids, but immunosuppressive agents may be required. Myocarditis that progresses to dilated cardiomyopathy with heart failure is frequently fatal without heart transplantation.

Special Implications for the Therapist 11-9

MYOCARDITIS

Preferred Practice Patterns:
6D: Impaired Aerobic Capacity/Endurance Associated With Cardiovascular Pump Dysfunction or Failure
Other patterns may apply depending on underlying disease (e.g., SLE, cancer).

Active myocarditis is considered a contraindication for therapy, because this condition can progress very quickly and stress must be avoided; each case is evaluated by the physician. Athletes in whom myocarditis is suspected or diagnosed should discontinue all sports for 6 months after onset of symptoms. Preparticipation evaluation of cardiac function is essential before resuming sports activities. An athlete can resume competing when ventricular function and cardiac dimensions return to normal and clinically significant arrhythmias are absent on ambulatory monitoring.[61] If an impairment of myocardial contractility is present, diastolic blood pressure may be elevated to maintain stroke volume. Disruptions leading to lethal cardiac arrhythmias cannot be predicted. See also Special Implications for the Therapist: Infective Endocarditis, 11-14 and Special Implications for the Therapist: Rheumatic Fever and Heart Disease, 11-15. ■

Cardiomyopathy
Definition and Overview.   Cardiomyopathy is actually part of a group of conditions affecting the heart muscle itself, so that contraction and relaxation of myocardial muscle fibers are impaired. Cardiomyopathies are not caused by other heart or systemic disease, so by definition, cardiomyopathy excludes structural and functional abnormalities caused by valvular disorders, CAD, hypertension, congenital defects, and pulmonary vascular disorders.

Cardiomyopathies are classified as dilated (most common), hypertrophic, or restrictive on the basis of general features of presentation and pathophysiology (Table 11-14). Considerable overlap can occur among these three classifications within the same person (see Pathogenesis).

Incidence and Risk Factors.   The cause of most cardiomyopathies is unknown; cardiomyopathy can affect persons of any age and is often seen in young adults in the second and third decades. The actual incidence is also unknown, but the disease may be more common than was previously realized. This increase in incidence may be attributed to two important variables: (1) improved technology that has allowed for more accurate evaluation of ventricular dimensions and ventricular wall movement and (2) an increased incidence of myocarditis, an important precursor to cardiomyopathy as a result of a wide variety of pathogens, toxins, and autoimmune reactions. Delayed-onset cardiotoxic effects of chemotherapeutic agents may appear as chronic cardiomyopathy. Risk factors for the development of this type of cardiomyopathy include increasing doses of chemotherapeutic agents and previous mediastinal radiation.[243] Doxorubicin HCl (Adriamycin) and daunorubicin HCl (Cerubidine) are the two agents recognized most often in association with dilated cardiomyopathy.

Dilated cardiomyopathy occurs most often in black men between ages 40 and 60 years. About one-half of the cases of dilated cardiomyopathy are idiopathic, and the remainder result from some known disease process (e.g., rheumatic fever, myasthenia gravis, progressive muscular dystrophy, hemochromatosis, amyloidosis, sarcoidosis). Risk factors for dilated cardiomyopathy may include obesity, long-term alcohol abuse, systemic hypertension, cigarette smoking, infections, and pregnancy.* *Hypertrophic cardiomyopathy* appears to be genetically transmitted as an autosomal dominant trait on chromosome 14, and *restrictive cardiomyopathy* occurs as a result of myocardial fibrosis (e.g., amyloidosis, sarcoidosis, hemochromatosis), hypertrophy, infiltration, or defect in myocardial relaxation.

Pathogenesis.   The exact pathogenesis of cardiomyopathy is unknown; the risk factors mentioned previously seem to lower the threshold for the development of cardiomyopathy. For example, heavy consumption of alcohol is thought to cause dilated cardiomyopathy through three mechanisms: direct toxic effect of alcohol or of its metabolites; effects of nutritional deficiencies, especially thiamine deficiency; and toxic effects of beverage additives, such as cobalt. Obesity produces an increase in total blood volume and cardiac output because of the high metabolic activity of excessive fat. In moderate to severe cases of obesity, this may lead to left ventricular dilation, increased left ventricular wall stress, and left ventricular diastolic dysfunction. Regardless of the underlying cause, dilated cardiomyopathy results from extensively damaged myocardial muscle fibers and is characterized by cardiac enlargement. The heart ejects blood less efficiently than nor-

*Peripartum cardiomyopathy is a rare but very serious disease that results in heart failure. It may appear for no apparent reason during the last month of pregnancy or shortly after delivery; incidence is higher among multiparous women older than 30 years, particularly those with malnutrition or preeclampsia. Estimates vary, but the occurrence may be 1 in every 1300 to 4000 deliveries. Maternal death from CHF, blood clots, and infection and stillbirth can occur. Symptoms of orthopnea, cough, palpitations, and high blood pressure may not occur until several weeks after delivery.

TABLE	11-14

Comparison of Cardiomyopathies

	TYPE OF CARDIOMYOPATHIES		
	DILATED	HYPERTROPHIC	RESTRICTIVE
Etiologic and risk factors	Alcoholism, pregnancy, infection, toxins, nutritional deficiency, hypertension, cigarette smoking, obesity, chemotherapy, connective tissue disorders Idiopathic	Inherited defect of muscle growth and development	Infiltrative disease Amyloidosis Sarcoidosis Hemochromatosis
Pathologic findings	Cardiac enlargement; myocardial fiber degeneration	Left ventricular hypertrophy; rigid walls	Endocardial scarring of the ventricles; rigid walls
Chamber size	Increased	Normal or decreased	Normal or decreased
Myocardial mass	Increased	Increased	Normal or increased
Endocardial thickness	Normal or increased	Increased	Increased
Contractility	Decreased	Increased or decreased	Normal or decreased
Clinical manifestations	Fatigue, weakness, chest pain, palpitations	Asymptomatic; sudden death; dyspnea, angina pectoris, fatigue, dizziness, palpitations; exercise intolerance	Exercise intolerance; dyspnea, fatigue; neck vein distention, peripheral edema, ascites
Cardiovascular complication	Left ventricular failure	Left ventricular failure	Right ventricular failure

Modified from Haak SW, Richardson SJ, Davey SS: Alterations of cardiovascular function. In McCance KL, Huether SE, editors: *Pathophysiology: the biologic basis for disease in adults and children*, ed 2, St Louis, 1994, Mosby, pp 1035, 1037.

mal, so that a large volume of blood remains in the left ventricle after systole, which results in ventricular dilation with enlargement and dilation of all four chambers and eventually leads to CHF (Fig. 11-16).

Hypertrophic cardiomyopathy is distinguished by inappropriate and excessive left ventricular hypertrophy (thickening of the interventricular septum) and normal or even enhanced cardiac muscle contractile function. Over time, the overgrowth of the wall leads to rigidity in the myocardium. The result is decreased diastolic functioning since the rigid myocardium cannot relax during the diastolic phase, reducing the amount of blood flowing into the ventricles. Restrictive cardiomyopathy is the least common form; it is identified by marked endocardial scarring (fibrosis) of the ventricles, and the resulting rigidity impairs diastolic filling.

Clinical Manifestations.

Generally, the symptoms of cardiomyopathy are the same as for heart failure (e.g., dyspnea, orthopnea, tachycardia, palpitations, peripheral edema, distended jugular vein). *Dilated cardiomyopathy* is characterized by fatigue and weakness; chest pain (unlike angina) may occur. Blood pressure is usually normal or low. *Hypertrophic cardiomyopathy* is frequently asymptomatic, sudden death being the presenting sign. The most common symptom is dyspnea caused by high pulmonary pressures produced by the elevated left ventricular diastolic pressure; symptoms are often exacerbated during strenuous exercise. *Restrictive cardiomyopathy* causes clinical manifestations related to decreasing cardiac output. As cardiac output falls and intraventricular pressures rise, signs of CHF appear. The earliest manifestations may include exercise intolerance, fatigue, and shortness of breath followed by other symptoms listed in Table 11-14.

Medical Management

Diagnosis and Treatment.   Diagnosis requires exclusion of other causes of cardiac dysfunction, especially causes of CHF and arrhythmias. Catheterization to assess arteries and valves, echocardiography, chest radiography, blood chemistries, and ECG are specific tests performed. Researchers continue to investigate ways to monitor people with heart failure and to devise noninvasive diagnostic techniques.

The specific treatment of cardiomyopathy is determined by the underlying cause and may include physical, dietary, pharmacologic, mechanical circulatory support, and surgical intervention including transplantation. Cardiac resynchronization therapy, the use of a pacemaker-like device to electrically stimulate both ventricles simultaneously (biventricular pacing), has been approved for use in CHF and is under investigation for use with dilated cardiomyopathy. Alternately, a cardiac support device called a "heart jacket" is under investigation for use in the United States for cardiomyopathy. This specially designed polyester material is stitched into place around the heart to prevent diseased heart muscle from further enlargement. Clinical safety trials are under way at the University of Pennsylvania.

Idiopathic dilated cardiomyopathy has no known cause; therefore there is no specific therapy. In contrast to the other forms of cardiomyopathy, the progression of myocardial dysfunction of dilated cardiomyopathy may be stopped or reversed if alcohol consumption is reduced or stopped early in the course of the disease. Beta-blockers have an important immunoregulatory role in modifying the dysregulated cytokine network and reducing myocardial contractility and workload.[175] Calcium-channel blocking agents (see Table 11-4) may be used to relieve symptoms and improve exercise intolerance. Restrictive cardiomyopathy has no specific treatment

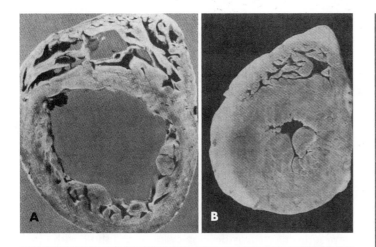

FIGURE 11-16 **A,** Cross-sectional view of dilated cardiomyopathy. **B,** Hypertrophied heart. (From Kinney M: *Comprehensive cardiac care,* ed 7, St Louis, 1991, Mosby, pp 346, 349.)

interventions. The goal is to control CHF through the use of diuretics, vasodilators, and salt restriction.

Prognosis. Seventy-five percent of persons diagnosed with idiopathic dilated cardiomyopathy die within 5 years after the onset of symptoms because diagnosis does not usually occur until advanced stages. Persons with hypertrophic cardiomyopathy can lead long, relatively asymptomatic lives; some people have a history of gradually progressive symptoms, but others experience sudden death, especially during exercise, as the initial diagnostic event. Restrictive cardiomyopathy may cause sudden death as a result of arrhythmia, or a more progressive course may occur, with eventual heart failure. Intervention rarely results in long-term improvement.

Many persons with various types of cardiomyopathy experience a stabilization or even an improvement in symptoms, but the end result of cardiomyopathy is sudden death or a fatal progression toward heart failure. No cure exists, outside of cardiac transplantation. Heart transplantation shows a 1-year survival rate of over 80% and a 3-year survival of 70% for dilated cardiomyopathy. The 1-year survival rate without transplant is 5%.

Special Implications for the Therapist **11-10**

CARDIOMYOPATHY

Preferred Practice Patterns:
6B: Impaired Aerobic Capacity/Endurance Associated With Deconditioning
6D: Impaired Aerobic Capacity/Endurance Associated With Cardiovascular Pump Dysfunction or Failure
Other patterns (e.g., musculoskeletal) may apply depending on the chronicity of the condition and level of physical activity.

Sudden death can occur, but the incidence is rare. It occurs more often in younger people who have cardiomyo-

pathy, and it may be avoided by eliminating strenuous exercise (e.g., running, competitive sports) when a diagnosis has been established. Rest improves cardiac function and reduces heart size. During the early stages of the disease, many people find it difficult to accept activity restrictions and need encouragement to follow guidelines for activity restriction. Clients should avoid poorly tolerated activities; combine rest with activity; understand that physical stress and emotional stress exacerbate the disease; learn correct breathing techniques, since Valsalva's maneuvers decrease the inflow of venous blood and impair outflow and should be avoided; and understand that alcohol depresses myocardial contractility and should be eliminated.

The therapist can provide valuable information regarding energy conservation techniques (see Box 8-2) to assist persons with continued independence in activities of daily living and possibly even to improve activity tolerance. This is especially true for the person awaiting a cardiac transplant. The therapist involved with athletes (of all ages) is advised to follow the American Heart Association's guidelines for preparticipation screening and identifying athletes at risk for sudden cardiac death.[61,153,154] Cardiomyopathy associated with cardiotoxicity following chemotherapy is often clinically silent because of the clients' low levels of physical activity. An evaluation to screen for potential cardiopulmonary dysfunction is essential with these clients. The evaluation should include an assessment of current physical activity levels and exercise tolerance and monitoring of heart rate and rhythm, blood pressure, respiratory responses, and any other signs and symptoms of exercise intolerance (e.g., dyspnea, fatigue, light-headedness or dizziness, pallor, palpitations, chest discomfort).[243] A scale that rates perceived exertion (see Table 11-13) is often useful during the evaluation and for establishing initial exercise guidelines toward improving endurance.

For the person who has been hospitalized and has not ambulated yet, the therapist will need to assess tolerance to activities in bed before ambulating. During activities, monitor pulse, respirations, blood pressure, and color. The heart rate, systolic blood pressure, and respiratory rate normally increase in proportion to the exercise (movement) intensity whereas the diastolic blood pressure changes minimally (+/− 10 mm Hg). Improved activity tolerance may be demonstrated by minimal change in pulse or blood pressure during activities with minimal fatigue after the activity. Pulse, respirations, and blood pressure should return to a normal range within 3 minutes of the end of the activity. Discontinue any activity that results in chest pain, severe dyspnea, cyanosis, dizziness, hypotension, or sustained tachycardia.

Abnormal responses include either blunted or excessive rises in heart rate or systolic blood pressure, excessive increases in diastolic blood pressure or respiratory rate, a fall in systolic blood pressure with increasing activity, or increasing irregularity of the pulse. These signs may be the result of cardiopulmonary toxicity or simply the result of deconditioning. Increasing irregularity in the pulse with pairs or runs of faster beats or more than six isolated irregular beats/min must be reported to the physician.[243] If the person is receiving diuretics, monitor for signs of too-vigorous diuresis (e.g., muscle cramps, orthostatic hypotension). If the person becomes hypotensive, use a supine position with legs elevated to increase venous return and to ensure cerebral blood flow. ■

Trauma

Nonpenetrating.   Any blunt chest trauma, which is especially common in steering wheel impact from an automobile accident, may produce myocardial contusion, resulting in myocardial hemorrhage with little if any myocardial scar once healing is complete. Large contusions may lead to myocardial scars, cardiac rupture, CHF, or formation of aneurysms.

The chest pain of myocardial contusion is similar to that of MI and is often confused with musculoskeletal pain from soft tissue consequences of chest trauma. Myocardial contusion is usually treated similarly to MI, with initial monitoring and subsequent progressive ambulation and cardiac rehabilitation (see Special Implications for the Therapist: Myocardial Infarction, 11-6).

Penetrating.   Penetrating cardiac injuries are most often due to external objects, such as bullets or knives, and sometimes from bony fragments secondary to chest injury. Iatrogenic causes of cardiac penetrating injury include perforation of the heart during catheterization and cardiac trauma from cardiopulmonary resuscitation. Complications include arrhythmias, aneurysm formation, death from infection (e.g., bacterial endocarditis or infection from a retained foreign body), a form of pericarditis associated with this type of injury, ventricular septal defects, and foreign body embolus.

Myocardial Neoplasms.

Tumors involving the heart are rare, but they may be primary or metastatic and benign or malignant. The most common primary tumor (usually benign) is a myxoma, arising most often from the endothelial surface of the left atrium; tumors located in other cardiac chambers account for 10% of myxomas. Other benign cardiac tumors (also rare) include lipoma, papilloma, fibroelastoma, rhabdomyoma, and fibroma. Malignant cardiac neoplasms may include angiosarcoma, rhabdomyosarcoma, mesothelioma, fibrosarcoma, and malignant lymphoma.

Metastases to the heart and pericardium are much more common than primary cardiac tumors and are generally associated with cancers of the lung and breast, melanoma, and lymphoma. Tumor may involve the heart by one of four pathways: retrograde lymphatic extension, hematogenous spread, direct contiguous extension, or transvenous extension. Metastatic involvement of the heart and pericardium may go unrecognized until autopsy. Impairment of cardiac function occurs in approximately 30% of cases and is usually attributed to pericardial effusion. The clinical presentation includes shortness of breath, cough, anterior thoracic pain, pleuritic chest pain, or peripheral edema. Cardiac neoplasms come to the attention of a therapist when (1) progressive interference with mitral valve function results in exercise intolerance or exertional dyspnea; (2) embolus causes a stroke; or (3) systemic manifestations occur, including muscle atrophy, arthralgias, malaise, or Raynaud's phenomenon.

Treatment is surgical excision with subsequent cardiac rehabilitation as required by the postoperative cardiovascular condition. Secondary tumors that have metastasized to the heart from elsewhere are not usually considered curable, have a poor prognosis, but are treated with radiation and chemotherapy.

◆ Congenital Heart Disease

Overview and Incidence.   Congenital heart disease is an anatomic defect in the heart that develops in utero during the first trimester and is present at birth. Over the past three decades, major advances have been made in the diagnosis and treatment of congenital heart disease resulting in many more children who have survived to adulthood with surgically corrected or uncorrected anomalies. Today, there are over 1 million adults with congenital heart conditions. Congenital heart disease affects about 8 of every 1000 babies born in the United States, making this the most common category of congenital structural malformation. Other than prematurity, it is the major cause of death in the first year of life. Children with congenital heart disease are also more likely to have extracardiac defects, such as tracheoesophageal fistula, diaphragmatic hernias, and renal abnormalities.

There are two categories of congenital heart disease: cyanotic and acyanotic (Table 11-15). In clinical practice this system of classification is problematic, because children with acyanotic defects may develop cyanosis and those with cyanotic defects may be pink and have more clinical signs of CHF. Cyanotic defects result from obstruction of blood flow to the lungs or mixing of desaturated blue venous blood with fully saturated red arterial blood within the chambers of the heart. Most acyanotic defects involve primarily left-to-right shunting through an abnormal opening.

Etiologic Factors.   Many congenital heart diseases have genetic causes with well-known chromosomal anomalies (e.g., trisomy 13, 18, 21; Turner's syndrome). Approximately 10% of all congenital heart defects are known to be associated with a single identified mutant gene or chromosomal abnormalities; the remaining causes are either unknown or are attributable to multiple factors, such as diabetes, alcohol consumption, viruses, maternal rubella infection during the first trimester, and drugs, such as thalidomide. In the case of atrial septal defect, most result from spontaneous genetic mutations although some are inherited. Patent ductus arteriosus occurs in pregnancies complicated by persistent perinatal hypoxemia or maternal rubella infection and among infants born at high altitude or prematurely.[30]

Pathogenesis.   The heart begins to form from a tubelike structure during the fourth week after conception. As development progresses, the tube lengthens and forms chambers, septa, and valves. Anything that interferes with this developmental process during the first 8 to 10 weeks of pregnancy can result in a congenital defect (Fig. 11-17).

Cyanotic.   In *transposition of the great vessels (TGV)*, no communication exists between systemic and pulmonary circulations so that the pulmonary artery leaves the left ventricle and the aorta exits from the right ventricle. In order for the infant with this condition to survive, there must be communication between the two circuits. In approximately one third of all cases, another associated defect occurs that permits intracardiac mixing (e.g., atrial septal defect, ventricular septal defect, patent ductus arteriosus), but two thirds have no other defect present and severe cyanosis develops.[31] *Tetralogy of Fallot (TOF)* consists of four classic defects: (1) pulmonary stenosis, (2) large ventricular septal defect (VSD), (3) aortic communication with both ventricles, and (4) right ventricular hypertrophy. *Tricuspid atresia* is a failure of the tricuspid valve to develop, with a lack of communication from the right atrium to the right ventricle. Blood flows through an atrial septal defect or a ductus arteriosus to the left side of the heart and through a ventricular septal defect to the right ventricle

TABLE	11-15

Congenital Heart Disease

DEFECT	INCIDENCE	CLINICAL MANIFESTATIONS	PROGNOSIS
Cyanotic			
Transposition of the great vessels	16%*; 3:1 male/female ratio	Depends on size and type of defects; cyanosis; CHF (newborn)	Improved surgical treatment provides excellent long-term outcome
Tetralogy of Fallot	10%-15%	*Infants:* acutely cyanotic at birth or progressive cyanosis first year	At risk for sudden lethal arrhythmias; mild obstruction progresses with age; reduced life expectancy
		Children: hypoxic events with tachypnea, increasing cyanosis, digital clubbing; poor growth and development; seizures, loss of consciousness, death possible	
		Adults: dyspnea, limited exercise tolerance	
Tricuspid atresia	<1%; relatively rare	Newborn cyanosis; tachycardia; dyspnea; digital clubbing (older child)	Unreported; depends on success of treatment
Acyanotic			
Ventricular septal defect	25%; single most common CHD; 25%-40% close spontaneously by age 2 yr; 90% close by age 10 yr	Asymptomatic with small defect; CHF (age 1-6 mo); history of frequent respiratory infections; poor growth and development; dyspnea, fatigue, and exercise intolerance (older child)	No physical restrictions
Atrial septal defect	10% children; 2:1 female/male ratio. Accounts for 33% of all CHD cases surviving to adulthood	*Older child:* asymptomatic; growth failure; CHF. *Adult:* fatigue or dyspnea on exertion	No physical restrictions if corrected; frequent complications in adults
Coarctation of the aorta	6%; 3:1 male/female ratio	High systolic blood pressure (BP) and bounding pulses in arms; weak or absent femoral pulses; cool lower extremities with lower BP	Good if survive to childhood; exercise testing recommended before participation in athletics; reduced life expectancy; increased risk of aortic dissection during pregnancy
		Infants: CHF	
		Children: headaches, fainting, epistaxis (hypertension); exercise intolerance, easy fatigability	
		Adults: asymptomatic or signs of hypertension (headache, epistaxis, dizziness, palpitations)	
Patent ductus arteriosus	12%; spontaneous closure in normal term infants by day 4; common in children born to mothers affected by rubella during first trimester; increased incidence in infants born at high altitudes (over 10,000 ft); present in 20%-60% of premature infants weighing <1500 g	*Children:* asymptomatic; CHF. *Adult:* if symptomatic: fatigue, dyspnea, palpitations	Closure may occur up to age 2 yr; normal life expectancy with small defect; aneurysm and rupture can occur; poor prognosis for large defect without transplantation
Aortic stenosis	5% of all CHD	Asymptomatic; exercise intolerance, dizziness, and chest pain with prolonged standing	Good with early detection and surgical treatment; exercise testing recommended before participation in athletics

CHF, congenital heart failure; *CHD,* coronary heart disease.
*Figures account for percentage of all congenital heart disease.

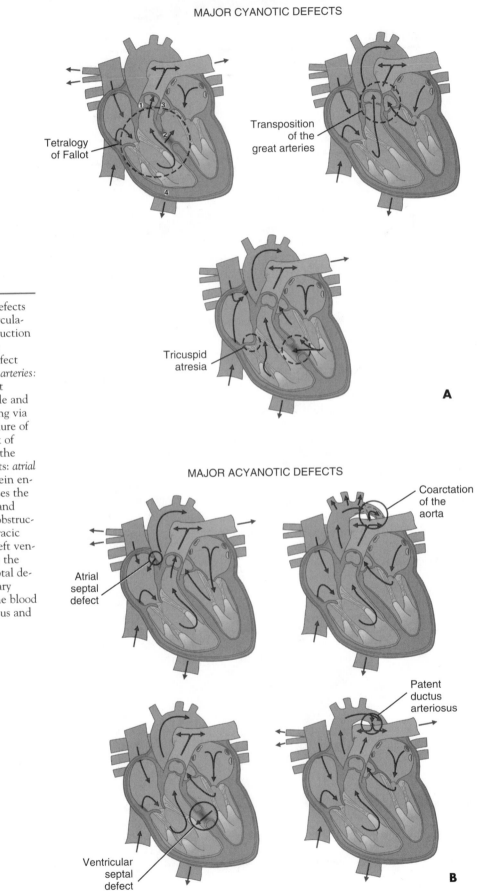

MAJOR CYANOTIC DEFECTS

Tetralogy of Fallot

Transposition of the great arteries

Tricuspid atresia

A

MAJOR ACYANOTIC DEFECTS

Atrial septal defect

Coarctation of the aorta

Patent ductus arteriosus

Ventricular septal defect

B

FIGURE **11-17** **A,** Major cyanotic defects (see Fig. 11-1 for normal structure and circulation of the heart): *tetralogy of Fallot:* obstruction of right ventricular outflow tract, blood is shunted through the ventricular septal defect from right to left; *transposition of the great arteries:* systemic venous blood returns to the right atrium and then goes to the right ventricle and on to the aorta instead of going to the lung via the pulmonary artery; *tricuspid atresia:* failure of the tricuspid valve to develop with a lack of communication from the right atrium to the right ventricle. **B,** Major acyanotic defects: *atrial septal defect:* blood from the pulmonary vein enters the left atrium, and some blood crosses the atrial septal defect into the right atrium and ventricle; *coarctation of the aorta:* severe obstruction of blood flow in the descending thoracic aorta; *ventricular septal defect:* when the left ventricle contracts, it ejects some blood into the aorta and some across the ventricular septal defect into the right ventricle and pulmonary artery; *patent ductus arteriosus:* some of the blood from the aorta crosses the ductus arteriosus and flows into the pulmonary artery.

and out to the lungs. There is complete mixing of unoxygenated and oxygenated blood in the left side of the heart, resulting in systemic desaturation and varying amounts of pulmonary obstruction.

Acyanotic.   *Ventricular septal defect* is an abnormal opening between the right and left ventricles that may vary in size from a small pinhole to complete absence of the septum, resulting in a common ventricle. Atrial septal defect (ASD) is an abnormal opening between the atria, allowing blood from the higher-pressure left atrium to flow into the lower-pressure right atrium. *Coarctation of the aorta* is a localized narrowing near the insertion of the ductus arteriosus, resulting in increased pressure proximal to the defect (head, upper extremities) and decreased pressure distal to the obstruction (body, lower extremities). *Patent ductus arteriosus* is a failure of the fetal ductus arteriosus (artery connecting the aorta and pulmonary artery) to close within the first weeks of life. The continued function of this vessel allows blood to flow from the high-pressure aorta to the low-pressure pulmonary artery, causing continuous flow from the aorta to the pulmonary artery (referred to as left-to-right shunting). A patent ductus arteriosus rarely closes spontaneously after infancy. *Aortic stenosis* is discussed later in this chapter in the section on Diseases Affecting the Heart Valves.

Clinical Manifestations.
The most common signs and symptoms include cyanosis and signs of CHF (e.g., dyspnea, pulmonary edema, fatigue). See Table 11-15 for clinical manifestations of each particular defect. Complications may include heart failure, pulmonary edema, pneumonia, hypoxia, and sudden death. There is often a risk of bacterial endocarditis and pulmonary vascular obstructive disease later in life.

Medical Management
Prevention and Diagnosis.   As whole genome sequencing continues to develop, identification of genetic mutations predisposing to congenital heart disease (CHD) may allow preventive measures by modulation of secondary genetic or environmental factors.[216] Until then, most forms of CHD can potentially be detected in utero with the routine use of ultrasonography. The prenatal diagnosis of a major cardiac malformation requires further assessment for extracardiac and chromosomal disorders. Conversely, diagnosis of Down syndrome (prenatally or postnatally) requires early cardiologic assessment for cardiac anomalies, most commonly atrioventricular and ventricular septal defects. Prenatal knowledge of cardiac anomalies allows for optimal perinatal and postnatal management. Prenatal screening for maternal rubella antibodies provides important information for further diagnostic testing. In cases where prenatal diagnosis does not occur and when there are no symptoms initially, cardiac anomalies can remain undetected for years and even decades. For example, a person with atrial septal defect may have normal sinus rhythm for the first three decades of life and then develop atrial fibrillation and supraventricular tachycardia.[31,32]

Clinical diagnosis begins with detection of signs and symptoms, auscultation, and detection of heart murmur. Transesophageal, Doppler color-flow echocardiography and now real-time 3D echocardiography provide a definitive diagnosis without invasive cardiac catheterization and angiography.

Treatment and Prognosis.   Remarkable innovations in medical and surgical approaches over the past several decades now allow for correction of major cardiac defects in children, even in early infancy. Prenatal (in utero) correction has not been accomplished as yet. Postnatally, curative or palliative (provides relief of symptoms) surgical correction is now available for more than 90% of persons with congenital heart disease. There is a clear trend toward complete correction of malformations replacing staged procedures to obtain initial palliation and delayed correction. The risk for most surgical procedures is low (between 1% and 5%). Gene transfer to create a patent ductus arteriosus in animal studies may lead the way for additional gene transfer techniques to be successful in humans in the future.

Special Implications for the Therapist   11-11

CONGENITAL HEART DISEASE

Preferred Practice Patterns:
5B: Impaired Neuromotor Development
6D: Impaired Aerobic Capacity/Endurance Associated With
*   Cardiovascular Pump Dysfunction or Failure*
Other patterns may apply depending on complications (e.g., pneumonia, heart failure).

Therapists need to be alert to signs of CHF in children with congenital heart disease and in infants with suspected congenital heart disease. Signs of CHF indicate a worsening clinical condition; the earlier these are detected, the sooner intervention can be initiated. (See also Special Implications for the Therapist: Congestive Heart Failure). The surgical procedures associated with the repair of congenital heart disease (e.g., bypass, deep hypothermia) are associated with an increased incidence of neurologic abnormalities. Neurodevelopmental deficits resulting from surgical repair of cardiac defects may include choreoathetosis, cerebral palsy, or hemiparesis.[85] Gross motor development can be negatively impacted by prolonged hospitalization, deficiencies in cardiovascular status, surgical techniques used to minimize blood loss, or any combination of these factors. The more complex the defect or defects and the more numerous open-heart surgeries required, the greater the risk for neurologic impairment.[227]

Most children with significant heart defects will have had heart surgery before they start school. In addition to a developmental assessment, the therapist should evaluate for soft tissue restriction at the site of the healed scar (either sternal or thoracic), which may affect breathing capacity. Physiologic response to therapy intervention can be assessed by observing skin color, respiratory effort, and behavioral response. Oxygen saturation monitors may not be helpful because these children have abnormally low readings as their baseline level.[227] Data on exercise capacity after specific types of surgical procedures are available.[213] In general, anyone who has had successful surgery is allowed unrestricted sports activity. Young children with unrepaired tetralogy of Fallot instinctively learn to squat, getting into the flat-footed baseball catcher's stance when they are fatigued. This posture increases the tension in the leg muscles, reduces

Continued

blood flow to the leg muscles, and raises peripheral resistance and blood pressure.

Twenty or thirty years ago, diagnosis of congenital defects was much more difficult, and many anomalies went undetected. Adults with undiagnosed congenital defects may develop exercise intolerance, shortness of breath, palpitations, blood pressure irregularities, or symptoms of CHF, which should alert the therapist of the need for medical referral. Exercise recommendations for children and adolescents with congenital malformations are available.[61] Care of pregnant women with congenital heart disease requires understanding of the specific congenital defect, the nature of previous surgical correction, and the presence of any complications or sequelae.[52] ■

DISEASE AFFECTING THE CARDIAC NERVOUS SYSTEM

◆ Arrhythmias: Disturbances of Rate or Rhythm

Definition and Overview.   The number of times the heart beats (rate) and the heart rhythm are generated and regulated by the sinoatrial (SA) node, the internal pacemaker located in the upper right portion of the heart. The signal from the SA node travels through the cardiac conduction system, first through the walls of the atria and then through the walls of the ventricles causing the atrial (supraventricular) and ventricular chambers of the heart to contract and relax at regular rates necessary to maintain circulation at different levels of activity. An arrhythmia (dysrhythmia) is a disturbance of heart rate or rhythm caused by an abnormal rate of electrical impulse generation by the SA node or the abnormal conduction of impulses.

Arrhythmias are usually classified according to their origin as ventricular or supraventricular (atrial), according to the pattern (fibrillation or flutter) or according to the speed or rate at which they occur (tachycardia or bradycardia). Arrhythmias vary in severity from mild, asymptomatic disturbances that require no intervention (e.g., sinus arrhythmia, in which the heart rate increases and decreases with respiration) to catastrophic ventricular fibrillation, which requires immediate resuscitation. The clinical significance depends on the effect on cardiac output and blood pressure, which is partially influenced by the site of origin.

Etiologic Factors and Incidence.   Arrhythmias may be congenital or may result from one of several factors, including hypertrophy of heart muscle fiber secondary to hypertension, previous MI, or valvular heart disease, or degeneration of conductive tissue that is necessary to maintain normal heart rhythm (called *sick sinus syndrome*). The prevalence of atrial fibrillation doubles with each advancing decade of age beginning at age 50 to 59 years with a statistically significant increase among men age 65 to 84 years, although this gap closes with advancing age and remains unexplained.[128,161] Improved cardiac care has increased the number of survivors of cardiac incidents who may experience subsequent complications, such as arrhythmias.

Cardiac arrhythmias are very common in the setting of heart failure, with atrial and ventricular arrhythmias often present in the same person. Arrhythmias can occur when a portion of the heart is temporarily deprived of oxygen, dis-

turbing the normal pathway of the heartbeat. Toxic doses of cardioactive drugs (e.g., digoxin and other cardiac glycosides), phenylpropanolamine found in some decongestants, alcohol and caffeine consumption, high fevers, and excessive production of thyroid hormone (hyperthyroidism) may also lead to arrhythmias. In many cases, particularly in younger people, there is no known or apparent cause.

Pathogenesis and Clinical Manifestations

Rate.   The adult heart beats an average of 60 to 100 beats/min; an arrhythmia is considered any significant deviation from the normal range. Whether change in heart rate (number of contractions of the cardiac ventricles per period of time) produces symptoms at rest or on exertion depends on the underlying state of the cardiac muscle and its ability to alter its stroke output to compensate.

Rate arrhythmias are of two basic types: tachycardia and bradycardia. Tachycardia occurs when the heart beats too fast (>100 beats/min). Tachycardia develops in the presence of increased sympathetic stimulation, such as occurs with fear, pain, emotion, exertion, or exercise; or with ingestion of artificial stimulants, such as caffeine, nicotine, and amphetamines. Tachycardia is also found in situations in which the demands for oxygen are increased, such as fever, CHF, infection, anemia, hemorrhage, myocardial injury, and hyperthyroidism. Usually the individual with tachycardia perceives no symptoms, and medical intervention is directed toward the underlying cause.

Bradycardia (less than 60 beats/min) is normal in well-trained athletes, but it is also common in individuals taking beta-blockers, those who have had traumatic brain injuries or brain tumors, and those experiencing increased vagal stimulation (e.g., from suctioning or vomiting) to the physiologic pacemaker. Organic disease of the sinus node, especially in older people and those with heart disease, can also cause sinus bradycardia. Bradycardia is usually asymptomatic, but when it is caused by a pathologic condition, the person may experience fatigue, dyspnea, syncope, dizziness, angina, or diaphoresis. Medical intervention is not usually required unless symptoms interfere with function or are drug- or angina-induced; atropine or a mechanical pacemaker can be used to reestablish a more normal heart rate.

Rhythm.   Arrhythmias as variations from the normal rhythm of the heart (especially the heartbeat) are detected when they become symptomatic or during monitoring for another cardiac condition. Abnormalities of cardiac rhythm and electrical conduction can be lethal (sudden cardiac death), symptomatic (syncope or near syncope, dizziness, chest pain, dyspnea, palpitations), or asymptomatic. They are dangerous because they reduce cardiac output so that perfusion of the brain or myocardium is impaired, or they tend to deteriorate into more serious arrhythmias with the same consequences.

The many different types of abnormal cardiac rhythms are usually classified according to their origin (atrial, ventricular), but only the most common ones are included here. Complete discussion of all other cardiac arrhythmias is available.[109] *Sinus arrhythmia* is an irregularity in rhythm that may be a normal variation in athletes, children, and older people or may be caused by an alteration in vagal stimulation. Sinus arrhythmia may be respiratory (increases and decreases with respiration) or nonrespiratory and associated with infection, drug toxicity (e.g., digoxin, morphine), or fever. Treatment for the respiratory type of sinus arrhythmia is not necessary; all other sinus arrhythmias are treated by providing intervention for the underlying cause.

Atrial fibrillation (AF) is the most common chronic arrhythmia. It is characterized by rapid, involuntary, irregular muscular contractions of the atrial myocardium—quivering or fluttering instead of contracting normally. Consequently, blood remains in the atria after they contract and the ventricles do not fill properly. The heart races, but blood flow may diminish, creating a drop in oxygen levels that results in symptoms of shortness of breath, palpitations, fatigue, and more rarely, fainting. Atrial fibrillation occurs most often as a secondary arrhythmia associated with rheumatic heart disease, dilated cardiomyopathy, atrial septal defect, hypertension, mitral valve prolapse, recurrent cardiac surgery, and hypertrophic cardiomyopathy (conditions that affect the atria). Secondary atrial fibrillation can also occur in people without cardiac disease but in the presence of a systemic abnormality that predisposes the individual to arrhythmia (e.g., hyperthyroidism, medications, diabetes, obesity, pneumonia, or alcohol intoxication or withdrawal). People with atrial fibrillation are prone to blood clots because blood components that remain in the atria aggregate and attract other components, triggering clot formation, often within 24 to 48 hours of the first abnormal contraction. Atrial fibrillation can result in congestive heart failure, cardiac ischemia, and arterial emboli that can result in an ischemic stroke.

Ventricular fibrillation is an electrical phenomenon that results in involuntary incoordinated muscular contractions of the ventricular muscle; it is a frequent cause of cardiac arrest. Treatment is directed toward depolarizing the muscle, thus ending the irregular contractions and allowing the heart to resume normal regular contractions.

Heart block is a disorder of the heartbeat caused by an interruption in the passage of impulses through the heart's electrical system. This may occur because the SA node misfires or the impulses it generates are not properly transmitted through the heart's conduction system. Heart blocks are differentiated into three types determined by ECG testing as first-degree, second-degree, or third-degree (complete) heart block. Causes include CAD, hypertension, myocarditis, and overdose of cardiac medications (e.g., digitalis, calcium-channel blockers, beta-blockers). Depending on the degree of the heart block, it can cause fatigue, dizziness, or fainting. Heart block can affect people at any age, but this condition primarily affects older people. Mild cases do not require intervention; medication and pacemakers are the two primary forms of management for symptomatic cases.

Sick sinus syndrome, or brady-tachy syndrome, is a complex cardiac arrhythmia and conduction disturbance that is associated with CAD or drug therapy (e.g., digitalis, calcium-channel blockers, beta-blockers, antiarrhythmics). Sick sinus syndrome as a result of degeneration of conductive tissue necessary to maintain normal heart rhythm occurs most often among older people. A variety of other heart diseases and other conditions (e.g., cardiomyopathy, sarcoidosis, amyloidosis) also may result in sinus node dysfunction. Sick sinus syndrome is characterized by bradycardia alone, bradycardia alternating with tachycardia, or bradycardia with atrioventricular block resulting in cerebral manifestations of lightheadedness, dizziness, and near or true syncope.

Sinus node dysfunction is suspected in the older adult experiencing episodes of syncope or near syncope, especially in the presence of heart palpitations. An accurate diagnosis is made with ECG, often requiring a 24-hour Holter monitor to document the arrhythmias described. Treatment for the symptomatic person varies according to the specific arrhythmia manifestations and may include antiarrhythmic agents alone or combined with a permanent-demand pacemaker or withdrawal of agents that may be responsible.

Medical Management

Diagnosis.   ECG is the most common test procedure to document arrhythmias, but if the person is not experiencing symptoms, the heartbeat may look normal. Tape-recorded ambulatory ECG may be used to document arrhythmias. The individual may use continuous monitoring (Holter monitoring; Fig. 11-18) recording all cardiac cycles over a prescribed period of time (usually 24 to 48 hours) or cardiac event monitoring recording ECG just when symptoms are perceived. Monitoring is especially helpful in recording sporadic arrhythmias that an office or stress-test ECG might miss. Monitoring may also be used by persons recovering from MIs, receiving antiarrhythmic medications, or using pacemakers. New pocket-sized devices to allow home monitoring are available; readings may be stored, and the device can be hooked up to the physician's ECG or diagnostic computer or transmitted over the telephone. For symptoms that occur rarely (e.g., once every 6 months), an insertable loop recorder can be used. This small device is implanted

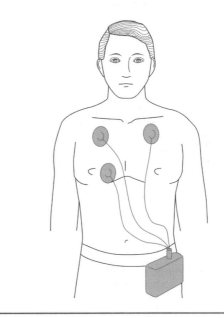

FIGURE   **11-18** External cardiac monitoring (a form of telemetry) may be used to evaluate effects of medical treatment and allows continuous (or pinpoint "event") observation of the heart's electrical activity in people with symptomatic arrhythmia or any cardiac abnormality that might lead to life-threatening arrhythmias. Various different types are used depending on the desired information. The standard three-electrode system consists of a positive electrode, negative electrode, and ground electrode; up to 12 leads may be used. The Holter monitor is usually strapped around the person's waist, securely but comfortably. If the belt is not snug enough, the weight of the monitor pulls on the electrodes.

under the skin in the chest using a local anesthetic. Monitoring units do not replace an ECG and should not be used without a physician's approval.

Transesophageal echocardiography (TEE) imaging study using an ultrasonic transducer mounted on the tip of a flexible instrument is used to detect cardiac emboli before medications are initiated to control rate and rhythm. If a serious arrhythmia is suspected, an electrophysiologic study (EPS) can be performed. This test is an invasive study that uses wires placed via catheterization to electronically stimulate the heart in an attempt to reproduce the arrhythmia.

Treatment. Normal heart rhythm returns spontaneously (called *cardioversion*) almost immediately in some cases, especially if there is no underlying heart disease. When conversion to normal rate and rhythm does not occur there are two major approaches to cardioversion: electrical and pharmacologic. The electrical method employs the use of a device called a *defibrillator* and is usually most effective and may require several weeks of anticoagulant therapy (warfarin) to reduce stroke risk. Pharmacologic treatment may include agents prolonging depolarization and/or other cardiovascular medications (see Table 11-4). If successful, cardioversion restores sinus rhythm and drug therapy is used to maintain normal heart rate and rhythm.

Some tachycardias can be treated with radio-wave ablation, a nonsurgical but invasive technique that uses catheterization to thread wires into the heart through which radio waves can be aimed at the heart tissue where the arrhythmia originates. The catheter-delivered quick bursts of current destroy the specific areas of heart muscle that are generating the abnormal electrical signals causing the arrhythmia. One complication of this technique is the potential destruction of the conducting system (the heart's own internal pacemaker), which necessitates surgical implantation of an artificial pacemaker for some people.

Pacemakers, implants designed to replace the heartbeat by delivering a battery-supplied electrical stimulus through leads attached to electrodes in contact with the heart, may be used in cases of bradycardia, heart block, or refractory tachycardia.* Pacemakers initiate the heartbeat when the heart's intrinsic conduction system fails or is unreliable. In the case of life-threatening arrhythmias (e.g., ventricular tachycardia, ventricular fibrillation) that do not respond to other types of intervention, a device called an implantable cardioverter-defibrillator (ICD) may be implanted. The cardioverter-defibrillator monitors the heart rhythm, and if the heart starts beating abnormally, it uses an electric shock to restore the normal sinus (heart) rhythm, something a pacemaker cannot do.

For people whose arrhythmias are resistant to pharmacologic therapy, another surgical intervention is available called the *maze procedure*. This procedure requires open-heart surgery and involves a series of mazelike cuts made in the atria and then sewn back together. The scar tissue that forms during the healing process blocks faulty circuits, preventing atrial fibrillation. Many people still need a pacemaker and drug

therapy to maintain normal rate and rhythm. A more refined version of this procedure (catheter maze) takes a percutaneous, nonsurgical, noninvasive approach using radiofrequency ablation to destroy tissue.

A new treatment intervention called *ventricular resynchronization therapy* is gaining recognition for the treatment of intraventricular conduction disturbances associated with CHF. This redesigned pacemaker resynchronizes the right and left ventricles so they pump at the same time, making the heart pump more forcefully instead of pumping faster (as occurs with a typical pacemaker or in the case of CHF when the heart beats faster to compensate for a weak pumping mechanism).[239]

Prognosis. Sudden cardiac arrest (sudden death) is responsible for 300,000 deaths annually and is often preceded by fatal heart dysrhythms in people who have no prior history of heart disease. In fact, new data from the Framingham Heart Study indicate that atrial fibrillation is independently associated with a substantially increased risk for death in both men and women even after adjustment for age and associated factors, such as hypertension, congestive heart failure, and stroke. Defibrillation within the first few minutes of cardiac arrest can save up to 50% of lives compared to an estimated 5% of sudden cardiac arrest victims in the United States who survive. Early defibrillation is the key to survival, and toward that end, emergency medical teams are using automatic external defibrillator (AED) portable units that use a computer program to sense whether a defibrillation shock is warranted and will initiate the shock.[188]

The most appropriate and effective drug or drug combination remains unknown, and side effects of long-term rate and rhythm control intervention (e.g., organ toxicity of the lung, liver, and thyroid; aggravation of a preexisting arrhythmia or developing a new arrhythmia instead of preventing it) may prevent long-term use of drug therapy. About 10% of affected individuals continue to have episodes despite treatment, and one-half who are treated have a recurrence within 6 months.

Special Implications for the Therapist 11-12

ARRHYTHMIAS

Preferred Practice Patterns:
5A: Primary Prevention/Risk Reduction for Loss of Balance and Falling
6D: Impaired Aerobic Capacity/Endurance Associated With Cardiovascular Pump Dysfunction or Failure

Anytime a person's pulse is abnormally slow, rapid, or irregular, especially in the presence of known cardiac involvement, documentation and notification of the physician are necessary. Predisposing factors for arrhythmias include fluid and electrolyte imbalance (see Chapter 4) and drug toxicity (see Table 11-4 and Special Implications for the Therapist: Cardiomyopathy, 11-10). To prevent postoperative cardiac arrhythmias, consult carefully with respiratory therapy personnel to provide adequate oxygen during activities that increase the heart's workload.

---

*This refers to a condition in which the heart is beating very quickly, but only a portion of those beats are functional; many more beats just echo or make a beat but without contractile force behind the blood flow. Functionally, the heartbeat is actually very slow.

Clients describing palpitations or similar phenomena may not be experiencing symptoms of arrhythmic heart disease. Palpitations can occur as a result of an overactive thyroid, secondary to caffeine sensitivity, as a side effect of some medications, from decreased estrogen levels, and through the use of drugs such as cocaine. Encourage the client to report any such symptoms to the physician if this has not already been brought to the physician's attention. See Special Implications for the Therapist: Signs and Symptoms of Cardiovascular Disease, 11-1.

It is the position of the American Physical Therapy Association that properly trained physical therapists should be authorized to perform advanced cardiac life support procedures to include cardiac monitoring for arrhythmia recognition and cardiac defibrillation.[13] Physical therapists exercise many people with a history of personal or family heart disease or known risk factors for cardiac disease potentially necessitating cardiopulmonary resuscitation. Public access to emergency defibrillation was signed into law (Cardiac Arrest Survival Act; HR 2498) in 2000 placing AEDs in federal buildings and providing nationwide Good Samaritan protection that exempts from liability anyone who renders emergency treatment with a defibrillator to save a life. Also signed into law was the Rural Access to Emergency Devices Act (SF 2528) authorizing $25 million in federal funds to help rural communities purchase AEDs and train people to use them. Clinics offering physical and occupational therapy services should have an AED on site at all times.[188]

Performing an assessment of falls for individuals with cardiac disease, especially for anyone with a personal or family history of arrhythmias, is highly recommended. Screening for syncope, assessing balance and fall risk, and falling prevention programs are important components of a therapist's evaluation. Evaluations of specific assessment and screening tests are available.[46,69,210,238]

Exercise and Arrhythmias

Exercise often increases arrhythmias because of the increase in activity of the sympathetic nervous system and the increase in circulating catecholamines. Exercise may induce cardiac arrhythmias under several specific conditions, including diuretic and digitalis therapy, or following recent ingestion of caffeine. Exercise-induced arrhythmias are generated by enhanced sympathetic tone, increased myocardial oxygen demand, or both. The therapist can be involved in preparticipation screening of all athletes for conditions that put them at risk for sudden cardiac death (see Special Implications for the Therapist: Cardiomyopathy, 11-10). At times, the arrhythmias may disappear with exercise and increased perfusion. Exercise recommendations for athletes with selected arrhythmias are available.[61]

Medications that are effective in controlling arrhythmias at rest may not be effective during exertion or stress. In addition, side effects of antiarrhythmic agents may be more apparent during exercise. For example, decreases in either exercise performance or blood pressure during exercise may occur. Because of their effects on the electrophysiologic characteristics of cardiac cells, these medications have the potential to cause abnormal rhythms. The effect of slowing the impulse through the myocardium may manifest itself during exercise as a partial or complete heart block.

Individuals with known arrhythmias and clients who are taking antiarrhythmic medications may need to be evaluated under conditions of graded exercise to ensure that the arrhythmia remains under control during activity. Monitoring heart rate and blood pressure during activity and palpation of peripheral pulses are essential in the absence of ECG. Continued monitoring and observation during the recovery period are also important because arrhythmias often occur during recovery rather than during peak exercise. If the exercise is stopped abruptly and the individual remains upright, pooling of blood in the lower body occurs. The decreased venous return and subsequent decreased blood flow to the heart may facilitate an irregular rhythm. By continuing to exercise at a low intensity during recovery, a sudden decrease in venous return is avoided.

For the client who is wearing or has worn a cardiac monitor (Holter, event, loop), the therapist must obtain the interpretation of the results to determine if modifications are needed in the person's activities. Anyone with life-threatening arrhythmias should not begin physical therapy activity until intervention for the arrhythmia is initiated and the condition is stabilized. Increasing frequency of arrhythmias developing with activity must be evaluated by the physician.[108]

Pacemaker

For the client wearing a pacemaker, the first weeks after surgery may be characterized by fatigue, during which time activity restrictions apply. Most people can drive, but strenuous activities using the arms (e.g., housework, golf, tennis, lifting more than 10 lb) are contraindicated. Once the incision is fully healed and the pacemaker is stable, scar mobilization is permissible. The usual precautions for scar mobilization apply, including mobilizing the tissue in the direction of the scar before using any cross-transverse techniques and mobilizing toward the scar rather than away from the scar to avoid overstretching the healing tissue.

Problems with pacemakers are uncommon, but any unusual deviation from the set heartbeat expected or the development of unusual symptoms, such as dyspnea, dizziness or lightheadedness, and syncope or near syncope, must be reported immediately to the physician. It is important that the therapist understand the underlying problem as well as the type of pacemaker the client is using before monitoring the client's response to an exercise program. More detailed information regarding types of pacemakers and pacemaker implantation is available[109]; see also information from pacemaker manufacturer. It should be noted that MRIs and prolonged exposure to electromagnetic waves are contraindicated in anyone who is pacemaker-dependent. Most exposures to electromagnetic interference are transient and pose no threat to people with pacemakers and implantable cardioverter-defibrillators. Concerns that cellular telephone radiation is linked to pacemaker or implantable cardioverter-defibrillator disruption have not been substantiated or proven clinically important (see the section on Physical Agents in Chapter 3).

Heart rate is limited to the programmed level, and individuals with fixed-rate ventricular synchronous devices require monitoring by blood pressure and perceived exertion scales, with close attention to symptoms of cerebral ischemia. Newer, improved pacemakers produce the cardiac output needed for exercise, making it possible for individuals with pacemakers to be physically active at work and during recreation. Exercise may be limited only by the underlying heart disease and left ventricular function. If the pacemaker recipient has undergone exercise testing safely, aerobic conditioning and endurance training can be initiated, although precaution is still advised regarding vigorous upper-body activities.

In some individuals who have suffered cardiac arrest and now have a pacemaker (or other implantable device), the re-

Continued

sponse to surviving cardiac arrest has been compared to post-traumatic stress disorder (PTSD; see discussion in Chapter 2) that can occur after a person experiences a traumatic event that is outside the realm of usual human experience. Depression, anxiety, difficulty concentrating, negative health beliefs, and increased somatic complaints may be present with or without persistent emotional disability and maladaptation to the event. The therapist should refer anyone suspected of having persistent depression or anxiety to the physician or mental health professional. ■

DISEASES AFFECTING THE HEART VALVES

Heart problems that occur secondary to impairment of valves may be caused by infection such as endocarditis, congenital deformity, or disease (e.g., rheumatic fever, coronary thrombosis). Three types of valve deformities may affect aortic, mitral, tricuspid, or pulmonic valves (Fig. 11-19): stenosis, insufficiency, or prolapse (see also the section on Congenital Heart Disease).

Stenosis is a narrowing or constriction that prevents the valve from opening fully and may be caused by scars or abnormal deposits on the leaflets. Valvular stenosis causes obstruction to blood flow, and the chamber behind the narrow valve must produce extra work to sustain cardiac output. *Insufficiency* (also referred to as *regurgitation*) occurs when the valve does not close properly and causes blood to flow back into the heart chamber. The heart gradually dilates in re-

sponse to the increased volume of work; severe degrees of incompetence are possible in the absence of symptoms. *Prolapse* affects only the mitral valve and occurs when enlarged leaflets bulge backward into the left atrium.

Valve conditions increase the workload of the heart and require the heart to pump harder to force blood through a stenosed valve or to maintain adequate flow if blood is seeping back. Initially the cardiovascular system compensates for the overload and the person remains asymptomatic, but eventually as stenosis or insufficiency progresses, cardiac muscle dysfunction and accompanying symptoms of heart failure (breathlessness, dyspnea) develop. Over the past 15 years, advances in surgical techniques and a better understanding of timing for surgical intervention have brought tremendous improvement in the clinical outcome of people with valvular heart disease, extending survival rates with less overall morbidity.[41]

The presence of CAD in clients with either mitral or aortic valve disease is a negative prognostic indicator; ischemic mitral regurgitation carries the worst prognosis with higher operative mortality and lower long-term survival compared with nonischemic cases.[41] Heart transplantation may be necessary when the risk of surgery is prohibitively high in some cases of valvular disease. Continued advances in noninvasive assessment (e.g., real-time 3D echocardiography) and noninvasive treatment (e.g., gene therapy, valves grown from blood vessel cells, and even valve self-repair with tissue engineering techniques) should improve the outlook for anyone with valvular heart disease in the years to come.

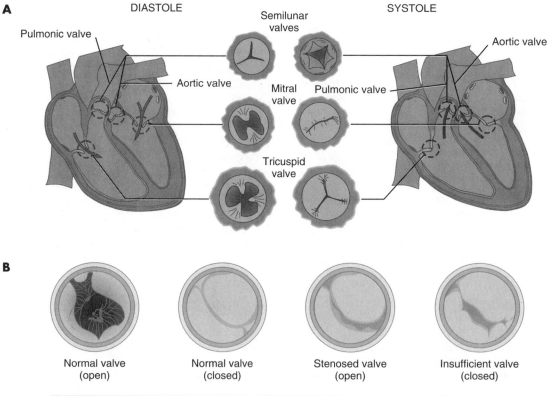

FIGURE **11-19** Valves of the heart. **A,** The pulmonic, aortic, mitral, and tricuspid valves are shown here as they appear during diastole (ventricular filling) and systole (ventricular contraction). **B,** Normal position of the valve leaflets, or cusps, when the valve is open and closed; fully open position of a stenosed valve; closed regurgitant valve showing abnormal opening for blood to flow back into.

◆ Mitral Stenosis

Etiologic Factors and Pathogenesis.   Mitral stenosis is a sequela of rheumatic heart disease that primarily affects women. Often a history of rheumatic fever is absent. Because the mitral valve is thickened, it opens in early diastole with a snap that is audible on auscultation and then closes slowly with a resultant murmur. The anterior and posterior leaflets are fixed like a funnel with an opening in the center, and they move together, rather than in opposite directions. When the valve has narrowed sufficiently, left atrial pressure rises to maintain normal flow across the valve and to maintain a normal cardiac output. This results in a pressure difference between the left atrium and the left ventricle during diastole.

Clinical Manifestations.   In mild cases, left atrial pressure and cardiac output remain normal, and the person is asymptomatic, perhaps until pregnancy or the development of atrial fibrillation, when dyspnea and orthopnea develop. In moderate stenosis, dyspnea and fatigue appear as the left atrial pressure rises and mechanical obstruction of filling of the left ventricle reduces cardiac output. With severe stenosis, left atrial pressure is high enough to produce pulmonary venous congestion at rest and reduce cardiac output with resulting dyspnea, fatigue, and right ventricular failure. Lying down at night further increases the pulmonary blood volume, causing orthopnea and paroxysmal nocturnal dyspnea.

Medical Management

Diagnosis, Treatment, and Prognosis.   Echocardiography is the most valuable technique for assessing mitral valve stenosis and providing information about the condition of the valve and left atrial size. Doppler techniques (measuring blood flow using ultrasound) can be used to determine the severity of the problem.

Because mitral stenosis may be asymptomatic, intervention is delayed until symptoms develop. Mitral stenosis may be present for a lifetime, with few or no symptoms, or it may become severe in a few years. The onset of atrial fibrillation accompanied by more severe symptoms may be treated pharmacologically (digoxin, antiarrhythmic agents, anticoagulants). Surgery may be indicated in the presence of uncontrollable pulmonary edema, severe dyspnea limiting function, pulmonary hypertension, arrhythmia, or systemic emboli uncontrolled by anticoagulation treatment. Surgical procedures include valve repair (commissurotomy to break apart the adherent leaves), replacement with an artificial valve, or balloon valvotomy. In many cases, balloon valvotomy provides excellent mechanical relief with prolonged benefit, unlike the poor results in aortic stenosis.[41] Operative mortality rates are low; problems associated with prosthetic valves may occur because of thrombosis, leaking, endocarditis, or degenerative changes in tissue valves.

◆ Mitral Regurgitation

Etiologic Factors and Pathogenesis.   Mitral regurgitation has many possible causes, but involvement of the mitral valve accounts for approximately one half of all cases. Other secondary causes include infective endocarditis (valve perforation), dilated cardiomyopathy, rheumatic disease, collagen vascular disease, rupture of the chordae tendineae, and, rarely, cardiac tumors. It is independently associated with female gender, lower body mass index, and older age. Evidence suggesting that mitral regurgitation may be induced by appetite suppressant medications has resulted in new research investigating the relationship of mitral regurgitation to obesity.[123]

During left ventricular systole, the mitral leaflets do not close normally, and blood is ejected into the left atrium as well as through the aortic valve. In acute regurgitation, left atrial pressure rises abruptly, possibly leading to pulmonary edema. When regurgitation is a chronic condition, the left atrium enlarges progressively; the degree of enlargement usually reflects the severity of regurgitation.

Clinical Manifestations.   Unfortunately, people with mitral regurgitation lack early warning signs and may remain asymptomatic until severe and often irreversible left ventricular dysfunction occurs. For many years the left ventricular end-diastolic pressure and the cardiac output may be normal at rest, even with considerable increase in left ventricular volume. Eventually, left ventricular overload may lead to left ventricular failure. People with mitral regurgitation experience exertional dyspnea (because of increased left atrial pressure) and exercise-induced fatigue (because of reduced cardiac output). Atrial fibrillation may also develop.

Medical Management

Diagnosis, Treatment, and Prognosis.   The diagnosis is primarily clinical (auscultation), but it can be confirmed and quantified by color Doppler echocardiography. Other testing procedures may include cardiac catheterization to assess the regurgitation, left ventricular function, and pulmonary artery pressure; coronary arteriography to determine the cause of the lesion and for preoperative evaluation; and nuclear medicine techniques to measure left ventricular function and estimate the severity of regurgitation.

Persons with chronic lesions who are asymptomatic require careful monitoring for left ventricular function and may require surgery even if no symptoms are present. Unlike stenosis, regurgitant lesions may progress insidiously, causing left ventricular damage before symptoms have developed. Surgical intervention may be recommended if left ventricular function is impaired or when activity becomes severely limited. Mitral valve repair has a lower operative mortality and a better late outcome than mitral valve replacement. Acute mitral regurgitation secondary to MI often requires emergency surgery, but the surgical risk is high and the outcome poor. Acute non–MI-related mitral regurgitation has a much better prognosis with postoperative survival after well-timed mitral valve repair. Indicators of poorer prognosis include mitral valve replacement, age more than 75 years, and the presence of CAD.[41]

◆ Mitral Valve Prolapse

Incidence and Etiologic Factors.   Mitral valve prolapse (MVP) has been described as a common disease with frequent complications. However, according to new data from the Framingham Heart Study, MVP is not as prevalent as previously reported (2.4% compared to previously reported 10% or higher) and affects men and women equally.[77] MVP is characterized by a slight variation in the shape or structure of the mitral (left atrioventricular) valve. This structural variation has many other names, including floppy valve syndrome, Barlow's syndrome,* myxomatous mitral valve syndrome, and click-murmur syndrome.

The cause remains unknown, although there may be a genetic component involving the angiotensin receptor gene resulting in autonomic or neuroendocrine dysfunction.[224] Results of family studies of people with mitral valve prolapse favor an autosomal dominant pattern of transmission for primary mitral valve prolapse with nearly 100% gene expression by females.[63] This condition usually occurs in isolation; however, it can be associated with a number of other conditions, such as Marfan's syndrome, rheumatic fever, endocarditis, myocarditis, atherosclerosis, SLE, muscular dystrophy, acromegaly, adult polycystic kidney disease, and cardiac sarcoidosis.

Pathogenesis. Mitral valve prolapse is a pathologic, anatomic, and physiologic abnormality of the mitral valve apparatus affecting mitral valve leaflet motion. Normally, when the lower part of the heart contracts, the mitral valve remains firm and prevents blood from leaking back into the upper chambers. In mitral valve prolapse, the slight variation in shape of the mitral valve allows one part of the valve, the leaflet, to billow back into the left atrium during contraction of the ventricle. One or both of the valve leaflets may bulge into the left atrium during ventricular systole. Usually the amount of blood that leaks back into the left atrium is not significant, but in a small number of people, it develops into mitral regurgitation. MVP is the most common cause of isolated mitral regurgitation.

The presence of symptoms linked to neuroendocrine dysfunctions or to the autonomic nervous system has led to the recognition of a pathologic condition known as *mitral valve prolapse syndrome (MVPS)*. Usually diagnosed by chance in asymptomatic individuals during routine tests, MVPS (prolapse with or without mitral regurgitation) has a high clinical incidence of neuropsychiatric symptoms (e.g., anxiety disorder, panic attacks, depression), as well as symptoms of autonomic dysfunction (e.g., postural hypotension, palpitations, cold hands and feet, shortness of breath, chest pain). As the autonomic nervous system is being formed in utero, the mitral valve is also being formed. If there is a slight variation in the structure of the heart valve, there is also a slight variation in the function or balance of the autonomic nervous system. The importance of recognizing that MVP may occur as an isolated disorder or with other coincident findings has led to the use of both terms.

Clinical Manifestations. More than 50% of all people with MVP are asymptomatic, another 40% experience occasional symptoms that are mildly to moderately uncomfortable, and only 1% suffer severe symptoms and lifestyle restrictions. Although the malformation occurs during gestation, it usually remains unnoticed until young adulthood. The person usually becomes aware of symptoms suddenly, and there does not appear to be any correlation between the severity of symptoms and the severity of the prolapse.

The most common triad of symptoms associated with MVP is profound fatigue that cannot be correlated with exercise or stress, palpitations, and dyspnea. Fatigue may not be related to exertion, but deconditioning from prolonged inactivity may

develop, further complicating the picture. The therapist is more likely to see the individual with MVP associated with connective tissue disorders or the MVPS with autonomic dysfunction. Frequently occurring musculoskeletal findings in clients with MVPS include joint hypermobility, temporomandibular joint (TMJ) syndrome, pectus excavatum, mild scoliosis, straight thoracic spine, and myalgias. The increased joint mobility that has been identified in a small proportion of persons with MVP does not appear to lead to either severe arthritis or frequent joint dislocations.[64]

Other symptoms associated with MVPS may include tremors, swelling of the extremities, sleep disturbances, low back pain, irritable bowel syndrome, excessive perspiration or inability to perspire, rashes, muscular fasciculations, visual changes or disturbances, difficulty in concentrating, memory lapses, and dizziness. Chest pain or discomfort may occur as a result of autonomic nervous system dysfunction (dysautonomia). The autonomic nervous system imbalance results in inadequate relaxation between respirations and eventually causes the chest wall muscles to go into spasm. The chest pain is sharp, lasts several seconds, and is usually felt to the left of the sternum. It is intermittent pain that may occur frequently for a few weeks and then disappear completely, only to return again some weeks later.

Medical Management
Diagnosis, Treatment, and Prognosis. MVP is often discovered during routine cardiac auscultation or when echocardiography is performed for another reason. It is characterized by a symptomatic clinical presentation and clicking noise on auscultation in late systole, with or without sounds of valvular leak (murmur). The mitral valve begins to prolapse when the reduction of left ventricular volume during systole reaches a critical point at which the valve leaflets no longer coapt (edges approximate together); at that instant, the click occurs and the murmur begins. Complete diagnostic (major and minor) criteria have been outlined elsewhere.[28] Echocardiography may be used to confirm the diagnosis, and ECG, event, or Holter monitoring (see Fig. 11-18) to show arrhythmias may be used.

Management includes reassurance; beta-blockers to control arrhythmias; an exercise program to improve overall cardiovascular function; counseling to eliminate caffeine, alcohol, and cigarette use; and administration of prophylactic antibiotics before any invasive procedure (including dental work, sigmoidoscopy) as prophylaxis against endocarditis. Rarely, surgical replacement of the valve may be recommended when severe structural problems are present that contribute to reduced activity or deterioration of left ventricular function from progression of MVP to mitral regurgitation.

MVP or MVPS is a benign condition in the vast majority of people. It is not life-threatening, and only rarely does it result in complications or significantly alter a person's lifestyle. Progressive mitral regurgitation with gradual increase in left atrial and left ventricular size, atrial fibrillation, pulmonary hypertension, and the development of congestive heart failure occurs in 10% to 15% of people with both murmurs and clicks. Men older than 50 years are most often affected.[28] According to new data available, people with MVP or MVPS are not at greater risk for heart failure, other forms of heart disease, or early death from stroke as was once thought.[77]

---

*Barlow's syndrome is a controversial clinical syndrome that may have as its only manifestation mitral valve prolapse without regurgitation.

◆ Aortic Stenosis

Etiologic Factors and Pathogenesis. Aortic stenosis is a disease of aging that is likely to become more prevalent as the proportion of older people in our population increases. It is most commonly caused by progressive valvular calcification either superimposed on a congenitally bicuspid valve or, in the older adult, involving a previously normal valve following rheumatic fever. Other risk factors for aortic stenosis are the same as those for heart disease and include obesity, a sedentary lifestyle, smoking, and high cholesterol. Factors affecting the progression of the disease remain uncertain. Over 80% of affected persons are men, and when women are affected, differences are noted (e.g., women with aortic stenosis have thicker ventricular walls reducing wall stress and higher ejection fractions)* that require different postoperative management (e.g., low cardiac output requiring volume expansion rather than the use of pressor agents).[41] Preschool and school-aged children are more likely to have a bicuspid valve; teenagers and young adults present with three leaflets, but these are partially fused.

Although the deformed valve is not stenotic at birth, it is subjected to abnormal hemodynamic stress, which may lead to thickening and calcification of the leaflets with reduced mobility. The orifice of the aortic valve narrows, causing increased resistance to blood flow from the left ventricle into the aorta. Outflow obstruction increases pressure within the left ventricle as it tries to eject blood through the narrow opening, causing decreased cardiac output, left ventricular hypertrophy, and pulmonary vascular congestion.

Clinical Manifestations. In adults, aortic stenosis is usually asymptomatic until the sixth (or later) decade. Characteristic sounds on auscultation may be heard, but cardiac output is maintained until the stenosis is severe and left ventricular failure, angina pectoris, or exertional syncope develops. The origin of exertional syncope in aortic stenosis remains controversial, perhaps caused by an exercise-induced decrease in total peripheral resistance, which is uncompensated because cardiac output is restricted by the stenotic valve. The most common sign of aortic stenosis is a systolic ejection murmur radiating to the neck (usually heard best in the aortic area). Sudden death may occur, even in previously asymptomatic individuals.

Medical Management

Diagnosis, Treatment, and Prognosis. The clinical assessment of aortic stenosis can be difficult, especially in the older person. Echo-Doppler (echocardiography with Doppler ultrasonography) is diagnostic in most cases. ECG may show left ventricular hypertrophy, and x-ray or fluoroscopy may show a calcified aortic valve. Coronary angiography may be necessary in older adults at risk for coronary disease before valve replacement.

Pharmacologic therapy has limited use in this condition. Surgical intervention is usually required for the symptomatic person and should be strongly considered for the asymptomatic person because of the risk of sudden death. Surgical procedures may include valve replacement with a mechanical prosthesis or bioprosthesis (made with biologic material) or using the pulmonary valve in place of the aortic valve and re-

placing the pulmonary valve with a homograft (Ross procedure). This latter procedure avoids a lifetime of anticoagulation therapy and the need for further surgery that occurs when a mechanical valve wears out. A less invasive alternative to aortic valve replacement, balloon valvuloplasty (splitting the stenotic valve with a balloon-tipped catheter that is introduced into the valve and inflated) has been used in treatment for aortic stenosis. Limited long-term success with less reliable and less durable outcomes has resulted in this procedure being considered palliative rather than curative. It may be useful in alleviating symptoms in people who are not candidates for aortic valve replacement because of other medical problems.

Adults with aortic stenosis who are asymptomatic have a normal life expectancy; they should receive prophylactic antibiotics against infective endocarditis. Once symptoms appear, the prognosis is poor without surgery but excellent with valve replacement even in the older adult, especially in the absence of coexisting illnesses.[41] The onset of angina, exercise-induced syncope, or cardiac failure represents a poor prognostic outcome resulting in death. Mortality rises to 10% after age 80 years. Bioprostheses may develop degenerative changes, requiring replacement in 2 to 20 years. This is quite variable and depends on the person's age at the time of implantation.

◆ Aortic Regurgitation (Insufficiency)

Etiologic Factors and Pathogenesis. In the past, aortic regurgitation occurred secondary to rheumatic fever, but antibiotics have reduced the number of rheumatic-related cases. Nonrheumatic causes account for most cases today, including congenitally bicuspid valves, infective endocarditis (valve destruction by bacteria), and hypertension. Aortic regurgitation may also occur secondary to aortic dissection with or without aortic aneurysm (see Fig. 11-24), ankylosing spondylitis, Reiter's syndrome, collagen vascular disease, syphilis, and Marfan's syndrome.

When cardiac systole ends, the aortic valve should completely prevent the flow of aortic blood back into the left ventricle. A leakage during diastole is referred to as *aortic regurgitation* or *aortic insufficiency*. When aortic regurgitation develops gradually, the left ventricle compensates by both dilation and enough hypertrophy to maintain a normal wall thickness/cavity ratio, thereby preventing development of symptoms. Eventually the left ventricle fails to stand up under the chronic overload, and symptoms develop.

Clinical Manifestations. Long-standing aortic regurgitation may remain asymptomatic even as the deformity increases, causing enlargement of the left ventricle. The large total stroke volume in aortic regurgitation produces a wide pulse pressure and systolic hypertension resulting in exertional dyspnea, fatigue, and excessive perspiration with exercise as the most frequent symptoms; paroxysmal nocturnal dyspnea and pulmonary edema may also occur. Angina pectoris or atypical chest pain may be present, but this is uncommon in the absence of CAD.

Medical Management

Diagnosis, Treatment, and Prognosis. Once aortic regurgitation is suspected on physical examination, echocardiography with Doppler examination of the aortic valve can help estimate its severity. Aortography during catheterization helps confirm the severity of the disease. Scintigraphic studies can

---

*The amount of blood the ventricle ejects is called the *ejection fraction*; the normal ejection fraction is about 60% to 75%. A decreased ejection fraction is a hallmark finding of ventricular failure.

quantify left ventricular function and functional reserve during exercise and provide a useful predictor of prognosis.

Acute aortic regurgitation may lead to left ventricular failure; surgical reconstruction or replacement of the valve (Ross procedure; see the section on Aortic Stenosis) is advisable before onset of permanent left ventricular damage (usually before ejection fraction falls below 55%), even in asymptomatic cases. Chronic regurgitation carries a poor prognosis without surgery when significant symptoms develop. Medical therapy may include vasodilators to reduce the severity of regurgitation and diuretics and digoxin to stabilize or improve symptoms.

◆ Tricuspid Stenosis and Regurgitation

Tricuspid stenosis occurs in people with severe mitral valve disease (usually rheumatic in origin) and is uncommon. Exercise testing and rehabilitation do not occur until after valve surgery. Tricuspid regurgitation may occur secondary to carcinoid syndrome, SLE, or infective endocarditis among injection drug users, and in the presence of mitral valve disease. Surgical repair is more common than valvular replacement for tricuspid valve disease.

Special Implications for the Therapist **11-13**

VALVULAR HEART DISEASE

Preferred Practice Patterns:
6B: *Impaired Aerobic Capacity/Endurance Associated With Deconditioning*
6D: *Impaired Aerobic Capacity/Endurance Associated With Cardiovascular Pump Dysfunction or Failure*

People with mild valvular malfunction have no symptoms and can usually exercise vigorously and take part in intense sports activities without adverse effects. Although exercise will not improve the mechanical function of a valve, improvement in submaximal cardiac capacity can occur. Exercise is usually stopped for the same reason as it is in healthy adults (i.e., when respiratory distress is obvious or when the person expresses a desire to stop). More than one valvular involvement is not uncommon in people with rheumatic valvular disease and in people who develop valvular regurgitation as a result of ventricular dilation. Usually symptoms and clinical course are determined by the predominant pathologic condition. When two valves are affected equally, symptoms are determined by the most proximally located valve. The combination of aortic regurgitation with mitral valve regurgitation is the most common, but the combination of mitral valve disease (either regurgitation or stenosis) with aortic stenosis is the most problematic.[206]

Exercise
Exercise testing for most people with valvular disease is of limited value. For example, there is poor correlation between the degree of mitral stenosis and the duration of symptom-limited treadmill exercise. However, exercise echocardiography performed on a stationary cycle can be a valuable means for determining left ventricular function in people during exercise.

Prescriptive exercise must be individualized based on the underlying pathologic condition, medical intervention, and condition of the person. General guidelines include exercise a minimum of 3 days per week with alternate days of rest to allow for maximum recuperation. Walking, biking, and swimming are acceptable exercise modalities, but weight training may be considered contraindicated in anyone who is symptomatic with shortness of breath or chest pain or discomfort. A perceived exertion between light and somewhat hard (rating of perceived exertion [RPE] of 11 to 14; see Table 11-13) is the goal, but the individual will usually begin with a much lighter workout and progress over time to this level.[206] Tolerance to symptoms and current exercise habits are important determinants in progressing an exercise program. Some people with valvular disease avoid physical activity as much as possible and never exercise to the point of developing any symptoms of dyspnea, fatigue, or muscular discomfort. These symptoms develop at light loads in people unaccustomed to any physical activity, regardless of the severity of the valvular disease. Other people force themselves to ignore mild (or even moderate to severe) symptoms to stay on the job or finish a task started.

Fatigue, weakness, and pallor are signs of an inadequate cardiac output for the demands of the exercise. These signs and symptoms are partly subjective, and it is a clinical decision as to how far to allow these people to continue exercising. Chest pain may indicate myocardial ischemia or pulmonary hypertension, or it may be a noncardiac symptom arising from the chest wall. Follow precautions for angina pectoris. Exercise should be stopped immediately when any signs of reduced cerebral blood flow develop, such as severe facial pallor, confusion, dizziness, heart palpitations, and unsteady gait. (See also Box 11-6 and Table 11-6.)

Pulmonary edema can be produced by exercising beyond a certain point in people with valvular disease, especially those with mitral stenosis. Pulmonary congestion induced by exercise may cause coughing rather than dyspnea, and exercise should be stopped if coughing becomes significant. Heart failure may occur secondary to chronic, progressive valvular disease. Slight puffiness of the ankles at the end of the day, nocturia, mild nocturnal dyspnea, unexpected weight gain, or more than the usual amount of fatigue can be minor symptoms that are passed over unless specifically sought. Such symptoms must be reported to the physician. (See also Special Implications for the Therapist: Congestive Heart Failure, 11-7.)

The status of the myocardium is another important variable in exercise impairment relative to valvular heart disease. Severe aortic regurgitation is well-tolerated for many years until myocardial weakness occurs. In all forms of heart disease, the healthy myocardium can compensate and maintain the systemic blood flow at or near normal levels for an extended period of time. For the client with valvular disease and myocardial disease or associated CAD, this compensation is not possible, and a lower exercise capacity results.

Stenosis
Valvular stenosis develops or progresses gradually, and because the normal valve orifice is larger than is necessary, stenosis is usually severe before exercise symptoms occur (i.e., a normal valve is larger than is needed for normal functioning and therefore has excess capacity). Stenosis only becomes symptomatic when the condition encroaches on critical cross-sectional diameter of the opening so that a doubling of the blood flow (from activity or exertion) across the valve quadruples the atrial pres-

sure. When the atrial pressure exceeds 25 mm Hg, dyspnea develops. The intensity of exertion associated with dyspnea does correlate with the magnitude of atrial pressure, providing a good indicator of the severity of stenosis. However, some people do not complain of dyspnea from lung congestion, only muscular fatigue on exertion as a result of a low cardiac output.

Stress testing may be performed before initiation of an exercise program; with or without those test results, clients should be monitored closely, possibly using the perceived exertion or dyspnea scales mentioned earlier in this chapter. Because of reduced cardiac output, muscle perfusion is reduced and lactate is produced at low workloads. Maximal heart rate may be reduced when dyspnea is the cause of premature termination of exercise. Exercise systolic blood pressure may reach only 130 mm Hg because of low output. Exercise capacity in clients with mitral stenosis can be improved by slowing heart rate and prolonging the diastolic filling period with the use of beta-blocking agents.

In the case of symptomatic aortic stenosis, clients are not candidates for exercise programs because of the danger of sudden death. Persons who are asymptomatic must be carefully screened before increasing their physical activity, and for most, exercise intensity should be mild. In people with impaired left ventricular function, cardiac output fails to increase normally with exercise, causing fatigue. Angina with exercise is a common symptom when the aortic stenosis is severe.

Regurgitation

Exercise capacity may be unaffected in cases of mild regurgitation. Mitral regurgitation increases when aortic blood pressure is increased, such as occurs during isometric contractions. Light to moderate rhythmic and repetitive exercise reduces peripheral resistance and is recommended in place of isotonic exercise, which increases the heart rate. Persons with aortic regurgitation caused by weakening of the aortic wall (Marfan's or Ehlers-Danlos syndromes) must avoid all strenuous exercise.

Prolapse

Most people with MVP can participate in all sports activities, including intense competitive sport. Exercise is a key component in the management of MVP (not to alter function of the prolapsed valve but to improve overall cardiovascular function), and although many clients are referred to an exercise physiologist, the physical therapist may also encounter requests for conditioning and exercise programs. Many times, symptoms of fatigue and dyspnea cause a person to limit physical activity, leading to deconditioning and contributing to a cycle of even more fatigue and shortness of breath.

Caution is advised in the use of weight training for the client with MVP; gradual buildup using light weights and increased repetitions is recommended. Some people with MVPS are prone to exercise-induced arrhythmias, which can (rarely) result in sudden death. Any time tachycardia develops in someone with known MVP, immediate medical referral is necessary.

Postoperative Considerations

Postoperative considerations are the same as for people who have had abdominal or cardiothoracic surgery (see the section on The Cardiac Client and Surgery in this chapter; see also Table 11-6 and Box 11-2). After uncomplicated valve ballooning, a return to normal activities is possible within 5 to 7 days. Gradual walking programs can be initiated at home for most people 10 days after surgery, or the client may enroll in a structured cardiac rehabilitation program. Cardiac rehabilitation postoperatively in people with valvular heart disease is similar to that of post-CABG clients. Care should be taken to avoid high-impact exercises or exercises with a risk of trauma in people who are receiving anticoagulation therapy to avoid hemarthrosis and bruising (see Tables 39-6 and 39-7).[206]

Exercise outcomes differ after aortic, mitral, and mitral/aortic valve surgery. The degree of improvement in exercise capacity depends on the degree of residual dysfunction, presence or absence of arrhythmia, age of the subject, and the effort made to improve exercise capacity. Functional capacity is substantially increased following aortic valve surgery but limited following mitral and mitral/aortic surgery possibly because of differences in oxygen uptake. As mentioned, for people with mitral stenosis, exercise provides an early warning system since the onset of dyspnea with strenuous exercise signals the beginning of clinical deterioration.[206] People with mechanical prosthetic valves receive lifelong anticoagulant therapy (not required for bioprostheses) and may not tolerate vigorous, weight-bearing activities. Mechanical prostheses have fixed openings that place some limitation, at least theoretically, on cardiac performance during maximal effort.[129] Because stress testing can be normal, exercise Doppler echocardiography has been used to help prescribe physical activity in clients with prosthetic valves. ■

◆ Infective Endocarditis

Infective, or bacterial, endocarditis is an infection of the endocardium, the lining inside the heart, including the heart valves, most commonly damaging the mitral valve, followed by the aortic and tricuspid valves. Bacterial endocarditis may involve normal valves but more often affects valves that have been damaged by some other previous pathologic process (e.g., rheumatic disease, congenital defects, cardiac surgery). It is categorized as either acute or subacute, depending on the clinical course, organisms, and condition of the valves. Endocarditis can occur at any age but rarely occurs in children; one half of all clients diagnosed are older than 60 years. Older adults may be at greater risk of endocarditis because valvular endocardial disruption is more common, immunity is impaired, and nutrition is poor. Endocarditis is more prevalent among men than women.

Etiologic and Risk Factors.   Endocarditis is frequently caused by bacteria (particularly streptococci or staphylococci) normally present in the mouth, respiratory system, or GI tract or as a result of abnormal growths on the closure lines of previously damaged valves (e.g., rheumatic disease).

In addition to previous valvular damage, persons with prosthetic heart valves, injection drug users, immunocompromised clients (including individuals receiving treatment for cancer), women who have had a suction abortion or pelvic infection related to intrauterine contraceptive devices, and postcardiac surgical clients are at high risk for developing endocarditis. Congenital heart disease and degenerative heart disease, such as calcific aortic stenosis, may also cause endocarditis.

Hospital-acquired infective endocarditis has become more common as a result of iatrogenic endocardial damage produced by surgery, intracardiac pressure-monitoring catheters, ventriculoatrial shunts, and hyperalimentation lines that reach the right atrium. Portals of entry for microorganisms are also provided by wounds, biopsy sites, pacemakers, IV and arterial catheters, indwelling urinary catheters, and intratracheal airways.

Pathogenesis.   As an infection, endocarditis causes inflammation of the cardiac endothelium with destruction of the connective tissue because of the action of the bacterial lytic enzymes. As these blood-borne microorganisms adhere to the endocardial surface, destruction of the connective tissue occurs as a result of the action of bacterial lytic enzymes. The surface endocardium becomes covered with fibrin and platelet thrombi that attract even more thrombogenic material. The result is the formation of wartlike growths called *vegetations*. These vegetations, consisting of fibrin and platelets, can break off from the valve, embolize, and cause septic infarction in the myocardium, kidney, brain, spleen, abdomen, or extremities. These thromboemboli contain bacteria that not only cause ischemic infarcts but also form new sites of infection transforming into microabscesses. Bacteria may further invade the valves causing intravalvular inflammation, destroying portions of the valves, and causing valve deformities.

Splinter hemorrhages of the nail beds may be caused by distal vasospasm, embolic events, or other local factors promoting engorgement and bleeding of the capillaries that lie right below the nail. The cause of digital clubbing is unclear, but perhaps platelet clumps lodge in the nail-bed capillaries of fingers and toes and release platelet-derived growth factor resulting in the pathologic changes of clubbed digits. Petechiae (small, red, nonblanching macules on the conjunctivae, palate, buccal mucosa, heels, shoulders, arms, legs, and upper chest) are thought to involve microemboli, but some have also suggested that immune complex vasculitis is the primary process.[126] Infective endocarditis of the right-side heart valves occurs commonly in injection drug users. Although a variety of hypotheses have been put forward to explain this phenomenon, no single explanation has been proven.

Clinical Manifestations.   Endocarditis can develop insidiously, with symptoms remaining undetected for months, or it can cause symptoms immediately, as in the case of acute bacterial endocarditis. Clinical manifestations can be divided into many groups (Table 11-16). It causes varying degrees of valvular dysfunction and may be associated with manifestations involving any number of organ systems, including lungs, eyes, kidneys, bones, joints, and central nervous system. The aortic valve is most frequently infected (20% to 40% of cases), with mitral valve infection present in 25% to 35% of cases and both valves infected in about 25% of cases. Neurologic signs and symptoms are predominant in about one third of all cases in those people over 60 years. The classic findings of fever, cardiac murmur, and petechial lesions of the skin, conjunctivae, and oral mucosa are not always present.

Up to 50% of people with infective endocarditis initially have musculoskeletal symptoms including arthralgia (most common), arthritis, low back pain, and myalgias. One half of these people will have only musculoskeletal symptoms without other manifestations of endocarditis. The early onset of joint pain and myalgia as the first sign of endocarditis is more likely if the person is older and has had a previously diagnosed heart murmur. Proximal joints are most often affected, especially the shoulder, followed by knee, hip, wrist, ankle, metatarsophalangeal and metacarpophalangeal joints, and acromioclavicular joints (order of declining incidence). Most often one or two joints are painful, and symptoms begin suddenly accompanied by warmth, tenderness, and redness. Symmetric arthralgia in the knees or ankles may lead to a diagnosis of rheumatoid arthritis (RA), but as a rule, morning stiffness is not as prevalent in clients with endocarditis as in those with RA or polymyalgia rheumatica. Bone and joint infections are particularly common among injection drug users. The most common sites of osteoarticular infections are the vertebrae and wrist, sternoclavicular, and sacroiliac joints, often with multiple joint involvement.[196]

Almost one third of clients with endocarditis have low back pain, which may be the primary symptom reported. Back pain is accompanied by decreased range of motion and spinal tenderness. Pain may affect only one side, and it may be limited to the paraspinal muscles. Endocarditis-induced back pain may be very similar to that associated with a herniated lumbar disk, since it radiates to the leg and may be accentuated by raising the leg or by sneezing, coughing, or laughing; however, neurologic deficits are usually absent in persons with endocarditis.

TABLE   11-16

Clinical Manifestations of Infective Endocarditis

Systemic Infection	Intravascular Involvement	Immunologic Reaction	Musculoskeletal	Neurologic
Fever	Chest pain	Arthralgia	Arthralgia	Confusion
Chills	Congestive heart failure	Proteinuria	Myalgias	Abscess
Sweats	Cold and painful extremities	Hematuria	Low-back pain	Cerebritis
Malaise	Clubbing	Acidosis		Meningitis
Weakness	Petechiae	Arthritis		Stroke (embolic or hemorrhagic)
Anorexia	Splinter hemorrhages			
Weight loss	Osler's nodes			
Cough				
Dyspnea				
Hemoptysis				

Endocarditis may produce destructive changes in the sacroiliac joint characterized by pain localized over the sacroiliac, probably as a result of seeding of the joint by septic emboli. Widespread diffuse myalgia may occur during periods of fever, but these are not appreciably different from the general myalgia seen in clients with other febrile illnesses. More commonly, myalgia is restricted to the calf or thigh. Bilateral or unilateral leg myalgias occur in approximately 10% to 15% of all persons with endocarditis.

The cause of back pain and leg myalgia associated with endocarditis has not been determined. Concurrent aseptic meningitis is a possible hypothesis; emboli that break off from the infected cardiac valves are supported by biopsy evidence of muscle necrosis or vasculitis in clients with endocarditis. Rarely, other musculoskeletal symptoms, such as osteomyelitis, tendinitis, hypertrophic osteoarthropathy, bone infarcts, and ischemic bone necrosis, may occur.

Medical Management
Diagnosis, Treatment, and Prognosis.
Infective endocarditis is often difficult to diagnose since it can present with a wide array of signs and symptoms, as well as a confusing clinical picture. Blood cultures to identify specific pathogens in the presence of septicemia are required to determine appropriate antibiotic therapy, which is the primary medical intervention. Other laboratory test results indicative of infectious endocarditis include elevated erythrocyte sedimentation rate, proteinuria, and hematuria. Echocardiography may be used to confirm the diagnosis and is useful in showing underlying valvular lesions and quantifying their severity. This test is not as useful in older adults because it is common to find echogenic areas around and on degenerative valves that are impossible to distinguish from the infective vegetations seen with infective endocarditis. Large masses on valves are much more diagnostic.

Although it is easily prevented (for the at-risk person) by taking antibiotics before and after procedures such as dental cleaning, genitourinary instrumentation, and open cardiovascular surgery, endocarditis is difficult to treat and can result in serious heart damage or death. Potential complications are many, including CHF and arterial, systemic, or pulmonary emboli. Therapy with antibiotics may be prolonged, and without complete treatment, relapse can occur up to 2 or more weeks after medical intervention. Surgical valve replacement may be necessary, depending on the response to treatment, sites of infection, recurrent infection, or infection of a prosthetic valve.

Special Implications for the Therapist   11-14

INFECTIVE ENDOCARDITIS

Preferred Practice Patterns:
6B: Impaired Aerobic Capacity/Endurance Associated With Deconditioning
6D: Impaired Aerobic Capacity/Endurance Associated With Cardiovascular Pump Dysfunction or Failure
In the presence of neurologic and/or musculoskeletal manifestations, other practice patterns may be appropriate (see Table 11-16).

Physical exertion beyond normal activities of daily living is usually limited for the person receiving antibiotic therapy for endocarditis and during the following weeks of recovery. The therapist is not likely to treat a person diagnosed during this acute phase of endocarditis. However, because early manifestations of endocarditis may be primarily peripheral (musculoskeletal or cutaneous) in nature, the therapist may be the first to recognize signs and symptoms of a systemic disorder. Splinter hemorrhages (dark red linear streaks resembling splinters under the nail bed), clubbing (see Fig. 14-4), petechiae, purplish red subcutaneous nodes on the finger and toe pads, and lesions on the thenar and hypothenar eminences of the palms, fingers, and sometimes the soles are present in up to 50% of affected individuals.[126] For any client with known risk factors or a recent history of endocarditis, the therapist must be alert for signs of endocarditis, indications of complications (easy fatigue associated with heart failure or peripheral emboli), lack of response to therapy intervention, or signs indicating relapse. Often, the client thinks the symptoms are recurrent bouts of the flu. ∎

◆ Rheumatic Fever and Heart Disease
Overview, Incidence, and Etiologic Factors.   Rheumatic fever is one form of endocarditis (infection), caused by streptococcal group A bacteria, that can be fatal or may lead to rheumatic heart disease (10% of cases), a chronic condition caused by scarring and deformity of the heart valves (Fig. 11-20). It is called rheumatic fever because two of the most common symptoms are fever and joint pain.

The infection generally starts with strep throat in children between ages 5 and 15 years and damages the heart in approximately 50% of cases. The aggressive use of specific antibiotics in the United States had effectively reduced the incidence of rheumatic fever to around 0.5 cases per 100,000 school-age children and removed it as the primary cause of valvular damage. However, between 1985 and 1987, a series of epidemics of rheumatic fever were reported in several widely diverse geographic regions of the continental United States, affecting children, young adults aged 18 to 30 years, and, occasionally, middle-aged persons. Currently, the prevalence and incidence of cases have not approximated the 1985 record, but they have remained above previous levels.

Pathogenesis.   The exact pathogenesis is unclear, but rheumatic fever produces a diffuse, proliferative, and exudative inflammatory process in the connective tissue of certain structures. The bacteria adhere to the oral and pharyngeal cells and then release its degradation products. Antigens to streptococcal cells bind to receptors on the heart, brain cells, muscles, and joints, which begins the autoimmune response; thus rheumatic fever is classified as an autoimmune disease. In the case of the heart valves, the inflammatory products cross react with cardiac proteins affecting cardiac valve tissue and myocardium. All layers of the heart (epicardium, endocardium, myocardium, pericardium) (see Fig. 11-1) may be involved, including the valves. Endocardial inflammation causes swelling of the valve leaflets, with secondary erosion along the lines of leaflet contact. Small, beadlike clumps of vegetation containing platelets and fibrin are deposited on eroded valvular

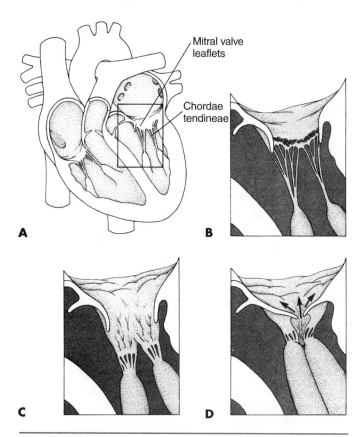

A

B

C

D

FIGURE **11-20** Cardiac valvular disease caused by rheumatic fever. **A,** Inflammation of the membrane over the mitral (and aortic) valves may cause edema and accumulation of fibrin and platelets on the chordae tendineae. **B,** This accumulation of inflammatory materials produces rheumatic vegetations that affect the support provided by the chordae tendineae to the atrioventricular valves. **C,** In this view, the mitral valve leaflets have become thickened with scar tissue and calcified. The chordae tendineae often fuse. **D,** As a result, the scarred valve fails to close tightly (mitral stenosis) and regurgitation or back-flow of blood into the atrium develops. Prolonged, severe stenosis with mitral regurgitation leads to symptoms of CHF. (Modified from Goodman CC, Snyder TE: *Differential diagnosis in physical therapy,* ed 3, Philadelphia, 2000, Saunders, p 110.)

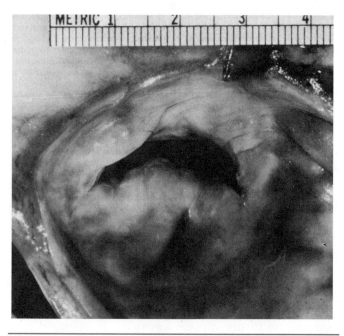

FIGURE **11-21** When viewed from the atrial aspect, a severely stenotic mitral valve has a narrowed orifice that has the appearance of a classic fish-mouth deformity. (From Kissane JM, editor: *Anderson's pathology,* St Louis, 1990, Mosby.)

tissue and on the chordae tendineae*; the mitral and aortic valves are most commonly affected. Over time, scarring and shortening of the involved structures occur, and the leaflets adhere to each other as the valves lose their elasticity. As many as 25% of clients will have mitral valvular disease 25 to 30 years later, with fibrosis and calcification of valves, fusion of commissures (union or junction between adjacent cusps of the heart valves) and chordae tendineae, and mitral stenosis with fish-mouth deformity (Fig. 11-21).

Clinical Manifestations. Although strep throat is the most common manifestation of the streptococcal virus, streptococcal infections can also affect the skin and, less com-

monly, the lungs. In some cases of strep throat the initial triggering sore throat or pharyngitis does not cause extreme illness, if any discomfort at all. However, the major manifestations of acute rheumatic fever are usually carditis, acute migratory polyarthritis, and chorea, which may occur singly or in combination. In the acute, full-blown sequelae, shortness of breath and increasing nocturnal cough also occur. A ring or crescent-shaped rash with clear centers on the skin of the limbs or trunk (erythema marginatum) is present in fewer than 2% of persons with an acute episode. Subcutaneous nodules may occur over bony prominences and along the extensor surfaces of the arms, heels, knees, or back of the head, but these do not interfere with joint function.

Carditis is most likely to occur in children and adolescents. Mitral or aortic semilunar valve dysfunction (see Pathogenesis) may result in a previously undetected murmur. Chest pain caused by pericardial inflammation and characteristic heart sounds may occur. *Polyarthritis* may develop in a child or young adult with acute rheumatic fever 2 to 3 weeks after an initial cold or sore throat. Sudden or gradual onset of painful migratory joint symptoms in knees, shoulders, feet, ankles, elbows, fingers, or neck; fever (99° to 103° F); palpitations; and fatigue are present. Malaise, weakness, weight loss, and anorexia may accompany the fever.

The migratory arthralgias usually involve two or more joints simultaneously or in succession and may last only 24 hours, or they may persist for several weeks. In adults, only a single joint may be affected. Joints that are sore and hot and contain fluid completely resolve, followed by acute synovitis, heat, synovial space tenderness, swelling, and effusion present in a different area the next day. The persistence of swelling, heat, and synovitis in a single joint or joints for more than 2 to 3 weeks is extremely unusual in acute rheumatic fever.

---

*Chordae are the tendinous cords connecting the two atrioventricular (AV) valves (the tricuspid valve between the right atrium and right ventricle and the mitral valve between the left atrium and left ventricle) to the appropriate papillary muscles in the heart ventricles; the chordae tendineae in effect anchor the valve leaflets. This support to the AV valves during ventricular systole helps prevent prolapse of the valve into the atrium.

TABLE	11-17	

Jones Criteria for Diagnosis of Rheumatic Fever (1992 Update)

MAJOR MANIFESTATIONS	MINOR MANIFESTATIONS	SUPPORTING EVIDENCE OF STREPTOCOCCAL INFECTION
Carditis	Previous rheumatic fever or rheumatic heart disease	Recent scarlet fever
Polyarthritis	Arthralgia	Positive throat culture for group A *Streptococcus*
Chorea	Fever	Other positive laboratory tests
Erythema marginatum	Elevated appearance of C-reactive protein	
Subcutaneous nodules	Leukocytosis	
	ECG changes	

From Dajani AS, Ayoub A, Burman FZ, et al: American Heart Association Medical/Scientific Statement: guidelines for the diagnosis of rheumatic fever: Jones criteria, 1992 update, *Circulation* 87:302-307, 1993.
ECG, Electrocardiogram.

Rheumatic *chorea* (also called Sydenham's chorea or St. Vitus' dance) occurs in 3% of cases 1 to 3 months after the streptococcal infection and is always preceded by polyarthritis. Chorea in a child, teenager, or young adult is almost always a manifestation of acute rheumatic fever.* The chorea develops as rapid, purposeless, nonrepetitive movements that may involve all muscles except the eyes. This pattern of movement may last for 1 week, several months, or even several years without permanent impairment of the central nervous system.

Medical Management
Diagnosis and Treatment. Late diagnosis can have serious consequences requiring immediate antibiotic and antiinflammatory treatment. Jones criteria are used as the basis for diagnosis (Table 11-17), and throat culture for group A streptococci is usually positive. Echocardiography combined with Doppler technology provides reliable hemodynamic and anatomic data in the assessment of rheumatic heart disease.

Aspirin may be used to treat the joint manifestations and as a general antiinflammatory agent. Corticosteroids are used when there is clear evidence of rheumatic carditis. Children with acute chorea are generally treated with some form of CNS depressant, such as phenobarbital. Commissurotomy and prosthetic valve replacement may be necessary for valvular dysfunction associated with chronic rheumatic disease.

Prognosis. Initial episodes of rheumatic fever last weeks to months, but 20% of children affected have recurrences within 5 years; relapses increase the risk of heart damage that leads to rheumatic heart disease, with mitral or aortic stenosis or insufficiency caused by progressive valve scarring. Mortality for acute rheumatic fever is low (1% to 2%), but persistent rheumatic activity with complications (enlarged heart, atrial fibrillation, arterial embolism, heart failure, pericarditis) is associated with long-term morbidity and mortality.

---

*Other causes of chorea are SLE, thyrotoxicosis, and cerebrovascular accident, but these are uncommon and unlikely in a child.

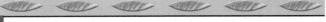

Special Implications for the Therapist   11-15

RHEUMATIC FEVER AND HEART DISEASE

Preferred Practice Patterns:
6B: Impaired Aerobic Capacity/Endurance Associated With Deconditioning
6D: Impaired Aerobic Capacity/Endurance Associated With Cardiovascular Pump Dysfunction or Failure
Other practice patterns may apply in the presence of polyarthritis or chorea.

The increased incidence of streptococcal group A bacteria in the adult population may result in cases of sudden or gradual onset of painful migratory joint symptoms affecting the knees, shoulders, feet, ankles, elbows, fingers, or neck. Anytime an adult presents with intermittent or migratory joint symptoms, the client's temperature must be taken. The therapist should ask about recent exposure to someone with strep throat, the recent history or presence of rash anywhere on the body, sore throat, or cold. The sore throat or cold symptoms may be mild enough that the person does not seek medical care of any kind. The presence of fever accompanied by a clinical presentation of migratory arthralgias or a positive history of recent illness described requires medical evaluation.

The risk of developing acute rheumatic fever following untreated tonsillopharyngitis is only 1% in the pediatric population, but as many as 25% of people affected by rheumatic fever develop mitral valve dysfunction 25 to 30 years later. Adults who experience exercise intolerance or exertional dyspnea of unknown cause and who have a previous history of childhood rheumatic fever may be experiencing the effects of mitral valve prolapse. Dyspnea associated with mitral valve prolapse is most commonly accompanied by fatigue and palpitations. This history in combination with this triad of symptoms requires evaluation by a physician.

In the case of a confirmed diagnosis of rheumatic fever–related mitral valve involvement, exercise will not improve the mechanical function of the valve, but improvement in cardiovascular function can occur. (See Special Implications for the Therapist: Valvular Heart Disease.) ∎

DISEASES AFFECTING THE PERICARDIUM

The pericardium consists of two layers: the inner visceral layer, which is attached to the epicardium; and an outer parietal layer (see Fig. 11-1). The pericardium stabilizes the heart in its anatomic position despite changes in body position and reduces excess friction between the heart and surrounding structures. It is composed of fibrous tissue that is loose enough to permit moderate changes in cardiac size but that cannot stretch fast enough to accommodate rapid dilation or accumulation of fluid without increasing intracardiac pressure.

The pericardium may be a primary site of disease and is often involved by processes that affect the heart; it may also be affected by diseases of the adjacent tissues. Pericardial diseases are common and have multiple causes. Three conditions primarily affect the pericardium: acute pericarditis, constrictive pericarditis, and pericardial effusion. These three diseases are grouped together for ease of understanding in the following section.

◆ Pericarditis

Definition and Overview.   Pericarditis or inflammation of the pericardium, the double-layer membrane surrounding the heart, may be a primary condition or may be secondary to a number of diseases and circumstances (Box 11-9). It may occur as a single acute event, or it may recur and become a chronic condition called *constrictive pericarditis* (uncommon).

BOX 11-9

Causes of Pericarditis

Idiopathic (85%)
Infections
  Viral (Coxsackie, influenza, Epstein-Barr, hepatitis, human immunodeficiency virus [HIV])
  Bacterial (tuberculosis, *Staphylococcus*, *Streptococcus*, *Meningococcus*, pneumonia)
  Parasitic
  Fungal
Myocardial injury
  Myocardial infarction (MI)
  Cardiac trauma: instrumentation; blunt or penetrating pericardium; rib fracture
  Post cardiac surgery
Hypersensitivity
  Collagen diseases: rheumatic fever, scleroderma, systemic lupus erythematosus (SLE), rheumatoid arthritis
  Drug reaction
  Radiation or cobalt therapy
Metabolic disorders
  Uremia
  Myxedema
Chronic anemia
Neoplasm
  Lymphoma, leukemia, lung or breast cancer
Aortic dissection
Graft-versus-host disease

Incidence and Etiologic Factors.   The most common types of pericarditis encountered by the therapist will be drug-induced or those present in association with autoimmune diseases (e.g., connective tissue disorders such as SLE, rheumatoid arthritis), postmyocardial infarction, with renal failure, after open-heart surgery, and after radiation therapy. Other types encountered less often include viral pericarditis (e.g., Epstein-Barr, hepatitis, human immunodeficiency virus [HIV]) and neoplastic pericarditis (from spread to the pericardium of adjacent lung cancer or invasion by breast cancer, leukemia, Hodgkin's disease, or lymphoma). Isolated cases of constrictive pericarditis as a manifestation of chronic graft-versus-host diseases after peripheral stem cell transplantation have been reported.[211]

Pathogenesis.   Many causes of pericarditis affect both the pericardium and the myocardium (myopericarditis) with varying degrees of cardiac dysfunction. Constrictive pericarditis is characterized by a fibrotic, thickened, and adherent pericardium that is compressing the heart. The heart becomes restricted in movement and function (cardiac tamponade). Diastolic filling of the heart is reduced, venous pressures are elevated, cardiac output is decreased, and eventual cardiac failure may result.

When fluid accumulates within the pericardial sac it is referred to as *pericardial effusion*. Blunt chest trauma or any cause of acute pericarditis can lead to pericardial effusion. Rapid distention or excessive fluid accumulation from this condition can also compress the heart and reduce ventricular filling and cardiac output.

Clinical Manifestations.   The presentation and course of pericarditis are determined by the underlying etiology. For example, pericarditis may occur 2 to 5 days after infarction as a result of an inflammatory reaction to myocardial necrosis, or it may occur within the first year after radiation initiates a fibrinous and fibrotic process in the pericardium. Often there is pleuritic chest pain that is made worse by lying down and by respiratory movements and is relieved by sitting upright or leaning forward. The pain is substernal and may radiate to the neck, shoulders, upper back, upper trapezius, left supraclavicular area, epigastrium, or down the left arm. Other symptoms may include fever, joint pain, dyspnea, or difficulty swallowing. Auscultation of the lower left sternal border where the pericardium lies close to the chest wall will produce a pericardial friction rub, a high-pitched scratch sound that may be heard at end-expiration. This sound is produced by the friction between the pericardial surfaces that results from inflammation and occurs during heart movement. Symptoms of constrictive pericarditis develop slowly and usually include progressive dyspnea, fatigue, weakness, peripheral edema, and ascites. Constrictive disease can lead to diastolic dysfunction and eventual heart failure.

Medical Management

Diagnosis.   Clinical examination, including clinical presentation, auscultation, and client history, may be diagnostic. A classic sign of pericarditis is the pericardial friction rub heard on auscultation. Other diagnostic tools include chest x-ray (showing enlarged cardiac shadow), characteristic ECG changes (showing evidence of an underlying inflammatory process), and laboratory studies (e.g., elevated sedimentation rate or elevated white blood count [nonspecific indicators of inflammation] and elevated cardiac enzymes [post MI]). Computed tomography (CT), magnetic resonance imaging (MRI), and echocardiography are modalities used for imaging the pericardium and pericardial disease.

Treatment.   New treatments for pericardial diseases are being developed as a result of modern imaging, new understanding of molecular biology, and immunology techniques. Comprehensive and systematic implementation of new techniques of pericardiocentesis, pericardial fluid analysis, pericardioscopy, epicardial and pericardial biopsy, as well as the application of new techniques for pericardial fluid and biopsy analyses have permitted early specific diagnosis, creating foundations for etiologic intervention in many cases. In cases of recurrent pericarditis resistant to conventional intervention and in the case of neoplastic pericarditis, intrapericardial application of medication has been proposed.[148]

Conventional treatment remains twofold, directed toward prevention of long-term complications and the underlying cause. For example, while treating the underlying infection (antibiotics for bacterial pericarditis), symptomatic treatment is provided for idiopathic, viral, or radiation pericarditis; antiinflammatory drugs are given for severe, acute pericarditis or pericarditis associated with connective tissue disorders; chemotherapy is given for neoplastic pericarditis; or dialysis is performed for uremic pericarditis. Analgesics may be prescribed for the pain and fever. Pericardiocentesis (surgical drainage with a needle catheter through a small subxiphoid incision) may be performed if cardiac compression from pericardial effusion does not resolve.

Treatment for constrictive pericarditis is both medical and surgical, including digitalis preparations, diuretics, sodium restriction, and pericardiectomy (surgical excision of the damaged pericardium).

Prognosis.   The prognosis in most cases of acute viral pericarditis is excellent when there is no (or only minimal) myocardial involvement, since this is frequently a self-limited disease. Without medical intervention, shock and death can occur from decreased cardiac output with cardiac involvement. Constrictive pericarditis is a progressive disease without spontaneous reversal of symptoms. Most people become progressively disabled over time. Surgical removal of the pericardium is associated with a high mortality rate when progressive calcification in the epicardium and dense adhesions or fibrosis between the pericardial layers are present.

Special Implications for the Therapist   **11-16**

PERICARDITIS

Preferred Practice Pattern:
6D: Impaired Aerobic Capacity/Endurance Associated With Cardiovascular Pump Dysfunction or Failure

Pericardial pain can masquerade as a musculoskeletal problem, presenting as just upper back, neck, or upper trapezius pain. In such cases, the pain may be diminished by holding the breath or aggravated by swallowing or neck or trunk movements, especially side bending or rotation. Pain is also aggravated by respiratory movements, such as deep breathing, coughing, and laughing. The therapist must screen for medical disease by assessing aggravating and relieving factors and by asking the client about a history of fever, chills, upper respiratory tract infection (recent cold or flu), weakness, heart disease, or recent MI (heart attack).

Special precautions depend on the underlying cause of the pericarditis. Mild cases require intervention per client tolerance, and the therapist observes for any symptoms of CHF. A mild pericarditis can quickly progress to a severe condition that requires medical evaluation. The clinician is referred to each individual section in this text representing the etiology of pericarditis for precautions. ■

DISEASES AFFECTING THE BLOOD VESSELS

Diseases of blood vessels observed in a therapy setting can include intestinal infarction, aneurysm, peripheral vascular disease (PVD), vascular neoplasm, and vascular malformation; only intestinal infarction will not be discussed here.

◆ Aneurysm

Definition and Overview.   An aneurysm is an abnormal stretching (dilation) in the wall of an artery, a vein, or the heart with a diameter that is at least 50% greater than normal. When the vessel wall becomes weakened from trauma, congenital vascular disease, infection, or atherosclerosis, a permanent saclike formation develops. A false aneurysm can occur when the wall of the blood vessel is ruptured and blood escapes into surrounding tissues, forming a clot (Fig. 11-22; see also Fig. 11-24).

Aneurysms are of various types (either arterial or venous) and are named according to the specific site of formation (Fig. 11-23). The most common site for an arterial aneurysm is the aorta, forming a thoracic aneurysm (which involves the ascending, transverse, or first part of the descending portion of the aorta) or an abdominal aneurysm (which generally involves the aorta between the renal arteries and iliac branches). *Thoracic aortic aneurysms* account for approximately 10% of all aortic aneurysms and occur most frequently in hypertensive men between the ages of 40 and 70 years. *Abdominal aortic aneurysms* occur about four times more often than thoracic aneurysms, and the incidence is increasing, probably because of the increasing number of adults over 65 years of age. *Peripheral arterial aneurysms* affect the femoral and popliteal arteries.

Incidence and Etiologic Factors.   Incidence increases with increasing age, usually beginning after age 50 years. Family members (parent, adult child, or sibling) of anyone with an aneurysm have a fourfold increased risk of aneurysm, and gene defects on chromosome 11 have been identified with some of the connective tissue disorders associated with aneurysm.[240] Other gene defects that cause isolated aneurysms have not been identified. Aneurysms occur much more often in men than in women, and one-half of affected persons are hypertensive.

Atherosclerosis or any injury to the middle or muscular layer of the arterial wall (tunica media) is responsible for most arterial aneurysms. Other less common causes of aneurysm in-

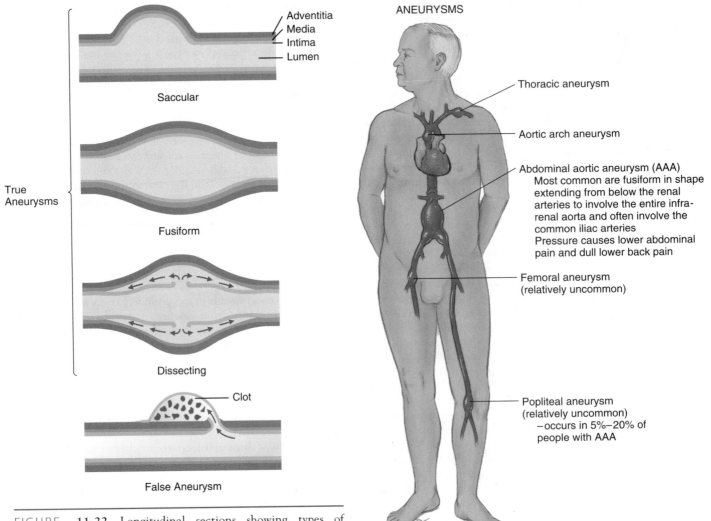

FIGURE **11-22** Longitudinal sections showing types of aneurysms. In a true aneurysm, layers of the vessel wall dilate in one of the following ways: saccular, a unilateral outpouching; fusiform, a bilateral outpouching; or dissecting, a bilateral outpouching in which layers of the vessel wall separate, with creation of a cavity. In a false aneurysm, the wall ruptures, and a blood clot is retained in an out-pouching of tissue.

FIGURE **11-23** Aneurysms are named according to the specific site of formation. Abdominal aortic aneurysms are the most common type; more than 95% of abdominal aortic aneurysms are located below the renal arteries and extend to the umbilicus, causing low back pain. (From Jarvis C: *Physical examination and health assessment*, ed 3, Philadelphia, 2000, Saunders, p 579.)

clude trauma (blunt or surgical), Marfan's disease (congenital defects of the arterial wall) and other hereditary abnormalities of connective tissue, and inflammatory diseases and infectious agents (bacterial infection, syphilis, polyarteritis). The emergence of HIV has been associated with a dramatic increase in the incidence of syphilis. Since syphilitic aortitis generally presents between 10 and 30 years after the primary infection, there may be an increased incidence of associated aneurysms in the coming years. Hypertension seems to enhance aneurysm formation.

Pathogenesis.   Plaque formation erodes the vessel wall predisposing the vessel to stretching of the inner and outer layers of the artery and formation of a sac. The stretching of the media produces infarct expansion, a weak and thin layer of necrotic muscle, and fibrous tissue that bulges with each systole. Abnormal proteolysis, the presence of elastolytic serum enzymes, and deficiencies of collagen and elastin have

been implicated as factors contributing to the development of these aneurysms.[137] With time, the aneurysm becomes more fibrotic, but it continues to bulge with each systole, thus acting as a reservoir for some of the stroke volume. In the case of thoracic aortic aneurysms, the shear force of elevated blood pressure causes a tear in the intima with rapid disruption and rupture of the aortic wall. Subsequent hemorrhage causes a lengthwise splitting of the arterial wall, creating a false vessel (Fig. 11-24), and a hematoma may form in either channel (i.e., the false or true lumen).

Clinical Manifestations.   Aneurysms may be asymptomatic; when they do occur, manifestations depend largely on the size and position of the aneurysm and its rate of growth. Substernal, back, neck, or jaw pain may occur as enlargement

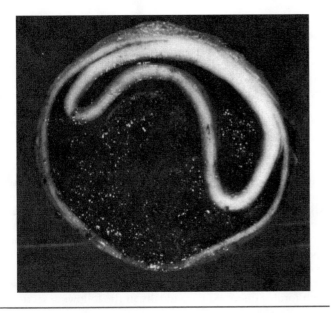

FIGURE   **11-24**   Dissecting aneurysm. Cross section of the aorta with dissecting aneurysm showing true aortic lumen (*above* and *right*) compressed by dissecting column of blood that separates the media and creates a false lumen. (From Kissane JM, editor: *Anderson's pathology*, St Louis, 1990, Mosby.)

of the aneurysm impinges adjacent structures. Dissection over the aortic arch and into the descending aorta may be experienced as extreme, sharp pain felt at the base of the neck or along the back into the interscapular areas. When pressure from a large volume of blood is placed on the trachea, esophagus, laryngeal nerve, lung, or superior vena cava, symptoms of dysphagia; hoarseness; edema of the neck, arms, or jaw and distended neck veins; and dyspnea and/or cough may occur, respectively.

Other signs and symptoms may be present in the case of *acute aortic dissection* as a result of compression of branches of the aorta. These include acute MI, reversible ischemic neurologic deficits, stroke, paraplegia, renal failure, intestinal ischemia, and ischemia of the arms and legs. Acute chest pain may also result from a nondissecting hematoma of the aorta or erosion of a penetrating atherosclerotic ulcer.[137]

In the case of an untreated *abdominal aortic aneurysm* expansion and rupture can occur in one of several places, including the peritoneal cavity, the mesentery, retroperitoneum, into the inferior vena cava, or into the duodenum or rectum. The most common site for an abdominal aortic aneurysm is just below the renal arteries, and it may involve the bifurcation of the aorta (see Fig. 11-23). Most abdominal aortic aneurysms are asymptomatic, but intermittent or constant pain in the form of mild to severe midabdominal or lower back discomfort is present in some form in 25% to 30% of cases. Groin or flank pain may be experienced because of increasing pressure on other structures. Early warning signs of an impending rupture may include abdominal heartbeat when lying down or a dull ache (intermittent or constant) in the midabdominal left flank or lower back. Rupture is most likely to occur in aneurysms that are 5 cm or larger, causing intense flank pain with referred pain to the back at the level of the rupture. Pain may radiate to the lower abdomen, groin, or genitalia. Back pain may be the only presenting symptom before rupture occurs.

The most common site for *peripheral arterial aneurysm* is the popliteal space in the lower extremities. Most are caused by atherosclerosis and occur bilaterally in men. Popliteal aneurysm presents as a pulsating mass, 2 cm or more in diameter, and causes ischemic symptoms in the lower limbs (e.g., intermittent claudication, rest pain, thrombosis and embolization resulting in gangrene). *Femoral aneurysm* presents as a pulsating mass in the femoral area on one or both sides.

Medical Management
Diagnosis.   Detection of abdominal and peripheral aneurysms often occurs when the physician palpates a pulsating mass during routine examination or when x-rays are taken for other purposes (although not all aortic aneurysms have abnormalities on chest radiography). Radiography, ultrasonography, echocardiography with color Doppler imaging, CT and MRI, arteriography, and aortography may be used for investigation.

Prevention and Treatment.   Annual examination to ensure early identification is recommended for family members (parent, adult child, or sibling) of anyone who has previously been diagnosed with an aortic aneurysm. Anyone with a family risk or signs of diseased arteries should take preventive measures, including smoking cessation, regular exercise, blood pressure control, and cholesterol management. Surgical intervention before rupture provides a good prognosis; at 5 cm, the risk of rupture exceeds the risk of repair. A new, less invasive procedure known as *endoluminal stent-graft* may offer an alternative to open abdominal surgery. Guided by angiographic imaging, a catheter is inserted through the femoral or brachial artery to the aneurysm. A balloon within the catheter is then inflated, pushing open the stent, which attaches with tiny hooks to healthy arterial wall above and below the aneurysm. This creates a channel for blood flow that bypasses the aneurysm.

Prognosis.   The standard open surgical approach to replace the diseased aorta is steadily improving but is still associated with high morbidity and substantial mortality rates. Myocardial infarction, respiratory failure, renal failure, and stroke are the principal causes of death and morbidity after surgical procedures performed on the thoracic aorta. At the same time, the endoluminal stent-graft comes with its own set of complications including fever, breakdown or migration of the device, leaks, and unknown durability. Further studies to improve treatment are needed. Aneurysm rupture is associated with a high mortality; frequently, aneurysms are discovered only at autopsy.

Special Implications for the Therapist   11-17

ANEURYSM

Preferred Practice Patterns:
  4J: Impaired Motor Function, Muscle Performance, Range of Motion, Gait, Locomotion, and Balance Associated With Amputation (peripheral aneurysm)
  5D: Impaired Motor Function and Sensory Integrity Associated With Nonprogressive Disorders of the Central Nervous System—Acquired in Adolescence or Adulthood
Continued

5I: Impaired Arousal, Range of Motion, and Motor Control Associated With Coma, Near Coma, or Vegetative State

Anyone with complications associated with an aneurysm is also at risk for pulmonary complications.

Since the prevalence of all diseases of the aorta increases with age and because the population in the United States is aging, it is expected that this condition will be encountered with increasing frequency. Knowledge of the natural history, familial history, and clinical features of this disorder may alert the therapist to the need for medical intervention. For the person who has had a surgically repaired aneurysm, activities are restricted and are only gradually reintroduced. The therapist may be involved in bedside exercises and early mobility, which are especially important to prevent thromboembolism as a result of venous stasis during prolonged bed rest and immobility.

Because of the invasiveness of open abdominal surgery, anyone undergoing this procedure is at high risk for pulmonary complications. Incisional pain and the use of abdominal musculature in coughing discourage the person from full inspirations as well as effective forceful hugging or coughing. The acute care therapist will utilize clinical techniques to assist with cough with pillows or towel rolls at the incisional site and forceful huffing (see description in Chapter 14).[109] Proper lifting techniques should be reviewed before discharge, even though the client will not be able to provide a return demonstration. Activities that require pushing, pulling, straining, or lifting more than 10 lb are restricted for 6 to 10 weeks postoperatively.

Anterior or abdominal soft tissue mobilization for persons with back pain who have postoperative abdominal scars may require indirect techniques. This precaution is especially true for the person with a previous abdominal aneurysm, the person with a known nonoperative aneurysm (<5 cm), or the person with a family history of aneurysm or an undiagnosed aneurysm. The therapist must always palpate the abdomen for a pulsating mass before performing anterior or abdominal therapy. It is possible to palpate the width of the pulse beginning at the abdominal midline and progressing laterally. The pulse should be characterized by a uniform width on either side of the abdominal midline until the umbilicus is reached, at which point the aortic bifurcation results in expansion of the pulse width. Throbbing pain that increases with exertion should alert the therapist to the need to monitor vital signs and palpate pulses. ∎

◆ Peripheral Vascular Disease

Although PVD is usually thought to refer to diseases of the blood vessels supplying the extremities, in fact, PVD actually encompasses pathologic conditions of blood vessels supplying the extremities and the major abdominal organs, most often apparent in the intestines and kidneys. PVD is organized based on the underlying pathologic finding (e.g., inflammatory, arterial occlusive, venous, or vasomotor disorders) (Table 11-18). Although the terms *peripheral arterial disease* (PAD) and *peripheral vascular disease* (PVD) are often used interchangeably, PVD is a broader, more encompassing grouping of disorders of both the arterial and venous blood vessels whereas PAD only refers to arterial blood vessels. PVD typically affects the legs more often than the arms, but upper extremity involvement is not uncommon.

Approximately 8 million Americans over age 60 years are affected by PVD with 20% of those people over age 70 years. Like coronary artery disease (CAD) and cerebrovascular disease (CVD), arterial occlusive forms of PVD are most common as a result of atherosclerosis. Intermittent claudication is the classic symptom of PAD. Like angina associated with CAD, intermittent claudication associated with PAD is predictable and nearly always develops after the same amount of exertion (e.g., walking a specific distance); generally occurs in the same area of the feet, legs, or buttocks; and usually improves rapidly with rest. Data from the Framingham Heart Study and other population studies indicate that intermittent claudication sharply increases in late middle age and is somewhat higher among men than women. In fact the true prevalence of PAD is at least five times higher than expected based on the reported prevalence of intermittent claudication.[55] Specific symptoms of the various forms of PVD depend on the underlying pathologic condition, blood vessels involved (arteries or veins), and location of the affected blood vessels; each form is discussed individually in the following sections.

Inflammatory Disorders. Inflammatory conditions of the blood vessels are often discussed as immunologic conditions because inflammation and damage to large and small vessels result in end-stage organ damage. Vasculitis (e.g., arteritis, such as polyarteritis nodosa and giant cell arteritis, Kawasaki disease) is the most commonly encountered inflammatory blood vessel disease in a therapy practice. Vasculitis is actually a group of disorders that share a common pathogenesis of inflammation of the blood vessels involving arteries, veins, or nerves resulting in narrowing or occlusion of the lumen or formation of aneurysms that can rupture. Vascular inflammation is a central feature of many rheumatic diseases, especially rheumatoid arthritis and scleroderma. (See also the section on Rheumatoid Vasculitis in Chapter 4.)

Vasculitis. Vasculitis can involve blood vessels of any size, type, or location and can affect any organ system, including the nervous systems; classification is usually according to the size of the predominant vessels involved (Table 11-19). Vasculitis may be acute or chronic with varying degrees of involvement. The distribution of lesions may be irregular and segmental rather than continuous. Neurologic manifestations of vasculitis can occur in conjunction with any of the vasculitides listed, affecting the peripheral nervous system (PNS) or the central nervous system (CNS). It may occur as an isolated peripheral nerve vasculitis (localized vasculitis). Numerous vasculitis diseases have been reported in association with HIV disease. The primary target organ involvement is usually muscle and nerve, skin, testicle, kidney, and less often, the CNS.

Immune (antibody-antigen) complexes to each disorder are deposited in the blood vessels resulting in varying symptoms, depending on the organs affected. In the case of vasculitic neuropathy, the formation of antibody-antigen complexes activates the complement cascade with generation of C3a and C5a (chemotactic agents that recruit polymorphonuclear [PMN] leukocytes to the vessel walls). Phagocytosis of the immune complexes takes place, and release of free radicals and proteolytic enzymes disrupts cell membranes and damages blood vessel walls. The complement cascade generates the formation of complement membrane attack complex that also contributes to endothelial damage (see dis-

TABLE   11-18

Peripheral Vascular Diseases

INFLAMMATORY DISORDERS	ARTERIAL OCCLUSIVE DISORDERS	VENOUS DISORDERS	VASOMOTOR DISORDERS
Vasculitis (see also Table 11-21) Polyarteritis nodosa Arteritis Allergic or hypersensitivity angiitis Kawasaki disease Thromboangiitis obliterans (Buerger's disease)	Arterial thrombosis/embolism Thromboangiitis obliterans Arteriosclerosis obliterans	Thrombophlebitis Varicose veins Chronic venous insufficiency	Raynaud's disease Complex regional pain syndrome (CRPS, formerly reflex sympathetic dystrophy [RSD])

TABLE   11-19

Vasculitis

VESSELS INVOLVED	VASCULITIDES	ORGAN SYSTEMS INVOLVED
Small vessels (arterioles, capillaries, venules)	Hypersensitivity vasculitis; drug-induced vasculitis Vasculitis associated with infections or other diseases	Skin, viscera, heart, synovium, GI tract According to underlying cause and involved structures
Medium-sized and small muscular vessels	Vasculitis associated with malignancy Thromboangiitis obliterans (Buerger's disease) Kawasaki disease (muscular arteries, rarely veins) Polyarteritis nodosa Vasculitis in rheumatic disease and connective tissue disorders Angiitis of the CNS Wegener's granulomatosis (uncommon)	Determined by site of malignancy Arteries and veins of digits and limbs Cardiac, iliac, renal, internal mammillary Aorta and its primary and secondary branches, renal and visceral arteries, muscle, testes, nerves Synovium, skin, nail beds CNS Local: nasal structures Systemic: lungs (upper and lower respiratory tracts), renal (glomerulonephritis), any organ can be involved
Large and medium-sized vessels	Takayasu's arteritis (rare) Giant cell (temporal) arteritis	Aorta and its primary branches, renal and visceral arteries Extracranial arteries of the head and neck; any other artery but less common
Peripheral nervous system	Localized vasculitis	Vasa nervosum at the level of the epineural arteries (i.e., blood vessels supplying the neural arch in the spinal axis)

GI, *Gastrointestinal;* CNS, *central nervous system.*

cussion in Chapter 5; see also Fig. 5-13). The resulting damage to endothelial cells results in thickening of the vessel wall, occlusion, and ischemia to the affected nerves with axonal degeneration and the resultant neuropathy.

Polyarteritis Nodosa

Overview and Etiologic Factors.   Polyarteritis nodosa refers to a condition consisting of multiple sites of inflammatory and destructive lesions in the arterial system; the lesions are small masses of tissue in the form of nodes or projections (nodosum). The cause of polyarteritis nodosa is unknown, although hepatitis B is present in 50% of cases, and polyarteritis occurs more commonly among IV drug abusers and other

groups who have a high prevalence of hepatitis B (see the section on Hepatitis B in Chapter 16). Any age can be affected, but it is more common among young men.

Clinical Manifestations.   Polyarteritis nodosa affects small and medium-sized blood vessels, resulting in a variety of clinical presentations depending on the specific site of the blood vessel involved. Some of the more likely symptoms include abrupt onset of fever, chills, tachycardia, arthralgia, and myositis with muscle tenderness.

Any organ of the body may be affected, but most often involved are the kidneys, heart, liver, GI tract, muscles, and testes. Abdominal pain, nausea, and vomiting are common with GI tract involvement. Pericarditis, myocarditis, arrhythmias, and myocardial infarction reflect cardiac involvement. Complications may include aneurysm, hemorrhage, thrombosis, and fibrosis leading to occlusion of the lumen. Multiple asymmetric neuropathies (motor and sensory distribution) can occur when vasculitis affects the arteries of the peripheral nerves (vasa nervorum). Paresthesias, pain, weakness, and sensory loss occur, involving several or many peripheral nerves simultaneously.

Medical Management
Diagnosis, Treatment, and Prognosis.   Diagnosis is made by characteristic laboratory findings, biopsy of symptomatic sites (especially muscle or nerve), and, possibly, visceral angiography. When CNS vasculitis is suspected, angiography is necessary because MRI and CT do not provide sufficient evidence to confirm the diagnosis.

Prolonged use of corticosteroids is necessary to control fever and constitutional symptoms while vascular lesions are healing. Immunosuppressants may be used in conjunction with steroids to improve survival; withdrawal from drugs is often followed by relapse. Treatment of polyarteritis nodosa associated with hepatitis B is more complicated because cytotoxic drugs used to treat the vasculitis can exacerbate the hepatic disease. Prognosis is poor without intervention, with a 5-year survival rate of only 20%. Pharmacologic therapy with corticosteroids increases survival to 50%, and steroids combined with immunosuppressive drugs have improved 5-year survival to 90%.

Arteritis
Overview and Incidence.   Arteritis, sometimes called giant cell arteritis (GCA) or cranial or temporal arteritis, is a vasculitis primarily involving multiple sites of temporal and cranial arteries (i.e., arteries of the head and neck and sometimes the aortic arch). It is the most common vasculitis in the United States and affects older people; the incidence increases with age after 50 years. Postmenopausal women are affected twice as often as men, especially for those individuals who have an arthritis-related disease called *polymyalgia rheumatica (PMR)*. Other risk factors identified in women include heart murmurs and smoking.

Etiologic Factors and Pathogenesis.   Most studies have shown an association of giant cell arteritis with a specific HLA allele, and tumor necrosis factor appears to influence the susceptibility to both GCA and PMR. There may be an infectious origin, but additional studies are necessary to clarify the genetic influence or susceptibility to these conditions. The molecular pathogenesis of GCA involves interleukin (IL-1), intercellular adhesion molecules, and other factors, but the exact pathogenesis remains unknown. The possible role of female sex hormones requires further investigation.

Immunologic research indicates an antigen-driven disease with local T-cell and macrophage activation in vessel walls with calcified atrophic media. The middle layer (tunica media) of the large and medium-sized arteries, particularly those blood vessels supplying blood to the head, is inflamed causing the arteries to swell and obstruct blood flow (stenosis); ischemic complications and secondary thrombosis may occur. Healing produces fibrosis of the arterial wall and the affected blood vessel becomes cordlike, thickened, and nodular, which can be observed externally when the temporal artery is involved.

Clinical Manifestations.   The onset of arteritis is usually sudden, with severe, continuous, unilateral, throbbing headache and temporal pain as the first symptoms with flulike symptoms or visual disturbances. The pain may radiate to the occipital area, face, or side of the neck. Visual disturbances range from blurring to diplopia to visual loss. Irreversible blindness may occur anywhere in the course of the disease from involvement of the ophthalmic artery. Other symptoms may include enlarged, tender temporal artery; scalp sensitivity; and jaw claudication (i.e., pain in response to chewing, talking, or swallowing) when involvement of the external carotid artery causes ischemia of the masseter muscles; the pain is relieved by rest. Approximately 40% of cases present with nonclassic symptoms of respiratory tract problems (most often dry cough), fever of unknown origin, painful paralysis of a shoulder (mononeuritis multiplex), or claudication of the arm with cold hands, arm weakness, and absent radial pulses.[130] Left untreated, the condition may lead to blindness and occasionally to a stroke, heart attack, or aortic dissection.

Medical Management
Diagnosis.   Early diagnosis is important to prevent blindness caused by obstruction of the ophthalmic arteries. Diagnosis is made by recognition of the presenting symptoms, and in some cases, arteritis follows polymyalgia rheumatica,* a similar condition (see Chapter 26). Biopsy of the temporal artery may be performed but is often negative given the focal (segmental) nature of the disease. Color ultrasonography of the temporal arteries detects characteristic signs of vasculitis with a high sensitivity and specificity even in the absence of clinical signs of vascular inflammation (helpful in diagnosing temporal arteritis in people with previously diagnosed PMR). People with extracranial giant cell arteritis (GCA) present with occlusive arterial lesions that may be detected with multiple imaging modalities: arteriography, intravenous angiography (IV-DSA), CT scanning, and magnetic resonance angiography (MRA). However, inflammation of the arterial wall cannot be detected by these means. Standard CT imaging with contrast enhancement and certain MR sequences as well as ultrasound permit identification of the edema and inflammation of the vessel wall. This is an important marker for active disease. Laboratory findings include elevated erythrocyte sedimentation rate (ESR), reflective of the underlying inflammatory process.

Treatment and Prognosis.   Treatment of arteritis to prevent blindness and other vascular complications is with oral antiinflammatory drugs (usually a corticosteroid such as prednisone), providing symptomatic relief in 3 to 5 days. Visual loss can be permanent if allowed to persist for several hours without adequate intervention. With proper intervention, arteritis is a self-limiting disease, usually resolving within 6 to 12 months. About 30% of affected individuals relapse in the first year of treatment during dose tapering. Alternative therapies of combined pharmacology with corticosteroids and

---

*Although giant cell arteritis and polymyalgia rheumatica may occur as separate entities, most epidemiologic surveys group these two conditions together as one disorder. These may be two forms of a common pathophysiologic process characterized by varying degrees of synovitis and arteritis. They may actually represent two points along a single disease continuum.

methotrexate may be more effective in controlling disease with fewer complications.[125]

Hypersensitivity Angiitis.

Hypersensitivity angiitis, a form of vasculitis, can occur at any age, but it most commonly affects children and young adults. The etiology is unknown, but the disease often follows an upper respiratory tract infection, and allergy or drug sensitivity plays a role in some cases. It is usually localized to the small vessels of the skin, first appearing on the lower extremities in a variety of possible lesions. A classic triad of symptoms occurs in 80% of cases that includes purpura (bruising and petechiae or round purplish red spots under the skin), arthritis, and abdominal pain. Inflammation and hemorrhage may occur in the synovium and CNS. Medical management (diagnosis, treatment, prognosis) is the same as for the other forms of vasculitis already discussed.

Kawasaki Disease

Overview and Etiologic Factors.   Kawasaki disease, also known as mucocutaneous lymph node syndrome, is an acute febrile illness associated with systemic (multiorgan) vasculitis. It can occur in any ethnic group but seems most prevalent in Asian populations (especially Japanese, with equal incidence in Japan and in the United States among Japanese or Japanese descendants). Children under the age of 5 years comprise 80% of all cases, and 20% develop cardiac complications that can be fatal. The etiology is unknown, but because seasonal and geographic outbreaks appear to occur, an infectious cause is suspected. Current etiologic theories center on an immunologic response to an infectious, toxic, or antigenic substance.[142]

Pathogenesis.   Substantial evidence suggests that immune activation has a role in the pathogenesis of Kawasaki syndrome. The principal area of pathologic findings is the cardiovascular system. Kawasaki disease progresses pathologically and clinically in stages. During the acute stage of the illness (first 2 weeks) vascular inflammation and immune activation within the arterioles, venules, and capillaries occur, which later progress (stage 2, weeks 2 to 4) to include the main coronary arteries, the heart, and the larger veins. The acute phase is also associated with the appearance of circulating antibodies that are cytotoxic against vascular endothelial cells; the presence of elevated anticardiac myosin autoantibodies may be involved in the myocardial damage that occurs in this phase. In the final stage the vessels develop scarring, intimal thickening, calcification, and formation of thrombi. If death occurs as a result of this disease (rare) it is usually the result of aneurysm, coronary thrombosis, or severe scar formation and stenosis of the main coronary artery.

Clinical Manifestations.   Clinical manifestations present in three phases: acute phase, subacute phase, and convalescent phase. In the *acute phase*, a sudden high fever (lasting over 5 days) that is unresponsive to antibiotics and antipyretics is followed by extreme irritability.

During the *subacute phase* (lasting approximately 25 days), the fever resolves, but the irritability persists along with other symptoms, such as anorexia, rash (exanthema) of the trunk and extremities with reddened palms and soles of the hands and feet, and subsequent desquamation (skin scales off) of the tips of the toes and fingers, peripheral edema of the hands and feet, cervical lymphadenopathy (usually unilateral), bilateral conjunctival infection without exudate, and changes in the oral mucous membranes (e.g., erythema, dryness and cracks or fissures of the lips, reddening or strawberry tongue). In one third of all cases, children develop arthralgias and GI tract symptoms, typically lasting about 2 weeks. Joint involvement may persist for as long as 3 months. During this subacute phase, the person is at risk for cardiac involvement, especially the development of myocarditis, pericarditis, and arteritis that predisposes to the formation of coronary artery aneurysm in nearly 25% of cases not treated within 10 days of fever onset.

The *convalescent phase* occurs 6 to 8 weeks after onset of Kawasaki disease and is characterized by a resolution of all clinical signs and symptoms. However, during this phase the blood values have not returned to normal. At the end of the convalescent phase, all values return to normal and the child has usually regained his or her usual temperament, energy, and appetite.

Medical Management

Diagnosis, Treatment, and Prognosis.   Early recognition and prompt management of the acute syndrome are critical. Diagnosis is made on the basis of clinical manifestations and associated laboratory tests (there are no specific laboratory tests for Kawasaki disease). Echocardiograms are useful in providing a baseline and for monitoring myocardial and coronary artery status. The introduction of high-dose intravenous immune globulin (IVIG) in combination with aspirin therapy to reduce fever and control inflammation and aneurysm formation has significantly reduced the prevalence of coronary artery abnormalities. The exact mechanism by which this treatment intervention reduces the vasculitis of acute Kawasaki syndrome has not been determined. Prognosis is good for recovery with intervention, although serious cardiovascular problems (e.g., coronary thrombosis, aneurysm) may occur later in persons with cardiac sequelae. Giant aneurysms (diameter exceeding 8 mm) have the worst prognosis, since these are unlikely to regress or resolve, with death common in this subgroup population. Occasionally, severe ischemic heart disease requires cardiac transplantation.[142]

Thromboangiitis Obliterans (Buerger's Disease)

Overview and Pathogenesis.   Thromboangiitis obliterans, also referred to as Buerger's disease, is a vasculitis (inflammatory and thrombotic process) affecting the peripheral blood vessels (both arteries and veins), primarily in the extremities. The cause is not known, but it is most often found in men younger than 40 years who smoke heavily, although the incidence in women is increasing. There has been some suggestion that unrecognized cocaine use may masquerade as Buerger's disease.[151]

The pathogenesis of thromboangiitis obliterans is unknown; general inflammatory concepts apply. The inflammatory lesions of the peripheral blood vessels are accompanied by thrombus formation and vasospasm occluding and eventually obliterating (destroying) small and medium-sized vessels of the feet and hands. Recent studies have linked elevated levels of homocysteine to Buerger's disease. Homocysteine has many potential effects: limits the bioavailability of nitric oxide, impairs endothelium-dependent vasorelaxation, increases oxidative stress, stimulates smooth-muscle-cell proliferation, alters the elastic properties of vessel walls, and generates a prethrombotic state through the activation of factor V.

Clinical Manifestations. Clinical manifestations of pain and tenderness of the affected part are caused by occlusion of the arteries, reduced blood flow, and subsequent reduced oxygenation. The symptoms are episodic and segmental, meaning that the symptoms come and go intermittently over time and appear in different asymmetric anatomic locations. The plantar, tibial, and digital vessels are most commonly affected in the lower leg and foot. Intermittent claudication centered in the arch of the foot or the palm of the hand is often the first symptom.

When the hands are affected, the digital, palmar, and ulnar arteries are most commonly involved. Pain at rest occurs with persistent ischemia of one or more digits. Other symptoms include edema, cold sensitivity, rubor (redness of the skin from dilated capillaries under the skin), cyanosis, and thin, shiny, hairless skin (trophic changes) from chronic ischemia. Paresthesias, diminished or absent posterior tibial and dorsalis pedis pulses, painful ischemic ulceration, and eventual gangrene may develop (see Fig. 11-26). Inflammatory superficial thrombophlebitis is common.

Medical Management

Diagnosis, Treatment, and Prognosis. Arteriography may be used in the diagnosis, but definitive diagnosis of thromboangiitis obliterans is determined by histologic examination of the blood vessels (microabscesses in the vessel wall) in a leg amputated for gangrene. Given the new findings that cocaine use may present very much like Buerger's disease, laboratory screening for drug use may be appropriate in some cases.[151]

Intervention should begin with cessation of smoking and avoidance of any environmental or secondhand smoke inhalation. All other treatment techniques are aimed at improving circulation to the foot or hand, including pharmacologic intervention (e.g., vasodilators, pain relief) and physical or occupational therapy (see also Medical Management: Atherosclerosis). Regional sympathetic ganglionectomy may produce vasodilation, ulcerations require wound care, and amputation (sometimes multiple) may be required when the individual is unable to quit smoking or when conservative care fails. With the recent finding of elevated levels of plasma homocysteine associated with Buerger's disease, screening for hyperhomocysteinemia and treatment of this condition have been recommended, especially to assess which clients may eventually require amputation. Since homocysteine is easily removed by pyridoxine and folic acid supplementation, this may become a new intervention strategy for Buerger's disease.

Thromboangiitis is not life-threatening, but it can result in progressive disability from pain and loss of function secondary to amputation. Cessation of smoking is the key determinant in prognosis.

Special Implications for the Therapist 11-18

INFLAMMATORY DISORDERS

Preferred Practice Patterns:
4A: Primary Prevention/Risk Reduction for Skeletal
*   Demineralization (Osteoporosis)*
5G: Impaired Motor Function and Sensory Integrity
*   Associated With Acute or Chronic Polyneuropathies*
*   (peripheral neuropathy)*
7A, 7D, 7E: (integumentary patterns) Associated With
*   Buerger's disease*

See also Special Implications for the Therapist: Peripheral Vascular Disease, 11-24. Additional practice patterns may be appropriate if there is CNS involvement.

Peripheral neuropathy is a well-known and frequently early manifestation of many vasculitis syndromes. The pattern of neuropathic involvement depends on the extent and temporal progression of the vasculitic process that produces ischemia. A severe, burning dysesthetic pain in the involved area is present in 70% to 80% of all cases. Other symptoms may include paresthesias and sensory deficit; severe proximal muscle weakness and muscular atrophy can occur secondary to the neuropathy. In the early phase, one nerve is affected and causes symptoms in one extremity (mononeuritis multiplex) but can involve other nerves as the disorder progresses. The therapist should watch for anyone with neuropathy who exhibits constitutional symptoms, such as fever, arthralgia, or skin involvement. This may herald a possible vasculitis syndrome and requires medical referral for accurate diagnosis. Early recognition of vasculitis can help prevent a poor outcome. Untreated or with a poor outcome to intervention, CNS involvement (e.g., encephalopathy, ischemic and hemorrhagic stroke, cranial nerve palsy) can occur late in the course of vasculitis.

When corticosteroids (e.g., prednisone alone or sometimes in combination with other medications) are used (e.g., in the case of vasculitic neuropathy), the therapist must be aware of the need for osteoporosis prevention and attend to the other potential side effects from the chronic use of these medications (see the section on Corticosteroids in Chapter 4). Alternative methods of pain control may be offered in a rehabilitation setting, such as biofeedback, transcutaneous electrical nerve stimulation (TENS), and physiologic modulation (e.g., using handheld temperature sensor to control autonomic nervous system function; see the section on Fibromyalgia in Chapter 6).

Vasculitis (Inflammatory Disease of Arteries and Veins)

The therapist's role in management of vasculitis may be primarily for relief of painful muscular and joint symptoms when present and in the prevention of functional loss in the case of neuropathies. For the client with thromboangiitis obliterans (Buerger's disease), exercise must be graded to avoid claudication and the client must be instructed in a home program for preventive skin care (see Table 11-22). Gangrene can occur as a result of prolonged ischemia from vessel obliteration; clients are typically treated for wound care and postoperatively after amputation. (See the section on Arteriosclerosis Obliterans below.)

Often a client with some other primary orthopedic or neurologic diagnosis has also been medically diagnosed with vasculitis (see the section on Rheumatoid Vasculitis in Chapter 4 and Special Implications for the Therapist boxes for clients with associated cardiovascular involvement, such as atherosclerosis, myocarditis, pericarditis, or aneurysm).

Arteritis

Early recognition and referral can prevent the serious complications associated with arteritis. Older adults who experience sudden or unexplained headaches, lingering flulike symptoms such as muscle aches (myalgia) and fatigue, persistent fever, unexplained weight loss, jaw pain when eating, or visual disturbances must be referred to their physician. This is especially true for anyone with a previous diagnosis of polymyalgia rheumatica (PMR). The use of corticosteroids can result in side effects such as osteoporosis and bone fractures, weight gain, diabetes, and high blood pressure (see complete discussion in Chapter 4). The client must be advised regarding an osteoporosis prevention program (see discussion in Chapter 23) and how to handle an increase in appetite. Remaining physically active and exercising are key components for both these issues. ■

Arterial Occlusive Diseases.   Occlusive diseases of the blood vessels are a common cause of disability and usually occur as a result of atherosclerosis. Other causes of arterial occlusion may include trauma, thrombus or embolism, vasculitis, vasomotor disorders such as Raynaud's and reflex sympathetic dystrophy (now called *complex regional pain syndrome*), arterial punctures, polycythemia, and chronic mechanical irritation of the subclavian artery being compressed by a cervical rib. For each individual case, see the discussion of the underlying cause of the occlusion to understand etiologic and risk factors and pathogenesis.

Atherosclerotic occlusive disease can also affect other vessels throughout the body other than the cardiac blood vessels. For example, occlusive disease affecting the intestines results in acute intestinal ischemia or ischemic colitis (see Chapter 15), depending on the location of the occlusion. Occlusive cerebrovascular disease (CVD) (see Chapter 31) as a result of atherosclerosis accounts for many episodes of weakness, dizziness, blurred vision, or sudden cerebrovascular accident

(CVA) or stroke. Extracranial arterial ischemia (e.g., common carotid bifurcation, vertebral artery) accounts for over one-half of these types of strokes.

Arterial Thrombosis and Embolism.   Occlusive diseases may be complicated by arterial thrombosis and embolism (Fig. 11-25). Chronic, incomplete arterial obstruction usually results in the development of collateral vessels before complete occlusion threatens circulation to the extremity. Arterial embolism is generally a complication of ischemic or rheumatic heart disease, with or without MI. Signs and symptoms of pain, numbness, coldness, tingling or changes in sensation, skin changes (pallor, mottling), weakness, and muscle spasm occur in the extremity distal to the block (Fig. 11-26). Treatment may include immediate or delayed embolectomy, anticoagulation therapy (e.g., heparin), and protection of the limb.

Thromboangiitis Obliterans (Buerger's Disease). Thromboangiitis obliterans is discussed as a vasculitis in a subsequent section (see Inflammatory Disorders) but is mentioned here as an occlusive disorder because the inflammatory lesions of the peripheral blood vessels are accompanied by thrombus formation and vasospasm occluding blood vessels.

Arteriosclerosis Obliterans (Peripheral Arterial Disease [PAD])

Definition and Overview.   Arteriosclerosis obliterans, defined as arteriosclerosis in which proliferation of the intima has caused complete obliteration of the lumen of the artery, is also known as atherosclerotic occlusive disease, chronic occlusive arterial disease, obliterative arteriosclerosis, and peripheral arterial disease (PAD). It is the most common arterial occlusive disease and accounts for about 95% of cases. It is

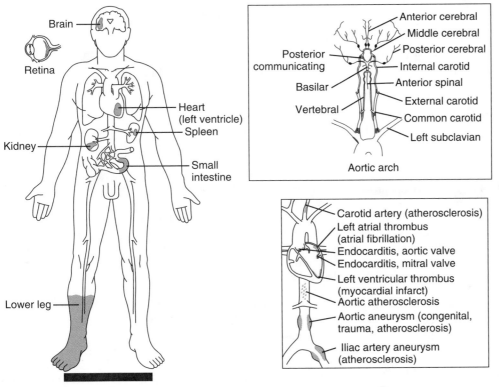

FIGURE **11-25 A,** Common sites of infarction from arterial emboli. **B,** Sources of arterial emboli.

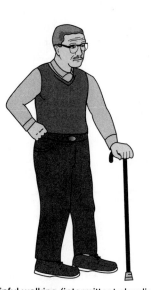

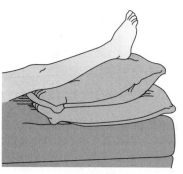

FIGURE **11-26** Signs and symptoms of arterial insufficiency.

Painful walking (intermittent claudication)

Elevated foot develops increased pallor

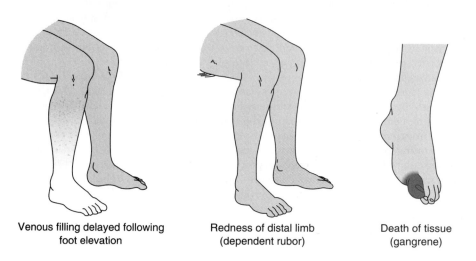

Venous filling delayed following foot elevation

Redness of distal limb (dependent rubor)

Death of tissue (gangrene)

a progressive disease that causes ischemic ulcers of the legs and feet and is most often seen in older clients, associated with diabetes mellitus.

Etiologic and Risk Factors.   Atherosclerosis as the underlying cause of occlusive disease, with its known etiologic and associated risk factors, is discussed earlier in the chapter. PAD correlates most strongly with cigarette smoking and either diabetes or impaired glucose tolerance. Other risk factors include male gender,* hypertension, low levels of high-density lipoprotein cholesterol, high levels of triglycerides, apolipoprotein B, lipoprotein (a), homocysteine, fibrinogen, and blood viscosity. Individuals with PAD are more likely to have coronary heart disease and cerebrovascular disease than those without PAD.[55]

Pathogenesis.   See also Atherosclerosis: Pathogenesis. Since peripheral disease is one expression of atherosclerosis, understanding the pathogenesis of atherosclerosis is important. The arterial narrowing or obstruction that occurs as a result of the atherosclerotic process reduces blood flow to the limbs during exercise or at rest. Muscular reactivity is also adversely affected in PAD. Prostacyclin and nitric oxide usually activate vascular relaxation. In PAD, these relaxation factors are reduced and constrictive factors such as endothelin increase. This imbalance of vascular reactivity contributes to decreased blood flow.[197]

Clinical Manifestations.   In peripheral vessels, claudication symptoms appear when the diameter of the vessel narrows by 50%. PAD affecting the lower extremities is primarily one of large- and medium-sized arteries and most frequently involves branch points and bifurcations. Symptoms of arterial occlusive disease usually occur distal to the narrowing or obstruction. Acute ischemia may present with some or all of the classical symptoms, such as pain, pallor, paresthesia, paralysis, and pulselessness. However, arteries can become significantly blocked without symptoms developing, a phenomenon referred to as *silent ischemia*. Even though silent ischemia is not associated with symptoms, it poses the same long-term sequelae and complications as overt ischemia and must be treated. It is strongly suspected when systolic blood pressure is lower at the ankle than at the arm (see further discussion of ankle/brachial index in this section).

*It has been reported that PAD is more prevalent in women than generally appreciated, but estimates vary greatly according to the diagnostic criteria applied. Prevalence and incidence rates do not differ significantly by gender, although incidence rates in women lag behind those in men in a pattern similar to that for coronary artery disease.[164]

Occlusive disease of the distal *aorta and iliac arteries* usually begins just proximal to the bifurcation of the common iliac arteries, causing changes in both lower extremities (Fig. 11-27; Table 11-20). Bilateral, progressive, intermittent claudication (pain, ache, or cramp in the muscles causing limping) is almost always present in the calf muscles and is usually present in the gluteal and quadriceps muscles presenting as buttock, thigh, and calf pain. The distance a person can walk before the onset of pain indicates the degree of circulatory inadequacy (e.g., two blocks or more is mild; one block is moderate; one-half block or less is severe). The primary symptom may only be a sense of weakness or tiredness in these same areas; both the pain and weakness or fatigue are relieved by rest.

Occlusive disease of the *femoral and popliteal arteries* usually occurs at the point at which the superficial femoral artery passes through the adductor magnus tendon into the popliteal space. Occlusion of these regions is also marked by intermittent claudication of the calf and foot that may radiate to the ipsilateral* popliteal region and lower thigh. There are definite changes of the affected lower leg and foot as listed in Table 11-20.

Occlusive disease of the *tibial and common peroneal arteries*, as well as the pedal vessels and small digital vessels, occurs slowly and progressively over months or years. The eventual outcome depends on the vessels that are occluded and the condition of the proximal and collateral vessels. Arterial ulcers may develop as a result of ischemia, usually located over a bony prominence on the toes or feet (e.g., metatarsal heads, heels, lateral malleoli). The skin is shiny and atrophic, and fissures and cracks are common. Pain at rest indicates more severe involvement, which may mimic deep venous thrombosis (DVT), but relief from the occlusive disease can sometimes be obtained by dangling the uncovered leg over the edge of the bed. This dependent position would increase symptoms of DVT, which is usually treated by leg elevation. Exercise may cause pedal pulses to disappear in some people. Sudden occlusion of the arteries, usually at the level of one of these smaller branches, results in gangrene. The necrotic tissue may become gangrenous and infected, requiring surgical intervention.

Occlusive arterial disease for the person with diabetes is further complicated by very slow healing, and healed areas may break down easily. In the case of diabetes mellitus (DM), diabetic neuropathy with diminished or absent sensation of the toes or feet often occurs, predisposing the person to injury or pressure ulcers that may progress because of poor blood flow and subsequent loss of sensation (Table 11-21) (see the section on Diabetes in Chapter 10). Amputation rate in people with diabetes is markedly higher than for those individuals with PAD without DM.

Medical Management

Diagnosis.   Diagnosis is based on client history and clinical examination. Diagnostic tools may include noninvasive vascular tests (e.g., ankle/brachial index, segmental limb pressures, pulse volume recordings, duplex ultrasonography) or, if invasive tests are required, arteriography with contrast or with magnetic resonance imaging. An in-depth discussion of the diagnosis and intervention strategies for chronic arterial insufficiency of the lower extremities is available.[9]

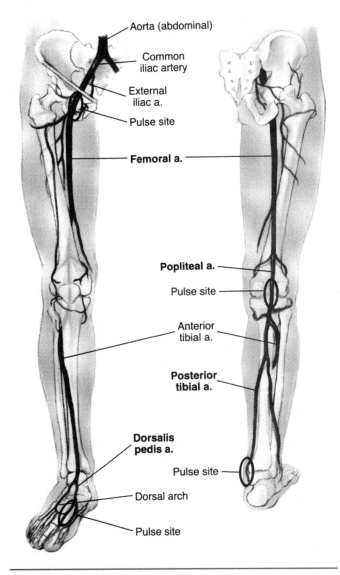

FIGURE **11-27** Arteries in the leg. The abdominal aorta branches (aortic bifurcation) into the right and left common iliac artery. This artery passes through the pelvic cavity and under the inguinal ligament to become the major artery supplying the leg, called the femoral artery. The femoral artery travels down the thigh until, at the lower thigh, it courses posteriorly, where it becomes the popliteal artery. Below the knee, the popliteal artery divides into the anterior tibial artery and posterior tibial artery. The anterior tibial artery travels down the front of the leg onto the dorsum of the foot, where it becomes the dorsalis pedis. In the back of the leg, the posterior tibial artery travels down behind the malleolus and forms the plantar arteries in the foot. (From Jarvis C: *Physical examination and health assessment*, ed 3, Philadelphia, 2000, Saunders, p 553.)

Prevention and Treatment.   Prevention is the key to reducing the incidence of PVD caused by atherosclerosis. Risk factor reduction and lifestyle measures are the first steps with smoking cessation (or not ever starting) as the single most effective prevention tool. A conservative approach to care that includes a program of dietary management to decrease cholesterol and fat, pain control, and daily physical training and exercise therapy to improve collateralization and function has been uniformly endorsed by experts in vas-

---

*Although symptoms occur ipsilateral to the occlusion anywhere distal to the bifurcation of the aorta, most people have bilateral disease and therefore bilateral symptoms.

TABLE 11-20

Arterial Occlusive Disease

SITE OF OCCLUSION	SIGNS AND SYMPTOMS

Aortic bifurcation	Sensory and motor deficits
	    Muscle weakness
	    Numbness (loss of sensation)
	    Paresthesias (burning, pricking)
	    Paralysis
	Intermittent claudication (lower back, gluteal muscles, quadriceps, calves; relieved by rest)
	Cold, pale legs with decreased or absent peripheral pulses

Iliac artery	Intermittent claudication (buttock, hip, thigh; relieved by rest) Diminished or absent femoral or distal pulses Impotence in males
Femoral and popliteal artery	Intermittent claudication (calf, foot; may radiate) Leg pallor and coolness Dependent rubor Blanching of feet on elevation No palpable pulses in ankles and feet Gangrene
Tibial and common peroneal artery	Intermittent claudication (calves; feet occasionally) Pain at rest (severe disease); possibly relieved by dangling affected leg Same skin and temperature changes in lower leg and foot as described above Pedal pulses absent; popliteal pulses may be present

cular disease.[9] Careful attention must be given to preventive skin care (Table 11-22) to avoid even minor injuries, infections, or ulcerations.

Low-dose aspirin may be administered as an antiplatelet agent, and pentoxifylline may be used to improve capillary blood flow. Cilostazol (Pletal), with its unique combination of antiplatelet, vasodilatory, and antithrombotic effects, has been added to the pharmacologic agents for use with PAD. Although there are frequent minor adverse effects (e.g., headache, diarrhea, palpitations) the improved results with this agent (e.g., increased maximal walking distance 28% to 100%, increased pain-free walking distance 45% to 96%) may warrant its use over pentoxifylline.[42] Statins used for the prevention of cardiovascular disease because of their antithrombotic properties have been shown effective in reducing the risk of DVT and may become useful in the primary and secondary prevention of DVT.[190]

Surgical intervention (revascularization procedures such as bypass graft or angioplastic treatment) is indicated if blood flow is compromised enough to produce symptoms of ischemic pain at rest, if tissue death has occurred, or if claudication interferes with essential activities or work. This decision is usually made after exercise therapy combined with risk factor modification has been unsuccessful in preventing this level of impairment and subsequent disability. Cessation of smoking may be required by the physician before surgery is considered. Persons with localized occlusions of the aorta and iliac arteries less than 10 cm in length, with relatively normal vessels proximally and distally, are good candidates for angioplasty or stenting (see Figs. 11-3 and 11-5). Conversely, people with multisegmented arterial disease with more involved symptoms are at greater risk of amputation. Endovascular intervention includes a variety of catheter-based surgical techniques that are being improved by laser techniques.

Prognosis. Arterial occlusive diseases are not life-threatening, but people with symptoms such as intermittent claudication often have a decreased quality of life because of mobility limitations. Symptoms of chronic arterial insufficiency progress slowly over time so that progressive disability from pain, ulceration, gangrene, and loss of function or limbs is more likely to occur than death as a result of peripheral occlusive diseases. On the other hand, because people with either asymptomatic or symptomatic PAD have widespread arterial disease, they have a significantly increased risk of stroke, MI, and cardiovascular death. Twenty percent of all individuals with PVD have a heart attack or stroke, and 30% of those have a 5-year mortality rate that climbs to 62% in men and 33% in women in 10 years.[9,121]

Special Implications for the Therapist **11-19**

ARTERIOSCLEROSIS OBLITERANS (Peripheral Arterial Disease)

See also Special Implications for the Therapist: Peripheral Vascular Disease, 11-24.

Arterial Tests and Measures

Until recently, exercise testing using a 12-degree grade at a preset speed of 2 mph was the current practice to assess for claudication associated with PAD, but limited reproducibility and limited sensitivity to change in exercise performance were serious problems. Graded treadmill protocols have been developed to test people with PAD that are highly reproducible and able to

Continued

TABLE	11-21

Comparison of Arterial, Venous, and Neuropathic Ulcers

	ARTERIAL ULCER	VENOUS ULCER	NEUROPATHIC (DIABETIC) ULCER
*Etiology**	Arteriosclerosis obliterans Atheroembolism Large- or medium-vessel atherosclerosis Raynaud's disease Diabetes mellitus Collagen disease Vasculitis	Valvular incompetence History of DVT Venous insufficiency accompanied by hypertension Peripheral incompetence; varicose veins	Diabetes mellitus; combination of arterial disease and peripheral neuropathy Repetitive unrecognized trauma
Location	Anywhere on leg or dorsum of foot or toes Bone prominences (anterior tibial) Lateral malleolus	Medial aspect of distal one third of lower extremity Behind medial malleolus	Same areas in which arterial ulcers appear, especially toes Areas where peripheral neuropathy occurs (pressure points on plantar aspect of foot, toes, heels)
Clinical Manifestations	Painful, especially with legs elevated Pulses poor quality or absent Intermittent claudication (exertional calf pain) Rest pain or nocturnal aching of foot or forefoot relieved by dependent dangling position Integumentary (trophic) changes Hair loss Thin, shiny skin Ischemia: pale, white skin color Areas of sluggish blood flow: Red-purple mottling Hypersensitivity to palpation History of minor nonhealing trauma	Not often painful; venous insufficiency can cause aching pain; more comfortable with legs elevated Normal arterial pulses Eczema or stasis dermatitis Edema Dark pigmentation	Classic symmetric ascending stocking-glove distribution of sensory loss (begins in feet and ascends to knees, then symptoms begin in the hands) May not be painful because of loss of sensation (e.g., neuropathic ulcers are painless or insensate when palpated) Some people experience unpleasant sensations (tingling or hypersensitivity to normally painless stimuli) Loss of vibratory sense and light touch Pulses may be present or diminished (arteries become calcified) Neuropathic foot is warm and dry Loss of vascular tone increases arteriovenous shunting and impairs blood flow necessary for wound healing; sepsis common Altered biomechanics and weight bearing
Wound Appearance	 Minimal exudate with dry necrosis Blanched wound base and periwound tissue	 Superficial Highly exudative Red wound base Irregular edges	Round, craterlike with elevated rim (see Fig. 9-26); diabetes hastens changes described in figure at left (arterial ulcer) Minimal drainage Frequently deep High infection rate

DVT, Deep vein thrombosis.
*Ulceration may also occur as a result of lymphatic disorders (see Chapter 12), skin cancer (see Chapter 9), metabolic abnormalities, and vasculitis (see Table 11-19).

TABLE	11-22

Guidelines for Skin Care and Protection

Temperature Protection

Nicotine causes vasoconstriction of the small vessels in the hands and feet; avoid all tobacco products.

Recognize and avoid other triggers that cause vasoconstriction (e.g., emotional distress, caffeine, cold or cough remedies that contain a decongestant).

Wear layers of clothing made of natural fibers, such as cotton, to draw moisture away from the skin; in cold weather, wear a hat and scarf because heat is lost through the scalp; silk is a good insulator, consider it for socks and long underwear.

Wear thick mittens, which are warmer than gloves, and socks purchased from an outdoor clothing or ski shop designed to wick moisture away while retaining body heat.

Avoid air conditioning; wear warmer clothes, layer light clothing, or wear a sweater or jacket in air conditioning; be careful when going into an air-conditioned environment after being out in the heat or vice versa.

Test water temperature before bathing or showering or have a member of the family test first; use other portion of the body to test if insensitivity exists in hand or foot.

Use a heating pad, hot water bottle, or an electric blanket to warm the sheets of your bed before getting into bed, but *do not* apply these directly to the skin and do not sleep with any electric device left on; if necessary wear light socks and mittens or gloves to bed. Do not soak hands or feet in hot water.

Keep household temperatures at a constant, even, and comfortable level.

Keep protective covering available at all times, even in the summer.

Avoid contact with extremes of temperature, such as oven, dishwasher (hot dishes), refrigerator, or freezer; wear thick oven mitts whenever reaching into the oven. Keep mittens or warm gloves by the refrigerator and freezer to prevent symptoms when reaching into it.

Wear rubber gloves whenever cleaning, washing dishes, or rinsing or peeling vegetables under water.

Avoid holding ice, ice-cold fruit, hot or cold drinks, or frozen foods; wear protective gloves whenever making contact with any of these items.

Skin Care

Take care of your skin, and give your hands and feet extra care and protection; examine hands and feet daily; at the first sign of bruising, skin changes (e.g., cracking, calluses, blisters, redness), swelling, infection, or ulcer, immediately contact a member of your health care team (e.g., nurse, physical therapist, physician). If vision is impaired, have a family member or health care professional inspect your hands and feet.

Circulation problems tend to create dry skin and delay healing; keep your skin clean and well-moisturized; wash with a mild, creamy, or moisturizing liquid soap or gel; clean carefully between fingers and toes; *do not* soak them.

Avoid perfumed lotions, and do not put lotion on sores or between toes.

Observe carefully for any activities that might put pressure on your fingertips, such as using a manual typewriter, playing a musical instrument (e.g., guitar, piano), and doing crafts or needlework.

Do not go barefoot indoors or outdoors; this includes getting up at night; avoid wearing open-toed shoes, pointy-toed shoes, high heels, or sandals; always wear absorbent socks or socks that wick perspiration away from skin; avoid nylon material (including pantyhose material); avoid stockings with seams or with mends; change socks or stockings daily.

Make sure shoes provide good support without being too tight, avoid shoes that cause excessive foot perspiration, and alternate shoes throughout the week (i.e., do not wear the same shoes every day). Do not wear shoes without socks or stockings.

Avoid hot tubs and prolonged baths; dry carefully between toes; water temperature should be between 90° and 95° F.

Use heel protectors, sheepskin, and other protective devices whenever recommended.

Other Tips

For Raynaud's disease or phenomenon, avoid situations that precipitate excitement, anxiety, or feelings of fear; teach yourself how to recognize early signs of these emotions and use relaxation techniques to reduce stress.

For Raynaud's disease or phenomenon, when you have an attack, gently rewarm fingers or toes as soon as possible; place your hands under your armpits, wiggle fingers or toes, or move or walk around to improve circulation; if possible, run warm (*not* hot) water over the affected body part until normal color returns.

Do not use razor blades; use electric razors.

Avoid medications and substances (e.g., nicotine; caffeine in chocolate, tea, coffee, and soft drinks) that can cause blood vessels to narrow; discuss all medications with your physician.

Maintain good circulation; do not stay in one position for more than 30 minutes; use breathing and stretching exercises whenever confined to a desk, chair, car, or bed for more than 30 minutes.

Do not wear constricting or tight clothing, especially tight socks; avoid elastic around wrists or ankles.

Do not wear jewelry, such as watches or bracelets, to bed at night.

Leave a night light on in dark areas; turn on lights in dark areas and hallways.

Do not sit with legs crossed because this can cause pressure on the nerves and blood vessels.

Avoid sunburn.

Do not scratch insect bites; do not scratch areas of itchy skin.

Do not do bathroom surgery on corns or calluses; do not use chemical agents for the removal of corns or calluses; see your physician.

Care of Nails

Use clippers, not scissors; *do not* use razor blades; cut toenails straight across, but file fingernails in a rounded fashion to the tips of your fingers.

Take care of your nails; use cuticle softener or moisturizing cream or lotion around cuticles; push the cuticles back very gently with a cotton swab soaked in cuticle remover; *do not* push cuticles back with a sharp object and *do not* cut the cuticles with scissors or nail clippers.

Use lamb's wool between overlapping toes.

evaluate change in exercise performance. Two widely used graded protocols maintain a walking speed of 2.0 mph, one with grade increases of 3.5% every 3 minutes, the other with grade increases of 2.0% every 2 minutes. As the individual walks on the treadmill, time to pain and maximal walking time are recorded. All people limited by claudication are reproducibly brought to maximal levels of discomfort using either of these protocols.[7]

Venous filling time provides a reasonable assessment of the general state of perfusion but requires patent venous valves to be a valid measure. Have the client assume a recumbent position and elevate the legs to facilitate venous drainage. When the veins have collapsed below the level of the skin, quickly bring the person to a sitting position with the legs hanging in a dependent position. The time necessary for the veins to fill to skin level is the venous filling time. A filling time greater than 25 seconds implies an increased risk of ulceration, infection, and poor wound healing.

The ankle/brachial index (ABI) (Box 11-10) is another measure of arterial perfusion at the level measured available to therapists for use in documenting the need for and benefit of a prescriptive exercise program. Blood pressures are measured both in the arm (brachial blood pressure) and the ankle with the client in a supine position for both measures. The ankle blood pressure may be auscultated using the dorsalis pedis pulse or posterior tibialis artery with the cuff placed above the ankle or using Doppler if available. The systolic ankle pressure is divided by the brachial systolic pressure. With increasing degrees of arterial narrowing, there is a progressive fall in systolic blood pressure distal to the sites of involvement. If both pressures are measured with the person in the supine position, and the vessels are unobstructed, the ratio of ankle to brachial pressures should be 1.0.[197] If flow to the lower extremity is decreased, the ratio will be less than 1.0. Based on two large population-based studies, the reference standard of ABI less than 0.90 at rest or less than 0.85 after exercise in adults older than 55 years indicates PAD.[74,199] ABI measurements may be of limited value in anyone with diabetes because calcification of the tibial and peroneal arteries may render them noncompressible.[9]

ABI can be measured before and after exercise to assess the dynamics of intermittent claudication. This can be accomplished by leaving the ankle pressure cuffs in place during the exercise. Once the walk is completed or pain develops, the person rapidly assumes a supine position and the ankle pressures are measured. At modest workloads, the healthy adult can maintain ankle systolic pressures at normal levels. If the exercise is strenuous, there may be a transient fall in systolic pressure that rapidly returns to baseline levels. In people with intermittent claudication, a different response is seen, even at low workload. If the person walks to the point of claudication, ankle systolic pressure falls precipitously, often to unrecordable levels, and will not return to baseline levels for several minutes. It is not necessary (and may be misleading) to measure arm systolic pressure after exercise since this will increase by an amount related to the workload and the most important variable is the extent to which ankle pressure falls and the time it takes to recover (i.e., the period of postexercise ischemia). In general, if ankle pressure falls by more than 20% of the baseline value and requires more than 3 minutes to recovery, the test is considered abnormal.[9,180]

Prescriptive Exercise

In prescribing an exercise program for someone with claudication secondary to occlusive disease, exercise tolerance must be determined. A training heart rate should be based on the exer-

cise tolerance test because persons with PVD frequently have CAD as well. Frequently, symptoms of claudication occur before training heart rate is reached, but the heart rate should be monitored and should not exceed the training heart rate, even in the absence of symptoms. Anginal chest pain is a red flag to decrease intensity.

A progressive conditioning program, including walking for fixed periods, is essential, even if the initial length of walking time is only 1 minute. Exercise can protect against atherothrombotic events by elevating tissue plasminogen activator (t-PA)[253]; improving peripheral circulation[83]; improving ambulatory function, endothelial-dependent dilation, and calf blood flow[29]; and favorably altering cardiovascular risk factor profile (e.g., improved lipid profile, reduced blood pressure), an important element in the management of peripheral arterial disease.[118]

The greatest improvement occurs with intermittent exercise to near-maximal pain progressing to a long-term (6 months or more) program of structured walking for at least 30 minutes three times weekly.[84] The most effective program begins with brisk treadmill walking at a pace that is comfortable for the individual until claudication begins followed by immediate rest and continued walking when the pain subsides. The therapist can direct the client to progress quickly to levels of exercise at maximal tolerable pain in order to obtain optimal symptomatic benefit over time. This pattern is repeated starting with intervals as short as 1 to 5 minutes, alternating with rest periods of sufficient duration to eliminate pain (usually 2 to 10 minutes). Without complicating factors, the individual is usually able to complete at least a 30- to 45-minute walk without pain or rest breaks within 6 to 8 weeks. Claudication is influenced by the speed, incline, and surface of the walk and should be modified whenever possible to improve exercise tolerance. Impairment measures, functional measures, quality of life assessment, and specific walking parameters are outlined in detail elsewhere.[197]

Altered gait pattern has been documented with PAD[82] with less time spent in the swing phase of the gait cycle and more time in double stance. This ambulatory pattern favors greater gait stability at the expense of greater walking speed and can be improved with exercise rehabilitation. People with intermittent claudication associated with PAD are also functionally limited by dorsiflexion weakness, impairing their ability to perform tasks requiring distal lower extremity strength.[201]

After exercise, numbness in the foot as well as pain in the calf may occur. The foot may be cold and pale, which is an indication that the circulation has been diverted to the arteriolar bed

Continued

of the leg muscles. Many people with claudication are already receiving beta-blockers for angina or hypertension (see also Special Implications for the Therapist: Angina Pectoris, 11-3 and Special Implications for the Therapist: Hypertension, 11-4). The main factor limiting success of exercise therapy is lack of client motivation. For this reason, the most successful programs combine regular, supervised outpatient sessions with home exercise programs; regularity rather than intensity should be stressed. Comorbid diseases, such as coronary artery disease or diabetes mellitus, and severity and location of arterial occlusive disease do not preclude successful response to prescriptive exercise. Unstable cardiopulmonary conditions require more careful consideration and collaboration with the health care team.[9]

Precautions

When arterial thrombosis or embolism is suspected, the affected limb must be protected by proper positioning below the horizontal plane and protective skin care provided. Heat or cold application and massage are contraindicated, and family members must also be notified of these restrictions. The home health therapist must be alert to the possibility of hot water bottles, heating pads, electric blankets, and hot foot soaks being used by the client without physician approval. This precaution is especially true for people with diabetic-associated peripheral neuropathies and for people with paraplegia. Encourage the person with vascular disease to prevent becoming chilled by keeping the thermostat at home set at 70° to 72° F and to avoid prolonged exposure to cold outdoors (e.g., prewarming the car, dressing properly in layers, especially protecting hands and feet). In addition, many people with PVD and diabetes mellitus have peripheral sensory neuropathy and are at greater risk for skin breakdown on the foot from weight-bearing activities such as walking or running (see Table 11-22). These individuals should participate in alternate forms of exercise (e.g., bicycling, swimming/aquatics) even though these exercises may not improve walking ability as much as a structured walking program.[165] ∎

Venous Diseases. Venous diseases can be acute or chronic; acute venous disease includes thrombophlebitis, and chronic venous disease includes varicose vein formation and chronic venous insufficiency.

Thrombophlebitis

Definition and Overview. Thrombophlebitis is a partial or complete occlusion of a vein by a thrombus (clot) with secondary inflammatory reaction in the wall of the vein. A venous thrombus is an intravascular collection of platelets, erythrocytes, leukocytes, and fibrin, the end result of the clotting cascade with the potential to produce significant morbidity and mortality.[229] There are two types of venous thrombosis: superficial (most commonly of the saphenous vein; Fig. 11-28) and deep (usually of the pelvis and lower extremities). Superficial venous thrombosis of the upper extremity can occur although it is much less common, usually in people with a systemic illness in the presence of an indwelling central venous catheter (e.g., used in the treatment of cancer), malignancy, and less often, hemodialysis.[152]

In the lower extremities, superficial venous thrombus is usually the result of varicose veins, is self-limiting, and is not a serious condition. Deep vein thrombus of the lower extremity may be either a calf vein or proximal thrombosis. Calf vein thrombosis is usually clinically silent and benign without

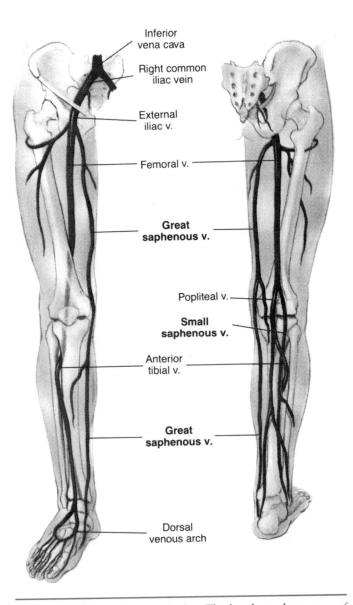

FIGURE 11-28 Veins in the leg. The legs have three types of veins: deep veins (femoral and popliteal) coursing alongside the deep arteries to conduct most of the venous return from the legs; superficial veins, the great and small saphenous veins; and perforators (not pictured), the connecting veins that join the two sets and route blood from the superficial into the deep veins. The great saphenous vein starts at the medial side of the dorsum of the foot and ascends in front of the medial malleolus, crossing the tibia obliquely and ascending along the medial side of the thigh. The small saphenous vein starts on the lateral side of the dorsum of the foot and ascends behind the lateral malleolus and up the back of the leg, where it joins the popliteal vein. (From Jarvis C: *Physical examination and health assessment*, ed 3, Philadelphia, 2000, Saunders, p 553.)

complications although silent calf vein thromboses can extend into more proximal veins and become pulmonary emboli (PEs; see the discussion in Chapter 14). Proximal thrombosis occurs in the popliteal, femoral, iliac veins, or the inferior vena cava, also with a greater risk of significant PE.[229]

Incidence and Etiologic and Risk Factors. DVT is the third most common cardiovascular disease after acute coronary artery episodes and cerebrovascular accidents, affecting

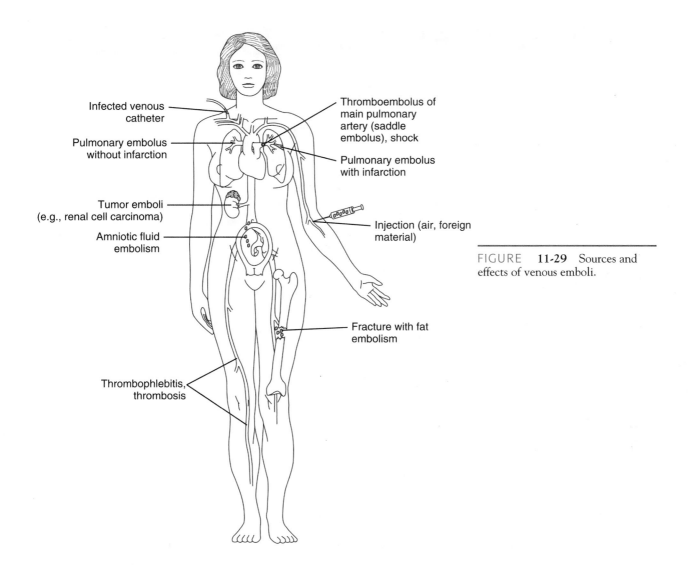

Infected venous catheter

Pulmonary embolus without infarction

Tumor emboli (e.g., renal cell carcinoma)

Amniotic fluid embolism

Thromboembolus of main pulmonary artery (saddle embolus), shock

Pulmonary embolus with infarction

Injection (air, foreign material)

Fracture with fat embolism

Thrombophlebitis, thrombosis

FIGURE   **11-29**   Sources and effects of venous emboli.

up to 2 million Americans annually.[168] Approximately 30% of all people (women more than men) undergoing major general surgical procedures* develop clinical manifestations of deep vein thrombophlebitis (DVT) up to 2 weeks postoperatively (Fig. 11-29). Substantial evidence indicates that the pathologic processes of venous (and arterial) thromboembolism involve both genetic and lifestyle influences. Scientific progress over the past decade has revealed a growing number of genetic factors present in more than 1% of the population that increase the relative risk of venous thrombosis between twofold and sevenfold. Several of these factors have been demonstrated to interact adversely with lifestyle influences, such as oral contraceptives and smoking.

Thrombus formation is usually attributed to venous stasis, hypercoagulability, or injury to the venous wall although other risk factors may be present (Table 11-23). It is commonly held that at least two of these three conditions must be present for thrombi to form. What were previously considered to be idiopathic causes of thrombosis now have been identified as abnormalities associated with thrombophilia, such as elevated levels of coagulation factors VIII and XI, a particular prothrombin mutation, elevated levels of homocysteine, and a syndrome of activated protein C resistance.[71] Acquired resistance to the anticoagulant action of activated protein C may be associated with the increased risk of venous thrombosis associated with pregnancy, hormone replacement therapy, the use of oral contraceptives, and possibly even in vitro fertilization.[57]

Pathogenesis.   Any trauma to the endothelium of the vein wall exposes subendothelial tissues to platelets in the venous blood, initiating thrombosis. Platelets on the vein wall attract the deposition of fibrin, leukocytes, and erythrocytes, forming a thrombus that may remain attached to the vessel wall or break off and become free-floating as an embolism. The embolus travels through the progressively enlarging venous vessels, through the right side of the heart to the progressively narrowing pulmonary artery where it may become lodged and occlude pulmonary circulation (pulmonary embolus [PE]).[229] If a thrombus occludes a major vein (e.g., femoral vein, vena cava, axillary vein), the venous pressure and volume rise distally. However, if a thrombus occludes a deep small vein (e.g., tibial, popliteal), collateral vessels develop and relieve the increased venous pressure and volume.

---

*High-risk surgical candidates have a history of recent venous thromboembolism or have undergone extensive pelvic or abdominal surgery for advanced malignancy, CABG, renal transplantation, splenectomy, or major orthopedic surgery to the lower limbs (e.g., hip or knee arthroplasty, surgery for fractured hip, tibial osteotomy).

TABLE	11-23

Risk Factors for Deep Venous Thrombosis (DVT)

Immobility (Venous Stasis)
Prolonged bed rest (e.g., burns, fracture)
Prolonged air travel
Neurologic disorder (e.g., spinal cord injury, stroke)
Cardiac failure
Absence of ankle muscle pump

Trauma (Venous Damage)
Varicose veins
Surgery
Local trauma (e.g., direct injury)
Intravenous injections
Fracture or dislocation
Childbirth and delivery
Sclerosing agents

Other
Diabetes mellitus
Genetic
Obesity
Previous deep vein thrombosis (DVT)
Buerger's disease
Age >60 yr
Idiopathic

Lifestyle
Hormonal status
• Oral contraceptive use
• Hormone replacement therapy
• Hormonal medications (e.g., tamoxifen, doxorubicin [Adriamycin])
• Pregnancy
• In vitro fertilization (?)
Smoking

Hypercoagulation
Hereditary thrombotic disorders
Neoplasm (especially viscera, ovary)
↑ Levels of coagulation factors (VIII, XI)
Prothrombin mutation
↑ Levels of homocysteine
Activated protein C syndrome

When the thrombus adheres to the vein wall, secondary inflammatory changes develop and the thrombus is eventually invaded by fibroblasts, resulting in scarring of the vein wall and destruction of the valves. Restoration of the central venous canal (recanalization) may occur as a result of the healing process. Although blood flow is restored through the vein, the valves do not recover function, resulting in back flow of blood and other secondary functional and anatomic problems (e.g., stasis, venous stasis ulcers, risk of another DVT, pulmonary embolism from recurrent DVT).

Clinical Manifestations. In the early stages, approximately one-half of the people with DVT are asymptomatic for any signs or symptoms in the affected extremity. The lower extremities are affected most often, but upper extremity venous thrombi can also develop, the latter usually presenting with edema of the involved extremity and without pain. When symptoms occur in the lower extremity, the client may report a dull ache, a tight feeling, or pain in the calf often misdiagnosed as some other cause of leg pain. When symptoms are reported in the entire extremity, the condition is more extensive. Thrombi may be present in both extremities, even though symptoms are unilateral.

Signs are often absent; when present, they may be variable and unreliable, consisting of slight swelling in the involved calf or ankle, slight fever, and, possibly, tachycardia. Any of these symptoms can occur without DVT, possibly associated with other vascular, inflammatory, musculoskeletal, or lymphatic conditions that produce signs and symp-

toms similar to those of DVT.[229] An asymmetric prominence of the subcutaneous vein pattern may be present, such as across the inguinal ligament, indicating an iliofemoral occlusion, or across the front of the shin, indicating a popliteal thrombosis. The skin of the leg and ankle on the affected side may be relatively warmer than on the unaffected side (check for temperature changes with the backs of the fingers). If venous obstruction is severe, the skin may be cyanotic. Pulmonary emboli (see Chapter 14), most often from the large, deep veins of the pelvis and legs, are the most devastating complication of DVT and can occur without apparent warning.

In the case of superficial thrombophlebitis, dull pain and local tenderness in the region of the involved vein may be accompanied by signs of superficial induration (firm or hard cord) and redness. Swelling and deep calf tenderness are only present when DVT has developed. Chills and high fever accompany iatrogenic phlebitis secondary to IV catheter insertion; tenderness (not redness) is an early sign of peripheral IV site phlebitis.

Medical Management
Diagnosis. History and clinical examination are followed by Doppler ultrasonography as a rapid screening procedure to detect thrombosis; small thrombi in calf veins are easily missed when collateral circulation exists. Venous duplex scanning has replaced contrast venography as the primary diagnostic test of DVT because it allows noninvasive visualization of the vein while simultaneously providing information on venous flow.

Homans' sign (Fig. 11-30) is still assessed during physical examination despite the fact that this test is insensitive, non-specific, and present in fewer than 30% of documented cases of DVT. In addition, more than one-half of all people with a positive Homans' sign do not have evidence of venous thrombosis. A positive Homans' sign can also occur with superficial phlebitis, Achilles tendinitis, and gastrocnemius and plantar muscle injury. Calf muscle strain or contusion may be difficult to differentiate from thrombophlebitis; further diagnostic testing may be required to determine the correct diagnosis. Occasionally, a ruptured Baker cyst may produce unilateral pain and swelling in the calf. A history of arthritis in the knee of the same leg and the disappearance of the popliteal cyst at the time symptoms develop are clues the physician can use to make the differentiation.

Prevention.   Primary prevention of DVT is important through the use of early ambulation for low-risk individuals and prophylactic use of anticoagulants (see Table 11-4) in people considered at high risk for venous thrombosis. The highest incidence of DVT occurs with abdominal, pelvic, hip, or knee surgery and open prostate procedures. Routine use of elastic stockings in all postoperative clients has been adopted in most hospitals, and many facilities use pneumatic pressure devices with on/off cycles applied for the first 24 hours after major surgery to mimic the calf pump.

Treatment.   The goals of DVT management are to prevent progression to pulmonary embolism, limit damage to the vein, and prevent another clot from forming. Current therapy is to administer low-dose heparin or a low–molecular weight heparin* followed by long-term oral anticoagulation (warfarin). Anticoagulation therapy for acute thrombophlebitis prevents enlargement of the thrombus and allows for further attachment of the thrombus to the vessel wall thereby preventing PE.[229]

Management of DVT changed dramatically with the introduction of low–molecular weight heparin used as a bridge to warfarin. This new medication is more effective than the previously used unfractionated heparin, has fewer major bleeding complications, and does not require laboratory monitoring of coagulation tests to adjust medications, allowing for earlier hospital discharge or treatment at home. However, anticoagulation therapy does not effectively address the need to restore venous function in the thrombosed veins. Recanalization of the involved veins occurs in less than 10% of all cases, even with adequate anticoagulation therapy and despite symptomatic and clinical improvement.

Formerly, symptomatic intervention included bed rest for 3 to 5 days to prevent emboli and pressure fluctuations in the venous system that occur with walking; elevation of the leg with the knee flexed until the edema and tenderness subsided; and continuous local application of heat to relieve venospasm, produce analgesia, and promote resolution of inflammation. Ambulation (while wearing elastic stockings) was permitted if local tenderness and swelling had resolved (usually after 7 days for calf thrombosis and 10 to 14 days for thigh or pelvic thrombosis). Today, routine practice is to authorize ambulation in all

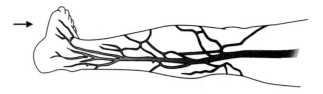

FIGURE   **11-30** Homans' sign, now considered an unreliable test for diagnosing DVT although still widely in use. Discomfort in the upper calf during gentle, forced dorsiflexion of the foot with the knee extended is a positive Homans' sign. This response may occur in the presence of thrombophlebitis as a result of the stretch imposed on the affected vessels. Homans' sign is not a specific finding in phlebitis because dorsiflexion may be painfully restricted with a variety of musculoskeletal conditions. Clinicians are encouraged to use available risk assessment scales in place of this test.[229]

cases of DVT after adequate anticoagulation has been administered (when the INR ratio is 2.0 to 3.0, usually after 48 hours)* if local symptoms and general condition permit. Elastic stockings must be worn whenever the person is ambulating or in the upright position. Local treatment (heat, elevation) can still be applied in the first week, and prolonged standing or sitting is still avoided for another 5 to 7 days.

For cases of massive DVT, thrombolysis, thrombectomy, and embolectomy (often performed in an interventional angiography laboratory) are being used with increasing skill and improved outcomes. New research is leading to the next generation of antithrombotic compounds such as direct coagulation factor inhibitors, tissue factor pathway inhibitors, the use of statins,[190] and gene therapy. Gene therapy for antithrombotic strategies can involve a number of different approaches, such as inhibition of coagulation factors, overexpression of anticoagulant factors, or modulation of endothelial biology to make thrombus formation or propagation unfavorable. Other investigators are looking at the systemic administration of recombinant tissue factor pathway inhibitor (TFPI) to decrease intimal hyperplasia after vascular injury and to suppress systemic mechanisms of blood coagulation and thrombosis.[258]

Prognosis.   DVTs that are not diagnosed can lead to life-threatening consequences, such as PE. With appropriate intervention and in the absence of complications, a return to normal health and activity can be expected within 1 to 3 weeks for the person with a calf DVT and within 6 weeks for the person with thigh or pelvic DVT. Prognosis depends on the size of the vessel involved, the presence of collateral circulation, and the underlying cause of the thrombosis (e.g., spinal cord injury, stroke, or neoplasm may prevent return to former health). Recurrence occurs in 5% of DVT cases and 1% of PE cases and may be related to risk factors listed in Table 11-23 or too short a time on anticoagulants. It remains unknown whether anticoagulant therapy should be extended for longer periods (>3 months), if lower intensity should be

---

*Low–molecular weight heparin has replaced unfractionated heparin because of a predictable pharmacokinetic profile, high bioavailability, a long plasma half-life, and an easy means of administration (subcutaneous injection) without the need to monitor activated partial thromboplastin time.[246]

*The concern in an acute care or rehabilitation setting is the increased risk of PE in clients who are aggressively mobilized too soon after a diagnosis of a DVT and before adequate anticoagulation has been administered. At least 48 to 72 hours of bed rest is considered prudent before returning a person with acute DVT to ambulation and physical therapy. A large cohort prospective study to assess the risk of PE with early mobilization has been recommended.[135]

recommended during this extension (i.e., with a target INR of less than 2.0), or if the benefits of extended anticoagulant therapy outweigh the risk of bleeding complications.

A potential long-term complication of DVT is venous stasis insufficiency (postphlebitic syndrome) when permanent damage to the vein has occurred; see the section on Chronic Venous Insufficiency in this chapter. Between 25% and 30% of people who had DVT treated with anticoagulants will develop some form of postthrombotic syndrome in the first 10 years following DVT. The National Institutes of Health are investigating the combined use of anticoagulants and thrombolytics to preserve the patency of the veins thereby reducing the frequency of post-thrombotic syndromes compared to anticoagulation therapy alone. Previously, the prohibitive cost, need for hospitalization, and procedural complications associated with thrombolytic therapy have prevented their use in proximal DVT.

Special Implications for the Therapist   11-20

THROMBOPHLEBITIS

Preferred Practice Patterns:
6A: Primary Prevention/Risk Reduction for
*   Cardiovascular/Pulmonary Disorders*
7A: Primary Prevention/Risk Reduction for Integumentary
*   Disorders*

Risk Assessment
Populations at risk (see Table 11-23), especially postoperative, postpartum, and immobilized clients, should be identified by the medical staff and observed carefully. Risk factor assessment scales (e.g., Autar DVT scale) for use in a therapy practice are available.[15,16,229] Using seven risk categories (i.e., increasing age, body mass index, immobility, special DVT risk, trauma, surgery, high-risk disease), the therapist can accurately predict and categorize each person's risk for venous thromboembolic disease as no risk (<10%), low risk (10%), moderate risk (11% to 40%), or high risk (>41%).[229]

The person at risk for DVT secondary to fracture and subsequent immobility involving a lower extremity cast should be carefully evaluated when the cast is removed. Normally, calf muscle atrophy is easily observed when the cast is removed. Normal calf size (less than 1-cm difference between left and right) without atrophy on cast removal may signal swelling associated with DVT. For the client with diagnosed thrombophlebitis, the therapist should monitor and report any signs of PE, such as chest pain, hemoptysis, cough, diaphoresis, dyspnea, and apprehension. Clients with a history of DVT may develop chronic venous insufficiency even years later and therefore must be monitored periodically for life.

Anyone receiving anticoagulant therapy (e.g., Coumadin [warfarin]) must be monitored for manifestations of bleeding, as evidenced by blood in the urine, in the stool, or along the gums or teeth; subcutaneous bruising; or back, pelvic, or flank pain. The presence of any of these signs or symptoms must be reported to the physician immediately. The risk for bleeding is increased with alcohol use, especially if there is concomitant liver disease, since alcohol also can potentiate warfarin. Many herbs have nat-

ural anticoagulant effects that can potentiate the effect of warfarin, and others can counteract its effect. Ginkgo biloba, garlic, dong quai, dan shen, and ginseng (commonly ingested herbs in supplemental form) should not be used or taken at the same time with warfarin. Anyone using these products should be encouraged to discuss medication dosage with the prescribing physician. Eating large quantities of vitamin K–rich foods can also interfere with the drug's anticoagulant effects, requiring careful monitoring of food intake while on warfarin.

Bleeding under the skin and easy bruising in response to the slightest trauma can occur when platelet production is altered. This condition necessitates extreme care in the therapy setting, especially any intervention requiring soft tissue mobilization, manual therapy, or the use of any equipment, including modalities and weight-training devices. (See the section on Platelets in Chapter 39; see also Tables 39-5, 39-6, and 39-7.) Rarely, skin necrosis associated with the use of warfarin occurs presenting as large hemorrhagic blisters on the breasts, buttocks, thighs, and penis requiring wound care management.

Prevention and Intervention
Prevention is the key to treatment of thrombophlebitis, both preventing thrombus formation and preventing thrombi becoming emboli. Preventive therapy can be tailored to the individual's level of risk and may include active and passive range of motion exercise, early ambulation for brief but regular periods whenever possible, coughing and deep-breathing exercises, and proper positioning. The person at risk must be taught the importance of avoiding one position for prolonged periods and to avoid pillows under the legs postoperatively to facilitate venous return. At the same time, elevation of the legs just above the level of the heart aids blood flow by gravitational force and prevents venous stasis as a contributing factor to the formation of new thrombi. Placing the foot of the bed in Trendelenburg's position (6-inch elevation with slight knee bend to prevent popliteal pressure) decreases venous pressure and helps relieve pain and edema. Prolonged sitting in a chair in the early postoperative period should be avoided.

After thrombosis of a deep calf vein, elastic support hose should be worn for at least 6 to 8 weeks or longer if risk assessment is moderate or high. Helping the client find easier ways to put the hose on and explaining the purpose may increase compliance in using the hose consistently and correctly. Support pantyhose may be an acceptable alternative for some people who have trouble putting on the compressive stockings or who live in very hot climates. The hypothesis for the use of compressive or elastic stockings is that the compressive force applied by the stocking causes the vessel wall to become applied to the thrombus, thereby keeping the thrombus in its location and preventing movement inside the blood vessel. Without the external compressive force of the stockings, once the person stands, increased hydrostatic pressure causes venous distention and permits the thrombus to become free-floating inside the vessel.[229] ∎

Varicose Veins
Definition and Incidence.   Varicose veins are an abnormal dilation of veins, usually the saphenous veins of the lower extremities, leading to tortuosity (twisting and turning) of the vessel, incompetence of the valves, and a propensity to thrombosis. Women are affected more often than men (secondary to pregnancy) with leg varicosities until age 70 years,

when the gender ratio disappears. Forty-one percent of women ages 40 to 50 years and 72% of women ages 60 to 70 years have varicose veins.[102] This condition most often develops between the ages of 30 and 50 years for all persons. A separate but similar condition called *spider veins* or *telangiectasia* (broken capillaries) results in fine-lined networks of red, blue, or purple veins usually on the thighs, calves, and ankles. The veins may form patterns resembling a sunburst, a spider web (see Fig. 9-2), or a tree with branches but can also appear as short, unconnected, or parallel lines.

Etiologic and Risk Factors.   Varicose veins may be an inherited trait, but it is unclear whether the valvular incompetence is secondary to defective valves in the saphenous veins or to a fundamental weakness of the walls of the vein leading to dilation of the vessel. Periods of high venous pressure associated with heavy lifting or prolonged sitting or standing are risk factors. Hormonal changes (e.g., pregnancy, menopause, hormonal therapy) often contribute to the development of this condition by relaxing the vein walls. Other risk factors include pressure associated with pregnancy or obesity, heart failure, hemorrhoids, constipation, esophageal varices, and hepatic cirrhosis. Risk factors for spider veins are similar (age, hormones, familial predisposition) but also include local injury (past or present).

Pathogenesis.   Blood returning to the heart from the legs must flow upward through the veins, against the pull of gravity. This blood is milked upward, principally by the massaging action of the muscles against the veins. To prevent the blood from flowing backward, the veins contain one-way valves located at intervals, which operate in pairs by closing to stop the reverse movement of the blood. The vessels most commonly affected by varicosities are located just beneath the skin superficial to the deep fascia and function without the kind of support deep veins of the legs receive from surrounding muscles. As the one-way valves become incompetent or the veins become more elastic, the veins engorge with stagnant blood and become pooled. Any condition accompanied by pressure changes places a strain on these veins, and the lack of pumping action of the lower leg muscles causes blood to pool. Other sites involved include the hemorrhoidal plexus of the rectum and anal canal (either inside or outside the anal sphincter), submucosal veins of the distal esophagus, and the scrotum (varicocele).

The weight of the blood continually pressing downward against the closed venous valves causes the veins to distend and eventually lose their elasticity. When several valves lose their ability to function properly, the blood collects in the veins, causing the veins to become swollen and distended. During pregnancy, the uterus may press against the veins coming from the lower extremities and prevent the free flow of returning blood. More force is required to push the blood through the veins, and the increased back-pressure can result in varicose veins.

Clinical Manifestations.   The clinical picture is not directly correlated with the severity of the varicosities; extensive varicose veins may be asymptomatic, but minimal varicosities may result in multiple symptoms. The development of varicose veins is usually gradual; the most common symptom reported is a dull, aching heaviness, tension, or feeling of fatigue brought on by periods of standing. Cramps of the lower legs may occur, especially at night, and elevation of the legs often provides relief. Itching from an associated dermatitis may also occur above the ankle.

The most visible sign of varicosities is the dilated, tortuous, elongated veins beneath the skin, which are usually readily visible when the person is standing (Fig. 11-31). Varicosities of long duration may be accompanied by secondary tissue changes, such as a brownish pigmentation of the skin and a thinning of the skin above the ankle. Swelling may also occur around the ankles. Untreated, the veins become thick and hard to the touch; impaired circulation and skin changes may lead to ulcers of the lower legs, especially around the ankles (see Table 11-21). (See also the section on Esophageal Varices in Chapter 15.) One of the most important distinctions between varicose veins and spider veins is that in some cases, varicose veins can result in thromboses (blood clots) and phlebitis (inflammation of the vein) or venous insufficiency ulcers. Spider veins are merely a cosmetic issue with no adverse effects.

Medical Management
Diagnosis.   The physician must distinguish between the symptoms of arteriosclerotic peripheral vascular disease, such as intermittent claudication and coldness of the feet, and symptoms of venous disease, because occlusive arterial disease usually contraindicates the operative management of varicosities below the knee. When the two conditions coexist, the reduced blood flow caused by the atherosclerosis may even improve the varicosities by reducing blood flow through the veins.

Visual inspection and palpation identify varicose veins of the legs, and Doppler ultrasonography or the duplex scanner is useful in detecting the location of incompetent valves. Endoscopy or radiographic diagnosis identifies esophageal varices, rectal examination or proctoscopy is used to diagnose hemorrhoids, and palpation identifies varicocele (scrotal swelling).

Treatment.   Treatment of mild varicose veins is conservative, consisting of periodic daily rest periods with feet elevated slightly above the heart. Client education as to the importance of promoting circulation is stressed, including instructions to make frequent changes in posture, a daily exercise program, and the appropriate use of properly fitting elastic stockings.

When varicosities have progressed past the stage at which conservative care is helpful, surgical intervention and compression sclerotherapy may be considered. In the past, surgical treatment of varicose veins consisted of removing the varicosities and the incompetent perforating veins (ligation and stripping), a procedure sometimes referred to as *stripping the veins* or *miniphlebectomy*. Other procedures for varicose veins have been developed including radiofrequency (radio waves used to seal off the vein), sclerotherapy (injections of a hardening, or sclerosing, solution; over several months' time, the injected veins atrophy and blood is channeled into other veins), and laser therapy (noninvasive use of near-infrared wavelengths). Ligation and stripping the greater saphenous vein prevent its use as a source for future coronary artery bypass grafts, motivating researchers to develop effective intervention techniques that salvage large veins.

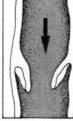

FIGURE 11-31 **A,** Diagrams of normal (*top*) and varicose (*bottom*) veins. **B,** Person with varicose veins. (**A** from O'Toole M, editor: *Miller-Keane encyclopedia and dictionary of medicine, nursing, and allied health*, ed 6, Philadelphia, 1997, Saunders, p 1702. **B** from Jarvis C: *Physical examination and health assessment*, Philadelphia, 1992, Saunders, p 660.)

NORMAL VEINS

Functional valves aid in flow of venous blood back to heart

(see enlargement at left)

A

VARICOSE VEINS

Failure of valves and pooling of blood in superficial veins

B

Oral dietary supplementation has been adopted by some individuals as an addition to traditional management of varicose veins. The loss of vascular integrity associated with the pathogenesis of both hemorrhoids and varicose veins may be aided by several botanical extracts shown to improve microcirculation, capillary flow, and vascular tone while strengthening the connective tissue of the perivascular substrate.[146]

Prognosis. Good results with relief of symptoms are usually possible in the majority of cases. Early conservative care for varicose veins during initial stages may help prevent the condition from worsening, but advanced disease may not be prevented from recurring even with surgical intervention or sclerotherapy. Although surgery for varicose veins can improve appearance, it may not reduce the physical discomfort, suggesting that most lower limb symptoms may have a nonvenous cause. A high mortality is associated with ruptured, bleeding esophageal varices (see Chapter 15).

already diagnosed with, varicose veins. Since excessive sitting or standing contributes to this condition, the therapist can individualize a program to help the person avoid static postures and utilize quick stretch or movement breaks coordinated with deep-breathing exercises. Over-the-counter pantyhose should be replaced with special compressive hose that do not constrict behind the knee, upper leg, waist, or groin. These should be worn as much as possible during the daytime hours (including during exercise for some people) but may be removed at night. After exercise and at the end of the day, instruct the individual to elevate the legs in a supported position above the level of the heart for 10 to 15 minutes. Encourage the person to practice good breathing techniques during this time. Aerobic exercise, strength training, or resistive exercises are encouraged, but high-impact activities, such as jogging or step aerobics, should be avoided. Brisk walking, cycling, cross-country skiing or Nordic track, rowing, and swimming are all good alternatives to high-impact activities. ■

Special Implications for the Therapist 11-21

VARICOSE VEINS

Preferred Practice Patterns:
6A: *Primary Prevention/Risk Reduction for Cardiovascular/Pulmonary Disorders*
7A: *Primary Prevention/Risk Reduction for Integumentary Disorders (other Integumentary patterns may apply depending on progression of disease or chronic complications)*

The therapist can be very instrumental in developing prescriptive exercise and preventive measures for anyone at risk for, or

Chronic Venous Insufficiency

Definition and Incidence. Chronic venous insufficiency (CVI), also known as postphlebitic syndrome and venous stasis, is defined as inadequate venous return over a long period of time. This condition follows most severe cases of DVT although it is possible to develop CVI without prior episodes of DVT. CVI may also occur as a result of leg trauma, varicose veins, and neoplastic obstruction of the pelvic veins. The long-term sequelae of CVI may be chronic leg ulcers accounting for the majority of vascular ulceration; incidence is expected to continue rising with the aging of America.[168]

Etiologic Factors and Pathogenesis. CVI occurs when damaged or destroyed valves in the veins result in decreased venous return, thereby increasing venous pressure and producing venous stasis. Without adequate valve function and in the absence of the calf muscle pump, blood flows in the veins bi-directionally, causing high ambulatory venous pressures in the calf veins (venous hypertension). Superficial veins and capillaries dilate in response to the venous hypertension. Red blood cells, proteins, and fluids leak out of the capillaries into interstitial spaces, producing edema and the reddish brown pigmentation characteristic of CVI.

Chronic pooling of blood in the veins of the lower extremities prevents adequate cellular oxygenation and removal of waste products. Any trauma, especially pressure, further lowers the oxygen supply by reducing blood flow into the area. Cell death occurs, and necrotic tissue develops into venous stasis ulcers. The cycle of reduced oxygenation, necrosis, and ulceration prevents damaged tissue from obtaining necessary nutrients, causing delayed healing and persistent ulceration. Poor circulation impairs immune and inflammatory responses, leaving venous stasis ulcers susceptible to infection.

Other contributing factors may include poor nutrition, immobility, and local trauma (past or present). A previous history of burns requiring skin grafts predisposes the individual to venous insufficiency. The area of the graft usually lacks superficial veins, properly functioning capillaries, or both, resulting in blood pooling in these areas. As a result previously burned areas and skin grafts in the lower extremity are susceptible to vascular ulceration.

Clinical Manifestations.   CVI is characterized by progressive edema of the leg; thickening, coarsening, and brownish pigmentation of skin around the ankles; and venous stasis ulceration (see Table 11-21). Venous insufficiency ulcers constitute approximately 80% of all lower extremity ulcers occurring most often above the medial malleolus where venous hypertension is greatest. These ulcers characteristically are shallow wounds with a white creamy to fibrous slough over a base of good granulation tissue. They generally produce little pain and a moderate to large amount of drainage. The wounds typically have irregular borders, partial to full thickness, often with signs of reepithelialization (e.g., pink or red granulation base). Frequently, moderate to severe edema is present in the limb; in long-standing cases, this edema becomes hardened to a dense, woody texture. The skin of the involved extremity is usually thin, shiny, dry, and cyanotic. Dermatitis and cellulitis may develop later in this condition.

Medical Management.   The physician will differentiate between CVI and other causes of edema and ulceration of the lower extremities using client history, clinical examination, and diagnostic tests to rule out or confirm superimposed acute phlebitis. Arterial and venous insufficiency may co-exist in the same person.

Treatment goals and techniques are as for varicose veins (increase in venous return, reduction of edema). Conventional methods of compression and rest and elevation (e.g., more frequent periods of leg elevation above the level of the heart are encouraged throughout the day with the foot of the bed elevated 6 inches at night) have been augmented by surgical intervention. Rapid progress in endovascular procedures with angioplasty and stenting has made it possible for the development of techniques to relieve obstruction and repair reflux in the deep veins. Venous stasis ulcers require ongoing treatment, usually involving the therapist (e.g., primary intervention for edema reduction and topical ulcer and wound care). More detailed information is available.[112,136,222,223] Researchers are developing bioengineered skin, a living human dermal replacement for the management of venous ulcers. See the section on Skin Transplantation in Chapter 20.

The prognosis is poor for resolution of CVI, with chronic venous stasis ulcers causing loss of function and progressive disability. Recurrent episodes of acute thrombophlebitis may occur, and noncompliance with the treatment program is common.

Special Implications for the Therapist   **11-22**

CHRONIC VENOUS INSUFFICIENCY

Preferred Practice Patterns:
6A: *Primary Prevention/Risk Reduction for*
       Cardiovascular/Pulmonary Disorders
7A: *Primary Prevention/Risk Reduction for Integumentary*
       Disorders (prevent complications of bed rest)
7B: *Impaired Integumentary Integrity Associated With*
       Superficial Skin Involvement (other Integumentary patterns may apply depending on progression of condition)

The therapist can be very instrumental in providing clients with venous insufficiency with education and prevention to avoid complications that can occur with vascular ulceration and chronic wounds. Formulating an exercise prescription; collaborating with a nutritionist; and understanding the underlying etiology, hemodynamics, co-morbidities, and principles of tissue repair are essential in developing a plan of care. Compression therapy (e.g., bandages, stockings, pumps) to promote venous return from peripheral veins to central circulation is an intervention modality often administered with CVI especially with venous leg ulcers; the therapist may also use Unna's boot (see Fig. 9-8). The presence of CHF is considered a precaution to the use of external compression and requires close collaboration between the physician and therapist.

An assessment of the legs should be performed frequently to observe for stasis ulcers, skin changes (e.g., color, texture, temperature), impaired growth of nails, and discrepancy in size of extremities, including observations and measurements for edema. In the home health setting, the client or family should be instructed to contact a member of the medical team if any edema or change in the condition of the extremity occurs. When a stasis ulcer of any size is detected, treatment is initiated. A wound care specialist (usually a physical therapist or a nurse) is a vital part of the health care team in the management of stasis ulcers. Specific wound care management is available elsewhere.[112,136,222,223] Whirlpool beyond an initial one or two treatments is contraindicated, because the increased blood volume and dependent position (underlying causes of wound) can make the edema worse. When pulsatile debridement devices are unavailable, limited hydrotherapy (maximal temperature 80° F) may be indicated to remove loose debris, and toxic antiseptics may be indicated to moisten dried exudate or to facilitate debridement.

The client should be advised to avoid prolonged standing and sitting; crossing the legs; sitting too high for feet to touch the floor or too deep, causing pressure against the popliteal space;

Continued

and wearing tight clothing (including girdles, elastic waistbands, or too tight jeans) or support hose or stockings that extend above the knee, which act as a tourniquet at the popliteal fossa. Thigh-high elastic stockings are recommended, but they must be worn properly to avoid bunching behind the knee.

Arterial obstruction in the presence of venous insufficiency may not be readily recognized. Wounds associated with CVI that do not demonstrate healing within 2 weeks of beginning wound care may undergo a noninvasive arterial Doppler study (ankle/brachial index) to determine the level of circulation. This index is the result of a vascular diagnostic test comparing the systolic blood pressure between the ankle and brachial pulses. An index result of 1.0 indicates an adequate arterial blood supply; an index less than 1.0 indicates insufficient blood flow to the distal regions for healing to occur (see Box 11-10). ■

BOX 11-11

Collagen Vascular Diseases

Ankylosing spondylitis
Dermatomyositis
Localized (cutaneous) scleroderma
Mixed connective tissue disease
Polyarteritis nodosa
Polymyalgia rheumatica
Polymyositis
Rheumatoid arthritis (RA)
Sjögren's syndrome
Systemic lupus erythematosus (SLE)
Systemic sclerosis (scleroderma)
Temporal arteritis

Vasomotor Disorders.   Vasomotor disorders of the blood vessels causing headaches and reflex sympathetic dystrophy (now classified as complex regional pain syndrome) are discussed in Chapters 36 and 38, respectively.

Raynaud's Disease and Raynaud's Phenomenon

Definition and Overview.   Intermittent episodes of small artery or arteriole constriction of the extremities causing temporary pallor and cyanosis of the digits (fingers more often than toes) and changes in skin temperature are called *Raynaud's phenomenon*. These episodes occur in response to cold temperature or strong emotion, such as anxiety or excitement. When this condition is a primary vasospastic disorder it is called (idiopathic) *Raynaud's disease*. If the disorder is secondary to another disease or underlying cause, the term Raynaud's phenomenon is used.

Incidence and Etiology Factors

Raynaud's Disease.   Eighty percent of persons with Raynaud's disease are women between the ages of 20 and 49 years. The exact etiology of Raynaud's disease remains unknown, but it appears to be caused by hypersensitivity of digital arteries to cold, release of serotonin, and genetic susceptibility to vasospasm. Raynaud's disease accounts for 65% of all people affected by this condition. Raynaud's disease is usually experienced as more annoying than medically serious.

Raynaud's Phenomenon.   Epidemiologists estimate that Raynaud's phenomenon is a problem for 10% to 20% of the general population; it affects women 20 times more frequently than men, usually between the ages of 15 and 40 years. Risk factors for Raynaud's phenomenon are different between men and women. The Framingham Offspring Study reports that age and smoking are associated with Raynaud's phenomenon in men only, whereas marital status and alcohol use were observed in women only. These findings suggest that different mechanisms influence the expression of Raynaud's phenomenon in men and women.[75] Raynaud's phenomenon as a condition secondary to another disease is often associated with Buerger's disease or connective tissue disorders (collagen vascular diseases), such as Sjögren's syndrome, scleroderma, polymyositis and dermatomyositis, mixed connective tissue disease, SLE, and rheumatoid arthritis (Box 11-11). Raynaud's phenomenon can be a sign of occult (hidden) neoplasm, especially suspected when it presents unilaterally.

Raynaud's phenomenon may also occur with change in temperature, such as occurs when going from a warm outside environment to an air-conditioned room. In addition, Raynaud's phenomenon may be associated with occlusive arterial diseases and neurogenic lesions, such as thoracic outlet syndrome, or with the effects of long-term exposure to cold (occupational or frostbite), trauma, or use of vibrating equipment such as jackhammers. Injuries to the small vessels of the hands may produce Raynaud's phenomenon. The trauma can be a result of repetitive stress that comes from using crutches for extended periods, typing on a computer keyboard, or even playing the piano.

Several medications (e.g., beta-blockers, ergot alkaloids prescribed for migraine headaches, antineoplastics used in chemotherapy) have also been implicated. Because nicotine causes small blood vessels to constrict, smoking can trigger attacks in persons who are predisposed to this phenomenon.

Pathogenesis and Clinical Manifestations.   Scientists theorize that Raynaud's phenomenon is associated with a disturbance in the control of vascular reflexes. Although the causes differ for Raynaud's disease and Raynaud's phenomenon, the clinical manifestations are the same, based on a pathogenesis of arterial vasospasm in the skin. It begins with the release of chemical messengers, which cause blood vessels to constrict and remain constricted. The flow of oxygenated blood to these areas is reduced, and the skin becomes pale and cold. The blood in the constricted vessels, which has released its oxygen to the tissues surrounding the vessels, pools in the tissues, producing a bluish or purplish color. In the case of fibromyalgia-associated Raynaud's phenomenon, symptoms may be the result of cold-induced spasms of the arteries caused by a problem in the autonomic nervous system control of the blood supply to the extremities. Altered or reduced numbers of alpha$_2$-adrenergic receptors on the platelets correlate with Raynaud's phenomenon in fibromyalgia-associated Raynaud's.[19] These receptors are involved in the functioning of the autonomic nervous system. This could explain why the cold-induced pain is significant but without skin color changes in this population.

In most cases, the skin color progresses from blue to white to red. First, ischemia from vasospastic attacks causes cyanosis, numbness, and the sensation of cold in the digits (thumbs usually remain unaffected). The affected tissues become numb or painful. For unknown reasons, the flow of chemical that triggered the process eventually stops. The vessels relax, and blood flow is restored. The skin becomes white (characterized by pallor) and then red (characterized by rubor) as the vasospasm subsides and the capillaries become engorged with oxygenated blood. Oxygen-rich blood returns to the area, and as it does so, the skin becomes warm and flushed. The person may experience throbbing, paresthesia, and slight swelling as this occurs.

Sensory changes, such as numbness, stiffness, diminished sensation, and aching pain, often accompany vasomotor manifestations. Initially, no abnormal findings are present between attacks, but over time, frequent, prolonged episodes of vasospasm causing ischemia interfere with cellular metabolism, causing the skin of the fingertips to thicken and the fingernails to become brittle. In severe, chronic Raynaud's phenomenon, the underlying condition may have produced scars in the vessels, reducing the vessel diameter and therefore blood flow. When attacks occur, they are often more severe, resulting in prolonged loss of blood to fingers and toes, which can produce painful skin ulcers; rarely, gangrene may develop. Episodes of Raynaud's disease are often bilateral, progressing distally to proximally along the digits. Raynaud's phenomenon may be unilateral, involving only one or two fingers, but this clinical presentation warrants a physician's differential diagnosis, since it can be associated with cancer (Fig. 11-32).

Medical Management
Diagnosis and Prognosis. Diagnosis is usually made by clinical presentation and past medical history. Raynaud's disease is diagnosed by a history of symptoms for at least 2 years with no progression and no evidence of underlying cause. Raynaud's disease must be differentiated from the numerous possible disorders associated with Raynaud's phenomenon. Untreated and uncontrolled Raynaud's may damage or destroy the affected digits. Rarely, necrosis, ulceration, and gangrene re-

sult. Even with intervention, the person with Raynaud's disease or phenomenon may experience disability and loss of function.

Prevention and Treatment. Treatment for *Raynaud's disease* is limited to prevention or alleviation of the vasospasm because no underlying cause or condition has been discovered although pharmacologic agents for primary and secondary Raynaud's phenomenon are under investigation. Clients are encouraged to avoid stimuli that trigger attacks, such as cool or cold temperatures, changes in temperature, and emotional stress, and to eliminate use of nicotine, which has a constricting effect on blood vessels. Physical or occupational therapy is often prescribed and should include client education about managing symptoms through protective skin care and cold protection (see Table 11-22), biofeedback, stress management and relaxation techniques, whirlpool or other gentle heat modalities, and exercise. Large movement arm circles in a windmill fashion can restore circulation in some people. The individual will have to experiment with the speed at which to move the arms; some people benefit from slow, gentle movement whereas others find greater success with fast rotations. Pharmacologic management may include vasodilators and nonaddicting analgesics for pain. Therapists can be instrumental in teaching physiologic modulation starting with hand warming. The use of a hand-held device to measure fingertip temperature combined with self-guided or audio-guided relaxation can be very effective and is available.[114]

When conservative care fails to relieve symptoms and the condition progresses clinically, sympathetic blocks followed by intensive therapy may be helpful. Sympathectomy may be necessary for persons who only temporarily benefit from the sympathetic blocks.

Treatment for *Raynaud's phenomenon* consists of appropriate treatment for the underlying condition or removing the stimulus causing vasospasm. The clinical care described for Raynaud's disease may also be of benefit. In addition, the use of antioxidants as an effective treatment of Raynaud's phenomenon as well as the role of therapeutic angiogenesis (regeneration of vessels) remains under investigation.

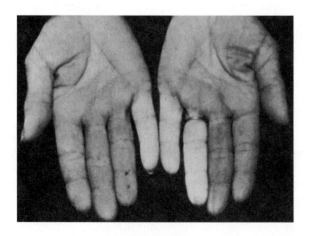

FIGURE **11-32** Raynaud's disease or phenomenon. White color (pallor) from arteriospasm and resulting deficit in blood supply may initially involve only one or two fingers, as shown here. Cold and numbness or pain may accompany the pallor or cyanosis stage. Subsequent episodes may involve the entire finger and may include all the fingers. Toes are affected in 40% of cases. (From Jarvis C: *Physical examination and health assessment*, ed 3, Philadelphia, 2000, Saunders, p 575.)

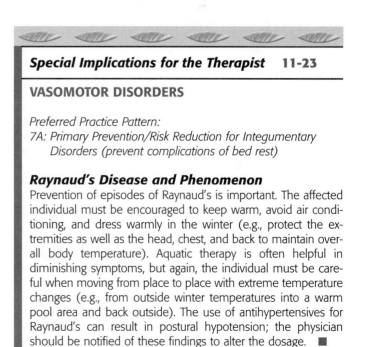

Special Implications for the Therapist 11-23

VASOMOTOR DISORDERS

Preferred Practice Pattern:
7A: Primary Prevention/Risk Reduction for Integumentary Disorders (prevent complications of bed rest)

Raynaud's Disease and Phenomenon
Prevention of episodes of Raynaud's is important. The affected individual must be encouraged to keep warm, avoid air conditioning, and dress warmly in the winter (e.g., protect the extremities as well as the head, chest, and back to maintain overall body temperature). Aquatic therapy is often helpful in diminishing symptoms, but again, the individual must be careful when moving from place to place with extreme temperature changes (e.g., from outside winter temperatures into a warm pool area and back outside). The use of antihypertensives for Raynaud's can result in postural hypotension; the physician should be notified of these findings to alter the dosage. ■

Special Implications for the Therapist   11-24

PERIPHERAL VASCULAR DISEASE

Preferred Practice Patterns:

4C: Impaired Muscle Performance

4J: Impaired Motor Function, Muscle Performance, Range of Motion, Gait, Locomotion, and Balance Associated With Amputation

6B: Impaired Aerobic Capacity/Endurance Associated With Deconditioning

6D: Impaired Aerobic Capacity/Endurance Associated With Cardiovascular Pump Dysfunction or Failure

7A: Primary Prevention/Risk Reduction for Integumentary Disorders (prevent complications of bed rest; other Integumentary patterns may apply depending on progression of disease and clinical manifestations)

Even though Special Implications for the Therapist boxes for each individual disease making up PVD have been presented, a brief overview or summary of PVD as a whole seems warranted and a reminder that because of the prevalence of atherosclerotic disease in anyone with PVD, heart rate and blood pressure should be monitored during the evaluative process and during initial interventions. This is especially important in cases of diabetes mellitus and anyone who has undergone an amputation, which implies severe disease. Notably, people with PAD may exhibit precipitous rises in blood pressure during exercise owing to the atherosclerotic process present and the diminished vascular bed.[243] Examination of the pedal pulses should be part of the physical examination for all clients older than 55 years, and measurement of the ABI is recommended for those who have diminished or nonpalpable pedal pulses but who do not have diabetes.[9] For the client with back pain, buttock pain, or leg pain of unknown or previously undiagnosed cause, screening for medical disease including assessment of risk factors, past medical history, and special tests and measures (e.g., bicycle test, palpation of pulses) is essential.[91,96]

PVD can be confusing, with the wide range of diseases affecting veins and arteries, the etiology of which is sometimes occlusive, sometimes inflammatory, and, occasionally, as in the case of Buerger's disease, both occlusive and inflammatory. The basic point to keep in mind is how arterial disease differs (significantly) from venous disease in clinical presentation, pathogenesis, and management. Focusing on the underlying etiologic factors is the key to choosing the most appropriate and effective intervention. For example, in the case of acute arterial disease, the tissues are not oxygenated and ischemia can result in local trauma or burns; gangrene can develop quickly. The goal is to increase oxygen without increasing demand or need for oxygen. Claudication occurs when the activity causes increased oxygen demand in an already compromised area.

During the acute phase of arterial ischemia rehabilitation, intervention and movement are minimized, heat and massage are contraindicated, and the person is instructed in the use of positions that will increase blood flow to the tissues involved (e.g., head elevated with legs slightly lower than the heart). Chronic arterial disease can be treated by the therapist concentrating on improving collateral circulation and increasing vasodilation. The role of exercise in peripheral arterial disease (especially in reducing claudication) has been well-documented[27] (see also the section on Arterial Occlusive Diseases in this chapter).

In venous disorders, the tissues are oxygenated but the blood is not moving, and stasis occurs. With venous occlusion, the skin is discolored rather than pale (ranging from angry red to deep blue-purple), edema is prominent, and pain is most marked at the site of occlusion, although extreme edema can render all the skin of the limb quite tender. The goal of therapy is to create compressive pumping forces to move fluid volume and reduce edema. For this reason, heat or cold, compressive stockings, massage, and activity (e.g., ankle pumps, heel slides, quad sets, ambulation) are part of the treatment protocol.

Further guidelines for exercise in the management of peripheral vascular disease are outlined elsewhere.[7,99] See also the previous section on Arteriosclerotic Obliterans (Peripheral Arterial Disease [PAD]). Modifying cardiovascular risk factors, improving exercise duration and decreasing claudication, preventing joint contractures and muscle atrophy, preventing skin ulcerations, promoting healing of any pressure ulcers, and improving quality of life are part of the therapy plan of care. In the case of lower extremity amputation the use of unweighted ambulation to reduce the physiologic demands of walking during early rehabilitation has been reported.[166] For people with vascular ulcers, improving the arterial supply or venous return will lessen pain, increase mobility, and allow ulcers to heal. Whenever ulcers are present, understanding the type of ulcer and underlying etiology will point to the best intervention. The assessment and therapeutic intervention of vascular wounds are beyond the scope of this text; the reader is referred to other more appropriate texts.[136,222,223] ■

◆ Vascular Neoplasms

Malignant vascular (i.e., involving the blood vessels) neoplasms are extremely rare and may include angiosarcoma, hemangiopericytoma, and Kaposi's sarcoma. *Angiosarcomas* (hemangiosarcomas) can occur in either gender and at any age, most commonly appearing as small, painless, red nodules on the skin, soft tissue, breast, bone, liver, and spleen. Almost one half of all people with angiosarcoma die of the disease. *Hemangiopericytoma* arises from the smooth muscle cells that are external to the walls of capillaries and arterioles. Most commonly located on the lower extremities and retroperitoneum (space between the peritoneum lining of the walls of the abdominal and pelvic cavities and the posterior abdominal wall) these tumors are composed of spindle cells with a rich vascular network. Metastasis to the lungs, bone, liver, and lymph nodes occurs in 10% to 50% of cases, but the majority of hemangiopericytomas are removed surgically without having invaded or metastasized.

Kaposi's sarcoma in association with AIDS most likely occurs as a result of loss of immunity. One form of the tumor resembles a simple hemangioma with tightly packed clusters of capillaries, most often visible on the skin. Although Kaposi's sarcoma is malignant and may be widespread in the body, it is not usually a cause of death.

◆ Arteriovenous Malformations

Arteriovenous malformations (AVMs) are congenital vascular malformations of the cerebral vasculature. AVMs are the result of localized maldevelopment of part of the primitive vascular plexus consisting of abnormal arteriovenous communications without intervening capillaries. There is a central tangled mass of fragile, abnormal blood vessels called the *nidus* that shunts blood from cerebral feeding arteries directly into cerebral veins. The loss of the normal capillary network between the high-pressure arterial system and the low-pressure venous system results in a faster flow and elevated pressure within the delicate vessels of the AVM. The lack of a gradient pressure system predisposes the lesion to rupture.

AVMs vary in size, ranging from massive lesions that are fed by multiple vessels to lesions too small to identify. Perfusion to adjacent brain tissue may be impaired because blood flow is diverted to the AVM, a phenomenon referred to as *vascular stealing*. AVMs may occur in any blood vessel, but the most common sites include the brain, GI tract, and skin. Approximately 10% of cases present with aneurysms. Small AVMs are more likely to bleed than large ones, and once bleeding occurs, repeated episodes are likely. Clinical presentation depends on the location of the malformation and may relate to hemorrhage from the malformation or an associated aneurysm or to cerebral ischemia caused by diversion or stasis of blood. Seizures, migrainelike headaches unresponsive to standard therapy, and progressive neurologic deficits may develop.

Diagnostic testing and planned intervention rely on cerebral angiography to show the AVM size, location, feeding vessels, nidus, and venous outflow vessels. Other tests may include MRI, x-rays, ultrasound, electroencephalogram (EEG), and arteriogram. Treatment options are individualized depending on the size and location of the lesion as well as any other surgical risks present. In the last 10 years, endovascular embolization and stereotactic radiosurgery (delivery of extremely precise doses of radiation to destroy abnormal blood vessels) have increased survival outcomes, especially for lesions previously considered inoperable or in cases of high surgical risk factors. Prognosis is guarded, since there is a 2% to 4% chance of hemorrhage with the concomitant risk of permanent neurologic deficit or even death.

Special Implications for the Therapist   11-25

ARTERIOVENOUS MALFORMATIONS

Generally, the individual with a known AVM is advised to avoid activities and exercise that can increase intracranial or blood pressure (see Box 15-1). Weight training and contact sports are contraindicated, and some physicians advise against high-aerobic exercise including running. Postoperative complications can include hemorrhage, seizures, nausea, vomiting, or headache, and symptomatic perilesional edema can occur up to 1 year after the procedure. Neurologic deficits vary but are usually transient; radiation-induced brain injury is rare. The radiation's effect begins immediately, but complete obliteration of the lesion can take up to 3 years, during which time the affected individual must continue to maintain a normal blood pressure. ■

◆ The Lymphatic Vessels

The lymphatic system (see also the section on The Lymphatic System in Chapter 12) is part of the circulatory system that collects excess tissue fluid and plasma that has leaked out of capillaries into the interstitial space and returns it to the bloodstream. The lymphatic system consists of lymphatic vessels and lymph nodes and functions to remove impurities from the circulatory system and to produce cells of the immune system (lymphocytes) that are vital in fighting bacteria and viruses. The lymph nodes are also part of the lymphoid system, the organs and tissues of the immune system. All the lymphoid organs link the hematologic and immune systems in that they are sites of residence, proliferation, differentiation, or function of lymphocytes and mononuclear phagocytes (mononuclear phagocyte system).

Disorders of the lymphatic system may result from inflammation of a lymphatic vessel (lymphangitis), inflammation of one or more lymph nodes (lymphadenitis), an increased amount of lymph (lymphedema), or enlargement of the lymph nodes (lymphadenopathy). There are also three forms of lymph vascular insufficiency that can occur. The first, *dynamic insufficiency*, occurs when the lymphatic load exceeds the lymphatic transport capacity. In this situation, the anatomy of the lymphatic system and its function are normal but are overwhelmed. A second form of insufficiency of the lymph vascular system is caused by a reduction of the lymphatic transport capacity below the level of a normal lymphatic protein load. This reduction results in low lymph flow failure called *mechanical insufficiency*. A third form of lymph vascular insufficiency occurs when the lymphatic system has a reduced transport capacity, leading to an overflowing of lymph. This form is called *safety valve insufficiency*. For a complete discussion of the lymphatic system, see Chapter 12.

OTHER CARDIAC CONSIDERATIONS

Despite the success of new immunosuppressive regimens and better results with transplantation, few people who are dying of heart failure will actually have the opportunity to receive a heart transplant. The mechanical technology may eventually allow selected persons to receive long-term (permanent) support as a substitute for cardiac transplantation. The recipient is often home in 6 weeks with follow-up home health care. In the future, studies may be done to determine the efficacy of removing the cardiac assistive device after prolonged heart rest provides cardiac recovery. Survival with the natural recovered heart may be possible in some people.

Researchers are actively pursuing tissue engineering to replace transplantation and mechanical devices (e.g., artificial heart, implanted cardiac assistive devices or other bridges to transplantation) to help keep people alive while they await heart transplant or as a replacement intervention for transplantation.

◆ The Cardiac Client and Surgery

Persons with previously diagnosed cardiac disease undergoing general or orthopedic surgery are at risk for additional postoperative complications. Anesthesia and surgery are often associated with marked fluctuations of heart rate and blood pressure, changes in intravascular volume, myocardial ischemia or depression, arrhythmias, decreased oxygenation, and increased sympathetic nervous system activity. In addition, changes in medications, surgical trauma, wound healing, infection, hemorrhage, and pulmonary insufficiency may overwhelm the diseased heart. All these factors place an additional stress on the cardiac client during the perioperative period.

Cardiac surgery via median sternotomy requires a longitudinal incision and disruption of the sternum. During the operative procedure, the bone is rewired with stainless steel wire and fixed with low separation strength and security of closure approximately 5% of norm (this increases to 90% of normal strength at 6 weeks for most people).[155] A single-lung transplantation requires a posterolateral thoracotomy, whereas a double-lung transplant requires bilateral anterior thoracotomies referred to as a "clam shell." In this latter procedure, the rib cage and sternum are lifted perpendicularly as the hood of a car would be lifted. The heart-lung procedure is still done by open sternotomy.

Complications following a sternotomy include mediastinitis, poor wound healing, chronic pain, posttraumatic stress disorder, and more rarely, brachial plexus injury. Risk factors for these complications may include obesity, osteoporosis, diabetes or other co-morbidities, women who have large breasts (the weight of both breasts puts additional traction on sutures), and client noncompliance or poor compliance. Efforts to develop a less invasive means of performing cardiac surgery may be possible with recent advances in technology, especially videoscopic visualization and the ability to provide myocardial protection. Surgeons are examining alternate techniques in hopes of reducing operative stress, postoperative pain, and postoperative recovery time. New procedures are being developed that eliminate the use of a sternotomy, such as the minithoracotomy or "keyhole" thoracotomy via a small incision that allows surgeons to operate on a beating heart. These alternate surgical techniques involve passing instruments through small incisions in the skin and muscle and between the ribs. Surgeons can suture bypass vessels around blocked coronary arteries without shutting down the heart and rerouting the blood through a bypass machine.

Special Implications for the Therapist   11-26

CARDIAC CLIENT AND SURGERY

Noncardiac Surgery

Therapy for people with cardiovascular disease undergoing orthopedic surgery or neurosurgery is only altered by the need for more deliberate and careful monitoring of the person's response to activity and exercise. Postoperative rehabilitation may take longer because of the underlying cardiac condition and any complications that may arise as a result of cardiovascular compromise. Careful observation for DVT must be ongoing during the first 1 to 3 weeks postoperatively. Anyone with polycythemia or thrombocytopenia is at increased risk for hemorrhage, necessitating additional special precautions (see Chapter 13).

Physical therapy initiated in the intensive care unit focuses on restoring mobility, increasing strength, and improving balance and reflexes; heel slides, ankle pumps, and bedside standing are included in the early postoperative protocol. Pulmonary hygiene and breathing exercises are essential to prevent atelec-

tasis (particularly left lower lobe atelectasis), especially in the case of implantation of an artificial heart, because of the location of the device. Frequent, slow, rhythmic reaching, turning, bending, and stretching of the trunk and all extremities many times throughout the day help alleviate the surgical pain-tension cycle and facilitate pulmonary function.

Cardiac Surgery

Progressive ambulation can be initiated as soon as the client can transfer. In the case of open-heart surgery, sternal precautions are standard postoperative orders (see Box 11-2; see also Special Implications for the Therapist, 20-6: Lung Transplantation); preventing separation of the sternum may require hand-held assistance in place of assistive devices (e.g., walker, quad cane) initially. It is important to know whether the chest has been closed; the skin may be closed, but the chest is not. Upper extremity precautions are determined by the physician according to the surgery that was performed and the status of the incision. When the chest is closed, shoulder flexion and abduction can proceed until the point of movement at the chest wall or rib cage. This rotation can cause a torque, and further motion must be limited at that point.

When the client can ambulate 1000 feet, the treadmill (1 mile/hr) or exercise cycle (0.5 RPEs [rating of perceived exertion]) can be used (see Table 11-13), usually around the fourth postoperative day if there are no complications. Whether to use the treadmill or bicycle is generally an individual decision made by the client based on personal preference; presence of orthopedic problems must be taken into consideration. Resistive elastic or small weights and aerobic training are introduced between 4 and 6 weeks postoperatively. Pushing or pulling activities and lifting more than 10 lb are contraindicated in the first 4 to 6 weeks.

Chest (and in women, breast) discomfort, shortness of breath, upper quadrant myalgia (chest, arms, neck, upper back), palpitations, low activity tolerance, mood swings, and localized swelling in the case of grafts taken from the leg are all commonly reported in the early days and weeks after cardiac surgery. These clinical manifestations are minimized but not completely eliminated with the less invasive "keyhole" (minithoracotomy) surgery performed in some facilities.

Exercise

The use of lower extremity–derived aerobic exercise to improve hemodynamics, normalize heart rate, improve oxygen uptake and delivery, and decrease diastolic blood pressure has been well-documented and discussed earlier in this chapter. Many of these individuals have not exercised in years and remain deconditioned or fearful of exercise. The therapist must firmly encourage active participation in a program of physical activity and exercise for anyone who has given up and chosen to remain sedentary. Exercise tolerance must be monitored closely during the early weeks after surgery. The therapist is encouraged to use perceived exertion scales, such as the dyspnea index or Borg scale (see Table 11-13), monitor changes in diastolic pressure, and rely on measurements of oxygen uptake to set exercise limits.

Psychosocial Considerations

Psychologic and emotional recovery from cardiac surgery is not always addressed or discussed. Recent research has documented that cardiac surgery is often accompanied by significant cognitive decline, especially memory loss (verbal and visual), planning tasks (visuoconstruction), and psychomotor speed.

Additional research is needed to determine if the observed cognitive decline is related to the surgery itself (e.g., effects of anesthesia, hypoperfusion associated with use of the heart-lung bypass machine, disruption of atherosclerotic plaque-forming emboli), normal aging in a population with cardiovascular risk factors, or a combination of these and other factors.[203-205]

Depression is commonly reported after CABG and after cardiac surgery in general. The majority of people who are depressed after cardiac surgery were depressed before surgery. There does not appear to be any correlation between depressed mood and cognitive decline after cardiac surgery, which suggests that depression alone cannot account for the cognitive decline. Since cardiac surgery is increasingly performed in older adults with more co-morbidity, identifying people at risk for adverse neurocognitive outcomes will be helpful in protecting them by modification of the surgical procedure or by more effective medical therapy.[157, 203-205] ∎

◆ Cardiogenic Shock

Shock is acute, severe circulatory failure associated with a variety of precipitating conditions. Regardless of the cause, shock is associated with marked reduction of blood flow to vital organs, eventually leading to cellular damage and death. See Table 13-1 for categories and causes of shock.

The therapist may see a client in one of three stages of shock. *Stage 1*, compensated hypotension, is characterized by reduced cardiac output that stimulates compensatory mechanisms that alter myocardial function and peripheral resistance. During this stage, the body tries to maintain circulation to vital organs such as the brain and the heart and clinical symptoms are minimal. Blood pressure may remain normotensive.

In *stage 2*, compensatory mechanisms for dealing with the low delivery of nutrients to the body are overwhelmed, and tissue perfusion is decreased. Early signs of cerebral, renal, and myocardial insufficiency are present. Cardiogenic shock (inadequate cardiac function) may result from disorders of the heart muscle, valves, or electrical pacing system. Shock associated with MI or other serious cardiac disease carries a high mortality rate. The therapist is only likely to see this type of client in a CCU setting. *Stage 3* is characterized by severe ischemia with damage to tissues by toxins and antigen-antibody reactions. The kidneys, liver, and lungs are especially susceptible; ischemia of the GI tract allows invasion by bacteria with subsequent infection.

Clinical manifestations of shock may include (in early stages) tachycardia, increased respiratory rate, and distended neck veins. In early septic shock (vascular shock caused by infection), there is hyperdynamic change with increased circulation so that the skin is warm and flushed and the pulse is bounding rather than weak. In the second phase of shock (late septic shock) hypofusion (reduced blood flow) occurs with cold skin and weak pulses; hypotension (systolic blood pressure of 90 mm Hg or less)*; mottled extremities with weak or absent peripheral pulses; and collapsed neck veins. This phase is usually irreversible; the client is unresponsive, and cardiovascular collapse eventually occurs.

Treatment is directed toward both the manifestations of shock and its cause.

---

*Some healthy adults may have blood pressure levels this low without ill effects or with only minor symptoms of orthostatic hypotension when changing positions quickly.

Special Implications for the Therapist   11-27

CARDIOGENIC SHOCK

Preferred Practice Pattern
6D: Impaired Aerobic Capacity/Endurance Associated With Cardiovascular Pump Dysfunction or Failure

The therapist in an acute care or home health setting may be working with a client who is demonstrating signs and symptoms of impending shock. Careful monitoring of vital signs and clinical observations will alert the therapist to the need for medical intervention (see early signs of shock listed in previous section). The client in question may demonstrate normal mental status or may become restless, agitated, and confused.

For the acute care therapist, people hospitalized with shock are critically ill and are usually unresponsive. Cardiopulmonary and musculoskeletal function as well as prevention of further complications will be the focus of the therapist. Treatment for the immobile person in shock, which is directed toward positioning, skin care, and pulmonary function, must be short in duration but effective, to avoid fatiguing the person. ∎

◆ The Cardiac Client and Pregnancy

Normal physiologic changes during pregnancy can exacerbate symptoms of underlying cardiac disease, even in previously asymptomatic individuals. The most common cardiovascular complications of pregnancy are peripartum cardiomyopathy, aortic dissection, and pregnancy-related hypertension. Peripartum cardiomyopathy or cardiomyopathy of pregnancy is discussed briefly earlier in the text (see the section on Cardiomyopathy). Pregnancy predisposes to aortic dissection, possibly because of the accompanying connective tissue changes. Dissection usually occurs near term or shortly postpartum in the arteries (including coronary arteries) or the aorta, and special implications are the same as for aneurysm.

◆ The Heart in Collagen Vascular Diseases

Collagen vascular diseases (now more commonly referred to as diffuse connective tissue disease) (Box 11-11) often involve the heart, although cardiac symptoms are usually less prominent than other manifestations of the disease.

Lupus Carditis.   SLE is a multisystem clinical illness (see Chapter 6) characterized by an inflammatory process that can target all parts of the heart, including the coronary arteries, pericardium, myocardium, endocardium, conducting system, and valves. Lupus cardiac involvement may include pericarditis, myocarditis, endocarditis, or a combination of the three. Cardiac disease can occur as a direct result of the autoimmune process responsible for SLE or secondary to hypertension, renal failure, hypercholesterolemia (excess serum cholesterol), drug therapy for SLE, and, more rarely, infection (infective carditis).

Pericarditis is the most frequent cardiac lesion associated with SLE, presenting with the characteristic substernal chest pain that varies with posture, becoming worse in recumbency and improving with sitting or bending forward. In some people, pericarditis may be the first manifestation of SLE.

Myocarditis (see also the section on Myocardial Disease) is a serious complication reported to occur in less than 10% of people with SLE. The simultaneous involvement of cardiac and skeletal muscle may occur more commonly than previously suspected. More sensitive diagnostic techniques now make early detection of occult myocarditis possible. Myocarditis in association with SLE occurs most often as left ventricular dysfunction and conduction abnormalities with varying degrees of heart block.

Lupus *endocarditis* occurs in up to 30% of persons affected by SLE. Major lesions associated with lupus endocarditis include the formation of multiple noninfectious wartlike elevations (verrucae) around or on the surface of the cardiac valves, most commonly the mitral and tricuspid valves. Other types of valvular disease associated with SLE include mitral and aortic regurgitation or stenosis.

Rheumatoid Arthritis. On rare occasions, the heart is involved as a part of rheumatoid arthritis (RA), a chronic, systemic, inflammatory disorder that can affect various organs but predominantly involves synovial tissues of joints (see Chapter 26). When the heart is affected, rheumatoid granulomatous inflammation with fibrinoid necrosis may occur in the pericardium, myocardium, or valves. Involvement of the heart in RA does not compromise cardiac function.

Ankylosing Spondylitis. Ankylosing spondylitis is a chronic, progressive inflammatory disorder affecting fibrous tissue primarily in the sacroiliac joints, spine, and large peripheral joints (see Chapter 26). A characteristic aortic valve lesion develops in as many as 10% of persons with long-standing ankylosing spondylitis. The aortic valve ring is dilated, and the valve cusps are scarred and shortened. The functional consequence is aortic regurgitation (see the section on Aortic Regurgitation [Insufficiency]).

Scleroderma. Scleroderma or systemic sclerosis is a rheumatic disease of the connective tissue characterized by hardening of the connective tissue (see Chapter 9). Involvement of the heart in persons with scleroderma is second only to renal disease as a cause of death in scleroderma. The myocardium exhibits intimal sclerosis (hardening) of small arteries, which leads to small infarctions and patchy fibrosis. As a result, CHF and arrhythmia are common. Cor pulmonale may occur secondary to interstitial fibrosis of the lungs, and hypertensive heart disease may occur as a result of renal involvement.

Polyarteritis Nodosa. Polyarteritis refers to a condition of multiple sites of inflammatory and destructive lesions in the arterial system; the lesions consist of small masses of tissue in the form of nodes or projections (nodosum) (see previous discussion in this chapter). The heart is involved in up to 75% of cases of polyarteritis nodosa. The necrotizing lesions of branches of the coronary arteries result in MI, arrhythmias, or heart block. Cardiac hypertrophy and failure secondary to renal vascular hypertension occur.

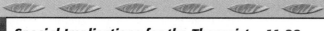

Special Implications for the Therapist   **11-28**

COLLAGEN VASCULAR DISEASES

Treatment of the collagen vascular diseases described must take into consideration the possibility of cardiac involvement. The physician has usually diagnosed concomitant cardiac disease, but complete health care records are not available to the therapist. If the therapist identifies signs or symptoms of cardiac origin, the client may be able to confirm previous diagnosis of the condition. In such cases, careful monitoring may be all that is required. However, the alert therapist may be the first health care provider to identify signs or symptoms of underlying dysfunction during onset, necessitating medical referral. (See each collagen vascular disease for discussion of individual implications.) ∎

◆ Cardiac Complications of Cancer and Cancer Treatment

Cardiovascular emergencies in oncology clients include all the usual cardiac problems, as well as complications of cancer and its therapy. Pericardial effusions and tamponade, cardiac masses, and extrinsic compression of the heart and great vessels by tumor masses, or fluid collections may all occur. Certain tumors may secrete mediators that are directly toxic to the heart. Tumors can also cause arrhythmias as a result of the mediators they secret or of direct mechanical irritation of the heart or pericardium. Cancer therapy is also associated with cardiac emergencies. Perioperative myocardial ischemia or infarction and arrhythmias may complicate surgery. Pericardial effusions and tamponade can follow surgery, radiation, or chemotherapy.

Chest radiation for any type of cancer (e.g., Hodgkin's disease, non-Hodgkin's lymphoma, esophageal cancer, lung cancer, breast cancer) exposes the heart (and lungs) to varying degrees and doses of radiation. Cardiac toxicity may occur following chest irradiation and the administration of many chemotherapeutic agents. Previous mediastinal radiation and increasing cumulative doses of chemotherapy or irradiation are known risk factors for the development of cardiotoxicity. Chemotherapy agents may prompt acute and chronic heart failure (e.g., anthracycline antibiotics, mitoxantrone, doxorubicin combined with paclitaxel used in the treatment of breast cancer)[183] or coronary spasm leading to angina, myocardial infarction, arrhythmias, or sudden death (e.g., 5-fluorouracil). Endocarditis also occurs in cancer clients with vascular access devices and immune compromise.

Recombinant technology has resulted in the development of biologic response modifiers, including the interferons, interleukins, and tumor necrosis factor, which also have some adverse cardiovascular effects. Hypotension and tachycardia are the most common problems although there have been some reports of myocardial ischemia and infarction. These adverse effects appear to be caused by significant alterations in fluid balance rather than any dysrhythmic or cardiotoxic properties of the drugs. Fortunately, many of the cardiac complications associated with chemotherapeutic agents and biologic response modifiers are transient and reversible.[109]

The most common manifestations of cardiotoxicity are cardiac arrhythmias or acute or chronic pericarditis. Other cardiac problems that may develop include blood pressure changes, thrombosis, electrocardiographic changes, myocardial fibrosis with a resultant restrictive cardiomyopathy, conduction disturbances, congestive heart failure, accelerated and radiation-induced CAD, and valvular dysfunction. These may occur during or shortly after treatment or within days or weeks after treatment; or they may not be apparent until months and sometimes years after completion of chemotherapy.[178]

Although only a small percentage of persons develop serious problems or obvious symptoms of cardiotoxicity, many people have functional limitations that are not clinically apparent because they are physically inactive. A number of risk factors may predispose someone to cardiotoxicity, including total daily dose, increasing cumulative dose, schedule of administration, concurrent administration of cardiotoxic agents, prior chemotherapy, mediastinal radiation, age (younger than 18 years or older than 70 years), female gender, history of preexisting cardiovascular disorders or other co-morbidities such as diabetes, and presence of electrolyte imbalances (e.g., hypokalemia, hypomagnesemia).[178]

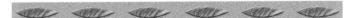

Special Implications for the Therapist   11-29

CARDIAC COMPLICATIONS OF CANCER TREATMENT

Any client referred to therapy who has completed oncologic treatment should be assessed for potential cardiac (and pulmonary) dysfunction, including questions about previous and current activity levels, evaluation of exercise tolerance or endurance, monitoring of heart rate and rhythm, blood pressure, and respiratory responses. Any symptoms of exercise intolerance (shortness of breath, light-headedness or dizziness, fatigue, pallor, palpitations, chest pain or discomfort) must be noted. (See also Special Implications for the Therapist: Cardiomyopathy, 11-10, and Special Implications for the Therapist: Pericarditis, 11-16.) Clients may be asymptomatic, with the only manifestation being electrocardiographic changes. Ideally, the oncology and cardiac team may recommend continuous cardiac monitoring with baseline and regular electrocardiographic and echocardiographic studies and measurement of serum electrolytes and cardiac enzymes for those individuals with risk factors or a history of cardiotoxicity. Specific exercise guidelines have also been outlined for the inclusion of gradual endurance training as a part of the treatment plan for anyone with cardiotoxicity secondary to oncologic treatment.[243] (See also the sections on Radiation Injuries in Chapter 4 and Cancer and Exercise in Chapter 8.)

Cardiotoxicity can be prevented by screening and modifying risk factors, aggressively monitoring for signs and symptoms as chemotherapy is administered, and continuing follow-up after completion of a course or the entire treatment. Cardioprotective agents are being developed with approval by the U.S. Food and Drug Administration (FDA), such as dexrazoxane for anthracycline chemotherapy.[178] ■

REFERENCES

1. Abou-Agag LH, Aikens ML, Tabengwa EM, et al: Polyphyenols increase t-PA and u-PA gene transcription in cultured human endothelial cells, *Alcohol Clin Exp Res* 25(2):155-162, 2001.
2. Agency for Health Care Policy and Research: *Clinical guideline no. 17: cardiac rehabilitation*, Columbia, Md, 1995. Copies are available for $8.00 from the U.S. Government Printing Office, [202] 512-1800. Order stock no. 01702600154-9. Also available on-line: HYPERLINK "http://text.nlm.nih.gov/" http://text.nlm.nih.gov/
3. Albert CM, Mittleman MA, Chae CU, et al: Triggering of sudden death from cardiac causes by vigorous exertion, *N Engl J Med* 343(19):1409-1411, 2000.
4. Albert MA, Ridker PM: The role of C-reactive protein in cardiovascular disease risk, *Curr Cardiol Rep* 1(2):99-104, 2000.
5. American College of Sports Medicine (ACSM): *Guidelines for exercise testing and prescription*, ed 6, Baltimore, 2000, Williams & Wilkins.
6. American College of Sports Medicine (ACSM): Position stand: the recommended quantity and quality of exercise for developing and maintaining cardiorespiratory and muscular fitness, and flexibility in healthy adults, *Med Sci Sports Exerc* 30(6):975-991, 1998.
7. American College of Sports Medicine (ACSM): *Resource manual for guidelines for exercise testing and prescription*, ed 3, Baltimore, 1998, American College of Sports Medicine.
8. American Heart Association: *2001 Heart and stroke statistical update*, Dallas, 2000, The Association. Available on-line: http://www.americanheart.org/statistics/index.html
9. American Heart Association: *Coronary heart disease and stroke remain the leading causes of death of women in America* Dallas, 2000, The Association. Available on-line: www.americanheart.org
10. American Heart Association: *Diagnosis and treatment of chronic arterial insufficiency of the lower extremities: a critical review*, Dallas, 2000, The Association. Available on-line: HYPERLINK "http://www.americanheart.org/Scientific/statements" www.americanheart.org/Scientific/statements
11. American Heart Association: Statement on exercise: benefits and recommendations for physical activity programs for all Americans, Dallas, 2000, The Association. Available on-line: HYPERLINK "http://www.americanheart.org/Scientific/statements/" www.americanheart.org/Scientific/statements/
12. American Heart Association: *Women, heart disease, and stroke statistics*, Dallas, 2000, The Association. Available on-line: HYPERLINK "http://www.americanheart.org" www.americanheart.org
13. American Physical Therapy Association (APTA): *House of Delegates policy no. 06-80-19-55, program 32*, 2001. Available on-line: HYPERLINK "http://www.apta.org" www.apta.org
14. Aspinall W: Clinical testing for the craniovertebral hypermobility syndrome, *J Orthop Sports Phys Ther* 12:180-181, 1989.
15. Autar R: Calculating patients' risk of deep vein thrombosis, *Br J Nurs* 7(1):7-12, 1998.
16. Autar R: Nursing assessment of clients at risk of deep vein thrombosis (DVT): the Autar DVT scale, *J Adv Nurs* 23(4):763-770, 1996.
17. Barsness GW: Enhanced external counterpulsation in unrevascularizable patients, *Curr Interven Cardiol Rep* 3(1):37-43, 2001.
18. Belardinelli R, Georgiou D, Cianci G, et al: Randomized, controlled trial of long-term moderate exercise training in chronic heart failure, *Circulation* 99:1173-1182, 1999.
19. Bennett R: FMS and Raynaud's phenomenon, *Fibromyalgia Network Newsletter*, April 1996. Available from P.O. Box 31750, Tucson, AZ 85751-1750. Phone: 1-800-853-2929. Available on-line: www.fmnetnews.com
20. Benton RE, Sale M, Flockhart DA, et al: Greater quinidine-induced QTc interval prolongation in women, *Clin Pharmacol* 67(4):413-418, 2000.
21. Bergholm R, Makimattila S, Valkonen M, et al: Intense physical training decreases circulating antioxidants and endothelium-dependent vasodilation in vivo, *Atherosclerosis* 145:341-349, 1999.
22. Blackwood AM, Sagnella GA, Cook DG, et al: Urinary calcium excretion, sodium intake and blood pressure in a multi-ethnic population: results of the Wandsworth Heart and Stroke Study, *J Hum Hypertens* 15(4):229-237, 2001.
23. Bleasdale-Barr KM, Mathias CJ: Neck and other muscle pains in autonomic failure: their association with orthostatic hypotension, *J R Soc Med* 91(7):344-359, 1998.
24. Braith RW: Exercise training in patients with CHF and heart transplant recipients, *Med Sci Sports Exerc* 30(10):S367-S378, 1998.
25. Braith RW, Vincent KR: Resistance exercise in the elderly person with cardiovascular disease, *Am J Geriatr Cardiol* 8(2):63-79, 1999.
26. Braith RW, Welsch MA, Feigenbaum MS, et al: Neuroendocrine activation in heart failure is modified by endurance exercise training, *J Am Coll Cardiol* 34(4):1170-1175, 1999.

27. Brandsma JW, Robeer BG, van den Heuvel S, et al: The effect of exercises on walking distance of patients with intermittent claudication: a study of randomized clinical trials, *Phys Ther* 78(3):278-288, 1998.

28. Braunwald E, Zipes DP, Libby P, editors: *Heart disease: a textbook of cardiovascular medicine*, ed 6, Philadelphia, 2001, Saunders.

29. Brendle DC, Joseph LJ, Corretti MC, et al: Effects of exercise rehabilitation on endothelial reactivity in older patients with peripheral arterial disease, *Am J Cardiol* 87(3):324-329, 2001.

30. Brickner ME, Hillis LD, Lange RA: Congenital heart disease in adults. I, *N Engl J Med* 342(4):256-263, 2000.

31. Brickner ME, Hillis LD, Lange RA: Congenital heart disease in adults. II, *N Engl J Med* 342(5):334-342, 2000.

32. Bron D, Asmis R: Vitamin E and the prevention of atherosclerosis, *Int J Vitamin Nutr Res* 71(1):18-24, 2001.

33. Brooks G: *Physiologic monitoring of patients during exercise*. Presentation at Combined Sections Pre-conference seminar, New Orleans, Feb 2, 2000.

34. Brown S, Norris J, Kraus W, et al: Effects of moderate exercise training in the absence of weight loss on cardiovascular risk factors in mildly obese subjects, *Clin Exer Physiol* 2(1):25-31, 2000.

35. Brown WV: The benefit of aggressive lipid lowering, *Atherosclerosis* 1(2):15-19, 2000.

36. Burkman RT: Oral contraceptives: current status, *Clin Obstet Gynecol* 44(1):62-72, 2001.

37. Cahalin LP: Cardiac muscle dysfunction. In Hillegass E, Sadowsky S, editors: *Essentials of cardiopulmonary physical therapy*, ed 2, Philadelphia, 2001, Saunders, pp 106-181.

38. Cahalin LP: Exercise training in heart failure: inpatient and outpatient considerations, *AACN Clin Issues* 9(2):225-243, 1998.

39. Cahalin LP: Heart failure, *Phys Ther* 76(5):516-533, 1996.

40. Cappuccio FP, Kalaitzidis R, Duneclift S, et al: Unraveling the links between calcium excretion, salt intake, hypertension, kidney stones, and bone metabolism, *J Nephrol* 13(3):169-177, 2000.

41. Carabello PJ, Heit JA, Atkinson EJ, et al: Long-term use of oral anticoagulants and the risk of fracture, *Arch Intern Med* 159:1750-1756, 1999.

42. Cariski AT: Cilostazol: a novel treatment option in intermittent claudication, *Int J Clin Pract Suppl* 119:11-18, 2001.

43. Centers for Disease Control and Prevention (CDC): *Health statistics*, 2000. Available on-line: HYPERLINK "http://www.cdc.gov" www.cdc.gov

44. Chae CU, Pfeffer MA, Glynn RJ, et al: Increased pulse pressure and risk of heart failure in the elderly, *JAMA* 281(7):634-639, 1999.

45. Chakraborti T, Mandal A, Mandal M, et al: Complement activation in heart diseases: role of oxidants, *Cell Signal* 12(9-10):607-617, 2000.

46. Chandler JM, Duncan PW: Balance and falls in the elderly: issues in evaluation and treatment. In Guccione AA, editor: *Geriatric physical therapy*, ed 2, St Louis, 2000, Mosby.

47. Chilton R: *New trends in cardiovascular disease*, Galveston, Texas, 2001, University of Texas Medical Branch.

48. Ciccone CD: *Pharmacology in rehabilitation*, ed 3, Philadelphia, 2001, Davis.

49. Ciesla N: State of the heart: cardiopulmonary PT in the '90s, *Phys Ther* 4(5):64-71, 1996.

50. Cole CR, Blackstone EH, Pashow FJ, et al: Heart-rate recovery immediately after exercise as a predictor of mortality, *N Engl J Med* 341(18):1351-1357, 1999.

51. Cole CR, Foody JM, Blackstone EH, et al: Heart rate recovery after submaximal exercise testing as a predictor of mortality in a cardiovascularly healthy cohort, *Ann Intern Med* 132(7):552-555, 2000.

52. Colman JM, Sermer M, Seaward PG, et al: Congenital heart disease in pregnancy, *Cardiol Rev* 8(3):166-173, 2000.

53. Colucci WS: Nesiritide for the treatment of decompensated heart failure, *J Card Fail* 7(1):92-100, 2001.

54. Cote P, Kreitz BG, Cassidy JD, et al: The validity of the extension-rotation test as a clinical screening procedure before neck manipulation: a secondary analysis, *J Manipulative Physiol Ther* 19(3):159-164, 1996.

55. Criqui MH, Denenberg JO, Langer RD, et al: The epidemiology of peripheral arterial disease: importance of identifying the population at risk, *Vasc Med* 2(3):221-226, 1997.

56. Crumlish CM, Bracken J, Hand MM, et al: When time is muscle, *Am J Nurs* 100(1):26-34, 2000.

57. Curvers J, Nienhuis SJ, Nap AW, et al: Activated protein C resistance during in vitro fertilization treatment, *Eur J Obstet Gynecol Reprod Biol* 95(2):222-224, 2001.

58. Davydov L, Cheng JW: The association of infection and coronary artery disease: an update, *Expert Opin Investig Drugs* 9(11):2505-2517, 2000.

59. Dean E: Preferred practice patterns in cardiopulmonary physical therapy: a guide to physiologic measures, *Cardiopulmonary Phys Ther* 10(4):124-134, 1999.

60. Deckelbaum RJ, Fisher EA, Winston M: AHA Conference Proceedings. Summary of a scientific conference on preventive nutrition: pediatrics to geriatrics, *Circulation* 100(4):450-456, 1999.

61. Del Rosario JD, Strong WB: The preparticipation cardiovascular evaluation of young athletes, *J Musculoskel Med* 16(8):445-459, 1999.

62. Denollet J, Brutsaert DL: Personality, disease severity, and the risk of long-term cardiac events in patients with a decreased ejection fraction after myocardial infarction, *Circulation* 97(2):128-129, 1998.

63. Devereux RB, Brown WT, Kramer-Fox R, et al: Inheritance of mitral valve prolapse: effect of age and sex on gene expression, *Ann Intern Med* 97:826-832, 1982.

64. Devereux RB, Kramer-Fox R, Brown WT, et al: Relation between clinical features of mitral valve prolapse syndrome and echocardiographically documented mitral valve prolapse, *J Am Coll Cardiol* 8:763-772, 1986.

65. Dhalla NS, Temsah RM, Netticadan R: Role of oxidative stress in cardiovascular diseases, *J Hypertens* 18(6):655-673, 2000.

66. Dickey RA, Feld S: The thyroid-cholesterol connection: an association between varying degrees of hypothyroidism and hypercholesterolemia in women, *J Womens Health Gend Based Med* 9(4):333-336, 2000.

67. Durand P, Prost M, Loreau N et al: Impaired homocysteine metabolism and atherothrombotic disease, *Lab Invest* 81(5):645-672, 2001.

68. Everson SA, Kaplan GA, Goldberg DE, et al: Hypertension incidence is predicted by high levels of hopelessness, *Hypertension* 35(2):561-567, 2000.

69. Fall risk: predicting vs. preventing, 2001. Available on-line: HYPERLINK "http://www.onbalance.com" www.onbalance.com

70. Fardy PS, Azzollini A, Magel JR, et al: Gender and ethnic differences in health behaviors and risk factors for coronary disease among urban teenagers: the PATH program, *J Gend Specif Med* 3(2):59-68, 2000.

71. Federman DG, Kirsner RS: An update on hypercoagulable disorders, *Arch Intern Med* 161(8):1051-1056, 2001.

72. Feldman MD, Sun B, Koci BJ: Stent-based gene therapy, *J Long Term Eff Med Implants* 10(1-2):47-68, 2000.

73. Ford E, Newman J, Deosaransingh K: Racial and ethnic differences in the use of cardiovascular procedures: findings from the California Cooperative Cardiovascular Project, *Am J Public Health* 90(7):1128-1134, 2000.

74. Fowlkes FG, Housley E, Cawood EH, et al: Edinburgh Artery Study: prevalence of asymptomatic and symptomatic peripheral arterial disease in the general population, *Int J Epidemiol* 30:384-392, 1991.

75. Fraenkel L, Zhang Y, Chaisson CE, et al: Different factors influencing the expression of Raynaud's phenomenon in men and women, *Arthritis Rheum* 42(2):306-310, 1999.

76. Francis GS: Pathophysiology of chronic heart failure, *Am J Med* 110(suppl 7A):37-46, 2001.

77. Freed LA, Levy D, Levine RA, et al: Prevalence and clinical outcome of mitral-valve prolapse, *N Engl J Med* 341(1):48-50, 1999.

78. Frownfelter D, Dean E, editors: *Principles and practices of cardiopulmonary physical therapy*, ed 4, St Louis, 2002, Mosby.

79. Fuchs FD, Chambless LE, Whelton PK, et al: Alcohol consumption and the incidence of hypertension: the atherosclerosis risk in communities study, *Hypertension* 37(5):1242-1250, 2001.

80. Fukuda K: Development of regenerative cardiomyocytes from mesenchymal stem cells for cardiovascular tissue engineering, *Artif Organs* 25(3):187-193, 2001.

81. Gan SC, Beaver SK, Houck PM, et al: Treatment of acute myocardial infarction and 30-day mortality among women and men, *N Engl J Med* 343(1):8-15, 2000.

82. Gardner AW, Forrester L, Smith GV: Altered gait profile in subjects with peripheral arterial disease, *Vasc Med* 6(1):31-34, 2001.

83. Gardner AW, Katzel LI, Sorkin JD, et al: Improved functional outcomes following exercise rehabilitation in patients with intermittent claudication, *J Gerontol A Biol Sci Med* 55(10):M570-M577, 2000.

84. Gardner AW, Poehlman ET: Exercise rehabilitation programs for the treatment of claudication pain, JAMA 274:975-980, 1995.

85. Gherpelli JLD, Azeka E, Riso A, et al: Choreoathetosis after cardiac surgery with hypothermia and extracorporeal circulation, Pediatr Neurol 19:113-118, 1998.

86. Gill TM, DiPietro L, Krumholz HM: Role of exercise stress testing and safety monitoring for older persons starting an exercise program, JAMA 284(3):342-349, 2000.

87. Gillum LA, Mamidipudi SK, Johnston SC: Ischemic stroke risk with oral contraceptives: a meta-analysis, JAMA 284(1):72-78, 2000.

88. Giri S, Thompson PD, Kiernan FJ, et al: Clinical and angiographic characteristics of exertion-related acute myocardial infarction, JAMA 282(18):1731-1736, 1999.

89. Glynn RJ, Chae GU, Guralnik JM, et al: Pulse pressure and mortality in older people, Arch Intern Med 160(18):2765-2772, 2000.

90. Goldberg JA: Aerobic and resistive exercise modify risk factors for coronary heart disease, Med Sci Sports Exerc 21:669-674, 1989.

91. Goodman CC, Snyder TE: Differential diagnosis in physical therapy, ed 3, Philadelphia, 2000, Saunders.

92. Goraya TY, Jacobsen SJ, Pellikka PA, et al: Prognostic value of treadmill exercise testing in elderly persons, Ann Intern Med 132(11):862-870, 2000.

93. Gorelick PB, Sacco RL, Smith DB, et al: Prevention of a first stroke: a review of guidelines and a multidisciplinary consensus statement from the National Stroke Association, JAMA 281(12):1112-1120, 1999.

94. Gottlieb S: Short, sharp bouts of exercise good for the heart, BMJ 321(7261):589, 2000.

95. Gottlieb S, Harpaz D, Shotan A, et al: Sex differences in management and outcome after acute myocardial infarction in the 1990s: a prospective observational community-based study, Circulation 102:2484-2490, 2000.

96. Gray JC: Case report: diagnosis of intermittent vascular claudication in a patient with a diagnosis of sciatica, Phys Ther 79(6):582-590, 1999.

97. Grubb BP, Kosinski DJ: Syncope resulting from autonomic insufficiency syndromes associated with orthostatic intolerance, Med Clin North Am 85(2):457-471, 2001.

98. Grundy SM, Balady GJ, Criqui MH, et al: Guide to primary prevention of cardiovascular diseases: a statement for healthcare professionals from the task force on risk reduction, Circulation 95:2329-2331, 1997.

99. Hall CM, Brody LT: Therapeutic exercise: moving towards function, ed 2, Philadelphia, 1998, Lippincott.

100. Harrington DM, Fong J, Sempos CT, et al: Comparison of the Heart and Estrogen/Progestin Replacement Study (HERS) cohort with women with coronary disease from National Health and Nutrition Examination Survey III (NHANES III), Am Heart J 136(1):115-124, 1998.

101. Harris KA, Holly RG: Physiological response to circuit weight training in borderline hypertensive subjects, Med Sci Sports Exerc 19:246-252, 1987.

102. Harvard Women's Health Watch (HWHW): Varicose veins, HWHW 8(11):5, 2000.

103. Hayase M, Woodbum KW, Perlroth J, et al: Photoangioplasty with local motexafin luteum delivery reduces macrophages in a rabbit post-balloon injury model, Cardiovasc Res 49(2):449-455, 2001.

104. Hayward CS, Webb CM, Collins P: Effect of sex hormones on cardiac mass, Lancet 357(9265):1354-1356, 2001.

105. Healthy People 2010: Healthy people objectives, 2001. Available on-line: HYPERLINK "http://www.health.gov/healthypeople/" www.health.gov/healthypeople/

106. Heiat A, Vaccarino V, Krumholz HM: An evidence-based assessment of federal guidelines for overweight and obesity as they apply to elderly persons, Arch Intern Med 161(9):1194-1203, 2001.

107. Helgason CM, Wolf PA: American Heart Association Prevention Conference IV: prevention and rehabilitation of stroke. Executive summary, Circulation 96:701-707, 1997.

108. Hillegass EA: Cardiovascular diagnostic tests and procedures. In Hillegass EA, Sadowsky HS, editors: Essentials of cardiopulmonary physical therapy, ed 2, Philadelphia, 2001, Saunders, pp 336-379.

109. Hillegass EA, Sadowsky HS, editors: Essentials of cardiopulmonary physical therapy, ed 2, Philadelphia, 2001, Saunders.

110. Hines LM, Stampfer MJ, Ma J, et al: Genetic variation in alcohol dehydrogenase and the beneficial effect of moderate alcohol consumption on myocardial infarction, N Engl J Med 344(8):549-555, 2001.

111. Hu FB, Stampfer MJ, Colditz GA, et al: Physical activity and risk of stroke in women, JAMA 283(22):2961-2967, 2000.

112. Hudson KD, Long L: Management of chronic venous ulcers, Phys Ther Case Rep 3(2):57-63, 2000.

113. Hulley S, Grady D, Bush T, et al: Heart and estrogen/progestin replacement study (HERS) research group: randomized trial of estrogen plus progestin for secondary prevention of coronary heart disease in postmenopausal women, JAMA 280:605-613, 1998.

114. Hulme J: Fibromyalgia: a handbook for self care & treatment, ed 3, Missoula, Mont, 2000, Phoenix Publishing Co.

115. Humphrey R, Arena R: Surgical innovations for chronic heart failure in the context of cardiopulmonary rehabilitation, Phys Ther 80(1):61-69, 2000.

116. Irion GL: Development of an inpatient cardiac rehabilitation program, Acute Care Perspectives 9(1):21-22, 2000.

117. Irwin S, Tecklin JS: Cardiopulmonary physical therapy, ed 4, St Louis, 2003, Mosby.

118. Izquierdo-Porrera AM, Gardner AW, et al: Effects of exercise rehabilitation on cardiovascular risk factors in older patients with peripheral arterial occlusive disease, J Vasc Surg 31(4):670-677, 2000.

119. Jairath N: Implications of gender differences on coronary artery disease risk reduction in women, AACN Clin Issues 12(1):17-28, 2001.

120. Johns Hopkins Medical Letter: Exercising toward recovery after a heart attack, 12(2):4-5, 2000.

121. Johns Hopkins Medical Letter: Peripheral vascular disease: walking toward a cure, 12(1):3, 2000.

122. Jolliffe JA, Rees K, Taylor RS, et al: Exercise-based rehabilitation for coronary heart disease (Cochrane Review), Cochrane Database Syst Rev 1:CD001800, 2001.

123. Jones EC, Devereux RB, Roman MJ, et al: Prevalence and correlates of mitral regurgitation in a population-based sample (the Strong Heart Study), Am J Cardiol 87(3):298-304, 2001.

124. Jones JW, Richman BW, Crigger NA, et al: Technique of transmyocardial revascularization: avoiding complications in high-risk patients, J Cardiovasc Surg 42(3):353-357, 2001.

125. Jover JA, Hernandez-Garcia C, Morado IC, et al: Combined treatment of giant-cell arteritis with methotrexate and prednisone: a randomized, double-blind, placebo-controlled trial, Ann Intern Med 134(2):106-114, 2001.

126. Kamath NV, Warner MR, Camisa C: Infective endocarditis: cutaneous clues to the diagnosis, Consultant 39(11):3085-3097, 1999.

127. Kannel WB: The Framingham Study: its 50-year legacy and future promise, J Athleroscler Thromb 6(2):60-66, 2000.

128. Kannel WB, Wolf PA, Benjamin EJ, et al: Prevalence, incidence, prognosis, and predisposing conditions for atrial fibrillation: population-based estimates, Am J Cardiol 82(8A):2N-9N, 1998.

129. Kavanagh T: Cardiac rehabilitation. In Goldberg L, Elliot DL: Exercise for prevention and treatment of illness, Philadelphia, 1994, Davis, pp 48-82.

130. Kelly J, Rudd AG: Giant cell arteritis presenting with arm claudication, Age Ageing 30(2):167-169, 2001.

131. Kenny RA, Dey AB: Syncope. In Tallis RC, Fillit HM, Brocklehurst JC, editors: Brocklehurst's textbook of geriatric medicine and gerontology, ed 5, New York, 1998, Churchill Livingstone, pp 455-473.

132. Keteyian SJ: Chronic heart failure and cardiac rehabilitation for the elderly: is it beneficial? Am J Geriatr Cardiol 8:80-86, 1999.

133. Kim JR, Oberman A, Fletcher GF, et al: Effect of exercise intensity and frequency on lipid levels in men with coronary heart disease: Training Level Comparison Trial, Am J Cardiol 87(8):942-946, 2001.

134. Kinney MR, Packa DR: Andreoli's comprehensive cardiac care, ed 8, St Louis, 1995, Mosby.

135. Kiser TS, Stefans VA: Pulmonary embolism in rehabilitation patients: relation to time before return to physical therapy after diagnosis of deep vein thrombosis, Arch Phys Med Rehabil 78:942-945, 1997.

136. Kloth L, McCullough JM: Wound healing: alternatives in management, ed 3, Philadelphia, 2001, Davis.

137. Kouchoukos NT, Dougenis D: Surgery in the thoracic aorta, N Engl J Med 336(26):1876-1888, 1997.

138. Lamont D, Parker L, White M, et al: Risk of cardiovascular disease measured by carotid intima-media thickness at age 49-51: life course study, BMJ 320(7230):273-278, 2000.

139. Lavie CJ, Milani RV: Cardiac rehabilitation and preventive cardiology in the elderly, *Cardiol Clin* 17(1):233-240, 1999.

140. Legato MJ: Gender and the heart: sex-specific differences in normal anatomy and physiology, *J Gend Specif Med* 3(7):15-18, 2000.

141. Legato MJ: *Gender specific aspects of human biology for the practicing physician*, Armonk, NY, 1997, Futura Publishing Co.

142. Leung DYM, Meissner HC: The many faces of Kawasaki syndrome, *Hosp Pract* 35(1):77-81, 2000.

143. Levy D, Wilson PWF: Atherosclerotic cardiovascular disease: an epidemiologic perspective. In Topol EJ, editor: *Comprehensive cardiovascular medicine*, Philadelphia, 1998, Lippincott-Raven Publishers, pp 27-43.

144. Luft FC: Molecular genetics of salt-sensitivity and hypertension, *Drug Metab Dispos* 29(4, pt 2):500-504, 2001.

145. Luskin FM: A review of mind-body therapies in the treatment of cardiovascular disease. I. Implications for the elderly, *Altern Ther Health Med* 4(3):46-61, 1998.

146. MacKay D: Hemorrhoids and varicose veins: a review of treatment options, *Altern Med Rev* 6(2):126-140, 2001.

147. Magee DJ: *Orthopedic physical assessment*, ed 4, Philadelphia, 2001, Harcourt Health Sciences.

148. Maisch B, Ristic AD, Seferovic PM: New directions in diagnosis and treatment of pericardial disease: a project of the Taskforce on Pericardial Disease of the World Heart Federation, *Herz* 25(8):794-798, 2000.

149. Maisel AS, Koon J, Krishnaswamy P, et al: Utility of B-natriuretic peptide as a rapid, point-of-care test for screening patients undergoing echocardiography to determine left ventricular dysfunction, *Am Heart J* 141(3):267-374, 2001.

150. Manson JAE, Hu FB, Rich-Edwards JW, et al: Brisk exercise reduces coronary risk in women, *N Engl J Med* 341:650-658, 1999.

151. Marder VJ, Mellinghoff IK: Cocaine and Buerger disease: is there a pathogenetic association? *Arch Intern Med* 160(13):2057-2060, 2000.

152. Marinella MA, Kathula SK, Markert RJ: Spectrum of upper-extremity deep venous thrombosis in a community teaching hospital, *Heart Lung* 29(2):113-117, 2000.

153. Maron BJ, Thompson PD, Puffer JC, et al: Cardiovascular preparticipation screening of competitive athletes: a statement for health professionals from the Sudden Death Committee, American Heart Association, *Circulation* 94(4):850-856, 1996.

154. Maron BJ, Thompson PD, Puffer JC, et al: Cardiovascular preparticipation screening of competitive athletes: addendum to a statement for health professionals from the Sudden Death Committee, American Heart Association, *Circulation* 97(22):2294, 1998.

155. Maxwell M: Personal communication. International Heart Institute, Missoula, Mont, 2001.

156. McCann ME: Sexual healing after heart attack, *Am J Nurs* 89(9):1133-1138, 1989.

157. McKhann GM, Borowicz LM, Goldsborough MA, et al: Depression and cognitive decline after coronary artery bypass grafting, *Lancet* 349(9061):1282-1284, 1997.

158. Meier CR: The possible role of infections in acute myocardial infarction, *Biomed Pharmacother* 53(9):397-404, 1999.

159. Menasche P, Hagege AA, Scorsin M, et al: Myoblast transplantation for heart failure, *Lancet* 357(9252):279-280, 2001.

160. Meyer K, Samek L, Schwaibold M, et al: Interval training in patients with severe chronic heart failure: analysis and recommendations for exercise procedures, *Med Sci Sports Exerc* 29(3):306-312, 1997.

161. Michelena HI, Ezekowitz MD: Atrial fibrillation: are there gender differences? *J Gend Specif Med* 3(6):44-49, 2000.

162. Moliterno DJ: No association between plasma lipoprotein (a) concentrations and the presence or absence of coronary atherosclerosis in African-Americans, *Arterioscler Thromb Vasc Biol* 15(7):850-855, 1995.

163. Morbidity and Morbidity Weekly Report (MMWR): Mortality from coronary heart disease and acute myocardial infarction—United States, 1998, *MMWR Morb Mortal Wkly Rep* 50(06):90-93, 2001.

164. Mosca L, Grundy SM, Judelson D, et al: AHA/ACC Scientific Statement: Consensus Panel Statement. Guide to preventive cardiology for women, *Circulation* 99(18):2480-2484, 1999.

165. Mueller MJ: Invited commentary: the effect of exercises on walking distance of patients with intermittent claudication, *Phys Ther* 78(3):286-288, 1998.

166. Mulcare JA, Jackson K, Petersen DR, et al: Physiological responses during unweighted ambulation of patients with transtibial amputation: a pilot study, *Phys Ther Case Rep* 2(3):99-103, 1999.

167. Muller JE: Triggering myocardial infarction by sexual activity: low absolute risk and prevention by regular physical exertion: determinants of Myocardial Infarction Onset Study investigators, *JAMA* 275(18):1405-1409, 1996.

168. National Center for Health Statistics (NCHS): Surveys and data: vital statistics, 2001. Available on-line: HYPERLINK "http://www.cdc.gov/nchs/default.htm" www.cdc.gov/nchs/default.htm

169. National Heart Attack Alert Program (NHAAP): HYPERLINK "http://www.nhlbi.nih.gov/health/prof/heart/index.htm#mi" www.nhlbi.nih.gov/health/prof/heart/index.htm#mi

170. National Institute of Diabetes and Digestive Kidney Diseases (NIDDKD): Overweight, obesity, and health risk: National Task Force on the Prevention and Treatment of Obesity, *Arch Intern Med* 160(7):898-904, 2000.

171. National Institutes of Health: *National Heart, Lung, and Blood Institute detection, evaluation, and treatment of high blood cholesterol in adults: adult treatment panel III (ATPIII) guidelines*, 2001. Available on-line: HYPERLINK "http://www.nhlbi.nih.gov" www.nhlbi.nih.gov

172. Nieto FJ, Young TB, Lind BK, et al: Association of sleep-disordered breathing, sleep apnea, and hypertension in a large community-based study: Sleep Heart Healthy Study, *JAMA* 283(14):1829-1836, 2000.

173. Nikol S, Huehns TY: Preclinical and clinical experience in vascular gene therapy: advantages over conservative/standard therapy, *J Invasive Cardiol* 13(4):333-338, 2001.

174. Nolan J, Fox KA: Heart rate variability and cardiac failure, *Heart* 81(5):561-562, 1999.

175. Ohtsuka T, Hamada M, Hiasa G, et al: Effect of beta-blockers on circulating levels of inflammatory and anti-inflammatory cytokines in patients with dilated cardiomyopathy, *J Am Coll Cardiol* 37(2):412-417, 2001.

176. O'Kane PD, Jackson G: Erectile dysfunction: is there silent obstructive coronary artery disease? *Int J Clin Pract* 55(3):219-220, 2001.

177. Orlic D, Kajstura J, Chimenti S, et al: Bone marrow cells regenerate infarcted myocardium, *Nature* 410(6829):640-641, 2001.

178. Pai VB, Nahata MC: Cardiotoxicity of chemotherapeutic agents: incidence, treatment, and prevention, *Drug Saf* 22(4):263-302, 2000.

179. Pandey DK, Labarthe DR, Goff DC, et al: Community-wide coronary heart disease mortality in Mexican Americans equals or exceeds that in non-Hispanic whites: the Corpus Christi Heart Project, *Am J Med* 110(2):147-148, 2001.

180. Papamichael CM, Lekakis JP, Stamatelopoulos KS, et al: Ankle-brachial index as a predictor of the extent of coronary atherosclerosis and cardiovascular events in patients with coronary artery disease, *Am J Cardiol* 86(6):615-618, 2000.

181. Pasternak RC: Cardiovascular disease prevention. I. What works—what doesn't? *Consultant* 39(11):2957-2963, 1999.

182. Pasternak RC: Cardiovascular disease prevention. II. What works—what doesn't? *Consultant* 39(11):2973-2984, 1999.

183. Perez EA: Doxorubicin and paclitaxel in the treatment of advanced breast cancer: efficacy and cardiac considerations, *Cancer Invest* 19(2):155-164, 2001.

184. Pescatello LS: Physical activity, cardiometabolic health and older adults: recent findings, *Sports Med* 28(5):315-323, 1999.

185. Pescatello LS, Miller B, Danias PG, et al: Dynamic exercise normalizes resting blood pressure in mildly hypertensive premenopausal women, *Am Heart J* 138(5, pt 1):916-921, 1999.

186. Pollock ML, Franklin BA, Balady GJ, et al: AHA Science Advisory. Resistance exercise in individuals with and without cardiovascular disease: benefits, rationale, safety, and prescription. An advisory from the Committee on Exercise, Rehabilitation, and Prevention, Council on Clinical Cardiology, American Heart Association; Position paper endorsed by the American College of Sports Medicine, *Circulation* 101(7):828-833, 2000.

187. Priebe HJ: The aged cardiovascular risk patient, *Br J Anaesth* 85(5):763-778, 2000.

188. Public Access Defibrillation League (PADL): *Cardiac Arrest Survivor's Act*, 2001. Available on-line: HYPERLINK "http://www.padl.org" www.padl.org

189. Rangarajan U, Kochar MS: Hypertension in women, *WMJ* 99(3):65-70, 2000.

190. Ray JG, Mamdani M, Tsuyuki RT, et al: Use of statins and the subsequent development of deep vein thrombosis, *Arch Intern Med* 161(11):1405-1410, 2001.

191. Rich MW: Heart failure in the 21st century: a cardiogeriatric syndrome, *J Gerontol A Biol Sci Med Sci* 56(2):M88-M96, 2001.

192. Rivett DA: The premanipulative vertebral artery testing protocol: a brief review, *Physiotherapy* 23:9-12, 1995.

193. Rivett DA, Sharples KJ, Milburn PD: Effect of premanipulative tests on vertebral artery and internal carotid artery blood flow: a pilot study, *J Manipulative Physiol Ther* 6:368-375, 1999.

194. Roffe C: Ageing of the heart, *Br J Biomed Sci* 55(2):136-148, 1998.

195. Rosenfeld AG: Women's risk of decision delay in acute myocardial infarction: implications for research and practice, *AACN Clin Issues* 12(1):29-39, 2001.

196. Sapico FL, Liquete JA, Sarma RJ: Bone and joint infections in patients with infective endocarditis: review of a 4 year experience, *Clin Infect Dis* 22:783-787, 1996.

197. Scherer S: Exercise in the patient with claudication, *Cardiopulmonary Phys Ther* 10(2):45-48, 1999.

198. Schiele F, Batur MK, Seronde MF, et al: *Cytomegalovirus, Chlamydia pneumoniae,* and *Helicobacter pylori* IgG antibodies and restenosis after stent implantation: an angiographic and intravascular ultrasound study, *Heart* 85(3):304-311, 2001.

199. Schroll M, Munck O: Estimation of peripheral arteriosclerotic disease by ankle blood pressure measurements in a population study of 60-year-old men and women, *J Chronic Dis* 34:261-269, 1981.

200. Schwartz JB: The electrocardiographic QT interval and its prolongation in response to medications: differences between men and women, *J Gend Specif Med* 3(5):25-28, 2000.

201. Scott-Okafor HR, Silver KK, Parker J, et al: Lower extremity strength deficits in peripheral arterial occlusive disease patients with intermittent claudication, *Angiology* 52(1):7-14, 2001.

202. Seals DR, Taylor JA, Ng AV, et al: Exercise and aging: autonomic control of the circulation, *Med Sci Sports Exerc* 26(5):568-576, 1994.

203. Selnes OA, Goldsborough MA, Borowicz LM, et al: Determinants of cognitive change after coronary artery bypass surgery: a multifactorial problem, *Ann Thorac Surg* 67(6):1669-1676, 1999.

204. Selnes OA, Goldsborough MA, Borowicz LM, et al: Neurobehavioural sequelae of cardiopulmonary bypass, *Lancet* 353(9164):1601-1606, 1999.

205. Selnes OA, Royall RM, Grega MA, et al: Cognitive changes 5 years after coronary artery bypass grafting: is there evidence of late decline? *Arch Neurol* 58(4):598-604, 2001.

206. Shankar K: *Exercise prescription,* Philadelphia, 1999, Hanley & Belfus.

207. Shaw DK, Deutsch DT, Bowling RJ: Efficacy of shoulder range of motion exercise in hospitalized patients after coronary artery bypass graft surgery, *Heart Lung* 19(3):321-322, 1990.

208. Shaw LJ, Hachamovitch R, Redberg RF: Current evidence on diagnostic testing in women with suspected coronary artery disease: choosing the appropriate test, *Cardiol Rev* 8(1):65-74, 2000.

209. Sherwood A, May CW, Siegel WC, et al: Ethnic differences in hemodynamic responses to stress in hypertensive men and women, *Am J Hypertens* 8:552-557, 1995.

210. Shumway-Cook A, Brauer S, Woollacott M: Predicting the probability for falls in community-dwelling older adults using the Timed Up & Go Test, *Phys Ther* 80(9):896-903, 2000.

211. Silberstein L, Davies A, Kelsey S, et al: Myositis, polyserositis, and constrictive pericarditis as manifestations of chronic graft-versus-host disease after peripheral stem cell transplantation, *Bone Marrow Transplant* 27(2):231-233, 2001.

212. Sixth Report of the Joint National Committee on Prevention, Detection, Evaluation and Treatment of High Blood Pressure, *Arch Intern Med* 157(21):2413-2446, 1997.

213. Skinner JS: *Exercise testing and exercise prescription for special cases,* ed 2, Philadelphia, 1993, Lea & Febiger.

214. Smit AA, Halliwill JR, Low PA, et al: Pathophysiological basis of orthostatic hypotension in autonomic failure, *J Physiol* 519(pt 1):1-10, 1999.

215. Springer S, Fife A, Lawson W, et al: Psychosocial effects of enhanced external counterpulsation in the angina patient: a second study, *Psychosomatics* 42(2):124-132, 2001.

216. Srivastava D: Genetic assembly of the heart: implications for congenital heart disease, *Annu Rev Physiol* 63:451-469, 2001.

217. Stamou SC, Corso PJ: Coronary revascularization without cardiopulmonary bypass in high-risk patients: a route to the future, *Ann Thorac Surg* 71(3):1056-1061, 2001.

218. Stewart KJ, McFarland LD, Weinhofer JJ, et al: Safety and efficacy of weight training soon after acute myocardial infarction, *J Cardiopulm Rehabil* 18:37-44, 1998.

219. Stone PH, Krantz DS, McMahon RP, et al: Relationship among mental stress-induced ischemia and ischemia during daily life during exercise: the psychophysiologic investigations of myocardial ischemia (PIMI) study, *J Am Coll Cardiol* 33(6):1476-1484, 1999.

220. Strong JP, Malcolm GT, McMahan CA, et al: Prevalence and extent of atherosclerosis in adolescents and young adults: implications for prevention from the Pathobiological Determinants of Atherosclerosis in Youth Study, *JAMA* 282(8):727-735, 1999.

221. Sundquist J, Winkleby MA, Pudaric S: Cardiovascular disease risk factors among older black, Mexican-American, and white women and men: an analysis of NHANES III, 1988-1994. Third National Health and Nutrition Examination Survey, *J Am Geriatr Soc* 49(2):109-116, 2001.

222. Sussman C: *The wound care patient education and resource manual,* Gaithersburg, Md, 1999, Aspen Publishers.

223. Sussman C, Bates-Jensen B, editors: *Wound care: a collaborative practice manual for physical therapists and nurses,* ed 2, Gaithersburg, Md, 2001, Aspen Publishers.

224. Szombathy T, Janoskuti L, Szalai C, et al: Angiotensin II type 1 receptor gene polymorphism and mitral valve prolapse syndrome, *Am Heart J* 139(1, pt 1):101-105, 2000.

225. Takazoe K, Ogawa H, Yasue H, et al: Increased plasminogen activator inhibitor activity and diabetes predict subsequent coronary events in patients with angina pectoris, *Ann Med* 33(3):206-212, 2001.

226. Takeyama J, Itoh H, Kato M, et al: Effects of physical training on the recovery of the autonomic nervous activity during exercise after coronary artery bypass grafting: effects of physical training after CABG, *Jpn Circ J* 64(11):809-813, 2000.

227. Tasso KH: Gross motor development of a child with multiple congenital heart defects, *Phys Ther Case Rep* 3(2):71-77, 2000.

228. Temizhan A, Dincer I, Pamir G, et al: Is there any effect of chronobiological changes on coronary angioplasty? *J Cardiovasc Risk* 8(1):15-19, 2001.

229. Tepper SH, McKeough DM: Deep venous thrombosis: risks, diagnosis, treatment interventions and prevention, *Acute Care Perspectives* 9(1):1-7, 2000.

230. Thiel H, Wallace K, Donut J, et al: Effect of various head and neck positions on vertebral artery blood flow, *Clin Biomechanics* 9:105-110, 1994.

231. Thomas CM, Pierzga JM, Kenney WL: Aerobic training and cutaneous vasodilation in young and older men, *J Appl Physiol* 86(5):1676-1686, 1999.

232. Tsikouris JP, Tsikouris AP: A review of available fibrin-specific thrombolytic agents used in acute myocardial infarction, *Pharmacotherapy* 21(2):207-217, 2001.

233. Tsuji T, Tamai H, Igaki K, et al: Biodegradable polymeric stents, *Curr Interven Cardiol Rep* 3(1):10-17, 2001.

234. Urano H, Ikeda H, Ueno T, et al: Enhanced external counterpulsation improves exercise tolerance, reduces exercise-induced myocardial ischemia and improves left ventricular diastolic filling in patients with coronary artery disease, *J Am Coll Cardiol* 37(1):93-99, 2001.

235. Vaccarino V, Holford TR, Krumholz HM: Pulse pressure and risk for myocardial infarction and heart failure in the elderly, *J Am Coll Cardiol* 36(1):130-138, 2000.

236. Vainio H, Bianchini F: Prevention of disease with pharmaceuticals, *Pharmacol Toxicol* 88(3):111-118, 2001.

237. Van Belle E, Ketelers R, Bauters C: Patency of percutaneous transluminal coronary angioplasty sites at 6-month angiographic follow-up: a key determinant of survival in diabetics after coronary balloon angioplasty, *Circulation* 103(9):1218-1224, 2001.

238. VanSwearingen JM, Brach JS: Making geriatric assessment work: selecting useful measures, *Phys Ther* 81(6):1233-1252, 2001.

239. Varma C, Camm AJ: Pacing for heart failure, *Lancet* 357(9264):1277-1283, 2001.

240. Vaughan CJ, Casey M, He J, et al: Identification of a chromosome 11q23.2-q24 locus for familial aortic aneurysm disease, a genetically heterogeneous disorder, *Circulation* 103(20):2469-2475, 2001.

241. Vliet EL: *Screaming to be heard: hormonal connections women suspect … and doctors ignore*, New York, 1995, M. Evans and Co.

242. Wannamethee SG, Shaper AG: Physical activity in the prevention of cardiovascular disease: an epidemiological perspective, *Sports Med* 31(2):101-114, 2001.

243. Watchie J: Cardiopulmonary complications of cancer treatment, *Clin Manage* 12:92-95, July/Aug 1992.

244. Watchie J: Cardiopulmonary implications of specific diseases. In Hillegass EA, Sadowsky HS, editors: *Essentials of cardiopulmonary physical therapy*, ed 2, Philadelphia, 2001, Saunders, pp 285-335.

245. Weaver WD, Cerqueira M, Hallstrom AP, et al: Prehospital-initiated vs. hospital-initiated thrombolytic therapy: the Myocardial Infarction Triage and Intervention Trial, *JAMA* 270(10):1211-1216, 1993.

246. Weitz JJ: Low-molecular-weight heparins, *N Engl J Med* 337:688-698, 1997.

247. Wenger NK: Lipid management and control of other coronary risk factors in the postmenopausal woman, *J Womens Health Gend Based Med* 9(3):235-243, 2000.

248. Wiley RL, Dunn CL, Cox RH, et al: Isometric exercise training lowers resting blood pressure, *Med Sci Sports Exerc* 24:749-754, 1992.

249. Williams JE, Paton CC, Siegler IC, et al: Anger proneness predicts coronary heart disease risk: prospective analysis from the atherosclerosis risk in communities (ARIC) study, *Circulation* 101(17):2034-2039, 2000.

250. Williams SG, Cooke GA, Wright DJ, et al: Disparate results of ACE inhibitor dosage on exercise capacity in heart failure: a reappraisal of vasodilator therapy and study design, *Int J Cardiol* 77(2-3):239-245, 2001.

251. Williams PT: Relationship of distance run per week to coronary heart disease risk factors in 8,283 male runners: the National Runners' Health Study, *Arch Intern Med* 157(2):191-198, 1997.

252. Wilson PW: Metabolic risk factors for coronary heart disease: current and future prospects, *Curr Opin Cardiol* 14:176-185, 1999.

253. Womack CJ, Ivey FM, Gardner AW, et al: Fibrinolytic response to acute exercise in patients with peripheral arterial disease, *Med Sci Sports Exerc* 33(2):214-219, 2001.

254. World Health Organization (WHO): 1999 World Health Organization—International Society of Hypertension guidelines for the management of hypertension, *J Hypertens* 17:151-183, 1999.

255. Young IS, Woodside JV: Antioxidants in health and disease, *J Clin Pathol* 54(3):176-186, 2001.

256. Zambetti M, Moliterni A, Materazzo C, et al: Long-term cardiac sequelae in operable breast cancer patients given adjuvant chemotherapy with or without doxorubicin and breast irradiation, *J Clin Oncol* 19(1):37-43, 2001.

257. Zieske AW, Malcolm GT, Strong JP: Pathobiological determinants of atherosclerosis in youth (PDAY) cardiovascular specimen and data library, *J La State Med Soc* 152(6):296-301, 2000.

258. Zoldhelyi P, Chen ZQ, Shelat HS, et al: Local gene transfer of tissue factor pathway inhibitor regulates intimal hyperplasia in atherosclerotic arteries, *Proc Natl Acad Sci USA* 98(7):4078-4083, 2001.

CHAPTER 12

THE LYMPHATIC SYSTEM

BONNIE LASINSKI

The lymphatic system, which develops embryologically from the venous system,* is a one-cycle system. The interstitial fluid that remains after the extracellular fluid is resorbed via the veins is taken up by the initial lymphatic vessels, into larger collecting vessels, into lymphatic trunks, and back into the right side of the heart via the lymphatic ducts that empty into the subclavian veins in the neck. This is a one-way, one-cycle system from the periphery to the central circulation. It is designed to help maintain fluid balance in the tissues, fight infection, and assist in the removal of cellular debris and waste products from the extracellular spaces. In many ways, it functions like the "sanitation" system of a major city. It is largely ignored and goes unnoticed until it is disrupted and the "garbage" (in the form of lymphedema) piles up. This drainage system is separate from the general circulatory system but is the conduit for returning tissue fluids to the circulatory system.[55]

The cardiovascular system is a two-cycle system of vessels with a pump (the heart) to move the fluid (blood) through arteries, capillaries, and cells and then back to the heart via the veins; the arterial and venous vessels comprise the two cycles. Fluid that leaves the arterial side of the capillary bed in a process called *ultrafiltration* nourishes the tissues and cells. Of the fluid volume that perfuses the tissues, 90% reenters the circulation via the venous capillary network (*reabsorption*) due to differences in concentration of fluid and protein in the tissues and in the venous end of the capillary network. The remaining 10% of extracellular tissue fluid and plasma proteins in the interstitial spaces must be returned to the heart via the lymphatic system.†

The lymphatic system is a pressure driven system based on the principles of osmotic diuresis. If the normal lymphatic transport mechanisms are disrupted (e.g., by scar tissue or reduced muscle pumping), significant accumulations of water and protein‡ can remain in the tissue spaces, resulting in latent, acute, or chronic lymphedema. The dynamics of fluid exchange in the tissues are controlled by the microcirculation unit consisting of the arterial and venous capillaries, the tissue channels; the proteolytic cells (macrophages) in the tissues; and the initial lymphatics (see the description of initial lymphatics in the next section).

ANATOMY AND PHYSIOLOGY

The lymphatic system is comprised of superficial and deep lymph vessels and nodes. Other lymphatic organs and tissues include the thymus, bone marrow, spleen, tonsils, and Peyer's patches of the small intestine. These perform important immune functions discussed in Chapter 6. Superficial vessels rely on an interaction of oncotic and hydrostatic pressures, muscle contraction, arterial pulsation, and gentle movement of the skin to move lymph fluid, whereas the deeper vessels, which generally parallel the venous system, contain smooth muscle and valves, and help prevent backflow.[12]

The lymphatic vessel network is an intricate one-way vessel system that serves to drain the 10% excess tissue fluid volume and plasma proteins that remain in the interstitium after normal capillary perfusion/filtration has taken place and return it to the central circulation via the large veins in the neck. All lymph fluid eventually passes through lymph nodes before emptying into the right lymphatic duct and the thoracic duct. The fluid is then returned to the bloodstream via the left and right subclavian veins.[55]

The anatomy of the lymphatic vessel system can be compared in some ways to the vein system on the leaves and stems of trees. The smallest vessels, or veins, are at the periphery of the tissues (leaves), and the diameter of these vessels gradually increases in the stem of the leaf, as the system progresses into larger and larger vessels (corresponding to deeper tissues) and continuing to progress to larger stems/branches of the tree until the trunk is reached. The smallest of lymphatic vessels (diameter 20 to 40 μm), called *lymphatic capillaries* or *pre-collectors*, begin as blind-ended sacs of endothelium just under the epidermis.[12,23] These are referred to as the *initial lymphatics* and are in close proximity with the venous and arterial capillaries* (Fig. 12-1).

The vessel walls of these initial lymphatics are one cell thick, formed by overlapping endothelial cells with many

---

*Two major theories exist of the embryologic origin of the lymphatic system: the *centrifugal* or venous budding theory and the *centripetal* theory. The centrifugal theory states that the lymphatic endothelium develops from the venous endothelium; the centripetal theory states that both systems (venous and lymphatic) develop from undifferentiated (stem type) mesenchymal cells. Advances in lymphangiogenesis research may clarify which theory is correct; this information will have great impact on genetic research and the eventual molecular treatment of lymphangiodysplasias.[58]

†Most protein molecule's diameters are too large to pass through openings in the endothelium of the venous capillaries. A small amount of protein, if broken down into smaller molecules by macrophages, can pass through the open junctions in the venous endothelium. However, the majority of extracellular protein must be transported via the lymphatic system. Although ten percent of the total fluid volume seems small, it can amount to two liters per day.

‡This protein is a result of cellular metabolism and is not related to food protein ingested.

---

*Terminology has changed over the years; the reader should be aware that initial lymphatic and lymphatic capillary refer to the same structure.

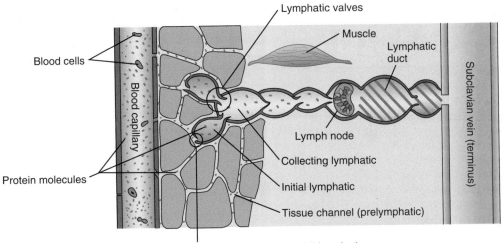

FIGURE   12-1   Anatomy of the lymphatic vessel system (schematic). This diagram shows the passage of protein (dots) in normal tissue from the blood capillary, through the tissue channels, into and through the lymphatic system, back to the venous system, and eventually emptying into the subclavian vein. Note that the protein molecules are not on the venous side of the diagram, because for the most part, these molecules are too large to pass through the openings in the venous endothelium. Also note that this is a schematic diagram and not drawn to scale; the lymphatic duct depicted emptying into the venous system (subclavian vein) is much deeper (under the fascia) than this two-dimensional illustration can portray. Various malfunctions are illustrated in Fig. 12-15. (From Casley-Smith JR, Casley-Smith JR: *Modern treatment for lymphoedema*, ed 5, Adelaide, Australia, 1997, Lymphoedema Association of Australia.)

loose junctions between cells opening and closing (Fig. 12-2). This action allows for movement of water and proteins into the vessel and prevents the escape of protein into the interstitium during the compression of the initial lymphatics. These cells are also in direct contact with the microfilaments of the surrounding connective tissues. They are connected to the tissue matrix by anchoring filaments that act as "guide wires" to pull the cell junctions open when the tissue pressure rises due to increased extracellular fluid volume[12] (Fig. 12-3). These vessels are arranged in a meshlike plexus; for every square millimeter of tissue, 7 mm of lymphatics are available to drain it.[11]

The initial lymphatics function as force-pumps powered by variations in total tissue pressure caused by movement, muscular contraction, respiration, and variations in external pressure caused by massage, gravity, change in position, and other similar factors. Without changes in total tissue pressure, these force-pumps cannot function, and fluid will accumulate in the interstitium, leading to edema.

◆ Microcirculation Unit

A brief discussion of Starling's theory of fluid dynamics is helpful to understand the microcirculation unit. In 1897, Starling proposed the mechanism governing fluid flow out of the blood capillaries into the tissues and back into the capillaries again. There are four pressures that are important in Starling's Law: (1) *plasma hydrostatic pressure*, the pressure inside the capillaries that decreases as fluid passes from the arterial to the venous side of the capillary loop; (2) *tissue hydrostatic pressure*, the pressure of fluid in the tissue channels (usually negative, or less than atmospheric pressure) that tends to pull fluid from the capillaries into the

tissues*; (3) *plasma colloidal osmotic pressure*, caused by plasma proteins, causes a siphon effect and fluid is pulled into the capillaries; (4) *tissue colloidal osmotic pressure*, pressure caused by plasma proteins in the tissues that causes a net movement of fluid into the tissues. All of these pressure systems determine how much fluid moves and where it moves within the body.

The laws of basic fluid dynamics dictate that fluid flows from an area of high pressure to an area of lower pressure until equilibrium is reached. Starling's law simplified means that fluid at the arterial end of the capillary will tend to flow into the tissue spaces because plasma (blood) hydrostatic pressure is higher at the arterial end compared with the tissue hydrostatic pressure (THP) of the tissues.

If all else is "normal," when the fluid reaches the venous side of the capillary, the plasma hydrostatic pressure will be lower than the plasma colloid (protein) osmotic pressure, and the fluid will be forced back into the venous side of the capillary. That accounts for about 90% of the fluid on the venous end of the capillary. Ten percent of net-ultrafiltrate must return to the central circulation via the lymphatics. If all is normal there, the initial lymphatics will take up that fluid, move it to the collecting lymphatics and larger lymphatic trunks, through regional lymph nodes, and eventually into the right lymphatic duct or the thoracic duct, and back into the vena cava (see Fig. 12-8).

In the presence of lymphatic dysfunction, some part or all of the 10% of fluid volume and the proteins will remain

---

*However, in edema, it can become positive and tend to keep fluid out of the tissues. This is the one "safety factor" that controls lymphedema (i.e., the fibrous tissue actually helps to increase tissue hydrostatic pressure [THP] and control the size of the limb to some extent).

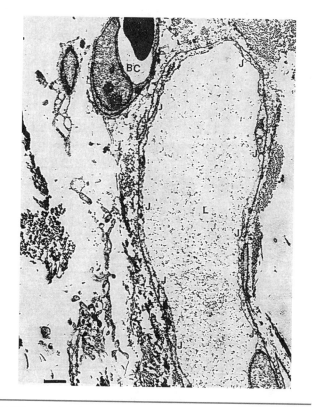

FIGURE **12-2** An initial lymphatic (*L*) in a quiescent (at rest or inactive) tissue. Many closed (narrow or tight) junctions (*J*) are evident. A blood capillary (*BC*) is shown for comparison of size, endothelial opacity, and other characteristics. The bar at the lower left (1μm) is provided to give the viewer size perspective. (From Casley-Smith JR, Casley-Smith JR: *Modern treatment for lymphoedema*, ed 5, Adelaide, Australia, 1997, Lymphoedema Association of Australia. Modified from Casely-Smith JR: *Br J Exp Path* 46:35-49, 1965.)

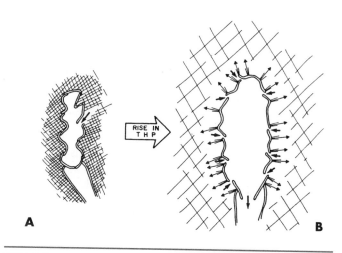

FIGURE **12-3** Effects of elevated tissue hydrostatic pressure (*THP*) on initial lymphatic functioning. **A,** Normal lymphatic vessel at a fairly low tissue hydrostatic pressure and normal lymphatic drainage. **B,** Tissue response to a tremendous increase in tissue hydrostatic pressure (represented by the large arrow). The swelling in the interstitial tissues pulls on the anchoring filaments, pulling and holding open the initial lymphatic endothelial junctions (thin arrows pointing outwards), allowing fluid to pour into the initial lymphatic in an attempt to reduce edema. In this way, in place of a few widely open junctions, there are many slightly open ones, through which fluid is forced (thicker arrows directed inward), down a hydrostatic pressure gradient. (From Casley-Smith JR, Casley-Smith JR: *Modern treatment for lymphoedema*, ed 5, Adelaide, Australia, 1997, Lymphoedema Association of Australia.)

trapped in the tissue spaces and cause lymphedema. With lymphedema, the challenge for the therapist is to effectively move that fluid back into functioning lymphatics and then into the central circulation. This model is a very gross simplification but can be helpful in understanding the basics of fluid dynamics in the capillary loop. Many other factors affect the tissues in addition to those mentioned above.[12,57]

Deeper in the dermis are *pre-collectors* (Fig. 12-4), which flow into *collecting lymphatics* located in the subcutaneous tissue (Fig. 12-5). The true collecting vessels have valves to prevent backflow and some muscle tissue in their walls to further enhance their pumping action.[12,57] Extrinsic muscle contraction or lymphatic drainage massage also increases this pumping action.

Collecting lymphatics do not form a plexus, but there can be connections between them. Their diameter gradually increases in size to form the *lymph trunks*, which lie near the deep fascia. Each segment of collecting lymphatic vessels between valves is called a *lymphangion* (Fig. 12-6). The muscle in the collecting lymphatic walls contracts rhythmically. Smooth muscle cells around the endothelial cell layer face the lumen of the vessel. These are innervated by the autonomic nervous system and contract on the average of 5 to 10 times per minute.[59] This "lymphangiomotoricity" combines with the contraction of the lymphangion itself, which is triggered by distention of the vessel wall. The greater is the stretch, the greater is the force of the contraction. If many lymphangions contract at once and outflow is obstructed (e.g., by scarred or radiated lymph nodal areas), pressure inside the vessel can reach as high as 100 mm Hg. High intravascular pressure fatigues the muscle wall, leading to ineffective smooth muscle contraction and ultimately to vessel failure. The walls dilate, preventing closure of valve flaps, and a backflow of lymph distal to the site of obstruction occurs, causing lymphedema. This is one plausible explanation for the fact that many individuals with a "limb at risk" develop lymphedema months or even years after their original surgery. For a time, the remaining lymphatics function marginally without evidence of clinical lymphedema, but these units become overtaxed, eventually the walls fatigue, and latent lymphedema progresses to acute and then to chronic lymphedema.

The lymph trunks in the extremities join into the larger lymph vessels of the trunk, which join to form the *thoracic duct* and the *right lymphatic duct* that pump the lymph into the central circulation at the left and right subclavian veins in the root of the neck. The lymphatic vessels are embedded in fatty tissue and accompany the chains of lymph nodes along the blood vessels.[23] This explains why injury to blood vessels in an area implies injury to lymphatic vessels in that area too, regardless of whether it is "unexpected" or "controlled" trauma, as in surgery.

As lymph flows from the periphery to the root of the limbs to the center of the body, it passes through many *lymph nodes*, which act as filters to cleanse the lymph of waste products and cellular debris. Vessels distal to nodes are called *afferent lymph vessels*. Vessels leaving lymph nodes for more proximal points

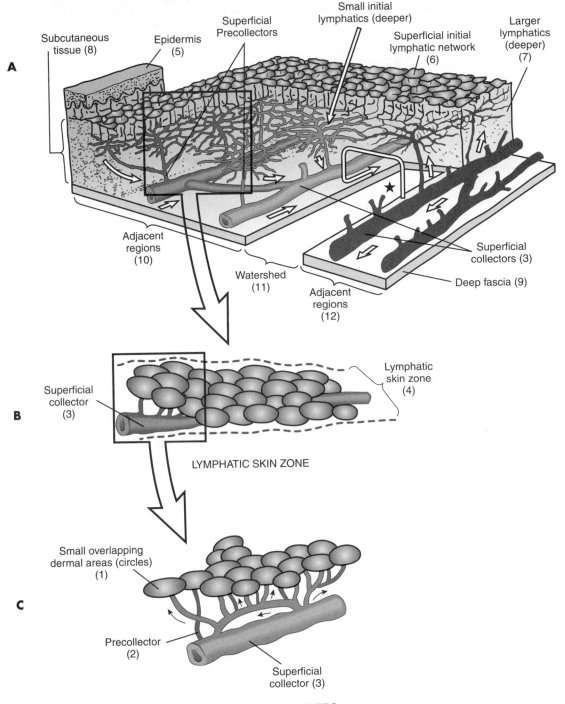

A

Subcutaneous tissue (8)

Epidermis (5)

Superficial Precollectors

Small initial lymphatics (deeper)

Superficial initial lymphatic network (6)

Larger lymphatics (deeper) (7)

Adjacent regions (10)

Watershed (11)

Adjacent regions (12)

Superficial collectors (3)

Deep fascia (9)

B

Superficial collector (3)

Lymphatic skin zone (4)

LYMPHATIC SKIN ZONE

C

Small overlapping dermal areas (circles) (1)

Precollector (2)

Superficial collector (3)

OVERLAPPING DERMAL LAYERS

FIGURE **12-4** Overview of the lymphatic drainage system. **A,** Overview of the lymphatic drainage paths from a skin region. The epidermis (5) is superficial to a superficial initial lymphatic network (6), which sends blindly ending vessels into the dermis and which is linked to the deep dermal plexus of larger initial lymphatics (7), in the subcutaneous tissue (8), by many connections. The superficial collecting lymphatics (3), which discharge into the larger ones (not shown), lie next to the deep fascia (9). A watershed (11) lies between two adjacent regions, (10 and 12), which drain in opposite directions (medium arrows). One of these is obstructed (red vessels). The deep and superficial initial lymphatic plexuses overlap across this watershed. These groups of cross-connections provide collateral drainage and are enlarged by manual massage. The large, U-shaped arrow (★) shows this path. **B,** Lymphatic skin zone (4) that extends along the length of a superficial collector (3). Certain areas of the skin drain into a specific superficial collector, which accounts for the clinical observation of lymphedema in portions of an extremity (e.g., pockets of extra swelling or asymmetrical edema). When a specific superficial collector is blocked (or if the deep collector into which it drains is blocked), the result is edema at that site. **C,** Shows small overlapping dermal areas (circles = 1), which drain into networks of initial lymphatics (not shown), which drain into small collecting lymphatics called *precollectors* (2) and then to larger *superficial collectors* (3). (From Casley-Smith JR, Casley-Smith JR: *Modern treatment for lymphoedema*, ed 5, Adelaide, Australia, 1997, Lymphoedema Association of Australia. Modified from Foldi M, Kubik S: *Lehrbuch der lymphologie fur mediziner und physiotherapeuter mit anhang: praktische linweise fur die physiotherape*, Stuttgart, Germany 1989, Gustav Fischer Verlag.)

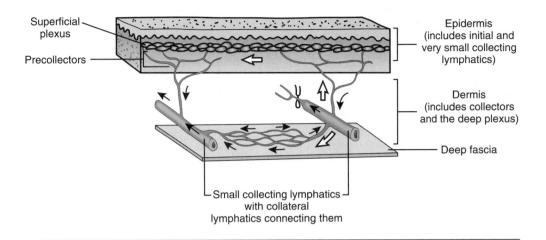

FIGURE   **12-5**   Collecting lymphatics. Lymphatics traverse through the epidermis, dermis, and deep fascia via lymphatics that increase in size as they go deeper into the tissues. Two layers of lymphatic plexuses are in the skin: the epidermis and dermis (layer just below the epidermis, formerly called the *corium*), which contains blood and lymphatic vessels, nerves, and nerve endings, glands, and hair follicles. Lymphatic vessels in the dermal layer can divert fluid from a blocked area and drain it into normally functioning area(s). In this illustration, one of the two larger collectors (on the right) is blocked; note the watershed between the blocked and the open collecting lymphatic. The lymph that would normally be transported along this blocked collector instead passes up into the superficial plexus and down into the deeper plexus formed by collaterals in the watershed area located just above the deep fascia. In these, the lymph passes to the nonblocked collector (on the left) and then drains into larger lymph vessels (not shown). When edema exists, the valve flaps in the collaterals are dilated and do not meet, thereby allowing lymph to move in either direction across these vessels (i.e., across the watershed). (From Casley-Smith JR, Casley-Smith JR: *Modern treatment for lymphoedema*, ed 5, Adelaide, Australia, 1997, Lymphoedema Association of Australia. Modified from Foldi M, Kubik S: *Lehrbuch der lymphologie fur mediziner und physiotherapeuter mit anhang: praktische linweise fur die physiotherape*, Stuttgart, Germany 1989, Gustav Fischer Verlag.)

FIGURE   **12-6**   The lymphangion. Many lymphangions may contract at once, but sometimes only one lymphangion is triggered. The pressure exerted by each lymphangion is usually a few mm Hg but can be over 100 mm Hg if outflow is obstructed and many units are contracting at once. Contraction is triggered by distention (i.e., greater filling creates greater force) but can be modified by humoral (including medications) and nervous factors. Pumping is greatly aided by varying total tissue pressure (TTP) (e.g., from adjacent muscles, respiration, manual lymphatic drainage), as previously mentioned in the text. (From Casley-Smith JR, Casley-Smith JR: *Modern treatment for lymphoedema*, ed 5, Adelaide, Australia, 1997, Lymphoedema Association of Australia.)

are called *efferent lymph vessels*. Lymph nodes also produce lymphocytes and macrophages, which are critical for immune function; destroy foreign bacteria, harmful viruses, and cancer cells; and filter waste products. Lymph nodes offer 100 times the normal resistance to flow of lymph within the lymphatic vessels themselves, which explains why they are often the sites of obstruction in lymphatic dysfunction.[12,28,57]

◆ Lymphatic Territories and Watersheds

The anatomy of the lymphatic system is a regional one. The body is divided into a series of lymph drainage territories called *lymphotomes*, which are bordered and separated by so-called "watershed" areas. The watershed areas are characterized by sparse collateral flow to adjacent lymphotomes,[6,29] but connections exist between lymphotomes in the superficial and deep plexuses and via collateral lymphatics between deep collectors in adjacent lymphotomes located just above the deep fascia. Under normal conditions, the lymph drains in different directions on either side of these watersheds (Fig. 12-7).

The trunk can be divided into four quadrants: the left and right thoracic lymphotomes and the left and right abdominal lymphotomes. The left and right thoracic lymphotomes drain into the ipsilateral axilla, as do the left and right upper extremities. Some individuals possess an auxiliary drainage pathway from the lateral aspect of the upper arm called the *deltoid-pectoral* or *cephalic chain*. This pathway drains directly into the ipsilateral subclavian nodal area, bypassing the axilla entirely. If present, an individual may be less likely to develop upper extremity lymphedema secondary to axillary disruption (surgical or by radiation), as this pathway may provide sufficient lymph transport capacity for the upper extremity. This pathway can be disrupted by supraclavicular radiation therapy sometimes used to treat recurrent cancer of the chest wall.[35]

The left and right abdominal lymphotomes drain into the left and right superficial inguinal nodes, respectively. Each leg and corresponding half of the lumbar, gluteal, and genital region drains to the ipsilateral superficial inguinal nodes. From there, fluid drains into the deep inguinal, pelvic and abdominal nodes, into the cisterna chyli, the thoracic duct, and to

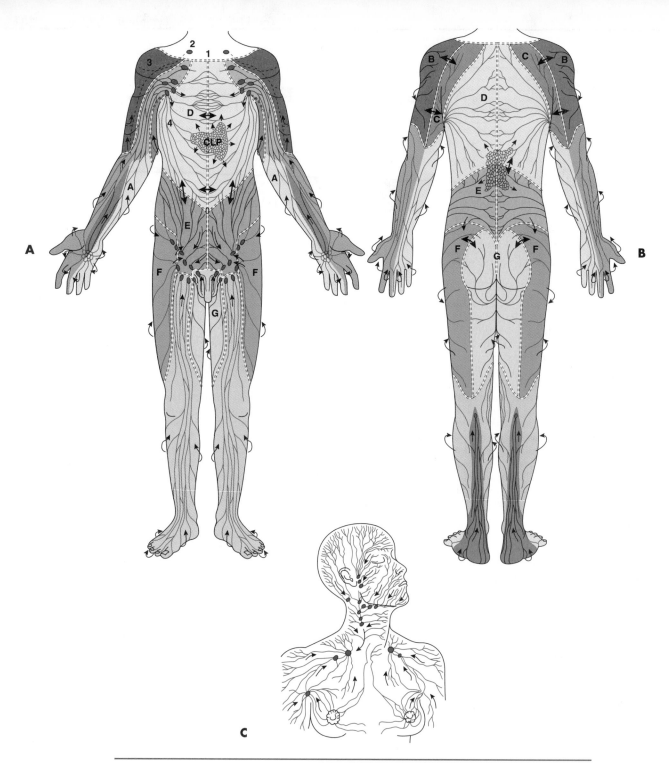

FIGURE 12-7 Regional lymphatic system. The dermal and subcutaneous lymph territories (lymphotomes are indicated by different shadings) of the lymphatic system are separated by watersheds marked by (= = = =). **A,** Anterior view. **B,** Posterior view. **C,** Head, neck, and breast. Arrows indicate the direction of the lymph flow. Normal drainage is away from the watershed, but collaterals cross the watershed (*thick double arrows*). When the main drainage paths from each of these regions are blocked, lymph (*thick single arrows*) has to be carried across the watersheds via collaterals and the plexuses. The cutaneous lymphatic plexus (*CLP*) is shown in the center of the chest only. It is filled from the tissues and covers the entire body; this is not shown to avoid confusion. These initial lymphatics fill superficial collectors, which drain into deep ones and then into the lymphatic trunks (*small arrows*). *Letters* designate various lymphotomes: *A,* forearm lymphotomes; *B,* lateral arm lymphotome; *C,* medial arm lymphotome; *D,* thoracic lymphotome; *E,* abdominal lymphotome; *F,* lateral thigh lymphotome; *G,* medial thigh lymphotome. The lymphotome of the external genitals and perineum is shown but unlabeled. Numbers refer to: *1.* mid-trunk watershed; *2.* supraclavicular nodes; *3.* lateral upper arm trunks ("cephalic" or deltoid trunks); *4.* axillo-inguinal anastomotic pathways. (From Casley-Smith JR, Casley-Smith JR: *Modern treatment for lymphoedema,* ed 5, Adelaide, Australia, 1997, Lymphoedema Association of Australia. Modified from Foldi M, Kubik S: *Lehrbuch der lymphologie fur mediziner und physiotherapeuter mit anhang: praktische linweise fur die physiotherape,* Stuttgart, Germany 1989, Gustav Fischer Verlag.)

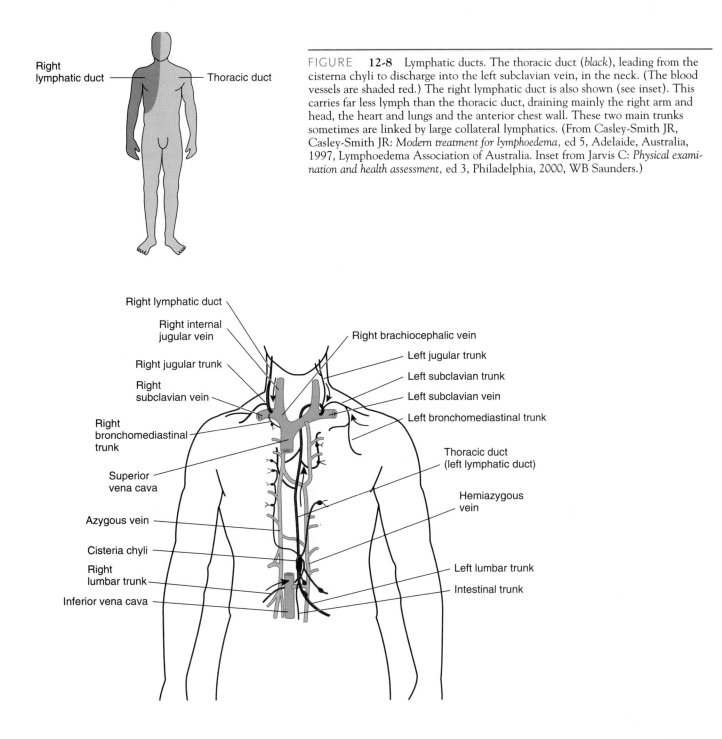

FIGURE   **12-8**   Lymphatic ducts. The thoracic duct (*black*), leading from the cisterna chyli to discharge into the left subclavian vein, in the neck. (The blood vessels are shaded red.) The right lymphatic duct is also shown (see inset). This carries far less lymph than the thoracic duct, draining mainly the right arm and head, the heart and lungs and the anterior chest wall. These two main trunks sometimes are linked by large collateral lymphatics. (From Casley-Smith JR, Casley-Smith JR: *Modern treatment for lymphoedema*, ed 5, Adelaide, Australia, 1997, Lymphoedema Association of Australia. Inset from Jarvis C: *Physical examination and health assessment*, ed 3, Philadelphia, 2000, WB Saunders.)

the left subclavian vein[12] (Fig. 12-8). Most of the lower leg drains via the femoral trunks, which run on the anterior thigh to the inguinal nodes, also draining the medial and lateral thigh lymphotomes. There is a small posterior lower leg lymphotome draining to the popliteal nodes by way of the dorsolateral trunks.

A midline watershed divides the head, neck, and face areas. The right side drains to the right cervical nodes and then to the right supraclavicular nodes; the left side drains to the left cervical nodes and then to the left supraclavicular nodes. The posterior aspect of the head and neck drain into the vertebral lymphatics that drain into the supraclavicular nodes on the ipsilateral side.[12,29]

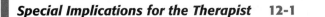

Special Implications for the Therapist   **12-1**

ANATOMY OF THE LYMPHATIC SYSTEM

It is important to realize that the right upper extremity and thoracic lymphotome drain into the right lymphatic duct and that the left upper extremity, left thoracic lymphotome, and both lower extremities, external genital areas, and abdominal lymphotomes drain into the left subclavian vein via the thoracic duct. Lymphatic obstruction/impairment affects the trunk quadrants and extremities. In addition to ex-

Continued

tremity edema, individuals may develop lymphedema of the breast, lateral trunk, abdomen, genitals, supra-pubic area, or buttocks.

Drainage can be changed from lymphotome to another by expelling lymph from an overloaded one toward a normal one even across two or three intermediate overloaded areas (see Fig. 12-5). This change in flow occurs through the most superficial plexus, which then drains into the deeper (but still very superficial) collectors and deep trunks. The deep trunks also have collaterals crossing the watersheds to accomplish this flow. It is the dilatation of the collectors and collaterals together with the superficial plexus that account for the success of the therapy intervention using lymphatic drainage as part of the program. Improper treatment of extremity edema without considering the impact of that treatment on the trunk quadrant adjacent to the limb/limbs involved can result in the development of truncal or genital edema, when none existed before intervention for the extremity edema.[8]

Lymph Nodes

Normal, healthy lymph nodes are soft and nonpalpable. Palpable lymph nodes do not always indicate serious or ongoing disease, but this determination requires an evaluation by a physician. Therapists may identify suspicious palpable lumps in a client who has already been examined by a physician. However, the therapy profession offers greater opportunity for identification of suspicious nodes, given the specificity of palpatory skills and techniques practiced by a therapist. For this reason, the therapist should not hesitate to return a client to the referring or primary physician for further evaluation.

Past medical history is extremely helpful in determining the urgency of referral. A suspicious, palpable node in the presence of a previous history of cancer warrants immediate medical referral. Supraclavicular and inguinal nodes are common metastatic sites for cancer. Nodes involved with metastatic cancer are usually hard and fixed to the underlying tissue. In acute infections, nodes are tender asymmetrically, enlarged, and matted together, and the overlying skin may be red and warm (erythematous). Changes in size (greater than 1 cm); shape (matted together); and consistency (rubbery or firm) of lymph nodes in more than one area or the presence of painless enlarged lymph nodes must be reported to the physician.

In the case of recent pharyngeal or dental infections, minor, residual enlargement of cervical nodes may be observed. Intraoral infection may also cause an inflamed cervical node. The therapist may first be alerted to this condition by a spasm of the sternocleidomastoid muscle causing neck pain. Palpation may appear to aggravate a primary spasm, as if the spasm were originating in the muscle, when in fact a lymph node under the muscle is the source of symptoms. In such cases, the past history is the key to quickly identifying the need for medical referral or follow-up care.

Lymphadenopathy in certain anatomic areas such as preauricular or postauricular (in front of or behind the ear); supraclavicular; deltopectoral; and pectoral regions are viewed by the medical community with greater suspicion because these areas are not usually enlarged as a result of local subclinical infections or trauma.[53] ◼

INFLAMMATION AND INFECTION IN THE LYMPHATIC SYSTEM

Disorders of the lymphatic system may result from *lymphangitis* (inflammation of a lymphatic vessel); *lymphadenitis* (inflammation of one or more lymph nodes); *lymphedema* (an increased amount of lymph fluid in the soft tissues); or *lymphadenopathy* (enlargement of the lymph nodes). Lymph nodes act as defense barriers and are secondarily involved in virtually all systemic infections and in many neoplastic disorders arising elsewhere in the body.

The specific node or nodes affected in an infectious disease depends on the location of the infection, the nature of the invading organism, and the severity of the disease. For example, infections involving the pharynx, salivary glands, and scalp often cause tender enlargement of the neck nodes, referred to as *reactive cervical lymphadenopathy*. *Generalized lymphadenopathy*, enlargement of two or three regionally separated lymph node groups, is usually due to inflammation, neoplasm, or immunologic reactions.

These two types of lymphadenopathy are normal reactions to infection that result in large and tender lymph nodes, but the node is not necessarily infected (warm or reddened, as with lymphadenitis). The presence of lymphadenopathy is usually more significant in people older than 50 years; lymphadenopathy in people under age 30 is usually due to benign causes, but this must be medically determined.

◆ Lymphedema

Definition.   Lymphedema is a swelling of the soft tissues that results from the accumulation of protein-rich fluid in the extracellular spaces. It is caused by decreased lymphatic transport capacity and/or increased lymphatic load and is most commonly seen in the extremities but can occur in the head, neck, abdomen, and genitalia.

Classification of Lymphedema.   Lymphedema is divided into two broad categories: primary (idiopathic) and secondary (acquired) lymphedema. In the past, primary lymphedema was classified as connatal,* if it appeared at birth, praecox if it appeared at puberty, or tarda if it developed after age 35.

The severity of lymphedema is graded using the International Society of Lymphology (ISL)'s Stage I, Stage II, and Lymphostatic Elephantiasis Stage III scale[3,22] (Box 12-1). Stage I lymphedema is soft, pits on pressure, and reverses with elevation. In the early stages, there is a chronic inflammatory response to the excessive protein in the interstitium. The subcutaneous tissues begin to fibrose, progressing the lymphedema from Stage I to II. In fact, a lymphedematous limb may be Stage II in the foot and ankle and Stage I in the thigh.

Stage II lymphedema is nonpitting and does not reduce on elevation of the limb, and clinical fibrosis is present. Skin changes such as eczema, warts, papillomas, and lymph fistulae are common in severe Stage II lymphedema. Chronic inflammation can lead to recurrent bacterial and fungal infections. The most severe Stage III lymphedema is

---

*The term *connatal* (present from birth) applies to most primary lymphedemas that are present at birth, rather than the term *congenital*, which implies a specific genetic abnormality.

BOX 12-1

Stages of Lymphedema

Stage I

Accumulation of protein-rich, pitting edema
Reversible with elevation; area affected may be normal size upon waking in the morning
Increases with activity, heat, and humidity

Stage II

Accumulation of protein-rich, nonpitting edema with connective scar tissue
Irreversible; does not resolve overnight; increasingly more difficult to pit
Clinical fibrosis is present
Skin changes present in severe Stage II

Stage III (Lymphostatic Elephantiasis)

Accumulation of protein-rich edema with significant increase in connective and scar tissue
Severe nonpitting fibrotic edema
Atrophic changes (hardening of dermal tissue, skin folds, skin papillomas, hyperkeratosis)

TABLE 12-1

Causes of Lymphedema

PRIMARY	SECONDARY*
Unknown	Filariasis
Hereditary	Primary or metastatic neoplasm (benign or malignant)
Developmental abnormality	
• Aplasia	Surgery (lymph node dissection or removal)
• Hypoplasia	Radiation treatment
• Hyperplasia	Chemotherapy
	Severe infection
	Other surgery (e.g., multiple abdominal/pelvic surgeries)
	Lipedema
	Chronic venous insufficiency
	Liposuction
	Crush injury
	Compound fracture
	Severe laceration
	Degloving skin injury
	Burns
	Morbid obesity
	Multiparity
	Paralysis
	Prolonged systemic use of cortisone (cortisone skin)
	HIV/AIDS
	Air travel (a "trigger" for those at risk; see Table 12-2)

* Listed in approximate descending order.

referred to as lymphostatic elephantiasis. This is characterized by severe nonpitting, fibrotic edema with atrophic skin changes such as thickened, leathery, keratotic skin, skinfolds with tissue flaps, warty protrusions, papillomas, and leaking lymph fistulae. Lymphangiomas (form of lymphangiectasia) may also be present.

Incidence. The exact incidence of primary lymphedema is unknown because many people remain undiagnosed or if diagnosed, treatment or follow-up care does not occur, and the condition remains unreported.[36] Approximately 15% of primary lymphedemas are present at birth (formerly called *connatal*). The most common form of primary lymphedema occurs from adolescence to midlife and accounts for 75% of primary lymphedema in a 4:1 ratio of females to males (formerly called *lymphedema praecox*). Of all primary lymphedema, 10% to 20% appears abruptly after age 35 (formerly called *lymphedema tarda*).[12] A small percentage of primary lymphedemas occur in association with rare genetic syndromes such as Milroy's (appears at birth) and Meige's (develops anywhere from early childhood to puberty) diseases, accounting for approximately 2% of primary lymphedemas.

The incidence of secondary lymphedema also remains an approximate figure. Presently, no detailed maps are available of the geographical distribution of secondary lymphedema caused by filariasis but distribution may be governed by climate with an estimated 420 million people exposed to this infection in Africa in the year 2000.[37] The WHO estimates 700,000 people in the Americas are affected today (including 400,000 in Haiti and 100,000 in the Dominican Republic). Clinical reports on the incidence of secondary lymphedema from other causes vary with an estimated 3 million new cases

in the United States each year; up to 30% of breast cancer survivors in the United States develop lymphedema sometime in their lifetime. The incidence increases after surgery and radiation when these procedures are combined.[15,21,41]

Etiologic Factors. The exact cause of *primary lymphedema* is unknown and cannot be linked to any significant traumatic event (Table 12-1). Primary lymphedema is most likely the result of lymphangiodysplasias or malformations of the lymphatic vessel present at birth (Fig. 12-9) but sometimes delayed in symptomatic presentation. Although a small percentage of primary lymphedemas are linked to genetic causes (e.g., Milroy's disease and Meige's Syndrome), most cases are not genetically linked and are more likely the result of some developmental abnormality in the fetus. A family history of lymphedema is present in only 10% to 20% of all people with primary lymphedema.[18]

Klippel-Trénaunay-Weber syndrome (KTWS) is a rare occurrence in embryonic development and is associated with numerous anomalies. These can include varicose veins, cavernous hemangioma of the skin, and hypertrophy of bones and soft tissues in one or several extremities. In addition, dysplasia of the lymphatic system and neurogenic and visceral vascular malformations can occur. The dysplasia of the lymphatics can result in lymphedema in the involved extremities[57] (Fig. 12-10).

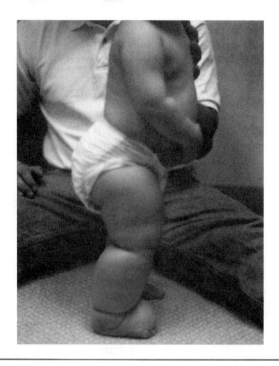

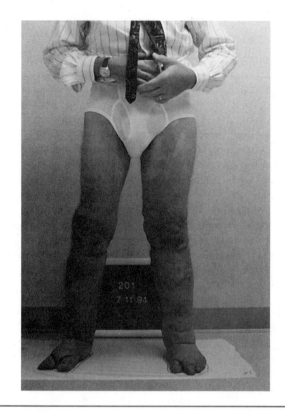

FIGURE   **12-9**   A 13-month-old with primary lymphedema of the right lower extremity, right buttock, and genital area since birth. (Courtesy Lymphedema Therapy, Woodbury, Long Island, New York, 2000.)

FIGURE   **12-10**   A 50-year-old man with Klippel-Trénaunay syndrome, a lymphangiodysplasia that caused lymphedema in both lower extremities. Note the skeletal abnormalities of the toes, the large hemangioma on the left thigh, and the venous varicosities in the lower legs. (Courtesy Lymphedema Therapy, Woodbury, Long Island, New York, 2000.)

Malformations of the lymphatic vessels associated with primary lymphedema can be divided into three types: aplastic, hypoplastic, and hyperplastic. *Aplasia* occurs when the lymphatic collectors are so few that they are considered "absent." Aplasia may also involve the absence of lymph capillaries that render the adequate collectors less functional. Aplasia is most often combined with hypoplasia; complete aplasia would result in tissues unable to support life. *Hypoplasia* refers to less than the normal expected number of lymph collectors in the affected region and may also occur when collectors present are unable to function as transport vessels. Hypoplasia represents the most common cause of primary lymphedema occurring in 75% of the cases. *Hyperplasia* accounts for 15% of primary cases and is characterized by grossly dilated and enlarged lymphatics that can become varicose. Hyperplasia can occur in the lymphatics of the superficial plexus of the skin or in the main lymph trunks. As a result of the overdilation of the vessels, the intralymphatic valve flaps do not seal, and a reflux of lymph occurs. When this occurs in the mesenteric/intestinal lymphatics, a reflux of chyle* from the intestines to distal areas also takes place—that is, the skin of the genitals, buttocks and thighs, or to the knee joint (Fig. 12-11). *Lymphangiectasia* refers to lymphatic hyperplasia in a deeper organ or localized area of a limb. Lymphangiomas and lymph cysts are forms of lymphangiectasia.

Secondary lymphedema occurs as the result of damage to otherwise normal lymphatic vessels/nodes from a known entity. The most common cause of secondary lymphedema worldwide is filariasis. Filariasis is a parasitic infection, carried by mosquitoes in endemic regions, often found in tropical climates (Africa, South America, India, Malaysia). The larvae of the worm are injected into the dermis with the mosquito bite. They pass into the initial lymphatics and larger collecting lymphatics and can grow to 20 cm in length and 1 to 2 cm in diameter as they mature into the adult worm forms. The adult male has a long tail that whips back and forth, damaging the fragile lymphatic walls. The greatest damage, however, is done after the worm dies, often 5 to 10 years after the initial infection. At that time, foreign proteins from the worm body cause severe local inflammatory reactions leading to severe fibrosis and scarring of the tissues, totally blocking the larger lymph collectors. This total blockage results in massive swelling distal to that collection site.[5,31,57]

In the United States and other regions of the world where the filaria parasite does not exist or has been eradicated, the most common cause of secondary lymphedema is invasive procedures used in the diagnosis and treatment of cancer. Regional lymph node dissection for diagnostic staging and eradication of tumor sites disrupts the lymphatic system. Radiation therapy, reconstructive or other surgical procedures, or the combination of these procedures are well-known contributing factors to the development of lymphedema.

Local radiation treatment after surgery for cancer increases the incidence of secondary lymphedema three times that of

---

*Chyle is the protein-rich, milky fluid taken up by the intestinal lymphatics during digestion, consisting of lymph and triglyceride fat in a stable emulsion, and conveyed by the thoracic duct to empty into the venous system.

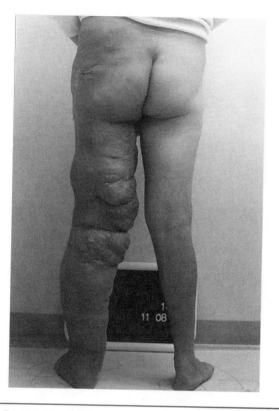

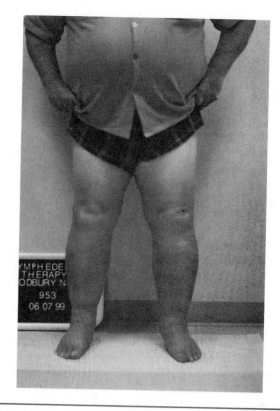

FIGURE 12-11 A 19-year-old male with primary lymphedema of the left lower extremity (onset age 8). Lymphedema progressed to involve the buttocks and genitalia after prolonged pneumatic compression pump usage. This young man had three microsurgical procedures (lympho-venous and lympho-lymphatic anastamoses) in an attempt to reduce the genital and extremity edema. In addition, he had two debulking surgeries, which also were unsuccessful in reducing the lymphedema. He developed chylous reflux and eventually had sclerotherapy to his leaking abdominal lymphatics, which was very successful in stopping the severe leakage of chyle from his scrotum, medial thigh, and buttock. The chyle-filled papules are visible on the posterior aspect of the thigh and calf. Notice the abnormal bulges and skinfolds on the posterior thigh, which result when the debulked areas fill in with edema fluid. (Courtesy Lymphedema Therapy, Woodbury, Long Island, New York, 2000.)

FIGURE 12-12 A 63-year-old man with lymphedema of both lower extremities, left greater than right. The swelling developed in the left leg 1 year after a coronary artery bypass graft (CABG) procedure when veins were harvested from the left leg. The swelling began in the right leg, worsened in the left leg, and progressed into the abdomen after radium seed implantation for prostate cancer. This man's marginal lymphatic system was overwhelmed by the "trauma" caused by the CABG procedure and the radium seed implantation procedure. (Courtesy Lymphedema Therapy, Woodbury, Long Island, New York, 2000.)

surgery alone, probably due to the increase in local tissue fibrosis that further impairs lymph flow through the remaining functioning lymphatic vessels.[12] If there is significant burning and blistering of the skin during radiation treatment, the risk of lymphedema is increased due to the decreased elasticity of the skin and subcutaneous tissues.[48]

Other causes of secondary lymphedema include bacterial or viral infection; multiple abdominal surgeries, particularly in the obese individual; any trauma or surgery that impairs the lymphatics; or repeated pregnancies (see Table 12-1). Liposuction, done for cosmetic reasons to enhance appearance, when performed on an individual with an asymptomatic but marginal lymphatic system can trigger lymphedema in the operative limb. Crush injuries, compound fractures, or severe lacerations/degloving injuries to the skin can significantly impair lymph flow. These types of injuries are also usually associated with damage to blood vessels. The damaged blood vessels leak fibrinogen, blocking the tissue channels and initial lymphatics and thus contributing to the development of lym-

phedema. Other known causes that have been reported associated with secondary lymphedema include chronic venous insufficiency,* paralysis, lipedema, skin thinned by cortisone (sometimes referred to as *cortisone skin*), and AIDS, particularly if Kaposi's sarcoma is present.[12]

Surgery is "controlled trauma," but it is trauma nevertheless; the more extensive the procedure, the more extensive is the trauma. Surgery in individuals with a marginal lymphatic system (where the lymph transport capacity equals the normal lymph load) can cause enough of an overload to trigger lymphedema. For example, an individual undergoing a triple coronary artery bypass graft (CABG) procedure with donor veins taken from the legs may develop chronic leg edema that is often misdiagnosed as venous insufficiency or "cardiac related." This is particularly true in the older, obese individual who has poor functional mobility. If the diagnosis of lymphedema is delayed or *never made* and is not addressed, the individual may not be able to succeed in postoperative rehabilitation (Fig. 12-12).

*Some medications used in the treatment of breast cancer (e.g., Tamoxifen, Adriamycin) have been associated with peripheral thrombophlebitis. These medications can cause blood clots resulting in deep vein thrombosis, venous insufficiency, and eventual secondary lymphedema.

In the past, most health care professionals knew about upper limb lymphedema secondary to axillary dissection for breast cancer, but many were not aware that an individual who had a CABG procedure or inguinal node dissection for melanoma of the foot, testicular, or prostate cancer, or pelvic/abdominal node dissection for gynecologic cancer was at risk for lymphedema of the leg. Anyone with postoperative leg edema after a fracture or total hip or knee replacement would not have been routinely evaluated for lymphedema 10 years ago. The combination of venous edema and lymphedema is often overlooked in the management of edema secondary to trauma. Many cases of chronic edema with recurrent infection and skin ulcerations are treated as pure venous edemas with poor results because the lymphatic component of the edema is not addressed.

Pathogenesis.   Lymphedema by definition is a low flow edema that occurs when the lymph transport capacity is inadequate to transport the normal volume of lymph. It is a failure of the safety valve mechanisms (Fig. 12-13). This can occur when the lymph load is normal but the lymph transport capacity is inadequate (*decreased absorption of lymph in lymph nodes*) or when there is an increase in the lymphatic load (e.g., fluid entering the tissues) and the transport capacity is inadequate (*subtotal lymphatic blockage*). In reality, the body adjusts the load if the capacity alters in response to changes in tissue hydrostatic pressure and other changes in homeostasis (*remaining lymphatics increase their pumping activity*), and conversely, the capacity can be adjusted if the load alters (*intralymphatic pressure increases*). When the safety valve mechanisms are no longer effective or become overwhelmed, the body's normal compensation is not enough, and lymphedema develops.

Lymphedema causes the lymphatic vessels to dilate; the valve flaps become incompetent (*dilation/lymph valvular insufficiency*), and the protein-rich lymphatic fluid refluxes to the tissue spaces (*perilymphatic tissues*). At first, a proliferation of initial lymphatic vessels occurs as the system tries to cope with the accumulation of lymphatic load. Lymph vessels can rejoin, or collateral lymphatics can develop to bypass the damaged area. In lymphedematous tissue, a state of chronic inflammation exists.[43]

This chronic inflammation leads to progressive tissue fibrosis, resulting in a state of relative hypoxia in the tissues, further impeding tissue oxygenation and contributing to a cycle of chronic inflammation and increased risk of infection. In either primary or secondary lymphedema, infection or delayed wound healing (the latter can be directly related to the low oxygen state caused by edema) will add to the high-protein edema. Infection in the tissues (cellulitis) or infection in the lymph vessels (lymphangitis) can cause progressive tissue fibrosis and/or scarring in the lymph vessels (*lymphangiosclerosis*).

Though some recanalization and collateralization of lymph vessels take place, lymphatic function remains compromised. An increase in the size of the tissue channels occurs with an increase in the distance for the oxygen to diffuse from the capillaries to the cells (Fig. 12-14). Gas exchange and metabolism of cellular waste products is impaired. Although the number of macrophages increases, their activity is decreased in the lymphedema fluid for reasons not clearly understood. Some theories suggest that the chronic lack of essential nutrients (e.g., oxygen) or perhaps a toxic

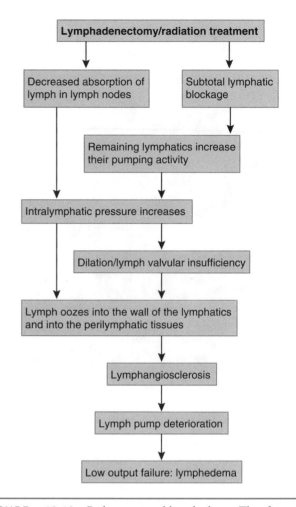

FIGURE   **12-13**   Pathogenesis of lymphedema. This flow chart follows the progression from an "at-risk" or latent phase of lymphedema to acute lymphedema following lymphadenectomy and/or radiation treatment to the nodal area. (Courtesy of Dr. Michael Földi, June 1999.)

factor produced by the stagnant proteins or the damaged tissues contribute to the deterioration of macrophage.[15,19] In chronic lymphedema, the muscle wall of the collecting lymphatics hypertrophies, reducing the effective pumping power of these vessels (*lymph pump deterioration*).

The effect of lymphedema on the blood vessels causes a proliferation of new small blood vessels and the development of arteriovenous anastomoses. These new small vessels may leak due to abnormal changes in total tissue pressure in the lymphedematous region, further overloading the area.

Proteins, fats, cellular waste products, and the 10% of tissue fluid volume that is not directly transported by the venous system have no alternative transport pathway from the interstitium to the venous system except via the lymphatic system. When this transport mechanism is impaired, lymphedema develops (Fig. 12-15, A). The impairment can be structural or functional.

Structural Impairment.   Aging or damaged blood vessels are associated with structural impairment as fibrin physically narrows or blocks tissue channels (Fig. 12-15, B). Hypoplasia of the collecting lymphatics is also associated with the patho-

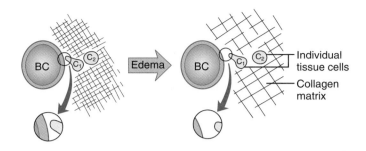

FIGURE 12-14 Reduction of gas (oxygen) exchange. Even a relatively minor amount of edema, which moves the fibers and individual tissue cells ($C1$, $C2$) apart by only a small amount can cause a great increase in the resistance to diffusion of gases (and other small lipid-soluble molecules) between the cells and the blood capillaries (*BC*). The magnified view of the distance between the BC and the tissue cell (representing the cell's oxygen supply) is greatly increased in the edematous state. The greater distance for oxygen to diffuse to nourish the cells will eventually lead to a hypoxic state. (From Casley-Smith JR, Casley-Smith JR: *Modern treatment for lymphoedema*, ed 5, Adelaide, Australia, 1997, Lymphoedema Association of Australia.)

genesis of structural lymphedema (Fig. 12-15, *C*). Primary lymphedema that manifests itself in puberty with a growth spurt and increase in tissue mass causes the body to outgrow or outstrip the capacity of the lymphatic system. The functioning vessels become overwhelmed, the walls fail, dilate, and result in valvular incompetence, causing increased peripheral intralymphatic pressures and peripheral lymphedema.

Structural lymphedema may also occur when the flaps of incompetent valves of the initial lymphatics (Fig. 12-15, *D*) no longer meet, allowing reflux of lymph to regions distal to the blockage. The initial lymphatics eventually dilate as well, their endothelial junctions remain open, and lymph refluxes to the tissues. Other causes of structural lymphedema include gaps and tears in the initial lymphatic walls associated with trauma and inflammation (Fig. 12-15, *E*), physical obstruction of collecting lymphatics (Fig. 12-15, *F*) associated with fibrosis, radiation therapy, tumor growth, surgical excision of lymphatics during tumor removal, and torn anchoring filaments (Fig. 12-15, *G*) associated with sudden acute edema. The latter may occur secondary to massive trauma or infection and can tear the microfilaments that connect the initial lymphatics to the interstitial tissues, resulting in the collapse of the initial lymphatics due to the high total tissue pressure.

In the case of lymphedema caused by filariasis, the adult worm blocks the vessel it is in. Damage to lymph vessels occurs due to the whiplike action of the constantly motile adult worms and the toxic effects of parasite secretory/excretory products. When the worm dies, the toxins released stimulate a granulomatous reaction with infiltration of plasma cells, eosinophils, and giant cells, further damaging the vessel and surrounding tissue as severe inflammation develops. Over time, repeated limb bacterial infections in previously damaged vessels may superimpose additional lymphatic damage.

Functional Impairment

Anything that causes a lack of variation in total tissue pressure (TTP) causes lymphedema. Bed rest, paralysis, or prolonged immobility (e.g., a long air flight) can severely limit changes in total tissue pressure.* It is this variation that contributes to a pressure gradient between the interstitial tissues and the intralymphatic pressure. Normally this pressure gradient stimulates the lymphangions to contract, which enhances the flow of lymph from the periphery to the center of the body. When the tissue pressure does not change or vary, the force pumps remain inactive.

Other factors contributing to functional impairment of the lymphatic system may include spasm of collecting lymphatics (e.g., lymphangiospasm caused by inflammation stimulating sympathetic nerves); paralysis of the collecting lymphatics (e.g., prolonged distention leading to fatigue and ultimately, failure); and impaired contraction of the collecting lymphatics caused by physical obstruction of fibrotic tissue surrounding lymphatic vessels. This type of functional impairment is common in severe Stage II lymphedema and lymphostatic elephantiasis. If collectors cannot pump, lymph refluxes peripherally, causing overdilation of initial lymphatics, valvular incompetence, lymphatic failure, and ultimately, lymphedema.

Clinical Manifestations. Primary or secondary lymphedema is characterized by clinical signs and symptoms caused by the effects of lymphedema on the lymphatics, body tissues, and blood vessels. Lymphedema resulting from filariasis is reversible in its early stages; secondary lymphedema can be transient if damage is minor. Secondary lymphedema can develop immediately postoperatively, weeks, months, or years after surgery.

Lymphedema can develop in any part of the body or limb(s). Signs or symptoms of lymphedema include a full sensation in the affected body part; a sensation of skin tightness; decreased flexibility in the hand, wrist, or ankle; difficulty fitting into clothing in one specific area; or ring, wristwatch, or bracelet tightness. In advanced cases, fistulas to the skin, joints, or gut may develop; these are portals of entry for bacteria to invade the skin and cause recurrent infection.

Physical impairments caused by lymphedema can include increased circumferential limb girth; postural changes; tremendous discomfort (heavy, aching, bursting sensations); neuromuscular deficits; and integumentary complications. These physical impairments can lead to functional limitations and disability along with the potential for psychosocial morbidity (e.g., social isolation, depression, suicide).[2]

Healing time is increased, and all this is occurring in a heavy, painful, clumsy limb that is more prone to injury due to its abnormally large size and decreased functional mobility. Risk of injury is increased, whereas oxygenation and metabolism of waste and cellular debris are decreased. This is a most dangerous environment. As the lymphedema progresses, atrophic skin changes can occur due to the low oxygen state, including loss of hair and sweat glands, formation of keratotic patches on the skin, and the development of papillomas (blisterlike outpocketings of the skin) that sometimes leak lymphatic fluid. Angiosarcoma (Stewart-Treves Syndrome) is a rare malignancy that can develop in an advanced, chronic lymphedema that is left untreated.

---

*A 1996 survey by the Lymphoedema Association of Australia reported an increase in the incidence of lymphedema and exacerbation of preexisting lymphedema after air flight.[16]

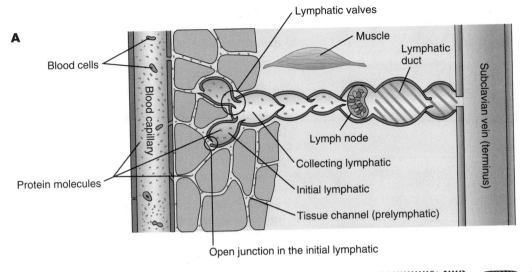

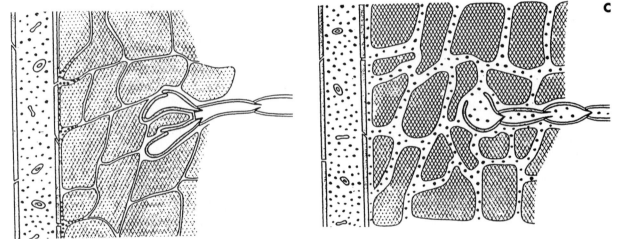

FIGURE 12-15 Low-flow, high-protein lymphedema caused by structural impairment. **A,** "Normal" tissue for comparison showing the passage of protein (*dots*) in normal tissue from the blood capillary, through the tissue channels, into and through the lymphatic system, and back to a vein. **B,** Altered interstitial tissue (e.g., too few or too narrow tissue channels). Notice that the prelymphatic channels are much narrower than in the normal tissue and the protein molecules are stacked up on the arterial side, unable to move easily through the narrow tissue channels, causing impaired lymph flow (and eventual tissue fibrosis). Inlet valves are closed because the endothelial cell junctions cannot open properly in fibrosed tissues contributing to poor lymph drainage. **C,** Abnormally few initial lymphatics. This may occur developmentally or because some of the vessels become blocked (e.g., by fibrin). In this case, too few initial lymphatics are evident. Notice the dilation of the prelymphatic channels, the greater concentration of protein molecules in the tissue channels, and the malformed inlet valve (From Casley-Smith JR, Casley-Smith JR: *Modern treatment for lymphoedema,* ed 5, Adelaide, Australia, 1997, Lymphoedema Association of Australia.)

Continued

Complications of Lymphedema

As lymphedema progresses, the dermal layer of the skin thickens, the skin itself dries and cracks, and ulcerations often develop. These ulcers do not heal due to the tension on the tissues from the edema and the decreased oxygen state, coupled with the subcutaneous fibrosis and chronic inflammation. As the skin and tissues stretch, skinfolds and tissue flaps can develop. These folds/flaps become breeding grounds for fungal and bacterial infections that further damage skin integrity, creating new portals of entry for the bacteria as the skin macerates and cracks. Chronic fungus (tinea) is common on the foot and toes of anyone with lymphedema of the legs, as well as in the groin and under the breast. This fungus can be difficult, if not impossible, to treat topically. If this tinea is not addressed during treatment, a successful outcome is not possible[12] (Fig. 12-16).

The progressive increase in girth and weight of the affected areas contributes to pathologic alterations in the gait pattern and decreases in functional range of motion and strength due to fatigue and inactivity. With increasing edema and subcutaneous fibrosis, tactile sensation and kinesthetic awareness are impaired, increasing the risk of injury to the affected areas.

If the edema progresses into the trunk quadrant adjacent to the lymphedematous limb, a further loss of trunk strength and function can occur. Some individuals, for example, must sleep in a recliner chair to prevent losing their independence,

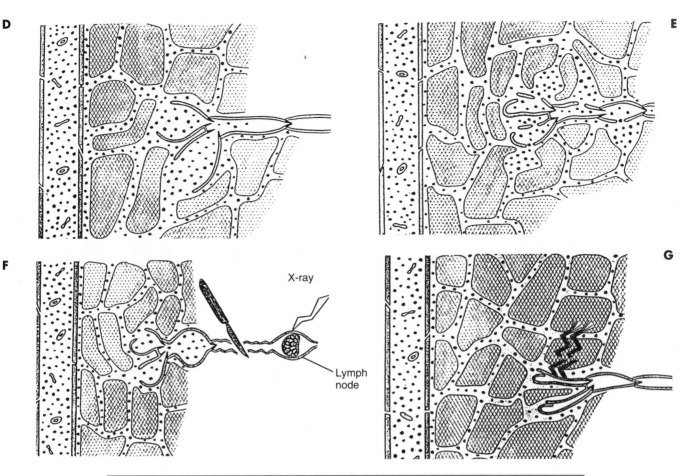

FIGURE 12-15—cont'd Low-flow, high-protein lymphedema caused by structural impairment. **D,** Malformations of the initial lymphatics preventing their inlet-valves from sealing; the pre-lymphatic tissue channels are dilated, a high-protein concentration exists there, and the tissue channels become dilated and stretched. This can happen in both primary and secondary lymphedema; in secondary lymphedema, it occurs after prolonged lymphostasis from a more proximal blockage. **E,** Injuries to the walls of the very fragile initial lymphatics. Lymph refluxes into the tissue channels causing them to dilate. The high concentration of protein in the extracellular tissues causes a chronic inflammatory response and greater risk of infection. Note the larger spaces between the tissues. This results in a larger distance for oxygen to diffuse and leads to tissue hypoxia. **F,** Iatrogenic factors (e.g., surgery, radiation, tumor growth) that damage the lymphatic ducts or larger vessels impair lymph flow from the periphery. When movement of lymph from the tissue channels into the initial lymphatics is impaired, the tissue channels dilate, lymph stasis occurs, and there is a high-protein concentration in the tissues with subsequent chronic inflammation, increased risk of infection, and progressive swelling of the limb. **G,** Anchoring filaments tearing away from the interstitial tissue. This occurs in severe edema from other causes (e.g., rapid swelling from acute lymphedema as a result of trauma can tear the anchoring filaments from the surrounding tissues). The initial lymphatics can no longer function as conduits, as they would normally. The lymphostasis this produces worsens the existing edema. (From Casley-Smith JR, Casley-Smith JR: *Modern treatment for lymphoedema*, ed 5, Adelaide, Australia, 1997, Lymphoedema Association of Australia.)

since they can no longer mobilize themselves and their heavy limbs in bed. A vicious cycle develops with decreasing mobility and strength leading to joint contractures, further increasing the risk to the already impaired skin integument. The limbs may be painful and hypersensitive, and the adjacent trunk quadrants may ache and throb. Balance may be impaired, and the individual may no longer be able to shower or bathe independently, due to fear of falling or inability to move the heavy limbs over the bath or shower ledge. Hygiene becomes a problem, further increasing the risk for fungal and bacterial infections.

Primary lymphedema is more common in females and affects the lower extremities most often. However, it is seen in males and in the upper extremities too.[10] Primary lymphedema can be present in many parts of the body, and if it is present from birth, the deep internal organs can be affected. Clinical cases of primary lymphedema of the lower extremities involve the buttocks, genitals, and intestines with reflux of intestinal chyle (chylous reflux/protein-losing enteropathy) through fistulae on the genitals, buttocks, and thighs (see Fig. 12-20).

This protein-losing enteropathy is a medical emergency. Severe protein loss can occur from this leakage of protein-rich

FIGURE   **12-16**   A 30-year-old male with spina bifida and lymphedema secondary to paralysis and unsuccessful plastic surgery with skin graft for a chronically itchy, 2-cm keratotic lesion on the left anterior ankle crease. **A,** Chronic ulceration complicated by fungal infection of the ulcer itself and the foot/toes. Note the hypertrophic fibrotic skin at the ankle and warty changes on the toes. **B,** After 4 weeks of CLT treatment (debridement of the ulcer was done daily in addition to the lymphatic drainage, compression bandaging, and other skin care). Exercise was not possible due to paralysis, deep abdominal breathing exercises and modified self-lymphatic drainage was taught and then practiced daily. Note that the wound healed completely and the infection resolved. (Courtesy of Lymphedema Therapy, Woodbury, Long Island, New York, 2000.)

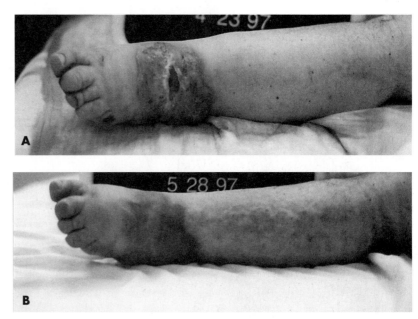

chyle from the intestinal lymphatics. Individuals with primary lymphedema who complain of abdominal bloating, chronic diarrhea, or intolerance of fatty foods may also experience fluid accumulation in the abdomen and genitals from the pressure of the fluid leaking from the intestinal lymphatics into the abdomen. In some cases, these clients are treated medically/surgically with sclerotherapy to seal off these leaking lymphatics in an attempt to halt the reflux of this fluid into the abdomen.

Surgical dissection/radiation therapy involving the cervical, supraclavicular, or mandibular lymph nodes can cause secondary head and neck edema. Significant edema of the head and neck can cause severe functional impairments in speech, swallowing, and respiration, in addition to the pain and psychologic trauma from cosmetic disfigurement. When scarring and lymphatic dysfunction is severe, treatment such as manual lymphatic drainage cannot always restore normal cosmesis; however, it can successfully reduce some of the edema, leading to improved function. For example, in individuals with severe edema of the throat and neck after surgery and radiation for tongue cancer, lymphatic drainage can reduce the swelling enough to allow the person to discontinue use of a tracheotomy tube previously considered permanent. Some clients are able to eat solid foods again; others with severe periorbital and lower facial edema may be able to open the eyes and read and watch television again. Although these are not "cures," they are great improvements in function that are important to individual quality of life.

Medical Management.   Remarkable progress has occurred in diagnosis and management of lymphedema in the United States since 1990. Ironically, this has occurred despite the incorrect prediction for those with breast cancer that the advent of breast-conserving lumpectomy would eliminate upper-extremity lymphedema so commonly seen in individuals postmastectomy. Many individuals who undergo lumpectomy receive axillary node dissection and radiation therapy too; these are the very factors that multiply an individual's risk of developing lymphedema. It has been re-

ported that a 3% incidence of lymphedema after sentinel lymph node biopsy (SLNB) alone increased to 17% when the client required an axillary dissection following the SLNB.[50] Thanks to advances in surgery and chemotherapy and the emphasis on early detection, many more individuals are surviving cancer for many years, living and functioning well with "limbs at risk" for lymphedema.

Diagnosis

Primary Lymphedema.   An easy to perform clinical test for determining primary lower-extremity lymphedema is Stemmer's sign, a thickened cutaneous fold of skin over the second toe, typically present in the early and differential diagnosis of a primary ascending lymphedema without false positive findings.* It appears in the late stages of the descending lymphedema[49] (Fig. 12-17).

Secondary Lymphedema.   The clinical diagnosis of secondary lymphedema is fairly straightforward in a limb at risk, when there is known disruption to the regional lymphatics (e.g., after axillary dissection/radiation for breast cancer or after inguinal node dissection/radiation for melanoma of the leg). A detailed medical history, including all surgical procedures and their chronology relative to the onset or worsening of the edema is the cornerstone of a successful lymphologic evaluation. In secondary lymphedema, most often, no other diagnostic tests are needed to confirm the diagnosis. A venous Doppler study of the edematous limb is often done to rule out a thrombus as the cause of the swelling. It is crucial to have recurrence of cancer firmly ruled out as the causative factor before initiating treatment for the lymphedema. Many oncologists will request a magnetic resonance imaging (MRI) or computed tomography (CT) scan of the chest for upper-extremity swelling or the pelvis and abdomen for lower-extremity swelling before initiating a referral for treatment of the lymphedema.

---

*Although it is possible to have a false negative Stemmer's sign, primary lymphedema is rarely accompanied by a false positive Stemmer's sign.

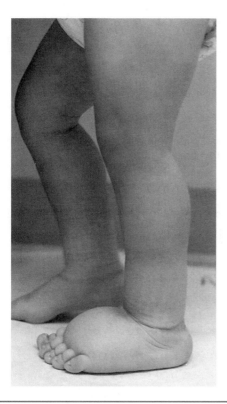

FIGURE 12-17 Stemmer's sign is clearly visible as a thickening of the skin folds of the toes of this 22-month-old child with a history of primary lymphedema of the left lower extremity diagnosed at birth. (Courtesy Lymphedema Therapy, Woodbury, Long Island, New York, 2000.)

Lymphedema may be the first sign of cancer recurrence even years after cancer treatment. The prospect of recurrent disease is a frightening one, but it must be ruled out. Malignant lymphedema (i.e., directly resulting from neoplasm blocking a major nodal region or lymph vessel) is usually more severe and progresses more rapidly than nonmalignant secondary lymphedema. It is often associated with severe pain and/or sensory/motor deficits, particularly in the upper extremity when the brachial plexus is involved. These symptoms must be differentiated from the pain and weakness of radiation plexopathy, which sometimes progresses more slowly, but causes the same type of functional deficits.

In cases of unexplained swelling, particularly in the lower extremities when no known trauma or surgery is evident, the clinical examination and history may not provide a definitive medical diagnosis. Although the MRI and CT scan will clearly show edema fluid in a limb or region, these tests do not give a description of lymphatic function. This type of information is obtained from a lymphoscintigram, a sophisticated nuclear medicine test (the cost is comparable to the MRI or CT scan) that outlines the major lymphatic trunks in a region and provides a functional description of how much tracer material is moved, how far, and in what unit of time, compared with the "normal" values of a person of similar height and weight.

The test involves subcutaneously injecting a small amount of radioactive tracer in the web spaces of the first and second digits of either the hands or feet. The client then performs a set of standard movements for a specific time period and ser-

ial radiographs are taken.* As the tracer is taken up by the lymphatics, it will outline the major lymph trunks and show the volume of tracer moved per unit of time. The presence of tracer reflux that goes back down a limb is called *dermal back-flow* and gives an indication of more proximal obstruction in the deeper lymphatic collectors. When the etiologic factors of edema are unclear, this test clearly shows the functional deficits in the lymphatics. It is especially helpful in ruling out secondary lymphedema in cases of lipedema with questionable lymphedema of the legs.

Treatment. The primary focus in a case of lymphedema triggered by a new or metastatic cancer is to treat the cancer first and then manage the lymphedema. Input on how to minimize exacerbation of the lymphedema during the cancer treatment is often well received, if given with the intent to provide comfort and function. Individuals are encouraged to undergo any treatment that they wish to pursue, without guilt or fear that it will worsen the lymphedema. They need to know the possibilities and risks, but should not be frightened from necessary treatment for the cancer by a well-meaning health care professional. On the other hand, the lymphedema should not be ignored. Management of the lymphedema must be coordinated with the medical team (e.g., medical oncologist, surgeon, radiation oncologist) and the client. This can avoid further overloading the person with additional appointments and adding more to their daily activities than they can handle.

No clear-cut pharmaceutical drug is available to treat lymphedema, although there is hope for a safe, effective medication that will lyse the protein accumulating in the obstructed area and speed the healing process. Clinical studies have shown that the benzopyrones (Coumarin, Venalot, Daflon, and their natural counterparts, the bioflavonoids, rutin, horse chestnut, and grapeseed extract)† have some effect on increasing proteolysis and increasing macrophage activity (remember that the macrophages become inactive in the lymphedema fluid and unable to perform their immune functions). This increased proteolysis helps to reduce the interstitial protein concentration, signaling the body to reabsorb more extracellular fluid, thereby reducing the lymphedema. These substances have been shown to soften fibrotic tissue and increase the healing of chronic ulcerations and bacterial infections in elephantiasis lymphedema, probably due to the activity of the macrophages, stimulating the immune response.[12,17,20,28,38,40,44]

Diuretics work well on sodium retention edemas but do not help lymphedema, yet they continue to be prescribed. Although it is true that taking large doses of diuretics will reduce total body fluid volume, these medications do not address the cause of the lymphedema (i.e., that the lymph load is exceeding the reduced lymph transport capacity).

---

*The amount of exposure from all the radiographs is approximately equal to one x-ray.

†The benzopyrones have not been approved by the Food and Drug Administration (FDA) in the United States, and the oral Coumarin was decertified in Australia due to several cases of death associated with liver problems. Other oral benzopyrones are still available in Switzerland, France, and Germany. Topical Coumarin powder and ointment is still available through compounding pharmacists in the United States. Bioflavonoid liquid and tablets have been available in U.S. health food stores for years. They are combined with various other compounds (known as the bioflavonoid complex) and necessitate taking a larger dose of the complex to receive the desired amount of bioflavonoid.

Furthermore, diuretics may move the "water" component of the lymphatic fluid, further concentrating the extracellular protein in the tissues increasing fibrosis. Moreover, chronic use of high-dose diuretics leaves the individual at great risk for developing electrolyte disturbances.

It should be mentioned here that some of the new nonsteroidal antiinflammatory drugs (NSAIDs) Cox-2 inhibitors (Celebrex, Vioxx) have a warning in the insert about leg edema being a possible side effect. This has been clinically reported in several cases with lymphedema and arthritis; the individual with arthritis may experience an increase in edema when taking these drugs.[5] Therapists must be aware of this possible side effect in anyone on these medications and not assume that increased edema is due, for example, to behavioral noncompliance or a problem with fit of a compression garment.

Surgery has been used to "treat" severe lymphedema in the past with limited success. It is still done today if an individual receives no benefit from conservative treatments or does not have access to these treatments. Although numerous surgical approaches have been proposed to treat chronic lymphedema of the extremity, none has been clinically successful.[36,45] Animal and cadaver studies continue investigating surgical techniques to resect tumors, reconstruct breast tissue, or perform liposuction that will prevent venous occlusion and subsequent lymphatic dysfunction.[32,33]

Many microsurgical procedures attempt to anastomose a lymph vessel or node with a vein or with another functioning lymph vessel or lymph node. The morbidity and mortality from these procedures is significant. These procedures often fail soon after the surgery, leaving the individual with more superficial scarring that further blocks collateral lymph flow from the obstructed limb.

Debulking procedures (e.g., the Charles operation) seek to physically remove the excess fibrosclerotic connective tissue. These operations create extensive longitudinal scars on the involved extremities. Long incisions are made in the skin and subcutaneous tissues are removed down to the muscle and bone; the skin flaps are reopposed and sutured in place. Although these procedures attempt to address the severely impaired cosmesis in the affected individuals, they do not address the cause of the impairment, which is decreased lymph transport capacity. This problem is unchanged by these procedures; over time, the limbs begin to swell again, often with disfiguring asymmetrical tissue flaps, large lymph cysts called *papillomata* (up to 6 to 8 cm in diameter) or warty protrusions on the skin (see Fig. 12-11).[12,29]

Reconstructive surgery after mastectomy is a very personal matter. Many procedures are available from the insertion of a tissue expander, followed later by the insertion of a permanent saline implant to the more extensive myocutaneous tissue flap procedures (i.e., transverse rectus abdominal muscle [TRAM] flap, free latissimus flap) involving transplanting flaps of muscle and skin to the breast area to form a more "natural" breast. The TRAM flap, which transplants the contralateral rectus abdominis muscle by tunneling it across the abdomen and up to the breast area involves extensive scarring in the suprapubic area from hip to hip, in addition to the individual scars on the breast area. The procedure usually consists of two other minor procedures, performed separately to tattoo the areola and create a nipple. The horizontal scar hip to hip effectively blocks a large area of collateral lymph flow from the ipsilateral

thoracic lymphotome through the abdominal lymphotome to the superficial inguinal nodes. This area of collateral lymph drainage is important for the treatment of ipsilateral upper extremity lymphedema that can develop after axillary dissection and mastectomy. In some cases, abdominal lymphedema develops after this procedure.*

The latissimus flap procedure also creates a long transverse scar on the ipsilateral posterolateral thorax, effectively blocking a large area of collateral lymph drainage from the upper extremity to the ipsilateral superficial inguinal nodes. This lymphatic pathway may be needed to treat an upper extremity lymphedema secondary to axillary dissection or radiation.

Prognosis. Left untreated, lymphedema is a progressive disease; current surgical and pharmacologic approaches do not affect a "cure." Lymphedema is a lifelong, chronic condition, but one that can be managed effectively with proper intervention, client education, and regular follow-up care.

---

*This should not be confused with *asymmetrical edema*, which may really be a hernia of the abdominal contents on the contralateral side where the abdominal muscle was removed. This occurs on rare occasions, but it must be medically diagnosed and surgically corrected.

Special Implications for the Therapist 12-2

LYMPHEDEMA

Preferred Practice Patterns:

Five integument patterns are based on the level of skin involvement. Formerly, a singular pattern related to lymphatic impairment was included as part of the Integumentary Paractice Patterns but has subsequently been moved to the section on Cardiovascular/Pulmonary practice. Additionally, reduced mobility and compounding psychosocial aspects may result in physical deconditioning described by practice pattern 6B. Clients who develop radiation fibrosis or surgical scars from cancer surgery may also be described by integument patterns involving partial- and full-thickness skin involvement. Practice patterns are dependent on clinical presentation; additional patterns may be appropriate depending on the underlying cause of the lymphedema but may include the following:

7A: Primary Prevention/Risk Reduction for Integumentary Disorders

7B: Impaired Integumentary Integrity Associated With Superficial Skin Involvement

7C: Impaired Integumentary Integrity Associated With Partial-Thickness Skin Involvement and Scar Formation

7D: Impaired Integumentary Integrity Associated With Full-Thickness Skin Involvement and Scar Formation

7E: Impaired Integumentary Integrity Associated With Skin Involvement Extending into Fascia, Muscle, or Bone and Scar Formation

6H: Impaired Circulation and Anthropometric Dimensions Associated With Lymphatic System Disorders

6B: Impaired Aerobic Capacity/Endurance Associated With Deconditioning

4B: Impaired Posture

4D: Impaired Joint Mobility, Motor Function, Muscle Performance, and Range of Motion Associated With Connective Tissue Dysfunction

4E: Impaired Joint Mobility, Motor Function, Muscle Performance, and Range of Motion Associated With Localized Inflammation

It is critical to advise those who are at risk for lymphedema of the signs and symptoms of lymphedema and to educate them on risk reduction strategies to minimize stress on their marginal lymphatic systems (Table 12-2). Great care must be taken to avoid further overloading an already compromised area by the application of various modalities or therapeutic exercises. For clients who are free of lymphedema but receiving radiation therapy, the radiated area must be observed carefully and consistently for any signs such as blistering; discoloration; erythema (redness); or increased skin temperature changes. Any of these can be indications of developing lymphedema.

Lymphodynamic insufficiency is a concern when treating lymphedema. Clients, particularly those with primary lymphedema of the lower extremities should be evaluated for abdominal and genital edema before undergoing any treatment to reduce the extremity lymphedema to avoid the complication of moving more fluid into an already overloaded abdominal area. Throughout the episode of care, observe the areas adjacent to the lymphedematous limb or region (the ipsilateral buttock, suprapubic/genital areas, ipsilateral breast/lateral trunk, the contralateral lower extremity in a case with pelvic/abdominal node obstruction) to insure that treatment of the peripheral lymphedema does not create lymphedema in adjacent lymph drainage areas. An increased risk of this fluid movement occurs when using gradient compression pump therapy to treat extremity lymphedema.*

Infection

Understanding the risk for infection is critical when evaluating and educating individuals with or at risk for lymphedema. These individuals are extremely prone to local infection from even a minor trauma, abrasion, or insect bite and must be educated in risk reduction and proper skin care to minimize their risk for recurrent infections.

Minor irritations, local areas of redness of the skin, and minor dermatitis reactions must be observed and treated aggressively to avoid progression to a major infection. In a therapy department, the treatment environment and all equipment must be meticulously cleaned.† Many people with lymphedema are unaware of the increased risk of infection or are lulled into complacency by health care professionals who tell them "not to worry" because antibiotics are available if an infection develops. Any infection further stresses the already overloaded regional lymphatic system, possibly scarring some of the remaining functioning lymphatic vessels and ultimately contributing to progressive and chronic lymphedema.

Any infection in a lymphedematous limb, even local, must be medically treated immediately without delay. Individuals must be instructed to contact the physician immediately or go to the emergency department, and they must advise the staff of the lymphedema diagnosis and the impending infection requiring antibiotics. Making this pronouncement firmly can save precious time, eliminating the need to request a referral from the infectious diseases department or obtaining cultures while the bacteria are multiplying and increasing in strength.

Orthopedic Lymphedema

Postsurgical lymphedema occurs after total knee or total hip replacement. If the individual is poorly mobile and had some degree of "swelling" in the legs preoperatively (often attributed to arthritis), the increase in edema postoperatively is often considered the normal sequelae for the procedure. Important loss of time in rehabilitation occurs for these people who are in pain and experience decreased range of motion and strength due to the increasing edema. When the edema is properly reduced and maintained, rehabilitation can progress quite well, provided that the therapist remembers the concept of limiting lymph load so as not to exceed the individual lymph transport capacity. This clinical skill comes with experience and constant monitoring in the early stages of activity to assess which activities increase the person's subjective feeling of "congestion and fullness" in the affected areas.

Heat modalities will increase superficial vasodilation and ultrafiltration, increasing edema and therefore should be avoided. Electrical stimulation, particularly waveforms and intensities that produce sustained tetanic muscle contractions should be used cautiously. Prolonged sustained tetanic muscle contractions (as opposed to rhythmic, reciprocal muscle contractions) can impair lymph flow in the area of skin overlying the muscle group, causing a retrograde edema distal to that site.

A past history of multiple abdominal or thoracic surgeries, vein stripping/sclerotherapy, and liposuction in the legs should remind the evaluating therapist to carefully assess signs and symptoms of lymphedema. A limb that was perceived as "less than perfect" can become a severely swollen, distorted limb, psychologically devastating the individual whose appearance was of paramount importance.

Evaluation

When evaluating an individual with suspected lymphedema (or the individual with unexplained edema of an extremity/extremities), cardiac, renal, thyroid, and arteriovenous disease must be ruled out medically. A detailed history must be taken, including past medical history, especially cancer; information about swelling; onset and progression; tests conducted to evaluate/diagnose the condition; chronology of all surgeries; vein stripping; bypass stents; and insertion or removal of ports for administration of chemotherapy, especially biological response modifiers, as these tend to cause high levels of fluid retention and metabolic dysfunction.

It is important to keep in mind that secondary lymphedema can be the result of an orthopedic surgery or trauma that further

---

*Excessive shear on the skin of a lymphedematous limb or a limb at risk from vigorous massage or from a compression pump exceeding 45 mm Hg compression can tear microfilaments and collapse the initial lymphatic walls, advancing a preexisting lymphedema or triggering lymphedema in a limb at risk.

†In a therapy setting, careful thought must be given even to everyday procedures. For example, a woman with mild Stage I upper extremity lymphedema, secondary to axillary dissection developed cellulitis in her involved extremity after receiving a week of treatment for her lymphedema. Treatment involved a skin care program using moisturizer. During treatment, the jar of moisturizing cream was always open on the counter, and the therapist dipped into the jar with a bare hand, applying the cream to the client's skin, returning to the jar several times with the same bare hand that had rubbed the cream on her arm. Although the skin on the arm was intact, the client was concerned that a possible link existed between her infection and the cream that was used on others, some of whom she noted had open wounds. Although no direct proof of the connection between this clinical practice and the client's infection is available, it is a reminder of the need to improve our infection control on *all* clients, regardless of their "level" of risk. (See the section on Infectious Diseases in Chapter 7 and the Standard Precautions in Appendix A.)

Continued

TABLE	12-2

Lifelong Precautions for Clients with Lymphedema

RISK	ACTIVITY
Infection	Maintain clean and dry skin; keep the skin supple by applying oil or bland cream; perfumed or fragranced lotions and creams can be irritating. A mild cleansing lotion such as Cetaphyl or Alpha Keri Oil is recommended. Moisturizers with a high petroleum content (i.e., first ingredient listed is mineral oil or petrolatum) will damage the rubber/latex fibers of compression garments; check with therapist/garment manufacturer regarding safe products to use under garments.
	When drying, be gentle but thorough. Make certain to dry in any creases and between the digits. Watch for moist, cracking skin between the toes as a sign of fungal infection that must be treated.
	No needle sticks, injections, vaccinations, acupuncture, electrolysis, or blood drawing on the involved extremity; NO exceptions can be taken to this guideline. If a technician is unsuccessful obtaining blood from the uninvolved arm, use legs or feet for blood drawing (unless these are at risk).
	Immediate treatment with cleansing, antibiotic ointment, and/or bandaging for all wounds no matter how minor (e.g., insect bites, paper cuts, hangnail, blister, burn); check often for signs of infection.
	Protect hands and feet at all times (e.g., socks and supportive footwear, rubber gloves for cleaning, long oven mitts, garden gloves for any outdoor work, thimble for sewing).
	Avoid harsh chemicals and abrasive compounds.
	Use extreme caution when cutting fingernails, toenails, or cuticles; creams are sometimes recommended for removing cuticles, but these are still chemicals and should not be used; use vegetable oil and gently push back cuticles with the pad of your finger, do NOT use a stick or nail file.
	Use electric razor to remove unwanted hair; never use a razor blade.
Circulatory compromise	No blood pressure measurements should be taken on the involved extremity.
	Avoid constricting jewelry and clothing, especially tight underwear, underwire brassieres, socks, or stockings; avoid elastic around neck, upper arm, wrists, fingers, ankles, and toes.
	Avoid lifting heavy weights or carrying heavy objects with the involved extremity; no heavy handbags with over-the-shoulder straps; be extremely cautious when lifting children, as they can make sudden and unexpected movements.
	Avoid repetitive limb movements against resistance (e.g., pushing, pulling, rubbing, scraping, or scrubbing) that could cause sudden, rapid blood flow through muscle and tissue.
	Maintain an ideal body weight with proper nutrition and low-salt, low-caffeine diet; avoid smoking, using recreational or illicit drugs, and drinking alcoholic beverages.
	Changes in pressure gradient during air travel require use of compression garments and low-salt diet.
	Avoid prolonged automobile travel; if travel is necessary; take frequent breaks and exercise other precautions (e.g., elevation, hydration, loose clothing, proper nutrition, compressive garment or bandages when recommended).
	Avoid overheating local body parts or rise in core body temperature: use pyrogenic medications, even with low-grade fever; avoid saunas, hot tubs, hot pads, hot packs, or tanning booths; close monitoring is required during extensive exercise or marathon running.
	Avoid sunburn; keep the limb protected from the sun; avoid tanning booths.
	Chemicals such as those used in the application of artificial fingernails may cause an edematous response in some people.
Stress to impaired lymphatic system	Avoid heavy breast prostheses after a mastectomy; too much pressure on the supraclavicular lymph nodes can slow and interrupt the lymphatic pathways.
	Do not overtire a limb at risk. If it starts to ache, lie down with it elevated. If your leg is involved, avoid prolonged sitting. It is better to lie down with the affected leg elevated than to sit with the leg elevated. Prolonged sitting can prevent lymphatic drainage through the gluteal region.
	As previously mentioned, avoid tight jewelry and clothing on the affected limb, especially if some swelling is present. Underpants, brassieres, jeans, shoes, or any other article of clothing with straps must be loose around the waist, thighs, and crotch. NO redness or indentation should be evident upon removal.
	Compression stockings/sleeves must not leave a compressive band at the ankle, knee, groin, or waist. It should not chafe at any point. If it does, obtain help from the therapist.

NOTE: For additional resources, see Box 12-2.
Modified from Boris M, Weindorf S, Lasinski B: Managing lymphedema: risk reduction strategies, *Lymphedema Ther*, New York, 2002, Woodbury.

disrupted marginal lymphatics. Individuals with extensive acute or chronic edema after trauma or surgery should be evaluated for lymphedema. Early intervention and management of this type of lymphedema can significantly minimize the complications of advanced, untreated lymphedema mentioned earlier.

In the case of a known history of cancer, lymphedema that does not respond to proper treatment may be caused by metastases blocking lymphatic flow. In such a case, treatment may result in proper lymphatic drainage but the results would be temporary and the lymph fluid would begin to build up again. The therapist must remain alert to this possibility.

Clinical evaluation includes a detailed description of skin integrity, using body diagrams, both anterior-posterior (AP) and lateral to draw unusual body contours; location and condition of scars, fibrotic areas, and open wounds; evidence of healed ulcerations; and the location of papillomas, warts, leaking edema and/or subcutaneous fibrosis, folliculitis, and palpable nodes in the axillary or inguinal areas. The presence of toe/nail fungus, presence or absence of pitting and subcutaneous fibrosis, presence or history of folliculitis, and palpable nodes in the axilla or inguinal areas should be noted. The presence or absence of pain, paresthesias, or other sensory impairments is documented. Using a visual analog scale of 0 to 10 is the easiest documentation for this assessment.

Photographs are helpful to detail changes in skin color and texture (high-speed film without flash is preferable to avoid distortion of color/shadows). Accurate circumferential measurements taken at fixed intervals with standardized positioning noted are often more helpful describing the limb segments than volumetric measurements that give a total difference in overall volume of the entire limb. Volumetric measurements are particularly helpful in cases of bilateral extremity edema when no "normal limb" can be used for comparison.

An accurate history of infections in the affected areas, how these were treated, and how they responded to treatment is critical. A chronological review of the person's previous treatments/interventions for lymphedema and the response to treatment is important.

Careful documentation of the individual's functional impairments related to the lymphedema is key to evaluating the outcome of any treatment that is recommended. Many individuals with chronic lymphedema have "learned to live with it" and often do not consider that they have a "limitation." Tactful questioning can uncover the many compensating mechanisms employed to get through the day.

Finally, the results of specific tests used to diagnose the edema should be reviewed. Venograms and lymphangiograms involve cut downs and the injection of dyes into the vessels (these have been known to sclerose and damage vessels) are no longer recommended by lymphologists. Lymphoscintigrams, useful to differentiate between venous edema, lipedema, and lymphedema, have already been discussed. Remember, that a combination of these conditions can coexist. Cases complicated by genetic lymphangiodysplasias need the intervention of an experienced lymphologist.[28,56]

Preoperative Evaluation

A preoperative screening evaluation should record baseline circumferential measurements of both operative and nonoperative extremities. Tissue texture, unusual limb asymmetries/contours, skin color, strength, and functional range of motion are recorded. Any sensory abnormalities or neurologic impairments are noted. Risk reduction techniques with emphasis on proper skin hygiene and recognition of the early signs of lymphedema and secondary infection are reviewed with the individual. A list of resources, including who to contact should a problem arise (and when available) is provided to the individual. Discussion of individual activities of daily living (ADLs) and brief task analysis of job and home can point to possible problem areas that may need to be modified to reduce the risk of triggering lymphedema from "overuse" of the postoperative extremity or re-

duce potential exposure to trauma, chemicals, excessive heat, or repetitive tasks.

Physical Therapy Intervention

Regardless of training approach to lymphedema, several overall components of intervention may be modified according to each individual client's needs: (1) manual lymphatic drainage; (2) short-stretch compression bandaging; (3) exercise; (4) compression garments; (5) education (e.g., basic anatomy, skin and nail care, self-massage, self-bandaging, garment care, infection management); (6) compression pumps; and (7) psychologic and emotional support. These components comprise a treatment approach referred to as *comprehensive lymphedema management** that is the same for all the combined manual lymphatic therapies and is carried out in two distinct phases: the initial intensive intervention phase and the optimization phase.

Initial Intensive Intervention Phase.   During this phase of treatment, daily intervention requiring maximum compliance is necessary to disperse lymph fluids through the superficial lymphatic vessel network and to prevent congestion of fluid in areas proximal to the compression bandages. Components of treatment include the following:

1. Meticulous skin care and treatment of any infections that may also include debridement of ulcers and wound care.
2. Lymphatic drainage: Variations exist in specific stroke and pressure techniques such as Vodder, Leduc, Foldi, Casley-Smith; however, all schools of thought work to decongest the trunk quadrants first before addressing the lymphedematous extremity, decongesting the proximal portions of the limb first and progressively working distally to the end of the limb with the direction of flow always toward the trunk. Special strokes are available for fibrotic areas.
3. The affected limb/limbs are then bandaged with short-stretch compression bandages during the initial treatment phase and fitted with a compression garment at the completion of treatment.
4. Each individual is instructed in specific self-care, self-massage techniques, and exercises that are modified for the individual. The basic principle is to enhance the lymphatic pumping and collateral lymph flow from the involved/impaired areas into adjacent, normally functioning areas and eventually into the trunk with return to the central circulation via the right lymphatic duct and the thoracic duct.[6,7]

Optimization Phase.   During this second phase, the individual home program is finalized, continuing with the components of comprehensive lymphedema management from the initial intervention phase now modified for each person according to the clinical presentation and individual needs. During this phase, customized pressure gradient elastic support garments may replace compression bandaging when the limb is normal or close to normal.

Components of Comprehensive Lymphedema Therapy. Considerable advances were made in the treatment of lymphedema after Kubik's detailed description of the regional

Continued

---

*Different countries use different acronyms for this treatment approach sometimes referred to as *complete decongestive therapy* (CDT); *combined decongestive physiotherapy* (CDP); *complex lymphedema therapy* (CLT); *decongestive lymphatic therapy* (DLT); or *complex physical therapy* (CPT). In the United States, the more common usage is CDP or CDT.

anatomy of the lymphatic system published in 1985 (see Fig. 12-7). Foldi and Foldi reported the successful results of their techniques referred to as *combined decongestive physiotherapy (CDP)* documenting 50% reductions in lymphedema after a 4-week course of daily CDP. Of those individuals, 50% maintained that reduction by adhering to a home program of self-manual lymph drainage (MLD); exercises; and continuous compression on the affected limb using compression garments/bandages.[26,27] Casley-Smith and Casley-Smith (1994) presented results of another conservative treatment referred to as *complex physical therapy (CPT),* reporting reductions of more than 60% in 618 lymphedematous limbs.

 Manual Lymph Drainage.   The concepts of MLD were first introduced in 1882 by von Winiwarter. These techniques were improved by Vodder in the 1930s[59] but were originally applied to improve the functioning of normal lymphatics. Moreover, the reductions in edema obtained with MLD in those early years were unable to be maintained due to lack of adequate compression bandages and garments. The Vodder techniques were modified by Asdonk and Leduc and later by Foldi and Casley-Smith.*[14] MLD, a gentle, manual treatment technique consisting of several basic strokes† is designed to improve the activity of intact lymph vessels by providing mild mechanical stretches on the wall of the lymph collectors.

 Compression Bandaging.   *Short-stretch compression bandages* applied to the lymphedematous extremity after lymphatic drainage help maintain the edema reduction achieved through the lymph drainage. Short-stretch bandages have minimal recoil and only stretch 70% of their "unstretched" length. They have a low resting pressure (i.e., when the bandaged limb is at rest, they exert minimal pressure on the skin), avoiding any skin ischemia or breakdown. Conversely, they have a high working pressure. When the muscles (in the bandaged limb) contract against the short-stretch bandage, the bandage provides a semirigid force, creating an increase in interstitial tissue fluid pressure, an increase in lymph uptake, and increased pumping of the collecting lymphatics. Therefore these bandages are comfortable when the limb is at rest, and greatly increase the transport of lymph when the limb is in motion.

Long-stretch compression bandages have a low working pressure and a high resting pressure—that is, they are not very effective in increasing the transport of lymph when the bandaged limb is moving and they can become dangerously tight when the limb is at rest, creating a tourniquet effect on the limb at rest. These are not the bandages of choice for the individual with lymphedema.

Proper bandaging techniques, using sufficient padding materials over bony prominences and to even out unusual limb contours, ensure that a gradient of pressure is achieved. This gradient must be greatest at the most distal point of the involved limb, gradually decreasing as the bandage layers reach the proximal portion of the limb. This gradient is particularly critical in limbs where large, balloonlike areas separated by a deep skinfold/ridge that can occur at a joint such as the ankle, knee, wrist, elbow. According to the Law of LaPlace, the pressure applied is inversely proportional to the radius of the limb segment bandaged—that is, the smaller the radius of the limb segment, the greater is the pressure applied by the bandage. For example, when bandaging an upper extremity with significant edema in the dorsum of the hand but a narrow wrist relative to the hand and forearm, the wrist area must be sufficiently padded to increase the radius (of the wrist limb segment) to be larger than the radius of the hand. If this is not done, the bandaging may actually cause an increase in the edema in the dorsum of the hand.[18]

A proper compression gradient achieved with short-stretch bandages can increase tissue pressure, improve the activity of the lymphangion, and increase the efficiency of the muscle pump in the involved limb. It not only maintains the reduction in the involved limb that was achieved through lymph drainage; it can actually increase that reduction by enhancing the muscle pump during activity. In addition, the application of varying densities of foam pieces or "chips," encased in adhesive gauze, stockinet, or fabric, applied under the compression bandages over fibrotic areas, can soften the fibrosis, allowing for further reduction of the limb.[18,56]

Compression bandaging is usually worn 24 hours during the initial intensive phase of treatment, removed only for bathing and lymph drainage, and immediately reapplied. After the initial treatment phase, the individual is able to maintain adequate compression during the day with a compression garment. Getting the individual to understand that they must maintain some form of nighttime compression is the key to success in the optimization phase of the program. The short-stretch bandages, because of their low resting pressure and "customized" fit, provide the optimal nighttime compression. The drawback to this is that self-bandaging is time consuming and difficult for the less mobile or obese individual or person with a very large, heavy limb. Several "compression alternatives" are now available for this purpose that use various fabric "sleeves" with foam padding and Velcro closures for easier application. Results of one clinical study reported that followed individuals who wore their compression garments day and night maintained their reductions during the optimization phase. No skin problems or tissue breakdown resulted from wearing the garments to bed. It should be noted, however, that most of the involved individuals had custom, low-elastic garments that were not measured and fitted until the involved limbs were fully reduced (plateau in reduction).[40]

 Exercise Guidelines.   Exercise activates muscle groups and joints in the affected extremity. Combining a specific exercise program for each individual with the use of sufficient compression facilitates the process of decongestion by using the natural pumping effect of the muscles to increase lymph flow while preventing limb refilling.

Most clinicians experienced in lymphedema treatment agree on basic guidelines for exercise. Any exercise program for the individual with lymphedema must follow the basic concepts of the combined approach—that is, work the trunk muscles first, followed by the limb girdle muscles, working from proximal to distal on the limb and finishing with trunk exercises and deep abdominal breathing to enhance flow through the thoracic duct. Exercise must always be performed with a compression gar-

---

*These major contributors have developed training programs to teach their methods. No standards are available in the United States for lymphedema training programs. LANA, a nonprofit organization composed of physicians, nurses, physical and occupational therapists and massage therapists who specialize in lymphedema management, has developed standards for lymphedema therapists in the United States. This will help ensure access to adequate treatment for all individuals living with lymphedema (for more informations, visit http://www.clt-lana.org).

†Some proponents of MLD advise against the use of the word *massage* (e.g., manual lymphatic massage or lymphatic drainage massage) because the term *massage* means "to knead." MLD does not have kneading elements and is generally applied suprafascially, whereas massage is usually applied to subfascial tissues.

ment or compression bandages on the involved limb(s) to enhance the variation in total tissue pressure to facilitate increased lymph flow. In addition, therapists must remember that lymph load must not exceed lymph transport capacity, or the exercise/activity will increase the lymphedema.

Certain activities are considered higher risk for exacerbating lymphedema, such as running, jogging, stair climbing machines, sports involving ballistic type movements of the involved limbs such as tennis and racquetball, and activities with risk of traumatic sprain/strain injuries (e.g., karate, soccer, football, hockey, and downhill skiing). Activities such as brisk walking, cycling, swimming, cross country skiing, and Tai Chi are lower risk activities. Although weight training is not contraindicated, the progression of the program must be carefully monitored to avoid overload of the limbs/trunk, causing lymph congestion and subsequent exacerbation of the lymphedema.

Simply stated, the greater the intensity of the exercise, the greater the oxygen demand. With increased oxygen demand comes increased blood flow to the muscles, which provides the oxygen to do the work. Signs of limb "overload" are aching; congested, full feeling; discomfort in the proximal lymph nodal area (axilla or inguinal areas); pain; throbbing; or change in skin color. If any of these signs or symptoms occurs, the activity should be discontinued and the limb should be elevated and a cold compress applied. Deep breathing exercises and some self-lymph drainage may help decongest the trunk and limbs and reduce the discomfort. The individual must learn to "listen" to his or her body and grade future activity accordingly to avoid overloading the system.

There has been little clinical work done addressing strenuous exercise and lymphedema. Miller (1997) reported a 38% decrease in limb lymphedema after a 4- to 6-week period in 40 individuals with upper extremity lymphedema secondary to breast cancer treatment.[39] These individuals followed a program of resistive exercise while wearing compression bandages on the affected limbs. Further studies are needed in this area.

Compression Garments. Compression garments were never designed to "treat and reduce" lymphedema but rather were meant to "hold" a limb that had already been reduced. Since lymphedema damages the elastic fibers of the skin, compression of the affected area is necessary to prevent reaccumulation of the lymphatic fluid.

Originally, compression garments were engineered to treat venous edema and were meant to be applied to the edema-free extremity before the individual got out of bed after a night of limb elevation. The same premise should apply to the lymphedematous extremity—that is, the edema must be reduced for the garment to work effectively. Care must be given to the fit and function of the myriad of fabrics, compression grades, and styles available with proper instruction given in donning and doffing. In addition, realistic expectations concerning these garments are a must to achieve client success and comfort.[7,12,28]

Education and Home Program. Education begins on the first day of therapy intervention and is an absolute essential part of both phases of the program. The clients must understand the pathophysiologic reasons why they are doing what they are doing for each component of therapy and carry this through on discharge into their home program. The success of any combined lymphedema treatment program hinges on compliance with the home maintenance program.

Client education includes instruction in the basic anatomy and physiology of the lymphatic system, the pathophysiology of

the individual's particular lymphedema, individual self-drainage pathways to follow during the exercise program, basic principles of the individual exercise program, the risk of infection and how to reduce that risk, wear and care instruction for compression bandages/garments, and individual skin care regimen. Hands-on instruction in self-bandaging techniques requires practice and patience but is essential for the individual to master. In the home maintenance phase after initial intensive treatment, skin care and risk reduction/management of infection is the single most important component of the home program. Psychologic support including support groups is a critical component of a comprehensive lymphedema management program.

Maintaining reductions of lymphedema has been documented with compliance to a home program of skin care, exercise with self-lymphatic drainage, and compression garment wear. Significant decrease in microlymphatic hypertension (measured by fluorescence microlymphography and lymph capillary pressure measurement); decrease in extremity lymphedema; and improvement in lymphoscintigraphic findings have been reported after a course of CPT.[30,34] Individuals with less than 100% compliance with the home program lose a portion of their reductions[7,24] (Figs. 12-18, 12-19, and 12-20).

Skin care. Generally, for most people, an hour per day spent on exercise and garment care is reasonable for this condition. It is reasonable to spend 20 minutes twice daily on exercise and self-massage and another 20 minutes with skin care and washing or caring for compression garments. The better the individual understands the pathophysiology of the lymphedema, the greater the compliance.

Instruction in skin care includes the use of low pH/neutral pH soaps, cleansers, and moisturizers; the proper care of nails on finger and toes (see Table 12-2 and Table 11-22); use of topical antibiotic or antifungal preparations; and instruction in skin hygiene and compression garment/bandage washing for good hygiene. The normal pH of healthy skin is acidic (less than 7.0) and accounts for the waterproof barrier of the skin surface. Repeated use of alkaline soaps and cleansers on the skin will result in the loss of this waterproof property, drying the skin and causing microscopic cracks in the skin surface, increasing the likelihood of bacterial invasion. The elements of a personal first aid kit including oral and topical over-the-counter or prescription antibiotics, adhesive bandages, and alcohol wipes are discussed. The client is instructed to carry this kit whenever traveling. For older adults, poorly mobile individuals, or the visually impaired person, a caregiver can be instructed in how to inspect the lymphedematous limb or area daily for signs of skin irritation/infection.

No absolute do's and don'ts are available, but people must be cautioned to prevent lymph overload in their work and home activities. Each individual must weigh the risk level of each activity and learn what is safe for him or her. Yet, typically, most time is spent in teaching the client self-massage, exercise, and bandaging techniques. Although consistency in using these techniques is very important, many people suffer exacerbation of the lymphedema from an infection or skin problem, necessitating removal of the compression garment. These incidents can be minimized if the individual knows what to look for and how to proceed when an infection occurs. Knowing the procedure for an emergency visit, who to contact and how to advocate for their own care within the medical system should be discussed and reviewed at the time of discharge and at subsequent follow-up visits.

Continued

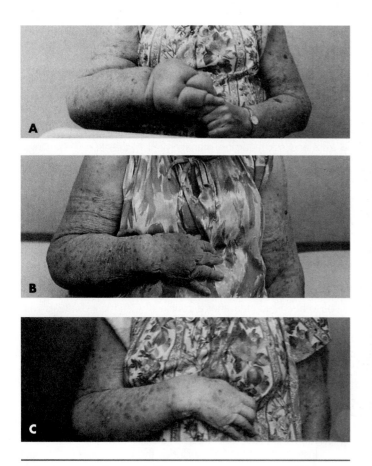

FIGURE 12-18 **A,** Before treatment: an 84-year-old woman with severe, elephantitic lymphedema of her right upper extremity for 20 years, secondary to surgery and radiation treatment for breast cancer 30 years ago. Her right hand was essentially nonfunctional. She needed assist in all areas of ADLs. **B,** After 20 CDT treatments, she has achieved a 77% reduction in the lymphedema in her right upper extremity and has begun to use her right hand functionally again. **C,** Four years post CDT treatment. She follows through with a home exercise program, skin care, and compression garment wear. She has not had any additional treatments other than the initial 20, and she has improved her reduction to almost 100% in the years posttreatment. She is more independent in ADLs and can even don her compression glove and sleeve with minimal assistance. (Courtesy Lymphedema Therapy, Woodbury, Long Island, New York, 2000.)

If an infection develops, a decision must be made whether to remove compression garments/bandages, discontinue any lymphatic drainage, and discontinue exercise until the infection is under control. Circumstances occur when an infection is diagnosed in the very early stages (e.g., minor erythema may be present without pain or fever), and the physician may recommend continuation of the compression garments if tolerated to avoid any significant increase in limb size. Every situation is individual and unique and requires consultation with the physician and the therapist before making any changes in the management program. Any sign or symptom of infection always requires immediate medical attention.

Guidelines for job and lifestyle modifications. The same principles for exercise apply to pacing/modifying work activities and activities of daily living to avoid overload. Affected individuals do not necessarily have to give up a job just because lymphedema has been diagnosed. Cooperative discussion may be helpful between the therapist, client, and the client's supervisor to implement simple task modifications insuring client safety and comfort at work. Some work requirements may have to be reduced, modified, or eliminated, and the supervisor should be aware of any special needs the employee may have (e.g., the need to wear compression garments and to protect them with constant changes of vinyl gloves throughout the day in a food service job, or the need for a hair stylist to rest with arm/arms elevated in between customers).

Successful management of lymphedema should mean greater "ability" for the individual, not "disability." It may be necessary to modify a workstation to provide more comfort for the individual with leg edema. Interactive education is the key to success. If the employer understands the problem of lymphedema and is assisted in providing a simple solution, everyone wins. For example, an individual with lower extremity lymphedema may need to get up from the workstation every hour and walk around for 5 minutes. A place to elevate the affected leg under the desk may be needed.

Requesting reasonable accommodations is an important goal, but sometimes, certain job tasks cannot be modified. For example, a nurse with significant upper extremity lymphedema may have difficulty getting assistance every time she needs to move and lift a patient. Constant lifting and positioning heavy patients can worsen an upper extremity lymphedema. In such cases, the decision rests with the individual whether a job change is needed or whether it will be necessary to stay and make the best of things.

Compression Pumps. Historically in the United States, a person with lymphedema was given a prescription for a compression garment and range-of-motion exercises. In some cases, treatment with a pneumatic compression pump was prescribed as the edema progressed. The degree and intensity of this treatment varied greatly due to lack of verified, long-term, scientific studies proving the efficacy of one treatment form over the other. Treatment with pneumatic compression consisted of placing the involved limb into a rubber sleeve that inflated with air from the pump, squeezing the limb, moving fluid proximally toward the trunk. Pumps available in single or multichamber models can apply pressures from 10 to 100 mm Hg; the walls of the superficial lymphatics can collapse with greater than 45 mm Hg pressure.[8,13,25]

In the presence of soft tissue injury, vigorous massage or the use of compression pumps at pressures higher than 45 mm Hg can cause severe damage to the walls of the initial lymphatic vessels (possibly by tearing the anchoring microfilaments mentioned earlier). This collapse of the initial lymphatic walls impairs lymphatic transport capacity and results in lymphedema and extravasation of lymphedema into an adjacent trunk quadrant.[8]

Atrophy or hypertrophy of the skin can further compromise lymphatic function due to the loss of elasticity. A network of collagen and elastin fibers surrounding the lymphatic system helps the skin respond to movement so any variable that can damage the lymph system of the skin (e.g., aging, chronic sun exposure, prolonged use of systemic steroids) compromises the response of the tissues to movement caused by massage or pneumatic compression. The resultant injury to the blood vessels and lymphatics causes fluid and protein to leak from the damaged vessels, setting up a chronic inflammatory response potentially leading to permanent fibrosclerotic changes.[48] These fibrosclerotic changes further compromise oxygen perfusion in the tissues, resulting in a repetitive cycle of hypoxia and chronic inflammation—the perfect environment for bacterial and fungal infections to

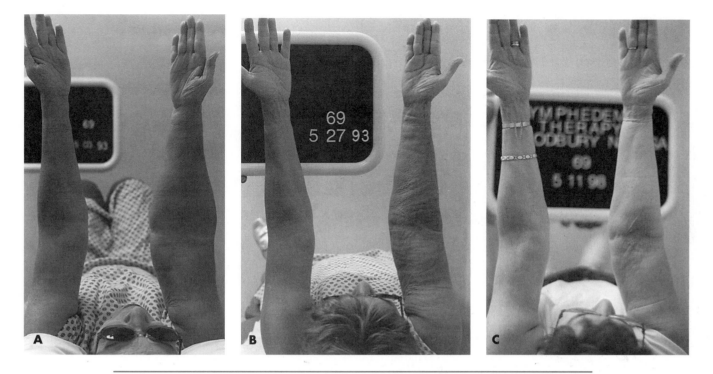

FIGURE   **12-19   A,** Before treatment, a 69-year-old woman with Stage II lymphedema of the right upper extremity of 20 years duration, secondary to breast cancer surgery and treatment. For the past few years, she has had recurrent cellulitis infections in the right arm with hospitalization several times per year to receive IV antibiotics. **B,** After 18 CDT treatments, she achieved a 57% reduction in the lymphedema in the right upper extremity. The wrinkling in her forearm/upper arm is from the compression bandaging, which was removed shortly before taking this photo. These wrinkles are only temporary. Note the significant reduction in lymphedema. **C,** Five years after CDT treatment. She has improved the reduction in the lymphedema of her right upper extremity to 64%. She has had no additional treatment for her lymphedema, but she follows her home program of self-massage, exercise, skin care, and compression garment wear. She has had only two cellulitis infections in the past 5 years that were treated successfully with only oral antibiotics. Note the reshaping of the forearm/upper arm since previous photos were taken. (Courtesy Lymphedema Therapy, Woodbury, Long Island, New York, 2000.)

flourish. In addition, pump treatment protocols require daily use for hours per day, physically and psychologically restricting the person who is "tied to the machine" for hours at a time.

Although the pneumatic pumps can be helpful in early Stage I lymphedema, when simple elevation overnight usually reduces the edema, they are less helpful in Stage II fibrotic lymphedema. Although the pumps increase the reabsorption of water by the venous system, they do not move the extracellular protein because these molecules are too large to enter the venous fenestrae. Proteins must be transported via the lymphatics. This is a situation that is a trigger to filter more fluid into the tissue spaces diluting the concentrated protein and ultimately increasing the edema. The higher protein concentration remaining in the tissues also causes the chronic inflammatory response discussed earlier, triggering the development of more subcutaneous fibrosis. The vicious cycle of lymphedema repeats itself. The chronic inflammatory response increases the individual's risk of developing secondary infections (cellulitis/lymphangiitis).

Psychosocial Considerations.   Great emphasis has been given to the myriad of physical symptoms and resulting impairments associated with lymphedema. Little is reported on the psychologic distress these individuals must suffer on a daily basis. People are curious about the change in size and shape of the affected limb. Individuals are faced with tremendous alterations in body image; many feel embarrassed. Some are scorned by a public perception that they are deformed or distorted. Those with severe leg lymphedema with chronic infections and ulcerations may leak lymphatic fluid from their limbs and experience public humiliation when people turn away from them in fear and ignorance. Affected individuals become prisoners in their own homes, too embarrassed or afraid to go out in public. Many are judged by others who do not understand "how this could happen" and why it was not "taken care of." Individuals living with lymphedema have experienced tremendous guilt and self-doubt in the past. Many people were told by numerous medical professionals, "There is nothing to be done; just learn to live with it." Even today, physicians and therapists in this country still tell individuals with lymphedema that nothing can be done except to "elevate the limb and wear loose long sleeves/pants."

Clinicians and researchers are realizing that individuals with lymphedema need tremendous psychologic support to cope with the problems associated with living with such a chronic condition.[42] Today, innovative lymphedema treatment programs offer support groups (Box 12-2). The National

Continued

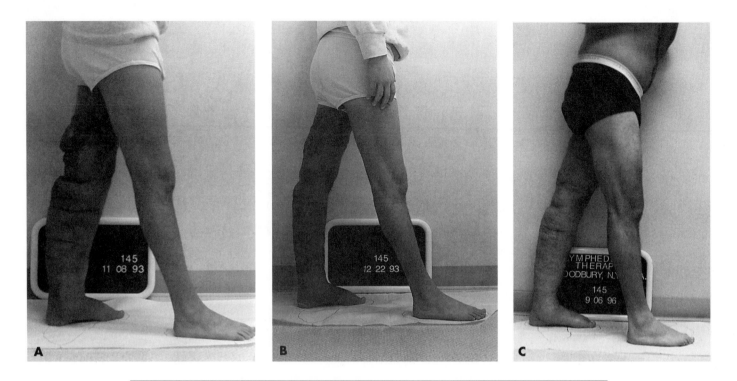

FIGURE   **12-20**   **A,** Before treatment: a 19-year-old male with severe Stage II primary lymphedema of the left lower extremity, progressing to the left buttock and genitals, with chylous reflux to the scrotum, buttock, and thigh. The onset of the edema was at age 8 (see Fig. 12-11). He spent most of his high-school years in and out of the hospital. In the 24 months before treatment, he was hospitalized 22 times for cellulitis in the left lower extremity and placed in the intensive care unit (ICU) with septic shock three times. **B,** After one course of CDT of 30 treatments interrupted by a 2-week hospitalization (1 week in ICU) for cellulitis of the left leg/buttock with severe chylous leakage from the scrotum, buttock, and thigh. This individual went into septic shock and needed hyperalimentation to treat the hypoproteinemia (that resulted from the chylous leakage) via a central venous line. Despite the massive increase in swelling and open areas on the posterior left thigh and buttock resulting from the cellulitis, he achieved a 67% reduction in the lymphedema of his left lower extremity with reductions in the abdominal, suprapubic, and genital swelling as well. **C,** Three years after CDT. Note that some increase in the girth of the left lower extremity has occurred, particularly in the areas just proximal and distal to the knee, where the tissues are lax from the original debulking surgery. These areas fill in quickly without compression. Some of the girth increase is due to weight gain, now that he no longer has recurrent cellulitis and the chylous reflux is under control. This young man, having spent his high-school years in and out of the hospital was able to complete his college degree and is pursuing a career in business, since his CDT treatment. He has made his lymphedema management home program a priority in his life and continues to maintain a 60% reduction in the lymphedema in his left lower extremity. (Courtesy Lymphedema Therapy, Woodbury, Long Island, New York, 2000.)

Lymphedema Network (NLN), an advocacy organization, hosts a biannual educational conference offering workshops and an opportunity to network with other affected individuals and health care providers who specialize in lymphology (the study of the lymphatic system). The Lymphoedema Association of Australia (LAA) is supporting a study of many interrelated issues that include individual self-perception; specifics regarding the lymphedema; functional limitations; psychosocial issues; reactions/support of friends, family, caregivers, health care professionals; and access to care, social services, and state financial assistance with supplies needed to treat and maintain lymphedema.

Great strides are being made in recognizing lymphedema as a condition that deserves to be acknowledged and treated early and aggressively. Theoretically, all clinicians know that psycho-logic support is crucial to success in managing a chronic illness or condition. However, having the practical applications in place to help the individual takes a tremendous commitment in personal time and financial resources. Nevertheless, a successful lymphedema treatment program must offer ongoing support and follow-up care. ■

◆ Lymphadenitis

Infections elsewhere in the body can lead to lymphadenopoathy as described previously. When the lymph node becomes overwhelmed by the infection, the lymph node itself can become infected, which is called *lymphadenitis*. Lymphadenitis can be classified as acute or chronic; acutely

BOX **12-2**

Important Resources in the Treatment of Lymphedema*

American Cancer Society

In 1998, the American Cancer Society sponsored an international meeting on breast cancer-related lymphedema in New York City. Lymphologists from all over the world met and discussed current diagnosis, treatment, management, resources, professional education, and advocacy. The results from that meeting are published in Lymphedema: results from a workshop on breast cancer, treatment-related lymphedema, and lymphedema resource guide, *Cancer: Interdiscipl Internat J Amer Can Society* 83:2775-2890, 1998. Available from the American Cancer Society (800) 231-5355.

American Physical Therapists Association (APTA): Oncology Section—Lymphedema Focus Group

Elizabeth Augustine, P.T.
(301) 402-3015
FAX: (301) 480-0669

International Society for Lymphology (ISL)

College of Medicine
University Medical Center
1510 North Campbell Avenue
Tucson, AZ 85724
(520) 626-6118
FAX: (520) 626-0822
www.u.arizona.edu/~witte/ISL.htm
A quarterly journal is available on international research on lymphedema.

Lymphoedema Association of Australia (LAA)

94 Cambridge Terrace
Malvern, SA 5061, Australia
(011) 61 (8) 8271-2198
FAX: (011) 61 (8) 8271-8776
Available at http://www.lymphoedema.org.au.

Lymphology Association of North America (LANA)

Available at http://www.clt-lana.org

Lymphatic Research Foundation

39 Poole Drive
Roslyn, New York 11576
(516) 625-9675
FAX (516) 625-9410
Available at http://www.lymphaticresearch.org.

Lymphovenous Canada

Lymphovenous News is published by Lymphophenous Association of Ontario.
Available at http://www.lymphovenous-canada.com.

National Lymphedema Network, Inc.

Latham Square
1611 Telegraph Avenue, Suite 1111
Oakland, CA 94612-2138
Hotline: (800) 541-3259
Direct: (510) 208-3200
FAX: (510) 208-3110
(800) 541-3259
Available at http://www.lymphnet.org.
A quarterly newsletter is available.

*The listing of any particular program or the omission of others does not denote support or preference for one method of lymphedema intervention over another. This list of resources is meant to guide the interested therapist to further information.

inflamed lymph nodes are most common locally in the cervical region in association with infections of the teeth or tonsils or in the axillary or inguinal regions secondary to infection of the extremities. In acute lymphadenitis, the lymph nodes are enlarged, tender, warm, and reddened. In the case of chronic lymphadenitis, long-standing infection from a variety of sources results in scarred lymph nodes with fibrous connective tissue replacement. The nodes are enlarged and firm to palpation but not warm or tender. The management of lymphadenitis is treatment of the underlying disorder.

◆ Lymphangitis

Lymphangitis, an acute inflammation of the subcutaneous lymphatic channels usually occurs as a result of hemolytic streptococci or staphylococci (or both) entering the lymphatic channels from an abrasion or local trauma, wound, or infection (usually cellulitis; see Chapter 9). The involvement of the lymphatics is often first observed as a red streak under the skin (referred to in layperson terms as *blood poisoning*), radiating from the infection site in the direction of the regional lymph nodes. The red streak may be very obvious, or it may be very faint and easily overlooked, especially in dark-skinned people. The nodes most commonly affected are submandibular, cervical, inguinal, and axillary, in that order. Involved nodes are usually tender and enlarged (greater than 3 cm).

Systemic manifestations may include fever, chills, malaise, and anorexia. Other symptoms may present in association with the underlying infection located elsewhere in the body. Bacteremia from any cause can result in suppurative arthritis (inflammatory with pus formation), osteomyelitis, peritonitis, meningitis, or visceral abscesses. When cellulitis results in lymphangitis, throbbing pain occurs at the site of bacterial invasion, and the client presents with a warm, edematous extremity (or possible scrotal lymphedema in males and occasionally vulvar lymphedema in females).

Medical Management of Lymphatic System Infection in the Intact Lymphatic System

Diagnosis. Lymphangitis may be confused with superficial thrombophlebitis, but the erythema associated with lymphangitis is first seen as a red streak under the skin radiating toward the regional lymph nodes (usually ascending proximally), whereas the erythema associated with thrombosis is usually over the thrombosed vein with local induration and inflammation. However, suppurative thrombophlebitis may develop if bacteria are introduced during IV therapy, especially when the needle or catheter is left in place for more than 48 hours. The physician will also differentiate cellulitis from soft tissue infections (e.g., gangrene, necrotizing fasciitis) that may require early and aggressive incision and resection of necrotic infected tissue.

Anyone with a history of vascular disease taking anticoagulant medication should have a Doppler and ultrasound to rule out deep venous thrombosis before being treated. Laboratory tests are often not required but may include blood culture (often positive for staphylococcal or streptococcal species) and culture and sensitivity studies on the wound exudate or pus.

Treatment and Prognosis. Prompt parenteral antibiotic therapy is mandatory because bacteremia and systemic toxicity develop rapidly once organisms reach the bloodstream via the thoracic duct. Antibiotic treatment may be accompanied by general measures such as heat, elevation, immobilization of the infected area, and analgesics for pain. Appropriate wound care may include drainage of the pus from an infected wound when it is clear that an abscess is associated with the site of initial infection. An area of cellulitis should not be excised, because the infection may be spread by attempted drainage when pus is not present. Treatment as described should be effective against invading bacteria within a few days.

Medical Management of Lymphatic System Infections in the Individual with an Impaired Lymphatic System: the Individual at Risk and the Individual with Lymphedema

Diagnosis. Confusion of cellulitis/lymphangitis with thrombophlebitis in the individual with lymphedema or at risk for lymphedema is common and has a disastrous impact on the severity of the lymphedema. An episode of cellulitis/lymphangitis often triggers the development of lymphedema in the individual who is at risk but has no clinical signs of edema. Improper, inadequate treatment of these infections can lead to chronic infection/inflammation and progression of the lymphedema.

The individual who has had regional lymph node dissection and/or radiation has an impaired immune response in the areas that drain to that regional nodal area. Consequently, infection can spread rapidly in those regions and any delay in treatment while awaiting blood cultures and vascular tests can cause progression of the infection.

The combination of the impaired nodal area and the inactivity of the macrophages in the lymphedematous region allow the bacteria to multiply rapidly, feeding on the high pro-

tein lymphedema fluid. It is not uncommon for a person to develop a high fever with shaking chills (105° F) within 30 minutes of "feeling ill" or "feeling an ache or pain" in the lymphedematous region. It is not acceptable for these people to "wait and see" and call their physician in a day or two. They must be seen and evaluated by a physician immediately to rule out thrombosis versus cellulitis/lymphangitis and initiate appropriate treatment immediately.

Treatment and Prognosis. Treatment of cellulitis/lymphangitis in the individual with lymphedema or at risk for lymphedema differs from treatment of these conditions in the individual with an intact lymphatic system. In the healthy individual,* heat is often prescribed as an adjunct to relieve pain in the inflamed area, whereas heat should *never* be applied on individuals with lymphedema or those at risk for developing lymphedema. This contraindication includes those individuals who have developed lymphedema following orthopedic surgeries.

Local heating will increase vasodilation and ultrafiltration of more fluid into the interstitial spaces, further overloading the decompensated lymphatic transport capacity, exacerbating the existing lymphedema, or possibly triggering lymphedema in the limb at risk, where no clinical lymphedema existed before the onset of the infection. Rest and immobilization of the involved areas are recommended measures. Cold can be applied to relieve pain. Experienced lymphologists initiate immediate oral antibiotic therapy, usually with high doses of broad-spectrum antibiotics and periodic medical monitoring in the first 48 to 72 hours to observe the area for spread of the infection. It is imperative that the original area of redness be outlined with indelible marker to check on the progress or regression of the infection.

If a poor response to the oral antibiotics is evident, hospitalization for intravenous (IV) antibiotics may be necessary. A local infection can progress to septic shock if not treated effectively. A common cause of recurrent cellulitis/lymphangitis is poor, inadequate treatment of a previous infection. A common complaint is recurrent infection in the same area of the same limb every 2 to 3 weeks. In fact, this is more likely the same infection that was never eradicated the first time. Cases like this often give a common history of administration of too short (3 to 5 days) or inadequate doses of oral antibiotics to treat the cellulitis/lymphangitis associated with lymphedema.

---

*In a healthy individual cellulitis and lymphangitis are relatively rare. Many cases of primary lymphedema are missed in young individuals who present with unexplained recurrent cellulitis in the absence of injury or trauma. Recurring cellulitis does not develop unless some underlying pathology is causing it (usually primary lymphedema).

Special Implications for the Therapist   12-3

LYMPHANGITIS

Preferred Practice Patterns:
7A: *Primary Prevention/Risk Reduction for Integumentary Disorders*
7B: *Impaired Integumentary Integrity Associated With Superficial Skin Involvement*

6H: Impaired Circulation and Anthropometric Dimensions Associated With Lymphatic System Disorders

Clinicians must remember the pathophysiology of lymphedema to understand the seriousness of these infections. Obviously, not every local infection will progress to septicemia. However, the risk is there, given the low oxygen state in the lymphedematous area, the limited response of the macrophages, and the diminished immune response in the individual with nodal dissection/irradiation or in the case of primary lymphedema, too few, fibrosed, or poorly developed nodes.

At the first sign of infection, the affected individual must seek medical consultation immediately and discontinue all current lymphedema treatment modalities, including manual lymphatic drainage, pumps, bandaging and garments, until the physician determines it is safe to resume. If the infection is treated early, some physicians may allow resumption of bandaging or garments as tolerated to avoid the limb ballooning out of control as the infection is resolving. This is determined on a case-by-case basis by the physician who is familiar with the individual, follows the individual's care closely, and provides emergency treatment as needed for that person. ■

◆ **Lipedema**

Overview and Etiologic Factors.   The term *lipedema* was first used by Allen and Hines[1] to describe a symmetrical "swelling" of both legs, extending from the hips to the ankles, caused by deposits of subcutaneous adipose tissue. The underlying etiologic factors of these fat deposits remains unknown. Although lipedema is not a disorder of the lymphatic system per se, it is often confused with bilateral lower-extremity lymphedema, thus the reason for discussing it in this chapter. It occurs almost exclusively in women, may have an associated family history (20% of cases), and is usually accompanied by hormonal disorders as well.[52] If present in a man, it is accompanied by massive hormonal disorder.

Fat in the lower extremities extends to the malleoli, often with flaps of tissue hanging over the foot. The feet are not affected; occasionally, lipedema is found in the arms. Typically, fatty bulges are in the medial proximal thigh and the medial distal thigh, just above the knee. Clinically, the affected individuals complain of pitting edema as the day progresses, which is relieved by prolonged elevation of the leg(s) overnight.[12,46,47]

Stages of Lipedema.   In stage I, the skin is still soft and regular, but nodular changes can be felt on palpation (Fig. 12-21). No color changes occur in the skin, and the subcutaneous tissues have a spongy feel, like a soft rubber doll. In stage II, the subcutaneous tissue becomes more nodular and tough. Large fatty lobules begin to form on the medial distal and proximal thigh and medial and lateral ankles just above the malleoli (Fig. 12-22). Pitting edema is common, increasing as the day progresses. The individual may report hypersensitivity over the anterior tibial area. Skin color changes occur in the lower leg, indicative of secondary lymphedema, which often occurs in later stage lipedema.

Pathophysiology of Lipedema.[52]   Many histologic and physiologic changes occur in lipedema. A decrease in the elasticity of the epidermis and subcutis also occurs. The basement

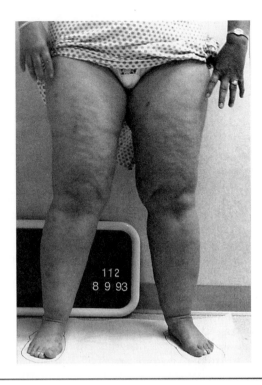

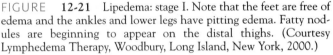

FIGURE   **12-21**   Lipedema: stage I. Note that the feet are free of edema and the ankles and lower legs have pitting edema. Fatty nodules are beginning to appear on the distal thighs. (Courtesy Lymphedema Therapy, Woodbury, Long Island, New York, 2000.)

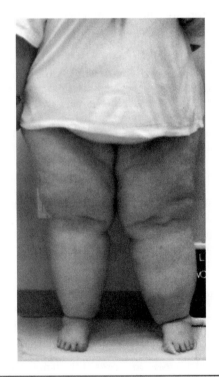

FIGURE   **12-22**   Lipedema: stage II. Note that obvious pitting edema on the dorsum of the feet is evident, and the tissues are beginning to hang over the medial and lateral ankles and above the knees. The discoloration at the anterodistal left lower leg is from a resolving cellulitis, secondary to the lymphedema that developed secondary to the lipedema. (Courtesy Lymphedema Therapy, Woodbury, Long Island, New York, 2000.)

membrane of vessels is thickened, and disturbances in vaso-motion take place. The veno-arterial reflex (VAR)* is disturbed, causing decreased vascular resistance, increased skin perfusion, and increased capillary filtration. Increased venous/blood capillary pressure causes increased ultrafiltration. These changes combined with the decreased efficiency of the calf muscle pump, results in both the dependent pitting edema seen in stage I and the secondary lymphedema that often complicates lipedema in its later stages.

Histologic changes seen in lipedema include a thinning of the epidermal layer, thickening of the subcutaneous tissue layer, fibrosis of arterioles, tearing of elastic fibers, dilated venules and capillaries, and hypertrophy and hyperplasia of fat cells. Clinical studies show enlargement of the prelymphatic channels[50] and defects in capillary perfusion.[56] Some authors have reported no alteration in lymphatic transport,[9] whereas others[4] have reported decreased lymph outflow in those individuals with lipedema. Foldi and Foldi (1993) reported an increase in fat cell growth during lymphostasis.[28]

Medical Management

Diagnosis.   The diagnosis of lipedema is difficult if the clinician is unfamiliar with this condition. Often, these people are told that they are "fat" and should just lose weight to resolve the problem. For reasons still unknown, the fatty tissue accompanying this condition cannot be significantly decreased by diet. It is not uncommon for a diagnosis of primary lymphedema to be made. This results in frustration for the person who then seeks out lymphedema therapy with poor results.

Several significant clinical differences between lipedema and bilateral primary lymphedema. The feet are not involved in lipedema; although they are edematous with a positive Stemmer's sign in lymphedema, Stemmer's sign is negative in lipedema (see Fig. 12-17). The "swelling" in lipedema is symmetrical, whereas in primary lymphedema, usually one limb is more involved than the other. The subcutaneous tissues feel rubbery in lipedema. In advanced Stage II lymphedema, significant subcutaneous fibrosis occurs, which feels firmer than lipedema.

Although incidences of cellulitis in Stage II lipedema, usually with a component of lymphedema as well, have been reported, the frequency of cellulitis in Stage II lymphedema is much higher. The time of onset of the "swelling" in lipedema is usually around puberty, and 90% of these cases have accompanying diagnoses of hormonal disturbance (thyroid, pituitary, or ovarian). This is usually not the case with primary lymphedema.

A lymphoscintigram may be helpful to differentiate between lymphedema and lipedema; however, results can be conflicting, as lymphedema often occurs to some degree in the later stages of lipedema, probably due to impairment of lymph flow caused by the pressure of fatty tissue. In fact, clinical cases of bilateral lower-extremity lymphedema in the morbidly obese individual are seen; the onset of the lymphedema occurs after body weight exceeds 350 to 400 pounds (lbs). It is plausible to suspect that the pressure of a large apron of abdominal fat can effectively block lymph flow through the inguinal area, causing the lymphedema, but the difference between these cases and lipedema is that obesity does not cause lipedema. Lipedema is caused by a hormonal imbalance resulting in excessive deposition of adipose tissue, most often in the lower extremities (see Figs. 12-21; 12-22), although it can occur in the upper extremities too.

Treatment and Prognosis.   No effective medical treatment for lipedema is available, and the prognosis is guarded; however, significant functional improvements are possible with good program compliance and therapy intervention. Medical management involves treating the hormonal disturbance as effectively as possible and providing nutritional guidance to avoid additional weight gain. Many of these individuals have endured years of ridicule because of their physical appearance and become recluses in their homes, further limiting their activity level. As lipedema progresses and the hypersensitivity increases, they feel less inclined to walk or exercise because of the pain. They inevitably gain more weight due to the inactivity and depression, often finding food their only comfort.

Special Implications for the Therapist   12-4

LIPEDEMA

Preferred Practice Patterns:
7A: Primary Prevention/Risk Reduction for Integumentary Disorders
7B: Impaired Integumentary Integrity Associated With Superficial Skin Involvement
6H is not selected because although impaired anthropometric measurements are evident, these are not caused by lymphatic system disorder.

The primary goal of therapy intervention in the person with lipedema is symptomatic relief and realistic improvement of trunk and lower extremity function. Application of the combined lymphedema treatments has shown some success in relieving the pain and hypersensitivity in the lower legs and improving general mobility. Usually, a lower level of compression is needed to support a lipedematous limb, compared with a lymphedematous limb of the same size and girth. This guideline applies to the compression garments too.

These individuals often require more padding under the compression bandages, particularly in the anterior tibial area. They do not tolerate the heavier, denser compression fabrics and usually require a lower-grade compression garment than someone with uncomplicated lymphedema. The therapist must remember, however, that later stage lipedema is often accompanied by lymphedema too, and the treatment and management must take that factor into consideration when recommending exercise and garments.

The main goals of intervention are to decrease pain and hypersensitivity, decrease the lymphedematous component of the disease, and assist the individual in maintaining and/or reducing adipose tissue through exercise and nutritional guidance.

---

*Under normal circumstances, the VAR is an important mechanism for the regulation of microcirculation and interstitial fluid exchange. It is measured as a ratio between skin perfusion in the supine versus the standing position using a laser Doppler flowmeter.

The compression garments can help decrease the adipose tissue with exercise and weight loss. The most difficult task is fitting the compression garments. They must be custom-made due to the large size of the individual and are often uncomfortable at the waist, particularly when sitting.

Making the radical change in daily activity level is most challenging for these individuals. Providing continued support and encouragement is important. Networking is helpful and is facilitated by offering a support group, even when held on an irregular, informal basis. An hour-long educational meeting, even if only offered three or four times per year, can provide a neutral meeting place for people to begin networking. Nothing can compare with the encouragement and hope that an individual with lipedema/lymphedema can derive from seeing and talking with someone else living with the same problem and hearing how others cope on a day-to-day basis. Therapists can learn some of the best guidance on exercise and coping with garments in a group like this. ■

REFERENCES

1. Allen EV, Hines EA: Lipedema of the legs, *Proc Staff Mayo Clinic* 15: 184-187, 1940.
2. Augustine E: Oncology section of the American Physical Therapy Association position statement—physical therapy: management of lymphedema in patients with a history of cancer, *Rehabil Oncol* 18(1): 9-12, 2000.
3. Bernas M, Witte CL, Witte MH: The diagnosis and treatment of peripheral lymphedema: draft revision of the 1995 Consensus Document of the International Society of Lymphology Executive Committee for Discussion at the September 3-7, 2001, XVIII International Congress of Lymphology in Genoa, Italy, *Lymphology* 34(2): 84-91, 2001.
4. Bilancini S et al: Functional lymphatic alterations in patients suffering from lipedema, *Angiology* 46:333-339, 1995.
5. Boris M: Personal communication, *Lymphedema therapy*, New York, 2000, Woodbury.
6. Boris M, Weindorf S, Lasinski, B: Lymphedema reduction by noninvasive complex lymphedema therapy, *Oncology* 8(9):95-106, 1994.
7. Boris M, Weindorf S, Lasinski, B: Persistence of lymphedema reduction after noninvasive complex lymphedema therapy, *Oncology* 11(1): 99-109, 1997.
8. Boris M, Weindorf S, Lasinski B: The risk of genital edema after external pump compression for lower limb lymphedema, *Lymphology* 31:15-20, 1998.
9. Brautigam P et al: Analysis of lymphatic drainage in various forms of leg edema using two compartment lymphoscintigraphy, *Lymphology* 31(2): 43-55, 1998.
10. Brunner U et al: Epidemiology and clinic of primary lymphoedema based on 500 cases. In Bollinger A, Partsch H, Wolf JHN, editors: *The initial lymphatics*, Stuttgart, Germany, 1985, Stuttgart Thieme.
11. Casley-Smith JR: The efficiency of the lymphatic system, *Lymphologie* 2:24-29, 1978.
12. Casley-Smith JR: There are many benzopyrones for lymphedema, *Lymphology* 30:38, 1997
13. Casley-Smith JR, Bjorlin M. Some parameters affecting the removal of oedema by massage—mechanical or manual. In Casley-Smith JR, Piller NB, editors: Progress in Lymphology X, Adelaide, Australia, 1985, University of Adelaide Press.
14. Casley-Smith JR et al: Treatment for lymphedema of the arm—the Casley-Smith method. A non-invasive method produces continued reduction, *Cancer* 83:2843-2860, 1998.
15. Casley-Smith JR, Casley-Smith JR: High-protein oedema and benzobyrones, Sydney and Baltimore, 1986, JB Lippincott.
16. Casley-Smith JR, Casley-Smith JR: Lymphedema initiated by aircraft flights, *Aviat Space Environ Med* 67:52-56, 1996.
17. Casley-Smith JR, Casley-Smith, JR: Lymphedema therapy in Australia; complex physical therapy, exercises and benzopyrones on over 600 limbs, *Lymphology* 27(Suppl):622-626, 1994.
18. Casley-Smith JR, Casley-Smith JR: Modern treatment for lymphoedema, Adelaide, Australia, 1997, Lymphoedema Association of Australia.
19. Casley-Smith JR, Gaffney RM: Excess plasma protein is a cause of chronic inflammation and lymphoedema. Quantitative electron microscopy, *J Pathology* 133:243-272, 1981.
20. Casley-Smith JR, Piller NB, Morgan RG: Treatment of lymphedema of the arms and legs with 5,6 benzo-alpha pyrone, *New Eng J Med* 329: 1158-1163, 1993.
21. Chua B, Ung O, Boyges J: *Toward optimal treatment of the axilla in early breast cancer*. Poster presented at ASCO, New Orleans, LA, May 19-21, 2000.
22. Consensus Document of the International Society of Lymphology Executive Committee: Diagnosis and treatment of peripheral lymphedema, *Lymphology* 28:113-117, 1995.
23. Darocxy J, Schingale FJ, Mortimer PS: Practical ambulant lymphology, Munich, 1996, Verlag Medical Concept Gemeinschaft mit beschraenkter.
24. Dickens S et al: Effective treatment of lymphedema of the extremities, *Arch Surg* 133:452-457, 1998.
25. Foldi E: Massage and damage to lymphatics, *Lymphology* 28(1):3, 1995.
26. Foldi E: Treatment of lymphedema and patient rehabilitation, *Anticancer Res* 18:2211-2212, 1998.
27. Foldi E, Foldi, M, Weissleder H: Conservative treatment of lymphedema of the limbs, *Angiology* 36:171-180, 1985.
28. Foldi M, Foldi E: Lymphoedema: methods of treatment and control. A guide for patients and therapists, Stuttgart, 1991, Gustav Fischer Verlag. (First English translation by Dr. Andrew C. Newell for the Lymphoedema Association of Victoria, Inc, Australia, March 1993.)
29. Foldi M, Kubik S: *Lehrbuch der lymphologie fur medizuner und physiotherapeuter: mit anhang, praktische hinweise fur die physiotherapie*, Stuttgart and New York, 1989, Gustav Fischer Verlag.
30. Franzeck UK, Spiegel I, Fischer M: Combined physical therapy for lymphedema evaluated by fluorescence microlymphography and lymph capillary pressure measurements, *J Vasc Res* 34:306-311, 1997.
31. Freedman DO: Filariasis. In Bennett JC, Plum F: Cecil textbook of medicine, ed 21, Philadelphia, 2000, WB Saunders.
32. Frick A et al: Liposuction technique and lymphatic lesions in lower legs: anatomic study to reduce risks, *Plast Reconstr Surg* 103(7):1868-1873, 1999.
33. Gabka CJ, Baumeister RG, Maiwald G: Advancements of breast conserving therapy by onco-plastic surgery in the management of breast cancer, *Anticancer Res* 18(3C):2219-2224, 1998.
34. Huang JH, Kwon JY, Lee KW: Changes in lymphatic function after complex physical therapy for lymphedema, *Lymphology* 32:15-21, 1999.
35. Leduc A, Caplan I, Leduc O: Lymphatic drainage of the upper limb: substitution lymphatic pathways, *Euro J Lymphol* 4:13;11-18, 1993.
36. Lerner R: Chronic lymphedema. In Chang JB, editor: Textbook of angiology, New York, 2000, Springer-Verlag.
37. Lindsay SW, Thomas CJ: Mapping and estimating the population at risk from lymphatic filariasis in Africa, *Trans R Soc Trop Med Hyg* 94(1): 37-45, 2000.
38. Loprinzi CL et al: Lack of effect of coumarin in women with lymphedema after treatment for breast cancer, *New Eng J Med* 340:346-350, 1999.
39. Miller LT: A theory to support the use of vigorous exercise in the reduction of breast cancer lymphedema, *Phys Ther* 7:5, 1997.
40. Mortimer PS, Badger C, Clarke I: A double-blind, randomized, parallel-group placebo-controlled trial of O-betahydroxyethyl-rutosides in chronic arm oedema resulting from breast cancer treatment, *Phlebology* 10:51-55, 1995.
41. Mortimer PS et al: The prevalence of arm lymphoedema following treatment for breast cancer, *Quart J Med*, 89:377, 1996.
42. Newman M, Brennan M, Passik S: Lymphedema complicated by pain and psychological distress: a case with complex treatment needs, *J Pain Sympt Manage* 12:376-379, 1996.
43. Olszewski WL, editor: *Lymph stasis: pathophysiology, diagnosis, and treatment*, London, 1991, Olszewski, WLCRC Press.
44. Pecking A et al: Efficacy of daflon 500 mg in the treatment of lymphedema (secondary to conventional therapy for breast cancer), *Angiology* 48:93-98, 1997.

45. Petrek J, Lerner R: Lymphedema. In Harris JR, Lippmann ME, Morrow M et al: *Diseases of the breast,* Philadelphia, 2000, Lippincott Williams and Wilkins.

46. Rank BK, Wong CSC: Lipoedema, *Austral-NZ J Surg* 35(3):165-169, 1966.

47. Rudkin GH, Miller TA: Lipedema: a clinical entity distinct from lymphedema, *Plast Reconstr Surg* 94:841-849, 1994.

48. Ryan TJ: The skin and its response to movement, *Lymphology* 31:128-129, 1998.

49. Stemmer R: Stemmer's sign—possibilities and limits of clinical diagnosis of lymphedema, *Wien Med Wochenschr* 149(2-4):85-86, 1999.

50. Sener S et al: Lymphedema after sentinel lymphadenectomy for breast carcinoma, *Cancer* 92(4): 748-752, 2001.

51. Stoberl CH, Partsch H, Urbanek A: Indirekte lymphographie beim lipodem. In Foldi E: *Odem perimed,* Erlangen, Germany, 1986.

52. Strossenreuther RHK: Die bahandlung des lipodems. In Foldi M, Kubik S: *Lehrbuch der lymphologie,* Stuttgart and New York, 1999, Gustav Fischer Verlag.

53. Swartz M: Cellulitis and subcutaneous tissue infections. In Mandell G, Bennett J, Dolin R, editors: *Principles and practice of infectious diseases,* ed 5, Philadelphia, 2000, Churchill Livingstone.

54. Taylor HM, Rose KE, Twycross RG: A double-blind clinical trial of hydroxy-ethylrutosides in obstructive arm lymphoedema, *Phlebology* 1(Suppl):22-28, 1993.

55. Tunkel R, Cohen S: Lymphedema management, *Rehabil Oncol* 18(1): 26-27, 2000.

56. Weinert V, Leeman S: Das lipodem, *Hautarzt* 42:484-486, 1991.

57. Weissleder H, Schuchardt C: Lymphedema: diagnosis and therapy, ed 2, Stuttgart, Germany 2001, Koln, Viavital Verlag GmbH.

58. Witte M: *New research perspectives: angiogenesis update 2000.* Presentation at the National Lymphedema Network conference, Orlando, Fla, September 2000.

59. Wittlinger H, Wittlinger G: *Textbook of Dr. Vodder's manual lymph drainage,* ed 4, vol 1-3, Brussels, 1992, Haug International

CHAPTER 13

THE HEMATOLOGIC SYSTEM

CATHERINE C. GOODMAN

*H*ematology is the branch of science that studies the form and structure of blood and blood-forming tissues. Two major components of blood are examined: plasma and formed elements (erythrocytes or red blood cells [RBCs], leukocytes or white blood cells [WBCs], and platelets or thrombocytes). Delivery of these formed elements throughout the body tissues is necessary for cellular metabolism, defense against injury and invading microorganisms, and acid-base balance. The formation and development of blood cells, which usually takes place in the red bone marrow, are controlled by hormones (specifically erythropoietin) and feedback mechanisms that maintain an ideal number of cells.

The hematologic system is integrated with the lymphatic and immune systems; for a complete understanding of these systems see Chapters 6 and 12. The lymph nodes are part of the lymphatic system but also part of the hematopoietic (blood-forming) system and the lymphoid system, which consists of organs and tissues of the immune system (see Fig. 6-3). Lymph fluid passes through these nodes, or valves, which are located in the lymph channels at 1- to 2-cm intervals. As the fluid passes through the nodes, it is purified of harmful bacteria and viruses. Networks of the lymphatic system are situated in several areas of the body and may be considered primary (thymus and bone marrow) or secondary (spleen, lymph nodes, tonsils, and Peyer's patches of the small intestine). All of the lymphoid organs link the hematologic and immune systems in that they are sites of residence, proliferation, differentiation, or function of lymphocytes* and mononuclear phagocytes (mononuclear phagocyte system).† For example, in the hematologic system, the lymphocytes of the spleen produce approximately a third of the antibody available to the immune system.

SIGNS AND SYMPTOMS OF HEMATOLOGIC DISORDERS

Disruption of the hematologic system results in circulatory disorders characterized by edema and congestion, infarction, thrombosis and embolism, lymphedema, and hypotension and shock (Box 13-1). *Edema* is the accumulation of excessive fluid within the interstitial tissues or within body cavities. *Congestion* is the accumulation of excessive blood within the blood vessels of an organ or tissue. The forms of lymphedema include cerebral edema, inflammatory edema, peripheral dependent edema, or pulmonary edema. Congestion may be localized, as with a venous thrombosis, or generalized, as with heart failure (e.g., congestive heart failure [CHF]), which results in congestion in the lungs, lower extremities, and abdominal viscera.

Infarction is a localized region of necrosis caused by reduction of arterial perfusion below a level required for cell viability. Such a situation occurs as a result of arterial obstruction due to atherosclerosis, arterial thrombosis, or embolism, when oxygen supply fails to meet the oxygen requirements of organs with end-arteries such as the gastrointestinal (GI) tract and heart and, less often, the kidneys and spleen. Cerebral cortical neurons (cerebral infarction) and myocardial cells (myocardial infarction) are most vulnerable to ischemia, although protective collateral blood flow develops in the heart through anastomoses.

A *thrombus* is a solid mass of clotted blood within an intact blood vessel or chamber of the heart. An *embolus* is a mass of solid, liquid, or gas that moves within a blood vessel to lodge at a site distant from its place of origin (see Fig. 11-25) Most emboli are thromboemboli. Thrombosis (development of a thrombus or clot) results from pathologic activation of the hemostatic mechanisms involving platelets, coagulation factors, and blood vessel walls. Endothelial injury, alteration in blood flow (stasis and turbulence), and hypercoagulability of the blood (e.g., protein abnormalities either primary or associated with cancers) promote thrombosis and thromboembolism.

Lymphedema, or chronic swelling of an area owing to accumulation of interstitial fluid (edema), occurs in hematolymphatic disorders secondary to obstruction of lymphatic vessels or lymph nodes. Obstruction may be of an inflammatory or mechanical nature from trauma, regional lymph node resection or irradiation, or extensive involvement of regional nodes by malignant disease. Women who have been treated surgically for breast cancer with lymph node dissection, mastectomy, and/or radiation therapy are at double the risk of developing lymphedema of the arm and/or chest wall (see Chapter 12). When the obstruction that slows the lymph fluid exceeds the pumping capacity of the system, the fluid accumulates in the tissues in the extremity, causing edema in one or more limbs. This accumulation of fluid may become a source for bacterial growth, leading to infection, fibrosis, and possible loss of functional limb use.

---

*Lymphocytes are any of the nonphagocytic leukocytes (WBCs) found in the blood, lymph, and lymphoid tissues that make up the body's immunologically competent cells. They are divided into two classes: B and T lymphocytes (see the section on leukocytosis in this chapter and Chapter 6).

†Macrophage and monocyte cells capable of ingesting microorganisms and other antigens.

BOX 13-1

Most Common Signs and Symptoms of Hematologic Disorders

Edema
- Lymphedema
- Cerebral edema
- Inflammatory edema
- Peripheral dependent edema
- Pulmonary edema

Congestion

Infarction (brain, heart, GI tract, kidney, spleen)

Thrombosis

Embolism

Shock
- Rapid, weak pulse (late phase)
- Hypotension (systolic blood pressure less than 90 mmHg)
- Cool, moist skin (late phase)
- Pallor
- Weak/absent peripheral pulses

TABLE 13-1

Etiologic Factors of Shock

Category of Shock	Causes
Hypovolemic	Hemorrhage (loss of blood, shock)
	Vomiting
	Diarrhea
	Dehydration secondary to:
	Decreased fluid intake
	Diabetes mellitus (diuresis during diabetic ketoacidosis or severe hyperglycemia)
	Diabetes insipidus
	Inadequate rehydration of long-distance runner
	Addison's disease
	Burns
	Pancreatitis, peritonitis, bowel obstruction
Cardiogenic	Arrhythmias
	Acute valvular dysfunction
	Acute myocardial infarction
	Severe congestive heart failure
	Cardiomyopathy
Obstructive	Massive pulmonary embolism
	Pulmonary hypertension
	Tension pneumothorax
	Obstructive valvular disease (aortic or mitral stenosis)
	Cardiac tumor (atrial myxoma)
Septic	Bacteremia; overwhelming infections
Neurogenic	Spinal cord injury
	Pain
	Trauma
	Vasodilator drugs

Shock occurs when the hypotensive changes diminish arterial blood circulation and thus decrease perfusion so that organs and tissues do not receive adequate oxygen to meet their metabolic needs. Shock may be classified by cause as hypovolemic; cardiogenic; obstructive; septic, which is also called *endotoxin shock, urosepsis,* or *sepsis;* or neurogenic (Table 13-1). Signs of shock include rapid, weak pulse; hypotension (systolic blood pressure of 90 mmHg or less); cool, pale, moist skin; and mottled extremities with weak or absent peripheral pulses.

In early septic shock, tachycardia accompanies increased circulation so that the skin is warm and flushed and the pulse is bounding rather than weak. In the second phase of shock (late septic shock), hypoperfusion (reduced blood flow) occurs, characterized by cold skin and weak pulses; this phase is usually irreversible and the client is unresponsive. Eventually, cardiovascular collapse follows severe hypotension.

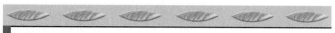

Special Implications for the Therapist 13-1

HEMATOLOGIC DISORDERS

Hematologic conditions alter the oxygen-carrying capacity of the blood and the constituents, structure, consistency, and flow of the blood. These changes can contribute to hypocoagulopathy or hypercoagulopathy, increased work of the heart and breathing, impaired tissue perfusion, and increased risk of thrombus. Hematologic abnormalities require that the results of the client's blood analysis and clotting factors be monitored so that therapy intervention can be modified to minimize risk.[16] Precautions and interventions for the client with lymphedema are discussed in Chapter 12 (see Table 12-2).

Exercise and Sports

Exercise training can induce blood volume expansion immediately (plasma volume) and over a period (erythrocyte volume) and is associated with healing, improved quality of life, and improved exercise capabilities in cases of anemia from hemorrhage, trauma, renal disease, and chronic diseases. The reestablishment of erythropoiesis through exercise and effect of exercise on blood volume in other groups remain unknown but are a potential area for further investigation and consideration in the clinical setting.[66]

Improvements in athletic performance using exogenous erythropoietin (referred to as "blood doping") have been documented as improvements in running time and maximal oxygen uptake. However, these effects are not without risk for increased blood viscosity and thrombosis with potentially fatal results. Until a definitive test is developed for detection of exogenous erythropoietin, the therapist must remain aware of this potential problem.[68]

Monitoring Vital Signs

Clients in whom shock develops may exhibit orthostatic changes in vital signs. A drop in systolic blood pressure of 10 to 20 mmHg or more, associated with an increase in pulse rate of more than 15 beats/min may indicate a depleted intravascular volume. The therapist is unlikely to see a client with acute hypovolemia; hypovolemia is more likely the result of dehydration as in the case of the long-distance runner or the client with severe diarrhea or slow GI tract bleeding. The aging population is especially vulnerable to development of unknown slow intestinal bleeding, especially with the use of aspirin or nonsteroidal antiinflammatory drugs (NSAIDs).

Clients with peripheral neuropathies or clients taking medications such as certain antihypertensive drugs may be normovolemic and experience an orthostatic fall in blood pressure, but without associated increase in pulse rate. The older client is likely to experience orthostatic changes as a natural consequence of aging. If any doubt exists, the client should be placed in the supine position with legs elevated to maximize cerebral blood flow. The Trendelenburg position, in which the head is lower than the rest of the body, is no longer used because of the increased difficulty of breathing in this position. ■

AGING AND THE HEMATOPOIETIC SYSTEM

Although blood composition changes little with age, the percentage of the marrow space occupied by hematopoietic (blood-forming) tissue declines progressively. The percentage of bone marrow fat is equal to the person's age, reaching a plateau at around age 50 years. Other changes include decreased total serum iron, total iron-binding capacity, and intestinal iron absorption but with increased total body and bone marrow iron; increased fragility of plasma membranes; a rise in fibrinogen and increased platelet adhesiveness*; red cell rigidity; and early activation of the coagulation system. The cumulative effect of these changes appears in the form of disturbed blood flow in older subjects leading to the development or aggravation of various circulatory disorders, especially hypertension, stroke, and diabetes. In addition, correlations found between hematologic changes and changes in behavioral patterns and some cognitive functions suggest that hematologic changes contribute to other changes associated with aging as well.[1]

Age-related changes in the peripheral blood include slightly decreased hemoglobin and hematocrit, although levels remain within the normal adult range. Low hemoglobin levels noted in aging adults can be caused by iron deficiency (usually via blood loss such as ulcer, telangiectasia, colon polyps, or cancer) or can be associated with a long-standing condition such as rheumatologic conditions often seen in a therapy practice (referred to as *anemia of chronic disease*). B$_{12}$, which is required to produce blood cells, and the subsequent development of anemia (resulting from a B$_{12}$ deficiency) with its hematologic, neurologic, and GI manifestations are discussed later in this chapter.

Aging is also associated with a decreased number of lymph nodes and diminished size of remaining nodes, decreased function of lymphocytes, and decline in cellular immunity owing to altered T-cell function (see the section on Effects of Aging on the Immune System in Chapter 6). The effect of ag-

ing on quantity, form, and structure of lymphocytes is not well documented.

BLOOD TRANSFUSIONS

Advances in treating hematologic/immunologic disorders through blood transfusions and bone marrow transplantation have provided new success in long-term treatment and a cure for some previously fatal disorders (see Chapter 20). Modern blood banking and transfusion medicine have developed techniques to administer only the blood component needed by the client, such as packed RBCs for anemia or platelets for bleeding disorders. Clients in a therapy setting who have undergone numerous surgical procedures (e.g., traumatic injuries) or elective orthopedic or cardiac procedures may also receive autologous blood transfusions (i.e., reinfusion of a person's own blood) when significant blood loss or hemorrhage occurs. The development of recombinant human erythropoietin (rHuEpo, EPO, or Epogen) with its ability to stimulate erythropoiesis and elevate RBCs has reduced the need for blood transfusion in a variety of clinical situations (e.g., hematologic malignancies, cancer-related anemia, or surgical procedures, especially joint arthroplasty and cardiac procedures).

Occasionally, complications of blood transfusion occur in the form of a posttransfusion reaction. Transfusion-related acute lung injury (TRALI), which is clinically similar to adult respiratory distress syndrome, occurs in approximately one of every 2000 transfusions.[39] With appropriate respiratory intervention, most people recover rapidly and without permanent pulmonary damage.[63] Other complications may include transmission of disease, iron overload, air embolism, and circulatory overload when blood is administered rapidly in large amounts. These complications are rare, but they occur most often in clients with either cardiac or renal disease, in whom they may cause flaccid paralysis, affecting the muscles of respiration and eventually the heart, leading to cardiac arrest. Delayed hemolytic transfusion reaction occurs in 1 out of 3200 transfusion when the RBCs are destroyed 2 to 10 days after a transfusion as a result of an RBC antibody not previously detected. Fever and anemia may present 2 to 10 days after the transfusion sometimes accompanied by jaundice and anemia-related dyspnea.

Transfusion as a source for hepatitis (B and C) has been reduced since the initiation of donor screening for the hepatitis antibody. People with hemophilia who received coagulation factor concentrates before 1984 have been at highest risk among transfusion recipients because of exposures to pooled blood products prepared from thousands of donors. The availability of nonhuman plasma factors has virtually eliminated the transmission of viruses among people with hemophilia.

The risk of human immunodeficiency virus (HIV) infection by transfusion is low overall, calculated at one in 1 million transfusions. The risk of HIV transmission by blood transfusion has been continually reduced through the elimination of high-risk individuals from blood donor pools and the use of more sensitive screening. Acquired immune deficiency syndrome (AIDS) has developed in a small percentage of people receiving transfusion of RBCs, platelets, or commercial coagulation factor concentrates. AIDS has also been reported in infants after neonatal exchange, but the majority of pediatric cases were associated with maternal transmission from mothers with HIV.

---

*Platelet morphology (form and structure) does not appear to change with age, but platelet count and function have been found to vary from normal to increased or decreased.

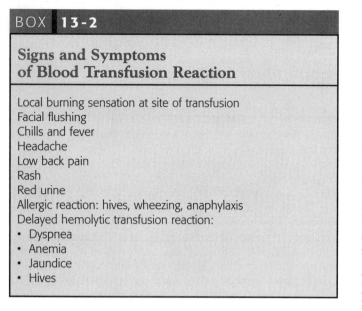

BOX 13-2

Signs and Symptoms of Blood Transfusion Reaction

Local burning sensation at site of transfusion
Facial flushing
Chills and fever
Headache
Low back pain
Rash
Red urine
Allergic reaction: hives, wheezing, anaphylaxis
Delayed hemolytic transfusion reaction:
• Dyspnea
• Anemia
• Jaundice
• Hives

Special Implications for the Therapist 13-2

BLOOD TRANSFUSIONS

Most blood transfusion reactions occur during the actual transfusion and are not of consequence to the therapist but when autologous transfusion is unavailable or inappropriate, the therapist must be alert for any signs of adverse reaction. Among the most common transfusion reactions are antigen-antibody reactions resulting from blood type incompatibility with clumping of cells, hemolysis, and release of cellular elements into the serum. Signs and symptoms indicating such a reaction are listed in Box 13-2. Occasionally, a client may develop a delayed allergic reaction observed as dyspnea or hives; the latter may be brought to the therapist's attention after local modality intervention. The therapist may also be the first to recognize early signs of hepatitis (jaundice), especially changes in sclerae or skin color or reported changes in urine (dark or tea-colored) and stools (light-colored or white). ■

DISORDERS OF IRON ABSORPTION

◆ Hemochromatosis

Hemochromatosis is an autosomal recessive hereditary disorder characterized by excessive iron absorption by the small intestine. The hemochromatosis gene has been located on chromosome 6, involving substitution of a protein responsible for regulation of iron metabolism. Affecting approximately three out of every 1000 people in the United States, hemochromatosis is present at birth but remains asymptomatic until the development of iron loading and onset of symptoms between ages 50 and 60 (sometimes as early as age 30). The prevalence is equal among men and women, but men experience symptoms eight times more often than women (menstruation helps to slow progression of the disorder). One in eight to 10 people is a carrier having inherited the gene from one parent.

Individuals with hemochromatosis lack an effective way to remove excess iron and the iron begins to accumulate in the liver, pancreas, skin, heart, and other organs. Excess iron accumulation in the body promotes oxidation and causes tissue injury and subsequent organ damage. Symptoms include weakness, fatigue, abdominal pain, arthralgia or arthritis, hepatomegaly, and darkened skin. Complications can include cirrhosis of the liver (a risk factor for liver cancer); diabetes mellitus; pulmonary involvement; cardiac myopathy; and impotence (males) or decreased libido (females) and sterility.

Diagnosis can be made by a simple genetic test based on family history. A liver biopsy is no longer necessary to establish the diagnosis but may be helpful when assessment of liver damage is required. In families where hemochromatosis has been previously diagnosed, all first-degree blood relatives should be screened for hemochromatosis. Newborns can be followed closely with blood tests for liver analysis and iron status. Monthly monitoring is required for those with known hemochromatosis. Treatment should begin early in the disease process when iron levels exceed normal values and liver function tests are outside the expected values. Medical intervention consists of therapeutic phlebotomy (i.e., medical blood letting) until a mild state of anemia occurs with iron saturation at less than 50% and ferritin level becomes less than 50 ng/mL. Affected individuals are instructed to avoid ingesting anything that is iron fortified and substances that enhance iron absorption such as alcohol and vitamin C.

The prognosis is good as long as the iron levels remain in the normal range of values and the disease has not affected the liver. If iron overload causes liver damage, phlebotomy cannot prevent progressive liver disease, and the disease can be fatal. When the liver tries to process the high levels of iron, toxic intermediates are developed, leading to further liver disease such as cirrhosis. Treatment with phlebotomy does not improve diabetes or arthritis associated with hemochromatosis.[70]

Special Implications for the Therapist 13-3

HEMOCHROMATOSIS

Preferred Practice Patterns:
4E: Impaired Joint Mobility, Motor Function, Muscle
Performance, and Range of Motion Associated
With Localized Inflammation

Arthropathy occurs in 40% to 60% of individuals with hemochromatosis and can be the first manifestation of the disease. The arthropathy associated with hemochromatosis is not reversible and often continues to progress even with effective medical intervention. Osteoarthritic manifestations are diverse with minimal joint inflammation at first. The affected individual may report twinges of pain on flexing the small joints of the hand, especially the second and third metacarpophalangeal (MCP) joints. Acute joint presentation can occur with progression that involves the large joints including the hips, knees, and shoulders accompanied by severe impairment and resulting disability. Hemochromatosis may be associated with calcium pyrophosphate dihydrate (CPPD) deposition disease. This presents as an acute inflammatory arthritis.[70]

Therapeutic intervention is essential in providing flexibility, strength, and proper alignment to promote function, prevent falls, and prevent the loss of independence in activities of daily living. The therapist can be very helpful in evaluating the need for assistive devices, orthotics, and splints toward these goals. ■

DISORDERS OF ERYTHROCYTES

◆ The Anemias

Definition.   Anemia is a reduction in the oxygen-carrying capacity of the blood owing to an abnormality in the quantity or quality of erythrocytes (RBCs). The World Health Organization (WHO) has defined anemia in terms of the level of hemoglobin: less than 14 g/100 mL for men and less than 12 g/100 mL for women. Different ranges exist for men and women, infants and growing children, and different metabolic and physiologic states.* Anemia is present if the hematocrit is less than 41% in adult males or 37% in adult females.

Overview.   Anemia is not a disease but is rather a symptom of many other disorders, such as dietary deficiency (nutritional anemia); acute or chronic blood loss (iron deficiency); congenital defects of hemoglobin (sickle cell diseases); exposure to industrial poisons, diseases of the bone marrow; chronic inflammatory, infectious, or neoplastic disease; or any other disorder that upsets the balance between blood loss through bleeding or destruction of blood cells and production of blood cells.

Many types and causes of anemia exist; not all are discussed in this text. The most common anemias observed in a therapy setting fall into four broad disease-related categories: (1) iron deficiency associated with chronic GI blood loss secondary to NSAID use; (2) chronic diseases or inflammatory diseases, such as rheumatoid arthritis (RA) or systemic lupus erythematosus (SLE); (3) nutritional conditions (e.g., malabsorption syndrome leading to vitamin B_{12}, folate, or iron deficiency; alcohol abuse leading to folate deficiency); (4) infectious diseases such as tuberculosis or AIDS; and (5) neoplastic disease or cancer (bone marrow failure). Anemia with neoplasia may be a complication of chemotherapy (e.g., Cisplatin, Carboplatin, Taxol) or as a consequence of radiation to the pelvis.

Anemias are classified according to etiologic factors (Table 13-2) or morphology (form/structure) (Box 13-3). Descriptions of anemias based on erythrocyte morphology refer to the size and hemoglobin content of the RBC. In some anemias, variations occur in size (e.g., anisocytosis) or shape (e.g., poikilocytosis) of erythrocytes.

Etiologic Factors and Pathogenesis.   Anemia results from (1) excessive blood loss, (2) increased destruction of erythrocytes, or (3) decreased production of erythrocytes. Anemia is the most common hematologic abnormality; only

---

*These normal values must be evaluated on an individual basis; normal levels may be inadequate if tissue oxygen delivery is impaired by pulmonary insufficiency, cardiac disorders, or an increase in hemoglobin oxygen affinity, whereas low levels may be appropriate if tissue oxygen requirements are decreased, as in the case of hypothyroidism.

TABLE	13-2

Causes of Anemia

EXCESSIVE BLOOD LOSS (HEMORRHAGE)

Trauma, wound
GI cancers
Telangiectasia
Bleeding peptic ulcer
Excessive menstruation
Bleeding hemorrhoids

DESTRUCTION OF ERYTHROCYTES (HEMOLYTIC)

Mechanical or autoimmune hemolysis
Hemoglobinopathies (e.g., sickle cell diseases)
Enzyme defects (e.g., glucose-6-phosphate dehydrogenase deficiency)
Parasites (e.g., malaria)
Hypersplenism
Hereditary spherocytosis

DECREASED PRODUCTION OF ERYTHROCYTES

Chronic diseases (e.g., rheumatoid arthritis, tuberculosis, cancer)
Nutritional deficiency (e.g., iron, vitamin B_{12}, alcohol abuse, folic acid deficiency)
Cellular maturational defects (e.g., thalassemias, cytotoxic or antineoplastic drugs)
↓Bone marrow stimulation (e.g., hypothyroidism, decreased erythropoietin production)
Bone marrow failure (e.g., leukemia, aplasia)
Bone marrow replacement (myelophthisis; usually replacement by neoplasm)
Inborn or acquired metabolic defect; myelodysplastic syndrome (sideroblastic anemia)

---

the anemias most commonly observed in a rehabilitation or therapy setting are discussed here, using the three etiologic categories from Table 13-2 as a guideline.

The underlying pathogenesis can be multifactorial and depends on the condition causing the anemia. A number of physiologic compensatory responses to anemia occur, depending on the rapidity of onset and duration of anemia and the condition of the individual. In acute onset anemia with severe loss of intravascular volume, peripheral vasoconstriction and central vasodilation occur to preserve blood flow to the vital organs. If the anemia persists, small vessel vasodilation will provide increased blood flow to ensure better tissue oxygenation. These vascular compensations result in decreased systemic vascular resistance, increased cardiac output, and tachycardia, resulting in a higher rate of delivery of oxygen-bearing erythrocytes to the tissues. Other compensatory mechanisms include a compensatory increase in plasma volume to maintain total blood volume and enhance tissue perfusion and stimulation of erythropoietin production to increase newerythrocyte production.

Excessive Blood Loss.   Excessive blood loss, as occurs with GI bleeding in the client with a history of long-term use of aspirin or NSAIDs, is the most commonly encountered

BOX 13-3

Anemia Classified by Morphology

Normocytic (normal size)
Macrocytic (abnormally large)
Microcytic (abnormally small)
Normochromic (normal amounts of hemoglobin)
Hyperchromic (high concentration of hemoglobin)
Hypochromic (low concentration of hemoglobin)
Anisocytosis (various sizes)
Poikilocytosis (various shapes)

cause of anemia seen in a therapy practice. Slow, chronic GI blood loss from medication or any GI disorder (e.g., peptic ulcers, hiatal hernia, gastritis, gastric carcinoma, hemorrhoids, diverticula, ulcerative colitis, colon polyps, colon cancer) can result in iron-deficiency anemia.

Destruction of Erythrocytes.
Destruction of erythrocytes (hemolysis; hemolytic) occurs primarily as a result of autoimmune conditions. This occurs when the immune system produces antibodies that clump (agglutinate) a person's own RBCs together. These are then recognized by the immune system as nonself or foreign bodies and are phagocytized in the spleen, thereby reducing the available RBCs (and available hemoglobin). Hemolytic anemia could be associated with SLE; lymphoproliferative diseases such as leukemia (chronic lymphocytic leukemia) and lymphoma; or immune-related thrombocytopenia (idiopathic thrombocytopenic purpura [ITP]). Medications such as penicillin, quinidine, quinine, and methyldopa can also cause autoimmune hemolytic anemia. Hemoglobinopathy-related anemias (e.g., sickle cell anemia, thalassemias) develop as a result of destroyed erythrocytes, but these diseases are discussed elsewhere in this chapter.

Decreased Production of Erythrocytes.
Chronic diseases such as RA, systemic lupus erythematosus, tuberculosis, or cancer may decrease production of erythrocytes. Anemia of chronic disease is characterized by modestly reduced RBC survival; the bone marrow fails to compensate for the slightly decreased RBC life span. Normally, iron is released from disintegrating RBCs and recirculates within the bloodstream. In the chronic inflammatory process, inflammatory cytokines* cause an increase of ferritin (an iron storage complex formed in the intestinal mucosa) in macrophages, thereby hindering release of iron. Failure to increase RBC production is largely caused by this trapping of iron within the reticuloendothelial system,† preventing its transfer to the bone marrow for use.

Nutritional deficiency as a cause of anemia can occur at any age. Iron, protein, vitamin B_{12}, and other vitamins and minerals are needed for the production of hemoglobin and the formation of erythrocytes. Growing children; lower socioeconomic groups; older adults (as a result of economic constraints, lack of interest in food preparation, and poor dentition); menstruating women, and pregnant women are the most common groups to develop iron deficiency anemia.

The most common cause of vitamin B_{12} deficiency is pernicious anemia. Loss of intrinsic factor may contribute to a vitamin B_{12} deficiency. In the case of pernicious anemia caused by a deficiency of vitamin B_{12}, poor diet rarely causes the vitamin deficiency; rather it is a result of defective intestinal absorption. After being ingested, vitamin B_{12} becomes bound to intrinsic factor, a protein secreted by gastric parietal cells. Any condition that destroys gastric parietal cells also results in decreased intrinsic factor, which is required for absorption of vitamin B_{12}.

Destruction of intrinsic factor production sites may occur with gastrectomy (see the section on Aging and the Gastrointestinal System in Chapter 15). Other causes of vitamin B_{12} deficiency include bacterial overgrowth in the lumen of the intestine (competes for vitamin B_{12}); surgical resection of the ileum (eliminates the site of vitamin B_{12} absorption), and, more rarely, dietary deficiency (e.g., strict vegetarian diet); tapeworm infection; and severe Crohn's disease. The latter condition can cause sufficient destruction of the ileum to retard vitamin B_{12} absorption.

Folic acid deficiency is a very common cause of decreased production of erythrocytes. Folic acid deficiency has many causes, but it usually results from inadequate dietary intake, chronic alcoholism, malabsorption syndromes, anorexia, and consumption of overcooked food. In anemia due to folic acid deficiency associated with alcoholism, high levels of alcohol in the blood partially block the response of the bone marrow to folic acid, which thereby interferes with erythropoiesis. The common occurrence of folic acid deficiency during the growth spurts of childhood and adolescence and during the third trimester of pregnancy is explained by the increased demands for folate required for DNA synthesis in these circumstances. Pregnant women need six times the normal amount of folic acid to meet the needs of the developing fetus. Long-term use of anticonvulsants (e.g., primidone, diphenylhydantoin, phenobarbital); antimetabolites administered for cancer and leukemia; and certain oral contraceptives may interfere with folate absorption.

Bone marrow disorders constitute the most likely source of anemia caused by decreased production of erythrocytes in a therapy practice. Aplastic anemia, marrow replacement with fibrotic tissue or tumor, acute leukemia, or infiltrative disease (e.g., lymphoma, myeloma, carcinoma) falls into this etiologic category. Anemias of radiation-induced bone marrow failure occur because the bone marrow stem cells are destroyed and mitosis (cell division) is inhibited, preventing the synthesis of RBCs. Antimetabolites used in cancer therapy also cause bone marrow failure by blocking the synthesis of purines or nucleic acids required for synthesis of protein within the cell. Because bone marrow transplantation may be curative for aplastic anemia, it is hypothesized that the defect associated with that type of anemia must be intrinsic to the hematopoietic cells, perhaps consisting of damage to the stem cells with a resultant inability to regenerate and repopulate the bone marrow.

---

*Cytokines, cell-derived chemicals that are secreted by various types of cells, act on other cells to stimulate or inhibit their function. Chemicals derived from lymphocytes are called *lymphokines*. Chemicals derived from lymphocytes that act on other WBCs are called *interleukins* (i.e., they interact between two types of leukocytes).

†The reticuloendothelial system is a network of cells and tissues found throughout the body, especially in the blood, general connective tissue, spleen, liver, lungs, bone marrow, and lymph nodes. Some of the reticuloendothelial cells found in the blood are concerned with blood cell formation and destruction, and the metabolism of iron and pigment. These cells have a significant role in inflammation and immunity.

Clinical Manifestations. Mild anemia often causes only minimal and usually vague symptoms such as fatigue until hemoglobin concentration and hematocrit fall below half of normal. As the anemia progresses, general signs and symptoms caused by the inability of anemic blood to supply the body tissues with enough oxygen may include weakness; dyspnea on exertion; easy fatigue; pallor or yellowness of skin, especially the palms of the hands, fingernails,* mucosa, and conjunctiva; tachycardia; increased angina in pre-existing coronary artery disease (CAD); leg ulcers (sickle cell); and, occasionally, koilonychia (Fig. 13-1).

Central nervous system (CNS) symptoms can develop in cases of severe pernicious anemia, whereas neuropathy is observed in early cases of B_{12} deficiency allowing for early identification. The findings typically consist of a symmetric sensory neuropathy that begins in the feet and lower legs, although rarely, it may involve the upper extremities, especially fine motor coordination of the hands. This upper extremity neuropathy may clinically manifest as problems with deteriorating handwriting. Affected individuals may also describe moderate pain or paresthesias of the extremities, especially the feet. The person may interpret the neuropathy as difficulty with locomotion, when, in fact, they are experiencing the loss of proprioception. The affected individual may need to hold onto the wall, countertops, or furniture at home due to difficulties maintaining balance. An associated positive Romberg sign may occur. Loss of motor function is a late manifestation of B_{12} deficiency. Although a symmetrical neuropathy is the usual pattern, B_{12} deficiency occasionally presents as a unilateral neuropathy and/or bilateral but asymmetrical neuropathy. Rarely, subacute degeneration of the spinal cord caused by vitamin B_{12} deficiency can occur in pernicious anemia, characterized by pyramidal and posterior column deficits. CNS manifestations may include headache, drowsiness, dizziness, fainting, slow thought processes, decreased attention span, apathy, depression, and irritability.

Complications depend on the specific type of anemia; severe anemia can cause heart failure and hypoxic damage to the liver and kidney, with all the signs and symptoms associated with either of those conditions. Anemia in the presence of any coronary obstruction results in low blood oxygen levels. The decreased oxygen perfusion of the heart precipitates angina more quickly and more often.

Medical Management

Diagnosis. The clinical picture cannot be depended on for confirmation of the suspected diagnosis because symptoms may not be recognized until hemoglobin concentration is reduced to half of normal. Personal and family history may point to congenital anemia, and a physical examination may elicit signs of primary hematologic diseases such as lymphadenopathy, hepatosplenomegaly, skin and mucosal changes, or bone tenderness. To determine the specific type of anemia present, the hematologist examines a peripheral blood smear and calculates red cell indices (and, in some cases, the rate of RBC

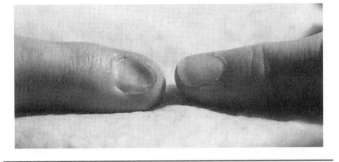

FIGURE **13-1** Normal nail on the right compared with nail on the left is referred to as *koilonychia* and sometimes called *spoon-shaped nails* or *spoon nails*. They are thin, depressed nails with lateral edges turned up and are concave from side to side. They may be idiopathic, congenital, or a hereditary trait and are occasionally due to iron deficiency anemia. (From Swartz, MH: *Textbook of physical diagnosis,* Philadelphia, 1988, WB Saunders, plate I[D]).

destruction). Laboratory diagnosis may include other measures such as a complete blood cell count (CBC); determination of serum iron; serum ferritin; and reticulocyte count. In the case of B_{12} deficiency, a level less than 300 pg/mL is an indication of early deficiency requiring treatment.

Treatment and Prognosis. Treatment of anemia is directed toward alleviating or controlling the causes, relieving the symptoms, and preventing complications. It is critical that the underlying cause of anemia be determined. For example, endoscopy to identify the source of GI blood loss for a client with a long-term history of NSAID use would indicate the need to stop taking the medication or prescribe the use of proton pump inhibitors (PPIs) (e.g., Prilosec, Aciphex, Prevacid); Cytotec; Carafate; or histamine blockers (H_2-blockers) such as Pepcid, Tagamet, and Zantac (see Chapter 15).

Treating the underlying cause can include bone marrow transplantation to replace damaged marrow; vitamin B_{12},* folic acid, or iron supplemental therapy for nutritional deficits or in the case of chronic blood loss; oxygen therapy to prevent hypoxia; corticosteroids and androgens to stimulate marrow to produce RBCs; splenectomy to decrease the destruction of RBCs; anti-T lymphocyte antibodies and other immunosuppressive agents for the treatment of aplastic anemia; and recombinant human erythropoietin (Epogen [EPO]) for the treatment of anemia related to chronic disease. The use of erythropoietin in the treatment of anemia associated with chronic renal failure and anemia secondary to zidovudine (AZT) therapy in people with HIV stimulates erythropoiesis and may elevate RBC counts enough to decrease the need for blood transfusions in these two groups.

The prognosis for anemia depends on the etiologic factors and potential treatment for the underlying cause. For example, the prognosis is good for anemia related to nutritional deficiency, but poor for hemolytic anemia. Likewise, treatment is aimed at correcting the underlying pathogenesis. Untreated or misdiagnosed B_{12} deficiency can be progressive, resulting in

---

*Pallor in dark-skinned people may be observed by the absence of the underlying red tones that normally give brown or black skin its luster. The brown-skinned individual demonstrates pallor with a more yellowish-brown color, and the black-skinned person appears ashen or gray.

*Parenteral treatment of B_{12} deficiency should be considered for those individuals with B_{12} levels less than 300 pg/mL due to irreversible neurologic deficits that can develop.[67]

irreversible neurologic damage. Anemia in the older adult (age 85 or older) is associated with an increased risk of death. Although anemia was once considered a normal consequence of aging, it is now recognized as a sign of other disease (e.g., hip fracture, RA, erosive gastritis, peptic ulcer, malnutrition, cirrhosis, ulcerative colitis [see Table 13-2]) in the older adult requiring further assessment.[34]

Special Implications for the Therapist   13-4

THE ANEMIAS

Preferred Practice Patterns:

Practice patterns depend on manifestations of clinical signs and symptoms, complications, and the system(s) affected (e.g., dyspnea, angina, tachycardia associated with cardiovascular/pulmonary system; peripheral neuropathy associated with the nervous system).

Exercise and Anemia

The impact of anemia on functional recovery in the acute care or rehabilitation setting and the theoretical risk of increased morbidity and mortality during prescribed therapeutic exercise has not been thoroughly investigated. Further study is indicated to examine the implications for anemia on functional recovery and cardiopulmonary complications during rehabilitation.[17] The following guidelines should be used until proven protocols are developed. Exercise for any anemic person should be approved by the physician. Diminished exercise tolerance may be expected in anyone with anemia along with easy fatigability, depending on the cause of the anemia. Increased physical activity increases the demand for oxygen, which may not be adequately available in the circulating blood. Pacing and training that distribute the intensity of the workload over time can be used to promote physiologic recovery.[16] For the sedentary aging adult, decreased activity can mask exercise intolerance; observe carefully for any changes in mental status.

The prevalence of iron deficiency anemia is likely to be higher in athletic populations and groups, especially in younger female athletes, than in sedentary individuals. In anemic individuals, iron deficiency decreases athletic performance and impairs immune function leading to other physiologic dysfunction. Although it is likely that blood losses secondary to exercise such as foot strike hemolysis or iron loss through sweat, may contribute to anemia, nonathletic causes must also be considered. Dietary choices explain much of a negative iron balance, but the GI and genitourinary systems must be evaluated for blood loss.[68] Evidence also exists for increased rates of RBC iron and whole-body iron turnover. The young female athlete may want to consult with medical or dietary consultants about the use of low-dose iron supplements during training.[5]

Research has shown that people with chronic renal failure who have severe anemia are able to exercise but must do so at a lower intensity than that of the normal population. The maximum oxygen consumption (VO_{2max}) for the anemic client is at least 20% less than that for the normal population. Exercise testing and prescribed exercise(s) in anemic clients must be initiated with extreme caution and should proceed very gradually to tolerance and/or perceived exertion levels.[20,57]

Precautions

Knowing the underlying cause of the anemia may be very helpful in identifying red flag symptoms indicating the need for alteration of the program or medical referral. For example, GI blood loss associated with NSAID use may worsen suddenly, precipitating a crisis in a therapy setting. It is not uncommon for clients to present with both anemia and cardiovascular disease, precipitating angina (see Special Implications for the Therapist, Angina, 11-3. Splenomegaly associated with some types of anemia requires precautions in performing soft tissue techniques in the left upper quadrant, especially up and under the rib cage; indirect techniques away from the spleen are indicated.

Bleeding under the skin and easy bruising in response to the slightest trauma often occur when platelet production is altered (thrombocytopenia) secondary to hypoplastic or aplastic anemia. This condition necessitates extreme care in the therapy setting, especially any intervention requiring manual therapy or the use of any equipment, including modalities and weight-training devices.

Decreased oxygen delivery to the skin results in impaired healing and loss of elasticity, delaying wound healing and healing of other musculoskeletal injuries. If the anemia is caused by vitamin B_{12} deficiency (e.g., pernicious anemia, pregnancy, hyperthyroidism), the nervous system is affected. Alteration of the structure and function of the peripheral nerves, spinal cord (myelin degeneration), and brain may occur. Paresthesias, especially numbness mimicking carpal tunnel syndrome; gait disturbances; extreme weakness; spasticity; and abnormal reflexes can result. Permanent neurologic damage unresponsive to vitamin B_{12} therapy can occur in extreme cases when intervention has been delayed.

Monitoring Vital Signs

Tachycardia may be the first change observed when monitoring vital signs, usually accompanied by a sense of fatigue, generalized weakness, loss of stamina, and exertional dyspnea. Systolic blood pressure may not be affected, but diastolic pressure may be lower than normal, with an associated increase in the resting pulse rate. Resting cardiac output is usually normal in people with anemia, but cardiac output increases with exercise more than in nonanemic people. As the anemia becomes more severe, resting cardiac output increases and exercise tolerance progressively decreases until dyspnea, tachycardia, and palpitations occur at rest. ■

DISORDERS OF LEUKOCYTES

Alterations in the blood leukocyte (WBC) concentration and in the relative proportions of the several leukocyte types are recognized as measures of the reaction of the body to disease processes and noxious agents. In many instances, these alterations give useful indications of the nature of the pathologic process and may be seen in association not only with acute infections but also with many chronic ailments treated by the therapist.

Leukocytes may be classified in three main groups: granulocytes (basophils, eosinophils, neutrophils); monocytes; and lymphocytes. *Granulocytes* (granular leukocytes) contain lysing agents within their granules that are capable of digesting various foreign materials. The main type of granulocyte is the neutrophil, also called the *polymorphmononuclear (PMN) leukocyte*; these are usually not found in normal "healthy" tissue and are referred to as the first line of hematologic defense against invading pathogens. However, besides the beneficial microbicidal activity of neutrophils, granulocytes are also involved in the pathophysiology of organ damage in ischemia/reperfusion, trauma, sepsis, or organ transplantation. *Monocytes* are the largest circulating blood cells and represent an immature cell until it leaves the blood and travels to the tissues. Once migrated, monocytes form macrophages when activated by foreign substances, such as bacteria. Monocytes/macrophages participate in chronic inflammation by synthesizing numerous mediators and eliminating various pathogens. *Lymphocytes* are known to intervene in immune responses such as secreting cytokines, killing cells, or the production of antibodies. Antibodies react with antigens, thus initiating the immune response to fight infection. The exact role or function of leukocytes during inflammatory processes remains the subject of considerable investigation.

◆ Leukocytosis

Leukocytosis, defined as a transient increase in the number of leukocytes in the blood, may occur as a result of a variety of causes (Box 13-4) and may also occur as a normal protective response to physiologic stressors such as strenuous exercise, emotional changes, temperature changes, anesthesia, surgery, pregnancy, and some drugs, toxins, and hormones. Leukocytosis develops within 1 or 2 hours after the onset of acute hemorrhage and is greater when the bleeding occurs internally (i.e., into the peritoneal cavity, pleural space, or joint cavity or as a result of a skull fracture with associated intracranial bleed or subarachnoid hemorrhage) than when the bleeding is external.

Leukocytosis is a common finding in and characterizes many infectious diseases recognized by a count of more than 10,000 WBCs/mm³ (see Table 39-2). Elevated WBC count in response to the serious underlying processes listed in Box 13-4 is referred to as "leukemoid reactions." Leukocytosis can be associated with an increase in circulating neutrophils (neutrophilia), recruited in large numbers early in the course of most bacterial infections and in the presence of rapidly growing neoplasms. When the liver, GI tract, or bone marrow is involved, the counts may be especially high. Some tumors can also release hormone-like substances that cause leukocytosis.

BOX 13-4

Causes of Leukocytosis

Acute appendicitis
Acute hemorrhage
Acute rheumatic fever
Bacterial infections
Inflammation or tissue necrosis (e.g., infarction, myositis, vasculitis)
Intoxication by chemicals
Metabolic intoxications (e.g., uremia, eclampsia, acidosis, gout)
Neoplasms (e.g., bronchogenic carcinoma, lymphoma, melanoma)
Pneumonia
Splenectomy

Clinical Manifestations.   Clinical signs and symptoms of leukocytosis are usually associated with symptoms of the conditions listed in Box 13-4 and may include fever, symptoms of localized or systemic infection, and symptoms of inflammation or trauma to tissue.

Medical Management
Diagnosis, Treatment, and Prognosis.   Major leukocyte functions are accomplished in the tissues so that the leukocytes in the blood are in transit from the site of production or storage to the tissues, even in normal people. Variations in the blood concentrations of each leukocyte type may be of brief duration and easily missed or may persist for days or weeks. Laboratory tests for detecting leukocyte abnormalities include total leukocyte count, leukocyte differential cell count (see Chapter 39), peripheral blood morphology, and bone marrow morphology.

Treatment is directed toward the underlying cause of the change in leukocytes and control of any infections. Prognosis is dependent on the etiology of the leukocytosis.

◆ Leukopenia

Leukopenia, or reduction of the number of leukocytes in the blood below 5000/mL (see Chapter 39), can be caused by a variety of factors such as anaphylactic shock, alcohol and nutritional deficiencies, splenomegaly, and SLE. It can occur in many forms of bone marrow failure, such as that following antineoplastic chemotherapy or radiation therapy*, in overwhelming infections, in dietary deficiencies, and in autoimmune diseases. People with leukemia, lymphoma, myeloma, and Hodgkin's disease have serious underlying immune deficiencies, which may contribute to the risk of infection associated with leukopenia. Unlike leukocytosis, leukopenia is never beneficial. As the leukocyte count decreases, the risk for infection increases.

Clinical Manifestations.   Clinical signs and symptoms of leukopenia may include sore throat, cough, high fever, chills, sweating, ulcerations of mucous membranes (e.g., mouth, rectum, vagina), frequent or painful urination, and persistent infections.

Medical Management
Diagnosis and Treatment.   As with leukocytosis, diagnosis is by laboratory testing for leukocyte abnormalities. Treatment is directed toward elimination of the cause of the reduced leukocytes and control of any infections. Pharmacologic therapy includes the use of antibiotics, antifungal agents, and colony-stimulating drugs such as filgrastim (Neupogen). This drug markedly assists in decreasing the incidence of infection in people who have received bone marrow-depressing antineoplastic agents.

---

*The risk of infection from leukopenia after bone marrow radiation has been reduced with continued improvements in medical treatment. The use of naturally occurring glycoproteins to help collect blood stem cells administered after chemotherapy reduces the duration of blood cell reduction and prevents the serious problems encountered in the past. These glycoproteins are hematopoietic growth factors called colony-stimulating factors (CSFs) or more specifically, granulocyte colony-stimulating facter (GCSF), or Neupogen. Growth factors move the stem cells from the bone marrow into the peripheral blood and can result in a temporary 10- to 100-fold increase in the numbers of circulating stem cells at the time of bone marrow recovery. Neupogen not only increases the number but also the function of granulocytes.

◆ Basophilia*

Basophils have a high content of heparin (anticoagulant) and histamine and have an important role in acute systemic allergic reactions. In the presence of bacteria or other infectious agents, the basophils erupt and distribute chemicals that trigger inflammation. At this point, neutrophils, eosinophils, or monocytes arrive to engulf or phagocytose the alien particle. Basophilia is primarily associated with myeloproliferative disorders (e.g., polycythemia rubra vera, agnogenic myeloid metaplasia, essential thrombocythemia, and chronic myelogenous leukemia [CML]).

◆ Eosinophilia

Eosinophils, usually active in the later stages of inflammation, have some phagocytic properties, but they are generally weaker than neutrophils. One of the primary functions of eosinophils is to surround and engulf antigen-antibody complexes formed during an allergic response. They are also able to defend against parasitic infections. *Eosinophilia* (abnormally large number of eosinophils in the blood) can occur as a result of allergic reactions such as asthma or hay fever, pernicious anemia, drug reactions, and neoplastic conditions, such as leukemia. Increased levels of eosinophils have been identified with *eosinophilia-myalgia syndrome,* a connective tissue disease induced by chemical exposure[15] or the ingestion of tryptophan taken for insomnia and back pain.

◆ Neutrophilia

Granulocytes assist in initiating the inflammatory response, and they defend the body against infectious agents by phagocytosing bacteria and other infectious substances. Generally, the neutrophils (the most plentiful of the granulocytes) are the first phagocytic cells to reach an infected area, followed by monocytes; neutrophils and monocytes work together to phagocytose all foreign material present.

Granulocytosis (an excess of granulocytes in the blood) or *neutrophilia* (increased number of neutrophils in the blood) are terms used to describe the early stages of infection or inflammation. The capacity of corticosteroids or alcohol to diminish the accumulation of neutrophils in inflamed areas may be due to their ability to reduce cell adherence.

The many potential causes of neutrophilia include inflammation or tissue necrosis (e.g., after surgery from tissue damage, severe burns, myocardial infarction, pneumonitis, rheumatic fever, RA); acute infection (e.g., *Staphylococcus, Streptococcus, Pneumococcus*); drug- or chemical-induced causes (e.g., epinephrine, steroids, heparin, histamine); metabolic causes (e.g., acidosis associated with diabetes, gout, thyroid storm, eclampsia); and neoplasms of the liver, GI tract, or bone marrow. Physiologic neutrophilia may also occur as a result of exercise, extreme heat/cold, third-trimester pregnancy, and emotional distress.

◆ Neutropenia

Neutropenia is the condition associated with a reduction in circulating neutrophils (less than 2000/mL). Bone marrow defects (failure to produce and release neutrophils at a normal rate) account for the majority of neutropenias. Failure of the marrow compartment can occur as a result of direct injury or from maturation defects of hematopoietic cells (the latter from nutritional deficiencies such as folate or vitamin B_{12} deficiencies). Neutropenia may occur in severe, prolonged infections (e.g., influenza, hepatitis B, malaria, measles, mumps, rubella) when production of granulocytes cannot keep up with demand or in the presence of decreased bone marrow production, such as with radiation, chemotherapy, leukemia, and myeloma. Carcinoma of the lung, breast, prostate, and stomach and malignant hematopoietic disorders can occupy enough of the medullary space to cause global marrow failure. Similarly, in specific myeloproliferative diseases and leukemias, bone marrow fibroblasts can proliferate significantly in the marrow and contribute to bone marrow failure. Immune-mediated bone marrow failure may cause neutropenia (e.g., rheumatic or autoimmune disease, acquired aplastic anemia). Increased destruction of neutrophils may also result in neutropenia (e.g., splenomegaly, hemodialysis).

◆ Lymphocytosis/Lymphocytopenia

Lymphocytosis is rare in acute bacterial infections and occurs most commonly in acute viral infections, especially those caused by the Epstein-Barr virus (EBV). Other causes include endocrine disorders (e.g., thyrotoxicosis, adrenal insufficiency) and malignancies (e.g., acute and chronic lymphocytic leukemia). Lymphocytopenia may be attributed to abnormalities of lymphocyte production associated with neoplasms and immune deficiencies and destruction of lymphocytes by drugs, viruses, or radiation, but the primary cause of lymphopenia is prednisone therapy. In some individuals no known cause is evident. Lymphocytopenia associated with heart failure and other acute illnesses may be caused by elevated levels of cortisol, but this is not yet well understood. For some people with AIDS, lymphocytopenia can be a major problem.

◆ Monocytosis

Monocytosis, an increase in monocytes, is most often seen in chronic infections such as tuberculosis, subacute endocarditis, Hodgkin's disease, and as a normal physiologic response in newborns. In malignant neoplasms, monocytosis is caused by anemia of chronic cancer. Monocytosis is present in more than 50% of people with collagen vascular disease (see Box 11-11). Monocytosis is usually seen in the late stages of recovery from bacterial infections, when monocytes are needed to phagocytose surviving microorganisms and debris.

Special Implications for the Therapist   **13-5**

LEUKOCYTES

It is important for the therapist to be aware of the client's most recent leukocyte (WBC) count before and during episodes of care if that person is immunosuppressed. At that time, the client is extremely susceptible to opportunistic infections and

---

*The remaining categories (e.g., basophilia/basopenia, eosinophilia/eosinopenia, neutrophilia/neutropenia, and so on) are all types of leukocytosis or leukopenia. The specific type is determined when the leukocyte differential (WBC count) determines the percentage of each type of granular and nongranular leukocyte.

severe complications. The importance of good handwashing (see Box 7-2) and hygiene practices cannot be overemphasized when treating immunocompromised clients. Some centers recommend that people with a WBC count of less than 1000/mm³ or a neutrophil count of less than 500/mm³ should wear a protective mask. Therapists should ensure that these people are provided with equipment that has been disinfected according to standard precautions (see Table 8-11 and Appendix A). ■

NEOPLASTIC DISEASES OF THE BLOOD AND LYMPH SYSTEMS

Hematologic malignancies include diseases in any hematologic tissue (e.g., bone marrow, spleen, thymus) that arise from changes in stem cells and metastases to the bone marrow. The primary hematologic disorders are the immunoproliferative diseases such as multiple myeloma and the myeloproliferative disorders, including polycythemia rubra vera; essential thrombocythemia; CML; and agnogenic myeloid metaplasia (AMM) (e.g., myelofibrosis; replacement of hematopoietic bone marrow with fibrous tissue). Evidence suggests that all of these diseases arise from single cell mutations specific to that disease. These cellular mutations produce malignant clones (genetically identical cells) that have a growth advantage over normal cells in the marrow.

Cancers arising from the major lymphoid cells of the body (lymph nodes and the spleen) are called *malignant lymphomas*. Origin of malignancy in this case is not the source of differentiation (i.e., lymphoma gets its name from the cells affected rather than from the origin of disease and is categorized as either Hodgkin's disease or non-Hodgkin's lymphoma).

◆ Bone Marrow and Stem Cell Transplantation

Bone marrow transplantation (BMT) is often a treatment choice for many of the neoplastic diseases of the blood and lymph systems. Both BMT and the more recent technique of stem cell transplantation are discussed in Chapter 20.

◆ The Leukemias

Leukemia is a malignant neoplasm of the blood-forming cells, specifically replacement of the bone marrow by a malignant clone (genetically identical cell) of lymphocytic or myelogenous cells. The disease may be acute or chronic, based on its natural course; acute leukemias have a rapid clinical course, resulting in death in a few months without treatment, whereas chronic leukemias have a more prolonged course. The four major types of leukemia are acute or chronic lymphocytic and acute or chronic myelogenous leukemia (Table 13-3).

When leukemia is classified according to its morphology (i.e., the predominant cell type and level of maturity), the following descriptors are used: *lympho-* for leukemias involving the lymphoid or lymphatic system; *myelo-* for leukemias of myeloid or bone marrow origin involving hematopoietic stem cells (see Fig. 20-5); *-blastic* and *acute* for leukemia involving immature (functionless) cells; and *-cytic* and *chronic* for leukemia involving mature cells. If classified immunologically, T-cell, B-cell, or null-cell leukemias are described.

Acute leukemia is an accumulation of neoplastic, immature lymphoid or myeloid cells in the bone marrow and peripheral blood, tissue invasion by these cells, and associated bone marrow failure. It is defined as more than 30% blasts in the bone marrow. *Chronic leukemia* is a neoplastic accumulation of mature lymphoid or myeloid elements of the blood that usually progresses more slowly than an acute leukemic process and permits the production of greater numbers of more mature, functional cells. With rapid proliferation of leukemic cells, the bone marrow becomes overcrowded with WBCs, which then spill over into the peripheral circulation. Crowding of the bone marrow by leukemic cells inhibits normal blood cell production. The three main symptoms that occur as a consequence of this infiltration and replacement process are (1)

TABLE	13-3

Overview of Leukemia

	ACUTE LYMPHOCYTIC LEUKEMIA (ALL)	CHRONIC LYMPHOCYTIC LEUKEMIA (CLL)	ACUTE MYELOGENOUS LEUKEMIA (AML)	CHRONIC MYELOGENOUS LEUKEMIA (CML)
Incidence (% of all leukemias)	20%	25%	40%	15%-20%
Adults	20%	100% (common)	85% (most common)	95%-100%
Children	80%-85% (most common)	NA	10%-20%	3
Age (yr)	Peak: 3-7 65+ (older adults)	50+	Any age; incidence increases with age from 45-80+	All ages
Etiologic factors	? Unknown; chromosomal abnormality; environmental factors; Down syndrome (high incidence)	Chromosomal abnormalities; slow accumulation of CLL lymphocytes	Benzene; alkylating agents; radiation; myeloproliferative disorders; aplastic anemia	Philadelphia chromosome; radiation exposure
Prognosis	Adults: 58% survival Children: 80% survival	71% survival Median survival: 6 yr	Poor even with treatment Adults: 10%-15% survival Children: 43% survival	Moderately progressive 32% survival

anemia and reduced tissue oxygenation from decreased erythrocytes, (2) *infection* from neutropenia as leukemic cells are functionally unable to defend the body against pathogens, and (3) *bleeding tendencies* from decreased platelet production (thrombocytopenia) (Fig. 13-2).

Leukemia is not limited to the bone marrow and peripheral blood. Abnormalities in one or more organ systems can result from the infiltration and replacement of any tissue of the body with nonfunctional leukemic cells or metabolic complications related to leukemia.

Leukemia is a complex disease that requires careful identification of the subtype for appropriate treatment. Molecular probes can be used to establish a morphologic diagnosis of acute or chronic leukemia and to predict a person's response to therapy. These analyses are sufficiently sensitive to detect one leukemic cell among 100,000 or even in 1 million normal cells. Because of this extreme sensitivity, molecular markers have generally been used to determine the presence or absence of a few leukemic cells remaining after intensive therapy, so-called *residual disease*.

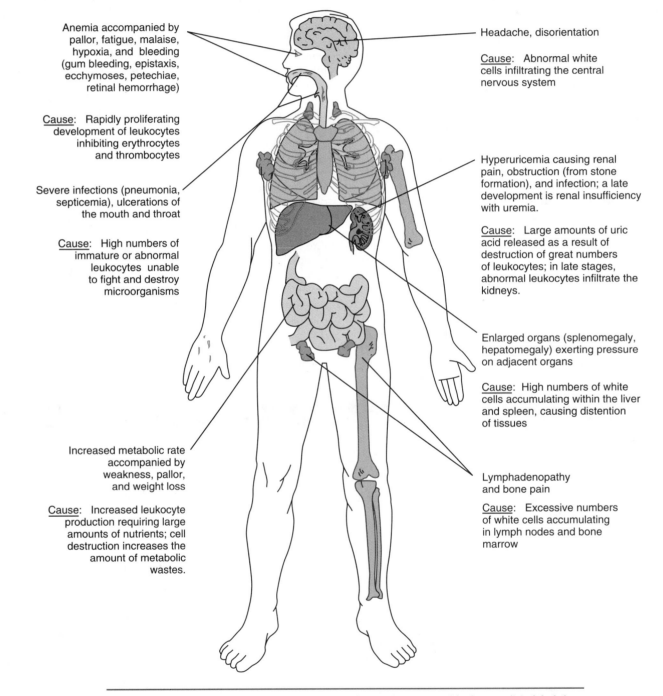

Anemia accompanied by pallor, fatigue, malaise, hypoxia, and bleeding (gum bleeding, epistaxis, ecchymoses, petechiae, retinal hemorrhage)

Cause: Rapidly proliferating development of leukocytes inhibiting erythrocytes and thrombocytes

Severe infections (pneumonia, septicemia), ulcerations of the mouth and throat

Cause: High numbers of immature or abnormal leukocytes unable to fight and destroy microorganisms

Increased metabolic rate accompanied by weakness, pallor, and weight loss

Cause: Increased leukocyte production requiring large amounts of nutrients; cell destruction increases the amount of metabolic wastes.

Headache, disorientation

Cause: Abnormal white cells infiltrating the central nervous system

Hyperuricemia causing renal pain, obstruction (from stone formation), and infection; a late development is renal insufficiency with uremia.

Cause: Large amounts of uric acid released as a result of destruction of great numbers of leukocytes; in late stages, abnormal leukocytes infiltrate the kidneys.

Enlarged organs (splenomegaly, hepatomegaly) exerting pressure on adjacent organs

Cause: High numbers of white cells accumulating within the liver and spleen, causing distention of tissues

Lymphadenopathy and bone pain

Cause: Excessive numbers of white cells accumulating in lymph nodes and bone marrow

FIGURE 13-2 Pathologic basis for the clinical manifestations of leukemia. (Modified from Black JM, Matassarin-Jacobs E, editors: *Luckmann and Sorensen's medical-surgical nursing*, ed 4, Philadelphia, 1993, WB Saunders.)

Over the last 25 years, death rates for leukemia have been falling significantly (57% decline) for children and more modestly for adults under 65 years. These declines in mortality reflect the advances made in the biologic and pathologic understanding of leukemia and subsequent treatment that is more specifically targeted at the molecular level. The aim of treatment is to bring about complete remission, or no evidence of the disease with return to normal blood and marrow cells without relapse. For leukemia, a complete remission that lasts 5 years after treatment often indicates a cure. Future clinical and laboratory investigation will likely lead to the development of new, even more effective treatments specifically for different subsets of leukemia. The development of new chemotherapeutic and biologic agents combined with refined dose and schedule and stem cell transplantation has already contributed to the clinical success of treatment.

◆ Acute Leukemia

Overview and Incidence. Acute leukemia is a rapidly progressive malignant disease of the bone marrow and blood that results in the accumulation of immature, functionless cells called *blast cells* in the marrow and blood that block the development of normal cell development. The two major forms of acute leukemia are *acute lymphocytic leukemia* (ALL) and *acute myelogenous leukemia* (AML). Lymphocytic leukemia involves the lymphocytes and lymphoid organs and myelogenous leukemia involves hematopoietic stem cells that differentiate into myeloid cells (monocytes, granulocytes, erythrocytes, and platelets).

Acute leukemia is primarily a disease of older adults, present equally between the genders. The incidence across all age groups is constant at 15 per 100,000 person, but begins to rise at age 45 years, and by age 80 years, incidence is approximately 160 per 100,000. AML constitutes 20% of all leukemias: 85% of adult acute leukemias and 20% of childhood leukemias. Of children with acute leukemia, 80% have the lymphocytic type (ALL). Even so, the incidence of acute lymphocytic leukemia is still four times higher in older adults than in children.

Etiologic and Risk Factors. The etiologic factors of acute leukemia are unknown in most cases. Most of the genetic defects that increase the likelihood of leukemia are acquired rather than inherited, but little is known about the environmental factors that induce these defects. The occurrence of certain leukemias early in childhood has led to the suggestion that changes in genes may be inherited or acquired in utero, but such changes have yet to be fully identified.

Predisposing environmental factors may include (1) exposure to ionizing radiation (e.g., atomic bomb survivors, diagnostic radiologists, or people with thymus enlargement, ankylosing spondylitis, or acne who received RT in the twentieth century); (2) occupational exposure to the chemical benzene*; (3) long-term, low-dose exposure to drugs, such as alkylating agents and nitrosourea used in chemotherapy; (4) presence of primary immune disorders; and (5) infection with the

human leukocyte virus (HTLV-1). Although these can be contributed to disease onset, most cases are not associated with any of these risk factors.[40]

Treatment-induced AML is the most commonly reported secondary cancer as a result of high doses of chemotherapy for Hodgkin's disease, multiple myeloma, and ovarian cancer. The most commonly found cytogenetic abnormalities associated with these types of induced leukemia are losses or deletions of chromosomes 5 and 7.[29]

Pathogenesis. Causal risk factors in combination with a genetic predisposition can alter nuclear deoxyribonucleic acid (DNA) in this disease. These DNA alterations result in leukemic cells that are unable to mature and respond to normal regulatory mechanisms. The molecular analysis of ALL has produced new insights into the pathogenesis of this disease at the molecular level. ALL, which accounts for 80% of all childhood leukemias, is caused by the malignant proliferation of precursor lymphocytes, called *lymphoblasts*. AML involves neoplastic proliferation of multipotent or committed hematopoietic precursor cells. In the case of therapy-related AML, alkylating agents (cytotoxic drugs and radiation) react directly with DNA and induce AML, primarily through partial chromosomal deletions or loss of whole chromosomes. The chromosome changes provide the altered cells with a proliferative advantage compared with normal cells.

Clinical Manifestations. Acute leukemia often presents as an apparent infection with an acute onset and high fever mimicking the flu (see Fig. 13-2). Bleeding due to platelet deficiency (thrombocytopenia) usually occurs in the skin and mucosal surfaces, manifested as gingival bleeding, epistaxis, mid-cycle menstrual bleeding, or heavy bleeding associated with menstruation.

Bone pain, especially of the sternum, ribs, and tibia, caused by expanded leukemic marrow and joint pain from leukemic infiltration or hemorrhage into a joint may be initial symptoms (more common finding in children than adults). Involvement of the synovium may lead to symptoms suggestive of a rheumatic disease, especially in children with ALL. Leukemic infiltration, hemorrhage into a joint, synovial reaction to an adjacent tumor mass, or crystal-induced synovitis may also result in arthritis symptoms. In the older adult, the disease can present insidiously with progressive weakness, pallor, a change in sense of well-being, and delirium.

Neurologic manifestations may be present at initial diagnosis of AML and occur with increasing frequency over time as a result of either leukemic infiltration or cerebral bleeding. Cranial nerve palsies most often involve the sixth and seventh cranial nerves. Headache, vomiting, papilledema, facial palsy, blurred vision, auditory disturbances, and meningeal irritation can occur if leukemic cells infiltrate the cerebral or spinal meninges. Because chemotherapeutic agents do not pass the blood-brain barrier, leukemia cells can grow easily in the brain.

Medical Management

Diagnosis. Leukemic cells react differently when exposed to various chemicals leading toward a histochemical diagnosis (e.g., chemical markers in the cells are used to differentiate between ALL and AML). Chromosomal studies are becoming an important tool in the differential diagnosis of ALL, and

---

*Benzene originates from cigarette smoke, gasoline, automobile emissions, and industrial pollution. Of benzene exposure that occurs in the environment, 70% is derived from vehicle exhaust emissions. The increase of environmental benzene has closely paralleled the rise in frequency of hematologic malignancies.[54]

cell-surface antigens have made it possible to further differentiate ALL into immunologic classes.

In the acutely ill client who presents with symptoms that indicate abnormal bone marrow function (infection, thrombocytopenia, anemia, bone pain), diagnosis is made by serologic examination and confirmed by bone marrow aspiration and biopsy. Peripheral blood smear, hemoglobin, platelet counts, and other blood tests are usually all abnormal. Lumbar puncture may be indicated if there is spinal fluid involvement.

Treatment. The diagnosis of acute leukemia is a medical emergency, especially if the WBC count is high (greater than 100,000/mL), placing the person at risk for cerebral hemorrhage caused by leukostasis (obstruction of and damage to blood vessels plugged with rigid blasts). Treatment decisions are based on protocol use developed by leukemia centers around the United States. AML has been treated initially with intensive combination chemotherapy, called *remission induction therapy,* to eradicate the neoplastic cells and restore normal hematopoiesis. Induction chemotherapy is followed by consolidation, which is sometimes followed by maintenance chemotherapy. Supportive care, including fluids, blood product replacement, and prompt treatment of infection with broad-spectrum antibiotics, may be required during the recovery period. Postinduction therapy may also include peripheral stem cell or bone marrow transplantation.

Prognosis. If left untreated, all leukemias are fatal. Leukemia is the most common cause of cancer death among men under age 40 and among women before age 20.[26] Over the last 30 years, a dramatic improvement has been seen in survival of individuals with leukemia, owing to the effectiveness of improved treatment. The use of stem cell transplantation from unrelated donors has grown in the past decade in part because of the expansion of the donor registry size although relapse-free survival remains limited in people with a large tumor burden at the time of transplantation.

Survival rate for children has improved from a 4-year survival rate of 4% in the 1960s to a 75% 5-year survival rate in the late 1990s. Five-year survival rate for adults is 44% and 30% achieve long-term disease-free survival.[26] Prognosis is less favorable if any of the following factors exist: (1) presentation in younger or older age groups, (2) male gender, (3) high leukocyte count (more than 100,000) at the time of diagnosis, (4) CNS involvement, and (5) chromosomal abnormalities.

◆ Chronic Leukemia

Chronic leukemia is a malignant disease of the bone marrow and blood that progresses slowly and permits numbers of more mature, functional cells to be made. Chronic leukemia has two major groups: chronic myelogenous leukemia (CML) and chronic lymphocytic leukemia (CLL) each with several subtypes. These are entirely different diseases and are presented separately. Other less common forms include prolymphocytic leukemia (terminal transformation of CLL); large lymphocytic leukemia; and hairy cell leukemia (also called leukemic reticuloendotheliosis, accounting for only 1% to 2% of adult leukemias).

Chronic Myelogenous Leukemia
Incidence and Etiologic Factors. CML results in increases in not only myeloid cells but also erythroid cells and platelets in peripheral blood and marked hyperplasia in the bone marrow. This type of leukemia accounts for 15% of all leukemias. Although the exact etiologic factors are unknown, the incidence of CML is increased in people with radiation exposure. It is the only form of leukemia with a known genetic predisposition (Philadelphia chromosome [Ph]). The specific genetic anomaly is a translocation that fuses the long arm of chromosome 22 to chromosome 9 in all three hematopoietic cell lines; this form of leukemia is more common in families, and especially those with immunologic abnormalities.

Pathogenesis. CML originates in the hematopoietic stem cell (i.e., this cell has the ability to develop into any one of several blood cells; see Fig. 20-5) and involves overproduction of myeloid (bone marrow) cells. The Ph chromosome (22) was the first consistent chromosomal anomaly identified in a cancer and is now detected in all cases of CML. In the case of the Ph chromosome associated with CML, two genes (*bcr* gene on chromosome 22 and *abl* gene on chromosome 9) are fused. This accidental fusion disrupts the normal pathway and results in the production of activated *bcr-abl* tyrosine kinase,* resulting in a dysregulated proliferation signal. The Ph chromosome is present in more than 95% of CML cases and 25% of cases of adult ALL, 10% of cases of childhood leukemia, and 5% of cases of AML.

Clinical Manifestations. Presenting signs and symptoms are often quite nonspecific. The most typical symptoms at presentation are fatigue, anorexia, and weight loss, although approximately 40% of affected individuals are asymptomatic. Splenomegaly is present in 50% of all cases. The natural history of CML is a progression from a benign chronic phase to a rapidly fatal blast crisis within 3 to 5 years. In contrast to the maturation of CML cells during the chronic phase, during a blast crisis, cells fail to mature and remain nonfunctional as in an acute leukemia.

Medical Management
Diagnosis. Abnormal bleeding and symptomatic splenomegaly are clinical signs pointing to CML, but CML must be differentiated from other myeloproliferative disease. As with other leukemias, laboratory findings, including blood and bone marrow testing, will assist in establishing the diagnosis. The Ph chromosome is almost invariably present and may be detected in either the peripheral blood or bone marrow.

Treatment and Prognosis. Stem cell transplantation remains the only curative therapy for CML (see Fig. 20-9), but many people with CML are not candidates requiring the development of alternative therapies. Recombinant human alpha-interferon in the chronic phase of CML may induce hematologic remission and suppress the Ph chromosome. Hydroxyurea and BuSulfan are also used to lower the neutrophil count in CML especially during the accelerated phase, which often precedes the onset of a blast crisis. CML is a moderately progressive form of leukemia; the chronic form eventually evolves into a more rapidly progressive phase, referred to as *accelerated phase* and ultimately a *blast crisis,* which is more resistant to treatment. This progression to acute

---

*Tyrosine kinase is an enzyme that is necessary for normal cell growth. In normal cells, the enzyme turns on and off as it should but in people with CML, this enzyme appears to be in the permanent "switched-on" state, eliminating the normal checks and balances on proliferation.

leukemia occurs at a median time around 3 to 4 years. Research for the treatment of CML using tyrosine kinase inhibitor (STI-571) as an anticancer drug based on the specific underlying molecular abnormality has demonstrated successful remission without serious side effects.[48] Combined research results from around the world are very encouraging for expanded treatment options for people with CML.[43,44]

Chronic Lymphocytic Leukemia
Incidence and Etiologic and Risk Factors.
CLL is the most common type of leukemia in Western society, accounting for 25% to 40% of all leukemias and increasing with advancing age. Of all affected people, 90% are older than 50 years, and men are affected twice as often as women. CLL may occur in as many as 3% of people over the age of 70. The cause of CLL is also unknown. Unlike other hematologic malignancies, no increased incidence occurs following radiation exposure, nor is there a known retroviral association. Chronic viral infections such as EBV are considered possible causes of chronic leukemia, and investigation continues to identify a possible viral cause. Some groups of people may have a genetic predisposition, but this has not been conclusively proven.[89]

Pathogenesis.
The molecular defect in CLL is unknown. Deletion of chromosome 12 is present in more than half of all people with CLL. Chromosome 14 abnormalities are also common with B-cell CLL, suggesting the presence of a tumor suppressor gene. These abnormalities correlate with a high leukocyte count and adverse response to treatment.[46] Cell division and apoptosis (programmed cell death) are the two major physiologic processes that control the size of cell populations. CLL arises as a result of the clonal expansion of B-lymphocytes in which a deregulation of apoptosis leads to prolonged cell survival. This process becomes even more exaggerated with increasing drug resistance, the usual cause of treatment failure in this condition.

Clinical Manifestations.
Chronic leukemia may be asymptomatic, or it may present with fatigue, or the initial presentation may be lymphadenopathy in the cervical, axillary, and supraclavicular areas. Other less common sites of involvement include the gut mucosa, lungs, skin, and bone. The most common initial symptoms are splenomegaly, extreme fatigue, malaise, weight loss, low-grade fever, night sweats, easy bruisability, bone pain, and decreased exercise tolerance. The duration of the chronic phase is about 3 years. In most people, a gradual transition occurs called the *accelerated phase* from the chronic to the acute phase over a median time of 3 to 4 years. Immune deficiency characterized by hypogammaglobulinemia is a major cause of opportunistic infections that complicate the disease course of more than 75% of clients.

Medical Management
Diagnosis.   Serologic examination and cytometry to evaluate antibodies and additional markers are used to make a histochemical diagnosis. Peripheral blood smear and other blood tests combined with bone marrow aspiration and biopsy confirm the diagnosis.

Treatment.   No known cure for CLL exists, and treatment is usually based on clinical staging. Until recently, initial stages of chronic leukemia were not treated because of drug resistance and the fact that complications of chemotherapy were more harmful than the leukemia. Treatment has been palliative during the symptomatic stage. The identification of the pathogenic pathways and points at which dysregulation of cell growth occurs is beginning to open up new therapeutic options where conventional cytotoxic chemotherapy has been unsuccessful. Additionally, the introduction of new active agents (e.g., purine analogues, monoclonal antibodies) has led to a renewed interest in clinical investigation of CLL.[83] The use of allogeneic transplant for the treatment of CLL has increased over the last years but remains a successful option in limited numbers of cases.

Prognosis.   CLL continues to be a fatal disease with a significant impact on life expectancy, but in the last few years a trend toward an improvement in overall survival has taken place. The chronic forms of leukemia usually remain stable for years and then transform to a more overtly malignant disease. Once the disease has progressed to the accelerated or blast phase, infection and hemorrhagic complications are major problems and survival is measured in months. Approximately 60% of young adults who have successful allogeneic bone marrow transplantation appear to be cured. Despite treatment advances, the median survival of CLL clients remains 4 to 6 years, but survival statistics in relation to changes in treatment approaches have not been evaluated yet.

Special Implications for the Therapist   13-6

LEUKEMIA

Preferred Practice Patterns:
Practice patterns are determined on an individual basis depending on clinical presentation and response to medical intervention or other treatment measures.

Precautions
The period after chemically induced remission is critical for each client who is now highly susceptible to spontaneous hemorrhage and defenseless against invading organisms. The usual precautions for thrombocytopenia and infection control must be adhered to strictly. The importance of strict handwashing technique (see Box 7-2) cannot be overemphasized. The therapist should be alert to any sign of infection and report any potential site of infection, such as mucosal ulceration, skin abrasion, or a tear (even a hangnail). Precautions are as for anemia, outlined earlier in this chapter.

Anticipating potential side effects of medications used in the treatment of leukemia can help the therapist better understand client reactions during the episode of care. Drug-induced mood changes, ranging from feelings of well-being and euphoria to depression and irritability, may occur; depression and irritability may also be associated with the cancer. Neuropathy with neurotoxic effects of chemotherapy is uncommon with the leukemias.

Joint Involvement
Arthralgias or arthritis occur in approximately 12% of adults with chronic leukemia, 13% of adults with acute leukemia,

Continued

and up to 60% of children with acute lymphoblastic leukemia. Articular symptoms are the result of leukemic infiltrates of the synovium, periosteum, or periarticular bone, or of secondary gout or hemarthrosis. Asymmetrical involvement of the large joints is most commonly observed. Pain that is disproportionate to the physical findings may occur, and joint symptoms are often transient. ∎

◆ Malignant Lymphomas

Lymphoma is a general term for cancers that develop in the lymphatic system. Lymphomas are divided into two distinct groups: Hodgkin's disease (HD) and non-Hodgkin's lymphoma (NHL). HD is distinguished from other lymphomas by the presence of a characteristic type of cell known as the Reed-Sternberg cell. All other types of lymphoma are called NHL.[4]

Hodgkin's disease is primarily a disease of young adults, but children and older adults can be affected. Incidence rates differ according to age with an overall incidence of approximately 2.6 per 100,000 (slightly lower for women). In the United States, about 7000 cases of Hodgkin's disease were diagnosed in 2002 compared with 53,900 cases of non-Hodgkin's disease. The overall incidence of Hodgkin's disease has remained stable for many years and represents 8% of all lymphomas.

In the past, NHL constituted only 3% of all malignancies in the United States and was uncommon except in groups with a predisposition. Recent recognition by epidemiologists and clinicians that the incidence of NHL has been undergoing a universal increase without identifiable cause has been reported. The incidence has doubled since the early 1970s among all age groups, except the very young; whites and blacks; both United States and international populations; and both genders.[26] NHLs are the most common neoplasm of adults between the ages of 20 and 40 years. The observed increases preceded that of HIV infection, but with the increasing incidence of AIDS, the number of cases of NHL has also sharply increased. Certain kinds of NHLs (lymphoblastic and Burkitt's) occur in children.

Hodgkin's Disease
Definition and Overview. Hodgkin's disease is an immunodeficiency disease of lymphoid tissue with the primary histologic finding of giant Reed-Sternberg cells in the lymph nodes. These cells are part of the tissue macrophage system and have twin nuclei and nucleoli that give them the appearance of owl eyes. The Reed-Sternberg cell is probably the malignant cell, with the surrounding cells representing tissue reaction. Although this malignancy originates in the lymphoid system and primarily involves the lymph nodes, it can metastasize to any tissue and often metastasizes to non-nodal or extralymphatic sites such as the spleen, liver, bone marrow, and lungs.

Hodgkin's disease is staged (determination of anatomic extent) according to the microscopic appearance of the involved lymph nodes, the extent and severity of the disorder, and the prognosis using the Ann Arbor staging classification (Table 13-4); it is not always possible to determine the primary tumor site. The stages are subdivided by the absence (A) or presence (B) of fever (more than 38° C [102° F]); night

---

TABLE	13-4

Ann Arbor Staging Classification for Hodgkin's Disease*

Stage I: Involvement of a single lymph node, group of nodes, or a single extralymphatic site I_E (e.g., spleen, thymus, Waldeyer's ring)

Stage II: Involvement of two or more lymph node regions on the same side of the diaphragm

Stage III: Involvement of lymph node regions or structures on both sides of the diaphragm; may include spleen or localized extranodal disease

Stage IV: Widespread extralymphatic involvement (liver, bone marrow, lung, skin)

---

*For all stages: A = asymptomatic; B = constitutional symptoms.

sweats; or weight loss (more than 10% of body weight in the last 6 months). At diagnosis, about 10% to 15% of clients will have disease limited to a single lymph node region (stage I), and another 10% to 15% of clients will have bone marrow or extensive extranodal disease (stage IV). The majority of people diagnosed with Hodgkin's disease will have stage II or III disease at presentation (70% to 80%).

Incidence and Risk Factors.   Hodgkin's disease peaks at two different ages: during the second to third decades and during the sixth to seventh decades; overall, a progressive increase in incidence occurs with advancing age. By age 80 years, the incidence is approximately 40 per 100,000. A greater incidence is seen in geographic bands, including the United States, the Netherlands, and Denmark. Although the exact cause of Hodgkin's disease remains under investigation, certain risk factors have been identified (Table 13-5).

Pathogenesis.   Overwhelming evidence exists that at least a substantial number of cases, if not all, of Hodgkin's disease represent monoclonal* B-cell disorders. Gene expression patterns can provide important clues to the pathogenesis of neoplastic diseases, including Hodgkin's disease. Hodgkin's disease is characterized by the abnormal expression of multiple cytokines, accounting for its unique clinicopathic features. Researchers continue to analyze the expression of chemokines† in tissues involved by Hodgkin's disease thus far demonstrating a significant role for chemokine expression in the pathogenesis of Hodgkin's disease. Lymph node tissue from people with Hodgkin's disease demonstrates elevated levels of interleukin (IL)-13, specifically expressed by

---

*Monoclonal or clonal refers to a population of cells derived from a single transformed (neoplastic) parent cell. The mutated cell with an alteration in its DNA forms an oncogene (mutated gene), leading to its transformation into a cancer-causing cell. The clone (cancer) is the total accumulation of cells that grow from the single mutated cell. All cancers (benign and malignant), including leukemia, lymphhoma, and myeloma, are all examples of monoclonal disorders that are derived from a single malignant cell.

†Chemokines are any of a group of low molecular weight cytokines (e.g., interleukins) identified on the basis of their ability to induce chemotaxis (cell movement; see Fig. 5-10) or chemokinesis (cell activity due to the presence of a chemical substance) in leukocytes in inflammation. Chemokines function as regulators of the immune system and may play roles in the circulatory and central nervous systems.

TABLE   13-5

Risk Factors for Malignant Lymphomas

NON-HODGKIN'S LYMPHOMA	HODGKIN'S DISEASE
Age (increased risk with increasing age)	
Gender (males more than females)	
Environmental Contaminants	
Herbicides and pesticides	*Environmental (?)*
Benzene	
Polychlorinated biphenyls (PCBs)	
Viral Infection	
Epstein-Barr/mononucleosis virus	Epstein-Barr/
Human T-lymphotrophic virus type I (HTLV)	mononucleosis virus
Human immunodeficiency virus (HIV)	
Immunocompromise/ immunodeficiency	
Chronic disease or illness; autoimmune diseases	Chronic disease or illness; autoimmune diseases
Immunosuppressants	Immunosuppressants
Cancer treatment with alkylating or cytotoxic agents	Cancer treatment with alkylating or cytotoxic agents
Inherited immune deficiencies (e.g., collagen vascular disease)	Systemic lupus erythematosus[73]
HIV	HIV
Acquired immunodeficiency syndrome (AIDS)	AIDS
Helicobacter pylori bacteria (gastric lymphoma)	Ulcerative colitis[58]
Methotrexate	Drug abuse
Obesity (women)[87]	Obesity (men)[87]

Hodgkin's lymphoma cell lines that may serve as an autocrine growth factor.[69] What induces the expression of these chemokines remains unresolved, but previous studies in mice have linked EBV with a pattern of chemokine response.[76] Modulation of the IL-13 signaling pathway may be a strategy for future treatment intervention.

Clinical Manifestations.   See Fig. 13-3.

Lymphatic System.   As normal lymphoid tissue is replaced by the malignant lymphoma, symptoms of Hodgkin's disease may develop, including painless swelling of lymph glands in the neck, armpit, or groin, persistent fatigue, recurrent high fever, night sweats, itching (pruritus), and weight loss. Asymptomatic lymphadenopathy (enlarged, firm, nontender, movable nodes) of the cervical (Fig. 13-4), axillary, inguinal, and retroperitoneal areas may be discovered on routine examination; but the constitutional symptoms of fever, night sweats, anorexia, or weight loss are present in about 40% of the population with lymphoma. Some clients report that lymph node tenderness increases with ingestion of alcohol.

Hodgkin's disease follows an anatomic distribution of nodal involvement, referred to as the *contiguous spread model*, so that a client with cervical adenopathy may also have supraclavicular or mediastinal adenopathy. Pelvic adenopathy or liver involvement is unlikely in the case of isolated cervical adenopathy. All symptoms occur with greater frequency in older clients and in people with a poor prognosis based on histologic findings. When enlarged lymph nodes obstruct or compress adjacent structures, local symptoms may occur, such as edema of the face, neck, or right arm from mediastinal node involvement. When enlarged lymph nodes obstruct the inferior vena cava, significant dependent edema of the lower extremities may occur.

Pulmonary System.   Pulmonary symptoms of nonproductive cough, dyspnea, chest pain, and cyanosis may occur secondary to mediastinal lymph node enlargement extending to the lung parenchyma with invasion of the pleura. Obstruction of the bile ducts as a result of liver damage causes bilirubin to accumulate in the blood and discolor the skin.

Central Nervous System.   Primary Hodgkin's disease limited to the CNS is exceedingly rare, and dissemination of disease to the CNS is uncommon.[8] Occasionally, spinal cord involvement may occur in the dorsal and lumbar regions, and compression of nerve roots of the brachial, lumbar, or sacral plexus can cause nerve root pain. Epidural involvement (also uncommon) causes back and neck pain with hyperreflexia. Extremity involvement is characterized by pain, nerve irritation, and obliteration of the pulse. Paraneoplastic neurologic syndromes may develop in Hodgkin's disease, usually with a lack of response of the paraneoplastic to treatment and poor prognosis for successful treatment of the Hodgkin's disease.

Progression of the disease results in immunodeficiency and infections. Without treatment, the entire node is replaced by malignant tissue with subsequent necrosis. Bone pain may occur from disease in the bone marrow, and as the bone marrow is replaced, pancytopenia (depression of all the cellular blood elements) and subsequent bleeding and infection develop. Tumor bulk may obstruct or invade vital organs, ultimately causing death.

Special Problems

Pregnancy and Hodgkin's disease.   Since the mean age at diagnosis of Hodgkin's disease is 32 years, it is not uncommon for women to develop Hodgkin's disease while pregnant. Diagnostic staging can be accomplished safely with magnetic resonance imaging (MRI) because it does not use ionizing radiation,[53] has no adverse impact on the natural course of Hodgkin's disease, and Hodgkin's disease has no effect on the course of gestation, delivery, or the incidence of prematurity or spontaneous abortions. The risk of metastatic involvement of the fetus by Hodgkin's disease is negligible.[62]

The management of Hodgkin's disease during pregnancy must be individualized. Many women have been successfully treated while pregnant without adverse effects on the fetus.[23] In cases of disease onset early in pregnancy, the recommendation may be made to consider a therapeutic abortion. Women presenting in later pregnancy are often able to have therapy delayed until after delivery or can undergo modified or standard combination chemotherapy and radiation therapy.[62] Antiretroviral treatment and prophylaxis for opportunistic in-

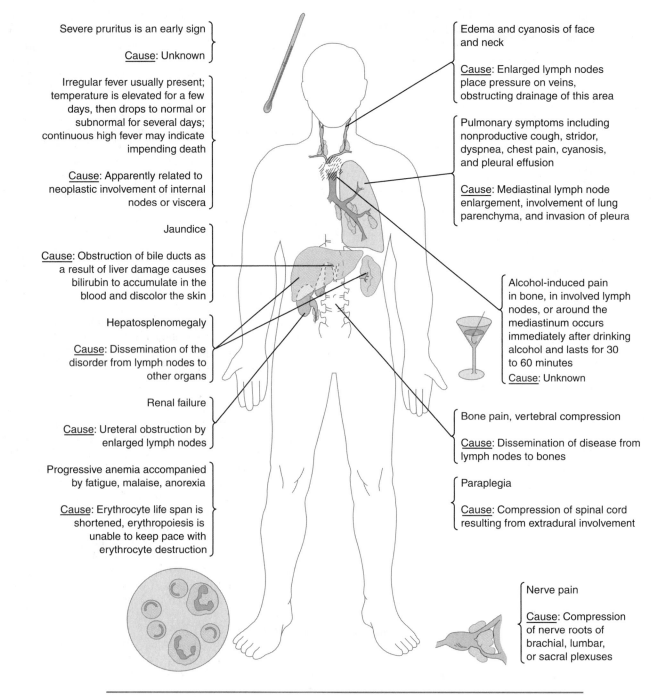

Severe pruritus is an early sign

Cause: Unknown

Irregular fever usually present; temperature is elevated for a few days, then drops to normal or subnormal for several days; continuous high fever may indicate impending death

Cause: Apparently related to neoplastic involvement of internal nodes or viscera

Jaundice

Cause: Obstruction of bile ducts as a result of liver damage causes bilirubin to accumulate in the blood and discolor the skin

Hepatosplenomegaly

Cause: Dissemination of the disorder from lymph nodes to other organs

Renal failure

Cause: Ureteral obstruction by enlarged lymph nodes

Progressive anemia accompanied by fatigue, malaise, anorexia

Cause: Erythrocyte life span is shortened, erythropoiesis is unable to keep pace with erythrocyte destruction

Edema and cyanosis of face and neck

Cause: Enlarged lymph nodes place pressure on veins, obstructing drainage of this area

Pulmonary symptoms including nonproductive cough, stridor, dyspnea, chest pain, cyanosis, and pleural effusion

Cause: Mediastinal lymph node enlargement, involvement of lung parenchyma, and invasion of pleura

Alcohol-induced pain in bone, in involved lymph nodes, or around the mediastinum occurs immediately after drinking alcohol and lasts for 30 to 60 minutes
Cause: Unknown

Bone pain, vertebral compression

Cause: Dissemination of disease from lymph nodes to bones

Paraplegia

Cause: Compression of spinal cord resulting from extradural involvement

Nerve pain

Cause: Compression of nerve roots of brachial, lumbar, or sacral plexuses

FIGURE   **13-3**   Pathologic basis for the clinical manifestations of Hodgkin's disease. (Modified from Black JM, Matassarin-Jacobs E, editors: *Luckmann and Sorensen's medical-surgical nursing,* ed 4, Philadelphia, 1993, WB Saunders.)

fection may also be administered.[36] With appropriate shielding, the estimated fetal dose of radiation can be reduced by 50% or more in most cases.[27] In nonpregnant women, to further reduce any risk, it is advisable to delay pregnancy for 12 months after completion of radiation therapy.[23]

Long-term semen banking is available for men whose future fertility may be compromised by suppression of spermatogenesis secondary to administration of chemo/radiotherapy treatment. Banking of a single ejaculate before chemo/radio-

therapy treatment may preserve potential fertility without compromising the oncology treatment.[32]

Hodgkin's Disease in the Older Adult.   This disease in the older person appears to have a different course when compared with that in younger clients. Older people tend to present with more advanced stages and a worse prognosis. Their health is often complicated by other medical problems, causing difficulty in tolerating aggressive chemotherapy. The prog-

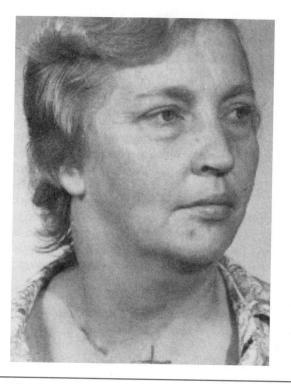

FIGURE   **13-4**   Enlarged cervical lymph node associated with Hodgkin's disease. (From del Regato J, Spjut HJ, Cox JD: *Cancer: diagnosis, treatment, and prognosis,* ed 6, St Louis, 1985, Mosby.)

nosis for the older person with Hodgkin's disease is worse, and treatment is more problematic.

Hodgkin's Disease in AIDS.

The incidence of Hodgkin's disease in young men is relatively high, irrespective of the AIDS epidemic, but HIV-positive clients are at increased risk, and those who develop Hodgkin's disease usually present with aggressive, advanced-stage disease and systemic symptoms. Treatment can produce long-term remissions but is poorly tolerated, and the incidence of opportunistic infections is increased. Overall survival is shortened by AIDS-related complications and refractory disease.

Medical Management

Diagnosis.   Diagnosis depends on identification of Reed-Sternberg cells in lymph node tissue or at other sites. Diagnosis may be delayed by several years owing to the insidious nature of lymphadenopathy. Because of the multiple organs that can be involved, diagnosis requires a complete physical examination in addition to routine blood chemistry profile and tests to determine the extent or the stage of the disease.

Accurate staging is essential for planning the treatment protocol and is accomplished with radiologic evaluation (e.g., computed axial tomography [CT] scan, lymphangiography [LAG], photon emission computed tomography [PET], scintigraphy); possible exploratory laparotomy with liver biopsy (if the findings will significantly alter stage and therapy); and multiple node biopsies. Needle biopsy is not adequate for diagnosis, as it does not yield sufficient tissue to exclude other diseases and to subclassify the disease; the excisional lymph node biopsy is required.

The Gallium scan (Gascan; scintigraphy) using radiotracer (Gallium-67) uptake is 85% to 90% accurate to predict residual disease after chemotherapy and is able to differentiate between active tumor tissue and fibrosis (uptake only occurs in viable lymphoma tissue not in fibrotic or necrotic tissue). CT scan may show a complete response, but if the Gallium scan is positive, that is an indication of recurrence or remission. PET imaging after treatment is used in favor of CT scanning.

Treatment.   Cure of Hodgkin's disease is the primary treatment goal through the use of radiation therapy, chemotherapy, and, in some cases, both. The specific treatment is guided by the stage of the disease at diagnosis. External-beam radiation therapy is used with stages I and II unless chemotherapy is required to shrink the bulk of disease before curative radiation therapy. Radiation therapy alone for stages I to III provides a 15- to 20-year survival rate of 90% to 95% and a relapse-free survival rate of 80%. Most relapses occur within the first 3 years after completing therapy, and late relapses are uncommon. More than half of the people who experience relapse after radiation therapy alone have disease that is curable with second-line standard chemotherapy.

Clinical stage III or IV is too widespread for successful radiation treatment only and requires treatment with chemotherapy. Two major goals are evident in advanced Hodgkin's disease: to improve the cure rate and to reduce acute and long-term toxicities. The optimal approach or program has not yet been determined but combination chemotherapy using ABVD (Adriamycin, bleomycin, vinblastine, and dacarbazine [DTIC]), sometimes followed by radiation therapy, is one of the best treatment programs for stage III or IV Hodgkin's disease. There is no acute leukemia from ABVD, a higher cure rate, and less sterility, although observation for heart and lung toxicity is required; used with mediastinal radiation therapy, ABVD may create early coronary artery disease and myocardial events. Today, 80% of people with advanced HD may be cured with a low rate of long-term toxicity.

New, more intensive chemotherapy regimens for advanced Hodgkin's disease using BEACOPP (bleomycin, etoposide, Adriamycin, cyclophosphamide, vincristine, procarbazine, prednisone) and Stanford V have demonstrated increased tumor response rates. New drug combinations are under investigation in several international trials.[77] For people with relapsed Hodgkin's disease after combination chemotherapy, current data support the use of high-dose chemotherapy with autologous stem cell transplantation. Biologic treatments such as cellular or monoclonal antibody-based therapies (e.g., rituximab) are still being developed.[33]

Prognosis.   Hodgkin's disease is now considered one of the most curable forms of cancer, and death rates have been decreasing since the early 1970s. Five-year survival rate is reportedly as high as 98% (but consistently reported as 90% to 95%) with successful treatment. The long-term prognosis for clients with Hodgkin's disease depends on several factors, including age at diagnosis (negative prognosticator: age above 50 years); disease stage at diagnosis; suitability of treatment administered; and rapidity of response to chemotherapy (failure to attain a temporary remission with first-line treatment is a poor prognostic sign). The presence of B (constitutional) symptoms (see Table 13-4) decreases the survival figures at each stage.

Despite significant advances in radiation techniques and combination chemotherapy, 20% to 30% of clients will be resistant to therapy or relapse after primary therapy. People who suffer relapse from primary radiation therapy (stage I to II) have a similar or even better prognosis than those with advanced stage (stage III to IV) disease treated with chemotherapy. The most important prognostic factors after relapse are the extent of disease at the time of relapse and age greater than 50 years. Older adults in advanced stages of disease are unable to tolerate maximal radiation and chemotherapy doses, which decreases their chances for survival. Treatment of older people may also be less effective, owing to a biologic difference in Hodgkin's disease in the aged adult.

Special Implications for the Therapist 13-7

HODGKIN'S DISEASE

Preferred Practice Patterns:
Other patterns may be appropriate depending on the client's age and complications present.
4B: Impaired Posture (bone pain)
4C: Impaired Muscle Performance
6B: Impaired Aerobic Capacity/Endurance Associated With Deconditioning
6H: Impaired Circulation and Anthropometric Dimensions Associated With Lymphatic System Disorders
7A: Primary Prevention/Risk Reduction for Integumentary Disorders (lymphedema; edema)

The therapist may palpate enlarged painless lymph nodes during a cervical, spine, shoulder, or hip examination. Lymph nodes are evaluated on the basis of size, consistency, mobility, and tenderness. Lymph nodes up to 1 cm in diameter of soft to firm consistency that move freely and easily without tenderness are considered within normal limits. Lymph nodes greater than 1 cm in diameter that are firm and rubbery in consistency or tender are considered suspicious. Enlarged lymph nodes associated with infection are more likely to be tender than slow-growing nodes associated with cancer. *Changes* in size, shape, tenderness, and consistency should raise a red flag. Supraclavicular nodes are common metastatic sites for occult lung, breast, and testicular cancers, whereas inguinal nodes implicate tumors arising in the legs, perineum, prostate, or gonads. The physician should be notified of these findings and the client advised to have the lymph nodes evaluated by the physician; in someone with a past medical history of cancer, immediate medical referral is necessary.

The therapist's role in lymphoma includes but is not limited to assessing and/or addressing (1) quality of life (QOL) issues including emotional and spiritual needs; (2) impairments, functional limitations, and disabilities; and (3) physical conditioning/deconditioning. Generalized weakness, decreased endurance, impaired mobility, altered kinesthetic awareness and balance, including unstable gait; respiratory impairment; involvement of the lymphatic system (lymphedema); and pain are only a few of the identified signs and symptoms of impairment common with this group of people. Requirements for infection control and treat-

ment subsequent to the cytotoxic effects on the CNS are outlined previously in the section on The Leukemias. Additionally, side effects of radiation and/or chemotherapy must be considered (see Chapter 4 and Table 8-8).

Depending on the results of the therapist's examination and evaluation, intervention strategies may include client and family education, pain management, mobility and gait training, therapeutic exercise, balance training, aerobic conditioning, respiratory rehabilitation, and lymphedema management. Monitoring vital signs is important and daily evaluation of lab values (e.g., hemoglobin, platelets, WBCs, hematocrit). See Tables 39-6 and 39-7 for planning or carrying out a therapy program.[4] ■

Non-Hodgkin's Lymphomas

Overview. Lymphomas, or non-Hodgkin's lymphoma (NHL), comprise a group of lymphoproliferative disorders that present as solid tumors arising from cells of the lymphatic system (lymphoid cells). Malignant transformation can occur at any stage of B- or T- lymphocyte differentiation; most lymphomas are the B-cell type. The lymph nodes are usually involved first, and any extranodal lymphoid tissue, particularly the spleen and thymus, and GI tract may also be involved. The bone marrow is commonly involved by lymphoma cells, but this is rarely the primary site of a lymphoma.

Lymphomas are classified according to cell size, growth pattern, T- and B-cell markers, and clinical grade (low grade, intermediate grade, or high grade). Nodular lymphomas are low grade, clinically indolent (slow-growing, painless, continually relapsing); intermediate lymphomas include mantle cell and poorly differentiated lymphocytic lymphomas; and high-grade lymphomas are clinically aggressive and include large cell immunoblastic, lymphoblastic, and Burkitt's lymphomas. Low-grade NHL eventually transforms to a more rapidly progressive form that is usually fatal. Clinical staging of NHL is done according to the same criteria for Hodgkin's disease with two exceptions: NHLs are more likely to present in an extranodal site, and the progression of the NHL does not follow the orderly anatomic progression typical of Hodgkin's disease. Stage I and II NHLs are rare, because the disease is much more likely to be disseminated at the time of diagnosis.

Etiologic and Risk Factors. Studies in the 1990s have linked NHL to two widespread environmental contaminants: exposure to benzene, which originates from cigarette smoke, gasoline, automobile emissions, and industrial pollution and polychlorinated biphenyls (PCBs) found throughout the food chain (highest in meats, dairy products, and fish).[28] More recently, one large study was unable to confirm the connection of benzene to lymphoma.[88] In people with HIV, the risk of developing NHL is more than 100 times greater than with noninfected people. Other predisposing risk factors for lymphoma are listed in Table 13-5.[61]

A wide variety of primary and secondary immunodeficiencies have been associated with an increased incidence of lymphomas. This phenomenon may reflect a decrease in the host's surveillance mechanism against transformed cells or be from prolonged exposure to oncogenic agents, such as EBV, as a consequence of failure to mount an adequate immune response.

The presence of *Helicobacter pylori* (bacteria) in the stomach lining is associated with the development of gastric lymphoma, but this comprises a very small proportion of cases.[40] Low-dose methotrexate therapy used for classic and juvenile RA carries an increased risk of lymphoproliferative disease.[9,14]

Pathogenesis.

Although the exact cause of NHL is unknown, studies using techniques of molecular biology have provided some clues to the pathogenesis of NHL. The malignant lymphomas develop from the malignant transformation of a single lymphocyte that is arrested at a specific stage of B or T lymphoid cell differentiation and begins to multiply, eventually crowding out healthy cells and creating tumors, which enlarge lymph nodes. Because immunosuppressed people have a greater incidence of the disease, an immune mechanism is suspected. Unlike in Hodgkin's disease, T-cell function is minimally affected (30%), but B-cell abnormalities are more common in NHL (70%). In children, virtually all malignant lymphomas are high-grade, aggressive neoplasms.

Clinical Manifestations.

The NHLs are variable in clinical presentation and course, varying from indolent disease to rapidly progressive disease. Lymphadenopathy is the first symptom of NHL with painless enlargement of isolated or generalized lymph nodes of the cervical, axillary, inguinal, and femoral (pelvic) chains. This development occurs slowly and progressively over an extended period (months to years).

Extranodal sites of involvement may include the nasopharynx; GI tract; bone (accompanied by bone pain); thyroid; testes; and soft tissue. Abdominal lymphoma may cause abdominal fullness, GI obstruction or bleeding, ascites, back pain, and leg swelling. NHL presenting as polyarthritis has been reported, and Sjögren's syndrome is associated with malignant lymphomas.[22,80] Constitutional symptoms, which may include fever, night sweats, pallor, fatigue, and weight loss, are present with high-grade lymphomas.

Primary CNS lymphoma is a NHL restricted to the nervous system; CNS lymphomas may or may not be AIDS-associated. Clients with HIV-associated NHL (HIV-NHL) CNS lymphoma present with clinical and radiographic findings, clinical characteristics, and prognosis substantially different from non–AIDS-associated CNS lymphoma. Neurologic manifestations associated with HIV-NHL include cerebral toxoplasmosis, abscesses, and infarctions, and prognosis is very poor.

Medical Management

Diagnosis.   Accurate diagnosis is important because of the other clinical conditions that can mimic malignant lymphomas (e.g. tuberculosis, SLE, lung and bone cancer). Molecular genetic techniques that take advantage of the clonal nature of this malignancy are now being applied to better characterize and diagnose the lymphomas. However, at the present time, a biopsy is still required to confirm the underlying cause of persistent enlargement of lymph nodes present on clinical examination. Chest x-ray and CT scan of the abdomen and pelvis may be helpful in staging. Spleen and bone marrow may be examined for staging, and peripheral blood may be tested, but blood abnormalities are not present until the disease is in an advanced stage.

The Gallium scan (Gascan; scintigraphy) using radiotracer (Gallium-67) uptake is 85% to 90% accurate to predict residual disease after chemotherapy and is able to differentiate between active tumor tissue and fibrosis (uptake only occurs in viable lymphoma tissue not in fibrotic or necrotic tissue). CT scan may show a complete response, but if the Gallium scan is positive, that is an indication of recurrence or remission. PET imaging after treatment is used in favor of CT scanning.

Treatment.   Aggressive chemotherapy is administered for high-grade lymphomas, and conservative therapy is used for low-grade lymphomas; localized disease may be treated with irradiation, whereas disseminated disease requires radiation and chemotherapy. The low-grade lymphomas are indolent and unaffected by therapy; treatment is palliative until the disease progresses, necessitating intervention (usually 1 to 3 years). Disseminated large-cell (intermediate grade) lymphomas are curable in 50% of cases using combination chemotherapy. Autologous BMT may be used for clients with high-risk aggressive lymphomas. Combined with aggressive chemotherapy, BMT (or stem cell transplant) can be curative even in older clients with NHL. For the individual with HIV-NHL, treatment is comprised of simultaneous combination chemotherapy and highly active antiretroviral therapy (HAART).[64] Researchers are investigating the use of autologous stem cell transplantation for selected individuals with HIV-NHL.

For most lymphomas, chemotherapy is palliative because of an inability to overcome drug resistance within the lymphoma cells; attempts at overcoming specific drug resistance mechanisms (e.g., multidrug resistance) have had limited success. A new therapeutic strategy combining the monoclonal antibody rituximab (Rituxan) with chemotherapy has produced high rates of response (up to 50%) and duration response of almost 1 full year for most B-cell NHLs.[84] Clinical studies suggest that rituximab may modulate the sensitivity of B-cell lymphoma to chemotherapy. This antibody therapy used before collecting stem cells may offer a means of purging peripheral blood stem cell grafts from contamination with neoplastic cells and also provide a posttransplantation immunotherapy.[24]

Recent clinical trials in lymphoma have investigated the use of antigen-presenting cells (APCs) for taking up, processing, and presenting tumor protein in a vaccine strategy. When macrophages are combined with rituximab (CD20 antibody), tumor cells are engulfed. This has led researchers to pursue the possibility of producing functional macrophages in large amounts as a new immune strategy to eradicate lymphoma.[13]

The optimal management of women with NHL who are pregnant requires special considerations because of the poor prognosis. Treatment during the first trimester is associated with significant risk to the developing fetus and should be avoided. Treatment during the second or third trimester should include standard chemotherapy despite the potential risk to the developing fetus.[62]

Prognosis.   Individuals with NHL survive for long periods when involvement is only regional. The presence of diffuse disease reduces survival time. The low-grade lymphomas are usually systemic and widespread, and cure cannot be achieved, whereas intermediate- and high-grade lymphomas are more likely to present as treatable and even curable localized disorders. The prognosis for people with high-grade lymphomas depends on their response to treatment.

Traditionally high-grade NHL associated with AIDS was associated with an extremely poor prognosis, but since the advent of antiretroviral therapy for HIV and with a multidisciplinary approach to complex AIDS cases involving malignancy, return to functional health has become possible for some individuals.[42] Prognostic indicators for decreased survival in HIV-NHL include age greater than 35 years, history of injection drug use, CD4 cell count less than 100/100 mL, a history of AIDS before the diagnosis of lymphoma, stage III or IV disease, and/or elevated lactate dehydrogenase (LDH) levels.[41]

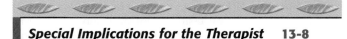

Special Implications for the Therapist 13-8

NON-HODGKIN'S LYMPHOMA

See Special Implications for the Therapist: Hodgkin's Disease, 13-7.
Preferred Practice Patterns:
See Hodgkin's Disease; neuromuscular patterns may be appropriate in NHL for lymphoma of the nervous system.

Although uncommon, the association between the use of methotrexate in RA and the development of lymphoma has been reported.[9,14] Anytime an individual receiving methotrexate for RA complains of back pain accompanied by constitutional symptoms and/or GI symptoms and/or the therapist palpates enlarged lymph nodes at any of the nodal sites, a medical referral is warranted. ■

Multiple Myeloma

Definition and Overview. Multiple myeloma (MM), also called *plasma cell myeloma,* is a primary malignant neoplasm of plasma cells arising most often in bone marrow. This bone tumor initially affects the bone marrow of the vertebrae, ribs, skull, pelvis, and femur. Later, organs such as the spleen, liver, and kidney are damaged. The extent, clinical course, complications, and sensitivity to treatment vary widely among affected people.

Incidence and Etiologic Factors. The incidence of MM has doubled in the past two decades with an annual incidence of approximately 14,400 cases in the United States.[26] MM occurs less often than the most common cancers (e.g., breast, lung, or colon), but its incidence is double that of Hodgkin's disease. This disease can develop at any age, but it peaks among people between age 50 and 70; black men are affected twice as often as white men. The incidence of MM in blacks is almost twice that in whites and is slightly more common in men than in women. Risk factors and the cause of multiple myeloma are unknown, but in the last decade, plasma cell malignancy has become another AIDS-associated neoplasm (possible link to human herpesvirus 8 [HHV-8]).

Pathogenesis. MM is characterized by the accumulation of monoclonal plasma cells, a differentiated form of B lymphocyte in the bone marrow that produces abnormally large amounts of one class of immunoglobulin (usually immunoglobulin G [IgG], occasionally IgA, and rarely any oth-

ers). The abnormal immunoglobulin produced by the malignant transformed plasma cell is called the *M-protein.* The M-protein is responsible for many of the clinical manifestations of the disease. Infiltration and destruction of organs, especially osteolysis of bone, by the neoplastic plasma cells result in pain. In addition to bone destruction, MM is characterized by disruption of RBC, leukocyte, and platelet production, which results from plasma cells crowding the bone marrow. Impaired production of these cell forms causes anemia, increased vulnerability to infection, and bleeding tendencies. Besides the malignant plasma cells, it has become clear that nonmalignant cells in the bone marrow also contribute to the development of this malignancy by the release of cytokines. Researchers are investigating the relationship of the human herpesvirus 8 (HHV-8) in the nonmalignant bone marrow cells as a possible link to the development of MM.[7]

Clinical Manifestations. The onset of MM is usually gradual and insidious. Presenting features in older adults (older than 75 years) are the same as those reported in younger people except for a higher rate of infection in the older population.[65] Many people pass through a long presymptomatic period called a monoclonal gammopathy of undetermined significance (MGUS) that lasts from 5 to 20 years. Eventually, serious infection (e.g., recurrent pneumonia, pyelonephritis, sepsis) develops in more than 75% of cases.

Skeletal. Most often, the initial symptom is bone pain, particularly at the sites containing red marrow (ribs, pelvis, spine, clavicles, skull, and humeri). Bone pain occurs when plasma cells infiltrate and replace the bone marrow with subsequent osteolytic lesions and destruction of bone. Bone loss, the major clinical manifestation of MM, often leads to pathologic fractures, spinal cord compression, osteolysis-induced hypercalcemia, and bone pain. Initially, the bone pain may be mild and intermittent or may develop suddenly as a severe pain in the back, rib, leg, or arm, which is often the result of an abrupt movement or effort that has caused a spontaneous (pathologic) bone fracture. The pain is often radicular and sharp to one or both sides and is aggravated by movement. Symptoms associated with bone pain usually subside within days to weeks after initiation of systemic chemotherapy, but if the disease progresses, more areas of bone destruction develop.

Renal. Renal impairment is a common complication of MM occurring in 50% of all cases at some stage in the disease process. The pathogenesis is multifactorial. Drainage of calcium and phosphorus from damaged bones eventually leads to the development of renal stones, particularly in immobilized clients. To rid the body of the excess calcium (hypercalcemia), the kidneys increase the output of urine, which can lead to serious dehydration if intake of fluids is inadequate. Hypercalcemia is a common presenting feature but less common after adequate chemotherapy. Symptoms of hypercalcemia may include confusion, increased urination, loss of appetite, abdominal pain, constipation, and vomiting (see the section on Hypercalcemia in Chapter 4). Eventually renal failure can occur.

Neurologic. Amyloidosis (deposits of insoluble fragments of a protein resembling starch) develops in approximately 10% of people with MM. These deposits cause tissues to become waxy and immobile and may affect nerves, muscles, and ligaments, especially the carpal tunnel area of the wrist. Carpal tunnel syndrome with pain, numbness, or tingling of the hands and fingers may develop. More serious neurologic complications may develop in 10% to 15% of clients with MM when vertebral body collapse or extradural extension of the tumor occurs. Spinal cord compression is usually observed early or in the late relapse phase of the disease. Back pain associated with spinal cord compression is usually present as the initial symptom, with radicular pain that is aggravated by coughing or sneezing. Motor or sensory loss and bowel/bladder dysfunction are signs of more extensive compression. Paraplegia is a late, irreversible event.

The association between MM and RA, Sjögren's syndrome, and other autoimmune diseases has been established, but it is not clear why this occurs.

Medical Management

Diagnosis.   In approximately 20% of people diagnosed with MM, screening laboratory studies may reveal an increased serum protein concentration indicating the disease. Plasma cells circulating in the peripheral blood can be detected by use of sensitive immunofluorescence, flow cytometric studies, or molecular genetic techniques. The detection of these cells is clinically important because they correlate with disease activity. As MM progresses, the plasma cells appear in greater numbers in the peripheral blood. The presence of abnormal immunoglobulin in the urine (Bence Jones protein) is also diagnostic of multiple myeloma. Diagnosis of bone lesions and spinal cord compression is made by radiographic evaluation.

Treatment.   All clients with MM should be monitored, but not all require treatment. Symptoms, physical findings, and laboratory data are taken into consideration. For many years, standard treatment for MM has been intermittent cycles of melphalan plus prednisone (MP) or a combination of alkylating agents when progression of disease occurs. Clinical results are good with temporary disease control in 50% of cases; relapse occurs, but event-free survival beyond 3 years and overall survival beyond 6 years is possible.[3] Newly developed third-generation high-potency bisphosphonates have been shown effective when used with chemotherapy not only on the improvement of bone lesions but also in decreasing the need for radiation, decreasing osteoporotic fractures, and improving survival in some people with myeloma (median survival is 1 year compared to 3 or 4 months with bone marrow transplant).[6,74] Bisphosphonates are potent inhibitors of osteoclastic activity (resorption) and exert an antitumor effect that is apoptotic and antiproliferative.[18]

The introduction of high-dose therapy with stem cell support has significantly improved the outcomes of MM with increased complete remission rate and extended disease-free and overall survival. Allogeneic (matched donor) bone marrow transplantation is possible for only 5% to 10% of people with MM who are younger than 60 years and have a human leukocyte antigen (HLA)-compatible sibling. The advantage of this type of BMT is that the graft contains no tumor cells that can provoke a relapse. However, there is a significant early and high rate of mortality (40%), and a risk of graft-versus-host disease (GVHD) and relapse is common. Autologous (harvested from recipient before the person is exposed to alkylating agents) bone marrow transplantation (ABMT) has broader

applicability because the age limit is higher and a matched donor is unnecessary. It is not suitable for people older than 70 years or who have major medical problems or relapsing disease. Eradication of MM may not occur, even with large doses of chemotherapy and irradiation, when infused ABMT or peripheral blood stem cells (PBSCT) have been contaminated by myeloma cells or their precursors, which will cause relapse. Treatment with vincristine; doxorubicin (Adriamycin); and dexamethasone (VAD) for 3 to 4 months and then collecting the peripheral blood stem cells is another option.[38]

Future treatment under investigation includes peripheral stem cell grafting, posttransplant immunotherapy, gene therapy, new drugs, development of oral bisphosphonates, new ways of delivering radiotherapy to specific sites, and radiopharmaceuticals that concentrate at involved marrow sites. The use of thalidomide for its ability to block the formation of new blood vessels that enable tumor growth in people with myeloma who relapse after high-dose chemotherapy is being investigated.[3] A tumor-specific vaccine for active immunization based on the myeloma protein (a unique tumor antigen) is also under investigation.[10]

Prognosis.   Despite 30 years of clinical trial research conducted by three major cooperative groups under the auspices of the National Cancer Institute, the prognosis for multiple myeloma (MM) has not markedly improved and it remains an incurable disease. Until the development of bisphosphonates, effective resistance of tumor cells to commonly employed cytotoxic drugs had been evident. For those people with MM who receive radiation or chemotherapy treatment, the median duration of remission is approximately 3 years, and the median survival is approximately 6 years. Long-term survival statistics using the combination of chemotherapy and bisphosphonates are not yet available. Positive factors for improved prognosis include the absence of chromosome 13 deletion, low β_2 microglobulin, and low C-reactive protein levels.[3]

If untreated, unstable MM can result in skeletal deformities, particularly of the ribs, sternum, and spine. Diffuse osteoporosis develops, accompanied by a negative calcium balance. Prognosis is affected by the presence of renal failure (poorer prognosis if present at the time of diagnosis), hypercalcemia, or extensive bony disease; infection and renal failure are the most common causes of death. A complete response or remission does not occur and eventually the disease progresses. Autotransplantation as currently performed is not curative in a substantial proportion of people treated. Future improvements with transplantation may be achieved by providing tumor-free grafts and posttransplant treatment aimed at eradicating minimal residual disease.

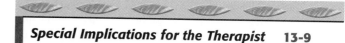

Special Implications for the Therapist   13-9

MULTIPLE MYELOMA

Preferred Practice Patterns:
*4A: Primary Prevention/Risk Reduction for Skeletal
    Demineralization (bone loss and osteoporosis)*
4B: Impaired Posture (skeletal deformity; bone pain)
4D: Impaired Joint Mobility, Motor Function, Muscle

Continued

Performance, and Range of Motion Associated With Connective Tissue Dysfunction (for those with arthritic component)

4G: Impaired Joint Mobility, Muscle Performance, and Range of Motion Associated With Fracture

5G: Impaired Motor Function and Sensory Integrity Associated With Acute or Chronic Polyneuropathies (carpal tunnel syndrome associated with local dissemination of neoplasm)

5H: Impaired Motor Function, Peripheral Nerve Integrity, and Sensory Integrity Associated with Nonprogressive Disorders of the Spinal Cord

Therapists can assist individuals with MM to manage both the disease and treatment-related symptoms, improve overall quality of life, and prevent further complications associated with decreased activity and exercise. Specific examination and evaluation can provide early recognition of complications, such as hypercalcemia and spinal cord compression. Any symptoms of hypercalcemia (see Clinical Manifestations in this section) must be reported to the physician; the client should seek immediate medical care, since this condition can be life-threatening. (For the client with amyloidosis, anemia, or renal failure, see the Special Implications for the Therapist for each of these conditions.) Adequate hydration and mobility help minimize the development of hypercalcemia.

The client with MM who develops signs of cord compression must be referred to the physician. Emergency MRI is required to locate the area of cord compression. A laminectomy may be required when spinal cord compression occurs but usually, immediate radiation and high-dose glucocorticoid therapy relieves the compression, avoiding the need for surgical intervention. Orthopedic back braces are generally poorly tolerated; however, newer lightweight supports with Velcro fasteners may be more useful. (For clients receiving BMT or PBSCT treatment, see the section on Transplantation in Chapter 20.) ∎

◆ Myeloproliferative Disorders

Uncontrolled expansion of all bone marrow elements results in a group of clinical conditions known as *myeloproliferative disorders*, which can be characterized as a malignant disease because increased production of bone marrow elements, such as erythroid, myeloid, and platelet lines, result from a neoplastic transformation of a hematopoietic stem cell or precursor cell that develops into a specific bone marrow cell.

The four diseases commonly grouped together as the myeloproliferative disorders are polycythemia vera, myelofibrosis or agnogenic myeloid metaplasia*, essential thrombocytopenia, and CML. These disorders are grouped together because the disease may evolve from one form into another; all of the myeloproliferative disorders may progress to acute myelogenous leukemia. Polycythemia rubra vera, thrombocytopenia, and CML are included in this text. Polycythemia is included because of the thrombosis or stroke associated as a complication, thrombocytopenia is included because of the risks during

exercise, and CML is covered because it is the most common myeloproliferative disorder, which was discussed previously.

Polycythemia Vera

Definition and Overview.   Polycythemia (rubra) vera, also known as erythrocytosis, is a neoplastic disease of the bone marrow stem cell primarily affecting the erythroid cells, which produce erythrocytes, but causing overproduction of all three hematopoietic cell lines. Polycythemia vera may be primary or secondary (see etiologic factors for differentiation); it is characterized by an elevated WBC count; platelet count and vitamin B_{12}; excessive number of erythrocytes leading to an increased concentration of hemoglobin; increased hematocrit (measure of the volume of packed RBCs); and increased hemoglobin level, basophilia, and a high leucine aminopeptidase (LAP; an intracellular enzyme) score.

Etiologic Factors and Pathogenesis.   Polycythemia is considered *primary* when caused by a precursor cell abnormality. The etiologic factors of primary polycythemia vera are attributed to benzene and other occupational exposures including radiation. It occurs in older people between 50 and 60 years, equally distributed between the genders. *Secondary* polycythemia is a physiologic condition resulting from a decreased oxygen supply to the tissues associated with high altitudes, heavy tobacco smoking, and chronic heart and lung disorders. In secondary polycythemia, the body attempts to compensate for the reduced oxygen by producing more hemoglobin and more erythrocytes.

Clinical Manifestations.   The increased concentration of erythrocytes causes increased blood viscosity with potential decreased cerebral blood flow, decreased cardiac output, and a tendency toward clotting (thrombosis) when the hematocrit level exceeds 60% (*therapeutic goal:* 42%). Clinically, symptoms are related to expanded blood volume, increased blood viscosity, and clogging of microcirculatory blood vessels. The client may demonstrate increased skin coloration (e.g., ruddy complexion of face, hands, feet, ears, and mucous membranes) and elevated blood pressure. Gout is sometimes a complication of secondary polycythemia, and a typical attack of acute gout may be the first symptom.*

The symptoms of both primary and secondary polycythemia are much the same; they are often insidious in onset and characterized by vague complaints, and diagnosis may not be made until a secondary complication, such as stroke or thrombosis, occurs. Other symptoms may include headache, dizziness, epistaxis, irritability, blurred vision, fainting, feeling of fullness in the head, disturbances of sensation in the hands and feet,† splenomegaly, general malaise and fatigue, backache, weight loss, easy bruising, and intolerable pruritus (itching), especially after bathing with warm water.

Medical Management

Diagnosis.   Diagnosis is made by history, examination, and laboratory analysis. WBC and platelet count are elevated in

---

*Myelofibrosis and agneogenic myeloid metaplasia are two names for the same neoplastic disorder that is characterized by replacement of the bone marrow by fibrous tissue (fibroblasts, collagen).

---

*The metabolic consequences of increased cell turnover associated with this condition result in increased waste products, including increased uric acid, which may lead to gout.

†Blockage of the capillaries supplying the digits of either the hands or feet may cause a peripheral vascular neuropathy with decreased sensation, burning numbness, or tingling. This same small blood vessel occlusion can also contribute to the development of cyanosis and clubbing of the digits. If untreated, the worst-case scenario may include gangrene requiring amputation.

most people with polycythemia vera and are normal in most people with secondary polycythemia. A specific test (chromium-labeled red cell mass) is used to distinguish between absolute polycythemia (increased red cell mass) and relative polycythemia (normal red cell mass but decreased plasma volume).

Treatment.   Treatment goals are to reduce erythrocytosis and blood volume, control symptoms, and prevent thrombosis. The primary treatment for polycythemia vera is myelosuppression with chemotherapy. The current choice of chemotherapy in polycythemia vera is the antimetabolite hydroxyurea, which does not appear to be associated with an increased incidence of acute leukemia. Phlebotomy to remove excess blood is a secondary treatment, but this is associated with thrombophilic complications, and it does not stop the rapid regeneration of erythrocytes possibly causing iron deficiency, necessitating supplemental iron administration. Treatment for secondary polycythemia is directed toward the underlying condition and treatment of symptoms, such as controlling the uric acid levels that produce gout.

Prognosis.   The prognosis for polycythemia vera is good, and median survival is 10 years with appropriate treatment. Without proper treatment, the mortality rate (18 months from the time of symptomatic onset) is 50%. The risk for stroke, myocardial infarction, and thromboembolism is high for people with this condition; thrombosis or hemorrhage is the major cause of death. Late in the course of this disease, bone marrow may be replaced with fibrous tissue (myelofibrosis); RBC production may decrease; and anemia and marked splenomegaly may develop.

Special Implications for the Therapist   13-10

POLYCYTHEMIA VERA

Preferred Practice Patterns:
4E: Impaired Joint Mobility, Motor Function, Muscle Performance, and Range of Motion Associated With Localized Inflammation (gout)
6A: Primary Prevention/Risk Reduction for Cardiovascular/Pulmonary Disorders (myocardial infarction and stroke prevention; thromboembolism)

Although polycythemia vera is associated with high altitudes, heavy smoking, and chronic heart conditions, clients with COPD have the highest potential risk for secondary polycythemia. Clients with chronic pulmonary conditions do not ventilate adequately, and the body attempts to compensate for the reduced oxygen by producing more RBCs.

Thrombosis occurs more often in clients with polycythemia, which requires the therapist to be alert to any possible signs of deep vein thrombosis (DVT) (see the section on thrombophlebitis in Chapter 11). Watch for complications such as hypervolemia, thrombocytosis, and signs of impending cerebrovascular accident (e.g., decreased sensation, numbness, transitory paralysis, fleeting blindness, headache, and epistaxis).

If the person has symptomatic splenomegaly, follow precautions for soft tissue techniques required in the left upper quadrant, especially up and under the rib cage. These procedures must be secondary or indirect techniques away from the spleen. ■

DISORDERS OF HEMOSTASIS

Hemostasis is the arrest of bleeding after blood vessel injury and involves the interaction among the blood vessel wall, the platelets, and the plasma coagulation proteins. Hemostasis results from the adhesion and aggregation capabilities of platelets to plug small breaks in blood vessels. Most physiologic and pathologic coagulation is initiated by the exposure of blood to tissue factor (previously called thromboplastin or coagulation factor III). Platelets release tissue factor (thromboplastin),* which converts prothrombin into thrombin in the first step of the coagulation mechanism. In the second step of the coagulation process, thrombin promotes the conversion of fibrinogen into fibrin.

Alterations of platelets and coagulation affect hemostasis, either by preventing hemostasis, as in the case of a bleeding or clotting disorder, or by causing hemostasis to occur when it is not needed, such as occurs in thromboembolic disease. Abnormalities in the number of circulating platelets, either an increase in the number of platelets, called *thrombocytosis*, or a decrease in the number of platelets, called *thrombocytopenia*, can interrupt normal blood coagulation and prevent hemostasis. Hemostasis requires normal platelet function and a platelet count between 150,000 and 450,000/mm³ in the peripheral blood. Bleeding caused by platelet disorders is characterized by mucosal and skin bleeding (petechiae), purpura,† and prolonged oozing of blood after trauma or surgery. Other common problems include epistaxis; gum bleeding; menorrhagia (excessive menstruation); and GI bleeding. Coagulation disorders caused by a deficiency of one or more clotting factors result in more serious bleeding such as deep muscle hematoma and spontaneous hemarthrosis.

◆ Thrombocytosis

Thrombocytosis, an increase in the number of circulating platelets (greater than 450,000/mm³), may be primary or secondary; it usually remains asymptomatic until the platelet count exceeds 1 million/mm³. Thrombocytosis may occur as a normal physiologic response (mobilization of platelets from the spleen or lung under the influence of epinephrine) to stress, infection, trauma, surgery, splenectomy, exercise, and ovulation. Abnormal thrombocytosis is caused by accelerated platelet production in the bone marrow.

Primary thrombocytosis (essential thrombocythemia) is a myeloproliferative disorder in which megakaryocytes (giant cell of the bone marrow) overproliferate in association with other conditions such as CML, polycythemia vera, and myelofibrosis (replacement of hematopoietic bone marrow with fibrous tissue). Blood viscosity is increased by the high platelet count, which causes intravascular clumping or thrombosis, particularly of peripheral blood vessels and especially in the fingers or toes. In severe episodes, thrombosis of hepatic,

---

*Tissue factor is found in places not normally exposed to blood flow, where the presence of blood is pathologic. It is present in significant amounts in the brain, subendothelium, smooth muscle, uterus, and epithelium. Tissue factor is not found in skeletal muscle or synovium, the usual locations for spontaneous bleeding in people with hemophilia.

†Purpura is a hemorrhagic condition that occurs when not enough normal platelets are available to plug damaged vessels or prevent leakage from even minor injury to normal capillaries. Purpura is characterized by movement of blood into the surrounding tissue (extravasation); under the skin; and through the mucous membranes, producing spontaneous ecchymoses (bruises) and petechiae (small, red patches) on the skin. When accompanied by a decrease in the circulating hematocrit, it is called *thrombocytopenic purpura*. In the acute form, bleeding can occur from any of the body orifices such as hematuria, nosebleed, vaginal bleeding, and bleeding gums.

mesenteric, or pulmonary vessels may occur. Other symptoms may include splenomegaly and easy bruising. Treatment may not be necessary or the condition may resolve with treatment of the underlying condition, as with secondary thrombocytosis. When thrombosis and hemorrhage occur, treatment with chemotherapy agents or phlebotomy is used to lower the platelet count.

Secondary thrombocytosis occurs after splenectomy because platelets that normally would be stored in the spleen remain in the circulating blood. The increase in platelets may be gradual, so that thrombocytosis does not occur for up to 3 weeks after splenectomy. Other forms of secondary (reactive) thrombocytosis occur as a result of conditions such as infection (e.g., tuberculosis); inflammatory disease (e.g., RA); and malignancy and resolve with treatment of the underlying pathology.

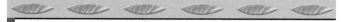

Special Implications for the Therapist 13-11

THROMBOCYTOSIS

The same precautions and screening for symptomatology apply for thrombocytosis as for deep vein thrombosis (see Chapter 11). Anyone who has had a splenectomy has increased susceptibility to infection. Observe carefully for any signs of infection (see Table 7-1). ■

◆ Thrombocytopenia

Thrombocytopenia, a decrease in the platelet count below 150,000/mm³ of blood, is caused by inadequate platelet production from the bone marrow, increased platelet destruction outside the bone marrow, or splenic sequestration (entrapment of blood and enlargement in the spleen). Thrombocytopenia is a common complication of leukemia or metastatic cancer (bone marrow infiltration) and aggressive cancer chemotherapy (cytotoxic agents). Thrombocytopenia may also be a presenting symptom of aplastic anemia (bone marrow failure); other causes are listed in Table 13-6.

Mucosal bleeding is the most common event and occurs by simply blowing the nose, but other sites of mucosal bleeding may include the nose, uterus, GI tract, urinary tract, respiratory tract, and brain (intracranial hemorrhage). Symptoms include epistaxis, petechiae and/or purpura in the skin (especially the legs) and oropharynx, easy bruising, melena, hematuria, excessive menstrual bleeding, and gingival bleeding.

Diagnosis requires the recognition of a bleeding disorder with laboratory examination of blood and bone marrow to confirm the suspected diagnosis. Treatment depends on the precipitating cause (e.g., splenectomy for splenic sequestration, treatment of underlying leukemia, or cessation of cytotoxic drugs until platelet count elevates). Other treatment methods for immune-related thrombocytopenia (e.g., idiopathic thrombocytopenic purpura [ITP]) may include use of corticosteroids (e.g., prednisone); attenuated androgens (danazol); and plasmapheresis, a procedure that removes blood from the body, separates the portion containing the

TABLE 13-6

Causes of Thrombocytopenia

Hypersplenism
Bone marrow failure or infiltration
   Radiation
   Aplastic anemia
   Leukemia
   Metastatic cancer
Cytotoxic or antineoplastic agents (chemotherapy)
Drug hypersensitivities (e.g., gold, sulfonamides, ethanol/alcohol, aspirin or other NSAIDs, quinidine, quinine, antibiotics [penicillins and cephalosporins])
Blood transfusions
Nutritional deficiency
Prosthetic heart valves (occurs only when there is a problem with the valve)
Viral and bacterial infections
Complication of heparin therapy
Autoantibody-mediated platelet injury (called idiopathic thrombocytopenic purpura)

NSAIDs, Nonsteroidal antiinflammatory drugs.

antiplatelet antibodies, and then returns the cleansed blood to the body. Transfusion usually occurs when the platelet count is less than 15,000/mm³ for secondary thrombocytopenia caused by acute leukemia treatment and severe complications of chemotherapy agents that cause thrombocytopenia (e.g., Gemzar, Adriamycin, high-dose Cytoxan, or Carboplatin).

The prognosis is variable depending on the underlying cause; it is poor when associated with leukemia or aplastic anemia but good with conditions amenable to treatment.

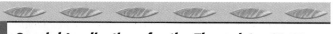

Special Implications for the Therapist 13-12

THROMBOCYTOPENIA

Preferred Practice Pattern:
4D: Impaired Joint Mobility, Motor Function, Muscle Performance, and Range of Motion Associated With Connective Tissue Dysfunction (hemarthropathy)

Thrombocytopenia can cause bleeding into the muscles or joints, and the therapist may encounter the severe consequences of this condition. The therapist must be alert for obvious skin or mucous membrane symptoms of thrombocytopenia, such as severe bruising, external hematomas, and the presence of petechiae. Such symptoms usually indicate a platelet level below 150,000/mm³. Instruct the client to watch for signs of thrombocytopenia, to immediately apply ice and pressure to any external bleeding site, and to avoid aspirin and aspirin-containing compounds without a physician's approval because of the risk of increased bleeding.

Strenuous exercise or any exercise that involves straining or bearing down could precipitate a hemorrhage, particularly of the eyes or brain. See Table 39-7 for specific exercise guidelines for thrombocytopenia. Exercise prescription is highly individualized and should take into account intensity, duration, and frequency that are appropriate for the individual's condition, age, and previous activity level.

Blood pressure cuffs and similar devices must be used with caution. When used, elastic support stockings must be thigh-high, never knee-high. Mechanical compression with a pneumatic pump and soft tissue mobilization are contraindicated unless approved by the physician. Anyone who has had a splenectomy has increased susceptibility to infection. Practice good handwashing (see Box 7-2) and observe carefully for any signs of infection (see Table 7-1). (See also Special Implications for the Therapist: Anemia, 13-4.) ■

◆ Effects of Aspirin and Other Nonsteroidal Antiinflammatory Drugs on Platelet Function

Acquired disorders of platelet function can occur through the use of aspirin and other NSAIDs that inactivate platelet cyclooxygenase. This key enzyme is required for the production of thromboxane A_2, a potent inducer of platelet aggregation and constrictor of arterial smooth muscle. A single dose of aspirin can suppress normal platelet aggregation for 48 hours or longer (up to a week) until newly formed platelets have been released. Platelets are anucleated and cannot synthesize new enzyme; once inactivated by aspirin or other NSAIDs, platelets remain inactive for the rest of their life span. Other NSAIDs have antiplatelet effects lasting less than 24 hours. The use of aspirin or an aspirin-containing compound is usually contraindicated before any surgical procedure. Symptoms from this phenomenon are mild and may consist of easy bruising and bleeding confined to the skin. Prolonged oozing after surgery involving dental or reconstructive plastic surgery may occur.

◆ Disseminated Intravascular Coagulation

Definition and Overview.   Disseminated intravascular coagulation (DIC), sometimes referred to as *consumption coagulopathy*, is a thrombotic disease caused by overactivation of the coagulation cascade (i.e., normal coagulation gone awry). It is an acquired disorder of platelet function, with diffuse or widespread coagulation occurring within arterioles and capillaries all over the body. DIC is actually a paradoxical condition in which clotting and hemorrhage occur simultaneously within the vascular system. Uncontrolled activation occurs of both the coagulation sequence, causing widespread formation of thromboses (clots) in the microcirculation, and the fibrinolytic system, leading to widespread deposition of fibrin in the circulation. Hemorrhage may occur from the kidneys, brain, adrenals, heart, and other organs.

Incidence and Etiologic Factors.   DIC is common, particularly after shock, sepsis, obstetric/gynecologic complications, leukemia and other neoplasms, and massive trauma. The oncology client may develop this syndrome as a result of either the neoplasm itself or of the treatment for the neoplasm. DIC may occur as a result of a variety of predisposing conditions that activate the clotting mechanisms (see Fig. 5-12).

Pathogenesis.   The development of DIC is generally characterized by complex pathologic processes with intravascular fibrin formation and inhibition of these same processes occurring simultaneously. Hypercoagulable reactions are mediated by cytokines, including tumor necrosis factor–alpha (TNF-α) and interleukin-6 (IL-6). Although fibrinolysis is activated in this process by the action of TNF-α, its activity is impaired by the inhibitory effect of plasminogen activator inhibitor-1.[75] The following three pathogenetic steps are observed and clearly illustrated in Fig. 5-12: (1) hemostasis is initiated by endothelial or tissue injury; (2) release of Factor XII or tissue thromboplastin (TTP); and (3) direct activation of factor X. *Damage to the endothelium* (e.g., from sepsis, hypoxia, cardiopulmonary arrest) can precipitate DIC by activating the intrinsic clotting pathway, whereas *tissue injury* (e.g., obstetric complications, malignant neoplasm, infection, burns) can precipitate DIC by activating the extrinsic pathway. *Release of Factor XII or TTP* in the circulation facilitates the *activation of factor X* (proteolytic effect).

Once either the clotting cascade (intrinsic or extrinsic) is stimulated, widespread coagulation occurs throughout the body, leading to thrombotic events within the vasculature. The normal inhibitory mechanisms become overwhelmed so that clotting can occur unrestricted. As a result of the widespread clotting that occurs, the clotting factors become used up and hemorrhage occurs. This leads to the two primary pathophysiologic alterations of DIC: thrombosis in the presence of hemorrhage.

Clinical Manifestations.   The tendency toward excessive bleeding can appear suddenly, with little warning, and can rapidly progress to severe or even fatal hemorrhage. Thrombosis may occur in various sites distant to the tumor or its metastases. Signs of DIC include continued bleeding from a venipuncture site, occult and internal bleeding, and, in some cases, profuse bleeding from all orifices. Other less obvious and more easily missed signs are generalized sweating, cold and mottled fingers and toes (due to capillary thrombi and hypoxia), and petechiae.

Medical Management

Diagnosis, Treatment, and Prognosis.   Diagnosis is made based on clinical presentation in combination with client history; the diagnosis is confirmed by laboratory blood tests (e.g., D-dimer test). Treatment is always directed toward the underlying cause and must be highly individualized according to the person's age, nature and origin of DIC, site and severity of hemorrhage or thrombosis, and other clinical parameters. The hemorrhagic or thrombotic symptoms may be alleviated by appropriate blood product replacement or anticoagulants, but the coagulopathy will continue until the causative process is reversed. Researchers are investigating strategies aimed at inhibiting coagulation activation with protein C and tissue factor-pathway inhibitor.

The mortality rate for DIC is no longer high with early recognition and treatment, but DIC does contribute to significant morbidity and some mortality as it occurs often with cancer. Acute DIC can be fatal depending on the response to treatment of the underlying sepsis or cardiovascular problem.

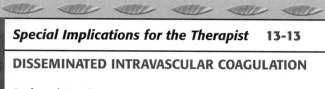

Special Implications for the Therapist 13-13

DISSEMINATED INTRAVASCULAR COAGULATION

Preferred Practice Patterns:
   Preferred practice patterns are not applicable in this condition. DIC is a medical problem that, when present as a comorbidity, requires consideration regarding precautions during any intervention, but it is not a condition requiring primary PT/OT intervention.

Clients with DIC are treated by the therapist in oncology or intensive care units (ICUs). DIC is either the consequence of malignancy or the end result of multisystem organ failure after trauma affecting multiple systems (e.g., severe trauma or burns). Clients are in critical condition and require bedside care. Care must be taken to avoid dislodging clots and causing new onset of bleeding. Monitor the results of serial blood studies, particularly hematocrit, hemoglobin, and coagulation times. To prevent injury, bed rest during bleeding episodes is required. ∎

◆ Sickle Cell Disease

Sickle cell disease (SCD) is a generic term for a group of inherited, autosomal recessive disorders characterized by the presence of an abnormal form of hemoglobin (hemoglobin S, or Hb S) within the erythrocytes. The presence of Hb S can cause RBCs to change from their usual biconcave disk shape to a crescent or sickle shape during deoxygenation. SCD occurs when a genetic mutation occurs so that almost all of the hemoglobin is abnormal. *Homozygous hemoglobin S* (HgbSS) occurs when an individual inherits two sickle cell genes with a substitution of valine for the normal glutamic acid of the beta globin chain of hemoglobin. *Heterozygous hemoglobin SC* (HgbSC) is the result of inheriting one sickle cell gene and one gene for another abnormal type of hemoglobin called C. Heterozygous *hemoglobin beta-thalassemia* (HgbSβ-thal) is the result of inheriting one sickle cell gene and one gene for a type of thalassemia, another inherited anemia. Beta thalassemias are caused by genetic mutations that abolish or reduce production of the beta globin subunit of hemoglobin.[60] Approximately three out of every 1000 black newborns and between 50,000 and 70,000 individuals in the United States have SCD; the number in Africa is correspondingly higher.[47]

The two primary pathophysiologic features of sickle cell disorders are chronic hemolytic anemia and vasoocclusion resulting in ischemic injury. Children with SCD are at increased risk for severe morbidity and mortality, especially during the first 3 years of life. When a sickled cell reoxygenates, the cell resumes a normal shape, but after repeated cycles of sickling and unsickling, the erythrocyte is permanently damaged and hemolyzes. This hemolysis is responsible for the anemia that is a hallmark of SCD. A brief discussion of thalassemias is presented, but only the most severe disorder, sickle cell anemia, is fully discussed in this text.

◆ Sickle Cell Anemia

The anemia associated with SCD is merely a result (symptom) of the disease and is not the disease itself. Consistent with this idea, the term *sickle cell disease* is used throughout the discussion of sickle cell anemia.

Definition and Incidence. Sickle cell anemia is a hereditary, chronic form of hemolytic anemia in which the rupture of erythrocytes (forming sickle cells) releases hemoglobin prematurely into the plasma, thereby reducing the delivery of oxygen to the tissues. It is a worldwide health problem, affecting many races, countries, and ethnic groups, and is the most common inherited hematologic disorder.

The WHO estimates that each year more than 250,000 babies are born worldwide with this inherited blood disorder. About one in 400 black newborns in the United States has sickle cell anemia, and one in 12 black Americans (8%) carries the sickle cell trait.[86] The disease is also prevalent in many Spanish-speaking regions of the world, such as South America, Cuba, and Central America, and among the Hispanic community in the United States.

Etiologic Factors. The cause of SCD and its worldwide incidence is the result of several factors. The sickle cell trait may have developed as a single genetic mutation that provided a selective advantage against severe forms of falciparum malaria. Anyone who carries the inherited trait for SCD but does not have the actual illness is protected against this form of malaria. In countries with malaria, children born with sickle cell trait survived and then passed the gene for SCD to their offspring. As populations migrated, the sickle cell trait and sickle cell anemia moved throughout the world. Several theories purport to explain the origination of SCD, but its actual origin is unknown. Four separate types of genetic mutations are known; each is related to the severity of illness and each is associated with a different geographic location, including different locations in Africa, eastern Saudi Arabia, and India.

Risk Factors. Because SCD is inherited as an autosomal recessive trait, both parents of an offspring must have the sickle hemoglobin gene. When both parents have sickle cell trait, they have a 25% chance with each pregnancy of having a child with sickle cell anemia. If one parent has sickle cell trait and the other has a beta-thalassemic disorder, they are at the same risk for having a child with a sickle beta-thalassemia syndrome. In couples in which one individual has sickle cell trait and one has hemoglobin C trait, the chance of having a child with Hb SC disease is also 25% with each pregnancy. If one parent has sickle cell anemia and the other has the sickle cell trait, the risk of having a child with sickle cell anemia is 50% (Fig. 13-5). Individuals with sickle cell trait can receive nondirective genetic counseling (i.e., counselees are given objective information without personal bias and without provision of specific recommendations) after hemoglobin electrophoresis and other measurements have been performed on each prospective parent.

SCD is characterized by a series of "crises"* that result from early destruction of the abnormal cells and obstruction of blood flow to the tissues. Stress from viral or bacterial infection, hy-

---

*Concern is evident about the use of the term *crises*, and some advocate the use of the word *episodes*, as adopted here. Clinicians may find that some affected individuals really prefer the term *crises*.

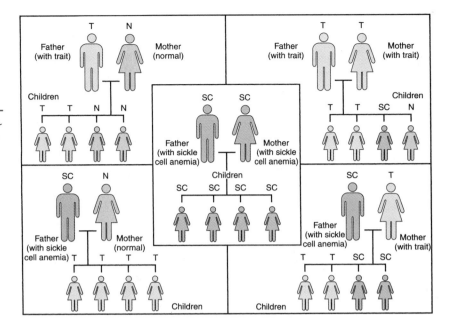

FIGURE **13-5** Statistical probabilities of inheriting sickle cell anemia. (From O'Toole MT: *Miller-Keane encyclopedia and dictionary of medicine, nursing, and allied health,* ed 6, Philadelphia, 1997, WB Saunders.)

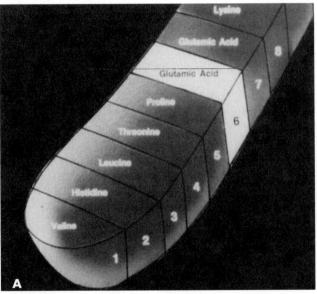

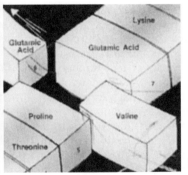

FIGURE **13-6**　A structural defect in the hemoglobin molecule (**A**). This single amino acid substitution from glutamic acid to valine at the sixth position in the beta chain of hemoglobin (**B**) has some devastating consequences. (From Gaston M: *Sickle cell anemia,* NIH Pub No 90-3058, Bethesda, Md, 1990, National Institutes of Health.)

poxia, dehydration, emotional disturbance, extreme temperatures (hot or cold), or fatigue may precipitate an episode. Additionally, episodes may be precipitated by the presence of acidosis; exposure to low oxygen tensions as a result of strenuous physical exertion, climbing to high altitudes, flying in nonpressurized planes, or undergoing anesthesia without receiving adequate oxygenation; pregnancy; trauma; and increased body temperature (fever). Any of these factors may shorten release time of oxygen, thereby precipitating an episode.

Pathogenesis.　The sickle cell defect occurs in hemoglobin, the oxygen-carrying constituent of erythrocytes. Hemoglobin contains four chains of amino acids, the compounds that make up proteins. Two of the amino acid chains are known as *alpha chains,* and two are called *beta chains.* In normal hemoglobin, the amino acid in the sixth position on the beta chains is glutamic acid. In people with SCD, the sixth po-

sition is occupied by another amino acid, valine (Fig. 13-6). Using DNA recombinant technology, the genetic locus for the beta globin has now been identified on chromosome 11.

This single point mutation of valine for glutamic acid results in a loss of two negative charges that causes surface abnormalities. The sickle hemoglobin transports oxygen normally, but after releasing oxygen, hemoglobin molecules that contain the beta chain defect stick to one another instead of remaining separate, and polymerize (change molecular arrangement), forming long, rigid rods or tubules inside RBCs. The rods cause the normally smooth, doughnut-shaped RBCs to take on a sickle or curved shape and to lose their vital ability to deform and squeeze through tiny blood vessels (Fig. 13-7). For a time, this sickling is reversible because the cells are reoxygenated in arterial blood; however, eventually, the change becomes irreversible. In the process of sickling and unsickling, the erythrocyte membrane becomes damaged.

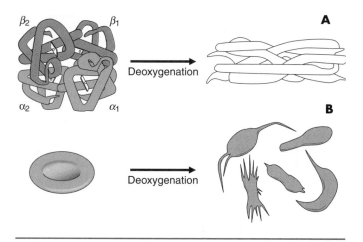

FIGURE   13-7   **A,** The molecular structure of hemoglobin (Hb) contains a pair of α polypeptide chains and a pair of β chains, each wrapped around a heme group (an iron atom in a porphyrin ring). The quaternary structure of the hemoglobin molecule enables it to carry up to four molecules of oxygen. **A,** In the folded beta chain molecule, the sixth position contacts the alpha chain. The amino acid substitution at the sixth position of the beta chain occurring in sickle cell anemia causes the hemoglobins to aggregate into long chains, altering the shape of the cell (Hb S). **B,** The change of the RBC from a biconcave disk to an elongated or crescent (sickle) shape occurs with deoxygenation.

The sickled cells, which become stiff and sticky, clog small blood vessels, depriving tissue from receiving an adequate blood supply. Under stress, oxygen is released too soon, and the cell sickles while it is in the capillary. Deoxygenation of sickle cells induces potassium (followed by water) efflux, which increases cell density and the tendency of HgbS to polymerize. The sickle cell also has a chemical on the cell surface that binds to blood vessel walls. As a result, these sickle-shaped, rigid, and sticky blood cells cannot pass through the capillaries, blocking the flow of blood.[60] Occlusion of the microcirculation increases hypoxia, which causes more erythrocytes to sickle; thus is a vicious circle precipitated, which is compounded in the presence of acidosis; dehydration; extreme temperatures; increased body temperature (fever); change in altitude; strenuous physical exertion; or emotional stress. This accumulation of sickled erythrocytes obstructing blood vessels produces tissue injury. The organs at greatest risk are those with venous sinuses, in which blood flow is slow and oxygen tension and pH are low (spleen, kidney, bone marrow) or those with a limited terminal arterial supply (eye, head of the femur). No tissue or organ is spared from this injury.

The earlier the oxygen is released, the more severe (clinically) the SCD; severity is related in part to normal fetal hemoglobin (Hb F). Average sickle red blood cells last only 10 to 20 days (normal is 120 days). The RBCs cannot be replaced fast enough, and anemia is the result. The release time can be shortened even more by the risk factors mentioned. Occlusion of small blood vessels throughout the body causes infarcts in the spleen, bone, kidney, and lung; bone marrow expands to compensate for increased RBC hemolysis, leading to osteoporosis and eventually osteosclerosis.

Clinical Manifestations.
Sickled erythrocytes cause severe hemolytic anemia and tend to occlude the microvasculature, resulting in both acute and chronic tissue injury.

Intravascular sickling and hemolysis can begin by 6 to 8 weeks of age, but clinical manifestations do not usually appear until the infant is at least 6 months old, at which time the postnatal decrease in Hb F, which inhibits sickling, and increased production of Hb S leads to the increased concentration of Hb S.

Acute manifestations of symptoms, called *crises* or *episodes*, usually fall into one of four categories: vasoocclusive or thrombotic, aplastic, sequestration, or rarely, hyperhemolytic (marked increase in red cell hemolysis associated with drugs or infections) (Fig. 13-8). Pain caused by the blockage of sickled RBCs forming sickle cell clots is the most common symptom of SCD, occurring unpredictably in any organ, bone, or joint of the body, wherever and whenever a blood clot develops. The frequency, duration, and intensity of the painful episodes vary widely (Table 13-7). Some people experience painful episodes only once a year; others may have as many as 15 to 20 episodes annually. The vasoocclusive episodes causing ischemic tissue damage may last 5 or 6 days, requiring hospitalization and subsiding gradually. Older clients more often report extremity and back pain during vascular episodes.

Aplastic crises or episodes caused by diminished RBCs result in profound anemia characterized by pallor, fatigue, jaundice, and irritability. This anemia occurs because sickled RBCs last only 10 to 20 days in the bloodstream, rather than the normal 120-day life span. The sickled RBCs are removed faster from the circulation than the bone marrow can produce them.

In sequestration episodes, sickled cells undergoing hemolysis in the spleen get trapped, causing blood pooling, infarction of splenic vessels, and splenomegaly. The spleen may become completely fibrotic, called *autosplenectomy*, owing to repeated blood vessel obstruction. Overwhelming infection may occur due to functional asplenia (i.e., the spleen is physically present but not functioning).

Complications.
Other complications include neurologic manifestations; hand-foot syndrome; renal involvement; bacterial infections (e.g., pneumococcal pneumonia, salmonella osteomyelitis); iron overload; cholelithiasis; chronic (nonhealing) leg ulcers (present in about 75% of older children or adults); retinopathy; and priapism (persistent penile erection). Hand-and-foot syndrome (dactylitis) occurs when a microinfarction (clot) occludes the blood vessels that supply the metacarpal and metatarsal bones, causing ischemia; it may be the infant's first problem caused by SCD. It presents with low-grade fever and symmetric, painful, diffuse, nonpitting edema in the hands and feet, extending to the fingers and toes (Fig. 13-9). This is a fairly common phenomenon seen almost exclusively in the young infant and child. Despite radiographic changes and swelling, the syndrome is almost always self-limiting, and bones usually heal without permanent deformity.

In the CNS, unlike other areas of the body, a tendency for sickle cell episodes to involve large vessels exists. Cerebrovascular accidents (CVAs) are a frequent, severe manifestation of SCD, most commonly occurring in the pediatric population. Careful neurologic examination often reveals hemiplegia or other mild neurologic deficits. MRI/magnetic resonance angiography (MRA) of the head and neck may show more extensive changes than are seen clinically, suggesting that silent strokes are not uncommon. Additionally, many cognitive effects from these microvasculature strokes result in learning problems.

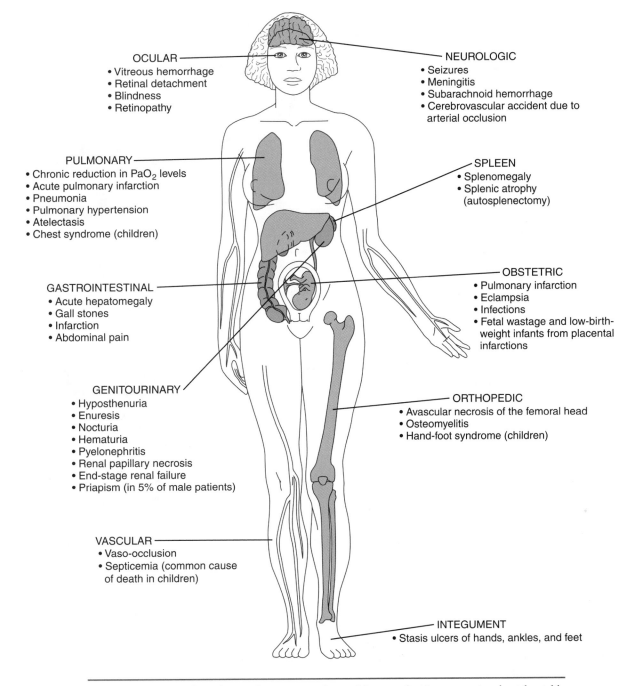

OCULAR
• Vitreous hemorrhage
• Retinal detachment
• Blindness
• Retinopathy

NEUROLOGIC
• Seizures
• Meningitis
• Subarachnoid hemorrhage
• Cerebrovascular accident due to arterial occlusion

PULMONARY
• Chronic reduction in PaO_2 levels
• Acute pulmonary infarction
• Pneumonia
• Pulmonary hypertension
• Atelectasis
• Chest syndrome (children)

SPLEEN
• Splenomegaly
• Splenic atrophy (autosplenectomy)

OBSTETRIC
• Pulmonary infarction
• Eclampsia
• Infections
• Fetal wastage and low-birth-weight infants from placental infarctions

GASTROINTESTINAL
• Acute hepatomegaly
• Gall stones
• Infarction
• Abdominal pain

GENITOURINARY
• Hyposthenuria
• Enuresis
• Nocturia
• Hematuria
• Pyelonephritis
• Renal papillary necrosis
• End-stage renal failure
• Priapism (in 5% of male patients)

ORTHOPEDIC
• Avascular necrosis of the femoral head
• Osteomyelitis
• Hand-foot syndrome (children)

VASCULAR
• Vaso-occlusion
• Septicemia (common cause of death in children)

INTEGUMENT
• Stasis ulcers of hands, ankles, and feet

FIGURE 13-8 Clinical manifestations and possible complications associated with sickle cell disease. These findings are a consequence of infarctions, anemia, hemolysis, and recurrent infections.

Acute chest syndrome is a common and potentially fatal combination of pneumonia and pulmonary infarction presenting with fever, cough, chest pain, and difficulty breathing. It is the second most common cause of hospitalization and leading cause of death. Pediatric cases are most often caused by infection, whereas pulmonary fat embolism is more common among adults. Clinical manifestations include pleuritic chest pain, fever, dyspnea, referred abdominal pain, cough, and hypoxia (Table 13-8). If pulmonary inflammation or infection affects the diaphragm, pain can be referred to the back or shoulder. Recurrent episodes of acute chest syndrome can result in chronic respiratory insufficiency.

Medical Management
Diagnosis. It is required in all the states in the United States that all infants are screened for SCD regardless of race or ethnic background (universal screening). This recommendation is based on several factors: (1) one out of every 200 Hispanic and 400 white children in Texas carries the sickle cell trait; (2) although SCD is more prevalent in certain racial and ethnic groups, it is not possible to define accurately an individual's heritage by physical appearance or surname; and (3) prophylactic penicillin and pneumococcal vaccination reduce both morbidity and mortality from pneumococcal infections in infants with sickle cell anemia and sickle-thalassemia.

TABLE 13-7

Clinical Manifestations of Sickle Cell Anemia

Pain
Abdominal
Chest
Headaches

Bone and Joint Crises
Low-grade fever
Extremity pain
Back pain
Periosteal pain
Joint pain, especially shoulder
　and hip

Vascular Complications
Cerebrovascular accidents
Chronic leg ulcers
Avascular necrosis of the
　femoral head
Bone infarcts

Pulmonary Crises
Bacterial pneumonia
Pulmonary infarction

Neurologic Manifestations
Convulsions
Drowsiness
Coma
Stiff neck
Paresthesias
Cranial nerve palsies
Blindness
Nystagmus

Hand-Foot Syndrome
Fever
Pain
Dactylitis

Splenic Sequestration Crisis
Liver and spleen enlargement
Spleen atrophy

Renal complications
Enuresis
Nocturia
Hematuria
Pyelonephritis
Renal papillary necrosis
End-stage renal failure (older
　adult population)

Modified from Goodman CC, Snyder TE: *Differential diagnosis in physical therapy,* ed 3, Philadelphia, 2000, WB Saunders, p. 186.

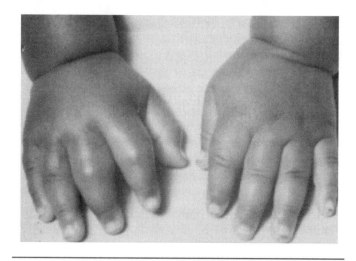

FIGURE　**13-9**　Dactylitis. Painful swelling of the hands or feet can occur when a clot forms in the hands or feet. This problem, known as *hand-and-foot syndrome,* occurs most often in children affected by SCD. (From Gaston M: *Sickle cell anemia,* NIH Pub No 90-3058, Bethesda, Md, 1990, National Institutes of Health.)

TABLE 13-8

Complications Associated with Pediatric Sickle Cell Anemia

CHEST SYNDROME	STROKE
Severe chest pain	Jerking or twitching of the face, legs, or arms
Fever of ≥38.8° C	Convulsions or seizures
(≥102° F)	Unusual or strange behavior
Very congested	Inability to move an arm and/or a leg
Cough	Ataxia or unsteady gait (do not assume
Dyspnea	these are guarding responses to pain)
Tachypnea	Stutter or slurred speech
Sternal or costal	Distal muscular weakness in the hands, feet,
retractions	or legs
	Changes in vision
	Severe, unrelieved headaches
	Severe vomiting

Screening targeted to specific racial and ethnic groups will therefore miss some affected infants, subjecting them to an increased risk of early mortality. Universal screening is the best, most reliable, and most cost-effective screening method to identify affected infants.[59] The cord blood of newborns is tested in the United States.

The diagnosis of sickle cell trait or any of the other sickle syndromes depends on the demonstration of sickling under reduced oxygen tension. A sickle turbidity test (Sickledex) can confirm the presence of Hb S in peripheral blood, and hemoglobin electrophoresis (separation and identification of hemoglobin under the influence of an applied electric field) is used to determine the amount of Hb S in erythrocytes. Electrophoresis is used to screen blood for sickle cell trait and will also detect SCD and heterozygosity (carrier state) for other hemoglobin disorders, such as Hb C. Because the HgbS and HgbC amino acid substitutions change the electrical charge of the protein, the migration patterns of the hemoglobin with electrophoresis result in distinct diagnostic patterns.[60]

Safe, accurate methods for performing prenatal diagnosis for SCD are possible as early as the tenth gestational week. Analyses of DNA from fetal cells obtained by amniocentesis or chorionic villus sampling can be performed at the sixteenth gestational week. The sickle and Hb C genes can be detected directly in fetal DNA samples, as can most Hb S β-thalassemia genes.

Treatment.　In the past decade, impressive progress has been made in directing treatment to the unique pathophysiology of SCDs. A large number of antisickling regimens are being investigated; although some have been shown to be effective in vitro, unacceptable toxicity prevents their use in humans at this time. Bone marrow transplantation cures SCD, but minimal availability and associated risks prevent its widespread use. In severe cases, bone marrow transplantation may be considered, and the data confirm that allogeneic bone marrow transplantation establishes normal erythropoiesis and is associated with improved growth and stable CNS imaging and pulmonary function in most recipients.[81] The event-free survival rate after allogeneic-matched sibling hematopoietic cell transplant for SCD is 82%.[31]

Supportive care is essential (e.g., rest, oxygen, administration of intravenous [IV] fluids and electrolytes, physical and occupational therapy for joint and bone involvement). Preventive measures (see Risk Factors) are used to reduce the incidence of episodes. Medications, such as analgesics or corticosteroids, are sometimes administered to relieve musculoskeletal pain.

Splenic or hepatic sequestration requires aggressive rehydration and transfusion. Exchange transfusions to reduce Hb S levels below 40% of total hemoglobin may be used therapeutically for neurologic, cardiac, or retinal symptoms; hypoxemia; severe prolonged or infarctive episodes; acute splenic sequestration in infants; and chronic leg ulcers. These transfusions also can be used prophylactically during pregnancy or before general anesthesia, but they carry the risk of hepatitis, red cell sensitization, hemosiderosis (increased iron storage), and transfusion reactions.

Prenatal and neonatal screening can identify this disorder and significantly reduce morbidity and mortality through the use of prophylactic antibiotics. Infants with documented SCD (sickle cell anemia or Hb S beta thalassemia) should be started on twice daily oral prophylactic penicillin as soon as possible, but not later than at 2 months of age. Drugs such as hydroxyurea (a cytotoxic drug), which stimulates Hb F production, are now being used as a treatment for sickle cell anemia and are considered safe in the pediatric population. Dramatic reduction of painful episodes, fewer hospitalizations, decreased need for transfusions, and fewer cases of acute chest syndrome occur with the use of hydroxyurea. Neutropenia is a potential side effect, requiring frequent monitoring.[35] The use of inhaled nitrous oxide (NO) to treat acute chest syndrome (ACS) is also under investigation because of its ability to prevent pulmonary hypertension and ventilation/perfusion mismatch. NO may confer some protection against polymerization of sickle hemoglobin and exert a reversible antiplatelet effect that may be beneficial in ACS. The onset of peripheral neuropathy associated with NO use in this population has delayed the final development of treatment protocols incorporating NO.[55,72]

Researchers are continuing to investigate the use of fetal hemoglobin as a treatment possibility. Fetal hemoglobin is produced during fetal development and for the first 6 months after birth. Hb F has some ability to prevent sickling and reduce hemolysis; some adults with SCD who naturally make substantial amounts of Hb F have less pain and better spleen function than others with SCD who do not have elevated levels of Hb F. Other researchers are investigating the use of erythropoietin (hormone produced by the kidneys that stimulates red cell production and increases HgbF levels in the red cells); drugs to reverse cellular dehydration (dehydration increases the rate of polymerization); and fetal cord blood transplantation (see Chapter 20).

Prognosis.   Historically, SCD has been associated with high mortality in early childhood due to overwhelming bacterial infections, splenic sequestration episodes, and the acute chest syndrome. Since the mid-1970s, comprehensive medical care has reduced morbidity and mortality in children with SCD, and currently, more than half of adults with SCD live beyond 50 years.

No cure for SCD is evident; it is a devastating condition with recurrent episodes leading to death at ages as young as 30

years. The sickle cell clots can be life-threatening, depending on their location. For example, a blood clot in the brain can cause a stroke. Recovery may be complete in some cases, but serious neurologic damage is more likely to occur, and repeated CVAs may lead to increased neurologic involvement, permanent paralysis, or death. Permanent damage from blood clots to the heart, kidney, lungs, liver, or eyes (blindness) can occur. Clients who survive until 50 years or older usually develop progressive renal damage with fatal uremia.

Special Implications for the Therapist   13-14

SICKLE CELL DISEASE

Preferred Practice Patterns:
4E: *Impaired Joint Mobility, Motor Function, Muscle Performance, and Range of Motion Associated With Localized Inflammation (joint effusion)*
4G: *Impaired Joint Mobility, Muscle Performance, and Range of Motion Associated With Fracture (aseptic necrosis)*
6A: *Primary Prevention/Risk Reduction for Cardiovascular/Pulmonary Disorders (emboli; stroke prevention)*
6B: *Impaired Aerobic Capacity/Endurance Associated With Deconditioning*
6F: *Impaired Ventilation and Respiration/Gas Exchange Associated With Respiratory Failure (pulmonary infarct, pneumonia, acute chest syndrome)*
7A: *Primary Prevention/Risk Reduction For Integumentary Disorders (chronic leg ulcers)*
7B: *Impaired Integumentary Integrity Associated With Superficial Skin Involvement (ulcers; possibly pattern 7C)*

It is important for the therapist to recognize signs of complications, especially signs of chest syndrome and stroke (see Table 13-8) and to provide client education about risks and risk prevention (e.g., importance of physical activity and/or mobility, prevention of pulmonary complications using breathing and incentive spirometry). Stroke is a relatively infrequent complication in the young infant; the median age for occurrence of stroke in children is 7 years. Splenic sequestration (entrapment of blood and enlargement in the spleen) can occur in children under age 6 with HgbSS and at any age with other types of SCD. Circulatory collapse and death can occur in less than 30 minutes. Any signs of weakness, abdominal pain, fatigue, dyspnea, tachycardia accompanied by pallor and hypotension require emergency medical attention. Client and family education should emphasize the importance of regularly scheduled medical evaluation for anyone receiving hydroxyurea. The risk of developing an undetected toxicity that can result in severe bone marrow depression must be explained. Outward signs of drug complications are rarely evident.

Exercise
The influence of the decreased oxygen availability associated with SCD on the cardiorespiratory and metabolic responses to endurance exercise has been examined in one study. Significantly lower exercise tolerance, significantly lower oxygen

Continued

consumption (VO$_2$), and minute ventilation were observed. These factors must be considered when prescribing exercise for this population.[56] During a sickle cell episode or crisis, the therapist may be involved in pain control or management. Precautions include avoiding stressors that can precipitate an episode, such as overexertion, dehydration, smoking, and exposure to cold or the use of cryotherapy for painful, swollen joints. (See Special Implications for the Therapist: Splenomegaly, 13-16 in this chapter.) Should a person with SCD experience an isolated musculoskeletal injury (e.g., sprained ankle) in the absence of any sickle cell episodes, careful application of ice can be undertaken.

Pain Management

People with SCD suffer both physically and psychosocially. They may describe feelings of helplessness against the disease and fear a premature death. Frequent hospitalizations and consequent job absences often result in stressful financial constraints. Depression is a common finding in this group of people. A program offering holistic treatment focuses on pharmacologic and nonpharmacologic strategies, offering the client multiple self-management options. The sickle cell pain can be successfully managed using whirlpool therapy at a slightly warmer temperature (102° F to 104° F), facilitating muscle relaxation through active movement in the water. The therapist should teach the client alternative methods of pain control such as the appropriate application of mild heat to painful areas or the use of visualization or relaxation techniques. Combined use of medications, psychologic support, relaxation techniques, biofeedback, and imagery is a useful intervention to lessen the effects of painful episodes.[30] Cognitive-behavioral therapy can be helpful in the management of sickle pain because of the high level of psychologic stress people with SCD experience.[78]

Joint effusions in SCD can occur secondary to long bone infarctions with extension of swelling, and septic arthritis. Clients with SCD may also have coexistent rheumatic or collagen vascular disease or osteoarthritis, necessitating careful evaluation to determine the presence of marked inflammation or fever before initiating intervention procedures. Teaching joint protection is important and may include assistive devices, equipment, or technology and pain-free strengthening exercises. Persistent thigh, buttock, or groin pain in anyone with known SCD may be an indication of aseptic necrosis of the femoral head. Blood supply to the hip is just adequate, even in healthy people, so the associated microvascular obstruction can leave the hip especially vulnerable to ischemia and necrosis. Up to 50% of sickle cell cases develop this condition. Total hip replacement may be indicated in cases in which severe structural damage occurs; sickle cell–related surgical complications most commonly include excessive intraoperative blood loss, postoperative hemorrhage, wound abscess, pulmonary complications, and transfusion reactions.[79]

Tolerance, Dependence, and Addiction

It is helpful if the client, family, and clinician understand the differences among tolerance, dependence, and addiction as they relate to the individual with SCD receiving or needing narcotic medications. Tolerance and dependence are both involuntary and predictable physiologic changes that develop with repeated administration of narcotics; these terms do not indicate the person is addicted. Tolerance occurs when, after repeated administration of a narcotic, larger doses are needed to obtain the same

effect. Dependence has occurred if withdrawal symptoms emerge when the narcotic is stopped abruptly. In either case, this means that once the medication is no longer needed, the dosage will have to be tapered down to avoid withdrawal symptoms. Addiction, although also based on physiologic changes associated with drug use, has a psychologic and behavioral component characterized by continuous craving for the substance. Addicted people will use a drug to relieve psychologic symptoms even after the physical pain is gone. The chronic use of narcotics for pain relief may lead to addictive use in vulnerable individuals, but even if someone is addicted, the pain should still be treated and narcotics should not be withheld if they are the drugs of choice for the pain condition. Ironically, undertreating the pain because of fear of fostering addiction actually encourages a pattern of drug-seeking and drug-hoarding behaviors.[25] ■

◆ Sickle Cell Trait

Sickle cell trait is not a disease but is rather a heterozygous condition in which the individual has the mutant gene from only one parent (β^s gene), and the normal gene (β^A globin gene), resulting in the production of both Hb S and Hb A with a predominance of Hb A (60%) over Hb S (40%). One in 12 black Americans (8%) has the sickle cell trait, and many other races and nationalities also carry the genetic defect. The gene has persisted because heterozygotes gain slight protection against falciparum malaria.

Under normal circumstances, sickle cell trait is rarely symptomatic; symptoms may occur with conditions associated with marked hypoxia and at high altitudes. No increased risk is evident for individuals with sickle cell trait who undergo general anesthesia, and a normal life expectancy is predicted. It was previously reported that no increased risk of sudden death was evident for those who participate in athletics, but a small number of cases have now been reported. However, it remains controversial whether the pathogenesis of these exercise-related deaths involved microvascular obstruction by sickled erythrocytes, since sickling can occur postmortem.[83] The recommendations are that athletes with sickle cell trait adhere to compliance with general guidelines for fluid replacement and acclimatization to hot conditions and altitude.[68]

◆ The Thalassemias

Definition. The thalassemias are a group of inherited, chronic hemolytic anemias predominantly affecting people of Mediterranean or southern Chinese ancestry (*thalassa* means sea, referring to early cases of SCD reported around the Mediterranean). American blacks and people from central Africa and southern Asia can also be affected by thalassemia.

Overview and Pathogenesis. The thalassemias are characterized by production of extremely thin, fragile erythrocytes, called *target cells*. Normal postnatal hemoglobin is composed of two alpha and two beta polypeptide chains (see Fig. 13-7). Unlike the alpha and beta polypeptide chains in sickle cell anemia, the polypeptide chains in the thalassemias are completely normal in structure, but they are insufficient in number because of a genetic alteration (e.g., deletion, nonsense mutation) that affects globin synthesis. The defective polypeptide unit is unbalanced and unstable and disintegrates, damaging RBCs and resulting in anemia.

Thalassemia is classified as alpha thalassemia or beta thalassemia because either alpha or beta chains can be affected by diminished synthesis. Beta thalassemia is more common and is the center of discussion in this section. It is called *classic thalassemia* or simply thalassemia. Some beta-thalassemia genes produce no beta globin chains and are termed *b'-thalassemia*. Other beta globin genes produce some beta globins, but in diminished quantities, and are termed *beta⁺ thalassemia*.

The severity of thalassemia depends on whether the affected client is homozygous or heterozygous for the thalassemia trait; homozygotes may develop *thalassemia major* (Cooley's anemia) or *thalassemia intermedia*, both characterized by profound anemia. Heterozygotes may develop *thalassemia minor* or *thalassemia trait*, characterized by mild anemia.

Clinical Manifestations.
The onset of thalassemia major is usually insidious and is not recognized until the latter half of infancy. The clinical manifestations of thalassemia are primarily attributable to (1) defective synthesis of hemoglobin, (2) structurally impaired RBCs, and (3) shortened life span of erythrocytes.

The symptoms of thalassemia major resemble those of other hemolytic anemias (e.g., jaundice, cholelithiasis, leg ulcers, and enlarged spleen). Bony changes can occur in older children if untreated. Ineffective erythropoiesis causes extreme expansion of marrow space into long bones, skull, and facial bones, causing a thickening of the cranium and a mongoloid appearance or facies. Extramedullary hematopoiesis in the liver, spleen, and around the spinal vertebrae may also develop. Growth abnormalities and cortical bone fragility result, with an increased rate of fractures. Thalassemia minor is usually asymptomatic, except for a mild anemia.

Medical Management
Diagnosis.   Diagnosis is by laboratory testing, and results may include target cells (abnormally thin, fragile cells) and other bizarrely shaped RBCs in the circulation and elevated serum bilirubin and fecal and urinary urobilinogen levels (from the severe hemolysis of abnormal cells). Electrophoresis is usually diagnostic when Hb F or Hb A is elevated.

Treatment.   Thalassemia minor is usually so mild that treatment is not required. Treatment for thalassemia major is by transfusion therapy; packed RBCs may be given on a regular transfusion schedule monthly or bimonthly, when the hemoglobin falls below 3 to 4 g/100 ml, or every 15 days to maintain the hemoglobin at 12 to 15 g/100 ml. When transfused cells are being rapidly destroyed by the spleen, splenectomy may be necessary. A major postsplenectomy complication may be severe and overwhelming infection requiring prophylactic antibiotics. Experimental approaches to therapy now include BMT and agents that increase Hb F production, such as 5-azacytidine and hydroxyurea (see Sickle Cell Anemia: Treatment). Gene therapy has been successful in animal (mice) studies.[21,45]

Repeated transfusions may result in iron overload, which may cause diabetes mellitus, hypofunction of the thyroid, parathyroid, and adrenal glands, and, eventually, myocardial hemosiderosis (accumulation of iron in the myocardium) and cardiac arrhythmias. Excessive iron can be somewhat removed from the blood by chelating agents, such as deferoxamine (Desferal), which binds iron ions to form water-soluble complexes that are removed by the kidneys.

Prognosis.   Thalassemia minor does not affect life expectancy, but clients who carry the thalassemia trait need genetic counseling. Until recently, the outlook for clients with thalassemia major has been poor, with lethal, severe hemolytic anemia and subsequent iron overload and dysfunction of almost all organ systems. Children are significantly delayed in growth and development; delay of puberty is universal, and many die before puberty. Treatment with blood transfusion and early chelation therapy has improved life expectancy from early puberty to early adulthood. Death from *hydrops fetalis* (the absence of all α globin production with progressive hemolysis causing fetal hypoxia, cardiac failure, generalized edema) can occur in homozygous α-thalassemia; it consistently results in stillbirth or death in utero.

◆ Hemophilia
Overview.   Hemophilia is a bleeding disorder inherited as a sex-linked autosomal recessive trait. This means that the genes involved are located on the X chromosome; males are affected because they have only one X chromosome, and females are the carriers in two thirds of all cases. It is the most common inherited coagulation (blood-clotting) disorder and is caused by an abnormality of plasma-clotting proteins necessary for blood coagulation. The two primary types of hemophilia are *hemophilia A*, or classic hemophilia (factor VIII deficiency, which constitutes 80% of all cases of hemophilia) and *hemophilia B*, or Christmas disease (factor IX deficiency, which affects about 15% of all people with hemophilia). Other less common deficiencies (such as deficiencies of clotting factors I, II, V, VII, X, or XIII) are transmitted autosomally and therefore affect males and females equally. These are not fully discussed in this text. Unless otherwise noted, hemophilia refers to both hemophilia A and B in this text.

Bleeding is prolonged in hemophilia, but the blood flow is not any faster than would occur in a normal person with the same injury. All affected individuals in a given family have the same change in their factor VIII or factor IX gene. Individually, the level of severity remains constant throughout a person's life and has the same severity in different members of the same family. The level of severity is dependent on the exact defect in the clotting factor gene and is classified according to the percentage of clotting factor (determined through blood tests)*: mild (5% to 50%); moderate (1% to 5%); and severe (<1%). For people with *mild* hemophilia (25% of all cases), spontaneous hemorrhages (bleeding occurs with no apparent cause) are rare, and joint and deep muscle bleeding are uncommon. Surgical, dental, or other injury or trauma precipitates symptoms that must be treated the same as for severe hemophilia. For those people with *moderate* hemophilia (15% of all people with hemophilia), spontaneous hemorrhage is not usually a problem, but major bleeding episodes can occur after minor trauma. People with *severe* hemophilia comprise 60% of people with hemophilia and may bleed spontaneously or with only slight trauma.

---

*Normal concentrations of coagulation factors are between 50% and 150%.

Incidence. A significant proportion of the American population is affected by hereditary defects in one or more of the clotting factors. Slightly more than 1% of the U.S. population has von Willebrand disease, and an additional 17,000 people are affected by hemophilia A or B (approximately 10,500 with hemophilia A, 3200 with hemophilia B).[12] Hemophilia primarily affects males from all races and socioeconomic groups.

Etiologic Factors. In this gender-linked (X chromosome) recessive disorder, the female carries the defective gene on one of the X chromosomes, and the male presents with the disease (Fig. 13-10). Every carrier has a one in four chance of having a child with hemophilia. Any male who inherits the defective X chromosome has hemophilia, but boys born to a father with hemophilia and a mother who is not a carrier will not have the disease. This is because boys get the X chromosome from the mother and Y chromosome from the father. The Y chromosome determines gender and does not contain genes for the production of clotting factors. Males with hemophilia transmit the gene to all of their daughters (girls receive one X chromosome from the father and one from the mother, which is called an *obligate carrier*) but to none of their sons (a father contributes the Y chromosome; a mother contributes the X chromosome). Although in two thirds of the cases of hemophilia a known family history is evident, this disorder can occur in families (approximately one third) without a previous history of blood-clotting disorders because of spontaneous genetic mutation.

Transmissible Diseases. Individuals, primarily those with severe hemophilia, who were treated before current purification techniques for factor concentrates (before 1986) may have been exposed to HIV. In 1991, approximately 70% of people with hemophilia had seroconverted to being positive for HIV, but since 1986, no further HIV transmission has occurred.

Transmission of hepatitis is equally serious, and about 90% of people with hemophilia who received clotting factor before the mid-1980s test positive for hepatitis C. Current improved methods of viral inactivation through pasteurization and solvent-treatment and monoclonal and recombinant technology have resulted in improved screening methods to identify donors with hepatitis and a reduced risk of hepatitis transmission. As of 1997, there have been no reports of hepatitis C transmission through clotting factor treated with these improved processes. Hepatitis B and D are also killed by these methods. Currently up to one third of individuals with a bleeding disorder and HCV are co-infected with HIV and everyone who was infected with HIV also contracted HCV.[51] Transmission of hepatitis A remains a risk for people with bleeding disorders who use plasma-derived products but can be prevented by immunization with a vaccine now available. All newborns with hemophilia are now receiving the hepatitis B vaccination series, but older clients usually have hepatitis B, with its long-term sequelae.

Women and Bleeding Disorders. The hemophilia community has recognized the needs of females affected by inherited bleeding disorders. Approximately 3000 women in the United States have an active bleeding disorder. Although hemophilia is rare in females, it can occur if the woman or girl has an altered clotting factor gene on both X chromosomes. This can happen if a girl is born to a father with hemophilia and a mother who is a carrier. One X chromosome with an altered hemophilia gene is inherited from a father with hemophilia or a mother who is a carrier and the other X chromosome acquires a new mutation in the hemophilia gene, or both X chromosomes acquire new mutations in the hemophilia gene. In some cases, girls are born with only one X chromosome. If this X chromosome carries the hemophilia gene, the child will have hemophilia. Most women with a bleeding disorder fall into one of three groups: (1) asymptomatic carriers, (2) those with von Willebrand disease (vWD) (see next section), and (3) those with a factor deficiency that is not a gender-linked defect.

Women with bleeding disorders experience excessive uterine bleeding during their menstrual cycle with possible oozing from the ovary after ovulation mid-cycle. Heavy menstrual flow is often the symptom that initiates a coagulation evaluation or more often is reported but not adequately diagnosed, as gynecologists only rarely (less than 1%) perform tests to confirm or exclude a bleeding disorder.[12,19] Cases have occurred in which a female carrier of the hemophilia gene has abnormal bleeding when the level of clotting factor is low

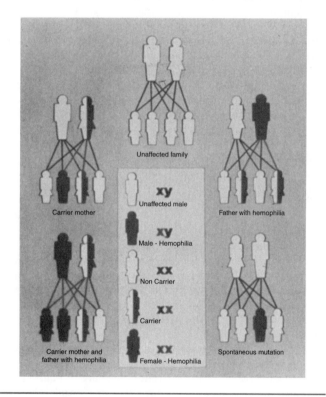

FIGURE 13-10 Inheritance patterns in hemophilia for all family members. A woman is definitely a carrier if she is (1) the biologic daughter of a man with hemophilia, (2) the biologic mother of more than one son with hemophilia, (3) the biologic mother of one hemophilic son and has at least one other blood relative with hemophilia. A woman may or may not be a carrier if she is (1) the biologic mother of one son with hemophilia, (2) the sister of a male with hemophilia, (3) an aunt, cousin, or niece of an affected male related through maternal ties, (4) the biologic grandmother of one son with hemophilia. (From *What you should know about bleeding disorders* [1997] and *What you should know about inheritance of hemophilia* [1998], New York, National Hemophilia Foundation).

enough to cause significant problems with coagulation, especially after trauma or surgery. Most women who have a bleeding disorder have vWD, but isolated cases of mild bleeding problems in carrier women may be caused by extreme expression of the affected gene. Abnormal bleeding from bruising; dental extractions; abortion or miscarriage; complications of pregnancy (e.g., placenta not delivered completely, episiotomy or tearing, prolonged postpartum hemorrhage); nosebleeds; and minor trauma (such as cuts with prolonged oozing) may be overlooked because of the misconception that bleeding disorders do not occur in women.

For more in-depth information, the reader is referred to materials specifically related to women and bleeding disorders available from the National Hemophilia Foundation.[85]

von Willebrand Disease.

vWD is a bleeding disorder that can closely mimic hemophilia but is caused by a defect in or shortage of a blood clotting protein called *von Willebrand factor (vWF)*. vWF carries factor VIII in the blood and helps factor VIII work properly, serving as a "bridge" between platelets and injury sites in the vessel walls by helping platelets get to the site of injury and protecting factor VIII from rapid proteolytic degradation. Although less widely known than hemophilia, vWD is actually the most common inherited bleeding disorder. vWD can be completely asymptomatic or can result in prolonged bleeding. vWD can be inherited from either parent (autosomal rather than gender-linked) and occurs equally in males and females.

Bleeding occurs primarily from mucous membranes (e.g., nosebleeds, gum bleeds, excessive bruising, GI bleeding, bleeding from tooth extraction, heavy menstrual bleeding, postoperative bleeding); joint bleeding is rare but can occur in severe cases. Individuals with vWD have a 50% chance of having children with the same disorder. The child will have one chromosome with the normal clotting gene and one with the vWD gene. Those who do not get the von Willebrand disease gene from their parents will be unaffected, as will their children. However, vWD can be the result of a spontaneous, new genetic mutation in any child; such a mutation can be passed on to offspring of either gender.

Treatment of vWD is dependent on the location of bleeding, type of vWD, and each person's response to therapies. Some people are treated with hormones (estrogen and progesterone) that raise levels of vWF. Mouth bleeds can be treated with application of various topical or oral medications. A synthetic hormone (desmopressin acetate [DDAVP]), administered intravenously, subcutaneously, or as a nasal spray, is effective in some people. Some people, depending on disease severity, receive plasma-derived factor VIII products (see Treatment in this section) that also contain vWF. Recombinant factor products do not contain vWF and are ineffective in controlling bleeding in vWD.

Pathogenesis.

At least 10 proteins called *clotting factors* in the blood must work in a precise order to make a blood clot. Hemophilia A, the most common of the congenital coagulation disorders, is due to a deficiency of the procoagulant protein factor VIII (antihemophilic factor [AHF]). AHF is produced by the liver and is necessary for the formation of thromboplastin in phase I of blood coagulation. Hemophilia B is caused by a defect in factor IX. The genetic pattern of hemophilia is very different from that of disorders such as SCD,

in which every affected individual has the identical genetic defect. The presence of such variable defects in the same gene accounts for the differences in severity of hemophilia. Many different genetic lesions cause factor VIII deficiency, such as gene deletions, with all or part of the gene missing, or missense and nonsense mutations, which cause the clotting factor to be made incorrectly or not at all; 25% to 30% of cases are due to new mutations. In the case of a carrier, some individuals have normal levels of clotting factors whereas others may have very low levels. This is due to the fact that in every cell of the body either the normal X chromosome or the affected X chromosome is randomly inactivated (turned off) in a process called *lyonization*. If the majority of the inactivated chromosomes are the normal X, then the levels of clotting factors may be very low, and such carriers may experience excessive bleeding.

New, sensitive methodologies have provided researchers information that the rate at which factor VIII gene mutations are occurring is rapidly increasing. Gene deletions and point mutations (a single base in the DNA is mutated to another base) are the two most common types of defects. Approximately 50 deletion mutations in the gene for factor VIII have been identified at the molecular level, and many independent deletion mutations in the factor IX gene have been found to be the cause of hemophilia B. Future studies should lead to the discovery of a wide range of defects as well as to potential new mutations. Advances in understanding of the protein will also provide new insights into the effects of particular mutations.

Clinical Manifestations.

Clinically, hemophilia A can only be distinguished from hemophilia B by specific factor assays. Spontaneous bleeding associated with hemophilia occurs with no apparent cause and is uncommon the first year of life, although bleeds can occur as a result of intramuscular injections, IV sites, and falls. Hematoma formation may result from injections or after firm holding, such as occurs when a child is held under the arms or by the elbow and lifted. Early signs and symptoms of hemophilia may include slow, persistent bleeding from circumcision, immunizations, and other minor trauma (e.g., cuts, scratches); excessive bruising from minor trauma; delayed hemorrhage (hours to days after injury) after a minor injury; severe hemorrhaging from the gums after dental extraction; bleeding after brushing teeth; severe nosebleeds; bleeding from the urinary or digestive tracts; and recurrent bleeding into subcutaneous tissue and muscles and around peripheral nerves and joints. Bruising; bleeding from the mouth, tongue, or frenulum; hematomas of the head; and hemarthrosis (bleeding into the joints) often occur during early ambulation. By age 3 to 4 years, 90% of children with severe hemophilia have had an episode of persistent bleeding not seen in mild cases.

Joint.   Bleeding into the joint spaces (hemarthrosis) is one of the most common clinical manifestations of hemophilia, affecting the synovial joints: knee, ankle, elbow, hip, shoulder, and wrist (in order of most common occurrence). Affected joints are referred to as "target" joints. Bleeding in the synovial joints of the feet, hands, temporomandibular joint, and spine is less common. Muscle hemorrhages can be more insidious and massive than joint bleeding and can occur anywhere, most commonly in the flexor muscle groups (e.g., iliopsoas, gastrocnemius, forearm flexors).

When blood is introduced into the joint, the joint becomes distended, causing swelling, pain, warmth, and stiffness. The synovial membrane responds by producing an increased number of synovial villi and vascular hyperplasia in an attempt to resorb the blood. The synovium responds to the blood as an irritant, releasing enzymes that break down RBCs and the cell byproducts (e.g., iron). This process causes the synovium to become hypertrophied with formation of fingerlike projections of tissue extending onto the articular surface. The mechanical trauma of normal weight-bearing motion may then impinge and further injure the pathologic synovium. Iron in the form of hemosiderin is deposited in the synovium, which impairs the production of synovial fluid. A vicious cycle is established as the synovium attempts to cleanse the joint of blood and debris, becoming more hypertrophic and susceptible to still further bleeding.[2] Erosive damage of the cartilage follows these changes in the synovium with narrowing of the joint space (Fig. 13-11), erosions at the joint margins, and

subchondral cyst formation. Collapse of the joint, joint sclerosis, and eventual spontaneous ankylosis may occur.

In later stages of joint degeneration, chronic pain, severe loss of motion, muscle atrophy, crepitus, and joint deformities occur. Despite advances in medical management, target joints can progress to advanced arthropathy. This is most commonly seen in people with severe hemophilia. The articular cartilage softens, turns brown (due to hemosiderin), and becomes pitted and fragmented. The inflamed synovium is thick and highly vascularized and can grow over the joint surfaces becoming pannus. Eventually, lesions in the deeper layers of cartilage result in subchondral bone breakdown and the formation of subchondral cysts. Osteophyte formation occurs along the edges of the joint (Tables 13-9 and 13-10). With the destruction of the cartilage, little to no joint space is left. This bone-on-bone contact can lead to significant pain, limitation of motion, joint malalignment, muscle atrophy, functional impairment, and disability. At this point, joint bleeds are rare. For the child, recurrent bleeds into the same joint can lead to growth abnormalities. The epiphyses where bone growth takes place are stimulated to grow in the presence of hyperemia caused by bleeding. Postural asymmetries may develop (e.g., leg length differences, angulatory deformities, bony enlargement at the affected joint).[2]

TABLE 13-9

Arnold-Hilgartner Hemophilic Arthropathy Stages

Staging scheme to classify joint changes seen on x-ray:

I   No skeletal abnormalities; soft tissue swelling

II   Osteoporosis and overgrowth of epiphysis; no erosions; no narrowing of cartilage space

III   Early subchondral bone cysts, squaring of the patella; intercondylar notch of distal femur and humerus widened; cartilage space remains preserved

IV   Finding of stage III more advanced; cartilage space narrowed significantly; cartilage destruction

V   End stage; fibrous joint contracture, loss of joint cartilage space, marked enlargement of the epiphyses, and substantial disorganization of the joints

From Arnold WD, Hilgartner MW: Hemophilic arthropathy, *J Bone Joint Surg Am* 59:287-305, 1977.

TABLE 13-10

Petterson Radiologic Classification of Hemophilic Arthropathy

TYPE OF CHANGE	FINDING	SCORE*
Osteoporosis	Absent	0
	Present	1
Enlarged epiphysis	Absent	0
	Present	1
Irregular subchondral surface	Absent	0
	Slight	1
	Pronounced	2
Narrowing of joint space	Absent	0
	< 50%	1
	> 50%	2
Subchondral cyst formation	Absent	0
	1 Cyst	1
	>1 Cyst	2
Erosions at joint margins	Absent	0
	Present	1
Incongruence between joint surfaces	Absent	0
	Slight	1
	Pronounced	2
Joint deformity (angulation and/or displacement between articulating bones)	Absent	0
	Slight	1
	Pronounced	2

From Anderson A, Holtzman TS, Masley J: *Physical therapy in bleeding disorders*, New York, 2000, National Hemophilia Foundation.

*NOTE: Possible total joint score is 0-13 points.

A joint scoring system based on radiographic findings used to classify and monitor joint changes and damage.

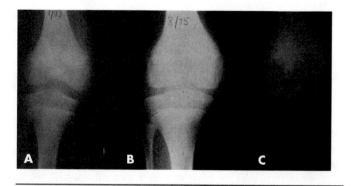

FIGURE **13-11** Stages of hemophilic arthropathy according to the Arnold-Hilgartner scale. **A,** Stage I (1973). **B,** Stage III (1975). **C,** Stage IV (1977). (Courtesy of Mountain States Regional Hemophilia Center, Colorado State Treatment Program, Denver, 1995.)

Muscle. Intramuscular hemorrhage that is visible in superficial areas such as the calf or forearm will also result in pain and limitation of motion of the affected part. Less obvious intramuscular hemorrhage such as occurs in the iliopsoas may result in groin pain, pain on extension of the hip, and reflexive flexion of the hip and thigh (see Figs. 15-10 and 15-11). Other signs and symptoms may include warmth, swelling, palpable hematoma, and neurologic signs such as numbness and tingling. A large iliopsoas hemorrhage can cause displacement of the kidney and ureter and can compress the neurovascular bundle including the femoral nerve with subsequent weakness; decreased sensation over the thigh and knee in the L2, -3, and -4 distribution; decreased or absent knee reflexes; temperature changes; and even permanent impairment. Iliopsoas bleeds are considered a medical emergency requiring immediate referral to a physician.

Nervous System. In general, compression of peripheral nerves and blood vessels by hematoma may result in severe pain, anesthesia of the innervated part, loss of perfusion, permanent nerve damage, and even paralysis. The femoral, ulnar, and median nerves are most commonly affected. CNS hemorrhage may include intracranial hemorrhage and rarely, intraspinal hemorrhage. Intracranial hemorrhages (ICH), or head bleeds inside the skull, in a newborn can occur regardless of the severity of hemophilia and may have long-term consequences such as paralysis, seizures, cerebral palsy, and other neurologic deficits. Although signs and symptoms of ICH may be dramatic (e.g., seizures or paralysis), often they are vague (e.g., crankiness or irritability, apnea or temporary cessation of breathing, tense and bulging fontanelle, lethargy, unequal size pupils, excessive vomiting, feeding difficulty) leading to a delay in diagnosis.

Inhibitors. Complications occur in 20% to 33% of people with moderately severe or severe factor VIII deficiency who develop inhibitors, or antibodies that destroy the infused factor. Inhibitors are much less frequent among people with hemophilia B or factor IX deficiency, affecting only 1% to 4%. The risk of developing an inhibitor does not remain the same during the lifetime of a person with hemophilia. Young children with severe hemophilia A are at the highest risk of inhibitor development after relatively few exposure days. Today's purification procedures provide factor concentrates that are safe in terms of inhibitor production and do not elicit higher rates of inhibitor production to either factor VIII or IX.

Medical Management

Diagnosis. Effective treatment of hemophilia is based on an accurate diagnosis of the deficient clotting factor and its level in the blood. Diagnosis is not always straightforward as a variety of factors can confound the test results (e.g., blood type, factor levels can be elevated by stress, hyperthyroidism, pregnancy and decreased in hypothyroidism). Additionally, cord blood sample at birth may have physiologically low levels of factor IX that only reach adult values by 3 to 6 months of age. Blood tests include assays for clotting factors, CBC (differential and platelets), and activated partial thromboplastin time (APTT). Other tests may be added depending on individual variables. It is also important for women in families of members with hemophilia to identify their carrier status through factor level analysis and DNA testing.

If possible, genetic studies to determine carrier status should be completed before pregnancy. However, prenatal diagnosis of hemophilia A and B is possible if a specific mutation has been found or if linkage studies have provided enough information about carrier status in the family. If one of these two criteria have been met, prenatal diagnosis can be performed through ultrasound at 14 to 16 weeks' gestation to determine the gender of the unborn child, or for 100% accurate diagnosis, chorionic villus sampling (CVS) at 10 to 11 weeks' pregnancy; amniocentesis at approximately 16 weeks' gestation; or percutaneous umbilical blood sampling (PUBS) at 18 weeks of pregnancy is required. The advantages and disadvantages of each test are reviewed in the literature.[37]

Treatment. Currently, no known cure or prenatal treatment for hemophilia exists. Gene therapy is still in experimental stages but appears very promising. When successful, gene therapy will deliver a normal (unaffected) copy of a gene into a target cell that contains a defective gene. Human trials are under way for hemophilia A and B using a variety of different delivery techniques. In fact, hemophilia is considered a model disease for treatment with gene therapy because it is caused by a single malfunctioning gene and only a small increase in clotting factor could provide a great benefit.

Until a medical cure is developed, primary goals for intervention in the case of bleeding episodes are to stop any bleeding that is occurring as quickly as possible and to infuse the missing factors until the bleeding stops. Treatment for severe forms of hemophilia is recommended to take place in specialized hemophilia treatment centers (HTCs) across the United States and its territories. In these centers, the specialized care required can be provided through a multidisciplinary team approach with appropriately trained and experienced health care providers. Treatment at an HTC has been shown to minimize disability, morbidity, and mortality.[12,71]

Factor replacement therapy, given intravenously, is currently the mainstay of hemophilia treatment. Treatment with infusion of the missing factor at a 40% to 50% level is recommended before minor surgery and dental extractions or in case of minor injury, and it may be recommended before physical or occupational therapy interventions. Infusion at 80% to 100% may be recommended before major surgery or in the case of head or abdominal trauma. Presently little or no data are available to direct the best intervention or management for women with bleeding disorders, and no consensus has been reached yet.

Permanent prophylaxis of recombinant factors for severe hemophilia (i.e., factor infusion given on a regularly scheduled basis) to maintain blood factor levels in the moderate range is widely accepted now. Standard treatment based on infusion of heat-treated factor VIII concentrates (human plasma-derived clotting factor) has now been replaced by administration of purified recombinant factor VIII products. Unlike human plasma-derived factors made from plasma pooled from thousands of donors, recombinant factor VIII is now derived from a nonhuman source. With recombinant factor, human viruses will not be easily transmitted through factor use, and the chance of any other contaminants being transmitted appears unlikely. Although the factor proteins themselves are not derived from human blood, all licensed recombinant factor VIII products contain albumin, which is derived from pooled human plasma, much the same way as plasma-derived factor products.[49] Product manufacturers are continuing to develop products with a higher recovery level and to increase the efficiency of the factor products (i.e., percent of factor protein that remains active in the blood after infusion; the higher the level of a factor product's recovery, the more efficient the product). The Food and Drug Administration (FDA) has approved an advanced recombinant, non–plasma-derived factor VIII product for the treatment of hemophilia A that does not contain albumin in its final formulation and that meets the criteria for safety, increased convenience, and increased efficacy.

Comprehensive medical management of hemophilia may involve the use of drugs to control pain in acute bleeding and chronic arthropathies. People with hemophilia cannot use the common pain reliever aspirin or any of its derivatives because these agents inhibit platelet function. More precisely, platelets do form an initial clot, but no factor VIII or IX is available to stabilize the clot. Some NSAIDs contain derivatives of aspirin and must be used cautiously. Corticosteroids are used occasionally for the treatment of chronic synovitis. Acetaminophen (Tylenol) is a suitable aspirin substitute for pain control, especially in children.

The treatment of chronic hepatitis (for those who received clotting factor before the mid-1980s) is a rapidly changing area of clinical practice. Treatment and prognosis for hepatitis are discussed in Chapter 16. Administration of hepatitis A vaccine (HAV) and hepatitis B vaccine (HBV) is recommended for anyone with chronic hepatitis C because of the potential for increased severity of acute hepatitis superimposed on existing liver disease. Younger children are now vaccinated against hepatitis A and B, but no vaccine is available for hepatitis C at this time. Liver transplantation is successful in people who have hemophilia with advanced liver disease but is often unavailable.

Physical therapy intervention (see Special Implications for the Therapist: Hemophilia, 13-15 in this chapter) has been effective in reducing the number of bleeding episodes through protective strengthening of the musculature surrounding affected joints, muscle reeducation, gait training, and client education. Physical therapy is used during episodes of acute hemorrhage to control pain and additional bleeding and to maintain positioning and prevent further deformity.

Prognosis.   Tremendous improvement has been made in carrier detection and prenatal diagnosis to provide early treatment and prevent complications. Gene therapy for hemophilia A and B, now in clinical trials, holds promise of a cure. Additionally, home infusion therapy provides immediate treatment with clotting factor for joint and muscle bleeds recognized early. Early treatment has significantly reduced the morbidity formerly associated with hemophilia.

Medical treatment prolongs life and improves quality of life associated with improved joint function, but HIV and hepatitis can significantly reduce longevity and quality of life. Fortunately, improvements in blood screening tests, more stringent donor exclusion criteria, improved viral inactivation methods, and the introduction of recombinant hemophilia therapies have combined to dramatically reduce the rate of new bloodborne viral infections among people with hemophilia, especially those children born in the last decade. However, since HIV was not isolated until 1984, approximately 9000 people with hemophilia (50% of all people with hemophilia) have become infected with HIV in the United

States, and another 2000 people who had hemophilia have already died of AIDS. Other virally transmitted diseases affecting people infused before 1984 include hepatitis B and C, cytomegalovirus (CMV), and EBV.

Special Implications for the Therapist   13-15

HEMOPHILIA

Preferred Practice Patterns:
4B: Impaired Posture (joint deformity)
4D: Impaired Joint Mobility, Motor Function, Muscle Performance, and Range of Motion Associated With Connective Tissue Dysfunction
5A: Primary Prevention/Risk Reduction for Loss of Balance and Falling
5C: Impaired Motor Function and Sensory Integrity Associated With Nonprogressive Disorders of the Central Nervous System: Congenital Origin or Acquired in Infancy or Childhood (CNS involvement)
5F: Impaired Peripheral Nerve Integrity and Muscle Performance Associated With Peripheral Nerve Injury (nerve compression)
6F: Impaired Ventilation and Respiration/Gas Exchange Associated With Respiratory Failure (coagulation defect)

Only a brief discussion of treatment for the adult or child with hemophilia can be included in this text. For a more detailed examination, evaluation, and interventions, the reader is referred to other more specific references.[2,11,50]

Hemophilia and Exercise

A regular exercise program, including appropriate sports activities and therapeutic strengthening and stretching exercises for affected extremities, is an important part of the comprehensive care of the individual with hemophilia. Exercise not only promotes physical wellness in the form of improved work capacity, it protects joints, enhances joint function, and is beneficial for decreasing the frequency of bleeds and has been shown to temporarily increase the levels of circulating clotting factor in individuals with a factor VIII deficiency.[52] Growing evidence suggests that exercise, coupled with a healthy diet, may boost the immune system of people with hemophilia who also have HIV and/or are living with hepatitis C.[82] The therapist can be very instrumental in helping the person with hemophilia to individualize an exercise or sports activity plan with specific but realistic goals and a schedule with alternating exercises (cross training).

An overall therapy program includes client education early on for family, client, school personnel, and coaches for prevention, conditioning, and wellness. Specific guidelines are available including all age levels from infants, toddlers, and preschoolers to adult, including sports safety information and the categorization of sports and activities by risk.[2,50] For older children and adolescents, selecting a sport with a good chance of success and adequate preparation (e.g., stretching and flexibility, conditioning including strength and weight training, endurance including an aerobic component, and possibly infusion before participation) for the sport is crucial. Although it is obvious that some bleeding may result from participation in a sport, fewer bleeding episodes occur when children engage in physical activities on a regular basis than when they are sedentary. When a particular sport or activity is often followed by bleeding, that activity should be reevaluated. A joint that requires multiple infusions to stop bleeding, remains symptomatic, or has persistent synovitis is not likely to withstand the stresses of a sport that relies on that joint.[50]

As orthopedic problems occur, a problem-oriented program is developed specific to the pathology. Generally, a therapy program includes exercises to strengthen muscles and improve coordination; methods to prevent and reduce deformity; methods to influence abnormal muscle tone and pathologic patterns of movement; techniques to decrease pain; functional training related to everyday activities; special techniques such as manual traction and mobilization; massage; and physiotechnical modalities such as cold, heat (including ultrasound), and electric modalities. Aquatic therapy is an excellent modality, especially for chronic arthropathy. The buoyancy of the water allows for ease of active movements across joints without the compressive force induced by gravity, thus decreasing pain. Water's density creates a resistive force to allow muscle strengthening, and the hydrostatic pressure can help reduce swelling.[2]

Specific Exercise Guidelines

The therapist and client must be alert to recognize any signs of early (first 24 to 48 hours) bleeding episodes (Table 13-11). Providing immediate factor replacement to stop the bleeding and following the RICE principle (Table 13-12) to promote comfort and healing are two goals for treating an acute joint (hemarthrosis) or muscle bleed (intramuscular hemorrhage). The joint range of motion can be measured during this acute episode in the pain-free range but should not be strength tested. Elastic wraps, splints, slings, and/or assistive devices may be necessary and a tolerance and/or weaning schedule established.[2] Initiation of exercise after a bleed must be delayed and rehabilitation progress is typically slower for individuals with factor VIII and factor IX deficiency who develop factor inhibitors. Prognosis for full return of function is diminished in such cases. In all cases of joint bleed, the use of heat is contraindicated; if used, hydrotherapy or aquatic intervention must be performed in comfortable but not hot temperatures to avoid blood vessel dilation.

When active bleeding stops, isometric muscle exercise should be initiated to prevent muscular atrophy. This exercise is especially critical with recurrent knee hemarthroses to prevent the visible atrophy of the quadriceps femoris muscle. As pain and edema diminish, the client should begin gentle active range-of-motion exercises followed by slowly progressing strengthening exercises when the joint is pain free through its full range. In the case of an iliopsoas bleed, when ambulation is resumed, crutches and toe touch weight bearing are initiated. Active movement should be performed in a pain-free range and progressed very slowly.[2]

For all muscles as the strengthening program is progressed, strengthening aids such as elastic bands or tubing and cuff weights can be used before transitioning to weight equipment. Preadolescents should avoid using high-weight lifting machines. Postbleed exercise should also take into consideration any damage that may have occurred to the joint, such as ligamentous or capsular stretching. Closed chain and other exercises to restore proprioception should be incorporated into the rehabilitation program.[2] As a prophylactic measure, clients with severe hemophilia generally need to infuse with clotting factor when participating in a strengthening program. With careful supervision and progression of the exercise program, the individual can progress to aerobic activities.

In some individuals, increased stress levels result in increased frequency of spontaneous bleeding. Biofeedback may be considered especially helpful for these clients who experience spontaneous bleeding during emotional upsets and periods of depression. Biofeedback can also be used for muscle retraining or relaxation techniques to control muscle spasm and allow range of motion.

Orthopedic/Surgical Interventions

At times, even with optimal infusion therapy and aggressive hemophilia care, a joint becomes a chronic problem. In such cases, orthopedic or surgical intervention may be indicated to alleviate pain and deformity and to restore the joint to a more functional state. This may include prescription for an orthosis or a splint or serial casting to increase range of motion.

Synovectomy (removal of the joint synovium) is recommended to stop a target joint from its cycle of bleeding. This pro-

Continued

TABLE	13-11

Clinical Signs and Symptoms of Hemophilia Bleeding Episodes

ACUTE HEMARTHROSIS	MUSCLE HEMORRHAGE	GASTROINTESTINAL INVOLVEMENT	CENTRAL NERVOUS SYSTEM INVOLVEMENT
Aura, tingling, or prickling sensation	Gradually intensifying pain	Abdominal pain and distention	Impaired judgment
Stiffening into the position of comfort (usually flexion)	Protective spasm of muscle	Melena (blood in stool)	Decreased visual and spatial awareness
Decreased range of motion	Limitation of movement at the surrounding joints	Hematemesis (vomiting blood)	Short-term memory deficits
Pain/tenderness	Muscle assumes a position of comfort (usually shortened)	Fever	Inappropriate behavior
Swelling	Loss of sensation	Low abdominal/groin pain due to bleeding into wall of large intestine or iliopsoas muscle	Motor deficits: spasticity, ataxia, abnormal gait, apraxia, decreased balance, loss of coordination
Protective muscle spasm		Hip flexion contracture due to spasm of the iliopsoas muscle secondary to retroperitoneal hemorrhage	
Increased warmth around joint			

Modified from Goodman CC, Snyder TE: *Differential diagnosis in physical therapy*, ed 3, Philadelphia, 2000, WB Saunders.

TABLE   **13-12**

Management of Joint and Muscle Bleeds

Joint: Acute Stage	Joint: Subacute Stage	Muscle
Factor replacement	Factor replacement (if indicated)	Factor replacement
R.I.C.E. (rest, ice, compression [applying pressure to the area for at least 10 to 15 minutes], and elevation [immobilization and elevating the body part above the heart level while applying the ice])	Progressive movement and exercises	R.I.C.E.
Pain-free movement	Wean splints and slings	Appropriate weight-bearing status; bed rest for iliopsoas bleed
Pain medication	Progressive weight-bearing	Progressive movement

Modified from Anderson A, Holtzman TS, Masley J: *Physical therapy in bleeding disorders*, New York, 2000, National Hemophilia Foundation.

cedure is not usually done to improve range of motion or to decrease pain, but rather to prevent further damage to the joint caused by bleeding. Arthroscopic synovectomy is best performed before joint degeneration has progressed beyond stage II on the Arnold-Hilgartner scale (see Table 13-9). Injection of a radioactive isotope (referred to as *isotopic synovectomy* or *synoviorthesis;* usually ^{32}P in the United States), which causes scarring to the synovium to arrest bleeding, is an alternate option. These procedures have unique advantages and disadvantages and may be more appropriate for one type of client than another.

Arthroplasty (joint replacement) is indicated when a joint shows end-stage damage and has become extremely painful. Client age, range of motion, and level of pain and function are determinants as to the timing of this procedure. Knees, hips, and shoulders are most commonly aided through arthroplasty with restoration of pain-free joint movement. *Arthrodesis* (joint fusion) may be performed in a joint with advanced, painful arthropathy untreatable by arthroplasty. Joint fusion can relieve or eliminate pain to provide improved quality of life, but it also causes permanent loss of joint motion. Arthrodesis can be a very effective way to provide the individual with a more stable base for weight-bearing activities.

Osteotomy (removal of a section of bone) may be done to correct angular deformities in a joint and may be considered before arthroplasty to reduce the stresses placed on a joint caused by poor alignment. Other less common interventions may include excision of a hemophilia pseudotumor or removal of cysts or exostoses.

The Person with Hemophilia and HIV. It is important for anyone with both these conditions to maintain optimal care of their musculoskeletal systems during and between bleeding episodes. It is especially important in the presence of chronic arthropathy and HIV or AIDS to maintain joint function through nonsurgical means, especially exercise. Surgery may be contraindicated if the risk of infection is too great (e.g., when the CD4 cell count is less than 200). Activities such as Tai Chi and yoga provide stretching; strengthening (including weight bearing); and a mild aerobic component. Aquatics or swimming must be approached with caution because of the potential for transmission of *cryptosporidiosis oocysts* that cause infection in immunocompromised individuals.[2] ■

ALTERATIONS IN SPLENIC FUNCTION

Most pathology of the spleen occurs as a result of disorders elsewhere in the body. When primary anatomic alterations cause splenomegaly (splenic enlargement), the underlying dysfunction may include splenic rupture (trauma); tumors; cysts; and vascular anomalies such as infarction (blockage) or aneurysm (dilation of blood vessel wall forming a sac). Hypersplenism, hyperactivity of the spleen, is the most common primary physiologic alteration. Hyposplenism, decreased function, may occur secondary to disease or removal of the spleen (splenectomy); congenital absence (asplenia) is rare.

◆ Splenomegaly
Etiologic Factors and Pathogenesis. The spleen's involvement in the lymphopoietic and mononuclear phagocyte systems predisposes it to multiple conditions causing splenomegaly. People of any age can be affected, but adults have a greater likelihood of developing any of the conditions associated with splenomegaly. The spleen may become enlarged by an increase in the number of cellular elements, by the deposition of extracellular material (as occurs in amyloidosis) or in the presence of extracellular hemopoiesis that accompanies reactive bone marrow disorders and neoplasm.

Splenic macrophages accumulate in chronic infections, hemolytic anemias, and storage diseases with a corresponding increase in the size of the spleen. Thickening of the arteries and central arterioles of the white pulp of the spleen occurs in SLE, and chronic passive congestion of the red pulp is common in people with portal hypertension due to cirrhosis, thrombosis of the portal or splenic veins, or right-sided heart failure. Congestive splenomegaly is characterized by slow passage of blood from the spleen and with more turbulence than when it enters.

Clinical Manifestations. A large palpable splenic mass in the left upper quadrant under the costal margin may be accompanied by pain during the acute phase of splenomegaly. The spleen is about a third the size of the liver and must be increased in size three times before it becomes palpable on examination. Other signs depend on the etiologic factors (e.g., ascites associated with cirrhosis, pallor with anemia, fever with infection). Lymphadenopathy (disease of the lymph nodes) often occurs with splenomegaly in association with any inflammatory or infectious condition.

Medical Management

Diagnosis, Treatment, and Prognosis.   Clinical diagnosis is based on history and physical examination, x-rays, ultrasound, or CT scan. Underlying hematologic disorder or infection may be confirmed with laboratory studies. Medical treatment depends on the underlying condition; a splenectomy may reverse anemia or other cytopenias (deficiency of any blood elements).

Special Implications for the Therapist   13-16

SPLENOMEGALY

Preferred Practice Patterns:
The therapist will consider the implications of splenomegaly during any planned intervention, but splenomegaly as a medical complication usually does not require the identification of practice pattern(s).

Because splenomegaly is often associated with conditions characterized by rapid destruction of blood cells, it is important to follow the usual precautions for anyone with poor clotting abilities (e.g., see Special Implications for the Therapist: The Anemias, 13-4). The client must be taught proper breathing techniques in conjunction with ways to avoid activities or positions that could traumatize the abdominal region or increase intracranial, intrathoracic, or intraabdominal pressure.

The person with a small or absent spleen is more susceptible to streptococcal infection, which calls for prevention techniques such as good handwashing (see Box 7-2 and Appendix A). ∎

REFERENCES

1. Ajmani RS, Rifkind JM: Hemorheological changes during human aging, *Gerontol* 44(2):111-120, 1998.
2. Anderson A, Holtzman TS, Masley J: *Physical therapy in bleeding disorders*, New York, 2000, National Hemophilia Foundation.
3. Barlogie B: High-dose therapy and innovative approaches to treatment of multiple myeloma, *Semin Hematol* 38(2)(Suppl 3):21-27, 2001.
4. Barnes L: Non-Hodgkin's lymphoma, *Rehabil Oncol* 18(2):14-16, 2000.
5. Beard J, Tobin B: Iron status and exercise, *Am J Clin Nutr* 72(Suppl 2):594S-597S, 2000.
6. Berenson JR et al: Zoledronic acid reduces skeletal-related events in patients with osteolytic metastases, *Cancer* 91(7):1191-1200, 2001.
7. Berenson JR, Sjak-Shie NN, Vescio RA: The role of human and viral cytokines in the pathogenesis of multiple myeloma, *Semin Cancer Biol* 10(5):383-391, 2000.
8. Biagi J et al: Primary Hodgkin's disease of the CNS in an immunocompetent patient: a case study and review of the literature, *Neuro-oncol* 2(4):239-243, 2000.
9. Braun-Moscovici Y et al: Methotrexate-treated arthritis and lymphoproliferative disease: coincidence only? *Clin Rheumatol* 20(1):80-82, 2001.
10. Butch AW, Kelly KA, Munchi NC: Dendritic cells derived from multiple myeloma patients efficiently internalize different classes of myeloma protein, *Exp Hematol* 29(1):85-92, 2001.
11. Buzzard B, Beeton K: *Physiotherapy management of hemophilia*, London, 2000, Blackwell Science.
12. Centers for Disease Control and Prevention: *White paper: recommendations for maintaining high quality care for persons with bleeding and clotting disorders*, Bethesda, Md, 2000, National Center for Infectious Disease.
13. Chaperot L et al: Differentiation of antigen-presenting cells (dendritic cells and macrophages) for therapeutic application in patients with lymphoma, *Leukemia* 14(9):1667-1677, 2001.
14. Dawson TM et al: Epstein-Barr virus, methotrexate, and lymphoma in patients with rheumatoid arthritis and primary Sjögren's syndrome: case series, *J Rheumatol* 28(1):47-53, 2001.
15. D'Cruz D: Autoimmune diseases associated with drugs, chemicals and environmental factors, *Toxicol Lett* 112-113:421-432, 2000.
16. Dean E: Oxygen transport deficits in systemic disease and implications for physical therapy, *Phys Ther* 77(2):187-202, 1997.
17. Diamond PT: Severe anemia: implications for functional recovery during rehabilitation, *Disabil Rehabil* 22(12):574-576, 2000.
18. Diel IJ, Solomayer EF, Bastert G: Biphosphonates and the prevention of metastasis: first evidences from preclinical and clinical studies, *Cancer* 88(Suppl 12):3080-3088, 2000.
19. Dilley A et al: von Willebrand disease and other inherited bleeding disorders in women with diagnosed menorrhagia, *Obstet Gynecol* 97(4):639, 2001.
20. Durstine JL et al: Physical activity for the chronically ill and disabled, *Sports Med* 30(3):207-219, 2000.
21. Dyall J et al: Lentivirus-transduced human monocyte-derived dendritic cells efficiently stimulate antigen-specific cytotoxic T lymphocytes, *Blood* 97(1):114-121, 2001.
22. Dybjer A et al: Seropositive polyarthritis and skin manifestations in T-prolymphocytic leukemia, *Leuk Lymphoma* 37(3-4):437-440, 2000.
23. Fenig E et al: Pregnancy and radiation, *Cancer Treat Rev* 27(1):1-7, 2001.
24. Flinn IW et al: Immunotherapy with rituximab during peripheral blood stem cell transplantation for non-Hodgkin's lymphoma, *Biol Blood Mar Transpl* 6(6):628-632, 2000.
25. Gorman K: Sickle cell disease, *Am J Nurs* 99(3):1-14, 1999. Available at: http://www.nursingcenter.com.
26. Greenlee RT et al: Cancer statistics, 2001, *CA Cancer J Clin* 51(1):15-36, 2001.
27. Greskovich JF, Macklis RM: Radiation therapy in pregnancy: risk calculation and risk minimization, *Semin Oncol* 27(6):633-645, 2000.
28. Hardell L et al: Some aspects of the etiology of non-Hodgkin's lymphoma, *Environ Health Perspect* 106(Suppl 2):679-681, 1998.
29. Harousseau JL: Leukemias induced by anticancer chemotherapies, *Bull Cancer* 86(11):929-938, 1999.
30. Hockey EG: *Personal communication*, Cleveland, Ohio, 2001, University Hospitals of Cleveland.
31. Hoppe CC, Walters MC: Bone marrow transplantation in sickle cell anemia, *Curr Opin Oncol* 13(2):85-90, 2001.
32. Horne G et al: Achieving pregnancy against the odds: successful implantation of frozen-thawed embryos generated by ICSI using spermatozoa banked prior to chemo/radiotherapy for Hodgkin's disease and acute leukemia, *Hum Reprod* 16(1):107-109, 2001.
33. Horwitz SM, Horning SJ: Advances in the treatment of Hodgkin's lymphoma, *Curr Opin Hematol* 7(4):235-240, 2000.
34. Izaks GJ, Westendorp RG, Knook DL: The definition of anemia in older persons, *JAMA* 281(18):1714-1717, 1999.
35. Kinney TR et al: Safety of hydroxyurea in children with sickle cell anemia: results of the HUG_KIDS Study, a phase I/II trial, *Blood* 94(5):1550-1554, 1999.
36. Klepfish A et al: Advanced Hodgkin's disease in a pregnant HIV seropositive woman: favorable mother and baby outcome following combined anticancer and antiretroviral therapy, *Am J Hematol* 63(1):57-58, 2000.
37. Koerner MA: Planning ahead: prenatal diagnosis of hemophilia A & B, *Hemaware Publication of the National Hemophilia Foundation*, January/February, 2000.
38. Kyle RA: Update on the treatment of multiple myeloma, *Oncologist* 6(2):119-124, 2001.
39. Lenahan SE et al: Transfusion-related acute lung injury secondary to biologically active mediators, *Arch Pathol Lab Med* 125(4):523-526, 2001.

40. Leukemia and Lymphoma Society: *About lymphoma and Hodgkin's disease; about leukemia,* 2000. Available at: http://www.leukemia-lymphoma.org/.

41. Levine AM: Acquired immunodeficiency syndrome-related lymphoma: clinical aspects, *Semin Oncol* 27(4):442-453, 2000.

42. Little RF et al: HIV-associated non-Hodgkin lymphoma: incidence, presentation, and prognosis, *JAMA* 285(14):1880-1885, 2001.

43. Mauro MJ, Druker BJ: Chronic myelogenous leukemia, *Curr Opin Oncol* 13(1):3-7, 2001.

44. Mauro MJ, Druker BJ: Sti571: a gene product-targeted therapy for leukemia, *Curr Oncol Rep* 3(3):223-227, 2001.

45. May C et al: Therapeutic haemoglobin synthesis in beta-thalassaemic mice expressing lentivirus-encoded human beta-globin, *Nature* 406(6791):82-86, 2000.

46. Migliazza A et al: Nuecleotide sequence, transcription map, and mutation analysis of the 13q14 chromosomal region deleted in B-cell chronic lymphocytic leukemia, *Blood* 97(7):2098-2104, 2001.

47. Morbidity and Mortality Weekly Report: Update: newborn screening for sickle cell disease, *MMWR* 49(32):729-731, 2000.

48. National Cancer Institute: Studies Document early success of STI-571, *J Natl Cancer Inst* 93(9):670, 2001.

49. National Hemophilia Foundation: *Bleeding disorders information,* 2001. Available at: http://www.hemophilia.org.

50. National Hemophilia Foundation: *Hemophilia, sports, and exercise,* New York, 1996, National Hemophilia Foundation.

51. National Hemophilia Foundation: Hepatitis updates, *Hemaware Publication of the National Hemophilia Foundation,* January/February 2000.

52. Nelson J: Hemophilia and exercise, *PT Magazine* 2:60-66, 1994.

53. Nicklas AH, Baker ME: Imaging strategies in the pregnant cancer patient, *Semin Oncol* 27(6):623-632, 2000.

54. O'Connor SR, Farmer PB, Lauder I: Benzene and non-Hodgkin's lymphoma, *J Pathol* 189(4):448-453, 1999.

55. Ogundipe O et al: Sickle cell disease and nitrous oxide-induced neuropathy, *Clin Lab Haematol* 21(6):409-412, 1999.

56. Oyono-Enguelle S et al: Cardiorespiratory and metabolic responses to exercise in HbSC sickle cell patients, *Med Sci Sports Exerc* 32(4):725-731, 2000.

57. Painter P et al: Low-functioning hemodialysis patients improve with exercise training, *Am J Kidney Dis* 36(3):600-608, 2000.

58. Palli D et al: Hodgkin's disease risk is increased in patients with ulcerative colitis, *Gastroenterol* 119(3):647-653, 2000.

59. Panepinto JA et al: Universal versus targeted screening of infants for sickle cell disease: a cost-effectiveness analysis, *J Pediatr* 136(2):201-208, 2000.

60. Pellett R: Sickle cell disease, *Rehabil Oncol* 18(2):10-13, 2000.

61. Persson B, Fredrickson M: Some risk factors for non-Hodgkin's lymphoma, *Int J Occup Med Environ Health* 12(2):135-142, 1999.

62. Pohlman B, Macklis RM: Lymphoma and pregnancy, *Semin Oncol* 27(6):657-666, 2000.

63. Popovsky MA: Transfusion-related acute lung injury, *Curr Opin Hematol* 7(6):402-407, 2000.

64. Ratner L et al: Chemotherapy for human immunodeficiency virus-associated non-Hodgkin's lymphoma in combination with highly active antiretroviral therapy, *J Clin Oncol* 19(8):2171-2178, 2001.

65. Rodon P et al: Multiple myeloma in elderly patients: presenting features and outcome, *Eur J Haematol* 66(1):11-17, 2001.

66. Sawka MN et al: Blood volume: importance and adaptations to exercise training, environmental stresses, and trauma/sickness, *Med Sci Sports Exerc* 32(2):332-348, 2000.

67. Schmidt, JL: *Personal communication,* Missoula, Mont, 2001, Community Physician Center.

68. Shaskey DJ, Green GA: Sports hematology, *Sports Med* 29(1):27-38, 2000.

69. Skinnider BF et al: Interleukin 13 and interleukin 13 receptor are frequently expressed by Hodgkin and Reed-Sternberg cells of Hodgkin lymphoma, *Blood* 97(1):250-255, 2001.

70. Sokolova Y: Acute shoulder pain and swelling in a 68-year-old man, *J Musc Med* 17(11):699-700, 2000.

71. Soucie JM et al: Mortality among males with hemophilia: relations with source of medical care. The Hemophilia Surveillance System Project Investigators, *Blood* 96(2):437-442, 2000.

72. Sullivan KJ et al: Nitric oxide successfully used to treat acute chest syndrome of sickle cell disease in a young adolescent, *Crit Care Med* 27(11):2563-2568, 1999.

73. Sultan SM, Ioannou Y, Isenberg DA: Is there an association of malignancy with systemic lupus erythematosus? An analysis of 276 patients under long-term review, *Rheumatol* (Oxford) 39(10):1147-52, 2000.

74. Takahashi R et al: A newly developed biphosphonate, YM529, is a potent apoptyosis inducer of human myeloma cells, *Leuk Res* 25(1):77-83, 2001.

75. ten Cate H: Pathophysiology of disseminated intravascular coagulation in sepsis, *Crit Care Med* 28(9 Suppl):S9-11, 2000.

76. Teruya-Feldstein J, Tosato G, Jaffe ES: The role of chemokines in Hodgkin's disease, *Leuk Lymphoma* 38(3-4):363-371, 2000.

77. Tesch H et al: Treatment of advanced stage Hodgkin's disease (German Hodgkin Study Group), *Oncology* 60(2):101-109, 2001.

78. Thomas VN: The role of cognitive-behavioral therapy in the management of pain in patients with sickle cell disease, *J Adv Nurs* 27:1002-1009, 1998.

79. Vichinsky EP et al: The perioperative complication rate of orthopedic surgery in sickle cell disease: report of the National Sickle Cell Surgery Study Group, *Am J Hematol* 62(3):129-138, 1999.

80. von Kempis J et al: Intravascular lymphoma presenting as symmetric polyarthritis, *Arthritis Rheum* 41(6):1126-1130, 1998.

81. Walters MC et al: Impact of bone marrow transplantation for symptomatic cell disease: an interim report, *Blood* 95(6):1918-1924, 2000.

82. Wang A, Frick N: HIV/AIDS updates: exercise may be even more beneficial than you think, *Hemaware Publication of the National Hemophilia Foundation,* New York, October, 2000.

83. Weiss MA: Novel treatment strategies in chronic lymphocytic leukemia, *Curr Oncol Rep* 3(3):217-222, 2001.

84. White CA, Weaver RL, Grillo-Lopez AJ: Antibody-targeted immunotherapy for treatment of malignancy, *Annu Rev Med* 52:125-145, 2001.

85. Williams J: *A guide for women and girls with bleeding disorders,* New York, 1998, National Hemophilia Foundation.

86. Wirthwein DP et al: Death due to microvascular occlusion in sickle-cell trait following physical exertion, *J Forensic Sci* 46(2):399-401, 2001.

87. Wolk A et al: A prospective study of obesity and cancer risk, *Cancer Causes Control* 12(1):13-21, 2001.

88. Wong O, Raabe GK: Non-Hodgkin's lymphoma and exposure to benzene in a multinational cohort of more than 308,000 petroleum workers, 1937 to 1996, *J Occup Environ Med* 42(5):554-568, 2000.

89. Yuille MR et al: Familial chronic lymphocytic leukemia: a survey and review of published studies, *Br J Haematol* 109(4):794-799, 2000.

CHAPTER 14

THE RESPIRATORY SYSTEM

CATHERINE C. GOODMAN

OVERVIEW

The respiratory system can be divided into three main portions: the upper airway, the lower airway, and the terminal alveoli (Fig. 14-1). The upper airway consists of the nasal cavities, sinuses, pharynx, tonsils, and larynx. The lower airway consists of the conducting airways, including the trachea, bronchi, and bronchioles (Fig. 14-2). The alveoli, or air sacs, at the end of the conducting airways in the lower respiratory tract are the primary lobules, sometimes called the *acini*, of the lung. The lungs are the major organs of respiration, providing gas exchange and thereby supplying the blood and body tissues with oxygen and disposing of waste carbon dioxide.

◆ Conditions Caused by Pulmonary Disease or Injury

Hypoxemia and pulmonary edema are two of the most common conditions caused by pulmonary disease or injury. *Hypoxemia*, deficient oxygenation of arterial blood, may lead to *hypoxia*, a broad term meaning diminished availability of oxygen to the body tissues. Hypoxemia is caused by respiratory alterations (Table 14-1), whereas hypoxia may occur anywhere in the body caused by alterations of other systems that have no relation to changes in the pulmonary system. Signs and symptoms of hypoxemia vary depending on the level of oxygenation in the blood (Table 14-2). Exercise testing may be performed to determine the degree of oxygen desaturation and/or hypoxemia that occurs on exertion. This testing requires analysis of arterial blood samples drawn with the subject at rest and at peak exercise. Continuous noninvasive measurement of arterial oxyhemoglobin saturation is usually determined by pulse oximetry.

Pulmonary edema, accumulation of fluid in the tissues and air spaces of the lung, is most commonly caused by heart disease, especially left ventricular failure, but it is also a complication of pulmonary disease and other systemic conditions. Pulmonary edema is discussed in detail later in the section on Parenchymal Disorders.

◆ Oxygen Transport Deficits in Systemic Disease

Although this chapter focuses on primary pulmonary impairment, pathologic conditions of every major organ system can have secondary effects on pulmonary (cardiovascular, cardiopulmonary) function and on the oxygen transport system. Such effects are of considerable clinical significance given

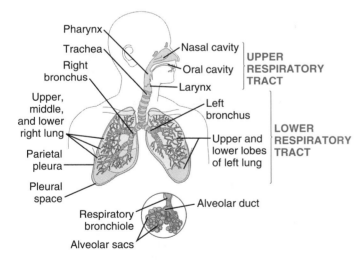

FIGURE 14-1 Structures of the upper and lower respiratory tracts. The upper respiratory tract consists of the nasal cavity, pharynx, and larynx; the lower respiratory tract includes the trachea, bronchi, and lungs. The circle shows the acinus, the terminal respiratory unit, which consists of the respiratory bronchioles, alveolar ducts, and alveolar sacs. This is the portion of the lungs where oxygen and carbon dioxide are exchanged.

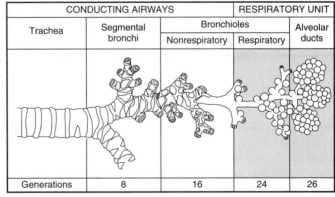

FIGURE 14-2 Structures of the lower airway. The first 16 generations of the airways branching in human lungs are purely conducting; transitional airways lead into the final respiratory zone consisting of alveoli where gas exchange takes place.

TABLE 14-1

Causes of Hypoxemia

MECHANISM	COMMON CLINICAL CAUSE
Ventilation/perfusion mismatch	Asthma
	Chronic bronchitis
	Pneumonia
Decreased oxygen content	High altitude
	Low oxygen content
	Enclosed breathing space (suffocation)
Hypoventilation	Lack of neurologic stimulation of the respiratory center
	Oversedation
	Drug overdose
	Neurologic damage
	Chronic obstructive pulmonary disease
Alveolocapillary diffusion abnormality	Emphysema
	Fibrosis
	Edema
Pulmonary shunting	Acute respiratory distress syndrome (ARDS)
	Hyaline membrane disease (ARDS in newborn)
	Atelectasis

Modified from McCance KL, Huether SE, editors: *Pathophysiology: the biologic basis for disease in adults and children*, ed 3, St Louis, 1998, Mosby—Year Book.

TABLE 14-2

Signs and Symptoms of Hypoxemia

Pao_2 (MM HG)	SIGNS AND SYMPTOMS
80-100	Normal
60-80	Moderate tachycardia, possible onset of respiratory distress, dyspnea on exertion
50-60	Malaise
	Light-headedness
	Nausea
	Vertigo
	Impaired judgment
	Incoordination
	Restlessness
35-50	Marked confusion
	Cardiac arrhythmias
	Labored respiration
25-35	Cardiac arrest
	Decreased renal blood flow
	Decreased urine output
	Lactic acidosis
	Lethargy
	Loss of consciousness
<25	Decreased minute ventilation* secondary to depression of the respiratory center

Modified from Frownfelter DL, Dean E: *Principles and practice of cardiopulmonary physical therapy*, ed 3, St Louis, 1996, Mosby–Year Book, p 237.
Pao_2, Partial pressure of arterial oxygen.
*The total expired volume of air per minute.

that they can be life-threatening and that therapy interventions usually stress the oxygen transport system even more. The resulting secondary effect may include a large range of pulmonary impairments, such as altered ventilation, perfusion, and ventilation/perfusion matching; reduced lung volumes, capacities, and flow rates; atelectasis; reduced surfactant production and distribution; impaired mucociliary transport; secretion accumulation; pulmonary aspiration; impaired lymphatic drainage; pulmonary edema; impaired coughing; respiratory muscle weakness or fatigue; and hypoxemia.[58]

The therapist must consider the possibility of secondary effects when assessing signs and symptoms of pulmonary disease in order to recognize the nature of the underlying etiologic factors. Making as specific a physical therapy diagnosis as possible enables the therapist to identify the most effective interventions in order to treat as specifically as possible.

◆ Signs and Symptoms of Pulmonary Disease

Pulmonary disease is often classified as acute or chronic, obstructive or restrictive, infectious or noninfectious, and is associated with many common signs and symptoms. The most common of these are cough and dyspnea. Other manifestations include chest pain, abnormal sputum, hemoptysis, cyanosis, digital clubbing, and altered breathing patterns (Box 14-1 and Table 14-3).

Cough. As a physiologic response, cough occurs frequently in healthy people, but a persistent dry cough may be caused by a tumor, congestion, or hypersensitive airways (allergies). A productive cough with purulent *sputum* may indicate infection, whereas a productive cough with nonpurulent sputum is nonspecific and just indicates irritation. *Hemoptysis* (coughing

BOX 14-1

Most Common Signs and Symptoms of Pulmonary Disease

Cough	Chest pain	Digital clubbing
Dyspnea	Hemoptysis	Altered breathing
Abnormal sputum	Cyanosis	patterns

and spitting blood) indicates a pathologic condition—infection, inflammation, abscess, tumor, or infarction.

Dyspnea. Shortness of breath (SOB; dyspnea) usually indicates inadequate ventilation or insufficient amounts of oxygen in the circulating blood. Dyspnea is usually caused by diffuse and extensive rather than focal pulmonary disease, pulmonary embolism being the exception. Factors contributing to the sensation of dyspnea include increased work of breathing (WOB), respiratory muscle fatigue, decreased breathing reserve, and strong emotions, particularly fear and anxiety. Dyspnea when the person is lying down is called *orthopnea* and is caused by redistribution of body water. Fluid shift leads to increased fluid in the lung, which leads to orthopnea. The abdominal contents also exert pressure on the diaphragm, decreasing the efficiency of the respiratory muscles.

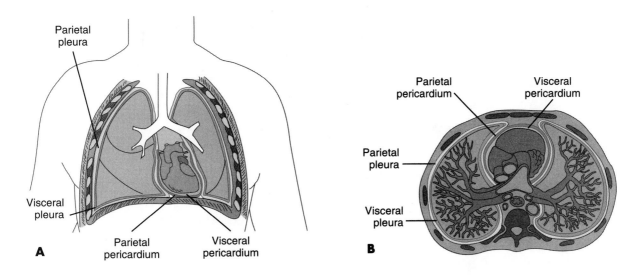

FIGURE   14-3   Chest cavity and associated structural linings shown in anterior, **A,** and cross-sectional, **B,** views. For instructional purposes the layers are depicted larger than actually found in the human body.

TABLE   **14-3**

Descriptions of Altered Breathing Patterns and Sounds

BREATHING PATTERN OR SOUND	DESCRIPTION
Apneustic	Gasping inspiration followed by short expiration
Biot's respiration (ataxia)	An irregular pattern of deep and shallow breaths; fast, deep breaths interspersed with abrupt pauses in breathing
Cheyne-Stokes respiration	Repeated cycle of deep breathing followed by shallow breaths or cessation of breathing
Hyperventilation	Abnormally prolonged and deep breathing
Hypoventilation	Reduction in the amount of air entering the pulmonary alveoli, which causes an increase in the arterial CO_2 level
Kussmaul's respiration	A distressing dyspnea characterized by increased respiratory rate (>20/min), increased depth of respiration, panting, and labored respiration typical or air hunger
Lateral-costal breathing	Chest becomes flattened anteriorly with excessive flaring of the lower ribs (supine position); minimal to no upper chest expansion or accessory muscle involvement with outward flaring of the lower rib cage instead; the person breathes into the lateral plane of respiration (gravity eliminated) because the weakened diaphragm and intercostal muscles cannot effectively oppose the force of gravity in the anterior plane; used to focus expansion in areas of the chest wall that have decreased expansion (e.g., spinal cord injury with atelectasis or pneumonia, asymmetric chest expansion with scoliosis)*
Paradoxical breathing (sometimes referred to as reverse breathing)	All or part of the chest wall falls in during inspiration; may be abdominal expansion during exhalation; can lead to a flattened anterior chest wall or pectus excavatum
Stridor	A shrill, harsh sound heard during inspiration in the presence of laryngeal obstruction
Wheezing	Breathing with a rasp or whistling sound resulting from constriction or obstruction of the throat, pharynx, trachea, or bronchi

*From Massery M: Personal communication, 2001.

Chest Pain.   Pulmonary pain patterns are usually localized in the substernal or chest region over involved lung fields, including the anterior aspect of the chest, side, or back. However, pulmonary pain can radiate to the neck, upper trapezius, costal margins, thoracic area of the back, scapulae, or shoulder. Shoulder pain caused by pulmonary involvement may radiate along the medial aspect of the arm mimicking other neuromuscular causes of neck or shoulder pain. Musculoskeletal causes of chest (wall) pain must be differentiated from pain of cardiac, pulmonary, epigastric, and breast origins.

Extensive disease may occur in the periphery of the lung without occurrence of pain until the process extends to the parietal pleura (Fig. 14-3). Pleural irritation then results in sharp, localized pain that is aggravated by any respiratory movement. Clients usually note that the pain is alleviated by

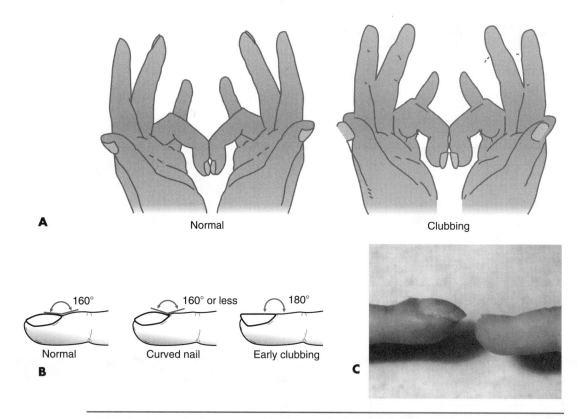

FIGURE **14-4** **A,** Assessment of clubbing by the Schamrath method. The client places the fingernails of opposite fingers together and holds them up to a light. If a diamond shape can be seen between the nails, there is no clubbing. **B,** The profile of the index finger is examined, and the angle of the nail base is noted; it should be about 160 degrees. The nail base is firm to palpation. Curved nails are a variation of normal with a convex profile and may look like clubbed nails, but the angle between the nail base and the nail is 160 degrees or less. In early clubbing, the angle straightens out to 180 degrees and the nail base feels spongy to palpation. **C,** Photograph of advanced clubbing of the finger (*left*) compared with normal finger (*right*). (From Swartz MH: *Textbook of physical diagnosis: history and examination*, Philadelphia, 1989, Saunders, plate IX [A].)

autosplinting, that is, lying on the affected side, which diminishes the movement of that side of the chest.[189,199]

Cyanosis. The presence of cyanosis, a bluish color of the skin and mucous membranes, depends on the oxygen saturation of arterial blood and the total amount of circulating hemoglobin. It is further differentiated as central or peripheral. Central cyanosis is best observed as a bluish discoloration in the oral mucous membranes, lips, and conjunctivae (i.e., the warmer, more central areas) and is most often associated with cardiac right-to-left shunts and pulmonary disease. Peripheral cyanosis is associated with decreased perfusion to the extremities, nail beds, and nose (i.e., the cooler, exposed areas) and is commonly caused by cold external temperature, anxiety, heart failure, or shock.

Clinically detectable cyanosis depends not only on oxygen saturation but also on the total amount of circulating hemoglobin that is bound to oxygen. Cyanosis can occur at varying levels of arterial oxygen saturation depending on the amount of circulating hemoglobin. For example, a child with severe anemia may not be cyanotic because all available hemoglobin is fully saturated with oxygen. However, a child with polycythemia may demonstrate signs of cyanosis because the overproduction of red blood cells (RBCs) results in increased

amounts of hemoglobin that are not fully saturated with oxygen. In some instances, however, such as in carbon monoxide poisoning, hemoglobin is bound with a substance other than oxygen. Cyanosis is not present since the hemoglobin is fully bound, but since the hemoglobin is not bound to oxygen, there is inadequate tissue oxygenation and potential tissue death. Arterial saturation in central cyanosis is usually decreased whereas arterial saturation may be normal in peripheral cyanosis. In the case of peripheral cyanosis, vasoconstriction with decreased blood supply rather than unsaturated blood is the underlying cause of symptoms.

Clubbing. Thickening and widening of the terminal phalanges of the fingers and toes result in a painless clublike appearance recognized by the loss of the angle between the nail and the nail bed (Fig. 14-4). Conditions that chronically interfere with tissue perfusion and nutrition may cause clubbing, including cystic fibrosis, lung cancer, bronchiectasis, pulmonary fibrosis, congenital heart disease, and lung abscess. Although 75% to 85% of clubbing is due to pulmonary disease and resultant hypoxia (diminished availability of blood to the body tissues), clubbing does not always indicate lung disease. It is sometimes present in heart disease and disorders of the liver and gastrointestinal tract.

TABLE	14-4

Breathing Patterns and Associated Conditions

HYPERVENTILATION	KUSSMAUL'S	CHEYNE-STOKES
Anxiety	Strenuous	Congestive heart
Acute head	exercise	failure
injury	Metabolic	Renal failure
Hypoxemia	acidosis	Meningitis
Fever		Drug overdose
		Increased in-
		tracranial
		pressure
		Infants (normal)
		Older people
		during sleep
		(normal)

HYPOVENTILATION	APNEUSTIC	BIOT'S (ATAXIA)
Fibromyalgia syndrome	Midpons lesion	Exercise
Chronic fatigue syndrome	Basilar artery	Shock
Sleep disorder	infarct	Cerebral hypoxia
Muscle fatigue		Heat stroke
Muscle weakness		Spinal meningitis
Malnutrition		Head injury
Neuromuscular disease		Brain abscess
Guillain-Barré		Encephalitis
Myasthenia gravis		
Poliomyelitis		
Amyotrophic lateral		
sclerosis (ALS)		
Pickwickian or obesity		
hypoventilation		
syndrome		
Severe kyphoscoliosis		

Altered Breathing Patterns.   Changes in the rate, depth, regularity, and effort of breathing occur in response to any condition affecting the pulmonary system (see Table 14-3). Breathing patterns can vary depending on the neuromuscular or neurologic disease or trauma (Table 14-4). In a large cross section of people and clinical disorders, hypoventilation is one of the most common changes in breathing patterns observed. Anything that can cause hypoxemia (e.g., fever, malnutrition, metabolic disturbance, decreased blood or oxygen supply) reduces energy supplies and results in respiratory muscle dysfunction and altered breathing patterns. When combined with skeletal muscle atonia associated with any neuromuscular cause, hypoventilation may further jeopardize the ventilatory pump.

Breathing pattern abnormalities seen with head trauma, brain abscess, diaphragmatic paralysis of chest wall muscles and thorax (e.g., generalized myopathy or neuropathy), heat stroke, spinal meningitis, and encephalitis can include *apneustic breathing, ataxic breathing,* or *Cheyne-Stokes respiration (CSR)*. Apneustic breathing localizes damage to the midpons and is most commonly due to a basilar artery infarct. Ataxic, or Biot's, breathing is caused by disruption of the respiratory rhythm generator in the medulla. CSR may be evident in the well older adult as well as in compromised clients. The most

common cause of CSR is severe congestive heart failure, but it can also occur with renal failure, meningitis, drug overdose, and increased intracranial pressure. It may be a normal breathing pattern in infants and older persons during sleep.

Spinal cord injuries above C3 result in loss of phrenic nerve innervation, necessitating a tracheostomy and ventilatory support.* Clients with generalized weakness, as in the Guillain-Barré syndrome, some myopathies or neuropathies, or incomplete spinal cord injuries, may show a tendency toward a specific breathing pattern called *lateral-costal breathing* (see Table 14-3).

---

*Throughout this chapter the term *ventilatory support* is used to refer to a variety of interventions, including mechanical ventilation via endotracheal intubation, noninvasive ventilatory support with continuous positive airway pressure (CPAP), positive end-expiratory pressure (PEEP), and bilevel positive airway pressure (BiPAP). See reference 75 for a complete description of the various means of ventilatory support.

Special Implications for the Therapist   14-1

SIGNS AND SYMPTOMS OF PULMONARY DISEASE

Many people with neuromusculoskeletal conditions as well as people with primary or secondary pulmonary impairments have the potential for oxygen transport deficits (and their sequelae discussed above), impaired ventilation, and altered breathing patterns. For each type of condition, the therapist must identify all the steps in the oxygen transport pathway that are affected so that intervention can be directed to the underlying problem as much as possible. Monitoring the cardiopulmonary status is important because many of the interventions provided by a therapist elicit an exercise stimulus and stress the oxygen transport system. Because impairment can result from diseases other than cardiopulmonary conditions, therapists in all settings need expertise in anticipating and detecting pulmonary dysfunction in the absence of primary pulmonary disease.[58] Recognizing abnormal responses to interventions is important in identifying the client who needs to be referred to another health care professional. For an excellent review of the oxygen transport deficits concept and more detailed implications by system, see reference 58.

Clinical observation of the client as he or she breathes is important (Table 14-5) and can alert the therapist to respiratory pathologic conditions. Assessment of the three muscle groups (abdominal and intercostal muscles and the diaphragm) involved in normal ventilatory function may be required. Enhancing motor performance and improving a client's functional level involve improving pulmonary potential. This can be accomplished using techniques to improve ventilation during therapy. The reader is referred to more specific texts for information about intervention techniques.[75,109]

High blood pressure in the pulmonary circulation (pulmonary hypertension) can cause pain during exercise that is often mistaken for cardiac pain (angina pectoris). For the therapist, musculoskeletal causes of chest pain must be differentiated from pain of cardiac, pulmonary, epigastric, and breast origins before treatment intervention begins.[94] The therapist involved in chest therapy and pulmonary rehabilitation must recognize precautions for and contraindications to therapy interventions in the medical client (Table 14-6). ■

TABLE 14-5

Clinical Inspection of the Respiratory System

Respiratory rate, depth, and effort of breathing
  Tachypnea
  Dyspnea
  Gasping respirations
Breathing pattern or sounds (see also Table 14-3)
  Cheyne-Stokes respiration
  Hyperventilation or hypoventilation
  Kussmaul's respiration
  Lateral-costal breathing
  Paradoxical breathing
  Prolonged expiration
  Pursed-lip breathing
  Wheezing
Cyanosis
Pallor or redness of skin during activity
Clubbing (toes, fingers)
Nicotine stains on fingers and hands
Retraction of intercostal, supraclavicular, or suprasternal spaces
Use of accessory muscles
Nasal flaring
Tracheal tug
Chest wall shape and deformity
  Barrel chest
  Pectus excavatum
  Pectus carinatum
  Kyphosis
  Scoliosis
Cough
Sputum: frothy; red-tinged, green, or yellow

AGING AND THE PULMONARY SYSTEM

Aging affects not only the physiologic functions of the lungs (ventilation, gas exchange) but also the ability of the respiratory system to defend itself. More than any other organ, the lung is susceptible to infectious processes and environmental and occupational pollutants (see the section on Environmental and Occupational Diseases in this chapter). These factors, combined with the normal aging process, contribute to the decline of lung function. Aging reduces the reserve capacity of virtually all pulmonary functions regardless of lifestyle although a sedentary lifestyle accelerates the decline in functional capacity.[136] Age-related alterations in the respiratory system are based on structural changes that lead to functional impairment of gas exchange.[230]

Reduction in diaphragmatic strength, decreased respiratory muscle strength and endurance, and subsequent increased work of breathing (WOB) requiring greater muscle oxygen consumption at any workload are observed with increasing age.[32] Many changes that occur with aging affect the lower airway, but in the upper airway the movement of the cilia slows and becomes less effective in sweeping away mucus and debris. This reduced ciliary action combined with the other changes noted predisposes the older client to increased respiratory infections.

Most adults attain maximal lung function (as measured by forced expiratory volume [FEV]) during their early 20s, but with

TABLE 14-6

Considerations for and Contraindications to Chest Therapy* in the Medical Client

CONSIDERATIONS	CONTRAINDICATIONS
Hemoptysis	Untreated tension pneumothorax; treat when chest tube has been inserted and client is stable
Fragile ribs (e.g., metastatic bone cancer, osteoporosis, flail chest, rib fractures, osteomyelitis of the ribs)	
Burns, open wounds, skin infections in thoracic area	Unstable cardiovascular system
Pulmonary edema, congestive heart failure	Hypotension
Large pleural effusion	Uncontrolled hypertension
Pulmonary embolism (controversial)†	Acute myocardial infarction
Symptomatic aneurysm or decrease in circulation of the main blood vessels	Arrhythmias
Platelet count between 20,000 and 50,000/mm³	Conditions prone to hemorrhage (platelet count <20,000/mm³ must have physician's approval)
Postoperatively	
Neurosurgery (positioning may cause increased intracranial pressure; can begin gentle breathing exercises)	
Esophageal anastomosis (gastric juices may affect suture line)	Unstabilized head and neck injury
Orthopedic clients who are limited in positioning	Intracranial pressure >20 mmHg
Recent spinal fusion	
Surgical complications (e.g., pericardial sac tear)	
Recent skin grafts or flaps	
Resected tumors (avoid tumor area)	
Recently placed pacemaker	
Older or nervous clients who become agitated or upset with therapy	
Acute spinal injury or recent spinal surgery, such as laminectomy (precaution: log-roll and position with care to maintain vertebral alignment)	

Modified from AARC clinical practice guideline: postural drainage therapy, *Respir Care* 36:1418-1426, 1991.
*Chest therapy refers to postural drainage including positioning and turning and may be accompanied by chest percussion and/or vibration.
†A question remains whether there may be a recurrence (repeat emboli in the medically unstable client, i.e., one whose blood level of anticoagulants is not yet adequate to prevent a possible second embolus from dislodging) with movement in positioning the client for postural drainage. However, allowing the client to lie still can contribute to the development of further venous stasis.

increasing age, especially after age 55 years, there is an overall decrease in the functional ability of the lungs to move air in and out. This decline peaks by age 75 years, falling to about 70% of our maximum. In the lower airways, symptomatic airway obstruction occurs especially in the presence of risk factors for chronic obstructive pulmonary disease (COPD). The lung tissue (parenchyma) changes in size and shape, becoming rounder with a loss of alveolar wall tissue and elastic tissue fibers in the alveolar walls. The reduced alveolar surface area and airways available for gas diffusion account for reduced lung function. The lung bases become less ventilated because of closing off of a number of airways. This increases the person's risk of dyspnea with exertion beyond the usual workload.

Respiratory muscle strength weakens in all people after age 40 years, and there is increased stiffness of the chest wall as the rib articulations and cartilage ossify and become less flexible. Other changes include the loss of elastic recoil of the lungs from a reduction of elastic fibers in the lung tissue, and alterations in gas exchange. All these changes contribute to the increased work of breathing, meaning that the older adult works harder for the same air exchange as the younger person. These changes are influenced by lifestyle and environmental factors, respiratory disease, and body size. The effects of age are not nearly as influential as the effects of smoking in causing a premature decline in lung function and in limiting the ability to exercise.

Pulmonary complications during anesthesia and the postoperative period are significantly increased in older adults with preexisting diseases. Loss of an effective cough reflex contributes to an increased susceptibility to pneumonia and postoperative atelectasis in the older population. Other contributing factors to the loss of an effective cough reflex include conditions more common in older age, such as reduced consciousness, use of sedatives, impaired esophageal motility, dysphagia, and neurologic diseases.

Special Implications for the Therapist   14-2

AGING AND THE PULMONARY SYSTEM

The therapist practicing in a geriatric setting needs to be knowledgeable about the normal consequences of aging to be able to identify the origin of and differences between impairments of aging and pathology. The ability to measure and discriminate between the process of aging and the sequelae of pathologic conditions (including consideration of the impact of comorbidities) is essential in the management of impairment and prevention of functional decline. Descriptions of the normal progressive decline of the respiratory system and the physiologic effects of pathologic conditions (both acute and chronic) as these conditions relate to the aging adult are available.[32,160] Appropriate test measures are available for this type of differential assessment.[100]

Pulmonary Capacity and Exercise

Although ventilatory and respiratory functions of older adults undergo a process of change related to aging that begins in early adulthood, it does not appear that healthy older people are limited by these changes in exercise capacity for activities that require moderate levels of VO_2. On the other hand, clients with obstructive lung disease have a significant loss of vital capacity and may experience shortness of breath at relatively low exercise intensities. In fact, the older person with obstructive lung disease may be limited in exercise by shortness of breath rather than by reduced cardiovascular capacity. The normal anatomic and physiologic changes associated with aging that reduce the

pulmonary reserve capacity of older adults combine with COPD pathology to exaggerate the pulmonary symptoms associated with aging.

Exercise capacity or exercise tolerance does decrease in the older adult as the Pao_2 (measure of oxygen in arterial blood) decreases. The level of habitual physical activity* is one factor favorably influencing O_2 delivery. The ability to deliver O_2 to the tissues is called maximal O_2 consumption, or VO_2 max. This measurement reflects the integration of three components of the delivery system that transports O_2 from the outside air to the working muscles: pulmonary ventilation, blood circulation, and muscle tissue. When the ventilation/perfusion imbalance is further compromised by age-associated reductions in cardiac output, the Pao_2 (and thus O_2 delivery) may be reduced even more.

Regular exercise can substantially slow the decline in maximal O_2 delivery caused by cardiovascular deconditioning related to age or lowered levels of habitual physical activity. Decreases in respiratory muscle strength and endurance occurring with age can be enhanced with exercise. Weight loss appears to alter static lung volumes, suggesting that some of the changes in lung function associated with aging may be due to the development of obesity and therefore modifiable with diet and exercise.[224] The total muscle mass decline with increasing age accounts for the age-related decrease in aerobic exercise capacity. A sedentary lifestyle is an additional key component to the reduced exercise capacity leading to deconditioning. This decrease in exercise capacity, whether caused by decline in muscle mass or decreased activity, can be slowed by exercise training. ■

INFECTIOUS AND INFLAMMATORY DISEASES

◆ Pneumonia

Overview and Etiologic Factors.   Pneumonia is an inflammation affecting the parenchyma of the lungs and can be caused by (1) a bacterial, viral, or mycoplasmal infection (organisms that have both viral and bacterial characteristics); (2) inhalation of toxic or caustic chemicals, smoke, dusts, or gases; or (3) aspiration of food, fluids, or vomitus. It may be primary or secondary, and it often follows influenza. The common feature of all types of pneumonia is an inflammatory pulmonary response to the offending organism or agent. This response may involve one or both lungs at the level of the lobe (lobar pneumonia) or more distally at the bronchioles and alveoli (bronchopneumonia).

Incidence.   Pneumonia is a commonly encountered disease with more than 1 million cases diagnosed each year, accounting for about 10% of admissions to adult medical services. It is a leading cause of death in the United States, claiming the lives of 40,000 Americans annually. Thirty percent of pneumonias are bacterial, especially prevalent in the older adult. Viral pneumonia, accounting for nearly one-half of all cases, is not usually life-threatening except in the immunocompromised person. The remaining 20% of all cases are caused by mycoplasma.

Risk Factors.   Infectious agents responsible for pneumonia are typically present in the upper respiratory tract and

---

*Daily physical activity can be assessed using the following categories: sedentary; sedentary with some daily activity; active through occupation or recreational activity; and trained athlete.

cause no harm unless resistance is lowered by some other factor. Many host conditions promote the growth of pathogenic organisms, but cigarette smoking (more than 20 cigarettes/day) is highly correlated with community-acquired pneumonia.[7] Pneumonia is also a frequent complication of acute respiratory infections, such as influenza and sinusitis. Other risk factors include chronic bronchitis, poorly controlled diabetes mellitus, uremia, dehydration, malnutrition, and prior existing critical illnesses, such as chronic renal failure, chronic lung disease, or acquired immunodeficiency syndrome (AIDS). In addition, the stress of hospitalization, confinement to an extended care facility or intensive care unit, surgery, tracheal intubation, treatment with antineoplastic chemotherapy or immunosuppressive drugs, and urinary incontinence promotes rapid colonization with pathogenic organisms.

Infants, older adults, people with profound disabilities or who are bedridden, and persons with altered consciousness (e.g., caused by alcoholic stupor, head injury, seizure disorder, drug overdose, general anesthesia) are most vulnerable. Inactivity and immobility causing pooling of normal secretions in the airways promote bacterial growth. People with severe periodontal disease, difficulty in swallowing, inability to take oral medications, or cough reflexes impaired by drugs, alcohol, or neuromuscular disease are at increased risk for the development of pneumonia as a result of aspiration.

Pathogenesis. Although a common disease, pneumonia is relatively rare in healthy people because of the effectiveness of the respiratory host defense system and the fact that healthy lungs are generally kept sterile below the first major bronchial divisions. In the compromised person, the normal release of biochemical mediators by alveolar macrophages as part of the inflammatory response does not eliminate invading pathogens. The multiplying microorganisms release damaging toxins stimulating full-scale inflammatory and immune responses with damaging side effects.

Endotoxins released by some microorganisms damage bronchial mucous and alveolocapillary membranes. Inflammation and edema cause the acini and terminal bronchioles to fill with infectious debris and exudate so that air cannot enter the alveoli, leading to ventilation/perfusion abnormalities and dyspnea. With the appearance of an inflammatory response, clinical illness usually occurs. Production of interleukin-1 (IL-1) and tumor necrosis factor by alveolar macrophages can contribute to many of the systemic effects of pneumonia, such as fever, chills, malaise, and myalgias (see Table 5-4).

Resolution of the infection with eventual healing occurs with successful containment of the pathogenic microorganisms. However, little is known about the actual processes that halt the acute inflammatory reaction in pneumonia and initiate recovery.

Aspiration Pneumonia. The risk of aspiration pneumonia occurs when anatomic defense mechanisms are impaired, such as occurs with seizures; depressed central nervous system (CNS); recurrent gastroesophageal reflux; neuromuscular disorders, especially with suck-swallow dysfunction; anatomic abnormalities (laryngeal cleft, tracheoesophageal fistula); and debilitating illnesses. Chronic aspiration often causes recurrent bouts of acute febrile pneumonia. Although any region may be affected, the right side, especially the right upper lobe

in the supine person, is commonly affected because of the anatomic configuration of the right main-stem bronchus.

Viral Pneumonia. Viral pneumonia is usually mild and self-limiting, often bilateral and panlobular but confined to the septa rather than the intraalveolar spaces as is more likely with bacterial pneumonia. Viral pneumonia can be a primary infection creating an ideal environment for a secondary bacterial infection, or it can be a complication of another viral illness, such as measles or chickenpox. The virus destroys ciliated epithelial cells and invades goblet cells and bronchial mucous glands. Bronchial walls become edematous and infiltrated with leukocytes. The destroyed bronchial epithelium sloughs throughout the respiratory tract, preventing mucociliary clearance.

Bacterial Pneumonia. Destruction of the respiratory epithelium by infection with the influenza virus may be one mechanism whereby influenza predisposes people to bacterial pneumonia. The lung parenchyma, especially the alveoli in the lower lobes, is the most common site of bacterial pneumonia. When bacteria reach the alveolar surfaces, most are rapidly ingested by phagocytes. Once phagocytosis has occurred, intracellular killing proceeds but at a slower rate for bacteria than for other particles. As the condition resolves, neutrophils degenerate and macrophages appear in the alveolar spaces, which ingest the fibrin threads, and the remaining bacteria in the respiratory bronchioles are then transported by lung lymphatics to regional lymph nodes. The infection is usually limited to one or two lobes.

Clinical Manifestations. Most cases of pneumonia are preceded by an upper respiratory infection, frequently viral. Signs and symptoms of pneumonia include sudden and sharp pleuritic chest pain aggravated by chest movement and accompanied by a hacking, productive cough with rust-colored or green, purulent sputum. Other symptoms include dyspnea, tachypnea accompanied by decreased chest excursion on the affected side, cyanosis, headache, fatigue, fever and chills, and generalized aches and myalgias that may extend to the thighs and calves. Older adults with bronchopneumonia have fewer symptoms than younger people, and 25% remain afebrile because of the changes in temperature regulation as part of the normal aging process. Associated changes in oxygenation may result in altered mental status (e.g., confusion) or loss of balance and subsequent falls as a result of the confusion.

Most cases of pneumonia are relatively mild and resolve within 1 to 2 weeks, although symptoms may linger for 1 or 2 more weeks (more typical of viral or mycoplasma pneumonia). If the infection develops slowly with a fever so low as to be unnoticeable the person may have what is referred to as "walking pneumonia." This form tends to last longer than any other form of pneumonia. Complications of pneumonia can include pleural effusion (fluid around the lung), empyema (pus in the pleural cavity), and more rarely, lung abscess.

Medical Management
Diagnosis. The clinical presentations of pneumonias caused by different pathogenic microorganisms overlap considerably, requiring microscopic examination of respiratory secretions in making a differential diagnosis. Gram stain,

color, odor, and cultures are part of the sputum analysis. A blood culture may help identify the bacteria, but bacterial counts are only positive in approximately 10% of bacterial pneumonias; 90% of bacterial pneumonias do not show a positive bacterial count. The U.S. Food and Drug Administration (FDA) has approved for marketing a simple, quick urine test (urinary antigen testing) for detecting *Streptococcus pneumoniae* that provides results in 15 minutes. Immediate test results allow specific treatment to begin right away thus controlling antibiotic overuse and antibiotic resistance with cost-effective targeted antibiotics. Results of the urine test should be confirmed with a culture. Research continues to develop new diagnostic techniques (e.g., polymerase chain reaction testing) to determine the microbiologic etiology of pneumonia.

Other diagnostic procedures may include chest films showing infiltrates that may involve a single lobe (lobar pneumonia from staphylococci) or may be more diffuse as in the case of bronchopneumonia (usually streptococci). Physical examination, including percussion and auscultation of the chest, may reveal signs of lung consolidation, such as dullness, inspiratory crackles, or bronchial breath sounds.

Treatment. The primary treatment for bacterial and mycoplasmic forms of pneumonia is antibiotic therapy along with rest and fluids. Treatment with specific antibiotics is based on the history and whether the pneumonia was community-acquired, hospital-acquired, or extended care facility–acquired and on the medical status and overall condition of the client (e.g., otherwise healthy or debilitated). Viral pneumonia is treated symptomatically unless secondary bacterial pneumonia develops. Hospitalization may be required for the immunocompromised client.

A vaccine is recommended for everyone age 65 years or older; for people with chronic disorders of the lungs, heart, liver, or kidneys; for individuals with poorly controlled diabetes mellitus; and for those with a compromised immune system or confined to a long-term care facility. Immunization can provide protection from pneumococcal disease for a period of 3 to 5 years in over 80% of vaccinated persons. A pneumococcal conjugate vaccine for routine use in infants and in high-risk children effective against invasive pneumococcal disease and to a lesser degree against otitis media and pneumonia has been licensed for use in the United States.[159,195] Because pneumonia is a common complication of the flu, the U.S. Centers for Disease Control and Protection (CDC) recommend annual flu vaccinations as well.

Prognosis. Community-acquired pneumonia remains a common and serious clinical problem despite the availability of potent antibiotics and aggressive supportive measures. It ranks sixth among the causes of death in the United States and currently accounts for almost 40% of hospital deaths. Ninety percent of those fatalities occur in people over age 65 years, largely owing to co-existing medical problems that weaken the immune system. Highly effective prevention and treatment methods can improve survival and reduce the likelihood of developing pneumonia, but one-half of older adults do not get vaccinations that could cut the death rate in one-half. The *Healthy People 2010* objective is to reduce hospitalization for immunization-preventable pneumonia to 8 per 10,000 in persons aged 65 years or older.

Special Implications for the Therapist **14-3**

PNEUMONIA

Preferred Practice Patterns:
6B: Impaired Aerobic Capacity/Endurance Associated With Deconditioning
6C: Impaired Ventilation, Respiration/Gas Exchange, and Aerobic Capacity/Endurance Associated With Airway Clearance Dysfunction
6F: Impaired Ventilation and Respiration/Gas Exchange Associated With Respiratory Failure

The Centers for Disease Control and Prevention (CDC) recommend adherence to Standard Precautions for clients with pneumonia. At the very least, careful hand washing by all personnel involved is essential for reducing the transmission of infectious agents. Adequate hydration and pulmonary hygiene, including deep breathing, coughing, and chest therapy, should be instituted in all clients hospitalized with pneumonia. Ventilatory support and supplemental oxygen may be needed to maintain adequate gas exchange in severely compromised clients. Preventive measures are important and include early ambulation in postoperative clients and postpartal women unless contraindicated. Proper positioning to prevent aspiration during the postoperative period and for all people who are immobilized or who have a poor gag reflex is important.

Occasionally, a lower lobe infection can irritate the diaphragmatic surface so that pain referred to the shoulder is the presenting symptom. For the client with a known diagnosis of pneumonia, the breathing pattern and the position assumed in bed can indicate the client's discomfort, reveal tachypnea, and demonstrate splinting of the chest to minimize pleuritic pain (i.e., lying on the affected side reduces the pleural rubbing that often causes discomfort).

Lobes affected by pneumonia will remain vulnerable to further infection for some time, especially in the bedridden, debilitated, or neuromuscularly compromised population. Chest physical therapy is not usually helpful in adults with uncomplicated pneumonias. However, the client, family, or caretakers should be instructed in breathing exercises and a positional rotation program with frequent positional changes to prevent secretions from accumulating in dependent positions and to optimize ventilation/perfusion matching. ■

◆ Pneumocystis Carinii Pneumonia

Definition and Incidence. *Pneumocystis carinii* pneumonia (PCP) is a progressive, often fatal pneumonia and represents the most frequently occurring opportunistic infection in persons with AIDS. Previously, the majority of people with AIDS developed PCP during the course of their illness, but this is much less common now with pharmacologic prophylaxis. PCP has been shown to be the first indicator of conversion from human immunodeficiency virus (HIV) infection to the designation of AIDS in 60% of cases.

Etiologic and Risk Factors. The origin of the organism is unknown. It is possibly acquired from the environment; infected humans; or animals, fungi, or protozoa. Other people at risk for the development of PCP include anyone who is immunosuppressed for organ transplantation, by chemotherapy for lymphoma or leukemia, by steroid therapy, or by malnutrition.

Pathogenesis and Clinical Manifestations.　　Infection begins with the attachment of the *Pneumocystis* trophozoite (the feeding stage of a sporozoan parasite) to the alveolar lining cell. The trophozoite feeds on the host cell, enlarges, and transforms into the cyst form that ruptures to release new trophozoites, repeating the cycle. If the process is uninterrupted by the immune system or antibiotic therapy, the affected alveoli progressively fill with organisms and proteinaceous fluid until consolidation disrupts gas exchange, slowly suffocating the person. The physiologic response to PCP includes fever, impaired gas exchange, and altered respiratory function. Symptoms of PCP develop slowly and present as fever and progressive dyspnea, accompanied by a nonproductive cough. Fatigue, tachypnea, weight loss, and other manifestations of underlying immunosuppressive disease may be present.

Medical Management
Diagnosis, Treatment, and Prognosis.　　Molecular techniques in the laboratory play an essential role in the microbiologic diagnosis of pneumonia in the immunocompromised person. Other diagnostic tools may include fiberoptic bronchoscopy to obtain respiratory specimens for testing and chest radiograph. Diagnosis is important because effective pharmacologic treatment is available.

Thanks to a worldwide collaborative effort among health care providers, academia, governments, and industry our knowledge about and treatment of infection caused by HIV have evolved from palliative care to the use of a chronic disease model where survival is measured by decades, not months or years.[108] Although pulmonary disease remains a major problem for people with HIV, prophylaxis against opportunistic infection in people with HIV has cut morbidity and mortality rates by 80%.[15] The increasing seroprevalence of HIV among women of reproductive age, the risks of vertical transmission of HIV, and the fact that PCP is the most common infection seen in people progressing to AIDS have led to recommendations for routine prenatal HIV infection counseling and testing.

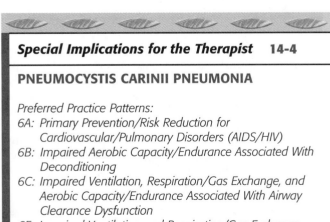

Special Implications for the Therapist　　**14-4**

PNEUMOCYSTIS CARINII PNEUMONIA

Preferred Practice Patterns:
6A: Primary Prevention/Risk Reduction for Cardiovascular/Pulmonary Disorders (AIDS/HIV)
6B: Impaired Aerobic Capacity/Endurance Associated With Deconditioning
6C: Impaired Ventilation, Respiration/Gas Exchange, and Aerobic Capacity/Endurance Associated With Airway Clearance Dysfunction
6F: Impaired Ventilation and Respiration/Gas Exchange Associated With Respiratory Failure

Carefully adhere to Standard Precautions to prevent contagion. Teach the client energy conservation techniques (see Box 8-2) as well as deep-breathing exercises. Expiratory air-flow reductions that persist after the acute infection resolves have been documented in cases of PCP (and bacterial pneumonia) in HIV-infected individuals. The clinical implications of these changes are unknown but may contribute to prolonged respiratory complaints and compromise in HIV-infected individuals who have had PCP.[156] See also Special Implications for the Therapist: Pneumonia, 14-3. ∎

◆ Pulmonary Tuberculosis
Definition.　　Tuberculosis (TB, formerly known as consumption) is an infectious, inflammatory systemic disease that affects the lungs and may disseminate to involve lymph nodes and other organs. It is caused by infection with *Mycobacterium tuberculosis* and is characterized by granulomas, caseous (resembling cheese) necrosis, and subsequent cavity formation. Latent infection is defined as harboring *Mycobacterium tuberculosis* without evidence of active infection; active infection is based on the presence of clinical and laboratory findings.

Overview.　　TB may be primary or secondary. The first or primary infection with the tubercle bacillus is usually asymptomatic and almost always (99%) remains quiet after the development of a hypersensitivity to the microorganism. The primary infection usually involves the middle or lower lung area with lesions consisting of exudation in the lung parenchyma. These lesions quickly become caseous and spread to the bronchopulmonary lymph nodes, where they gain access to the bloodstream and predispose the person to the subsequent development of chronic pulmonary and extrapulmonary TB at a later time.

Secondary TB develops as a result of either endogenous or exogenous reinfection by the tubercle bacillus. This is the most common form of clinical TB. Reactivated TB usually causes abnormalities in the upper lobes of one or both lungs. In the United States, development of secondary TB is almost always the result of endogenous reinfection that occurs when the primary lesion becomes active as a result of debilitation or lowered resistance.

Incidence.　　Despite improved methods of detection and treatment, TB remains a global health problem with the highest rates in Southeast Asia, sub-Saharan Africa, and eastern Europe. Before the development of anti-TB drugs in the late 1940s, TB was the leading cause of death in the United States. Drug therapy, along with improvements in public health and general living standards, resulted in a marked decline in incidence. However, recent influxes of immigrants from developing Third World nations, rising homeless populations, prolonged life span, and the emergence of HIV led to an increase in reported cases in the mid-1980s, reversing a 40-year period of decline. Overall, between 1985 and 1992 there was a 20% increase in new TB cases in the United States. Now, after years of rising TB infection rates, the United States has started to see a decrease in the annual number of cases (current incidence is 6.8 cases per 100,000 U.S-born individuals).[64, 154] However, the incidence of TB among foreign-born persons in the United States including the number of cases of multidrug-resistant TB has continued to rise annually, and there remains a huge reservoir of individuals who are infected.[205]

Multidrug-resistant TB has emerged as a major infectious disease problem throughout the world. The infected individual begins taking the prescribed medication, feels better, and discontinues taking the drugs normally required to be taken 6 to 9 months. The disease flares back up months later and is now resistant to the medications, and the person passes it along as a new drug-resistant strain characterized by mutations in existing genes.[74] The AIDS pandemic, the increased incidence of TB in populations without easy access to anti-TB medications (e.g., homeless people, economically disadvantaged people), the deterioration of the public health infrastructure, interruptions in the drug supply, and inadequate training of health care providers in the epidemiology of TB are some factors contributing to the increased incidence of multidrug-resistant TB.

Risk Factors.   Although TB can affect anyone, certain segments of the population have an increased risk of contracting the disease, particularly those with HIV infection and people age 65 years and older. The latter constitute nearly one-half of the newly diagnosed cases of TB in the United States and most cases of reactivation of dormant mycobacteria. Other groups at risk include (1) economically disadvantaged or homeless people living in overcrowded conditions, frequently ethnic groups, such as Hispanics, Native Americans, and Asian/Pacific Islanders; (2) immigrants from Southeast Asia, Ethiopia, Eastern Europe, Mexico, and Latin America*; (3) clients dependent on injection drugs, alcohol, or other drugs associated with malnutrition, debilitation, and poor health; (4) infants and children under the age of 5 years; (5) current or past prison inmates; (6) people with diabetes mellitus; (7) people with end-stage renal disease; and (8) others who are immunocompromised (not only those who are HIV infected but also those who are malnourished, organ transplant recipients, anyone receiving cancer chemotherapy or prolonged corticosteroid therapy). Limited access to health care because of socioeconomic status or illegal alien status and sociocultural differences contribute to delays in seeking care and influence adherence to treatment, contributing to the rise in TB among ethnic groups, especially along the U.S.-Mexican border.[154]

Risk associated with processing contaminated medical waste has been reported,[123] and the first documented case of cadaver-to-embalmer (mortician) TB has occurred, possibly by exposure to infectious aerosols generated during the aspiration of blood and other body fluids from the cadaver.[201] Staff members of laboratories and necropsy rooms are estimated to be between 100 and 200 times more likely than the general public to develop TB by the inhalation of the bacilli in aerosols or dried material, by injuries (e.g., cuts and accidental inoculations with infected instruments), and by contact with infected materials and surfaces. Necropsies on individuals with undiagnosed TB in life present a potential hazard to pathologists, technicians, and medical students involved in postmortem examinations.[54]

Environmental factors that enhance transmission include contact between susceptible persons and an infectious person in relatively small, enclosed spaces (e.g., evidence of limited transmission during extended airline, train, or bus travel has been documented)[131,155]; inadequate ventilation that results in insufficient dilution or removal of infectious droplet nuclei (e.g., older buildings such as hospitals, prisons, government buildings, universities); and recirculation of air containing infectious droplet nuclei. Adequate ventilation is the most important measure to reduce the infectiousness of the environment. Mycobacteria are susceptible to ultraviolet irradiation (i.e., sunshine), so outdoor transmission of infection rarely occurs.

Etiologic Factors.   The causative agent is the tubercle bacillus (Fig. 14-5), commonly transmitted in the United States by inhalation of infected airborne particles, known as droplet nuclei, which are produced when the infected persons sneeze, laugh, speak, sing, or cough. Casual contact or brief exposure to a few bacilli will not result in transmission of sufficient bacilli to infect a person. Rather, household contact of many months is required for transmission. Genetic factors determining susceptibility and resistance to the infection are suspected but have not been proven. In some other parts of the world, bovine TB carried by unpasteurized milk and other dairy products from tuberculous cattle is more prevalent.

The tubercle bacillus is capable of surviving for months in sputum that is not exposed to sunlight. Within the body it can lie dormant for decades and then become reactivated years after an initial infection. This secondary TB infection (endogenous reinfection) can occur at any time the person's resistance is lowered (e.g., alcoholism, immunosuppression, silicosis, advancing age, cancer). The older people of today were children when transmission of tubercle bacilli occurred more often. Now reactivation of the disease is developing in their later years with an increasing portion of older adults who have never been infected acquiring new infections in extended care facilities.

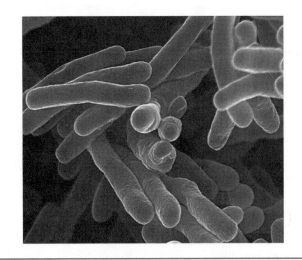

FIGURE   **14-5**   Tuberculosis bacteria. (Courtesy National Institute of Allergy and Infectious Diseases, National Institutes of Health, Bethesda, Md, 2001.)

---

*The Institute of Medicine (IOM) estimates that more than one-half of all TB cases in the United States will soon be attributable to foreign-born residents. The IOM has published a report calling for TB screening of all U.S. immigrants to prevent a predicted resurgence of the disease in the United States.[117]

Pathogenesis.   Once a susceptible person inhales droplet nuclei containing M. *tuberculosis* and bacilli become established in the alveoli of the lungs, a proliferation of epithelial cells surrounds and encapsulates the multiplying bacilli in an attempt to wall off the invading organisms, thus forming a typical tubercle. Two to ten weeks after initial human infection with the bacilli, acquired cell-mediated immunity usually limits further multiplication and spread of the TB bacilli.

No one yet knows how the TB bacterium does its damage. M. *tuberculosis* has no known endotoxins or exotoxins so there is no immediate host response to the infection. The organisms grow for 2 to 12 weeks until they reach a number sufficient to elicit a cellular immune response that can be detected by a reaction to the tuberculin skin test.

The organisms tend to be localized or focused at sites of infection. In persons with intact cell-mediated immunity, collections of activated T cells and macrophages form granulomas that limit multiplication and spread of the organism rendering the infection inactive, or *latent*. For the majority of individuals with an intact immune system, latent infection is clinically and radiographically undetected; a positive tuberculin skin test result is the only indication that infection has taken place. Individuals with latent TB infection but not active disease are not infectious and cannot transmit the organism. When residual lesions are visible on chest radiograph these sites remain potential lesions for reactivation.

If, however, the infection is not controlled by the immune defenses, the person develops symptoms of progressive primary TB. The granulomas become necrotic in the center and eventually produce fibrosis and calcification of the tissues. Tubercle bacilli can spread to other parts of the body by way of the lymphatics to the hilar lymph nodes and then through the bloodstream to more distant sites, producing a condition called *miliary* (evenly distributed small nodules) *tuberculosis*, most common in people 50 years or older and in very young children with unstable or underdeveloped immune systems. Erosion of blood vessels by the primary lesion can cause a large number of bacilli to enter the circulatory system, where they are carried to all areas of the body and may lodge in any organ, especially the kidneys, bone growth plates, lymph nodes, and meninges. Untreated, these tiny lesions spread and produce large areas of infection (e.g., TB pneumonia, tubercular meningitis).

Researchers have recently identified a segment of deoxyribonucleic acid (DNA) that allows the TB organism to invade macrophages, where they lie dormant for years before leaving the macrophage cells to invade the lungs or other parts of the body. Finding this genetic fragment may provide information needed to block the microorganisms from entering human cells. The DNA fingerprint identified probably represents only one of several mechanisms that permit the TB transmission and invasion.[105]

Clinical Manifestations.   Most symptoms associated with

TB do not appear in the early, most curable stage of the disease, but a skin test administered would be positive. Often symptoms are delayed until 1 year or more after initial exposure to the bacilli. Symptoms suggestive of TB include productive cough of more than 3 weeks' duration, especially when accompanied by other symptoms such as weight loss, fever, night sweats, fatigue, malaise, and anorexia. Rales may be heard in the area of lung involvement as well as bronchial breath sounds if there is lung consolidation.

Complications associated with TB can include bronchopleural fistulae, esophagopleural fistulae, pleurisy with effusion, tuberculous pneumonia or laryngitis, and sudden lung atelectasis indicating that a deep tuberculous cavity in the lung has perforated or created an opening into the pleural cavity, allowing air and infected material to flow to it. Extrapulmonary involvement (e.g., abdominal, pericardial, genitourinary, lymph node, central nervous system, or skeletal TB) increases in frequency in the presence of declining immunocompetency. Extrapulmonary TB occurs alone (i.e., without pulmonary involvement) in one-third of HIV-infected persons and in another one-third of HIV-infected persons with pulmonary involvement.[12]

Tuberculous involvement of the brain and spinal cord (extrapulmonary TB) is a common neurologic disorder in developing countries and has recently shown resurgence when associated with HIV. In tuberculous meningitis the process is located primarily at the base of the brain, and symptoms include those related to cranial nerve involvement as well as headache, decreased level of consciousness, and neck stiffness. Tuberculous meningitis is associated with high morbidity and mortality. Tuberculous spondylitis (Pott's disease), a rare complication of extrapulmonary TB, is discussed in Chapter 24.

Medical Management

Prevention.   Preventing the transmission of tuberculosis is essential by using such simple measures as covering the mouth and nose with a tissue when coughing and sneezing, reducing the number of organisms excreted into the air. However, preventive and therapeutic interventions must address not only the bacillus but also the financial, nutritional, and employment status of those people at risk. Adequate room ventilation and preventing overcrowding such as in homeless shelters and prisons are well-known preventive measures, but the complications of preventing this infection in many high-risk groups are considerable. For example, should control efforts among the poor emphasize the amelioration of social problems or merely the ingestion of appropriate antibiotics? Involuntary isolation is no longer acceptable, and directly observed therapy (i.e., the client receives the antibiotics under the supervision of an outreach worker) may be a violation of civil rights. How are individuals' civil liberties and the public health best balanced? How should health professionals address the problem of the noncompliant individual? The complex issues surrounding TB in the United States remain an unresolved challenge at this time.*

The term *preventive drug therapy* has been changed to *treatment of latent TB infection (LTBI)*. The failure of vaccination with BCG (bacille Calmette-Guérin), a freeze-dried preparation of a live, attenuated strain of *Mycobacterium bovi*, to control the global TB epidemic and the spread of multidrug resistance has resulted in renewed research efforts to develop a better vaccine. Recent advances in molecular microbiology, gene therapy, and immunobiology with the complete sequencing of the M. *tuberculosis* genome marked a turning point in TB vaccine research.[61,62]

---

*For an interesting and insightful look at these and other issues related to TB, the reader is referred to Lerner BH: *Contagion and confinement: controlling tuberculosis along the skid row*, Baltimore, 1998, Johns Hopkins University Press..

Diagnosis.   Recent advances in molecular techniques for the diagnosis of TB have improved the accuracy and speed of laboratory diagnosis in symptomatic people. Fortunately, some of these improved tools are appropriate for low-income settings and may help integrate new diagnostic tools into national TB control programs.[173] Diagnostic measures for identifying TB currently include history, physical examination, tuberculin skin test, chest radiograph, and microscopic examination and culture of sputum. The tuberculin skin test determines whether the body's immune response has been activated by the presence of the bacillus. The skin and other tissue become sensitized to the protein part of the tubercle bacilli. A positive reaction causes a swelling or hardness at the site of infection and develops 3 to 10 weeks after the initial infection. A positive skin test reaction indicates the presence of a TB infection but does not show whether the infection is dormant or is causing a clinical illness. Other diagnostic methods, such as bronchoscopy or biopsy, may be indicated in some cases.

Because of the dormant properties of the tubercle bacillus, anyone infected with TB should have periodic TB testing performed. In the case of someone with known TB, the skin test will always be positive, requiring periodic screening* with chest x-ray studies. The tuberculin skin test is the only method currently available that demonstrates infection with *M. tuberculosis* in the absence of active TB, although newer methods are under development.[51] The future direction of research to improve current diagnostic tests is based on the identification of the *M. tuberculosis* genome (described in 1998), developing highly specific diagnostic reagents, and the production of new vaccines.[13]

Treatment.   The American Thoracic Society and the Centers for Disease Control and Prevention[12] have published guidelines for the treatment of TB infection. These guidelines should contribute to improved TB control worldwide and to TB elimination in the United States.[49] Once diagnosed, all cases of active disease are treated, and certain cases of inactive disease are treated prophylactically. Treatment may be initiated with only a positive skin test even if chest film and sputum analyses show no evidence of the disease. In this way, the disease is less likely to reactivate later in life when the immune system is more likely to be compromised.

Pharmacologic treatment through medication is the primary treatment of choice and renders the infection noncontagious and nonsymptomatic. These agents work by inhibiting cell wall biosynthesis, but the intracellular response that occurs is complex and poorly understood at this time. New drug treatments now include combinations of all primary anti-TB medications (e.g., rifampin; isoniazid; pyrazinamide [Rifater], ethambutol) taken in one dose to replace the traditional treatment requiring multiple drugs daily. Treatment is problematic with homeless people and people who abuse alcohol and use injection drugs because this population is often noncompliant with the recommended 6- to 9-month treatment regimen. Multidrug-resistant TB has further complicated treatment. Treatment of resistant mycobacteria or the complications of TB frequently requires pneumonectomy.

Chemotherapy using a variety of chemical agents may be used, and often two or more drugs are used simultaneously to prevent the emergence of drug-resistant mutants. Immune amplifiers, such as interferon-gamma (IFN-gamma), interleukin-2 (IL-2), and interleukin-12 (IL-12), are being tested as possible treatment alternatives. Treatment regimens do not differ for pulmonary and extrapulmonary TB.

Prognosis.   Pulmonary TB is a major cause of morbidity and mortality worldwide, resulting in the greatest number of deaths from any one single infectious agent. This trend is due in part to increasing numbers of individuals co-infected with HIV and TB. Untreated, TB is 50% to 80% fatal, and the median time period to death is 2½ years. HIV-related death from TB represents one-third of all AIDS-related deaths.[233] Mortality from multidrug-resistant TB is high in all affected persons both those who are infected with HIV and persons free of HIV. Noncompletion of treatment (especially among inner-city residents and homeless people) presents an additional factor in the prognosis and subsequent failure to eradicate TB.

Special Implications for the Therapist   14-5

PULMONARY TUBERCULOSIS

Preferred Practice Patterns:
6A: *Primary Prevention/Risk Reduction for Cardiovascular/Pulmonary Disorders (AIDS/HIV)*
6B: *Impaired Aerobic Capacity/Endurance Associated With Deconditioning*
6C: *Impaired Ventilation, Respiration/Gas Exchange, and Aerobic Capacity/Endurance Associated With Airway Clearance Dysfunction*
6F: *Impaired Ventilation and Respiration/Gas Exchange Associated With Respiratory Failure*

Various other practice patterns may be appropriate in the case of extrapulmonary TB depending on the associated complications (e.g., 6H for lymph node involvement; 7C, 7D, 7E for integumentary [skin] involvement; 4A, 4B, 4G, and other patterns for musculoskeletal involvement; 5F for cranial nerve involvement; 5C, 5D for meningitis).

Health care workers should be alert at all times to the need for preventing TB transmission when cough-inducing procedures are being performed but especially in cases of known TB or HIV infection. Isolation measures for anyone who may be dispersing *M. tuberculosis* must be taken both in the acute care setting and in outpatient areas. If there is a high degree of suspicion or proven TB, clients should be cared for in negative-pressure isolation rooms while undergoing assessment and/or treatment. Procedures that may generate infectious aerosols should be carried out in similarly ventilated rooms. Precautions must be followed by all health care personnel having contact with clients diagnosed with TB (Table 14-7; see also Appendix A).

For the therapist evaluating a client with pulmonary TB, a thorough chest assessment and musculoskeletal evaluation should be performed. Chest expansion may be decreased because of diffuse fibrotic changes in progressive disease. Tracheal

Continued

---

*Previously an annual examination was recommended, but currently screening is based on symptomatic presentation (if asymptomatic, testing is not required) and job exposure (i.e., those health care workers treating persons with active TB or AIDS or HIV infection are at increased risk of exposure).

TABLE	14-7

Guidelines for Therapists for Preventing Transmission of Tuberculosis (TB)

All new employees (and student therapists) should be screened with the tuberculin skin test.

Doors to isolation rooms must be kept closed.

Clients infected with TB must cover mouth and nose with tissues when coughing, sneezing, or laughing.

Cough-inducing procedures should not be performed on TB clients unless absolutely necessary; such procedures should be performed using local exhaust, in a high-efficiency particulate air (HEPA)—filtered booth or individual TB isolation room. After completion of treatment, such persons should remain in the booth or enclosure until the cough subsides.

Clients must wear a mask when leaving the room.

Anyone entering the room must wear a protective mask, called a HEPA respirator, properly.

Therapists must be adequately trained in the use and disposal of masks and should use a particulate respirator (PR, a special mask)* whenever the client is undergoing cough-inducement or aerosol-generating procedures.

The therapist must check the condition of both the face piece and face seal each time the PR is worn.

Gloves are worn when touching infective material.

Disinfect the stethoscope between treatment sessions.

Staff and employees attending clients in all settings must be tested for TB: every 6 mo for high-risk therapists; other personnel annually.

Hand washing is required before and after contact with the client.

Isolation precautions must be continued until a clinical and bacteriologic response to medical treatment has been demonstrated.

Environmental surfaces (e.g., walls, crutches, bed rails, walkers) are not associated with transmission of infections; only routine cleaning of such items is required.

Therapists with current pulmonary or laryngeal TB should be excluded from work until adequate treatment is instituted, cough is resolved, and sputum is free of bacilli on three consecutive smears.

All TB control recommendations for inpatient facilities apply to hospices and home health services.

Home health personnel can reinforce client education about the importance of taking medications as prescribed unless adverse effects are observed.

From Guidelines for preventing the transmission of M. *tuberculosis* in health-care facilities, 1994, *MMWR Morb Mortal Wkly Rep* 43(RR-13):1-132, 1994. (This document remains the most recent recommendations at the time of this publication.)

*There are several types of face masks designated as particulate respirators; all National Institute for Occupational Safety and Health (NIOSH)–certified respirators are acceptable protection for health care workers against *Mycobacterium tuberculosis*. The respiratory protection standard set by the Occupational Safety and Health Administration (OSHA) requires a NIOSH-certified respirator; when such a respirator is used, the law requires that a training and fit-test program be present.

deviation may be present if there is a significant loss of volume in the upper lobes. Postural adaptations may have developed in late stages of the disease because of poor breathing patterns.[81] Other areas of assessment should include overall posture, gait, muscle strength, balance, and functional mobility. The therapist is referred to *The Guide* for examination guidelines along with considerations for evaluation and plan of care.

People with TB typically have a poor nutritional status and a progressive weight loss that may have secondary effects on the musculoskeletal system, such as postural defects and trigger point irritability. The effects of isolation result in disuse atrophy and cardiopulmonary and physical deconditioning, including progressive dyspnea. Finding the balance between exercise and clinical limitations is always a challenge for the therapist, and specific research related to exercise and the client with TB is only in the preliminary stages. Specific guidelines for evaluation of medical status during exercise are offered by Galantino and Bishop.[81]

Side effects of the medication can lead to peripheral neuritis that may be brought to the attention of the therapist. This and any other complication, such as hepatitis, hemoptysis, optic neuritis, or purpura, should be reported to the physician. Extrapulmonary TB is much less common than pulmonary TB. Treatment of Pott's disease follows the same chemotherapy regimen, with prompt response. Immobilization and avoidance of weight bearing may be required to relieve pain, with attention to maintaining strength and range of motion (see further discussion in Chapter 24).

For the Health Care Worker

For the health care worker who is exposed to TB and develops active disease, treatment will yield a "cure" if the appropriate pharmacologic intervention is followed for the full course prescribed, usually a minimum of 6 months. A cure simply means the active TB will not likely recur, but the person can be reexposed and reinfected. Treatment failure (not taking enough medication or for long enough duration) is a more likely outcome than reinfection/redisease because treatment compliance (i.e., noncompliance) is a much bigger problem. A person with active disease who misses 2 weeks of treatment must restart the entire course and risks the development of drug-resistant infection. After 2 weeks on effective medication, more than 85% of people with positive sputum cultures convert to a noninfectious status. Although the individual is no longer considered infectious, a minimum of 6 months is required before the disease is considered cured.

If the health care worker is exposed and infected but does not develop active disease (approximately 90% of all cases), there is a 10% lifetime risk that active disease can develop; one-half of that risk takes place in the first 2 years. That 10% risk can be reduced to approximately a 1% risk if a single prophylactic medication is taken properly for 6 months. In such cases, the individual is considered a "TB reactor" and will always skin test positive for TB. These individuals will require TB clearance in order to work in health care settings, schools, or other similar settings. Clearance is provided via medical documentation of treatment and with a letter from the attending physician.

> The TB bacterium must be inhaled and cannot be transmitted by physical contact with extrapulmonary sites unless the organism is expelled, aerosolized, and then inhaled. Although unusual, this type of situation may be encountered during wound care involving the integument and should be approached with appropriate Standard Precautions. ■

◆ Lung Abscess

Definition.   Described as a localized accumulation of purulent exudate within the lung, an abscess usually develops as a complication of pneumonia, especially aspiration and staphylococcal pneumonia. This can occur when bacteria are aspirated from the oropharynx along with foreign material or vomitus, or it can occur from septic embolus from a heart valve. Septic pulmonary emboli from staphylococcal endocarditis of the tricuspid or pulmonary valves are most often a complication of the use of illicit injection drugs. An abscess may also form when a neoplasm becomes necrotic and contains purulent material that does not drain from the area because of partial or complete obstruction.

Risk Factors.   Aspiration associated with alcoholism is the single most common condition predisposing to lung abscess. Other predisposed persons include those with altered levels of consciousness because of drug or alcohol use as mentioned, seizures, general anesthesia, lung cancer, or CNS disease; impaired gag reflex as a result of esophageal disease or neurologic disorders; poor dentition and periodontal care; and tracheal or nasogastric tubes, which disrupt the mechanical defenses of the airways.

Pathogenesis and Clinical Manifestations.   As with all abscesses, a lung abscess is a natural defense mechanism in which the body attempts to localize an infection and wall off the microorganisms so these cannot spread throughout the body. As the microorganisms destroy the local parenchymal tissue (including alveoli, airways, and blood vessels), an inflammatory process causes alveoli to fill with fluid, pus, and microorganisms (*consolidation*). Death and decay of consolidated tissue may progress proximally until the abscess drains into the bronchus, spreading the infection to other parts of the lung and forming cavities (*cavitation*).

Clinical signs and symptoms of abscess formation almost always include cough productive of foul-smelling sputum and persistent fever. Other characteristic features include chills, dyspnea, pleuritic chest pain, cyanosis, and clubbing of fingernails, which can develop over a short period of time. Cavitation causes severe cough with copious amounts of purulent sputum and sometimes hemoptysis.

Medical Management

Diagnosis.   The radiographic appearance of a thick-walled solitary cavity surrounded by consolidation suggests lung abscess but must be differentiated from other possible lesions. Cavitary lesions in the apex of the upper lobes are frequently due to TB rather than bacterial abscess. Sputum analysis and culture, bronchoscopy, or ultrasound-guided transthoracic needle biopsy may be diagnostic; the latter diagnostic procedure also permits successful drainage of pulmonary abscesses.

Treatment and Prognosis.   Treatment includes specific antibiotics and good nutrition. Chest physical therapy may be helpful if the abscess communicates with the main-stem bronchi; percussion helps promote drainage of associated secretions. Other measures are similar to the treatment of pneumonia. Bronchoscopy may be used to drain the abscess. Prognosis is good if antibiotics can treat the underlying cause, leaving only a residual lung scar. However, mortality remains in the range of 5% to 10% and is influenced by the severity of the primary disease that initially caused consolidation, the client's general state of health, and the promptness of treatment.[161]

◆ Pneumonitis

Pneumonitis, an acute inflammation of lung tissue usually caused by infections, is discussed in this chapter (see Environmental and Occupational Diseases) under its most common presentation as Hypersensitivity Pneumonitis. Other causes of pneumonitis include lupus pneumonitis associated with systemic lupus erythematosus (SLE), aspiration pneumonitis associated with inspiration of acidic gastric fluid, obstructive pneumonitis associated with lung cancer, and interstitial pneumonitis associated with AIDS. Consolidation with impaired gas exchange may occur in the involved lung tissue but with successful inactivation of the infecting agent, resolution occurs with restoration of normal lung structure.

◆ Acute Bronchitis

Acute bronchitis is an inflammation of the trachea and bronchi (tracheobronchial tree) that is of short duration (1 to 3 weeks) and self-limiting with few pulmonary signs. It may result from chemical irritation such as smoke, fumes, or gas, or it may occur with viral infections such as influenza, measles, chickenpox, or whooping cough. These predisposing conditions may become apparent during the therapist's interview with the client.

Symptoms of acute bronchitis include the early symptoms of an upper respiratory infection or a common cold, which progress to fever, a dry, irritating cough caused by transient hyperresponsiveness, sore throat, possible laryngitis, and chest pain from the effort of coughing. Later the cough becomes more productive of purulent sputum, followed by wheezing. There may be constitutional symptoms including moderate fever with accompanying chills, back pain, muscle pain and soreness, and headache. Clients with viral bronchitis present with a nonproductive cough that frequently occurs in paroxysms and is aggravated by cold, dry, or dusty air. Bacterial bronchitis (common in clients with chronic obstructive pulmonary disease [COPD]) causes retrosternal (behind the sternum) pain that is aggravated by coughing.

Treatment is conservative and symptomatic with cough suppressants, rest, humidity, and nutrition and hydration. Seasonal vaccination of people with recurrent bouts of bronchitis reduces the number and severity of exacerbations over the winter months.[73] The use of antibiotics for acute bronchitis remains controversial and is not recommended although some researchers report that antibiotics appear to have a modest beneficial effect.[25] Prognosis is usually good with treatment, and although acute bronchitis is usually mild, it can become complicated in people with chronic lung or heart disease and in older adults because they are more susceptible to secondary infections. Pneumonia is a critical complication.

OBSTRUCTIVE DISEASES

◆ Chronic Obstructive Pulmonary Disease

Definition. Chronic obstructive pulmonary disease (COPD), also called chronic obstructive lung disease, refers to a number of disorders that affect movement of air in and out of the lungs, particularly within the small airways. The most important of these disorders are obstructive bronchitis, emphysema, and chronic, unremitting asthma. Although these three diseases share a common obstructive component and can occur independently, they most commonly co-exist requiring differing treatment and having different prognoses.

Incidence and Risk Factors. COPD is second only to heart disease as a cause of disability in adults under 65 years of age and is the third leading cause of death worldwide following the trend of increasing prevalence of lung cancer. Nearly 16 million people in the United States are diagnosed with COPD (14 million with chronic bronchitis and 2 million with emphysema). COPD is almost always caused by exposure to environmental irritants especially smoking, the most common cause of COPD; this condition rarely occurs in nonsmokers. As with all chronic diseases, the prevalence of COPD is strongly associated with age and usually presents at age 55 to 60 years. More men are affected than women, but the incidence in women is increasing with the concomitant increase in smoking by women. Because smoking is the major cause of both emphysema and chronic bronchitis these two conditions often occur together.

Morbidity and mortality rates for COPD increase with the effects of exposure to irritating gases, dusts, or allergens; chronic irritation; and pollution in urban environments. Other contributing factors include chronic respiratory infections (e.g., sinusitis), periodontal disease,[188] the aging process, heredity, and genetic predisposition.

Pathogenesis and Clinical Manifestations. The pathogenesis and clinical manifestations of each component of COPD (i.e., chronic obstructive bronchitis, emphysema, asthma) are discussed separately in their respective sections. A broad overview of COPD is shown in Fig. 14-6.

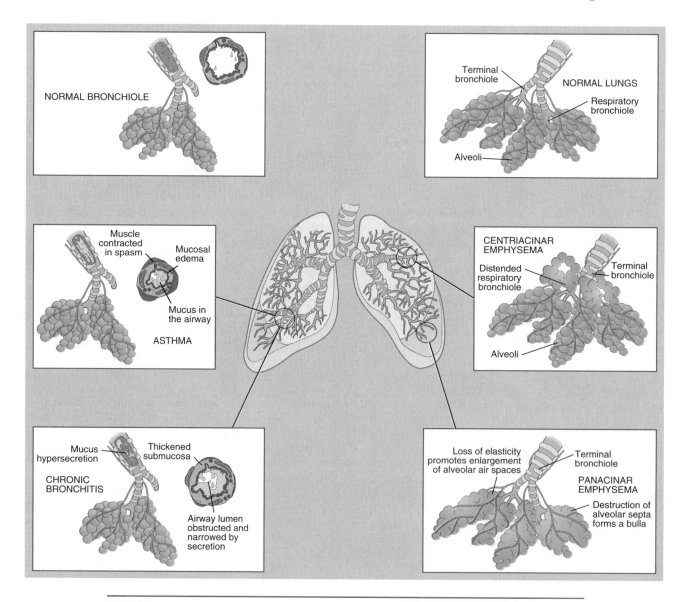

FIGURE 14-6 What happens in chronic obstructive lung disease/chronic air-flow limitation (COPD).

Medical Management

Diagnosis. Physical examination and air-flow limitation on pulmonary function testing (see Table 39-19) are assessment tools in determining the presence and extent of COPD. A simple and inexpensive portable spirometer permits such testing in the outpatient setting but may also be conducted in a respiratory lab with a computerized spirometer. The spirometer measures the maximal velocity of air that can be blown out of the lungs; that is, it is a measure of the efficiency of how much air goes into the lungs and how fast it is expired. More than a 10% difference measured before and after activity or before and after medication (a bronchodilator) is considered diagnostic of COPD (especially asthma). Predicted values based on age, height, and body weight are compared to actual values to determine the numeric (%) comparison.

History, clinical examination, x-ray studies, and laboratory findings usually enable the physician to distinguish COPD from other obstructive pulmonary disorders, such as bronchiectasis, adult cystic fibrosis (CF), and central airway obstruction. Thoracic computed tomography (CT) scanning may detect emphysema not apparent on the chest film, but it is very costly and rarely indicated for this purpose. Most cases of emphysema involve a history of cigarette smoking, chronic cough and sputum production, and dyspnea.

Laboratory analysis may include blood gas measurements to indicate the level of functional impairment or the presence of hypoxemia or hypercapnia (excess carbon dioxide in blood), sputum culture, or presence of immunoglobulin E (IgE) antibodies against specific allergens. Skin testing for allergens that trigger attacks is most useful in young clients with extrinsic asthma.

Treatment. The successful management of COPD requires a multifaceted approach that includes smoking cessation, pharmacologic management, pulmonary hygiene, exercise, control of complications, avoiding irritants, psychologic support, and dietary management. The main goals for the client with COPD are to improve oxygenation and decrease carbon dioxide retention. These are accomplished by (1) reducing airway edema secondary to inflammation (asthma) through the use of bronchodilator medication, (2) facilitating the elimination of bronchial secretions, (3) preventing and treating respiratory infection, (4) increasing exercise tolerance, (5) controlling complications, (6) avoiding airway irritants and allergens, and (7) relieving anxiety and treating depression, which often accompany COPD.

Common classifications of medications used in the treatment of COPD include oral or inhaled bronchodilators, antiinflammatory agents, antibiotics, mucolytic expectorants, mast cell membrane stabilizers, and antihistamines (Table 14-8). Systemic corticosteroids are of some help in acute exacerbations of COPD but do not produce any long-term benefit.[165] The benefits of pneumococcal vaccine have been proven (decreased mortality and hospitalization), and vaccination is recommended for all people with COPD. Annual prophylactic vaccination against influenza is also recommended. Narcotics, tranquilizers, and sedatives are used with caution because these depress the respiratory center. Research to improve the pharmacologic treatment includes investigation of multiple mediator antagonists, antiinflammatories with better delivery of the medication and lower side effects, and induced repair of alveolar tissue.[69]

People with PaO_2 of 55 to 59 mmHg or less (determined by arterial blood gases [ABGs]) with signs of tissue hypoxemia (see Table 14-2) are considered for long-term oxygen therapy. Oxygen therapy is also considered for those who desaturate during sleep or exercise. These guidelines have been adopted by Medicare as reimbursement criteria and have also been endorsed by the American Thoracic Society. Oxygen supplementation (sometimes referred to as limited supplementation based on symptoms [$LSSO_2$]) during exertion may alleviate dyspnea and increase exercise tolerance,[134] but this is not a standard outcome in all studies.[82] Continued research is needed to investigate more specific parameters in the use of supplemental oxygen.

TABLE 14-8

Pharmacotherapy for COPD

EMPHYSEMA, CHRONIC BRONCHITIS	ASTHMA	CYSTIC FIBROSIS
Mucolytic expectorants, inhaled (decrease viscosity of respiratory secretions)		Mucolytic expectorants, inhaled
Bronchodilators	Bronchodilators	Bronchodilators
Beta$_2$-adrenergic agonist	Beta$_2$-adrenergic agonist	
Anticholinergics (antagonize bronchial secretions)	Leukotriene antagonists	
Methylxanthines	Anticholinergics	
	Methylxanthines	
	Antihistamines in mild asthma (second generation, nonsedating)	
Use of corticosteroids being reevaluated	Prophylactic, antiinflammatory agents	Antiinflammatory agents
	Corticosteroids, inhaled	Systemic oral corticosteroids
	Cromolyn sodium (mast cell stabilizer)	High-dose ibuprofen
		Antibiotic reagents (inhaled and/or oral)

Courtesy Susan Queen, P.T., Ph. D., University of Kentucky, Lexington, 2001.
COPD, Chronic obstructive pulmonary disease.

Surgical treatment for COPD is uncommon and controversial, but lung-volume reduction surgery (LVRS; bilateral pneumectomy or removal of large bullae that compress the lung and add to dead space) may reduce the lung volume, relieve thoracic distention, and improve respiratory mechanics. LVRS may be a possible alternative treatment to lung transplantation for selected individuals with end-stage disease. Successful LVRS delays the need for lung transplantation and offers better conditions for transplantation at a later time.[221] A multicenter, prospective, randomized study has been established by the National Heart, Lung and Blood Institute called the National Emphysema Treatment Trial to study the medical management, including pulmonary rehabilitation, in COPD. The primary objectives will be to examine effects on pulmonary function, compare surgical techniques, and identify the role of LVRS in caring for individuals with advanced COPD.[71] Lung transplantation in COPD is still in its infancy stages. It appears that bilateral lung transplantation is associated with superior lung function, exercise tolerance, and a trend toward enhanced survival. Single-lung transplantation is still the most common type given the limited donor lungs and remains the preferred alternative for all other candidates.[176]

Prognosis. The prognosis for chronic bronchitis and emphysema is poor because these are chronic, progressive, and debilitating diseases. The death rate from COPD has increased 22% in the last decade, especially among older men, and the mortality rate 10 years after diagnosis is greater than 50%. COPD is largely preventable, and many believe that early recognition of small airway obstruction with appropriate treatment and cessation of smoking may prevent relentless progression of this disease. Early treatment of airway infections and vaccination against influenza and pneumococcal disease may provide symptomatic improvement but have no effect on the progression of the disease. There is no cure for COPD, but oxygen therapy has been shown to increase the survival rate.

Special Implications for the Therapist 14-6

CHRONIC OBSTRUCTIVE PULMONARY DISEASE

Preferred Practice Patterns:
6A: Primary Prevention/Risk Reduction for Cardiovascular/Pulmonary Disorders (tobacco disorder)
6B: Impaired Aerobic Capacity/Endurance Associated With Deconditioning
6C: Impaired Ventilation, Respiration/Gas Exchange, and Aerobic Capacity/Endurance Associated With Airway Clearance Dysfunction
6E: Impaired Ventilation and Respiration/Gas Exchange Associated With Ventilatory Pump Dysfunction or Failure
6F: Impaired Ventilation and Respiration/Gas Exchange Associated With Respiratory Failure

Pulmonary Rehabilitation
The pulmonary rehabilitation program model contains many intervention components beyond just chest physical therapy and exercise, including (but not limited to) assessment, education, optimization of medical therapy, psychosocial support, and nutritional therapy.[9] Chest physical therapy remains a standard adjunct to treatment of COPD, including breathing exercises, postural drainage, physical training, a program to improve posture, and strengthening of respiratory musculature. For the motivated child with asthma, breathing exercises and controlled breathing are of value in preventing overinflation, improving the strength of respiratory muscles and the efficiency of the cough, and reducing the work of breathing (WOB).

People with COPD often adopt a sedentary lifestyle leading to progressive deconditioning. Deconditioning will lead to progressive deterioration in limb muscle function that could adversely affect exercise capacity. The cost and benefits of pulmonary rehabilitation for people with COPD have been well-documented. Although there is little evidence that rehabilitation efforts can result in improved pulmonary function or arterial blood gases, many controlled and repetitive measured studies have demonstrated that programs that include exercise retraining can result in significant benefits, such as reduced hospitalizations, increased exercise tolerance, reduced dyspnea, improved skills in using inspiratory muscle training devices, increased independent activities of daily living (ADL) skills, and increased sense of well-being and quality of life.

Clients with COPD must be encouraged to remain active, with specific attention directed toward activities they enjoy. Training in pacing and energy conservation (see Box 8-2) allows even those with limited exercise tolerance to increase their daily activities. To strengthen the muscles of respiration, teach the person with COPD to take slow, deep breaths. To prevent early airway collapse during exhalation teach exhalation through pursed lips. Pursed-lip breathing helps slow the respiratory rate and open the airways during exhalation. Instruct the client to inhale through the nose and exhale with the lips pursed in a whistling or kissing position. Each inhalation should take about 4 seconds and each exhalation about 6 seconds. To help mobilize secretions, teach effective coughing techniques using diaphragmatic breathing. If secretions are thick, urge the client to drink fluids throughout the day.

The traditional approach of caring for people with chronic respiratory disease has been to rely on pulmonary function tests to quantify the severity and to assess response to therapy. However, people with chronic air-flow obstruction report disabling dyspnea when performing seemingly trivial tasks (e.g., activity with unsupported arms). Some muscles of the upper torso and shoulder girdle share both a respiratory and a positional function for the arms, resulting in functional limitations in many clients with lung disease during unsupported upper extremity activities. Simple arm elevation results in significant increases in metabolic and ventilatory requirements in clients with long-term air-flow limitations. The impact of these symptoms (and others) on an individual's quality of life (QOL) suggests that the therapist include an assessment of QOL issues when performing an evaluation. Pulmonary rehabilitation that includes upper extremity training (progressive resistance exercises [PREs]) reduces metabolic and ventilatory requirements for arm elevation. This type of program may allow clients with COPD to perform sustained upper extremity activities with less dyspnea.[67] Measuring QOL and how QOL has changed in response to pulmonary rehabilitation may provide the therapist with an additional outcome parameter. Various measures of health status have been investigated and are available.[41,76,145,196]

Exercise

Exercise limitation is a common and disturbing manifestation of COPD caused by multiple interrelated anatomic and physiologic disturbances. Exercise tolerance can be improved despite the presence of fixed structural abnormalities in the lung. Only a weak correlation between degree of airway obstruction and exercise tolerance has been shown suggesting that factors other than lung function impairment (e.g., deconditioning, peripheral muscle dysfunction) play a predominant role in limiting exercise capacity in people with COPD. In fact, recent work suggests that inspiratory capacity is a more powerful predictor of exercise tolerance than FEV_1 or forced vital capacity (FVC).[150] Research to determine the effect of inspiratory muscle training on exercise tolerance is under way.

Specific exercise training, alone or as part of a comprehensive pulmonary rehabilitation program including exercise training, breathing exercises, optimal medical treatment, psychosocial-spiritual support and health education, improves exercise endurance and, to a lesser degree, improves the maximal tolerated workload of the individual with COPD. As mentioned, pulmonary rehabilitation also improves QOL in terms of dyspnea, fatigue, and emotional state. Exercise training and pulmonary rehabilitation should be considered for all clients lacking contraindications who experience exercise intolerance despite optimal medical therapy.[33]

Lower-extremity training should be included routinely in the exercise prescription. The choice of type and intensity of training should be based primarily on the individual's baseline functional status, symptoms, needs, and long-term goals. Progressively increased walking is the most common form of exercise for COPD. Swimming is a preferred exercise option for clients with bronchial asthma (see following discussion). Therapists working with these clients should encourage them to maintain hydration by drinking fluids (including before, during, and after exercise) to prevent mucous plugs from hardening and to take medications as prescribed. When tolerated, high-intensity (continuous or interval) short-term training may lead to greater improvements in QOL and aerobic fitness than low-intensity training of longer duration, but it is not absolutely necessary to achieve gains in exercise endurance.[33,77]

Ventilatory muscle training should be included for anyone who continues to experience exercise limitation and breathlessness despite medical therapy and general exercise reconditioning. Exercise tolerance may improve following exercise training (including weight training)[52] because of gains in aerobic fitness or peripheral muscle strength,[146] enhanced mechanical skill and efficiency of exercise, improvements in respiratory muscle function, breathing pattern, or lung hyperinflation. Exercise training can also reduce anxiety, fear, and dyspnea previously associated with exercise in the deconditioned person.

Muscle weakness in stable COPD does not affect all muscles the same. For example, proximal upper limb muscle strength may be impaired more than distal upper limb muscle strength, peripheral muscle may be limited mainly by endurance capacity, and the diaphragm muscle may be altered structurally (e.g., changes in muscle length and configuration affecting the mechanical force and action)[46] and limited in strength capacity. These alterations in different muscle types require individual assessment and exercise prescription.[96,97]

Gains made in exercise tolerance, peripheral and respiratory muscle strength, and quality of life can last up to 2 years following a limited duration (6- to 12-week) rehabilitation program.[33,207] The optimal duration for an exercise program remains unknown; a 7-week course provides greater benefits than a 4-week course in terms of improvements in health status. Further studies in this area are needed.[98] Three training sessions per week improve exercise performance and health status, whereas a program consisting of two sessions per week for 8 weeks may not be effective in people with moderate COPD.[182] Maximally intense exercise sustained over 45 minutes daily 5 days per week for 6 weeks has been reported more effective in endurance training than exercise of a moderate intensity.[86] Other considerations for exercise training in chronic lung disease are available.[44]

Monitoring Vital Signs

Use a pulse oximeter to monitor oxygen saturation, keeping levels at 90% or above by adjusting supplemental oxygen levels, adjusting activity level, and practicing physiologic modulation or "quieting." Altering physiologic responses using principles of self-induced biofeedback and breathing techniques may be able to help some clients self-regulate oxygen saturation levels (see reference 116 for a description of these techniques). Although rare, some people with COPD retain CO_2 and have a depressed hypoxic drive requiring low oxygen levels to stimulate the respiratory drive. In such cases the upward adjustment of supplemental oxygen levels must be monitored very carefully; increasing total oxygen administered via nasal canula higher than 1 to 2 liters requires careful monitoring of the respiratory system (e.g., respiratory rate, breathing pattern), documentation, and consultation with other members of the pulmonary rehabilitation team.

Using a pulse oximeter can help the therapist and client observe for a decrease in oxygen saturation before hypoxemia occurs. Blood pressure and pulse should be observed at rest and in response to exercise, especially in anyone with COPD and cardiac arrhythmias. Most people with COPD who have mild arrhythmias at rest do not tend to have increased arrhythmias during exercise. Arrhythmias may disappear with exercise and increased perfusion. See also the section on Exercise and Arrhythmias in Chapter 11.

In people with expanded lung volumes because of air trapping such as occurs in COPD (especially emphysema), the first heart sound is best heard under the sternal area (put the scope in the client's left epigastric area) rather than the apical or mitral area. The hyperinflation of the lungs causes the heart to elongate, displacing the left ventricle downward and medially. Lung sounds are also changed because the loss of interstitial elasticity and the presence of interalveolar septa lead to air trapping with increased volume of air in the lungs. Air pockets are poor transmitters of vibrations; thus vocal fremitus (the client whispers "99, 99, 99"), breath sounds, and the whispered and spoken voice are impaired or absent on auscultation. This absence of the vesicular quality of lung sounds is distinctive and may be heard before radiographic evidence of COPD.*

A peak flowmeter, a home monitoring device to measure fast expiratory flow, can be used to determine how compromised a client may be compared to the normal values for that person. This may be a useful measure in determining

Continued

---

* On the other hand, when there is fluid in the lung or lungs, consolidation, or collapse (e.g., atelectasis), whispered words are heard perfectly and clearly. This is the earliest sign of atelectasis.

response to therapy intervention and documenting measurable outcomes.

Exercise and Medications

The majority of pulmonary medications are used to promote bronchodilation and improve alveolar ventilation and oxygenation and are delivered as an aerosol spray through a device called a *metered-dose inhaler (MDI).* Older adults sometimes have difficulty using an inhaler because of arthritis or other medical problems that impair hand/breath coordination. Proper technique is important to ensure delivery of the medication to the desired location (Box 14-2). When medications are properly used, their effects should improve an individual's ability to exercise and more effectively obtain the benefits of training. However, the many side effects of pulmonary medications may interfere with normal adaptations to habitual exercise so that exercise tolerance and conditioning may not occur.[39] For example, corticosteroids mask or impede the beneficial effects of exercise. Anyone with pulmonary disease taking prolonged corticosteroids may develop steroid myopathy (see Chapter 4) and muscular atrophy not only in the peripheral skeletal muscles but also in the muscle fibers of the diaphragm. Animal studies also suggest that severe undernutrition causes a decrease in muscle energy status contributing to diaphragmatic fatigue.[135] Some investigators are exploring the use of anabolic hormone supplementation and growth hormones in COPD therapy against losses in muscle from long-term corticosteroid use.[43, 223] ■

◆ Chronic Obstructive Bronchitis

Definition and Overview.   *Chronic bronchitis* is clinically defined as a condition of productive cough lasting for at least 3 months (usually the winter months) per year for 2 consecutive years. If obstructive lung disease characterized by a decreased FEV_1/FVC ratio* less than 75% is combined with chronic cough, chronic obstructive bronchitis is diagnosed. Initially, only the larger bronchi are involved, but eventually all airways become obstructed, especially during expiration.

Risk Factors and Pathogenesis.   Chronic bronchitis is characterized by inflammation and scarring of the bronchial lining. This inflammation obstructs air flow to and from the lungs and increases mucous production. Irritants such as cigarette smoke, long-term dust inhalation, or air pollution cause mucous hypersecretion and hypertrophy (increased number and size) of mucus-producing cells in the large bronchi. The swollen mucous membrane and thick sputum obstruct the airways, causing wheezing and a subsequent cough as the person tries to clear the airways. In addition, impaired ciliary function reduces mucous clearance and increases client susceptibility to infection. Infection results in even more mucous production with bronchial wall inflammation and thickening.

As airways collapse, air is trapped in the distal portion of the lung causing reduced alveolar ventilation, hypoxia, and acidosis. This downward spiral continues since the client now

---

*FEV_1 is the forced expiratory volume, a measure of the greatest volume of air a person can exhale during forced expiration; the subscript is added to indicate the percentage of the vital capacity that can be expired in 1 second. FVC is forced vital capacity, a measure of the greatest volume of air that can be expelled when a person performs a rapid, forced expiratory maneuver. This usually takes about 5 seconds.

has poor tissue oxygenation (hypoxemia and resultant decreased PaO_2) and an abnormal ventilation/perfusion (V/Q) ratio. As compensation for the hypoxemia, polycythemia (overproduction of erythrocytes) occurs. Cyanosis results from insufficient arterial oxygenation and peripheral edema from ventricular failure. If left untreated, hypoxemia will lead to cor pulmonale and congestive heart failure.

Clinical Manifestations.   The symptoms of chronic bronchitis are persistent cough and sputum production (worse in the morning and evening than at midday). The increased secretion from the bronchial mucosa and obstruction of the respiratory passages interfere with the flow of air to and from the lungs. The result is shortness of breath, prolonged expiration, persistent coughing with expectoration, and recurrent infection (Fig. 14-7). Infection may be accompanied by fever and malaise.

Over time, reduced chest expansion, wheezing, cyanosis, and decreased exercise tolerance develop. In addition, the obstruction present results in decreased alveolar ventilation and increased partial pressure of arterial carbon dioxide ($PaCO_2$). Hypoxemia (deficient oxygenation of the blood) leads to polycythemia (overproduction of erythrocytes) and cyanosis. If not reversed, hypoxemia leads to pulmonary hypertension and eventually cor pulmonale and congestive heart failure. Severe disability or death is the final clinical picture.

Medical Management.   See Medical Management and Special Implications for the Therapist: Chronic Obstructive Pulmonary Disease, 14-6 in the previous section.

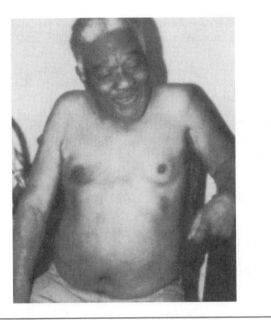

FIGURE 14-7 The person with chronic bronchitis may develop cyanosis and pulmonary edema causing a characteristic look. The person's shoulders are raised and muscles are tensed from shortness of breath and the increased work of breathing. In addition, slight gynecomastia (breast development) and petechiae present in the midsternal area are both side effects of large-dose oral corticosteroid therapy. (From Kersten LD: *Comprehensive respiratory nursing,* Philadelphia, 1989, Saunders.)

◆ Emphysema

Definition and Overview. *Emphysema* is defined as a pathologic accumulation of air in tissues, particularly in the lungs, and is found in the lungs of most people with COPD. There are three types of emphysema (see Fig. 14-6). *Centrilobular* emphysema, the most common type, produces destruction in the bronchioles, usually in the upper lung regions. Inflammation develops in the bronchioles, but usually the alveolar sac (distal to respiratory bronchioles) remains intact. *Panlobular* emphysema destroys the air spaces of the entire acinus and most commonly involves the lower lung. These two forms of emphysema, collectively called centriacinar emphysema, occur most often in smokers. Paraseptal (panacinar) emphysema destroys the alveoli in the lower lobes of the lungs resulting in isolated blebs along the lung periphery. *Paraseptal* emphysema is believed to be the likely cause of spontaneous pneumothorax.

Etiologic Factors. Cigarette smoking is the major etiologic factor in the development of emphysema and has been shown to increase the numbers of alveolar macrophages and neutrophils in the lung,* enhance protease† release, and im-

---

*Neutrophils, the most numerous type of leukocytes (white blood cells), increase dramatically in number in response to infection and inflammation. However, neutrophils not only kill invading organisms but also may damage host tissues when there are too many.

†Proteases, or proteolytic enzymes, are enzymes that destroy cells and proteins. The airway goblet cells and serous cells of bronchial glands normally secrete a protein called *secretory leukoprotease inhibitor,* which is capable of inhibiting neutrophils. The cellular interactions associated with smoking result in inactivation of protease inhibitors. This results in an imbalance between proteases and antiproteases (in favor of proteases), allowing even more cellular destruction than warranted by the inflammatory process already present.

pair the activity of antiproteases. However, other factors such as heredity must determine susceptibility to emphysema, because less than 10% to 15% of people who smoke develop clinical evidence of airway obstruction.

In many cases, emphysema occurs as a result of prolonged respiratory difficulties, such as chronic bronchitis that has caused partial obstruction of the smaller divisions of the bronchi. Emphysema can also occur without serious preceding respiratory problems as in the case of a defect in the elastic tissue of the lungs or in older persons whose lungs have lost their natural elasticity.

A small number of clients with COPD have an inherited deficiency of alpha$_1$-antitrypsin (AAT), a protective protein. AAT deficiency is suspected in persons who develop emphysema before age 40 years and in nonsmokers who develop the disease. Panacinar emphysema occurs in the older adult and in clients with AAT deficiency.

Pathogenesis. Emphysema is a disorder in which destruction of elastin protein in the lung that normally maintains the strength of the alveolar walls leads to permanent enlargement of the acini. Eventually the loss of elasticity in the lung tissue causes narrowing or collapse of the bronchioles so that inspired air becomes trapped in the lungs, making breathing difficult, especially during the expiratory phase. Obstruction results from changes in lung tissues, rather than from mucous production as in chronic bronchitis (which is why steroids are usually not helpful in this condition).

The permanent overdistention of the air spaces with destruction of the walls (septa) between the alveoli is accompanied by partial airway collapse and loss of elastic recoil. Pockets of air form between the alveolar spaces (blebs) and within the lung parenchyma (bullae). This process leads to increased ventilatory dead space, or areas that do not participate in gas or blood exchange. The work of breathing (WOB) is increased because there is less functional lung tissue for exchange of oxygen and carbon dioxide. As the disease progresses, there is increasing dyspnea and pulmonary infection. Eventually, cor pulmonale (right-sided congestive heart failure) develops.

In centrilobular emphysema the destruction of the lung is uneven and originates around the airways. The membranous bronchioles are thicker, narrower, and more reactive than in panlobular emphysema. Lung compliance is low or normal and does not relate to the extent of the emphysema (i.e., not to the losses of elastic recoil), but rather the decrease in air flow is related mainly to the degree of airway abnormality. In contrast, panlobular emphysema is characterized by even destruction of the lung and the small airways appear less narrowed and less inflamed than in centrilobular emphysema. Lung compliance is increased and is related to the extent of the emphysema; the decrease in air flow is primarily associated with the loss of elastic recoil rather than with the abnormalities in the airways.[55]

At the molecular and microvascular levels protease-antiprotease (associated with alpha$_1$-antitrypsin deficiency emphysema) and oxidant-antioxidant theories continue under investigation as theories relate to impaired reparative mechanisms in the causation of emphysema. Oxidative damage by free radicals, which is the basis for the free radical theory of aging (see discussion in Chapter 5), identifies cigarette smoke as the main source of oxidants contributing to epithelial damage associated with smoking-induced emphysema. Determining the mechanisms regulating the antioxidant responses is critical to understanding the role of oxidants in the pathogenesis of smoking-induced lung disease and to developing future strategies for antioxidant therapy.[193]

Clinical Manifestations. At first symptoms may be apparent only during physical exertion, but eventually marked exertional dyspnea progresses to dyspnea at rest. This occurs as a result of the irreversible destruction reducing elasticity of the lungs and increasing the effort to exhale trapped air. Cough is uncommon, with little sputum production. The client is often thin, has tachypnea with prolonged expiration, and must use accessory muscles for ventilation. To increase lung capacity, the client often leans forward with arms braced on the knees supporting the shoulders and chest. The combined effects of trapped air and alveolar distention change the size and shape of the client's chest, causing a barrel chest and increased expiratory effort. The normal arterial oxygen levels and dyspnea give clients a classic appearance (Fig. 14-8).

Persons with emphysema have high rates of anxiety associated with dyspnea or fear of dyspnea, claustrophobia, depression, malnutrition, insomnia, and respiratory failure and are prone to pneumonia, congestive heart failure, and pulmonary embolism. As emphysema progresses, there is a loss of surface area available for gas exchange. In the final stages, cardiac complications, especially enlargement and dilation of the right ventricle, may develop. The overloaded heart reaches its limit of muscular compensation and begins to fail (cor pulmonale).

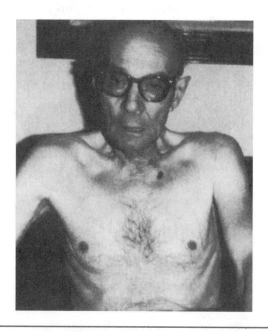

FIGURE **14-8** The person with emphysema presents with classic findings. Use of respiratory accessory (intercostal, neck, shoulder) muscles and cachectic appearance (wasting caused by ill health) reflect two factors: (1) shortness of breath, the most disturbing symptom, and (2) the tremendous increased work of breathing necessary to increase ventilation and maintain normal arterial blood gases. (From Kersten LD: *Comprehensive respiratory nursing,* Philadelphia, 1989, Saunders.)

Medical Management
Diagnosis and Treatment. Diagnosis is made on the basis of history (usually cigarette smoking), physical examination, chest film, and pulmonary function tests. The most important factor in the treatment of emphysema is cessation of smoking. Human lungs benefit no matter when someone quits smoking (see Table 2-3); quitting smoking is the most effective way of preventing lung function decline caused by emphysema (and chronic bronchitis). Pursed-lip breathing causes resistance to outflow at the lips, which in turn maintains intrabronchial pressure and improves the mixture of gases in the lungs. This type of breathing should be encouraged to help the client get rid of the stale air trapped in the lungs.

See also Chronic Obstructive Pulmonary Disease: Medical Management and Special Implications for the Therapist: Chronic Obstructive Pulmonary Disease, 14-6.

◆ Asthma
Definition and Overview. Asthma is defined as a reversible obstructive lung disease caused by increased reaction of the airways to various stimuli. It is a chronic inflammatory condition with acute exacerbations and characterized as a complex disorder involving biochemical, autonomic, immunologic, infectious, endocrine, and psychologic factors in varying degrees in different individuals. This condition can be divided into two main types according to causative factors: extrinsic (allergic) and intrinsic (nonallergic), but other recognized categories include adult-onset, exercise-induced, aspirin-sensitive, *Aspergillus* hypersensitivity, and occupational (Table 14-9).

Incidence and Risk Factors. Asthma as one component of COPD is the most common chronic disease in adults (10% incidence) and children (5% incidence), and the prevalence, morbidity, and mortality of asthma are increasing in the United States. The incidence of asthma cases and asthma deaths is increasing nationwide, but the reason for the increase is unknown. Explanations may include increased accuracy of medical diagnosis and increased chart documentation among physicians along with increased prevalence as average life expectancy increases. Air pollution, airtight homes, and windowless offices may also be risk factors contributing to the significant rise in incidence.

Asthma can occur at any age, although it is more likely to occur for the first time before the age of 5 years. In childhood, it is three times more common and more severe in boys; however, after puberty, the incidence in the genders is equal although monthly variations in asthma episodes seem to be correlated with estrogen levels for women.[45,232] Children with lower birth weight (<5½ pounds at birth) and prematurity (>3 weeks premature) are more susceptible to the effects of ozone (air pollution) compared with children who are born full term or full weight.[157] It is estimated that asthma goes unrecognized as an adverse factor affecting performance in 1 in 10 adolescent athletes.

Asthma is found most often in urban, industrialized settings; in colder climates; and among the urban disadvantaged population (areas of poverty). Asthma is more prevalent and more severe among black children, but this is not due to race or to low income per se but rather to demographic location because all children living in an urban setting are at increased risk for asthma.[5] Overcrowded living conditions with repeated exposure to cigarette smoke, dust, cockroaches, and mold and where

TABLE 14-9

Types of Asthma

CLASSIFICATION	TRIGGERS
Extrinsic	Immunoglobulin E (IgE)—mediated external allergens Foods; sulfite additives (wines) Indoor and outdoor pollutants, including ozone, smoke, exhaust Pollen, dust, molds Animal dander, feathers
Intrinsic	Unknown; secondary to respiratory infections
Adult-onset	Unknown
Exercise-induced	Alteration in airway temperature and humidity; mediator release
Aspirin-sensitive (associated with nasal polyps)	Aspirin and other nonsteroidal antiinflammatory drugs
Allergic broncho-pulmonary aspergillosis	Hypersensitivity to *Aspergillus* species
Occupational	Metal salts (platinum, chrome, nickel) Antibiotic powder (penicillin, sulfathiazole, tetracycline) Toluene diisocyanate (TDI) Flour Wood dusts Cotton dust (byssinosis) Animal proteins Smoke inhalation (firefighters) Latex-induced (see Box 3-5)

use of a gas stove or oven is used for heat may be contributing factors.[140] Alcoholic drinks, particularly wines, appear to be important triggers for asthmatic responses. Sensitivity to the sulfite additives and salicylates present in wine seems likely to play an important role in these reactions.[208]

Some questions have been raised about the association between obesity and asthma. Data from the Nurses Health Study II show that obesity increases women's risk of developing adult-onset asthma. The higher the body mass index (BMI), the greater the risk of developing asthma.[40] Other groups (e.g., children, all adults) have also been studied for an association between these two conditions but without a clear etiologic link. Whether there is an immunologic mechanism, hormonal link (excess estrogen in adipose tissue), reduction in air flow because of obesity, gastroesophageal reflux with bronchospasm, diet or nutritional basis, or some other connection remains undetermined. Co-morbidity of asthma and obesity may complicate the treatment of either condition, and prevention of obesity should be encouraged for children with asthma.[67]

Etiologic Factors. Asthma occurs in families, which indicates that it is an inherited disorder. Asthma is influenced by two genetic tendencies: one associated with the capacity to develop allergies (atopy) and the other with the tendency to develop hyperresponsiveness of the airways independent of atopy. Apparently, environmental factors interact with inherited factors to cause attacks of bronchospasm. Asthma can develop when predisposed persons are infected by viruses or exposed to allergens or pollutants.

Extrinsic asthma, also known as atopic or allergic asthma, is due to an allergy to specific triggers; usually the offending allergens are foods or environmental antigens suspended in the air in the form of pollen, dust, molds, smoke, automobile exhaust, and animal dander. In this type of asthma, mast cells, sensitized by IgE antibodies, degranulate and release bronchoactive mediators following exposure to a specific antigen. More than one-half of the cases of asthma in children and young adults are of this type.

Intrinsic asthma, or nonallergic asthma, has no known allergic cause or trigger, has an adult onset (usually over 40 years of age), and is most often secondary to chronic or recurrent infections of the bronchi, sinuses, or tonsils and adenoids. This type of asthma may develop from a hypersensitivity to the bacteria, or more commonly, viruses causing the infection. Other factors precipitating intrinsic asthma include drugs (aspirin, beta-adrenergic antagonists), environmental irritants (occupational chemicals, air pollution), cold dry air, exercise, and emotional stress.

Occupational asthma is defined as variable narrowing of airways, causally related to exposure in the working environment to specific airborne dusts, gases, acids, molds, dyes, vapors, or fumes. Many of these substances are very common and not ordinarily considered hazardous. Only a small proportion of exposed workers develop occupational asthma, but it has received considerable attention recently as the most frequent occupational lung disease worldwide. New substances and processes involving new chemicals have increased dramatically in the last two decades, and there is little information about "safe" levels of exposure that protect all workers.[23] High-risk occupations for asthma include farmers, animal handlers, and agricultural workers; painters; plastics and rubber workers; cleaners and homemakers (especially if cooking is done with a gas stove); textile workers; metal workers; and bakers, millers, and other food processors. Exposure to biologic dusts and gases and fumes can cause a 30% to 50% increased risk of asthma.

Pathogenesis. The airways are the site of an inflammatory response consisting of cellular infiltration, epithelial disruption, mucosal edema, and mucous plugging (Fig. 14-9). The release of inflammatory mediators produces bronchial smooth muscle spasm, vascular congestion, increased vascular permeability, edema formation, production of thick, tenacious mucus, and impaired mucociliary function. Several mediators also cause thickening of airway walls and increased contractile response of bronchial smooth muscles. These changes in the bronchial musculature, combined with the epithelial cell damage caused by eosinophil infiltration, result in the airway hyperresponsiveness characteristic of asthma.

Once the airway is in spasm, mucus plugs the airway, trapping distal air. Ventilation/perfusion mismatch, hypoxemia, obstructed expiratory flow, and increased workload of breathing follow. Most attacks of asthmatic bronchospasm are short-lived, with freedom from symptoms between episodes, although airway inflammation is present, even in asymptomatic persons. Excessive airway narrowing occurs when the smooth muscle shortens (not necessarily to an abnormal degree). The relationship between the mechanical and contractile proper-

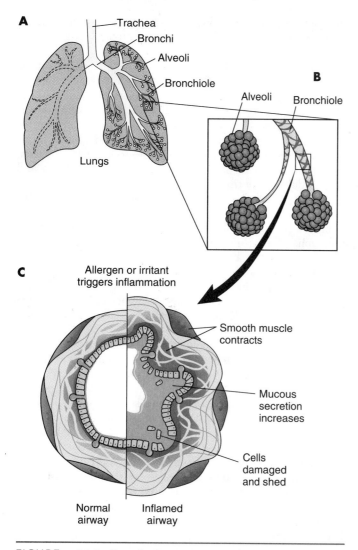

FIGURE   **14-9** Bronchiole response in asthma. **A,** Air is distributed throughout the lungs via small airways called *bronchioles.* **B,** Healthy bronchioles accommodate a constant flow of air when open and relaxed. **C,** In asthma, exposure to an allergen or irritant triggers inflammation causing constriction of the smooth muscle surrounding the bronchus (bronchospasm). The airway tissue swells; this edema of the mucous membrane further narrows airways with production of excess mucus also interfering with breathing.

ties of smooth muscle and lung volume and how these interact to determine smooth muscle length are the subject of new research. The relative importance of smooth muscle area and mechanical properties, altered airway structure, and airway inflammation in asthma is not yet determined.[119]

An out-of-balance immune system with abnormal or inadequately regulated CD+ T-cell immune response contributes to the underlying process that drives and maintains the asthmatic inflammatory process, but it remains unknown what contributes to this immune system dysfunction.[152] As mentioned in the section on etiologic factors, genetics, viruses, fungi, heavy metals, nutrition, and pollution have all been suggested. Researchers are also investigating the possibility of underlying neurogenic mechanisms that may contribute to the pathogenesis and pathophysiology of asthma.[50,184] Investigations include determination of the linkages among psychosocial factors and behavioral, neural, endocrine, and immune processes in the role of asthma. It has been shown that health-related behaviors, demographic factors, and psychosocial factors influence susceptibility to and severity of exacerbation of asthma.[132,197]

Clinical Manifestations.   Clinical signs and symptoms of asthma differ in presentation (Table 14-10), degree (Table 14-11), and frequency among clients, and although current symptoms are the most important concern of affected people, they reflect the current level of asthma control more than underlying disease severity.[168] During full remission, clients are asymptomatic and pulmonary function tests are normal.

At the beginning of an attack, there is a sensation of chest constriction, inspiratory and expiratory wheezing, nonproductive coughing, prolonged expiration, tachycardia, and tachypnea. Secondary bronchospasm is marked by recurrent attacks of dyspnea, with wheezing caused by the spasmodic constriction of the bronchi. Other symptoms may include fatigue, a tickle in the back of the throat accompanied by a cough in an attempt to clear the airways, and nostril flaring (advanced). The person usually assumes a classic sitting or squatting position to reduce venous return, leaning forward so as to use all the accessory muscles of respiration. The skin is usually pale and moist with perspiration, but in a severe attack there may be cyanosis of the lips and nail beds. In the early stages of the attack coughing may be dry, but as the attack progresses, the cough becomes more productive of a thick, tenacious, mucoid sputum. The nocturnal worsening of asthma is a common feature of this disease, and although many potential mechanisms for such a sleep-related effect have been proposed, no single factor or group of factors has been proved.[21]

An acute attack that cannot be altered with routine care is called *status asthmaticus.* This is a medical emergency requiring more vigorous measures and despite treatment can be fatal. With severe bronchospasm, the workload of breathing increases 5 to 10 times, which can lead to acute cor pulmonale. When air is trapped, a severe paradoxical pulse develops as venous return is obstructed; blood pressure drops over 10 mm Hg during inspiration. Pneumothorax occasionally develops. If status asthmaticus continues, hypoxemia worsens and acidosis begins. If the condition is untreated or not reversed, respiratory or cardiac arrest will occur. An acute asthma episode may constitute a medical emergency requiring emergency pharmacologic management.

Medical Management
Diagnosis.   Pulse oximetry, pulmonary function studies, arterial blood gas (ABG) analysis, complete blood count with differential, and chest films may be used in assessing for both the presence and the severity of asthma (see Chapter 39 for a description of and reference values for these tests). Inexpensive but reliable spirometer testing can be used to obtain evidence of the bronchial hyperreactivity associated with asthma. Diagnosis may be delayed in older clients who have other illnesses that cause similar symptoms or who attribute their breathlessness to the effects of aging and respond to the onset of asthma by limiting their activities to avoid eliciting symptoms. The diagnosis of occupational asthma is usually based on history of a temporal association between exposure and the onset of symptoms and objective evidence that these symptoms are related to air-flow limitation.

TABLE 14-10

Clinical Manifestations of Bronchial Asthma

Cough

Hacking, paroxysmal, exhausting, irritative, involuntary, nonproductive

Becomes rattling and productive of frothy, clear, gelatinous sputum

Main or only symptom

Tickle in the back of the throat accompanied by a cough

Respiratory-Related Signs

Shortness of breath; may occur at rest

Prolonged expiratory phase

Audible wheeze on inspiration and expiration or on expiration only; never on inspiration only

Often appears pale

May have a malar flush and red ears

Lips deep dark red color

May progress to cyanosis of nail beds, around mouth and lips

Restlessness

Apprehension

Anxious facial expression

Itching around nose, eyes, throat, chin, scalp

Respiratory-Related Signs—cont'd

Sweating may be prominent as attack progresses

May sit upright with shoulders in a hunched-over position, hands on the bed or chair, and arms braced (older children)

Speaks with short, panting broken phrases

Chest

Coarse, loud breath sounds (may become quiet or silent if severe)

Prolonged expiration

Generalized inspiratory and expiratory wheezing; increasingly high-pitched

With Repeated Episodes

Barrel chest

Elevated shoulders

Use of accessory muscles of respiration

Skin retraction (clavicles, ribs, sternum)

Facial appearance: flattened malar bones, circles beneath the eyes, narrow nose, prominent upper teeth, nostrils flaring

Modified from Wong DL: *Whaley and Wong's essentials of pediatric nursing,* ed 5, St Louis, 1997, Mosby–Year Book.

TABLE 14-11

Stages of Asthma

STAGE	SYMPTOMS
Mild	Symptoms reverse with cessation of activity; daytime symptoms ≤2 times/wk; nighttime symptoms ≤2 times/mo; inhaled medication as needed (not usually daily)
Moderate	Audible wheezing Use of accessory muscles of respiration Leaning forward to catch breath Daily (but not continual) daytime symptoms requiring short-acting inhalant and long-term treatment Episodes ≥2 times/wk; nighttime symptoms ≥ 4 times/mo
Severe	Blue lips and fingernails Tachypnea (30-40 breaths/min) despite cessation of activity Cyanosis-induced seizures Skin and rib retraction Activity limited; frequent daytime and nighttime episodes, sometimes continual

Prevention. Heavier emphasis on teaching self-management and especially prevention for anyone with asthma is recommended by the American Academy of Allergy, Asthma, and Immunology. An excellent daily asthma management plan is available.[8] *Healthy People 2010* has identified 11 objectives specifically related to this condition including increasing the proportion of people with asthma who receive formal education as part of their management program (see *Healthy People 2010:* http://health.gov/healthypeople/).

Treatment. Identifying specific allergens for each individual and avoidance of asthma triggers, combined with the use of two classes of medications (bronchodilators, antiinflammatory agents; see Table 14-8), have been recommended in the management of asthma.* Most people require bronchodilator therapy to control symptoms by activating beta-agonist receptors on smooth muscle cells in the respiratory tract, thereby relaxing the bronchial muscle and opening the airways; those with mild symptoms may use metered-dose inhaler (MDI) devices to administer sympathomimetic bronchodilators on an as-needed basis.

People who experience moderate to severe asthma may require daily administration of antiinflammatory agents such as corticosteroids to prevent asthma attacks. Antiinflammatory drugs have a preventive action by interrupting the development of bronchial inflammation. They may also modify or terminate ongoing inflammatory reactions in the airways. It is important that people with asthma know the difference between medications that must be taken daily to prevent asthma symptoms and medications that relieve symptoms once they begin. Low-dose corticosteroid inhalants are recommended to reduce the risk of side effects (e.g., reduced growth in chil-

---

*In the past asthma was thought to be caused by spasms of the muscles surrounding the airways between the trachea and lungs and therefore treated first with bronchodilator drugs to widen the constricted airways and ease symptoms. It is now clear that asthma attacks are actually episodic flareups of chronic inflammation in the lining of the airways necessitating the use of inhaled antiinflammatories to suppress the underlying inflammation and allow the airways to heal.

dren, ocular effects, death, osteoporosis) from prolonged use.[203] A new class of antiinflammatory medications known as *leukotriene modifiers* is now available; these work by blocking the activity of chemicals called *leukotrienes* that are involved in airway inflammation (see further discussion in Chapter 5).

Oxygen metabolites (free radicals) may play a direct or indirect role in the modulation of airway inflammation. Excessive superoxide and hydroxyl radical production accompanied by significantly lower free radical scavengers in asthma (the latter even during rest) endorses the correlation between disease severity and oxygen radical production in people with asthma.[194] Research efforts to investigate the use of dietary or micronutrient antioxidants and other alternative/complementary treatment of asthma (e.g., yoga, chiropractic, acupuncture, biofeedback, massage) are under way, with a range of findings reported for the use of these interventions. Although some researchers suggest that antioxidant nutrients (especially obtained from food sources such as fruits and vegetables) appear necessary in asthma treatment,[147,152,163] others report that people with asthma may have a diminished capacity to restore the antioxidant defenses, making the use of antioxidants questionable in this population.[174]

Genetic treatment is also under investigation. Several drug companies are developing drugs that damp down the entire asthmatic response.[83] Recombinant monoclonal antibody vaccine that blocks the release of histamine and other substances in cases of allergic asthma has been shown to improve health-related quality of life and reduce dosage of inhaled corticosteroids in children with mild to moderate asthma.[65] Gene transfer into the airway cells to block mediator proteins (signal transducer activator of transcription [STAT]) from setting off an immune response or too strong an immune response in the asthma pathway is also under investigation.[68,187]

Prognosis.   The outlook for clients with *bronchial asthma* is excellent despite the recent increase in the death rate. Childhood asthma may disappear, but only about one-quarter of the children with asthma become symptom-free when their airways reach adult size. This condition persists beyond childhood in 85% of women and in 72% of men.[11] Adult asthma may progress to COPD, but studies indicate that the majority of people with asthma do not experience decline in pulmonary mechanics or appear to be at risk for reduced life expectancy.[148] Attention to general health measures and use of pharmacologic agents permit control of symptoms in nearly all cases. *Status asthmaticus* can result in respiratory or cardiac arrest and possible death (see previous discussion). If ventilation becomes necessary, prognosis for recovery is poorer.

Special Implications for the Therapist   14-7

ASTHMA

Preferred Practice Patterns:
6B: Impaired Aerobic Capacity/Endurance Associated With Deconditioning
6C: Impaired Ventilation, Respiration/Gas Exchange, and Aerobic Capacity/Endurance Associated With Airway Clearance Dysfunction

6E: Impaired Ventilation and Respiration/Gas Exchange Associated With Ventilatory Pump Dysfunction or Failure
6F: Impaired Ventilation and Respiration/Gas Exchange Associated With Respiratory Failure

Many people with asthma do not even know they have the disease. Some think they simply have chronic bronchitis, colds, or allergies. Anyone who reports coughing or a feeling of tightness in the chest when others smoke nearby and especially anyone who gasps for breath after exercise should be referred to a physician for evaluation of these symptoms.

Exercise-Induced Asthma

Exercise-induced bronchospasm (EIB), or exercise-induced asthma (EIA), does not represent a unique syndrome but rather an example of the airway hyperactivity common to all persons with asthma. EIA is an acute, reversible, usually self-terminating airway obstruction that develops 5 to 15 minutes after strenuous exercise when the person no longer breathes through the nose, warming and humidifying the air, but opens the mouth. Breathing cold, dry air through the mouth degranulates mast cells that release bronchoconstrictive mediators inducing EIB. EIB/EIA lasts 15 to 60 minutes after the onset.

Coughing is the most common symptom of EIA, but other symptoms include chest tightness, wheezing, and shortness of breath. The affected (but undiagnosed) individual may comment, "I am more out of shape than I thought." This should be a red flag for the therapist to consider the possibility of asthma and need for medical diagnosis and intervention. If an asthma attack should occur during therapy, first assess the severity of the attack. Place the person in the high Fowler's position and encourage diaphragmatic and pursed-lip breathing. If the client has an inhaler available, provide whatever assistance is necessary for that person to self-administer the medication. Help the person to relax while assessing the person's response to the medication.

Usually the episode subsides spontaneously in 30 to 60 minutes. The severity of an attack increases as the exercise becomes increasingly strenuous. The problem is rare in activities that require only short bursts of energy (e.g., baseball, sprints, gymnastics, skiing) compared with those that involve endurance exercise (e.g., soccer, basketball, distance running or biking). Swimming, even long-distance swimming, is well-tolerated by people with EIA, partly because they are breathing air fully saturated with moisture, but the type of breathing required may also play a role. Exhaling under water, which is essentially pursed-lip breathing, is of benefit because it prolongs each expiration and increases the end-expiratory pressure within the respiratory tree.

Exercise and Medication

Bronchospasm can occur during exercise (especially in exercise-induced asthma) if the person with asthma has a low oxygen blood level before exercise. For this reason, it is helpful to take bronchodilators by MDI 20 to 30 minutes before exercise, performing mild stretching and warm-up exercises during that time period to avoid bronchospasm with higher workload exercise. Increased exercise should be accompanied by good bronchodilator coverage to promote bronchodilation and improve alveolar ventilation and oxygenation. Exercise guidelines for adults with asthma can be modified from recommendations for children with asthma (Table 14-12).

TABLE	14-12

Exercise Guidelines for Children With Asthma

RECOMMENDATION	BENEFIT
General exercise, school-based physical education	Maintains motor function, strength, stamina, and coordination; prevents or reverses side effects of medication (e.g., corticosteroids) Raises threshold for strenuous exercise before mouth breathing and EIB occur
Low-impact exercise (aerobics, weight training, stationary bike)	Permits exercise without increased bronchospasm
Warm-up before aerobic activity	Helps control airway reactivity; gradually desensitizes mast cells, reducing release of bronchoconstrictive mediators
Exercise in a trigger-free environment (i.e., avoid cold, pollution, or increased pollen outdoors; exercise indoors; avoid tobacco smoke; swimming program is ideal)	Prevents bronchospasm; controls symptoms
Take prescribed medication properly before exercise or activity producing bronchospasm	Prevents bronchospasm
Monitor FEV_1/FVC ratio before, during, and after physical activity* Decrease of 10% requires slowing activity Drop of 15%-20% from initial measurement requires cessation of exercise	Determines whether shortness of breath is due to exercise or if air flow is decreasing because of bronchospasm

EIB, Exercise-induced bronchospasm; FEV_1/FVC, ratio of forced expiratory volume in 1 sec to forced vital capacity.
*Peak flowmeters can be used to obtain this information. Determine the child's normal range of lung function by having the child blow in the meter in the morning and evening for 1 wk. The average level measured varies from person to person and is influenced by gender and height. Testing should establish a peak flow protocol against which lung function can be compared to determine if deterioration has occurred.

Many clients have found that using their inhalers in this way before exercise permits them to exercise without onset of symptoms. Proper administration of an MDI is essential (see Box 14-2). The first dose induces dilation of the larger, central bronchial tubes, relaxing smooth muscles in the airways; the second dose dilates the bronchioles (smaller airways). Metabolism of certain drugs administered can be altered by exercise, tobacco, marijuana, or phenobarbital (all of which increase drug metabolism). Cimetidine (Tagamet), erythromycin, or the presence of a viral infection may decrease drug metabolism. If a client develops signs of asthma or any bronchial reactivity during the exercise, the physician must be informed. Medication dosage can then be altered to maintain optimal physical performance. Excessive use of inhaled beta-adrenergic agents (using three or more full canisters monthly) requires physician referral for further evaluation. Common manifestations of drug-induced (theophylline) toxicity include nausea, vomiting, tremors, anxiety, tachycardia and arrhythmias, and hypotension. The use of nonsteroidal antiinflammatory drugs (NSAIDs), including aspirin, in older people with asthma should be avoided if possible because the drug interactions can cause increased bronchospasm in susceptible individuals.

Some athletes do not achieve the control needed for the performance demands of competition. The effectiveness of short-acting medications and medications in general for asthma varies widely among people with asthma while exercising. The preventive benefits of each medication dose may wane after taking a new drug for several weeks. Any athlete with asthma who cannot perform at the levels desired or expected because of asthma symptoms should be advised to review medications and medication use with the physician.

Medication and Bone Density

Long-term use of inhaled corticosteroids in the management of moderate to severe asthma is associated with decreased bone mineral density and associated increased risk of fractures, particularly in high-risk postmenopausal women (i.e., those not receiving hormone replacement therapy).[31, 225] All people receiving glucocorticoid therapy (e.g., prednisolone) at doses of 7.5 mg/day or more for 6 months or longer should discuss with their physician the use of low-dose inhaled corticosteroids, assessment of bone mineral density, and preventive therapies (e.g., biphosphonates, calcium supplementation, vitamin D).[166] The physical therapist can be very instrumental in providing education for the prevention and intervention for the treatment of osteopenia and osteoporosis. See the section on Osteoporosis in Chapter 23.

Monitoring Vital Signs

Monitoring vital signs can alert the therapist to important changes in bronchopulmonary function. Developing or increasing tachypnea may indicate worsening asthma; tachycardia may indicate worsening asthma or drug toxicity. Other signs of toxicity, such as diarrhea, headache, and vomiting, may be misinterpreted as influenza. Hypertensive blood pressure readings may indicate asthma-related hypoxemia. Auscultate the lungs frequently, noting the degree of wheezing and the quality of air movement. In this way, any change in respiratory status will be more readily perceived. If the client does not have a productive cough in the presence of rhonchi (dry rattling in the bronchial tube), teach effective coughing techniques.

Status Asthmaticus

Therapy can augment the medical management of the client with status asthmaticus. In coordination with the individual's

Continued

medications, the therapist helps to remove secretions; promotes relaxed, more efficient breathing; enhances ventilation/perfusion matching; reduces hypoxemia; and teaches the client to coordinate relaxed breathing with general body movement. Caution needs to be observed to avoid stimuli that bring on bronchospasm and deterioration (e.g., aggressive percussion, forced expiration maneuvers, aggressive bag ventilation, or manual hyperinflation with an intubated individual). Certain body positions may have to be avoided because of client intolerance or exacerbation of symptoms in those positions.[58]

Immediate medical care is recommended for anyone with asthma who is struggling to breathe with no improvement in 15 to 20 minutes after initial treatment with medications or who is hunched over and unable to straighten up or resume activity after medication dosage. The presence of blue or gray lips or nail beds is another indication of the need for medical attention. ■

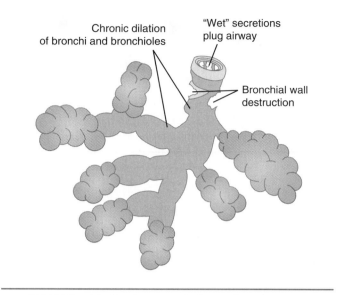

FIGURE   **14-10**   Airway pathology in bronchiectasis.

◆ Bronchiectasis

Definition.   Bronchiectasis is a progressive form of obstructive lung disease characterized by irreversible destruction and dilation of airways generally associated with chronic bacterial infections. Clinically, it is considered an extreme form of bronchitis. Abnormal and permanent dilation of the bronchi and bronchioles develops when the supporting structures (bronchial walls) are weakened by chronic inflammatory changes associated with secondary infection.

Incidence and Etiologic and Risk Factors.   The incidence of bronchiectasis is low in the United States because of improved control of bronchopulmonary infections. However, any condition producing a narrowing of the lumen of the bronchioles may create bronchiectasis, including TB, adenoviral infections, and pneumonia. Bronchiectasis also develops in people with immunodeficiencies involving humoral immunity, recurrent aspiration, and abnormal mucociliary clearance (immotile cilia syndromes). Cystic fibrosis causes about one-half of all cases of bronchiectasis. Sinusitis, dextrocardia (heart located on right side of chest), Kartagener's syndrome (alterations in ciliary activity), defective development of bronchial cartilage (Williams-Campbell syndrome), and endobronchial tumor predispose a person to bronchiectasis.

Pathogenesis.   Although bronchiectasis has been viewed as a progressive disease of destruction and dilation of the medium and large airways, there is now evidence of the importance of the small airways in the pathogenesis of this condition. Chronic inflammation of the bronchial wall by mononuclear cells is common to all types of bronchiectasis. Abnormal bronchial dilation characteristic of bronchiectasis is accompanied by accumulation of wet secretions that plug the airway and cause bronchospasm, producing even more purulent mucus. A vicious cycle of bacteria-provoked inflammatory lung damage occurs with irreversible destruction or fragmentation of the bronchial wall and resultant fibrosis further obstructing and obliterating the bronchial lumen (Fig. 14-10). In response to these changes, large anastomoses develop between the bronchial and pulmonary blood vessels to increase the blood flow through the bronchial circulation. These anastomoses are responsible for the hemoptysis present in persons with bronchiectasis.

Clinical Manifestations.   The most immediate symptom of bronchiectasis is persistent coughing, with large amounts of purulent sputum production (worse in the morning). Weight loss, anemia, and other systemic manifestations, such as low-grade fever, hemoptysis, fatigue, weakness, nasal congestion, and drainage from sinusitis, are also common. Clubbing may occur, and the breath and sputum may become foul-smelling with advanced disease. Complications such as an abnormality in ventilation/perfusion and resultant hypoxemia may occur. There is a known correlation between bronchiectasis and rheumatoid arthritis, but the exact mechanism for this remains unknown.

Medical Management

Diagnosis.   Imaging studies (e.g., high-resolution CT scan) have become increasingly accurate in depicting the features of early bronchiectasis. Ultrafast and multislice CT scans have increased the value of CT as a diagnostic tool by reducing the need for sedation or anesthesia. Other diagnostic tests include x-ray studies, laboratory tests including sweat chloride test for CF, electron microscopy of bronchial biopsy for immotile cilia, and sputum culture analyses.

Treatment.   The goals of treatment are removal of secretions and prevention of infection. The principal treatment is pulmonary physical therapy, bronchodilators, and antibiotics selected on the basis of sputum smears and cultures. Hydration is important, and oxygen may be administered. Surgical resection is reserved for the few clients with localized bronchiectasis and adequate pulmonary function who fail to respond to conservative management or for the person with massive hemoptysis. Long-term care is the same as for any person with COPD.

Prognosis.   The morbidity and mortality associated with bronchiectasis have declined markedly in industrialized nations, but prevalence remains high in Pacific and Asian countries. The overall prognosis is often poor, and although bronchiectasis is usually localized to a lung lobe or segment, persistent, nonresolving infection may cause the disorder to spread to other parts of the same lung. Complications of bronchiectasis include recurrent pneumonia, lung abscesses, metastatic infections in other organs (e.g., brain abscess), and respiratory failure. Good pulmonary hygiene and avoidance of infectious complications in the involved areas may reverse some cases of bronchiectasis.

Special Implications for the Therapist   14-8

BRONCHIECTASIS

Preferred Practice Patterns:
6B: *Impaired Aerobic Capacity/Endurance Associated With*
      Deconditioning
6C: *Impaired Ventilation, Respiration/Gas Exchange, and*
      Aerobic Capacity/Endurance Associated With Airway
      Clearance Dysfunction
6F: *Impaired Ventilation and Respiration/Gas Exchange*
      Associated With Respiratory Failure

The effects of bronchopulmonary hygiene physical therapy (chest therapy, chest physical therapy) to improve pulmonary function in bronchiectasis remain inconclusive.[125] The beneficial effects of chest therapy to mobilize secretions and improve pulmonary clearance (e.g., sputum production, radioaerosol clearance) in the treatment of bronchiectasis have been documented in one small study.[124] In many settings, chest therapy for the person with bronchiectasis is administered routinely on the basis of diagnosis rather than specific clinical criteria. Further research to clarify bronchopulmonary hygiene physical therapy or chest therapy outcomes is necessary and may provide the therapist with clinical goals other than secretion mobilization.

The selection of techniques to include in a chest therapy regimen varies among institutions as well as among practitioners and may include postural drainage and chest percussion of involved lobes performed several times per day. Family members can be instructed in how to provide this care at home. Directed coughing and breathing exercises to promote good ventilation and removal of secretions should follow positional or percussive therapy. The best times to do this are early morning and several hours after eating the final meal; these techniques just before bedtime may result in increased coughing and prevent the person from sleeping. For an excellent review of the use of chest physical therapy in the acute care setting see reference 51. ■

◆ Bronchiolitis

Definition and Overview.   Bronchiolitis is a commonly occurring, acute, diffuse, and often severe inflammation of the lower airways (bronchioles) in children under 2 years caused by a viral infection. Although acute infectious bronchiolitis has not been recognized as a distinct entity in adults, bronchiolitis obliterans does occur. Bronchiolitis was once classified as a type of chronic interstitial pneumonia and referred to as "small airways disease"; progress in pathology has provided more specific and even etiology-directed diagnoses that reflect the individual reaction patterns observed. Bronchiolitis obliterans in the adult is now considered acute or chronic with identification of these special forms (e.g., obliterative, eosinophilic bronchiolitis in asthma, necrotizing bronchiolitis in viral infection, or toxic fume bronchiolitis following exposure to noxious gases and the development of chemical pneumonitis).[178]

Bronchiolitis obliterans is the most important clinical complication in heart-lung transplant recipients and may represent a form of allograft rejection; it is a rare complication of allogeneic (human-to-human) bone marrow transplantation. Bronchiolitis obliterans may occur in association with rheumatoid arthritis, polymyositis, and dermatomyositis. Penicillamine therapy has been implicated as a possible cause of bronchiolitis obliterans in clients with rheumatoid arthritis.

Incidence and Etiologic Factors.   Bronchiolitis obliterans in adults usually occurs with chronic bronchitis; bronchiolitis in children is associated with pulmonary infections, such as respiratory syncytial virus (RSV), parainfluenza viruses, adenoviruses, or pertussis (whooping cough), or associated with measles. Primarily present in winter and spring, it is easily spread by hand-to-nose or nose-to-eye transmission. *Exudative bronchiolitis*, inflammation of the bronchioles with exudation of gray tenacious sputum, is often associated with asthma.

Pathogenesis and Clinical Manifestations.   Variable degrees of obstruction occur in response to infection as the bronchiolar mucosa swells and the lumina fill with mucus and exudate. These changes occur as the walls of the bronchi and bronchioles are infiltrated with inflammatory cells. Hyperinflation, obstructive emphysema from partial obstruction, and patchy areas of atelectasis may occur distal to the inflammatory lesion as the disease progresses.

Bronchiolitis begins as a simple upper respiratory infection (URI) with serous nasal discharge and mild fever. Cough, respiratory distress, and cyanosis occur initially, followed by a brief period of improvement. Dyspnea, paroxysmal cough, sputum production, and wheezing with marked use of accessory muscles follow as the disease progresses. Apnea may be the first indicator of RSV infection in very young infants. Severe disease may be followed by a rise in arterial carbon dioxide tension ($PaCO_2$) (hypercapnia), leading to respiratory acidosis and hypoxemia.

Medical Management
Diagnosis and Treatment.   Diagnosis is made on the basis of clinical findings, age, the season, and the epidemiology of the community. On chest radiographs this condition is difficult to differentiate from bacterial pneumonia. RSV can be positively identified using an enzyme-linked immunosorbent assay (ELISA) from direct aspiration of nasal secretions.

There is no specific treatment for bronchiolitis, and medical therapy is controversial. Treatment modalities may include steroids, humidified air, hydration, and physical therapy for postural drainage, coughing, and deep-breathing exercises. Antibiotics may be used initially when a bacterial cause of illness has not been ruled out or for secondary infections. Mist therapy combined with oxygen by hood or tent to alleviate dyspnea and hypoxia may be used with children.

Prognosis.   The disease lasts about 3 to 10 days, and the majority of cases can be managed at home with a good prognosis. Hospitalization may be necessary for anyone with complicating conditions such as underlying lung or heart disease, associated debilitated states, poor hydration, or questionable care at home. Some children deteriorate rapidly and die within weeks; others may follow a more long-term course. In the adult, the acute form usually has a good prognosis, but the prognosis for chronic bronchiolitis obliterans is poor, as in COPD.

Special Implications for the Therapist 14-9

BRONCHIOLITIS

Preferred Practice Patterns:
6B: Impaired Aerobic Capacity/Endurance Associated With Deconditioning
6C: Impaired Ventilation, Respiration/Gas Exchange, and Aerobic Capacity/Endurance Associated With Airway Clearance Dysfunction
6F: Impaired Ventilation and Respiration/Gas Exchange Associated With Respiratory Failure

RSV is the most common cause of pediatric acute bronchiolitis and pneumonia (see the section on RSV in Chapter 7). For this reason, any staff member with evidence of URI serves as a potential reservoir of RSV and should be excluded from direct contact with high-risk infants. All persons who come within 3 feet of an RSV client must wear a gown and mask with an eye shield and keep hands away from the face, especially the eyes, nose, and mouth. Hands must be washed before and after caring for any client and after handling potentially contaminated client care equipment. Standard Precautions (see Appendix A) must be strictly carried out.

Because RSV is readily transmitted by close contact with personnel, families, and other children both by direct contact (especially lifting or holding) and through contact with objects handled by the child, precautions against cross infection are important. The primary routes of inoculation for the organisms are large-droplet inhalation through the nose and eyes. When contact is made with mucous discharge or drainage from the eye, nose, or mouth, the therapist is reminded to wear an exterior hospital gown and to discard the gown (or change clothing) when leaving. Pregnant female personnel or visitors should be advised of the risk of potential physical defects in the developing embryo from contact with RSV. Prevention of RSV may be possible in the future with active maternal immunization during pregnancy providing passive immunity of infants.[66,87] ■

◆ Sleep-Disordered Breathing

Definition. Sleep-disordered breathing comprises a collection of syndromes characterized by breathing abnormalities during sleep that result in intermittently disrupted gas exchange and in sleep interruption. Sleep-disordered breathing includes Cheyne-Stokes respiration, hypoventilation syndromes with and without chronic lung disease, heavy snoring with daytime sleepiness (upper airway resistance syndrome), and sleep apnea. The most common and only one discussed here, *sleep apnea syndrome*, is defined as significant daytime symptoms (e.g., sleepiness) in conjunction with evidence of sleep-related upper airway obstruction and sleep disturbance.[27]

There are three types of sleep apnea: central, obstructive, and mixed. *Central apnea* is caused by altered chemosensitivity and cerebral respiratory control. In this type of apnea, the brain fails to send the appropriate signals to the respiratory muscles to initiate breathing and there is no diaphragmatic movement and no air flow. This is seen in infants less than 40 weeks' conceptual age and in people with neurologic disorders (e.g., tumors, brain infarcts, diffuse encephalopathies). The most dramatic presentation is the person with repetitive apneas during sleep, accompanied by extreme daytime sleepiness. *Obstructive apnea*, the most commonly diagnosed form of sleep apnea, is characterized by respiratory effort without air flow because of upper airway obstruction. *Mixed apnea* is a central apnea that is immediately followed by an obstructive event.

Incidence. Sleep apnea syndrome occurs twice as often in obese males between 25 and 55 years. Numerous theories to explain this variable are under investigation, but a single causative factor has not been identified.[175,214,231] At least 4% of the general adult population is affected (estimated between 12 and 18 million people), with a growing recognition of affected individuals and an observed dramatic increase in the older population. The incidence of obstructive sleep apnea may be much higher because the signs and symptoms of chronic sleep disruption are often overlooked or misdiagnosed in spite of their debilitating consequences.

Etiologic and Risk Factors. Obstructive apnea is due to partial or complete pharyngeal collapse during sleep, leading to either reduction (hypopnea) or cessation (apnea) of breathing. The main cause is upper body obesity (present in 70% of adult cases), especially a large neck circumference. A neck circumference greater than 16 inches for a woman or greater than 17 inches in a man correlates with an increased risk for this disorder.[210] People with anatomically narrowed upper airways, such as occur in micrognathia; macroglossia (large tongue); obesity; and adenoid, uvula, elongated soft palate, or tonsillar hypertrophy are predisposed to the development of obstructive sleep apnea. Other risk factors include increasing age; genetic factors (sleep-disordered breathing clusters in families); neurologic disorders; smoking; and cardiopulmonary dysfunctions, such as hypertension, moderate to severe heart failure (including cor pulmonale), calcification of carotid arteries, chronic bronchitis, or cardiac dysrhythmia. Alcohol or sedatives before sleeping may precipitate or worsen the condition.

Pathogenesis. There are several hypotheses as to the pathogenesis of sleep apnea syndrome. Collapse or obstruction of the airway may occur with the inhibition of muscle tone that characterizes rapid eye movement (REM) sleep. When loss of normal pharyngeal muscle tone allows the larynx to collapse passively during inspiration, upper airway obstruction occurs and prevents effective ventilation. By definition, apnea is a complete cessation of ventilation and therefore is precipitated by complete pharyngeal collapse whereas hypopnea results from partial pharyngeal closure and is manifested by a substantial reduction in, but not a cessation of, breathing. Both conditions can lead to substantial hypoxia and hypercapnia with arousal from sleep required to reestablish airway patency and a resumption of ventilation. This cycle of recurrent pharyngeal collapse with subsequent arousal from sleep leads to the primary symptoms of daytime somnolence.[72]

Clinical Manifestations.
The frequent interruptions of deep, restorative sleep often lead to daytime (including morning) sluggishness and headaches, daytime fatigue, excessive daytime sleepiness, cognitive impairment, recent weight gain, and sexual impotence. Bed partners usually report loud cyclic snoring with periods of silence (breath cessation), restlessness, frequent episodes of waking up gasping, and often thrashing movements of the extremities during sleep. Neurocognitive effects may include personality changes; irritability, hyperactivity, and depression*; judgment impairment or poor school performance; domestic, work-related, or automobile accidents; memory loss; and difficulty concentrating. Fragmented sleep with its repetitive cycles of snoring, airway collapse, and arousal may cause hypertension in some people, and sleep-disordered breathing may be a risk factor for cardiovascular involvement, including angina pectoris, acute myocardial infarction, cardiac arrhythmias, and ischemic stroke.[35,172]

Medical Management
Diagnosis.
Diagnosis may be made using sleep monitoring devices, radiologic imaging, laboratory assays, questionnaires, and clinical signs and symptoms, but the most reliable test to confirm the diagnosis is overnight polysomnography (i.e., monitoring the subject during sleep for periods of apnea and lowered blood oxygen saturation). The physician must differentiate sleep apnea syndrome from seizure disorder, narcolepsy, or psychiatric depression. A hemoglobin level is obtained, and thyroid function tests are performed.

Treatment.
Obstructive and mixed types of sleep apnea syndrome can be treated. Since many clients with sleep apnea are overweight, weight loss is recommended. Weight loss may be curative, but only a small percentage of people maintain their weight loss and symptoms return with weight gain. Therefore alternative interventions have been developed, and the most common treatment for obstructive sleep apnea is nasal continuous positive airway pressure (CPAP), used during sleep. The positive pressure from the CPAP pumps open the airway and prevents it from obstructing, but this treatment technique may not be tolerated by some people and adherence to its use is only about 40%.[143]

Surgery is recommended if an airway obstruction can be determined as the cause of the sleep apnea. Neurogenic causes of sleep apnea are more difficult to control. Oral appliances inserted into the mouth at bedtime to hold the jaw forward and prevent pharyngeal occlusion are regulated by the FDA, but little clinical testing has been done to determine the efficacy and safety of these devices.[191] Medications to stimulate breathing have not been beneficial, and alcohol and hypnotic medications should be avoided. In a limited number of cases, administration of oxygen during the night is helpful, but polysomnography must be used to assess the effects of oxygen therapy.[162]

---

*Neurocognitive effects of apnea may also cause a mood disorder leading to an erroneous diagnosis of dysthymia; treatment with standard antidepressant medications may exacerbate the condition.[229]

Prognosis.
Evidence indicates that chronic, heavy snoring may be associated with increased long-term cardiovascular and neurophysiologic morbidity. Cardiac and vascular morbidity may include systemic hypertension, cardiac arrhythmias, pulmonary hypertension, cor pulmonale, left ventricular dysfunction, stroke, and sudden death. Recognition and appropriate treatment of obstructive sleep apnea and related disorders will often significantly enhance the client's quality of life, overall health, productivity, and safety on the highway.[183]

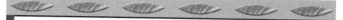

Special Implications for the Therapist 14-10

SLEEP-DISORDERED BREATHING: APNEA

Preferred Practice Patterns:
6A: Primary Prevention/Risk Reduction for Cardiovascular/Pulmonary Disorders (apnea is a risk factor for cardiovascular involvement)
6C: Impaired Ventilation, Respiration/Gas Exchange, and Aerobic Capacity/Endurance Associated With Airway Clearance Dysfunction

Currently, there is very little research on the effects of pulmonary rehabilitation in persons with sleep apnea. Results from one study showed positive exercise training responses with decreased ratings of shortness of breath, suggesting that pulmonary rehabilitation may be an effective intervention to consider in persons with obstructive sleep apnea.[164] Because of the possible cardiovascular complications associated with clients who have obstructive sleep apnea, vital signs should be monitored before, during, and after submaximal or maximal exercise. The client should not be left in the supine position for prolonged periods of time, even while awake.

There are some reports of sleep apnea in association with cervical lesions (e.g., osteophytes caused by diffuse idiopathic skeletal hyperostosis [DISH]),[114] as well as rheumatoid arthritis complicated with temporomandibular joint destruction and cervical involvement.[169] As this syndrome is studied more closely, a definitive correlation between cervical lesions and sleep disturbances may be documented. Physical therapy may be explored in developing treatment protocols when the musculoskeletal structures of the mandible contribute to the problem. ■

RESTRICTIVE LUNG DISEASE

Overview.
Restrictive lung disorders are a major category of pulmonary problems including any condition that limits lung expansion. Pulmonary function tests are characterized by a decrease in lung volume or total lung capacity. There are many causes of restrictive lung diseases that are covered in other sections of this chapter or book. More than 100 identified interstitial lung diseases can cause restrictive lung disease. Extrapulmonary causes may include neurologic (e.g., head or spinal cord injury, amyotrophic lateral sclerosis, myasthenia gravis, Guillain-Barré syndrome, muscular dystrophy, poliomyelitis) and neuromuscular (e.g., ankylosing spondylitis,

kyphosis or scoliosis, chest wall injury or deformity) disorders, obesity, or obstructive sleep disorders.

Clinical Manifestations. Clinical presentation varies according to the cause of the restrictive disorder. Generally, clients with restrictive lung disease exhibit a rapid, shallow respiratory pattern. Chronic hyperventilation occurs in an effort to overcome the effects of reduced lung volume and compliance. Exertional dyspnea progresses to dyspnea at rest. As the disease progresses, respiratory muscle fatigue may occur, leading to inadequate alveolar ventilation and carbon dioxide retention. Hypoxemia is a common finding, especially in the later stages of restrictive disease.

Medical Management
Treatment and Prognosis. The management of restrictive lung disease is based in part on the underlying cause. Treatment goals are oriented toward adequate oxygenation, maintaining an airway, and obtaining maximal function. For example, persons with spinal deformities may be helped with corrective surgery and obese persons may experience improved breathing after weight loss. Corticosteroids may help control inflammation and reduce further impairment, but previously damaged alveolocapillary units cannot be regenerated or replaced. Some clients with end-stage disease may be candidates for single-lung transplantation. Most restrictive lung diseases are not reversible, and the disease progresses to include pulmonary hypertension, cor pulmonale, severe decreased oxygenation, and eventual ventilatory failure.

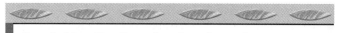

Special Implications for the Therapist **14-11**

RESTRICTIVE LUNG DISEASE

Preferred Practice Pattern:
6E: Impaired Ventilation and Respiration/Gas Exchange
*   *Associated With Ventilatory Pump Dysfunction or Failure*

A primary problem for clients with restrictive lung disease secondary to generalized weakness and neuromuscular disease is ineffective cough. Pulmonary physical therapy to facilitate cough and effective dislodging of secretions to the central airways may be exhausting for the client. Rest periods must be incorporated in the treatment. A person with restrictive lung disease will be more adversely affected by the restriction on lung function in the recumbent position, emphasizing the importance of routine positioning for immobile clients and active or active-assisted movements whenever possible. ∎

◆ **Pulmonary Fibrosis**
Definition and Overview. Pulmonary fibrosis (also known as interstitial lung disease) is a general term that refers to a variety of disorders in which chronic inflammation of lung tissue leads to progressive scarring (fibrosis) of the lungs, predominantly fibroblasts and small blood vessels that progressively remove and replace normal tissue.

Etiologic and Risk Factors. Two-thirds of cases of pulmonary fibrosis are *idiopathic pulmonary fibrosis* (cause unknown). In the remaining one-third, fibrosis in the lung is caused by healing scar tissue after active disease such as TB, systemic sclerosis, or adult respiratory distress syndrome (ARDS) or following inhalation of harmful particles, such as moldy hay, metal dust, coal dust, or asbestos. Other risk factors include some infections and connective tissue diseases such as rheumatoid arthritis or systemic lupus erythematosus; certain drugs, particularly some chemotherapy agents; and in rare cases, genetic or familial predisposition. Thoracic radiation (e.g., postmastectomy irradiation of the chest wall and regional lymphatics in clients with breast cancer) may result in pericarditis and pneumonitis, which can progress to pulmonary fibrosis weeks, or even months, after radiation treatments have ended (see the section on Radiation Lung Disease in Chapter 4).

Pathogenesis and Clinical Manifestations. Fibroblast proliferation (fibrosis) irreversibly distorts and shrinks the lung lobe at the alveolar level and causes a marked loss of lung compliance. The lung becomes stiff and difficult to ventilate with decreased diffusing capacity of the alveolocapillary membrane, causing hypoxemia. There does not appear to be an inflammatory process but rather abnormal wound healing in response to multiple, microscopic sites of ongoing alveolar epithelial injury and fibrosis.[192] The course of pulmonary fibrosis varies, with early symptoms such as shortness of breath and a dry cough potentially progressing to further complications.

Treatment and Prognosis. Treatment usually begins with corticosteroids to reduce lung inflammation; other anti-inflammatories may be tried if steroids fail to achieve the desired results. The clinical course of people with pulmonary fibrosis and rheumatoid arthritis is chronic and progressive. Response to treatment is unpredictable, and the overall prognosis is poor with median survival time less than 4 years.[88]

Special Implications for the Therapist **14-12**

PULMONARY FIBROSIS

Preferred Practice Pattern:
6E: Impaired Ventilation and Respiration/Gas Exchange
*   *Associated With Ventilatory Pump Dysfunction or Failure*

One of the most common late effects of chest irradiation is pulmonary fibrosis, which may not occur for months to years after radiation to the thorax. The total dose of radiation and the size of the treatment portal determine the severity of this condition. The changes in pulmonary function are usually a progressive decline in lung volumes and a decrease in lung compliance and diffusing capacity. As doses increase, the frequency of pulmonary fibrosis increases, but with improved dosage fractionation, most people die from the cancer before these complications develop. Physical therapy intervention depends on clinical presentation following the appropriate preferred practice pattern or patterns. ∎

◆ Systemic Sclerosis Lung Disease

Definition.   Systemic sclerosis (SS), or scleroderma, is an autoimmune disease of connective tissue characterized by excessive collagen deposition in the skin and internal organs, particularly the lungs. This condition is discussed in detail in Chapter 9.

Incidence.   Clinically, more than one-half of all people with SS develop interstitial lung disease, although autopsy results suggest a prevalence of 75%. The lungs, owing to a rich vascular supply and abundant connective tissue, are a frequent target organ (second to the esophagus in visceral involvement). Skin changes generally precede visceral alterations, and lung involvement rarely presents symptoms at first, but eventually pulmonary symptoms develop.

Pathogenesis and Clinical Manifestations.   Oxidative stress contributes to disease progression by a rapid degeneration of endothelial cell function in SS. Daily episodes of hypoxia-reperfusion injury produce free radicals (see Fig. 5-2) that cause endothelial damage, intimal thickening, and fibrosis along with inactivation of antioxidant enzymes.[80] There are two types of pulmonary involvement including infiltration of the lungs and/or pulmonary artery hypertension associated with these endothelial changes in the arterioles and capillaries. Lung biopsy of early lesions shows capillary congestion, hypercellularity of alveolar walls, increased fibrous tissue in the alveolar septa, and interstitial edema with fibrosis. As a result, initial symptoms of dyspnea on exertion and nonproductive cough develop. As fibroblast proliferation and collagen deposition progress, fibrosis of the alveolar wall occurs and the capillaries are obliterated. Clinically, the client demonstrates more severe dyspnea and has a greater risk of deterioration in pulmonary function.

Medical Management

Diagnosis.   Traditional tests such as pulmonary function tests and chest radiographs are insensitive and not predictive of outcome. Thin-section CT is very sensitive for early diagnosis of SS lung involvement, and some investigators use bronchoalveolar lavage to identify alveolitis in clients with SS.

Treatment.   Successful treatment of SS pulmonary disease remains an area for further development. Pharmacologic treatment using low-dose prednisone (as opposed to high-dose corticosteroids used with idiopathic pulmonary fibrosis) is recommended because of the possible association of high-dose corticosteroids with renal failure in clients with SS. Cyclophosphamide, an antineoplastic alkylating agent, has been used to treat interstitial lung disease in people with SS and remains under investigation.[218] Identifying the cycle of oxidative stress and antioxidant inactivation may result in treatment by supplementation of antioxidants and different kinds of drugs with antioxidant properties.[80] New investigations conclude that lung transplantation is a viable option for carefully selected individuals with scleroderma-related lung disease.[185] Stem cell transplantation, a very aggressive form of immunosuppression, is also under investigation.[79]

Prognosis.   SS lung disease is unpredictable and may be a mild, prolonged course, but as the pulmonary fibrosis advances, cor pulmonale characterized by peripheral edema may develop, progressing rapidly to respiratory failure and death. Lung disease is becoming the most frequent cause of death from SS.

Special Implications for the Therapist   14-13

SYSTEMIC SCLEROSIS LUNG DISEASE

Preferred Practice Patterns:
    Patterns may vary depending on degree of pulmonary involvement and response to treatment. See also Special Implications for the Therapist: Systemic Sclerosis, 9-13.
6B: *Impaired Aerobic Capacity/Endurance Associated With Deconditioning*
6E: *Impaired Ventilation and Respiration/Gas Exchange Associated With Ventilatory Pump Dysfunction or Failure (pulmonary fibrosis)*
6F: *Impaired Ventilation and Respiration/Gas Exchange Associated With Respiratory Failure*

The effectiveness of a pulmonary rehabilitation program with SS lung disease remains unknown and warrants research investigation. Therapy implications and interventions should be based on general principles regarding pulmonary involvement and specific clinical presentation. ■

◆ Chest Wall Disease or Injury

Chest or thoracic trauma ranges from superficial wounds such as contusions and abrasions to life-threatening tension pneumothorax. Flail chest occurs as a result of sternum or multiple rib fracture. By definition, a flail chest consists of fractures of two or more adjacent ribs on the same side, and possibly the sternum, with each bone fractured into two or more segments. The fractured rib segments are detached (free-floating) from the rest of the chest wall.

Clinical Manifestations.   It is common for a fractured rib end to tear the pleura and lung surface, thereby producing hemopneumothorax. Fractures of this type result in instability of a portion of the chest wall, causing paradoxical movement of the chest with breathing. During inspiration, the unstable portion of the chest wall moves (or falls) inward, and during expiration the chest wall moves outward with unequal chest expansion impairing movement of gas in and out of the lungs (Fig. 14-11), promoting atelectasis and impairing pulmonary drainage. Fractured ribs can also lacerate abdominal organs, the brachial plexus, and blood vessels. Other clinical manifestations of flail chest include excruciating pain, severe dyspnea, hypoventilation, cyanosis, and hypoxemia, leading to respiratory failure without the appropriate intervention.

Medical Management.   Initial treatment follows the ABCs of emergency treatment (*airway, breathing, circulation*) to treat the pneumothorax, thereby enabling the person to breathe deeply and to effectively clear secretions. Treatment

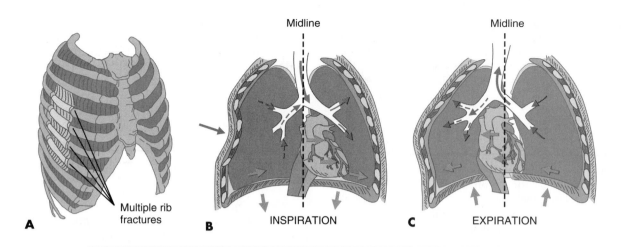

A Multiple rib fractures   **B** INSPIRATION   **C** EXPIRATION

FIGURE   **14-11**   Flail chest. Arrows indicate air movement or structural movement. **A,** A flail chest consists of fractured rib segments that are detached (free-floating) from the rest of the chest wall. **B,** On inspiration, the flail segment of ribs is sucked inward. The affected lung and mediastinal structures shift to the unaffected side. This compromises the amount of inspired air in the unaffected lung. **C,** On expiration, the flail segment of ribs bellows outward. The affected lung and mediastinal structures shift to the affected side with the diaphragm elevated on that side (not shown). Some air within the lungs is shunted back and forth between the lungs instead of passing through the upper airway.

for any cardiovascular collapse is then followed by pain control. Continuous positive airway pressure (CPAP) may be used to enhance lung expansion. Treatment may require internal fixation by controlled mechanical ventilation until the chest wall has stabilized, which may take 14 to 21 days or more. Whenever pulmonary function is adequate, intubation is avoided to help reduce infection, the most common complication associated with morbidity and mortality in clients with flail chest. Pharmacologic treatment may include muscle relaxants or musculoskeletal paralyzing agents (e.g., pancuronium bromide) to reduce the risk of separation of the healing costochondral junctions. *Hemothorax,* blood in the pleural cavity following chest trauma, must be removed through a chest tube. The tube is usually positioned in the sixth intercostal space in the posterior axillary line.

Older adults are more likely to have co-morbid conditions and less likely to tolerate traumatic respiratory compromise. Age and its effects on the body are the strongest predictor of outcome with flail chest, and increasing age is associated with increased complications and mortality.[4]

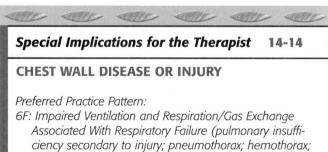

Special Implications for the Therapist   14-14

CHEST WALL DISEASE OR INJURY

Preferred Practice Pattern:
6F: Impaired Ventilation and Respiration/Gas Exchange
  Associated With Respiratory Failure (pulmonary insufficiency secondary to injury; pneumothorax; hemothorax; pulmonary collapse)

See also the section on Pneumothorax and Special Implications for the Therapist: Pneumothorax, 14-26.

The emergency room therapist is the most likely therapist to evaluate and treat someone with a flail chest although this varies by geographic region. Once the person has been stabilized and moved to the acute care setting, therapists may come into contact with this person during the recovery period. Manual techniques such as chest physical therapy may be used, but the presence of a lung contusion directs medical intervention more toward mobilizing blood secretions. Chest therapy may have a role in facilitating chest tube drainage but must be used carefully in the presence of any rib fractures. Percussion and vibration techniques are contraindicated directly over fractures but can be used over other lung segments. Rib or chest taping and ultrasound over the site of the fracture should not be used. Once the fractures have healed, rib mobilization and soft tissue mobilization for the intercostals may be necessary to restore normal respiratory movements.

Frequent turning and position changes, as well as deep-breathing and coughing exercises, are important. A semi-Fowler's position may help with lung reexpansion necessary to prevent atelectasis. In the case of flail chest from injury, simultaneous cardiac damage may have occurred, necessitating the same care as for a person who has suffered a myocardial infarction (see Special Implications for the Therapist: Myocardial Infarction, 11-6).

Sternal fractures associated with clinically silent myocardial contusion are best visualized on chest CT, but scapular fractures are often overlooked when only supine chest radiographs are performed. The therapist may recognize a suspicious clinical presentation (e.g., loss of scapular-humeral motion, symptoms out of proportion to the injury, development of previously undocumented large hematomas) suggesting the need for more definitive medical diagnosis. In the case of scapular fracture, once the fracture is healed the therapist may become involved in restoration of movement and strength. ■

ENVIRONMENTAL AND OCCUPATIONAL DISEASES

The relationship between occupations and disease has been observed, studied, and documented for many years. An in-depth discussion of this broad topic is included in Chapter 3. This chapter discusses only environmental and occupational diseases related to the lung. Occupational diseases can be divided into three major categories: (1) inorganic dusts (pneumoconioses), (2) organic dusts (hypersensitivity pneumonitis), and (3) fumes, gases, and smoke inhalation. These three categories have pathologic characteristics in common, including involvement of the pulmonary parenchyma with a fibrotic response.

◆ Pneumoconiosis

Overview.   Any group of lung diseases resulting from inhalation of particles of industrial substances, particularly inorganic dusts such as that from iron ore or coal, with permanent deposition of substantial amounts of such particles in the lung is included in the generic term of *pneumoconiosis* (dusty lungs). Clinically common pneumoconioses include coal workers' pneumoconiosis, silicosis, and asbestosis. Other types of pneumoconiosis include talc, beryllium lung disease (berylliosis), aluminum pneumoconiosis, cadmium workers' disease, and siderosis (inhalation of iron or other metallic particles). Farmers in dry-climate regions exposed to respirable dust (inorganic agricultural dusts) during farming activities (e.g., plowing, tilling) and toxic gases (e.g., from animal confinement) may develop chronic bronchitis, hypersensitivity pneumonitis, and pulmonary fibrosis.

Incidence and Etiologic Factors.   Obviously occurring in occupational groups, pneumoconiosis is most common among miners, sandblasters, stonecutters, asbestos workers, insulators, and agriculture workers. There is an increasing incidence with age because of cumulative effects of exposure, but overall incidence of diseases caused by mineral dust has declined recently in postindustrial countries. Instead there is a rise in occupational asthma and illnesses caused by exposure in new office buildings and hospitals.[26]

Silicosis, formerly called potters' asthma, stonecutters' cough, miners' mold, and grinders' rot, is most likely to be contracted in today's industrial jobs involving sandblasting in tunnels, hard-rock mining (extraction and processing of ores), and preparation and use of sand. It can occur in anyone habitually exposed (usually over a period of 10 years) to the dust contained in silica, and any miner is subject to it. Usually, silicosis is associated with extensive or prolonged inhalation of free silica (silicon dioxide) particles in the crystalline form of quartz.

Risk Factors.   Higher-risk workplaces are those with obvious dust, smoke, or vapor or those in which there is spraying, painting, or drying of coated surfaces. Heavier exposure occurs when there is friction, grinding, heat, or blasting; when very small particles are generated; and in enclosed spaces. Not all clients exposed to occupational inhalants will develop lung disease. Harmful effects depend on the (1) type of exposure; (2) duration and intensity of exposure; (3) presence of underlying pulmonary disease; (4) smoking history; and (5) particle size and water solubility of the inhalant. The larger the particle, the lower the probability of its reaching the lower respira-

tory tract; highly water-soluble inhalants tend to dissolve and react in the upper respiratory tract, whereas poorly soluble substances may travel as far as the alveoli.

The risk of lung cancer in those who both smoke and are exposed to asbestosis is increased in a multiplicative way.[28] Exposure to significant amounts of asbestos is most common when asbestos materials are disturbed during renovation, repair, or demolition of older buildings containing asbestos materials. Exposure while washing clothes soiled with these toxic substances has caused mesothelioma (malignancy associated with asbestos exposure) and berylliosis (beryllium lung disease associated with exposure to beryllium used in the manufacture of fluorescent lamps before 1950). Beryllium is used today as a metal in structural materials employed in aerospace industries, in the manufacture of industrial ceramics, and in atomic reactors, so exposure is still possible.

Pathogenesis.   Dust particles (indestructible mineral fibers) that are not filtered out by the nasociliary mechanism or mucociliary escalator may be deposited anywhere in the respiratory tract and lungs, especially the small airways and alveoli. Each disease has its own pathogenesis, but in general the most dangerous dust particles measure $2 \mu m$ or less and are deposited in the smallest bronchioles and the acini (see Fig. 14-2). The particles are ingested by alveolar macrophages, and most of the phagocytosed particles ascend to the mucociliary lining and are expectorated or swallowed. Some migrate into the interstitium of the lung and then into the lymphatics. These indestructible mineral fibers can actually pierce the lung cells. In response to the continued presence of these fibers and to the cell damage, activated macrophages secrete fibroblast-stimulating factor, which in turn mediates excessive fibrosis (i.e., the thickening and scarring of lung tissue that occur around the mineral fiber).

In *coal workers' pneumoconiosis*, ingestion of inhaled coal dust* by alveolar macrophages leads to the formation of coal macules, which appear on the radiograph as diffuse small opacities (or white areas) in the upper lung. In the pathogenesis of *silicosis*, groups of silicon hydroxide on the surface of the particles form hydrogen bonds with phospholipids and proteins, an interaction that is presumed to damage cellular membranes and thereby kill the macrophage. The dead macrophages release free silica particles and fibrogenic factors. The released silica is then reingested by macrophages, and the process is amplified. Between 10 and 40 years after initial exposure to silica, small rounded opacities called *silicotic nodules* form throughout the lung. These fibrotic nodules scar the lungs and make them receptive to further complications (e.g., TB, bronchitis, emphysema).

Asbestosis is characterized by inhalation of asbestos fibers, a fibrous magnesium and calcium silicate nonburning compound used in roofing materials, insulation for electric circuits, brake linings, and many other products that must be fire-resistant. As with the other pneumoconioses, asbestos particles are engulfed by macrophages. Once activated, macrophages then release inflammatory mediators resulting in nodular interstitial fibrosis that can be seen on radiographs along with thickened pleura. After an interval of 10 to 20 years between exposure and fur-

---

*Anthracite or hard coal is associated with a higher incidence of black lung than is bituminous or soft coal.

ther complications, calcified pleural plaques on the dome of the diaphragm or lateral chest wall develop. The lower portions of the lungs are more often involved than the upper portions in asbestosis. How asbestos causes mesothelioma is unclear; the formation of oxygen free radicals by macrophages can be a cause of chromosomal damage, or there may be a growth factor that governs individual susceptibility to mineral fiber–induced mesothelioma. Other mechanisms of oncogenesis have been proposed but remain unconfirmed.[47,180]

Clinical Manifestations.   Symptoms of pneumoconioses from dust exposure include progressive dyspnea, chest pain, chronic cough, and expectoration of mucus containing the offending particles. In rare cases, rheumatoid arthritis co-existing primarily with coal workers' pneumoconiosis but also with silicosis and asbestosis causes *Caplan's syndrome,* a condition characterized by the presence of rheumatoid nodules in the periphery of the lung. Long-term exposure to acid and other substances produces ulceration and perforation of the septum, whereas nickel and certain wood dusts cause nasal carcinoma.

Work-related asthma can be an exacerbation of asthma that was previously subclinical or in remission (work-aggravated asthma), a new onset of asthma caused by a sensitizing exposure (asthma with latency), or asthma that results from a single heavy exposure to a potent respiratory irritant (referred to as asthma without latency, irritant asthma, or reactive airways dysfunction syndrome). Symptoms are as discussed in the section on Asthma in this chapter.

Simple silicosis is usually asymptomatic and has no effect on routine pulmonary function tests. As the disease progresses, mucus tinged with blood, loss of appetite, chest pain, and general weakness may occur. In complicated silicosis, dyspnea and obstructive and restrictive lung dysfunction occur. Asbestosis is characterized by dyspnea, inspiratory crackles (on auscultation), and sometimes clubbing and cyanosis. As in the case of the other pneumoconioses, the simple or uncomplicated form of coal workers' pneumoconiosis is uncommon, but the chronic form is often associated with chronic bronchitis and infections.

Medical Management
Diagnosis.   Identifying a workplace-related cause of disease is important because it can lead to cure and to prevention for others. The recognition of occupational causes can be difficult because of the latency period, delayed responses that occur at home either after work or years after exposure. Diagnosis is by history of exposure (which may be minimal with asbestosis and far removed in time from the onset of disease; the person may even be unaware of the exposure), sputum cytology, lung biopsy, chest film showing nodular or interstitial fibrosis, and pulmonary function studies. Other pulmonary imaging techniques used in conjunction with the initial chest radiograph include conventional CT, high-resolution CT, and gallium scintigraphy. High-resolution CT scanning is the best imaging method in asbestosis because of its ability to detect parenchymal fibrosis and define the presence of co-existing pleural plaques. There may be a potential benefit of scanning for early detection of lung cancer, but this remains controversial at this time (see the section on Lung Cancer: Diagnosis in this chapter).

Prevention and Treatment.   Prevention is the first line of defense against occupational diseases. Workplace-based education, preemployment screening, yearly physical examina-

tions, surveillance and exposure reduction, and elimination of the pathogen are essential components of a strategy to prevent occupational lung disorders. Precautions such as the use of face masks, protective clothing, and proper ventilation are essential. Regular chest films are recommended for all workers exposed to silica as a means of early detection. In 1971, asbestos became the first material to be regulated by the U.S. Occupational Safety and Health Administration (OSHA). The Environmental Protection Agency has proposed a total ban, but there remains much controversy over the lack of scientific basis for this policy.

There is no standard treatment for these diseases. The dust deposits are permanent so treatment is directed toward relief of symptoms. Corticosteroids may produce some improvement in silicosis. Although there is no cure for any of the pneumoconioses, the complications of chronic bronchitis and cor pulmonale must be treated. When lung neoplasm occurs, surgical removal and therapeutic modalities such as radiotherapy or chemotherapy may be employed, but research results remain controversial as to whether these methods improve survival; to date, no standard systemic chemotherapy has been adopted.[180,186]

Prognosis.   The devastating feature of pneumoconioses is that there may be no obvious symptoms until the disease is in an advanced state. Once fully developed, prognosis is poor for most occupational lung diseases, with progressive and disabling results. Simple silicosis is not ordinarily associated with significant respiratory dysfunction unless complicated by emphysema and chronic bronchitis from cigarette smoking. Although now uncommon, acute silicosis resulting from heavy exposure to silica rarely responds to treatment and progresses rapidly over a few years when it occurs. The increased incidence of TB among people with silicosis presents an additional negative factor to the prognosis.

Exposure to asbestos, radon, silica, chromium, cadmium, nickel, arsenic, and beryllium may result in neoplasm. The relationship between silica and lung cancer has been under recent debate,[106] but both bronchogenic carcinoma and mesotheliomas of the pleura and peritoneum have been linked to asbestos. The exposure typically occurs 20 years before the development of bronchogenic carcinoma and approximately 30 to 40 years before the appearance of mesothelioma. The disease culminates in the sixth decade with few cases occurring before age 40 years. Mesothelioma is terminal with no effective treatment. Coal workers' pneumoconiosis was once thought to cause severe disability, but it is now clear that black lung causes minor impairment of pulmonary function at its worst. When coal miners have severe air-flow obstruction, it is usually due to smoking.

Special Implications for the Therapist   **14-15**

PNEUMOCONIOSES

Preferred Practice Patterns:
    Other pulmonary pathologic conditions frequently occur in conjunction with pneumoconioses. Preferred practice patterns for chronic bronchitis, cor pulmonale, lung cancer, emphysema, or tuberculosis may also apply.

6C: Impaired Ventilation, Respiration/Gas Exchange, and Aerobic Capacity/Endurance Associated With Airway Clearance Dysfunction

6E: Impaired Ventilation and Respiration/Gas Exchange Associated With Ventilatory Pump Dysfunction or Failure

New materials are being introduced into the workplace at a faster rate than their potential toxicities can be evaluated despite the fact that many have a pathologic effect on the pulmonary system. The possibility of occupational lung disease should be considered whenever a working or retired person has unexplained respiratory illness.

Steam inhalation and chest physical therapy techniques, such as controlled coughing and segmental bronchial drainage with chest percussion and vibration, help clear secretions. Exercise tolerance must be increased slowly over a long period beginning with increasing regular activities of daily living. Daily activities should be planned carefully to conserve energy (see Box 8-2), to decrease the work of breathing, and to afford frequent rest periods. Progression from increasing tolerance for daily activities to a conditioning program may precede an actual exercise program. In severe cases, oxygen may be necessary for any increase in activity level or exercise and the person may not progress beyond self-care skills. ■

◆ Hypersensitivity Pneumonitis

Exposure to organic dusts may result in hypersensitivity pneumonitis, also called extrinsic allergic alveolitis. The alveoli and distal airways are most often involved as a result of inhalation of organic dusts and active chemicals. Most of the diseases are named according to the specific antigen or occupation and involve organic materials such as molds (e.g., mushroom compost, moldy hay, sugar cane, or logs left unprotected from moisture), fungal spores (e.g., stagnant water in air conditioners and central heating units), plant fibers or wood dust (particularly redwood and maple), cork dust, coffee beans, bird feathers, hydroxyurea (cytotoxic agent), and serum.

Regardless of the specific antigen involved in the pathogenesis of hypersensitivity pneumonitis, the pathologic alterations in the lung are similar. A combination of immune complex–mediated and T cell–mediated hypersensitivity reactions occurs, although the exact mechanism of these processes is still unknown. Host factors such as cigarette smoking and the presence of some HLA proteins also play an important role in the development or suppression of the disease. Most characteristic is the presence of scattered, poorly formed granulomas that contain foreign body giant cells. Mild fibrosis may occur, usually in the alveolar walls.

The diagnosis of hypersensitivity pneumonitis of an organic origin is made by history of exposure, pulmonary function studies, and clinical manifestations, which commonly include abrupt onset of dyspnea, fever, chills, and a nonproductive cough. The symptoms typically remit within 24 to 48 hours but return on reexposure and with time may become chronic. Initially, symptoms can be reversed by removing the worker from the exposure (the only adequate treatment), by modifying the materials-handling process, or by using protective clothing and masks. Hypersensitivity pneumonitis may present as acute, subacute, or chronic pulmonary disease depending on the frequency and intensity of exposure to the antigen. The prognosis is poor with repeated exposure to these organic dusts, resulting in nonreversible interstitial fibrosis.

◆ Noxious Gases, Fumes, and Smoke Inhalation

Exposure to toxic gases and fumes is an increasing problem in modern industrial society. Any time oxygen in the air is replaced by another toxic or nontoxic agent, asphyxia (deficient blood oxygen; increased carbon dioxide in blood and tissues) occurs. Such is the case when products manufactured from synthetic compounds are heated at high temperatures releasing fumes. For example, workers who use heating elements to seal meat in plastic wrappers and workers involved in the manufacture of plastics and packaging materials made of polyvinyl chlorides are exposed to these fumes.

The most common mechanism of injury is local irritation, the specific type and extent depending on the type and concentration of gas and the duration of exposure. For example, highly soluble gases such as ammonia rapidly injure the mucous membranes of the eye and upper airway, causing an intense burning pain in the eyes, nose, and throat. Insoluble gases, such as nitrogen dioxide, encountered by farmers, cause diffuse lung injury.

Metal fume fever is a systemic response to inhalation of certain metal dusts and fumes, such as zinc oxide used in galvanizing iron, the manufacture of brass, and chrome and copper plating. Symptoms include fever/chills, cough, dyspnea, thirst, metallic taste, salivation, myalgias, headache, and malaise. *Polymer fume fever*, associated with heating of polymers, may cause similar symptoms. With brief exposures, the symptoms associated with these two syndromes are self-limiting, but prolonged exposure results in chronic cough, hemoptysis, and impairment of pulmonary function associated with a wide range of lung pathologic conditions.

Chemical pneumonitis can result from exposure to toxic fumes. The acute reaction may produce diffuse lung injury characterized by air space disease typical of pulmonary edema. In its chronic form, bronchiolitis obliterans develops.

Smoke inhalation injury produces direct mucosal injury secondary to hot gases, tissue anoxia caused by combustion products, and asphyxia as oxygen is consumed by fire. Thermal injury seen in the upper airway is characterized by edema and obstruction. Incomplete combustion of industrial compounds produces ammonia, acrolein, sulfur dioxide, and other substances in today's fires.

Environmental tobacco smoke (ETS), or exposure to secondhand smoke among nonsmokers, is widespread. Home and workplace environments are major sources of exposure. A total of 15 million children are estimated to be exposed to secondhand smoke in their homes annually. ETS increases the risk of heart disease and respiratory infections in children, increases the risk of lung cancer by a factor of 2 to 3, and is responsible for an estimated 3000 cancer deaths of adult nonsmokers annually.[103]

Infants born to women exposed to ETS during pregnancy have an increased chance of decreased birth weight and intrauterine growth retardation.[107] Prenatal exposure to mainstream smoke from the mother and even to ETS from the mother has been shown to change fetal lung development and cause air-flow obstruction, airway hyperresponsiveness, and early development of asthma and allergy.[121] Newborns, infants, and children under the age of 2 years are at high risk for cardiovascular effects if they are exposed to household ETS during this time. Endothelial cells of the blood vessels damaged as a result of exposure to passive smoking can be measured during the first decade of life. ETS over a period of more than 10 years changes the intima/media ratio by enhancing the thickness of the vessel wall. Other possible effects of involuntary smoking among children may include middle ear disease, lower respiratory infections, and sudden infant death syndrome.[212]

ETS is associated with rhinitis symptoms of runny nose and nasal congestion in some people and is associated with decreased flow in the airways, bronchial hyperresponsiveness, and increased respiratory infections.[89] Other symptoms following exposure to sidestream tobacco smoke may include headache, chest discomfort or tightness, and cough. See also the section on Lung Cancer in this chapter.

◆ Near Drowning

Definition.   Near drowning refers to surviving (24 hours or longer) the physiologic effects of hypoxemia and acidosis that result from submersion in fluid. Near drowning occurs in three forms: (1) dry drowning, inhalation of little or no fluid with minimal lung injury because of laryngeal spasm (10% to 15% of cases); (2) wet drowning, aspiration of fluid with asphyxia or secondary changes caused by aspiration (85%); and (3) recurrence of respiratory distress secondary to aspiration pneumonia or pulmonary edema within 1 to 2 days after a near-drowning incident. Recovery is rapid if respiration and circulation are restored before permanent neurologic damage occurs. Death may occur from asphyxia secondary to reflex laryngospasm and glottic closure.

Incidence and Risk Factors.   Unintentional drowning is the second leading cause of death in those under 15 years old and the third leading cause of accidental death among all age-groups. Nearly 80% of drowning victims are males; other risk factors include epilepsy, mental retardation, heart attack, head or spinal cord injury at the time of the accident, failure to use personal flotation devices, increased use of hot tubs and spas, and lack of proper swimming training or overestimation of endurance by those who can swim. Alcohol consumption while swimming or boating is involved in about 25% to 50% of adolescent and adult deaths associated with water recreation and is a major contributing factor in up to 50% of drownings among adolescent boys.[48]

Pathogenesis.   The complications of near drowning fall into two categories: the effects of prolonged *anoxia* on the brain and kidney, which as end organs may experience complications that are irreversible (determining the final prognosis), and acute lung injury from *aspiration* of fluids. When aspiration accompanies drowning, severe pulmonary injury often occurs, resulting in persistent arterial hypoxia and metabolic acidosis even after ventilation has been restored.

In the past, a distinction was made between the effects of saltwater and freshwater drowning (e.g., cardiovascular function, changes in blood volume and serum electrolyte concentrations), but it is now known that hypoxia is the most important determinant of survival in human near drowning regardless of the type of water involved. Regardless of the amount of water aspirated, the duration of submersion and the water temperature determine the pathologic events. Hypoxia

results in global cell damage; different cells tolerate variable lengths of anoxia. Neurons, especially cerebral cells, sustain irreversible damage after 4 to 6 minutes of submersion. The heart and lungs can survive up to 30 minutes. The extent of CNS injury tends to correlate with the duration of hypoxia, but hypothermia accompanying the incident is associated with changes in neurotransmitter release (glutamate, dopamine) and may reduce the cerebral oxygen requirements and help reduce CNS injury. For a detailed review of cold-water submersion, its mechanisms, and its effects the reader is referred to other sources.[84]

Clinical Manifestations.   The clinical features in near drowning are variable, and the person may be unconscious, semiconscious, or awake but apprehensive. Pulmonary and neurologic symptoms predominate with cough, tachypnea, and possible development of ARDS (see discussion in this chapter) with progressive respiratory failure. Other pulmonary complications include pulmonary edema, bacterial pneumonia, pneumothorax, or pneumomediastinum secondary to resuscitation efforts. Fever occurs in the presence of aspiration during the first 24 hours but can occur later in the presence of infection.

Early neurologic manifestations include seizures, especially during resuscitative measures, and altered mental status, including agitation, combativeness, or coma. Speech, motor, or visual abnormalities may occur and may improve gradually and resolve over several months.

Medical Management

Prevention.   Prevention of drowning and near-drowning events is a vital part of education. The Centers For Disease Control and Prevention (CDC) recommend mandating and enforcing legal limits for blood alcohol levels during water recreation activities, public education about the danger of combining alcohol (and other substances) with water recreation, restricting the sale of alcohol at water recreation facilities, and eliminating advertisements that encourage alcohol use during boating. Additional safeguard techniques for prevention of drowning among children are available.[48]

Treatment.   Improved training in cardiopulmonary resuscitation (CPR) has resulted in survival of the majority of near-drowning victims who live long enough to receive hospital care. Restoration of ventilation and circulation by means of resuscitation at the scene of the accident is the primary goal of treatment to restore oxygen delivery and prevent further hypoxic damage. Other treatment is largely supportive, with antibiotics for pulmonary infection, maintenance of fluid and electrolyte balance, possible transfusion for significant anemia, and management of acute renal failure.

Comatose near-drowning victims frequently have elevated intracranial pressure caused by cerebral edema and loss of cerebrovascular autoregulation. Reduction of cerebral blood flow adds ischemic injury to already damaged brain tissue. In order to reserve cerebral function in such cases, cerebral resuscitation (controlled hyperventilation; deliberate hypothermia; use of barbiturates, glucocorticoids, and diuretics) may be utilized.

Prognosis.   The prognosis depends in large part on the extent and duration of the hypoxic episode. People have survived as long as 70 minutes of immersion with complete recovery, but up to 20% of all near-drowning victims will have permanent sequelae, many of which are ultimately fatal. If laryngospasm is finally overcome and the person aspirates water or if aspiration of vomitus occurs during resuscitative measures, prognosis is worse than without these complications. Other unfavorable prognostic indicators include first blood pH values below 7, low rectal temperature on admission to the hospital, abnormal electroencephalogram (EEG), deterioration of room air oxygen saturation, and degree of EEG disturbance. Coincident head trauma or subdural hematoma presents an additional prognostic complication. Neurologic injury is the most serious and least reversible complication in those persons successfully resuscitated. Little, if anything, has been shown to help, and it carries a grave prognosis.

Special Implications for the Therapist   14-16

NEAR DROWNING

Preferred Practice Patterns:
   Other nonpulmonary components associated with near drowning are included in the neuromuscular patterns (5B, 5C, 5D, 5I).
7A: Primary Prevention/Risk Reduction for Integumentary Disorders (pressure ulcers)
6C: Impaired Ventilation, Respiration/Gas Exchange, and Aerobic Capacity/Endurance Associated With Airway Clearance Dysfunction
6F: Impaired Ventilation and Respiration/Gas Exchange Associated With Respiratory Failure

All near-drowning victims should be admitted to a hospital inpatient setting for observation over 24 to 48 hours because of the possibility of delayed drowning syndrome with confusion, substernal pain, and adventitious breath sounds (rales or rhonchi). The therapist is often involved early on in the case management, providing bedside care much the same as for a person with traumatic brain injury or spinal cord injury. It is not uncommon for a near-drowning accident to be associated with either traumatic brain injury or spinal cord injury.

Evaluate cardiopulmonary status, monitor vital signs, and observe respirations. Chest physical therapy may be necessary. To facilitate breathing, elevate the head of the bed slightly if possible; observe for signs of infection (see Table 7-1); and check for any areas of skin pressure or factors precipitating pressure ulcers. Provide passive or active-assistive exercise according to the person's functional abilities, and progress as quickly as possible given the medical status.

In the rehabilitation setting, large doses of steroids are administered early in the treatment of some cases of spinal cord injury to control cerebral or spinal cord edema. Suppression of the inflammatory reaction in persons receiving large doses of steroids may be so complete as to mask the clinical signs and symptoms of major diseases, perforation of a peptic ulcer, or spread of infection. See also the section on Corticosteroids in Chapter 4. ∎

CONGENITAL DISORDERS

◆ Cystic Fibrosis

Definition and Overview.   CF is an inherited disorder of ion transport (sodium and chloride) in the exocrine glands affecting the hepatic, digestive, male reproductive (the vas deferens is functionally disrupted in nearly all cases), and respiratory systems (Fig. 14-12). The basic defect predisposes to chronic bacterial airway infections, and almost all persons develop obstructive lung disease associated with chronic infection that leads to progressive loss of pulmonary function.

Incidence.   CF is the most common inherited genetic disease in the white population, affecting approximately 30,000 children and young adults (equal gender distribution) in the United States. More than 1000 new cases are diagnosed each year. The disease is inherited as an autosomal recessive trait, meaning that both parents must be carriers so that the child inherits a defective gene from each one. In the United States, 5% of the population, or 12 million people, carry a single copy of the CF gene. Each time two carriers conceive a child, there is a 25% chance (1:4) that the child will have CF, a 50% (1:2) chance that the child will be a carrier, and a 25% chance that the child will be a noncarrier.

Etiologic Factors.   In recent years there have been major advances in understanding the genetics of the disease. In 1985, the CF gene was located on the long arm of chromosome 7. In 1989, the gene for CF was cloned* and abnormalities in the CF transmembrane conductance regulator (CFTR) protein were attributed to CF. In healthy people, this CFTR protein provides a channel by which chloride (a component of salt) can pass in and out of the plasma membrane of many epithelial cells, including those of the kidney, gut, and conducting airways. Clients with CF have a defective copy of the gene that normally enables cells to construct that channel. As a result, salt accumulates in the cells lining the lungs and digestive tissues, making the surrounding mucus abnormally thick and sticky. More than 70% of individuals with CF have a deletion of three contiguous base pairs resulting in the loss of a single amino acid (phenylalanine) making the membrane of airway epithelia impermeable to chloride.[63,216]

Today, affected children are studied using polymerase chain reaction (PCR) techniques to search for identifiable mutations. Over 300 mutations in the CF gene affecting the CFTR protein have been described, but not all of the mutations have been identified, so mass screening cannot yet identify individuals carrying the gene for CF who would otherwise test negative.

Pathogenesis.   Much about the complex pathogenesis of CF is still unknown, but it does appear that this impermeability of epithelial cells to chloride results in (1) dehydrated and increased viscosity of mucous gland secretions, primarily in the lungs, pancreas, intestine, and sweat glands; (2) elevation of sweat electrolytes (sodium chloride); and (3) pancreatic enzyme insufficiency. The dehydration resulting in thick, viscous mucous gland secretions causes the

---

*Clones are identical copies of genes used to study the DNA sequence that allows scientists to determine the nature and function of the protein encoded by the gene. Cloning opens up the possibility of gene therapy for a disorder.

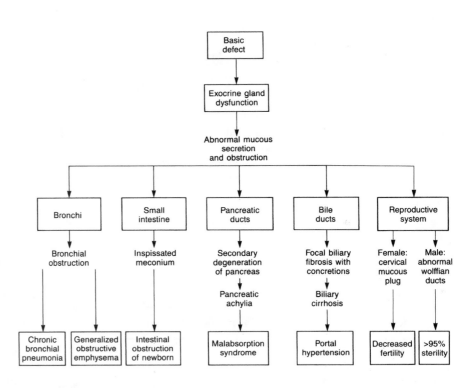

FIGURE 14-12 Various effects of exocrine gland dysfunction in cystic fibrosis. (From Wong DL: *Whaley and Wong's essentials of pediatric nursing*, ed 4, St Louis, 1993, Mosby, p 743.)

TABLE	14-13

Respiratory Diseases: Summary of Differences

DISEASE	PRIMARY AREA AFFECTED	RESULT
Acute bronchitis	Membrane lining bronchial tubes	Inflammation of lining
Bronchiectasis	Bronchial tubes (bronchi or air passages)	Bronchial dilation with inflammation
Pneumonia	Alveoli (air sacs)	Causative agent invades alveoli with resultant outpouring from lung capillaries into air spaces and continued healing process
Chronic bronchitis	Larger bronchi initially; all airways eventually	Increased mucous production (number and size) causing airway obstruction
Emphysema	Air spaces beyond terminal bronchioles (alveoli)	Breakdown of alveolar walls; air spaces enlarged
Asthma	Bronchioles (small airways)	Bronchioles obstructed by muscle spasm, swelling of mucosa, thick secretions
Cystic fibrosis	Bronchioles	Bronchioles become obstructed and obliterated; later, larger airways become involved
		Mucous plugs cling to airway walls, leading to bronchitis, bronchiectasis, atelectasis, pneumonia, or pulmonary abscess

From Goodman CC, Snyder TE: *Differential diagnosis in physical therapy*, ed 3, Philadelphia, 2000, Saunders.

mechanical obstruction responsible for the multiple clinical manifestations of CF. Bronchial and bronchiolar obstruction by the abnormal mucus predisposes the lung to infection and causes patchy atelectasis with hyperinflation. The disease progresses from mucous plugging and inflammation of small airways (bronchiolitis) to bronchitis, followed by bronchiectasis, pneumonia, fibrosis, and the formation of large cystic dilations that involve all bronchi. A summary of differences among these various respiratory diseases is provided (Table 14-13).

New findings about how specific molecules signal the onset of inflammation and tissue-damaging enzymes and how these chemicals all interact are adding to the knowledge base of CF pathophysiology. For example, in CF lungs, a decreased level of nitric oxide (NO), a chemical that decreases inflammation, may be explained by the loss of an enzyme needed to produce NO. Several laboratories are working to identify how a defect in CFTR causes the loss of NO or of the needed enzymes. The inflammatory response against bacteria in the airways of individuals with CF involves the generation of reactive oxygen species (formation of free radicals) leading to further inflammation and tissue damage. Without the necessary NO, a vicious cycle of inflammatory-immune processes and bacteria survival persists. Restoring the balance of oxidants and antioxidants could restore health in the CF lung.

New data on the structure of CFTR, including the size and shape of the channel through which the chloride must pass, how to stabilize the channel and increase the time it stays open, and the life cycle of this protein, are being used to provide scientists with ideas for new treatments. Other researchers are investigating why the CF lung is so receptive to the onslaught of infection by examining the role of defensin and other bacterial-killing molecules in the CF airway and the inhibition of these antimicrobial peptides by high salt concentrations.

Clinical Manifestations.   The consistent finding of abnormally high sodium and chloride concentrations in the sweat is a unique characteristic of CF. Parents frequently ob-serve that their infants taste salty when they kiss them. Almost all clinical manifestations of CF are a result of over-production of extremely viscous mucus and deficiency of pancreatic enzymes. A complete list of clinical manifestations by organ and in order of progression is given in Table 14-14. Recurrent pneumothorax, hemoptysis, pulmonary hypertension, and cor pulmonale are serious and life-threatening complications of severe and diffuse CF pulmonary disease.

Pancreas.   Approximately 90% of clients have pancreatic insufficiency with thick secretions blocking the pancreatic ducts causing dilation of the small lobes of the pancreas, degeneration, and eventual progressive fibrosis throughout. The blockage also prevents essential pancreatic enzymes from reaching the duodenum, thus impairing digestion and absorption of nutrients. Clinically, this process results in bulky, frothy (undigested fats because of a lack of amylase and tryptase enzymes), foul-smelling stools (decomposition of proteins producing compounds such as hydrogen sulfide and am-

---

TABLE 14-14

Clinical Manifestations of Cystic Fibrosis

Early Stages
Persistent coughing
Sputum production
Persistent wheezing
Recurrent infection
Excessive appetite, poor
  weight gain
Salty skin and sweat
Bulky, foul-smelling stools

Pulmonary
  Initial
Wheezy respirations
Dry, nonproductive cough
  Progressive Involvement
Increased dyspnea
Decreased exercise tolerance
Paroxysmal cough
Tachypnea
Obstructive emphysema
Patchy areas of atelectasis
Nasal polyps, chronic sinusitis
  Advanced Stage
Barrel chest
Kyphosis
Pectus carinatum
Cyanosis
Clubbing (fingers and toes)
Recurrent bronchitis
Recurrent bronchopneumonia
Pneumothorax
Hemoptysis
Right-sided heart failure
  secondary to pulmonary
  hypertension

Gastrointestinal
Voracious appetite (early)
Anorexia (late)
Weight loss
Failure to thrive or grow;
  protein-calorie malnutrition
Distended abdomen
Thin extremities
Sallow (yellowish) skin
Acute gastroesophageal reflux
  (GERD)
Intussusception

Distal Intestinal Obstruction
  Syndrome (Meconium Ileus)
Abdominal distention
Colicky, abdominal pain
Vomiting
Failure to pass stools
  (constipation)
Rapid development of dehydration
Anemia

Liver
Cirrhosis
Portal hypertension

Pancreatic
Large, bulky, loose, frothy, foul-smelling stools
  (pancreatic enzyme insufficiency)
Fat-soluble vitamin deficiency (vitamins A, D, E, K)
Recurrent pancreatitis
Iron deficiency anemia
Malnutrition
Diabetes mellitus

Genitourinary
Male urogenital abnormalities
Delay in sexual development
Sterility (all males); infertility (some females)

Musculoskeletal
Marked tissue wasting, muscle atrophy
Myalgia
Osteoarthropathy (adult)
Rheumatoid arthritis (adult)
Osteopenia/osteoporosis (adult)

monia). As the life expectancy for people with CF has improved, the incidence of glucose intolerance and CF-related diabetes has increased because pancreatic damage can eventually affect the beta cells. Hyperglycemia may adversely influence nutritional status and weight, pulmonary function, and development of late microvascular complications.[220]

Gastrointestinal.   The earliest manifestation of CF, *meconium ileus* (sometimes referred to as distal intestinal obstruction syndrome), is present in approximately 10% to 15% of newborns with CF; the small intestine is blocked with thick, puttylike, tenacious meconium. Prolapse of the rectum is the most common gastrointestinal complication associated with CF, occurring most often in infancy and childhood. Children of all ages with CF are susceptible to intestinal obstruction from thickened, dried, or impacted stools (inspissated meconium). Advances in investigative techniques have led to increasing reports of Crohn's disease and ischemic bowel disease in persons with CF. Prolonged administration of excessive doses of pancreatic enzymes is associated with the development of fibrosing colonopathy. To avoid this complication, current recommendation for a daily dose of pancreatic enzymes for most people with CF is below 10,000 units of lipase per kilogram per day. Poor nutrition and weight loss are common as a result of malabsorption, inadequate oral intake, early satiety, and increased utilization of calories.

Pulmonary.   Chronic cough and purulent sputum production are symptomatic of lung involvement. The child is unable to expectorate the mucus because of its increased viscosity. This retained mucus provides an excellent medium for bacterial growth, placing the individual at increased risk for infection. Reduced oxygen–carbon dioxide exchange causes variable degrees of hypoxia, clubbing (see Fig. 14-4), cyanosis, hypercapnia, and resultant acidosis. Chronic pulmonary infection and malabsorption lead to secondary manifestations of barrel chest, pectus carinatum, and kyphosis.

The most common complication of CF is an exacerbation of pulmonary disease requiring medical and physical therapy intervention. Early warning signs (Box 14-3) must be recognized and treatment initiated (referred to as a "tune-up"), preferably at home but sometimes in the hospital. Respiratory failure is a frequent complication of severe pulmonary disease in persons with CF and is the most common cause of CF-related deaths.

Genitourinary.   Genitourinary manifestations are primarily related to reproduction; infertility is universal in men and common in women. The vas deferens may be absent bilaterally, or if present it is usually obstructed so that although sperm production is normal, there are no sperm in the semen (azoospermia). Women experience decreased fertility because thick mucus in the cervical canal prevents conception. As the disease progresses, there is also an increased incidence of amenorrhea.

Musculoskeletal.   Muscle pain is reported and may be alleviated with proper nutrition and exercise although this is based on anecdotal information and has not been verified in studies. Decreased bone mineral density and bone mineral content are common at all ages in CF, attributed to multifactorial causes (e.g., nutrition, exposure to glucocor-

---

BOX 14-3

Signs and Symptoms of Pulmonary Exacerbation in Cystic Fibrosis

Increased cough
Increased sputum production and/or a change in appearance of sputum
Fever
Weight loss
School or work absenteeism (because of illness)
Increased respiratory rate and/or work of breathing (WOB)
New findings on chest examination (e.g., rales, wheezing, crackles)
Decreased exercise tolerance
Decrease in FEV_1 of 10% or more from baseline value within past 3 months
Decrease in hemoglobin saturation of 10% or more from baseline value within past 3 months
New finding(s) on chest x-ray

From Cystic Fibrosis Foundation: *Clinical practice guidelines for cystic fibrosis,* Bethesda, Md, 1997, The Foundation, pp 1-53, Appendices I-XI.

---

ticoid therapy, gonadal dysfunction, age, body mass, activity). Spinal consequences of bone loss include excessive kyphosis and neck and back pain.[170] Lung transplant is also associated with increased osteoporosis from long-term immunosuppression.

Hypertrophic pulmonary osteoarthropathy occurs with increasing frequency with increasing age and severity of disease. This condition is accompanied by clubbing of the fingers and toes, arthritis, painful periosteal new bone formation (especially over the tibia), and swelling of the wrists, elbows, knees, or ankles. The periostitis is observed radiographically in the diaphysis of the tubular bones and may be a single layer or a solid cloaking of the bone. Separately and usually without association with other manifestations of CF, attacks of episodic arthritis accompanied by severe joint pain, stiffness, rash, and fever may occur intermittently but repeatedly. Arthritis in CF is one of three types: CF arthritis (cause unknown but may relate to immune complex mechanisms), hypertrophic osteoarthropathy, and arthritis caused by co-existent conditions and drug reactions.[170]

Medical Management

Diagnosis. Now that the gene responsible for CF has been identified, prenatal diagnosis and screening of carriers are possible as part of genetic counseling. The tests only detect mutations already observed but account for 70% of all CF carriers. Screening practices vary widely among genetic centers, and routine screening procedures are not employed at this time; testing is reserved for families in which there is a member affected with CF. Prepregnancy genetic testing that involves DNA analysis of oocytes is available for couples at risk for having children with CF.

About one-half of all children with CF present in infancy with failure to thrive, respiratory compromise, or both. The age at presentation can vary, and some people are not diagnosed until adulthood. CF is traditionally diagnosed using the sweat test; a positive test occurs when the sodium chloride concentration is greater than 60 mEq/L (reference value: 40 mEq/L). Although elevated sweat electrolytes are associated with other conditions, a positive sweat test coupled with the clinical picture usually confirms the diagnosis. The test should be performed at a certified CF center and repeated a second time. Genotype analysis (performed prenatally or postnatally) can be a useful adjunct but is not the sole diagnostic criterion for CF.

Pancreatic elastase-1 (EL-1), a marker of exocrine pancreatic insufficiency in CF, can be measured in feces. EL-1 is a specific human protease synthesized by the acinar cells of the pancreas and is a reliable test of pancreatic sufficiency over the age of 2 weeks. This test can be used to rule out the diagnosis of CF, to confirm the need for pancreatic enzymes, and for annual monitoring of pancreatic-sufficient individuals to detect the onset of pancreatic insufficiency.[38,141]

Pulmonary function tests are performed in adolescents and adults to measure and monitor lung function over time (see Table 39-19). These tests are used to classify the severity of baseline lung disease. Almost all measures are based on the flow of air into and out of the lungs in a given period of time. The two most common lung function measures are FEV_1 (forced expiratory volume in 1 second) and FVC (forced vital capacity). These tests should be repeated two to four times each year for adults to assess the effectiveness of treatment; pulmonary function declines with progressive lung disease.

Diabetes mellitus should be identified early by screening with a glucose tolerance test from the age of 15 years and treated with insulin, dietary management, and exercise from the time of diagnosis of diabetes. The degree of glucose intolerance may be a strong determinant of future lung decline in individuals with CF suggesting a relationship between insulin deficiency and clinical deterioration.[151]

Treatment. A multidisciplinary approach must be taken in treating CF toward the goal of promoting a normal life for the individual. The treatment of CF depends on the stage of the disease and which organs are involved. Medical management is oriented toward alleviating symptoms and includes the use of antibiotics, aggressive pulmonary therapy with drugs (mucolytics) to thin mucous secretions, chest physical therapy, supplemental oxygen, and adequate hydration and enhanced nutrition with pancreatic enzymes administered before or with meals.

Drug therapy for CF has been primarily directed at prophylaxis and treatment of infections with antibiotics and supplementing digestive enzymes and vitamins. Pharmacotherapy (see Table 14-8) to date has included broad-spectrum antimicrobials to protect the respiratory epithelium from damage, aerosolized antibiotics (e.g., tobramycin) that deliver a more concentrated dose directly to the site of infection, and aggressive nutritional management with microencapsulated pancreatic enzymes. Other pharmacologic treatment may include sympathomimetics to control bronchospasm, parasympatholytics to offset smooth muscle constriction and bronchodilation, inhaled antiinflammatory agents to decrease the amount of inflammation in the airways, and mucolytics to thin mucous secretions. Recombinant human deoxyribonuclease I (rhDNAase I) or Dornase alfa, a mucolytic, is used to reduce sputum viscosity and increase mucociliary clearance.

Administered 30 minutes before chest therapy treatments, these combined treatment interventions improve the quality of life for people with CF by decreasing their hypoxemia and reducing their dyspnea. The end result is improved sleep patterns, increased activity, and improved nutritional status.

High-dose ibuprofen (the generic name for the drug found in Advil, Motrin, and Nuprin) may be used to slow the deterioration of the lungs by reducing inflammation and breaking the cycle of mucous buildup, infection, and inflammatory destruction. A totally implantable venous intravenous access device (TIVAD) for adults is under investigation in other countries as a means of providing effective long-term intravenous access for those individuals requiring intermittent antibiotics. The risks of mechanical failure, sepsis, and thrombosis have made this device more successful when inserted and cared for at a CF center.[129]

The identification of the mutated CF gene in 1989 has been followed by the first phase of gene therapy in 1993 to correct the basic defect in CF cells, rather than relying on treatment of the symptoms. Finding a way to deliver the normal copy of the gene into the lung or intrahepatic biliary epithelial cells with adequate gene expression remains a challenge. It is possible that delivery through an aerosolized technique will incorporate sufficient quantities of the CFTR gene into the cells to offset the presence of the abnormal protein. The expectation is that the normal CFTR will reverse the physiologic defect in CF cells. Other clinical trials are investigating the possibility of bypassing the defective CFTR altogether, developing drugs to transport chloride in the lung via a different route, eliminating elastase (a neutrophil product that damages the lung), and studying the effects of interleukin-10, a naturally occurring protein in the lung that limits inflammation.[137]

In the future, current therapeutic measures, such as intravenous antimicrobial treatment, will be improved by the additional delivery of new drugs to the bronchial tree by aerosol. Antibiotics, as well as protease inhibitors delivered by aerosol, should help to prevent damage by infection and inflammation and increase the probability of successful somatic gene therapy in this disease.

Double-lung or heart-lung transplants have been attempted on children with CF with advanced pulmonary vascular disease and who are severely disabled by dyspnea and hypoxia. Long-term survival has yet to be determined, but improved quality of life has been achieved. The new lungs do not acquire the CF ion transport abnormalities but are subject to the usual posttransplant complications. CF problems in other organ systems persist and may be worsened by some of the immunosuppressive regimens.[228] CNS complications occur more frequently in CF transplant recipients than other lung transplant recipients.[92] Studies of exercise performance in lung transplant recipients with end-stage CF report that exercise performance improves after transplantation but remains well below normal.[167]

Prognosis. The prognosis has steadily improved over the past 20 years, so that the median survival is now 32 years; more than 50% of children with CF live into adulthood. This increased survival is primarily due to continuous multidisciplinary care provided by specialists in CF centers, aggressive antibiotic therapy, and improved nutrition and pulmonary function, two main prognostic factors for improved survival.[144]

Children whose presenting symptoms were gastrointestinal at diagnosis have a good clinical course; those whose initial symptoms at diagnosis were pulmonary frequently demonstrate subsequent clinical deterioration. Pulmonary failure is still the most common cause of death. Males have a more favorable prognosis than females. New agents and gene therapy may substantially change the morbidity and mortality of this disease with continued improved survival time.

Special Implications for the Therapist   14-17

CYSTIC FIBROSIS

Preferred Practice Patterns:
4A: Primary Prevention/Risk Reduction for Skeletal Demineralization
6C: Impaired Ventilation, Respiration/Gas Exchange, and Aerobic Capacity/Endurance Associated With Airway Clearance Dysfunction
6E: Impaired Ventilation and Respiration/Gas Exchange Associated With Ventilatory Pump Dysfunction or Failure
6F: Impaired Ventilation and Respiration/Gas Exchange Associated With Respiratory Failure

Chest Physical Therapy

The therapist will be involved with postural drainage and chest physical therapy carried out several times per day or as often as the child is able to tolerate it without undue fatigue. Chest therapy should not be performed before or immediately after meals, so treatment must be scheduled to avoid mealtimes. Aerosol therapy to deliver medication to the lower respiratory tract should be administered just before chest therapy to maximize the effectiveness of both treatments. Breathing exercises, improving posture, mobilizing the thorax through active exercise, and manual therapy are part of promoting good breathing patterns and improving inspiratory muscle endurance. Specifics of chest physical therapy for this population are beyond the scope of this text; the reader is referred to more detailed materials available.[56,57,70]

The many difficulties surrounding percussion and postural drainage (e.g., poor compliance, time consuming, requires the assistance of a trained individual) have resulted in the development of alternative therapies for mucous clearance that can be accomplished without the assistance of another caregiver. Each of these techniques (e.g., autogenic drainage, positive expiratory pressure [PEP], Flutter® valve therapy) requires a certain level of compliance, motivation, understanding, neuromuscular function, and breath control. The therapist is very instrumental in evaluating each individual's needs, motivation, abilities, resources, and preferences in determining the best intervention or interventions to use.

Autogenic drainage and PEP help the individual to move the mucus up to the larger airways where it can be coughed out more easily. Autogenic drainage comprises a series of sequential breathing exercises designed to clear the small, medium, and large airways in that order. The PEP device maintains pressure in the lungs, keeping the airways open and allowing air to get behind the mucus. The air flowing through the device helps to "blow" the mucus to the large airways. This air flow combined with the "huff" cough routine (three to five forced air expirations making a huff sound followed by coughing, repeating this cycle for 15 minutes) helps the individual to cough up the mucus.

The Flutter® valve is similar to the PEP device but utilizes a stainless steel ball that vibrates, alternately opening and closing the device's air hole pulsing air back into the airways (Fig. 14-13). Current practice is to use one of the devices (PEP or Flutter® valve) followed by autogenic breathing techniques. The total treatment time is about 15 minutes and can be carried out independently by some children and most adolescents and adults with mild to moderate disease who can follow the directions and control their breathing. Preliminary studies on the Flutter® device suggest that Flutter® valve therapy is an acceptable alternative to standard chest physical therapy and may be more effective than postural drainage in prolonging the ability to raise secretions. Sputum production increased significantly 30 minutes after the end of treatment, and 1 hour after the end of treatment it was significantly greater than the amount produced following postural drainage.[22,93] The results of one study regarding the effects of inspiratory muscle training in individuals with CF have been reported but are too preliminary to discuss here.[59] Continued research is needed to clarify the effects of each intervention method on pulmonary function and exercise tolerance.

The development of an airway clearance vest provides mucous clearance to those individuals who lack the ability to perform the simpler techniques and is especially helpful with children (although the cost may be prohibitive). The device consists of an inflatable vest attached to an air pulse generator (Fig. 14-14). The generator, a compressor-like device, rapidly inflates and deflates the vest, gently compressing and releasing the chest wall to create air flow within the lungs. This device treats all lobes simultaneously for the duration of the time it is activated. This process moves mucus toward the larger airways where it can be cleared by coughing. The effectiveness of this mechanized device has been supported by the limited research published to date.[139,190]

Nutrition

Malnutrition and deterioration of lung function are closely interrelated and interdependent in the child with CF. Each affects the other, leading to a spiral decline in both. The occurrence of mal-

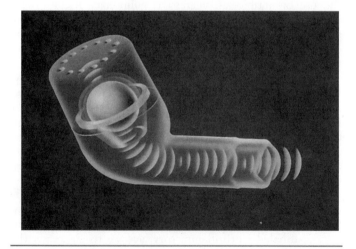

FIGURE **14-13** The Flutter® mucus clearance device. The Flutter® device can be used in anyone with chronic obstructive pulmonary disease. (Courtesy Axcan Scandipharm, Inc., Birmingham, Ala, 2001.)

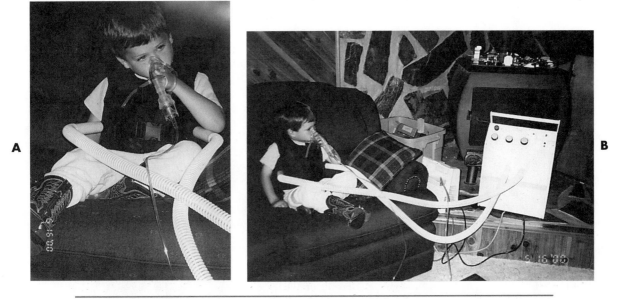

FIGURE 14-14   **A,** Four-year-old wearing ABI (American Biosystems, Incorporated) Vest®
to self-administer chest physical therapy. The vest can accommodate a child as young as 2 years old
and is worn 30 minutes twice each day. Medications used to open airways and relax bronchospasms
are administered through a nebulizer during the first 10 minutes of treatment, and the machine automatically shuts off every 10 minutes to allow the person to clear secretions. **B,** A foot-pad control
mechanism (not shown) can be used to manually stop the machine anytime to allow the client to
cough and clear mucus. Any position can be assumed, and at this age, the child can do everything
himself. This device promotes compliance and is accompanied by reduced use of medications and
infections. (Courtesy Kerry Resch, Missoula, Mont, 2001.)

nutrition during childhood seems to be associated with impaired growth and repair of the airway walls. In children, when growth in body length occurs, good nutrition is associated with better lung function. When adequate nutrition is combined with physical training and aerobic exercise, improved body weight, respiratory muscle function, lung function, and exercise tolerance occur with increases in both respiratory and other muscle mass.[104]

Exercise

Increasingly, exercise and sport are being advanced as core components of treatment for individuals with CF of all ages. A large portfolio of exercise literature has already established that supervised exercise programs enhance fitness (and thereby improve survival), increase sputum clearance, delay the onset of dyspnea, delay declines in pulmonary function, prevent decrease in bone density,[215] enhance cellular immune response,[29] and increase feelings of well-being, thereby potentially improving self-image, self-confidence, and quality of life for the person with CF. Reduced systemic oxygen extraction is an important factor limiting exercise in many individuals with CF, but the specific parameters of this limitation remain unknown and probably vary from person to person.[158,167]

The therapist can be very instrumental in providing client and family education about the importance of combining good nutrition and exercise/activity. The therapist helps each individual develop an exercise routine that includes strengthening, stretching, aerobic, and endurance components with special attention to breathing exercises to aerate all areas of the lungs. Weight loss with exercise is of special concern in this population, especially for the individual with CF and diabetes mellitus. Energy expenditure may be higher than usual for individuals with CF and

diabetes during periods of recovery from mild exercise or activity because of increased work of breathing consistent with higher ventilatory requirements.[213] This requires careful collaboration among client/family, therapist, and nutritionist.

Individuals with CF awaiting a transplant must remain as active as possible; whenever possible, the therapist can design a safe but effective exercise program. If significant oxygen desaturation or severe breathlessness limits activity, then exercise on a treadmill, stationary bike, or even a stationary device for seated pedaling is recommended with supplemental oxygen supplied at sufficient flow to match minute ventilatory requirements.[215]

Athletes With Cystic Fibrosis

For those individuals who are able and interested in participating in sports (Fig. 14-15), special considerations must be addressed. Calorie intake and maintaining weight, nutrition, and fluid and electrolyte balance are major concerns. Each individual must be assessed, evaluated, and monitored carefully. The therapist, family, and nutritionist can work together to minimize exercise and nutrition-induced complications. The information presented here is only a general guideline and may need to be modified for individual needs, metabolism, personal health, level and type of sports participation, and so on.

During the off-training season, the individual (especially children and adolescents) will need to eat one and one-half times the protein and calories of an athlete who does not have CF in order to maintain weight. During the sport season, calorie intake must be increased with the goal of maintaining weight. Hyponatremia (deficiency of sodium in the blood; see discussion in Chapter 4) can be a serious problem for athletes with CF who excrete three to five times the sodium (in sweat) of an

Continued

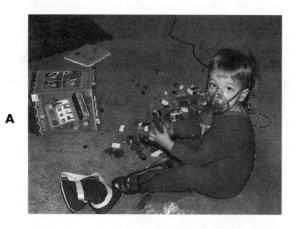

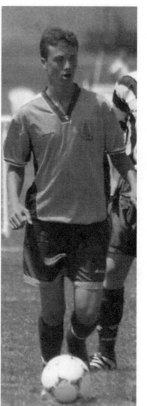

FIGURE   **14-15   A,** Eighteen-month-old shortly after diagnosis; face mask is a nebulizer (device designed to create and throw an aerosol) that is delivering albuterol (bronchodilator). **B,** This same individual in 1999 at age 15 years (6 feet tall; 145 pounds) competing in a regional soccer tournament. (Courtesy Kevin Hanson, Helena, Mont, 2001.)

athlete without CF during sports participation. This situation combined with increased intake of water further dilutes the sodium levels in the body. Sodium loss combined with losses of potassium and magnesium can result in life-threatening situations for these individuals. Some guidelines for these athletes include weighing before and after exercise and considering the loss as a loss of fluids accompanied by electrolytes; replacing fluid loss with electrolytes (e.g., drinks such as Gatorade, Recharge) instead of water; taking an appropriate number of salt tablets; and eating a meal with sodium-, potassium-, and magnesium-rich foods.

Sporting activity should not be undertaken during infective exacerbations. Sports that carry a medical risk for people with CF (e.g., bungee and parachute jumping, skiing, scuba diving) should be avoided. Individuals with CF who have portal hypertension with significant enlargement of the spleen and liver should be advised against contact sports such as rugby and football, in addition to bungee and parachute jumping. Skiing for anyone with CF who is already hypoxic is not advised; episodes of acute right-sided heart failure brought on by a combination of altitude and unaccustomed strenuous anaerobic and aerobic exercise have been reported. Scuba diving is contraindicated for anyone with lung disease if there is any evidence of air trapping. On ascent, the air expands increasing the risk of developing a pneumothorax.[215]

Adults With Cystic Fibrosis

As individuals with CF survive longer into adulthood, the unique needs of this population group are being considered. Achieving an ideal nutritional status is an integral part of management of people with CF, but how these requirements change as the individual ages remains unknown. Emphasis is continually placed on dietary intake and weight; the effects of this on eating behavior and self-perceptions are under investigation.[1] Other concerns include the effects of long-term use of pancreatic enzymes, osteoporosis associated with late-stage CF and its complications of increased fracture rates and severe kyphosis,[14] the effects of hormonal changes in relation to the menstrual cycle on lung function,[122] psychosocial-spiritual issues,[112] and infertility issues.[115]   ◼

PARENCHYMAL DISORDERS

◆ Atelectasis

Definition.   Atelectasis is the collapse of normally expanded and aerated lung tissue at any structural level (e.g., lung parenchyma, alveoli, pleura, chest wall, bronchi) involving all or part of the lung. Most cases are categorized as obstructive-absorptive or compressive.

Etiologic Factors and Pathogenesis.   The primary cause of atelectasis is obstruction of the bronchus serving the affected area. If a bronchus is obstructed (e.g., tumors, mucus, foreign material), atelectasis occurs as air in the alveoli is slowly absorbed into the bloodstream with subsequent collapse of the alveoli. Atelectasis can also develop when there is interference with the natural forces that promote lung expansion (e.g., hypoventilation associated with decreased motion or decreased pulmonary expansion such as occurs with paralysis, pleural disease, diaphragmatic disease, or masses in the thorax). Failure to breathe deeply postoperatively (i.e., because of muscular guarding and splinting from pain or discomfort with an upper abdominal, chest, or sternal incision), oversedation, immobility, coma, or neuromuscular disease can also interfere with the natural forces that promote lung expansion, leading to atelectasis.

Insufficient pulmonary surfactant, such as occurs in respiratory distress syndrome, inhalation of anesthesia, high concentrations of oxygen, lung contusion, aspiration of gastric contents or smoke inhalation, or increased elastic recoil as a result of interstitial fibrosis (e.g., silicosis, asbestosis, radiation pneumonitis), can also interfere with lung distention. When atelectasis is caused by inhalation of concentrated oxygen or anesthetic agents, quick absorption of these gases into the bloodstream can lead to collapse of alveoli in dependent portions of the lung.

Although atelectasis is usually caused by bronchial obstruction, direct compression can also cause it. The compressive type is due to air (pneumothorax), blood (hemothorax), or fluid (hydrothorax) filling the pleural space. Abdominal distention that presses on a portion of the lung can also collapse alveoli causing atelectasis. *Right middle lobe syndrome* refers to atelectasis secondary to compression of the bronchus to the right middle lobe by lymph nodes containing metastatic cancer.

Clinical Manifestations.   When sudden obstruction of the bronchus occurs, there may be dyspnea, tachypnea, cyanosis, elevation of temperature, drop in blood pressure, substernal retractions, or shock. In the chronic form of atelectasis, the client may be asymptomatic with gradual onset of dyspnea and weakness.

Medical Management
Diagnosis.   Atelectasis is suspected in penetrating or other chest injuries. X-ray examination may show a shadow in the area of collapse. If an entire lobe is collapsed, the radiograph will show the trachea, heart, and mediastinum deviated toward the collapsed area, with the diaphragm elevated on that side (see Figs. 14-11 and 14-19). Chest auscultation and physical assessment add to the clinical diagnostic picture. Blood gas measurements may show decreased oxygen saturation.

Treatment and Prognosis.   Once atelectasis occurs, treatment is directed toward removing the cause whenever possible. Suctioning or bronchoscopy may be employed to remove airway obstruction. Chronic atelectasis may require surgical removal of the affected segment or lobe of lung. Antibiotics are used to combat infection accompanying secondary atelectasis. Reexpansion of the lung is often possible, but the final prognosis depends on the underlying disease.

Special Implications for the Therapist **14-18**

ATELECTASIS

Preferred Practice Patterns:
    See also Special Implications for the Therapist: Pneumothorax, 14-26 and Special Implications for the Therapist: Chest Wall Disease or Injury, 14-14.

6B: Impaired Aerobic Capacity/Endurance Associated With Deconditioning
6C: Impaired Ventilation, Respiration/Gas Exchange, and Aerobic Capacity/Endurance Associated With Airway Clearance Dysfunction
6F: Impaired Ventilation and Respiration/Gas Exchange Associated With Respiratory Failure

Atelectasis is a postoperative complication of thoracic or high abdominal surgery. Left lower lobe atelectasis can occur following cardiac surgery. Within a few hours after surgery, atelectasis becomes increasingly resistant to reinflation. This complication is exacerbated in people receiving narcotics. One of the underlying goals of acute care therapy is to prevent atelectasis in the high-risk client. Diminished respiratory movement as a result of postoperative pain is often addressed by the therapist. Frequent, gentle position changes, deep breathing, coughing, and early ambulation help promote drainage of all lung segments.

Deep breathing and effective coughing enhance lung expansion and prevent airway obstruction. Deep breathing is beneficial because it promotes the ciliary clearance of secretions, stabilizes the alveoli by redistributing surfactant, and permits collateral ventilation of the alveoli, through Kohn's pores in the alveolar septa. Kohn's pores, which open only during deep breathing, allow air to pass from well-ventilated alveoli to obstructed alveoli, minimizing their tendency to collapse and facilitating removal of the obstruction. To minimize postoperative pain during deep-breathing and coughing exercises, teach the client to hold a pillow tightly over the incision. ■

◆ Pulmonary Edema
Definition and Incidence.   Pulmonary edema or pulmonary congestion is an excessive fluid in the lungs that may accumulate in the interstitial tissue, in the air spaces (alveoli), or in both. Pulmonary edema is a common complication of many disease processes. It occurs at any age but with increasing incidence in older people with heart failure.

Etiologic and Risk Factors.   Most cases of pulmonary edema are due to left ventricular failure (see Fig. 11-12, A), acute hypertension, or mitral valve disease, but noncardiac conditions, especially kidney or liver disorders prone to the development of sodium and water retention, can also produce pulmonary edema. Noncardiac causes of pulmonary edema include intravenous narcotics, increased intracerebral pressure, high altitude, sepsis, medications, inhalation of smoke or toxins (e.g., ammonia), transfusion reactions, shock, and disseminated intravascular coagulation. Other risk factors include hyperaldosteronism, Cushing's syndrome, use of glucocorticoids, and use of hypotonic fluids to irrigate nasogastric tubes. Pulmonary edema itself is a major predisposing factor in the development of pneumonia that complicates heart failure and ARDS.

Pathogenesis.   Pulmonary edema occurs when the pulmonary vasculature fills with fluid that leaks into the alveolar spaces, decreasing the space available for gas exchange. Normally the lung is kept dry by lymphatic

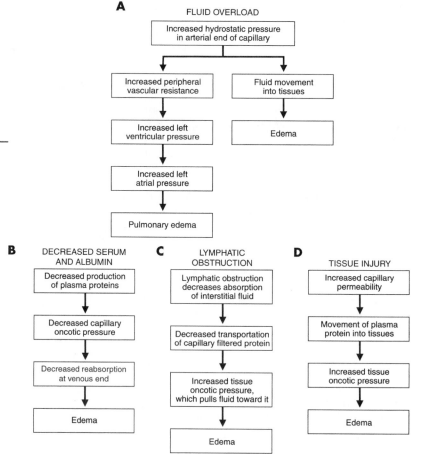

FIGURE   **14-16**   Mechanisms of pulmonary edema
formation. **A,** Fluid overload. **B,** Decreased serum and
albumin. **C,** Lymphatic obstruction. **D,** Tissue injury.
(From Black JM, Matassarin-Jacobs E, editors:
Luckmann and Sorensen's medical-surgical nursing, ed 5,
Philadelphia, 1997, Saunders, p 286.)

drainage and a balance among capillary hydrostatic pressure, capillary oncotic pressure, and capillary permeability. Pulmonary edema develops as a result of (1) fluid overload, (2) decreased serum and albumin, (3) lymphatic obstruction, and (4) disruption of capillary permeability (tissue injury) (Fig. 14-16).

Fluid Overload.   When the filling pressures on the left side of the heart increase, pulmonary capillary hydrostatic pressure increases. If it surpasses the oncotic pressure that holds fluid in the capillaries, fluid is drawn from capillaries in the lungs into the interstitial space. Normally, the lymphatic system removes this fluid from the lungs, but if the flow of fluid into the interstitium exceeds the ability of the lymphatic system to remove it, fluid overload and consequently pulmonary edema develop.* When osmotic pressure in the venous end of

the capillary exceeds interstitial pressure, fluid cannot return to the bloodstream and peripheral and pulmonary edema may result. Fluid overload may also occur from decreased sodium and water excretion associated with renal disorders.

As the fluid pressure increases in the tissues, it also increases in the left ventricle, which increases pressure in the left atrium. The disturbed pressure gradient results in less forward flow, resulting in pulmonary edema. Pulmonary edema is commonly seen when the left side of the heart is distended and fails to pump adequately (e.g., myocardial ischemia or infarction, mitral or aortic valve damage). In atrial fibrillation, the left atrium may be unable to efficiently pump blood into the left ventricle, resulting in fluid pooling and subsequent edema. If the right side of the heart fails, peripheral edema occurs through the same process. Left-sided heart failure leads to right-sided failure (and vice versa), so both pulmonary and peripheral edema may exist simultaneously.

Decreased Serum and Albumin.   In the case of liver cirrhosis, the serum protein and albumin levels are reduced in the vascular fluids. These changes result in less fluid reabsorption from the tissue spaces, and peripheral edema and ascites occur.

Lymphatic Obstruction.   When lymphatic channels are obstructed, tissue oncotic pressure rises and results in edema. This obstruction can occur as a result of tumor infiltration but

---

*A brief review of this concept may be necessary for an understanding of many pulmonary conditions. For an in-depth discussion the reader is referred to Guyton AC: *Human physiology and mechanisms of disease,* ed 6, Philadelphia, 1997, Saunders. Fluid movement in the lung (as in all vessels) is governed by vascular permeability and the balance of the hydrostatic and oncotic pressures across the capillary endothelium as described by Starling's equation. Hydrostatic forces favor fluid filtration, whereas oncotic pressure promotes reabsorption. Normally, filtration forces dominate and fluid continuously moves from the vascular space into the interstitium. Extravascular water does not accumulate because the lung lymphatics effectively remove the filtered fluid and return it to the circulation. When the capacity of the lymphatic system is exceeded, if the rate of fluid filtration exceeds its functional capabilities, water accumulates in the loose interstitial tissues around the airways, pulmonary arteries, and, eventually, the alveolar walls (alveolar edema).

most often occurs in association with cardiogenic causes of pulmonary edema. When hemodynamic alterations (changes in the movement of blood and the forces involved) in the heart increase the perfusion pressure in the pulmonary capillaries, effective lymphatic drainage is blocked.

Tissue Injury. Disruption of capillary permeability is the cause of pulmonary edema in acute lung injury associated with ARDS, inhalation of toxic gases, aspiration of gastric contents, viral infections, and uremia. In these conditions, destruction of endothelial cells or disruption of the tight junctions between them alters capillary permeability (see Figs. 5-8 and 5-9).

Clinical Manifestations. Clinical manifestations of pulmonary edema occur in stages. During the initial stage, clients may be asymptomatic or they may complain of restlessness and anxiety and the feeling that they are developing a common cold. Other signs include a persistent cough, slight dyspnea, diaphoresis, and intolerance to exercise. As fluid continues to fill the pulmonary interstitial spaces, the dyspnea becomes more acute, respirations increase in rate, and there is audible wheezing. If the edema is severe, the cough becomes productive of frothy sputum tinged with blood, giving it a pinkish hue. If the condition persists, the person becomes less responsive and consciousness decreases.

Medical Management
Diagnosis. Pulmonary edema is usually recognized by its characteristic clinical presentation. Cardiogenic pulmonary edema is differentiated from noncardiac causes by the history and physical examination; an underlying cardiac abnormality can usually be detected clinically or by the electrocardiogram (ECG), chest film, or echocardiogram. A chest film may show increased vascular pattern, increased opacity of the lung, especially at the bases, and pleural effusion. There are no specific laboratory tests diagnostic of pulmonary edema; when the condition progresses enough to cause liver involvement the physician may observe the hepatojugular reflex (positional or palpatory pressure on the liver results in distention of the jugular vein). Blood gas measurements indicate the degree of functional impairment, and sputum cultures may indicate accompanying infection.

Prevention and Treatment. Prevention is a key component with persons at increased risk for the development of pulmonary edema. Preventive measures may be as simple as lowering salt intake or pharmacologic treatment such as the use of digoxin and diuretics. Once pulmonary edema has been diagnosed, treatment is aimed at enhancing gas exchange, reducing fluid overload, and strengthening and slowing the heartbeat. Oxygen by mask or through ventilatory support is used along with diuretics, diet, and fluid restriction to remove excess alveolar fluid. Morphine to relieve anxiety and reduce the effort of breathing may be used for people who do not have narcotic-induced pulmonary edema. Other pharmacologic-based treatment may be used to help dilate the bronchi and increase cardiac output, strengthen contractions of the heart, and increase cardiac output.

Prognosis. The prognosis depends on the underlying condition. The presence of pulmonary edema is a medical emergency requiring immediate intervention to prevent further respiratory distress. It is often reversible with clinical management.

Special Implications for the Therapist 14-19

PULMONARY EDEMA

Preferred Practice Patterns:
6B: Impaired Aerobic Capacity/Endurance Associated With Deconditioning
6C: Impaired Ventilation, Respiration/Gas Exchange, and Aerobic Capacity/Endurance Associated With Airway Clearance Dysfunction
6F: Impaired Ventilation and Respiration/Gas Exchange Associated With Respiratory Failure

Symptoms of pulmonary edema that may come to the therapist's attention include engorged neck and hand veins (because of peripheral vascular fluid overload), pitting edema of the extremities, and, of course, the paroxysmal nocturnal dyspnea so common with this condition. One of the first signs of dyspnea may be an increased difficulty breathing when lying down, relieved by sitting up (orthopnea). Pulmonary edema can become life-threatening within minutes requiring immediate action by the therapist to get medical assistance for this person. Jugular vein distention may occur with liver involvement. Positional or palpatory pressure on the liver may result in right upper quadrant or right shoulder pain as well as jugular vein distention. The distention may be best observed with the person positioned sitting 30 to 45 degrees up from a fully supine position. Any liver involvement requires precautions when performing any soft tissue mobilization techniques to the anterior part of the abdomen, including the diaphragm. Indirect techniques or mobilization away from the liver is recommended.

When working with a client already diagnosed with pulmonary edema, the sitting (high Fowler's) position is preferred with legs dangling over the side of the bed or plinth. This facilitates respiration and reduces venous return. Monitor for decreased respiratory drive (less than 12 breaths per minute is significant), which should be documented and reported immediately. If oxygen is being administered, the therapist monitors the oxyhemoglobin saturation levels and titrates oxygen accordingly. It may be necessary to increase oxygen levels before exercise, but respiratory rate and breathing pattern must be monitored. The client may be taking nitroglycerin sublingually, which will further increase vasodilation and decrease ventricular preload. Monitor blood pressure closely, and observe for signs of hypotension because nitroglycerin can drop blood pressure dangerously. The therapist should consult with nursing or respiratory staff for any special considerations for each individual client.

Gradual exercise intolerance usually occurs as the dyspnea progresses. The client may comment about weight gain or difficulty fastening clothes. Check for peripheral edema in the immobile or bedridden client. In this group of people, edema can occur in the sacral hollow rather than in the feet and legs, because the sacrum is the lowest place on the trunk. Care must be taken to prevent pressure ulcers in this area. ∎

◆ Acute Respiratory Distress Syndrome

Definition. ARDS is a form of acute respiratory failure following a systemic or pulmonary insult. It is also called adult respiratory distress syndrome, shock lung, wet lung, stiff lung, hyaline membrane disease (adult or newborn), posttraumatic lung, or diffuse alveolar damage (DAD). It is often a fatal complication of serious illness (e.g., sepsis), trauma, or major surgery.

Incidence. ARDS has only been identified within the last 25 years, affecting a reported 150,000 people per year in the United States. This figure has been challenged, and part of the reason for the uncertainty of numbers is the lack of uniform definitions for ARDS and the heterogeneity of diseases underlying ARDS. The incidence has increased as improvements in intensive care have allowed more people to survive the catastrophic illnesses that precede ARDS. Any age can be affected, but often young adults with traumatic injuries develop ARDS.

Etiologic and Risk Factors. ARDS occurs as a result of injury to the lung by a variety of unrelated causes; the most common are listed in Table 14-15.

Pathogenesis. Alveolocapillary units, alveolar spaces, alveolar walls, and lungs are the site of initial damage (thus the name *diffuse alveolar damage*). Although the mechanism of lung injury varies with the cause, damage to capillary endothelial cells and alveolar epithelial cells is common in ARDS regardless of cause. Damage to these cells inactivates surfactant and allows fluids, proteins, and blood cells to leak from the capillary bed into the pulmonary interstitium and alveoli. The increased vascular permeability and inactivation of surfactant lead to interstitial and alveolar pulmonary edema and alveolar collapse.

TABLE	14-15

Causes of Acute (Adult) Respiratory Distress Syndrome (ARDS)*

Severe trauma (e.g., multiple bone fractures)
Septic shock
Pancreatitis
Cardiopulmonary bypass surgery
Diffuse pulmonary infection
Burns
High concentrations of supplemental oxygen
Aspiration of gastric contents
Massive blood transfusions
Embolism: fat, thrombus, amniotic fluid, venous air
Near drowning
Radiation therapy
Inhalation of smoke or toxic fumes
Thrombotic thrombocytopenic purpura
Indirect: chemical mediators released in response to systemic disorders (e.g., viral infections, pneumonia)
Drugs (e.g., aspirin, narcotics, lidocaine, phenylbutazone, hydrochlorothiazide, most chemotherapeutic and cytotoxic agents)

*Listed in order of decreasing frequency.

Pulmonary edema decreases lung compliance and impairs oxygen transport. The loss of surfactant leads to atelectasis and further impairment in lung compliance and oxygen transport (gas exchange). These are only the pulmonary manifestations of what is now recognized as a more systemic process called *multiple organ dysfunction syndrome (MODS)*, formerly called *multiple organ failure (MOF)*. See Chapter 4 for a discussion of MODS.

Clinical Manifestations. The clinical presentation is relatively uniform regardless of cause and occurs within 12 to 48 hours of the initiating event. The earliest sign of ARDS is usually an increased respiratory rate characterized by shallow, rapid breathing. Pulmonary edema caused by alveolar filling with exudate causes solidification of the tissue (consolidation). The subsequent alveolar collapse decreases lung compliance, causing dyspnea, hyperventilation, and the changes observed on chest radiographs (Fig. 14-17).

As breathing becomes increasingly difficult, the individual may gasp for air and exhibit intercostal, clavicular, or sternal retractions and cyanosis. Unless the underlying disease is reversed rapidly, especially in the presence of sepsis (toxins in the blood), the condition quickly progresses to full-blown MODS involving kidneys, liver, gut, CNS, and the cardiovascular system.

Medical Management

Diagnosis. Since ARDS is a collection of symptoms rather than a specific disease, differential diagnosis is through a process of diagnostic elimination. Cardiogenic pulmonary edema and bacterial pneumonia must be ruled out because there are specific treatments for those disorders. By definition, respiratory failure in the proper clinical setting (history, physical findings) constitutes ARDS. Physical examination, blood gas analysis to assess the severity of hypoxemia, microbiologic cultures to identify or exclude infection, and radiographs may be part of the diagnostic process.

Treatment. Specific treatment is administered for any underlying conditions (e.g., sepsis, pneumonia). Otherwise, treatment is based on early detection, and treatment goals are supportive and toward prevention of complications. Supportive therapy to maintain adequate blood oxygen levels may include administration of humidified oxygen by a tight-fitting face mask allowing for CPAP. Traditional ventilator management of ARDS emphasized normalization of blood gases and promoted high rates of further lung damage. It is now known that overdistention and cyclic inflation of injured lung can exacerbate lung injury and promote systemic inflammation. Mechanical ventilation with positive end-expiratory pressure (PEEP) can minimize these effects.[85] New strategies for protective ventilation (e.g., low-volume ventilation, permissive hypercapnia, prone positioning combined with airway pressure release ventilation [APRV]) have reduced ARDS mortality.[111,209] Sedation to reduce anxiety and restlessness during ventilation is required in some cases. If tachypnea, restlessness, or respirations out of phase with the ventilator (bucking) cannot be managed by sedation, pharmacologic paralysis may be induced.

Many studies are under way investigating new methods of prevention or treatment of ARDS, including inhalation of nitric oxide, intravascular oxygenators implanted in the vena cava to improve systemic oxygenation, and extracorporeal

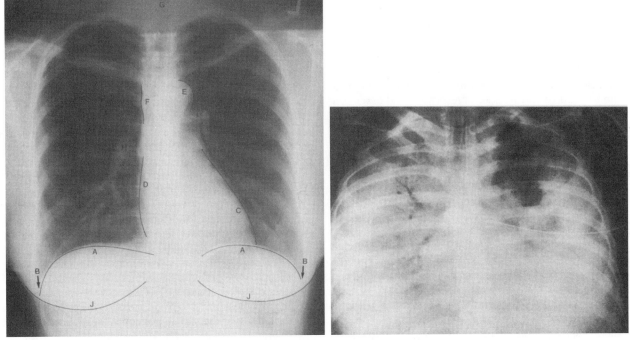

FIGURE   **14-17**   **A,** Normal chest film taken from a posteroanterior (PA) view. The backward L in the upper right corner is placed on the film to indicate the left side of the chest. Some anatomic structures can be seen on the x-ray study and are outlined: *A*, diaphragm; *B*, costophrenic angle; *C*, left ventricle, *D*, right atrium; *E*, aortic arch; *F*, superior vena cava; *G*, trachea; *H*, right bronchus; *I*, left bronchus; *J*, breast shadows. **B,** This chest film shows massive consolidation from pulmonary edema associated with acute (adult) respiratory distress syndrome (ARDS) following multisystem trauma. (**A** from Black JM, Matassarin-Jacobs E, editors: *Luckmann and Sorensen's medical-surgical nursing,* ed 4, Philadelphia, 1993, Saunders, p 935. **B** from Fraser RG, Paré JA, Paré PD, et al: *Diagnosis of diseases of the chest,* ed 3, Philadelphia, 1990, Saunders.)

membrane oxygenation, which fully replaces lung function. Prophylactic immunotherapy, antibodies against endotoxin, and inhibition of various inflammatory mediators are among the possibilities being tested. Tracheal gas insufflation, an adjunct to mechanical ventilation, allows ventilation of the central airway while carbon dioxide is cleared and may help reduce the amount of peak airway pressure required to maintain blood oxygen levels. This technique is under investigation and may be used routinely when commercially available systems are developed.[128]

Prognosis.   The final outcome is difficult to predict at the onset of disease, but associated multiorgan dysfunction and uncontrolled infection contribute to the mortality rate for ARDS of 50% to 70%. The major cause of death in ARDS is nonpulmonary MODS, often with sepsis. If ARDS is accompanied by sepsis, the mortality rate may reach 90%. Median survival in such cases is 2 weeks. The mortality rate increases with age, and clients older than 60 years of age have a mortality rate as high as 90%.

Most survivors are asymptomatic within a few months and have almost normal lung function 1 year after the acute illness. Lung fibrosis is the most common post-ARDS complication; the fibrosis may resolve completely, may result in respiratory dysfunction and, in some cases, pulmonary hypertension, or may result in death.

Special Implications for the Therapist   **14-20**

ACUTE (ADULT) RESPIRATORY DISTRESS SYNDROME

Preferred Practice Patterns:
    See also Special Implications for the Therapist: Atelectasis, 14-18 and Special Implications for the Therapist: Pulmonary Edema, 14-19.
6B: Impaired Aerobic Capacity/Endurance Associated With Deconditioning (pulmonary edema; progression to multisystem failure)
6C: Impaired Ventilation, Respiration/Gas Exchange, and Aerobic Capacity/Endurance Associated With Airway Clearance Dysfunction
6F: Impaired Ventilation and Respiration/Gas Exchange Associated With Respiratory Failure (pulmonary edema; atelectasis)
6G: Impaired Ventilation, Respiration/Gas Exchange, and Aerobic Capacity/Endurance Associated With Respiratory Failure in the Neonate
7A: Primary Prevention/Risk Reduction for Integumentary Disorders (pressure ulcers in the case of ventilatory support and/or prone positioning)

Continued

ARDS requires careful monitoring and supportive care; one case study even suggests 24-hour access to physical therapy intervention in acute respiratory failure as a means of avoiding invasive medical procedures. Timely physical therapy interventions improve gas exchange and reverse pathologic progression, thereby curtailing or avoiding artificial ventilation.[226] Assess the client's respiratory status frequently, and observe for retractions on inspiration, the use of accessory muscles of respiration, and developing or worsening dyspnea. On auscultation, listen for adventitious (rales or rhonchi) or diminished breath sounds and report any clear, frothy sputum that may indicate pulmonary edema.

Closely monitor heart rate and blood pressure watching for arrhythmias (see Special Implications for the Therapist: Arrhythmias, 11-12) that may result from hypoxemia, acid-base disturbances, or electrolyte imbalance. With pulmonary artery catheterization, know the desired pulmonary capillary wedge pressure (PCWP)* level and check the readings; report any significant elevations (see Table 39-20) or changes in waveform that indicate the catheter has become wedged. Empty condensation from the tubing of the ventilator to ensure maximal oxygen delivery during therapy.

Some areas of the lungs are well-ventilated but not well-perfused, whereas other areas are well-perfused but not well-ventilated. Position changes can encourage lung expansion by redistributing fluid in the lungs. Oxygenation in clients with ARDS may sometimes be improved by turning them from the supine to the prone position, dramatically reducing pulmonary dead space and improving aeration. This change takes the weight off (and improves ventilation in) the posterior regions of the lungs while promoting perfusion in the anterior aspects. The net result is a better ventilation/perfusion match (V/Q), an expansion of atelectatic alveoli, and increased functional residual lung capacity.

Caregivers may be reluctant to use the prone position. The therapist can be very instrumental in providing education on this topic. Selection criteria for this type of positioning may include individuals receiving ventilatory support at an oxygen concentration greater than 50%, with poor arterial blood gas levels (ABGs) and PEEP of 10 to 15 mm Hg or higher. Prone positioning should be considered if routine ventilator management has not been enough to improve the ventilatory status in an individual who is already pharmacologically immobilized or sedated (sedation is a requirement for prone positioning).

The client should be turned as far as possible on the abdomen; a 270-degree turn can improve oxygenation in some individuals, but ideally the full prone position is optimal. The person can be turned almost fully prone and supported with two or three pillows to help protect the airway, permit visualization, and allow suctioning as necessary. The better the person responds to the prone position, the longer that position can be maintained, and tolerance may build up with repeated use of the position. It is the repeated change from supine to prone positioning that redistributes pulmonary fluid and improves aeration and oxygenation overall.

Before turning, identify all invasive lines and bring them above the person's waist and over the head; lines inserted in the groin area can be moved over to the side that will remain nondependent. Taking these precautions will reduce the chances that the lines will get kinked or dislodged. One person is in charge of the person's airway during the turning, supporting the client's head and watching the intravenous lines. Any side-port line of a pulmonary artery catheter must be monitored especially carefully because it is closest to the client and more likely to kink. When the turn is completed, this same clinician turns the client's head to one side, making sure the airway is visible and open. Extra pillows or foam/gel pads may be needed to make room for the airway and increase comfort level. The dependent shoulder should be positioned with the elbow directly to the side and the hand facing up toward the head to prevent dislocation. A pad around the mouth to absorb bronchial secretions will decrease the potential for eye contamination.

The prone position promotes secretion removal by propelling secretions toward the upper airways. It also makes it easy to perform back care and help maintain sacral and heel skin integrity. Disadvantages include the potential for facial skin irritation (especially on the forehead), loss of important vascular accesses, and difficulty performing CPR if required. Blood pressure may drop after the turn but should stabilize within a few minutes; unstable blood pressure will necessitate returning the person to the supine position. Other indicators of poor position tolerance include a decline in SaO_2, SvO_2, or the tidal volume over time.[60] ■

◆ Postoperative Respiratory Failure

Postoperative respiratory failure can result in the same pathophysiologic and clinical manifestations as ARDS but without the severe progression to MODS (see previous discussion of ARDS). Risk factors include surgical procedures of the thorax or abdomen, limited cardiac reserve, chronic renal failure, chronic hepatic disease, infection, period of hypotension during surgery, sepsis, and smoking, especially in the presence of preexisting lung disease. In the pediatric population, a difficult respiratory course may result in necrotizing enterocolitis, a postoperative gastrointestinal complication related to ischemia of the bowel. This condition occurs when oxygen depletion in the heart or brain causes blood to be shunted away from less vital organs, such as the intestine.

The most common postoperative pulmonary problems include atelectasis, pneumonia, pulmonary edema, and pulmonary emboli. Prevention of any of these problems involves frequent turning, deep breathing, humidified air to loosen secretions, antibiotics for infection as appropriate, supplemental oxygen for hypoxemia, and early ambulation.

If respiratory failure develops, mechanical ventilation may be required, and treatment is very similar to that for ARDS.

◆ Sarcoidosis

Definition. Sarcoidosis is a systemic disease of unknown cause involving any organ that is characterized by granulomatous inflammation present diffusely throughout the body. These granulomas consist of a collection of macrophages surrounded by lymphocytes taking a nodular form. The lungs and lymph nodes are most commonly involved. In fact, granulomatous inflammation of the lung is present in 90% of clients with sarcoidosis. Secondary sites include the skin, eyes, liver, spleen, heart, and small bones in the hands and feet.

---

*Pulmonary artery catheterization measures left ventricular pressure and diastolic pressure. PCWP can indicate left ventricular failure coinciding with the onset of pulmonary congestion and pulmonary edema. PCWP can also register insufficient volume and pressure in the left ventricle indicating hypovolemic shock in other conditions.

Incidence.   Sarcoidosis occurs predominantly in the third and fourth decades (between the ages of 20 and 40 years) and has a slightly higher incidence in women than men. It is present worldwide with some interesting differences in prevalence among ethnic groups. It is 14 times more frequent in blacks in the southern United States.

Etiologic Factors and Pathogenesis.   The etiologic factors and pathogenesis of sarcoidosis are unknown, but there appears to be an exaggerated cellular immune response on the part of the helper T-lymphocytes to a foreign antigen whose identity remains unclear. Increasing evidence points to a triggering agent that may be genetic, infectious (bacterial or viral), immunologic, or toxic. Abnormalities of immune function, as well as autoantibody production, including rheumatoid factor and antinuclear antibodies, are seen in sarcoidosis and in connective tissue diseases, suggesting a common immunopathogenetic mechanism.

A series of interactions between the excessive accumulation of T-lymphocytes and monocytes and macrophages leads to the formation of noncaseating (i.e., do not undergo necrotic degeneration) granulomas in the lung and other organs characteristic of the disease. Granuloma formation may regress with therapy or as a result of the disease's natural course but may also progress to fibrosis and restrictive lung disease.

Clinical Manifestations.   Sarcoidosis can affect any organ, including bones, joints, muscles, and vessels. Lungs and thoracic lymph nodes are most often involved with acute or insidious respiratory problems sometimes accompanied by symptoms affecting the skin, eyes, or other organs. The diverse manifestations of this disorder lend support to the hypothesis that sarcoidosis has more than one cause. The clinical impact of sarcoidosis is directly related to the extent of granulomatous inflammation and its effect on the function of vital organs.

Pulmonary sarcoidosis has a variable natural course from an asymptomatic state to a progressive life-threatening condition. Signs and symptoms may develop over a period of a few weeks to a few months and include dyspnea, cough, fever, malaise, weight loss, skin lesions (Fig. 14-18), and erythema nodosum (multiple, tender, nonulcerating nodules). This condition may be entirely asymptomatic presenting with abnormal findings on routine chest radiographs. Respiratory symptoms of dry cough and dyspnea without constitutional symptoms* occur in over one-half of all people with sarcoidosis, and up to 15% develop progressive fibrosis. Chest pain, hemoptysis, or pneumothorax may be present.

Sarcoidosis may present with extrapulmonary symptoms referable to bone marrow, skin, eyes, cranial nerves or peripheral nerves (neurosarcoidosis), liver, or heart (Table 14-16). Neurosarcoidosis is an uncommon but severe and sometimes life-threatening manifestation of sarcoidosis occurring in 5% to 15% of cases. Sarcoidosis appears to be associated with a significantly increased risk for cancer in affected organs (e.g., skin, liver, lymphoma, lung). Chronic inflammation is the mediator of this risk.[16]

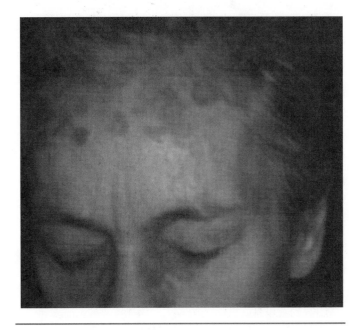

FIGURE   14-18   Cutaneous sarcoidal granuloma associated with sarcoidosis. This extrapulmonary sign (present in approximately 10% to 35% of documented systemic sarcoidosis cases) results from the presence of the granulomas in the tissues. The most common presentation is papular lesions noted on the head and neck, particularly the periorbital region, although they may appear in other areas of the body (including scars). The papules may be flesh-colored, red, or slightly hyperpigmented as shown here. In blacks, the papules may be hypopigmented. (From *J Musculoskel Med* 12:73-74, 1995 [case study].)

Medical Management

Diagnosis.   There is no specific test other than history for sarcoidosis so diagnosis is based on clinical examination, radiographic and laboratory test findings, and biopsy of easily accessible granulomas (e.g., skin lesions, salivary gland, palpable lymph nodes). When lung involvement is suspected, further testing may be required and new imaging techniques improve detection. Other granulomatous diseases (e.g., TB, berylliosis, lymphoma, carcinoma, fungal disease) must be ruled out.

CNS involvement in sarcoidosis poses a difficult diagnostic problem. Although neurologic involvement may occur long before the onset of symptoms, contrast-enhanced CT does not always reveal parenchymal and meningeal involvement.

Treatment.   Treatment may not be required, especially in those clients who are asymptomatic; short-term (<6 months) use of inhaled steroids may improve symptoms especially in people who mainly have cough. The long-term use of corticosteroids is the treatment of choice for those clients who have impaired lung function with pulmonary granulomas. Corticosteroids are quite effective in reducing the acute granulomatous inflammation, but their efficacy in altering the long-term prognosis is unproven so this therapy is reserved for people with severe or progressive pulmonary symptoms or pulmonary dysfunction.[126] Other agents, such as methotrexate, chloroquine, indomethacin, and azathioprine, are used for symptomatic skin involvement.

People with sarcoidosis who smoke are encouraged to quit because smoking aggravates impaired lung function

---

*Constitutional symptoms refer to symptoms of systemic illness, including fatigue, weakness, malaise, weight loss, sweating, and fever.

TABLE 14-16

Clinical Manifestations of Sarcoidosis

Pulmonary
Asymptomatic with abnormal chest film
Gradually progressive cough and shortness of breath
Pulmonary fibrosis with pulmonary insufficiency
Laryngeal and endobronchial obstruction

Extrapulmonary
Löfgren's syndrome: fever, arthralgias, bilateral hilar adenopathy, erythema nodosum
Heerfordt's syndrome (uveoparotid fever): fever, swelling of parotid gland and uveal tracts, seventh cranial nerve palsy
Erythema nodosum
Peripheral lymphadenopathy/splenomegaly
Lymphoma
Eyes: excessive tearing, swelling, uveitis, iritis, glaucoma, cataracts
Skin: nodules or skin plaques (see Fig. 14-18); skin cancer
Central nervous system: cranial nerve palsies, subacute meningitis, diabetes insipidus
Joints: polyarticular and monarticular arthritis
Bones: punched-out cystic lesions in phalangeal and metacarpal bones
Heart: paroxysmal arrhythmias, conduction disturbances, congestive heart failure, sudden death
Kidney: hypercalcemia with nephrocalcinosis or nephrolithiasis
Liver: granulomatous hepatitis, liver cancer

and promotes osteoporosis. Management of osteoporosis in this population requires special attention because there is often an underlying disorder in calcium metabolism that results in hypercalciuria and hypercalcemia. Prolonged exposure to direct sunlight should be avoided because vitamin D aids absorption of calcium, which can contribute to elevated serum and urinary calcium levels and the formation of kidney stones.

In cases of end-stage sarcoidosis, lung transplantation has been proven successful. Selection of clients with pulmonary sarcoidosis for transplantation requires that medical therapy, including the use of corticosteroids and alternative medications, has been exhausted and that other contraindicated variables are not present (see the section on Lung Transplantation in Chapter 20). Sarcoidosis frequently recurs in the allograft but rarely causes symptoms or pulmonary dysfunction.[127]

Prognosis. The prognosis is usually favorable, with complete resolution of symptoms and chest radiographic changes within 1 to 2 years. Most clients do not manifest clinically significant sequelae. However, because sarcoidosis is a multisystem disease that can cause complex problems, it can have a variable prognosis ranging from spontaneous remissions to progressive lung disease with pulmonary fibrosis in active sarcoidosis. In such cases, respiratory insufficiency and cor pulmonale may eventually occur. In 65% to 70% of cases there are no residual manifestations, 20% are left with permanent lung or ocular changes, and 10% of all cases die. Active sarcoidosis responds well to the administration of corticosteroids.

Special Implications for the Therapist 14-21

SARCOIDOSIS

Preferred Practice Patterns:
4A: Primary Prevention/Risk Reduction for Skeletal Demineralization (prolonged use of corticosteroids)
6E: Impaired Ventilation and Respiration/Gas Exchange Associated With Ventilatory Pump Dysfunction or Failure (progressive pulmonary fibrosis)
6F: Impaired Ventilation and Respiration/Gas Exchange Associated With Respiratory Failure (hemothorax)
6H: Impaired Circulation and Anthropometric Dimensions Associated With Lymphatic System Disorders
In the case of extrapulmonary manifestations of sarcoidosis (e.g., skin, cranial or peripheral nerve, heart involvement) other practice patterns may be identified.

There is a distinct arthritic component associated with sarcoidosis, variously reported in 10% to 35% of people who develop extrapulmonary involvement. The knees or ankles are the most common sites of acute arthritis. Distribution of joint involvement is usually polyarticular and symmetric, and the arthritis is commonly self-limiting after several weeks or months. Occasionally, the arthritis is recurrent or chronic, but even then, joint destruction and deformity are rare. Treatment of arthritis in sarcoidosis is usually as for any other form of arthritis. The arthritic symptoms may develop early as the first manifestation of the disease or late in the disease and are usually accompanied by erythema nodosum. When further complicated by bilateral hilar adenopathy (enlargement of hilum or roots of the lung where the main bronchi enter the lungs), this triad of symptoms is called *Löfgren's syndrome.* Recurrent Löfgren's syndrome is extremely rare and is usually self-limiting.

Therapists should be alert to any presenting signs or symptoms of increased disease activity associated with sarcoidosis since medical vigilance with attention to new symptoms is important in the management of sarcoidosis. This disease presents in many and diverse patterns, but observe especially for exertional dyspnea that progresses to dyspnea at rest, chest pain, joint swelling, or increased fatigue and malaise reducing the client's functional level or ability to participate in therapy. Muscle involvement and bone involvement are frequently underdiagnosed. Symptoms of muscle weakness, aches, tenderness, and fatigue, often accompanied by neurogenic atrophy, may indicate sarcoid myositis.[24]

Cranial nerve palsies (especially facial palsy), multiple mononeuropathy, and less commonly, symmetric polyneuropathy may all occur. Symmetric polyneuropathy can affect either motor or sensory fibers solely or both disproportionately. An unusual combination of neurologic deficits affecting the CNS or peripheral nerves (or both) suggests sarcoidosis and should be evaluated medically. Improvement of neurologic function may occur with the use of corticosteroids. For clients receiving steroid therapy, increased side effects of the medication should be reported to the physician. For example, long-term use of steroids lowers resistance to infection, may induce diabetes and myopathy, and is associated with weight gain, loss of potassium in the urine, and gastric irritation (see the section on Corticosteroids in Chapter 4 and Tables 4-7 and 4-8). ■

◆ Lung Cancer

Overview.   Lung cancer, a malignancy of the epithelium of the respiratory tract, is the most frequent cause of cancer death in the United States. The term *lung cancer*, also known as *bronchogenic carcinoma*, excludes other pulmonary tumors, such as sarcomas, lymphomas, blastomas, hematomas, and mesotheliomas.

Types of Lung Cancer.   At least a dozen different types of tumors are included under the broad heading of lung cancer. Clinically, lung cancers are classified as small cell lung cancer (SCLC, 20% of all lung cancers) and non-SCLC (NSCLC, 80% of all lung cancers). Within these two broad categories, there are four major types of primary malignant lung tumors: SCLC includes small cell carcinoma (oat cell carcinoma); NSCLC includes squamous cell carcinoma, adenocarcinoma, and large cell carcinoma. The characteristics of these four lung cancers are summarized in Table 14-17.

Incidence.   Lung cancer remains the leading cause of cancer death in the United States and one of the world's leading causes of preventable death. More people die of lung cancer than of colon, breast, and prostate cancer combined. In 1987, lung cancer overtook breast cancer to become the most common cause of death from cancer among women in the United States. Among women, both incidence and mortality continue to rise although incidence rates appear to have slowed in the last decade.[99,107] Approximately 3000 adolescents start smoking every day, with 4.5 million children and adolescents now smoking cigarettes and another 1 million using smokeless tobacco, suggesting that future statistics may not change for the better.[171]

The encouraging news is that as a result of a decline in smoking by men beginning around 1960 (and possibly the long-term benefits of reductions in tobacco carcinogens in cigarettes), the incidence and mortality rates in males have been decreasing.[120] It is hypothesized that similar smoking cessation among women will have the same positive results, but mortality rates are not expected to peak until 2010. Deaths from lung cancer increase at ages 35 to 44 years with a sharp increase between ages 45 and 55 years. Incidence continues to increase up until age 74 years, after which the incidence levels off and decreases among the very old.

Risk Factors.   Lung cancer can be traced to an environmental risk factor in the majority of cases, as reflected in the vast number of genetic alterations discovered in lung tumors with a pathogenesis believed to be mediated by carcinogen exposure.[6] The primary risk factor for lung cancer predominantly centers on cigarette smoking but also includes occupational and environmental exposures, geographic location (e.g., large industrial cities and urban areas of southern states have the highest rates), age, family history, nutrition, and the presence or previous history of lung disease.

Cigarette Smoking.   Cigarette smoking (more than 20 cigarettes per day) remains the greatest risk factor for lung cancer; 85% to 90% of all lung cancers occur in smokers although remarkably, fewer than 20% of cigarette smokers develop lung cancer. The relative risk of lung cancer increases with the number of cigarettes smoked per day and the number of years of smoking history. The people at highest risk began smoking in their teens, inhale deeply, and smoke at least one-half pack per day. The number of pack years is calculated by multiplying

TABLE	14-17

Characteristics of Lung Cancer

TUMOR TYPE	INCIDENCE	GROWTH RATE	METASTASIS	TREATMENT
Small Cell Lung Cancer (SCLC)				
Small cell (oat cell)	20%-25%	Very rapid	Very early; to mediastinum or distal area of lung	Combination chemotherapy and radiation therapy; surgical resectability is poor
Non-Small Cell Lung Cancer (NSCLC)				
Squamous cell (epidermal)	30%	Slow	Localized; metastasis not common or occurs late, usually to hilar lymph nodes, adrenals, liver	Surgical resectability is good if stage I or II. Chemotherapy and radiation therapy for all stages are under continued investigation
Adenocarcinoma	30%-35%* (some reports 35%-40%)	Slow to moderate	Early; metastasis throughout lung and brain or to other organs	Surgical resectability is good if localized stage I or II. Chemotherapy or chemoradiation and surgery may be combined for stage III
Large cell (anaplastic)	10%-15%	Rapid	Early and widespread metastasis to kidney, liver, adrenals	Surgical resectability is poor if involvement is widespread; better prognosis if stage I or II. Chemotherapy of limited use; radiation therapy is palliative

From Statistical data from the U.S. Department of Health and Human Services. Publication No. 96-691. Washington, D.C., 1996.
*A major histologic change has occurred over the last three decades as the most common cell type has shifted from squamous cell to adenocarcinoma. This shift appears to be the result of physiochemical changes in the late twentieth century smoke (e.g., increased levels of tobacco-specific nitrosamines).[17]

the packs of cigarettes consumed per day by the number of years of smoking. Lung cancer increases proportionately to the history of packs smoked per year and also depends on other variables, such as time of breath holding, amount of cigarette smoked, and size of puff. The risk for dying of lung cancer is 20 times higher among people who smoke two or more packs of cigarettes per day than among those who do not smoke. Smoking is a major cause of cancers of the oropharynx and bladder among women. Evidence is also strong that women who smoke have increased risks for liver, colorectal, and cervical cancer and cancers of the pancreas and kidney. There is also an increased risk for stroke, death from ruptured abdominal aortic aneurysm, and peripheral vascular disease among smokers compared to nonsmokers.[107] For other effects of smoking see the section on Tobacco in Chapter 2.

Former smokers have about one-half the risk for dying from lung cancer than do current smokers (see Table 2-3). Compared with current smokers, the risk for lung and bronchus cancer among former smokers declines as the duration of abstinence lengthens, with risk reduction becoming evident within 5 years of cessation.[153]* The statistics point to the fact that lung cancer is the most preventable of all cancers. The elimination of cigarette smoking would virtually eliminate SCLC. Smoking cessation also appears to slow the rate of progression of carotid atherosclerosis.

There are approximately 50 known carcinogens and promoting substances found in tobacco smoke; the major causal agents of lung cancer are the polynuclear aromatic hydrocarbons (PAHs) and tobacco-specific N-nitrosamines. Tobacco smoking also results in increased exposure to ethylene oxide, aromatic amines, and other agents that cause damage to DNA.[113] For this reason, the risk of lung cancer is increased in a smoker who is also exposed to other carcinogenic agents, such as radioactive isotopes, polycyclic aromatic hydrocarbons and arsenicals, vinyl chloride, metallurgic ores, and mustard gas.

Marijuana. Marijuana contains many of the same organic and inorganic compounds that are carcinogens, co-carcinogens, or tumor promoters found in tobacco smoke. Marijuana produces inflammation, edema, and cell injury in the tracheobronchial mucosa of smokers and contributes to oxidative stress, a precursor for DNA mutations. Although several experimental and epidemiologic studies suggest marijuana use as a possible cause of cancers, this issue remains controversial.[78] In users under 40 years of age, cannabis is suspected to increase the risk of squamous cell carcinoma of the upper aerodigestive tract, particularly of the tongue, larynx, and possibly lung.[42]

Environmental Tobacco Smoke. In 1992 the U.S. Environmental Protection Agency declared secondhand smoke (ETS) (i.e., "passive smoking" or smoke inhaled from the environment surrounding an active smoker) to be a human carcinogen. ETS increases the relative risk for lung cancer about 1.5-fold (as compared with 20 to 30 times greater among lifetime smokers compared with nonsmokers).[10] There are no

known safe levels of secondhand smoke. This exposure increases the risk for the children and partners of smokers and becomes an occupational hazard in individuals working in bars, restaurants, or other places that are not smoke-free. See previous section on Environmental Tobacco Smoke in this chapter.

Occupational Exposure. Studies on whether occupational factors increase the risk of cancer development in the nonsmoker are limited in number but confirm that certain occupational exposures are associated with an increased risk for lung cancer among both male and female nonsmokers.[177] The inhalation of asbestos fibers is associated with higher cancer risks for both smokers and nonsmokers although the rate is considerably higher for smokers. The rate of lung cancer in people who live in urban areas is 2.3 times greater than that of those living in rural areas, possibly implicating air pollution as a risk factor in lung cancer. The exact role of air pollution is still unknown, but known carcinogens continue to be released into outdoor air from industrial sources, power plants, and motor vehicles; epidemiologic research provides some evidence for an association between air pollution and lung cancer.[53] Indoor exposure to radon, a product of uranium and radium produced from the decomposition of rocks and soil (more common in some parts of the United States), is a known carcinogen capable of damaging lung DNA. Other sources of radon exposure include radioactive waste and underground mines; exposure to tobacco smoke multiplies the risk of concurrent exposure to radon.

Other occupational or environmental risk factors associated with lung cancer include diesel exhaust, benzopyrenes, silica, formaldehyde, copper, chromium, cadmium, arsenic, alkylating compounds, sulfur dioxide, and ionizing radiation.

Previous Lung Disease. The presence of other lung diseases, such as pulmonary fibrosis, scleroderma, and sarcoidosis, may increase the risk of developing lung cancer. COPD or fibrosis of the lungs inhibits the clearance of carcinogens from the lungs, thereby increasing the risk of alteration of DNA with resultant malignant cell growth.

Nutrition. Other risk factors include low consumption of fruits and vegetables, reduced physical activity, increased dietary fat (especially diets high in saturated or animal fat and cholesterol), and high alcohol intake.[20] Surprisingly, three large-scale clinical trials have determined that beta-carotene supplementation in heavy smokers increases the risk for lung cancer. The mechanism for this carcinogenic action remains unknown.[95,179]

Genetic Susceptibility. Several published studies suggest that lung cancer can aggregate in some families; it has been hypothesized that the defect in the body's ability to defend against the carcinogens in tobacco smoke may be inherited.[227] A first-degree smoking relative of an individual with lung cancer has an increased risk of developing lung cancer. This predilection may be due to a genetic predisposition, but the trait (lung cancer) may be expressed only in the presence of its major predisposing factor (i.e., tobacco). Carcinogenic chemicals may induce genomic instability either directly or indirectly through inflammatory processes in the lung epithelial cells. Lung cancer is used as a model for the study of the interplay between genetic factors and environmental exposure since the primary etiology is well-established.[102] De-

---

*Most studies suggest that smokers of strictly pipes and cigars experience some increase in risk of lung cancer compared with nonsmokers dependent on the amount smoked and the depth of inhalation. The cancer mortality rates for pipe and cigar smokers are about equal to those of cigarette smokers for cancer of the larynx, oral cavity, and esophagus.[30]

velopments in molecular biology have led to the investigation of biologic markers that may increase predisposition to smoking-related carcinogenesis. In the future lung cancer screening may be possible by using specific biomarkers.[219]

Pathogenesis.   As mentioned, there is a clear relationship between cigarette smoking and the development of SCLC. The effects of smoking include structural, functional, malignant, and toxic changes. DNA-mutating agents in cigarettes produce alterations in both oncogenes and tumor suppressor genes. Understanding of the molecular pathology of lung cancer is advancing rapidly with several specific genes and chromosomal regions being identified. Lung cancer appears to require many mutations in both dominant and recessive oncogenes before they become invasive. Several genetic and epigenetic changes are common to all lung cancer histologic types, whereas others appear to be tumor type specific. The sequence of changes remains unknown.[222]

All lung cancers are thought to arise from a common bronchial precursor cell, with differentiation then proceeding along various histologic pathways from poorly differentiated small cell cancer to the more intermediate undifferentiated large cell tumors, to the more differentiated adenocarcinomas and squamous cell tumors. Perhaps the histologic changes (thickening of bronchial epithelium, damage to and loss of protective cilia, mucous gland hypertrophy and hypersecretion of mucus, alveolar cell rupture) that occur more frequently in long-term smokers than nonsmokers predispose the lungs to changes. This results in a multistep process involving the development of hyperplasia, metaplasia, dysplasia, carcinoma in situ, invasive carcinoma, and metastatic carcinoma. As the details of the carcinogenic process are unraveled, one goal is to identify intermediate (preneoplastic) markers of exposure and inherent predisposition that will help assess the risk of lung cancer and allow for early detection.

Small Cell Lung Cancer.   When the cells become so dense that there is almost no cytoplasm present and the cells are compressed into an ovoid mass, the tumor is called small cell carcinoma or oat cell carcinoma. SCLC develops most often in the bronchial submucosa, the layer of tissue beneath the epithelium, and tends to be located centrally, most often near the hilum of the lung. These tumors can produce hormones that stimulate their own growth and the rapid growth of neighboring cells and cause bronchial obstruction and pneumonia with early intralymphatic invasion. Lymphatic and distant metastases are usually present at the time of diagnosis.

Non–Small Cell Lung Cancer.   Squamous cell carcinomas arise in the central portion of the lung near the hilum, projecting into the major or segmental bronchi. Although these tumors tend to grow rapidly, they often remain located within the thoracic cavity, making curative treatment more likely compared with other NSCLC types. These tumors may be difficult to differentiate from TB or an abscess because they often undergo central cavitation (formation of a cavity or hollow space).

Adenocarcinoma, the most common form of lung cancer in the United States, tends to arise in the periphery, usually in the upper lobes at different levels of the bronchial tree. An individual tumor may reflect the cell structure of any part of the respiratory mucosa from the large bronchi to the smallest bronchioles. Because of this, adenocarcinoma refers to a het-

erogeneous group of neoplasms that have in common the formation of glandlike structures. Adenocarcinoma is further subdivided into four categories: acinar, papillary, bronchioloalveolar, and solid carcinoma. Increasing incidence of adenocarcinoma cell type lung cancer is currently attributed to changes in smoking patterns (e.g., deeper and more intense inhalation) in response to reduced tar and nicotine in cigarettes. Presumably, the excess volume inhaled to satisfy addictive needs for nicotine delivers increased amounts of carcinogens and toxins to the peripheral areas of the lungs.[200]

Large cell carcinomas are so poorly differentiated that they cannot be classified with the other three categories above and require special diagnostic testing procedures to differentiate from other lung pathologic conditions.

Clinical Manifestations.   Symptoms of early-stage, localized lung cancer do not differ much from pulmonary symptoms associated with chronic smoking (e.g., cough, dyspnea, sputum production), so the person does not seek medical attention. Symptoms may depend on the location within the pulmonary system, whether centrally located, peripheral, or in the apices of the lungs. Systemic symptoms, such as anorexia, fatigue, weakness, and weight loss, are common, especially with advanced disease (metastases). Bone pain associated with bone metastasis is common; other symptoms resulting from metastases depend on the site of involvement (e.g., hepatomegaly and jaundice with liver metastasis; seizures, headaches, confusion, or focal neurologic signs with brain metastasis). Other symptoms of late disease include productive cough with hemoptysis, wheezing, chest pain, hoarseness, and nerve disorders as a result of local tumor invasion.

Small Cell Lung Cancer.   Signs and symptoms of SCLC depend on the size and location of the tumor and the presence and extent of metastases. Because SCLCs most commonly arise in the central endobronchial location in people who are almost exclusively long-term smokers, typical symptoms are a result of obstructed air flow and consist of persistent, new, or changing cough, dyspnea, stridor, wheezing, hemoptysis, and chest pain.[34] Intercostal retractions on inspiration and bulging intercostal spaces on expiration indicate obstruction. As obstruction increases, bronchopulmonary infection (obstructive pneumonitis) often occurs distal to the obstruction. Centrally located tumors cause chest pain with perivascular nerve or peribronchial involvement that can refer pain to the shoulder, scapula, upper back, or arm.

SCLC is (more often than NSCLC) associated with several paraneoplastic syndromes, including ectopic hormone production (adrenocorticotropic hormone [ACTH]) with Cushing's syndrome, production of hormones by tumors of nonendocrine origin, or production of an inappropriate hormone (antidiuretic hormone) by an endocrine gland. Neuroendocrine cells containing neurosecretory granules exist throughout the tracheobronchial tree. This phenomenon is important because resulting signs and symptoms may be the first manifestation of underlying cancer. See Special Implications for the Therapist box in this section; see also the section on Paraneoplastic Syndromes in Chapter 8.

Non–Small Cell Lung Cancer.   The less common peripheral pulmonary tumors (large cell) often do not produce signs or symptoms until disease progression produces localized, sharp, and severe pleural pain increased on inspiration, limiting lung expansion; cough and dyspnea are present. Pleural effusion may develop and limit lung expansion even more. Tumors in the apex of the lung, called *Pancoast's tumors*, occur both in squamous cell and adenocarcinomatous cancers. Symptoms do not occur until the tumors invade the brachial plexus (see Special Implications for the Therapist box in this section). Destruction of the first and second ribs can occur. Paralysis, elevation of the hemidiaphragm, and dyspnea secondary to phrenic nerve involvement can also occur. Other manifestations may include digital clubbing, skin changes, joint swelling associated with hypertrophic pulmonary osteoarthropathy (see previous discussion of this condition in the section on Cystic Fibrosis), decreased or absent breath sounds on auscultation, or pleural rub (inflammatory response to invading tumor).

Metastasis. The rich supply of blood vessels and lymphatics in the lungs allows the disease to metastasize rapidly.[34] Lung cancers spread by direct extension, lymphatic invasion, and blood-borne metastases. Tumors spread by direct invasion in the bronchus of origin; others may invade the bronchial wall and circle and obstruct the airway. Intrapulmonary spread may lead to compression of lung structures other than airways, such as blood or lymph vessels, alveoli, and nerves. Direct extension through the pleura can result in spread over the surface of the lung, chest wall, or diaphragm. Carcinomas of the lung of all types metastasize most frequently to the regional lymph nodes, particularly the hilar and mediastinal nodes. Supraclavicular, cervical, and abdominal channels may also be invaded. Tumors originating in the lower lobes tend to spread through the lymph channels.

Lung cancer generally has a widespread pattern of hematogenous metastases. This is due to the invasion of the pulmonary vascular system. After tumor cells enter the pulmonary venous system, they can be carried through the heart and disseminated systemically. Tumor emboli can become lodged in areas of organ systems where vessels become too narrow for their passage or where blood flow is reduced. The most frequent site of extranodal metastases is the adrenal gland. Lung cancer can also metastasize to the brain, bone, and liver before presenting symptomatically. Brain metastases constitute nearly one-third of all observed recurrences in people with resected NSCLC of the adenocarcinoma type. Metastases to the brain usually result in CNS symptoms of confusion, gait disturbances, headaches, or personality changes.

Tumor spread intrathoracically to the mediastinum and beyond can produce superior vena cava (SVC) syndrome with swelling of the face, neck, and arms and neck and thoracic vein distention more common in the early morning or after being recumbent for several hours. SVC syndrome is usually a sign of advanced disease. If left untreated, SVC syndrome results in cerebral edema and possible death. Increased intracranial pressure, headaches, dizziness, visual disturbances, and alteration in mental status are signs of progressive compression. Cardiac metastasis can occur and results in arrhythmias, congestive heart failure, and pericardial tamponade.

As a form of secondary malignancy, the lungs are the most frequent site of metastases from other types of cancer. Any tumor cell dislodged from a primary neoplasm can find its way into the circulation or lymphatics, which are filtered by the lungs. Carcinomas of the kidney, breast, pancreas, colon, and uterus are especially likely to metastasize to the lungs.

Medical Management

Diagnosis. Most early lung cancers are detected on routine chest film in clients presenting for unrelated medical conditions without pulmonary symptoms. Unfortunately, chest radiograph, the standard mode of detection, is not sensitive enough to show tumors when they are small and operable. Two new diagnostic tools are now available in nuclear medicine to allow noninvasive testing. The first is a chest scan called low-dose spiral computed tomography (CT), and the second is a new lung scan (lung imaging fluorescence endoscope [LIFE]) recently approved by the FDA that can literally light up cancerous (and preinvasive cancerous) cells using intravenously administered radioactive tracer that attaches to these cells. When the person is imaged with a special camera, the cancer cells show up as bright spots. A positive result would still need to be confirmed by biopsy. There are some concerns with the chest scan fast CT first mentioned (e.g., cost, false-positive findings, unnecessary biopsies of small benign tumors) although the availability of this type of diagnostic procedure may bring about annual screening for lung cancer for those at risk. However, mass screening for lung cancer with CT is not currently advocated because to date no randomized population trial has demonstrated a significant reduction in lung carcinoma mortality as a result of any screening intervention.[3,202]

Without the low-dose CT chest scan, diagnosis is usually established on sputum cytology for participants in a lung cancer detection program or on bronchoscopy in persons presenting with hemoptysis and a normal chest film. Localization of occult lung tumors is done by fiberoptic bronchoscopy that allows examination to the sixth or seventh branch of the bronchial tree. CT scans are routinely done to assess for metastasis to the mediastinum, liver, and adrenals. Other routine procedures include evaluation of serum chemistry values to look for electrolyte abnormalities (see Chapter 4), especially those associated with paraneoplastic syndrome (see Chapter 8), evaluation of renal and hepatic function, hematologic profiles, and ECG analysis. In addition, the development of sputum-based cellular diagnostics for the detection of early-stage lung cancer is under investigation. The presence of biomarkers in bronchial epithelial cells is highly associated with the development of lung cancer. Finding this early airway-confined phase of lung cancer may allow for the development of new management approaches for very early-stage lung cancer (e.g., aerosolized chemoprevention).[110]

Staging. NSCLC of the lung is staged at the time of initial presentation and used to estimate the person's prognosis and to determine intervention. The tumor, nodes, metastasis (TNM) staging system is used (see explanation in Chapter 8) and provides the basis for selecting cases for resection. Tumors confined to the lung without any metastases, regional or distant, are classified as stage I, and tumors associated with only hilar or peribronchial lymph node involvement (N1) are classified as stage II. Locally advanced tumors with mediastinal or cervical lymph node metastases and those with extension to the chest wall, mediastinum, diaphragm, or carina are classified as stage III tumors. Finally, tumors presenting with distant metastases (M1) are classified as stage IV.

SCLC is usually not considered a surgical disease requiring staging but rather is designated as limited or extensive disease. Limited disease is defined by involvement of one lung, the mediastinum, and either or both ipsilateral and contralateral supraclavicular lymph nodes (i.e., disease that can be encompassed in a single radiation therapy port). Spread beyond the lung, mediastinum, and supraclavicular lymph nodes is considered extensive disease.

Prevention.   Prevention is the key to eliminating or at least reducing the need for treatment of lung cancer. Targeted state and federal antitobacco programs have contributed to significant drops in cigarette consumption.[20] *Healthy People 2010* has set a goal of reducing the lung cancer mortality rate from 57.6 per 100,000 population (1998 figure) to 44.9 per 100,000 population representing a 22% improvement. *Healthy People 2010* has outlined a systematic approach to health improvement that includes methods for lung cancer prevention through prevention of tobacco use and tobacco addiction in all age-groups, ethnic groups, and socioeconomic groups. For details see *Healthy People 2010* (www.health.gov/healthypeople/).

Other strategies for lung cancer prevention include chemoprevention (i.e., administration of agents, usually drugs but also nutraceuticals or nutritional supplements, before the diagnosis of invasive cancer to absorb free oxygen radicals and to block or reverse carcinogenesis), adopting a diet high in fruits and vegetables, and reduction of ETS. The importance of vitamin C as an antioxidant protection has been demonstrated for nonsmokers exposed to ETS[118]; and vitamins A, C, and E are proposed as risk modulators with a protective effect.[219] Reduction or prevention of occupational exposure may be achieved through a combination of approaches including toxicologic testing of new compounds before marketing them, application of industrial hygiene techniques, industry regulation, and epidemiologic surveillance.

Treatment.   Awareness of the influence of growth factors, oncogenes, and tumor suppressor genes as well as signal transduction and angiogenesis pathways on the natural history of cancer cells has led to attempts to develop new molecular-based strategies directed at interrupting tumor cell growth. Treatments using monoclonal antibodies, inhibitors, antiangiogenic substances, and gene transfer and alteration are under investigation.[37] In the meantime current treatment with new agents used in combination as well as when combined with radiation has led to an improved response rate in the treatment of some lung cancers.[36]

Small Cell Lung Cancer.   Surgical resection in the treatment of SCLC is not usually considered and when used, seems most effective for clients in the early stages of SCLC, after combination chemotherapy, which is the cornerstone of treatment for all stages of this disease, resulting in high response rates (65% to 85%).[130] For clients with more advanced disease, surgery causes unnecessary risk and stress, with no valid benefits. Laser therapy is a surgical treatment used when the tumor mass is causing nonresectable bronchial obstructions and when accessible by bronchoscope.

SCLC is quite sensitive to radiation therapy, which, in conjunction with chemotherapy, is now routinely administered to those with limited disease. Those with extensive disease usually receive combination chemotherapy initially. Other treatment options depend on the clinical manifestations and client needs (e.g., radiation therapy may be administered to the brain, bone, spine, or other sites of metastasis). In the future, tumor growth may be halted by replacement or substitution of mutated tumor suppressor gene functions or biochemical modulation of oncogene products. New forms of immunotherapy may also be targeted specifically toward mutant oncogenes in cancer cells.

Non–Small Cell Lung Cancer.   During the past 15 years treatment of stage III NSCLC has evolved considerably because of improvements in client selection, staging, and combined modality therapy. Results of several clinical trials suggest that induction chemotherapy or chemoradiation and surgical resection are superior to surgery alone, although the optimal induction regimen has not yet been defined. Trials are under way to determine whether chemoradiation and surgical resection lead to better survival than chemotherapy and radiation alone. Future studies will assess ways to combine radiation and novel chemotherapeutic agents and will identify molecular abnormalities that predict response to induction therapy.[149] Current data do not support adjuvant (postoperative) chemotherapy for stage I disease. Approach to stage IV disease is palliative and depends on location and extent of disease and clinical manifestations. For example, clients who develop spinal cord compromise secondary to metastatic disease can be palliated effectively with short-course external-beam radiotherapy.[138] Those who have lost bowel or bladder function (or both) or who present with flaccid paralysis are unlikely to regain significant organ function, although many with intact neurologic function may realize a short-term benefit in terms of quality of life.[206]

Prognosis.   The curability of lung cancer remains poor because by the time lung cancer is detected, invasion and metastasis have already occurred. The prognosis is influenced by the stage of the disease at presentation, the cell type, the treatment that can be given, and the status of the client at the time of diagnosis (e.g., people who are ambulatory respond to treatment better than those who are confined to bed more than 50% of the time). Other factors associated with poor prognosis include weight loss of more than 10% of body weight in 6 months and generalized weakness. Overall 5-year survival rate among older blacks with NSCLC is significantly lower compared with whites, largely explained by lower rates of surgical treatment.[18]

The new low-dose CT screening may change the future mortality of lung cancer by detecting even small lung tumors at an early, treatable stage. Currently, with treatment, only 14% of people with lung cancer survive beyond 5 years after diagnosis, but if caught early, lung cancer can be cured up to 70% of the time. Survival without treatment is rarely possible, and most untreated persons die within 1 year of diagnosis, with a median survival of less than 6 months. Curative treatment requires effective control of the primary tumor before metastasis occurs. Radiation therapy when used alone has been unsuccessful in attaining long-term survival. Chemotherapy is usually combined with surgery or irradiation for more advanced tumors. Once metastasis has occurred, surgical therapy is limited and treatment is palliative.

Other factors thought to confer poor prognosis include male gender, age older than 70 years, prior chemotherapy, elevated serum lactic dehydrogenase levels, low serum sodium, and elevated alkaline phosphatase levels (see Tables 39-14 and 39-15).

Special Implications for the Therapist 14-22

LUNG CANCER

Preferred Practice Patterns:

Symptoms resulting from metastases and corresponding practice patterns depend on the site of involvement but may include musculoskeletal patterns for bone metastases, neuromuscular patterns for nerve disorders such as brachial plexus compression caused by local invasion, and lymphatic compression secondary to intrapulmonary spread.

6A: *Primary Prevention/Risk Reduction for Cardiovascular/Pulmonary Disorders (tobacco disorder)*

6B: *Impaired Aerobic Capacity/Endurance Associated With Deconditioning*

6C: *Impaired Ventilation, Respiration/Gas Exchange, and Aerobic Capacity/Endurance Associated With Airway Clearance Dysfunction (asbestosis; obstructive disease)*

6E: *Impaired Ventilation and Respiration/Gas Exchange Associated With Ventilatory Pump Dysfunction or Failure (obstructive disease)*

6F: *Impaired Ventilation and Respiration/Gas Exchange Associated With Respiratory Failure (obstructive disease)*

7A: *Primary Prevention/Risk Reduction for Integumentary Disorders (skin breakdown; late-stage cancer)*

The effective management of short- and long-term side effects from lung cancer and its treatment is essential for rehabilitation. Increasing the therapist's knowledge of psychosocial-spiritual effects in these cases assists the therapist in planning appropriate intervention programs and promoting the optimal use of resources. If clients and their families can overcome treatment barriers, they will be more motivated toward achieving increased and sustained independence and quality of life. The therapist can be very helpful in teaching clients with lung cancer nonpharmacologic means of pain relief and energy conservation techniques while providing an optimal rest schedule and activity program in accordance with the degree of pulmonary involvement.

Effective breathing and coughing techniques should be taught and reinforced. Cigarette smoking should be discouraged. Numerous surveys have shown that the majority of current smokers demonstrate a desire to stop smoking and that intervention through smoking-cessation programs can be successful. The Agency for Health Care Policy and Research (AHCPR), which is now called the Agency for HealthCare Research and Quality (AHRQ), has recommended specific guidelines with intervention strategies to assist health care providers in giving smokers consistent and effective smoking-cessation guidelines. Every therapy and rehabilitation department should have information available about local smoking-cessation programs and a listing of local physicians willing to help anyone who expresses a desire to cease smoking.

Metastasis

Metastatic spread of pulmonary tumors to the long bones and to the vertebral column, especially the thoracic vertebrae, is common, occurring in as many as 50% of all cases. Local metastases by direct extension may involve the chest wall and may even erode the first and second ribs and associated vertebrae, causing bone pain and paravertebral pain associated with involvement of sympathetic nerve ganglia. Subsequently, chest, shoulder, arm, or back pain can be the presenting symptom but usually with accompanying pulmonary symptoms. The client may not associate the musculoskeletal symptoms with the pulmonary symptoms, so the therapist must always remember to screen for medical disease. Cases of lung cancer and shoulder pain for which no local cause could be found have been reported, and in each case radiotherapy to the ipsilateral mediastinum eliminated symptoms. Pain referred from intrathoracic involvement of the phrenic nerve is the suspected underlying pain mechanism.[133] Anytime the client fails to progress or improve in therapy, return to the physician is recommended for further diagnostic evaluation.

Spinal cord compression from extradural metastases of lung cancer usually occurs from direct extension of vertebral metastases. Back pain is often the first sign and may occur as progressive back pain 6 months before the diagnosis is made. The pain may be constant and aggravated by Valsalva's maneuver, sneezing or coughing, movement, and lying down and diminished by sitting up. Weakness, sensory loss, and a positive Babinski's reflex may be observed. Radiation is usually the treatment of choice for epidural metastases from lung cancer. Neurosurgical intervention may be indicated if the area of compression has been previously irradiated to maximal tolerance. Surgical decompression may also be indicated if neurologic deterioration occurs during the initiation of radiation therapy. The treatment field extends two vertebral bodies above and below the level of blockage. Corticosteroids are prescribed to reduce swelling and inflammation around the cord.[34]

Apical (Pancoast's) tumors do not usually cause symptoms while confined to the pulmonary parenchyma, but once they extend into the surrounding structures, the brachial plexus (C8 to T1) may become involved, presenting as a form of thoracic outlet syndrome. This nerve involvement produces sharp pleuritic pain in the axilla, shoulder (radiating in an ulnar nerve distribution down the arm), and subscapular area of the affected side, with atrophy and weakness of the upper extremity muscles. Invasion of the cervical sympathetic plexus may cause *Horner's syndrome* with unilateral miosis, ptosis, and absence of sweating on the affected side of the face and neck. Treatment for these two conditions may combine surgery with radiation. Local anesthetics administered through an axillary catheter placed in the brachial plexus for intractable neuropathic pain have also been reported; this approach is reversible and may be preferable to destructive procedures, such as cordotomy.[211] Therapy intervention for the thoracic outlet syndrome is an important part of the palliative treatment for this condition (see also the section on Thoracic Outlet Syndrome in Chapter 38).

Trigger points of the serratus anterior muscle also mimic the distribution of pain caused by C8 nerve root compression and must be ruled out by palpation, lack of neurologic deficits, and possible elimination with appropriate trigger point therapy. Pancoast's tumors may also masquerade as subacromial bursitis.

Paraneoplastic Syndromes

Paraneoplastic syndromes (remote effects of a malignancy; see discussion in Chapter 8) occur in 10% to 20% of lung cancer clients. These usually result from the secretion of hormones by the tumor acting on target organs producing a variety of symptoms, most commonly hypercalcemia, digital clubbing, osteoarthropathies, or rheumatologic disorders, such as polymyositis, lupus, and dermatomyositis. Occasionally, symptoms of paraneoplastic syndrome occur before detection of the primary lung tumor or as the first sign of recurrence presenting as a neuromusculoskeletal condition.[94] For example, hypertrophic osteoarthropathy with joint involvement may be diagnosed as arthritis without recognition of the underlying lung cancer. Digital clubbing is almost always present (or developing), sometimes with neurovascular changes of the hands and feet and usually with a previous history of cancer to alert the therapist. Treatment of the underlying cancer provides the most significant improvement of these syndromes because the underlying cause of the hormone secretion is the carcinoma itself.

Chemotherapy and Radiation Treatment

Clients undergoing chemotherapy, radiation therapy, or a combination of both and their family members must work closely with members of the multidisciplinary health team to obtain the information and emotional support they need. It is important that therapists have knowledge of side effects associated with different antineoplastic interventions and anticipate toxicities. For example, side effects of chemotherapy, including nausea and vomiting, require careful scheduling of therapy to optimize treatment success. In the presence of cancer pain, pain medication should be timed to allow maximal comfort during therapy (e.g., approximately 30 to 60 minutes before therapy).

Loss of appetite with accompanying weight loss may result in muscle weakness and decreased physical endurance requiring more frequent rest periods. The therapist may be able to assist the client with reduced functional status exhibiting other symptoms, such as dyspnea and fatigue, by teaching diaphragmatic breathing techniques, use of relaxation techniques for overused respiratory accessory muscles, and positioning for easing the work of breathing (e.g., sitting upright leaning forward slightly with elbows resting on knees).

Energy conservation (see Box 8-2) should be addressed by teaching the client to schedule strenuous activities at times of day when energy levels are the highest, alternating strenuous tasks with easier ones, using frequent rest breaks, planning activities to minimize the use of stairs or walking long distances, and workload reduction (encourage the client to perform elective tasks, especially household chores, less often and in the sitting position whenever possible). Monitoring platelet, hematocrit, and hemoglobin levels can help guide the therapist and client in establishing activity level (see Tables 39-6 and 39-7). Vital signs should be monitored before and after periods of increased activity; heart and lung sounds and oxygen saturation should be monitored during activity. Observe for signs of extreme fatigue, chest pain, or diaphoresis.

Other concerns addressed by the therapist may include regaining strength and endurance following chemotherapy or radiation therapy, mobility training for those clients with gait and balance disturbances, instruction for sleeping postures and bed mobility for clients with bone pain from metastasis,

and in late-stage cancer, prevention or treatment of contractures or skin breakdown. Helping the client recognize short-term and long-term side effects associated with treatment before these effects become life-threatening is essential (see Table 8-8). ■

DISORDERS OF THE PULMONARY VASCULATURE

◆ Pulmonary Embolism and Infarct

Definition and Incidence.   Pulmonary embolism (PE) is the lodging of a blood clot in a pulmonary artery with subsequent obstruction of blood supply to the lung parenchyma. Although a blood clot is the most common cause of occlusion, air, fat, bone marrow (e.g., fracture), foreign intravenous material, vegetations on heart valves that develop with endocarditis, amniotic fluid, and tumor cells (tumor emboli) can also embolize and occlude the pulmonary vessels.

PE is common, and in the United States the incidence is estimated at approximately 650,000 cases annually. It is the most common cause of sudden death in the hospitalized population. The overall incidence of PE appears to be declining, probably because of better treatment of established deep vein thrombosis (DVT) and increased use of thromboprophylaxis.

Etiologic and Risk Factors.   The most common cause of PE is DVT originating in the proximal deep venous system of the lower legs, but PE encompasses embolism from many sources, including air, bone marrow, arthroplasty cement, amniotic fluid, tumor, and sepsis.* Three major physiologic risk factors linked with PE are (1) *blood stasis* (e.g., immobilization caused by prolonged trips or spinal cord injury; bed rest, such as with burn cases, pneumonia, or obstetric and gynecologic clients; fracture care with casting or pinning; and older or obese populations); (2) *endothelial injury* (local trauma) secondary to surgical procedures (even as late as 1 month postoperatively), trauma, or fractures of the legs or pelvis; and (3) *hypercoagulable states* (e.g., oral contraceptive use, cancer, and hereditary thrombotic disorders).

Other clinical risk factors for PE include age over 60 years, obesity, heavy cigarette smoking, high blood pressure, congestive heart failure, trauma, previous history of thromboembolism, malignancy (neoplastic cells can generate thrombin or synthesize various procoagulants), infection, prolonged inactivity, paralysis, pregnancy, estrogen use (e.g., oral contraceptives, hormone replacement therapy), clotting abnormalities, and fractures of the hip or femur. Although diabetes mellitus has been traditionally considered a risk factor for PE, the Nurses' Health Study showed no association between PE and high cholesterol levels or diabetes.[91]

Pathogenesis.   Any level of the pulmonary artery, from the main trunk to the distal branches, is a site for emboli to lodge. Each embolus is a cylindrical mass of fresh or organizing thrombus comprised of alternating bands of red cells, fib-

---

*Before the introduction of routine prophylaxis with heparin (now low—molecular weight heparin [LMWH]) or warfarin sodium (Coumadin), the incidence of DVT following hip fracture, total hip replacement, or other surgeries involving the abdomen, pelvis, prostate, hip, or knee was extremely high.

rin strands, and leukocytes with a rim of fibroblasts at the periphery. PE ranges from incidental and clinically insignificant to massive embolism and sudden death.

The embolism causes an area of blockage, but actual pulmonary infarction (emboli arising within the lung) is uncommon because of the dual circulation of the lungs. Primary PE leads to ventilation/perfusion mismatch, which leads to hypoxia, but the bronchial arteries bringing in oxygenated blood will keep the lungs from infarction. The greater concern is that a clot will embolize to the pulmonary arteries from the popliteal or iliofemoral vein (approximately 50%) or from the calf veins (less than 5%). Either way, PE and DVT should be considered part of the same pathologic process, and in fact studies showed that a large percentage of people with DVT but no symptoms of PE also had evidence of PE on lung scanning. Conversely people with PE often have abnormalities on ultrasonographic studies of leg veins.[90]

Discharge of thrombus into the pulmonary artery with mechanical obstruction of the pulmonary vascular bed causes vasoconstriction as a result of vasoactive mediators released by activated platelets, increased pulmonary vascular resistance, pulmonary hypertension, and right ventricular failure (in severe cases).

Clinical Manifestations. Clients may be asymptomatic in the presence of small thromboemboli. The clinical findings in acute pulmonary thromboembolism depend on the size of the embolus and the individual's preexisting cardiopulmonary status. PE as a result of DVT can occur without warning. The DVT can become a thromboembolism by becoming dislodged from the venous wall, traveling through the venous return to the lungs, thus becoming a PE.

A *DVT* may present up to 2 weeks postoperatively as tenderness, leg pain, swelling (a difference in leg circumference of 1.4 cm in men and 1.2 cm in women is significant), and warmth. One exception to this presentation is the person who has been immobilized for a prolonged period in a cast. Removal of the cast normally presents with a leg that would measure less in circumference (muscle atrophy) than the uninvolved leg. Equal leg circumference should be a clinical red flag for medical evaluation.

DVT from any cause may be accompanied by a positive Homans' sign (deep calf pain on slow dorsiflexion of the foot or gentle squeezing of the affected calf; see Fig. 11-30), but Homans' sign is not specific for this condition because it also occurs with Achilles tendinitis and gastrocnemius and plantar muscle injury. Only one-half of the people with DVT experience pain with this test in the presence of a thrombus.

Other signs of DVT may include subcutaneous venous distention, discoloration, a palpable cord (superficial thrombus),* and pain on placement of a blood pressure cuff around the calf (considerable pain with the cuff inflated to 160 to 180 mm Hg). At least 50% of the cases of DVT are symptomatic, but in up to 30% of clients with clinical evidence of DVT or PE, no DVT is demonstrable.

Signs and symptoms of *PE* are present but nonspecific and vary greatly, depending on the extent to which the lung is in-

volved, the size of the clot, and the general medical condition of the individual. Sudden death may be the presentation, but dyspnea, pleuritic chest pain, apprehension, and persistent cough are the most common symptoms. Inflammatory reaction of the lung parenchyma or ischemia caused by obstruction of small pulmonary arterial branches causes pleuritic chest pain that is sudden in onset and aggravated by breathing. Other symptoms include hemoptysis, diaphoresis, tachypnea, and fever. The presence of hemoptysis indicates that alveolar damage has occurred.

Medical Management

Diagnosis. PE is difficult to diagnose because the signs and symptoms are nonspecific. PE may mimic (and even coexist with) pneumonia, congestive heart failure, pericarditis, myocardial infarction, pneumothorax, anxiety, pneumothorax, and even rib fractures. The physician must also differentiate conditions that can mimic thromboembolism to the calf, such as cellulitis, muscle strain or rupture, lymphangitis, and rupture of a Baker's cyst. Circumstances such as the onset of chest pain or dyspnea in hospitalized, postsurgical, or trauma cases are highly suspicious of PE. Clinical evaluation, nonimaging laboratory tests, and imaging tests are used to make the diagnosis.

Because the history and physical examination are neither sensitive nor specific in detecting thrombi in the deep veins of the lower extremities, duplex ultrasonography became the mainstay of diagnosis. Other specific tests included ventilation/perfusion (V/Q) scan or compression ultrasonography; the latter for the detection of DVT provides an effective noninvasive diagnostic technique. More recently, a new spiral CT technique has begun to replace pulmonary angiography because of its ability to directly visualize the pulmonary emboli. The major disadvantage of spiral CT is its inability to visualize beyond fourth-order branches of the pulmonary artery so that small distal emboli are not seen. Studies to investigate the use of magnetic resonance imaging (MRI) or magnetic resonance angiography (MRA) are ongoing.

Prevention and Treatment. The management of DVT and PE has changed dramatically in the last few years. Given the mortality of PE and the difficulties involved in its clinical diagnosis, prevention of DVT and PE is crucial. Primary prevention of DVT through the prophylactic use of anticoagulants is important for persons undergoing total hip replacement, major knee surgery, abdominal or pelvic surgery, prostate surgery, and neurosurgery. In fact, anyone hospitalized should be evaluated for risk of PE and placed on prophylaxis as appropriate.

Low–molecular weight (LMW) heparin (anticoagulant now replacing unfractionated heparin) is the most common agent for prophylaxis because it prolongs the clotting time and allows the body time to resolve the existing clot, thereby preventing further development of the thrombus; it does not reduce the immediate embolic risk or enhance clot lysis. LMW heparins have fewer major bleeding complications and do not require laboratory monitoring of coagulation tests to adjust medications. The U.S. FDA has approved outpatient treatment of DVT with the LMW heparin enoxaparin as a bridge to warfarin. Warfarin (Coumadin), an oral anticoagulant, is used simultaneously with heparin or during the transition from intravenous to oral anticoagulant with a targeted activated

---

*The femoral vein, which is part of the larger deep system of veins, may be palpable along the inner aspect of the thigh extending from the knee to the groin. This is distinguishable from a superficial phlebitis, which is usually superficial, localized, and limited in length to a small area.

partial thromboplastin time of 1.5 to 2.5 times the baseline value and an international normalized ratio of 2 to 3 (see discussion in Chapter 39). Prophylaxis and treatment with these medications for PE and DVT are different (see further discussion in the section on Thrombophlebitis in Chapter 11).

Thrombolytic therapy (a controversial, expensive treatment used with massive embolism) to lyse pulmonary thromboemboli in situ is accomplished through the use of thrombolytic agents such as streptokinase, urokinase, recombinant tissue plasminogen activator, and newer agents reteplase, saruplase, and recombinant staphylokinase that enhance fibrinolysis by activating plasminogen, generating plasmin. Plasmin directly lyses thrombi both in the pulmonary artery and in the venous circulation and has a secondary anticoagulant effect. Successfully utilized, pulmonary embolism thrombolysis reverses right-sided heart failure rapidly and safely. Based on new understanding of the pathogenesis of PE, acute massive pulmonary embolism may be treated in the future with antagonists to pulmonary constrictors or with direct pulmonary vasodilators.[198]

Surgical implantation of a filter in the vena cava may be used to prevent PE by filtering the blood and preventing clots from moving past the screen. There is an increased risk of caval occlusion and dependent edema as a result of obstruction of the filter with this procedure. Other procedures used in the case of massive DVT or hemodynamically unstable PE may include thrombectomy and embolectomy performed surgically in an angiography laboratory.

Prognosis.   PE is the primary cause of death for as many as 100,000 people each year (perhaps double that amount) and a contributory factor in another 100,000 deaths annually. About 10% of victims die within the first hour, but prognosis for survivors (depending on underlying disease and on proper diagnosis and treatment) is generally favorable. Clients with PE who have cancer, congestive heart failure, or chronic lung disease have a higher risk of dying within 1 year than do clients with isolated PE.

Small emboli resolve without serious morbidity, but large or multiple emboli (especially in the presence of severe underlying cardiac or pulmonary disease) have a poorer prognosis. PE may recur despite LMW heparin therapy, most commonly in people with massive PE or in whom anticoagulant therapy has been inadequate. PE is the leading cause of pregnancy-related mortality in the United States.

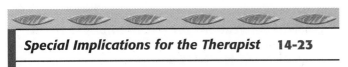

Special Implications for the Therapist   **14-23**

PULMONARY EMBOLISM AND INFARCTION

Preferred Practice Pattern:
6F: Impaired Ventilation and Respiration/Gas Exchange Associated With Respiratory Failure

A careful review of the client's medical history may alert the therapist to the presence of predisposing factors for the development of a PE. Frequent changing of position, exercise, the use of graduated-compression stockings, devices that provide intermittent pneumatic compression, and early ambulation are necessary to prevent thrombosis and embolism; sudden and extreme movements should be avoided. Under no circumstances should the legs be massaged to relieve muscle cramps, especially when the pain is located in the calf and the person has not been up and about.

Restrictive clothing, crossing the legs, and prolonged sitting or standing should be avoided. Elevating the legs, bending the bed at the knees, or propping pillows under the knees can produce venous stasis and should be done with caution to avoid severe flexion of the hips, which will slow blood flow and increase the risk of new thrombi.

After a PE or in the case of total hip replacement, treatment with anticoagulation continues for those at high risk of recurrence. Anyone taking anticoagulants should be monitored carefully for signs of bleeding, such as bloody stool, blood in urine, vaginal bleeding, bloody gums or nose, or large ecchymoses. If the person mentions any of these symptoms to the therapist, the client should be instructed to contact the physician immediately. Medications should not be changed without the physician's approval; the use of additional medications, especially over-the-counter preparations for colds, headaches, rheumatic pain, and so on, must be approved by the physician. See also Special Implications for the Therapist: Peripheral Vascular Disease, 11-24. ■

◆ Pulmonary Hypertension

Definition and Incidence.   Pulmonary hypertension is high blood pressure in the pulmonary arteries defined as a rise in pulmonary artery pressure of 5 to 10 mm Hg above normal (normal is 15 to 18 mm Hg).* Pulmonary hypertension may be *primary* or *secondary*; primary includes elevated pulmonary vascular resistance in the absence of other disease of the heart or lungs.

Primary pulmonary hypertension (PPH) is rare, that is, 1 or 2 cases per 1 million in the United States except in individuals using appetite suppressants, in which case the incidence may be as high as 25 to 50 cases per 1 million per year.[2] PPH occurs most commonly in young and middle-aged women (pregnant women have the highest mortality). It may have no known cause (idiopathic) although familial disease (the gene for familial PPH has been discovered) accounts for approximately 10% of cases. Secondary hypertension occurs as a complication of another disease, usually a respiratory (e.g., COPD) or cardiovascular disorder (especially left-sided heart failure in the older adult).

Pathogenesis.   PPH is characterized by diffuse narrowing of the pulmonary arterioles caused by hypertrophy of smooth muscle in the vessel walls and formation of fibrous lesions around the vessels. The underlying cause of these changes is unknown, but looking beyond simple pulmonary vasoconstriction, it is now recognized that defects in endothelial function, pulmonary vascular smooth muscle cells, and circulating blood factors may all be involved in the pathogenesis and pro-

---

*There is no definitive set of values used to diagnose pulmonary hypertension, but the National Institutes for Health (NIH) require a resting mean artery pressure of more than 25 mm Hg at rest and 30 mm Hg during exercise.

gression of PPH. Endothelial-cell injury may result in an imbalance in endothelium-derived mediators (too many "bad" mediators). Impaired endothelium release may account for reduced production of nitrous oxide (NO), a vasodilator, from the airways resulting in vasoconstriction. Defects in ion-channel activity in smooth muscle cells in the pulmonary artery also may contribute to vasoconstriction and vascular proliferation.[19] These changes force the heart to work harder and weaken the muscles in the pulmonary artery (and its branches) until elevated blood pressure in the lungs leads to right-sided heart failure (cor pulmonale).

Secondary pulmonary hypertension is caused by any respiratory or cardiovascular disorder that increases the volume or pressure of blood entering the pulmonary arteries or narrows or obstructs the pulmonary arteries. Increased volume or pressure overloads the pulmonary circulation whereas narrowing or obstruction elevates the blood pressure by increasing resistance to flow within the lungs.

If hypertension persists, hypertrophy occurs in the medial smooth muscle layer of the arterioles. The larger arteries stiffen, and hypertension progresses until pulmonary artery pressure equals systemic blood pressure. The result is right ventricular hypertrophy and eventual cor pulmonale.

Clinical Manifestations. Signs and symptoms of secondary pulmonary hypertension are difficult to recognize in the early stages when the symptoms of the underlying disease are more prominent. When pulmonary artery pressure is equal to systemic blood pressure, pulmonary hypertension may be detected. The most common symptoms of primary or secondary pulmonary hypertension are atypical cardiorespiratory symptoms, such as fatigue, chest discomfort or pain, tachypnea, syncope, cyanosis, and unexplained shortness of breath, beginning with exercise and later occurring with minimal activity or at rest.

Medical Management

Diagnosis. PPH can be difficult to diagnose, and there is usually a delay of 1 to 2 years between onset of symptoms and diagnosis. Sometimes the first indication of pulmonary hypertension is seen on a chest radiograph or ECG. The x-ray study may show rib scalloping (erosion of the inferior aspect of the ribs) from dilation of the arteries supplying the ribs. A reading of right ventricular hypertrophy (RVH) on the ECG report also indicates pulmonary hypertension.

The physician must differentiate PPH from chronic pulmonary heart disease (cor pulmonale), recurrent pulmonary emboli, mitral stenosis, and congenital heart disease. Exclusion of secondary causes is performed by echocardiography and lung scanning and sometimes by pulmonary angiogram. A chest film will show some characteristic changes, such as enlarged main pulmonary arteries with reduced peripheral branches, but is not diagnostic alone. Diagnosis of pulmonary hypertension can only be made with right-sided heart catheterization.

Treatment. Until recently, there had been only a limited number of therapies available to treat PPH. Over the years improved understanding of the molecular and cellular basis for this disease has allowed for the development of targeted approaches to treatment, bringing renewed optimism in the management of a disease previously considered untreatable.

Researchers are actively seeking ways to replace the "good" or inhibit the "bad" endothelial-derived mediators that contribute to the development of pulmonary vasculopathy. Continuous intravenous infusion of prostacyclin $PG1_2$ (esoprostenol [Flolan], a potent arteriole vasodilator) is used to dilate pulmonary arteries. This has been shown to improve exercise tolerance and pulmonary hemodynamics in both primary and secondary forms of pulmonary hypertension. It is the only treatment approved by the U.S. FDA at this time for PPH and pulmonary hypertension caused by scleroderma. Trials evaluating inhaled, subcutaneous, and oral delivery of prostacyclin are currently under way.[19] Other treatment approaches under investigation include gene therapy and focus on pathogenetic factors outside the pulmonary endothelium (e.g., potassium channel defect favoring vasoconstriction and cell proliferation, role of elastase, circulating blood factors contributing to blood thrombosis). Secondary pulmonary hypertension is also treated by treating the underlying cause.

Heart-lung transplantation is being used more often for PPH with improved results because of the availability of cyclosporin to prevent rejection. Candidates for heart-lung transplants are usually in the advanced stages of the disease with predicted survival at less than 1 year. Usually these individuals have failed to respond to vasodilator drugs.

Prognosis. The progression of PPH varies for each affected individual, but prognosis is poor without heart-lung transplantation. Some individuals may live 5 to 6 years from the time of diagnosis, but most people have a downhill course over a shorter period of time (2 to 3 years) with a fatal outcome. The cause of death is usually right ventricular failure or sudden death; sudden death occurs late in the disease process. Mortality in the United States has increased notably since 1979 although survival has improved in PPH with the advent of treatment with prostacyclin. Some portion of this reported increase may be related to improvements in diagnostic recognition, and some data suggest that the disease may be more common in the older population than has been previously recognized and reported.[142]

Secondary pulmonary hypertension can be reversed if the underlying disorder is successfully treated. If the hypertension has persisted long enough for the medial smooth muscle layer to hypertrophy, secondary pulmonary hypertension is no longer reversible.

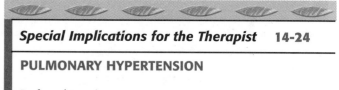

Special Implications for the Therapist **14-24**

PULMONARY HYPERTENSION

Preferred Practice Pattern:
6D: Impaired Aerobic Capacity/Endurance Associated With Cardiovascular Pump Dysfunction or Failure

Impairment of exercise performance is associated with pulmonary hypertension because pulmonary vascular resistance and pulmonary artery pressure increase dramatically with exercise. There may be impaired heart rate kinetics during exercise with corresponding impaired cardiac output response and slow recovery of the heart.[181] For these reasons, clients with pulmonary hypertension must be closely monitored when participating in activities or therapy that requires increased physical stress. See Appendix B, Guidelines for Activity and Exercise, and Table 39-20.

Maintenance of adequate systemic blood pressure is essential, and the therapist must be familiar with the medications used and potential side effects, especially if blood pressure is altered pharmacologically. Inhaled nitrous oxide, an endogenous vasodilator, increases oxygen consumption at the same workload during exercise, thereby improving exercise capacity. Ambulatory nitrous oxide inhalation therapy may be recommended in the future to improve exercise capacity for people with pulmonary hypertension.[101,217]

Secondary pulmonary hypertension may occur in clients with connective tissue diseases such as scleroderma because the disease affects the vasculature of several organs, including the lungs (pulmonary fibrosis) and kidneys. The arterioles usually demonstrate intimal proliferation with progressive luminal occlusion. The development of hypertension often indicates the onset of an accelerated scleroderma renal crisis. Medical treatment is toward control of the blood pressure. ■

◆ Cor Pulmonale

Definition and Incidence.   Cor pulmonale, also called pulmonary heart disease, is the enlargement of the right ventricle secondary to pulmonary hypertension that occurs in diseases of the thorax, lung, and pulmonary circulation. It is a term that describes the pathologic effects of lung dysfunction as it affects the right side of the heart. Right-sided heart dysfunction secondary to left-sided heart failure, vascular dysfunction, or congenital heart disease is excluded in the definition of cor pulmonale.

Chronic cor pulmonale occurs most frequently in adult male smokers, although the incidence in women is increasing as heavy smoking in females becomes more prevalent. The actual prevalence of cor pulmonale is difficult to determine because cor pulmonale does not occur in all cases of chronic lung disease and because routine physical examination and laboratory tests are relatively insensitive to the presence of pulmonary hypertension. It has been estimated that cor pulmonale accounts for 5% to 10% of organic heart disease.

Etiologic and Risk Factors.   Pulmonary vascular diseases and respiratory diseases (e.g., emphysema, chronic bronchitis) are the primary causes of cor pulmonale. Emphysema and chronic bronchitis cause over 50% of cases of cor pulmonale in the United States. When a PE has been sufficiently massive to obstruct 60% to 75% of the pulmonary circulation, acute cor pulmonale can occur, but cor pulmonale can also be caused by COPD.

Cor pulmonale can also develop under conditions of sustained elevations in intrathoracic pressure associated with mechanical ventilation (and PEEP). The intrathoracic vessels narrow, leading to reduced cardiac output and possible cor pulmonale. Chronic widespread vasculitis, such as occurs in association with the collagen vascular disorders (e.g., rheumatoid arthritis, systemic lupus erythematosus [SLE], dermatomyositis, polymyositis, Sjögren's syndrome, CREST syndrome accompanying scleroderma), can also cause chronic cor pul-

monale. Occasionally, widespread radiation pneumonitis can be the underlying cause of cor pulmonale.

Other (uncommon) causes include pneumoconiosis, pulmonary fibrosis, kyphoscoliosis, pickwickian syndrome, lymphangitic infiltration from metastatic carcinoma, and obliterative pulmonary capillary changes that cause vasoconstriction and later, hypertension. The feature common to all these conditions that predisposes to cor pulmonale is hypoxia.

Pathogenesis.   Sustained elevation in pulmonary arterial hypertension is thought to be mediated through two pathophysiologic vascular mechanisms: persistent vasoconstriction and vascular structural remodeling. The combination of these processes causes vascular luminal narrowing and vessel obliteration. These factors reduce pulmonary vascular surface area to the critical degree necessary for the development of pulmonary hypertension. As pulmonary hypertension creates long-term pressure overload in the right ventricle, cor pulmonale develops. Normally, the ventricle is a thin-walled (heart) muscle able to meet an increase in volume and pressure, but long-term pressure overload from hypertension causes the tissue to hypertrophy. In the case of acute cor pulmonale caused by emboli, loosely adherent, soft thrombus forms undetected in the veins of the legs or pelvis (phlebothrombosis or thrombophlebitis). The thrombus suddenly breaks loose and lodges at or near the bifurcation of the main pulmonary artery. Whether caused by ventricular hypertrophy or embolic obstruction, there is a marked fall in pressure necessary to drive blood through the compromised vascular bed since the right ventricle is compromised.

Clinical Manifestations.   Evidence of cor pulmonale may be obscured by primary respiratory disease and appear only during exercise testing. The heart appears normal at rest, but with exercise, cardiac output falls and the ECG shows right ventricular hypertrophy. The predominant symptoms are related to the pulmonary disorder and include chronic productive cough, exertional dyspnea, wheezing respirations, easy fatigability, and weakness.

Sudden severe, central chest pain can occur caused by acute dilation of the root of the pulmonary artery and secondary to right ventricular ischemia. The person may collapse, often with loss of consciousness, and death may occur within minutes if the thrombus is large and does not dislodge. If the thrombus is small or moves more peripherally in response to pounding on the chest or chest compression during resuscitation, acute cor pulmonale develops rather than sudden death.

Low cardiac output causes pallor, sweating, hypotension, anxiety, impaired consciousness, and a rapid pulse of small amplitude. The specific signs associated with cor pulmonale include exercise-induced peripheral cyanosis, clubbing (see Fig. 14-4), distended neck veins, and bilateral dependent edema.

Medical Management

Diagnosis.   Diagnosis is made on the basis of physical examination, radiologic studies, and ECG or echocardiogram, sometimes both. Pulmonary function tests usually confirm the underlying lung disease. Laboratory findings may include polycythemia present in cor pulmonale secondary to COPD. The diagnosis of acute cor pulmonale may be difficult to confirm in light of the emergency procedures required to manage the acute life-threatening situation. Physical examination may not reveal any specific diagnostic signs, and the ECG and chest film may not be diagnostic in the early stages of cor pulmonale.

Treatment.   The primary goal of medical treatment is to reduce the workload of the right ventricle. This is accomplished by lowering pulmonary artery pressure, as in the treatment of pulmonary hypertension. Oxygen administration, salt and fluid restriction, and diuretics are essential along with treatment of the underlying chronic pulmonary disease while at the same time relieving the hypoxemia, hypercapnia, or acidosis. Surgical removal of embolic material is a controversial procedure performed only when a confirmed diagnosis of massive PE with accessible thrombus in the main pulmonary artery or its branches is available. There is no specific surgical treatment available for most causes of chronic cor pulmonale. Heart-lung transplantation for clients with primary pulmonary hypertension is a proven therapy in the early stages of development.

Prognosis.   Since cor pulmonale generally occurs late during the course of COPD and other irreversible disease, the prognosis is poor. Once congestive signs appear, the average life expectancy is 2 to 5 years, but survival is significantly longer when uncomplicated emphysema is the cause. Although cor pulmonale can be caused by obstructive and restrictive lung diseases, restrictive lung diseases have a lower life expectancy once they reach the stage of cor pulmonale.

Special Implications for the Therapist   **14-25**

COR PULMONALE

Preferred Practice Patterns:
6B: Impaired Aerobic Capacity/Endurance Associated With Deconditioning
6D: Impaired Aerobic Capacity/Endurance Associated With Cardiovascular Pump Dysfunction or Failure
7A: Primary Prevention/Risk Reduction for Integumentary Disorders

Those people who are bedridden must be repositioned frequently to prevent atelectasis (and skin breakdown). Breathing exercises should be carried out frequently throughout the day. Diaphragmatic and pursed-lip breathing exercises should be reviewed for anyone with COPD. Teach the client (or family member) how to detect edema in the lower extremities, especially the ankles, by pressing the skin over the shins for 1 to 2 seconds, looking for a lasting finger impression. Watch for signs of digitalis toxicity (see Table 11-4), such as complaints of anorexia, nausea, vomiting, or yellow halos around visual images.

Since pulmonary infection exacerbates COPD and cor pulmonale, all health care workers must practice careful hand washing and follow Standard Precautions. Early signs of infection (e.g., increased sputum production, change in sputum color, chest pain or chest tightness, fever) must be reported to the physician immediately. Watch for signs of respiratory failure, such as change in pulse rate; deep, labored respirations; and increased fatigue produced by exertion. ■

◆ Collagen Vascular Disease

Collagen vascular diseases, now more commonly referred to as diffuse connective tissue diseases (see Box 11-11), are often associated with pulmonary manifestations, including exudative pleural effusion, pulmonary nodules, rheumatoid nodules in association with coal workers' pneumoconiosis (Caplan's syndrome), interstitial fibrosis, and pulmonary vasculitis.

All these pulmonary conditions have been associated with rheumatoid arthritis; all except the nodules and pleural effusion have been seen with SL; and pleuritis and pneumonitis have been observed in Sjögren's syndrome, polymyositis, and dermatomyositis. Pulmonary fibrosis or pulmonary hypertension or both are commonly part of the clinical picture associated with scleroderma. Polymyalgia rheumatica and temporal arteritis may demonstrate granulomatous inflammation of the pulmonary parenchyma.

Approximately one-half of clients with SLE develop lung disease, primarily pleuritis, pleural effusion, or acute pneumonitis. Pulmonary involvement may not be evident clinically, but pulmonary function tests reveal abnormalities in many persons with SLE. Lupus pneumonitis causes recurrent episodes of fever, dyspnea, and cough. Interstitial pneumonitis leading to fibrosis occurs in a small proportion of people with SLE; the inflammatory phase may respond to treatment, whereas the fibrosis does not. Occasionally, pulmonary hypertension develops. Rarely are ARDS and massive intraalveolar hemorrhage fatal pulmonary complications.

Interstitial lung disease can develop before joint involvement becomes evident in rheumatoid arthritis, particularly in men. People with rheumatoid arthritis who are receiving treatment with methotrexate or gold may develop interstitial lung disease that represents a drug hypersensitivity. Penicillamine therapy in clients with rheumatoid arthritis has been implicated in causing bronchiolitis obliterans.

Bilateral upper lobe fibrosis may develop late in ankylosing spondylitis. Lung involvement varies in systemic sclerosis, but there is radiographic evidence of pulmonary disease in a majority of clients. Cutaneous scleroderma can involve the anterior chest wall and abdomen, causing restrictive lung function. General dryness and lack of airway secretions cause the major problems of hoarseness, cough, and bronchitis in Sjögren's syndrome, and interstitial lung disease is possible. Only 5% to 10% of clients with polymyositis and dermatomyositis develop interstitial lung disease, but weakness of respiratory muscles contributing to aspiration pneumonitis is common.

DISORDERS OF THE PLEURAL SPACE

◆ Pneumothorax

Definition.   Pneumothorax is an accumulation of air or gas in the pleural cavity caused by a defect in the visceral pleura or chest wall. The result is collapse of the lung on the affected side. There are several types of pneumothorax, including spontaneous, tension, open, traumatic, and iatrogenic (Fig. 14-19).

Incidence and Risk Factors.   Pneumothorax is common, especially with trauma or after medical procedures

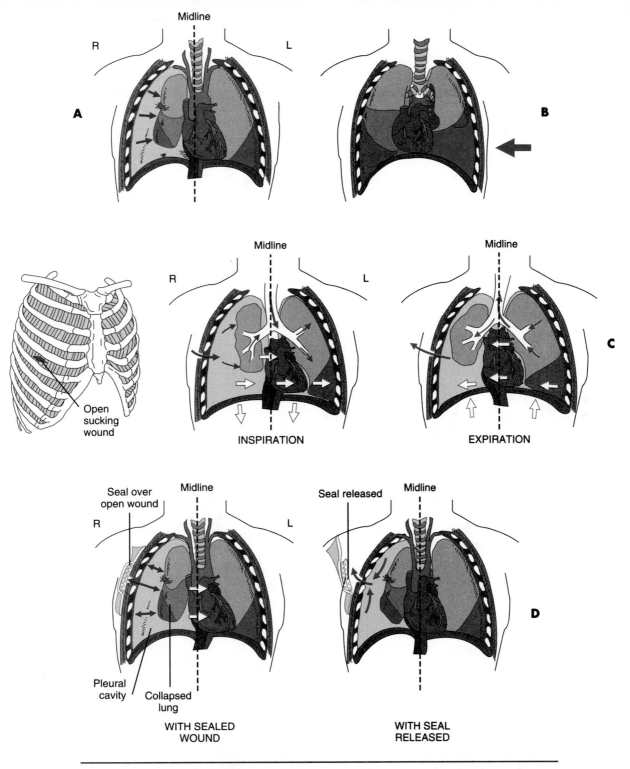

FIGURE 14-19 **A,** Pneumothorax. Lung collapses as air gathers in the pleural space between the parietal and visceral pleurae. **B,** Massive hemothorax, blood in the pleural space (*arrow*) below the left lung, causing collapse of lung tissue. **C,** Open pneumothorax (sucking chest wound). *Solid arrows,* Air movement; *open arrows,* structural movement. A chest wall wound connects the pleural space with atmospheric air. During inspiration, atmospheric air is sucked into the pleural space through the chest wall wound. Positive pressure in the pleural space collapses the lung on the affected side and pushes the mediastinal contents toward the unaffected side. This reduces the volume of air in the unaffected side considerably. During expiration, air escapes through the chest wall wound, lessening positive pressure in the affected side and allowing the mediastinal contents to swing back toward the affected side. Movement of mediastinal structure from side to side is called mediastinal flutter. **D,** Tension pneumothorax. If an open pneumothorax is covered (e.g., with a dressing), it forms a seal, and tension pneumothorax with a mediastinal shift develops. A tear in lung structure continues to allow air into the pleural space. As positive pressure builds in the pleural space, the affected lung collapses, and the mediastinal contents shift to the unaffected side. Tension pneumothorax is corrected by removing the seal (i.e., dressing), allowing air trapped in the pleural space to escape.

(e.g., mechanical ventilation, central line insertion) or surgical procedures in the thorax, head, neck, and abdomen that puncture the chest wall or occasionally after dental procedures involving pressurized air forced into the surrounding connective tissue in a person at risk. Following chest trauma, both air and blood are likely to escape into the pleural space. This is called *hemopneumothorax.* Pneumothorax can develop at any age; spontaneous pneumothorax is especially common in tall, slender boys and men between the ages of 10 and 30 years (rarely in men over 40 years). Smoking appears to increase the risk of primary spontaneous pneumothorax in men by as much as a factor of 20 in a dose-dependent manner (i.e., chances increase as number of cigarettes smoked increases). Pneumothorax can occur with a variety of primary or metastasized lung tumors, but this is an uncommon cause. A single case of CPR training causing a minimally symptomatic pneumothorax has been reported.[204]

Pathogenesis.   When air enters the pleural cavity the lung collapses and a separation between the visceral and parietal pleurae (see Fig. 14-3) occurs destroying the negative pressure of the pleural space. This disruption in the normal equilibrium between the forces of elastic recoil and the chest wall causes the lung to recoil by collapsing toward the hilum. The result is shortness of breath and mediastinal shift toward the unaffected side compressing the opposite lung. The causative pleural defect may be in the visceral pleura (lung lining) or the parietal pleura (chest wall lining). The pleural space fills with air, and the lung becomes atelectatic with collapsed alveolar air spaces.

Spontaneous pneumothorax occurs when there is an opening on the surface of the lung allowing leakage of air from the airways or lung parenchyma into the pleural cavity. Most often this happens when an emphysematous bleb (blisterlike formation) or bulla (larger vesicle) or other weakened area on the lung ruptures. The majority of people with spontaneous pneumothorax have subpleural bullae that are most likely induced by the degradation of elastic fibers in the lung caused by the smoking-related influx of neutrophils and macrophages. Spontaneous pneumothorax can occur during sleep, at rest, or during exercise and can progress to become a tension pneumothorax.

Tension pneumothorax is a dangerous form of pneumothorax that occurs when air in the pleural space cannot escape through the rupture and cannot regain entry into the bronchus. In tension pneumothorax, the site of pleural rupture acts as a one-way valve, permitting air to enter on inspiration but preventing its escape by closing up during expiration. Under these conditions, continuously increasing air pressure in the pleural cavity may cause progressive collapse of the lung tissue. Air pressure in the pleural space pushes against the already recoiled lung, causing compression atelectasis, and against the mediastinum, compressing and displacing the heart and great vessels. Venous return and cardiac output decrease.

Open pneumothorax occurs when air pressure in the pleural space equals barometric pressure because air that is drawn into the pleural space during inspiration (through the damaged chest wall and parietal pleura or through the parietal pleura and damaged visceral pleura) is forced back out during expiration.

Traumatic pneumothorax is a secondary pneumothorax with the entry of air directly through the chest wall or by laceration of the lung caused by penetrating or nonpenetrating chest trauma, such as a rib fracture, stab, or bullet wound that tears the pleura. Bleb or bulla rupture associated with COPD can also introduce air into the pleural space. Other causes of this type of pneumothorax include TB, sarcoidosis, lung abscess, ARDS, and PCP. The pathogenesis is similar to spontaneous pneumothorax.

Iatrogenic pneumothorax develops as a result of direct puncture or laceration of the visceral pleura during attempts at central line placement, percutaneous lung aspiration, thoracentesis, or closed pleural biopsy. Direct alveolar distention can occur with anesthesia, CPR, or mechanical ventilation with PEEP.

Clinical Manifestations.   Dyspnea is the first and primary symptom of pneumothorax, but other symptoms may include a sudden sharp pleural chest pain, fall in blood pressure, weak and rapid pulse, and cessation of normal respiratory movements on the affected side of the chest. If the pneumothorax is large or if there is a tension pneumothorax, it may push the mediastinum toward the unaffected lung, causing the chest to appear asymmetric. The pain may be referred to the ipsilateral shoulder (corresponding shoulder on the same side as the pneumothorax), across the chest, or over the abdomen.

Clinical manifestations of tension pneumothorax include severe hypoxemia, dyspnea, and hypotension (low blood pressure) in addition to the other signs and symptoms of pneumothorax already mentioned. Increased intrathoracic pressure from a tension pneumothorax may result in neck vein distention. Untreated tension pneumothorax may quickly produce life-threatening shock and bradycardia.

Medical Management
Diagnosis and Treatment.   Diagnosis is made by chest film. There are no specific laboratory tests, but blood gas measurements indicate the degree of respiratory impairment. Depending on the size of the pneumothorax, no specific treatment is required for spontaneous pneumothorax beyond bed rest and the administration of oxygen to relieve dyspnea. Repair or closure of the pleural defect with evacuation of air from the pleural space is rarely necessary, but emergency aspiration of air via intercostal chest tube may be required in tension pneumothorax when progressive collapse of the lung tissue occurs. Surgery is occasionally required to control bleeding, remove large volumes of blood clots, and treat coexisting complications of trauma.

It is not a good idea to travel by airplane or to have pulmonary function tests performed (e.g., cystic fibrosis) for at least 2 weeks after a pneumothorax has healed. Encouraging smoking cessation is essential.

Prognosis.   There is a low mortality rate with idiopathic pneumothorax, but a corresponding 15% mortality rate for pneumothorax associated with underlying lung disease. From 30% to 50% of affected persons experience a recurrence, and after one recurrence, subsequent episodes are much more likely. The physiologic events associated with tension pneumothorax are life-threatening, requiring immediate treatment.

Special Implications for the Therapist 14-26

PNEUMOTHORAX

Preferred Practice Pattern:
6F: Impaired Ventilation and Respiration/Gas Exchange
Associated With Respiratory Failure

In the case of trauma (e.g., motor vehicle accident, assault, traumatic falls) the presence of undiagnosed nondisplaced rib fractures or rib fragments must be considered when getting a person up for the first time. The client's movements and the action of parasternal intercostal muscles can displace the rib causing puncture of the lung or penetrating aortic injury. When getting someone up for the first time, monitor vital signs, especially blood pressure and pulse, and request emergency medical help immediately anytime someone with this type of history demonstrates sudden shoulder or chest pain, altered breathing pattern, or drop of blood pressure accompanied by weak and fast pulse, pallor, dyspnea, or extreme anxiety. See also Special Implications for the Therapist: Chest Wall Disease or Injury, 14-14. ■

◆ Pleurisy

Definition and Etiologic Factors.   Pleurisy (pleuritis) is an inflammation of the pleura caused by infection, injury (e.g., rib fracture), or tumor. It may be a complication of lung disease, particularly of pneumonia, but also of TB, lung abscesses, influenza, SLE, rheumatoid arthritis, or pulmonary infarction.

Clinical Manifestations.   The symptoms develop suddenly, usually with a sharp, sticking chest pain that is worse on inspiration, coughing, sneezing, or movement associated with deep inspiration. Other symptoms may include cough, fever, chills, and rapid shallow breathing (tachypnea). The visceral pleura is insensitive; pain results from inflammation of the parietal pleura. Because the latter is innervated by the intercostal nerves, chest pain is usually felt over the site of the pleuritis, but pain may be referred to the lower chest wall, abdomen, neck, upper trapezius muscle, and shoulder. On auscultation, a pleural rub can be heard (sound caused by the rubbing together of the visceral and costal pleurae).

Pathogenesis.   There are two types of pleurisy: wet and dry. The membranous pleura that encases each lung is composed of two close-fitting layers; between these layers is a lubricating fluid. If the fluid content remains unchanged by the disease, the pleurisy is said to be dry. If the fluid increases abnormally, it is a wet pleurisy, or pleurisy with effusion (Fig. 14-20). Inflammation of the part of the pleura that covers the diaphragm is called *diaphragmatic pleurisy* and occurs secondary to pneumonia. When the central portion of the diaphragmatic pleura is irritated, sharp pain may be referred to the neck, upper trapezius, or shoulder. Stimulation of the peripheral portions of the diaphragmatic pleura results in sharp pain felt along the costal margins, which can be referred to the lumbar region by the lower thoracic somatic nerves (Fig. 14-21).

Wet pleurisy is less likely to cause pain because there usually is no chafing. The fluid may interfere with breathing by compressing the lung. If the excess fluid of wet pleurisy becomes infected with formation of pus, the condition is known as *purulent pleurisy* or *empyema*. Pleurisy causes pleurae to become reddened and covered with an exudate of lymph, fibrin, and cellular elements and may lead to pleural effusion.

In *dry pleurisy*, the two layers of membrane may become congested and swollen and rub against each other, which is painful. Although only the outer layer causes pain (the inner layer has no pain nerves), the pain may be severe enough to require the use of a strong analgesic.

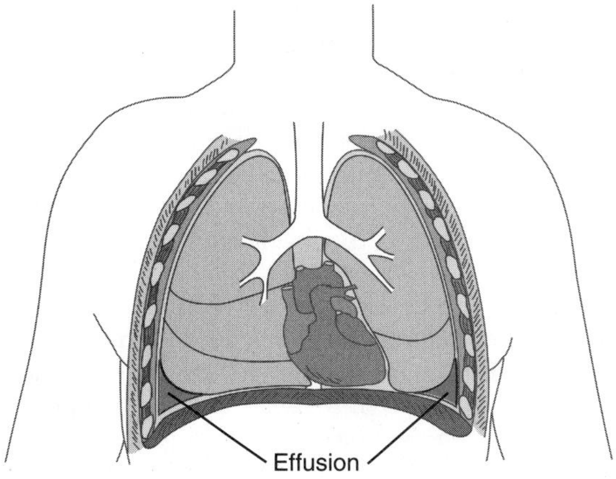

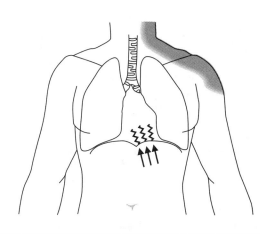

FIGURE **14-20** *Pleural effusion,* a collection of fluid in the pleural space between the membrane encasing the lung and the membrane lining the thoracic cavity, as seen on upright x-ray examination. *Pleurisy* (pleuritis) is an inflammation of the visceral and parietal pleurae. When there is an abnormal increase in the lubricating fluid between these two layers, it is called pleurisy with effusion.

FIGURE **14-21** Diaphragmatic pleurisy. Irritation of the peritoneal (outside) or pleural (inside) surface of the central area of the diaphragm refers sharp pain to the neck, supraclavicular fossa, and upper trapezius muscle. The pain pattern is ipsilateral to the area of irritation. Irritation to the peripheral portion of the diaphragm refers sharp pain to the costal margins and lumbar region (not shown).

Medical Management. Treatment is usually with aspirin and time or, if the pleurisy is severe and unresponsive, NSAIDs. Antibiotics may be prescribed for a specific infection. Sclerosing therapy for chronic or recurrent pleurisy may be recommended.

Special Implications for the Therapist **14-27**

PLEURISY

Preferred Practice Patterns:
6C: *Impaired Ventilation, Respiration/Gas Exchange, and Aerobic Capacity/Endurance Associated With Airway Clearance Dysfunction*
6F: *Impaired Ventilation and Respiration/Gas Exchange Associated With Respiratory Failure*

Bed rest is an important part of the care plan for the client with pleurisy. Therapy in the acute care setting should be coordinated to provide as much uninterrupted rest as possible. Breathing and coughing exercises are important but often avoided because of the pain these respiratory movements cause. To minimize discomfort, apply firm pressure with hands or a pillow to the site of the pain during deep breathing and coughing. ■

◆ **Pleural Effusion**

Definition. Pleural effusion is the collection of fluid in the pleural space (between the membrane encasing the lung and the membrane lining the thoracic cavity) where there is normally only a small amount of fluid to prevent friction as the lung expands and deflates (see Fig. 14-20). Pleural fluid normally seeps continually into the pleural space from the capillaries lining the parietal pleura and is then reabsorbed by the visceral pleural capillaries and lymphatics.

Incidence and Etiologic Factors. The causes of pleural effusions are best considered in terms of the underlying pathophysiology: *transudates* caused by abnormalities of hydrostatic or osmotic pressure (e.g., congestive heart failure, cirrhosis with ascites, nephrotic syndrome, peritoneal dialysis) and *exudates** resulting from increased permeability or trauma (e.g., infection, primary or secondary malignancy, PE, trauma including surgical trauma [e.g., cardiotomy]). Any condition that interferes with either the secretion or drainage of this fluid will lead to pleural effusion. Pleural effusion is common with heart failure and lymphatic obstruction caused by neoplasm.

Less common causes include drug-induced effusion, pancreatitis, collagen vascular diseases (SLE, rheumatoid arthri-

*An exudate is a fluid with a high content of protein and cellular debris that has escaped from blood vessels and has been deposited in tissues or on tissue surfaces, usually as a result of inflammation. A transudate is a fluid substance that has passed through a membrane or has been forced out from a tissue; in contrast to an exudate, a transudate is characterized by high fluidity and a low content of protein, cells, or solid matter derived from cells. (See discussion in Chapter 5 and Figs. 5-8 and 5-9.)

tis), intraabdominal abscess, or esophageal perforation. A person of any age can be affected, but it is more common in the older adult owing to the increased incidence of heart failure and cancer.

Pathogenesis. The most common mechanism of pleural effusion is migration of fluids and other blood components through the walls of intact capillaries bordering the pleura. When stimulated by biochemical mediators of inflammation, junctions in the capillary endothelium separate slightly, enabling leukocytes and plasma proteins to migrate out into affected tissues. Rupture of a blood vessel or leakage of blood from an injured vessel causes a form of pleural effusion called hemothorax (see Fig. 14-20).

Malignancy effusion is usually a local effect of the tumor, such as lymphatic obstruction or bronchial obstruction with pneumonia or atelectasis. Lymphatic blockage from any cause can result in drainage of the contents of lymphatic vessels into the pleural space. It can also be a result of systemic effects of tumor elsewhere, but in either case malignant cells in the pleural effusion of a person with lung cancer indicate an inoperable situation.

Clinical Manifestations. Clinical manifestations of pleural effusion will depend on the amount of fluid present and the degree of lung compression. A small amount of effusion may be discovered only by chest x-ray examination. Large effusions cause clinical manifestations related to their volume and the rate at which they accumulate in the pleural space causing restriction of lung expansion. Clients usually present with dyspnea on exertion that becomes progressive. They may develop nonspecific chest discomfort; sometimes the chest pain is pleuritic, a sharp, stabbing pain exacerbated by coughing or breathing and changes in position. Other symptoms characteristic of the underlying cause of pleural effusion may be the primary clinical picture (e.g., weight loss and fever with TB or cancer, signs of heart failure).

Medical Management

Diagnosis. Examination of the pleural fluid via transthoracic aspiration biopsy (surgical puncture and drainage of the thoracic cavity) includes analysis of pH; specific gravity; protein; stains and cultures for bacteria, TB, and fungi; eosinophilia count; and glucose concentration to aid in the differential diagnosis. Chest pain must be differentiated from pain of pericardial or musculoskeletal origin. Chest radiographs and physical examination with possible CT scan are necessary components of the diagnostic process.

Treatment. Treatment may not be required when the individual is asymptomatic, or if the client is only mildly symptomatic, transthoracic aspiration may be all that is necessary. In the case of an underlying disease process (e.g., congestive heart failure or renal pathologic findings associated with transudates), treatment is aimed toward that condition. Drainage of the fluid for exudate-caused effusion provides symptomatic improvement but does not significantly alter lung volumes or gas exchange. Removal of fluid associated with malignancy is considered only if the individual is symptomatic and could benefit from aspiration. Repeated aspiration is avoided since significant protein loss can occur and the fluid reaccumulates in 1 to 3 days.

Some (exudate) pleural effusions resolve with antibiotic therapy. Recurrent (exudate) pleural effusions may be treated by pleurectomy (surgically stripping the parietal pleura away from the visceral pleura) and pleurodesis (sclerosing substance introduced into the pleural space to create an inflammatory response that scleroses tissues together). Both these procedures have negative effects that must be taken into consideration.

Prognosis.   Prognosis depends on the underlying disease; in cancer, recurrent pleural effusion may be associated with the terminal stage of disease. Tumor-related effusion generally implies a poor prognosis.

Special Implications for the Therapist   14-28

PLEURAL EFFUSION

Preferred Practice Pattern:
6F: Impaired Ventilation and Respiration/Gas Exchange Associated With Respiratory Failure

After transthoracic aspiration, encourage deep-breathing exercises to promote lung expansion and watch for respiratory distress or pneumothorax (sudden onset of dyspnea, cyanosis). In the presence of a chest tube prevent kinking by carefully coiling the tubing on top of the bed and securing it to the bed linen, leaving room for the client to turn. Position changes must be performed carefully to avoid disturbing the surgical site or the chest tube. The therapist may apply firm support with both hands to the surgical site and chest tube area to help lessen muscle pull and pain as the client coughs. If the person has open drainage through a rib resection or intercostal tube, use hand and dressing precautions.

Small pleural effusions (<500 ml) frequently have minimal findings on physical exam. Effusions with 500 to 1500 ml demonstrate dullness to percussion, diminished breath sounds, and reduced tactile and vocal fremitus over the involved hemithorax. Effusions greater than 1500 ml will present with concomitant atelectasis, demonstrate bronchial or tracheal breath sounds, and sound like the bleating of a goat on auscultation (referred to as egophony) with inspiratory lag on the affected side. ∎

◆ Pleural Empyema

Pleural empyema (infected pleural effusion) is an accumulation of pus that occurs occasionally as a complication of pleurisy or some other respiratory disease, usually pneumonia. It is a normal response to infection but may also occur following external contamination (penetrating trauma, chest tube placement, or other surgical procedure) or esophageal perforation.

Symptoms include dyspnea, coughing, ipsilateral pleural chest or shoulder pain, malaise, tachycardia, cough, and fever. In addition to chest films, transthoracic aspiration biopsy may be done to confirm the diagnosis and determine the specific causative organism. The condition is treated with intercostal chest tube drainage, antibiotics, rest, and sedative cough mixtures. See Special Implications for the Therapist: Pleural Effusion, 14-28.

REFERENCES

1. Abbott J, Conway S, Etherington C, et al: Perceived body image and eating behavior in young adults with cystic fibrosis and their healthy peers, *J Behav Med* 23(6):501-507, 2000.
2. Abenhaim L, Moride Y, Brenot F, et al: Appetite-suppressant drugs and the risk of primary pulmonary hypertension: International Primary Pulmonary Hypertension Study Group, *N Engl J Med* 335:609-615, 1996.
3. Aberle DR, Gamsu G, Henschke CI, et al: A consensus statement of the Society of Thoracic Radiology: screening for lung cancer with helical computed tomography, *J Thorac Imaging* 16(1):65-68, 2001.
4. Albaugh G, Kann B, Puc MM, et al: Age-adjusted outcomes in traumatic flail chest injuries in the elderly, *Am Surg* 66(10):978-981, 2000.
5. Aligne AC, Auinger P, Byrd RS, et al: Risk factors for pediatric asthma: contributions of poverty, race, and urban residence, *Am J Respir Crit Care Med* 162(3, pt 1):873-877, 2000.
6. Almand B, Carbone DP: Biological considerations in lung cancer, *Cancer Treat Res* 105:1-30, 2001.
7. Almirall J, Gonsalez CA, Balanzo X, et al: Proportion of community acquired pneumonia cases attributable to tobacco smoking, *Chest* 116(2):375-379, 1999.
8. American Academy of Allergy, Asthma and Immunology (AAAI): *Guidelines for the diagnosis and management of asthma*. National Asthma Education and Prevention Program: Clinical Practice Guidelines, Expert Panel Report 2. Publication no. 97-4051, Bethesda, Md, 1997, National Institutes for Health (NIH). On-line, 1999: www.aaaai.org
9. American College of Sports Medicine (ACSM): *ACSM's resource manual for guidelines for exercise testing and prescription*, ed 3, Philadelphia, 1998, Lippincott Williams & Wilkins.
10. American Institute for Cancer Research (AICR): *Food, nutrition, and the prevention of cancer: a global perspective*, Washington, DC, 1997.
11. American Lung Association (ALA): American Lung Association fact sheet: asthma in adults (on-line), Jan 2001: www.lungusa.org/asthma
12. American Thoracic Society (ATS) and Centers for Disease Control and Prevention (CDC): Targeted tuberculin testing and treatment of latent tuberculosis infection, *Am J Respir Crit Care Med* 161:1376-1395, 2000.
13. Andersen P, Munk ME, Pollock JM, et al: Specific immune-based diagnosis of tuberculosis, *Lancet* 356(9235):1048-1049, 2000.
14. Aris RM, Renner JB, Winders AD, et al: Increased rate of fractures and severe kyphosis: sequelae of living into adulthood with cystic fibrosis, *Ann Intern Med* 128(3):186-193, 1998.
15. Ashley EA, Johnson MA, Lipman MC: Human immunodeficiency virus and respiratory infection, *Curr Opin Pulm Med* 6(3):240-245, 2000.
16. Askling J, Grunewalk J, Eklund A, et al: Increased risk for cancer following sarcoidosis, *Am J Respir Crit Care Med* 160(5, pt 1):1668-1672, 1999.
17. Austin JHM, Stellman SD, Pearson GDN: Screening for lung cancer, *N Engl J Med* 344(12):935-936, 2001.
18. Bach PB, Cramer LD, Warren JL, et al: Racial differences in the treatment of early-stage lung cancer, *N Engl J Med* 341(16):1198-1205, 1999.
19. Bailey CL, Channick RN, Rubin LJ: A new era in the treatment of primary pulmonary hypertension, *Heart* 85(3):251-252, 2001.
20. Bal DG: Commentary on "European Consensus Statement on Lung Cancer," *CA Cancer J Clin* 48(3):165-166, 1998.
21. Ballard RD: Sleep, respiratory physiology, and nocturnal asthma, *Chronobiol Int* 16(5):565-580, 1999.
22. Ballone A, Lascioli R, Raschi S, et al: Chest physical therapy in patients with acute exacerbation of chronic bronchitis: effectiveness of three methods, *Arch Phys Med Rehabil* 81:558-560, 2000.
23. Banks DE, Tarlo SM: Important issues in occupational asthma, *Curr Opin Pulm Med* 6(1):37-42, 2000.
24. Barnard J, Newman LS: Sarcoidosis: immunology, rheumatic involvement, and therapeutics, *Curr Opin Rheumatol* 13(1):84-91, 2001.
25. Becker L, Glazier R, McIsaac W, et al: Antibiotics for acute bronchitis, *Cochrane Database Syst Rev* 79(2):CD000245, 2000.
26. Beckett WS: Occupational respiratory diseases, *N Engl J Med* 342(6):406-413, 2000.
27. Bennett LS: Adult obstructive sleep apnoea syndrome, *J Royal Coll Phys Lond* 33(5):439-444, 1999.
28. Billings CG, Howard P: Asbestos exposure, lung cancer and asbestosis, *Monaldi Arch Chest Dis* 55(2):151-156, 2000.

29. Boas SR, Danduran MJ, McColley SA, et al: Immune modulation following aerobic exercise in children with cystic fibrosis, *Int J Sports Med* 21(4):294-301, 2000.

30. Boffetta P, Pershagen G, Jockel KH, et al: Cigar and pipe smoking and lung cancer risk: a multicenter study from Europe, *J Natl Cancer Inst* 91(8):697-701, 1999.

31. Bonala SB, Reddy BM, Silverman BA, et al: Bone mineral density in women with asthma on long-term inhaled corticosteroid therapy, *Ann Allergy Asthma Immunol* 85(6, pt 1):495-500, 2000.

32. Bourgeois MC, Zadai CC: Impaired ventilation and respiration in the older adult. In Guccione AA, editor: *Geriatric physical therapy*, ed 2, St Louis, 2000, Mosby, pp 226-244.

33. Bourjeily G, Rochester CL: Exercise training in chronic obstructive pulmonary disease, *Clin Chest Med* 21(4):763-781, 2000.

34. Bressler TR: Small cell lung cancer. In Miaskowski C, Buchsel P: *Oncology nursing: assessment and clinical care*, St Louis, 1999, Mosby, pp 1301-1329.

35. Brouwers FM, Lenders JW: Sleep disordered breathing and hypertension, *N Engl J Med* 343(13):967, 2000.

36. Bunn PA, Kelly K: New combinations in the treatment of lung cancer: a time for optimism, *Chest* 117(4, suppl 1):138S-143S, 2000.

37. Bunn PA, Soriano A, Johnson G, et al: New therapeutic strategies for lung cancer: biology and molecular biology come of age, *Chest* 117 (4, suppl 1):163S-168S, 2000.

38. Cade A, Walters MP, McGinley N, et al: Evaluation of fecal pancreatic elastase-1 as a measure of pancreatic exocrine function in children with cystic fibrosis, *Pediatr Pulmonol* 29(3):167-168, 2000.

39. Cahalin LP, Sadowsky HS: Pulmonary medications, *Phys Ther* 75: 397-414, 1995.

40. Camargo CA, Weiss ST, Zhang S, et al: Prospective study of body mass index, weight change, and risk of adult-onset asthma in women, *Arch Intern Med* 159(21):2582-2588, 1999.

41. Camp PG, Appleton J, Reid WD: Quality of life after pulmonary rehabilitation: assessing change using quantitative and qualitative methods, *Phys Ther* 80(10):986-995, 2000.

42. Carriot F, Sasco AJ: Cannabis and cancer, *Rev Epidemiol Sante Publique* 48(5):473-483, 2000.

43. Casaburi R: Skeletal muscle function in COPD, *Chest* 117(5, suppl 1):267S-271S, 2000.

44. Casaburi R: Special considerations for exercise training in chronic lung disease. In *American College of Sports Medicine (ACSM) resource manual for guidelines for exercise testing and prescription*, ed 3, Philadelphia, 1998, Lippincott Williams & Wilkins, pp 334-339.

45. Case AM, Reid RL: Menstrual cycle effects on common medical conditions, *Compr Ther* 27(1):65-71, 2001.

46. Cassart M, Estenne M: The respiratory muscles in emphysema: the effects of thoracic distension, *Rev Mal Respir* 17(2):449-457, 2000.

47. Castranova V, Vallyathan V: Silicosis and coal workers' pneumoconiosis, *Environ Health Perspect* 108(suppl 4, no. 2):675-684, 2000.

48. Centers for Disease Control and Prevention (CDC): Drowning prevention (on-line), 2001: www.cdc.gov/ncipc/factsheets/drown.htm

49. Chaisson RE: New developments in the treatment of latent tuberculosis, *Int J Tuberc Lung Dis* 4 (12, suppl 2):S176-S181, 2000.

50. Chu HW, Kraft M, Krause JE, et al: Substance P and its receptor neurokinin 1 expression in asthmatic airways, *J Allergy Clin Immunol* 106(4):713-722, 2000.

51. Ciesla N: Chest physical therapy for patients in the intensive care unit, *Phys Ther* 76(6):609-625, 1996.

52. Clark CJ, Cochrane LM, Mackay E, et al: Skeletal muscle strength and endurance in patients with mild COPD and the effects of weight training, *Eur Respir J* 15(1):92-97, 2000.

53. Cohen AJ: Outdoor air pollution and lung cancer, *Environ Health Perspect* 108(suppl 4):743-750, 2000.

54. Collins CH, Grange JM: Tuberculosis acquired in laboratories and necropsy rooms, *Commun Dis Public Health* 2:161-167, 1999.

55. Cosio MG, Cosio Piqueras MG: Pathology of emphysema in chronic obstructive pulmonary disease, *Monaldi Arch Chest Dis* 55(2):124-129, 2000

56. Cystic Fibrosis Foundation (CFF): *Clinical practice guidelines for cystic fibrosis*, Bethesda, Md, 1997 (available for $100.00).

57. Cystic Fibrosis Foundation (CFF): *An introduction to chest physical therapy*, Bethesda, Md, 1997 (free publication).

58. Dean E: Oxygen transport deficits in systemic diseases and implications for physical therapy, *Phys Ther* 77(2):187-202, 1997.

59. deJong W, van Aalderen WM, Kraan J, et al: Inspiratory muscle training in patients with cystic fibrosis, *Respir Med* 95(1):31-36, 2001.

60. Dirkes SM, Dickinson SP: Common questions about prone positioning for ARDS, *Am J Nurs* 98(6):16JJ-16PP, 1998.

61. Doherty TM, Andersen P: Tuberculosis vaccines: developmental work and the future, *Curr Opin Pulm Med* 6(3):203-208, 2000.

62. Dreher D, Kok M, Pechere JC, et al: New strategies against an old plague: genetically engineered tuberculosis vaccines, *Schweiz Med Wochenschr* 130(50):1995-1999, 2000.

63. Drumm ML, Collins FS: Molecular biology of cystic fibrosis, *Mol Genet Med* 3:33-38, 1993.

64. Dye C, Scheele S, Dolin P, et al: Consensus statement. Global burden of tuberculosis: estimated incidence, prevalence, and mortality by country. WHO Global Surveillance and Monitoring Project, *JAMA* 282(7):677-686, 1999.

65. Easthope S, Jarvis B: Omalizumab, *Drugs* 61(2):253-260, 261, 2001.

66. Englund JA: Prevention strategies for respiratory syncytial virus: passive and active immunization, *J Pediatr* 135(2, pt 2):38-44, 1999.

67. Epstein SK, Celli BR, Martinez FJ, et al: Arm training reduces the VO2 and VE cost of unsupported arm exercise and elevation in chronic obstructive pulmonary disease, *J Cardiopulm Rehabil* 17(3):171-177, 1997.

68. Esnault S, Malter JS: Minute quantities of granulocyte-macrophage colony-stimulating factor prolong eosinophil survival, *J Interferon Cytokine Res* 21(2):117-124, 2001.

69. Ferguson GT: Update on pharmacologic therapy for chronic obstructive pulmonary disease, *Clin Chest Med* 21(4):723-738, 2000.

70. Fiel SB, Palys B, Sufian B, et al: *Growing older with CF: a handbook for adults*, Brussels, 1997, Scienta Healthcare Education, Solvay Pharmaceuticals.

71. Flaherty KR, Martinez FJ: Lung volume reduction surgery for emphysema, *Clin Chest Med* 21(4):819-848, 2000.

72. Fogel RB, White DP: Obstructive sleep apnea, *Adv Intern Med* 45:351-389, 2000.

73. Foxwell AR, Cripps AW: Haemophilus influenzae oral vaccination against acute bronchitis, *Cochrane Database Syst Rev* 79(2):CD001958, 2000.

74. Frothingham R: Mycobacteria: treatment approaches and mechanisms of resistance, *J Med Liban* 48(4):248-254, 2000.

75. Frownfelter D, Dean E: *Principles and practice of cardiopulmonary physical therapy*, ed 4, St Louis, 2002, Mosby.

76. Fuchs-Climent D, Le Gallais D, Varray A, et al: Factor analysis of quality of life, dyspnea, and physiologic variables in patients with chronic obstructive pulmonary disease before and after rehabilitation, *Am J Phys Med Rehabil* 80(2):113-120, 2001.

77. Fuchs-Climent D, Le Gallais D, Varray A, et al: Quality of life and exercise tolerance in chronic obstructive pulmonary disease: effects of a short and intensive inpatient rehabilitation program, *Am J Phys Med Rehabil* 78:330-335, 1999.

78. Fung M, Gallagher C, Machtay M: Lung and aero-digestive cancers in young marijuana smokers, *Tumori* 85(2):140-142, 1999.

79. Furst DE: Rational therapy in the treatment of systemic sclerosis, *Curr Opin Rheumatol* 12(6):540-544, 2000.

80. Gabriele S, Alberto P, Sergio G, et al: Emerging potentials for an antioxidant therapy as a new approach to the treatment of systemic sclerosis, *Toxicology* 155(1-3):1-15, 2000.

81. Galantino ML, Bishop KL: The new TB, *PT Magazine* 2(2):53-60, 1994.

82. Garrod R, Paul EA, Wedzicha JA: Supplemental oxygen during pulmonary rehabilitation in patients with COPD with exercise hypoxemia, *Thorax* 55(7):539-543, 2000.

83. Gauvreau GM, Wood LJ, Sehmi R, et al: The effects of inhaled budesonide on circulating eosinophil progenitors and their expression of cytokines after allergen challenge in subjects with atopic asthma, *Am J Respir Crit Care Med* 162(6):2139-2144, 2000.

84. Giesbrecht GG: Cold stress, near drowning and accidental hypothermia: a review, *Aviat Space Environ Med* 71(7):733-752, 2000.

85. Gillette MA, Hess DR: Ventilator-induced lung injury and the evolution of lung-protective strategies in acute respiratory distress syndrome, *Respir Care* 46(2):130-148, 2001.

86. Gimenez M, Servera E, Vergara P, et al: Endurance training in patients with chronic obstructive pulmonary disease: a comparison of high versus moderate intensity, *Arch Phys Med Rehabil* 81(1):102-109, 2000.

87. Glezen WP, Alpers M: Maternal immunization, *Clin Infect Dis* 28(2):219-224, 1999.

88. Gochuico BR: Potential pathogenesis and clinical aspects of pulmonary fibrosis associated with rheumatoid arthritis, *Am J Med Sci* 321(1): 83-88, 2001.

89. Gold DR: Environmental tobacco smoke, indoor allergens, and childhood asthma, *Environ Health Perspect* 108(suppl 4, no. 8):643-651, 2000.

90. Goldhaber SZ: Pulmonary embolism, *N Engl J Med* 339(2):93-104,1998.

91. Goldhaber SZ, Grodstein F, Stampfer MJ, et al: A prospective study of risk factors for pulmonary embolism in women, *JAMA* 277:642-645, 1997.

92. Goldstein AB, Goldstein LS, Perl MK, et al: Cystic fibrosis patients with and without central nervous system complications following lung transplantation, *Pediatr Pulmonol* 30(3):203-206, 2000.

93. Gondor M, Nixon PA, Mutich R, et al: Comparison of Flutter® device and chest physical therapy in the treatment of cystic fibrosis pulmonary exacerbation, *Pediatr Pulmonol* 28(4):255-260, 1999.

94. Goodman CC, Snyder TE: *Differential diagnosis in physical therapy*, ed 3, Philadelphia, 2000, Saunders.

95. Goodman GE: Prevention of lung cancer, *Crit Rev Oncol Hematol* 33(3):187-197, 2000.

96. Gosker HR, Wouters EF, van der Vusse GJ, et al: Skeletal muscle dysfunction in chronic obstructive pulmonary disease and chronic heart failure: underlying mechanisms and therapy perspectives, *Am J Clin Nutr* 71(5):1033-1047, 2000.

97. Gosselink R, Troosters T, Decramer M: Distribution of muscle weakness in patients with stable chronic obstructive pulmonary disease, *J Cardiopulm Rehabil* 20(6):353-360, 2000.

98. Green RH, Singh SJ, Williams J, et al: A randomized controlled trial of four weeks versus seven weeks of pulmonary rehabilitation in chronic obstructive pulmonary disease, *Thorax* 56(2):143-145, 2001.

99. Greenlee RT, Hill-Harmon MB, Murray T, et al: Cancer statistics, 2001, *CA Cancer J Clin* 51(1):15-36, 2001.

100. Guccione AA, editor: *Geriatric physical therapy*, ed 2, St Louis, 2000, Mosby, pp 226-244.

101. Hasuda T, Satoh T, Shimouchi A, et al: Improvement in exercise capacity with nitric oxide inhalation in patients with precapillary pulmonary hypertension, *Circulation* 101(17):2066-2070, 2000.

102. Haugen A, Ryberg D, Mollerup S, et al: Gene-environment interactions in human lung cancer, *Toxicol Lett* 112-113(9):233-237, 2000.

103. *Healthy People 2010: understanding and improving health: impact of poor air quality (tobacco smoke)* (on-line), 2000: www.health.gov/healthypeople/

104. Heijerman HG: Chronic obstructive lung disease and respiratory muscle function: the role of nutrition and exercise training in cystic fibrosis, *Respir Med* 87(suppl B):49-51, 1993.

105. Hennessey KA, Schulte JM, Valway SE, et al: Using DNA fingerprinting to detect transmission of Mycobacterium tuberculosis among AIDS patients in two health-care facilities in Puerto Rico, *South Med J* 93(8):777-782, 2000.

106. Hessel PA, Gamble JF, Gee JB, et al: Silica, silicosis, and lung cancer: a response to a recent working group report, *J Occup Environ Med* 42(7):704-720, 2000.

107. HHS (U.S. Department of Health and Human Services): *Women and smoking: a report of the Surgeon General*, Atlanta, 2001, U.S. Department of Health and Human Services, CDC, National Center for Chronic Disease Prevention and Health Promotion, Office on Smoking and Health.

108. Hildalgo JA, MacArthur RD, Crane LR: An overview of HIV infection and AIDS: etiology, pathogenesis, diagnosis, epidemiology, and occupational exposure, *Semin Thorac Cardiovasc Surg* 12(2):130-139, 2000.

109. Hillegass E, Sadowsky HS: *Essentials of cardiopulmonary physical therapy*, ed 2, Philadelphia, 2001, Harcourt Health Sciences.

110. Hirsch FR, Franklin WA, Gazdar AF, et al: Early detection of lung cancer: clinical perspectives of recent advances in biology and radiology, *Clin Cancer Res* 7(1):5-22, 2001.

111. Hirvela ER: Advances in the management of acute respiratory distress syndrome: protective ventilation, *Arch Surg* 135(2):126-135, 2000.

112. Hodson ME: Treatment of cystic fibrosis in the adult, *Respiration* 67(6):595-607, 2000.

113. Hoffman D, Djordjevic MV, Hoffman I: The changing cigarette, *Prev Med* 26(4):427-434, 1997.

114. Hughes TA, Wiles CM, Lawrie BW, Smith AP: Case report: dysphagia and sleep apnoea associated with cervical osteophytes due to diffuse idiopathic skeletal hyperostosis, *J Neurol Neurosurg Psychiatry* 57:384, 1994.

115. Hull SC, Kass NE: Adults with cystic fibrosis and (in)fertility: how has the health care system responded? *J Androl* 21(6):809-813, 2000.

116. Hulme J: *Fibromyalgia: a handbook for self care & treatment*, ed 3, Missoula, Montana, 2000, Phoenix Publishing, pp 108-114.

117. Institute of Medicine (IOM): Ending neglect: the elimination of tuberculosis in the United States (on-line), 2000: www.nationalacademies.org

118. Jacobs RA: Passive smoking induces oxidant damage preventable by vitamin C, *Nutr Rev* 58(8):239-241, 2000.

119. James A, Carroll, N: Airway smooth muscle in health and disease; methods of measurement and relation to function, *Eur Respir J* 15(4):782-789, 2000.

120. Jemal A, Chu KC, Tarone RE: Recent trends in lung cancer mortality in the United States, *J Natl Cancer Inst* 93(4):277-283, 2001.

121 Joad JP: Smoking and pediatric respiratory health, *Clin Chest Med* 21(1):37-46, 2000.

122. Johannesson M, Ludviksdottir D, Janson C: Lung function changes in relation to menstrual cycle in females with cystic fibrosis, *Respir Med* 94(11):1043-1046, 2000.

123. Johnson KR, Braden CR, Cairns KL, et al: Transmission of Mycobacterium tuberculosis from medical waste, *JAMA* 284(13):1683-1688, 2000.

124. Jones A, Rowe BH: Bronchopulmonary hygiene physical therapy in bronchiectasis and chronic obstructive pulmonary disease: a systematic review, *Heart Lung* 29(2):125-135, 2000.

125. Jones A, Rowe BH: Bronchopulmonary hygiene physical therapy for chronic obstructive pulmonary disease and bronchiectasis, *Cochrane Database Syst Rev* 5(2):CD000045, 2000.

126. Judson MA: Clinical aspects of pulmonary sarcoidosis, *JSC Med Assoc* 96(1):9-17, 2000.

127. Judson MA: Lung transplantation for pulmonary sarcoidosis, *Eur Respir J* 11(3):738-844, 1998.

128. Kacmarek RM: Complications of tracheal gas insufflation, *Respir Care* 46(2):167-176, 2001.

129. Kariyawasam HH, Pepper JR, Hodson ME, et al: Experience of totally implantable venous access devices (TIV Ads) in adults with cystic fibrosis over a 13-year period, *Respir Med* 94(12):1161-1165, 2000.

130. Kelly K: New chemotherapy agents for small cell lung cancer, *Chest* 117(4, suppl 1):156S-162S, 2000.

131. Kenyon TA: Transmission of multidrug-resistant *Mycobacterium tuberculosis* during a long airplane flight, *N Engl J Med* 334(15):933-938, 1996.

132. Kern-Buell CL, McGrady AV, Conran PB, et al: Asthma severity, psychophysiological indicators of arousal and immune function in asthma patients undergoing biofeedback-assisted relaxation, *Appl Psychophysiol Biofeedback* 25(2):79-91, 2000.

133. Khaw PY, Ball DL: Relief of non-metastatic shoulder pain with mediastinal radiotherapy in patients with lung cancer, *Lung Cancer* 28(1): 51-54, 2000.

134. Knower MT, Dunagan DP, Adair NE, et al: Baseline oxygen saturation predicts exercise desaturation below prescription threshold in patients with chronic obstructive pulmonary disease, *Arch Intern Med* 161(5):732-736, 2001.

135. Koerts-de Lang E, Schols AM, Rooyackers OE, et al: Different effects of corticosteroid-induced muscle wasting compared with undernutrition on rat diaphragm energy metabolism, *Eur J Appl Physiol* 82(5-6): 493-498, 2000.

136. Kohrt WM, Brown M: Endurance training of the older adult. In Guccione AA, editor: *Geriatric physical therapy*, ed 2, St Louis, 2000, Mosby, pp 245-258.

137. Konstan MW: *CF clinical trials—a status report*, Bethesda, Maryland, 2000, Cystic Fibrosis Foundation.

138. Kovner F, Spigel S, Rider I, et al: Radiation therapy of metastatic spinal cord compression: multidisciplinary team diagnosis and treatment, *J Neurooncol* 42:85-92, 1999.

139. Langenderfer B: Alternatives to percussion and postural drainage: a review of mucus clearance therapies: percussion and postural drainage, autogenic drainage, positive expiratory pressure, flutter valve, intrapulmonary percussive ventilation, and high-frequency chest compression with the ThAIRapy Vest, *J Cardiopulm Rehabil* 18(4):283-289, 1998.

140. Lanphear BP, Aligne CA, Auinger P, et al: Residential exposures associated with asthma in US children, *Pediatrics* 107(3):505-511, 2001.

141. Leus J, Van Biervliet S, Robberecht E: Detection and follow up of exocrine pancreatic insufficiency in cystic fibrosis: a review, *Eur J Pediatr* 159(8):563-568, 2000.

142. Lilienfeld DE, Rubin LJ: Mortality from primary pulmonary hypertension in the United States, 1979-1996, *Chest* 117(3):796-800, 2000.

143. Loube DI: Technologic advances in the treatment of obstructive sleep apnea syndrome, *Chest* 116(5):1426-1433, 1999.

144. Mahadeva R, Webb K, Westerbeek RC, et al: Clinical outcome in relation to care in centers specializing in cystic fibrosis: cross sectional study, *BMJ* 316:1771-1775, 1998.

145. Mahler DA: How should health-related quality of life be assessed in patients with COPD? *Chest* 117(2, suppl):54S-57S, 2000.

146. Maltais F, LeBlanc P, Jobin J, et al: Peripheral muscle dysfunction in chronic obstructive pulmonary disease, *Clin Chest Med* 21(4):665-677, 2000.

147. McDermott JH: Antioxidant nutrients: current dietary recommendations and research update, *J Am Pharm Assoc* 40(6):785-799, 2000.

148. McFadden ER: Natural history of chronic asthma and its long-term effects on pulmonary function, *J Allergy Clin Immunol* 105(2, pt 2):S535-S539, 2000.

149. Meko J, Rusch VW: Neoadjuvant therapy and surgical resection for locally advanced non-small cell lung cancer, *Semin Radiat Oncol* 10(4):324-332, 2000.

150. Milic-Emili J: Inspiratory capacity and exercise tolerance in chronic obstructive pulmonary disease, *Can Respir J* 7(3):282-285, 2000.

151. Milla CE, Warwick WJ, Moran A: Trends in pulmonary function in patients with cystic fibrosis correlate with the degree of glucose intolerance at baseline, *Am J Respir Crit Care Med* 162(3, pt 1):891-895, 2000.

152. Miller AL: The etiologies, pathophysiology, and alternative/complementary treatment of asthma, *Altern Med Rev* 6(1):20-47, 2001.

153. MMWR (Morbidity and Mortality Weekly Report): Declines in lung cancer rates, *MMWR Morb Mortal Wkly Rep* 49(47):1066-1069, 2000.

154. MMWR (Morbidity and Mortality Weekly Report): Preventing and controlling tuberculosis along the U.S.-Mexican border, *MMWR Morb Mortal Wkly Rep* 50(RR1):1-27, 2001.

155. Moore M, Valway SE, Ihle W, et al: A train passenger with pulmonary tuberculosis: evidence of limited transmission during travel, *Clin Infect Dis* 28(1):52-56, 1999.

156. Morris AM, Huang L, Bacchetti P, et al: Permanent declines in pulmonary function following pneumonia in human immunodeficiency virus-infected persons: the Pulmonary Complications of HIV Infection Study Group, *Am J Respir Crit Care* 162(2, pt 1):612-616, 2000.

157. Mortimer KM, Tager IB, Dockery DW, et al: The effect of ozone on inner-city children with asthma: identification of susceptible subgroups, *Am J Respir Crit Care Med* 162(5):1838-1845, 2000.

158. Moser C, Tirakitsoontorn P, Nussbaum E, et al: Muscle size and cardiorespiratory response to exercise in cystic fibrosis, *Am J Respir Crit Care Med* 162(5):1823-1827, 2000.

159. Mulholland EK: Conjugate pneumococcal vaccines: an overview, *Med J Aust* 173(suppl 9):S48-S50, 2000.

160. Murray JF, Nadel J: *Textbook of respiratory medicine*, ed 3, Philadelphia, 2000, Saunders.

161. Mwandumba HC, Beeching NJ: Pyogenic lung infections: factors for predicting clinical outcome of lung abscess and thoracic empyema, *Curr Opin Pulm Med* 6(3):234-239, 2000.

162. National Institutes of Health (NIH): Sleep apnea (on-line), 2001: www.nih.gov/

163. Neuman I, Nahum H, Ben-Amotz A: Reduction of exercise-induced asthma oxidative stress by lycopene, a natural antioxidant, *Allergy* 55(12):1184-1189, 2000.

164. Nielsen KE, Knipper JS, Lane-Gipson NK, et al: Selected outcomes of pulmonary rehabilitation in persons with OSA, *Phys Ther* 80(5):S5, 2000 (abstract).

165. Niewoehner DE, Erbland ML, Deupree RH, et al: Effect of systemic glucocorticoids on exacerbations of chronic obstructive pulmonary disease, *N Engl J Med* 340:1941-1947, 1999.

166. Nishimura J, Ikuyama S: Glucocorticoid-induced osteoporosis: pathogenesis and management, *J Bone Miner Metab* 18(6):350-352, 2000.

167. Oelberg DA, Systrom DM, Markowitz DH, et al: Exercise performance in cystic fibrosis before and after bilateral lung transplantation, *J Heart Lung Transplant* 17(11):1104-1112, 1998.

168. Osborne ML, Vollmer WM, Pedula KL, et al: Lack of correlation of symptoms with specialist-assessed long-term asthma severity, *Chest* 115(1):85-91, 1999.

169. Oyama T, Okuda Y, Oyama H, et al: Sleep apnea syndrome in rheumatoid arthritis (RA) patients complicated with cervical and temporomandibular lesions, *Ryumachi* 35(1):3-8, 1995.

170. Parasa RB, Maffulli N: Musculoskeletal involvement in cystic fibrosis, *Bull Hosp Jt Dis* 58(1):37-44, 1999.

171. Patel DR, Homnick DN: Pulmonary effects of smoking, *Adolesc Med* 11(3):567-576, 2000.

172. Peppard PE, Young T, Palta M, et al: Prospective study of the association between sleep-disordered breathing and hypertension, *N Engl J Med* 342(190):1378-1384, 2000.

173. Perkins MD: New diagnostic tools for tuberculosis, *Int J Tuberc Lung Dis* 4(12, suppl 2):S182-S188, 2000.

174. Picado C, Deulofeu R, Lleonart R, et al: Dietary micronutrients/antioxidants and their relationship with bronchial asthma severity, *Allergy* 56(1):43-49, 2001.

175. Pillar G, Malhotra A, Fogel R, et al: Airway mechanics and ventilation in response to resistive loading during sleep: influence of gender, *Am J Respir Crit Care Med* 162(5):1627-1632, 2000.

176. Pochettino A, Kotloff RM, Rosengard BR, et al: Bilateral versus single lung transplantation for chronic obstructive pulmonary disease: intermediate-term results, *Ann Thorac Surg* 70(6):1813-1818, 2000.

177. Pohlabeln H, Boffetta P, Ahrens W, et al: Occupational risks for lung cancer among nonsmokers, *Epidemiology* 11(5):532-538, 2000.

178. Popper HH: Bronchiolitis, an update, *Virchows Arch* 437(5):471-481, 2000.

179. Pryor WA, Stahl W, Rock CL: Beta carotene: from biochemistry to clinical trials, *Nutr Rev* 58(2, pt 1):39-53, 2000.

180. Ramaell M, Van Meerbeeck J, Van Marck E: Mesothelioma, current insights, *Cancer J* 7(5) (on-line), 2000. www.cancer.org/eprise/main/doc root/PUB/content/PUB_3_3_CA

181. Riley MS, Porszasz J, Engelen MP, et al: Responses to constant work rate bicycle ergometry exercise in primary pulmonary hypertension: the effect of inhaled nitric oxid, *J Am Coll Cardiol* 36(2):547-556, 2000.

182. Ringbaek TJ, Broendum E, Hemmingsen L, et al: Rehabilitation of patients with chronic obstructive pulmonary disease: exercise twice a week is not sufficient! *Respir Med* 94(2):150-154, 2000.

183. Rodenstein DO: Sleep apnoea syndrome: the health economics point of view, *Monaldi Arch Chest Dis* 55(5):404-410, 2000.

184. Rogers DF: Motor control of airway goblet cells and glands, *Respir Physiol* 125(1-2):129-144, 2001.

185. Rosas V, Conte JV, Yang SC, et al: Lung transplantation and systemic sclerosis, *Ann Transplant* 5(3):38-43, 2000.

186. Rusch V, Saltz L, Venkatraman E, et al: A phase II trial of pleurectomy/decortication followed by intrapleural and systemic chemotherapy for malignant pleural mesothelioma, *J Clin Oncol* 12(6):1156-1163, 1994.

187. Sampath D, Castro M, Look DC, et al: Constitutive activation of an epithelial signal transducer and activator of transcription (STAT) pathway in asthma, *J Clin Invest* 103(9):1353-1361, 1999.

188. Scannapieco FA, Ho AW: Potential associations between chronic respiratory disease and periodontal disease: analysis of National Health and Nutrition Examination Survey III, *J Periodontol* 72(1):50-56, 2001.

189. Scharf SM: History and physical examination. In Baum GL, Wolinsky E, editors: *Textbook of pulmonary diseases*, ed 5, Boston, 1989, Little, Brown, pp 213-226.

190. Scherer TA, Barandun J, Marinez E, et al: Effect of high-frequency oral airway and chest wall oscillation and conventional chest physical therapy on expectoration in patients with stable cystic fibrosis, *Chest* 113(4):1019-1027, 1998.

191. Schoem SR: Oral appliances for the treatment of snoring and obstructive sleep, *Otolaryngol Head Neck Surg* 122(2):259-262, 2000.

192. Selman M, King TE, Pardo A: Idiopathic pulmonary fibrosis: prevailing and evolving hypotheses about its pathogenesis and implications for therapy, *Ann Intern Med* 134(2):136-151, 2001.

193. Sethi JM, Rochester CL: Smoking and chronic obstructive pulmonary disease, *Clin Chest Med* 21(1):67-86, 2000.

194. Shanmugasundaram KR, Kumar SS, Rajajee S: Excessive free radical generation in the blood of children suffering from asthma, *Clin Chim Acta* 305(102):107-114, 2001.

195. Shinefield HR, Black S: Efficacy of pneumococcal conjugate vaccines in large scale field trials, *Pediatr Infect Dis J* 19(4):394-397, 2000.

196. Singh SJ, Sodergren SC, Hyland ME, et al: A comparison of three disease-specific and two generic health-status measures to evaluate the outcome of pulmonary rehabilitation in COPD, *Respir Med* 95(1):71-77, 2001.

197. Smith A, Nicholson K: Psychosocial factors, respiratory viruses and exacerbation of asthma, *Psychoneuroendocrinology* 26(4):411-420, 2001.

198. Smulders YM: Pathophysiology and treatment of haemodynamic instability in acute pulmonary embolism: the pivotal role of pulmonary vasoconstriction, *Cardiovasc Res* 48(1):23-33, 2000.

199. Snider GL: History and physical examination. In Baum GL, Wolinsky E, editors: *Textbook of pulmonary diseases,* ed 5, vol I, Boston, 1994, Little, Brown, pp 243-271.

200. Stellman SD, Muscat JE, Hoffmann D, et al: Impact of filter cigarette smoking on lung cancer histology, *Prev Med* 26(4):451-456, 1997.

201. Sterling TR, Pope DS, Bishai WR, et al: Transmission of *Mycobacterium tuberculosis* from a cadaver to an embalmer, *N Engl J Med* 342(4):246-248, 2000.

202. Strauss GM: Randomized population trials and screening for lung cancer: breaking the cure barrier, *Cancer* 89(11, suppl):2399-2421, 2000.

203. Suissa S, Ernst P, Benayoun S, et al: Low-dose inhaled corticosteroids and the prevention of death from asthma, *N Engl J Med* 343(5):332-336, 2000.

204. Sullivan F, Avstreih D: Pneumothorax during CPR training: case report and review of the CPR literature, *Prehospital Disaster Med* 15(1):64-69, 2000.

205. Talbot EA, Moore M, McCray E, et al: Tuberculosis among foreign-born persons in the United States, 1993-1998, *JAMA* 284(22):2894-2900, 2000.

206. Thomas CR, Williams TE, Cobos E, et al: Lung cancer. In Lenhard RE, Osteen RT, Gansler T: *Clinical oncology,* Atlanta, 2001, American Cancer Society, pp 269-295.

207. Troosters T, Gosselink R, Decramer M: Short- and long-term effects of outpatient rehabilitation in patients with chronic obstructive pulmonary disease: a randomized trial, *Am J Med* 109(3):207-212, 2000.

208. Vally H, de Klerk N, Thompson PJ: Alcoholic drinks: important triggers for asthma, *J Allergy Clin Immunol* 105(3):462-467.

209. Varpula T, Pettila V, Nieminen H, et al: Airway pressure release ventilation and prone positioning in severe acute respiratory distress syndrome, *Acta Anaesthesiol Scand* 45(3):340-344, 2001.

210. Victor LD: Obstructive sleep apnea, *Am Fam Physician* 60(8):2279-2283, 1999.

211. Vranken JH, Zuurmond WW, de Lange JJ: Continuous brachial plexus block as treatment for the Pancoast syndrome, *Clin J Pain* 16(4):327-333, 2000.

212. Wahlgren DR, Hovell MF, Meltzer EO, et al: Involuntary smoking and asthma, *Curr Opin Pulm Med* 6(1):31-36, 2000.

213. Ward SA, Tomezsko JL, Holsclaw DS, et al: Energy expenditure and substrate utilization in adults with cystic fibrosis and diabetes mellitus, *Am J Clin Nutr* 69(5):913-919, 1999.

214. Ware JC, McBrayer RH, Scott JA: Influence of sex and age on duration and frequency of sleep apnea events, *Sleep* 23(2):165-170, 2000.

215. Webb AK, Dodd ME: Exercise and sport in cystic fibrosis: benefits and risks, *Br J Sports Med* 33(2):77-78, 1999.

216. Welsh MJ, Denning GM, Ostedgaard LS, Anderson MP: Dysfunction of CFTR bearing the delta F508 mutation, *J Cell Sci Suppl* 17:235-239, 1993.

217. Wensel R, Opitz CF, Ewert R, et al: Effects of iloprost inhalation on exercise capacity and ventilatory efficiency in patients with primary pulmonary hypertension, *Circulation* 101(20):2388-2392, 2000.

218. White B, Moore WC, Wigley FM, et al: Cyclophosphamide is associated with pulmonary function and survival benefit in patients with scleroderma and alveolitis, *Ann Intern Med* 132(12):947-954, 2000.

219. Williams MD, Sandler AB: The epidemiology of lung cancer, *Cancer Treat Res* 105(1):31-52, 2001.

220. Wilson DC, Kalnins D, Stewart C, et al: Challenges in the dietary treatment of cystic fibrosis related diabetes mellitus, *Clin Nutr* 19(2):87-93, 2000.

221. Wisser W, Deviatko E, Simon-Kupilik N, et al: Lung transplantation following lung volume reduction surgery, *J Heart Lung Transplant* 19(5):480-487, 2000.

222. Wistuba II, Gazdar AF: Molecular pathology of lung cancer, *Verh Dtsch Ges Pathol* 84(4):96-105, 2000.

223. Wolfe R, Ferrando A, Sheffield-Moore M, et al: Testosterone and muscle protein metabolism, *Mayo Clin Proc* 75(suppl):S55-S59, 2000.

224. Womack CJ, Harris Dl, Katzel LI, et al: Weight loss, not aerobic exercise improves pulmonary function in older obese men, *J Gerontol A Biol Sci Med Sci* 55(8):M453-M457, 2000.

225. Wong CA, Walsh LJ, Smith CJ, et al: Inhaled corticosteroid use and bone-mineral density in patients with asthma, *Lancet* 355(9213):1399-1403, 2000.

226. Wong WP: Physical therapy for a patient in acute respiratory failure, *Phys Ther* 80(7):662-670, 2000.

227. Wood ME, Kelly K, Mullineaux LG, et al: The inherited nature of lung cancer: a pilot study, *Lung Cancer* 30(2):135-144, 2000.

228. Yankaskas JR, Aris R: Outpatient care of the cystic fibrosis patient after lung transplantation, *Curr Opin Pulm Med* 6(6):551-557, 2000.

229. Yantis MA: Identifying depression as a symptom of sleep apnea, *J Psychosoc Nurs Ment Health Serv* 37(10):28-34, 1999.

230. Zaugg M, Lucchinetti E: Respiratory function in the elderly, *Anesthesiol Clin North Am* 18(1):47-58, 2000.

231. Zhou XS, Shahabuddin S, Zahn BR, et al: Effect of gender on the development of hypocapnic apnea/hypopnea during NREM sleep, *J Appl Physiol* 89(1):192-199, 2000.

232. Zimmerman JL, Woodruff PG, Clark S, et al: Relation between phase of menstrual cycle and emergency department visits for acute asthma, *Am J Respir Crit Care* 162(2, pt 1):512-515, 2000.

233. Zumula A, Malon P, Henderson J, et al: Impact of HIV infection on tuberculosis, *Postgrad Med J* 76(895):259-268, 2000.

CHAPTER 15

THE GASTROINTESTINAL SYSTEM

CATHERINE C. GOODMAN

The gastrointestinal (GI) tract consists of upper and lower segments with separate functions. The upper GI tract includes the mouth, esophagus, stomach, and duodenum and aids in the ingestion and digestion of food. The lower GI tract includes the small and large intestines (Fig. 15-1). The small intestine accomplishes digestion and absorption of nutrients, whereas the large intestine absorbs water and electrolytes, storing waste products of digestion until elimination.

The enteric nervous system (ENS) has become the focus of new research and discoveries in a new area of study referred to as *psychoneuroimmunology* with a subspecialty of clinical gastroenterology called *neurogastroenterology*. Insight into the connections among emotions, brain function, and GI function have revolutionized our thinking about the so-called "mind-body connection." New information is being discovered about the sensory functions of the intestine and how neural, hormonal, and immune signals interact. More than 30 chemicals of different classes (neuropeptides) transmit instructions to the brain, and all these chemicals are represented in the enteric nervous system. Representatives of all the major categories of immune cells are found in the gut or can be recruited rapidly from the circulation in response to an inflammatory stimulus. The constant presence of these neurotransmitters and neuromodulators in the bowel suggests that emotional expression or active coping generates a balance in the neuropeptide-receptor network and physiologic healing beginning in the GI system. For an in-depth discussion of the enteric nervous system and an understanding of the chemicals that transmit emotions throughout the body, see references 27 and 51 and the section on Psychoneuroimmunology in Chapter 2.

Scientists continue to study influences of the nervous system on immune and inflammatory responses in the mucosal surfaces of the intestines along with the innervation of the immune system and the molecular communication pathways as these relate to emotions and thoughts and the GI system. The gut immune system has 70% to 80% of the body's immune cells, and the protective blocking action of the secretory response in the gut is crucial to the integrity of the GI tract immune function and host defense. Studies suggest that the development and expression of the regional immune system of the GI tract is independent of systemic immunity. Nutrients have fundamental and regulatory influences on the immune response of the GI tract and therefore on host defense. Reduction of normal bacteria in the gut after antibiotic treatment or in the presence of infection may interfere with the nutrients available for immune function in the GI tract.[19]

New understanding of intestinal disorders and new approaches to the management of these disorders are expected in the next decade.[6]

SIGNS AND SYMPTOMS OF GASTROINTESTINAL DISEASE

Clinical manifestations of GI disease can be caused by a variety of underlying conditions or disorders. The primary condition may be of GI origin, but some GI symptoms are part of a collection of systemic symptoms called *constitutional symptoms* and may be associated with any systemic condition (Table 15-1).

Nausea occurs when nerve endings in the stomach and other parts of the body are irritated and usually precedes vomiting. Intense pain in any part of the body can produce nausea as a result of the nausea-vomiting mechanism of the involuntary autonomic nervous system. Nausea can be caused by strong emotions and may accompany psychologic disorders, a variety of systemic disorders (e.g., acute myocardial infarction, diabetic acidosis, migraine, hepatobiliary and pancreatic disorders, Menière's syndrome, and GI disorders), and drugs such as morphine, codeine, excess alcohol, anesthetics, and anticancer drugs.

Vomiting may be caused by anything that precipitates nausea. Complications of vomiting include fluid and electrolyte imbalances, pulmonary aspiration of vomitus, gastroesophageal mucosal tear (Mallory-Weiss syndrome), malnutrition, and rupture of the esophagus.

Diarrhea (abnormal frequency or volume of stools) results in poor absorption of water and nutritive elements and electrolytes, fluid volume deficit, and acidosis as a result of bicarbonate depletion (see Chapter 4). Other systemic effects of prolonged diarrhea are dehydration, electrolyte imbalance, and weight loss. The causes of diarrhea are many and varied (Table 15-2). Drug-induced diarrhea, most commonly associated with antibiotics, may not develop until 2 to 3 weeks after first ingestion of an antibiotic, but if the onset of diarrhea coincides with the use of drugs, it may resolve when the drug is discontinued.

Anorexia, diminished appetite or aversion to food, is a nonspecific symptom often associated with nausea, vomiting, and sometimes diarrhea. It may be associated with disorders of other organ systems, including cancer, heart disease, and renal disease. *Anorexia-cachexia*, a systemic response to cancer, occurs as a result of increased metabolic rate caused by the tumor cells and metabolites produced and released by tumor

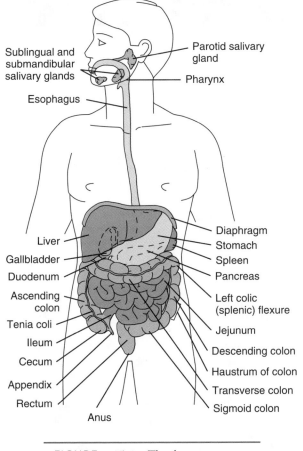

FIGURE   15-1   The digestive system.

TABLE 15-1

Clinical Manifestations of Gastrointestinal Disease

GASTROINTESTINAL SIGNS AND SYMPTOMS	CONSTITUTIONAL SYMPTOMS	GI SIGNS AND SYMPTOMS ASSOCIATED WITH STRENUOUS EXERCISE
Nausea and vomiting	Nausea	Fecal urgency; diarrhea
Diarrhea	Vomiting	Abdominal cramps
Anorexia	Diarrhea	Belching
Constipation	Malaise	Nausea and vomiting
Dysphagia	Fatigue	Heartburn
Achalasia	Fever	
Heartburn	Night sweats	
Abdominal pain	Pallor	
Gastrointestinal bleeding	Diaphoresis	
Hematemesis	Dizziness	
Melena		
Hematochezia		
Fecal incontinence		

---

cells into the bloodstream. These effects of tumor cells stimulate the satiety center in the hypothalamus and produce appetite loss, gross alterations of metabolic patterns, and a profound systemic condition referred to as anorexia-cachexia. A downward spiral of symptoms occurs with appetite loss leading to malnutrition, weight loss, muscular weakness, and a negative nitrogen balance that contributes to the development of cachectic wasting.

Constipation is a condition in which fecal matter is too hard to pass easily or in which bowel movements are so infrequent that discomfort and other symptoms interfere with daily activities. Constipation may occur as a result of many other factors such as diet, dehydration (including lack of fluid intake), side effects of medication, acute or chronic diseases of the digestive system, inactivity or prolonged bed rest, emotional stress, personality, and lack of exercise (see Table 15-2). Although constipation often is described as a condition of old age, it is probably multifactorial caused more often by lifestyle factors than by physiologic decline. Lifelong bowel habits, current diet, lack of fluid intake, and immobility are likely causes of constipation in the older adult (older than 65 years).[21] People with mechanical low back pain may develop constipation as a result of muscle guarding and splinting that causes reduced bowel motility. Pressure on sacral nerves from stored fecal content may cause an aching discomfort in the sacrum, buttocks, or thighs.[28]

Dysphagia (difficulty swallowing) produces the sensation that food is stuck somewhere in the throat or chest (esophagus). Dysphagia may be a symptom of many other disorders including neurologic conditions (e.g., stroke, Alzheimer's, Parkinson's); local trauma and muscle damage (including physical assault); or mechanical obstruction. Obstruction may be *intrinsic*, originating in the wall of the esophageal lumen (e.g., tumors, strictures, outpouchings called *diverticula*), or *extrinsic*, outside the esophageal lumen, such as a tumor or swelling that prevents the passage of food. Dysphagia caused by swelling can occur as a side effect of certain types of drugs such as antidepressants, antihypertensives, and asthma medications.

Achalasia is a failure to relax the smooth muscle fibers of the GI tract. This especially occurs as a result of failure of the lower esophageal sphincter to relax normally with swallowing. The affected person reports a feeling of fullness in the sternal region and progressive dysphagia. Although the cause of achalasia is not known, the loss or absence of ganglion cells in the myenteric plexus* of the esophagus appears to be a part of the cause. Anxiety and emotional tension aggravate the condition and precipitate the attacks. Progression of the condition results in dilation of the esophagus and loss of peristalsis in the lower two thirds of the esophagus.

Heartburn, dyspepsia, pyrosis, or indigestion, a burning sensation in the esophagus usually felt in the midline below the sternum in the region of the heart, are often symptoms of gastroesophageal reflux and occur when acidic contents of the stomach move backward or regurgitate into the esophagus. The presence of a hiatal hernia; ingestion of certain foods;† drugs such as alcohol and aspirin; and movements such as lifting, stooping, or bending over after a large meal may bring on

---

*The myenteric plexus is the nerve plexus lying in the muscular layers of the esophagus, stomach, and intestines.

†Certain foods act as muscle relaxants. For example, chocolate contains four substances that can relax the lower esophageal sphincter: caffeine, theobromine, theophylline, and fat. Fat-rich foods lower sphincter muscle pressure by release of cholecystokinin from the upper intestinal mucosa. Fat also delays emptying of the stomach, giving more opportunity for this effect to occur. Other implicated foods include spicy and highly seasoned foods, onions, alcohol, peppermint, and spearmint.

TABLE	15-2

Causes of Diarrhea and Constipation

	DIARRHEA	CONSTIPATION
Neurogenic	Irritable bowel syndrome Diabetic enteropathy Hyperthyroidism Caffeine	Irritable bowel syndrome Central nervous system lesions (e.g., multiple sclerosis, Parkinson's) Dementia Spinal cord tumors or lesions Atony
Muscular	Muscular incompetence Electrolyte imbalance Endocrine disorder Alcohol, wine	Muscular dystrophy (Duchenne's) Electrolyte imbalance Endocrine disorder Severe malnutrition (e.g., eating disorders, cancer) Inactivity; back injury/pain
Mechanical	Incomplete obstruction (e.g., neoplasm, adhesions, stenosis) Postoperative effect (e.g., gastrectomy, ileal bypass, intestinal resection, cholecystectomy) Diverticulitis	Bowel obstruction Extraalimentary tumors Pregnancy Colostomy

Other	Diet (including food allergy, lactose intolerance, food
	    additives)
	Medications (including over-the-counter drugs and
	    laxative abuse)
	Malabsorption
	Infectious/inflammatory (including pelvic inflammatory
	    disease)
	Strenuous exercise
		Diet (especially lack of dietary bulk or fiber, iron
		    compounds)
		Medications (including over-the-counter drugs)
		Rectal lesions (e.g., anal fissure, hemorrhoids, abscess,
		    rectocele, stenosis, ulcerative proctitis)
		Psychologic variables (e.g., mental illness; busy lifestyle,
		    or ignoring the urge)

heartburn. Indigestion also may be a potential manifestation of angina associated with coronary artery disease.

Emotional stress can stimulate the vagus nerve, which controls the secretory and motility functions of the stomach. Stimulation of this cranial nerve causes the stomach to churn, increases the flow of various gastric juices, and causes contraction and spasm of the pylorus (opening of the stomach into the duodenum). If some of the stomach contents are displaced into the esophagus during this nervous activity, heartburn can occur.

Abdominal pain accompanies a large number of GI diseases and may be mechanical, inflammatory, ischemic, or referred. *Mechanical pain* occurs by stretching the wall of a hollow organ or the capsule of a solid organ. *Inflammatory pain* occurs via the release of mediators such as prostaglandins, histamine, and serotonin or bradykinin stimulating sensory nerve endings. *Ischemic pain* occurs as tissue metabolites are released in the area of diminished blood flow. *Referred pain* usually is well localized and may be associated with hyperalgesia and muscle guarding. Pain from the spine also can be referred to the abdomen, usually as a result of nerve root irritation or compression. This type of neuromusculoskeletal pain referred to the abdomen is characteristically associated with hyperesthesia over the involved spinal dermatomes and is intensified by motions such as coughing, sneezing, or straining.

GI bleeding may be characterized by coffee-ground emesis (blood that has been in contact with gastric acid), hematemesis (vomiting of bright-red blood), melena (black, tarry stools), or hematochezia (bleeding from the rectum, or maroon-colored stools), depending on the location of the lesion. Bleeding may not be clinically obvious to the client and may be diagnosed only by further testing.

The major causes of upper GI bleeding in the therapy population are erosive gastritis common in (1) severely ill people with major trauma or systemic illness, burns, or head injury; (2) peptic ulcers; (3) nonsteroidal antiinflammatory drugs (NSAIDs) such as aspirin or ibuprofen; and (4) chronic alcohol use. Drugs such as warfarin, heparin, and aspirin used as anticoagulants in the treatment of pulmonary emboli, venous thrombus, or valvular abnormalities can contribute to or exacerbate gastric erosion and subsequent bleeding.

Accumulation of blood in the GI tract is irritating and increases peristalsis, causing nausea, vomiting, or diarrhea with possible referred pain to the shoulder or back. The digestion of proteins originating from massive upper GI bleeding is reflected by an increase in blood urea nitrogen (BUN) (see Table 39-11). Other complications include fatigue, postural hypotension, tachycardia, weakness, or shortness of breath on exertion. Slow, chronic blood loss may result in iron deficiency anemia.

BOX 15-1

Causes of Increased Intraabdominal Pressure

Lifting	Obesity
Straining	Congestive heart failure
Bending over	Low-fiber diet
Prolonged sitting or standing	Constipation (see Table 15-2)
Chronic or forceful cough	Delayed bowel movement
Pregnancy	Vigorous exercise
Ascites	

fluoroscopy showing the position of the stomach in relation to the diaphragm. These tests may both be necessary to confirm the diagnosis because the hernia may slide down when the person is placed in the upright position for the radiograph. The primary treatment remains symptomatic control through the use of antacids and elevating the head of the bed. Treatment is essentially the same for gastroesophageal reflux disease (GERD) (see the section on Gastroesophageal Reflux Disease in this chapter). The prognosis is good overall with recurrences expected.

Special Implications for the Therapist   15-2

HIATAL HERNIA

For any client with a known hiatal hernia, the flat supine position and any exercises requiring the Valsalva maneuver (which increases intraabdominal pressure) should be avoided during therapy intervention. Before discharge, the client must be warned against activities that cause increased intraabdominal pressure and given safe lifting instructions. A slow return to function over the next 6 to 8 weeks is advised. Postoperatively (after surgical repair of the hernia using the thoracic approach), the client may have chest tubes in place requiring careful observation of the tubes during turning and repositioning and chest physical therapy to prevent pulmonary complications. ■

◆ Gastroesophageal Reflux Disease

Definition. Gastroesophageal reflux disease (GERD), or esophagitis, may be defined as an inflammation of the esophagus, which may be the result of reflux (backward flow) of infectious agents, chemical irritants, physical agents such as radiation and nasogastric intubation, or gastric juices. Reflux esophagitis is the most common type, with backward or return flow of the stomach and duodenal contents into the esophagus. Other types of esophagitis, such as infectious esophagitis, may occur with immunosuppression resulting from viral, bacterial, fungal, or parasitic organisms. Chemical esophagitis is usually a result of accidental poisoning in children or attempted suicide in adults. External irradiation for the treat-

ment of thoracic cancers may include portions of the esophagus and lead to esophagitis and stricture.

Incidence and Etiologic Factors. Although any age can be affected, this condition has an increasing incidence with increasing age. It is estimated that 10% of the population has daily symptoms of GERD and as much as one third of the population has monthly symptoms. A reduction in the pressure of the lower esophageal sphincter (LES), increased gastric pressure, or gastric contents located near the gastroesophageal junction can contribute to the development of esophageal reflux. A wide range of foods and lifestyle factors can contribute to GERD[47] (Table 15-3). Reflux is often associated with a sliding hiatal hernia, also called a *diaphragmatic hernia* (see Fig. 15-3). Smooth muscle relaxants used for cardiac conditions, such as beta-adrenergics, aminophylline, nitrates, and calcium channel blockers may contribute to incompetence of the LES. *Helicobacter pylori* infection does not cause GERD and may even protect certain susceptible individuals from developing GERD and its complications.[23]

Pathogenesis. Normally, a high-pressure zone exists around the gastroesophageal sphincter, which permits the passage of food and liquids but prevents reflux. Any of the predisposing factors listed in Table 15-3 may alter the pressure around the LES, resulting in reflux. Hydrochloric acid or gastric and duodenal contents containing bile acid and pancreatic juice coming in contact with the walls of the esophagus cause inflammation and mucosal ulcerations that may bleed. Subsequent granulation tissue causes scarring that frequently develops into esophageal strictures that narrow the esophagus, making swallowing difficult.

Clinical Manifestations. Heartburn, reflux, dysphagia, and painful swallowing are the primary symptoms of esophagitis. Pain usually is described as a burning sensation that moves up and down and may radiate to the back, neck, or jaw. Heartburn most often occurs 30 to 60 minutes after a meal and is produced by contact of regurgitated contents with the inflamed esophageal mucosa. Dysphagia is an indication of narrowing of the lumen, usually as a result of edema, spasm, or esophageal strictures. Aggravating factors include recumbency, bending, and meals; relief is obtained with antacids or baking soda, standing and walking, fluids, and avoidance of predisposing factors.

Reflux in the absence of esophagitis may be asymptomatic or accompanied by a sour taste in the mouth; severe reflux may reach the pharynx and mouth and result in laryngitis and morning hoarseness. Pulmonary aspiration can occur in people who are incapacitated (e.g., neurologically impaired); recurrent pulmonary aspiration can cause aspiration pneumonia, pulmonary fibrosis, or chronic asthma.

Medical Management
Diagnosis and Prognosis. Diagnostic tools include history, endoscopy, barium radiography, and *H. pylori* and esophageal pH testing. A full diagnostic evaluation is not always required when history and current symptoms clearly point to esophagitis; a therapeutic trial of treatment in mild cases may be diagnostic in itself. Response to nitroglycerin may help the physician differentiate between esophagitis and angina pectoris, but the response is not always diagnostic be-

TABLE 15-3

Causes of Gastroesophageal Reflux Disease

DECREASED PRESSURE OF LOWER ESOPHAGEAL SPHINCTER	INCREASED GASTRIC PRESSURE	GASTRIC CONTENTS NEAR JUNCTION
Foods: chocolate, peppermint, fatty foods, citrus products (including tomatoes), spicy foods, garlic, onions	Food (protein)	Recumbency
Beverages: coffee (including decaf), carbonated drinks, alcohol	Pregnancy (increased abdominal pressure)	Increased intra-abdominal pressure
Caffeine	Obesity	
Nicotine or cigarette smoke	Ascites	
Central nervous system depressants (e.g., morphine, diazepam)	Tight clothing; Spandex; pantyhose	
Other medications (e.g., calcium channel blockers, dopamine, theophylline, tricyclic antidepressants)	Back supports	
Estrogen therapy	Antacids	
Nasogastric intubation	Histamines	
Scleroderma		
Prolonged vomiting		
Surgical resection (destroys sphincter)		
Position (right side-lying; sitting)		
Pregnancy (last trimester: increased progesterone relaxes sphincter)		

cause nitroglycerin also can relieve esophageal spasm and some women with angina improve with antacids rather than nitroglycerin. Prognosis is good for reflux esophagitis with complete symptom resolution, but often variable for the chemical type and poor for infectious esophagitis. GERD can contribute to asthma and vocal cord inflammation and people who have uncontrolled acid reflux are at increased risk of developing esophageal cancer.[30]

Treatment. The first line treatment is now acid-suppressing inhibitors (PPIs) (e.g., Prilosec, Aciphex, Prevacid) for the healing of erosive gastroesophageal reflux disease and maintenance of healed erosive GERD. These medications shut off the chemical pump that transports acid into the stomach. Two new, minimally invasive surgical procedures have been approved by the FDA; these tighten up the lower esophageal sphincter. These procedures allow the majority of people to stop taking all GERD medications, including PPIs.

Lifestyle modifications also may be recommended including wearing loose clothing; dietary restrictions; avoiding caffeine, nicotine, alcohol, salicylates, and NSAIDs; remaining upright at least 3 hours after meals; avoiding meals near bedtime or naptime; elevation of the head of the bed to reduce nocturnal reflux and enhance esophageal acid clearance; weight loss, if obese (this last recommendation has not been confirmed by clinical studies).

Uncomplicated cases of esophagitis and typical symptoms of heartburn and regurgitation may be treated with two types of over-the-counter drugs: antacids (e.g., preparations such as calcium carbonate–magnesium carbonate [Mylanta]; or magnesium hydroxide–aluminum hydroxide [Maalox]; or histamine blockers (H_2-blockers) such as Pepcid, Tagamet, and Zantac. Antacids neutralize stomach acid, whereas histamine blockers prevent acid secretion. The goal of antacids is quick symptom relief, whereas the goal of histamine blockers is

long-term cure. Drinking fluids between meals (not with meals) helps reduce the likelihood of reflux; chewing gum to stimulate saliva helps neutralize gastric acid that is refluxing from the stomach into the lower esophagus.

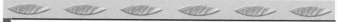

Special Implications for the Therapist   15-3

GASTROESOPHAGEAL REFLUX DISEASE

Clients with GERD are often treated in a therapy practice or rehabilitation setting for orthopedic and other conditions. Occasionally, GERD presents with atypical head and neck symptoms (e.g., sensation of a lump in the throat) without heartburn. People with GERD may have trouble exercising because physical activity can worsen symptoms. In fact, GERD induced by strenuous exercise is extremely common among athletes. The degree of reflux is greater in activities with more body agitation (e.g., running, aerobics) than in swimming or biking. Strenuous exercise inhibits both gastric and small-intestinal emptying, which may contribute to GERD. This combined with the potential for relaxation of the gastroesophageal sphincter suggest the importance of avoiding high-calorie meals or fatty foods (or other triggers) immediately before exercising to avoid or minimize exercise-related GERD.[68] The therapist can be instrumental in providing education and encouragement, essential to the lifestyle modifications necessary to this condition, and assist the person to implement changes related to diet and exercise.

Any intervention requiring a supine position should be scheduled before meals and avoided just after eating. Modification of position toward a more upright posture may be required if symptoms persist during therapy. Consider a trial of the exercises to strengthen the muscles around the esophageal sphincter (see Fig. 15-2). For nocturnal reflux, encourage the individual to sleep on the left side with a pillow in place to maintain this position. Right sidelying makes it easier for acid to flow into the esophagus because of the effect of gravity on the esophagus (the lower esophagus bends to the left and this straightens out with right sidelying).[36] See Special Implications for the Therapist: Hiatal Hernia, 15-2. Activities that increase intraabdominal pressure; constipation, which often accompanies back pain and other conditions (see Table 15-2); and tight clothing must be avoided.

With postoperative complications, chest physical therapy may be indicated. In addition, coughing and bronchospasm can result from a vagally mediated reflex secondary to refluxed acid contents in the esophagus. The therapist also may observe reflux in clients who have chronic bronchitis, asthma, and pulmonary fibrosis. The presence of GERD requires careful positioning to promote drainage of secretions without causing reflux. This is more readily accomplished when the stomach is empty. Positioning clients with gastrointestinal dysfunction for breathing control and coughing maneuvers requires special attention to minimize the risk of aspiration. Although head-up positions minimize reflux by reducing intraabdominal pressure, they can promote aspiration of pharyngeal contents. Sidelying positions (especially left sidelying) prevent regurgitation and aspiration and promote oropharyngeal accumulations and ease of suctioning.[20]

Polypharmacy (the use of multiple medications for a single disorder or for co-morbidities) can result in significant toxicity and drug interactions when taken with medications for acid-related diseases. Any new or unusual symptoms reported to the therapist should be documented with physician notification. Alternately, anyone with GI dysfunction is at risk for impaired metabolism due to evacuation of medicine, improper absorption, or both. Monitoring GI status and medication responses is essential in conjunction with the individual's response to therapy intervention.[20] ∎

◆ Mallory-Weiss Syndrome

Mallory-Weiss syndrome (MWS) is mucosal laceration of the lower end of the esophagus accompanied by bleeding. The most common cause is severe retching and vomiting as a result of alcohol abuse, eating disorders such as bulimia, or in the case of a viral syndrome. Other conditions such as pregnancy, migraine, hiatal hernia, gastric ulcer, biliary disease, and various medications have been associated with MWS. Any event that suddenly raises transabdominal pressure in exercise or lifting can cause such a tear. Diagnosis is made on endoscopy, and when treatment is necessary, fluid replacement and blood transfusion and H_2-receptor antagonists may be administered. Endoscopic ligation may be required if bleeding cannot be brought under control.

◆ Scleroderma Esophagus

Esophageal involvement is common in people with progressive systemic sclerosis caused by the CREST syndrome (calcinosis, Raynaud's phenomenon, esophageal motility disorder, sclerodactyly, and telangiectasia; see the section on Systemic Sclerosis in Chapter 9). The esophageal lesions in systemic sclerosis consist of muscular atrophy of the smooth muscle portion, with weakness of contraction in the lower two thirds

of the esophagus and incompetence of the LES. Symptoms include dysphagia to solids and to liquids in the recumbent position. Heartburn and regurgitation occur in the presence of gastroesophageal reflux and esophagitis. Currently, no effective treatment exists for the motor difficulty, but reflux esophagitis and its complications are treated aggressively as described earlier. Exercises described in Fig. 15-2 remain under investigation for this type of condition but may be beneficial.[24]

◆ Neoplasm

Overview and Risk Factors.   Histologically, two types of esophageal cancer exist: squamous cell and adenocarcinoma. Esophageal cancer is relatively uncommon, but the incidence of adenocarcinoma is rising possibly as a result of *H. pylori* eradication in GERD. Esophageal cancer is known for its marked variation by geographic region, ethnic background, and gender. In the United States, adenocarcinoma of the esophagus most frequently affects middle-aged white men, whereas squamous cell cancer is much more common in blacks associated with alcohol and tobacco use.[10]

The presence of other esophageal disease such as hiatal hernia, reflux, Barrett's esophagus, rings, webs, diverticula, stricture from lye ingestion, achalasia, and other head and neck cancers increases the risk of developing esophageal cancer. Gastroesophageal reflux is highly correlated with an increased risk of esophageal adenocarcinoma (but not squamous cell carcinoma of the esophagus).[30]

Etiologic Factors and Pathogenesis.   Chronic inadequate nutrition can impair both the structure and function of the esophagus. Nutritional deprivation, particularly deficiencies of vitamin A and zinc, results in mucosal changes increasing the vulnerability of esophageal mucosa to neoplastic changes. Any change in esophageal function that permits food and drink to remain in the esophagus for prolonged periods of time can result in ulceration and metaplasia. Chronic exposure to irritants such as alcohol and tobacco (inhaled or chewed)* also can cause neoplastic transformation. Tumors may be obstructive causing circumferential compression or ulceration with bleeding. Distant metastases also may occur, most commonly involving the liver and lung, but almost any organ can be involved.

Barrett's esophagus is a premalignant condition in which the normal squamous epithelium of the esophagus is replaced by metaplastic epithelium predisposing the individual to esophageal adenocarcinoma. The progression of Barrett's metaplasia to adenocarcinoma is associated with several changes in gene structure, gene expression, and protein structure. Researchers are identifying some of the molecular alterations in hopes of finding markers for early cancer detection or prognostication.[69]

Clinical Manifestations.   Dysphagia with or without pain is the predominant symptom of this condition and may not occur until the diameter of the lumen of the esophagus is reduced 30% to 50%. Pain associated with dysphagia usually

---

*Nitrosamines are powerful carcinogens involved as causative agents of cancers of the lung, oral cavity, esophagus, and pancreas associated with the use of tobacco products. Chronic stimulation of nicotinic receptors by nicotine and nitrosamines in smokers is one of the molecular events responsible for stimulation of cell proliferation and ultimately neoplasms.

is described as pressure-like and may radiate posteriorly between the scapulae. Heartburn initiated by lying down is the most common type of pain. Constant retrosternal chest pain that radiates to the back may occur in the presence of mediastinal extension or spinal nerve compression. Other signs and symptoms include anorexia and weight loss, hoarseness resulting from laryngeal nerve compression, and tracheoesophageal fistula causing cough and recurrent pneumonia.

Medical Management

Diagnosis and Treatment. Diagnosis is made by endoscopy with cytology and biopsy. After diagnosis, staging of the disease is performed with chest and abdominal computed tomography (CT) scanning or, if available, endoscopic ultrasonography to determine the most appropriate treatment. Neoplasms are classified as resectable with curative intent, resectable but not curable, and not resectable and not curable. The presence of distant metastases, invasion of the mediastinal muscularis or pleural invasion, or distant lymph node involvement excludes a curative resection. Curative surgery is esophageal reconstruction, which may improve the ability to eat and may prevent local tumor complications. The use of preoperative chemotherapy with radiation is under investigation. Unresectable disease or poor operative candidates may receive radiation therapy, which provides short-term relief of symptoms. Combinations of esophageal brachytherapy, external beam radiation, and multidrug combination chemotherapy are under clinical investigation; the use of brachytherapy appears to be associated with severe toxicity and the development of fistulas.[25]

Prognosis. Endoscopic surveillance can detect esophageal adenocarcinomas when they are early and curable, but most of these neoplasms are detected at an advanced stage. Carcinoma of the esophagus has one of the lowest possibilities of cure, with 5-year survival rates estimated to be approximately 10% overall and median survival of less than 10 months. The first symptoms of esophageal cancer are not usually apparent until the tumor involves the entire esophageal circumference. More important, the tumor by that time has often invaded the deeper layers of the esophagus and adjacent structures and is unresectable. Esophageal cancer metastasizes rapidly and given the continuous nature of lymphatic vessels in the area, removal of lymph nodes with the tumor is impossible, contributing to the poor prognosis.

Special Implications for the Therapist 15-4

ESOPHAGEAL CANCER

Preferred Practice Pattern:
6H: Impaired Circulation and Anthropometric Dimensions Associated With Lymphatic System Disorders

Lymphatic vessels of the esophagus are continuous with mediastinal structures and drain to the lymph nodes from the neck of the celiac axis. Metastasis is via this lymphatic drainage with tumors of the upper esophagus metastasizing to the cervical, internal jugular, and supraclavicular nodes. During an upper-

quarter screening examination the therapist may identify changes in lymph nodes, requiring medical referral. The usual precautions regarding clients with cancer apply to neoplasms of the GI system. The primary concern is the side effects of chemotherapy-induced bone marrow suppression. An exercise regimen including aerobic exercise at a minimal level enhances the immune system and is incorporated whenever possible. See also the section in Chapter 8: Cancer and Exercise. ∎

◆ Esophageal Varices

Esophageal varices are dilated veins in the lower third of the esophagus immediately beneath the mucosa (see Fig. 16-4). Dilation occurs in the presence of portal hypertension, usually secondary to cirrhosis of the liver. All the blood from the intestine drains via the portal vein to the liver before passing into the general circulation. Therefore any disease of the liver or portal vein that obstructs the flow of blood will cause expanding force pressure. The normal anatomic reaction to this condition is to decompress the portal venous system by opening up bypass veins (collaterals), most commonly around the lower esophagus and stomach. When blood flow can no longer be counterbalanced by the variceal wall tension the dilated veins (varices) rupture and bleed. Rupture and hemorrhage are common when portal pressure causes the varices to reach a size greater than 5 mm in diameter.

Variceal bleeding usually presents with painless but massive hematemesis with or without melena. Associated signs range from mild postural tachycardia to profound shock, depending on the extent of blood loss and degree of hypovolemia (decreased amount of blood in the body). The clinical picture is frequently consistent with chronic liver disease.

Diagnosis requires differentiation from peptic ulcer, gastritis, and other bleeding sources, often simultaneous conditions in people with cirrhosis secondary to alcoholism. Diagnosis is made by fiberoptic endoscopy. Bleeding varices constitute one of the most common causes of death among people with cirrhosis and other disorders associated with portal hypertension; therefore prevention and treatment are very important to prevent and replace blood loss and maintain intravascular volume.

About half of all episodes of variceal hemorrhage cease without intervention, although a high risk of rebleeding exists. Various prophylactic and therapeutic approaches to management include pharmacologic agents and endoscopic interventions such as band ligation or sclerotherapy (the injection of hardening agents). For bleeding not controlled with these methods a stent may be placed between the hepatic vein and the intrahepatic portion of the portal vein (transjugular intrahepatic portosystemic shunt [TIPS]).[33] This procedure provides a means of lowering portal pressure. Liver transplantation may be considered in cases unresponsive to treatment.[29]

Special Implications for the Therapist 15-5

ESOPHAGEAL VARICES

Preferred Practice Pattern:
7A: Primary Prevention/Risk Reduction for Integumentary Disorders

The primary concerns in therapy are to avoid causing rupture of varices and proper handling of clients with known GI bleeding. Carefully instruct the client in proper lifting techniques and avoid any activities that will increase intraabdominal pressure (see Box 15-1). See also Special Implications for the Therapist: Anemias, 13-4, and the section on Portal Hypertension in Chapter 16. For the client with known esophageal varices, observe closely for signs of behavioral or personality changes. Report increasing stupor, lethargy, hallucinations, or neuromuscular dysfunction. Watch for asterixis (involuntary jerking movements), a sign of developing hepatic encephalopathy (see Fig. 16-1).

To assess fluid retention, inspect the ankles and sacrum for dependent edema. To prevent skin breakdown associated with edema and pruritus, caution the client and family members caring for that person to avoid using soap when bathing and to use moisturizing cleansing agents instead. Precautions must be taken to handle the client gently, turning and repositioning often to keep the skin intact. Rest and good nutrition will conserve energy and decrease metabolic demands on the liver. ■

◆ Congenital
Tracheoesophageal Fistula

Overview. Tracheoesophageal fistula (TEF) is the most common esophageal anomaly and one of the most common congenital defects, occurring in approximately 1 in 4000 live births with equal gender distribution. In this disorder, the esophagus fails to develop as a continuous passage and abnormal communication between the lower portion of the esophagus and trachea occurs, often combined with some form of esophageal atresia, a condition in which the esophagus ends in a blind pouch (Fig. 15-4). Other associated conditions include congenital heart disease, prematurity, and the VATER complex (*v*ertebral defects, imperforate *a*nus, *t*racheoesophageal fistula, and *r*adial and *r*enal dysplasia).

Etiologic Factors and Pathogenesis. As a congenital malformation, the cause is unknown, but abnormalities are postulated to arise from defective differentiation as the trachea separates from the esophagus during the fourth to sixth weeks of embryonic development. Defective growth of endodermal cells leads to atresia (closure or absence of a normal body opening or tubular structure). In 90% of cases, the esophagus ends in a blind pouch with communication between the distal esophagus and the trachea. Less often, the proximal esophagus communicates with the trachea, or the esophagus is continuous in an H-type fistula.

Clinical Manifestations. The blind end of the proximal esophagus has a capacity of only a few milliliters, so as the infant with esophageal atresia swallows oral secretions, the pouch fills and overflows into the pharynx resulting in excessive drooling and, occasionally, aspiration. If a fistula connects the trachea with the distal esophagus, the abdomen fills with air and becomes distended, which may interfere with breathing. If the fistula connects the proximal esophagus to the trachea, the first feeding after birth will signal a problem. As the infant swallows, the blind end of the esophagus and the mouth fill with fluid that is aspirated into the lungs when the infant tries to take a breath. This triggers a protective cough and the choke reflex with intermittent cyanosis.

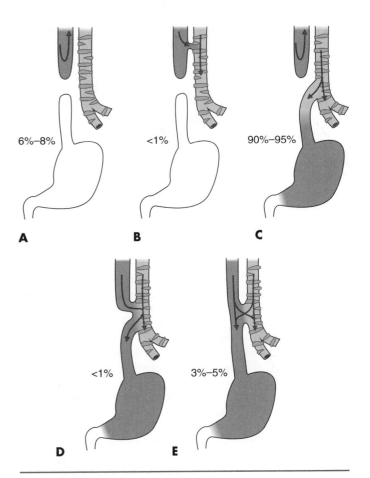

FIGURE 15-4 Five types of esophageal atresia and tracheoesophageal fistula. **A,** Simple esophageal atresia. Proximal and distal esophagus end in blind pouches. Nothing enters the stomach; regurgitated food and fluid may enter the lungs. **B,** Proximal and distal esophageal segments ends in blind pouches, and a fistula connects the proximal esophagus to the trachea. Nothing enters the stomach; food and fluid enter the lungs. **C,** Proximal esophagus ends in a blind pouch, and a fistula connects the trachea to the distal esophagus. Air enters the stomach; regurgitated gastric secretions enter the lungs through the fistula. **D,** Fistula connects both proximal and distal esophageal segments to the trachea. Air, food, and fluid enter the stomach and lungs. **E,** Simple tracheoesophageal fistula between otherwise normal esophagus and trachea. Air, food, and fluid enter the stomach and lungs. Between 90% and 95% of esophageal anomalies are type C; 6% to 8% are type A; 3% to 5% are type E; and less than 1% are type B or D.

Coughing, choking, and cyanosis are called the three Cs of TEF and may occur especially with the H-type fistula, which may not be diagnosed for weeks to months after birth.

Medical Management

Diagnosis, Treatment, and Prognosis. Esophageal anomalies are usually diagnosed at birth on the basis of clinical manifestations, but new technology is making in utero diagnosis more readily available. Occasionally this condition escapes detection until adulthood when recurrent pulmonary infections call attention to it. Confirmation of the non–H type is made by passing a catheter into the esophagus with radiographs of the chest and abdomen taken with the tube in place to show the level of the blind pouch. Fluoroscopy using radiopaque fluid also may be used to establish the diagnosis.

Surgical treatment to restore esophageal continuity and eliminate the fistula usually is performed shortly after birth. Surgical procedures may be performed in stages for infants who are premature, have multiple anomalies, or are in poor health. Antibiotics are instituted early owing to the certainty of aspiration pneumonia.

Without early diagnosis and treatment this condition is rapidly fatal. Early detection prevents feedings, which could cause aspiration and its complications. The survival rate is nearly 100% in full-term infants without severe respiratory distress or other anomalies. In premature, low–birth-weight infants with associated anomalies, the incidence of complications is high. The overall mortality rate is 10% to 15%.

THE STOMACH

◆ Gastritis

Definition and Incidence. Gastritis, inflammation of the lining of the stomach (gastric mucosa), is not a single disease but represents a group of the most common stomach disorders. Gastric erosions by definition are limited to the mucosa and do not extend beneath the muscularis mucosae. Based on clinical features, gastritis can be classified as *acute* or *chronic*. Other classifications may be made according to clinical, endoscopic, radiographic, or pathologic criteria. *Acute gastritis* may be hemorrhagic or acute-erosive, reflecting the presence of bleeding from the gastric mucosa. Gastric erosions and sites of hemorrhage may be distributed diffusely throughout the gastric mucosa or localized to the body of the stomach.

Chronic gastritis has two forms classified as types A and B. Type A gastritis is the less common form of chronic gastritis, associated with pernicious anemia, and is possibly an autoimmune disorder. The most severe type of chronic gastritis, chronic fundal gastritis, occurs in association with autoimmune diseases such as diabetes, Addison's disease, and thyroid disease, also suggesting an autoimmune mechanism. Type B, the more common form of chronic gastritis, is caused by chronic bacterial infection by *Helicobacter pylori*.

Etiologic Factors. Acute erosive gastritis may develop without apparent cause but is more likely to occur in association with serious illness or with various medications such as aspirin or other NSAIDs, that can produce acute gastric mucosal erosions. GI complications occur only in a small percentage of people taking NSAIDs, but the widespread use of these agents results in a substantial number of people affected. Most susceptible persons are those 65 years of age or older, especially those who have a history of ulcer disease. Other risk factors include taking NSAIDs longer than 3 months, taking high-dose or multiple NSAIDs, and concurrent corticosteroid therapy. Acute erosive gastritis associated with physiologic stress, often referred to as *stress-induced gastritis*, is associated with hospitalization for severe life-threatening disease, central nervous system (CNS) injury, or trauma (particularly burns but also renal failure, mechanical ventilation, sepsis, and hepatic failure).

No persuasive evidence exists that acute gastric mucosal injury associated with stress, alcohol, aspirin, or other NSAIDs progresses to chronic gastritis. *H. pylori* is a primary risk factor in the development of chronic gastritis, but other risk factors include aging, vitamin deficiencies, abnormalities of the gastric juice, hiatal hernia, or a combination of any of these.

Pathogenesis. Agents known to injure the gastric mucosa (e.g., *H. pylori*, aspirin or other NSAIDs, bile acids, pancreatic enzymes, alcohol) alter the mucosal defense mechanism leading to *acute gastritis*. The mechanism of mucosal injury is unclear and probably multifactorial. The most commonly accepted theory for agent-induced mucosal injury is the suppression of endogenous prostaglandins that normally stimulate the protective secretion of mucus.

The pathogenesis of *chronic gastritis* has three phases. Superficial gastritis is the initial stage with inflammation limited to the upper epithelial half of the gastric mucosa. Atrophic gastritis, the second stage, takes place as the inflammatory process extends to the deep portions of the mucosa with progressive distortion and destruction of the gastric glands. Pepsinogen, hydrochloric acid, and intrinsic factor* are diminished, and the feedback mechanism that normally inhibits gastrin secretions is impaired, causing elevated plasma levels of gastrin. The final stage, gastric atrophy, involves a profound loss of the glandular structures with thinning of the mucosa.

Clinical Manifestations. The most noticeable symptom of acute gastritis is epigastric pain with a feeling of abdominal distention, loss of appetite, and nausea. Pain is much less common with erosive gastritis than with ulcer disease; painless GI hemorrhage is frequently the only clinical manifestation. Additional symptoms may include heartburn, low-grade fever, and vomiting. Occult (no visible evidence) GI bleeding commonly occurs, especially in cases of trauma and in people taking aspirin or other NSAIDs. Chronic gastritis may be asymptomatic, or pain may occur after eating accompanied by indigestion.

Medical Management

Diagnosis, Treatment, and Prognosis. The diagnosis of gastritis may be made by a careful history, but confirmation is made by upper endoscopic examination, possibly including biopsy because epigastric pain may be due to peptic ulcer, gastroesophageal reflux, gastric cancer, biliary tract disease, food poisoning, and viral gastroenteritis.

Management of this condition requires avoidance of identified irritating substances (e.g., caffeine, nicotine, alcohol) combined with the use of proton pump inhibitors (PPIs), antacids, and/or H_2-blocking agents to block or reduce gastric acid secretion and minimize stomach acidity. Vitamin B_{12} is administered to correct pernicious anemia when it develops secondary to chronic gastritis. Because people taking NSAIDs and those in intensive care units have a high incidence of erosive gastritis, preventive therapy may be used to reduce mucosal injury.

Prognosis is good for both acute and chronic gastritis, especially with removal of the predisposing factor for acute gastritis. The risk of gastric cancer is known to be high in people with chronic gastritis and particularly in those with atrophic gastritis.

---

*As mentioned under Aging and the Gastrointestinal System, IF is a glycoprotein secreted by the gastric glands that plays an important role in the absorption of vitamin B_{12}. IF deficiency resulting in vitamin B_{12} deficiency may lead to pernicious anemia.

◆ Peptic Ulcer Disease

Definition and Overview.   An ulcer is a break in the protective mucosal lining exposing submucosal areas to gastric secretions. The word *peptic* refers to pepsin, a proteolytic enzyme, the principal digestive component of gastric juice, which acts as a catalyst in the chemical breakdown of protein. Acute lesions of the mucosa that do not extend through the muscularis mucosae are referred to as *erosions*. Chronic ulcers involve the muscular coat, destroying the musculature and replacing it with permanent scar tissue at the site of healing. Ulcers extending to the muscularis mucosae damage blood vessels, causing hemorrhage (Fig. 15-5).

Two kinds of peptic ulcer exist: the *gastric ulcer* (GU), which affects the lining of the stomach and the *duodenal ulcer* (DU), which occurs in the duodenum. DUs are two to three times more common than GUs although these ulcers can coexist. About 95% of DUs occur in the duodenal bulb or cap. About 60% of benign GUs are located at or near the lesser curvature and most frequently on the posterior wall (Fig. 15-6).

Stress ulcers, or secondary ulcers, occur in response to prolonged psychologic or physiologic stress (e.g., severe trauma, surgery, extensive burns, brain injury), causing an upset in the aggressive-defensive balance (see the section on Pathogenesis

of Peptic Ulcer Disease). For example, gastric mucosal changes develop within 72 hours in 80% of clients with greater than 35% burns. The mechanism causing stress ulcers is unknown but probably involves ischemia of the gastric mucosa, which has large oxygen requirements and low gastric pH (high acidity). These ulcers differ pathologically and clinically from peptic ulcer with very few symptoms and are painless until perforation and hemorrhage occur.

Incidence.   The population of the United States experiences about 500,000 new cases of peptic ulcer and 4 million ulcer recurrences per year. Up to 10% of the American population will develop an ulcer at some time in their life. Older age groups, especially middle-aged and older adults, are more likely to develop GUs; the peak incidence for GUs is in the sixth decade. Approximately 10% to 20% of people with GUs also have DUs. DUs are the most common with an average age at onset in the mid-30s, although DUs can occur at any time (including infancy). In the past, men were more likely than women to develop gastric and duodenal ulcers, but now equal distribution exists between the genders and the overall frequency of DU has been decreasing in the United States, especially in males.

Etiologic and Risk Factors.   In 90% of all ulcers (as well as for chronic gastritis), *Helicobacter pylori* infection is the most important risk factor for and cause of this condition. Gastric ulcers also can be caused by the effects of nonsteroidal antiinflammatory drugs (NSAIDs), and a connection between these two risk factors has been proposed, but this remains unproved.[39] The long-term use of NSAIDs has deleterious effects on the entire GI tract, from the esophagus to the colon, although the most obvious clinical effect is on the gastroduodenal mucosa. The exact mechanism remains unknown, but theoretically these drugs break down the mucous membrane that protects the GI tract by inhibiting the synthesis of gastric mucosal prostaglandins.* This interference with normal mucosal protective mechanisms leads to local injury by allowing stomach acids to dissolve the intestine (for further discussion of the systemic effects of NSAIDs, see Chapter 4; see also Table 4-3 for a list of commonly used NSAIDs).

---

*Prostaglandins have two types of actions: inhibition of acid secretion and enhancement of mucosal resistance to injury by mechanisms independent of acid secretory inhibition, the latter phenomenon being called *cytoprotection*.

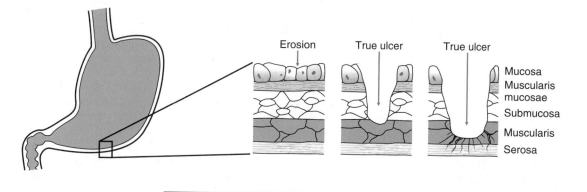

FIGURE   **15-5**   Lesions caused by peptic ulcer disease.

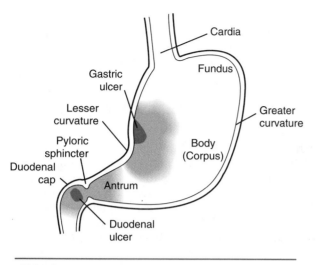

FIGURE **15-6** Most common sites of peptic ulcers.

The majority of recent studies have not found tobacco use or alcohol consumption to be risk factors for *H. pylori* infection although adequate nutritional status, especially frequent consumption of fruits and vegetables and vitamin C appear to be protective.[9] Although *H. pylori* has been identified as a major cause of ulcer disease, not all infected people develop ulcers. This fact suggests that other factors (e.g., lifestyle, psychologic stress) may be critical to the development of ulcers in some people. Individuals with multiple stressors, poor coping skills, and persistent anxiety and depression in the presence of recurrent ulcers lend support to the hypothesis that physiologic changes leading to ulcer can occur secondary to psychologic stress.[48]

Pathogenesis.　Peptic ulcer develops when an unfavorable balance exists between gastric acid and pepsin secretion (aggressive factors) and factors that compromise mucosal defense or mucosal resistance to injury or ulceration. In the pathogenesis of GUs, defective mucosal defense appears to be the major contributing factor, either defective gastric mucosal resistance or direct gastric mucosal injury. In contrast, for DUs evidence favors the importance of relative gastric hypersecretion.

The presence of the *H. pylori* infection induces various humoral and cellular immunities in the gastric mucosa, but the mechanism of *H. pylori*–induced gastroduodenal diseases remains unknown. Prolonged impaired and excessive immuno-inflammatory responses with destruction of the mucosal barrier system appear to be the underlying mechanism for tissue injury.[46] In the case of emotional stress, an increase in gastric secretion, blood supply, and gastric motility by irritation of the vagal nerve stimulates the thalamus. The sympathetic nervous system then causes the blood vessels in the duodenum to constrict, making the mucosa more vulnerable to trauma from gastric acid and pepsin secretion. Multiple chemical, neural, and hormonal factors participate in regulation of gastric acid secretion, making ulcer development a multifactorial process in such cases.

Clinical Manifestations.　The classic symptom of peptic ulcer is epigastric pain described as burning, gnawing, cramping, or aching near the xiphoid, coming in waves that last several minutes. Distention of the duodenal bulb produces epigastric pain, which may radiate to the back. Perforation of the posterior duodenal wall causes steady midline pain in the thoracic spine from T6 to T10 with radiation to the right upper quadrant. The daily pattern of pain is related to the secretion of acid and the presence of food in the stomach (e.g., the presence of food may cause GU pain whereas pain occurs 1 to 3 hours after meals with DUs). Other symptoms include nausea, loss of appetite, and sometimes weight loss. Symptoms may occur for 3 or 4 days or weeks, subsiding only to reappear weeks or months later.

Many people report symptoms outside the classic presentation of DU. Some people are asymptomatic until complications occur; this is especially typical in the older adult as weakened abdominal muscles and diminished pain perception mask early symptoms or present as nonspecific indicators such as mental confusion. Complications may include hemorrhage, perforation, and obstruction accompanied by unremitting pain. Symptoms depend on the severity of the hemorrhage. In mild bleeding, slight weakness and diaphoresis may be the only symptoms. Signs of bleeding include bright-red blood in the vomitus, coffee-ground vomitus, and melena (black, tarry stools).

Medical Management
Diagnosis.　Ulcers are diagnosed on the basis of symptoms and history, although the history is not as characteristic for GU as it is for DU. Appropriate use of one of the many new tests to diagnose *H. pylori* (e.g., serology, urease breath testing, saliva test, biopsy, and culture) can identify those individuals likely to benefit from antimicrobial treatment. Other tests may include barium radiographic examination and gastroscopy (endoscope passed into the stomach) used to determine the site of bleeding and to differentiate between benign and malignant ulcerations.

Prevention and Treatment.　Whether or not anyone who has had an ulcer or chronic indigestion should be tested and treated for *H. pylori* before starting long-term NSAID therapy remains a point of controversy. Using a protective agent with the NSAID may be recommended, especially if long-term use of the NSAID is needed. The smallest effective dose of NSAIDs is recommended, and clients must be warned against adding over-the-counter NSAIDs to a prescription dose.

The primary goals of medical treatment of peptic ulcers are (1) relief of symptoms, (2) promotion of healing, (3) prevention of complications, and (4) prevention of recurrences. Each person responds differently to different treatment modalities, requiring individual treatment planning. In general, GUs tend to heal more slowly than DUs. Antimicrobials (antibiotics) are used in the treatment of *H. pylori* along with proton pump inhibitors, antacids, and histamine H_2-blocking agents (stomach acid suppression or blockers; see discussion of GERD: Treatment) to allow the ulcer to heal completely. There does not appear to be lifelong immunity from *H. pylori* once infected; researchers are working on vaccine development.[65]

No substantial evidence supports dietary modifications as a treatment approach to peptic ulcers although adequate nutrition may be preventive.[9] Bland diets, soft diets, milk and cream diets, diets free of spices or fruit juices have no known effect in reducing gastric acid secretion, relieving symptoms, or promoting ulcer healing. Foods that seem to aggravate a person's symptoms most likely should be avoided. Coffee, caffeinated or not, stimulates gastric acid secretion and should be avoided. Researchers have reported that exercise at least three times a week greatly reduces the risk of GI bleeding. More strenuous forms of exercise such as swimming and bicycling do not provide greater protection from GI bleeding than do more moderate exercises such as walking.[14,49]

Surgical intervention is required for perforation because gastric and intestinal contents spilling into the peritoneal cavity can cause chemical peritonitis, bacterial septicemia, and hypovolemic shock. Peristalsis diminishes and paralytic ileus develops. Outlet obstruction caused by scarring of the duodenum or caudal portion of the stomach may also require surgery.

Prognosis. Prognosis is usually good and medical management can adequately control ulcers unless massive hemorrhage or perforation occurs, which carries a high mortality. Both duodenal and gastric ulcers tend to have a chronic course with remissions and exacerbations. Benign GUs should heal completely within 3 months of treatment. Well-controlled, double-blind studies have shown that curing *H. pylori* usually results in curing DU disease; however, antimicrobial resistance is largely responsible for treatment failure.

Special Implications for the Therapist **15-7**

PEPTIC ULCER DISEASE

Ulcer presentation without pain occurs more frequently in older, aging adults and in persons taking NSAIDs for painful musculoskeletal conditions, especially arthritis. Anyone with this type of medical history should be monitored for signs and symptoms of bleeding. Observe color (pallor), activity or exercise tolerance, and fatigue level. Monitoring vital signs for systolic blood pressure under 100 mm Hg, pulse rate greater than 100 beats per minute, or a 10 mm Hg or more drop in blood pressure with position changes accompanied by increased pulse rate may signal bleeding. Any client complaining of GI symptoms should be encouraged to report these findings to his or her physician. Musculoskeletal symptoms may recur after discontinuing the NSAIDs owing to the masking effects of these drugs. Once the drug is discontinued, painful symptoms may return in the presence of continued underlying ulcer disease. Medical follow-up is required in such situations.

Peptic ulcers located on the posterior wall of the stomach or duodenum can perforate and hemorrhage, causing back pain as the only presenting symptom. Occasionally ulcer pain radiates to the midthoracic back and right upper quadrant, including the right shoulder. Right shoulder pain alone may occur as a result of blood in the peritoneal cavity from perforation and hemorrhage. When back pain appears to be the only presenting symptom, a careful history may reveal alternating or concomitant GI symptoms such as vomiting of bright-red blood or coffee-ground vomitus. Back pain relieved by antacids is an indication of GI involvement and must be reported to the physician as well as any other indication of shoulder or back pain with accompanying gastrointestinal involvement.

For the competitive athlete, during the acute episode, anxiety and nervousness may increase gastric secretions. This effect in combination with poor nutrition (often the athlete has not eaten at all) requires careful monitoring and maximizing the use of medications and food intake with the performance schedule. For the average adult uninvolved in competitive sports, regular exercise as part of stress reduction is essential during remission. ∎

◆ Gastric Cancer

Primary Gastric Lymphoma. The stomach is a common site for extranodal disease associated with lymphoma, but primary lymphoma of the stomach is relatively uncommon. Occurring most often during the sixth decade of life, it is characterized by epigastric pain, early satiety, and fatigue. Clinically, primary gastric lymphoma does not differ significantly in its presentation from adenocarcinoma.

Gastric Adenocarcinoma

Definition and Incidence. Adenocarcinoma, a malignant neoplasm arising from the gastric mucosa, constitutes more than 90% of the malignant tumors of the stomach. In 2001, 21,700 new cases of stomach cancer were diagnosed in the United States and 12,800 Americans died from this disease.[31] This reflects a continued significant decline in incidence for unknown reasons but most likely attributed to improved sanitation and drinking water decreasing transmission of the *H. pylori* bacteria. Men over the age of 40 years are most likely to develop this disease, with a sharp increase in incidence after 50 years.

Etiologic and Risk Factors. Chronic gastritis with intestinal metaplasia, possibly secondary to chronic *H. Pylori* infection, is a strong risk factor for gastric cancer especially when combined with family history of gastric cancer. Other nonenvironmental risk factors include individual susceptibility, pernicious anemia, which causes atrophy of the gastric mucosa in the same locations where gastric tumors arise, type A blood, gastrectomy, gastric polyps, dietary factors such as smoked fish and meat containing benzopyrene, and nitrosamines produced endogenously in chronic gastritis.

Pathogenesis. Gastric carcinoma is a multistep and multifactorial process beginning with *H. pylori* in most cases, but the underlying mechanisms remain to be defined. The most common site for adenocarcinomas appears to be the glands of the stomach mucosa located in the distal portion of the stomach on the lesser curvature of the prepyloric antrum (see Fig. 15-6). Duodenal reflux and insufficient acid secretion may contribute to intestinal metaplasia. The reflux contains caustic bile salts that destroy the normally protective mucosal barrier in the stomach. Insufficient acid secretion by the atrophic mucosa creates an alkaline environment that permits bacteria to multiply and act on nitrates. The resulting increase in nitrosamines damages the DNA of mucosal cells further, promoting metaplasia and neoplasia.

Clinical Manifestations. The clinical presentation of gastric carcinoma depends on a variety of factors, including the morphologic characteristics of the tumor (e.g., infiltrating vs. ulcerating), size of the tumor, presence of gastric outlet obstruction, and metastatic vs. nonmetastatic disease. Early stages of gastric cancer may be asymptomatic or present with vague symptoms of indigestion, anorexia, and weight loss similar to peptic ulcer because ulceration can occur with gastric carcinoma.

Medical Management

Diagnosis. Diagnosis may be delayed by the fact that symptomatic relief can be obtained from early GI symptoms using over-the-counter medications. The choice of diagnostic tests depends on the clinical manifestation at the time of presentation. Endoscopy with cytologic brushings and biopsies of suspicious lesions are highly sensitive for detecting gastric carcinoma. In areas of high incidence, screening upper endoscopy is performed to detect early gastric carcinoma. Once the diagnosis has been made, staging to determine the local extent of disease and the presence of nodal or distant metastases must be done. Staging is accomplished through the use of liver chemistry tests, abdominal imaging studies (e.g., CT scan), and biopsy of suspected lymph nodes.

Treatment. Surgical therapy is still the treatment of choice for primary gastric adenocarcinoma. Despite many attempts, the postoperative strategies of adjuvant chemotherapy have been ineffective. Multimodality treatment consisting of preoperative chemotherapy and surgery may provide improved results if endoscopic ultrasonography and staging laparoscopy provide early identification of locally advanced tumors. Prevention using eradication of H. pylori is recommended only in individuals with high risk of cancer at this time.

Prognosis. Prognosis depends on the degree of gastric wall penetration, the presence of lymph node metastases, and the location of the primary site. Screening programs in other countries detect approximately 40% of tumors early with a 5-year survival rate of more than 60%. Without screening, the prognosis is poor because symptoms do not occur until the tumor has penetrated muscle layers of the stomach, spread to local tissue by direct extension in the abdominal cavity, metastasized via the lymphatic system, or created a paraneoplastic manifestation (e.g., Trousseau's syndrome,* dermatomyositis, and acanthosis nigricans†). Metastatic gastric carcinoma is currently incurable. Surgical resection is only possible in one third of gastric cancers. Of those people in whom surgical resection is a possibility, 20% survive 10 years.

(Virchow's) lymph node, or the client may point out an umbilical nodule.

After surgery, position changes every 2 hours, deep breathing, coughing, and incentive spirometry (handheld device used to provide visual feedback for voluntary maximal inspiration) may be used to prevent pulmonary complications. The semi-Fowler position (head of the bed raised 6 to 12 inches with knees slightly flexed) facilitates breathing and drainage after any type of gastrectomy. ■

◆ Congenital

Pyloric Stenosis

Definition and Overview. Pyloric stenosis (PS) is an obstruction at the pyloric sphincter (the sphincter at the distal opening of the stomach into the duodenum). The pyloric sphincter is a ring of muscles that serve to close the opening from the stomach into the intestine (Fig. 15-7). Obstruction occurs as a congenital condition, or in adults the most common cause is ulcer disease. When present as a congenital condition, it is known as *hypertrophic PS* caused by hypertrophy of the sphincter and is one of the most common surgical disorders of early infancy.

Incidence and Etiologic Factors. The cause of congenital hypertrophy of the pyloric sphincter is unknown. White males are affected more commonly than females in a 4:1 ratio. It is more likely to occur in a full-term infant than in a premature infant, especially the first-born child. Siblings, offspring of affected persons, and fathers and sons are at increased risk of developing PS (genetic predisposition). Prophylactic administration of erythromycin to newborns exposed to neonatal pertussis has been reported as a possible causal role in infantile pyloric stenosis.[13] The role of H. pylori as a cause of infantile hypertrophic pyloric stenosis is under investigation.[50]

Increased third-trimester maternal gastric secretion associated with maternal stress-related factors increases the likelihood of PS in the infant. PS may also be associated with other congenital conditions such as Turner's syndrome, trisomy 18, intestinal malrotation, esophageal and duodenal atresia, and anorectal anomalies.

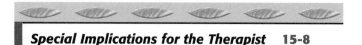

Special Implications for the Therapist 15-8

GASTRIC CANCER

Epigastric or back pain, possibly relieved by antacids, is a frequent complaint that the physician must differentiate from peptic ulcer disease. Generally the first manifestations of carcinoma are caused by distant metastasis when the condition is quite advanced. The therapist may palpate the left supraclavicular

---

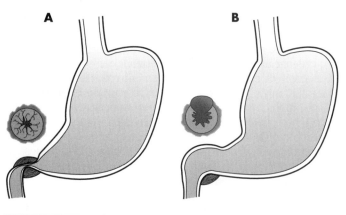

FIGURE 15-7 Hypertrophic pyloric stenosis. **A,** Enlarged muscular area nearly obliterates the pyloric channel. **B,** Longitudinal surgical division of muscle down to the submucosa or the placement of an expandable stent (not shown) establishes an adequate passageway.

---

*Spontaneous peripheral venous thrombosis of the upper and lower extremities that occurs in association with visceral carcinoma.

†A skin condition associated with an internal carcinoma characterized by diffuse thickening of the skin with gray, brown, or black pigmentation, usually in body folds such as the axillae.

The incidence of adult idiopathic PS is unknown but is considered rare. Although many physicians believe this condition is secondary to local disease, others think the condition in adults is the same entity as that observed in infants and children, but in a milder form and later in appearance.

Pathogenesis. The histologic and anatomic abnormalities in adult PS are indistinguishable from those in the infantile form. Individual fibers of the pyloric sphincter thicken or hypertrophy, so the entire sphincter is grossly enlarged and inelastic. Hyperplasia of the pyloric muscle occurs because of the extra peristaltic effort required to force the gastric contents through the narrow opening into the duodenum. This hypertrophy and hyperplasia form a palpable nodule severely narrowing the pyloric canal between the stomach and the duodenum, causing partial obstruction. Over time, inflammation and edema further reduce the size of the lumen, progressing to complete obstruction preventing food from passing from the stomach to the small intestine. Progressive obstruction results in complications of malnutrition and fluid and electrolyte abnormalities.

Clinical Manifestations. Projectile vomiting* is the most common and dramatic early symptom and may occur at birth. Overall, the age of onset and pattern of vomiting varies, but usually regurgitation or occasional projectile vomiting develops around the second to fourth week after birth. Projectile vomiting quickly leads to dehydration and lethargy with rapid progression to complete obstruction and the accompanying complications of malnutrition, weakness, wasting, weight loss, and fluid and electrolyte imbalances. The palpable nodule is firm, movable, about the size of an olive, and felt in the right upper quadrant in approximately 80% of all infants with PS. Persistent or episodic symptoms in some adults may extend from infancy with nausea and vomiting, epigastric pain, weight loss, and anorexia most commonly present. In contrast to congenital PS in the infant, the abdominal mass that occurs in adult PS is too small to be palpable.

Medical Management

Diagnosis, Treatment, and Prognosis. In infancy, diagnosis is usually by history and recognition of the clinical presentation. Ultrasound imaging is so accurate for the diagnosis of pyloric stenosis that it has replaced the upper GI series in most institutions. Some infants are treated with antispasmodic drugs to relax the pylorospasm and nutritional management, including refeeding the infant after vomiting, hoping that the pylorus spontaneously opens by 6 to 8 months of age. Surgical repair, including endoscopic balloon dilations, pyloromyotomy (local resection of the involved region of the pylorus), and pyloroplasty, is the standard medical treatment with a very high success rate for the infant and the adult (see Fig. 15-7). Placement of a stent at the site of obstruction is gaining popularity as an alternative intervention procedure. Postoperative vomiting is not uncommon in the pediatric population, especially during the first 24 to 48 hours. Complications include persistent pyloric obstruction; partial, superficial, or total wound separation (dehiscence); or in the case of stent implantation, stent migration.

---

*Projectile vomiting describes forcible vomiting that ejects vomitus 1 foot or more when in a supine position and 3 to 4 feet when in an upright or side-lying position.

THE INTESTINES

◆ Malabsorption Syndrome
Definition and Overview. Malabsorption syndrome is a group of disorders (celiac disease, cystic fibrosis, Crohn's disease, chronic pancreatitis, pancreatic carcinoma, pernicious anemia, short-gut syndrome) characterized by reduced intestinal absorption of dietary components and excessive loss of nutrients in the stool. Traditionally, malabsorption disorders have been classified as *maldigestion* (failure of the chemical processes of digestion) or *malabsorption* (failure of the intestinal mucosa to absorb the digested nutrients). Nutrients most commonly malabsorbed include fat, fatty acids or bile salts, calories (fat, protein, carbohydrates), iron, vitamin B_{12}, folic acid, calcium, vitamin D, magnesium, potassium, vitamin K, water, and lactose (sugar in milk).

Both conditions can occur separately or together simultaneously. *Digestive defects* include cystic fibrosis, in which pancreatic enzymes are absent, biliary or liver diseases with altered bile flow, and lactase deficiency, in which a congenital or secondary lactose intolerance occurs. *Absorptive defects* may be primary such as celiac disease or secondary to inflammatory disease of the bowel with the concomitant accelerated bowel motility and impaired absorption (e.g., ulcerative colitis, Crohn's disease).

Etiologic Factors and Pathogenesis. Clients in a therapy practice affected by malabsorption most often include people who develop gastroenteritis secondary to NSAID use, fibrosis caused by progressive systemic sclerosis or radiation injury, drug-induced malabsorption, exocrine deficiency of the pancreas caused by diabetes mellitus, and short-gut syndrome. Short-gut syndrome (short-bowel syndrome) is the malabsorptive state that often follows extensive resection of the small intestine or more rarely, congenital shortening of the bowel structures. Hyperabsorption of substances (e.g., vitamin D, calcium) also can occur with the intake of excessive amounts of calcium carbonate (Tums) for acid indigestion.

Generally, maldigestion is caused by deficiencies of enzymes (e.g., pancreatic lipase) and specific defects (e.g., poor digestion, lactose intolerance). Inadequate secretion of bile salts (e.g., advanced liver disease, obstruction of the common bile duct) and inadequate reabsorption of bile in the ileum also contribute to maldigestion. In the case of inadequate absorption, food is fully digested but not adequately absorbed. This situation occurs when the absorptive surface is normal but inadequate, or adequate but not functioning normally. This problem occurs within the mucosal cell and may be highly specific owing to a gene defect. Malabsorption syndrome also can be caused by a digestive defect, a mucosal abnormality, or lymphatic obstruction and can be a generalized malabsorption or an isolated malabsorption of a particular nutrient.

Clinical Manifestations. Early manifestations of malabsorption are progressive and not easily noticed by the person affected. Weight loss, fatigue, depression, and abdominal bloating are early symptoms. A change in bowel habits may occur with production of bulky, malodorous oil–covered stools (steatorrhea) that are difficult to flush. Excessive nocturnal reabsorption of intestinal fluids may cause nocturia. A gluten-related skin disorder, dermatitis herpetiformis, also may be present.

Other common signs and symptoms include explosive diarrhea, chronic diarrhea, abdominal cramps and bloating, indigestion, and flatulence. Late manifestations caused by nutritional deficiencies secondary to the malabsorption may include muscle wasting owing to diminished muscle mass, changes in bone mineral density secondary to impaired absorption of calcium, phosphate, and/or vitamin D, low blood pressure, and abdominal distention with active bowel sounds.

Any cause of decreased intrinsic factor can result in decreased absorption of vitamin B_{12} resulting in pernicious anemia. Other clinical findings are dependent on the particular condition or specific nutrient involved. The therapist is most likely to see the symptoms listed in Table 15-4.

Medical Management

Diagnosis. Differentiation among the various causes of malabsorption is important in determination of the specific treatment. A large number of diagnostic tests are available (e.g., fecal fat analysis for fat malabsorption, oral tolerance tests and measurement of breath hydrogen for lactose intolerance, other breath tests to detect the presence of compounds produced by intraluminal bacteria). Specific tests are also available to assess pancreatic insufficiency. Biopsy of the small intestinal mucosa may be necessary. Sometimes clinical trials for treatable conditions are diagnostic (e.g., gluten-free diet for celiac disease, antibiotics for bacterial overgrowth, use of over-the-counter preparations of lactase enzyme for lactose intolerance).

Treatment and Prognosis. Therapy depends on the underlying condition such as avoidance of gluten for celiac disease or replacement of pancreatic enzymes for pancreatic insufficiency (cystic fibrosis). Probiotics, live microbial food supplements that beneficially affect the host by improving intestinal microbial balance, alleviating lactose intolerance, and enhancing immune function are being investigated in the treatment of malabsorption syndromes (and other gastrointestinal-related conditions).[37] Muscular twitching and tetany are treated with calcium phosphate or gluconate administered orally or intravenously. In severe cases total parenteral nutrition (TPN)* may be the only treatment option,

---

*Parenteral nutrition (sometimes called *hyperalimentation*) is a technique for meeting a person's nutritional needs by means of intravenous feedings, allowing bowel rest. Nutrition by intravenous feeding is administered via a central venous catheter, usually inserted into the superior vena cava and may be TPN or supplemental. TPN also may be given peripherally for short periods of time.

as in the case of reduced absorptive surface (e.g., short-gut syndrome).

The prognosis is good for any of these conditions if the underlying defect can be corrected. A slightly higher incidence of non–Hodgkin's lymphoma in adult life may occur with untreated gluten-sensitive enteropathy. Anyone who develops GI symptoms while in remission on a gluten-free diet should be evaluated for cancer.

People with celiac disease have a greater risk of developing other related immune system disorders. Genes that make a person more susceptible to celiac disease also are known to be connected with autoimmune disorders, including insulin-dependent diabetes mellitus (IDDM, type 1), systemic lupus erythematosus, Sjögren's syndrome, scleroderma, autoimmune chronic active hepatitis, Graves' disease, Addison's disease, and myasthenia gravis.

Special Implications for the Therapist   15-9

MALABSORPTION SYNDROME

Preferred Practice Patterns:
4A: Primary Prevention/Risk Reduction for Skeletal Demineralization
4C: Impaired Muscle Performance (decreased muscle mass; muscle atrophy)
5E: Impaired Motor Function and Sensory Integrity Associated With Progressive Disorders of the Central Nervous System
5F: Impaired Peripheral Nerve Integrity and Muscle Performance Associated With Peripheral Nerve Injury (carpal tunnel syndrome associated with vitamin B_{12} deficiency)

In the rehabilitation setting or for the acute care client who has not been eating solid foods, diarrhea may develop when the person begins to reestablish a normal diet. Prolonged viral conditions can wash out the enzymes normally present in the columnar epithelial cells. Reestablishing normal eating may require additional time to restore the enzymatic homeostasis in the intestines. Paresthesias, muscle weakness, and muscle wasting accompanied by fatigue and weight loss can be signs of malnutrition (e.g., eating disorders) or malabsorbed fat, protein,

---

TABLE	15-4

Symptoms Associated With Malabsorption

SYMPTOMS	MALABSORBED NUTRIENTS
Muscle weakness, muscle wasting, paresthesias	Generalized malnutrition; fat, protein, carbohydrates
Osteomalacia	Fat, protein, carbohydrates, iron, water; vitamins A, D, K
Tetany, paresthesias, Trousseau's sign, Chvostek's sign	Calcium, vitamin D, magnesium, potassium
Numbness and tingling; neurologic damage	Vitamin B_{12}, vitamin B
Bone pain, fractures, skeletal deformities	Calcium, vitamin D, protein
Muscle spasms	Electrolyte imbalance, calcium, pregnancy
Easy bleeding or bruising	Vitamin K
Generalized swelling	Protein

or carbohydrates. Malabsorption of calcium, vitamin D, magnesium, and potassium can cause paresthesias, tetany, and positive Trousseau's and Chvostek's signs* (see Figs. 4-2 and 4-3). Other effects of malabsorption syndrome possibly seen in a therapy setting include muscle spasms caused by electrolyte imbalance (especially low calcium) and pregnancy, easy bleeding or bruising as a result of a vitamin K deficiency, and generalized swelling caused by protein depletion (see Table 15-4).

Malabsorption of calcium, vitamin D, and protein can cause bone pain with pathologic (compression) fractures and skeletal deformities. In fact, 20% of osteoporosis is osteomalacia secondary to decreased absorption of vitamin D (see discussions of osteomalacia and osteoporosis in Chapter 23).[62] On the other hand, excessive absorption of vitamin D and calcium through the use of calcium carbonate for acid indigestion should be evaluated by a physician; these antacids may be used by women to obtain the daily 1500 mg calcium requirement as protection against osteoporosis. The therapist can direct education and intervention toward prevention and treatment of these related conditions.

Physicians may recommend vitamin B_{12} or other B vitamin supplements for people with carpal tunnel syndrome. Malabsorption of these essential vitamins alters the structure and disrupts the function of the peripheral nerves, spinal cord, and brain and can cause numbness and tingling and permanent neurologic damage unresponsive to vitamin B_{12} therapy in extreme cases. ∎

for 1 to 3 hours in a person over 45 years of age who has peripheral vascular disease points to a diagnosis of intestinal ischemia. Arteriography may be performed if the person is a good candidate for surgery.

Special Implications for the Therapist   15-10

INTESTINAL ISCHEMIA

Preferred Practice Patterns:
6B: *Impaired Aerobic Capacity/Endurance Associated With Deconditioning (peripheral vascular disease, unspecified); see also the section on PVD in Chapter 11*
7A: *Primary Prevention/Risk Reduction for Integumentary Disorders*

Intestinal angina as a result of atherosclerotic plaque–induced ischemia can result in intermittent back pain (usually at the thoracolumbar junction) with exertion. Clinical presentation combined with past medical history, the presence of coronary artery disease risk factors (see Table 11-2), and the presence of peripheral vascular disease may alert the therapist to the need for a medical referral if the client has not been medically diagnosed. ∎

◆ Vascular Diseases

Blood is supplied to the bowel by the celiac and superior and inferior mesenteric arteries. These arteries have anastomotic intercommunications at the head of the pancreas and along the transverse bowel. Obstruction of blood flow can occur as a result of atherosclerotic occlusive lesions or embolism.

Intestinal Ischemia.   *Acute intestinal ischemia* results from embolic occlusions of the visceral branches of the abdominal aorta, generally in people with valvular heart disease, atrial fibrillation, or left ventricular thrombus. Other causes include thrombosis of one or more visceral vessels involved with arteriosclerotic occlusive changes or nonocclusive mesenteric vascular insufficiency in people with congestive heart failure receiving recently instituted digitalis.

Symptoms of acute intestinal ischemia include rapid onset of crampy or steady epigastric or periumbilical abdominal pain combined with minimal or no findings on abdominal examination and a high leukocyte count. Angiography of the superior mesenteric artery is essential to early diagnosis. If occlusion is present, laparotomy is performed to reestablish blood flow to the intestine if possible and to remove necrotic bowel if some viable bowel exists.

Atherosclerotic plaque of the superior mesenteric, celiac, and inferior mesenteric arteries causes a significant decrease in blood flow to the intestines resulting in chronic intestinal ischemia. Symptoms of epigastric or periumbilical pains lasting

◆ Bacterial Infections

Botulism.   Botulism, once considered a rare disease, has become a serious public health problem. The Centers for Disease Control and Prevention report that each year 76 million people get sick, more than 300,000 are hospitalized, and 5000 deaths occur as a result of foodborne illnesses, primarily among the very young, the older adult, and the immunocompromised.[41] It is estimated that only a fraction of the people who experience gastrointestinal tract symptoms from foodborne illnesses actually seek medical care. Recent changes in human demographics, food preferences, changes in food production and distribution systems, microbial adaptation, and lack of support for public health resources have led to the emergence of novel in addition to traditional foodborne diseases. Increasing travel and trade opportunities have increased the risk of contracting and spreading foodborne illness locally, regionally, and globally.[43]

Only foodborne botulism is discussed here; see Chapter 38 for a complete discussion of the effects of botulism on the peripheral nervous system. Most cases of foodborne illness or death are caused by unknown or unidentified microorganisms. Botulism is caused by known agents; most result from *Escherichia coli* and *Campylobacter*, *Listeria*, and *Salmonella* species linked to milk, shellfish, unpasteurized apple cider, eggs, fish, meats, and some fruits.[42] Once ingested these neurotoxins resist gastric digestion and proteolytic enzymes and are readily absorbed into the blood from the proximal small intestine. Minute amounts of circulating toxin reach the cholinergic nerve endings at the myoneural junction and bind to the presynaptic nerve terminals. Flaccid paralysis is caused by inhibition of acetylcholine release from cholinergic terminals at the motor end plate. A predilection exists for the cra-

---

*Trousseau's sign is an indication of tetany seen as carpal spasm elicited by compressing the upper arm (as occurs when taking a blood pressure measurement). Chvostek's sign is a spasm of the facial muscles elicited by tapping the facial nerve in the region of the parotid gland; it is seen in tetany.

nial nerves with progression caudally and symmetrically to the trunk and extremities.

In addition to GI symptoms of prolonged bloody diarrhea leading to dehydration, weight loss, fever, nausea, and severe abdominal pain, early neurologic involvement includes motor weakness, paresthesias, and cranial nerve palsies with visual changes (double vision or diplopia, and intolerance to light, or photophobia), ptosis, dysarthria or dysphagia, difficulty breathing, and impaired swallowing. No sensory changes occur. Motor weakness of the face and neck muscles can progress to involve the diaphragm, accessory muscles of breathing, and extremities. Vomiting, abdominal pain, back pain, headache, and constipation may occur before or after the onset of paralysis. The usual secondary effects of flaccid motor paralysis can occur, such as severe muscle wasting, pressure ulcers, and aspiration pneumonia.

Toxin identification is made by stool or serum analysis or cultures of the organism. Electromyography is confirmatory* and necessary to differentiate this condition from myasthenia gravis or Guillain-Barré syndrome. Selection of appropriate treatment depends on identification of the responsible pathogen if possible and determining if specific therapy is available. Immediate administration of antitoxin prevents further binding of free botulism to the presynaptic endings. Many episodes of acute gastroenteritis are self-limiting and require fluid replacement and supportive care. Untreated food botulism can be fatal within 24 hours of toxin ingestion. Respiratory failure caused by rapid onset of respiratory muscle weakness is a complication that is often fatal.

Special Implications for the Therapist   15-11

BOTULISM

Preferred Practice Patterns:
5E: Impaired Motor Function and Sensory Integrity Associated With Progressive Disorders of the Central Nervous System
5F: Impaired Peripheral Nerve Integrity and Muscle Performance Associated With Peripheral Nerve Injury (Cranial Nerve Involvement)
7A: Primary Prevention/Risk Reduction for Integumentary Disorders (risk of pressure ulcers secondary to flaccid motor paralysis)

The sudden onset of rapidly progressive symptoms associated with botulism is most likely to be reported to a physician rather than to a therapist. However, presentation of acute symmetric cranial nerve impairment (ptosis, diplopia, dysarthria), followed by descending weakness or paralysis of the muscles in the extremities or trunk with or without back pain, and dyspnea from respiratory muscle paralysis, requires immediate medical referral. After the acute onset and initiation of medical treatment, treatment is as for cranial nerve palsy. In mild to moderate cases, clients experience a gradual recovery of muscle strength that can take as long as a year after disease onset; in severe cases, a 40% mortality rate exists. ■

---

*Nerve conduction velocities are normal but action potentials are decreased with a supramaximal stimulus. Facilitation is found after repetitive stimulation at high frequency.

◆ Inflammatory Bowel Disease

Overview and Definition.   Inflammatory bowel disease (IBD) refers to two inflammatory conditions: Crohn's disease (CD) and ulcerative colitis (UC) (Table 15-5). *Crohn's disease* is a chronic lifelong inflammatory disorder that can affect any segment of the intestinal tract (intestine or ileum, large intestine or colon) and even tissues in other organs. It can affect all layers of the intestine and is characterized by diseased areas of intestine with normal intestine between ("skip" areas) with periods of exacerbation and remission. CD is also referred to as *regional enteritis, regional ileitis, terminal ileitis,* or *granulomatous colitis,* depending on the location of the inflammation.

Ulcerative colitis is a chronic inflammatory disorder of the mucosa and submucosa of the colon in a continuous manner without skips. It is characterized by chronic diarrhea and rectal bleeding with ulceration. It may be referred to as ulcerative proctitis (involving the rectum only) or pancolitis (involving the entire colon).

Incidence and Etiologic Factors.   Both CD and UC are bowel disorders of unknown cause involving genetic and immunologic influences on the GI tract's ability to distinguish foreign from self-antigens. These two conditions can occur in all age groups and affect both genders equally; incidence peaks between the ages of 15 and 35, but Crohn's disease does occur in later decades usually after age 50. An estimated 1 million Americans are affected by IBD with equal distribution between these two conditions.[18]

Although these disorders tend to occur in families, no single genetic marker (i.e., histocompatibility antigen) has been identified yet, preventing early identification of susceptible individuals. Inflammatory bowel conditions are considered to be autoimmune diseases in which either the antibodies or other defense mechanisms are directed against the body. A possible correlation between the onset of disease with life stresses and poor adaptation to those stresses is cited in the majority of literature regarding IBD, but this has not been proved conclusively. More likely, these factors exacerbate the illness but are not a cause of the condition. Autoimmune disorders such as systemic lupus erythematosus and fibromyalgia often accompany IBD.

A growing number of reports have demonstrated a disorder of autonomic function in subgroups of people with functional bowel disorders. Altered autonomic balance (low vagal tone, increased sympathetic activity) may alter visceral perception. Autonomic dysfunction may represent the physiologic pathway accounting for many of the extraintestinal symptoms and frequent GI problems encountered by people with other disorders such as chronic fatigue and fibromyalgia.[66]

Pathogenesis.   Two features distinguish CD from UC. In CD, inflammation usually involves all layers of the bowel wall, referred to as *transmural inflammatory disease,* and the inflammatory process is discontinuous so that segments of inflamed areas are separated by normal tissue in a skip pattern. The transverse colon is affected in half of all cases; other more common sites include the small bowel, colon, and anorectal region. In UC, involvement extends uniformly and continuously, usually starting from the distal part of the rectum.

Inflammation accompanying CD produces thickened, edematous tissue, and chronic inflammation leads to ulcerations, which produce fissures that extend the inflammation into lymphoid tissue. Mesenteric* lymph nodes often are enlarged, firm, and matted together. The lesions are granulomatous (epithelioid cells rimmed by lymphocytes) with projections of inflamed tissue surrounded by fibrous scarring narrowing the intestinal lumen. A combination of the granulomas (nodular swelling), ulceration, and fibrosis results in a cobblestone appearance of the mucosal surface of the colon (Fig. 15-8).

Inflammation of the mucosa associated with UC results in small erosions and subsequent ulcerations with eventual abscess formation and necrosis (Fig. 15-9). Destruction of the mucosa causes bleeding, cramping pain, bowel frequency, and large volumes of watery diarrhea owing to decreased absorption and decreased transit time of intestinal contents through the colon.

Clinical Manifestations.   Clinically, these disorders are characterized by recurrent inflammatory involvement of intestinal segments with diverse clinical manifestations often resulting in a chronic, unpredictable course. For comparison of specific signs and symptoms, see Table 15-5.

Arthritis and Inflammatory Intestinal Diseases.   The
theory that an immune mechanism may be involved in the development of IBD is based in part on the presence of extraintestinal manifestations involving the hematologic, dermatologic, renal, ocular, hepatobiliary, and musculoskeletal systems. Tumor necrosis factor (TNF), an inflammatory cytokine produced by the cells of the immune system, may be implicated in the pathophysiology of Crohn's disease and rheumatoid arthritis. It would appear that proinflammatory and immune-regulatory cytokines are upregulated in the mucosa of individuals with IBD. This knowledge has opened up new avenues of treatment pursuing monoclonal antibodies directed against TNF.

Polyarthritis, migratory arthralgias, and redness of the skin (erythema nodosum) are the most common musculoskeletal/integument impairments. Joint involvement ranging from arthralgia only to acute arthritis is a common finding in IBD (in 25% of clients with IBD). Intestinal arthritis is usually peripheral, monoarticular, affecting the knee, ankle, or wrist, but it can affect any joint and more than one joint. Spondylitis and sacroiliitis also can occur. Joints of the lower extremities are affected more often than those of the upper extremities, and asymmetric inflammation of the proximal interphalangeal joints of the toes is particularly suggestive of enteropathic arthritis.[5] Acute arthritis associated with chronic IBD comes and goes, occurring during the course of the bowel disease or preceding repeat episodes of bowel symptoms by 1 to 2 weeks. The onset of arthritis occurs abruptly and reaches a peak within 48 to 72 hours manifesting as pain, erythema, swelling, and limited range of motion. Peripheral arthritis is usually self-limited, resolves within several months as the underlying disease is treated and without permanent sequelae or joint deformities. Spinal disease runs a course independent of the bowel disease and does not necessarily improve with medical treatment of the underlying IBD.

Pathologically, the synovitis is nonspecific without crystals or evidence of infection. Tests for specific forms of arthritis

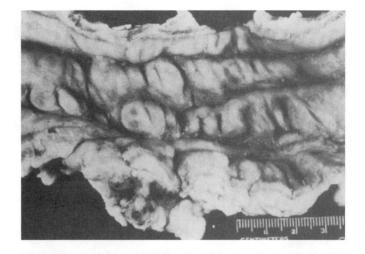

FIGURE **15-8** Crohn's disease. The mucosal surface of the colon displays a cobblestone appearance owing to the presence of linear ulcerations and edema and inflammation of the intervening tissue. (From Marshak R, Lindner A: *Radiology of the small intestine*, Philadelphia, 1976, WB Saunders.)

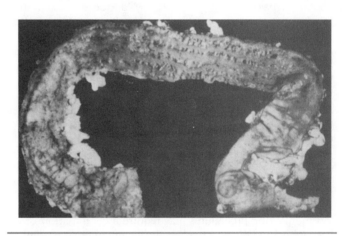

FIGURE **15-9** Ulcerative colitis. Prominent erythema and ulceration affecting the whole colon. (From Sleisenger MH, Fordtran JS, editors: *Gastrointestinal disease*, ed 5, Philadelphia, 1993, WB Saunders, p 1310.)

(e.g., rheumatoid factor and antinuclear antibody) are usually negative; HLA-B27 (*human leukocyte antigen*) is positive* (see explanation of HLA in Chapter 6; see also Table 39-17). Treatment of intestinal arthritis is toward control of the underlying intestinal inflammation; treatment of AS associated with IBD is the same as for idiopathic AS.

Medical Management
Diagnosis and Treatment.   Because no specifically distinctive characteristic features or specific diagnostic tests exist, the diagnosis of CD and UC remains one of exclusion based on medical history and clinical presentation. Diagnostic

---

*The mesentery is a membranous peritoneal fold attaching the small intestine to the dorsal abdominal wall.

*A statistical association has been shown between HLA-B27 and the development of AS.

TABLE	15-5

Comparison of the Characteristics of Crohn's Disease and Ulcerative Colitis

CHARACTERISTICS	CROHN'S DISEASE	ULCERATIVE COLITIS
Incidence		
Age at onset	Any age; 10-30 yr most common	Any age; 10-40 yr most common
Family history	20% to 25%	20%
Gender (prevalence)	Equal in women and men	Equal in women and men
Cancer risk	Increased; early detection best means of prevention	Increased; preventable with bowel resection
Pathogenesis		
Location of lesions	Any segment; usually small or large intestine	Large intestine; rectum
Skip lesions	Common	Absent
Inflammation and ulceration	Entire intestinal wall involved	Mucosal/submucosal layers involved
Granulomas	Typical	Uncommon
Thickened bowel wall	Typical	Uncommon
Narrowed lumen and obstruction	Typical	Uncommon
Fissures and fistulas	Common	Absent
Clinical Manifestations		
Abdominal pain	Mild to severe; common	Mild to severe; less frequent
Diarrhea	May be absent; moderate	Typical; often severe; chronic
Bloody stools	Uncommon	Typical
Abdominal mass	Common; right lower quadrant	Uncommon
Anorexia	Can be severe	Mild or moderate
Weight loss	Can be severe	Mild to moderate
Skin rashes	Common, mild	Common, mild
Joint pain	Common, mild to moderate	Common, mild to moderate
Growth retardation (pediatric)	Often marked	Usually mild
Clinical course	Remissions and exacerbations	Remissions and exacerbations

Modified from Huether SE, McCance KL: Alterations in digestive function. In McCance KL, Huether SE, editors: *Pathophysiology: the biologic basis for disease in adults and children*, St Louis, 1994, Mosby, p 1341.

and monitoring procedures may require a combination of radiographic modalities. Microscopically, granulomas present in CD (but not present in UC) distinguish CD from UC.

Current treatment is directed toward symptomatic relief and control of the disease process on an individual basis. Some treatment measures may include diet and nutrition, symptomatic medications such as antidiarrheals or antispasmodics, or specific drug therapy (e.g., immune modifiers, antibiotics, corticosteroids, aminosalicylates). People with Crohn's disease often have relapses; current investigations are looking for better treatments to maintain remission. A broad range of cytokine-based therapies directed at the mucosa and enteric flora are currently being tested (e.g., anti–tumor necrosis factor, infliximab/Remicade/cA2) in addition to growth hormone, a new glucocorticoid (budesonide), methotrexate, and other agents.[63,70]

Hospitalization may be required in the case of severe, unremitting disease with complications. Surgical resection of the colon, colostomy, or ileostomy may be performed for toxic megacolon or if medical intervention is unsuccessful with complications such as fistula, abscess, or for relief of obstruction. Treatment refractoriness including physiologic resistance to treatment may have its origin in specific individual immunologic peculiarities; researchers are investigating immunologic, biochemical, and clinical parameters to identify a reliable marker predictive of treatment response.[26]

Prognosis. CD is an incurable, chronic, and sometimes debilitating disease with a known increased risk of intestinal cancer in people who develop this condition at a young age of onset (less than 30 years of age). Surgical removal of the diseased bowel does not prevent bowel cancer in CD, so screening of stool specimens and periodic colonoscopic examination and biopsy are required for early detection. With proper medical and surgical treatment, the majority of people are able to cope with this disease and its complications. Few people die as a direct consequence of CD. The mortality rate (5% to 10%) increases with the duration of the disease.

Like CD, UC is a chronic, occasionally debilitating disease. However, it can be cured by colon resection, although this is not always the best course of action. The clinical course is variable but recurrent with long periods of remission possible. Approximately 85% of clients with UC have mild to moderate intermittent disease managed without hospitalization. The remaining 15% demonstrate a full-blown course involving the entire colon, severe diarrhea, and systemic signs and symptoms. A 20% mortality rate exists during the first 10 years of UC when complications occur. Also like CD, 10 years of chronic attacks of UC can predispose the colon to meta-plastic changes leading to colon cancer, but unlike CD, in UC, removal of the affected bowel can prevent bowel cancer.

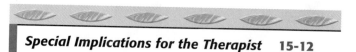

Special Implications for the Therapist   15-12

INFLAMMATORY BOWEL DISEASE

Preferred Practice Patterns:
4A: Primary Prevention/Risk Reduction for Skeletal Demineralization
4D: Impaired Joint Mobility, Motor Function, Muscle Performance, and Range of Motion Associated With Connective Tissue Dysfunction (arthritic component)
4E: Impaired Joint Mobility, Motor Function, Muscle Performance, and Range of Motion Associated With Localized Inflammation (ankylosing spondylitis; psoas abscess)
4F: Impaired Joint Mobility, Motor Function, Muscle Performance, Range of Motion, and Reflex Integrity Associated With Spinal Disorders (ankylosing spondylitis)

When terminal ileum involvement in CD produces periumbilical pain, referred pain to the corresponding low back is possible. Pain of the ileum is intermittent and perceived in the lower right quadrant with possible associated iliopsoas abscess or ureteral obstruction from an inflammatory mass causing hip, thigh, or knee pain, often with an antalgic gait. Specific objective tests are available to rule out systemic origin of hip, thigh, or knee pain (Figs. 15-10 and 15-11; see also Fig. 15-17).

Approximately 25% of all clients with IBD may present with migratory arthralgias, monarthritis, polyarthritis, or sacroiliitis. The joint problems and gastrointestinal disorders may appear simultaneously, the joint problems may manifest first (sometimes even years before bowel symptoms), or intestinal symptoms present along with articular symptoms but are disregarded as part of the whole picture by the client. Any time a client presents with low back, hip, or sacroiliac pain of unknown origin, the therapist must screen for medical disease by asking a few simple questions about the presence of accompanying intestinal symptoms, known personal or family history for IBD, and possible relief of symptoms after passing stool or gas.[28] Joint problems usually respond to treatment of the underlying bowel disease but in some cases require separate management. Interventions for the musculoskeletal involvement follows the usual protocols for each area affected.

The therapist must always know what medications clients are taking so that the first sign of possible side effects will be recognized and the physician alerted. Corticosteroids are an important and effective drug for treating moderate and severe IBD but carry with them all of the complications of prolonged high-dose steroid therapy (see Table 4-7).

People with IBD are known to have low bone mineral content and a high prevalence of osteoporosis. The pathogenesis is not completely understood but is considered multifactorial at this time including possible genetic factors,[61] malabsorption, corticosteroid use, and deficiency of fat-soluble vitamins, among them vitamin K necessary for calcium binding to bone.[60] Low

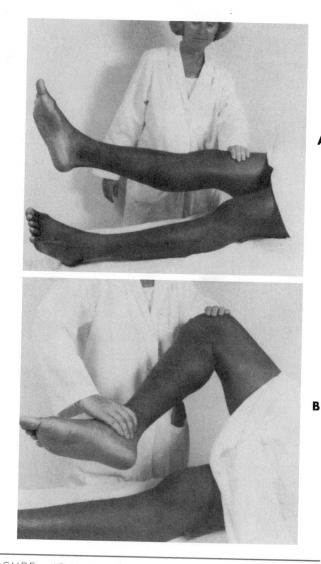

FIGURE **15-10** Muscle tests. **A,** Iliopsoas muscle test. With the client supine, instruct the client to lift the right leg straight up; apply resistance to the distal thigh as the client tries to hold the leg up. When the test is negative, the client feels no change; when the test is positive (i.e., the iliopsoas muscle is inflamed or abscessed), pain is felt in the right lower quadrant. **B,** Obturator muscle test. With the client supine, perform active assisted motion, flexing at the hip and knee; hold the ankle and rotate the leg internally and externally. A negative or normal response is no pain; a positive test for inflamed obturator muscle is right lower quadrant (abdominal) pain. (From Jarvis C: *Physical examination and health assessment,* ed 3, Philadelphia, 2000, WB Saunders, p 608.)

bone mineral density (BMD) may be more characteristic of CD than of UC, but no consistent differentiation has been made between CD and UC in this regard.[59] The therapist can provide osteoporosis education and prevention for clients with IBD. See the section on Osteoporosis in Chapter 23.

Hydration and nutrition are always long-term concerns with clients who have UC or CD. The client must be observed for any signs of dehydration (e.g., dry lips, hands, headache, brittle hair, incoordination, disorientation; see Box 4-6), in addition to any increase or pathologic change in symptoms. Any increase in painful symptoms or increased stool output or stool frequency must be reported to the physician.

Continued

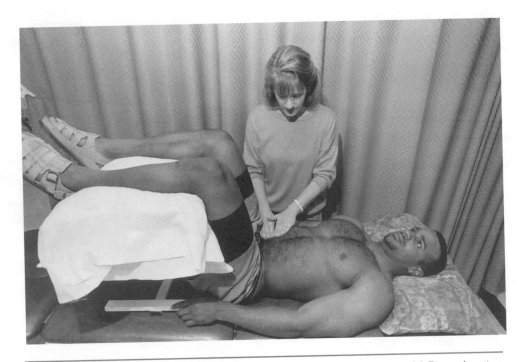

FIGURE   15-11   Palpating the iliopsoas muscle.   In addition to assessing McBurney's point, the examiner may also palpate the iliopsoas muscle by placing the client in a supine position with the hips and knees both flexed 90 degrees, and with the lower legs resting on a firm surface (a traction table stool works well for this; pillows under the lower legs may be necessary to obtain the full position). Palpate approximately one third the distance from the anterior superior iliac spine toward the umbilicus; it may be necessary to ask the client to initiate hip flexion on that side to help isolate the muscle and avoid palpating the bowel. A positive test for iliopsoas abscess produces right lower quadrant (abdominal) pain; alternatively, palpation may produce back pain or local muscular pain from a shortened or tight muscle indicating the need for soft tissue mobilization (STM) and stretching of the iliopsoas muscle. STM in this area would be contraindicated in the presence of any abdominal or pelvic inflammatory process involving the iliopsoas muscle until the infection has been treated with complete resolution.

People with IBD may have a characteristic personality susceptible to emotional stresses, which precipitate or exacerbate their symptoms. Studies investigating the effects of emotional words on the digestive tract in cases of irritable bowel syndrome (a separate entity from IBD; see following discussion of IBS) also may represent the same response in IBD, but this has not been substantiated yet. Preliminary data (in cases of irritable bowel syndrome) demonstrates a change in rectal tone during exposure to angry, sad, or anxious words.[78] Additionally, the chronic nature of IBD affecting persons in the prime of life often results in feelings of anger, anxiety, and possible depression. These emotions are important factors in the client's response to treatment and in modifying the overall course of the disease. See also Chapter 2 for an understanding of biopsychosocial aspects of disease. ■

◆ Antibiotic-Associated Colitis

Antibiotics can suppress normal GI flora, the bacteria usually residing within the lumen of the intestine, thus allowing yeasts and molds to flourish. Other kinds of microorganisms can replace normal GI flora suppressed by antibiotic therapy such as *Clostridium difficile*, the major cause of colitis in people with antibiotic-associated diarrhea. Although nearly all antibiotics have been associated with this syndrome, drugs such as clindamycin, ampicillin, and the cephalosporins commonly are implicated.

Clostridium difficile is not invasive but replaces normal GI flora by producing toxins that damage the colonic mucosa. *C. difficile* toxins compromise the epithelial cell barrier by at least two pathophysiologic pathways involving complex interactions between immune and inflammatory cells.[52] The overgrowth of *C. difficile* causes lesions described as raised, exudative, necrotic, and inflammatory plaques. These plaques attach to the mucosal surface of the small intestine or colon, or both, giving this condition the name *pseudomembranous enterocolitis* (PMC). When the lesions are restricted to the small intestine, the term *pseudomembranous enteritis* is applied.

Onset of symptoms (primarily voluminous, watery diarrhea, but also abdominal cramps and tenderness and fever) occurs during early administration or within 4 weeks after the drug has been discontinued. Complications of untreated illness include dehydration with accompanying electrolyte imbalance, perforation, toxic megacolon, and death.

Diagnosis is made by a stool test for *C. difficile* toxin or other laboratory tests. Discontinuation of the antibiotics is usually enough to relieve symptoms, but antimicrobial agents such as metronidazole or the more expensive vancomycin are prescribed to treat the *C. difficile*. Supportive measures may include administration of intravenous fluids to correct fluid losses, electrolyte imbalance, and hypoalbuminemia. Recurrence of symptoms is common when treatment is discontinued or in the case of vancomycin-resistant organisms, requiring retreatment, or in some cases, careful medical observation. In severe disease, mortality rates can be as high as 30%.

Special Implications for the Therapist   15-13

ANTIBIOTIC-ASSOCIATED COLITIS

The primary concern with any client experiencing excessive watery diarrhea is fluid and electrolyte imbalance. See the implications previously discussed in Chapter 4. Because the onset of this condition may occur up to 1 month after the antibiotic has been discontinued, the client may not recognize the association between current GI symptoms and previous medications. Anytime someone taking antibiotics or recently completing a course of antibiotics develops GI symptoms especially with joint and/or muscle involvement, encourage physician notification.

Reactive arthritis occurring after *C. difficile* infection is most common with colitis associated with antibiotic therapy. *Reactive arthritis* is defined as the occurrence of an acute, aseptic, inflammatory arthropathy arising after an infectious process, but at a site remote from the primary infection. The arthritis typically involves the large and medium joints of the lower extremities and first manifests 1 to 4 weeks after the infectious insult (see Chapter 24). Reactive arthritis may include some, but not all, of the three features associated with Reiter's syndrome and is often designated incomplete Reiter's syndrome. ■

◆ Irritable Bowel Syndrome

Definition and Incidence.   Irritable bowel syndrome (IBS) is a group of symptoms that represent the most common disorder of the GI system. IBS has been referred to as nervous indigestion, functional dyspepsia, spastic colon, nervous colon, and irritable colon, but because of the absence of inflammation, it should not be confused with colitis, Crohn's disease, or other inflammatory diseases of the intestinal tract. IBS is a chronic condition and is not limited to the colon but can occur anywhere in the small and large intestines. Women are more often affected than men, especially in early adulthood, but IBS can occur in either gender at any age.

Etiologic Factors and Pathogenesis.   IBS is considered a "functional" disorder because the symptoms cannot be attributed to any identifiable abnormality of the bowel (structural or biochemical). IBS is characterized by abnormal intestinal contractions presumably as a result of the digestive tract's reaction to emotions, stress, and certain chemicals in particular foods. Episodes of emotional stress, fatigue, smoking, alcohol intake, or eating (especially a large meal with high fat content, roughage, or fruit) do not cause but rather trigger symptoms. Intolerance of lactose and other sugars may account for IBS in some people.

Messages from the central nervous system are processed in the intestine by an elaborate neural network. New studies investigating the effects of emotional words on the digestive tract substantiate the close interaction among mind, brain, and gut. Preliminary data demonstrate an increase in intestinal contractions and change in rectal tone during exposure to angry, sad, or anxious words. These changes in intestinal motor function may influence brain perception.[7,8]

At the same time, in some cases of IBS pain and discomfort are not accompanied by changes in GI motility, suggesting an increased internal sensitivity, that is, enhanced sensation and perception of what is happening in the digestive tract referred to as "enhanced visceral nociception." In such cases it may be that the internal pain threshold is lowered for reasons that remain unclear. Scientists continue to explore the brain-gut connection to better understand IBS and other functional GI disorders.

Clinical Manifestations.   Symptoms of IBS usually begin in young adulthood and persist intermittently throughout life with variable periods of remission. A generally accepted definition of IBS requires at least 3 months of abdominal pain that is relieved by a bowel movement and at least three of the following symptoms (present at least 25% of the time): abdominal bloating or distention, passage of mucus, changes in stool form (hard or loose and watery), alterations in stool frequency, or difficulty in passing a movement. Diarrhea, constipation, or alternating diarrhea and constipation with abdominal cramps and pain are common. Rapid alterations in the speed of bowel movement create an obstruction to the natural flow of stool and gas. The resultant pressure buildup in the bowel produces the pain and spasm reported.

Pain may be steady or intermittent, and there may be a dull deep discomfort with sharp cramps in the morning or after eating. The typical pain pattern consists of lower left quadrant abdominal pain accompanied by constipation and diarrhea. Other symptoms may include nausea and vomiting, anorexia, foul breath, sour stomach, and flatus.

Medical Management
Diagnosis, Treatment, and Prognosis.   Diagnosis is based on a classic history. Sigmoidoscopy often reveals marked spasm and mucus in the colonic lumen and frequently provokes a spontaneous exacerbation of symptoms. Laboratory studies include a complete blood count and stool examination to rule out lactose intolerance and the presence of occult blood, parasites, and pathogenic bacteria. GI films may show altered motility without other evidence of abnormalities. Other radiologic modalities may be employed to diagnose this condition.

Treatment is aimed at relieving abdominal discomfort, stabilizing bowel habits, and altering underlying causes of the syndrome. Lifestyle changes (especially dietary changes), medications, and psychotherapy have been advocated. Dietary exclusion of milk and milk products may be helpful for those people with lactose intolerance. Increased dietary fiber, use of bulking agents such as psyllium preparations, and avoidance of alcohol, tobacco, and GI stimulants such as caffeine-containing beverages often are recommended.

A stress reduction program with a regular program of relaxation techniques and exercise in conjunction with psychotherapy and biofeedback training may be effective for some people. Medications may include antianxiety or antidepressant drugs, and anticholinergic agents before meals to help control symptoms. Alternative therapy, including peppermint oil (capsule form) and other natural substances (e.g., chamomile, rosemary, valerian, ginger), has antispasmodic effects and may relieve cramping.

IBS is not a life-threatening disorder, and prognosis is good for controlling symptoms through diet, medication, regular physical activity, and stress management. No known relationship exists between IBS and malignancy of the bowel.

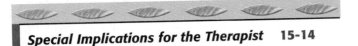

Special Implications for the Therapist 15-14

IRRITABLE BOWEL SYNDROME

Regular physical activity helps relieve stress and assists in bowel function, particularly in people who experience constipation. The therapist should encourage anyone with IBS to continue with the prescribed rehabilitation intervention program during symptomatic periods. Therapists must be alert to the person with IBS who has developed breath-holding patterns or hyperventilation in response to stress. Teaching proper breathing is important for all daily activities, especially during exercise and relaxation techniques. See Chapter 2.

For therapists working in the field of women's health, a known correlation exists between a history of (childhood or adult) emotional or sexual abuse and neurologic and functional (or organic) gastrointestinal disorders.[3,53] The first step in effective intervention is recognizing these individuals. Many articles are available to help the therapist incorporate this type of evaluation including the APTA Guidelines for Recognizing and Providing Care for Victims of Domestic Violence.[4,16,35] More must be done in this area to offer therapists guidelines and intervention management skills when sexual abuse has been part of the history. ■

◆ Diverticular Disease

See also the section on Meckel's Diverticulum.

Definition and Incidence. *Diverticular disease* is the term used to describe diverticulosis (uncomplicated disease) and diverticulitis (disease complicated by inflammation). Diverticulosis refers to the presence of outpouchings (diverticula) in the wall of the colon or small intestine, a condition in which the mucosa and submucosa herniate through the muscular layers of the colon (Fig. 15-12) to form outpouchings containing feces (Fig. 15-13). When food particles or feces become trapped in the diverticula and the pockets become infected and inflamed diverticulitis develops. This acquired deformity of the colon is rarely reversible and usually asymptomatic. The most common site is the sigmoid colon (95% of cases) because of the high pressures in this area required to move stool into the rectum, but any segment of the colon may be involved.

Diverticular disease is common and increasing in incidence in westernized countries because of low-fiber diets, present in approximately 10% of people in the United States. Incidence increases after age 60 and in obese individuals. The disease is present in as many as half of all adults over 65 years in the United States.

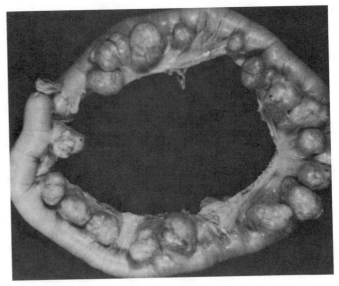

FIGURE 15-12 Multiple diverticula in resected section of the colon. Weak spots in the muscle layers of the intestinal wall permit the mucosa to bulge outward (herniate) into the pelvic cavity. (From Rosai J: *Ackerman's surgical pathology*, ed 7, St Louis, 1989, Mosby.)

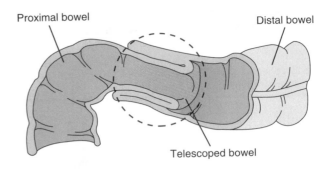

FIGURE 15-13 Intussusception. A portion of the bowel telescopes into adjacent (usually distal) bowel.

Etiologic and Risk Factors. Causes of diverticular disease include atrophy or weakness of the bowel muscle, increased intraluminal pressure, obesity, and chronic constipation. Disturbances of the pelvic floor in women are particular risk factors for constipation leading to diverticular disease. Some people are born with diverticula, probably resulting from an inherited defect in the muscular wall of the intestines, but the majority of people who have diverticulosis develop it with age, indicating that both heredity and lifestyle play a role. Use of NSAIDs and acetaminophen, the active ingredient in Tylenol, may be associated with diverticular disease. Further studies are under way to verify this potential link.[2]

The current hypothesis as to the primary cause (and major risk factor) of diverticular disease is a low-fiber diet, which decreases stool bulk and predisposes individuals to constipation. The subsequent increased intraluminal pressure pushes the mucosa through connective tissue, weakening bowel muscle. In addition to a low-fiber diet as a major risk factor, ingestion of poorly digested foods that can block the opening of the diverticulum and cause inflammation also may contribute to the development of diverticular disease. Such foods as corn, popcorn, and foods with tiny seeds (e.g. cucumbers, tomatoes, berries) have been implicated, but this remains a controversial issue.

Pathogenesis.   Diverticula form at weak points in the colon wall, usually where arteries penetrate the muscularis to nourish the mucosal layer. Changes in the connective tissue of the gut wall contribute to the diminished resistance of the intestinal wall. The circular and longitudinal muscles (taeniae coli) surrounding the diverticula become thickened and hypertrophy as a result of age–related changes in collagen and progressive deposition of elastin in longitudinal muscle. Increased contraction of these muscles is required when hard, compact stools form in the absence of adequate fiber, but decreased neurons in the distal colon associated with aging result in disorders of neuromuscular function and impaired evacuation compounding the problem. Increased intraluminal pressure then increases the herniation. Over a person's lifetime, diverticula may increase in number and size but only rarely extend to other portions of the colon.

Diverticulitis occurs when undigested food blocks the diverticulum (blind outpouchings), decreasing blood supply to the blood vessels penetrating the internal circular layer of bowel muscularis. This phenomenon leaves the bowel at risk for invasion by bacteria into the diverticulum and subsequent inflammation. The inflamed area becomes congested with blood and may bleed. Diverticulitis can lead to perforation when the trapped mass in the diverticula erodes the bowel wall. Chronic diverticulitis can result in increased scarring and narrowing of the bowel lumen, potentially leading to obstruction.

Clinical Manifestations.   Diverticular disease is asymptomatic in 80% of people affected. More commonly, these individuals report passing fresh blood and clots and experience a sense of urgency to defecate. When diverticula become inflamed, diverticulitis develops, and the person experiences episodic or constant, severe abdominal pain located in the left quadrant or midabdominal region, often with extension into the back. The mechanism of pain is probably increased tension in the colonic wall with an associated rise in intraluminal pressure. Other symptoms may include pelvic pain in women, constipation alternating with diarrhea, increased flatus, fever, sudden onset of painless rectal bleeding, and anemia in the presence of chronic blood loss. Eating and increased intraabdominal pressure increase pain (see Box 15-1), whereas temporary partial or complete relief may follow a bowel movement or passage of flatus.

Medical Management

Diagnosis, Treatment, and Prognosis.   Barium enema studies show the characteristic diverticula; colonoscopy and sigmoidoscopy also may provide diagnostic information, and a CT scan may sometimes reveal the inflamed colon segment. No specific laboratory tests exist, but fecal examination for occult blood may be positive, and anemia may be identified. Stool cultures may be used to exclude bacterial or parasitic infections.

Insights on the pathophysiology and mechanisms of neural injury may lead to more specific treatment in the future (e.g.,

serotonergic agents and neurotrophins), but for now, treatment is directed at relieving symptoms and preventing diverticulitis. This is accomplished primarily through dietary changes with adherence to a high-fiber diet, prevention of constipation with bran and bulk laxatives, and exercise during periods of remission. Acute diverticulitis may require antibiotics and complete rest of the colon accomplished by nasogastric tube feedings and parenteral fluids until the inflammatory process has been resolved. Bleeding is a rare complication of diverticulosis and usually is self-limited; but in approximately 10% of people with bleeding diverticula, the hemorrhage is severe enough to require hospitalization, blood transfusion, and possible surgical removal of the affected part of the colon and possible temporary colostomy.

Prognosis is good for the person with known diverticular disease, especially when prevention of diverticulitis is possible by consuming a high-fiber diet and avoiding indigestible foods. If the diverticulum is not blocked and infected or inflamed (diverticulitis), the person may be asymptomatic. If the trapped fecal material (fecaliths) does not liquefy and drain from the diverticulum, diverticulitis develops.

Special Implications for the Therapist   15-15

DIVERTICULAR DISEASE

Exercise is an important treatment component during periods of remission. The therapist is instrumental in helping establish an appropriate exercise program. Throughout all activity and exercise, clients with diverticular disease must be careful to avoid activities that increase intraabdominal pressure (see Box 15-1) to avoid further herniation. The therapist can provide valuable information regarding appropriate body mechanics and techniques to reduce intraabdominal pressure for all activities.

Back pain can occur as a symptom of this disease. Anyone with back pain of nontraumatic or unknown origin must be screened for medical disease, including possible GI involvement. If infection occurs and penetrates the pelvic floor or retroperitoneal tissues (i.e., those organs outside the peritoneum such as the kidneys, pancreas, colon, and pancreas), abscesses may result causing isolated referred hip or thigh pain. A variety of objective test procedures may be employed by the therapist to assess for iliopsoas abscess formation (see Figs. 15-10 and Fig. 15-11), including palpation of McBurney's point (see Fig. 15-16), assessment of rebound tenderness (see Fig. 15-17), the iliopsoas muscle test, the obturator test, and palpation of the iliopsoas muscle (see Figs. 15-10 and 15-11). ∎

◆ Neoplasms

Intestinal Polyps.   A growth or mass protruding into the intestinal lumen from any area of mucous membrane can be termed a *polyp*. Polyps are either *neoplastic* or *nonneoplastic*. Adenomatous (benign neoplastic) polyps of the intestine usually develop during middle age, and more than two thirds of the population over 65 years old have at least one polyp. Until a polyp becomes large enough to obstruct the intestine, no symptoms are discernible. Early symptoms may be lower abdominal cramping pain, diarrhea with rectal bleeding, and passage of mucus.

Nonneoplastic polyps include adenomatous and hyperplastic and are usually asymptomatic although inflammatory polyps may present with symptoms of the underlying inflammatory bowel disease usually present (e.g., UC or CD). Treatment is not always required; polyps associated with rectal bleeding may be removed through a proctoscope. Adenomatous polyps may be a risk factor for the development of adenocarcinomas (colorectal cancer); therefore, regardless of the clinical manifestations, adenomatous polyps are removed (by polypectomy, usually performed through a sigmoidoscope or colonoscope; large polyps may require removal by laparotomy). Hyperplastic polyps do not progress to become cancerous.

Contrary to previous beliefs, studies have now shown that high-fiber diets do not reduce the risk of recurrent colorectal adenomas in people who have had at least one precancerous polyp already removed. Researchers continue to question whether high-fiber diets can slow the development of adenomas.[58]

Benign Tumors.   The most common benign tumors of the small intestine are adenomas, leiomyomas, and lipomas. Benign tumors of the small intestine rarely become malignant, may be symptomatic, or may be incidental findings at operation or autopsy. *Adenomas* account for 25% of all benign bowel tumors and are usually asymptomatic, although bleeding and intussusception (see the section on Mechanical Obstruction in this chapter) are occasional complications. *Leiomyomas* are smooth muscle tumors that can occur at any location in the intestine but are most common in the jejunum. They usually are associated with bleeding when they protrude into the lumen where necrosis of tumor tissue and ulceration of the mucosa occur. Obstruction is uncommon, but intussusception or volvulus (Figs. 15-13 and 15-14) may occur. Surgical removal of large leiomyomas is recommended because of the bleeding and the increased risk of malignancy with increasing size. *Lipomas* are fatty tumors that occur throughout the length of the small intestine but occur most

frequently in the distal ileum. When symptomatic, the presenting symptom is obstruction resulting from tumor size, causing intussusception. Other complications may include ulceration and bleeding of the overlying mucosa and subsequent sequelae.

Malignant Tumors.   The most common malignant tumors of the small intestine are metastatic through direct extension from adjacent organs (e.g., stomach, pancreas, colon). Adenocarcinoma and primary lymphoma account for the majority of bowel malignancy. Other types of colorectal cancer, including melanoma and fibrosarcoma, and other types of sarcoma are rare and are not discussed further in this book.

Adenocarcinoma

Overview and Incidence.   Adenocarcinoma of the colon and rectum (colorectal cancer) is the third most commonly diagnosed cancer and the second leading cause of cancer death among men in the United States; third in women after lung and breast cancer, except after age 75 when colorectal cancer is responsible for more deaths than breast cancer. Incidence increases with age, starting at 40 years, and occurs slightly more often in men and in populations of high socioeconomic status, possibly owing to dietary factors. Colorectal tumors are staged using the Dukes' classification (Table 15-6). Overall incidence and mortality rates are on the decline, possibly indicating that advances in diagnosis and treatment are making an impact.

Etiologic and Risk Factors.   The cause of colon cancer is unknown, although a number of environmental and familial factors have been considered. Genetic syndromes are more likely to occur before age 40 and make up less than 6% of all colorectal cancers. Known risk factors associated with increased risk of colonic cancer include increasing age, male gender, adenomatous polyps, ulcerative colitis, Crohn's disease, cancer elsewhere in the body (especially reproductive or breast cancer in women), familial history of colon cancer or familial adenomatous polyps (FAP), sedentary lifestyle, and immunodeficiency disease. Anyone who has first-degree relatives diagnosed with colon or rectal adenoma is twice as likely to develop colon cancer as those with no history of such cancer in the immediate family. The risk is even higher if the relative was under 50 years at the time of diagnosis.

Cigarette smoking may increase the risk of colorectal cancer but data collected suggest a lag time of at least 35 years for

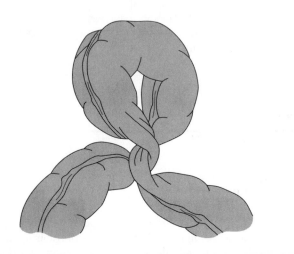

TABLE	15-6

Dukes' Staging of Colorectal Tumors

Stage A	Cancer limited to the bowel wall; mucosal involvement only
Stage B	Cancer extending through the bowel wall; local invasion without penetration of the serous membrane
Stage C	Involvement of regional lymph nodes, with or without extension into the bowel wall
Stage D	Distant metastases regardless of primary tumor size

tobacco-induced tumors to develop. Geographic distributions of highest incidence coincide with regional diets low in fiber and high in animal fat and protein; people who emigrate tend to acquire the risk characteristics of their new environment. About 75% of all colorectal cancer occurs in people with no known predisposing factors; in such cases, the lifetime risk of developing this type of cancer is about 5%.

Colon cancer incidence and mortality rates are lower in females compared with males, and numerous epidemiologic studies suggest that estrogen replacement therapy reduces cancer risk in postmenopausal women.[12] It is not clear how estrogen acts to reduce fatal colon cancer risk. One theory is that it lowers the concentration of bile acids, perhaps creating an environment that is hostile to the growth of cancer cells in the colon; another is that estrogen acts directly on the lining of the colon to suppress tumor growth.

Pathogenesis.   Most colorectal cancers have a long preinvasive phase, growing slowly during invasion. More than 95% of colorectal cancers are adenocarcinomas that arise from glandular cells that line the mucosa of the colon and rectum. This disease appears to begin with benign lesions (adenomatous polyps) containing abnormal but not malignant cells. Some benign polyps may regress and disappear over time but most continue to undergo changes that change them into malignant tumors. This process is thought to be due to a series of genetic mutations within the cells. The accumulation of molecular genetic alterations involves activation of oncogenes, inactivation of tumor-suppressor genes, and abnormalities in genes involved in DNA repair (see Chapter 8). Hormones stimulating the rate of cell turnover and excessive free radical formation and oxidation also may play a role in colon carcinogenesis.[38] Untreated tumors can grow into the wall of the colon. The lymphatic channels are located underneath the muscularis mucosae so that the lesions must extend across this layer before metastasis can occur.

Clinical Manifestations.   Colon carcinoma has few early warning signs, as is the case with esophageal and stomach cancer. When symptoms do present, they present according to whether the lesion is in the right or left side of the colon. A persistent change in bowel habits is the single most consistent symptom for either side. Bright-red blood from the rectum is a cardinal sign of colon cancer but must be differentiated from diverticulosis, which is also a common cause of painless bright-red blood. Other symptoms may include persistent stomach pain, diarrhea, or constipation; many cases of colon cancer are asymptomatic until metastasis has occurred. Complications include intestinal obstruction, bleeding, perforation, anemia, ascites, distant metastases, to the liver most commonly, but also to the lungs, bone, and brain.

Medical Management
Prevention.   Evidence exists that reductions in colorectal cancer morbidity and mortality can be achieved through detection and treatment of early-stage cancer and the identification and removal of adenomatous polyps, the precursors of colorectal cancer. Regular screening examinations (e.g., annual stool-sample test to check for blood, sigmoidoscopy and digital rectal exam every 5 to 10 years) are recommended for adults over 50 years and for younger people with a family history of the disease. Colonoscopy is the primary screening test that involves inserting a snakelike scope into the rectum and large bowel to detect tiny polyps before they develop into cancer. The nature of this test prevents participation in the colorectal cancer screening process such that investigators are working to develop alternative screening tests. Advances in computed tomography (CT) technology and computer capabilities have contributed to the development of a new imaging modality for colorectal lesions called *CT colonography* or *virtual colonoscopy*. This is a rapid, minimally invasive, and painless procedure that inserts a tiny probe just 4 centimeters into the rectum. This screening technique may not be sensitive enough and does not identify flat lesions at all requiring continued development of the technology before it can be applied as a standard procedure.[56,64]

Other preventive strategies include altering modifiable risk factors such as sedentary lifestyle, high-fat diet, and cigarette smoking. Evidence for a protective role of physical activity and exercise in colon and rectal cancer has been reported.[17] The role of a high-fiber diet in preventing colon cancer remains unclear although its benefits for other diseases remain undisputed. Cancer chemoprevention (pharmacologic, nutritional supplemental interventions applied before cancer occurrence) is the next step in attempting to inhibit or reverse the tumorigenic process in colorectal cancer, especially the heritable syndromes.[32,57] Taking aspirin or other nonsteroidal antiinflammatories (NSAIDs) daily for 20 years can reduce the risk of colon cancer by nearly one half. A possible mechanism of this benefit is decreased prostaglandin production, achieved through inhibition of cyclooxygenase (COX) activity.[40,67] Understanding the neoplastic events at the molecular level may provide more definitive preventative information in the coming decade.

Diagnosis.   Carcinoma of the colon should be suspected in anyone over the age of 40 who presents with occult blood in the stool, iron-deficiency anemia, overt rectal bleeding, or alteration in bowel habits, especially if associated with abdominal discomfort or any of the risk factors mentioned earlier. Physical examination of the abdomen to detect liver enlargement and ascites is followed by palpation of appropriate lymph nodes. Diagnostic procedures include rectal examination, sigmoidoscopy, proctoscopy, colonoscopy with biopsy of lesion, CT scan, and barium enema studies. Laboratory diagnostic tests may include a screening test for occult fecal blood and a blood test for carcinoembryonic antigen (CEA), detected in some individuals with colorectal carcinoma. CEA is one of the most widely used tumor markers worldwide primarily in GI cancers, especially colorectal malignancy. It is of little use in detecting early colorectal cancer, but high preoperative concentrations of CEA correlate with adverse prognosis and serial CEA measurements can detect recurrent cancer in asymptomatic clients.[22]

Treatment.   Surgical removal of the tumor is the mainstay of colorectal cancer treatment. Adjuvant chemotherapy may be administered, depending on the results of the staging process, to treat metastatic disease; radiation therapy is helpful for rectal carcinoma. Radiation therapy may be given before surgery to reduce the tumor size or alter the malignant cells to prevent tumor survival after surgery. Tumors in the distal rectum may require resection of the entire rectum with subsequent permanent colostomy. Given the link between adenomatous polyps and cancer, emphasis is on prevention through screening for colonic polyps and carcinomas.

Prognosis. Colorectal cancer survival is related closely to the clinical and pathologic stage of the disease at diagnosis. Approximately 65% present with advanced disease. The 5-year survival for cancer limited to the bowel wall at the time of diagnosis approaches 90% but drops to 35% to 60% when lymph nodes are involved and less than 10% with metastatic disease to distant organs such as the liver.[1] Local recurrence can occur if special operative precautions to prevent implantation of malignant cells are not followed. CEA is a marker for recurrent tumor and should be monitored every 6 months to improve survival. Routine follow-up colonoscopy also is recommended.

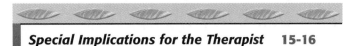

Special Implications for the Therapist 15-16

ADENOCARCINOMA OF THE COLON AND RECTUM

Tumors of the rectum can spread through the rectal wall to the prostate in men and the vagina in women. Prostate involvement can cause dull, vague, aching pain in the sacral or lumbar spine regions. See Special Implications for the Therapist: Prostate Cancer, 18-3. Pelvic, hip, or low back pain may occur with extension to the vagina in women.

Systemic and pulmonary metastases occur through the hemorrhoidal plexus, which drains into the vena cava. Subsequent chest, shoulder, arm, or back pain can occur, usually accompanied by pulmonary symptoms; see also Special Implications for the Therapist: Lung Cancer, 14-22. Liver metastasis occurs after invasion of the mesenteric veins from the left colon or the superior veins from the right colon, which empty into the portal circulation; see also the section on Hepatic Encephalopathy in Chapter 16. Any time a person with low back pain reports simultaneous or alternating abdominal pain at the same level as the back pain, or GI symptoms associated with back pain, a medical referral is required.

Anemia caused by intestinal bleeding associated with colon cancer requires special consideration. See Special Implications for the Therapist: Anemias, 13-4. ■

Primary Intestinal Lymphoma

Primary intestinal lymphoma originates in nodules of lymphoid tissue within the bowel wall and accounts for 15% of small bowel cancers in the United States and two thirds of such cancers in undeveloped countries. Primary lymphoma is the most common form of presentation for gastrointestinal lymphomas, and the stomach is one of the most frequent sites of extranodal lymphoma. The cause of primary lymphoma is unknown, although chronic *H. pylori* infection is associated strongly with the development of primary intestinal lymphoma of the mucosa-associated lymphoid tissue (MALT) type.[44] An apparent causal relationship exists between lymphoma and chronic inflammatory intestinal conditions such as celiac disease, possibly because of the persistent activation of lym-

phocytes in the bowel. The risk of intestinal lymphoma is also increased in conditions of immunodeficiency after treatment with immunosuppressive drugs. The mechanisms by which malignant transformation occurs remain under investigation.

Signs and symptoms may include chronic abdominal pain, diarrhea, clubbing of the fingers, weight loss, and occult bleeding. Intestinal obstruction, intussusception, and perforation with massive hemorrhage and peritonitis are possible complications.

Clinical diagnosis is by radiographic studies of the small intestine, CT or magnetic resonance imaging (MRI) scans, and endoscopic ultrasonography. Combined-modality therapy with chemotherapy followed by radiation therapy is used for large-cell lymphoma and eradication of *H. pylori* (associated with complete remission in nearly 80% of low-grade MALT lymphoma in an early clinical stage) and radiation therapy alone for later stages of MALT lymphoma. With these improved treatment modalities primary lymphoma has become a highly curable disease. Surgical resection for small, local involvement is possible, but the role of surgery has come into question with increasing knowledge of intestinal lymphoma pathogenesis and with new therapeutic approaches described. The overall prognosis is much less favorable when extraintestinal spread occurs (5-year survival rate is less than 10%). When the disease is localized and confined to the small intestine, it does not recur after surgical removal in more than half the cases, but the disease is usually too diffuse to permit surgery.

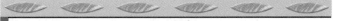

Special Implications for the Therapist 15-17

PRIMARY INTESTINAL LYMPHOMA

Special considerations relate to any complications present with this condition such as anemia from intestinal bleeding or complications associated with chemotherapy and radiation therapy. See Special Implications for the Therapist: Oncology, 8-1. ■

◆ Obstructive Disease

Anything that reduces the size of the gastric outlet, preventing the normal flow of chyme and delaying gastric emptying, can cause an obstruction of the bowel. Delayed gastric emptying may be secondary to obstruction of the stomach or secondary to an inability to generate effective propulsive forces (peristalsis). Obstruction of the intestines can occur as a result of (1) organic disease, (2) mechanical obstruction, or (3) functional obstruction (Table 15-7).

Organic Disease
Clinical Manifestations. Distention develops accompanied by colicky, cramping pain and tenderness in the periumbilical area progressively becoming constant. Vomiting occurs as a reflex associated with the waves of pain. Constipation develops into obstipation (intractable constipation) as fecal obstruction builds up in the distal bowel. Propulsion of gas through the intestines causes a rumbling noise called *borborygmus*, and the person is aware of intestinal movement. Constitutional symptoms such as low-grade fever, perspira-

TABLE 15-7

Causes of Intestinal Obstruction

Organic Disease	Mechanical	Functional
Ulcers	Postoperative	Postoperative
Strictures	adhesions	Drugs
Gallstones	Intussusception	Anticholinergics
Neoplasms	Volvulus	Beta-adrenergics
Granulomatous	External hernia	Opiates
processes		Electrolyte imbalance
Viral infections		Metabolic disorders
Scleroderma		Diabetes mellitus
Polymyositis		Hypoparathyroidism
Brainstem tumors		Pregnancy
Gastroesophageal		Vagotomy
reflux		Anorexia nervosa
Vascular occlusion		Spinal cord injury
Mesenteric		Vertebral fracture
infarction		Pneumonitis
Abdominal angina		

Many of the organic and functional classes do not cause obstruction as much as these cause ileus with reduced or absent peristalsis. The presentation is the same but the cause and treatment are different.

tion, tachycardia, and dehydration may accompany this condition. The affected individual is restless, changing position frequently because of the constant pain.

Signs of dehydration, hypovolemia, and metabolic acidosis may be seen within 24 hours of complete obstruction. Impaired blood supply to the bowel results in necrosis and strangulation. Strangulation is characterized by fever, leukocytosis, peritoneal signs, or blood in the feces. Further complications may develop such as perforation, peritonitis, and sepsis. In debilitated persons, distention of the abdomen can be severe enough to compress the diaphragm, decreasing lung compliance and resulting in atelectasis and pneumonia.

Pathogenesis.   Gases and fluids accumulate proximal to the obstruction causing abdominal distention. The body's response to distention is temporarily increased peristalsis as the bowel attempts to force the material through the obstructed area. The distention also decreases the intestine's ability to absorb water and electrolytes, which are further imbalanced by vomiting. If the obstruction is at the pylorus or high in the small intestine, metabolic alkalosis develops as a result of vomiting and excessive loss of hydrogen ions. With prolonged obstruction or obstruction lower in the intestine, metabolic acidosis is more likely to occur because bicarbonate from pancreatic secretions and bile cannot be reabsorbed.

Medical Management

Diagnosis, Treatment, and Prognosis.   Diagnosis requires differentiation of obstruction from other acute abdominal conditions such as inflammation and perforation of a viscus, renal or gallbladder colic, obstruction from other causes, vascular disease, and torsion of an organ, as occurs with an ovarian cyst. Abdominal radiography is the most useful diag-

nostic tool, and laboratory findings may reveal electrolyte disturbances associated with vomiting and dehydration.

Supportive care to alleviate pain and symptoms and to facilitate passage of flatus and feces is instituted toward the goals of restoration of bowel function and prevention of surgical intervention. Intestinal intubation (insertion of a tube into the intestinal lumen to decompress the lumen and break up the obstruction) may relieve obstruction without surgery. Complete obstruction of the intestine is surgically resected; immediate surgery is required in the case of strangulation. Prognosis varies with the underlying cause; strangulation increases the mortality rate to 25%.

Special Implications for the Therapist   15-18

ORGANIC OBSTRUCTIVE DISEASE

The therapist may see this client in an acute care setting for ambulation after the obstructive incident has been treated. Dehydration is the primary concern, requiring monitoring of vital signs and symptoms (e.g., dry lips, hands, headache, brittle hair, incoordination, disorientation; see Box 4-6) along with encouragement of fluid intake throughout therapy. Movement and activity, along with deep-breathing exercises, help promote abdominal relaxation and restore bowel function. ■

Mechanical Obstruction

Adhesions.   Adhesions are the most common cause of small and large intestine obstruction caused by fibrous scars formed after abdominal surgery. These fibrous bands of scar tissue can loop over the bowel, either mechanically obstructing the bowel by constricting it or the fibrous band can become the axis around which the bowel can twist (volvulus). Peritonitis may cause obstruction by kinking or angulating the bowel or by directly compressing the lumen.

Intussusception.   Intussusception is a telescoping of the bowel on itself, that is, one part of the intestine prolapses into the lumen of an immediately adjacent section (see Fig. 15-13). A reported link between the rotavirus vaccine and intussusception in infants and young children is under investigation.[45] In adults the leading point of an intussusception is often a lesion in the bowel wall, such as Meckel's diverticulum or a tumor. Once the leading point is entrapped, peristalsis drives it forward, dragging the mesentery into the enveloping lumen. As the two walls of the intestine press against each other, inflammation, edema, and decreased venous return and venous stasis occur. Untreated, necrosis and gangrene develop.

Clinical manifestations in adults are as listed for obstruction; complications in children include prolonged ischemia and subsequent necrosis with eventual perforation, peritonitis, and sepsis. Usually, diagnostic testing includes rectal examination, abdominal radiograph, and barium enema. The barium enema may be part of the diagnosis and treatment as the force of the flowing barium is usually enough to push the invaginated bowel into its normal position. If the hydrostatic reduction is unsuccessful (in 30% to 40% of cases), surgical reduction of the intussusception and resection of any nonviable intestine are performed. The prognosis for children and adults with this condition is good if treated.

Volvulus. Volvulus is a torsion of a loop of intestine twisted on its mesentery, kinking the bowel and interrupting the blood supply (Fig. 15-14). The cause of this phenomenon is usually a congenital abnormality such as a malrotation of the bowel that allows excess mobility of the bowel loops and predisposes the intestine to volvulus. Other focal points for a stationary object about which the bowel twists are tumors or Meckel's diverticulum. Treatment to decompress the bowel by inserting a long tube to release the pressure against the proximal end of the loop is tried first. If successful, the bowel volvulus relaxes. If unsuccessful, surgical intervention is sometimes required.

Hernia

Definition and Incidence. A hernia is an acquired or congenital abnormal protrusion of part of an organ or tissue through the structure normally containing it. One-half million Americans each year have repair of a groin hernia. Hernias can occur at any age in men or women and most frequently occur in the abdominal cavity as a result of a congenital or acquired weakness of abdominal musculature. Weakness can occur as part of the aging process contributing to acquired hernias. As people age, muscular tissues become infiltrated by adipose and connective tissues, resulting in weakness. The most common types of hernias are *inguinal* (direct and indirect), *femoral, umbilical,* and *incisional* or *ventral* (Fig. 15-15). Hiatal hernia is discussed earlier in this chapter.

Etiologic and Risk Factors. When muscular weakness (congenital or acquired) is accompanied by obesity, pregnancy, heavy lifting, coughing, surgical incision, or traumatic injuries from blunt pressure, the risk of developing a hernia increases. Often, herniation is the result of a multifactorial process involving one or more of these factors. For example, herniation can occur when increased abdominal pressure in a postoperative or posttraumatic injury is aggravated by nutritional or metabolic factors that result in poor wound healing and defective or poor collagen synthesis. Many other possible combinations of risk factors exist (Table 15-8).

Structural abnormalities account for most congenital hernias, but congenital factors do not explain the increased incidence of hernias (e.g., the direct inguinal type) in advancing age groups. Predisposing factors are equally important such as situational stress (e.g., repetitive local trauma, strenuous physical activities); degenerative changes associated with increased abdominal pressure; the wear and tear of living; multiparity (women); and altered collagen synthesis in middle age. Sudden stress, as occurs in abdominal trauma or industrial accidents, also may contribute to the development of a hernia with or without an underlying congenital defect.

Pathogenesis. Structural and biochemical abnormalities and abnormalities of local collagen metabolism have been proposed as factors in the eventual appearance of a hernia. Other biologic factors can affect the balance between collagen synthesis and lysis, eventually leading to the development of herniation. For example, any condition such as renal failure, diabetes mellitus, malnutrition, vitamin or mineral deficiencies, underlying systemic disease, altered immunity, or resistance to infection that can impair a person's ability to generate the proteinaceous constituents of collagen can alter collagen metabolism.

Inguinal hernias account for about 75% of all hernias. They occur in the groin when a sac formed from the peritoneum and containing a portion of the intestine pushes either directly outward through the weakest point in the abdominal wall (direct hernia) or downward through the internal inguinal ring into the inguinal canal through which the testes descend into the scrotum during infancy (males) or to the labia (females) (indirect hernia). The direct hernias occur most often as a result of a deficient number of transversus abdominis aponeurotic fibers at a site called *Hesselbach's triangle,* the area between the pubic ramus and the musculofascial components in the lower abdominal wall. The direct inguinal hernia is more common in the older adult, especially in an area that is congenitally weak because of a deficient number of muscle fibers. The indirect inguinal hernia is most common in infants, young people, and males, the last because it follows the tract that develops when the testes descend into the scrotum before birth. A wide space at the inguinal ligament also can contribute to the development of an inguinal hernia.

Femoral hernia is a protrusion of a loop of intestine into the femoral canal, a tubular passageway into the thigh that carries nerves and blood vessels. The pathologic anatomy present is an enlarged femoral ring with a correspondingly narrowed transversus abdominis aponeurosis. This type occurs more often in multiparous women, acquired as a result of increased intraabdominal pressure gradually forcing more and more preperitoneal fat into the femoral canal, enlarging the femoral ring.

The pathology of *umbilical hernias* is caused by increased abdominal pressure (see discussion of risk factors) exerted against a thinning of the umbilical ring and fascia. *Incisional hernia* occurs postoperatively (see discussion of risk factors) when the transected fibers are unable to form collagen links strong enough to hold the edges of the wound together.

Clinical Manifestations. The most common manifestation of a hernia of any type is an intermittent or persistent bulge, accompanied by intermittent or persistent pain. Inguinal hernia usually begins as a small, marble-sized soft lump under the skin. At first it is painless and can be reduced by pushing it back in place. As pressure from the abdominal contents pushes against the weak abdominal wall, the size of the lump formed by the hernia increases, requiring surgical repair (herniorrhaphy).

The pain associated with simple hernias depends on the involved structures and whether these are compressed or irritated. The pain usually is localized and sharp, aggravated by changes in position, by physical exertion, during a bowel movement or by any activity causing the Valsalva maneuver (bearing down with increased intraabdominal pressure), and relieved by cessation of the physical activity that precipitated it. It may radiate from the groin to the ipsilateral thigh, flank, or hypogastrium (lowest middle abdominal region). In the female, painful symptoms may be aggravated by the onset of menstruation.

The ilioinguinal nerve penetrates the abdominal wall cranially and somewhat laterally to the deep inguinal ring, passing the transverse and internal oblique muscles stepwise. Neuralgic pain may occur when the dull inguinal hernial pain causes a local reflex increase of tone in the internal oblique and transverse muscles of the abdomen. As the nerve passes

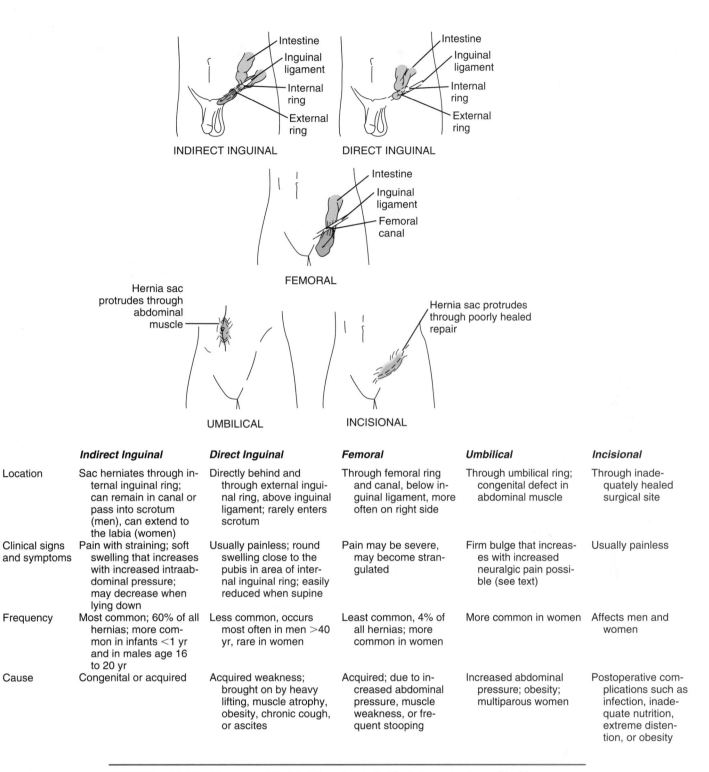

	Indirect Inguinal	*Direct Inguinal*	*Femoral*	*Umbilical*	*Incisional*
Location	Sac herniates through internal inguinal ring; can remain in canal or pass into scrotum (men), can extend to the labia (women)	Directly behind and through external inguinal ring, above inguinal ligament; rarely enters scrotum	Through femoral ring and canal, below inguinal ligament, more often on right side	Through umbilical ring; congenital defect in abdominal muscle	Through inadequately healed surgical site
Clinical signs and symptoms	Pain with straining; soft swelling that increases with increased intraabdominal pressure; may decrease when lying down	Usually painless; round swelling close to the pubis in area of internal inguinal ring; easily reduced when supine	Pain may be severe, may become strangulated	Firm bulge that increases with increased neuralgic pain possible (see text)	Usually painless
Frequency	Most common; 60% of all hernias; more common in infants <1 yr and in males age 16 to 20 yr	Less common, occurs most often in men >40 yr, rare in women	Least common, 4% of all hernias; more common in women	More common in women	Affects men and women
Cause	Congenital or acquired	Acquired weakness; brought on by heavy lifting, muscle atrophy, obesity, chronic cough, or ascites	Acquired; due to increased abdominal pressure, muscle weakness, or frequent stooping	Increased abdominal pressure; obesity; multiparous women	Postoperative complications such as infection, inadequate nutrition, extreme distention, or obesity

FIGURE   **15-15**   Hernias.   (Modified from Jarvis C: *Physical examination and health assessment,* ed 3, Philadelphia, 2000, WB Saunders, p 779.)

these muscles in steps, it may be exposed to pressure, giving rise to pain of the neuralgic type. Ilioinguinal or femoral neuritis caused by nerve entrapment from sutures, adhesions, or the actual formation of a symptomatic neuroma after section of a nerve in this region can occur. These conditions usually resolve spontaneously without specific treatment, but therapy in conjunction with local nerve blocks may be indicated if symptoms persist after the first postoperative month.

Genitofemoral neuralgia (causalgia) occurs less commonly but results in severe pain and paresthesia (or hyperesthesia) in the distribution of the genitofemoral nerve. Radiation of pain to the genitalia and upper thigh may occur and pain is aggravated by walking, stooping, or hyperextending the hip. Recumbency and flexion of the thigh may relieve painful symptoms. This condition requires neurectomy for pain relief.

TABLE 15-8

Risk Factors for Hernias

INGUINAL	FEMORAL	UMBILICAL	INCISIONAL
Advanced age	Pregnancy (multiparous)	Infants	Poor wound healing
Prematurity		Low birth weight	Infection
Positive family history		African descent	Inadequate nutrition
Abdominal wall defects		Congenital hypothyroidism	Abdominal distention
Undescended testis		Mucopolysaccharidoses	Obesity
Connective tissue disorders		Down syndrome	Prolonged use of steroids
Cystic fibrosis		Obesity	Advanced age
Shunt for hydrocephalus		Pregnancy	Immunosuppression
Ascites		Ascites	Postoperative pulmonary complications (coughing, straining)
			Type of incision (vertical)

When the contents of the hernial sac can be replaced into the abdominal cavity by manipulation, the hernia is said to be *reducible*. Hernias that cannot be reduced or replaced by manipulation are referred to as *irreducible* and *incarcerated*. Complications occur when the protruding organ is constricted to the extent that circulation is impaired (strangulated hernia) or when the protruding organs encroach on and impair the function of other structures. When a hernia contains incarcerated or strangulated structures, the pain becomes persistent and often is associated with systemic signs or symptoms such as elevated temperature, tachycardia, vomiting, and abdominal distention.

Medical Management

Diagnosis, Treatment, and Prognosis. History and physical examination remain the most important aspects of diagnosis for all types of hernia; there may be a past history of hernia. The diagnosis of umbilical hernia is usually obvious because of protrusion of the umbilicus confirmed by palpation of the involved structures.

Various supports and trusses are available to contain hernias, but these offer only a temporary solution and do not prevent the hernia from getting bigger with associated complications. Surgical repair is the only curative treatment. The use of strapping techniques is not recommended, because the tape used may lead to ulceration of the thin skin covering the hernia and eventual rupture.

Prognosis varies with the type of hernia and accompanying complications. The incidence of incarceration is about 10% in indirect inguinal hernia and 20% in femoral hernia. Umbilical hernia in adults has a high morbidity and mortality associated with incarceration.

Special Implications for the Therapist 15-19

HERNIA

Preferred Practice Pattern:
6H: Impaired Circulation and Anthropometric Dimensions
Associated With Lymphatic System Disorders

Early diagnosis is important in preventing incarceration and strangulation. Any client experiencing chronic cough, pregnancy, or back, hip, groin, or sacroiliac pain should be asked, "Have you ever been told you have a hernia, or do you think you have a hernia now?" For the client recovering from surgical repair of a hernia, heavy lifting and straining should be avoided for 4 to 6 weeks after surgery. Substance abusers and cigarette smokers have an additional risk factor for delayed wound healing and dehiscence. Transient anesthesia of the skin beneath the hernial incision is a possible postoperative phenomenon. Whether in the presence of an uncorrected hernia or postoperatively, the client should avoid activities and positions that produce painful symptoms associated with the hernia.

The therapist should be aware of two complications that may occur in clients wearing a truss. In the client with a small hernia the pressure of the overlying truss on a protruding hernial mass enhances the chances of strangulation by obstructing lymphatic and venous drainage. In a person with a large direct inguinal hernia, the constant overlying pressure of the truss pad on the margins of the hernial defect eventually leads to atrophy of the fascial aponeurotic structures, enlarging the hernial opening and promoting growth of the hernia, thus making subsequent surgical repair more difficult. Any time a person chooses to wear a truss without prior physician evaluation, the therapist is advised to encourage that client to seek medical advice.

Although uncommon, psoas abscess still can be confused with a hernia. The therapist may perform evaluative tests to rule out a psoas abscess, but the physician must differentiate between an abscess and a hernia; see the iliopsoas and obturator muscle tests (see Fig. 15-10), iliopsoas palpation (see Fig. 15-11), and McBurney's point (Fig. 15-16). Psoas abscess is often softer than a femoral hernia and has ill-defined borders, in contrast to the more sharply defined margins of the hernia. The major differentiating feature is the fact that a psoas abscess lies lateral to the femoral artery, not medial to it, as is the case for the femoral hernia.

Whereas most people do well after surgical repair, some have persistent postoperative pain or discomfort. If a person has had a previous inguinal hernial repair and now presents with painful groin or thigh pain, the physician must differentiate between ilioinguinal nerve entrapment and neuroma of a branch of the nerve severed previously. Any person (especially an older

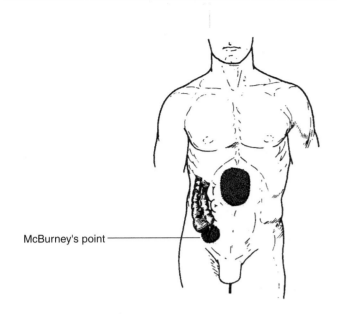

McBurney's point

FIGURE 15-16 Pain areas associated with appendicitis, including McBurney's point. Tenderness upon palpation of this point is indicative of appendicitis. With the client supine and legs extended, isolate the anterior superior iliac spine and the umbilicus, then gently palpate approximately one half the distance between those two points. A positive test produces painful symptoms in the right lower quadrant. (Modified from O'Toole M, editor: *Miller-Keane encyclopedia and dictionary of medicine, nursing, and allied health,* ed 6, Philadelphia, 1997, WB Saunders, p 119.)

client) with a known hernia complaining of pain, nausea, vomiting, or other new symptom in the anatomic vicinity of the hernia should report these symptoms to the physician to rule out a systemic condition unrelated to the herniation.

Congenital muscle weakness complicated by the additional risk factors of obesity and increased intraabdominal pressure should be identified and treated. Educate clients in proper lifting techniques and precautions to avoid heavy lifting and straining, which reduces intraabdominal pressure as an additional risk factor for the development of hernias and aids in preventing worsening of an already existing hernia. The mouth-open position as a reminder to breathe properly and to prevent increased intraabdominal pressure is essential during all lifting procedures. Obesity as a cause of increased intraabdominal pressure may be addressed by weight control through exercise (see Special Implications for the Therapist: Obesity, 2-4).

Special care must be taken when treating the client who has a vertical incision. When a vertical incision transects fascial aponeurotic fibers, the incision is made perpendicular to the direction of those fibers. Simple muscle contraction, as in coughing, straining, or turning over in bed, tends to distract the wound edges. Laparoscopic repair will likely eliminate this type of surgical incision. ■

Functional Obstruction
Adynamic or Paralytic Ileus.   Adynamic or paralytic ileus is a neurogenic or muscular impairment of peristalsis that can cause functional intestinal obstruction. The term "functional obstruction" is somewhat of a misnomer in that the intestine is not blocked or plugged so much as peristalsis stops

and movement of intestinal contents stops or is slowed down considerably. This condition has a variety of causes (see Table 15-7), most commonly occurring after abdominal surgery when the bowel ceases to function for a limited period of time (several hours to several days). Paralytic ileus is a common sequela of spinal cord injury. Neurogenic impairment also may occur after abdominal procedures in which the surgeon handles the bowel extensively or after surgery involving the retroperitoneal area.

Clinical manifestations include mild to moderate abdominal pain that tends to be continuous rather than colicky, as with mechanical obstruction. Borborygmus and bowel sounds are absent. Dehydration with prolonged vomiting and massive generalized abdominal distention may occur. The diagnosis is suspected in the presence of a precipitating condition and signs and symptoms of obstruction in the absence of bowel sounds. Diagnosis is confirmed by radiography of the abdomen and barium enema to rule out organic obstruction.

Most cases of adynamic ileus respond to restricted oral intake with gradual reintroduction of foods as bowel function returns. Severe and prolonged ileus may require complete elimination of food and fluids and aspiration of gastric secretions by suctioning until the bowel begins to function again. In such cases, parenteral nutrition is utilized to reintroduce fluids and electrolytes. Prognosis depends on the underlying cause of adynamic ileus. Removal of the cause may result in resolution of the ileus. Intubation with a rectal tube or colonoscope to decompress a dilated colon may be successful in returning bowel function but is not a commonly performed procedure.

Special Implications for the Therapist   **15-20**

ADYNAMIC OR PARALYTIC ILEUS

Anterior lumbar fusion procedures may indirectly cause a functional ileus when the client is unable to ambulate early or remains immobile and inactive for any reason. The therapist may use transcutaneous electrical nerve stimulation (TENS) in the acute care setting for the short term to assist in pain control and to encourage mobility. Increased activity stimulates movement of air out of the bowel and helps prevent constipation and the subsequent development of a functional ileus. ■

Congenital
Intestinal atresia and stenosis, although rare, are the most frequent causes of neonatal intestinal obstruction. Either condition is diagnosed on the basis of persistent vomiting of bile-containing fluid during the first 24 hours after birth. Surgical correction is usually successful, but coexistent anomalies often exist and complicate treatment.

Stenosis and Atresia.   *Stenosis* is a narrowing of a canal, in this case the small intestine. Intestinal atresia refers to defects caused by the incomplete formation of a lumen, in this case the tubular portion of the intestine. Many hollow organs

originate as strands and cords of cells, the centers of which are programmed to die, thus forming a central cavity or lumen.

Most cases of intestinal atresia are characterized by complete occlusion of the lumen, which was not fully established in embryogenesis. Meconium ileus (accumulation of meconium in the small intestine causing neonatal intestinal obstruction) accounts for 25% of all cases, and cystic fibrosis accounts for another 10%. Intestinal atresia may have several forms: multiple intestinal occlusions giving the appearance of a string of sausages, disconnected blind ends, blind proximal and distal sacs joined by a cord, or a thin transluminal diaphragm across the opening. All forms require surgical intervention with good prognosis for recovery.

Meckel's Diverticulum.

Meckel's diverticulum is an outpouching of the bowel located at the ileum of the small intestine, near the ileocecal valve. It occurs because of failure of destruction of the vitelline duct, an embryonic communication between the midgut and the yolk sac. Meckel's diverticulum is the most common congenital malformation of the GI tract, present in 2% of the population. Males are affected more often than females in a 2:1 ratio with accompanying complications in the same ratio.

Meckel's diverticulum may be asymptomatic or symptoms may include abdominal pain similar to other conditions such as appendicitis, Crohn's disease, and peptic ulcer disease. Common complications associated with Meckel's diverticulum include bleeding or hemorrhage from peptic ulceration of the ileum adjacent to the ectopic gastric mucosa; intestinal obstruction; diverticulitis that mimics appendicitis; and perforation caused by peptic ulceration in the diverticulum or in the ileum.

Diagnosis is made usually during the first 2 years but may go undetected into adulthood when it is discovered on autopsy or during laparotomy for an unrelated condition. The diagnosis is made usually based on history, physical examination, and radionuclide scan. Prognosis is good with surgical resection to remove the diverticulum. Severe hemorrhage must be treated before surgery to correct hypovolemic shock through the administration of blood transfusion, intravenous fluids, and oxygen.

THE APPENDIX

◆ Appendicitis

Definition and Incidence.   Appendicitis is an inflammation of the vermiform appendix that often results in necrosis and perforation with subsequent localized or generalized peritonitis. On the basis of operative findings and histologic appearance, acute appendicitis is classified as simple, gangrenous, or perforated. It is the most common disease of the appendix, occurring at any age, with the peak incidence among men in their second and third decades. The overall incidence is declining for unknown reasons, possibly as a result of increased dietary fiber intake in recent years or improved hygiene and fewer intestinal infections associated with indoor plumbing.

Etiologic Factors.   Approximately half of all cases of acute appendicitis have no known cause. At least one third are caused by obstruction preventing normal drainage. Obstruction may occur as a result of tumor, foreign body such as fecal material (fecalith) lodged in the lumen of the appendix,

parasites (e.g., intestinal worms), or lymphoid hyperplasia. Because the appendix is chiefly lymphatic tissue, an infection that produces enlarged lymph nodes elsewhere in the body also can increase the glandular tissue in the appendix and obstruct its lumen. Other causes include Crohn's disease of the terminal ileum, ulcerative colitis when it spreads to the mucosa of the appendix, and tuberculous enteritis.

Pathogenesis.   Classically, appendicitis is believed to develop primarily from obstruction of the lumen and secondarily from bacterial infection. When the long, narrow appendiceal lumen becomes obstructed, inflammation begins in the mucosa, with swelling and hyperemia of the vermiform appendix. As secretions distend the obstructed appendix, the intraluminal pressure rises and eventually exceeds the venous pressure, causing venous stasis and ischemia. The accumulation of neutrophils produces microabscesses, and arterial thromboses aggravate the ischemia. The infected necrotic wall becomes gangrenous and may perforate, often in 24 to 48 hours. The mucosa ulcerates and permits invasion by intestinal bacteria. *Escherichia coli* and other bacteria multiply and cause inflammation and infection that spread to the peritoneal cavity unless the body's defenses are able to overcome the infection or the appendix is removed before it ruptures.

Clinical Manifestations.   The presenting symptoms of acute appendicitis occur in a classic sequence of abdominal (epigastric, periumbilical, or right lower quadrant) pain accompanied by anorexia, nausea, vomiting, and low-grade fever in adults (children tend to have higher fevers). Women may experience acute pelvic pain that must be differentiated from other causes of pelvic pain (e.g., ectopic pregnancy, diverticulitis, incarcerated hernia, kidney stones). Pain associated with appendicitis is constant and may shift within 12 hours of symptom onset to the right lower quadrant with point tenderness over the site of the appendix at McBurney's point, a point between 1½ and 2 inches superomedial to the anterior superior iliac spine, on a line joining that process and the umbilicus (see Fig. 15-16). Aggravating factors include anything that increases intraabdominal pressure (see Box 15-1) such as coughing, walking, laughing, and bending over. Older adults frequently have few or no symptoms with minimal fever and only slight tenderness until perforation occurs.

Atypical Appendicitis.

Many cases of appendicitis are atypical because of the position of the appendix, the person's age, or the presence of associated conditions, such as pregnancy. The person may not recognize the need for medical attention but may report symptoms to the therapist. Early recognition of the need for medical evaluation is imperative.

Retrocecal appendicitis and *retroilieal appendicitis* may occur when the inflamed appendix is shielded from the anterior abdominal wall by the overlying cecum and ileum. The pain seems less intense, less localized, and less discomfort occurs with walking or coughing. The pain may not shift as expected from the epigastrium to the right lower quadrant.

Pelvic appendicitis may begin with pain in the epigastrium but quickly settles in the lower abdomen, commonly localized to the left side for an unknown reason. The absence of abdominal tenderness may be deceptive, but the physician will elicit this symptom on pelvic examination. *Appendicitis in the immunosuppressed* individual presents as abdominal pain and fever without leukocytosis, but concern about other causes usually delays recognition.

Appendicitis in the aging adult is usually vague with minimal pain and only slight temperature elevation. Abdominal tenderness is present and localized to the right lower quadrant but is deceptively mild. *Appendicitis in pregnancy* does not present a diagnostic problem in the first trimester but later in gestation may be confused as an obstetric condition. Displacement of the appendix by the enlarged uterus may result in tenderness in the right subcostal area or adjacent to the umbilicus.

Medical Management

Diagnosis.   Acute appendicitis must be diagnosed early to prevent perforation, abscess formation, and postoperative complications but is not always easy to make. Although the clinical diagnosis may be straightforward in people who present with classic signs and symptoms, atypical presentations require the physician to differentiate appendicitis from a large variety of GI, genitourinary, and gynecologic conditions. A careful history and thorough physical examination are the primary diagnostic tools. An elevated white blood cell count ($>20,000/mm^3$; leukocytosis), suggests ruptured appendix and peritonitis. Helical computer tomography and ultrasonography are highly accurate diagnostic tools. Histologic examination of the resected appendix is used to confirm the diagnosis, and at least 10% of appendices resected are normal.

Treatment and Prognosis.   Appendectomy, or surgical removal of the vermiform appendix, is performed as soon as possible. Antibiotics are administered preoperatively in the presence of systemic symptoms or when surgery is unavailable. With accurate diagnosis and early surgical removal, mortality and morbidity rates are less than 1%. Prognosis is good unless diagnosis is delayed and perforation occurs (rarely during the first 8 hours of symptomatic presentation). Perforation with complications such as peritonitis, hypovolemia, and septic shock has a poor prognosis. Perforation is more likely in infants under 2 years of age and in adults over 60 years.

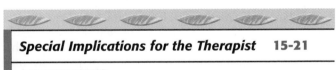

Special Implications for the Therapist   15-21

APPENDICITIS

When appendicitis is atypical the client may not recognize the need for medical attention but may report the symptoms to the therapist. Early recognition of the need for medical referral is important. In an athletic training or physical therapy setting, appendicitis may present with symptoms of right thigh, groin (testicular) pain, pelvic pain, or referred pain to the hip.

In addition to screening for the presence of constitutional symptoms, a variety of objective test procedures may be employed by the therapist. Ask the client to cough: localization of painful symptoms to the site of the appendix is typical. Perform the iliopsoas muscle test and the obturator muscle test (see Fig. 15-10), palpate the iliopsoas muscle (see Fig. 15-11), palpate McBurney's point (see Fig. 15-16), and assess for rebound tenderness (Fig. 15-17). If any of these tests is positive for reproduction of symptoms in the right lower quadrant, a medical re-

ferral is necessary. If appendicitis is suspected, medical attention must be immediate. The client should be instructed to lie down and remain as quiet as possible, taking nothing by mouth (including water); heat is contraindicated. ■

THE PERITONEUM

◆ Peritonitis

Overview.   Peritonitis, or inflammation of the serous membrane lining the walls of the abdominal cavity, is caused by a number of situations that introduce microorganisms into the peritoneal cavity. Peritonitis that occurs spontaneously is called *primary peritonitis*. Peritonitis as a consequence of trauma, surgery, or peritoneal contamination by bowel contents (e.g., perforated duodenal ulcer or appendix) is referred to as *secondary peritonitis*.

Etiologic Factors.   Specific causes of peritonitis are many and varied. Primary peritonitis is associated with ascites and chronic liver disease or the nephrotic syndrome. Secondary peritonitis occurs as a result of inflammation of abdominal organs, irritating substances from a perforated gallbladder or gastric ulcer, rupture of a cyst, or irritation from blood, as in cases of internal bleeding.

Secondary peritonitis may be classified as bacterial, chemical, or metastatic. *Bacterial peritonitis* is caused by bacterial infection (*E. coli*, bacteroides, staphylococcus, streptococcus, pneumococcus, gonococcus) introduced most commonly by perforation of a viscus. Such perforation can occur in the case of appendicitis, an ulcer, a bowel infarct, colonic diverticulum, chronic peritoneal dialysis at the site of catheter exit, and urinary infection. These

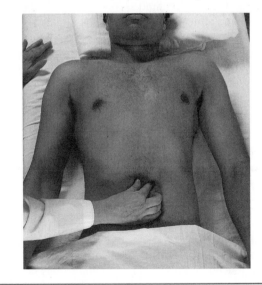

FIGURE   **15-17** Rebound tenderness (Blumberg sign). Assess for rebound tenderness by pressing down slowly and deeply at an abdominal site away from the painful area. Quickly lifting the examiner's hand allows the indented structures to rebound suddenly. A normal or negative response is no pain on release of pressure. Pain on release of pressure confirms rebound tenderness, a reliable sign of peritoneal inflammation. Perform this test at the end of the examination because it can cause severe pain and muscle rigidity. (From Jarvis C: *Physical examination and health assessment,* ed 3, Philadelphia, 2000, WB Saunders, p 607.)

bacterial organisms spread quickly throughout the abdominal cavity and may enter the bloodstream from the peritoneum, causing life-threatening septicemia.

Chemical peritonitis is a noninfectious inflammation caused by bile leakage, usually from a perforated gallbladder, but sometimes from a needle biopsy of the liver, or any breach in the GI wall that allows GI contents to spill into the abdominal cavity. Once bacteria enter the abdominal cavity, then chemical peritonitis progresses quickly and develops into bacterial peritonitis. Other causes include substances such as gastric acid, blood, or foreign material introduced by surgery (e.g., talc), and acute pancreatitis, which releases and activates lipolytic and proteolytic enzymes. *Metastatic peritonitis* occurs when neoplasm perforates the viscus of the stomach and tumor cells infiltrate the peritoneum.

Pathogenesis. Once the inflammatory process has begun, a fibrinopurulent exudate covers the peritoneal surface. The exudate becomes organized and fibrotic, forming adhesions and causing obstruction. When a perforation drains contaminants into the peritoneal cavity, the ability of the peritoneum to combat the inflammatory process is overpowered. The entire surface of the peritoneum may be involved (generalized peritonitis) or only specific sites (localized). When the pelvic peritoneum is involved, pelvic peritonitis (also called *pelvic inflammatory disease*) occurs.

Peritonitis creates severe systemic effects. Circulatory alterations, fluid shifts, and respiratory problems can cause critical fluid and electrolyte imbalances. The circulatory system undergoes great stress from several sources. The inflammatory response shunts extra blood to the inflamed area of the bowel to combat the infection. Peristaltic activity of the bowel ceases. Fluids and air are retained within its lumen, raising pressure and increasing fluid secretion into the bowel; circulating volume diminishes.

Clinical Manifestations. Peritonitis presents as an acute abdomen with severe abdominal pain; the abdomen becomes rigid (involuntary guarding) and sensitive to the touch. Nausea, vomiting, and high fever follow. Complications may include paralytic ileus (diminished to absent peristalsis) and septic shock. A peritoneal abscess develops if the perforation becomes self-encased or walled off. Antibiotic therapy may mask or delay the recognition of signs of abscess. In persons with underlying ascites, the signs and symptoms of peritonitis may be more subtle, with fever as the only manifestation of infection, or possibly nausea, vomiting, nonspecific abdominal pain, or altered mental status.

Medical Management
Diagnosis, Treatment, and Prognosis. Abdominal films, barium enema, and an abdominal tap may be used in the differential diagnosis of peritonitis. Peritonitis should be treated immediately to control infection; preserve the barrier to further microbial invasion; minimize the effects of paralytic ileus; and correct fluid, electrolyte, and nutritional disorders.

If peritonitis is advanced and surgery is contraindicated because of shock and circulatory failure, oral fluids are prohibited and intravenous fluids are necessary for replacement of electrolyte and protein losses. A long intestinal tube is inserted through the nose into the intestine to reduce pressure within the bowel. Once the infection has become walled off

and the client's condition improves, surgical drainage and repair can be attempted.

Despite treatment with antibiotics, surgical drainage and debridement, and supportive measures, generalized peritonitis is still associated with a mortality rate of 50% and is especially dangerous in the older adult. Individuals recovering from an episode of bacterial peritonitis should be considered as potential candidates for liver transplantation.

Special Implications for the Therapist 15-22

PERITONITIS

Special considerations associated with peritonitis are related to the underlying cause (e.g., liver or kidney disease, postoperative, cancer) and resultant complications (e.g., fluid and electrolyte imbalance, pulmonary compromise). The client with peritonitis usually is hospitalized and undergoing medical treatment. The therapist should be familiar with implications associated with the underlying cause and any complications present.

Vital signs should be regularly monitored (see Appendix B) and a semi-Fowler's position used to help the client breathe deeply with less pain to prevent pulmonary complications. Position changes must be accomplished with extreme caution because the slightest movement intensifies the pain. Watch for signs of dehiscence (separation of layers of a surgical wound) such as the person reporting that something broke loose or gave way inside. Follow all safety measures such as keeping the side rails up on the bed if fever and pain disorient the client. ◼

THE RECTUM

◆ Rectal Fissure

A rectal or anal fissure is an ulceration or tear of the lining of the anal canal, usually on the posterior wall. An acute fissure occurs as a result of excessive tissue stretching or tearing such as childbirth or passage of a large, hard bowel movement through the area. The skin tear is very fragile and tends to reopen easily with the next bowel movement prompting the person to avoid going to the bathroom for days. Neglecting the "call of the stool" can result in constipation and further exacerbation of the problem especially in the presence of risk factors for constipation (see the section on Constipation in this chapter).

Anal fissures frequently heal within a month or two when treated with a combination of bran and bulk laxatives or stool softeners, sitz baths, and emollient suppositories. Chronic fissures are usually secondary to a tight rectal sphincter or infectious material retained in the anal sinuses. Sharp pain, followed by burning, accompanies defecation. Other symptoms include mucus, an external skin tag at the anus (sentinel pile), and itching.

◆ Rectal Abscesses and Fistulas

Anal abscesses and fistulas can occur as a result of an infected anal gland, fissure, or prolapsed hemorrhoid and are most common in people with Crohn's disease. The infection can cause pus, mucus, and blood to drain from the anus. Fistulas (abnormal channels to the body's surface) may form spontaneously to drain the abscesses. Swelling, pain, and throbbing exacerbated by sitting or walking are the primary symptoms and may heal with time or may be treated with surgical drainage with or without antibiotics.

◆ Hemorrhoids

Hemorrhoids, or piles, are varicose veins in the perianal region and may be internal or external. Hemorrhoids are fairly common, affecting as many as half of all adults more than 50 years of age. This condition is associated especially with anything that increases intraabdominal pressure (see Box 15-1) such as pregnancy, pelvic congestion or pelvic venous disease, congestive heart failure, prolonged sitting or standing, low-fiber diet, obesity, diarrhea, and delaying a bowel movement when the urge presents itself.

Internal hemorrhoids usually are noticed first when a small amount of bleeding occurs during passage of stool especially if straining occurs during a bowel movement. Internal hemorrhoids are asymptomatic (rectal tissue lacks nerve fibers) except in the presence of an anal fissure, thrombosis, or strangulation of the varicose vein. In the case of strangulation straining can cause an internal hemorrhoid to protrude (prolapse) from the anus. The blood supply is cut off by the anal sphincter causing local discomfort and possible itching. This can result in thrombosis when blood within the hemorrhoid clots.

External hemorrhoids bleed (bright-red blood) if the hemorrhoid is injured or ulcerated and are very painful because they form in nerve-rich tissue outside the anal canal. Other manifestations include pressure, rectal itching, irritation, and a palpable mass. Severe bleeding or mild bleeding repeatedly from prolonged trauma to the vein during defecation can cause iron-deficiency anemia.

Internal hemorrhoids may require ligation, sclerosing, laser surgery, or cryosurgery to destroy the affected tissue. In the case of advanced chronic hemorrhoids, recurrent bleeding and anemia may necessitate surgery (hemorrhoidectomy). *External hemorrhoids* can be treated with local application of topical medications, sitz baths, high-fiber diet, and avoidance of constipation and other causes of increased intraabdominal pressure. A stool softener or psyllium preparation may be used when a modified diet is unsuccessful in eliminating constipation. Local topical preparations for hemorrhoids are used to reduce pain or itching.

Special Implications for the Therapist   **15-23**

THE RECTUM

Therapists may be involved with clients with pelvic pain and/or pelvic floor dysfunction accompanied by chronic rectal conditions. The client may have a history of sexual assault/abuse and/or anal intercourse. These individuals experience severe muscle spasm of the sphincter resulting in groin or pelvic pain and trigger points of the pelvic floor and gluteal muscles. Any anorectal symptoms (e.g., change in bowel habits, rectal pain,

bleeding) that have not been reported to the physician or are changing in pattern must be evaluated by a physician.

Clients involved in any activity requiring increased abdominal support or causing increased intraabdominal pressure should be questioned as to the presence of hemorrhoids. For clients with hemorrhoids postoperatively, prone positioning or sidelying supported with pillows between the knees and ankles is preferred. Supine positioning and sitting for brief periods can be accomplished with a rubber air ring under the buttocks for support. Movement, exercise, drinking plenty of fluids, and heeding the call of nature are important in the prevention of constipation-induced hemorrhoids. ■

REFERENCES

1. AHCPR (Agency for Health Care Policy and Research): Colorectal cancer screening: summary, http://www.ahcpr.gov, 2001.
2. Aldoori WH, Giovannucci EL, Rimm EB et al: Use of acetaminophen and nonsteroidal antiinflammatory drug: a prospective study and the risk of symptomatic diverticular disease in men, *Arch Fam Med* 7(3):262-3, 1998.
3. Ali A, Toner BB, Stuckless N, et al: Emotional abuse, self-blame, and self-silencing in women with irritable bowel syndrome, *Psychosom Med* 62(1):76-82, 2000.
4. American Physical Therapy Association (APTA): Guidelines for recognizing and providing care for victims of domestic violence, No. P-138, Alexandria, Va, 1997 APTA.
5. Anderson M, Robinson M: Watching for—and managing—joint problems in inflammatory bowel disease, *J Musculo Med* 13(11):28-34, 1996.
6. Befus AD, Mathison R, Davison J: Integration of neuro-endocrine immune responses in defense of mucosal surfaces, *Am J Trop Med Hyg* 60(4):26-34, 1999.
7. Blomhoff S, Spetalen S, Jacobsen MB, et al: Intestinal reactivity to words with emotional content and brain information processing in irritable bowel syndrome, *Dig Dis Sci* 45(6):1160-5, 2000.
8. Blomhoff S, Spetalen S, Jacobsen MB, et al: Rectal tone and brain information processing in irritable bowel syndrome, *Dig Dis Sci* 45(6):1153-9, 2000.
9. Brown LM: Helicobacter pylori: epidemiology and routes of transmission, *Epidemiol Rev* 22(2):283-97, 2000.
10. Burdick JS: Esophageal cancer prevention, cure, and palliation, *Semin Gastrointes Dis* 11(3):124-33, 2000.
11. Camilleri M, Lee JS, Viramontes B, et al: Insights into the pathophysiology and mechanisms of constipation, irritable bowel syndrome, and diverticulosis in older people, *J Am Geriatr Soc* 48(9):1142-50, 2000.
12. Campbell-Thompson M, Lynch IJ, Bhardwaj B: Expression of estrogen (ER) subtypes and Erbeta isoforms in colon cancer, *Cancer Res* 61(2):632-40, 2001.
13. CDC (Centers for Disease Control and Prevention): Hypertrophic pyloric stenosis in infants following pertussis prophylaxis with erythromycin, *J Am Med Assoc* 283(4):471-2, 2000.
14. Cheng Y, Macera CA, Davis Dr, et al: Does physical activity reduce the risk of developing peptic ulcers? *Br J Sports Med* 34(2):116-21, 2000.
15. Christensen J, Miftakhov R: Hiatus hernia: a review of evidence for its origin in esophageal longitudinal muscle dysfuntion, *Am J Med* 108(Suppl 4a):3S-7S, 2000.
16. Clark TJ, McKenna LS, Jewell MJ: Physical therapists' recognition of battered women in clinical settings, *Phys Ther* 76(1):12-9, 1996.
17. Colbert LH, Hartman TJ, Malila N, et al: Physical activity in relation to cancer of the colon and rectum in a cohort of male smokers, *Cancer Epidemiol Biomarkers Prev* 10(3):265-8, 2001.
18. Crohn's & Colitis Foundation of America (CCFA): Questions and Answers about Crohn's Disease and Ulcerative Colitis, http://www.ccfa.org, 2001.
19. Cunningham-Rundles S, Lin DH: Nutrition and the immune system of the gut, *Nutrition* 14(7-8):573-9, 1998.
20. Dean E: Oxygen transport deficits in systemic diseases and implications for physical therapy, *Phys Ther* 77(2):187-202, 1997.

21. De Lillo AR, Rose S: Functional bowel disorders in the geriatric patient: constipation, fecal impaction, and fecal incontinence, *Am J Gastroenterol* 95(4):901-5, 2000.

22. Duffy MJ: Carcinoembryonic antigen as a marker for colorectal cancer: is it clinically useful? *Clin Chem* 47(4):624-30, 2001.

23. Falk GW: GERD and H. pylori: is there a link? *Semin Gastrointest Dis* 12(1):16-25, 2001.

24. Ferdjallah M, Wertsch JJ, Shaker R: Spectral analysis of surface electromyography (EMG) of upper esophageal sphincter-opening muscles during head lift exercise, *J Rehabil Res Dev* 37(3):335-40, 2000.

25. Gaspar LE, Winter K, Kocha WI, et al: A phase I/II study of external beam radiation, brachytherapy, and concurrent chemotherapy for patients with localized carcinoma of the esophagus (Radiation Therapy Oncology Study Group 9207): final report, *Cancer* 88(5):988-95, 2000.

26. Gelbmann CM: Prediction of treatment refractoriness in ulcerative colitis and Crohn's disease—do we have reliable markers? *Inflamm Bowel Dis* 6(2):123-31, 2000.

27. Gershon MD: *The second brain: a groundbreaking new understanding of nervous disorders of the stomach and intestines*, New York, 1999, Harperperennial Library.

28. Goodman CC, Snyder TE: *Differential diagnosis in physical therapy*, ed 3, Philadelphia, 2000, WB Saunders.

29. Gow PJ, Chapman RW: Modern management of oesophageal varices, *Postgrad Med J* 77(904):75-81, 2001.

30. Green JA, Amaro R, Barkin JS: Symptomatic gastroesophageal reflux as a risk factor for esophageal adenocarcinoma, *Dig Dis Sci* 45(12):2367-8, 2000.

31. Greenlee RT, Hill-Harmon MB, Murray T, et al: Cancer statistics, 2001, *CA Cancer J Clin* 51(1):15-36, 2001.

32. Hawk E, Lubet R, Limburg P: Chemoprevention in hereditary colorectal cancer syndromes, *Cancer* 86(11 Suppl):2551-63, 1999.

33. Hegab AM, Luketic VA: Bleeding esophageal varices. How to treat this dreaded complication of portal hypertension, *Postgrad Med* 109(2):75-6, 81-6, 89, 2001.

34. Johns Hopkins Medical Letter: Do you need a B₁₂ boost? 10(4):6, 1998.

35. Johnson C: Handling the hurt: physical therapy and domestic violence, *Phys Ther* 5(1):52-64, 1997.

36. Khoury RM, Camacho-Lobato L, Katz PO, et al: Influence of spontaneous sleep positions on nighttime recumbent reflux in patients with gastroesophageal reflux disease, *Am J Gastroenterol* 94(8):2069-73, 1999.

37. Kopp-Hoolihan L: Prophylactic and therapeutic uses of probiotics: a review, *J Am Diet Assoc* 101(2):229-38, 2001.

38. Kountouras J, Boura P, Lygidakis NJ: New concepts of molecular biology for colon carcinogenesis, *Hepatogastroenterology* 35:1291-7, 2000.

39. Lazzaroni M, Bianchi PG: Nonsteroidal anti-inflammatory drug gastrophathy and *Helicobacter pylori*: the search for an improbable consensus, *Am J Med* 110(1A):50S-4S, 2001.

40. Lynch PM: COX-2 inhibition in clinical cancer prevention, *Oncology* 15(3 Suppl 5):21-6, 2001.

41. Mead P, Slutsker L, Dietz V, et al: Food-related illness and death in the United States, *Emerg Infect Dis* 5:607-9, 1999.

42. MMWR (Mortality and Morbidity Weekly Report): Diagnosis and management of foodborne illnesses, *MMWR* 50(RR02): 1-69, 2001.

43. MMWR (Mortality and Morbidity Weekly Report): Preliminary FoodNet Data on the Incidence of Foodborne Illnesses—Selected Sites, United States, 2000, 50(13):241-6, 2001.

44. Morgner A, Bayerdorffer E, Neubauer A, et al: Gastric MALT lymphoma and its relationship to *Helicobacter pylori* infection: management and pathogenesis of the disease, *Microsco Res Tech* 48(6):349-56, 2000.

45. Murphy TV, Gargiullo PM, Massoudi MS, et al: Intussusception among infants given an oral rotavirus vaccine, *New Engl J Med* 344(8):564-72, 2001.

46. Nagura H, Ohtani H, Sasano H, et al: The immuno-inflammatory mechanism for tissue injury in inflammatory bowel disease and *Helicobacter pylori*–infected chronic active gastritis. Roles of the mucosal immune system, *Digestion* 63 Suppl 1:12-21, 2001.

47. Oliveria SA, Christos PJ, Talley NJ, et al: Heartburn risk factors, knowledge, and prevention strategies: a population-based survey of individuals with heartburn, *Arch Intern Med* 159(14):1592-8, 1999.

48. Overmier JB, Murison R: Anxiety and helplessness in the face of stress predisposes, precipitates, and sustains gastric ulceration, *Behav Brain Res* 110(1-2):161-74, 2000.

49. Pahor M, Guralnik JM, Salive ME, et al: Physical activity and risk of severe gastrointestinal hemorrhage in older persons, *J Am Med Assoc* 272:595-9, 1994.

50. Paulozzi LJ: Is *Helicobacter pylori* a cause of infantile hypertrophic pyloric stenosis? *Med Hypotheses* 55(2):119-25, 2000.

51. Pert C: *Molecules of emotion: Why you feel the way you feel*, New York, 1999, Simon & Schuster.

52. Pothoulakis C, Lamont JT: Microbes and microbial toxins: paradigms for microbial-mucosal interactions. II. The integrated response of the intestine to *Clostridium difficile* toxins, *Am J Physiol Gastrointest Liver Physiol* 280(2):G178-83, 2001.

53. Reilly J, Baker GA, Rhodes J, et al: The association of sexual and physical abuse with somatization: characteristics of patients presenting with irritable bowel syndrome and non-epileptic attack disorder, *Psychol Med* 29(2):399-406, 1999.

54. Roberfroid MB: Prebiotics and probiotics: are they functional foods? *Am J Clin Nutr* 71(6 Suppl):1682S-7S, 2000.

55. Rose SJ, Rothstein JM: Muscle mutability: general concepts and adaptations to altered patterns of use, *Phys Ther* 62:1773, 1982.

56. Rubin DT, Dachman AH: Virtual colonoscopy: a novel imaging modality for colorectal cancer, *Curr Oncol Rep* 3(2):88-93, 2001.

57. Sandler RS, Halabi S, Kaplan EB, et al: Use of vitamins, minerals, and nutritional supplements by participants in a chemoprevention trial, *Cancer* 91(5):1040-5, 2001.

58. Schatzkin A, Lanza E, Corle D, et al: Lack of effect of a low-fat, high-fiber diet on the recurrence of colorectal adenomas. Polyp Prevention Trial Study Group, *N Eng J Med* 342(16):1149-55, 2000.

59. Schoon EJ, Blok BM, Geerling BJ, et al: Bone mineral density in patients with recently diagnosed inflammatory bowel disease, *Gastroenterology* 119(5):1203-8, 2000.

60. Schoon EJ, Muller MC, Vermeer C, et al: Low serum and bone vitamin K status in patients with longstanding Crohn's disease: another pathogenetic factor of osteoporosis in Crohn's disease? *Gut* 48(4):448, 2001.

61. Schulte CM, Dignass AU, Goebell H, et al: Genetic factors determine extent of bone loss in inflammatory bowel disease, *Gastroenterology* 119(4):909-920, 2000.

62. Semrad CE: Bone mass and gastrointestinal disease, *Ann NY Acad Sci* 904:564-70, 2000.

63. Shanahan F: Inflammatory bowel disease: immunodiagnostics, immunotherapeutics, and ecotherapeutics, *Gastroenterology* 120(3): 622-35, 2001.

64. Spinzi G, Belloni G, Martegani A, et al: Computed tomographic colonography and conventional colonoscopy for colon diseases: a prospective blinded study, *Am J Gastroenterol* 96(2):394-400, 2001.

65. Sutton P: Helicobacter pylori vaccines and mechanisms of effective immunity: is mucus the key? *Immunol Cell Biol* 79(1):67-73, 2001.

66. Tougas G: The autonomic nervous system function in functional bowel disorders, *Gut* 47 (Suppl 4):78-80, 2000.

67. Vainio H, Bianchini F: Prevention of disease with pharmaceuticals, *Pharmacol Toxicol* 88(3):111-8, 2001.

68. Vanagunas A: Managing gastrointestinal problems in athletes, *J Musculoskel Med* 16(7):405-15, 1999.

69. Wijnhoven BP, Tilanus HW, Dinjens WN: Molecular biology and Barrett's adenocarcinoma, *Ann Surg* 233(3):322-37, 2001.

70. Yang YX, Lichtenstein GR: Methotrexate for the maintenance of remission in Crohn's disease, *Gastroenterology* 120(6):1553-5, 2001.

CHAPTER 16

THE HEPATIC, PANCREATIC, AND BILIARY SYSTEMS

CATHERINE C. GOODMAN

*T*he *liver* has more than 500 separate functions, such as the conversion and excretion of bilirubin (red bile pigment, an end-product of heme from hemoglobin in red blood cells [RBCs]). The liver is the sole source of albumin and other plasma proteins and also produces 500 to 1500 mL of bile each day. Other important functions of the liver include production of clotting factors and storage of vitamins. The liver and gut are the key organs in nutrient absorption and metabolism; nutrients bind to toxins in this pathway and aid in eliminating these toxins from the body. The liver contributes to a functional immune system by reducing the amount of toxins that could impair the gut lining, which in turn helps prevent the entry of bacteria and viruses into the system. Bile acids, drugs, chemicals, and toxins undergo extensive enterohepatic circulation during the processes of metabolism. The liver also filters all of the blood from the gastrointestinal system and is therefore the primary organ for metastasis of intestinal cancer.

The *pancreas* is both an exocrine and an endocrine gland. Its primary function in digestion is exocrine secretion of digestive enzymes and pancreatic juices, transported through the pancreatic duct to the duodenum. Proteins, carbohydrates, and fats are broken down in the duodenum, aided by pancreatic and other secretions, which also help to neutralize the acidic substances passed from the stomach to the duodenum. The endocrine function involves the secretion of glucagon and insulin by islet of Langerhans cells for the regulation of carbohydrate metabolism. Pancreatic disease may result in a variety of clinical presentations depending on whether the exocrine or endocrine function has been impaired.

The *gallbladder*, acting as a reservoir for bile, stores and concentrates the bile during fasting periods and then contracts to expel the bile into the duodenum in response to the arrival of food. Bile helps in alkalinizing the intestinal contents and plays a role in the emulsification, absorption, and digestion of fat. The signal for the gallbladder to contract comes from the release of cholecystokinin, a hormone released into the bloodstream from the wall of the duodenum and upper small intestine.

SIGNS AND SYMPTOMS OF HEPATIC DISEASE

Primary signs and symptoms of liver diseases vary and can include gastrointestinal (GI) symptoms, edema/ascites, dark urine, light-colored or clay-colored feces, and right upper ab-

dominal pain (Box 16-1). Impairment of the liver can result in *hepatic failure* when either the mass of liver cells is sufficiently diminished or their function is impaired as a result of cirrhosis, liver cancer, or infection and/or inflammation. Hepatic failure does not refer to one specific morphologic change but rather to a clinical syndrome that includes hepatic encephalopathy, renal failure (hepatorenal syndrome), endocrine changes, and jaundice.

Dark urine and *light stools* occur in association with jaundice (yellow pigmentation of skin, sclerae, and mucous membranes) (see the section on Jaundice later in this chapter) when the serum bilirubin level increases from normal (0.1 to 1.0 mg/dL) to a value of 2 or 3 mg/dL. Any damage to the liver impairs bilirubin metabolism from the blood. Normally, bile converted from bilirubin causes brown coloration of the stool. Light-colored (almost white) stools and urine the color of tea or cola indicate an inability of the liver or biliary system to excrete bilirubin properly.

Skin changes associated with the hepatic system include jaundice, pallor, and orange or green skin. When bilirubin reaches levels of 2 to 3 mg/dL, the sclera of the eye takes on a yellow hue. When bilirubin level reaches 5 to 6 mg/dL, the skin becomes yellow. The changes described here in urine, stool, or skin color may be caused by hepatitis, gallbladder disease, and/or pancreatic cancer blocking the bile duct, hepatotoxic medications, or cirrhosis. Other skin changes may include bruising, spider angiomas, and palmar erythema.

Spider angiomas (arterial spider, spider telangiectasis, vascular spider) are branched dilations of the superficial capillaries, which may be vascular manifestations of increased estrogen levels (hyperestrogenism) (see Fig. 9-2). Spider angiomas and palmar erythema both occur in the presence of liver impairment as a result of increased estrogen levels normally metabolized by the liver. *Palmar erythema* (warm redness of the skin over the palms, also called *liver palms*) especially affects the hypothenar and thenar eminences and pulps of the finger. The soles of the feet may be similarly affected. The person may complain of throbbing, tingling palms.

Neurologic symptoms such as confusion, sleep disturbances, muscle tremors, hyperreactive reflexes, and asterixis (see following discussion) may occur. When liver dysfunction results in increased serum ammonia and urea levels, peripheral nerve function can be impaired. Ammonia from the intestine (produced by protein breakdown) is normally transformed by the liver to urea, glutamine, and asparagine, which are then excreted by the renal system. When the liver does not metabolize and detoxify ammonia, ammonia is transported to the brain,

Most Common Signs and Symptoms of Hepatic Disease

Gastrointestinal symptoms (see Table 15-1)
Edema/ascites
Dark urine
Light- or clay-colored stools
Right upper quadrant abdominal pain
Skin changes
    Jaundice
    Bruising
    Spider angioma
    Palmar erythema
Neurologic involvement
    Confusion
    Sleep disturbances
    Muscle tremors
    Hyperreactive reflexes
    Asterixis
Musculoskeletal pain (see text for sites)
Hepatic osteodystrophy
Hepatic failure
    Hepatic encephalopathy
    Renal failure (hepatorenal syndrome)
    Endocrine changes
    Jaundice
Portal hypertension

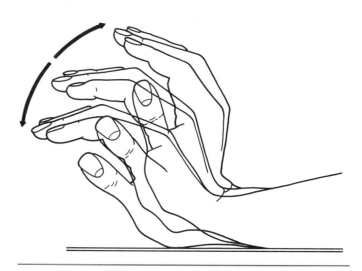

FIGURE 16-1 Flapping tremor. The flapping tremor elicited by attempted wrist extension while the forearm is fixed is the most common neurologic abnormality associated with liver failure. It can also be observed in uremia, respiratory failure, and severe heart failure. The tremor is absent at rest, decreased by intentional movement, and maximal on sustained posture. It is usually bilateral, although one side may be affected more than the other. (From Sherlock S, Dooley J: *Diseases of the liver and biliary system*, ed 9, Oxford, 1993, Blackwell Scientific Publications, p 89.)

where it reacts with glutamate (excitatory neurotransmitter) to produce glutamine. The reduction of brain glutamate impairs neurotransmission, leading to altered CNS metabolism and function. Asterixis and numbness or tingling (misinterpreted as carpal tunnel syndrome) can occur as a result of this ammonia abnormality, causing intrinsic nerve pathology.

Asterixis, also called *flapping tremors* or *liver flap*, is a motor disturbance; specifically, it is the inability to maintain wrist extension with forward flexion of the upper extremities. A test for asterixis is asking the client to extend the wrist and hand with the rest of the arm supported on a firm surface or with the arms held out in front of the body. Observe for quick, irregular extensions and flexions of the wrist and fingers (Fig. 16-1). Altered neurotransmission, in the form of impaired inflow of joint and other afferent information to the brainstem reticular formation, causes the movement dysfunction.

Musculoskeletal locations of pain associated with the hepatic and biliary systems include thoracic pain between scapulae, right shoulder, right upper trapezius, right interscapular, or right subscapular areas. Sympathetic fibers from the biliary system are connected through the celiac and splanchnic (visceral) plexuses to the hepatic fibers in the region of the dorsal spine. These connections account for the intercostal and radiating interscapular pain that accompanies gallbladder disease. Although the innervation is bilateral, most of the biliary fibers reach the cord through the right splanchnic nerves, producing pain in the right shoulder.

Hepatic osteodystrophy, abnormal development of bone, can occur in all forms of cholestasis (bile flow suppression) and hepatocellular disease, especially in the alcoholic. Bone pain may occur especially in the presence of osteomalacia or, more often, osteoporosis. Hepatic osteoporosis is secondary to osteoblastic dysfunction rather than to excessive bone resorption.* Vertebral wedging, vertebral crush fractures, and kyphosis can be severe; decalcification of the rib cage and pseudofractures† occur frequently. Osteoporosis associated with primary biliary cirrhosis and primary sclerosing cholangitis parallels the severity of liver disease rather than the duration. Painful osteoarthropathy may develop in the wrists and ankles as a nonspecific complication of chronic liver disease.

Portal hypertension, ascites, and *hepatic encephalopathy* are three other major symptoms of liver disease that are discussed in greater depth in this chapter as distinct clinical conditions.

Special Implications for the Therapist 16-1

SIGNS AND SYMPTOMS OF HEPATIC DISEASE

Any client presenting with undiagnosed or untreated jaundice must be referred to the physician for follow-up. Active, intense exercise should be avoided when the liver is compromised

---

*The pathogenesis is probably complex, and factors include calcium malabsorption, alcohol, corticosteroid therapy, estrogen deficiency in the postmenopausal woman, and vitamin D deficiency with secondary hyperparathyroidism.

†Pseudofractures or Looser's zones are narrow lines of radiolucency (areas of darkness on x-ray film) usually oriented perpendicular to the bone surface. This may represent a stress fracture that has been repaired by the laying down of inadequately mineralized osteoid, or these sites may occur as a result of mechanical erosion caused by arterial pulsations, as arteries frequently overlie sites of pseudofractures.

(i.e., during jaundice or any other active liver disease), because the cornerstone of medical treatment and promotion of healing of the liver is rest. (See also Special Implications for the Therapist: Jaundice, 16-2; Portal Hypertension, 16-9; Ascites, 16-10; and Hepatic Encephalopathy, 16-11.)

An increased risk of coagulopathy (decreased clotting ability) also occurs with liver disease, necessitating precautions. Easy bruising and bleeding under the skin or into the joints in response to the slightest trauma can occur when coagulation is impaired. This condition necessitates extreme care in the therapy setting, especially with any intervention requiring manual therapy or the use of any equipment, including modalities, resistive exercise or weight-training devices, and potentially the use of gait belts.

The most common neurologic abnormality associated with liver failure (called liver flap or asterixis) (see Fig. 16-1) also can be observed in uremia, respiratory failure, and severe heart failure. The rapid flexion extension movements at the metacarpophalangeal and wrist joints often are accompanied by lateral movements of the digits. Sometimes movement of arms, neck, and jaws; protruding tongue; retracted mouth; and tightly closed eyelids are involved, and the gait is ataxic. The tremor is absent at rest, decreased by intentional movement, and maximal on sustained posture. It is usually bilateral, although not bilaterally synchronous, and one side may be affected more than the other. It may be observed by gentle elevation of a limb or by the client's gripping the therapist's hand. In coma, the tremor disappears. ∎

AGING AND THE HEPATIC SYSTEM

The *liver* decreases in size and weight with advancing age requiring more time to process substances, medications, and alcohol. Liver function test results, such as levels of aspartate transaminase (AST), alanine transaminase (ALT), gammaglutamyl transpeptidase (GGTP), alkaline phosphatase, and total serum bilirubin (see Chapter 39), remain unchanged and within normal limits established for the adult. However, these tests often measure hepatic damage rather than overall function; abnormal values for these tests in older adults reflect disease rather than the effects of aging. The decreased liver weight is accompanied by diminished blood flow; this combination of decreased liver mass and blood flow may account for some changes in drug elimination observed in the older adult.* In the past, adjusting dosage downward based on hepatic function related to aging has not been considered necessary. However, emerging data on the use of pharmacologic agents in the older population suggest that the administration of many agents (especially chemotherapeutic agents in increasing use) may be affected by physiologic changes occurring with age. Dose adjustments to compensate for pharmacokinetic and pharmacodynamic changes that occur in the older adult are being studied and adjustments for specific drugs presented.[29]

---

*Many factors may influence drug metabolism in the older adult, including changes in body composition, decline in renal function, alterations in serum albumin levels (drugs such as sulfonamides and salicylates compete with bilirubin for binding sites on albumin, a transport plasma protein), individual variability, poor compliance, lack of understanding of drug therapy, presence of other systemic illnesses, and taking multiple drugs simultaneously (drug-drug interaction).

The liver itself becomes more fibrotic, but this change is not synonymous with pathologic cirrhotic changes. On autopsy, a buildup of brown pigment is seen, which is a result of accumulated unexcretable metabolic residue (end-stage metabolic products of lipids and proteins) acquired over a lifetime; no apparent physiologic significance has been identified with this pigment. Changes in liver oxidative status and function and the activity of the enzymatic antioxidant defense system as well as the influence of aging on the susceptibility of the hepatic system to hepatotoxins remain the focus of ongoing animal studies.[41]

Other studies are bringing to light the effects of physiologic age-related changes in the hepatic system such as the significance of growth hormone synthesis by the hepatic system responsible for maintaining various body tissues (e.g., bones, muscles, cardiovascular system, immune system, central nervous system). Researchers are particularly interested in examining whether treatment with exogenous growth hormone can retard or reverse hepatic age-related changes in body structure and function.[3]

The *pancreas* undergoes structural changes, such as fibrosis, fatty acid deposits, and atrophy, but the pancreas has a large reserve capacity, and 90% of its function would have to be lost before any observable dysfunction occurs. Much remains unknown about the *gallbladder* in the aging process, but aging apparently has little effect on gallbladder size, contractility, or function. The gallbladder releases less bile into the liver, allowing more time for gallstones to develop. There is some evidence that moderate and vigorous physical activity enhances the function of the gallbladder as measured by reduced risk of gallbladder removal in physically active women.[27]

HEALING IN THE HEPATIC SYSTEM

In general, older organs may not adapt to injury as well as younger organs, so severe hepatic illnesses (e.g., severe hepatitis) may not be tolerated as well by the older person. Delayed or impaired tissue repair may require longer time for recovery of homeostasis. Chronic liver disease is associated with intrapulmonary shunting and reduced pulmonary vascular function. Pulmonary edema occurs secondary to hepatic encephalopathy. Vascular changes in the lungs have been well documented in people with chronic liver disease and reflect the importance of the liver in the control of vasoactive substances that regulate normal fluid balance, including lung fluids.[6]

Liver injury is followed by complete parenchymal regeneration, the formation of scars, or a combination of both. The outcome depends on the extent and chronicity of the insult. Chronic hepatic injury, such as chronic viral hepatitis or alcoholic liver injury, destroys the extracellular matrix framework. This type of destruction results in a combination of regenerated nodules separated by bands of fibrous connective tissue (fibrosis), which is termed *cirrhosis*. Orthotopic liver transplantation has become an established therapy for end-stage liver disease (e.g., cirrhosis caused by alcoholism, hepatitis C), acute liver failure, and primary biliary cirrhosis or primary sclerosing cholangitis, as well as for nonalcoholic cirrhosis and hepatic or biliary malignancy. Biliary atresia is the most common indication for pediatric liver transplantation. Theoretically, anyone with advanced, irreversible liver disease with certain mortality may be considered for a liver transplant provided the disease could be corrected by liver transplantation (see Table 20-6).

Current animal research is centered on identifying and harvesting specific stem cells from the bone marrow that under special conditions will convert into functioning liver tissue. In human research, a new procedure called *hepatocyte transplantation* is being pioneered. In this procedure billions of donor liver cells are injected by intravenous infusion into the blood with the hope that the cells will correct life-threatening liver problems that would otherwise require a liver transplant. Other research efforts are working toward the development of bioartificial devices for liver support. An effective temporary liver support system could improve the chance of survival with or without a transplant as the final treatment (see Chapter 20).

LIVER

◆ Jaundice (Icterus)

Overview and Incidence. Jaundice or icterus is not a disease but is rather a common symptom of many different diseases and disorders. It is characterized by yellow discoloration of the skin, sclerae, mucous membranes, and excretions owing to staining of tissues by the bile pigment bilirubin (hyperbilirubinemia). Jaundice can occur at any age in any person with no predilection for gender; jaundice is one of the most common health care problems in neonates, occurring in 15% to 20% of all newborns.

Risk Factors. Risk factors for the development of jaundice are listed in Box 16-2. Jaundice in the postoperative client is not uncommon and may be a potentially serious complication of surgery and anesthesia. Jaundice associated with cancerous biliary obstruction increases with age. Clinical management of jaundice is complicated by anything that can damage the liver, including stress, hypoxemia, blood loss, infection, and administration of multiple drugs. Drug-induced liver disease is a common cause of jaundice in older persons (see Table 16-5). In most cases, drug toxicity stops when the agent is withdrawn.

BOX 16-2

Risk Factors for Jaundice

Consumption of raw shellfish
Contact with jaundiced persons (see Transmission, Table 16-2): persons on dialysis, drug abusers, homosexuals, or prostitutes
History of jaundice, hepatitis, anemia, splenectomy, or cholecystectomy
Injections within the last 6 months for drug use/abuse, tattoo (inscription or removal), blood or plasma transfusion
Neonate/newborn
Occupation or employment involving alcohol consumption
Place of origin: Mediterranean, Africa, Far East
Recent travel to areas where hepatitis is present at all times (endemic)
Surgery/anesthesia

Etiologic Factors and Pathogenesis. Jaundice may be classified according to the location of the pathologic change as *prehepatic*, *hepatic*, or *posthepatic*; causes of each state are listed in Table 16-1. In the prehepatic state, bilirubin increases before it reaches the liver as a result of its overrelease, usually secondary to hemolysis (destruction) of RBCs. Hepatic jaundice results in bilirubin increase when pathology within the liver parenchyma impairs the liver's ability to adequately excrete bilirubin. Posthepatic (obstructive) jaundice occurs when bile duct obstruction impairs bilirubin transport after the bilirubin leaves the liver. Gallstones in the common bile duct are the most common cause of obstructive jaundice; cancer of the pancreas is also relatively common, particularly in older persons.

About 4 mg/kg of bilirubin is produced each day, 80% to 85% of which is derived from the catabolism of the heme of hemoglobin in worn out or defective RBCs and subsequent conversion to bilirubin. The remaining 15% to 20% of bilirubin is derived from the destruction of maturing but ineffective erythroid cells in the bone marrow. Normally, the liver cells excrete the bilirubin, but if the liver is diseased, flow of bile is obstructed, or destruction of erythrocytes is excessive, the bilirubin accumulates in the blood. The bilirubin binds with albumin, which transports it from the blood plasma to the liver, forming a complex known as *unconjugated bilirubin*. Unconjugated bilirubin cannot be excreted in the urine or bile, but it is easily taken up by fatty tissue and the brain. Bilirubin is easily bound to elastic tissue, such as the skin, blood vessels, sclerae, and synovium, which in turn become icteric (jaundiced or yellow).

Once the unconjugated bilirubin reaches the liver, it joins with glucuronic acid to form conjugated bilirubin. Conjugation transforms bilirubin from a lipid-soluble substance that can cross biologic membranes to a water-soluble substance that can be excreted in the bile or converted to urobilinogen, a yellow pigment that is subsequently excreted in the urine, giving normal urine its characteristic color. As a result of this pathologic process, jaundice may be categorized according to whether the bilirubin is primarily unconjugated or conjugated, which indicates whether the increase in bilirubin occurs before, at, or after it reaches the liver.

Clinical Manifestations. Jaundice is the predominant sign of hyperbilirubinemia, and it becomes obvious when bilirubin levels exceed 2.0 to 2.5 mg/dL, with yellowing of the sclerae of the eyes. When bilirubin level reaches 5 to 6 mg/dL, the skin becomes yellow. *Unconjugated hyperbilirubinemia* (indicating prehepatic pathology) may present as weakness or abdominal or back pain with acute hemolytic crisis. Stool and urine color are normal, but mild jaundice is observed in the skin, sclerae, or mucous membranes.

Conjugated hyperbilirubinemia (indicating hepatic or posthepatic pathology) may be asymptomatic when associated with factors that stop or suppress bile flow (cholestasis); in the case of intermittent cholestasis, symptoms may include light-colored stools, malaise, and pruritus (itching) from the deposition of bile salts in the skin. Conjugated hyperbilirubinemia associated with hepatocellular disease may be accompanied by malaise, anorexia, low-grade fever, and right upper quadrant discomfort. Dark urine, jaundice, vascular spiders, white nailbed, loss of sexual hair, palmar erythema, yellow plaque spots on eyelids (xanthelasma), asterixis, or fetor hepaticus

TABLE	16-1

Classification Of Jaundice

PREHEPATIC	HEPATIC	POSTHEPATIC
Hemolytic blood transfusion reaction	Bacterial toxins	Bile duct strictures
Blood incompatibility (mother and infant)	Hepatitis	Gallstones
Autoimmune hemolytic anemia	Liver congestion	Pancreatic stones
Severe burns	Cirrhosis	Pancreatitis
Defective albumin binding	Metastatic cancer	Tumors of the ducts or adjacent structures
Sickle cell disease	Prolonged use of medications (toxic metabolites) metabolized by the liver	
Hemolytic drugs	Anorexia	
	Physiologic jaundice of the newborn	
	Primary biliary cirrhosis	

(musty, sweet breath odor resulting from the liver's inability to metabolize the amino acid methionine) may be present, depending on the cause, severity, and chronicity of liver dysfunction (see Fig. 16-3). Jaundice associated with hepatitis is described as the icteric stage (see Table 16-4).

Conjugated hyperbilirubinemia associated with biliary obstruction presents with right upper quadrant colicky pain, weight loss (carcinoma), jaundice, dark urine, and light-colored stools. Signs and symptoms may be intermittent when caused by stone or tumor.

Medical Management

Diagnosis.　A careful history and physical examination are important in determining the nature and cause of jaundice. Past medical history of drug or alcohol use, exposure to persons with infectious hepatitis, recurrent abdominal pain and nausea (gallstones), and preexisting liver disease are helpful clues as to the (infectious) cause of jaundice.

Specific urine and blood serum testing is used to determine the level of bilirubin and whether it is conjugated or unconjugated pointing to a prehepatic, hepatic, or posthepatic condition. Because bilirubin has to be conjugated in order to be excreted, and conjugation occurs in the liver, high levels of unconjugated bilirubin indicate a prehepatic problem (i.e., the bilirubin has not reached the liver to be conjugated) (see Table 16-1). High levels of conjugated bilirubin indicate that the bilirubin has passed through the liver, pointing to improper excretion of bilirubin from the liver or obstructed flow of bile outside the liver.

Other conditions may be demonstrated using ultrasonography, computed tomographic (CT) scan, or magnetic resonance imaging (MRI). Percutaneous liver biopsy may also be used to determine the cause and extent of hepatocellular dysfunction; liver biopsy performed under ultrasound or CT may be performed when metastatic disease or hepatic mass is suspected.

Treatment and Prognosis.

Treatment is determined by the underlying cause of the jaundice (e.g., surgery for obstructive jaundice, medical management [rest and supportive measures] for hepatitis, withdrawal of cholestatic drug, phototherapy for neonate). Likewise, prognosis depends on the underlying disease. The reader is referred to the Prognosis section for the individual disease or condition causing the jaundice. Once the underlying cause has been treated, jaundice fades slowly over 3 to 4 weeks, leaving the client looking particularly pale and washed out.

Special Implications for the Therapist　16-2

JAUNDICE (ICTERUS)

With successful treatment of the underlying cause, jaundice usually begins to resolve within 4 to 6 weeks. After this time, activity and exercise can be resumed or increased per individual tolerance, depending on the overall medical condition and presence of any complications. The return of normal stool and urine colors is an indication of resolution. (See also Special Implications: Signs and Symptoms of Hepatic Disease, 16-1.)　■

◆ Hepatitis

Hepatitis is an acute or chronic inflammation of the liver caused by a virus, a chemical, a drug reaction, or alcohol abuse. Classifications of hepatitis discussed in this text are listed in Box 16-3. Six different identifiable hepatitis viruses (A, B, C, D, E, and G)* are responsible for more than 95% of all viral-induced cases worldwide. Other viral causes of hepatitis include Epstein-Barr virus (mononucleosis), herpes simplex virus types I and II, varicella-zoster virus, measles, or cytomegalovirus (CMV). Hepatitis owing to any cause produces very similar symptoms and usually requires a careful client history to establish the diagnosis.

People with mild-to-moderate acute hepatitis rarely require hospitalization. The emphasis is on preventing the spread of infectious agents and avoiding further liver damage when the underlying cause is drug-induced or toxic hepatitis. Persons with fulminant hepatitis (of severe, sudden intensity;

---

*The letter F was not skipped; it represents the Fulminant form of hepatitis, the generic term for any rapidly progressing form of liver inflammation resulting in hepatic encephalopathy within a few weeks of developing infection. Fulminant hepatitis is not strictly viral-induced but can develop as a result of any form of hepatitis.

Hepatitis Classifications

Viral
Toxic
Autoimmune or idiopathic
Alcoholic

sometimes fatal) require special management because of the rapid progression of the disease and the potential need for urgent liver transplantation.

Chronic Hepatitis. Chronic hepatitis comprises several diseases that are grouped together because they have common clinical manifestations and are all marked by chronic necroinflammatory injury that can lead insidiously to cirrhosis and end-stage liver disease. The disease is defined as chronic with evidence of ongoing injury for 6 months or more.[32]

Previously, chronic hepatitis was classified as either chronic persistent hepatitis (CPH) or chronic active hepatitis (CHP), but recent advances in understanding of the causes and natural history of this type of liver injury have led to the elimination of these terms. Now chronic hepatitis is described in diagnostic terms that include the etiology, degree of active inflammation and injury (i.e., grade: mild, moderate, severe or I, II, III), and the degree of scarring or how advanced the process is (i.e., stage: I, II, III; IV represents cirrhosis). Stages of disease are usually irreversible.

Chronic hepatitis has multiple causes including viruses, medications, metabolic abnormalities, and autoimmune disorders. Despite extensive testing, some cases cannot be attributed to any known cause and are probably the result of as yet unidentified viruses. Hepatitis B (with or without hepatitis D), hepatitis C, and hepatitis G can progress to chronic hepatitis. Most people with chronic hepatitis are asymptomatic, and when symptoms occur these are nonspecific and mild with fatigue, malaise, loss of appetite, polyarthralgias, and intermittent right upper quadrant discomfort. Some people report sleep disturbances or difficulty in concentrating. Symptoms of advanced disease or an acute exacerbation include nausea, poor appetite, weight loss, muscle weakness, itching, dark urine, and jaundice. Once cirrhosis is present, weakness, weight loss, abdominal swelling, edema, easy bruising, muscle wasting and weakness, gastrointestinal bleeding, and hepatic encephalopathy with mental confusion may arise.

The diagnosis of chronic viral hepatitis is based on serologic testing. The strict definition of chronic hepatitis (from any cause) is based upon histologic features of hepatocellular necrosis and chronic inflammatory cell infiltration in the liver, but the diagnosis can usually be made from clinical features and blood test results alone. Liver biopsy is important to assess the severity of underlying liver disease (grade and stage) and to determine the need for antiviral treatment. The treatment for chronic viral hepatitis has improved substantially in the last decade and depends on the underlying cause and grade and stage of disease. With the advances currently being made in the fields of antiviral and immunomodulatory therapeutics, it is anticipated that the considerable progress made in treating these diseases over the past decade will continue in the future.[32]

The prognosis in chronic hepatitis is variable depending on the development of cirrhosis and other complications such as hepatocellular carcinoma. Male gender, moderate to severe alcohol consumption, and other coexistent liver disorders are the factors that increase the rate of progression to cirrhosis; HCV is the major risk factor of development of liver cancer. The 5-year survival rate for compensated cirrhosis is greater than 90%, but the prognosis and survival rate for decompensation (characterized by development of variceal bleeding, ascites, and hepatic encephalopathy) are extremely poor. Progression of chronic hepatitis to decompensated cirrhosis is an indication for liver transplantation.

Fulminant Hepatitis. Fulminant hepatitis is the generic term for any rapidly progressing form of liver inflammation that results in hepatic encephalopathy (confusion, stupor, and coma) within a few weeks of developing infection. This type of hepatitis is rare, occurring in less than 1% of persons with acute viral hepatitis, but can be fatal. Alcohol is the most common hepatotoxin but exposure to other hepatotoxins, such as acetaminophen (analgesic accounting for 20% to 25% of all cases of fulminant hepatitis),[28] isoniazid (antitubercular drug), halothane (anesthetic), valproic acid (anticonvulsant), mushroom toxins, or carbon tetrachloride also may contribute to this condition. In addition to liver failure, numerous complications can occur, including additional infection, cerebral edema, hypoglycemia, coagulation defects, GI hemorrhage, electrolyte disturbances with ascites, cardiorespiratory insufficiency, and renal insufficiency.

Diagnosis is made in the presence of a combination of hepatic encephalopathy, acute liver disease (elevated serum bilirubin and transaminase levels), and liver failure. Treatment is supportive, because the underlying etiologic factors of liver failure are rarely treatable short of liver transplantation. Prognosis is determined in part by the cause of the condition. Persons with fulminant hepatitis from HAV or acetaminophen overdose are more likely to recover spontaneously than are those with idiosyncratic drug-induced liver failure (see Table 16-5), HBV, or idiopathic fulminant liver failure without liver transplantation. Short-term prognosis without liver transplantation is very poor, and the mortality rate is high (80%). Despite the poor prognosis, complete recovery can occur as a result of liver cell regeneration with recovery of liver function. The development of effective artificial liver support devices may prolong the time available to find a donor liver or to allow the native liver to regenerate.

Viral Hepatitis[5]

Overview. Each of the recognized hepatitis viruses belongs to a different virus family, and each has a unique epidemiology. Characteristics of these strains of viruses are presented in Table 16-2. The identification of the specific virus is made difficult by the fact that a long incubation period often occurs between acquisition of the infection and development of the first symptoms. The incubation period for HAV is 2 to 7 weeks, 2 to 6 months for HBV, and 1 to 2 weeks for HCV. Not all causative agents have been identified, and because hepatitis can be easily spread before symptoms appear, morbidity is high in terms of loss of time from school or work. More than half, and possibly as many as 90%, of all cases go unreported because symptoms are mild or even subclinical.

TABLE	16-2

Types of Viral Hepatitis

	HEPATITIS A	HEPATITIS B	HEPATITIS C	HEPATITIS D	HEPATITIS E
Incidence	Less than 30,000 cases reported to CDC in 2000; reduced incidence with introduction of hepatitis vaccine A	Reduced incidence; 150,000 new acute cases in the United States (2000); 1 million carriers	Transfusion-related cases decreasing with blood screening but increased incidence expected related to risk behaviors in the 1960s and 1970s; 4 million infected	Uncommon in United States; most common in drug addicts, sexually active young adults, individuals receiving multiple transfusions	Epidemic in developing countries; rare in US; risk greatest to persons traveling to endemic regions
Morbidity	Results in acute infection only; does not progress to chronic hepatitis or cirrhosis; small risk of fulminant hepatitis; lifetime immunity	Most common cause of chronic hepatitis and liver cancer; second major cause of cirrhosis in the United States after alcohol abuse	Accounts for 60% to 70% of all chronic hepatitis; 30% of chronic cases progress to cirrhosis; associated with liver cancer	Most severe form of viral hepatitis; frequently progresses to chronic active hepatitis or death; mortality rate 2% to 20%	Causes acute self-limiting infection; does not progress to chronic hepatitis; high mortality in pregnant women, 10% mortality
Transmission	Fecal-oral route; spread by feces, saliva, and contaminated food and water	Parenteral Sexual contact Vertical Unidentified exposure	Parenteral Unidentified exposure	Parenteral Sexual contact Same as B; requires co-infection with HBV to produce	Same as A; fecal-oral (contamination of water)
Treatment	Immune globulin before or within 2 weeks of exposure; supportive; most people recover within 6 to 10 wk	Alpha interferon and lamivudine for chronic HBV; effective in 40% cases; HBIG for exposed, unvaccinated persons	Combination therapy (interferon, ribavirin) in select cases	Interferon alfa–2b can inhibit HDV replication but effect ends when therapy ends	None; preventive measures
Diagnosis	Blood test to identify antibody; anti-HAV; IgM	Blood test to identify antigen and antibodies; HBsAg; HBeAg; HbcAg	Blood test to identify antibody; does not distinguish between current and past infection; anti-HCV Limited use of nucleic acid test (polymerase chain reaction)	Blood test to detect antigen and antibody; anti-HDV	Blood test to detect anti-HEV IgM antibodies
Vaccine	Vaccine available; combined HAV and HBV vaccine available (Twinrix)	Vaccines available; combined HAV and HBV vaccine available	None available	Immunization against hepatitis B can prevent hepatitis D infection	Recombinant vaccines, IgM antibodies under investigation

Hepatitis E and G are rare in the United States and therefore not included.
From Centers for Disease Control and Prevention (CDC): National Center for Infectious Diseases (online): http://www.cdc.gov/ncidod/diseases/hepatitis, 2001.

Hepatitis A (HAV), formerly known as infectious hepatitis, most commonly affects children and young adults, although persons of any age are susceptible. A second peak incidence occurs in older persons who travel to parts of the world where the risk of HAV is increased. HAV is often spread in environments characterized by poor sanitation and overcrowding, such as day care centers, correctional facilities, military train-

ing sites, and schools (Table 16-3). The primary mode of transmission is the oral-fecal route*; major outbreaks of HAV

---

*The oral-fecal route of transmission is primarily from poor or improper handwashing and personal hygiene, particularly after using the bathroom and then handling food for public consumption. This route of transmission also may occur through the shared used of oral utensils, such as straws, silverware, and toothbrushes.

occur when people consume water or shellfish from sewage-contaminated waters. HAV is rarely transmitted through transfused blood, and little placental transmission occurs, although the antibody is often detected in infants of infected mothers.

HAV is highly contagious, with the peak time of viral excretion and contamination occurring during the 1-week period *before* the onset of symptoms of jaundice. Thus the greatest danger of infection is during the incubation period, when a person is unaware that the virus is present. The illness can last from 4 to 8 weeks; it generally lasts longer and is more severe in persons older than 40 years.

Hepatitis B (HBV), formerly called *serum hepatitis*, is transmitted parenterally* through needle sticks, sexual relations, intravenous drug use, sharing needles, blood transfusions or blood products (e.g., clotting factor), dialysis, and perinatal (vertical) transmission from mother to child. Drug use and intimate contact with another person with hepatitis B are the two most frequent sources of hepatitis B virus (HBV). Because

---

*Parenteral refers to transmission in some other mode than via the alimentary canal (enteric system), such as by injection subcutaneous, intramuscular, intraorbital, intracapsular, intraspinal, intrasternal, or intravenous.

TABLE	16-3

Risk Factors for Hepatitis

HAV	HBV	HBC	HCD	HEV
Household contacts or sexual contacts of infected persons	Injection drug use	Current or previously used injected illegal drugs (even if only 1 or 2 times years ago); intranasal cocaine use with shared equipment	Same as B	Same as A
Unprotected homosexual/ bisexual activity	Unprotected homosexual/bisexual activity; persons with multiple sex partners or diagnosis of sexually transmitted disease			
Injection/non-injection illegal drug users (regional outbreaks reported)	Incarceration in correctional facilities—adults and youth (drug use, unsafe sexual practices)	Received blood transfusion or organ transplant before July 1992 or blood clotting products made before 1987		
Living in areas with increased rates of HAV (children at greatest risk)	Certain ethnic groups and adoptive families with adoptees from these areas: Asia, South America, South Africa, Mexico, Eastern and Mediterranean Europe			
Travel to areas where HAV is endemic	Travel to high-risk areas			
Tattoo inscription or removal; body or ear piercing with shared or unsterile needles	Occupational risk*: morticians, dental workers, emergency medical technicians, firefighters, health care workers in contact with body fluid or blood	Tattooing/body piercing as a risk factor for HCV has not been completely evaluated in the United States but does not appear likely		
	Liver transplant recipient	Evidence of liver disease; liver transplant recipient		
	Infants born to mothers with HBV	Infants born to HCV-infected mothers (low risk; 5%)		
	Immunocompromised individuals; receiving/administering chronic kidney dialysis (clients/staff)	Long-term kidney dialysis (clients/staff)		
Blood clotting factor disorder (slight increase in risk	Multiple blood product or blood transfusions before July 1992			

*HBV can survive in dried blood at least 1 week.

From Centers for Disease Control and Prevention (CDC): National Center for Infectious Diseases (online): http://www.cdc.gov/ncidod/diseases/hepatitis, 2001.

HBV can be transmitted through heterosexual or homosexual intercourse, it is considered a sexually transmitted disease.

Hepatitis C virus (HCV), formerly post-transfusion non-A, non-B hepatitis associated with blood transfusion, is now most commonly associated with parenteral drug use, although HCV is also a problem in the bleeding disorders community. As with HAV, the period of infectivity begins before onset of symptoms, and the person may become a lifetime carrier of this virus. Clinically, HCV is very similar to HBV and often is asymptomatic; the acute HCV infection is usually mild. Chronic hepatitis C varies greatly in its course and outcome from asymptomatic with normal liver function to mild degree of liver injury and overall good prognosis to severe symptomatic hepatitis C with complications of cirrhosis and end-stage liver disease.

Hepatitis D (delta virus, HDV) is a defective single-stranded RNA that presents as a coinfection or superinfection of hepatitis B. This virus requires HBsAg for its replication, so only individuals with hepatitis B are at risk for hepatitis D. Risk factors and transmission mode are the same as for HBV; parenteral drug users have a high incidence of HDV. The symptoms of HDV are similar to those of HBV except that clients are more likely to have fulminant hepatitis and to develop chronic active hepatitis and cirrhosis.

Hepatitis E (HEV), previously known as enteric non-A, non-B hepatitis, is transmitted by contaminated water via the oral-fecal route and clinically resembles HAV. It is believed to be nonfatal although it has been clearly associated with liver damage. A 20% to 25% mortality rate exists in pregnant women.[1] This virus tends to occur in poor socioeconomic conditions, primarily occurs in developing countries, and is rare in the United States. No specific treatment is available for HEV, but ensuring clean drinking water remains the best preventive strategy.

Hepatitis G (HGV) is most prevalent in African countries. It is parenterally transmitted, although vertical and sexual transmission are well documented. It may cause acute or chronic infection, but little information about this viral cause of hepatitis is known.[47] HGV has been identified as the causative agent of approximately 20% of posttransfusion hepatitis cases and approximately 15% of community-acquired hepatitis cases that are not caused by HAV. Although present in liver tissue, pathogenicity to the liver has not been proved.

Incidence and Risk Factors.

Each year approximately 500,000 Americans are infected with some form of hepatitis virus; annually about 15,000 persons die from its complications. HAV is the predominant type of hepatitis among persons younger than 15 years; 70% of hepatitis B cases and 58% of hepatitis C cases are reported in the 20- to 39-year age group. Prevalence of HBV infection is more than four times higher among blacks, Hispanics, American Indians, and Alaskan Natives than among whites.[35] Prevalence varies most according to risk factors for acquisition, so for parenterally transmitted hepatitis (B, C, D, G), the highest rates are among persons with direct percutaneous blood exposures, such as intravenous drug users.

Whereas HAV is usually eliminated from the body by the time jaundice appears, the body is not always able to rid itself of HBV, and the virus can persist in body fluids indefinitely. The carrier state occurs in 90% to 95% of infected neonates, 20% of older children, and 1% to 10% of adults; approximately 1 to 1.25 million persons are chronic carriers of HBV. Men are more likely than women to develop the carrier state; immunosuppressed individuals are also at increased risk. Transfusion as a source for HBV is now ranked last among known sources for HBV infection since the initiation of donor screening for hepatitis B core antibody (anti-HBc) started in 1987.

HCV accounts for 25% of acute viral hepatitis and 90% of cases of posttransfusion hepatitis. A blood-screening test for HCV has reduced the numbers of blood transfusion-related cases of this virus by 50% in the United States. Currently 60% of the new cases of HCV occur among intravenous drug users sharing needles. See Table 16-3 for other risk factors. Currently, up to one third of individuals with a bleeding disorder are coinfected with HIV and everyone with a bleeding disorder who was infected with HIV also contracted HCV. The incidence of symptomatic hepatitis C is expected to increase in the coming decades among "baby boomers" who experimented with or used injection drugs, donated blood for money, or shared straws to snort cocaine in the past.

People undergoing chronic hemodialysis are at high risk for HBV/HCV infection because the process of hemodialysis requires vascular access for prolonged periods. In an environment where multiple clients receive dialysis concurrently, repeated opportunities exist for person-to-person transmission of infectious agents, directly or indirectly via contaminated devices, equipment and supplies, environmental surfaces, or hands of personnel. Furthermore, individuals receiving hemodialysis are immunosuppressed, which increases their susceptibility to infection, and they require frequent hospitalizations and surgery, which increases their opportunities for exposure to nosocomial infections.[36] HBV is relatively stable in the environment and remains viable for at least 7 days on environmental surfaces at room temperature. HBsAg has been detected in dialysis centers on clamps, scissors, dialysis machine control knobs, and doorknobs. Thus blood-contaminated surfaces that are not routinely cleaned and disinfected represent a reservoir for HBV transmission. Dialysis staff members can transfer virus to clients from contaminated surfaces by their hands or gloves or through use of contaminated equipment and supplies.[36]

Pathogenesis.

The pathology of hepatitis is similar to that of other viral infections. The primary target of the hepatitis virus is the hepatocyte. Once inside the cell, the virus replicates and causes hepatocellular injury. Hepatic cell necrosis, scarring, Kupffer cell hyperplasia, and infiltration by mononuclear phagocytes occur with varying severity in response to the virus.

The injured liver cells are recognized as being "foreign" and are targeted by the immune system. Killer T lymphocytes are activated and destroy infected hepatocytes as part of the cell-mediated immune system response. If this process is self-limiting (e.g., Hepatitis A and E), the hepatocellular damage is minimal and the liver fully regenerates after the initial damage. However, if liver inflammation and injury persist as chronic hepatitis (e.g., Hepatitis B, C, D, and G) the chronic inflammatory response may cause irreparable damage to the liver, leading to cirrhosis or even hepatocellular carcinoma.

Clinical Manifestations. Classic symptoms of hepatitis are the same, regardless of the responsible virus. Most individuals present with malaise, fatigue, mild fever, nausea, vomiting, anorexia, right upper quadrant discomfort, and occasionally diarrhea. Tobacco users may report losing interest or experiencing aversion to tobacco. Clinical jaundice, dark urine, and clay-colored stools also may be observed. Some people may develop extrahepatic manifestations (more frequent in chronic HCV than in B or D) including neuropathy, arthralgias, myalgias, pruritus, vascular spiders (angiomas), palmar erythema, Hashimoto's thyroid disease, diabetes mellitus, corneal ulceration, idiopathic thrombocytopenia, and fibromyalgia. A small number of people with HCV may develop one of several rheumatic diseases (e.g., polyarthritis, rheumatoid arthritis, Sjögren's syndrome, systemic lupus erythematosus).

Hepatitis occurs in three stages: the initial or preicteric stage, the icteric or jaundice stage, and the recovery period (Table 16-4). During the *initial* or *preicteric* stage (sometimes also referred to as the *prodromal stage*), the urine darkens and the stool lightens as less bilirubin is conjugated and excreted. Asymptomatic viral hepatitis is common, and many cases are not diagnosed because the symptoms mimic the flu or may be too mild to visit a health care professional.

The *icteric stage* of clinical illness is characterized by the appearance of jaundice, which peaks in 1 to 2 weeks and may persists for 6 to 8 weeks. During this stage, the acuteness of the inflammation subsides. Persons who have been treated with human immune serum globulin (ISG) may not develop hepatitis. The *recovery stage* or period of convalescence lasts for 3 to 4 months, during which time the person generally feels well but fatigues easily. Chronic hepatitis may begin at this time.

Medical Management

Prevention. Prevention takes place at three levels: primary, secondary, and tertiary. Primary prevention involves primary immunization (HAV, HBV), education regarding food preparation and proper handwashing, avoiding needle punctures by contaminated needles (or other similar infective material), practicing protective sex or avoiding sexual contact during the period of HBV surface antigen positivity. Secondary prevention involves passive immunization following exposure to HAV or HBV, travel precautions when visiting areas where hepatitis is endemic (e.g., avoid drinking unbottled water or beverages served with ice, avoid eating foods rinsed in contaminated water such as fruits and vegetables, and avoid eating shellfish). Tertiary prevention involves education to those infected about preventing possible infectivity to others and self-care during active infection (e.g., avoid strenuous activity and ingestion of hepatotoxins such as alcohol and acetaminophen; some advocate alternative treatment such as herbs, acupuncture, and dietary measures).

Hepatitis A. Preventive measures include HAV vaccine for persons 2 years of age and older, standard precautions, and immune globulin (a preparation of antibodies) during the period of incubation following exposure. When an infection begins, the body produces gamma-globulin that includes antibodies to fight the infection. In some cases, after the infection has been eliminated, enough immune globulin remains in the body to prevent a recurrence of that particular infection, providing lifetime immunity. If the therapy is administered within 2 weeks of exposure to the HAV infection, it bolsters the person's own antibody production and provides 6 to 8 weeks of passive (temporary) immunity. HAV vaccine is recommended (before exposure) for anyone wishing to obtain immunity or who is at risk for infection (e.g., persons traveling to areas with intermediate to high rates of endemic hepatitis A, persons living in communities with high endemic rates or periodic outbreaks of HAV infection, men who have sex with men or who are bisexual and their partners of either gender, and clients with chronic liver disease).[35]

Hepatitis B. Hepatitis B is a preventable disease achieved by administering the combined hepatitis A and B vaccine (Twinrix) in three doses over a period of 6 months.

TABLE	16-4

Stages of Hepatitis

INITIAL/PREICTERIC (3 TO 10 DAYS, UP TO 3 WEEKS)	ICTERIC (VARIABLE; 1 TO 3 WEEKS)	RECOVERY (3 TO 4 MONTHS)
Dark urine	Jaundice	Return of appetite
Light stools	GI symptoms subside	Resolution of serum bilirubin and amino
Vague GI symptoms	Liver decreases in size and	transferase elevations
Constitutional symptoms	tenderness	Clearance of virus
Fatigue	Enlarged spleen	Convalescence; easily fatigued
Malaise	Enlarged postcervical lymph	
Weight loss	nodes	
Anorexia	Neutralizing antibodies appear	
Nausea/vomiting		
Diarrhea		
Aversion to food, alcohol, cigarette smoke		
Enlarged and tender liver		
Rash, hives		
Intermittent pruritus (itching)		
Arthralgias		

Lifelong protective immunity develops in 95% of healthy adults. In the unvaccinated person, hepatitis B immune globulin (HBIG) should be administered within 24 hours of the exposure, followed by the HBV series at 0, 1, and 6 months. Immunity to hepatitis B also confers immunity to hepatitis D; therefore, hepatitis B vaccination is recommended for preexposure immunization prophylaxis.

Once individuals begin to engage in behaviors associated with the high-risk groups, they may become infected before vaccine can be given. A major obstacle in eliminating HBV is identifying persons and vaccinating them before they become infected. For this reason, in the United States it is now recommended that all infants, health care workers,* and persons in the high-risk category for HBV receive the HBV vaccine. Children younger than 5 years of age, if infected, have a high risk of becoming HBV carriers. Testing to identify pregnant women who are HbsAg positive† and providing their infants with immunoprophylaxis effectively prevents HBV transmission during the perinatal period. The World Health Organization (WHO) has recommended that all countries integrate HBV vaccination into their national immunization programs, and much progress has been made toward the goal to control, eliminate, and eradicate hepatitis in the coming generations.[54]

Hepatitis C.   Currently, no vaccine is available to prevent this (RNA) virus, because of the rapidity of HCV mutations in adaptation to the environment[25] and no immunoglobulin is effective in treating exposure. The only means of preventing new cases of hepatitis C are to screen the blood supply, encourage health care professionals to take precautions when handling blood and body fluids, and educate people about high-risk behaviors.

Diagnosis.   In addition to the history and clinical examination, serologic and molecular testing help provide an accurate diagnosis. Serodiagnosis may be helpful in detecting the presence of viral markers that indicate the cause of acute viral hepatitis (see Table 16-2). Molecular testing developed in the last decade (nucleic acid testing [NAT]) can directly detect rapidly and accurately the presence of enteric (and other) microorganisms. The most widely used of these methods is the polymerase chain reaction (PCR) to detect the hepatitis B/C virus.‡[33] Researchers are working to develop improved molecular techniques for increased diagnostic precision for all the hepatitis viruses.[34] Other laboratory tests provide biochemical indicators of HCV infection (e.g., elevated alanine, aspartate aminotransferase). Transaminases (enzymes normally present in hepatocytes) are released from the acutely damaged hepatocytes, and serum transaminase levels rise, often to levels exceeding normal levels by 20-fold. Bilirubinuria and an elevated serum bilirubin level are usually found. Liver function tests (see Table 39-15) can indicate other viral liver diseases, drug toxicity, or alcoholic hepatitis.

Viral load does not correlate with the severity of the hepatitis or with a poor prognosis (as it seems to in HIV infection), but viral load does correlate with the likelihood of a response to antiviral therapy. None of the serodiagnostic tests are able to determine the current extent of liver damage; a liver biopsy provides information about the severity of disease and establishes grading and degree of fibrosis but is only necessary in the case of chronic hepatitis.

Treatment.   Treatment options have expanded and prevention methods are available for two of the six viruses although no cure is available for the four viruses that are responsible for chronic liver disease (Hepatitis B, C, D, G). The development of new antiviral agents that inhibit steps in the viral replication process is under investigation.[38] Any hepatic irritants such as alcohol or chemicals (e.g., occupational exposure to carbon tetrachloride) must be avoided in all types of hepatitis.

Hepatitis A.   Treatment is primarily symptomatic, and bed rest is recommended for persons who are jaundiced to avoid complications from liver damage. Hospitalization may be required for excessive vomiting and subsequent fluid and electrolyte imbalance. During the anorexic period, the client may receive nutritional supplements and, possibly, intravenous glucose infusions.

Hepatitis B.   Current data indicate that the combination use of alpha interferon* and lamivudine (Epivir, reverse transcriptase inhibitor) is effective in approximately 40% of adults who have chronic infection to achieve virologic, biochemical, and histologic remission. This drug combination diminishes the disease progression but does not provide a "cure" or elimination of the virus. Relapse on cessation of treatment is common, and significant side effects of this medication are reported.

Hepatitis C.   Therapy for hepatitis C is a rapidly changing area of clinical practice. Combination therapy with interferon and ribavirin (Virazole, a nucleoside analogue) is being used in select cases with chronic HCV clients who are at risk for progression to cirrhosis (e.g., persistently elevated ALT levels, liver biopsy indicative of inflammation or fibrosis) although this is successful in reducing inflammation in only half of all cases.† Those individuals with less severe histologic changes or with compensated cirrhosis (i.e., without jaundice, ascites, variceal hemorrhage, or encephalopathy) may not benefit from antiviral treatment and must be assessed on a case-by-case basis. Many potential side effects and contraindications exist to the use of interferon (e.g., pregnancy, younger than 18 years or older than 60 years, hyperthyroidism, major depressive illness, autoimmune disease, organ transplant recipient, active substance or alcohol abuse) that prevent this

---

*According to the Occupational Safety and Health Administration (OSHA) Bloodborne Pathogen Standard (1991), hepatitis B vaccination must be offered to all employees within 10 days of employment. Records related to this vaccination must be maintained. Employees who decline vaccination must sign a standardized declination form.

†The HBsAg is a core protein antigen of the HBV present in the nuclei of infected cells. Presence of HBsAg in the blood usually indicates the individual is infectious. HBc antibodies appear during the acute infection but do not protect against reinfection.

‡At the time of this writing, the nucleic amplification methods of identifying hepatitis RNA are available in only a limited number of research laboratories. FDA had not yet approved these tests for diagnostic purposes; they are used most commonly for clients being managed with antiviral therapy.

---

*Interferon (recombinant DNA) is a genetically engineered copy of a naturally occurring protein that acts as an antiviral agent. It has multiple biologic effects on cells of diverse origin including antiviral, immunomodulatory, and antiproliferative activities.

†The FDA has also approved a new drug (Rebetron) that combines alpha-interferon with ribavirin using a new technology that cloaks it from the immune system so it stays active longer. Rebetron has not been compared directly yet with combination therapy (ribavirin added to alpha interferon).

treatment from being applied to all individuals with HCV infection. Administration of HAV and HBV vaccine is recommended for anyone with chronic hepatitis C because of the potential for increased severity of acute hepatitis superimposed on existing liver disease.[48]

Prognosis.   Prognosis varies with each type. A substantial proportion of hepatitis B morbidity and mortality that occurs in the health care setting can be prevented by vaccinating health care workers against HBV. In addition, health care workers must practice infection control measures (see Appendix A). Other prophylactic strategies are based on avoidance of high-risk behavior and use of immune globulin.

Hepatitis A.   HAV is rarely fatal and does not lead to chronic hepatitis or cirrhosis. Most people recover fully and become immune to HAV. Relapse may occur, characterized by arthralgia with positive rheumatoid factor (RF) as a common laboratory finding. Fulminant hepatitis resulting in death develops in a very small percentage of people with HAV (0.1%).

Hepatitis B.   In adults with normal immune status, most (94% to 98%) recover completely from newly acquired HBV infections, eliminating virus from the blood and producing neutralizing antibody that creates immunity from future infection. Approximately 10% of infected persons become lifetime carriers of HBV. In immunosuppressed persons (including hemodialysis clients), infants, and young children, most newly acquired HBV infections result in chronic infection. Although the consequences of acute hepatitis B can be severe, most of the serious sequelae associated with the disease occur in persons in whom chronic infection develops. Although persons with chronic HBV infection are often asymptomatic, chronic liver disease develops in two thirds of these persons, and approximately 15% to 25% die prematurely from cirrhosis or liver cancer.[36] Orthotopic liver transplantation for cirrhosis caused by HBV is a possible treatment but has a poor prognosis because of almost universal reinfection.

Hepatitis C.   Only 15% of the people infected with HCV clear the virus from the liver. The remaining 85% develop chronic disease, although chronic hepatitis C is usually well tolerated with few symptoms or signs of liver disease despite 20 years or more of infection. When HCV continues to attack liver cells beyond a 6-month period, causing liver inflammation and scarring (cirrhosis), liver failure can occur; 60% to 80% of all cases progress to cirrhosis. Hepatitis C is the primary etiology of chronic liver disease in the United States and the leading cause of hepatocellular cancer and liver transplantation. As mentioned, incidence of chronic hepatitis C with its associated morbidity and mortality is expected to triple in the next decade. The progression of HCV may be accelerated if a person is also infected with the acquired immunodeficiency syndrome (AIDS) virus. HIV/HCV coinfection among individuals with bleeding disorders results in mortality; more than 5000 people have died, and the numbers continue to climb.[39]

Hepatitis D.   Hepatitis D by itself appears to be relatively harmless, but it has a high morbidity and mortality rapidly leading to hepatic failure and cirrhosis when it accompanies hepatitis B.

Special Implications for the Therapist   16-3

VIRAL HEPATITIS

See also Special Implications for the Therapist: Bloodborne Viral Pathogens, 7-6.

Preferred Practice Patterns:
Practice patterns are dependent upon clinical presentation. Although extrahepatic manifestations occur such as neuropathy and skin, joint, and/or bone involvement, these are usually unresponsive to physical therapy intervention and resolve gradually with medical intervention for the underlying cause (hepatitis). Exceptions occur such as in the case of required wound care or management of rheumatic diseases or fibromyalgia.

Any direct contact with blood or body fluids of clients with hepatitis B or C requires the administration of immune globulin, a preparation of antibodies, in the early incubation period. Therapists at risk for contact with HBV because of their close contact with the blood or body fluids of carriers should receive active immunization against HBV. All therapists should follow standard precautions at all times to protect themselves and must wear personal protective equipment whenever appropriate. Such gear should never be worn in the car or laundered at home to avoid contamination of those sites. Enteric precautions are required when caring for individuals with type A or E hepatitis. Any therapist working in dialysis units or providing wound care should review infectious control guidelines available.[36] For the therapist who has been diagnosed with viral hepatitis, recommendations and work restrictions for HCWs are discussed in Chapter 7; see Table 7-6.

Studies dealing with the natural history of acute hepatitis have provided perspective on the frequency of skin and joint manifestations. More than a third of the adults studied had joint pains during the course of the illness. The frequency of arthralgia as a symptom associated with hepatitis increases with age. Joint pains affected only 18% of children, compared with 45% of adults older than 30 years. No known studies have been published regarding the benefit of physical therapy in providing symptomatic joint relief until these symptoms resolve as the person recovers from the underlying pathology. In the case of a client with undiagnosed hepatitis presenting with joint symptoms, the systemically derived arthralgia will not respond to therapy. Any time intervention fails to provide symptomatic relief or resolution of symptoms, the results must be reported to the physician for further follow-up evaluation.

Overall, in the recovery process, adequate rest to conserve energy is important. The affected individual is encouraged to gradually return to pre-illness levels of activity. Fatigue associated with the anicteric phase of hepatitis may interfere with activities of daily living and may persist even after the jaundice resolves. A careful balance of activity is important to avoid weakness secondary to prolonged bed rest; a reasonable activity level is more conducive to recovery than is enforced bed rest. Whenever possible, rehabilitation intervention or increased activity should not be scheduled right after meals.

Watch for signs of fluid shift, such as weight gain and orthostasis; dehydration; pneumonia; vascular problems; pressure ulcers; and any signs of recurrence. After the diagnosis of viral hepatitis has been established, the affected individual should have regular medical checkups for at least 1 year and should avoid using any alcohol or over-the-counter drugs during this period.

Alpha interferon (antiviral used in the treatment of some hepatitis) has bone marrow suppressive effects requiring careful monitoring of platelet or neutrophil count (see Tables 39-6 and 39-7). Other side effects of combination therapy may include increased fatigue, increased muscle pain and potential inflammatory myopathy, headaches, local skin irritation (site of injection), irritability and depression, hair loss, itching, sinusitis, and cough. These symptoms usually subside in the first few weeks of treatment; prolonged or intolerable side effects must be reported to the physician.

HBV and the Athlete

Great concern is often expressed over the possibility of contagion among athletes in competitive sports, particularly sports with person-to-person contact. Infectious agents such as human immunodeficiency and other viruses, bacteria, and even fungi have been examined. No cases of HIV or hepatitis C transmission resulting from sports participation have been reported, but two cases of hepatitis B transmission through exposure to blood during sports participation have been documented.

For most of the infections considered, the athlete is more at risk during activities off the playing field than while competing. Inclusion of immunizations against measles and hepatitis B as a prerequisite to participation would eliminate these two diseases from the list of dangers to athletes (and all individuals). Education, rather than regulations, is the best approach in considering the risks to athletes from contagious diseases.[8] Although risk of bloodborne pathogen infection during sports is exceedingly small, good hygiene practices concerning blood are still important. The American Academy of Pediatrics (AAP) has made recommendations to minimize the risk of bloodborne pathogen transmission in the context of athletic events and has issued safety precautions. The therapist in this type of setting is encouraged to review these guidelines.[2]

No evidence has been reported that intense, highly competitive training is harmful for the asymptomatic HBV-infected person, whether the disease is acute or chronic. Therefore the presence of HBV infection does not contraindicate participation in sports or athletic activities; decisions regarding play are made according to clinical signs and symptoms such as fatigue, fever, or organomegaly. Chronic HBV infection with evidence of organ impairment requires reduction in intensity and duration of activity. ■

Toxic Hepatitis

Overview and Etiologic Factors.
Toxic hepatitis is a form of nonviral liver inflammation that occurs secondary to exposure to certain chemicals, drugs, and most recently, herbal preparations and other botanicals (sometimes referred to as neutraceuticals) used alone or in combination with prescription drugs for self-medication without supervision.[50] More than 600 medicinal agents, chemicals, and herbal remedies are recognized as producing hepatic injury.*[28] Specific chemical hepato-

---

*For example, any of the following herbal products (chaparral, comfrey, germander, jin bu huan, mistletoe, nutmeg, ragwort, sassafras, senna, or tansy) can cause liver-related complications (ranging from acute hepatitis and jaundice to cirrhosis and death from liver failure) in anyone with an underlying liver disease.

TABLE	16-5

Causes of Chemical and Drug-Induced Hepatitis

DOSE-RELATED	IDIOSYNCRATIC
Acetaminophen* (Tylenol) (analgesic; suicide attempt)	Alpha-methyldopa (antihypertensive)
Alcohol	Halothane (anesthetic)
Amanita phalloides (poisonous mushroom)	Isoniazid (antitubercular)
Anabolic steroids	Minocycline (antibiotic)
Aspirin	Monoamine oxidase inhibitors (antidepressant)
Benzene, toluene	
Carbon tetrachloride	Nitrofurantoin
Chloroform (anesthetic)	Phenytoin (Dilantin) (anticonvulsant)
Methotrexate (antineoplastic agent)	Rifampin (antitubercular)
Oral contraceptives	Quinidine (antiarrhythmic)
Organic pesticides	Sulfonamides (antibiotic)
Penicillin	Sulindac (NSAID)
Tetracyclines (antibiotic)	Valproate (anticonvulsant)
Trichloroethylene	
Vinyl chloride	

*Acetaminophen is Tylenol and is not an NSAID. It has no antiinflammatory properties, only analgesic and antipyretic uses. It has no relationship to ibuprofen.

toxins may include alcohol, acetaminophen (Tylenol), carbon tetrachloride,* trichloroethylene, derivatives of benzene and toluene, organic pesticides, poisonous mushrooms (*Amanita phalloides* and related species, rare in the United States but more common in Europe), and vinyl chloride. Industrial toxins require rigorous safety precautions and ongoing monitoring to minimize the risk to industrial workers, but despite these guidelines, occupational hepatotoxicity is on the rise, as a result of the modern development of many new chemicals.

Drug-induced hepatitis occurs after the administration of one of various drugs and appears to be increasing reflecting the increasing number of new agents that have been introduced into clinical practice over the past several decades.[28] Substances that act as hepatotoxins may be categorized according to whether the hepatotoxic reaction is dose-related and predictable or idiosyncratic (i.e., unpredictable hypersensitivity reaction) (Table 16-5). Some drugs, such as oral contraceptives, may impair liver function and produce jaundice without causing necrosis, fatty infiltration of liver cells, or a hypersensitivity reaction. By far the most common drug-induced liver failure is acetaminophen because of its availability, which makes possible the chronic ingestion of therapeutic dosages or overdose as a means of suicide.

A host of factors may enhance susceptibility to drug-induced liver disease including age, gender, obesity, diabetes mellitus or other comorbidities, malnutrition, and other preexisting liver diseases. Anyone with cirrhosis and impaired liver

---

*Carbon tetrachloride was the most common industrial chemical considered an occupational inhalation poison until it was banned in most countries.

function may have altered metabolism of certain agents adding another risk factor for hepatic injury. Alcohol combined with other substances/medications may cause hepatic injury.

Pathogenesis. Acute hepatic necrosis occurs when depletion of glutathione stores (nonessential amino acid occurring in proteins) in the liver allows the metabolized drug, chemical, or other substance to bind with the liver rather than with the amino acid. Sensitive persons may be predisposed to idiosyncratic reactions either because they possess different metabolic pathways from those of the general population or because they are unusually sensitive to a uniform pharmacologic effect of the drug or other substance other than the desired therapeutic response.

Clinical Manifestations. Toxic reactions are often difficult to identify, because the majority occur in acutely ill people who may be receiving a number of different drugs over a short period of time. Liver necrosis occurs within 2 or 3 days after acute exposure to a dose-related hepatotoxin. Several weeks may pass before manifestations of a reaction occurs. Clinical manifestations vary with the severity of liver damage and the causative agent. Some compounds can produce mild, subtle damage without any acute illness. In most individuals, symptoms resemble those of acute viral hepatitis and may include anorexia, nausea, and vomiting; fatigue and malaise; jaundice; dark urine; clay-colored stools; headache, dizziness, and drowsiness (carbon tetrachloride poisoning); and fever, rash, arthralgias, and epigastric or right upper quadrant pain (halothane anesthetic). Complications of unrecognized or untreated toxic hepatitis may include cirrhosis or renal failure.

Medical Management

Treatment and Prognosis. Treatment consists of removal of causative agent, rest, and alleviation of side effects. Gastric emptying is used to eliminate acetaminophen intoxication. Once a substance has caused liver damage, this substance (as well as chemically similar compounds) must be avoided for life. Reexposure to this compound is likely to cause the same symptoms with an increased risk of more severe liver damage on the second or third exposure. Industrial workers exposed to chemicals are encouraged to have regular medical examinations and blood tests, even if they are asymptomatic.

Special Implications for the Therapist 16-4

TOXIC HEPATITIS

Preferred Practice Patterns:
See Viral Hepatitis

Therapists should be alert to the possibility of drug toxicity or drug reactions in clients taking multiple medications or reactions in people who are combining prescription medications or over-the-counter medications with herbal supplements/neutraceuticals. Many people do not consider over-the-counter drugs as medications and may take the same drug with different names or combine over-the-counter drugs with prescription medications. People with memory loss or short-term memory deficits may

take multiple doses in a short amount of time because they cannot remember when or whether they took their medication. Other guiding principles for the recovery process are as mentioned for viral hepatitis. ■

Autoimmune Hepatitis

Overview. Autoimmune hepatitis sometimes referred to as idiopathic chronic hepatitis is a chronic inflammatory disorder of the liver of unknown cause. It is characterized by the presence of autoantibodies, high levels of serum immunoglobulins, and frequent association with other autoimmune diseases. Autoimmune hepatitis is one of the three major autoimmune liver diseases, along with primary biliary cirrhosis and primary sclerosing cholangitis. Variant forms of autoimmune hepatitis have been termed "overlap syndromes" because they share features of several liver diseases.

The International Autoimmune Hepatitis Group has classified two types of autoimmune hepatitis: type 1 or classic autoimmune hepatitis and type 2 or autoimmune hepatitis. Both forms are more common among women than men and have similar clinical and serum biochemical features. Two peaks of incidence occur: one between the ages of 15 and 25 and the other around the time of menopause (between the ages of 45 and 60). Type 2 is found largely in Europe, affecting girls or young women.[32]

Etiologic Factors and Pathogenesis. The cause and pathogenesis of autoimmune hepatitis are not known. The disease appears to occur among genetically predisposed individuals upon exposure to as yet unidentified noxious environmental agents triggering an autoimmune process directed at liver antigens. It appears to be a self-perpetuating inflammatory process within the liver mediated by immunologic mechanisms characterized by inadequate immunoregulation and untempered antibody production against normal hepatocytes.

Clinical Manifestations. Autoimmune hepatitis is represented by a wide spectrum of clinical manifestations first presenting with jaundice and fatigue. It tends to be more severe and rapid in onset than chronic hepatitis B, is usually progressive, and leads to end-stage liver disease if not treated with immunosuppression. Systemic manifestations include arthralgia, acne, and amenorrhea. Other symptoms may include fever, malaise, recurrent or persistent jaundice, rash, or gynecomastia (breast development in the male). Pleurisy, pericarditis, or ulcerative colitis may be part of the client's history. Signs of chronic liver disease may be present, such as spider angiomas, palmar erythema, digital clubbing, and hepatosplenomegaly.

Medical Management

Diagnosis, Treatment, and Prognosis. Laboratory and histologic findings help determine the diagnosis. This disease responds rapidly to corticosteroid therapy. Prednisone alone or in combination with azathioprine (Imuran), an immunosuppressant drug that has a direct, antiinflammatory effect, induces clinical, biochemical, and histologic remission in 75% of people. Corticosteroid or immunosuppressive therapy usually is continued indefinitely although withdrawal with careful monitoring is achieved in some cases. Relapses occur in

40% to 50% of cases after cessation of therapy, and fatal flares of disease can occur weeks to months after stopping treatment; repeat treatment is required, and remission usually follows. Prognosis depends on the stage of disease at the time of diagnosis and initiation of therapy but is generally good for those individuals who respond quickly to the immunosuppressive therapy. People with autoimmune hepatitis that progresses to end-stage liver disease have excellent survival rates following liver transplantation.[10]

Special Implications for the Therapist   16-5

AUTOIMMUNE HEPATITIS

Preferred Practice Patterns:
See Viral Hepatitis

Management of a client who has an autoimmune disease with liver involvement is a challenge. Energy conservation and maintaining quiet body functions during active liver disease must be balanced by activities to prevent musculoskeletal deconditioning with accompanying loss of strength, flexibility, and/or mobility. ■

◆ Alcoholic Liver Disease

Alcohol abuse is the most common cause of liver disease in the Western world, resulting in alcoholic hepatitis and cirrhosis. Much progress has been made in the understanding of the pathogenesis of alcoholic liver disease (ALD), resulting in improvement of prevention and therapy, with promising prospects for even more effective treatments. New understanding of the nutritional deficiencies induced by alcohol has brought to light the need to supplement S-adenosylmethionine (SAMe) and polyenylphosphatidylcholine (PPC) in the presence of significant liver disease. Clinical trials are ongoing in people with ALD regarding these nutritional/antioxidant therapies along with studies of antifibrotics, antiinflammatory medications, other antioxidants, liver transplantation in alcoholics who have brought their alcoholism under control, and the development of agents that oppose alcohol craving.[30]

Alcoholic Hepatitis.   Alcoholic hepatitis can be an acute or chronic inflammation of the liver caused by parenchymal necrosis as a result of heavy alcohol ingestion. It is potentially reversible but is also the most frequent cause of cirrhosis, which is not reversible and is potentially fatal. The specific mechanism by which liver damage is sustained has not been fully determined. Immune-mediated hepatic damage is suspected in the pathogenesis of alcoholic hepatitis. Neutrophil accumulation is relatively unique to alcoholic injury (in most forms of hepatitis, mononuclear cells predominate) and may contribute to hepatocellular injury.

Unfortunately, many people with progressive liver damage have few symptoms until the disease is advanced; initial symptoms are those of the complications of cirrhosis (e.g., ascites, esophageal varices, and encephalopathy). If such is the case, irreversible liver damage has already occurred. Anorexia, nausea, vomiting, weight loss, jaundice, and abdominal pain are common presenting symptoms. Liver pain is rare despite the inflammation and parenchymal damage, because the liver parenchyma is relatively free of nerve fibers. Mild pain and tenderness may occur over the abdomen, sometimes mistaken for indigestion. Fever is common, but persons with alcoholic liver disease are also prone to development of infections (e.g., pneumonia, urinary tract infection, infection of the peritoneal cavity), which could account for the fever. Cutaneous signs of chronic liver disease may be present, including spider angiomas, palmar erythema, loss of body hair, and gynecomastia.

Diagnosis includes a history of excessive, prolonged alcohol intake, but this information may not be available. Liver biopsy reveals a typical fatty-appearing liver associated with cirrhosis, and laboratory studies may show anemia, elevated WBC count, leukocytosis, elevated serum bilirubin, and prolonged prothrombin time. Treatment of acute alcoholic hepatitis is supportive, with high-carbohydrate diet, vitamin supplementation, parenteral fluids, and corticosteroids in people with severe alcoholic hepatitis when the diagnosis is certain and severity criteria are met.

Alcoholic hepatitis carries a poor prognosis if the person continues to drink alcohol. Frequently, the disease will stabilize if the person stops drinking. The person's condition can revert to normal, but it more commonly either progresses to cirrhosis or runs a rapid course to hepatic failure and death. Cirrhosis is often already present at the time of diagnosis, complicated by the development of ascites, encephalopathy, GI bleeding from varices, and deteriorating renal function. Evidence of coagulopathy, ascites, hepatorenal syndrome, or encephalopathy is a poor prognostic sign.

Special Implications for the Therapist   16-6

ALCOHOLIC HEPATITIS

Preferred Practice Patterns:
See Viral Hepatitis

Follow the same guidelines regarding liver protection as are discussed in Special Implications for the Therapist: Viral Hepatitis, 16-3. Increased susceptibility to infections requires careful handwashing before treating this client. (See also Special Implications for the Therapist: Cirrhosis, 16-7.) The presence of coagulopathy requires additional precautions. See the discussion, Special Implications for the Therapist: Signs and Symptoms of Hepatic Disease, 16-1. ■

Cirrhosis

Overview and Etiologic Factors.   Cirrhosis of the liver is actually a group of chronic end-stage diseases of the liver resulting from a variety of chronic inflammatory, toxic, metabolic, or congestive damage. There are many potential causes of cirrhosis (e.g., drugs, hepatitis, hereditary metabolic diseases, primary biliary cirrhosis), but alcohol abuse and hepatitis C are the most common causes in the Western world. Only 10% to 15% of clients with chronic alcoholism develop cirrhosis; however, more than 65% of all cases of cirrhosis are related to alcohol. In other words, not all alcoholism results in cirrhosis, but most cirrhosis is caused by alcohol. Men are more likely to develop Laënnec's (alcoholic) cirrhosis, but women develop cirrhosis earlier.* Cirrhosis is the fourth leading cause of death in persons between 35 and 54 years of age. It is the ninth leading cause of death overall in the United States.

Pathogenesis and Clinical Manifestations.

Cirrhosis is characterized by a combination of two lesions, fibrosis and regeneration nodules. Pathologically the normal microscopic lobular architecture of the liver is lost as inflammation results in necrosis of parenchymal tissue, which is replaced with fibrous bands of connective tissue (Fig. 16-2). These fibrous bands eventually constrict and partition the organ into irregular nodules. Fibrous scarring distorts the liver and causes it to

---

*Women are more vulnerable to the effects of alcohol than men. Women produce substantially less of the gastric enzyme alcohol dehydrogenase, which breaks down ethanol in the stomach. As a result, women absorb 75% more alcohol into the bloodstream. Other effects and gender differences are discussed further in Chapter 2.

shrink, and biliary channels may be altered or obstructed, producing jaundice. Scarring also may distort the vascular bed, leading to portal hypertension and intrahepatic shunting. Portal hypertension causes a reverse flow of blood and enlargement of the esophageal, umbilical, and superior rectus veins. Subsequent bleeding varices, ascites, and incomplete clearing of metabolic wastes such as ammonia can lead to encephalopathy. Other possible mechanisms in the pathogenesis of alcoholic fibrosis involve free-radical generation (see Fig. 5-2) by alternative pathways of ethanol metabolism (the so-called microsomal enzyme oxidizing system) and many of the cytokines prominent in other forms of liver injury, including tumor necrosis factor, interleukin-1, PDGF, and TGF-beta.

The signs and symptoms of cirrhosis (see Fig. 16-2; Fig. 16-3) are multiple and varied, representing interference with four major functions of the liver: (1) storage and release of blood to maintain adequate circulating volume, (2) metabolism of nutrients and detoxification of poisons absorbed from the intestines, (3) regulation of fluid and electrolyte balance, and (4) production of clotting factors. Individuals with cir-

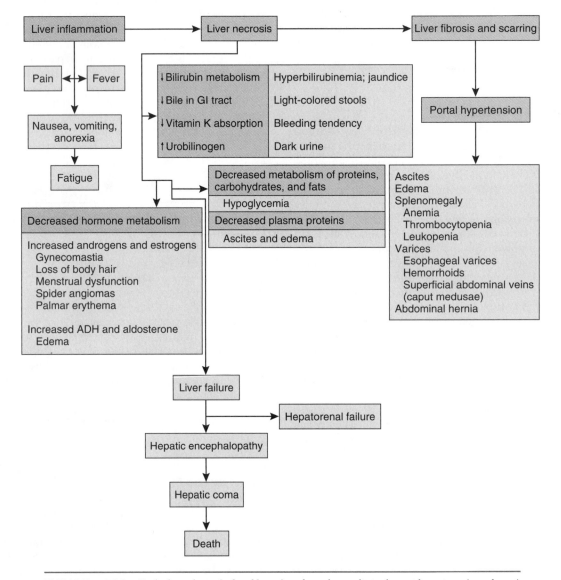

FIGURE   16-2   Pathologic basis (*colored boxes*) and resultant clinical manifestations (*gray boxes*) associated with cirrhosis of the liver.

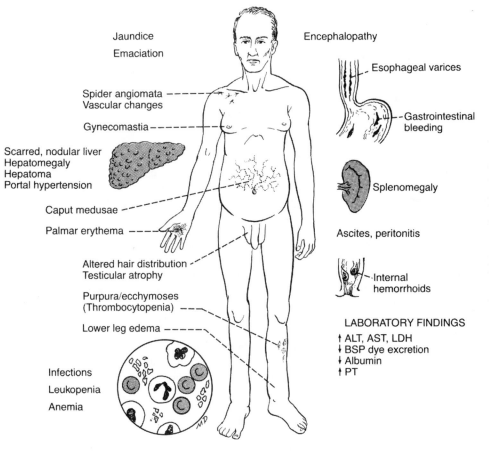

Jaundice
Emaciation

Spider angiomata
Vascular changes

Gynecomastia

Scarred, nodular liver
Hepatomegaly
Hepatoma
Portal hypertension

Caput medusae

Palmar erythema

Altered hair distribution
Testicular atrophy

Purpura/ecchymoses
(Thrombocytopenia)

Lower leg edema

Infections
Leukopenia
Anemia

Encephalopathy

Esophageal varices

Gastrointestinal
bleeding

Splenomegaly

Ascites, peritonitis

Internal
hemorrhoids

LABORATORY FINDINGS
↑ ALT, AST, LDH
↓ BSP dye excretion
↓ Albumin
↑ PT

FIGURE 16-3 Liver cirrhosis. Clinical presentation and laboratory findings associated with liver cirrhosis. *ALT,* alanine aminotransferase; *AST,* aspartate aminotransferase; *LDH,* lactate dehydrogenase; *BSP,* sulfobromophthalein; *PT,* prothrombin time. (From Black JM, Matassarin-Jacobs E, editors: *Medical-surgical nursing: clinical management for continuity of care,* ed 5, Philadelphia, 1997, WB Saunders, p 1879.)

rhosis who are asymptomatic and show little clinical evidence of hepatocellular dysfunction are said to have *well-compensated cirrhosis.* As evidence of complications develops, the clinical condition is referred to as *decompensated cirrhosis.*

Medical Management

Diagnosis.   The presence of cirrhosis may remain undetected until autopsy. Laboratory results are used to evaluate liver function (see Table 39-15). Impaired hepatocellular function is revealed by elevated liver serum enzymes, reduced dye excretion, hypoalbuminemia, and elevated prothrombin time. Liver biopsy is the most specific diagnostic test and provides information as to the extent of the disease.

Treatment.   Cirrhosis has no cure. Medical management of the client with any type of cirrhosis is supportive, with a view toward maximization of liver function, prevention of infection, and control of complications. Whenever possible, the primary causative agent for the cirrhosis is removed (e.g., abstinence from alcohol). A nutritious diet and adequate rest are essential to minimize trauma risk and to maximize regeneration in this progressive, degenerative disorder. Complications are treated individually (see the sections on Portal Hypertension, Ascites, and Hepatic Encephalopathy in this chapter).

Prognosis.   Cirrhosis develops slowly over a period of years. Its severity and rate of progression depend on the cause. In established cases with severe hepatic dysfunction, only 50% survive 2 years and 35% survive 5 years. Hematemesis, jaundice, and ascites are unfavorable signs. Liver failure and

cirrhosis are indications for liver transplantation or possibly the use of a bioartificial device to extend the time available for organ donation or liver regeneration. A 6-month period of abstinence may be required for the person with alcoholic cirrhosis before transplantation. Without transplantation hepatocellular carcinoma is a common complication and prognosis is poor, although survival may be prolonged.

Special Implications for the Therapist   16-7

CIRRHOSIS

Preferred Practice Patterns:
4A: Primary Prevention/Risk Reduction for Skeletal Demineralization (osteoporosis)
4B: Impaired Posture (osteoporosis)
4C: Impaired Muscle Performance (osteoporosis; alcoholic myopathy)
5A: Primary Prevention/Risk Reduction for Loss of Balance and Falling
6D: Impaired Aerobic Capacity/Endurance Associated With Cardiovascular Pump Dysfunction or Failure (chronic alcoholic myopathy: cardiomyopathy)

(See also Special Implications for Portal Hypertension, Ascites, Hepatitis, Encephalopathy, Anemia, Splenomegaly, Esophageal
Continued

Varices, Renal Failure, or Liver Transplantation according to the client's condition.)

One of the most common symptoms associated with cirrhosis is ascites, an accumulation of fluid in the peritoneal cavity surrounding the intestines. The distention often occurs very slowly over a number of weeks or months and may be associated with bilateral edema of the feet and ankles. The client may be unable to put on a pair of shoes, preferring to leave the shoes unlaced or to wear slippers. In a home health or inpatient hospital setting, this change in dress may not be as noticeable as in a private practice or outpatient clinic. It is always important to remain alert to these potential signs of fluid retention and to ask about any changes in health status or weight gain.

Detection of blood loss in the form of hematemesis, tarry stools, bleeding gums, frequent and heavy nosebleeds, or excessive bruising must be reported to the physician. Preventing increased intraabdominal pressure (see Box 15-1) and preventing injury owing to falls require client education regarding safety precautions.

Alcohol causes whole-body and tissue-specific changes in protein metabolism. Chronic alcohol use increases nitrogen excretion and reduces skeletal muscle protein synthesis with concomitant loss of lean tissue mass. Loss of skeletal collagen contributes to alcohol-related osteoporosis. The loss of skeletal muscle protein (i.e., chronic alcoholic myopathy) occurs in up to two thirds of all chronic alcohol users. Protein turnover changes in organs such as the heart have important implications for cardiovascular function and morbidity. Most clients with cirrhosis have significantly reduced aerobic capacity, although the exact mechanism for this has not been proved.[9,43]

Rest to reduce metabolic demands on the liver and to increase circulation often is recommended for clients with cirrhosis. Frequent rests during therapy and avoiding unnecessary fatigue are also important. Exercise limitation in cirrhosis is typically attributed to cirrhotic myopathy without impaired oxygen utilization. Chronic alcoholic myopathy affecting the proximal muscles is usually mild and results in muscle atrophy and measurable decrease in muscle strength. The therapist must remain alert to any potential medical complications in any client regardless of the physical therapy diagnosis. ∎

Primary Biliary Cirrhosis

Overview and Etiologic Factors.
Primary biliary cirrhosis (PBC) is a slowly progressive (irreversible), chronic liver disease that causes inflammatory destruction of the small intrahepatic bile ducts, bile acid buildup, cirrhosis, and ultimately, liver failure. An autoimmune attack against the bile duct is probably an important pathogenetic element but the precipitating event and contribution of genetic and environmental factors are not known. The disease is associated with other autoimmune disorders, including sicca complex, CREST syndrome, rheumatoid arthritis, scleroderma, Sjögren's syndrome, systemic lupus erythematosus, thyroiditis, pernicious anemia, and renal tubular acidosis. A strong female preponderance (10:1) exists, affecting primarily women between 30 and 65 years. Although it is most common in whites from North America and Europe, cases have occurred in all races. Prevalence appears to be increasing in Western populations, but the cause is unknown.

Pathogenesis.
The pathologic progression of PBC is divided into four successive stages referred to as Stages I to IV. The initial lesion (Stage I) involves attack on bile duct epithelium by cytotoxic T cells; autoantibodies are present, which supports a suspected autoimmune basis. Antigenic alterations occur in the membranes of the bile duct epithelial cells, which appear to be an inviting target for sensitized cytotoxic T-lymphocytes, but the reasons for this sensitization and the mechanism of T-lymphocyte activation remain unknown. In stage I the lobular parenchyma remains normal, but segmental bile duct injury occurs, with irregular, hyperplastic changes in the bile duct epithelium. Necrosis and ulceration of the epithelium commonly occur at this stage.

Stages II and III are characterized by bile ductal proliferation and early cholestasis (stoppage or suppression of bile flow). As a result of the destructive inflammatory process that is characteristic of stage I, small bile ducts are obliterated and scarring occurs in the medium-sized ducts with chronic inflammation of the portal tracts. As the inflammation process subsides, fibrosis and distortion of the normal liver architecture occur. The disease terminates as end-stage liver disease (i.e., cirrhosis) in stage IV, as fibrotic nodules replace the liver tissue.

Clinical Manifestations.
Initially, many people with PBC are asymptomatic whereas others present with advanced disease and its complications. Some of the early symptoms such as fatigue, dry eyes or mouth, and pruritus are overlooked or ignored. Other symptoms may include nausea or frequent indigestion; burning, pins-and-needles sensations, or prickling of the eyes; GI bleeding; right upper quadrant pain (posterior); joint or bone pain, and muscle cramping. Complications include cirrhosis (and its complications, especially ascites, portal hypertension, and liver failure), malabsorption with steatorrhea (impairment of excretion of bile into the intestine), osteoporosis, and osteomalacia owing to malabsorption of vitamin D and calcium. Signs of advanced PBC include dark urine, pale stools, easy bruising or bleeding, increased skin pigmentation (resembling a deep tan), and jaundice. Toxic levels of ammonia, the result of decreased liver function and buildup of decomposing nitrogenous materials such as proteins, may cause encephalopathy with symptoms ranging in severity from lethargy to coma.

Medical Management
Diagnosis and Treatment. Diagnosis is often sought by the client because of fatigue or pruritus. Liver function tests and blood serum analysis are diagnostic; liver biopsy may be used to confirm the diagnosis and is essential to establish the stage of the disease. The course of the disease is variable, and early diagnosis is important to identify individuals with rapidly progressing disease to initiate therapeutic measures and evaluate the necessity of liver transplantation.

Many people with PBC are now treated with ursodeoxycholic acid (UDCA), a bile acid taken in capsules, which may reduce the concentration of toxic bile acids and has been shown to improve tests of liver function. UDCA does not retard disease progression and has no specific antifibrotic effect although the drug clearly improves survival free of liver transplantation in people with moderate or severe (but not mild) disease.[23,24] Clinical trials are under way to test other drugs and combinations of medications that will be more effective in preventing biliary cirrhosis and improve liver function.[15]

Cholestyramine and rifampin help control pruritus by binding with bile salts in the intestine. Replacement of vitamins A, K, and D may be required in cases in which steatorrhea is present, especially if it is aggravated by drugs for the pruritus. PBC-associated osteoporosis is more common in advanced disease and the principles of management for postmenopausal osteoporosis also apply in liver disease.[55] Liver transplantation is the only proven therapy for advanced primary biliary cirrhosis and should be considered sooner rather than later. Immunosuppression following organ transplantation is a major risk factor for bone loss and the complications of osteoporosis.

Prognosis.   PBC usually follows a progressive, indolent (painless, slow growing) course, with life expectancy being approximately 5 to 10 years after diagnosis. Death is usually a result of hepatic failure or complications of portal hypertension associated with cirrhosis. Survival is impaired even in asymptomatic individuals, emphasizing the need for treatment in hopes of delaying the onset of late-stage disease. A serum bilirubin value of more than 10 mg/dL (normal range is 0.1 mg/dL to 1.0 mg/dL) is an accurate indicator of impending liver failure and used in determining optimal timing for liver transplantation; evaluation for liver transplantation is initiated when the bilirubin level rises above 3 mg/dL and the person develops jaundice. With liver transplantation, 1-year survival is 75%, with a projected 5-year survival of more than 65%.

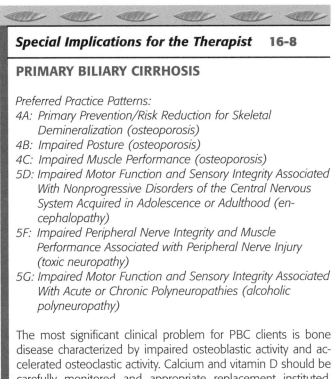

Special Implications for the Therapist   **16-8**

PRIMARY BILIARY CIRRHOSIS

Preferred Practice Patterns:
4A: Primary Prevention/Risk Reduction for Skeletal Demineralization (osteoporosis)
4B: Impaired Posture (osteoporosis)
4C: Impaired Muscle Performance (osteoporosis)
5D: Impaired Motor Function and Sensory Integrity Associated With Nonprogressive Disorders of the Central Nervous System Acquired in Adolescence or Adulthood (encephalopathy)
5F: Impaired Peripheral Nerve Integrity and Muscle Performance Associated with Peripheral Nerve Injury (toxic neuropathy)
5G: Impaired Motor Function and Sensory Integrity Associated With Acute or Chronic Polyneuropathies (alcoholic polyneuropathy)

The most significant clinical problem for PBC clients is bone disease characterized by impaired osteoblastic activity and accelerated osteoclastic activity. Calcium and vitamin D should be carefully monitored and appropriate replacement instituted. Physical activity following an osteoporosis protocol should be encouraged but with proper pacing and energy conservation. (See also Special Implications for the Therapist 16-1: Signs and Symptoms of Hepatic Disease and Liver Transplantation, 20-3 and Osteoporosis and Osteomalacia [Chapter 23].)

Occasionally, sensory neuropathy (xanthomatous neuropathy) of the hands and/or feet may occur as a result of increased serum cholesterol levels and an abnormal lipoprotein X. Cholesterol-laden macrophages accumulate in the subcutaneous tissues and create local lesions, termed xanthomas, around the eyelids and over skin, tendons, nerves, joints, and other locations. Treatment and precautions are as listed for this condition associated with diabetes mellitus or other etiologies (see Special Implications for the Therapist: Diabetes Mellitus, 10-15).   ■

Portal Hypertension
Definition and Overview.   Portal hypertension is abnormally high blood pressure in the portal venous system (Fig. 16-4); it occurs commonly, especially with cirrhosis, as a result of obstruction of the portal blood flow. This obstruction may be located in the portal vein (prehepatic), within the hepatic lobule (intrahepatic), or in the hepatic vein (posthepatic). Normal blood pressure in this system is 3 to 5 mm Hg; portal hypertension is characterized by pressure greater than 25 mm Hg.

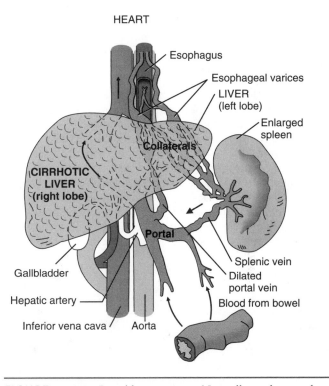

FIGURE   **16-4**   Portal hypertension. Normally, in the portal venous system (consisting of the portal veins, sinusoids, and hepatic veins), the portal veins carry blood from the GI tract, gallbladder, pancreas, and spleen to the liver. Veins collecting from these sites form the splenic vein and superior and inferior mesenteric veins, which in turn, merge to create the portal vein. Portal hypertension occurs when portal venous pressure exceeds the pressure in the nonportal abdominal veins (e.g., inferior vena cava) by at least 5 mm Hg. As portal pressure rises, increased resistance to blood flow causes blood pooling in the spleen and the development of collateral channels formed in an effort to equalize pressures between these two venous systems. These collateral vessels or varices bypass the liver and cause large, tortuous veins, especially in the esophagus (*esophageal varices*).

Incidence and Etiologic Factors. Portal hypertension can occur at any age, depending on the cause. Most cases affect adults and are caused by alcoholic cirrhosis. Other causes include portal vein obstruction by a thrombus, tumor, or sarcoidosis; infection; Budd-Chiari syndrome and other venoocclusive disease; splenomegaly; surgical trauma; pancreatitis; and inadequate decompression via varices (esophageal, retroperitoneal, periumbilical, or hemorrhoidal).

Pathogenesis and Clinical Manifestations. As described, any condition or cause of obstruction to the blood flow through the portal system or vena cava results in resistance to portal blood flow and the resultant development of portal hypertension. High pressure in the portal veins causes collateral vessels to enlarge between the portal veins and the systemic veins, where blood pressure is considerably lower. Collateral veins in the esophagus, anterior abdominal wall, and rectum enable blood to bypass the obstructed portal vessels. High pressure and increased flow volume through these collateral veins result in further problems, such as varices, splenomegaly, ascites, and hepatic encephalopathy.

Varices are distended, tortuous, collateral veins produced by the prolonged elevation of pressure in these collateral veins (see Fig. 16-4). The vomiting of blood from bleeding esophageal varices is the most common clinical manifestation of portal hypertension. Anemia may develop from the prolonged slow bleeding associated with varices or rupture. In addition to anemia, the prolonged bleeding also can lead to increased toxic wastes (such as ammonia, because blood is a protein) and subsequent sequelae (e.g., hepatic encephalopathy, altered peripheral nervous system function). Distended collateral veins may radiate over the abdomen, giving rise to the description *caput medusae* (Medusa's head) (Fig. 16-5). Hepatic vein thrombosis presents acutely with abdominal pain, liver enlargement, ascites, and jaundice.

Splenomegaly (enlargement of the spleen) is caused by increased pressure in the splenic vein, which branches from the portal vein. *Ascites* is caused by increased pressure forcing water and solids out of the tributaries of the portal vein into the peritoneal cavity. *Hepatic encephalopathy* occurs when blood that is shunted through collateral vessels to the systemic veins bypasses the liver, where toxins, hormones, and other harmful substances are normally removed. The presence of toxic substances (e.g., ammonia) in the blood reaching the brain results in hepatic encephalopathy.

Medical Management

Diagnosis, Treatment, and Prognosis. Diagnosis of portal hypertension is often made at the time of variceal bleeding and is assessed by ultrasonography, abdominal CT, or upper endoscopy. The individual usually has a history of jaundice, hepatitis, or alcoholism. Liver function tests may be abnormal, and liver biopsy may determine the etiology.

Treatment usually addresses complications, especially pharmacologic management of bleeding varices, endoscopic ligation of the bleeding varices, or, occasionally, emergency surgery. In the person who is a potential candidate for liver transplantation, too ill for major surgery, or who has continued bleeding despite endoscopic therapy, placing a transjugular intrahepatic portasystemic stent-shunt (TIPSS) is an alternative to surgery. The shunt creates a channel through the liver into which a stent is placed that decompresses the portal circulation. Ruptured varices are associated with a high mortality rate (30% to 60%). Recurrent bleeding esophageal varices are a poor prognostic indicator. Most clients die within 1 to 2 years from complications of bleeding varices or hepatic failure.

Special Implications for the Therapist 16-9

PORTAL HYPERTENSION

Preferred Practice Patterns:
Patterns will depend upon complications associated with portal hypertension. For example, some people with varices develop anemia or toxic neuropathy, whereas others may develop ascites and encephalopathy. The therapist should refer to the practice patterns for each of those (or other) conditions on an individual basis.

Portal pressure in individuals is dynamic with highest pressures during the night, after eating, and in response to coughing, sneezing, and exercise. Such variations may combine with local factors in vessel walls to contribute to a pressure surge that can lead to a variceal bleed. The therapist can teach the individual how to modify and reduce pressure, especially anything that increases intraabdominal pressure (see Box 15-1) such as coughing, straining at stool, or improper lifting. Any therapy program for a client with known varices must take this factor into account when presenting active or active-assisted exercises, or unsupported gait training. (See also the section on Esophageal Varices and Anemia.)[12] ∎

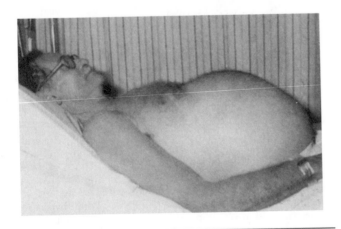

FIGURE 16-5 Ascites in an individual with cirrhosis. Distended abdomen, dilated upper abdominal veins, and inverted umbilicus are classic manifestations. Peripheral edema associated with developing ascites may be observed first by the therapist. (From Swartz MH: *Textbook of physical diagnosis*, Philadelphia, 1989, WB Saunders, plate XII.)

Ascites

Definition and Overview. Ascites is the abnormal accumulation of serous (edematous) fluid within the peritoneal cavity, the potential space between the lining of the liver and the lining of the abdominal cavity. Ascites is most often caused by cirrhosis, but other diseases associated with ascites include heart failure, constrictive pericarditis, abdominal malignancies, nephrotic syndrome, and malnutrition.

Pathogenesis.   The mechanisms of ascites caused by cirrhosis are complex, and several factors contribute to the development of ascites: (1) portal hypertension, resulting in increased plasma and lymphatic hydrostatic pressures; (2) hypoalbuminemia, resulting in decreased oncotic pressure; and (3) hyperaldosteronism, resulting in sodium and water retention. Portal hypertension and reduced serum albumin levels cause capillary hydrostatic pressure to exceed capillary osmotic pressure. This imbalance tends to push water into the peritoneal cavity. Portal hypertension also increases the production of hepatic lymph, which weeps into the peritoneal cavity. Decreased metabolic function of the liver results in the reduced albumin synthesis mentioned as well as in an accumulation of hormones that regulate sodium and water balance. As ascites sequesters more and more bodily fluid, the kidneys respond by retaining sodium and water, which expands plasma volume and thereby accelerates portal hypertension and further formation of ascites.

Clinical Manifestations.   Ascites becomes clinically detectable when more than 500 ml has accumulated, causing weight gain, abdominal distention (with a downward protruding umbilicus), increased abdominal girth, and, eventually, peripheral edema (see Fig. 16-5). Dyspnea with increased respiratory rate occurs when the fluid displaces the diaphragm or when defects in the diaphragm allow ascites to pass into the pleural cavity, decreasing lung capacity. Complications include hepatorenal syndrome and bacterial peritonitis. Hepatorenal syndrome, a form of functional renal failure, occurs when liver function is compromised, which is usually progressive and fatal. Bacterial peritonitis (infection of the ascitic fluid) can be asymptomatic or accompanied by fever, chills, abdominal pain, and tenderness.

Medical Management

Diagnosis.   Diagnosis of ascites is usually based on clinical manifestations in the presence of liver disease. Paracentesis may be used to aspirate ascitic fluid for bacterial culture, biochemical analysis, and microscopic examination, but this procedure may cause peritonitis and is not used as much as in the past. Abdominal x-rays, abdominal ultrasonography, and CT scan may locate fluid in the peritoneal cavity.

Treatment.   Depending upon the underlying cause of fluid retention nonsurgical medical management of ascites includes restriction of sodium intake, administration of diuretics, and restriction of fluids (in some cases). Electrolytes must be monitored carefully with supplementation of potassium and chloride if necessary (see Chapter 4). Review of current medications is required with withdrawal of any that inhibit prostaglandin synthesis and thus impair renal sodium excretion (e.g., aspirin and other NSAIDs). Surgical intervention has included paracentesis (sometimes repeated but with increased risk of bacterial peritonitis) and the insertion of a stent placed between the hepatic vein and the intrahepatic portion of the portal vein (transjugular intrahepatic portosystemic stent-shunt [TIPSS]).[16]

Prognosis.   Resolution of ascites may be dramatic after treatment intervention, but 25% of persons with cirrhosis-associated ascites still die within 1 year depending on the status of liver function and ability to control the ascites. The presence of bacterial peritonitis is an ominous complication of late-stage liver disease with a 2-year survival rate of less than 50%. Liver transplantation remains the most successful therapy for liver disease underlying ascites but is not always readily available.

Special Implications for the Therapist   16-10

ASCITES

Preferred Practice Patterns:
See Cirrhosis.
6A: Primary Prevention/Risk Reduction for Cardiovascular/Pulmonary Disorders (prevention of pneumonia/atelectasis)
6E: Impaired Ventilation and Respiration/Gas Exchange Associated With Ventilatory Pump Dysfunction or Failure (decreased lung capacity; elevated diaphragm)
6H: Impaired Circulation and Anthropometric Dimensions Associated With Lymphatic System Disorders (lymphedema)
7A: Primary Prevention/Risk Reduction for Integumentary Disorders (peripheral edema; lymphedema)

Most people with ascites are more comfortable in a high Fowler's position (head of the bed raised 18 to 20 inches above the level with the knees elevated). Breathing techniques are important to maintain adequate respiratory function and to prevent the development of atelectasis or pneumonia. The homebound person who has ascites should be monitored for the possible development of bacterial peritonitis. Onset of fever, chills, abdominal pain, and tenderness should be reported to the physician.

Decreases in serum albumin* associated with the development of ascites are accompanied by a parallel decrease in oncotic pressure in blood vessels causing peripheral edema. This edema may mask muscle wasting that occurs when the body does not have an adequate intake of protein to maintain structure and facilitate wound healing. The client must be encouraged to change position to maintain integrity of the skin and promote circulation. Small pillows or folded towels can be used to support the rib cage and the bulging flank while the client is lying on his or her side.

The abdominal distention associated with ascites may develop very slowly over a number of weeks or months and may be accompanied by bilateral edema of the feet and ankles. The client may be unable to put on a pair of shoes, preferring to leave the shoes unlaced or to wear slippers. In a home health, inpatient hospital, or nursing home setting, this change in dress

Continued

---

*Persons with serum albumin levels between 2.5 and 3.5 g/dl are at moderate risk of malnutrition, and those whose levels are 2.5 g/dl or less are at great risk (see Table 39-15). Because albumin binds to calcium, serum albumin levels drop when serum calcium levels are low.

may not be as noticeable as in a private practice an outpatient clinic. It is always important to remain alert to these potential signs of fluid retention and to ask about any changes in health status or weight gain.

Fluid intake and output are usually carefully measured and restricted, so in any setting the therapist is encouraged to know the individual's limits and to participate in reporting measurements as well. This is especially important because clients frequently ask the therapist for fluids in response to perceived exertion or increased exertion after exercise or ambulation. The person who is noncompliant or in denial requests fluids because of the false belief that fluids provided but not recorded do not count. For the homebound client, who is receiving diuretics, the bedroom should be close to the bathroom. ■

Hepatic Encephalopathy

Definition and Overview.   Hepatic encephalopathy or hepatic coma refers to a variety of neurologic signs and symptoms in persons with chronic liver failure or in whom portal circulation is impaired. This neuropsychiatric syndrome can occur secondary to acute or chronic liver disease. *Acute hepatic encephalopathy* occurs as a result of fulminant hepatic failure; cerebral edema resulting in coma is common with high mortality. *Chronic hepatic encephalopathy* usually occurs with chronic liver disease and is often reversible.

Risk Factors.   Any disease or condition of the liver that destroys liver parenchyma or causes abnormal shunting of blood around the liver tissue may predispose the client to hepatic encephalopathy. When cirrhosis progresses, portal hypertension may occur (see text for discussion of cirrhosis and portal hypertension) with possible subsequent hemorrhage. In addition to GI bleeding, other factors that may precipitate or severely aggravate hepatic encephalopathy in clients with severe liver disease include constipation, diuretics, infection, increased dietary protein, and CNS-depressant drugs, such as alcohol, benzodiazepines (e.g., Librium, Valium, Dalmane, Tranxene), and opiates.

Pathogenesis.   The known etiology of this disorder is the liver's inability to metabolize ammonia, but the exact pathogenesis of hepatic encephalopathy remains unclear. Protein (food)- and gut-derived (GI bleed) toxins normally are taken up and detoxified by the liver. When these toxins are no longer absorbed into the portal vein and removed from the blood by the liver because of hepatocyte dysfunction, they pass directly to the brain, where they have direct harmful effects on the nervous system. Reduced hepatic function or bypass of blood around the liver results in rising ammonia levels that are toxic to central and peripheral nervous system function. Additionally, as blood ammonia levels rise, many unusual compounds, such as octopamine, begin to form and serve as false neurotransmitters in the CNS.

It is possible that specific causes of hepatic encephalopathy do not exist at all, but rather brain function is affected to a certain degree by the *various* consequences of liver failure (e.g., accumulation of neuroactive compounds and neurotoxins, changes in the metabolism of amino acids, decreased availability of energy fuels and circulatory changes) finally precipitating the syndrome of hepatic encephalopathy.

Clinical Manifestations.   Clinical manifestations of hepatic encephalopathy vary depending on the severity of neurologic involvement. Four stages of development occur as the ammonia level increases in the blood with the clinical features listed in Table 16-6. Flapping tremors (asterixis; see Fig. 16-1) and numbness/tingling (mimicking carpal tunnel syndrome) are common early (stage I) symptoms associated with this condition. Subtle personality changes listed in stage I may include disorientation or confusion, euphoria or depression, forgetfulness, and slurred speech. Minor lapses in memory and inability to concentrate, slurred speech, and confusional episodes may be transient or permanent and are usually more noticeable to the affected person than to the outside observer. As this condition progresses, the person develops a sleep disorder or may become unconscious. This sequence may occur over a period of many months (chronic encephalopathy) or may develop rapidly in days or weeks as in the case of fulminant hepatic failure (acute encephalopathy).

The motor apraxia in stage II can be best observed by keeping a record of the client's handwriting and drawings of simple shapes, such as a circle, square, triangle, and rectangle. Progressive deterioration is apparent in these handwriting samples. In stage III, the person is most likely hospitalized or

---

TABLE	16-6

Stages of Hepatic Encephalopathy

STAGE I (PRODROMAL)	STAGE II (IMPENDING)	STAGE III (AROUSAL)	STAGE IV (COMATOSE)
Slight personality changes	Tremor progresses to asterixis	Hyperventilation	No asterixis
Slight tremor	Resistance to passive movement	Marked confusion	Positive Babinski's reflex
Bilateral numbness/tingling	Myoclonus	Abusive and violent	Hepatic fetor
Muscular incoordination	Lethargy	Noisy, incoherent speech	
Impaired handwriting	Unusual behavior	Asterixis (liver flap)	
Sleep disturbances	Apraxia	Muscle rigidity	
	Ataxia	Positive Babinski's reflex	
		Hyperactive deep tendon reflexes	

Modified from Goodman CC, Snyder TE: *Differential diagnosis in physical therapy*, ed 3, Philadelphia, 2000, WB Saunders, p 272.

homebound with hospice care and can still be aroused. Stage IV is a comatose state from which the person cannot be aroused and can respond only to painful stimulus. Hepatic fetor is a musty, sweet odor of the breath caused by the liver's inability to metabolize the amino acid methionine.

Medical Management

Diagnosis, Treatment, and Prognosis.   Diagnosis of hepatic encephalopathy is based on history of liver disease and clinical manifestations. No specific diagnostic test is available, but electroencephalography (EEG) and blood chemistry tests are used to confirm the diagnosis.

Because protein is the source of the toxins, many of the symptoms can be improved by eliminating any sources of protein (i.e., stopping any internal bleeding and restricting dietary protein). Pharmacologic treatment may include antibiotics (neomycin) to reduce bacterial production of ammonia. Lactulose, a bowel cathartic (causes evacuation) also may be used to increase gastric acid, another means of effectively killing the naturally occurring bacteria that survive in the intestines and produce ammonia.

More extreme measures may include peritoneal dialysis and exchange transfusions to remove and replace most of the person's blood. Liver transplantation may be performed for cases of fulminant liver failure. Without intervention, mortality is high, as the person's condition progresses into coma with hepatic failure.

Special Implications for the Therapist   16-11

HEPATIC ENCEPHALOPATHY

Preferred Practice Patterns:
See also Anemia, Ascites.
5A: Primary Prevention/Risk Reduction for Loss of Balance and Falling
5E: Impaired Motor Function and Sensory Integrity Associated With Progressive Disorders of the Central Nervous System (alcoholic ataxia)
5G: Impaired Motor Function and Sensory Integrity Associated With Acute or Chronic Polyneuropathies
5I: Impaired Arousal, Range of Motion, and Motor Control Associated With Coma, Near Coma, or Vegetative State
7A: Primary Prevention/Risk Reduction for Integumentary Disorders (pressure ulcer secondary to malnutrition, immobility, edema)

The inpatient or homebound client with impending hepatic coma has difficulty ambulating and is extremely unsteady. Protective measures must be taken against falls and seizures. The home health therapist must be alert for any report of GI bleeding that will result in protein accumulation in the GI tract, exacerbating this condition (e.g., blood in stools or black, tarry stools). The client should be following a low-protein diet.

The physician may prescribe lactulose to decrease ammonia in the bowel, but diarrhea may be a side effect. The client experiencing prolonged diarrhea should be encouraged to report this information to the physician for possible follow-up. A reduced dosage may be required to prevent further electrolyte imbalance. (See the section on Electrolyte Imbalance in Chapter 4.)

The immobile client who lacks reflexes is vulnerable to numerous complications requiring attention to the prevention of pneumonia and skin breakdown. Skin breakdown in a client who is malnourished from liver disease and is immobile, jaundiced, and edematous can occur in less than 24 hours. Careful attention to skin care, passive exercise, and frequent changes in position are required.

Rest between activities is advocated, and strenuous exercise is to be avoided. The therapist should watch for (and immediately report) signs of anemia (e.g., reduced hemoglobin, weakness, dyspnea on exertion, easy fatigability, skin pallor, tachycardia; see the section on Anemia in Chapter 11), infection (see Table 7-1), and GI bleeding (e.g., melena, hematemesis, easy bruising). ■

Intrahepatic Cholestasis of Pregnancy.   Intrahepatic cholestasis (suppression of bile flow) of pregnancy is a familial disorder characterized by pruritus and cholestatic jaundice; it usually occurs in the last trimester of each pregnancy and promptly resolves after delivery. A variant of this condition, without jaundice, is referred to as *pruritus gravidarum*. Of the women who develop pregnancy-induced intrahepatic cholestasis, 50% have other family members who have experienced jaundice during pregnancy or after the use of oral contraceptives. Women who have experienced cholestatic jaundice of pregnancy should avoid all contraceptives because of a high risk of disease recurrence.

The increase in gonadal and placental hormones during pregnancy is most likely responsible for the cholestasis in susceptible women. Maternal health is unaffected by this condition, but the effects on the unborn child can be serious, including fetal distress, stillbirth, prematurity, and an increased risk of intracranial hemorrhage during delivery. No effects are apparent on the liver of the mother other than centrilobular cholestasis at the time of the pregnancy.

Vascular Disease of the Liver.   *Congestive heart failure* is the major cause of liver congestion, especially in the Western world, where ischemic heart disease is so prevalent. Backward congestion of the liver and the decreased perfusion of the liver secondary to decline in cardiac output result in abnormal liver function tests. Hepatic encephalopathy may contribute to the altered mentation seen with severe congestive heart failure. Decreased cerebral perfusion, hypoxemia, and electrolyte imbalance are usually the major contributors to the confused state that can be seen in people with severe congestive heart failure.

Shock from any cause results in decreased perfusion of the liver and often leads to ischemic necrosis of the centrilobular hepatocytes.

Infarction of the liver is uncommon, but occlusion of the portal vein or the hepatic artery or its branches can occur as a result of embolism, polyarteritis nodosum, unknown cause, or accidental surgical ligation. Thrombosis interrupts the portal blood flow through the sinusoids, which allows a backflow of venous blood into the sinusoids that results in liver congestion. (See the section on Portal Hypertension in this chapter.)

Liver Neoplasms. Hepatic neoplasms can be divided into three groups: benign neoplasms, primary malignant neoplasms, and metastatic malignant neoplasms. Cancer arising from the liver itself is called *primary;* liver cancer that has spread from somewhere else is labeled *secondary.* Primary liver tumors may arise from hepatocytes, connective tissue, blood vessels, or bile ducts and are either benign or malignant (Table 16-7). Primary malignant cancer is almost always found in a cirrhotic liver and is considered a late complication of cirrhosis. Benign and malignant neoplasms occur in women taking oral contraceptives.

A few rare tumors arise from the bile ducts within the liver and are associated with certain hormonal drugs and cancers. These *cholangiocarcinomas* are discussed later in the chapter.

Benign Neoplasms

Liver Hemangioma. About 2% of autopsied livers contain hemangiomas, making this lesion the most common benign liver tumor. It is of unknown etiology and occurs in all age groups, more commonly among women. The pathology is similar to that of hemangiomas anywhere in the body; it is a solitary, blood-filled mass of variable size and can be located anywhere in the liver. Areas of thrombosis are common, and older lesions may begin to calcify. The end stage is a fibrous scar.

Most hepatic hemangiomas are asymptomatic until they become large enough to cause a sense of fullness or upper abdominal pain. Hepatomegaly or an abdominal mass is the most common physical finding. About 10% of clients with clinically detectable lesions are febrile. Hepatic hemangiomas are often discovered coincidentally on CT scan, by MRI, or during laparotomy; otherwise radiographic arteriography or dynamic radionuclide scanning is used to make the diagnosis. Needle aspiration or biopsy is avoided because of the risk of hemorrhage.

Treatment is not usually recommended, because most hepatic hemangiomas have a benign course with negligible risk of malignancy and minimal chance of spontaneous hemorrhage. Surgical resection may be performed if the hemangioma is consistently symptomatic, producing pain or fever, or if the tumor is large enough for traumatic rupture to be considered a risk (e.g., a palpable lesion in an athlete).

TABLE	16-7

Classification of Primary Liver Neoplasms

ORIGIN	BENIGN	MALIGNANT
Hepatocytes	Adenoma	Hepatocellular carcinoma
Connective tissue	Fibroma	Sarcoma
Blood vessels	Hemangioma	Hemangioendothelioma
Bile ducts	Cholangioma	Carcinoma

From Matassarin-Jacobs E, Strasburg K: Nursing care of clients with hepatic disorders. In Black JM, Matassarin-Jacobs E, editors: *Medical-surgical nursing: clinical management for continuity of care,* ed 5, Philadelphia, 1997, WB Saunders, p 1896.

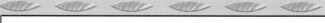

Special Implications for the Therapist **16-12**

LIVER HEMANGIOMA

Most liver hemangiomas are small and found incidentally and require no special precautions. In the case of a known large liver hemangioma, the client must be cautioned to avoid activities and positions that will increase intraabdominal pressure to avoid risk of rupture (see Box 15-1). For the same reason, throughout therapy and especially during exercise, the client must be instructed in proper breathing techniques. ■

Liver Adenomas. Liver cell adenomas occur most commonly in the third and fourth decades, almost exclusively in women. The incidence of benign hepatic cell tumors, called *adenomas,* is increasing, possibly in association with environmental estrogens, estrogens in oral contraceptives used by women, or the use of androgens in the case of liver adenomas in men. Although classified as benign tumors, they are highly vascular and carry a risk for rupture and subsequent hemorrhage. The clinical presentation is often one of acute abdominal disease because of necrosis of the tumor with hemorrhage. Pain, fever, and circulatory collapse occur in the presence of hemorrhage.

Most of these adenomas are evaluated with MRI or CT. Liver function test results are usually within normal limits. The treatment for benign adenomas is dependent on the underlying cause. Hormone-dependent tumors may resolve with cessation of the oral contraceptives or androgens. Surgical excision (or hepatic lobectomy in the case of acute hemorrhage) of the involved liver segment is indicated in the absence of hormonally induced tumor. Prognosis is excellent; although malignant transformation can occur, it is a rare phenomenon.

Special Implications for the Therapist **16-13**

LIVER ADENOMAS

The therapist is most likely to see this client postoperatively after the danger of rupture and hemorrhage has passed. Standard postoperative protocols are usually sufficient. ■

Liver Malignant Neoplasms
Primary Hepatocellular Carcinoma

Overview and Incidence. Hepatocellular carcinoma (HCC or HCCa) constitutes about 90% to 95% of primary liver cancers in adults. In many countries including the United States, a definite increase in the incidence of HCC has been reported, largely attributable to the increasing incidence of hepatitis C infection.[37] Although HCC can develop at any age, in the Western world, incidence increases at age 60 years, occurs more frequently in men, and appears to be closely associated with cirrhosis. Geographic variations exist in the United States with significantly higher death rates reported in western, southern, and central states.

Etiologic and Risk Factors.   Epidemiologic and laboratory studies have firmly established a strong and specific association between HBV (any form, even HBV carrier state) and hepatitis C and hepatocellular carcinoma. These viruses act either as a carcinogen or as a co-carcinogen in chronically infected hepatocytes. Interestingly, hepatitis B may be noncirrhotic when HCC develops, but hepatitis C increases the risk only after cirrhosis develops.

Evidence also points to a link between ethanol abuse and hepatocellular carcinoma, probably mediated by its capacity to induce cirrhosis. Other risk factors include gender (men have three to eight times greater risk), increasing age (more than 60 years), certain mycotoxins*, anabolic steroids, long-term oral contraceptive use,† polyvinylchloride, and nitrosamines. In addition, metabolic conditions such as hemochromatosis, alpha$_1$-antitrypsin deficiency, Wilson's disease, and glycogen storage diseases have been linked by epidemiologic study more than by a direct causal relationship. Rarely, hepatobiliary complications occur in women using oral contraceptive agents. Women with current or previous benign or malignant hepatic tumors should not take oral contraceptives.

Pathogenesis and Clinical Manifestations.   The exact events leading to malignant transformation of the hepatic cell remain unknown. HBV appears to be an oncogenic virus that can integrate its viral DNA sequences into the cellular genome. This integration appears to be a necessary step for the mentioned transformation. Histologically, hepatocellular carcinoma is made up of cords or sheets of cells that resemble the hepatic parenchyma. Blood vessels such as portal or hepatic veins are commonly involved by tumor.

Clients with primary (benign and malignant) and secondary (metastatic) tumors often present with a similar clinical picture. Symptoms may be vague initially with minor temperature elevation and GI symptoms. Common clinical manifestations include jaundice, right upper quadrant pain, right shoulder pain, abdominal mass or distention, weight loss, diarrhea or constipation, and nausea. Complications may include cachexia, tumor rupture, thrombosis of portal or hepatic vein, tumor embolism, portal hypertension with esophageal varices, ascites, hepatic failure, and widespread metastases.

Medical Management

Diagnosis.   Serum levels of alpha-fetoprotein are high in up to 60% of cases (400 ng/ml compared with the normal adult level of 10 ng/ml) but are not absolutely diagnostic. Tumors detected or suspected at the time of alpha-fetoprotein measurement or ultrasonography are further examined. HBsAg is present in a majority of cases in endemic areas, whereas in the United States anti-HCV is found in up to 40% of cases. Liver biopsy is diagnostic, and endoscopic ultrasonography can detect hepatocellular carcinomas of 1 cm, offering the advantage of allowing guided percutaneous biopsy or aspiration cytology. Dynamic CT scanning with intravenous contrast material may also demonstrate lesions as small as 1 cm. Final diagnosis is based on histologic findings in resected hepatic tumors, biopsy specimens, or on the radiologic findings of hepatic arteriography.

Prevention and Treatment.   The use of vaccination to prevent infection with hepatitis B is expected to reduce the incidence of hepatocellular carcinoma associated with HBV. This is the only malignancy for which effective immunization is available. In the meantime, early screening of high-risk populations and detection remain the key to successful treatment of this malignancy. Surgical resection (partial or total hepatectomy) has been the primary treatment if no nodal involvement or distant spread is present.

Newer treatment techniques for unresectable hepatocellular carcinoma to reduce tumor size now include transarterial chemoembolization (angiography to embolize the tumor arterial supply) and percutaneous ethanol injection (alcohol injection into the tumor). Radiofrequency ablation, cryosurgery,* and hepatic artery infusion chemotherapy are advanced procedures providing increasingly better outcomes over time for unresectable liver cancer. Pilot programs exploring the effectiveness of combining these techniques are under way.[17,44] Other areas of ongoing investigation include regional gene therapy and interference with tumor growth by inhibition of angiogenesis. Liver transplantation is a possible treatment option for clients with decompensating cirrhosis (see the section on Pathogenesis of Cirrhosis in this chapter) and a small hepatocellular carcinoma confined to the liver.

Prognosis.   Untreated HCC has a very poor prognosis, especially in clients with multiple tumor nodules. Factors affecting the prognosis favorably include early detection, tumor size (less than 5 cm), tumor location, presence of a tumor capsule, well-differentiated tumor, lack of vascular invasion, and absence of cirrhosis. Successful treatment with liver resection has increased 5-year survival rates to 35%. Tumor resection in the presence of cirrhosis is accompanied by risk of tumor recurrence or death from the remaining underlying liver dysfunction. If treatment fails to eradicate the tumor process, the expected survival is no more than 4 to 6 months.

Special Implications for the Therapist   16-14

PRIMARY HEPATOCELLULAR CARCINOMA

Preferred Practice Patterns:
6E: Impaired Ventilation and Respiration/Gas Exchange
     Associated With Ventilatory Pump Dysfunction or Failure
     (elevated diaphragm)

Continued

---

*The most significant mycotoxins are the aflatoxins, particularly those produced by *Aspergillus flavus*, a fungus from mold found in wheat, soybeans, corn, rice, oats, peanuts, milk, and cheese.

†This risk factor increases with higher dosage, longer duration of use, and older age.

*Cryosurgery involves penetrating a tumor within the liver with a probe, which the surgeon guides by watching an ultrasound monitor. When the probe reaches the center of the tumor, liquid nitrogen is pumped in to freeze it. Freezing continues until the frozen portion extends to 1 cm beyond the borders of the tumor. The tumor is then thawed and refrozen. This procedure cannot be performed where there is cirrhosis or where the tumor is too close to a critical blood vessel.

7A: Primary Prevention/Risk Reduction for Integumentary Disorders (edema)

Liver tumors that cause elevation of the diaphragm can cause right shoulder pain or symptoms of respiratory involvement. Peripheral edema associated with developing ascites may be observed first by the therapist (see the section on Ascites in this chapter). As the tumor grows, pain may radiate to the back (mid-thoracic region). Paraneoplastic syndromes (see Chapter 8) resulting from ectopic hormone may occur including polycythemia, hypoglycemia, and hypercalcemia. (See Special Implications for the Therapist: Oncology, 8-1). ■

Metastatic Malignant Tumors.   The liver is one of the most common sites of metastasis from other primary cancers (e.g., colorectal, stomach, pancreas, esophagus, lung, breast, melanoma, Hodgkin's disease, and non-Hodgkin's lymphoma). Metastatic tumors occur 20 times more often than primary liver tumors and constitute the bulk of hepatic malignancy. As with other types of cancers, secondary liver cancer can occur as a result of local invasion from neighboring organs, lymphatic spread, spread across body cavities, and spread via the vascular system. The liver filters blood from anywhere else in the body, but because all blood from the digestive organs passes through the liver before joining the general circulation, the liver is the first organ to filter cancer cells released from the stomach, intestine, or pancreas.

Metastatic tumors to the liver originating in some organs (e.g., stomach, lung) never give rise to hepatic symptoms, whereas others produce hepatic symptoms or jaundice with less than 60% replacement of the liver. Certain tumors (colon, breast, melanoma) typically replace 90% of the liver before jaundice develops. Melanomas are associated with such minimal tissue reaction that almost complete hepatic replacement occurs before hepatic symptoms develop. Clinical manifestations, diagnosis, and treatment are as for the primary (original) neoplasm. Experimental and clinical data show evidence of a correlation between elevated blood levels of carcinoembryonic antigen (CEA) and the development of liver metastases from colorectal carcinomas. A cause-effect relationship between these two observations has not been identified. Investigations continue to explore the use of tumor markers and the clinical usefulness of CEA throughout the different stages of management in both animal and human studies. Treatment is as for unresectable liver cancer; see the section on Hepatocellular Carcinoma in this chapter.

Other ongoing research is investigating the use of a totally implantable pump for hepatic arterial infusion (HAI) therapy for those with unresectable hepatic metastases and for post-hepatic resection. This enables oncologists to give much higher doses of chemotherapy directly into the blood supply of the tumors as well as use a continuous infusion schedule. This approach may offer more successful treatment of people with metastatic colorectal carcinoma to the hepatic system.[20,21]

Liver Abscess.   Liver abscess most often occurs among individuals with other underlying disorders. Most common underlying causes include *bacterial cholangitis* secondary to obstruction of the bile ducts by stone or stricture; *portal vein bacteremia* secondary to bacterial seeding via the portal vein from infected viscera following bowel inflammation or organ perforation; *liver flukes*, a parasitic infestation; or *amebiasis*, an infestation with amebae from tropical or subtropical areas. Other predisposing factors are diabetes mellitus, infected hepatic cysts, metastatic liver tumors with secondary infection, and diverticulitis. Pyogenic (pus-filled) abscesses may be single or multiple; liver cirrhosis is a strong risk factor for single pyogenic liver abscess, and multiple abscesses often arise from a biliary source of infection.

Clinical manifestations are commonly right-sided abdominal and right shoulder pain, nausea, vomiting, rapid weight loss, high fever, and diaphoresis. The liver's close proximity to the base of the right lung may contribute to the development of right pleural effusion. Complications of hepatic abscess relate to rupture and direct spread of infection. Pleuropulmonary involvement from the rupture of an abscess through the diaphragm, and peritonitis from leakage into the abdominal cavity can occur.

Diagnosis is accomplished by a variety of possible tests including liver function tests, chest roentgenograms, contrast-enhanced CT scan of the abdomen, ultrasonography of the right upper quadrant, liver scan, or arteriography. Treatment may consist of antimicrobial therapy alone or percutaneous aspiration of the abscess with antimicrobial therapy. Surgery may be required to relieve biliary tract obstruction and to drain abscesses that do not respond to percutaneous drainage and antibiotics.

Unrecognized and untreated, pyogenic liver abscess is universally fatal. The mortality from hepatic abscess in treated cases remains high, ranging from 40% to 80%. Amebic abscesses are an exception; when treated, the mortality rate is less than 3%. Early diagnosis and aggressive treatment can significantly reduce the mortality in some cases. Specific antibiotics are required whenever abscess is caused by amebic infestation.

Special Implications for the Therapist   16-15

LIVER ABSCESS

Preferred Practice Patterns:
6E: *Impaired Ventilation and Respiration/Gas Exchange Associated With Ventilatory Pump Dysfunction or Failure (decreased lung capacity; elevated diaphragm)*
6F: *Impaired Ventilation and Respiration/Gas Exchange Associated With Respiratory Failure (pleural effusion)*
7A: *Primary Prevention/Risk Reduction for Integumentary Disorders (high fever; immobility)*

Clients with liver abscess are very ill and usually are seen only by the therapist assigned to an intensive care unit team. In such situations, vital signs are assessed regularly to detect high fever and rapid pulse, which are early signs of sepsis (a common complication). Movement, coughing, and deep breathing are important to prevent or limit pulmonary complications related to hepatic abscess, and skin care in the presence of high fever is essential. Careful disposal of feces and careful handwashing to avoid transmission are required when abscess is caused by amebic infestation. ■

Liver Injuries.   *Toxic liver injury* can occur as a result of drugs or from occupational exposure to chemicals and toxins. Hepatotoxic chemicals produce liver cell necrosis, a consequence of the metabolism of the compound by the oxidase system of the liver. Agents responsible for toxic liver injury include yellow phosphorus, carbon tetrachloride, phalloidin (mushroom toxin), and acetaminophen (analgesic). Reye's syndrome in children may be related to aspirin toxicity. In addition to jaundice, other symptoms of liver toxicity may occur (e.g., cholestasis, chronic hepatitis). Toxic liver injury produces toxic hepatitis (discussed earlier in the chapter). The prognosis is usually good if the toxin is withdrawn and never reintroduced. Whatever drug is responsible, it is well documented that liver toxicity becomes more severe with advancing age.

Liver injury by trauma may be either penetrating or blunt, leading to laceration and hemorrhage. Penetrating injuries are usually knife or missile wounds (gunshot). A knife wound leaves a sharp clear incision, whereas gunshot wounds enter and exit with greater damage. Blunt trauma from a fall or from hitting a steering wheel has varying effects, from small hematomas to large lacerations as a result of severe impact forces.

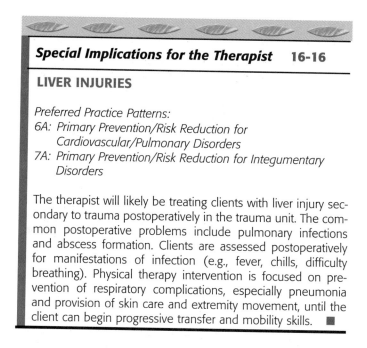

Special Implications for the Therapist   16-16

LIVER INJURIES

Preferred Practice Patterns:
6A: *Primary Prevention/Risk Reduction for Cardiovascular/Pulmonary Disorders*
7A: *Primary Prevention/Risk Reduction for Integumentary Disorders*

The therapist will likely be treating clients with liver injury secondary to trauma postoperatively in the trauma unit. The common postoperative problems include pulmonary infections and abscess formation. Clients are assessed postoperatively for manifestations of infection (e.g., fever, chills, difficulty breathing). Physical therapy intervention is focused on prevention of respiratory complications, especially pneumonia and provision of skin care and extremity movement, until the client can begin progressive transfer and mobility skills. ■

PANCREAS

◆ Diabetes Mellitus
The pancreas has dual functions, acting as both an endocrine gland in secreting hormones insulin and glucagon and as an exocrine gland in producing digestive enzymes. The cells of the pancreas that function in the endocrine capacity are the islets of Langerhans, constituting 1% to 2% of the pancreatic mass. Defective endocrine function of the pancreas resulting in ineffective insulin (whether deficient or defective in action within the body) characterizes diabetes mellitus (see Chapter 10).

◆ Pancreatitis
Pancreatitis is a potentially serious inflammation of the pancreas that may result in autodigestion of the pancreas by its own enzymes. Pancreatitis may be acute or chronic; the acute form is brief, usually mild, and reversible, whereas the chronic form is recurrent or persisting. Approximately 15% of all cases of acute pancreatitis develop into chronic pancreatitis.

Acute Pancreatitis
Incidence and Etiologic Factors.   Acute pancreatitis can arise from a variety of etiologic factors; it can occur in association with one of several other clinical conditions (Box 16-4) or as the result of an unknown cause (10% to 20%). The incidence varies with the circumstances and age of the affected person; incidence increases after age 55 years. In metropolitan areas, affected people tend to be younger, and alcoholism is the most common etiology. In rural areas and in geriatric clients, gallstones predominate as a cause.

Pathogenesis.   Acute pancreatitis is thought to result from escape of activated pancreatic enzymes from acinar cells* into surrounding tissues. The exact pathogenesis is unknown, but it may include edema or obstruction of the ampulla of Vater (e.g., stone; Fig. 16-6) with resultant reflux of bile into pancreatic ducts or direct injury to the acinar cells, which allows leakage of pancreatic enzymes into pancreatic tissue. Enzyme activation breaks down tissue and cell membranes, causing pathologic changes varying from acute connective tissue edema and cellular infiltration with subsequent

---

*Acinus is the smallest functional unit of the liver; the term also is used to refer to a terminal respiratory unit (*pulmonary acinus*).

BOX 16-4

Conditions Associated With Acute Pancreatitis

*Alcoholism
Autoimmune diseases
Cystic fibrosis
*Gallstones
Hereditary (familial) pancreatitis
Hypercalcemia
Hyperlipidemia
Infection
Ischemia
Medications (oral contraceptives, antibiotics, AZT)
Neoplasm
Peptic ulcers
Postoperative inflammation
Pregnancy (third trimester)
Trauma (including ischemia/perfusion that occurs during some surgical procedures)
Vasculitis
Viral infections

*Most common causes.

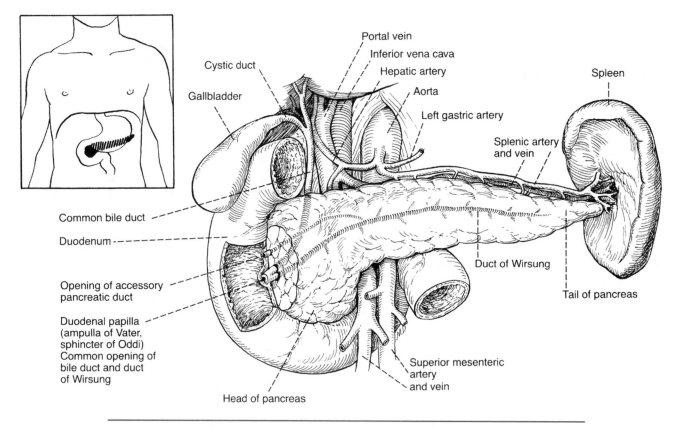

FIGURE 16-6 The pancreas. The pancreas (located behind the stomach) and gallbladder are anterior to the L1-3 vertebral bodies. Attaching to the duodenum to the right the pancreas extends horizontally across to the spleen in the left abdomen, coming in contact with the duodenum, kidneys, liver, and spleen. Obstruction of either the hepatic or common bile duct by stone or spasm blocks the exit of bile from the liver, where it is formed, and prevents bile from ejecting into the duodenum. (From Black JM, Matassarin-Jacobs E, editors: *Luckmann and Sorensen's medical-surgical nursing*, ed 4, Philadelphia, 1993, WB Saunders, p 1681.)

scarring to necrosis of the acinar cells, hemorrhage from necrotic blood vessels, and intrahepatic and extrahepatic fat necrosis. Autodigestion and inflammation of all or part of the pancreas may occur, resulting in the formation of a soaplike substance that binds with calcium. Increased intracellular calcium concentration also mediates acinar cell damage.

Oxygen-derived free radicals and many cytokines (e.g., interleukin 1, IL-6, IL-8, tumor necrosis factor, platelet activating factor; see the section on Cytokines, Chapter 5) are considered to be principal mediators in the transformation of acute pancreatitis from a local inflammatory process into a multiorgan illness.[4,46] Other organs, such as the lungs and kidneys, can be affected by pancreatic enzymes and toxins entering into the retroperitoneal lymphatics and bloodstream. These systemic effects are major causes of morbidity and mortality.

Clinical Manifestations. Symptoms in clients presenting with acute pancreatitis can vary from mild, nonspecific abdominal pain to profound shock with coma and, ultimately, death. Gallstone-associated pancreatitis typically produces symptoms after a large meal. Abdominal pain begins abruptly in the mid-epigastrium, increases in intensity for several hours, and can last from days to more than a week. The pain is caused by edema, which distends the pancreatic ducts and

capsule; chemical irritation and inflammation of the peritoneum from leaking pancreatic enzymes and toxins; and irritation or obstruction of the biliary tract. Pancreatic pain has a penetrating quality and radiates to the upper back or thoracolumbar junction because of the retroperitoneal location of the pancreas. Pain is made worse by walking and lying supine and is relieved by sitting and leaning forward or left sidelying in the fetal position.

Other common symptoms include nausea and vomiting, fever and sweating, tachycardia, malaise and weakness, and mild jaundice from impingement on the common bile duct. Symptoms are often preceded by a heavy meal or excessive alcohol consumption. Complications may include shock, acute (adult) respiratory distress syndrome (ARDS), acute renal failure, hypercalcemia, pancreatic pseudocysts,* abscess, or chemical or septic peritonitis. Tetany may develop as a result of calcium deposition in areas of fat necrosis, leading to reduced calcium levels or as a decreased response to parathormone (parathyroid hormone).

---

*A pseudocyst is a liquefied collection of necrotic debris and pancreatic enzymes surrounded by a rim of pancreatic tissue or adjacent tissues; it contains no true epithelial lining. Complications of pseudocysts include infection, bleeding, and rupture into the peritoneum.

Medical Management

Diagnosis.   Diagnosis is based on clinical presentation and clinical studies, including abdominal x-ray, ultrasound for the diagnosis of gallstones, CT scan to evaluate the pancreas (possibly serial examinations if symptoms fail to resolve with treatment), and laboratory studies. Early in the disease (within 24 to 72 hours), pancreatic digestive enzymes released from injured acinar cells into the blood result in elevated serum amylase and lipase levels, which are diagnostic for acute pancreatitis. Urine amylase level is also elevated, which is significant in the diagnosis. The ratio of amylase clearance to creatinine clearance by the kidney increases significantly in cases of pancreatitis. Anyone with hereditary pancreatitis should be periodically screened for pancreatic cancer, and those with chronic pancreatitis involving endocrine function must be evaluated for the presence of diabetes.

Treatment.   For most persons, acute pancreatitis is a mild disease that subsides spontaneously within several days. Treatment for pancreatitis is largely symptomatic and is designed to provide rest for the pancreas by stopping the process of autodigestion. Oral foods and fluids may be withheld to decrease pancreatic secretions, with gradual reintroduction of clear liquids and progression to a regular low-fat diet per tolerance. Nasogastric suction may be required to relieve pain and prevent paralytic ileus in individuals with nausea and vomiting. Analgesics, fluid management, and cessation of alcohol intake are essential components of medical treatment. Calcium gluconate is given intravenously in the presence of hypocalcemia with tetany. Long-term parenteral feeding may be required for protracted cases. Surgical intervention is indicated in the presence of cholelithiasis (removal of gallstones) or pancreatic necrosis. The pathogenesis of pancreatitis is not understood well enough to develop a specific therapy to stop the inflammatory cascade, and gene therapy for hereditary pancreatitis is beyond current technologic capabilities but may be a future treatment option.

Prognosis.   Prognosis depends on the severity of the condition; treatment produces varying results, but the clinical course follows a self-limited pattern, resolving within 2 weeks in up to 90% of cases. Many people, especially those with gallstone pancreatitis, improve rapidly, but recurrences are common in alcoholic pancreatitis. Complications of shock and ARDS develop in approximately 10% of cases, resulting in lengthy hospitalizations and high mortality.

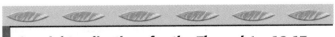

Special Implications for the Therapist   16-17

ACUTE PANCREATITIS

Preferred Practice Patterns:
See Acute (Adult) Respiratory Distress Syndrome (Chapter 14), Tetany (Chapter 4).

The therapist is most likely to see acute pancreatitis either when the early presentation is back pain (undiagnosed) or when ARDS develops as a complication, necessitating assisted respi-

ration and pulmonary care. Pancreatic inflammation and scarring occurring as part of the acute pancreatic process can result in decreased spinal extension, especially of the thoracolumbar junction. This problem is difficult to treat and requires the therapist to make reasonable goals (e.g., maintain function and current range of motion), especially when the pancreatitis is in an active, ongoing phase. Even with client compliance with treatment intervention and subsiding of inflammation, the residual scarring is difficult to reach or affect with mobilization techniques and continues to reduce mechanical motion.

Back pain associated with acute pancreatitis may be accompanied by GI symptoms such as diarrhea, pain after a meal, anorexia, and unexplained weight loss. The client may not see any connection between GI symptoms and back pain and may not report the additional symptoms. The pain may be relieved by heat initially (decreases muscular tension); preferred positions include leaning forward, sitting up, or lying motionless on the left side in a fetal-flexed position. Promoting comfort and rest as part of the medical rehabilitation process may necessitate teaching the client positioning (side-lying, knee-chest position with a pillow pressed against the abdomen, or sitting with the trunk flexed may be helpful) and relaxation techniques.

For the client who is restricted from eating or drinking anything to rest the GI tract and decrease pancreatic stimulation, even ice chips can stimulate enzymes and increase pain. In such cases, the therapist must be careful not to give in to the client's repeated requests for food, water, or ice chips unless approved by nursing or medical staff. Clients with acute pancreatitis are allowed to resume oral intake when all abdominal pain and tenderness have resolved. (See also Chapter 4 for care of the client with fluid or electrolyte imbalance.) ∎

Chronic Pancreatitis

Incidence.   The distribution of idiopathic chronic pancreatitis is bimodal, with a juvenile form of the disease occurring in young persons (mean age, 25 years) and a second distribution peak at age 60 years. Chronic pancreatitis is caused by long-standing alcohol abuse in more than 90% of adult cases; cases in children are related to cystic fibrosis.

Pathogenesis.   Structural or functional impairment of the pancreas leads to chronic pancreatitis. Progressive destruction of the pancreas occurs with resulting irregular fibrosis and chronic inflammation. Functional obstruction of the pancreatic duct may be caused by mechanical obstruction (e.g., cancer, cystic fibrosis mucus). Although the etiologic role of alcohol is well established, the mechanism by which it causes pancreatitis is unclear. Alcohol stimulates precipitation of protein plugs in the ducts, which serve as the point of origin (nidus) for subsequent calculi. These stones obstruct the ductal system, leading to progressive necrosis and scarring.

The fact that chronic pancreatitis is often characterized by intermittent acute attacks followed by periods of quiescence suggests that in many persons the pathogenesis involves repeated bouts of acute pancreatitis followed by scarring. In persons without a history of acute episodes, the pathogenesis of chronic pancreatitis may relate to persistent necrosis and insidious scarring, similar to the progression of cirrhosis of the liver.

Clinical Manifestations. In clients with alcohol-associated pancreatitis, epigastric and left upper quadrant pain often begins 12 to 48 hours after an episode of excessive alcohol consumption. Pain eventually may become almost continuous, and referred upper left lumbar pain with muscle guarding may occur. Attacks may last only a few hours or as long as 2 weeks, and symptoms are similar to those of acute pancreatitis with additional symptoms of weight loss, flatulence, diarrhea owing to loss of enzymes, or constipation. Chronic pancreatitis is characterized by an irreversible destruction of the exocrine and endocrine pancreatic parenchyma leading to malabsorption and diabetes (loss of islet cell function).

Medical Management. Clinical history in the presence of typical findings on examination is correlated with laboratory studies and imaging (e.g., abdominal films, ultrasound, upper GI tract series, endoscopy) to make the diagnosis. In contrast to acute pancreatitis, chronic pancreatitis does not usually produce an elevated amylase level unless associated with a distinct attack. Calcium levels may be decreased, but unlike the case with acute pancreatitis, this does not lead to tetany.

The treatment of chronic pancreatitis is directed toward prevention of further pancreatic injury, pain relief, and replacement of lost endocrine/exocrine function. In the case of cystic fibrosis and for selected individuals with alcoholic pancreatitis, oral enzyme replacements are taken before and during meals to correct enzyme deficiencies and to prevent malabsorption. Cessation of alcohol intake is essential in the management of chronic pancreatitis; insulin may be required in the case of islet cell dysfunction. Surgical drainage for persistent pseudocysts as well as surgical intervention to eliminate obstruction of the bile ducts may be indicated.

Chronic pancreatitis is a serious disease, often leading to chronic disability. Chronic pancreatitis associated with cystic fibrosis may produce death secondary to lung infection. Alcohol-related chronic pancreatitis has a poor prognosis without alcohol cessation. For those persons who cannot be helped by treatment, addiction to narcotics is a frequent result. Clients with chronic pancreatitis who undergo total pancreas resection inevitably become diabetic unless they receive islet autotransplantation (a newly developing procedure).[45]

Special Implications for the Therapist   16-18

CHRONIC PANCREATITIS

Preferred Practice Patterns:
Patterns associated with chronic pancreatitis are determined by the presence of associated complications such as diabetes, neuropathy, osteoporosis, and complications of alcoholism (e.g., malnutrition, cirrhosis, ascites). Each client must be assessed individually.

Back pain in the upper thoracic area or pain at the thoracolumbar junction may be the presenting symptom for some individuals with chronic pancreatitis, but past medical history including the presence of pancreatitis should raise a red flag suggesting careful screening required in these cases. People with alcohol-related chronic pancreatitis often have peripheral neuropathy.

The clinical presentation with aggravating and relieving factors (e.g., alcohol consumption, food intake, positional changes noted) or failure to improve with therapy intervention adds additional red flag symptoms.[13]

The person with known pancreatitis and/or pancreatectomy may need monitoring of vital signs and/or blood glucose levels depending on complications present. Education about the effects of malabsorption and associated osteoporosis should be included. See also Special Implications for the Therapist: Malabsorption, 15-9. ■

◆ Pancreatic Cancer

Overview and Incidence. Pancreatic cancer represents the fourth leading cause of cancer mortality in the United States with more than 29,700 deaths each year.[19] Most pancreatic neoplasms (90%) arise from exocrine cells in the ducts and are called *ductal adenocarcinoma* (65% in the proximal or head of the pancreas, 15% in the pancreas body and tail, 20% diffuse involvement of the entire gland). These are the focus of the discussion here. The remaining primary pancreatic neoplasms include cystic neoplasms involving the entire pancreas and islet cell tumors affecting the endocrine portion of the pancreas. Pancreatic lymphomas are rare but respond dramatically to chemotherapy and metastatic tumors can spread to the pancreas via hematogenous or lymphatic means.

From 1930 until 1980, the incidence of pancreatic cancer doubled and then peaked in the 1980s. The reason(s) for this remain unknown. Pancreatic cancer is more common in black men than in whites, occurs in the Western world most often, and has a peak incidence in the seventh and eighth decades.

Etiologic and Risk Factors. Clear evidence of increased risk of pancreatic cancer has been shown related to advancing age, tobacco use, male gender, previous peptic ulcer surgery and cholecystectomy, and among Jews and blacks. The presence of diabetes mellitus (especially in women), chronic pancreatitis, and prior gastrectomy may be contributing factors. No support exists for any direct effect from exposure to radiation, socioeconomic status, alcohol intake, or coffee consumption, although these risk factors remain under investigation.[31] Although unusual, a genetic predisposition to pancreatic cancer has been documented. Gene mutations and other acquired chromosomal abnormalities are being recognized with increasing frequency. How mutations or abnormalities in gene expression relate to the pathogenesis of pancreatic cancer remains unknown.

Pathogenesis. Molecularly, a large number of pancreatic adenocarcinomas have been examined for genetic alterations in cancer-causing genes (e.g., tumor suppressor genes, oncogenes, DNA mismatch repair genes; see Chapter 8) but data remain limited and inconclusive at this time. The role of various polypeptide growth factors and their receptors in the regulation of pancreatic cancer is also under investigation. Microscopically, ductal adenocarcinomas contain infiltrative glands of various sizes and shapes surrounded by dense, reactive fibrous tissue. Many ductal adenocarcinomas infiltrate into vascular spaces, lymphatic spaces, and perineural spaces. Pancreatic cancer appears to progress from flat ductal lesions to papillary ductal lesions without irregularities then with irregularities (atypia) and finally to infiltrating adenocarcinoma. The existence of such a progression suggests that it may be possible to detect a curable precursor lesion and early cancer with a molecular test in the future.[31]

Clinical Manifestations.   The clinical features of pancreatic cancer are initially nonspecific and vague, which contribute to the delay in diagnosis. Early symptoms include anorexia, nausea, weight loss, and abdominal discomfort. Pain is a common symptom of pancreatic carcinoma and may become intractable later in the progression of disease. At first, epigastric pain radiating to the back (thoracic) or back pain alone, and jaundice with pruritus occur, the latter when there is obstruction of the biliary tree. Radiating pain associated with carcinoma of the body and tail of the pancreas localizes in the left lumbar region. Sitting up and leaning forward may provide some relief initially and usually indicate that the lesion has spread beyond the pancreas and is inoperable. Advanced cases may experience cachexia, muscle wasting, and ascites.

Metastasis.   Pancreatic ductal adenocarcinomas metastasize via the hematologic and lymphatic systems to the liver, peritoneum, lungs and pleura, and to the adrenal glands. These metastasized tumors may grow by direct extension causing further involvement of the duodenum, stomach, spleen, and colon. Tumors of the body and tail of the pancreas are twice as likely to metastasize to the peritoneum compared with tumors in the head of the pancreas.

Medical Management
Diagnosis.   With the expanding knowledge of cell biology and nuclear control of cellular proliferation, strategies for screening (or directed treatment) are not far off. At the present time, no single diagnostic test exists, but rather a range of serologic and radiologic studies are available for evaluation and staging of this disease. Anyone with jaundice may be evaluated by ultrasound or contrast-enhanced spiral computed tomography (CT). Magnetic resonance cholangiopancreatography (MRCP) is a newer noninvasive technique used to visualize both the bile duct and the pancreatic duct.

The TNM staging system (for tumor, node, metastases) (see Chapter 8) classifies pancreatic carcinoma according to tumor size, extent of local invasion, presence or absence of regional lymph node metastases, and presence or absence of distant nonnodal metastatic disease. Preoperative staging provides information required for determining surgical resectability and prognosis.

Treatment.   Management of symptoms such as obstructive jaundice, duodenal obstruction, and back pain is often difficult. Palliative therapy may be operative or nonoperative to provide significant relief of symptoms. The use of biliary stents through the obstructing lesion to alleviate jaundice provides some relief. Pancreatic resection and reconstruction currently provide the only opportunity for cure. Despite sophisticated preoperative staging methods, many people with adenocarcinoma of the pancreatic head that appears to be resectable preoperatively are found to have metastatic or locally invasive disease at laparotomy, precluding resection. Combined-modality treatment with chemotherapy and radiation therapy after curative resection provides symptomatic relief and prolongs survival in some cases. When tumors of the pancreas cannot be removed, a surgical biliary bypass operation or nonoperative biliary stenting to relieve jaundice without removing the tumor have been shown to be equally effective but with no improvement in long-term survival.[31]

Pharmacology for pain control may include nonnarcotic oral analgesics (e.g., NSAIDs, Tylenol) initially, with later introduction of narcotics and other adjuvant drugs (e.g., tricyclic antidepressants). Percutaneous chemical splanchnicectomy (destruction of the splanchnic nerve) may be used for the nonoperative treatment of pain, to reduce the need for oral narcotics.

Prognosis.   The overall prognosis for pancreatic carcinoma is very poor with a mortality rate of nearly 100%. Despite advances in diagnostic technology that have shortened the interval between onset of symptoms and definitive treatment, no appreciable impact on survival has occurred. Operative resection offers the only hope for cure, but fewer than 15% of clients have resectable disease at the time of diagnosis; 5-year survival after curative resection has improved to 20%. Once distant metastases are established, survival is so limited that a conservative therapeutic approach is followed.[31] Return of hepatic function following relief of obstruction is variable. Bile secretion may return to normal within hours; immunologic dysfunction may take weeks to normalize; jaundice characteristically improves dramatically within the first several days but may not disappear for weeks, and some of the other symptoms such as pruritus, loss of appetite, and malaise correct within hours or days following relief of the obstruction.

Special Implications for the Therapist   16-19

PANCREATIC CANCER

Preferred Practice Patterns (associated with intractable referred back pain):
4B: Impaired Posture
4C: Impaired Muscle Performance
4F: Impaired Joint Mobility, Motor Function, Muscle Performance, Range of Motion, and Reflex Integrity Associated With Spinal Disorders

Vague back pain may be the first symptomatic presentation, and cervical lymphadenopathy (called Virchow's node) may be the first sign of distant metastases. The therapist is most likely to palpate an enlarged supraclavicular lymph node (usually left-sided), a finding that should always alert the therapist to the need to screen for medical disease. Paraneoplastic syndrome (see Chapter 8) associated with pancreatic carcinoma may present as neuromyopathy, dermatomyositis, or thrombophlebitis associated with abnormalities in blood coagulation (coagulopathy). The presence of coagulopathy represents a precaution in the administration of certain therapeutic interventions. See Special Implications for the Therapist: Signs and Symptoms of Hepatic Disease, 16-1.

The therapist is most likely to be involved with the client with diagnosed pancreatic cancer who experiences intractable back pain. Referral to chronic pain clinics or hospice centers likely includes physical therapy services. Repeated nerve blocks may be
Continued

performed after a reasonable effort to manage pain through the use of transcutaneous electrical nerve stimulation (TENS), biofeedback, analgesics, or other pain control techniques. Indwelling infusion pumps implanted to deliver analgesics directly to the site of visceral afferent nerves in the epidural or intrathecal spaces may be used for short periods (i.e., 1 to 3 months). ◼

◆ Cystic Fibrosis

Cystic fibrosis is a disease of the exocrine glands that results in the production of excessive, thick mucus that obstructs the digestive and respiratory systems. When the disease was first being differentiated from other conditions, it was given the name cystic fibrosis of the pancreas, because cysts and scar tissue on the pancreas were observed during autopsy. This term describes a secondary rather than primary characteristic (indepth discussion of this disorder is found in Chapter 14).

BILIARY

See Table 16-8.

◆ Cholelithiasis (Gallstones)

Definition and Overview. Cholelithiasis is the formation or presence of gallstones that remain in the lumen of the gallbladder or are ejected with bile into the cystic duct. Gallstones are stonelike masses called calculi (singular: calculus) that form in the gallbladder as a result of changes in the normal components of bile. Two types are classified according to composition: 75% consist primarily of cholesterol (cholesterol stones), whereas 25% are composed of bilirubin salts (e.g., calcium bilirubinate and other calcium salts), called pigment stones. Chronic cholecystitis (gallbladder or cystic duct inflammation) may accompany cholelithiasis when gallstones become lodged in the cystic duct and obstruct the flow of bile in and out of the gallbladder.

Incidence. Gallstones, the most common cause of biliary tract disease in the United States, occur increasingly with advancing age, so that gallstones are present in 20% of men and 35% of women by age 65 years. In the United States, an estimated 15 to 20 million people have gallstones. About 25 years ago, the typical person with gallstones was described as a fat, fair, fertile, flatulent, forty, female. As the incidence of gallstones continues to increase, this descriptor no longer strictly applies. For example, very elderly people with associated conditions such as heart and lung disease develop gallstones as a complication.

Etiologic and Risk Factors. Specific risk factors for the development of gallstones are listed in Box 16-5. Fasting overnight for 14 hours or more (presumably skipping breakfast) has been associated with a higher rate of gallstones. Without the stimulation of food, the gallbladder does not put out enough solubilizing bile acids that keep cholesterol dissolved and unable to form stones. Adequate calcium and vitamin C may reduce the risk of gallbladder disease,[49] but whether risk for gallbladder disease can be reduced by altering intake of a specific dietary factor has not been established.[52] Lifestyle and diet alone do not account for the variation within high incidence areas, and even excessive cholesterol in the bile probably requires another particle or substance to trigger gallstone formation.

TABLE 16-8

Biliary Tract Terminology

TERM	DEFINITION
Chole-	Pertaining to bile
Cholang-	Pertaining to bile ducts
Cholangiography	X-ray study of bile ducts
Cholangitis	Inflammation of bile duct
Cholecyst-	Pertaining to the gallbladder
Cholecystectomy	Removal of gallbladder
Cholecystitis	Inflammation of gallbladder
Cholecystography	X-ray study of gallbladder
Cholecystostomy	Incision and drainage of gallbladder
Choledocho-	Pertaining to common bile duct
Choledocholithiasis	Stones in common bile duct
Choledochostomy	Exploration of common bile duct
Cholelith-	Gallstones
Cholelithiasis	Presence of gallstones
Cholescintigraphy	Radionuclide imaging of biliary system
Cholestasis	Stoppage or suppression of bile flow

Modified from Kallsen C: Nursing care of clients with biliary and exocrine pancreatic disorders. In Black JM, Matassarin-Jacobs E, editors: *Medical-surgical nursing: clinical management for continuity of care*, ed 5, Philadelphia, 1997, WB Saunders, p 1908.

Elevated estrogen levels associated with gallstones may occur during the last trimester of pregnancy, when gallbladder stasis reduces precipitation of cholesterol from the gallbladder and/or possibly some chemical alteration of bile. Other estrogen-associated causes of gallstones include use of oral contraceptives, postmenopausal therapy, or multiparity (two or more pregnancies resulting in viable offspring).[53]

The formation of gallstones does not appear to be related to smoking or alcohol intake. Genetic predisposition is difficult to establish, because the disease is very common in the general population, but studies in mice and in humans have identified genetic factors that may predispose some people to cholesterol gallstones.[22] Two known familial-related causes of gallstones are American Indian ancestry (specifically Pima Indian) and hemolytic anemia (e.g., congenital spherocytosis and sickle cell anemia), which can cause pigment stones.

Pathogenesis. Gallstones form when the tenuous balance of solubility of biliary lipids tips in favor of precipitation of cholesterol, unconjugated bilirubin, or bacterial degradation products of biliary lipids. Approximately 80% of all gallstones are made of cholesterol; the remaining 20% are made of bile pigment. Gallstones most often develop when the bile necessary for digestion of fats and stored in the gallbladder becomes oversaturated with cholesterol. Cholesterol is usually in a liquid state but when excess amounts of it enter the bile, it may become insoluble and precipitate out to form a stone. In most persons, many of whom do not develop gallstones, bile contains more cholesterol than can be maintained in stable solution; in other words, it is supersaturated with cholesterol.

The combination of metabolic alterations in hepatic cholesterol secretion with changes in gallbladder motility results

Risk Factors Associated With Gallstones

Age (increasing incidence with increasing age)
Gender (female-male ratio = 3:1)
Genetic factors
Bacterial infection
Decreased physical activity
Elevated estrogen levels
  Pregnancy
  Use of oral contraceptives
  Estrogen replacement therapy (ERT)
High bile cholesterol
  Obesity
  Diabetes mellitus
  Hyperlipidemia
  Rheumatoid arthritis
Low levels of bile salts
  Hydroxylase deficiency
  Malabsorption
Diet
  High-fat, high-calorie foods
  Very low-calorie, rapid weight loss diets
  Prolonged fasting
  Inadequate calcium, vitamin C (under investigation)
Liver disease
American Indian ancestry (Pima Indian)
Hemolytic anemia (pigment stones)

in the production of cholesterol crystals and the formation of gallstones. When the stone passes from the gallbladder into the ducts linking the gallbladder to the small intestine, liver, or pancreas, it may create a painful obstruction resulting in a type of abdominal pain called biliary colic. Although the chemical imbalance causing cholesterol stones to form has been identified, the cause of the imbalance remains undetermined. In obese individuals, the mechanism appears to involve cholesterol synthesis, whereas in people who are not obese, decreased secretion of bile acids seems to be the key.

Pigmented gallstones are formed by supersaturation of bile with calcium hydrogen bilirubinate, the acid calcium salt of unconjugated bilirubin (see the section on Jaundice in this chapter). The formation of pigmented stones is associated with biliary infection and increased amounts of unconjugated bilirubin in bile rather than gallbladder hypomotility present with cholesterol stones. The unconjugated bilirubin precipitates in the gallbladder or bile ducts to form stones.

Clinical Manifestations.   Most gallstones are asymptomatic; approximately 30% cause painful symptoms. Obstruction of the cystic duct (see Fig. 16-6) distends the gallbladder while the muscles in the duct wall contract trying to expel the stones, producing abdominal pain (biliary colic). The pain of biliary colic may be intermittent or steady; it is usually severe and is located in the right upper quadrant just below or slightly to the right of the sternum with abdominal tenderness, muscle guarding, and rebound pain. Painful symp-

toms often radiate to the mid-upper back, below or between the scapulae or just to the right shoulder.* Episodes can last from 20 minutes to several hours and may develop daily or as infrequently as once every few years.

Other symptoms are vague, including heartburn, belching, flatulence, epigastric discomfort, and food intolerance (especially for fats and cabbage). Gallstones in the older adult may not cause pain, fever, or jaundice but rather, mental confusion and shakiness may be the only manifestations of gallstones. Serious complications occur in 20% of cases when a stone becomes lodged in the lower end of the common bile duct, causing inflammation (cholangitis) leading to bacterial infection and jaundice (indicating the stone is in the common bile duct). Sometimes acute pancreatitis develops when the duct from the pancreas that joins the common bile duct also becomes blocked (see Fig. 16-6). About 15% of clients with gallstones also have stones in the common bile duct (choledocholithiasis).

Medical Management

Diagnosis.   Diagnosis is based on the history, physical examination, and radiographic evaluation (stones containing calcium show up on plain x-ray). In the past, oral cholecystogram was used for imaging of the stones, but this has been replaced by abdominal ultrasonography. Ultrasonography demonstrates gallstones in more than 95% of cases. Other more specialized radiography may be required to differentiate cholelithiasis from other causes of extrahepatic biliary obstruction, such as intravenous cholangiography (dye-enhanced x-ray imaging of the bile duct) and endoscopic or percutaneous cholangiography.

Treatment.   No treatment is the usual recommendation for anyone with asymptomatic gallstones except in the case of women with rheumatoid arthritis. The high incidence of gallstones in this population suggests that early noninvasive intervention with bile-desaturating agents may prevent the development of cholecystitis or gallbladder cancer.[18] In all individuals with mild or moderate symptoms, a low-fat diet can often relieve symptoms and when combined with ursodeoxycholic acid administration seems to have a protective role in preventing the development of biliary cholesterol crystals.[11] Lipid-lowering medications and other pharmacologic agents are under investigation for the treatment of gallstones. Laparoscopic cholecystectomy has replaced open cholecystectomy as the treatment of choice for symptomatic gallbladder disease. When the gallbladder is removed, bile drains directly from the liver into the intestine eliminating the opportunity for stone formation.

Prognosis.   Cholelithiasis is the fifth leading cause of hospitalization among adults and accounts for 90% of all gallbladder and duct diseases. However, the prognosis with medical treatment is usually good, depending on the severity of disease, presence of complications (especially infection), and response to antibiotics. Cholecystectomy in the older population has a higher risk for injury related to anesthesia, pain medications, and, sometimes, the response to the trauma of surgery. Gallstones may be a risk factor for gallbladder cancer, but this is a rare tumor that is easily detected by radiographic modalities.

---

*Radiating pain to the mid-back and scapula occurs owing to splanchnic (visceral) fibers synapsing with adjacent phrenic nerve fibers (major branch of the cervical plexus innervating the diaphragm).

Special Implications for the Therapist   16-20

CHOLELITHIASIS (GALLSTONES)

Physical activity may play an important role in the prevention of symptomatic gallstone disease in up to a third of all cases. Based on a limited number of studies, increasing exercise to 30 minutes of endurance-type training five times per week is recommended.[26,27] When the gallbladder has been removed (or is blocked by a stone) a small amount of less concentrated bile is still secreted into the intestine. The loss of a gallbladder itself does not appear to have an impact on physical activity and exercise.

In the past, gallbladder removal required a significant incision with muscle disruption, scarring, and, frequently, postoperative back pain associated with the formation of deep scar tissue. Now the closed procedure (laparoscopic cholecystectomy) can be performed as outpatient (day) surgery without these complications. Air introduced into the abdomen during this operative technique is removed after the procedure thereby reducing the postoperative abdominal pain. However, many individuals still experience referred pain to the right shoulder for 24 to 48 hours. Deep breathing, physical movement and activity as tolerated, and application of a heating pad to the abdomen (if approved by the surgeon) can help ease the discomfort.

The usual postoperative exercises (e.g., breathing, turning, coughing, wound splinting, compressive stockings, leg exercises) for any surgical procedure apply, especially in case of complications. Early activity helps to prevent pooling of blood in the lower extremities and subsequent development of thrombosis. Early activity also assists the return of intestinal motility, so the client is encouraged to begin progressive movement and ambulation as soon as possible. ■

◆ Choledocholithiasis

Defined as calculi in the common bile duct, choledocholithiasis occurs in 15% of persons with gallstones and has the same etiology and pathogenesis. The percentage rises with age, and the incidence in older adults may be as high as 50%. Common duct stones usually originate in the gallbladder, but they also may form spontaneously in the common duct and can therefore occur after a person has had a cholecystectomy. Stones that occur in the absence of a gallbladder are referred to as *primary common duct stones*.

Approximately 30% to 40% of duct stones are asymptomatic when no obstruction exists. When symptomatic, duct stones may produce severe and persistent biliary colic (see the section on Clinical Manifestations of Cholelithiasis in this chapter) accompanied by chills and fever, obstructive jaundice, cholangitis (bile duct inflammation*), pancreatitis, or a combination of these.

Diagnosis is based on clinical picture and radiologic or endoscopic evidence of dilated bile ducts, ductal stones, or impaired bile flow. Endoscopic retrograde cholangiopancreatography (ERCP)† provides the most direct and accurate means of determining the cause, location, and extent of obstruction in the symptomatic client. If the obstruction is thought to be due

to a stone, ERCP is the procedure of choice, because it permits endoscopic sphincterotomy, which opens the sphincter of Oddi (see Fig. 16-6) and allows passage of gallstones up to 1 cm in size. Alternately, endoscopic sphincterotomy and stone extraction may be combined with laparoscopic cholecystectomy. Medical management includes antibiotic therapy when cholangitis is present.

A high mortality (50%), caused by rapidly developing and fatal sepsis, occurs when common bile duct stones (choledocholithiasis) are accompanied by inflammation of the bile duct (cholangitis).

Special Implications for the Therapist   16-21

CHOLEDOCHOLITHIASIS

Special considerations for the therapist are the same as for the client with cholelithiasis. When choledocholithiasis occurs in the absence of a gallbladder (primary common duct stones), the presenting symptom can be shoulder pain. The therapist must be alert to this possibility in anyone who has had a cholecystectomy. (See also the section on Obstructive Jaundice in this chapter.) ■

◆ Cholecystitis

Cholecystitis, or inflammation of the gallbladder, may be acute or chronic and occurs as a result of impaction of gallstones in the cystic duct (see Fig. 16-6) causing obstruction to bile flow and painful distention of the gallbladder. The acute form is most common during middle age, whereas the chronic form is most common among older adults.

Gallbladder inflammation causes prolonged pain characterized as steady right upper quadrant abdominal pain with abdominal tenderness, muscle guarding, and rebound pain. Upper quadrant pain often radiates to the upper back (between the scapulae) and into the right scapula or right shoulder. Accompanying GI symptoms usually include nausea, anorexia, and vomiting and there may be signs of visceral parietal or peritoneal inflammation (e.g., pain worse with movement and locally tender to touch). Gallbladder attacks are usually caused by gallbladder and/or cystic duct and/or bile duct distention as the stone causes obstruction to the flow of bile.

Diagnosis is made on the basis of clinical history, examination, laboratory findings, and imaging. The WBC count is usually elevated (12,000 to 15,000/ml). Total serum bilirubin, serum aminotransferase, and alkaline phosphatase levels are often elevated in the acute disease, but they are normal or minimally elevated in the chronic form. X-ray films of the abdomen show radiopaque gallstones in 15% of cases. Right upper quadrant abdominal ultrasound may show the presence of gallstones, but it is not specific for acute cholecystitis (much higher sensitivity for cholelithiasis). Radionuclide scanning (hepatobiliary imaging, also known as hepato-iminodiacetic acid [HIDA] scan)* is useful in demonstrating an obstructed

---

*The combination of pain, fever and chills, and jaundice is referred to as *Charcot's triad*, the classic picture of cholangitis.

†ERCP consists of introduction of radiopaque medium into the biliary system by percutaneous puncture of a bile duct to provide x-ray examination of the bile ducts.

---

*The client swallows a long, thin, lighted flexible tube connected to a computer and a monitor. A special dye is injected that stains the bile ducts, making them more visible. Any stone detected can be removed immediately. The same information can be obtained by passing a thin needle into the abdominal wall through which dye is injected into the ducts, a procedure called *percutaneous transhepatic cholangiography*.

cystic duct; if the gallbladder fills with the isotope, acute cholecystitis is unlikely, but filling of the bile duct strongly suggests a positive diagnosis.

Laparoscopic cholecystectomy (gallbladder resection) often is performed during the first hospitalization for acute cholecystitis although the exact timing depends on the surgeon's judgment; the presence of complications may delay surgery. Prognosis for both acute and chronic cholecystitis is good with medical intervention. Acute attacks may resolve spontaneously, but recurrences are common requiring cholecystectomy. Complications can be serious and usually are associated with infection and sepsis. The mortality of acute cholecystitis is 5% to 10% for clients older than 60 years with serious associated diseases.

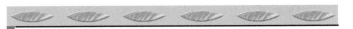

Special Implications for the Therapist 16-22

CHOLECYSTITIS

Special considerations for the therapist are the same as for the client with cholelithiasis (see also the section on Obstructive Jaundice in this chapter). It is possible for a person to develop acholelithiasis cholecystitis, or inflammation of the gallbladder without gallstones. The therapist may see a clinical picture typical of gallbladder disease, including mid-upper back or scapular pain (below or between the scapulae) or right shoulder pain associated with right upper quadrant abdominal pain. Close questioning may reveal accompanying associated GI signs and symptoms.

The person may have been evaluated for gallbladder disease, but ultrasonography does not always show small stones. Unless further and more elaborate testing has been performed to examine gallbladder function, the individual may end up in therapy for treatment of the affected musculoskeletal areas. Lack of results from therapy and/or progression of symptoms corresponding to progression of disease requires further medical follow-up. ■

◆ Primary Biliary Cirrhosis
(See Primary Biliary Cirrhosis, earlier in this chapter, in the Cirrhosis section.)

◆ Sclerosing Cholangitis
Sclerosing cholangitis is a chronic inflammatory disease of the intrahepatic and extrahepatic bile ducts of unknown etiologic factors. It has been linked to altered immunity, toxins, and infectious agents, and is thought to have possible genetic etiologic factors. Approximately two thirds of cases occur in clients 20 to 40 years of age and the incidence is rising; it has a higher incidence in men and is often seen in association with ulcerative colitis.

The inflammatory process associated with this disease results in fibrosis and thickening of the ductal walls and multiple concentric strictures. This fibrosing process narrows and eventually obstructs the intrahepatic and extrahepatic bile ducts; the basic mechanisms of disease pathogenesis in PSC remain unknown. Symptomatic presentation usually includes pruritus and jaundice accompanied by fatigue, anorexia, and weight loss. Vague upper abdominal pain may be present.

Diagnosis is made on the basis of clinical findings confirmed by ERCP or liver biopsy; magnetic resonance cholangiopancreatography (MRCP) is a newer noninvasive diagnostic technique available. Many clinical trials of medical therapy have been conducted, but none have demonstrated significant efficacy. Progress has been made in the area of orthotopic liver transplantation. Immunosuppressive treatment with corticosteroids has had little effect in changing the course of this disease; clinical trials are exploring the use of cyclosporin A, methotrexate, and ursodeoxycholic acid (UDCA) alone or in combination. UDCA has been shown to improve liver histology and survival in people with primary biliary cirrhosis and has a beneficial effect in PSC when combined with endoscopic dilation of major duct stenosis.[51] The goal of treatment is to treat people as early as possible to prevent progression to the advanced stages of this disease.

The prognosis is poor owing to the progressive nature of this disease, with gradual development of cirrhosis, portal hypertension, and death from hepatic failure without liver transplantation. Clients with this condition are predisposed to the development of cholangiocarcinoma, occurring in 10% to 15% of all cases.[42] Liver transplantation is the only therapeutic option for people with end stage liver disease resulting from this disorder. The results of transplantation for PSC are excellent with 1-year survival rates of 90% to 97% and 5-year survival rates of 80% to 85%. Recurrence of PSC after liver transplantation is common but appears to have little effect on survival. The results of liver transplantation for people with cholangiocarcinoma remain poor.[14]

Special Implications for the Therapist 16-23

SCLEROSING CHOLANGITIS

Special considerations for the therapist are the same as for the client with Cholelithiasis (see also the section on Obstructive Jaundice, this chapter). ■

◆ Neoplasms of the Gallbladder and Biliary Tract
Benign Neoplasms.   Biliary neoplasms, whether benign or malignant, are rare. *Papillomas* are the most common benign tumors affecting the gallbladder or common bile duct; they may be single or multiple and often are associated with gallstones. Benign tumors of the common bile duct are more clinically significant because they can obstruct biliary flow and cause obstructive jaundice. *Adenomas*, benign epithelial tumors, may be premalignant based on the observation that adenocarcinoma occurs in as many as 50% to 80% of persons with adenoma. Treatment is usually removal by cholecystectomy, because most lesions that are found cause symptoms and are possibly premalignant.

Malignant Neoplasms.   *Adenocarcinoma of the gallbladder* is the most common malignant lesion of the biliary tract (90% of cases), but it only accounts for 5% of all cancers at the time of autopsy. Predisposing factors include age over 60 years, female sex, gallstones, obesity, high carbohydrate intake, ulcerative colitis, and ethnic origin (Japanese, Japanese-American, Mexicans, Mexican-American, certain American Indian tribes, native Alaskan, and Bolivian). Workers in the textile, rubber, and metal-fabricating industries may have an increased incidence, and AIDS has been associated with cancers throughout the entire biliary tract. However, despite all of these known risk factors, many cases of gallbladder cancer occur in people without obvious risk factors.[7]

Bile duct cancer is the second most common biliary tract malignancy; it occurs predominantly in men. Gallstones are also present in 70% of all cases, but primary sclerosing cholangitis also has an associated increased incidence of bile duct cancer. Spread of cancer, whether originating in the gallbladder or bile duct, occurs by direct extension into the liver or to the peritoneal surface, and it may do so before symptoms develop. Other metastatic sites include the lymph nodes, lung, bone, and adrenal glands.

Clinical presentation of malignant gallbladder diseases depends on the stage of disease and the location and extent of the lesion, but it is often insidious. By the time the tumor becomes symptomatic, it is almost invariably incurable. Symptoms most often mimic gallstone disease (acute and chronic cholecystitis). Right upper quadrant pain radiating to the upper back is the most common symptom (75% of cases), with weight loss, progressive (obstructive) jaundice, anorexia, and right upper quadrant mass occurring in 40% to 50% of cases. Pruritus and skin excoriations are commonly associated with the presence of jaundice.

Prevention through screening of populations at risk (e.g., people with sclerosing cholangitis, intraductal stones, cystic diseases) may be able to offer preventive strategies and prophylactic or early intervention. Diagnosis is often made unexpectedly during surgery. Most gallbladder cancers have caused significant clinical problems at the time of diagnosis. The most helpful diagnostic studies before surgery include endoscopic ultrasonography, cholangiography, computed tomography, and MRI.

Treatment varies; it may include radical resection if the tumor is well localized without metastases, stenting of duct obstruction (obstructive jaundice) for unresectable tumor, and chemotherapy or radiation for local control and pain relief. Prognosis is poor even with treatment, and few people survive more than 6 months after diagnosis; the 5-year survival rate varies between 10% and 45%.[7]

Special Implications for the Therapist 16-24

GALLBLADDER AND BILIARY TRACT NEOPLASM

Special considerations for the therapist are the same as for the client with cholelithiasis. (See also the section on Obstructive Jaundice in this chapter.) See also Special Implications for the Therapist: Oncology, 8-1. ∎

REFERENCES

1. Aggarwal R, Krawczynski K: Hepatitis E: an overview and recent advances in clinical and laboratory research, *J Gastroenterol Hepatol* 15(1):9-20, 2000.
2. American Academy of Pediatrics (AAP): Human immunodeficiency virus and other blood-borne viral pathogens in the athletic setting. Committee on Sports Medicine and Fitness, *Pediatrics* 104(6):1400-3, 1999.
3. Arvat E, Broglio F, Ghigo E: Insulin-like growth factor I: implications in aging, *Drugs Aging* 16(1):29-40, 2000.
4. Bhatia M, Brady M, Shokuhi S, et al: Inflammatory mediators in acute pancreatitis, *J Pathol* 190(2):117-25, 2000.
5. Centers for Disease Control and Prevention (CDC): National Center for Infectious Diseases: Viral Hepatitis A, online www.cdc.gov/nci_dod/diseases/hepatitis, 2001.
6. Dean E: Oxygen transport deficits in systemic disease and implications for physical therapy, *Physical Therapy* 77(2):187-202, 1997.
7. De Groen PC, Gores, GJ, LaRusso NF, et al: Biliary tract cancers, *New Engl J Med* 341(18):1368-78, 1999.
8. Dorman JM: Contagious diseases in competitive sport: what are the risks? *J Am Coll Health* 49(3):105-9, 2000.
9. Epstein SK, Ciubotaru RL, Zilberberg MD, et al: Analysis of impaired exercise capacity in patients with cirrhosis, *Dig Dis Sci* 43(8):1701-7, 1998.
10. Faust TW: Recurrent primary biliary cirrhosis, primary sclerosing cholangitis, and autoimmune hepatitis after transplantation, *Semin Liver Dis* 20(4):481-95, 2000.
11. Festi D, Colecchia A, Larocca A, et al: Review: low caloric intake and gall-bladder motor function, *Aliment Pharmacol Ther* 14 (Suppl 2):51-3, 2000.
12. Garcia-Pagan JC, Feu F, Castells A, et al: Exercise, circadian variations of portal pressure and variceal hemorrhage in patients with cirrhosis, *Gastroenterology* 111:1300-6, 1996.
13. Goodman CC, Snyder TE: *Differential diagnosis in physical therapy*, ed 3, Philadelphia, 2000, WB Saunders.
14. Gow PJ, Chapman RW: Liver transplantation for primary sclerosing cholangitis, *Liver* 20(2):97-103, 2000.
15. Heathcote EJ: Management of primary biliary cirrhosis. The American Association for the Study of Liver Diseases practice guidelines, *Hepatology* 31(4):1005-13, 2000.
16. Hegab AM, Luketic VA: Bleeding esophageal varices. How to treat this dreaded complication of portal hypertension, *Postgrad Med* 109(2):75-6, 81-6, 89, 2001.
17. Heslin MJ, Medina-Franco H, Parker M, et al: Colorectal hepatic metastases: resection, local ablation, and hepatic artery infusion pump are associated with prolonged survival, *Arch Surg* 136(3):318-23, 2001.
18. Ito S, Hasegawa H, Nozawa S, et al: Gallstones in patients with rheumatoid arthritis, *J Rheumatol* 26:1458-66, 1999.
19. Jemal A, Thomas A: Cancer statistics 2002, *CA Cancer J Clin* 52(1):23-47, 2002.
20. Kemeny MM: The surgical aspects of the totally implantable hepatic artery infusion pump, *Arch Surg* 136(3):348-52, 2001.
21. Koea JB, Kemeny N: Hepatic artery infusion chemotherapy for metastatic colorectal carcinoma, *Semin Surg Oncol* 19(2):125-34, 2000.
22. Ko CW, Lee SP: Gallstone formation. Local factors, *Gastroenterol Clin North Am* 28(1):99-115, 1999.
23. Kumar D, Tandon RK: Use of ursodeoxycholic acid in liver diseases, *J Gastroenterol Hepatol* 16(1):3-14, 2001.
24. Lazaridis KN, Lindor KD: Management of primary biliary cirrhosis: from diagnosis to end-stage disease, *Curr Gastroenterol Rep* 2(2):94-8, 2000.
25. Lechmann M, Liang TJ: Vaccine development for hepatitis C, *Semin Liver Dis* 20(2):211-26, 2000.
26. Leitzmann MF, Giovannucci EL, Rimm EB, et al: The relation of physical activity to risk for symptomatic gallstone disease in men, *Ann Intern Med* 128(6):417-25, 1998.
27. Leitzmann MF, Rimm EB, Willett WC, et al: Physical activity reduces risk for cholecystectomy in women, *N Engl J Med* 341:777-84, 1999.
28. Lewis JH: Drug-induced liver disease, *Med Clin North Am* 84(5):1275-311, 2000.

29. Lichtman SM, Skirvin JA: Pharmacology of antineoplastic agents in older cancer patients, *Oncology (Huntingt)* 14(12):1743-55, 2000.

30. Lieber CS: Alcoholic liver disease: new insights in pathogenesis lead to new treatments, *J Hepatol* 32(1 Suppl):113-28, 2000.

31. Lillemoe KD, Yeo CJ, Cameron JL: Pancreatic cancer: state-of-the-art care, *CA Cancer J Clin* 50(4):241-68, 2000.

32. Lindsay KL, Hoofnagle JH: Chronic hepatitis. In Goldman et al: *Cecil textbook of medicine*, ed 21, Philadelphia, 2000, WB Saunders, pp 790-7.

33. Louie M, Louie L, Simor AE: The role of DNA amplification technology in the diagnosis of infectious diseases, *CMAJ* 163(3):301-9, 2000.

34. Modahl LE, Lai MM: Hepatitis delta virus: the molecular basis of laboratory diagnosis, *Crit Rev Clin Lab Sci* 37(1):45-92, 2000.

35. Morbidity and Mortality Weekly Report (MMWR): Prevention of Hepatitis A through active or passive immunization: recommendations of the Advisory Committee on Immunization Practices (ACIP): 48(No. RR-12):1-54, 1999.

36. Morbidity and Mortality Weekly Report (MMWR): Recommendations for preventing transmission of infections among chronic hemodialysis patients, *MMWR* 50(RR-05):1-43, 2001.

37. Nakakura EK, Choti MA: Management of hepatocellular carcinoma, *Oncology (Huntingt)* 14(7):1085-98, 2000.

38. National Digestive Diseases Information Clearinghouse (NIDDK): Chronic hepatitis C: current disease management. NIH Publication No. 99-4230 (online www.niddk.nih.gov/health), 2001.

39. National Hemophilia Foundation (NHF): Hepatitis updates. Hemaware January/February New York, New York, 2000, p 53.

40. OSHA/US Department of Labor: Occupational exposure to bloodborne pathogens: Final rule, *Fed Register* 56:64004, 1991.

41. Palomero J, Galan AI, Munoz ME, et al: Effects of aging on the susceptibility to the toxic effects of cyclosporin A in rats. Changes in liver glutathione and antioxidant enzymes, *Free Radic Biol Med* 30(8):836-45, 2001.

42. Prall RT, Lindor KD, Wiesner RH, et al: Current therapies and clinical controversies in the management of primary schlerosing cholangitis, *Curr Gastroenterol Rep* 2(2):99-103, 2000.

43. Preedy VR, Reilly ME, Patel VB, et al: Protein metabolism in alcoholism: effects on specific tissues and the whole body, *Nutrition* 15 (7-8):604-8, 1999.

44. Rivoire M, De Cian F, Meeus P, et al: Cryosurgery as a means to improve surgical treatment of patients with multiple unresectable liver metastases, *Anticancer Res* 20(5C):3785-90, 2000.

45. Robertson RP, Lanz KJ, Sutherland DE, et al: Prevention of diabetes for up to 13 years by autoislet transplantation after pancreatectomy for chronic pancreatitis, *Diabetes* 50(1):47-50, 2001.

46. Sakorafas GH, Tsiotou AG: Etiology and pathogenesis of acute pancreatitis: current concepts, *J Clin Gastroenterol* 30(4):343-56, 2000.

47. Sathar M, Soni P, York D: GB virus C/hepatitis G virus (GBV-C/HGV): still looking for a disease, *Int J Exp Patho* 81(5):305-22, 2000.

48. Siddiqui F, Mutchnick M, Kinzie J, et al: Prevalence of hepatitis A virus and hepatitis B virus immunity in patients with polymerase chain reaction-confirmed hepatitis C: implications for vaccination strategy, *Am J Gastroenterol* 96(3):858-63, 2001.

49. Simon JA, Hudes ES: Serum ascorbic acid and gallbladder disease prevalence among US adults: the Third National Health and Nutrition Examination Survey (NHANES III), *Arch Intern Med* 160(7):931-36, 2000.

50. Stickel F, Egerer G, Seitz HK: Hepatotoxicity of botanicals, *Public Health Nutr* 3(2):113-24, 2000.

51. Stiehl A, Benz C, Sauer P: Primary sclerosing cholangitis, *Can J Gastroenterol* 14(4):311-5, 2000.

52. Tseng M, Everhart JE, Sandler RS: Dietary intake and gallbladder diseases: a review, *Public Health Nutr* 2(2):161-72, 1999.

53. Uhler ML, Marks JW, Judd HL: Estrogen replacement therapy and gallbladder disease in postmenopausal women, *Menopause* 7(3):162-7, 2000.

54. Van Damme P: Hepatitis B: vaccination programmes in Europe—an update, *Vaccine* 19(17-19):2375-9, 2001.

55. Wolfhagen FH, van Buuren HR, Vleggaar FP, et al: Management of osteoporosis in primary biliary cirrhosis, *Baillieres Best Pract Res Clin Gastroenterol* 14(4):629-41, 2000.

CHAPTER 17

THE RENAL AND UROLOGIC SYSTEMS

WILLIAM G. BOISSONNAULT AND CATHERINE C. GOODMAN

The structures associated with the excretion of urine are (1) the kidneys and ureters, comprising the *upper urinary tract,* and (2) the bladder and urethra of the *lower urinary tract* structures (Fig. 17-1). The kidneys serve as both an endocrine organ and a target of endocrine action, with the aim of controlling mineral and water balance. The kidneys' main function is to filter waste products and remove excess fluid from the blood. Every day the kidneys filter 200 quarts of fluid; about 2 quarts leave the body in the form of urine, and the remainder is retained in the body. These filtration and storage functions associated with excretion expose the kidney and bladder to carcinogens for extended periods, increasing the risk of cancer developing in these organs compared with the other urinary tract structures. In addition, the urethra of females lies close to the vaginal and rectal openings, allowing for relative ease of bacterial transport and increased risk of infection. The shorter urethra in females also contributes to the increased incidence of urinary tract infections (UTIs) in females.

Therapists have an important role on the medical team for primary intervention of a number of renal/urinary tract disorders such as urinary incontinence (UI) and overactive bladder and for those on dialysis or having postrenal transplant. UI afflicts a significant percentage of the geriatric population, and UTIs rank second only to upper respiratory tract infections in incidence of bacterial infections. Therapists encounter these two disorders often as common co-morbidities in the clinical arena.

The presence of UTI increases the risk of infection developing elsewhere. This could occur while the therapist is treating someone for a knee injury or postcerebral vascular accident. Recognizing clinical signs and symptoms of renal/urologic problems (Box 17-1) will facilitate medical referral. Understanding how these diseases and the prescribed medical treatment can influence rehabilitative efforts is essential to help ensure a positive functional outcome.

AGING AND THE RENAL/UROLOGIC SYSTEM

Aging is accompanied by a gradual reduction of blood flow to the kidneys, coupled with a reduction in nephrons (the units that extract wastes from the blood and concentrate them in the urine; see Fig. 17-5). As a result the kidneys become less efficient at removing waste from the blood, and the volume of urine increases somewhat with age. A tendency toward greater renal vasoconstriction in the older adult is evident, as compared with young individuals. This occurs as a result of

mental stress, in physiologic circumstances such as physical exercise, or in disease manifestations such as the effective circulatory volume depletion that develops in heart failure.[78]

Renal system changes that occur with aging cause alterations in the functional balance of fluid and electrolytes so that sodium regulation is not as effective. Older people are at greater risk for developing hyponatremia (reduced sodium in the blood), affecting the musculoskeletal system (see Chapter 4). Changes typical of the aging kidney are also accelerated when hypertension overlaps the physiologic renal process because both aging and hypertension affect the same structure (i.e., the glomeruli).

A reduction in bladder capacity increases the number of times an individual urinates in a day and also the urinary timetable changes. Although the kidneys produce most of the urine during the day in young people, a shift to night production over time makes one or two nocturnal trips to the bathroom commonplace after age 60.

Although specific age-related anatomic changes have not been associated with urinary tract disease, certain age groups (e.g., older adults) are at significant risk of developing a variety of disorders. Hormonal changes in women, combined with the aging properties of the connective tissues, fascia, or collagen fibers contribute to pelvic floor disorders. Transient ischemic attacks (TIAs) and strokes may result in mild to severe deficits or fluctuations in muscle tone affecting the pelvic floor muscles.

The effect of multiple medications, conditions such as benign prostatic hyperplasia (BPH) and pelvic floor disorders and the incidence of pelvic surgeries and catheterization in the older population all increase the risk of developing urinary tract disease. A large number of adults over age 60 are incontinent, and many older adults require dependent living situations because of this disorder. Considering the percentage of the rehabilitation population made up by the older adult, therapists will continue to be involved in the treatment of renal/urologic disorders.

INFECTIONS

◆ Urinary Tract Infections

Common infections of the urinary tract develop in either the upper or lower urinary tract. Lower urinary tract infections include cystitis (bladder infection) or urethritis (urethra). Symptoms of UTIs depend on the location of the infection in either the upper or lower urinary tract (infection rarely occurs in both simultaneously).

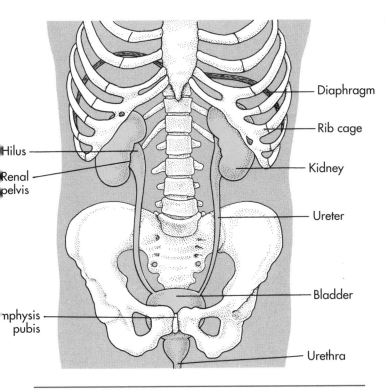

FIGURE   **17-1**   Structure and function of the renal/urologic system. The kidneys are located in the posterior upper abdominal cavity in the retroperitoneal space (behind the peritoneum) at the vertebral level of T12 to L2. The upper portion of the kidney is in contact with the diaphragm and moves with respiration. The lower urinary tract consists of the bladder and urethra. The bladder, a membranous, muscular sac, is located directly behind the symphysis pubis and is used for storage and excretion of urine. From the renal pelvis, urine is moved by peristalsis to the ureters and into the bladder. The urethra serves as a channel through which urine is passed from the bladder to the outside of the body. (From Goodman CC, Snyder TE: *Differential diagnosis in physical therapy,* ed 3, Philadelphia, 2000, WB Saunders.)

Incidence.   UTIs are very common in the general population and especially the geriatric populations. By age 24, one third of women have had at least one physician-diagnosed UTI that is treated with prescription medication.[29] Approximately 20% of women and 10% of men living at home have bacteriuria. For those living in skilled nursing facilities, assisted living, or extended care facilities the prevalence of infection is even higher: 25% for women and 20% for men.[2]

Up to 5% of female and 1% to 2% of male children experience UTIs. In addition, recurrent UTIs can occur in up to 80% of children who experience uncomplicated infection. Risk factors for this condition include premature birth, the presence of urinary tract abnormalities such as neurogenic bladder and systemic or immunologic disease, and a family history of UTI.

Etiologic and Risk Factors.   The cause of chronic infections, especially interstitial cystitis (IC) or bladder infections, remains unknown. Many theories have been proposed, but no single hypothesis has proven correct. The most likely cause is autoimmunity, based on the presence of immunoglobulin deposits in the bladder and the presence of serum antibladder an-

BOX 17-1

Most Common Signs and Symptoms of Urinary Tract Problems

Urinary frequency
Urinary urgency
Nocturia
Pain (shoulder, back, flank, pelvis, lower abdomen)
Costovertebral tenderness
Fever and chills
Hyperesthesia of dermatomes
Dysuria
Hematuria
Pyuria
Dyspareunia

BOX 17-2

Risk Factors for Urinary Tract Infections

Age
Immobility/inactivity (impaired bladder emptying)
Instrumentation and urinary catheterization
Frequently catheterized neurogenic bladder
Atonic bladder (spinal cord injury; diabetic neuropathy)
Increased sexual activity
Use of diaphragm (contraceptive device) or spermicide-coated condoms
Uncircumcised penis (first year of life)
Obstruction
• Renal calculi
• Prostatic hyperplasia
• Malformations or urinary tract abnormalities
Constipation (see Table 15-2)
Women greater than men (see explanation in text)
• Anatomic variations
• Surgical or natural menopause without hormone replacement therapy
• Pregnancy
Kidney transplantation
Diabetes mellitus
Partners of Viagra users*
Sexually transmitted disease (STD) (urethritis)

*This is most likely the result of increased frequency of intercourse in women over the age of 35 who are more likely to also experience vaginal dryness.

tibodies. Other proposed etiologic factors include lymphatic and/or vascular obstruction, dysfunctional bladder epithelium, neurogenic disorders, allergic responses, and genetic origin.

Numerous risk factors are evident for UTIs (Box 17-2), but urinary tract instrumentation and urinary catheterization are the most common predisposing factors. Older adults are at higher risk for these risk factors and UTIs in general. Reasons for this include general immobility or inactivity, which causes impaired bladder emptying; bladder ischemia resulting from urine retention; urinary outflow obstruction from renal calculi and prostatic hyperplasia; postmenopausal vaginitis; constipation; and diminished bactericidal activity of prostatic secretions. Urinary obstruction results in urinary stasis and reflux may be a source for bacteria to gain access to the kidney(s). People with diabetes are more prone to infection because of the associated glycosuria that provides a fertile medium for bacterial growth.

Adult women are at greater risk of developing UTI than men for several reasons. As mentioned, the urethra in females is shorter and also close to the entrances to the vagina and rectum. The bacteria that result in most UTIs are acquired from the large bowel. The urethral meatus is close to the fecal reservoir and rectum. Sexually active women are at higher risk of developing UTIs because it is thought that sexual intercourse can influence the movement of bacteria in the direction of the bladder. This again is due to the proximity of the urethral meatus and vagina. UTIs are more common during pregnancy. The increased risk is due to dilation of the upper urinary system, reduction of the peristaltic activity of the ureters, and displacement of the urinary bladder, which moves to a more abdominal position, thus further affecting the ureteral position. Effects of estrogen decline as a result of a hysterectomy and/or oophorectomy and during the perimenopausal and postmenopausal years may also contribute to increased risk of infection and incontinence.

Pathogenesis.

The bacteria most often responsible for UTI are gram-negative organisms, with *Escherichia coli* accounting for 80% of urinary tract pathogens. *Pseudomonas*, *Staphylococcus*, and *Candida* are more common in anyone undergoing invasive instrumental investigations and in children with urogenital abnormalities. Routes of entry of bacteria into the urinary tract can be ascending (up the urethra into the bladder); bloodborne (bacteria in the bloodstream); or lymphatic (uncommon).

Clinical Manifestations.

Classic features of UTIs are evident in older children and adults and include frequency, urgency, dysuria, nocturia, or in children, enuresis. The individual may notice cloudy, bloody, or foul-smelling urine and a burning or painful sensation during urination or intercourse. Pain may be noted in the suprapubic, lower abdominal, groin, or flank areas, depending on the location of the infection. If the diaphragm is irritated, as in the case of kidney involvement, ipsilateral shoulder or lumbar back pain may occur. Fever, chills, and malaise may also be present. The clinical manifestations in older adults can be varied and somewhat surprising. The expected complaints of fever, chills, and sweats may be absent. Flank pain, urgency, frequency, and incontinence are potential symptoms but may not be present until the infection is well advanced.

Medical Management

Prevention. UTIs can be prevented in some cases by drinking at least eight 8-ounce glasses of water each day; urinating right after sexual intercourse; for females, wiping from the front to back after urination so that bacteria from the anal area are not pushed into the urethra; changing sanitary pads often during menstruation; refraining from using perfumed toilet paper, heavily scented soap, or powders in the vaginal area; and washing the genital area with warm water before sexual activity to minimize the chance that bacteria can be introduced. For those women using a diaphragm for birth con-

trol, making sure it is properly fitted and inserted with clean hands is an important preventive step.

Certain foods are considered potent bladder irritants, and some health care professionals recommend that the following items be eliminated or at least reduced in those individuals with chronic infections: caffeine; alcohol; tobacco (nicotine); chocolate; spices and spicy foods; acidic foods (e.g., tomatoes, citrus fruits); artificial sweeteners; sharp cheeses; coffee; tea; carbonated beverages; and chemical preservatives (found in many foods and beverages). Keeping a dietary diary correlated with symptoms may help identify food sources of bladder irritation.

Diagnosis and Treatment.

The diagnosis of UTI is typically made based on history and urinalysis. A bacterial count of greater than 100,000 organisms per milliliter of urine is a commonly accepted criterion for diagnosis. Besides the bacterial count, the urine leukocyte count is also used. Ultrasound, radiographs, computed tomography (CT) scans, and renal scans may be used to identify contributing factors such as obstruction. The communication difficulties that occur with older adults can delay detection of this disease.

Postvoid residual (PVR) and more complex tests such as voiding cystourethrography (VCUG) (upper urinary system) and urodynamic testing with and without fluoroscopy determination may be recommended for anyone at risk for urinary retention. Whenever possible, ultrasound assessment, rather than urinary catheterization, is recommended for the PVR.

Antibiotic agents are typically used to treat acute infections, and in some cases, prophylactic antibiotics are used daily; in the case of sexual intercourse as a precipitating factor, women may be advised to take antibiotics just after sex, not on a daily basis.[56] Increased fluid intake may also help relieve symptoms and signs and is often used as an adjunct to pharmacologic treatment. *Lactobacillus acidophilus*, a probiotic supplement of live, active organisms, may be recommended for anyone taking antibiotics to replace the naturally occurring bacteria in the intestines and to prevent candidiasis (yeast growth). A vaccine to prevent recurrent urinary infections of the bladder has proved successful in mice and is currently being tested in clinical trials. The use of hormone replacement therapy for chronic, recurrent infections in postmenopausal women is also under investigation.

Special Implications for the Therapist   17-1

URINARY TRACT INFECTIONS

Preferred Practice Patterns:
5B: Impaired Posture
*5D: Impaired Joint Mobility, Motor Function, Muscle
    Performance, and Range of Motion Associated With
    Connective Tissue Dysfunction*

Depending on the severity of the infection, the person with an UTI may not be able to participate fully in a rehabilitation program until the disease is brought under control. If the client begins to complain of nausea or vomiting, has a fever greater than 102° F (39° C), or the therapist notes a change in mental status (most often confusion), immediate contact with the client's physician is warranted. These may be indications for hospital admission.

Awareness of the symptoms and signs associated with this disease may allow the therapist to recognize the onset of infection in its early stages. The initial symptoms may be subtle enough that the client is not alarmed to the point that he or she visits a physician. Early detection and treatment of this disorder are important to prevent possible permanent structural damage. In the case of insidious onset of back or shoulder pain, especially with a recent history of any infection, a medical screening examination may be warranted.

UTIs also increase the risk of development of infection elsewhere in the body, including osteomyelitis, pleurisy, and pericarditis. Therapists should also always be aware of their role in infection prevention and minimize their involvement as a risk factor (see Boxes 7-2 and 7-4).

In the case of the individual with recurrent, chronic infections such as inflammatory IC, intervention by a physical therapist will address any deficits in the musculoskeletal system as noted by the evaluation, postural dysfunction, increased or decreased range of motion, and decreased strength. A crucial aspect to evaluation and intervention is the condition of the soft tissue, especially in the lower quadrant. Restrictions are commonly found in people with IC involving the muscles that attach to the pelvis (e.g., adductors, gluteals, obturator internus and externus, piriformis, abdominals, and iliopsoas). A trigger point evaluation is essential in determining the presence of somatovisceral responses contributing to frequency and urgency. Specific passive and active stretching exercises and muscle reeducation activities are progressed according to the individual's response to the soft tissue interventions. Modalities such as biofeedback, ultrasound, and electrical stimulation along with behavioral techniques (e.g., for reducing frequency and urgency) may be employed.[42] More specific intervention guidelines are available.[35,36,75,84] ■

◆ Pyelonephritis

Overview. Pyelonephritis is an infectious, inflammatory disease involving the kidney parenchyma and renal pelvis. The disease can be acute or chronic. Acute pyelonephritis is typically related to a bacterial infection. Chronic pyelonephritis is a tubulointerstitial disorder marked by progressive, gross, and irregular scarring and deformation of the calices and overlying parenchyma. The anatomic changes can lead to insufficient renal function. Chronic pyelonephritis may be responsible for up to 25% of the population with end-stage renal disease.

Etiologic and Risk Factors. Gram-negative bacteria such as *Escherichia coli*, and *Proteus*, *Klebsiella*, *Enterobacter*, and *Pseudomonas* species are the most common agents associated with acute pyelonephritis. Infection may also be associated with chronic disease but when present, is superimposed on either obstruction, vesicoureteral reflux,* or both.

The majority of cases of acute pyelonephritis are associated with ascending UTIs (see Box 17-2). In other cases, pyelonephritis can stem from bloodborne pathogens associated with infection elsewhere. People with bacterial endocarditis and miliary tuberculosis are susceptible to kidney involvement. In addition, immunocompromised people are at risk for fungi seeding the kidney.

Pathogenesis. Although urine is typically sterile, the distal end of the urethra is commonly colonized by bacterial flora. As described under Risk Factors, bacteria can be transported to the urinary bladder in many ways. After urination, the subsequent passage of sterile urine from the kidneys to the bladder dilutes any bacteria that may have entered the bladder. If the residual urine volume is increased, as with an atonic bladder, an accumulation of insufficiently diluted bacteria can occur. Bacteria in the bladder urine typically do not gain access to the ureters for a variety of anatomic reasons. However, people with an abnormally short passage of the ureter within the bladder muscle wall and an angle of ureter insertion into the bladder wall that is more perpendicular are at risk for reflux of urine into the ureter itself. This reflux can be of sufficient force to carry the urine and the accompanying bacteria into the renal pelvis and calices.

Clinical Manifestations. The onset of symptoms and signs associated with acute pyelonephritis is usually abrupt. The complaints may include fever, chills, malaise, headache, and back pain. The person may also complain of tenderness over the costovertebral angle (Murphy's sign). Also, often present are symptoms of bladder irritation, including dysuria, urinary frequency, and urgency.

Medical Management
Diagnosis and Treatment. The presence of the above symptoms calls for laboratory testing. Urinalysis will reveal pyuria, bacteriuria, and varying degrees of hematuria. A urine culture will demonstrate heavy growth of the bacterial agent. In addition, the blood count may show leukocytosis.

If the infection is severe enough or if complicating factors are present, hospital admission may be required for treatment. Typically, however, the condition is treated with an appropriate antibiotic medication with supplemental probiotics (*Lactobacillus acidophilus*) advised. Symptoms typically begin disappearing within several days. If the person does not show improvement within 48 to 72 hours, contact with the physician is warranted.

RENAL DISORDERS

◆ Cancer
Renal Cell Carcinoma
Overview and Incidence. Adult kidney neoplasms account for approximately 2% of all cancers. Renal cell carcinoma (RCC) is the most common adult renal neoplasm accounting for approximately 80% to 90% of renal tumors, and its incidence is rising. This disease can also occur in children and young adults. RCC occurs twice as often in males as in females, with a peak range of incidence between 60 to 70 years. The term *renal cell carcinoma* is based on the cell of origin, the nephron, consisting of the renal corpuscle, the proximal convoluted tubule, the nephronic loop, and the distal convoluted tubule.

---

*Urine is forced from the urinary bladder into the ureters and kidneys.

Etiologic and Risk Factors. Although a genetic basis is strongly suggested and several genes have been implicated, no single etiologic agent has been identified. Both genetic and environmental factors are implicated. RCC has been linked with von Hippel-Lindau (VHL) disease, which is an autosomal dominant hereditary disorder. This disease is linked to a defect of a gene on chromosome 3. Defects of this chromosome have also been demonstrated in people with renal cell carcinoma.

Tobacco smoking and obesity are established risk factors for RCC. Other risk factors include hypertension (diuretic use),[70] reduced consumption of fruits and vegetables, increased red meat intake, and occupational exposure to substances such as solvents and asbestos.[32,79]

Pathogenesis. The oncogenic mechanisms of renal cell carcinoma are becoming clearer with recent advances in molecular biology, but the exact mechanism remains unknown. Tumorigenic pathways differ among the different types of RCCs. RCCs are of four histologic subtypes: (1) clear cell, (2) granular cell, (3) papillary adenocarcinoma, and (4) the sarcomatoid variant. The tumors may be solid or focally cystic and demonstrate focal hemorrhage and necrosis.

Clinical Manifestations. Kidney cancers are generally silent during the early stages. Symptoms associated with metastasis are often the initial manifestations. The client may develop a cough or convulsions secondary to metastasis to the lungs or brain or an onset of back pain may occur secondary to a pathologic fracture.

The classic triad associated with renal cancers consists of hematuria, abdominal or flank pain, and a palpable abdominal mass. This combination of findings, however, occurs only in approximately 10% of cases. When it does occur, it carries a poor prognosis. Hematuria is the single most common presenting finding, occurring in up to 50% of cases. In the early stages of this disease the hematuria may be intermittent and microscopic. Other findings include flank pain, weight loss, anemia, abdominal mass, and fever.

Potentially confusing the clinical presentation of this condition is the fact that RCCs are a source of ectopic hormone production. Hypertension, hyperparathyroidism, and erythrocytosis can result via this mechanism. Metastasis most often occurs to the lungs and the skeletal system.

Medical Management

Prevention. Mass screening with the purpose of detecting RCC at its earliest stage is not recommended at this time, but screening focused on certain risk groups is advocated. Further research is needed to identify avoidable risks, develop effective chemoprevention, and recognize individuals at risk.[79]

Diagnosis. The primary feature of RCC is the renal parenchymal mass, which can be detected by a variety of imaging modalities. The widespread availability of abdominal ultrasound, magnetic resonance imaging (MRI), and CT scanning has increased the diagnosis of incidental renal tumors. Determining whether the mass is benign or malignant is often difficult, requiring surgical removal before a definitive diagnosis can be made. If hematuria is present, intravenous

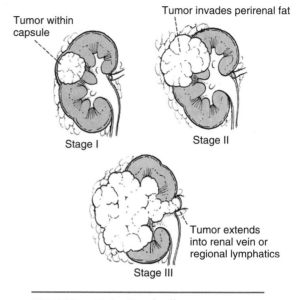

FIGURE **17-2** Renal cell carcinoma stages.

pyelography (IVP)* may be the initial procedure to identify renal abnormalities. Ultrasonography can be used to further evaluate the renal parenchyma, detecting small tumors (less than 1 cm). The advantage of the CT scan is that the greatest renal anatomic detail is obtained and also details of neighboring organs such as liver, colon, spleen, and lymphatics will also be available.

Staging. The TNM system for staging is used for this disease. Organ-confined lesions are associated with a 90% 5-year survival rate. If the disease has penetrated the renal capsule and invaded Gerota's fascia† or has spread into the regional lymph nodes, the prognosis is poor (Fig. 17-2).

Treatment. Surgery, including radical nephrectomy and regional lymph node dissection, is the treatment of choice for all resectable tumors. For clients with a solitary kidney or abnormal renal function, partial nephrectomy may be performed, but this approach carries a risk of tumor recurrence as a result of unrecognized satellite lesions or premalignant lesions that might have been present at the time of surgery. No single chemotherapeutic agent has been identified to have significant results with this disease. New research has shown that peripheral blood stem cells from a healthy sibling donor can induce regression in people with metastatic RCC who have had no response to conventional immunotherapy.[11]

Prognosis. Although occurring less often than prostate and bladder cancer, RCC is actually the most malignant urologic disease resulting in death in more than 35% of all cases.[79] Survival in RCC is related to pathologic stage,

---

*IVP is a radiographic test, which allows for evaluation of the kidneys, ureters, and bladder. A dye injected into the bloodstream is filtered and secreted by the renal tubules. The IVP provides information, including renal size function, position, the presence of calculi, masses, and congenital variants.

†Gerota's fascia is a fibroareolar tissue surrounding the kidney and perirenal fat.

grade, vascular invasion, deoxyribonucleic acid (DNA) content, and histologic pattern of the tumor. Small incidental tumors have an excellent prognosis and require minimal (if any) postoperative management. The involvement of regional lymph nodes and metastasis to the ipsilateral adrenal gland are poor prognostic indicators; metastatic RCC remains highly resistant to systemic therapy. Early detection and advances in surgical techniques will continue to improve the prognosis.

Special Implications for the Therapist   17-2

RENAL CELL CARCINOMA

Therapists working primarily with the geriatric population need to be aware of the symptoms and signs of this disease. Questions in the history related to hematuria, unexplained weight loss, fatigue, fever, and malaise are important, regardless of the reason for the physical therapy care. Awareness of new onset of unexplained abdominal, flank, or back pain; cough; or other signs of pulmonary involvement should raise concern on the therapist's part and warrants communication with a physician. In addition, RCC is the most common metastatic tumor to the sternum. An onset of sternal pain or a mass in someone with a history of RCC should be brought to the physician's attention.

The extensive abdominal and thoracic surgical sites may produce scarring that affects the client's posture and ability to move, increasing mechanical stress on the musculoskeletal system. Myofascial and soft tissue mobilization of the abdominal and thoracic regions may be of benefit to these people. If a history of abnormal renal function in addition to the cancer is evident, additional precautions may need to be taken by the therapist. See the section on Chronic Renal Failure later in this chapter. ■

Wilms' Tumor

Overview, Incidence, and Risk Factors.   Wilms' tumor, or nephroblastoma, is the most common malignant neoplasm in children. Approximately 500 new cases are reported annually in the United States. Age is the primary risk factor. The disease most commonly occurs during the first 7 years of life, with approximately 75% of cases occurring in children under the age of 5. The peak incidence occurs between the ages of 3 and 4, and the tumor occurs equally in boys and girls.

Etiologic Factors and Pathogenesis.   Molecular genetics plays an important role in the cause of Wilms' tumor. The biologic signaling pathways determining the origin of Wilms' tumor are complex, and several genes in several loci may be involved. The most well-known and studied gene of the Wilms' tumor is the WT1 suppressor gene, a complex protein that is an essential regulator of kidney development; mutations in this gene result in the formation of tumors. Other genetic alterations such as the genetic alteration on the short arm of chromosome 11p13 that inactivates one or several tumor suppressor genes are under investigation.[46]

The tumor arises from embryonic renal precursors. Wilms' tumor is distinguished by vascular invasion and displacement of structures, characterized by multiple subcapsular masses. Grossly, the tumor appears to be fleshy but may have areas of necrosis that lead to cavity formation. A unique mixture of primitive cells is often evident, and highly differentiated tubular cells resembling embryonic glomeruli and tubules are also apparent. The tumor occurs bilaterally in 10% of cases.

Clinical Manifestations.   The most common presenting feature is a large abdominal mass. Up to 30% of children may complain of abdominal pain, whereas hematuria may occur in up to 15% to 20% of cases. Symptoms associated with hypertension may occur in up to 50% of children. Lastly, fever, anorexia, and nausea and vomiting may be part of the presentation.

Medical Management

Diagnosis.   Abdominal ultrasonography helps define the cystic or solid nature of the mass and helps determine whether the renal vein or vena cava is involved. Excretory urography is also diagnostic. Chest films are indicated to determine whether metastasis has occurred to the pulmonary system. CT scan of the abdomen is helpful in determining the extent of the tumor but can be difficult to perform with small children.

Treatment.   Surgical resection of the tumor is the primary treatment regardless of the stage of the disease. An abdominal surgical approach is generally used to allow for bilateral exploration and confirmation of the extent of the disease. Regional lymphadenectomy is carried out, as lymph node involvement strongly affects the prognosis. Chemotherapy is also used for all stages of the disease, including preoperatively, with radiation therapy being added to the treatment regimen for stage III and IV disease. (See Chapter 8 for the side effects associated with chemotherapy and radiation therapy.) Wilms' tumor may recur after 9 to 11 years.

Prognosis.   Prognosis depends on the histologic appearance of the lesion, stage of the disease, and age of the child. More than 80% of people with Wilms' tumor can be cured using multimodal therapy.[16] A poor prognosis is indicated by invasion of the mass beyond the renal capsule and by anaplasia of the tumor, which is manifested by nuclear enlargement and hyperchromasia with atypical mitotic figures. Children under age 2 tend to have a better prognosis with a 2-year survival rate of up to 73%.

◆ Renal Cystic Disease
Overview.   A renal cyst is a cavity filled with fluid or renal tubular elements making up a semisolid material. The cyst may also be a segment of a dilated nephron. The presence of these cysts can lead to degeneration of renal tissue and obstruction of tubular flow. Renal cysts vary in size considerably, ranging from microscopic to several centimeters in diameter, and can be single or multiple and unilateral or bilateral.

The four types of renal cystic disease are (1) polycystic kidney disease, (2) medullary sponge kidney, (3) acquired cystic disease, and (4) single or multiple cysts. Simple renal cysts are the most common. They are usually less than 1 cm in diameter and do not often produce symptoms or compromise renal function.

Incidence. Polycystic kidney disease is one of the most common hereditary disorders in the United States, affecting more than 500,000 Americans. Polycystic kidney disease, with the onset in infancy, is usually associated with autosomal recessive inheritance and with the onset in adults is usually associated with autosomal dominant inheritance. Approximately 10% of people who develop end-stage renal disease (ESRD) have autosomal dominant polycystic kidney disease.

Etiologic and Risk Factors. In general, renal cystic disease is thought to develop from either tubular obstructions, which increase intratubular pressure, or from renal tubule basement membrane changes that would allow dilatation. The autosomal dominant disease results from a defect on the short arm of chromosome 16. People who inherit this gene defect are likely to develop the disorder. Regarding autosomal dominant polycystic kidney disease, a positive family history is noted in approximately 75% of cases. A history of UTIs and kidney stones is also a frequent finding.

Pathogenesis. Renal cysts can occur at any point along the nephron. Once the dilation of the tubule occurs forming the cyst, local fluid accumulation results in gradual but continued growth of the lesion. The tubular dilatation can occur from tubular obstruction, which elevates pressure, or from a defective and highly compliant basement membrane. The expanding cysts can eventually compromise the intrinsic renal vascular system, which can obstruct tubular flow and result in degeneration of the renal parenchyma.

Clinical Manifestations. The simple or solitary cysts are usually asymptomatic and found incidentally on routine urographic examination. Symptoms associated with autosomal dominant disease may include pain, hematuria, fever, and hypertension. Abdominal or flank pain is associated with bleeding into the cyst or growth of the cyst. Most of these clients will have enlarged kidneys that are palpable abdominally. The hematuria can be gross or microscopic. Rupture of a cyst usually accounts for the gross hematuria. Fever can be related to an infected cyst secondary to an ascending UTI. The hypertension is caused by compression of the intrarenal blood vessels and the resultant activation of the renin-angiotensin system.

Medical Management
Diagnosis. Most simple cysts are discovered on routine urographic examination. Often, urinalysis detects hematuria and proteinuria, or the clinical examination may reveal enlarged, palpable kidneys. The primary concern is to determine if a malignancy is present. Ultrasonography and CT scanning help determine this. At times, tissue biopsy or surgical exploration is necessary to make the definitive diagnosis.

Treatment. If a simple or solitary cyst is found, observation and periodic reassessment are standard procedure. If polycystic kidney disease is present, treatment is primarily supportive. Treating the hypertension and implementing a low-protein diet may slow the development of renal failure but will not prevent it from occurring.

Special Implications for the Therapist **17-3**

RENAL CYSTIC DISEASE

When treating a client with a history of renal cystic disease, therapists should be aware of symptoms and signs suggesting that the condition is worsening. The presence of any of these clinical findings warrants referral to a physician. An awareness that this population is at risk for hypertension and UTI and at increased risk of developing cerebral and aortic aneurysms and mitral valve problems is also necessary. The presentation of any symptoms or signs suggestive of the presence of these conditions again warrants referral to a physician. Lastly, the fact the kidneys may be enlarged can account for atypical findings on palpation. ■

◆ **Renal Calculi**
Overview. Urinary stone disease is the third most common urinary tract disorder, exceeded only by infections and prostate disease. A majority of the stones develop in the kidneys and are designated by the term *nephrolithiasis*. Once the stones move out of the kidney into the ureter, they are referred to as *ureteral stones*. The calculi are crystalline, ranging from popcorn-kernel shapes to jagged starbursts, and can cause urinary obstruction. Urinary obstruction typically occurs at one of the following three sites: (1) the ureteropelvic junction, (2) where the ureter crosses over the iliac vessels, and (3) at the ureterovesical junction (Fig. 17-3). The four basic types of stones are calcium, magnesium ammonium phosphate, uric acid, and cystine. Of kidney stones, 80% to 90% are composed of calcium.

Etiologic Factors. In most instances, the presence of a renal stone is associated with an increased blood level and urinary excretion of the principal component. An example of how this occurs is increased intestinal absorption of calcium and decreased reabsorption in the proximal tubules of the kidney.

Risk Factors. A wide variety of risk factors are associated with urinary calculi, including gender, age, geography, climate, diet, genetics, and environment. The primary age span for the initial presentation of the disease is 30 to 50 years of age. Men are more often affected than women by a ratio of 4:1 until the sixth or seventh decade when the incidence increases in women. A higher incidence of renal calculi occurs in industrialized countries and areas noted for high temperatures and humidity. The incidence of this disease is highest in the hot summer months.

Excess intake of supplemental calcium, oxalate, and purines can increase the incidence of stones, whereas adequate fluid intake and bran ingestion can help prevent calculi formation. Consistently sleeping on one side of the body may make the weight-bearing side more prone to kidney stones. Although the exact pathophysiology of the association between sleep posture and recurrent unilateral stone disease remains unknown, sleep posture may alter renal hemodynamics during sleep and promote stone formation.[73] Obesity is associ-

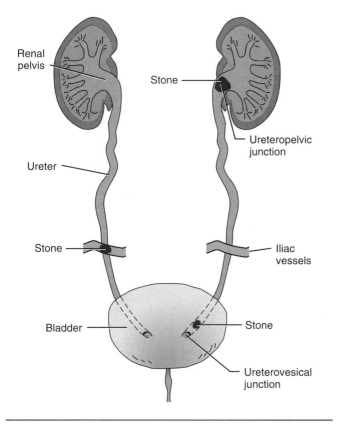

Renal
pelvis

Stone

Ureteropelvic
junction

Ureter

Stone

Iliac
vessels

Bladder

Stone

Ureterovesical
junction

FIGURE   **17-3**   The three common sites of urinary obstruction secondary to renal calculi.

ated with an increased incidence of urinary stone episodes in women but not in men.[66]

Pathogenesis.   High concentration of calcium in the kidney has long been believed to be part of the cause of stones, but new research suggests than many stones may have an infectious origin, caused by tiny bacteria called nanobacteria. Nonobacteria are small intracellular bacteria found in human kidney stones, capable of forming a calcium phosphate shell that serves as a crystallization center for renal calculi formation. Nanobacteria are hypothesized to be the initial nidi on which a kidney stone is built up, at a rate dependent on the supersaturation status of the urine. Those individuals with both nanobacteria and diminished defenses against stone formation (i.e., genetic factors, diet, and drinking habits) could be at increased risk for stone formation.[39]

Clinical Manifestations.   *Renal colic* is the term used to describe the pain associated with urinary tract obstruction; pain usually occurs once the stone has moved out of the kidney into the ureter. Acute, excruciating flank and upper outer abdominal quadrant pain is the classic complaint. The pain may also radiate into the lower abdominal, bladder, and perineal areas, including the scrotum in males and labia in females. Nausea and vomiting; urinary urgency and frequency; blood in the urine; and cool, clammy skin may also be present.

Medical Management
Diagnosis.   A variety of tests are used to diagnose this disease. Approximately 90% of calculi are radiopaque, making

them visible on an abdominal radiograph. Noncontrast helical CT scanning is the first-line imaging test for renal colic. Other traditional imaging tests (e.g., ultrasonography and IVP) are also important in the management of stone disease. Hematuria, infection, the presence of stone-forming crystals, and urine pH can be determined on urinalysis. Excretory urography allows for visualization of the urinary collecting and drainage system by the use of a contrast medium before the abdominal film.

Treatment.   A majority of stones 5 to 6 mm in diameter (a little smaller than the width of a pencil eraser) will pass spontaneously; this can take a few hours to even a few months. Pain medication and antibiotic therapy (if infection is present) are commonly administered during the initial 6-week period. Onset of a fever during this period is a medical emergency, requiring prompt drainage by catheterization or a percutaneous nephrostomy tube. If spontaneous passage does not occur, more aggressive intervention is used.

In situ extracorporeal shock wave lithotripsy (ESWL) is the first-line treatment in most people when intervention is required. ESWL uses the transmission of shock waves (a type of sound wave) to break the calculi into fragments. Since the soft tissues of the body have similar densities the shock waves pass through these structures with low attenuation. When the shock wave encounters a boundary between substances of differing acoustic density (i.e., a calculus in the ureter), high compressive forces are generated causing a breakdown of the stone. The goal is to reduce the diameter to the point where spontaneous passage of the stone occurs. This technology continues to be updated and improved. Other more invasive procedures may be used, including ureteroscopy, percutaneous nephrolithotomy, or surgical stone removal (least common approach).

Prevention.   Recurrence of calculi is common in up to 50% of people within 5 years if preventive steps are not taken. Appropriate preventive measures are determined by the cause of the stone formation. Adequate fluid intake is essential to the prevention of stones and recurrences by reducing the saturation of stone-forming crystals. In fact, choice of beverage may make a difference in some people with a significantly decreased risk with consumption of coffee (caffeinated and decaffeinated); tea; beer; and wine and increased risk with apple juice and grapefruit juice.[18,19,55] Although biochemical and epidemiologic data suggest that high sodium, animal protein, and sucrose intake increase the risk of stones, no clinical demonstration indicates that dietary changes reduce the recurrence of stones.[14]

Clients with calcium oxalate calculi are required to reduce their intake of foods high in oxalate, including spinach, cocoa, chocolate, pecans, and peanuts, or to eat calcium and oxalates together because the two compounds bind in the stomach and are expelled in the stool. If the stones are associated with underlying disease such as hyperparathyroidism, the co-morbidity must be effectively treated. Undue restrictions in calcium intake may be detrimental both for stone recurrences and bone mineralization; therefore "adequate" calcium intake (800 to 1000 mg/day, which varies by geography and age) should be encouraged but only in food, as supplemental calcium appears to increase the risk of stones for susceptible people.[14]

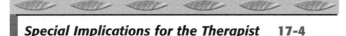

Special Implications for the Therapist   17-4

RENAL CALCULI

If the classic symptoms are present, the renal colic associated with the calculi will not be confused with pain from mechanical dysfunction. The condition, however, may be manifested by symptoms that are intermittent and not severe. Depending on where the urinary collecting system is obstructed, the condition may be manifested solely by unilateral back pain, ranging from the thoracolumbar junction to the iliac crest. The therapist needs to be vigilant for complaints of urinary dysfunction and risk factors associated with this disease. Murphy's percussion test can be performed to determine the need for medical referral.

If working with someone who is concurrently being treated conservatively for renal calculi, the therapist must be vigilant for complaints of fever, chills, or sweats. An onset of these symptoms warrants immediate communication with the physician. ■

◆ Chronic Renal Failure

Overview.   Chronic renal failure (sometimes referred to as *renal insufficiency* or *kidney failure*) can be attributed to a variety of conditions that result in permanent loss of nephrons. The loss of nephrons results in progressive deterioration of glomerular filtration, tubular reabsorption, and endocrine functions of the kidneys. The progressive inability of the kidneys to function eventually results in uncompensated renal failure with significant systemic effects, influencing all the other body systems.

Incidence.   In the early 1970s, U.S. governmental support for dialysis and transplantation began. The number of patients with end-stage renal disease (ESRD) treated by maintenance hemodialysis in the United States has increased sharply during the past 30 years. In 1999, more than 3000 hemodialysis centers had greater than 190,000 chronic hemodialysis patients and more than 60,000 staff members. The technologic advances in dialysis and transplantation have resulted in improved outcomes for those with renal disease. Even so, more than 50,000 Americans die each year because of kidney disease, and more than 260,000 experience chronic kidney failure and need an artificial kidney machine (dialysis) or organ transplantation to survive.[54]

Etiologic and Risk Factors.   The presence of a number of diseases can account for destruction of nephrons, but diabetes mellitus and controlled or poorly controlled high blood pressure* are the two leading causes of chronic renal failure. Other disorders contributing to the development of kidney failure include urinary tract obstruction and infection; hereditary defects of the kidneys; polycystic kidneys; glomerular disorders (e.g., glomerulonephritis); and systemic lupus erythematosus (SLE).

---

*Renovascular disease (e.g., renovascular hypertension) results from renal arterial obstruction caused most commonly by atherosclerosis.

An increased risk of renal disease is also associated with over-the-counter (OTC) analgesic drug use. Heavy average intake (more than one pill per day) and medium-to-high cumulative intake (1000 or more pills in a lifetime) of acetaminophen double the odds of developing end-stage renal disease (ESRD). In addition, high cumulative intake of nonsteroidal antiinflammatory drugs (NSAIDs) (5000 or more pills in a lifetime) increased the risk of developing the disease.[65] Nephropathy is caused by the excessive consumption of analgesic mixtures containing at least two antipyretic analgesics combined with caffeine and/or codeine.[26]

Age is also a factor, since adults 65 and older account for a large percentage of newly diagnosed conditions. This is linked with the age-related reduced glomerular filtration rate (GFR) and the often-present concurrent medical diseases in the older adult. The reduced GFR also increases the susceptibility of older people to the harmful effects of nephrotoxic drugs.

Pathogenesis.   Owing to the loss of nephrons, renal failure is marked by the kidneys' inability to adequately remove metabolic waste products from the blood and to regulate fluid, electrolyte, and pH balance of extracellular fluids. The rate of nephron destruction can vary considerably, occurring over a period of several months to many years. Typically, four stages mark the progression of chronic renal failure: (1) diminished renal reserve, (2) renal insufficiency, (3) renal failure, and (4) end-stage renal disease (ESRD).

In the *first stage*, diminished renal reserve, the GFR is approximately 50% of normal. During this stage, no overt symptoms of impaired renal function are evident. Depending on the health of the person, the kidneys have tremendous adaptive and compensatory capabilities, accounting for the delay in symptoms. The unaffected nephrons undergo structural and physiologic hypertrophy in an attempt to make up for those nephrons that are no longer functioning. During this stage, blood urea nitrogen (BUN) and creatinine levels are normal.

The *second stage*, renal insufficiency, is manifested by a reduction in GFR to approximately 20% to 35% of normal. During this stage, azotemia (abnormally high level of nitrogenous waste in the blood); anemia; and hypertension can appear. The *third stage* is renal failure. This occurs when the GFR is less than 20% to 25% of normal. At these levels the kidneys cannot regulate volume and solute composition. This inability leads to edema, metabolic acidosis, and hypercalcemia. Neurologic, gastrointestinal, and cardiovascular complications now become a part of the clinical manifestations of this disease.

The *fourth stage*, end-stage renal disease, occurs when about 90% of kidney function has been lost and the GFR is less than 5% of normal. The complications noted in the first three stages are magnified by the continued progressive loss of kidney function. Uremia (urea and other wastes in the blood) is the term used to describe the clinical manifestations of this stage. Virtually all body systems are involved, with a multitude of symptoms and signs being present. Besides the physiologic changes that are occurring, anatomic changes are also evident. The mass of the kidneys is generally reduced, and histologic investigation reveals a reduction in renal capillaries and scarring of the glomeruli. In addition, atrophy and fibrosis are evident in the kidney tubules. During this final stage, survival is dependent on dialysis or transplantation.

Clinical Manifestations. Chronic renal failure is marked by a multitude of symptoms and signs. The onset of these findings is typically very gradual and subtle, often resulting in a delay in diagnosis. Table 17-1 summarizes the systemic effects associated with chronic renal failure. When the kidneys can no longer draw off excess water, wastes, and salt, the tissues swell and toxins accumulate, resulting in the most typical cluster of symptoms: nausea, vomiting, loss of appetite, fatigue, increased blood pressure, itching, decreased urinary output, swelling of the face and feet, and mental dullness or slowed thinking.

Hematologic. Anemia is the most significant hematologic problem associated with chronic renal failure. Controlling the production of red blood cells is the hormone erythropoietin primarily produced by the kidneys. Renal failure leads to decreased erythropoietin production, resulting in subsequent decrease in red blood cell (RBC) numbers. In addition, the RBCs that are produced have a shortened life span. (See Chapter 13 for additional information regarding anemia; administration of recombinant erythropoietin used to correct the anemia may be key to the prevention of other co-morbidities, and administration of erythropoietin has also been shown to improve exercise capacity in renal disease.)[77] Up to 20% of those with chronic renal failure have a tendency to bleed and bruise easily related to impaired platelet function.

Cardiovascular. Cardiovascular diseases often occur in those with chronic renal failure and are the leading cause of death in dialysis recipients. Renovascular hypertension often appears early in the course of this disease because of increased renin production and excess extracellular fluid volume. Owing to the immunologic complications associated with chronic renal failure, infections can more easily occur, potentially leading to pericarditis. Retrosternal pain can be a result of pericarditis. Congestive heart failure is another common problem in dialysis recipients.

Gastrointestinal. Gastrointestinal system complaints occur often in uremia. High concentrations of ammonia and increased gastric acid secretion can contribute to the nausea and vomiting and the metallic taste in the mouth. The resul-

tant depressed appetite contributes to malnutrition, fatigue, weakness, and malaise. Malnutrition has a high prevalence in cases of terminal kidney disease, partly as a result of the therapeutic restriction on calories and proteins but also because of the metabolic reactions typical with this disease and to anorexia. In addition, alterations in the metabolism of calcium, phosphorus, and potassium can result in electrolyte imbalances (see Chapter 4).

Musculoskeletal. The skeletal changes associated with chronic renal failure are common and occur early in the disease secondary to abnormalities in calcium, phosphate, and vitamin D metabolism. Kidney disease impairs the GFR. Subsequently, the body retains phosphate and loses calcium. A drop in serum calcium signals a cascade of events starting with the release of parathyroid hormone, which signals the body to increase calcium resorption from bone to make up the loss. The reduced calcium and phosphate levels in bone lead to renal osteodystrophy,* characterized by varying degrees of osteomalacia, osteosclerosis, osteoporosis, and soft tissue and vascular calcification (Fig. 17-4). Bone reabsorption occurs in several locations (subperiosteal, subchondral, trabecular, endosteal, and subligamentous).

In addition to bone demineralization, this process also leads to calcification deposits. After dialysis is initiated, a rapid rise in calcium levels occurs, preceding a fall in phosphate levels. Metastatic calcification is the result, affecting the eyes (conjunctivitis); muscle; muscular lining of arteries; skin (pruritus, or intense itching); and periarticular soft tissues. The prevalence of calcifications increases with the duration of hemodialysis. Muscle, joint, and bone pain can be severe with resultant bone deformities and fractures. Tissue calcifications can be lethal if they develop in cerebral, coronary, or pulmonary vessels.

Other musculoskeletal manifestations attributable to chronic renal insufficiency include destructive spondyloarthropathy, tendon rupture, crystal deposition, infection,

---

*Renal osteodystrophy is a type of rickets formerly called renal rickets and sometimes referred to as azotemic osteodystrophy. Although uncommon at one time, the incidence has risen with increased survival of people with renal disease on dialysis.

TABLE	17-1

Chronic Renal Failure: Summary of Clinical Manifestations

SYSTEM	MANIFESTATIONS
General	Fatigue, weakness, decreased alertness, inability to concentrate
Skin	Pallor, ecchymosis, pruritus, dry skin and mucous membranes, thin/brittle fingernails, urine odor on skin
Hematologic	Anemia, tendency to bleed easily
Body fluids	Polyuria, nocturia, dehydration, hyperkalemia, metabolic acidosis, hypocalcemia, hyperphosphatemia
Eye, ear, nose, throat	Metallic taste in mouth, nosebleeds, urinous breath, pale conjunctiva
Pulmonary	Dyspnea, rales, pleural effusion
Cardiovascular	Dyspnea on exertion, hypertension, friction rub, retrosternal pain on inspiration
Gastrointestinal	Anorexia, nausea, vomiting, hiccups, gastrointestinal bleeding
Genitourinary	Impotence, amenorrhea, loss of libido
Skeletal	Osteomalacia, osteoporosis, bone pain, fracture, metastatic calcification of soft tissues, edema
Neurologic	Recent memory loss, coma, seizures, muscle tremors, paresthesias, muscle weakness, restless legs, cramping

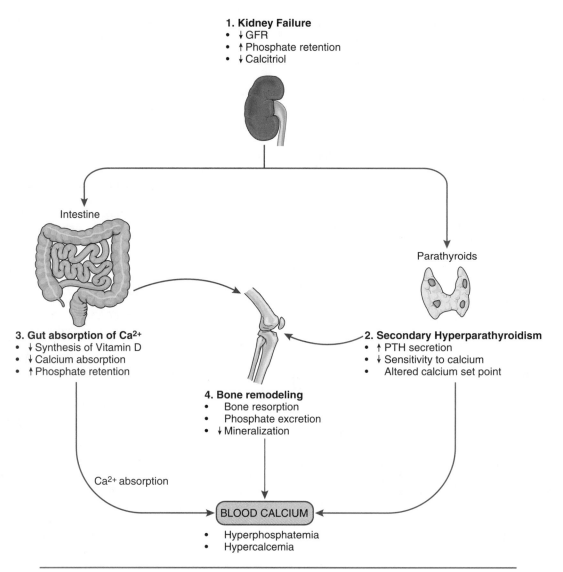

1. Kidney Failure
- ↓ GFR
- ↑ Phosphate retention
- ↓ Calcitriol

Intestine

Parathyroids

3. Gut absorption of Ca²⁺
- ↓ Synthesis of Vitamin D
- ↓ Calcium absorption
- ↑ Phosphate retention

2. Secondary Hyperparathyroidism
- ↑ PTH secretion
- ↓ Sensitivity to calcium
- Altered calcium set point

4. Bone remodeling
- Bone resorption
- Phosphate excretion
- ↓ Mineralization

Ca²⁺ absorption

BLOOD CALCIUM
- Hyperphosphatemia
- Hypercalcemia

FIGURE 17-4 Mechanisms of altered bone turnover. (1) Renal osteodystrophy can be viewed as the result of a vicious cycle that begins with moderate to severe renal failure. As the glomerular filtration rate (GFR) decreases, phosphate excretion decreases, and calcium elimination increases. (2) The body attempts to compensate for the loss of calcitriol and reduced calcium absorption by increasing parathyroid hormone secretion (PTH). PTH mobilizes calcium from the bones (bone reabsorption) and facilitates phosphate excretion. This release of calcium and phosphate into the blood results in hyperphosphatemia and hypercalcemia. (3) As kidney failure progresses, the damaged kidneys can no longer convert vitamin D to its active form and without active vitamin D, calcium absorption in the intestines is decreased and paradoxically facilitates phosphate retention. (4) Thus the normal process of bone mineralization with calcium and phosphate is impaired. Demineralization of the bone frees more calcium and phosphorus into the blood. As the disease progresses even more, the parathyroid gland may become unresponsive to the normal feedback system and continues to produce parathyroid hormone, causing acceleration of renal osteodystrophy.

and avascular necrosis. These changes are less common than those in renal osteodystrophy and are more often seen in people who have undergone long-term hemodialysis or renal transplantation.

Neurologic. Alteration of central nervous system (CNS) and peripheral nervous system (PNS) function often occurs with chronic renal failure associated with uremia. CNS involvement (uremic encephalopathy) is manifested by recent memory loss, inability to concentrate, perceptual errors, and decreased alertness. Uremic toxins contribute to atrophy and

demyelination of both sensory and motor nerves of the PNS. The lower extremities are much more commonly affected than the upper extremities; neurologic changes are typically symmetrical and can also be manifested as peripheral neuropathy or restless leg syndrome, which is more pronounced at rest.

Medical Management
Prevention. The ultimate goal and mission of the National Kidney Foundation is the eradication of diseases of the kidney. Toward that end, *Healthy People 2010* has identified several goals related to kidney failure, including (1) re-

duce kidney failure due to diabetes; (2) increase the proportion of people with chronic kidney failure who receive a transplant within 3 years of registration on the waiting list; (3) increase the proportion of people with chronic kidney failure who receive counseling on nutrition, treatment choices, and cardiovascular care 12 months before the start of renal replacement therapy; (4) reduce deaths from cardiovascular disease in persons with chronic kidney failure; and (5) reduce the rate of new cases of end-stage renal disease (ESRD).[33]

Since diabetic nephropathy is the leading cause of kidney failure in the United States, prevention strategies and risk factor modification related to glycemic control, prevention of hypertension, coronary artery disease, physical inactivity, and reducing or eliminating tobacco-related behaviors (e.g., smoking) are a large part of the prevention of renal disease. In the future, pancreas transplantation may become a part of diabetes prevention and therefore end-stage renal disease (ESRD) prevention.[74]

Diagnosis.   In addition to the symptoms and signs associated with this disease, documentation of elevated BUN and serum creatinine values leads to the diagnosis of renal failure. Imaging modalities are also used to support a diagnosis of chronic renal failure. The finding of bilateral small kidneys (less than 10 cm) by ultrasonography is supportive of the diagnosis. This disease is also marked by subperiosteal reabsorption along the radial borders of the digits of the hand. This finding confirms hyperparathyroidism, which would have to have been present for at least 1 year to be demonstrable. A variety of biochemical and radiologic techniques are available to assist in the diagnosis and monitoring of renal osteodystrophy. Measurement of serum parathyroid hormone remains the single most useful biochemical test in predicting bone histology in an individual.

Treatment.   The treatment of chronic renal failure falls under two categories: conservative management and renal replacement therapy. The goals of conservative care are to slow the deterioration of the remaining renal function and to assist the body in its fight to compensate for the existing condition. Renal replacement therapy consists of dialysis or renal transplantation. The stage of the disease will determine which of the treatment approaches will be instituted.

Conservative management consists of a wide variety of interventions. In the case of renal artery (atherosclerotic) stenosis, renal artery angioplasty with stent placement may be used. Treating hypertension and carefully managed nutrition and supplements are vital for these clients. For example, proteins are broken down to form nitrogenous wastes, which adds to the problem of azotemia, or phosphorus (normally removed by the kidneys) can build up in the blood, contributing to loss of calcium and bone. The use of oral and intravenous (IV) calcitriol to suppress parathyroid hormone is standard practice.

The development of recombinant human erythropoietin for treatment of anemia in clients with renal disease has increased hematocrit levels and improved appetite, energy levels, exercise capacity,[77] sexual function, and skin characteristics. Early and aggressive treatment of hypocalcemia and hyperphosphatemia is vital to slowing the concurrent osteodystrophy. Phosphate-binding antacids, calcium supplements, and doses of vitamin D are often prescribed. Pharmacologic agents such as angiotensin-converting enzyme, which inhibits the release of renin and blocks the conversion of angiotensin I to an-

giotensin II; calcium antagonists; beta blockers; and some alpha blockers (see Table 11-4)[54] may be used to control renovascular hypertension and reduce proteinuria.

Renal replacement therapy (dialysis or transplantation) is the treatment of choice for end-stage renal disease (ESRD). The decision is based on the client's age, general health, donor availability, and personal preference. Dialysis can take the form of hemodialysis (HD) or peritoneal dialysis (PD) (also referred to as *continuous ambulatory peritoneal dialysis [CAPD]* and *continuous cycling peritoneal dialysis [CCPD]*). HD typically requires three sessions per week for 3 to 4 hours per session. The blood flows from an artery, through the dialysis machine chambers, and then back to the body's venous system, with the waste products and excess electrolytes diffusing into the dialyzing solution. The individual must travel to a renal center for this treatment and remains relatively immobile throughout the session.

PD relies on the same principles as HD but can be done independently at home. A catheter is implanted in the peritoneal cavity, and sterile dialyzing solution is instilled and then drained over a specific period. This process is completed four times daily. With CAPD/CCPD, fewer dietary restrictions and dramatic symptom swings associated with HD occur. Potential complications of PD include infection, catheter malfunction, dehydration, hyperglycemia, and hernia. Peritonitis is the most serious potential complication.

The steady improvement in the outcome of renal allografts has made kidney transplantation the treatment of choice for many people with chronic renal failure. Donor availability limits the number of transplants performed. In adults, the renal graft is placed extraperitoneally in the iliac fossa through an oblique lower abdominal incision. In small children, the graft is located retroperitoneally with a midline abdominal incision. Complications of the procedures include renal artery thrombosis, urinary leak, and lymphocele. For further discussion, see Chapter 20.

Prognosis.   Despite significant advances in technologic and pharmacologic interventions, the current annual mortality rate of people with end-stage renal disease (ESRD) in the United States is about 24%.[54] Cardiovascular diseases remain the number one cause of death in all categories of renal disease, including chronic renal insufficiency, end-stage renal disease (ESRD) on dialysis, and the renal transplant recipient. This is most likely due to the presence of multiple cardiovascular risk factors (e.g., hypertension, abnormal lipids, smoking, dietary factors).[48]

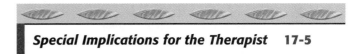

Special Implications for the Therapist   17-5

CHRONIC RENAL FAILURE

Preferred Practice Patterns:
4A: Primary Prevention/Risk Reduction for Skeletal Demineralization (osteodystrophy)
4C: Impaired Muscle Performance
4D: Impaired Joint Mobility, Motor Function, Muscle Performance, and Range of Motion Associated With Connective Tissue Dysfunction (tendon rupture)

Continued

5A: Primary Prevention/Risk Reduction for Loss of Balance and Falling (myopathy)

5D: Impaired Motor Function and Sensory Integrity Associated With Nonprogressive Disorders of the Central Nervous System—Acquired in Adolescence or Adulthood (uremic encephalopathy)

5G: Impaired Motor Function and Sensory Integrity Associated With Acute or Chronic Polyneuropathies

Other practice patterns may apply depending on developing associated conditions such as congestive heart failure, anemia, edema, and so on.

Therapists must be aware that several specific renal syndromes may be induced by the interaction of NSAIDs and analgesics (see Table 4-3) on renal function. Although the nephrotoxicity is relatively low, the increased availability of these medications as OTC products and the concentration of people taking NSAIDs/analgesics in a rehabilitation setting are factors contributing to a larger percentage of these people coming into contact with a therapist. Older adults are especially susceptible and more likely to use these agents. Additionally, NSAID-related renal involvement is probably underrecognized and with the Food and Drug Administration (FDA) approval of OTC sale of NSAIDs (e.g., naproxen sodium, ketoprofen, ibuprofen), incidence may increase in the coming years. Any time a client reports a history of prolonged and regular NSAID/analgesic use and renal symptoms, medical evaluation is required.

Physical therapy care of people with chronic renal failure has increased significantly in the past 20 years. Treating people with a diagnosis of chronic renal failure can be extremely challenging because of malnutrition, side effects of medications, and the number of body systems involved. The decreased alertness, inability to concentrate, and short-term memory deficits interfere with following instructions, including transfers, exercises, body mechanics, and so on. Adverse effects of some of the medications used for renovascular hypertension may include angioedema (i.e., swelling around the face, mouth, or throat), requiring immediate medical attention. Clients should be taught to rise slowly, dangling the legs and feet before standing, and to report any unusual swelling.

Reliance on the assistance of family and other health care providers is often necessary. The fatigue and general weakness may dictate that the therapist provide rest periods during a rehabilitation session. The potential osteodystrophy requires modification of evaluation and intervention techniques including osteoporosis education and prevention (see Special Implications for the Therapist: Osteoporosis, 23-1).

A number of potential renal transplantation complications that the therapist should be aware of include hypertension, lipid disorders, hepatitis, cancer, tendinopathies, and osteopenia (see the section on Transplantation in Chapter 20). Lastly, corticosteroids appear to be the primary factor in the impaired bone formation associated with graft recipients (see Chapter 4).

Dialysis[37,63]

Complications of dialysis are multiple and varied. Fluid shifts during dialysis can contribute to adverse neuromuscular and hemodynamic consequences that must be reported so that adjustments can be made in the dialysis fluid (dialysate). Symptoms of increased thirst and weight gain are common, and the weight gain and abdominal distention, especially with CAPD/CCCP, may cause extreme distress in the individual.

Depression among people on dialysis may be more common than is currently recognized, often masquerading as functional impairment, anorexia, or noncompliance. Impaired libido, impotence, infertility, dysfunctional uterine bleeding, amenorrhea, and anovulation are very common. Altered platelet function results in bleeding tendencies in anyone with uremia and the therapist is advised to follow the precautions listed in Tables 39-6 and 39-7.

People on dialysis have increased susceptibility to infection by various pathogens because they are immunosuppressed, and the dialysis process requires vascular access for prolonged periods of time. Infection of the vascular access site is a major concern because signs and symptoms of local infection are often absent early on. Careful monitoring for infection or inflammation is warranted with early medical referral. Standard precautions are essential for the individual in a dialysis unit, those individuals dialyzing and handling the equipment at home, and for the treating therapist.

Contact transmission can be prevented by hand hygiene (i.e., hand washing or use of a waterless hand rub); glove use; and disinfection of environmental surfaces. Of these, hand hygiene is the most important. In addition, nonsterile disposable gloves provide a protective barrier for workers' hands, preventing them from becoming soiled or contaminated, and reduce the likelihood that microorganisms present on the hands of personnel will be transmitted to clients. However, even with glove use, hand washing is needed because pathogens deposited on the outer surface of gloves can be detected on hands after glove removal, possibly because of holes or defects in the gloves, leakage at the wrist, or contamination of hands during glove removal.[10]

During progressive renal failure, catabolism and anorexia lead to loss of lean body mass but fluid retention at the same time, and weight gain can mask the loss of body mass. Malnutrition, anemia, and this loss of body mass can result in significant losses in muscle strength requiring careful assessment and rehabilitation. The mixed sensory and motor peripheral neuropathy common in people with uremia often improves symptomatically with adequate dialysis. Muscle mass will also improve with consistently good dialysis and nutrition.

Fluid retention also results in hypertension at the beginning of dialysis; alternately, dialysis can result in hypotension. The therapist should ask the client about the dialysis schedule and encourage the individual not to miss any treatment. Younger clients and those who have recently started dialysis are more likely to miss treatments. This may be reflected in rising blood pressure and elevated pulse rate. Monitoring vital signs and laboratory values is essential throughout the rehabilitative process.

Chest and back pain can occur during the early days of dialysis referred to as *first-use syndrome*. Delayed hypersensitivity reactions with mild itching and urticaria may be reported to (or observed by) the therapist. Maintaining the dialysis access site for the fistula or catheter may be difficult, requiring extreme caution during any rehabilitation or exercise intervention. Ischemia of the arm (or leg, depending on the location of the fistula) may be the first indication of thrombosis and subsequent stenosis. Any of these signs and symptoms should be reported to the renal staff.

For the individual with chronic renal failure, myopathies, neuropathies, and reduced muscle mass, carrying and lifting the bag of dialysate can be difficult. Strength training, balance, and mobility are key components of a home exercise program for the person using CAPD/CCCD. Exercise can be performed before, during, or after renal or peritoneal dialysis. When exercise is performed after dialysis, blood chemistry levels will be at their optimum, although fatigue may be a factor. Exercise during dialysis may be an option for some and usually improves the efficiency of dialysis because of better mobilization of dependent fluids, but most people do not choose this option.

Laboratory Values

Renal failure causes metabolic waste products to accumulate in the blood, which can be measured to assess renal function. The two most commonly measured waste products are serum creatinine and BUN. Changes in creatinine and BUN levels do not usually contraindicate physical or occupational therapy intervention but other test measures are important. Depressed serum albumin levels reflect poor nutritional status and these lab values should be monitored whenever available (see the section on Renal Function Tests in Chapter 39 and Table 39-11).

Renal Failure and Exercise

Limited research available has shown that impaired oxygen transport plays a role in limiting exercise in anyone with chronic renal failure, especially once dialysis begins.[68] Adults with chronic renal failure often show signs and symptoms of anemia, fatigue, wasting, and reduced work capacity with concomitant findings of reduced cardiac performance and muscle mass.[38] Functional capacity in people on dialysis is typically more than two standard deviations below the age- and gender-predicted norm and is often far lower, sometimes barely enough to carry out activities of daily living (ADLs). A prescriptive program of regular activity and exercise can improve physical functioning, exercise tolerance, and health-related quality of life.[51,60,61]

End-stage renal disease (ESRD) is characterized by compromised autonomic function associated with cardiac mortality; this is particularly prevalent in people with diabetes. Autonomic dysfunction may limit maximal age-predicted heart rates by as much as 20 to 40 beats/min. Therefore when prescribing exercise intensity, the perceived exertion rating may be a better choice for monitoring exercise.[47] Exercise has been identified as a factor associated with improved autonomic cardiac function in end-stage renal disease (ESRD).[9] Exercise prescription for anyone with chronic disease and/or disability must take these factors into consideration.

A timely and effective rehabilitation program can improve quality of life, endurance, and functional abilities toward greater independence. For the individual on dialysis, the most important independent quality of life predictor is the usual level of exercise activity. The person's perception of physical functioning as it relates to quality of life is important because these variables can be the focus for intervention strategies to prevent early deterioration in dialysis.[43]

The individual's clinical condition (and response to exercise) provides the greatest guidance in determining exercise or physical activity mode, intensity, frequency, and duration. With numerous medical problems associated with end-stage renal disease (ESRD), a major concern before initiating an exercise program is physiologic stability. Many of the risks of exercise are related more to exacerbation of co-morbid conditions (e.g., arthritis, diabetes, hypertension) than to the kidney disease itself. Exercise might cause a potassium efflux from exercising muscles and may elevate blood levels, although the possibility of exercise-induced hyperkalemia and resultant cardiac arrhyth-

mias is small. Serum potassium levels must be controlled before exercise, and should not be greater than 5 milliequivalents per liter (mEq/L). Individuals with uncontrolled blood chemistries should avoid weight training.

Some sources recommend exercise during dialysis[59,62] and the day after dialysis, since a greater chance of instability is evident before *renal* dialysis (PD is usually done daily and is easiest with an empty abdomen for mechanical reasons). People on dialysis may have a low-exercise capacity, with approximately half that of healthy individuals matched to age and gender. This corresponds to approximately 3 to 5 MET (one MET is equal to energy expenditure at rest; ADLs require 1.5 to 5 MET). A review of specific prescription principles, including weight-training guidelines, for individuals with chronic disease and specifically, renal disease is available.[25,47,51]

Exercise may help control blood pressure, especially in those individuals who are hypertensive. Blood pressure should be monitored in the arm opposite the arteriovenous shunt before exercise. If blood pressure is greater than 200/100 mm Hg, the individual should not exercise. Anyone with diabetes should be monitored for hypoglycemia or sudden drops in blood glucose levels. In addition, the kidney is essential in the production of vitamin D, which is necessary for calcium absorption. Exercise training ameliorates the enhanced muscle protein degradation associated with chronic renal failure. Anyone undergoing dialysis will be monitored for bone disease; strengthening exercises can help bone density, and bone density studies can provide outcome-based evidence of the value of exercise in these clients. In the case of polycystic kidney disease moderate exercise in animal models was considered safe but did not alter bone mineral density. Additional research in this area is needed, since other benefits may be derived from exercise in this and other kidney-diseased populations.[20] ■

◆ Inflammatory Glomerular Lesions

Overview. *Glomerulonephritis* is the term used to describe a group of diseases that damages the kidney's filtering units (glomeruli). It is the third leading cause of end stage kidney disease in the United States. The glomeruli are tufts of capillaries connecting the afferent and efferent arterioles of the nephron (Fig. 17-5). The capillaries are supported by a stalk made up of mesangial cells and a basement membrane and are arranged in lobules. The circulating blood is filtered in the glomeruli, with the urine filtrate being an end product. Glomerulonephritis accounts for approximately 50% of those who require dialysis.

The two categories of glomerular disease are the nephrotic and nephritic syndromes. Nephrotic syndrome is not a specific kidney disease but rather occurs as a result of any disease that causes damage to the kidney-filtering units such as diabetes, vasculitis, and lupus. Nephrotic syndrome can be caused by nephritis, which affects only the kidney. Nephrotic syndrome affects the integrity of the glomerular capillary membrane; nephrotic syndrome results in an inflammatory response within the glomeruli.

Etiologic Factors.   Most cases of primary glomerular disease and many cases of secondary disease have an immune origin. Two different immune mechanisms have been suggested, including (1) injury secondary to deposition of soluble circulating antigen-antibody complexes in the glomeruli and (2) injury secondary to antibodies reacting with insoluble fixed glomeru-

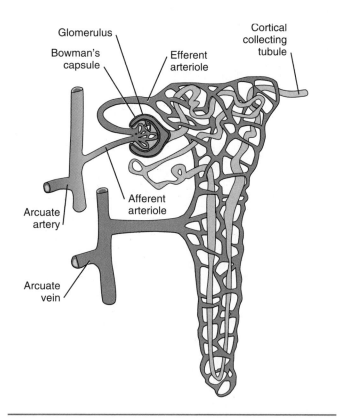

FIGURE 17-5 Components of the nephron. The afferent arteriole carries blood to the glomerulus for filtration through Bowman's capsule and the renal tubular system.

lar antigens. The antigen of the immune complexes can be endogenous as with DNA in systemic lupus erythematosus. The antigen can also be exogenous as in streptococcal membrane antigens in poststreptococcal glomerulonephritis.

Risk Factors. The presence of a variety of common disorders can significantly increase the risk of glomerular damage. Approximately 55% of those with type 1 diabetes mellitus (formerly insulin-dependent diabetes) and 30% of those with type 2 diabetes mellitus (formerly non-insulin-dependent diabetes) develop end-stage kidney disease. The glomerulus is the primary component of the kidney affected by diabetic neuropathy. Besides diabetes and systemic lupus erythematosus, hypertension is also associated with glomerular disease.

The nephrotic syndrome can occur at any age. In children the disease is most prevalent between 1.5 and 4 years of age. Boys are more commonly involved than girls, but the gender distribution is roughly equal in the adult population.

Pathogenesis. Whether the antigens are endogenous or exogenous, the antigen-antibody complex is formed in the circulation and becomes trapped in the glomerular membrane as the blood is being filtered. Injury to the glomerular membrane can occur through cell lysis or chemotaxis. Leukocytes are then drawn into the area. If the inciting antigen is short-lived, the inflammatory process is acute but then subsides. If the antigen is being chronically produced, the recurrent inflammatory reactions lead to chronic glomerulonephritis.

The histologic changes associated with glomerular disease include proliferative, sclerotic, and membranous changes. A lo-

cal increase in both the cellular (proliferative) and noncellular (sclerotic) components of the glomerulus occurs, as does an increase in the thickness of the glomerular capillary wall (membranous). These changes adversely affect the glomerular filtration mechanism and alter capillary permeability. Increased glomerular capillary permeability results in proteinuria, hematuria, pyuria, oliguria, edema, hypertension, and azotemia.

Proteinuria occurs when damage to the glomeruli allows protein normally kept in the plasma to leak into the urine in large amounts reducing the amount of protein in the blood. Since the protein in the blood helps keep fluid in the bloodstream, some of this fluid (transudate, see Fig. 5-8) leaks out of the bloodstream into the tissues, causing swelling. For a review of the inflammatory response, see the section on Inflammation in Chapter 5.

Clinical Manifestations. Typically, the earlier stages of glomerular disease are marked by the absence of overt symptoms. The usual initial manifestation of the nephrotic syndrome is generalized edema. The edema can be severe enough to be disabling. Proteinuria may also cause the urine to foam as protein is lost in the urine. The nephritic syndrome is typically marked by hematuria with bloody-tinged or brown urine visible in some cases. The damaged capillary walls allow RBCs to become part of the urine filtrate. In addition, pyuria, oliguria, hypertension, and nocturia are associated with this condition.

Medical Management

Diagnosis. Owing to the lack of symptoms in the early stages of glomerulonephritis the disease is often found incidentally by urinalysis or elevated blood pressure readings. Urinalysis may reveal proteinuria, hematuria, and pyuria, while blood analysis will reveal azotemia. Renal ultrasound and biopsy may be used, depending on the initial presenting symptoms and signs.

Treatment. The management of this condition is multifaceted and may depend on the underlying disease. Some of the kidney diseases that cause nephrotic syndrome are treatable with medications, but others have no known effective treatment. To prevent protein malnutrition, nutritional counseling is recommended. Restricted dietary salt intake is vital in the management of edema. These clients also typically need diuretics. A low-fat diet with a general weight control and exercise program are essential if hypercholesterolemia and hypertriglyceridemia are present. Lastly, dialysis and transplantation may be necessary for those in the late stages of glomerulonephritis (see the section on Chronic Renal Failure in this chapter).

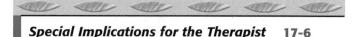

Special Implications for the Therapist **17-6**

INFLAMMATORY GLOMERULAR LESIONS

Therapists working with clients with a diagnosis of diabetes, SLE, vasculitis, and hypertension need to be aware of the association of glomerulonephritis and these disorders. Being vigilant for the clinical manifestations of glomerulonephritis (e.g., edema, hypertension, hematuria, oliguria) is important, and their presence warrants referral of the client to a physician. An awareness of the side effects associated with diuretics is also important. Potential side effects include muscle weakness, fatigue, muscle cramps, headaches, and depression, all of which can interfere with the rehabilitation program. (See Chapter 4 for additional information regarding diuretics; see also Table 11-4.) The onset of any of these complaints also warrants communication with a physician. Finally, many clients with glomerulonephritis progress to chronic renal failure. ■

DISORDERS OF THE BLADDER AND URETHRA

◆ Bladder Cancer

Overview and Incidence.   As the fourth leading cause of cancer in men and seventh leading cause of cancer death in the United States, bladder cancer is more common than is generally appreciated. Approximately 95% of urinary tract cancers occur in the bladder and are the most common urinary tract cancer in women. A majority of primary bladder cancers involve the bladder epithelium; the remaining 5% of urinary tract cancers occur in the renal pelvis and ureter. Overall incidence of bladder cancer is increasing in industrialized countries.

Etiologic and Risk Factors.   The cause of bladder cancer is unknown, but the carcinogens stored in the bladder and excreted in the urine have been linked to environmental factors, and susceptibility genes have been identified.[71] Although numerous risk factors have been identified (Box 17-3), many people with bladder cancer have no known carcinogens or risk factors.[13]

BOX **17-3**

Risk Factors for Bladder Cancer

Male gender
Age 50 and older
Cigarette smoking
Occupational exposures
• Combustion gas (e.g., diesel exhaust, asphalt fumes)
• Arsenic
• Dyes
• Benzidine
• Chemotherapeutic agents (e.g., phosphoramide mustards)
European descent
Western industrialized nation
History of chronic bladder infections, bladder stones, or previous tumors
Under investigation
• Gene-environment interaction
• Ingestion of red meat
• Chlorination byproducts in drinking water
• Regular intake of laxatives
• Daily consumption of 3 L or more of cold drinks
• Coffee
• Diabetes mellitus
• Hair dyes

Transitional cell carcinoma of the bladder was one of the earliest cancers to be linked with environmental hazards. A markedly higher incidence of bladder cancer has been documented in industries such as aniline dye industry and leather, rubber, diesel fuel, and paint manufacturing. Men are affected two to four times more often than women, and 80% of the population is 50 years of age and older, pointing to a delayed response.

Cigarette smoking has also been associated with a significant risk of developing bladder cancer. One of the first noted bladder carcinogens, 2-naphthylamine, is absorbed from unfiltered cigarette smoke. Cigarette smoking may be responsible for as many as 50% of male cases and 33% of female cases.[12,49] The relationship between coffee and bladder cancer remains controversial despite decades of research. Multiple studies with varying results have not been able to clear up this issue.[76] However, in general, reduced fluid intake may be a risk factor because reduced urinary frequency increases the time of contact between carcinogens and the bladder epithelium.[50]

Pathogenesis.   Tumors of the urinary collecting system can arise from epithelial, mesenchymal, or hematopoietic tissues, but the majority of bladder cancers arise from the epithelium. Approximately 90% to 98% of these cancers are transitional cell carcinomas with squamous cell carcinomas and adenocarcinomas making up the remainder. Bladder cancer is believed to develop through reversible premalignant stages followed by irreversible steps, ending in invasive cancer that can give rise to distant metastases. Variations in the clinical course suggest that different forms of bladder cancer develop along different molecular pathways, leading to tumor presentations of various malignant potential.[83]

The systemic absorption of environmental carcinogens, including cigarette smoke, followed by urinary excretion exposes the urinary epithelium to concentrated levels of the agents for prolonged periods. This interaction of the urine-soluble carcinogens with the epithelium is known as contact chemical carcinogenesis. The precise molecular events leading to the formation of bladder cancer are not known.

Clinical Manifestations.   Hematuria is the most common sign of bladder cancer. Gross hematuria is present in up to 75% to 80% of people with this condition, and microscopic hematuria is present in a majority of the remainder. The onset of hematuria is often sudden and frequently intermittent; the degree of hematuria is not related to the volume of tumor or its stage.[22] The intermittent pattern can result in a delay in diagnosis. Other signs of voiding dysfunction may also be present, including frequency, urgency, and dysuria.

In the presence of metastatic disease, back pain secondary to bony invasion or involvement of the periaortic lymph nodes may occur. Supraclavicular lymphadenopathy and hepatomegaly may also occur. Lymphedema of the lower extremities may occur secondary to locally advanced masses or pelvic lymph node involvement.

Medical Management
Diagnosis.   Bladder cancer is seldom recognized in its preclinical stage but rather is detected at cystoscopy and almost never recognized as an incidental finding. The diagnosis may be confirmed by transurethral resection or biopsy. The first diagnostic determination is whether the tumor is superfi-

cial or muscle invasive. More elaborate staging techniques (e.g., bone scan, ultrasonography, IVP) are only used for muscle-invasive bladder cancer because it is very rare for metastases to be associated with superficial disease. Confirmation is obtained with cystoscopy and transurethral resection. An abdominal CT scan, bone scan, and chest film can be used to investigate potential spread of the disease.

A number of urine-based markers, including telomerase (see Chapter 8), are under investigation for their potential usefulness in diagnosing transitional cell cancer and in monitoring for recurrence.[41]

Staging.   A staging scheme based on the progressive depth of involvement of the bladder wall by the tumor has been used to assign treatment and to assess outcomes and prognosis. Using the tumor, node, metastasis (TNM) method of staging, tumors confined to the papillary epithelial layer are classified as stage Ta, and flat in situ carcinomas are classified as Tis. Tumors that have penetrated the basement membrane and infiltrated into the submucosal lamina propria are classified as stage T1. Muscle-invasive tumors, depending on whether superficial or deep muscle invasion has taken place, are classified as T2 or T3a. Invasion of the bladder wall may obstruct the ureter, causing hydroureter. Tumors that have invaded the perivesical fat are classified as stage T3b. Tumors invading the pelvic viscera (e.g., the prostatic stroma, rectum, uterus, vagina, pelvic side walls) are classified as stage T4 (Fig. 17-6). Distant sites of metastasis include the liver, lung, and bone.

Prevention.   Approximately half of all bladder cancers in men are the result of cigarette smoking, and a large portion of the remainder are caused by industrial or agricultural carcinogens. Reducing exposure to these carcinogens would lower the incidence of this type of malignancy. Large total fluid intake may reduce the risk of bladder cancer by reducing the time of contact between carcinogens and the bladder epithelium.[6,50] Chemoprevention through the use of vitamins (A, B_6, C, and E) and zinc, combined with immunotherapy has been shown to reduce the long-term recurrence of bladder cancer by 40%.[45] Increasing consumption of fruits and vegetables and taking supplemental vitamins may be beneficial in reducing the incidence of bladder cancer.[44]

Early detection of bladder cancer when still superficial can reduce mortality. Evidence does suggest that screening men at risk who are older than 50 years can significantly lower the incidence of invasive disease and the mortality. Improved urinary markers will help improve screening programs.

Treatment.   Treatment of bladder cancer is determined on the basis of clinical and histologic findings and depends on the extent of the lesion and the person's general health. For treatment management, bladder cancer is distinguished as (1) superficial tumor with high risk of progression and recurrence (transurethral resection is standard for superficial bladder cancer in conjunction with bacille Calmette-Guérin [BCG] immunotherapy) and (2) muscle-invasive tumors (radical treatment is required and organ preservation as an alternative to standard radical cystectomy remains under investigation).

More advanced cancer requires resection of the pelvic lymph nodes. In men, the prostate and seminal vesicles may also be removed; in women, the uterus may be removed.

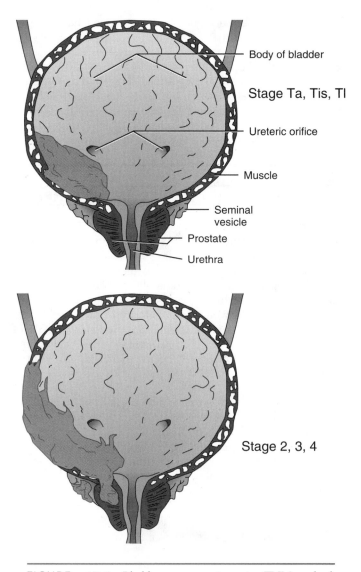

Stage Ta, Tis, TI

— Body of bladder

— Ureteric orifice

— Muscle

— Seminal vesicle

— Prostate

— Urethra

Stage 2, 3, 4

FIGURE   **17-6**   Bladder cancer staging using TNM method.

Radiotherapy in conjunction with concurrent chemotherapy is carried out, followed by salvage cystectomy in cases of residual tumor.[24] Radiotherapy alone or in a combination with chemotherapy remains the treatment of choice in cases of recurrent and/or metastatic bladder cancer.

Salvage cystectomy and bladder transplantation remain treatment options under continued investigation. In the future, understanding the pathogenesis of bladder cancer might lead to a more precise identification of particular tumors with regard to individualized strategies for treatment and prophylaxis.[83]

Prognosis.   Despite the continued increase in the number of new cases occurring each year, the mortality attributed to bladder cancer has remained relatively constant. Stage, grade, and possibly p53 status (see Chapter 8) of the tumor are prognostic indicators for local failure.[72] Bladder cancer is highly sensitive to chemotherapy and immunotherapy but also has a high incidence of local recurrence usually within the first 2 years. Approximately 30% of cases develop metastasis during the course of the disease, and 50% of individuals with muscle-invasive disease at the time of diagnosis already have distant metastases.[44] Although rare, long-term survival with recurrent cancer can be achieved in some individuals. Continued improvements in the management of bladder cancer will improve the prognosis in the future.

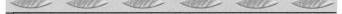

Special Implications for the Therapist   17-7

BLADDER CANCER

The risk of severe late-radiation sequelae is low (less than 5%), and about 75% of long-term survivors maintain a normally functioning bladder.[24] The therapist may likely treat those individuals who have residual bladder control problems. The high rate of cancer recurrence requires therapists to be vigilant in observing for the onset or return of symptoms and signs suggestive of urogenital system disease or metastatic spread. Anyone reporting visible blood in the urine must be evaluated further by a physician. ■

◆ Neurogenic Bladder Disorders

Overview.   The sensorimotor innervation of the urinary bladder can be interrupted at multiple levels, resulting in urinary dysfunction. Neurologic lesions above the sacral micturition reflex center level typically result in spastic bladder dysfunction. Reflex neurogenic bladder, spastic neurogenic bladder, cord bladder, and uninhibited bladder are terms used to describe neurogenic disorders that result in spastic bladder dysfunction. Neurogenic lesions at the level of the sacral micturition reflex center or affecting the peripheral innervation of the bladder typically result in flaccid bladder dysfunction.

Neurogenic bladder disorders can result in a variety of bladder abnormalities. These include diminished bladder capacity, a constricted external bladder sphincter, an atonic bladder that is unable to contract, a hyperactive detrusor (bladder) muscle, and loss of perception of bladder fullness. The inability of the bladder to function normally can lead to serious complications such as ascending UTIs; vesicoureteral reflux, which can seriously impair kidney function; and urinary calculi.

Etiologic Factors.   The common disorders that can result in spastic bladder dysfunction include cerebrovascular accident, dementia, Parkinson's, multiple sclerosis, and brain tumors. Spastic bladder dysfunction can also occur secondary to spinal cord lesions such as spinal cord injury, herniated intervertebral disk, vascular lesions, spinal cord tumors, and myelitis. Local pelvic irritation can result in spasm of the external bladder sphincter, impairing urinary function. The local irritation can occur in the presence of vaginitis, perineal inflammation, urethral inflammation, and chronic prostatitis. Flaccid bladder dysfunction can be secondary to meningomyelocele, spina bifida, diabetes mellitus, and anxiety or depression.

Pathogenesis.   The type of bladder disorder that occurs is dependent on the underlying cause. After a stroke or in the early stages of multiple sclerosis, an uninhibited bladder can develop. The sacral reflex arc and sensation are retained, the urine stream is normal, but the bladder capacity is diminished secondary to increased detrusor muscle tone and spasticity.

Conditions that affect the micturition center in the brainstem or impair reflex activity between the micturition center and the spinal cord can affect the coordinated activity of the detrusor muscle and the external bladder sphincter. This event is termed *detrusor-sphincter dyssynergia*. The external sphincter tightens during micturition as the detrusor muscle is contracting, resulting in increased intravesicular pressure and vesicoureteral reflux.

Immediately after a spinal cord injury, all reflexes are depressed. During this phase, the urinary bladder is atonic. Catheterization is essential to prevent overdistention of the bladder. One to 2 months after injury the reflexes become hyperactive. Frequent, spontaneous detrusor muscle contractions result in a small, hyperactive bladder. The act of voiding is interrupted, involuntary, or incomplete. In addition, high pressure voiding can cause vesicoureteral reflux and renal damage.

Diabetic bladder neuropathy occurs in 43% to 87% of people with type 1 diabetes mellitus.[30] Initially, the sensory supply of the bladder is affected, resulting in decreased urinary frequency. Then urinary hesitancy, weakness of stream, dribbling, and a sensation of the bladder not being fully emptied occurs. Vesicoureteral reflux and ascending UTIs are potential complications.

Clinical Manifestations.   Neurogenic bladder dysfunction is manifested by partial or complete urinary retention, incontinence, urgency, or frequent urination.

Medical Management

Diagnosis.   Numerous urologic tests are used to assess the anatomic and physiologic status of the bladder and associated structures. Serial cystometrograms provide an index of detrusor functional capacity, and cystourethroscopic evaluation determines the degree of bladder outlet obstruction. IV urography, ultrasonography, and cystosonography help assess the anatomic status of the bladder. Urodynamic evaluation to assess bladder function includes voiding flow rates, sphincter electromyograms (EMGs), and urethral pressure profile studies.

Treatment.   The primary goals of treatment include preventing incontinence, bladder overdistention, UTIs, and renal damage. Treatment modalities include catheterization, bladder training, surgery, and pharmacologic bladder manipulation.

Catheterization is a commonly employed intervention. Permanent indwelling catheters are used in people who are debilitated and have urinary retention or incontinence. In addition, if conservative or surgical options for treatment of incontinence are not feasible, permanent indwelling catheters may be used. Although a medical necessity in certain situations, permanent indwelling catheters also carry a risk. UTIs, urethral irritation, epididymo-orchitis, pyelonephritis, renal calculi, and cancer have all been associated with the use of permanent indwelling catheters in people with spinal cord injury.[21,82]

Intermittent catheterization is used to treat urinary retention and prevents bladder overdistention when performed at 3- to 4-hour intervals. Advantages of intermittent versus permanent catheterization include decreased urethral irritation and periodic bladder distention, which maintains some degree of muscle tone. Intermittent catheterization is often used in conjunction with pharmacologic intervention.

Medications are used to relax the external sphincter, decrease the outflow resistance of the internal sphincter, and alter the muscle tone of the bladder. Pharmacologic muscle relaxants such as diazepam (Valium) and baclofen (Lioresal) are used to decrease external sphincter tone. Parasympathomimetic drugs (except bethanechol chloride [Urecholine]) can increase bladder muscle tone, and anticholinergic drugs (except propantheline bromide [Pro-Banthine]) will decrease detrusor muscle tone and increase bladder capacity.

A variety of surgical interventions for neurogenic bladder exist. Sphincterectomy or transurethral resection of the bladder neck is performed in men with prostatic hyperplasia. Reconstruction of the sphincter, nerve resection, and urinary diversion are also surgical options. Resection of the sacral reflex nerves and of the pudendal nerve that controls the external sphincter can be done when spasticity is present.

Lastly, bladder-training methods are designed to enhance bladder function and prevent complications. Adequate fluid intake is essential for the prevention of infection and overconcentrated urine. With a hyperreflexive bladder or detrusor-sphincter dyssynergia the abnormally concentrated urine can stimulate afferent nerve endings, exacerbating the bladder disorder. This could increase vesicular pressures, vesicoureteral reflux, and overflow incontinence. Fluid intake must be controlled and monitored to prevent bladder distention. Biofeedback techniques using EMG or cystometry help the person control external sphincter function or increase intravesicular pressure sufficiently to overcome outflow resistance.

Special Implications for the Therapist   17-8

NEUROGENIC BLADDER DISORDERS

Preferred Practice Patterns:
See also Special Implications for the Therapist: Urinary Incontinence, 17-9.
5C: *Impaired Motor Function and Sensory Integrity Associated With Nonprogressive Disorders of the Central Nervous System—Congenital Origin or Acquired in Infancy or Childhood*
5D: *Impaired Motor Function and Sensory Integrity Associated With Nonprogressive Disorders of the Central Nervous System—Acquired in Adolescence or Adulthood*
5F: *Impaired Peripheral Nerve Integrity and Muscle Performance Associated With Peripheral Nerve Injury (flaccid bladder)*
5H: *Impaired Motor Function, Peripheral Nerve Integrity, and Sensory Integrity Associated With Nonprogressive Disorders of the Spinal Cord*

Therapists provide care for many people who have sustained spinal cord injuries and cerebrovascular accidents or who have myelomeningocele, multiple sclerosis, and brain tumors. Neurogenic bladder disorders are usually only one of the com-

plications associated with these conditions, but familiarity with this complication is important. The potential for UTIs, renal calculi, and renal damage is high in those with neurogenic bladder disorders. Familiarity with the signs and symptoms associated with these potential diseases is a necessity. The development of any of these co-morbidities can interfere with the rehabilitation process. Several medical conditions such as UTI, diabetes, congestive heart failure, bladder cancer, and enlarged prostate can be mistaken for a bladder control problem. Detection of any of these symptoms warrants communication with a physician.

Incontinence associated with any of the bladder conditions discussed here can be greatly improved and even eliminated in many people through a program of exercise and behavioral intervention. Specific guidelines are available.[35,36,75,80] ∎

◆ Urinary Incontinence
See the section on Pelvic Floor Disorders in Chapter 19.

Definition and Overview.   *Urinary incontinence* (UI) may be defined as an involuntary loss of urine that is sufficient to be a problem and occurs most often when bladder pressure exceeds sphincter resistance.[27] The following four categories can be used to classify UI:

1. *Functional incontinence* includes people who have normal urine control but who have difficulty reaching a toilet in time because of muscle or joint dysfunction.
2. *Stress incontinence* is the loss of urine during activities that increase intraabdominal pressure such as coughing, lifting, or laughing.
3. *Urge incontinence* is the sudden unexpected urge to urinate and the uncontrolled loss of urine. Urge incontinence is often related to reduced bladder capacity or detrusor instability (the latter is also referred to as *overactive bladder, hyperreflexive bladder, detrusor-sphincter dyssynergia,* or *detrusor hyperreflexia*).
4. *Overflow incontinence* is the constant leaking of urine from a bladder that is full but unable to empty. Some people can have more than one type of incontinence (most often stress and urge incontinence together), known as *mixed incontinence.*

UI is common, yet the condition is poorly understood, underdiagnosed, and often inadequately treated. Many people are embarrassed to acknowledge that they are incontinent. Only 20% to 50% of incontinent adults seek medical care.[81] Others regard incontinence as part of the normal aging process. The economic price tag associated with UI is estimated to be greater than $8 billion per year in the United States. Incontinence can be a significant contributory factor related to pressure sores, UTIs, institutionalization, depression, and isolation.

Prevalence.   UI is more prevalent in women than men and in the aging over the young. The prevalence of UI was first reported in 1988 at the National Institutes of Health Consensus Conference on Adult Urinary Incontinence. At that time, an estimated 10 million adults in the United States experienced incontinence, including 15% to 30% of the community-dwelling older adult and more than 50% of nursing home residents.[15] Others cite a range of 13 to 25 million individuals in the United States.[27] In fact, it is estimated that 50% of all admissions to skilled nursing facilities today are a direct result of UI, and another large portion of affected individuals are homebound.

Since the first Consensus Conference, an increased awareness of and focus on the problem of UI has come about. Until recently, the impact of UI on working women employed full time, a population generally characterized as healthy, has not been the focus of research. One survey at a large university center reported 21% of the women surveyed (age 18 and older) reported UI at least monthly.[28] Lastly, 28% of nulliparous elite college athletes reported urine loss while participating in their sport.[57]

Risk Factors.   A wide range of factors can contribute to the increased risk of developing UI (Box 17-4). In women, weakness or damage to the pelvic floor musculature (see Figs. 19-5 and 19-6), which changes the posterior ureterovesical angle, may occur secondary to normal aging, childbirth, or pelvic surgery. With the loss of this angle, any activity that places caudal pressure on the bladder results in involuntary flow of urine. These activities include coughing, laughing, sneezing, and lifting, all of which increase intraabdominal pressure (see Box 15-1). Overflow incontinence can occur as a result of conditions that cause urethral or bladder neck obstruction, such as BPH (see Chapter 18); fecal impaction; or organ prolapse (see Figs. 19-7 and 19-8).

Consistent evidence shows that frequency of UI increases with age, but little information is available on the frequency of different types of incontinence in different ages. A variety of factors may contribute to this phenomenon. Pelvic relaxation disorders such as what survivors of childhood or adult sexual assault (men and women) may experience can contribute to the development of incontinence. Menopause contributes to increased incontinence, and hormone replacement therapy does not seem to be a cure, although it may help in some cases. For men, BPH, prostatectomy, dementia, impaired mobility, and medications are the most common risk factors for UI.

Medications commonly prescribed for other illnesses and disease in older adult age groups can also increase the risk of incontinence. These pharmacologic agents can interfere with conscious inhibition of voiding, induce a quick diuresis, induce urinary retention, and reduce urethral resistance to the point of stress incontinence. Tranquilizers and sedatives may impair awareness of the usual cues related to urinary urgency and may also depress the cerebral corticoregulatory tract affecting detrusor muscle activity. Drugs producing anticholinergic side effects (e.g., major tranquilizers and antiparkinsonian agents) may cause urinary retention because of failure of bladder contraction.

Inadequate fluid intake and known bladder irritants (e.g., caffeine, acidic or citrus and spicy foods, alcohol) can also contribute to the development of UI. The bladder responds to fluid volume by expanding or contracting. Reduced fluid intake causes the bladder to shrink; less fluid means more concentrated urine irritating the bladder and less fluid results in a smaller bladder causing more frequent messages to the brain to toilet. Constipation may cause urethral obstruction and overflow incontinence. These clients will also be at risk for UTIs resulting in bladder irritability and an increased risk of incontinence. Lastly, as older adults lose their mobility and manual dexterity secondary to a multitude of ailments, including

---

BOX 17-4

Risk Factors for Urinary Incontinence

Altered local anatomy and physiology
  Anatomic fault
  Pelvic floor muscle weakness (e.g., normal aging; pregnancy/multiple pregnancies; prolonged childbirth/delivery [vaginal or cesarean section]; episiotomy; large gestational weight; any pelvic surgery including prostatectomy for men)
  Congenital sphincter muscle weakness or damaged sphincter muscle
  Pudendal nerve damage (e.g., childbirth trauma, pelvic surgery, radiation)
Neurologic disorder (e.g., myelomeningocele, multiple sclerosis, brain injury, Parkinson's, cerebral palsy, spinal cord injury, stroke)
High-impact physical activities
Restrictive clothing, restraints
Psychogenic (e.g., childhood and/or adult sexual trauma for both males and females, negative sexual experiences, emotional stress)
History of BPH
Constipation, fecal impaction
Tobacco use
Urinary tract infections
Medications
  Diuretics
  Tranquilizers, sedatives
  Hypertensives
  Alpha-adrenergic blockers (antihistamines, decongestants)
  Antiparkinson agents
  Tricyclic antidepressants
Decreased estrogen (deficiency)
Bladder irritation
  UTI
  Caffeine
  Alcohol
  Citrus fruits (acidic)
  Perfumed products (e.g., bubble bath, toilet paper, feminine hygiene products)
Inadequate fluid intake
Loss of ADL skills for toileting
Decreased or impaired mobility
Impaired cognitive function
Radiation therapy
Obesity

BPH, Benign prostatic hyperplasia; *UTI,* urinary tract infection.

---

arthritis, getting to the bathroom or commode in a timely fashion and manipulating clothing become increasingly difficult.

Less defined but under investigation is the role of ethnicity; menopausal status; history of gynecologic surgery; body mass index (i.e., obesity); smoking; and coffee and alcohol consumption on the risk of UI. Obesity is a common condition among women in developed countries and is believed to have a major impact on stress incontinence. The proposed mechanisms for this association include the increased intraabdominal pressures that adversely stress the pelvic floor and the effect of obesity on the neuromuscular function of the genitourinary tract.[17]

Pathogenesis and Clinical Manifestations.

Incontinence most often occurs when bladder pressure is greater than urethral sphincter pressure with general signs and symptoms of wet clothes or wet adult diaper, bedwetting, and/or direct observation of urine loss. *Functional incontinence* is the consequence of chronic impairments of physical or cognitive function and does not have a pathophysiologic origin. It is manifested similarly to urge incontinence.

Urge incontinence is often caused by involuntary bladder (detrusor) spasms and is associated with both increased frequency and urgency. It is often associated with neurologic conditions such as stroke, multiple sclerosis, advanced diabetes, spinal cord injury, senile dementia, or Alzheimer's. In the case of UI associated with a dyssynergistic or incoordinated bladder, (1) the bladder wall contracts while the ring-like sphincter that circles the urethral outlet remains closed,* resulting in a sense of urgency followed by hesitancy in the beginning of the void, or (2) the bladder wall relaxes while the sphincter remains open, resulting in dribbling or incontinence. It is characterized by leakage (sometimes large volume accidents) after a precipitant urge to urinate; events such as trying to insert a key in the door, running hands under water (or hearing running water), or passing by a bathroom.

Stress incontinence results from weakness or loss of tone in the pelvic floor muscles, urethral sphincter failure, hypermobility of the ureterovesical junction, and damage to the pudendal nerve (e.g., tumor, childbirth). It is accompanied by leakage that is coincident with increases in intraabdominal pressure (e.g., coughing, sneezing, laughing, bending, high-impact physical activity or exercise). Someone with mixed urge and stress incontinence may exhibit signs of both types. Other clinical manifestations, depending on the underlying pathology, may include constant dribbling, leakage without warning, frequency, urgency, nocturia, hesitancy, weak stream, or straining to void. Prolapsed bladder, uterus, and/or bowel may accompany or contribute to leakage especially when caused by multiple pregnancies and deliveries.

Overflow incontinence is usually the result of a neurologic problem such as hypotonic or underactive detrusor secondary to drugs, fecal impaction, diabetes, lower spinal cord injury, or multiple sclerosis. It can also occur as the result of obstruction (e.g., prostatic hyperplasia, genital prolapse, or surgical overcorrection of urethral detachment in women). In this situation, intravascular pressure will exceed the maximal urethral pressure as the bladder distends. Overflow incontinence is characterized by a variety of signs and symptoms, including frequent or constant dribbling, urge or stress incontinence signs and symptoms, or urinary urgency and frequent urination.

Medical Management

Prevention.   Preventive education is the key to eliminating a large majority of incontinence. Many health care professionals advocate early education to adolescent girls and young women before becoming pregnant. Prepartum and postpartum pelvic floor muscle training has been shown to have immediate and long-term effects in preventing incontinence, improving quality of life, and improving sexual dysfunction.[4,52,53]

Proper instruction in pelvic floor exercise emphasizing both fast-twitch and slow-twitch muscle fibers is an important part of prevention. Brief, verbal or written instruction in performing a Kegel pelvic muscle contraction is not adequate preparation as measured in more than 50% of cases investigated.[7] A properly performed "Kegel" exercise should result in a significant increase in the force of the urethral closure without an appreciable Valsalva's effort. Improperly done, the Kegel technique can potentially promote incontinence. A trained practitioner such as a physical therapist can provide assessment and training with necessary biofeedback to ensure the success of a properly performed exercise program.

Avoiding constipation through proper nutrition, adequate hydration, and responding to the need to toilet should be part of health curriculum in schools. The therapist can be very instrumental in establishing screening programs for all ages to assess for risk factors for UI or for the presence of incontinence and teaching proper lifting techniques, lifestyle management, behavioral techniques, and pelvic floor protection during increased abdominal pressure (e.g., lifting, laughing, coughing, sneezing, vomiting). Anyone experiencing leaking during exercise needs a prescriptive exercise program both for the leaking and modifying the exercise that precipitates the leaking.

Diagnosis.   Urinating more than eight times a day and/or two or more times a night and a sudden overwhelming urge to urinate are symptoms of urgency often associated with urge incontinence. A history of urgency accompanied by sudden involuntary voiding of urine is the hallmark diagnostic sign of UI. Normal bladder control is a minimum of 2 hours and usually gauged as 3 to 5 hours without toileting. Since UI is related to a wide variety of disorders and factors, a detailed investigation may be necessary to determine the cause(s). An important part of this investigation is a voiding diary to determine the frequency, timing, and amount of voiding and to assess the numerous other factors potentially associated with incontinence.[27]

A careful history will investigate medication usage, prescribed and OTC; past and current illnesses; and surgical and birth histories. Urinalysis and urodynamic evaluation are important to rule out the presence of diseases such as UTI, diabetes, bladder cancer, and others and to assess bladder and sphincter function, respectively.

Cystometry is used to assess bladder capacity, sensation, voluntary control, and contractility. Cystometry consists of filling the bladder with water or carbon dioxide and recording changes in intravesicular pressure. When stress incontinence is suspected, provocative stress testing is carried out. The client is asked to cough vigorously while the examiner observes for urine loss. The test is initially done in the lithotomy position but if negative, is repeated in a standing position.[27] Dynamic MRI is being investigated to study specific aspects of voiding associated with stress incontinence.[3,34]

---

*Normally, the bladder is designed to hold a pint of urine for several hours. As it fills, the detrusor muscle relaxes to allow the bladder to stretch and accommodate more urine; the sphincter contracts to prevent urine from escaping through the urethra. Pelvic floor muscles also support the base of the bladder and close off the bladder end of the urethra, further blocking the flow of urine. When the bladder is full, a message to get to the bathroom is received, at which time the sphincter and pelvic muscles relax, allowing urine to flow into the urethra while the detrusor muscle contracts to squeeze the urine out of the bladder.

Treatment. Management of UI depends on the type of incontinence and the person's age and general health but usually falls into one of three categories: behavioral, pharmacologic, and surgical. Behavioral intervention is considered the first line of treatment for pelvic muscle rehabilitation and includes a combination of lifestyle and dietary changes, prescriptive exercises including Kegel exercises and Beyond Kegel™ exercises,[36] pelvic floor electrical stimulation, biofeedback therapy, support devices such as pessaries,* and vaginal weight training. A new technology using noninvasive pulsed magnetic fields (extracorporeal magnetic innervation) has been developed and tested in clinical trials for pelvic floor muscle strengthening. Preliminary studies demonstrated as much as a 77% improvement after 6 weeks with 45% remaining improved at 18 weeks.[31] The FDA has approved this therapy for stress, urge, and mixed incontinence. Long-term outcomes are unknown; further studies are under way.

Stress Incontinence. Stress incontinence can be treated by physiotherapeutic, surgical, and pharmacologic interventions, singly or in combination. A pessary may be recommended for women who only leak during one activity such as playing tennis or high-intensity aerobics. Medications used to relieve urge incontinence may include estrogen replacement therapy (ERT); alpha-adrenergic blockers (e.g., phenylpropanolamine) to increase bladder outlet/sphincteric tone; and combination therapy with tricyclic antidepressant agents and antidiuretic hormone. Surgery may be used to correct a cystocele or alter the position of the bladder neck; collagen injections may be administered to increase sphincteric resistance. A bladder neck suspension procedure is used to prevent the bladder neck from displacing caudally when straining.

Urge Incontinence. Various interventions are used to treat urge incontinence, with the primary focus being behavioral modification; exercise therapy; bladder retraining; stress reduction; dietary changes (e.g., eliminating known bladder irritants including caffeine, acidic or citrus and spicy foods, alcohol); and pharmacologic therapy. Recommended medications for urge incontinence include antispasmodics, anticholinergics, ERT, and tricyclic antidepressants.

Other forms of treatment include catheterization, penile clamps, disposable urethral plug, urine collection devices, and surgically implanted artificial sphincters and bladder generators. A generator implanted in the abdominal wall sends impulses to the nerves that control the bladder functioning similarly to a heart pacemaker. Careful diagnosis to determine the type of incontinence and the underlying cause will allow for the proper choice of interventions.

Overflow Incontinence. Medical intervention may use pharmacotherapy (alpha-adrenergic antagonists, cholinergic agonists); clean, intermittent catheterization; and possibly surgery (e.g., bladder pacemaker, stricture dilation, prostatectomy, anterior vaginal repair), depending on the etiologic factors.

---

*Pessaries are devices inserted into the vagina that are designed to support the bladder and bladder neck. These devices come in a variety of shapes and sizes and are made of flexible or rigid silicone, latex, or acrylic. Some pessaries can stay in the vagina for up to 3 months before being removed, cleaned, and replaced; others are used just during exercise or sexual intercourse. A properly fitted pessary should not interfere with bowel or bladder function and should not be uncomfortable.

Special Implications for the Therapist   17-9

URINARY INCONTINENCE

See the section on Pelvic Floor Disorders in Chapter 19.
Preferred Practice Patterns:
   Selection of the most appropriate practice patterns depends in part on the underlying etiologic factors and pathogenesis of the UI.
4C: *Impaired Muscle Performance*
4D: *Impaired Joint Mobility, Motor Function, Muscle Performance, and Range of Motion Associated With Connective Tissue Dysfunction*
4I: *Impaired Joint Mobility, Motor Function, Muscle Performance, and Range of Motion Associated With Bony or Soft Tissue Surgery*
5B: *Impaired Neuromotor Development (spina bifida, myelomeningocele)*
5C: *Impaired Motor Function and Sensory Integrity Associated With Nonprogressive Disorders of the Central Nervous System—Congenital Origin or Acquired in Infancy or Childhood*
5F: *Impaired Peripheral Nerve Integrity and Muscle Performance Associated With Peripheral Nerve Injury (pudendal nerve injury)*
5H: *Impaired Motor Function, Peripheral Nerve Integrity, and Sensory Integrity Associated With Nonprogressive Disorders of the Spinal Cord*
7A: *Primary Prevention/Risk Reduction for Integumentary Disorders*

Therapists have an important direct role in the assessment and treatment intervention of UI. Physical therapy guides the rehabilitation of muscle imbalance and pelvic alignment and promotes pelvic muscle awareness and function through biofeedback, electrostimulation, therapeutic exercise, and a behavioral management approach.[8] The pelvic rehabilitation program is designed to prevent recurrence of the impairment and to restore bowel, bladder, sexual, and supportive muscle functioning.[67] Quality of life issues can be assessed using the Urge Impact Scale (URIS) for older people with urge incontinence.[23]

For some clients seen by therapists who do not specialize in pelvic floor rehabilitation, UI will be a co-morbidity or a condition that has yet to be evaluated. Many adults think that incontinence is an inevitable part of aging and do not report the problem. Any perimenopausal or postmenopausal woman; any woman who has been pregnant; anyone (male or female) over the age of 60 (earlier if prostate or bladder infection or cancer is evident); or any case of multiple risk factors should be screened for UI. Anyone with onset of incontinence with concomitant cervical spine pain (even without a history of trauma or known cause) may be experiencing cervical disc protrusion, requiring additional screening and evaluation. Additionally, the possibility of genitourinary disorders as a result of sexual abuse or assault exists and requires careful assessment.

The generally positive rapport that develops between client and therapist may facilitate the acknowledgment that UI exists and uncover the potential underlying risk factors. Specific questions should be included in the history to help bring this information to light such as the following:

Continued

Do you leak urine when you lift, cough, sneeze, or stand up?
Do you get up at night to urinate (how often)?
Do you go to the bathroom more often than every 2 to 3 hours?
How much water do you drink in a waking day?
Are you constipated?

The therapist may be in a position to direct the person to the appropriate physician for evaluation. Successful intervention in UI may enhance rehabilitation efforts geared to improve the client's physical and social activity level. A variety of examination, evaluation, and diagnosis tools and management options are available.[27,35,36,64,75,80,84] The National Association for Continence (http://www.nafc.org) also offers a wide variety of information, and the Women's Health Section of the American Physical Therapy Association offers a broad range of information and courses on incontinence specific to the physical therapist.

For an internal pelvic floor assessment, including a manual muscle test and assessment of trigger points, a consent-to-treat form is recommended. This form should include an explanation of the internal examination and specifically addresses the client's right to refuse or stop the evaluation at any time. Some clinicians offer to have a third person in the room during the assessment, either a friend or relative of the client's or another woman from the health care facility. Any unspoken behaviors or indication of discomfort on the part of the client should prompt the physical therapist to stop and communicate with the client before continuing or discontinuing. Issues of childhood incest or sexual assault or adult sexual issues may be a significant contributing factor, requiring combined pelvic muscle rehabilitation and psychotherapy or sexual abuse counseling.

Understanding the use of medications and potential side effects for these conditions is essential; many of the same medications used to treat incontinence can also cause incontinence if used inappropriately. Medications to treat other conditions can have side effects that cause incontinence. A concise listing of this information is available.[36]

Exercise and Incontinence

Studies to verify the effectiveness of exercise programs to strengthen pelvic muscles administered by nurses have provided evidence-based protocols.[69] Several references for physical therapy-based intervention approaches are also available,[4,52,53] but further research documentation of outcomes is needed.

Comparison of biofeedback and exercise programs administered by physical therapists showed equal effectiveness in reducing nocturnal urinary frequency and improved subjective outcome; only the group receiving physical therapy experienced reduced daytime urinary frequency.[58]

Although pelvic floor muscle exercises have proven effective in the short term, long-term noncompliance may hamper continued success. Predictors of compliance may include amount of urinary loss per wet episode and individual perception of the ability to do the exercises as recommended under various circumstances. This information should be taken into consideration during the education portion of any home program. Further studies to determine components of adherence behavior are needed.[1]

Stress Incontinence. Exercises can be performed to retrain and strengthen the pelvic floor musculature. This type of exercise has been advocated for decades.[40] Exercise manage-

ment including adductor and obturator assist and quick flick* exercises can help develop adequate sphincteric function and improve bladder and bladder outlet position in the pelvis. Restoring normal pelvic floor strength and bladder control is essential before resuming vigorous physical activity or exercise. The therapist is very instrumental in teaching contraction of the appropriate muscles (e.g., the pelvic diaphragm, urogenital diaphragm, and external sphincter muscles) without muscle contraction in the anal area or of the gluteal muscles and with complete relaxation of the pelvic muscles between contractions.

Physiologic quieting including hand warming, diaphragmatic breathing, and body/mind quieting can be used to normalize bladder function and autonomic nervous system innervation of bladder and bowel.[36] With verbal and manual cues, biofeedback (auditory, visual or electronic); physiologic quieting; and electromyography (EMG) (surface or intravaginal), the client can be taught to disassociate pelvic floor muscle activity from other hip and pelvic muscle activity and to maintain pelvic floor muscle tone while avoiding a Valsalva's maneuver. Weighted vaginal cones and electrical stimulation can also be used to rehabilitate the pelvic floor.

Urge Incontinence. Continence requires the ability to inhibit automatic detrusor contractions and pelvic floor exercises facilitate the use of urge inhibition techniques. The bladder needs to be trained to respond to a specific voiding schedule. Clients void at scheduled intervals to suppress the micturition reflux, increase bladder capacity, and decrease urinary frequency. The initial retraining interval is usually 60 minutes. The voiding intervals are increased by 15- to 60-minute extensions using urge inhibition if it occurs too soon. Success is marked by voiding at 3- to 4-hour intervals; continence (perhaps measured by number of pads used); minimal sensory symptoms; and functional capacity (minimum of 300 cc of urine or 8 or more seconds of a steady urine stream). Biofeedback (visual, auditory, or electronic) and physiologic quieting (e.g., diaphragmatic breathing) can also be used to train the client to inhibit abdominal muscle activity and bladder contractions, thereby reducing detrusor pressure.[81]

An episode of urge incontinence at least once a week increases the risk of fractures by 34% because of falls at night. Early diagnosis and appropriate treatment of urge incontinence may decrease the risk of fracture.[5] The therapist can be very instrumental in performing a home assessment for the older adult with urge incontinence. Placing strategically located nightlights near the bed, hallway to the bathroom, and bathroom and removing objects along the path (e.g., throw rugs) are essential preventive steps to take. For the individual with incontinence and postural orthostatic hypotension, low blood pressure (or even hypertensives with the potential for hypotension as a side effect) and rising from bed quickly at night can also result in falls. Assessing for this complication and teaching prevention measures are recommended (see the section on Orthostatic [Postural] Hypotension in Chapter 11). ■

---

*A "quick flick" exercise is the quick contract followed by release with full relaxation of the pelvic muscles while the gluteals, abdominals, adductors, and obturator internus muscles remain relaxed. Quick flicks are designed to improve the strength and function of the fast-acting fibers, primarily of the urogenital diaphragm and external sphincter muscles. These fibers are important for prevention of leaking during coughing, sneezing, lifting, and pulling because these fibers act with speed and intensity to maintain urinary control.[36]

REFERENCES

1. Alewijnse D et al: Predictors of intention to adhere to physiotherapy among women with urinary incontinence, *Health Educ Res* 16(2): 173-186, 2001.

2. Baldassare JS, Kaye D: Special problems of urinary tract infection in the elderly, *Med Clin North Am* 75:375-390, 1991.

3. Bo K et al: Dynamic MRI of the pelvic floor muscles in an upright sitting position, *Neurourol Urodyn* 20(2):167-174, 2001.

4. Bo K, Talseth T, Vinsnes A: Randomized controlled trial on the effect of pelvic floor muscle training on quality of life and sexual problems in genuine stress incontinent women, *Acta Obstet Gynecol Scand* 79(7): 598-603, 2000.

5. Brown JS et al: Urinary incontinence: does it increase risk for falls and fractures? Study of Osteoporotic Fractures Research Group, *J Am Geriatr Soc* 48(7):847-848, 2000.

6. Bruemmer B et al: Fluid intake and incidence of bladder cancer among middle-aged men and women in a three-county area of western Washington, *Nutr Cancer* 29(2):163-168, 1997.

7. Bump RC et al: Assessment of Kegel pelvic muscle exercise performance after brief verbal instruction, *Am J Obstet Gynecol* 165(2): 322-327, 1991.

8. Burgio KL et al: Behavioral vs. drug treatment for urge urinary incontinence in older women, *JAMA* 280(23):1995-2000, 1998.

9. Cashion AK et al: Heart rate variability, mortality, and exercise in patients with end-stage renal disease, *Prog Transplant* 10(1):10-16, 2000.

10. Centers for Disease Control and Prevention (CDC): National Center for Infectious Diseases: Viral Hepatitis, 2001. Available at http://www.cdc.gov/ncidod/diseases/hepatitis.

11. Childs R et al: Regression of metastatic renal-cell carcinoma after non-myeloablative allogeneic peripheral-blood stem-cell transplantation, *N Engl J Med* 343(11):750-758, 2000.

12. Chiu BC et al: Cigarette smoking and risk of bladder, pancreas, kidney, and colorectal cancers in Iowa, *Ann Epidemiol* 11(1):28-37, 2001.

13. Cohen SM, Shirai T, Steineck G: Epidemiology and etiology of premalignant and malignant urothelial changes, *Scand J Urol Nephrol Suppl* 205:105-115, 2000.

14. Colussi G et al: Medical prevention and treatment of urinary stones, *J Nephrol* 13:S65-S70, 2000.

15. Consensus Conference: Urinary incontinence in adults, *JAMA* 261:2685-2690, 1989.

16. Coppes MJ, Pritchard-Jones K: Principles of Wilms' tumor biology, *Urol Clin North Am* 27(3):423-433, 2000.

17. Cummings JM, Rodning CB: Urinary stress incontinence among obese women: review of pathophysiology therapy, *Int Urogynecol J Pelvic Flood Dysfunct* 11(1):41-44, 2000.

18. Curhan GC et al: Prospective study of beverage use and the risk of kidney stones, *Am J Epidemiol* 143(3):240-247, 1996.

19. Curhan GC et al: Beverage use and risk for kidney stones in women, *Ann Intern Med* 129(11):913, 1998.

20. Darnley MJ, DiMarco NM, Aukema HM: Safety of chronic exercise in a rat model of kidney disease, *Med Sci Sports Exer* 32(3):576-580, 2000.

21. Delnay KM et al: Bladder histological changes associated with chronic indwelling urinary catheter, *J Urol* 161(4):1106-1109, 1999.

22. Droller MJ: Bladder cancer: state-of-the-art care, *CA: Cancer J Clin* 48(5):269-284, 1998.

23. DuBeau CE, Kiely DK, Resnick NM: Quality of life impact of urge incontinence in older persons: a new measure and conceptual structure, *J Am Geriatr Soc* 47(8):989-994, 1999.

24. Dunst J et al: Bladder preservation in muscle-invasive bladder cancer by conservative surgery and radiochemotherapy, *Semin Surg Oncol* 20(1): 24-32, 2001.

25. Durstine JL et al: Physical activity for the chronically ill and disabled, *Sports Med* 30(3):207-219, 2000.

26. Elseviers MM, De Broe ME: Analgesic abuse in the elderly. Renal sequelae and management, *Drugs Aging* 12(5):391-400, 1998.

27. Fantl JA et al: Urinary incontinence in adults: acute and chronic management. Clinical Practice Guideline No 2, 1996 Update, Rockville, Md, US Department of Health and Human Services, Public Health Service, Agency for Health Care Policy and Research (AHCPR Pub No. 96-0682), March 1996.

28. Fitzgerald ST et al: Urinary incontinence. Impact on working women, *AAOHN J* 48(3):112-118, 2000.

29. Foxman B et al: Urinary tract infections: self-reported incidence and associated costs, *Ann Epidemiol* 10(8):509-515, 2000.

30. Frimodt-Miller C: Diabetic cystopathy: epidemiology and related disorders, *Ann Intern Med* 92:318, 1980.

31. Galloway NT et al: Update on extracorporeal magnetic innervation (ExMI) therapy for stress urinary incontinence, *Urology* 56(6 Suppl 1):82-86, 2000.

32. Godley PA, Ataga KI: Renal cell carcinoma, *Curr Opin Oncol* 12(3):260-264, 2000.

33. Healthy People 2010: Chronic kidney disease-objectives, 2001. Available at http://health.gov/healthypeople/.

34. Hedlund H et al: The clinical value of dynamic magnetic resonance imaging in normal and incontinent women: a preliminary study on micturition, *Scand J Urol Nephrol Suppl* 207:87-91, 2001.

35. Hulme J: *Beyond Kegels book II: a clinician's guide*, Missoula, Mont, 1999, Phoenix Publishing.

36. Hulme J: *Geriatric incontinence: a behavioral and exercise approach to treatment*, Missoula, Mont, 1999, Phoenix Publishing.

37. Ifudu O: Care of patients undergoing hemodialysis, *N Engl J Med* 339(15):1054-1062, 1998.

38. Jensen PB et al: Changes in cardiac muscle mass and function in hemodialysis patients during growth hormone treatment, *Clin Nephrol* 53(1):25-32, 2000.

39. Kajander EO et al: Nanobacteria: controversial pathogens in nephrolithiasis and polycystic kidney disease, *Curr Opin Nephrol Hypertens* 10(3):445-452, 2001.

40. Kegel AH: Progressive resistance exercises in the functional restoration of the perineal muscles, *Am J Obstet Gynecol* 56:238, 1948.

41. Konety BR, Getzenberg RH: Urine-based markers of urological malignancy, *J Urol* 165(2):600-611, 2001.

42. Kotarinos R: Interstitial cystitis, *J OB/GYN PT* 18(4):5-7, 1994.

43. Kutner NG, Zhang R, McClellan WM: Patient-reported quality of life early in dialysis treatment: effects associated with usual exercise activity, *Nephrol Nurs J* 27(4):357-367, 2000.

44. Lamm DL: Bladder cancer: twenty years of progress and the challenges that remain, *CA: Cancer J Clin* 48(5):263-268, 1998.

45. Lamm DL et al: Megadose vitamins in bladder cancer: a double-blind clinical trial, *J Urol* 151:21-26, 1994.

46. Lee SB, Haber DA: Wilms' tumor and the WI1 gene, *Exp Cell Res* 264(1):74-99, 2001.

47. Leutholtz BC, Ripoll I: *Exercise and disease management*, Boca Raton, Fla, 1999, CRC Press.

48. Mailloux LU: Hypertension in chronic renal failure and ESRD: prevalence, pathophysiology, and outcomes, *Semin Nephrol* 21(2): 146-156, 2001.

49. Marcus PM et al: Cigarette smoking, N-acetyltransferase 2 acetylation status and bladder cancer risk: a case-series meta-analysis of a gene-environment interaction, *Cancer Epidemiol Biomarkers Prev* 9(5): 461-467, 2000.

50. Michaud DS et al: Fluid intake and the risk of bladder cancer in men, *N Engl J Med* 340(18):1390-1397, 1999.

51. Moore GE: Exercise prescription in renal failure. In Shankar K, editor: *Exercise prescription*, Philadelphia, 1999, Hanley and Belfus.

52. Morkved S, Bo K: Effect of postpartum pelvic floor muscle training in prevention and treatment of urinary incontinence: a one-year follow up, *BJOG* 107(8):1022-1028, 2000.

53. Morkved S, Bo K: The effect of postpartum pelvic floor muscle exercise in the prevention and treatment of urinary incontinence, *Int Urogynecol J Pelvic Floor Dysfunct* 8(4):217-222, 1997.

54. National Kidney Foundation: About kidney disease, 2000. Available at http:www.kidney.org/general/about disease/.

55. National Kidney Foundation: Amount and choice of beverages can affect risk of kidney stones, 2000. Available at http://www.kidney.org/general/news/beverages.cfm.

56. National Kidney Foundation: Women with recurrent UTIs can self-treat (news release), 2000. Available at http://www.kidney.org/general/news/womenuti.cfm.

57. Nygaard IE et al: Urinary incontinence in elite nulliparous athletes, *Obstet Gynecol* 84:183-187, 1994.

58. Pages IH et al: Comparative analysis of biofeedback and physical therapy for treatment of urinary stress incontinence in women, *Am J Phys Med Rehabil* 80(7):494-502, 2001.

59. Painter PL: Exercise training during hemodialysis: rates of participation, *Dial Transpl* 17:165-168, 1988.

60. Painter PL et al: Low-functioning hemodialysis patients improve with exercise training, *Am J Kidney Dis* 36(3):600-608, 2000.

61. Painter PL et al: Physical functioning and health related quality of life changes with exercise training in hemodialysis patients, *Am J Kidney Dis* 35(3):482-492, 2000.

62. Painter PL et al: Effects of exercise training during hemodialysis, *Nephron* 43:87-92, 1986.

63. Pastan S, Bailey J: Dialysis therapy, *N Engl J Med* 338(20):1428-1437, 1998.

64. Pauls J: Urinary incontinence and impairment of the pelvic floor in the older adult. In Guccione AA, editor: *Geriatric physical therapy*, ed 2, St Louis, 2000, Mosby.

65. Perneger TV, Whelton PK, Klag MJ: Risk of kidney failure associated with the use of acetaminophen, aspirin and nonsteroidal anti-inflammatory drugs, *N Engl J Med* 331:1675-1679, 1994.

66. Powell CR et al: Impact of body weight on urinary electrolytes in urinary stone formers, *Urology* 55(6):825-830, 2000.

67. Press J, Lawler M, Smith JC: Physical medicine and rehabilitation, *JAMA* 282(10):925-926, 1999.

68. Sala E et al: Impaired muscle oxygen transfer in patients with chronic renal failure, *Am J Physiol Regul Integr Comp Physiol* 280(4):R1240-1248, 2001.

69. Sampselle CM et al: Continence for women: a test of AWHONN's evidence-based protocol in clinical practice, *J Wound Ostomy Continence Nurs* 27(2):109-117, 2000.

70. Schmeider RE, Delles C, Messerli FH: Diuretic therapy and the risk for renal cell carcinoma, *J Nephrol* 13(5):343-346, 2000.

71. Schnakenberg E et al: Susceptibility genes: GSTM1 and GSTM3 as genetic risk factors in bladder cancer, *Cytogenetic Cell Genet* 91(1-4):234-238, 2000.

72. Schuster TG, Smith DC, Montie JE: Pelvic recurrences post-cystectomy: current treatment strategies, *Semin Urol Oncol* 19(1):45-50, 2001.

73. Shekarriz B, Lu HF, Stoller ML: Correlation of unilateral urolithiasis with sleep posture, *J Urol* 165(4):1085-1087, 2001.

74. Stegall MD et al: Pancreas transplantation for the prevention of diabetic nephropathy, *Mayo Clin Proc* 75(1):49-56, 2000.

75. Stephenson R, O'Connor LJ: *Obstetric and gynecologic care in physical therapy*, ed 2, Thorofare, NJ, 2000, Slack.

76. Tavani A, La Vecchia C: Coffee and cancer: a review of epidemiological studies, 1990-1999, *Eur J Cancer Prev* 9(4):241-256, 2000.

77. Tsakiris D: Morbidity and mortality reduction associated with the use of erythropoietin, *Nephron* 85(Suppl 1):2-8, 2000.

78. Ungar A et al: Changes in renal autacoids and hemodynamics associated with aging and isolated systolic hypertension, *Prostaglandins Other Lipid Mediat* 62(2):117-133, 2000.

79. Van Poppel H et al: Precancerous lesions in the kidney, *Scand J Urol Nephrol Suppl* 205:136-165, 2000.

80. Wallace K, Sandalcidi D: Urinary incontinence step by step, 2001. Available at http://www.progressivetherapeutics.com or (888) 340-1500.

81. Weinberger MW: Conservative treatment of urinary incontinence, *Clin Obstet Gynecol* 38:175-188, 1995.

82. West DA et al: Role of chronic catheterization in the development of bladder cancer in patients with spinal cord injury, *Urology* 53(2):292-297, 1999.

83. Wiijkstrom H et al: Prevention and treatment of urologic premalignant and malignant tumors, *Scand J Urol Nephrol Suppl* 205:116-135, 2000.

84. Wilder E, editor: *Gynecologic physical therapy manual*, Alexandria, Washington, D.C., 1997, Women's Health Section of the American Physical Therapy Association. Available at http://www.apta.org.

CHAPTER 18

THE MALE GENITAL/REPRODUCTIVE SYSTEM

WILLIAM G. BOISSONNAULT AND CATHERINE C. GOODMAN

The male genital or reproductive system is made up of the testes, epididymis, vas deferens, seminal vesicles, prostate gland, and penis (Fig. 18-1). These structures are susceptible to inflammatory disorders, neoplasms, and structural defects. Unless treating individuals with urinary incontinence, therapists do not typically treat people for primary reproductive system disease, but because of the incidence and nature of these disorders, an understanding of their clinical presentation is essential.

Prostate cancer is the most common cancer in males in the United States, and testicular cancer, although relatively rare, is on the rise and the most common cancer in males age 15 to 35 years. Benign prostatic hyperplasia (BPH) is one of the most common disorders of the aging male population. Owing to the high incidence of these diseases, therapists will see clients with such a history, and the disorder or prescribed medical treatment could have a profound effect on the client's clinical presentation and response to treatment.

The initial presenting symptom for some of these disorders could be back pain, a condition for which physical therapy care is often sought. An awareness of other symptoms, besides pain, and signs associated with urogenital system diseases may alert the therapist to other origins of the back pain. The presence of such symptoms warrants communication with a physician regarding the client's status. Therapists have long been taught to ask clients with back pain questions regarding sexual function, the concern being the possible presence of cauda equina syndrome. An awareness of the more probable causes of sexual dysfunction help the therapist determine the relevance and potentially urgent nature of a client's complaints. The disorders discussed in this chapter are those of the highest incidence or of greatest implications for therapists.

AGING AND THE MALE REPRODUCTIVE SYSTEM

The reproductive system undergoes degenerative changes associated with aging that can affect sexual function. The testes become smaller, with thickening of the seminiferous tubules impeding sperm production; the prostate gland enlarges, potentially affecting urine outflow; and sclerotic changes occur in the local blood vessels, possibly resulting in sexual dysfunction (erectile dysfunction [ED]/impotence).

The age-related decrease in male sex hormone levels (androgen deficiency) also has significant local and systemic effects. Protein synthesis, salt and water balance, bone growth, and homeostasis and cardiovascular function are all under the influence of these hormones. A decline in bioavailable testosterone has been clearly correlated with age-related memory changes, decreasing sexual interest, and physical changes, including decreased strength, body mass, and bone density.[38]

DISORDERS OF THE PROSTATE

◆ Prostatitis

Overview. Inflammation of the prostate gland can be acute or chronic and bacterial or nonbacterial. These conditions are typically preceded by lower urinary tract infections (UTIs) (see Chapter 17). Therapists are least likely to encounter problems associated with acute prostatitis as the symptoms are usually severe enough that physician contact is initiated by the client (or family) and rehabilitation is typically placed on hold until the antibiotic therapy is successful. On the other hand, therapists are likely to encounter chronic bacterial prostatitis, which is a much more subtle disorder, and complete resolution with treatment is often difficult to obtain.

Incidence and Risk Factors. Prostatitis affects millions of men and about half of all men have at least one episode during their lifetime. The prevalence is highest among men in their 40s and older men especially prone to UTI develop prostatitis. Although generally occurring with much higher frequency in women than men, UTIs are among the more common infections, afflicting the male population secondary to bladder outlet obstruction associated with BPH. As the infection ascends through the urogenital system the prostate can become involved. Besides a history of UTI and BPH, recent urethral catheterization or instrumentation and multiple sexual partners increase the risk of developing prostatitis. Some men find that stress, emotional factors, alcohol, spicy foods, or caffeine triggers episodes. Lastly, poorly controlled diabetes mellitus increases the risk of UTI and prostatitis developing because the increased urine glucose provides the substrate for bacterial growth.

Etiologic Factors and Pathogenesis. The most common form of prostate inflammation is nonbacterial prostatitis. The underlying cause of nonbacterial prostatitis is unknown, but one possible cause is intraprostatic urine reflux. The urine reflux is theorized to cause a chemical prostatitis or to initiate an immunologic response to the urine. Autoimmunity may play a role in chronic prostatitis, since up to one third of men

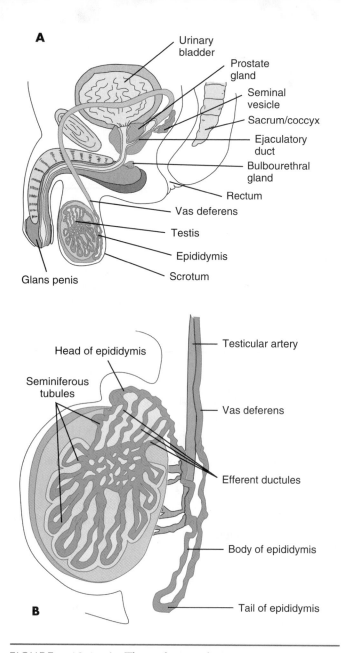

A, The male reproductive system. **B,** Internal structure of the testis and relationship of the testis to the epididymis. (From Guyton AC: *Anatomy and physiology*, Philadelphia, 1985, Saunders College Publishing.)

Labels for A:
Urinary bladder
Prostate gland
Seminal vesicle
Sacrum/coccyx
Ejaculatory duct
Bulbourethral gland
Rectum
Vas deferens
Testis
Epididymis
Scrotum
Glans penis

Labels for B:
Head of epididymis
Seminiferous tubules
Testicular artery
Vas deferens
Efferent ductules
Body of epididymis
Tail of epididymis

FIGURE 18-1

Ureaplasma species, chlamydiae, and mycoplasmata are possible etiologic factors.

Clinical Manifestations. See Table 18-1 for a summary of symptoms associated with nonbacterial prostatitis, chronic bacterial prostatitis, and acute bacterial prostatitis. Acute prostatitis occurs suddenly with severe symptoms. Fever, chills, and UTI are typical, along with pelvic discomfort. Blood in the urine, urinary retention, and urinary blockage are frequent, and there may be a steep rise in prostate antigen (PSA), a marker for prostate cancer. If not treated, acute prostatitis may become chronic. Men who experience chronic prostatitis (bacterial or nonbacterial) are plagued by persistent low-grade symptoms with flareups of pelvic pain and voiding problems and a marked decline in sexual function and emotional well-being. The pelvic pain is usually located behind the scrotum or in the perineum, the area between the rectum and testicles. This pain is usually made worse by sitting down and may be relieved by ejaculation. Pain in the tip of the penis may be experienced.

Medical Management
Diagnosis. Urinalysis, analysis of an expressed prostatic specimen, and a digital rectal examination (DRE) are used to establish a diagnosis of prostatitis. The DRE may reveal a swollen, tender, and warm prostate. Computed tomography (CT) and transrectal ultrasound are used if a prostatic abscess is suspected. Prostatitis is differentiated in part from BPH and prostate cancer by the presence of pain (rarely present in BPH or cancer) and by age (more than half of all men with prostatitis are younger than 45).

Treatment. Because the cause of nonbacterial prostatitis is unknown, treatment is often given to simply provide symptom control and relief. Antiinflammatory medications are administered. Antibiotics, fluoroquinolone, and antifungal agents may also be given. For unknown reasons, about half of

with prostatitis have elevated levels of specific molecules that regulate the inflammatory response. Another hypothesis is that many of the men affected have a pelvic floor spasm associated with undiagnosed pelvic floor disorder mimicking prostatitis. The National Institutes of Health (NIH) is funding several prostatitis studies to examine this further.

The most commonly found pathogens associated with chronic bacterial infections are the gram-negative enterobacteria such as *Escherichia coli*, *Proteus mirabilis*, *Klebsiella pneumoniae*, and *Pseudomonas aeruginosa*. The pathogens associated with acute bacterial prostatitis include *E. coli*, pseudomonads, staphylococci, and streptococci. Although controversial, other infectious agents such as gonococci,

TABLE 18-1

Clinical Manifestations of Prostatitis

ACUTE	NONBACTERIAL	CHRONIC BACTERIAL
Urinary	Urinary	Urinary
Frequency	Frequency	Frequency
Urgency	Urgency	Urgency
Nocturia	Dysuria	Dysuria
Dysuria	Impotence	Myalgia
Urethral discharge	Decreased libido	Arthralgia
High fever	Pain	Pain
Chills	Low back	Low back
Malaise	Rectal	Rectal
Myalgia	Scrotal	
Arthralgia		
Pain		
Lower abdominal		
Rectal		
Low back		
Sacral		
Groin/pelvis		

men with nonbacterial prostatitis respond to antibiotics; antibiotics are used to treat bacterial prostatitis.

Treatment of chronic bacterial prostatitis can be equally as difficult, as the antibiotic agents have difficulty penetrating the chronically inflamed prostate. Drug therapy of 4 to 6 months' duration may be used in an attempt to treat this infection. Transurethral prostatectomy (TURP) may be indicated if the disease is not cured with medications.

Special Implications for the Therapist   **18-1**

PROSTATITIS

When treating people at risk for developing prostatitis, therapists need to be vigilant for the onset of symptoms listed in Table 18-1. The symptoms may be subtle initially or difficult to ascertain because of communication difficulties common in the aging adult. The fact that therapy may extend over a number of weeks may allow the therapist to detect the subtle changes and initiate contact with the primary physician.

In young people with back pain, the thought of visceral disease accounting for the back pain is not always at the forefront. Prostatitis can be the cause of back pain of unknown cause in young males. The presence of any of the symptoms listed in Table 18-1, along with the onset of back pain, should raise concern.

When rehabilitating someone with a history of chronic bacterial prostatitis, therapists need to be aware of symptoms associated with UTIs. Many of these men experience recurrent UTIs as the prostatic bacteria continue to invade the bladder. The waxing and waning of symptoms may interfere with the client's compliance with a rehabilitation program. Reassurance that prostatitis is not a warning sign of cancer may be helpful. Bicycle seats can aggravate prostatitis so a recumbent bicycle is recommended, as this puts less pressure on the groin. ■

◆ Benign Prostatic Hyperplasia

Overview.   Benign prostatic hyperplasia is an age-related nonmalignant enlargement of the prostate gland.

Incidence and Risk Factors.   Of men age 50 and older, 75% experience symptoms of prostate enlargement.[56] The disease is rarely noted in men under age 40 and tends to occur after age 50.

Besides age, geography and ethnicity are important factors in the incidence of this disease. BPH is found most often in the United States and western Europe and least often in the Far East. The incidence of BPH is also higher in blacks than in whites. Drinking moderate amounts (one to three drinks per day) is associated with a reduced risk of BPH, and cigarette smoking increases the risk for BPH-like symptoms, possibly because bladder irritation caused by cigarette smoke may heighten the urgency and frequency of urination.

Pathogenesis.   Although the cause is unknown, changes in hormone balance associated with aging may be responsible for the development of BPH. Although commonly referred to as *benign prostatic hypertrophy*, the pathologic changes are marked by *hyperplasia*, not hypertrophy. Multiple prostatic nodules develop, resulting from the proliferation of epithelial cells, smooth muscle cells, and stromal fibroblasts of the gland. These nodules initially develop in the periurethral region of the prostate as opposed to the periphery of the gland (Fig. 18-2). The lumen of the urethra becomes progressively narrowed.

Regarding hormonal balance and aging, both androgens and estrogens contribute to the hyperplasia of this condition. Dihydrotestosterone (DHT), the biologically active metabolite of testosterone, is thought to be the primary mediator of hyperplasia, whereas estrogens sensitize the prostatic tissue to the growth-producing effects of DHT. The increased levels of estrogen that occur with aging may enhance the action of androgens at this point in the life cycle.

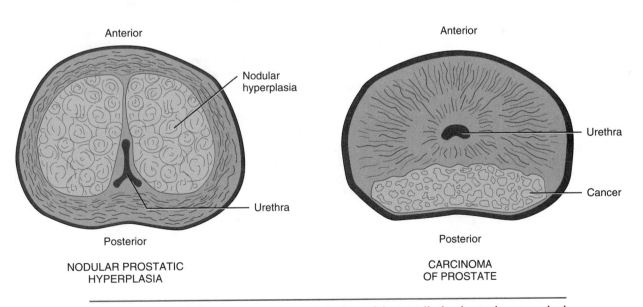

Anterior

Nodular
hyperplasia

Urethra

Posterior

**NODULAR PROSTATIC
HYPERPLASIA**

Anterior

Urethra

Cancer

Posterior

**CARCINOMA
OF PROSTATE**

FIGURE   **18-2**   In benign prostatic hyperplasia the nodules initially develop in the periurethral region, compressing the urethra. Cancer of the prostate typically develops initially in the periphery of the gland.

Clinical Manifestations. The clinical presentation of BPH is related to secondary involvement of the urethra. The nodular hyperplasia results in a narrowing of the urethra, producing urinary outflow obstruction. The client may note a decreased caliber and force of the urine stream and difficulty initiating or continuing the urine stream so that only small amounts of urine are released. In addition, residual urine in the bladder results in urinary frequency, which is particularly troublesome at night (nocturia). As the urethral obstruction progresses, the risk of developing UTIs, marked bladder distention with destructive bladder wall changes, hydroureter,* and hydronephrosis† increases (Fig. 18-3). Ultimately, renal failure and death may occur if treatment is not initiated. Other urinary symptoms associated with the later stages of the disease include urge incontinence, terminal urinary dribbling, urgency, hematuria, and dysuria.

Medical Management
Diagnosis.
Correlation of the history, palpation findings, and urodynamic test results (flow rate and force of stream) typically give rise to the diagnosis of BPH and indicate the choice of treatment. Regarding palpation, the bladder may be palpable as urinary retention progresses. In addition, a smooth, rubbery enlargement of the prostate may be noted during DRE, although the perceived size of the prostate does not always correlate with the degree of urethral compression.

The most commonly employed urodynamic test for the assessment of BPH is uroflowmetry. The urine flow rate and the force of the urine stream are measured.‡ Uroflowmetry by itself is a screening modality, not diagnostic, because the urinary obstruction could be occurring at sites other than at the prostate gland. In addition, diagnostic ultrasound and abdominal radiographs may be used to evaluate the size and length of the urethra, the size and configuration of the prostate, and the bladder capacity.

Treatment.
If symptoms related to BPH are mild, the condition is often just monitored because the clinical status of the disorder may stabilize or even improve. Aggressive treatment is indicated, however, if the more severe symptoms of obstruction develop. Symptoms suggesting advanced disease include urine retention, incontinence, hematuria, and chronic UTIs. The goals of treatment include providing client comfort and avoiding serious renal damage. For those with moderate to severe symptoms, the two medical treatment approaches for BPH are surgical and pharmacologic.

The goal of surgical intervention is to alleviate the obstruction to urine flow. Transurethral resection of the prostate (TURP)§ has been the most commonly employed procedure, with approximately 400,000 surgeries done annually. TURP is very successful in relieving symptoms and im-

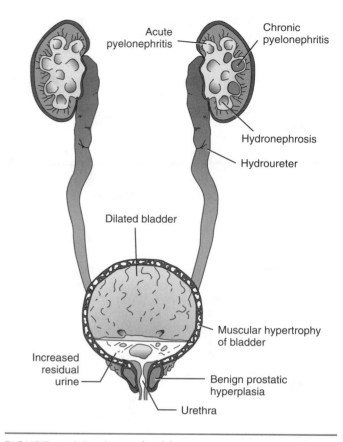

Acute pyelonephritis
Chronic pyelonephritis
Hydronephrosis
Hydroureter
Dilated bladder
Muscular hypertrophy of bladder
Increased residual urine
Benign prostatic hyperplasia
Urethra

FIGURE 18-3 A cascade of destructive events potentially associated with advanced benign prostatic hyperplasia. Viewing Fig. 18-1, *A,* the relationship of the prostate located at the base of the bladder, surrounding a part of the urethra can be visualized. As the prostate enlarges, the urethra becomes obstructed, interfering with the normal flow of urine.

proving quality of life, but some drawbacks are evident (e.g., requires a general anesthetic and hospital stay and may be accompanied by side effects of bleeding, incontinence, impotence, or retrograde ejaculation in which an ejaculation goes back into the bladder). An alternative technique is transurethral incision of the prostate (TUIP).* TURP is preferable, with a large gland, severe and recurrent gross hematuria, and prostatitis, where the goal is to remove infected tissue and calculi.

Pharmacologic agents can also be used to treat BPH by shrinking glandular tissue (5-alpha-reductase inhibitors)† and relaxing smooth muscle tissue of the prostate, bladder neck, and urethra (alpha-adrenergic blockers). The alpha-adrenergic receptors are located in the muscle fibers of the adenoma and prostate capsule. The resultant smooth muscle relaxation decreases pressure on the urethra, enhancing urinary flow. Phytopharmaceuticals (e.g., substrates from the saw palmetto plant) for the management of BPH represents up to 80% of all

---

*The ureteral wall becomes severely stretched secondary to the bladder outflow obstruction, which increases the pressure in a retrograde direction. The ureteral wall can become stretched to the point where it loses the ability to undergo peristaltic contractions.

†Urine-filled dilation of the renal pelvis and calices. Destruction of renal tissue may occur.

‡It is generally agreed that a peak urine flow rate of less than 10 ml/sec is suggestive of obstruction.

§A long tube with a miniature camera on the tip is threaded up the urethra into the bladder, allowing visual inspection of both of these structures. When the excess prostate tissue is identified, a surgical instrument is threaded through this tube, and resection is performed.

---

*In the case of TUIP, incisions in the muscle wall of the prostate and bladder neck allow for an outward expansion of the gland, relieving some of the pressure on the urethra.

†The 5-alpha-reductase inhibitors address the hormonal causes of BPH by preventing an enzyme called *5-alpha-reductase* from converting testosterone into DHT (DHT prompts glandular tissue to develop). As a result, the prostate shrinks by as much as 20%. This is a gradual process that can take up to a year to obtain maximum benefit.

prescriptions in many European countries.[30] Studies in the United States have shown significant effects of saw palmetto on epithelial contraction, urinary flow rates, and improved symptoms compared with placebos.[16,35]

Androgen suppression drug therapy can also be used to block the synthesis and action of testosterone, including DHT. A 20% to 30% reduction in prostate volume can be noted. This can result in a lessening of the severity of symptoms and improvement in the objective criteria related to urinary obstruction although this can take 3 to 6 months.

Thermotherapy either by transurethral microwave therapy (TUMT) (e.g., Prostatron) or laser surgery through laser-induced thermotherapy (LITT) has been developed over the past 10 years to provide effective alternatives to surgical management. Thermotherapy removes prostatic tissue, especially in the case of small-size BPH and in the presence of risk factors such as heart disease or anticoagulation therapy. This modality restores spontaneous urine flow by destroying diseased prostate tissue. Specifically, TUMT causes necrotic lesions within the adenoma and induces apoptosis in benign human prostatic stromal cells.

The potential advantages of these procedures over TURP and TUIP are shorter operative time usually without hospitalization, minimal bleeding, and decreased incidence of postoperative retrograde ejaculation and bladder neck contracture. Potential disadvantages include postoperative urinary retention, no tissue being available for histologic study, and less than optimal prospects for treating large lesions. This technique may be associated with a high recurrence rate requiring additional treatment.[66] In the case of laser, the larger is the lesion, the more passes are required, increasing the associated risks.[68] The introduction of an integrated system of computer, robotics, and laser technology for prostate resection may be the intervention of the future.[24]

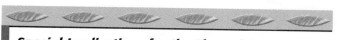

Special Implications for the Therapist   18-2

BENIGN PROSTATIC HYPERPLASIA

Preferred Practice Pattern:
5A: Primary Prevention/Risk Reduction for Loss of Balance and Falling (side effect of medication)
   See the Preferred Practice Patterns associated with urinary incontinence in this chapter.

Therapists conducting a past medical history with men over the age of 50 can easily include a series of four questions to help identify the presence of urologic involvement: (1) Do you urinate often, especially during the night? (2) Do you have trouble starting or continuing your urine? (3) Do you have weak flow of urine or interrupted urine stream? and (4) Does it feel like your bladder is not emptying completely? A *yes* answer to any of these questions warrants further medical evaluation. Painful urination, blood in the urine, or unexplained lower back, pelvis, hip, or upper thigh pain in the presence of any of these symptoms requires medical referral.

Surgical procedures for BPH carry the risk of complications such as impotence and retrograde ejaculation. Unexplained re-

ports of sexual dysfunction warrant communication with a physician. If the person notes sexual dysfunction and has a history of the above procedures, then ask him periodically about changes in sexual function. If there appears to be a worsening, communication with a physician would again be warranted.

Pharmacologic agents used to treat BPH are associated with numerous side effects. These include impotence, loss of libido, gynecomastia, drowsiness, dizziness, tachycardia, and postural hypotension. The therapist can advise clients about the possibility of falls from dizziness and loss of balance associated with these medications and take steps to institute a falls prevention program when appropriate (see the Special Implications for the Therapist: Orthostatic [Postural] Hypotension in Chapter 11). Any change or new onset of symptoms should be reported to the physician. ■

◆ Prostate Cancer

Overview.   Adenocarcinoma of the prostate accounts for 98% of primary prostatic tumors. Prostate cancer usually starts in the outer portion of the prostate and spreads inwardly and then beyond the gland with metastases in more advanced stages. Ductal and transitional cell carcinomas make up the remainder of the tumors.

Incidence.   Prostate cancer, the most common visceral malignancy in American men, is the second most common cause of male death from cancer. The number of new cases of prostate cancer in the last decade represents an increase of 200%.[28] One in six American men is at a lifetime risk of prostate cancer with approximately 189,000 men newly diagnosed in 2002.

Autopsy studies indicate that occult prostate cancer is present in 25% of men age 60 to 69, in 40% of men age 70 to 79, and in more than 50% of men age 80 and older.[53] Men less than 50 years old make up less than 1% of those with prostate cancer. Prostate cancer incidence and mortality vary strikingly among ethnic and national groups with a particular propensity for African Americans.[12]

Risk Factors.   Box 18-1 lists risk factors related to prostate cancer. Prostate cancer is a disease of the aging male, but evidence exists that genetic, environmental, and social factors jointly and in combination contribute to observed differences in various populations. Geographically, the highest frequencies of prostate cancer are found in the United States and north-

BOX   **18-1**

Risk Factors for Prostate Cancer

Age > 50 years
African American
Geography (United States and Scandinavian countries)
Family history; inherited gene mutation
Environmental exposure to cadmium
High-fat diet
Alcohol consumption

western Europe (Scandinavian countries), whereas the lowest are found in Mexico, Greece, and Japan. African Americans have twice the risk of non-Hispanic whites, which is attributed to traditional socioeconomic, clinical, and pathologic factors.[25]

Although no genetic marker has been found, a familial history of prostate cancer is a risk factor. An eightfold increase in risk has been estimated for men who have both a first- and second-degree relative with the disease.[57] If a close relative has prostate cancer, a man's risk of the disease doubles; with two relatives, his risk increases fivefold; and with three close relatives, the risk is about 97%.[43] In addition, mortality from prostate cancer is believed to be three times greater in relatives of men with prostate cancer compared with those without such a family history.

Exposure to cadmium through welding, electroplating, alkaline battery production, farming, typesetting, and ship fitting places men at higher risk of prostate cancer. Lastly, high dietary fat intake has been correlated with prostate cancer.[19,45]

Etiologic Factors and Pathogenesis.

Although the precise cause of prostate cancer is unknown, a strong endocrine system link is theorized. Androgens in particular have been implicated based on the androgenic control of normal growth and development of the prostate and the fact that males castrated before puberty do not develop prostate cancer or BPH. In addition, the responsiveness of prostate cancer to surgical castration and estrogen therapy supports this theory. The higher incidence of cancer in blacks is correlated with a 15% higher serum testosterone level in blacks.[10]

Although it is difficult to identify genes that predispose to prostate cancer due to late age at diagnosis, a prostate cancer susceptibility locus has been identified, along with linkage to a locus on chromosome 17p. However, this gene is only responsible for between 2% and 5% of all prostate cancers, suggesting that additional genes contribute to this disease.[44,62] A new cDNA fragment (C13) has been identified that is downregulated in malignant prostate tissues, suggesting that this gene encodes a protein that may have tumor- or metastasis-suppressing function in prostate tissue.[54] Further studies in this area are underway.

Most prostatic adenocarcinomas are characterized by small- to moderate-size disorganized glands that infiltrate the stroma of the prostate. The tumors are more likely to develop initially in the periphery of the prostate, unlike BPH, where the pathologic changes typically originate close to the urethra (see Fig. 18-2). The cancer invades adjacent local structures such as the seminal vesicles and urinary bladder and spreads to the musculoskeletal system, particularly the axial skeleton, and lungs. Lymphatic metastasis may involve the obturator, iliac, and periaortic lymph nodes, extending up through the thoracic duct (see Fig. 12-8).

The mechanism underlying the *organ-specific* metastasis of prostate cancer cells to the bone is still poorly understood. Whether the cells only invade the bone and proliferate there or whether they invade many tissues but survive mainly in the bone is unclear; this concept is referred to as *seed and soil*. New research suggests that osteonectin, a small protein found in bone marrow attracts prostate cancer cells to bone and once, attracted, stimulates the cells to invade bone. These findings suggest that antibodies to osteonectin could reduce the invasiveness of prostate cancer (and breast cancer) and offer a potential way of preventing the spread of prostate cancer to the bone.[27]

Clinical Manifestations.

The clinical presentation of prostate cancer is extremely variable and may be completely asymptomatic until the disease is advanced. In many men the disease is noted incidentally on DRE or discovered in fragments of prostatic tissue removed through TURP for BPH. Depending on the size and location of the lesion, the initial presenting symptom could be related to urinary obstruction, onset of pain, or constitutional symptoms such as fatigue and weight loss.

The urinary obstruction symptoms associated with cancer are similar to those associated with BPH but typically present in later stages of the disease compared with BPH. Cancer originating in the subcapsular region of the prostate as opposed to the periurethral area would account for this difference. The obstructive symptoms include urinary urgency, frequency, hesitancy, dysuria, hematuria, difficulty initiating or continuing the urine stream, and decreased urine stream. Blood in the ejaculate may also be noted.

Bony metastasis occurs via lymphatics to adjacent structures and pelvic nodes in the majority of people with metastatic disease. The axial skeleton is affected more than the appendicular skeleton, especially the spine, ribs, sternum, femur, and pelvis. Of the primary tumors that metastasize to the spine, prostate lesions rank fourth behind breast, lung, and myeloma. Prostate cancer can also metastasize to the lungs and liver. Pain complaints associated with prostate cancer can vary tremendously. A dull, vague ache may be noted in the rectal, sacral, or lumbar spine region, and the individual may have difficulty walking. The sacral and lumbar pain is typically associated with bony metastasis. Pain may be noted in the thoracic and shoulder girdle areas secondary to lymphatic spread of the disease or again secondary to local bony metastasis. Lastly, symptoms such as fatigue, weight loss, anemia, and dyspnea have all been attributed to metastatic spread of the disease.

Medical Management

Prevention. Recommendations for early detection include DRE and PSA serum assay after age 50. The study of cancer chemoprevention (the use of agents to slow progression of, reverse, or inhibit carcinogenesis) is ongoing in the area of prostate cancer because prostate cancer growth is known to depend on androgen. Blocking androgen at the cellular level may be a treatment intervention of the future.[23,65] Data supports the use of antiandrogens in the prevention of prostate cancer, although the toxicity of these agents (gynecomastia, gastrointestinal disturbance) poses concerns for the current application in all men.[4] Studies of predictive factors, biomarkers for chemoprevention, or agents that can interrupt the development of prostate cancer are under investigation.[65]

An inverse relationship has been observed between dietary intake of lycopene and the risk of prostate cancer. Vitamin E and selenium have also been shown to reduce prostate cancer incidence.[14] Vitamin and lycopene supplementation (and other antioxidants) may be another form of effective chemoprevention that is currently under investigation.[31,34]

Finally, although exercise can suppress androgen production and may thus decrease the risk of prostate cancer, epidemiologic studies assessing this relationship do not support the hypothesis that increased physical activity reduces the risk of prostate cancer.[33]

Diagnosis. The diagnosis of prostate cancer is made by a variety of tests, including DRE, transrectal ultrasound, serum PSA assay, and radiographic imaging modalities. Ultimately, tissue biopsy is performed to confirm the diagnosis.

The DRE may reveal a hardened, fixed structure or a diffusely undulated gland. A limitation to this procedure is that typically, only the posterior and lateral aspects of the prostate can be palpated. An ultrasound probe (transrectal ultrasound [TRUS]) can be performed by inserting a small ultrasound probe into the rectum. The sound waves emitted by the probe produce a video or photographic image of the prostate. These images help guide a thin needle through the rectum to the gland for a biopsy and staging (TRUS-guided biopsy). The use of positron emission tomography (PET) as a noninvasive means of detecting prostate cancer is under investigation.[5]

The PSA assay is now an important part of the screening process. PSA is a glycoprotein produced exclusively in the cytoplasm of benign and malignant prostatic cells. A normal assay value is anything less than or equal to 4 ng/ml; this should not rise more than 0.75 ng/dl per year. The average prostatic cancer produces approximately 10 times the PSA a normal prostate gland does. However, PSA values bounce around on a daily basis and an elevated PSA assay (between 4 and 10 ng/ml) may also be related to prostatitis, BPH, prostatic infarcts and prostatic biopsy and surgery. Therefore, an elevated PSA is organ-specific but is not diagnostic by itself. Lastly, the PSA may be false-negative in up to 30% of cases with localized prostate cancer.

Radiographic imaging modalities are also utilized for staging of the disease. Magnetic resonance imaging (MRI) allows for evaluation of the prostate gland and regional lymph nodes. Lymph node involvement must typically be advanced (nodes larger than 1 cm) to be demonstrable. Radiographs may detect metastatic lesions, but the radionuclide bone scan, although not diagnostic, is a more sensitive modality for detection of a metabolically active lesion.

A relatively new testing method, known as *reverse transcription-polymerase chain reaction (RT-PCR)* is now available and is capable of testing tiny markers that cancer cells carry when they spread to lymph nodes. This test is able to detect cancer previously undetected with standard tests and may also be able to assist in the detection of cancer cells in the surgical margins after radical prostatectomy.[29,59]

Staging. The Whitmore-Jewett staging system is the one most commonly used. The spread of prostate cancer has been divided into four stages, A through D (Fig. 18-4). The stage of the disease at the time of the diagnosis helps dictate the course of treatment. Alternately, a ranking called the *Gleason score,* which rates the tumor from 1 (slow growing) to 6 (very fast growing), may be used to determine the aggressiveness of the cancer tumor and the suitability of treatment.

Treatment. The medical treatment of prostate cancer depends on the man's age, health, the stage of the disease, and personal preferences. Many uncertainties surround the issue of treating prostate cancer because of the inability to differentiate tumors that will progress from those that will remain unchanged. More men appear to die with prostate cancer than from it.[21] No randomized controlled trials have demonstrated the superiority of one treatment over another in terms of survival, although differences in complications vary. The

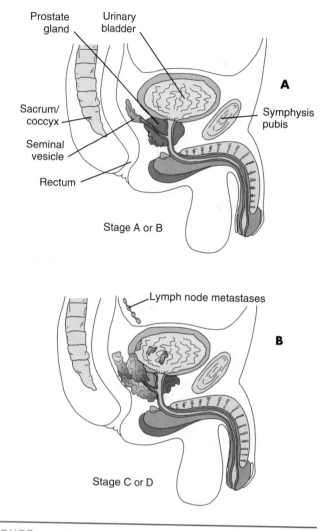

FIGURE   18-4   Prostate cancer: clinical staging. **A,** The tumor has not spread beyond the gland's capsule in stages A and B. **B,** In stage C the tumor has spread into adjacent tissues; in stage D the disease has spread into the lymphatic system and beyond.

American Urologic Association advocates a presentation of all options for the individual to consider. Once the cancer treatment has begun, most clients are reevaluated every 3 to 6 months. At follow-up visits, symptoms of urinary obstruction and pain are investigated. DRE and a PSA assay are carried out, and prostatic acid phosphatase levels are measured. Other tests may be routinely ordered depending on the individual's status.

The most commonly used, effective treatments include observation; radical prostatectomy; radiation (external beam or brachytherapy); and hormonal therapy. Unless relatively young, men with early stage A disease may be simply monitored because prostate cancer can be an indolent disease. These cancers rarely progress during the initial 5 years after diagnosis but do progress in 10% to 25% of clients 10 years after diagnosis.[2,11] Generally, however, men with a life expectancy of 10 years or more and with disease diagnosed in later stage A or B undergo radical prostatectomy and possibly radiation therapy.

Radical prostatectomy involves removal of the prostate, seminal vesicles, and a portion of the bladder neck and assures that the original source of the cancer is removed. The conventional surgical approach can be retropubic or perineal, but a newer technique commonly performed in France is gaining use in the United States. Using a laparoscopic approach provides a significantly magnified televised view of the surgical area minimizes the potential nerve damage common to traditional prostatectomy.[17,20]

The retropubic approach involves an incision from the pubic symphysis to the umbilicus and allows for staging pelvic lymphadenectomy. The primary postoperative complications with conventional surgery are infection; urinary incontinence (e.g., detrusor instability with small bladder capacity, pudendal nerve denervation); ED/impotence, excessive bleeding; and rectal injury with fecal incontinence. Potency may return gradually over the course of a year; however, after these procedures, as many as one third of men have incontinence or urinary frequency beyond 1 year, and an even greater number continue to experience ED.

Radiation therapy may be used to treat localized prostatic lesions, as an adjunctive treatment after radical prostatectomy or for palliative effects in the presence of widespread disease. Relief of pain and improvement in symptoms associated with urethral obstruction are possible benefits of this treatment modality. Radiation therapy is most often used with stage C disease because many men have occult pelvic lymph node metastases. The radiation therapy can be administered daily by external beam radiation over a number of weeks (usually up to two months). A new technique of external beam radiation called *three-dimensional (3D) conformal radiation* makes it easier to focus and shape the radiation beam (intensity modulation) so that it is less likely to hit other organs, thereby reducing rectal and bladder toxicity. This advanced technology is not yet available universally.[49,71]

For men with small, nonaggressive tumors, brachytherapy may be the preferred treatment. Brachytherapy is administered by a single injection of radioactive seeds directly into the prostate delivering a constant, highly concentrated, yet confined dose of radiation to the tissue in and immediately around the tumor. The prostate absorbs almost all of the radiation so that nerves and other tissues of the surrounding structures of the rectum, bladder, and urethra are spared with fewer complications like ED or incontinence. With technologic advances, brachytherapy now has similar cure rates for localized cancer as radiation and radical prostatectomy. More specific details about the selection, use, administration, and side effects of these two treatment tools are available.[52]

Hormone therapy is the treatment of choice in the presence of stage D disease, the goal being androgen deprivation. Testosterone stimulates prostate cancer growth, so by blocking its production, hormonal therapy shrinks or slows the progression of prostate tumors. Since the testes produce 95% of the circulating testosterone, orchiectomy is the primary method of manipulating hormone levels. A second option, estrogen therapy, is used less often because of adverse effects including impotence, gynecomastia, loss of libido, bloating, and pedal edema. Hormonal therapy is not usually advocated for newly diagnosed, locally contained prostate cancer because of its adverse effects (e.g., bone deterioration, decreased libido, mood changes, anemia). Additionally, serious cardiovascular disease, including stroke, heart attack, and deep venous thrombosis, can be associated with estrogen therapy in anyone at high risk.

Clinical trials are under way to investigate the development of a vaccine that fights prostate cancer by means of immunomodulation.[64] Researchers are able to trick the human immune system into recognizing cancerous prostate cells as foreign invaders by genetically engineering the individual's own cells and injecting them back into the body. This is done by harvesting prostate cancer cells, irradiating them, treating them with autologous granulocyte-macrophage colony-stimulating hormone (GM-CSF), and reintroducing them into the body. Results so far indicate that both T-cell and B-cell immune responses to human prostate cancer can be generated.[55]

Prognosis. Multiple sources of data show that prostate cancer incidence rates rose after the introduction of PSA testing. The average age at diagnosis has fallen, the proportion of advanced stage tumors has declined, the proportion of moderately differentiated tumors has increased, and a decline in mortality began in the United States in 1991.[42] Death occurs in less than 10% of all cases. Men with small or nonaggressive tumors are more likely to be cancer free than men with large or aggressive tumors. Seed implants are more successful for men whose pretreatment level of PSA is below 10 ng/ml. Without any treatment at all, men with the least aggressive prostate cancers face only a 4% to 7% risk of dying from prostate cancer within 15 years of diagnosis.[1]

The rate of relapse in men with pathologic evidence of pelvic lymph node involvement is high (more than 50%, although some studies report as high as 90%) within 5 years of local treatment. Lymph node involvement occurs in 15% to 20% of men with localized prostate cancer that exhibits high-risk features (as defined by tumor size, serum PSA level, and Gleason score).[13] Finally, prostate cancer is sometimes referred to as a "two-decade disease" because it often returns 10 to 20 years after successful local therapy, which is one reason why some physicians advocate radical prostatectomy. Metastatic prostate cancer remains a lethal disease, although new treatment strategies are being developed and incorporated into clinical trials that may improve survival rates.[26]

Postoperatively, after radical prostatectomy, incontinence is 100% when the catheter is removed, but urinary control is regained for most men within the first 6 to 8 weeks. Men can speed recovery of urinary function and reduce the likelihood of remaining incontinent by correctly exercising the pelvic floor exercises.[67] Any incontinence 12 months or more after surgery and rehabilitation may require additional medical intervention such as collagen injection (a sclerosing agent to "tighten up" the sphincter) or placement of an artificial urinary sphincter.

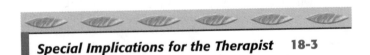

Special Implications for the Therapist 18-3

PROSTATE CANCER

Preferred Practice Patterns:
4A: *Primary Prevention/Risk Reduction for Skeletal Demineralization (hormonal therapy)*
4B: *Impaired Posture*
4C: *Impaired Muscle Performance*

4F: Impaired Joint Mobility, Motor Function, Muscle Performance, Range of Motion, and Reflex Integrity Associated With Spinal Disorders (metastases)

5A: Primary Prevention/Risk Reduction for Loss of Balance and Falling

5F: Impaired Peripheral Nerve Integrity and Muscle Performance Associated With Peripheral Nerve Injury

Screening for Medical Disease

Investigating the symptoms or signs associated with any prostate condition provides the therapist with the baseline information needed to monitor the client's status. For example, if the client experiences difficulty with initiating the urine stream, continuing the stream of flow, urinary frequency, or dribbling or continuous leaking, the therapist should periodically ask if there has been a change regarding the urinary dysfunction.

Considering the number of aging adult men seen in a rehabilitative setting and the incidence of prostate disease, therapists are seeing a number of clients with preexisting prostate conditions. Pain is often the primary or only symptom associated with prostate disease. If the pain is located in the thoracic, lumbar, or sacral area, the client may seek care from a therapist, thinking the pain is of mechanical origin. Metastatic spread of the disease to the axial skeleton or the periaortic lymph nodes may account for these complaints. If the back pain does not present in a mechanical fashion (based on history and physical examination findings) or the person notes urologic dysfunction, referral to a physician is warranted. A previous history of prostate cancer in any man with current reports of shoulder, back, groin, or hip pain of unknown cause must be screened for medical disease. Age over 50, past history of cancer, and unknown cause of musculoskeletal pain or symptoms are three red flags that warrant further medical investigation.

Postoperative Considerations

In a radical prostatectomy, the urogenital anatomy is significantly altered, the bladder neck or the internal sphincter may be surgically excised, and the prostate and a portion of the urethra are removed, compromising the pressure resistance normally provided by the urethra. Next, the bladder is reattached to the remaining urethra. Pelvic floor rehabilitation must be aimed at both the slow twitch fibers of the rhabdosphincter (external urethral sphincter) that maintain resistance and the fast twitch fibers of the pelvic floor muscles that can tighten quickly to prevent leakage during increased intraabdominal pressure (e.g., laughing, coughing, lifting) (see Box 15-1).

In the case of urinary incontinence, knowing the type of incontinence and the amount of leaking assists in prioritizing a treatment protocol. For example, dribbling after the completion of urinating indicates dysfunction of the external urethral sphincter or detrusor instability (excessive bladder contractions). Exercise and physiologic quieting (see Chapter 17) are often effective if innervation is intact. Pelvic floor reeducation has been shown effective in returning men to being functionally dry or completely continent after radical prostatectomy and should be recommended as a first-line option.[67]

If continuous urine flow occurs months after the surgery, "stove pipe urethra" may be diagnosed, and medical intervention is required. If urine flow is difficult to initiate or flow is weak, an overactive puborectalis muscle, a stricture, or decreased bladder contractions may be evident. Exercise, biofeedback, and

medication are treatment options to relax the pelvic musculature and improve detrusor contraction strength.

If no improvement has taken place with an appropriate rehabilitation program or if the symptoms are getting worse, the client should be referred to the physician who is managing the prostate condition. Knowledge of other potential symptoms associated with prostate conditions provide the basis for a screening checklist the therapist could use periodically while treating the individual. Once again, if an onset of new symptoms is noted, referral to the physician is warranted.

Metastases to the pelvic lymph nodes can cause lumbar plexopathy and swelling due to compression of veins and/or lymphatics. The development of lymphedema may be related to smoking, stage of cancer, and radiation therapy. The therapist has an important role in screening men for risk of lymphedema and early recognition/intervention of this condition.[8]

Complications of Medical Treatment

Important implications exist related to the commonly employed treatment approaches to the various prostate conditions. Complications associated with radical prostatectomy procedures include infection, incontinence, and impotence. If the therapist is seeing someone who has undergone such a procedure, being vigilant for symptoms associated with infection is necessary for months after the surgery. If the client reports malaise, fever, chills, sweats, or sudden worsening of symptoms, communication with the physician is warranted. The surgery may account for the individual's complaints of incontinence and impotence. The average time to achieve continence is 3 weeks with virtually all individuals being continent within 6 months. Postoperative impotence occurs in 70% of men who undergo retropubic prostatectomy. Potency can be spared in 70% to 80% with nerve sparing in young men.

Although reduced in recent years, delayed complications of radiation therapy can occur with increasing problems from 6 to 24 months postradiation.[22] Diarrhea; gastrointestinal (GI) or urinary bleeding; irritative voiding symptoms; impotence; and tenesmus (painful spasm of the anal sphincter with straining) are all possible complications. The presence of these problems could interfere with a rehabilitation program, slowing progress. A recent onset or worsening of any of these complications should be brought to the physician's attention.

Multiple potential side effects are associated with endocrine or hormonal manipulation (Box 18-2). Decrease in bone mass

Continued

BOX 18-2

Side Effects of Hormonal Manipulation

Decreased bone density, osteoporosis
Loss of libido
Impotence
Hot flashes
Gynecomastia
Bloating and pedal edema
Nausea and vomiting
Diarrhea
Weight gain/redistribution
Myocardial infarction, cerebrovascular accident, deep venous thrombosis

and increase in bone turnover with a concomitant increased risk of fracture has been documented in men receiving androgen deprivation (antiandrogen) therapy.[58] The therapist can institute an osteoporosis prevention plan for anyone receiving this treatment. As with the complications associated with surgical procedures and radiation therapy, these problems may interfere with rehabilitation, altering the prognosis. Knowing the individual is being treated with endocrine manipulative therapy and being familiar with the side effects can lessen alarm on the therapist's part if the client reports any of these symptoms. If symptoms or signs of myocardial infarct, cerebral vascular accident, or deep venous thrombosis develop, immediate referral to a physician is warranted (see Chapter 11). ■

DISORDERS OF THE TESTES

◆ Orchitis

Overview and Etiologic Factors.   Orchitis is inflammation of the testis, can be acute or chronic, and is often associated with epididymitis. Gram-negative bacteria and *Chlamydia trachomatis* are the usual infectious agents.

Incidence and Risk Factors.   Anyone with primary infections of the genitourinary tract or infections in other body regions (e.g., pneumonia, scarlet fever) is at risk of developing orchitis. Sexually active males with multiple partners are at higher risk of developing genitourinary infections. Males 10 years of age and older who have parotitis (mumps) are also at risk of developing orchitis. The incidence of orchitis in this group can be as high as 25% to 33%.[18] Men with indwelling catheters are also at higher risk of developing orchitis secondary to genitourinary tract infection.

Pathogenesis and Clinical Manifestations.   Orchitis is often secondary to UTIs. The bloodstream and lymphatics are then the route of spread from other body areas to the testes. Systemic infections such as pneumonia, scarlet fever, and parotitis use the same routes to spread to the testes.

Orchitis is marked by testicular pain and swelling. Pain may also be noted in the lower abdominal area. Fever and malaise can be present, but symptoms of urinary dysfunction are usually absent.

Medical Management

Diagnosis.   Physical examination reveals a tender and swollen testicle. Laboratory tests revealing an elevated white blood cell (WBC) count and urinalysis are an important component of the diagnostic process.

Treatment.   See the section on Epididymitis and Special Implications for the Therapist: Epididymitis and Testicular Torsion in this chapter.

◆ Epididymitis

Overview and Risk Factors.   Epididymitis is an inflammation of the epididymis. The two primary types of epididymitis are sexually and nonsexually transmitted infections. Males typically under the age of 40 who are sexually active with multiple partners are at higher risk of developing genitourinary disease that can lead to epididymitis. Iatrogenic

sources of infection include cystoscopy and indwelling catheters. In the older male population, this condition can be precipitated by prostatitis and UTIs.

Pathogenesis and Etiologic Factors.   Epididymitis is typically caused by bacterial pathogens. The sexually transmitted infections leading to epididymitis are associated with urethritis. In the nonsexually transmitted infections, urine-containing pathogens may be forced up the ejaculatory ducts, through the vas deferens, and into the epididymis. Pressure associated with voiding and physical strain can force the urine from the urethra. Infection originating elsewhere in the body can spread to the epididymis via the lymphatics of the spermatic cord. Congenital urinary tract abnormalities can lead to epididymitis in children.

Clinical Manifestations.   Epididymitis may be associated with pain, urinary dysfunction, fever, and urethral discharge. Unilateral scrotal pain is common, but pain may also be noted in the lower abdominal, groin, or hip adductor muscle areas. When bacteriuria is present, urinary frequency and urgency and dysuria can occur. When the epididymitis is related to sexually transmitted disease, urethritis and urethral discharge are present concurrently. Lastly, local scrotal erythema and swelling are associated with epididymitis.

Medical Management

Diagnosis.   In addition to the findings noted under Clinical Manifestations, urinalysis, urethral smear, and urine culture are important for the diagnosis of epididymitis. An elevated WBC count is also usually present.

Treatment.   During the acute phase, treatment includes bed rest; scrotal elevation and support; nonsteroidal antiinflammatory drugs (NSAIDs); or antibiotics. Hospitalization may be necessary if signs of sepsis or abscess formation are present or if the pain is severe. Once treatment has been initiated, a significant decrease in pain should be noted within a week, but the scrotal edema may be present for 2 to 3 months. (See the sections on epididymitis and testicular torsion.)

◆ Testicular Torsion

Overview.   Testicular torsion is an abnormal twisting of the spermatic cord as the testis rotates within the tunica vaginalis. The torsion can occur intra- or extravaginally, but intravaginal torsion is the more common. This condition is a surgical emergency. Early diagnosis and treatment is imperative to save the testis.

Etiologic Factors.   Torsion of the spermatic cord is often associated with congenital abnormalities. These include absence of the scrotal ligaments, incomplete descent of the testis, and a high attachment of the tunica vaginalis. Increased mobility of the testis and epididymis within the tunica vaginalis facilitate twisting of the spermatic cord. Testicular torsion can also occur after heavy physical activity.

Incidence and Risk Factors.   Intravaginal torsion most often occurs in males 8 to 18 years of age. The condition is rarely seen after age 30. The extravaginal torsions occur primarily in neonates. A firm, painless scrotal mass is discovered shortly after birth.

Pathogenesis.   The spermatic cord contains the vas deferens and the nerve and blood supply for the scrotal contents. If the torsion is severe enough to occlude the arterial supply, infarction of testicular germ cells can quickly occur. Intravaginal torsions are often precipitated by congenital abnormalities. These anomalies allow for rotation of the testis around the spermatic cord, or the torsion may occur between the testis and epididymis. Extravaginal torsion occurs most often during the fetal descent of the testes, before the tunica adheres to the scrotal wall. This allows the testis and fascial tunica to rotate around the spermatic cord above the level of the tunica vaginalis.

Clinical Manifestations.   An abrupt onset of scrotal pain and then swelling suggests testicular torsion. The pain may extend up into the inguinal area. Nausea, vomiting, and tachycardia may be present.

Medical Management
Diagnosis.   Diagnosis can be difficult and misdiagnosis of epididymitis can delay treatment resulting in testicular loss.[37] Physical examination reveals a firm, tender testis that is often positioned high in the scrotum. Erythema and scrotal edema may be present. The cremasteric reflex is often absent. Color and power Doppler sonography makes it possible to identify the absence of perfusion in the affected testis. Scintigraphy (radionuclide scanning) remains an acceptable diagnostic alternative in evaluation testicular torsion when color Doppler is unavailable or inadequate.[48] A urinalysis is performed to help rule out infection.

Treatment.   Testicular torsion is considered a urologic emergency. Once the diagnosis of testicular torsion is made, emergency surgery is performed. The procedure includes detorsion, and if the testis is deemed nonviable, then an orchiectomy is performed. The duration of the torsion is critical regarding salvage of the testis. If the surgery is performed within 3 hours of onset, a greater than 80% salvage rate occurs. The salvage rate drops to 20% if more than 12 hours passes before the surgery.

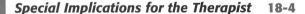

Special Implications for the Therapist   **18-4**

TESTICULAR TORSION

Pain extending into the groin and scrotum can occasionally be referred from muscle or joint structures, but if a client notes the onset of scrotal pain, immediate communication with a physician is warranted. Ask the client if he has noted scrotal swelling or tenderness; feels feverish or nauseated; has any difficulties with urination, including urgency, frequency, or dysuria; or has noted any urethral discharge. If the scrotal or groin pain is associated with musculoskeletal dysfunction, it can be expected that the therapist could alter the symptoms by mechanically stressing a component of the musculoskeletal system. ■

◆ **Testicular Cancer**
Overview.   Primary testicular tumors are divided into two histogenetic categories. Germ cell tumors (origin in the primordial germ cells) make up more than 95% of testicular tumors, whereas tumors of stromal or sex cord origin make up a majority of the remaining neoplasms. Metastatic tumors to the testis are uncommon, although involvement by lymphoma may occur in older men.

Incidence.   Although relatively rare, testicular cancer is the most common cancer in the 15- to 35-year-old male age group and second most common malignancy from age 35 to 39 with a white-to-black incidence ratio of 5 to 1. Approximately 7500 new cases of testicular cancer were estimated to occur in the United States in 2002, accounting for approximately 3% of male urogenital cancers.[28]

Etiologic and Risk Factors.   Although the cause is unknown, congenital and acquired factors have been associated with the development of testicular cancer; familial clustering has been observed particularly among siblings.[9,15] The first susceptibility gene for testicular cancer has been located and named TGCT1 on the long arm of chromosome X, inherited from the mother; its presence increases a man's risk of testicular cancer by up to 50 times.[50]

The most significant factor in testicular cancer is the association of cryptorchidism (the testes not descending into the scrotum). The incidence of testicular cancer is 35 times higher in males with a cryptoid testis. Regardless of whether this condition is caused by pre- or postnatal environmental exposures (e.g., endocrine-mimicking environmental pollutants, pesticides, industrial chemicals, or chemical contaminants in drinking water), it remains a topic of debate.

Other risk factors still under investigation may include mothers who took exogenous estrogen during pregnancy (diethylstilbestrol)[60,61]; scrotal trauma[41]; exposure to high levels of radiofrequency/microwave radiation in radar technicians[51]; first-born sons[69]; and nonidentical twins. Lastly, a history of infertility or infection has been associated with an increased risk of developing testicular cancer, although a causal relationship has not been established.

Pathogenesis.   Since germ cell tumors make up the vast majority of testicular cancers, the following discussion focuses solely on such tumors. Carcinoma in situ usually becomes an invasive germ cell tumor in a median period of approximately 5 years.[3] The neoplastic transformation of a germ cell results in either a seminoma, an undifferentiated tumor, or a nonseminomatous tumor composed of embryonal carcinoma teratoma, choriocarcinoma, or yolk-sac carcinoma (endodermal-sinus tumor). Seminomas are the most common testicular cancers, accounting for approximately 40% to 50% of germ cell tumors and most often appearing in the fourth decade of life. Seminomas appear as a solid, gray-white growth and are rarely necrotic or cystic. The entire testis can be replaced by the tumor.

The incidence of nonseminomas peaks in the third decade of life and hemorrhage, necrosis, or cystic changes are more common. Yolk-sac tumors are the most common germ cell tumors of infants. These tumors result in enlarged testes, which appear grossly as poorly defined lobulated masses. Focal areas of hemorrhage are common.

Clinical Manifestations. The most common initial sign of testicular cancer is enlargement of the testis with diffuse testicular pain, swelling, hardness, or some combination of these findings. The condition may go undetected if no pain is experienced and the male is not periodically performing testicular self-examination. The enlargement may be accompanied by an ache in the abdomen or scrotum or a sensation of heaviness in the scrotum. Metastasis, although with little or no local change, is noted in the scrotum.

Retroperitoneal primary tumors may present with back pain (psoas muscle invasion). Metastatic testicular cancer can present as back pain (may be the primary presenting complaint), abdominal mass, hemoptysis, or neck or supraclavicular adenopathy. Up to 21% of men with testicular germ cell cancer have back pain as the primary presenting symptoms.[6] A significant delay occurs in diagnosis of testicular cancer in these men compared with men who also had symptomatic unilateral testicular enlargement.

Pain may be the sole presenting symptom in metastasis to the retroperitoneal, cervical, and supraclavicular lymphatic chains. Since the testis embryologically originates in the genital ridge and descends during fetal life through the abdomen and inguinal canal into the scrotum, the primary lymphatic and vascular drainage of the testis is to the retroperitoneal lymph nodes and the renal or great vessels, respectively. Approximately 20% of all cases have involved lymph nodes.[3]

Occurring during the prime of life for most men and potentially affecting sexual and reproductive capabilities, testicular cancer has a major emotional impact.

Medical Management

Prevention. No known preventive strategies exist but teaching and promoting testicular self-examination as a technique for early detection of this disease is recommended.[7] Since survival is dependent on early detection, men should be encouraged to practice testicular self-examination at least every 6 months. For optimal effect, health education programs need to take into account complexities such as cultural diversity, if men are to heed vital, and in some cases, life-sustaining advice.

Diagnosis. A thorough urologic history and physical examination are the basis for making a diagnosis of testicular cancer. A painless testicular mass is highly suggestive of testicular cancer. Transillumination of the scrotum may also reveal a testicular mass. Serum tumor markers (e.g., alpha-fetoprotein, human chorionic gonadotropin [hCG], and lactate dehydrogenase) are increased in 40% to 60% of all cases and may be used to guide treatment and follow-up. Testicular ultrasound is used to differentiate a variety of scrotal disorders besides cancer (e.g., epididymitis, orchitis, hydrocele, or hematocele). The modalities used to assess metastatic spread include CT scans and MRI.

Staging. Clinical staging is based on the TNM classification system: stage I, or tumor confined to the testis, epididymis, or spermatic cord; stage II, which has spread to the retroperitoneal lymph nodes and divided into A, B, and C according to the size of the nodes; and stage III, which is distant metastasis or high serum tumor-marker values.

Treatment. Management of testicular cancer has changed substantially in the last 20 years, primarily because of the abil-

ity of cisplatin-containing combination chemotherapy to cure advanced disease. Once diagnosed, stage I, IIA, or IIB disease is treated with radical inguinal orchiectomy, followed by radiation to the retroperitoneal and ipsilateral pelvic lymph nodes. Sperm collection and cryopreservation before the initiation of therapy is a developing reproductive technology. Only a few sperm are needed for successful in vitro fertilization.[70]

Chemotherapy is used in cases of relapse after radiation therapy. The recommendation of which therapies to include is based on pathologic findings from the orchiectomy and results of the CT and MRI procedures. Nerve-sparing retroperitoneal lymph node dissection is often used to treat stage II seminomas and nonseminoma germ cell tumors. Initial combination chemotherapy is required in cases of advanced disease, but considerable debate is ongoing regarding the need for orchidectomy or node dissection before chemotherapy in cases of metastases.

Prognosis. With early detection, more than 90% of men with newly diagnosed germ-cell tumors are cured; delay in diagnosis correlates with a higher stage at presentation for treatment.[3] One confounding factor related to the diagnosis being delayed is the potential lack of perceptible testicular changes while the disease spreads.

Long-term sequelae of cisplatin use may include leukemia, cardiovascular events, and reports that circulating cisplatin can be detected in the plasma as long as 20 years after treatment.[39,47]

Special Implications for the Therapist 18-5

TESTICULAR CANCER

Preferred Practice Patterns:
4B: Impaired Posture (postoperative)
6E: Impaired Ventilation and Respiration/Gas Exchange Associated With Ventilatory Pump Dysfunction or Failure (pulmonary fibrosis)
6H: Impaired Circulation and Anthropometric Dimensions Associated With Lymphatic System Disorders (lymphatic dissection)
Other practice patterns may be appropriate depending on complications from treatment.

Therapists need to be aware of the potential signs and symptoms related to this disease because clients may be seen by the therapist for other conditions before the cancer is diagnosed. The most likely scenario is someone with thoracic or lumbar pain secondary to undiagnosed lymph node adenopathy or someone with low lumbar pain that radiates around the iliac crest to the groin. Low lumbar and iliac crest pain may be secondary to biomechanical dysfunction, whereas the groin pain could be secondary to the cancer. Correlation of findings from the history and physical examination and the client's response to treatment may raise suspicion, warranting communication with a physician.

An awareness of the location of superficial lymph nodes is also important for the therapist (see Fig. 12-7). Observation of a mass or even a filling-in of the concavity normally found in the left supraclavicular region should alert the therapist to palpate this area. Palpation of a nodule warrants a referral to a physician. A positive iliopsoas sign (see Figs. 15-10 and 15-11) also requires medical referral.

Surgical treatment of testicular cancer also holds implications for the therapist. Postoperatively, lymph node dissection can result in compromised lymphatic flow and resultant lymphedema (see Chapter 12). The surgical scars related to orchiectomy and retroperitoneal lymph node dissection may affect the person's posture or movement mechanics of the trunk, pelvis, and hip regions. Other potential adverse effects of the surgery include sexual dysfunction infertility, such as occurs with retrograde ejaculation or failure to ejaculate. Serious adverse effects of combination chemotherapy include neuromuscular toxic effects, death from myelosuppression, pulmonary fibrosis, and Raynaud's syndrome. See Treatment and Special Implications for the Therapist: Prostate Cancer for a description of the side effects of radiation and chemotherapy. ■

IMPOTENCE

Overview.   Impotence, also termed *erectile dysfunction (ED)* is a general term that refers to the inability to achieve, keep, or sustain an erection sufficient for satisfactory sexual performance and may include a problem with libido, penile erection, ejaculation, or orgasm.

Incidence and Risk Factors.   The prevalence of ED in various community studies has varied from as low of 7% to as high as 52% and has a definite correlation with increasing age. Incidence data are scarce, but a recent study of white males in the United States described an incidence of 26 cases per 1000 man-years. Epidemiologic studies of ethnic groups in the United States are not available at this time. Risk factors for ED include certain medications; chronic diseases, particularly neurologic conditions and diabetes mellitus; and smoking.[32,63] (Box 18-3).

Etiologic Factors.   Impotence may be organic or psychogenic. Approximately 50% to 80% of men seeking treatment for sexual dysfunction have an organic lesion. The ratio

---

BOX	18-3

Risk Factors for Impotence

Age
Smoking
Medical history
• Diabetes mellitus
• Coronary heart disease
• Hypothyroidism
• Hypopituitarism
• Hypertension
• Chronic uremia
• Neuromuscular disease
• Psychiatric disorders
• Multiple sclerosis
• Chronic alcoholism

Surgical history
• Transurethral procedures
• Aortoiliac procedures
• Proctocolectomy
• Abdominoperineal resection
Medications
• Antihypertensives
• Tranquilizers
• Amphetamines

---

of organic to psychogenic lesions is directly proportional to age. In 70% of men less than 35 years old, the cause is psychogenic. In 85% of men over the age of 50, the cause is organic. Conditions that can impede blood flow (e.g., atherosclerosis, medications) or impair nerve transmission (e.g., diabetes, surgery) are the most common organic causes.[36,40] The psychogenic factors include anxiety, fear, depression, stress, fatigue, and so on.

Pathogenesis.   Numerous factors and structures can influence the process of sexual function and dysfunction. Coordinated interaction between regulatory centers in the diencephalon, brainstem, and spinal cord are required for sexual function. In addition, the end organs of the vascular and nerve tree of the penis, the smooth muscle of the corpora cavernosa, the skeletal muscle of the penis, and the accessory sex glands all have important roles in sexual function. Normally, sexual stimulation triggers the arteries in the penis to widen and the smooth muscle to relax. Blood moves into the spongy smooth muscle while the penile veins constrict to keep the penis engorged and rigid.

It is beyond the scope of this textbook to cover all of the possible mechanisms leading to sexual dysfunction, but some examples follow. Neurogenic ED can result from surgical or traumatic injury to the autonomic or somatic penile innervation. The other possible neurologic mechanism is microscopic neuropathy with breakdown of cholinergic, adrenergic, noncholinergic, or nonadrenergic neurotransmission. Individuals with diabetes mellitus experience change in the ultrastructure of the cavernous nerves arising from the S2-S4 spinal nerves. These changes include diffuse thickening of the Schwann cells and perineural basement membranes.

ED can be a hemodynamic event and can warn of ischemic heart disease in some men. Conditions resulting in arterial insufficiency can also result in local penile changes. Researchers may eventually call impotence a "penile stress test" that can be as predictive as a treadmill exercise stress test for atherosclerosis and subsequent peripheral vascular disease.[46]

Clinical Manifestations.   Manifestations of sexual dysfunction include inability to have or maintain penile erection, inability to achieve orgasm, infertility, and dyspareunia. Most men (and their partners) experience significant feelings of emotional distress and/or depression associated with sexual dysfunction and subsequent infertility. Quality-of-life issues are an important aspect of this disorder.

Medical Management

Diagnosis.   Owing to the sheer number of possible etiologic factors, a definitive diagnosis related to impotence can be difficult. Differentiating between an organic versus psychogenic cause is the initial challenge. The nocturnal penile tumescence test, which monitors the incidence of nocturnal erections, helps with this distinction. Men with psychogenic impotence will have nocturnal erections, whereas those with an organic lesion will not. Arteriography is the standard test for vascular diagnostic testing, but ultrasonography is also used to assess the vascular integrity of the genital area.

Treatment.   Medical treatment for impotence varies depending on the cause. Pharmacologic treatment with Viagra has become the new first-line treatment for anyone without heart disease. Other products are being developed for ED such as alprostadil (now a topical gel applied to the head of the penis), previously only available as an injection into the penile tissue or inserted into the urethra as a small suppository. Testosterone injections are an option for men with documented androgen deficiency. Injection of vasoactive substances directly into the penis may also be used. Penile prosthetic devices can be implanted surgically and men with arterial and venous deficiencies are candidates for vascular reconstruction procedures. Erections can be achieved mechanically with a vacuum pump device. Lastly, psychologic counseling is indicated for those with a psychogenic basis for the impotence.

Special Implications for the Therapist   18-6

IMPOTENCE

Therapists ask clients with back pain about the presence of sexual dysfunction as part of the screening for cauda equina syndrome. Many people who answer "yes" to these questions may have a preexisting condition that accounts for the impotence. Sexual dysfunction may be a postoperative complication related to some of the procedures described earlier in this chapter. If the person notes a sudden change in sexual function, communication with a physician is warranted.

Prescriptive exercise is often recommended for the individual with intact nerve innervation and vascular supply. Kegel's and Beyond Kegel's™ and "quick flicks" (see Chapter 17) may be helpful. ■

REFERENCES

1. Albertsen PC et al: Competing risk analysis of men aged 55 to 74 years at diagnosis managed conservatively for clinically localized prostate cancer, JAMA 280:975-980, 1998.
2. Blute ML, Zincke H, Farrow GM: Long term follow-up of young patients with stage A adenocarcinoma of the prostate, J Urol 136:840-843, 1986.
3. Bosl GJ, Motzer RJ: Testicular germ-cell cancer, N Engl J Med 337(4):242-253, 1997.
4. Bostwick DG, Qian J: Effect of androgen deprivation therapy on prostatic intraepithelial neoplasia, Urology 58(2 Suppl 1):91-93, 2001.
5. Brush JP: Positron emission tomography in urological malignancy, Curr Opin Urol 11(2):175-179, 2001.
6. Cantwell B, Mannix KA, Harris AL: Back pain: a presentation of metastatic testicular germ cell tumors, Lancet 1:262-264, 1987.
7. Cook R: Teaching and promoting testicular self-examination, Nurs Stand 14(24):48-51, 2000.
8. Cotthoff A, Goff K, Kelly DG: The incidence of lymphedema following treatment for prostate cancer: a retrospective study (abstract), Phys Ther 8(5):A23, 2001.
9. Dong C, Hemminiki K: Modification of cancer risks in offspring by sibling and parental cancers from 2,112,616 nuclear families, Int J Cancer 92(1):144-150, 2001.
10. Edelstein R, Babayan R: Managing prostate cancer. Part I: localized disease, Hosp Pract 28(4):61-78, 1993.
11. Epstein JI, Paull G, Eggleston JC, Walsh PC: Prognosis of untreated stage A1 prostatic carcinoma: a study of 94 cases with extended follow-up, J Urol 136:837-839, 1986.
12. Farkas A, Marcella S, Rhoads GG: Ethnic and racial differences in prostate cancer incidence and mortality, Ethn Dis 10(1):69-75, 2000.
13. Ferrari AC et al: Prospective analysis of prostate-antigen specific markers in pelvic lymph nodes of patients with high-risk prostate cancer, J Natl Cancer Inst 89(20):1498-1504, 1997.
14. Fleshner NE, Kucuk O: Antioxidant dietary supplements: rationale and current status as chemopreventive agents for prostate cancer, Urology 57(4 Suppl 1):90-94, 2001.
15. Forman D et al: Familial testicular cancer: a report of the UK family register, estimation of risk and an HLA class 1 sib-pair analysis, Br J Cancer 65:255-262, 1992.
16. Gerber GS: Saw palmetto for the treatment of men with lower urinary tract symptoms, J Urol 163(5):1408-1412, 2000.
17. Gill IS, Zippe CD: Laparoscopic radical prostatectomy: technique, Urol Clin North Am 28(2):423-436, 2001.
18. Gillenwater JY et al: Adult and pediatric urology, ed 2, St Louis, 1991, Mosby.
19. Giovannucci E: A prospective study of dietary fat and risk of prostate cancer, J Natl Cancer Inst 271:498, 1994.
20. Guillonneau B et al: Laparoscopic radical prostatectomy: assessment after 240 procedures, Urol Clin North Am 28(1):189-202, 2001.
21. Hamdy FC: Prognostic and predictive factors in prostate cancer, Cancer Treat Rev 27(3):143-151, 2001.
22. Hamilton AS et al: Health outcomes after external-beam radiation therapy for clinically localized prostate cancer: results from the Prostate Cancer Outcomes Study, J Clin Oncol 19(9):2517-2526, 2001.
23. Han M, Nelson JB: Non-steroidal anti-androgens in prostate cancer: current treatment practice, Expert Opin Pharmacother 1(3):443-449, 2000.
24. Ho G et al: Experimental study of transurethral robotic laser resection of the prostate using the LaserTrode lightguide, J Biomed Opt 6(2):244-251, 2001.
25. Hoffman RM et al: Racial and ethnic differences in advanced-stage prostate cancer: the Prostate Cancer Outcomes Study, J Natl Cancer Inst 93(5):388-395, 2001.
26. Hussain A, Dawson N: Management of advanced/metastatic prostate cancer: 2000 update, Oncology (Huntington) 14(12):1677-1688, 2000.
27. Jacob K et al: Osteonectin promotes prostate cancer cell migration and invasion: a possible mechanism for metastasis to bone, Cancer Res 59(17):4453-4457, 1999.
28. Jemal A et al: Cancer statistics, 2002. CA: Cancer J Clin 2:23-47, 2002.
29. Kantoff PW et al: Prognostic significance of reverse transcriptase polymerase chain reaction for prostate-specific antigen in men with hormone-refractory prostate cancer, J Clin Oncol 19(12):3025-3028, 2001.
30. Koch E: Extracts from fruits of saw palmetto and roots of stinging nettle: viable alternatives in the medical treatment of benign prostatic hyperplasia and associated lower urinary tract symptoms, Planta Med 67(6):489-500, 2001.
31. Kucuk O et al: Phase II randomized clinical trial of lycopene supplementation before radical prostatectomy, Cancer Epidemiol Biomarkers Prev 10(8):861-868, 2001.
32. Lewis RW: Epidemiology of erectile dysfunction, Urol Clin North Am 28(2):209-216, 2001.
33. Liu S et al: A prospective study of physical activity and risk of prostate cancer in U.S. physicians, Int J Epidemiol 29(1):29-35, 2000.
34. Lu QY et al: Inverse associations between plasma lycopene and other carotenoids and prostate cancer, Cancer Epidemiol Biomarkers Prev 10(7):749-756, 2001.
35. Marks LS et al: Effects of saw palmetto herbal blend in men with symptomatic benign prostatic hyperplasia, J Urol 163(5):1451-1456, 2000.
36. Masters WH: Sex and aging: expectations and reality, Hosp Pract 175-198, 1986.
37. Matteson JR et al: Medicolegal aspects of testicular torsion, Urology 57(4):783-786, 2001.
38. Meacham RB: Andorgen replacement in the aging man, Infect Urol 14(2):30, 2001.
39. Meinardi MT et al: Cardiovascular morbidity in long-term survivors of metastatic testicular cancer, J Clin Oncol 18(8):1725-1732, 2000.
40. Mellinger BC, Weiss J: Sexual dysfunction in the elderly male, Am Urol Assoc Update Ser 11:146-152, 1992.

41. Merzenich H et al: Sorting the hype from the facts in testicular cancer: is testicular cancer related to trauma? *J Urol* 164(6):2143-2144, 2000.

42. Mettlin C: Impact of screening on prostate cancer rates and trends, *Microsc Tes Tech* 51(5):415-418, 2000.

43. National Prostate Cancer Coalition: Facts and statistics: prostate cancer, 2001. Available at http://www.4npcc.org.

44. Neuhausen SL et al: Prostate cancer susceptibility locus HPC1 in Utah high-risk pedigrees, *Hum Mol Genet* 8(13):2437-2442, 1999.

45. Newcomer LM et al: The association of fatty acids with prostate cancer risk, *Prostate* 47(4):262-268, 2001.

46. O'Kane PD, Jackson G: Erectile dysfunction: is there silent obstructive coronary artery disease? *Int J Clin Pract* 55(3):219-220, 2001.

47. Oliver RT: Testicular cancer, *Curr Opin Ocol* 13(3):191-198, 2001.

48. Pavlica P, Barozzi L: Imaging of the acute scrotum, *Eur Radiol* 11(2): 220-228, 2001.

49. Perez CA et al: New trends in prostatic cancer research. Three-dimensional conformal radiation therapy (3-D CRT), brachytherapy, and new therapeutic modalities, *Rays* 25(3):331-343, 2000.

50. Rapley EA et al: Localization to Xq27 of a susceptibility gene for testicular germ-cell tumours, *Nat Genet* 24(2):197-200, 2000.

51. Richter E et al: Cancer in radar technicians exposed to radiofrequency/ microwave radiation: sentinel episodes, *Int J Occup Environ Health* 6(3): 187-193, 2000.

52. Roach M: Three-dimensional conformal external beam radiotherapy or brachytherapy: which is the "best alternative" to radical prostatectomy? *CA: Cancer J Clin* 50(6):344-347, 2000.

53. Scardino PT: Early detection of prostate cancer, *Urol Clin North Am* 16:635-655, 1989.

54. Schmidt U, Fiedler U, Pilarsky CP: Identification of a novel gene on chromosome 12 between BRCA-2 and RP-1, *Prostate* 47(2): 91-101, 2001.

55. Simons JW et al: Induction of immunity to prostate cancer antigens: results of a clinical trial of vaccination with irradiated autologous prostate tumor cells engineered to secrete granulocyte-macrophage colony-stimulating factor using ex vivo gene transfer, *Cancer Res* 61(6): 2736-2743, 2001.

56. Smith RH, Wake R, Soloway MS: Benign prostatic hyperplasia: a universal problem among aging men, *Postgrad Med* 83(6):79, 1988.

57. Steinber GD et al: The familial aggregation of prostate cancer: a case control study (Abstract), *J Urol* 143:131A, 1990.

58. Stoch SA, Parker RA, Chen L: Bone loss in men with prostate cancer treated with gonadotropin-releasing hormone agonists, *J Clin Endocrin Metabol* 86(6):2787-2791, 2001.

59. Straub B et al: Reverse transcriptase-polymerase chain reaction for prostate-specific antigen in the molecular staging of pelvic surgical margins after radical prostatectomy, *Urology* 57(5):1006-1011, 2001.

60. Strohsnitter WC et al: Cancer risk in men exposed in utero to diethylstilbestrol, *J Natl Cancer Inst* 93(7):545-551, 2001.

61. Swan SH: Intrauterine exposure to diethylstilbestrol: long-term effects in humans, *APMIS* 108(12):793-804, 2000.

62. Tavtigian SV et al: A candidate prostate cancer susceptibility gene at chromosome 17p, *Nat Genet* 27(2):172-180, 2001.

63. Tengs TO, Osgood ND: The link between smoking and impotence: two decades of evidence, *Prev Med* 32(6):447-452, 2001.

64. Tjoa BA et al: Dendritic cell-based immunotherapy for prostate cancer, *CA: Cancer J Clin* 49:117-128, 1999.

65. Trump DL et al: Androgen antagonists: potential role in prostate cancer prevention, *Urology* 57(4 Suppl 1): 64-67, 2001.

66. Tsai YS et al: Transurethral microwave thermotherapy for symptomatic benign prostatic hyperplasia: long-term durability with postcare, *Eur Urol* 39(6):688-694, 2001.

67. Van Kampen M et al: Effect of pelvic-floor re-education on duration and degree of incontinence after radical prostatectomy: a randomized controlled trial, *Lancet* 355(9198):98-102, 2000.

68. Volpe MA, Fromer D, Kaplan SA: Holmium and interstitial lasers for the treatment of benign prostatic hyperplasia: a laser revival, *Curr Opin Urol* 11(1):43-48, 2001.

69. Weir HK et al: Pre-natal and peri-natal exposures and risk of testicular germ-cell cancer, *Int J Cancer* 87(3):438-443, 2000.

70. Zapalka DM, Redmon JB, Pryor JL: A survey of oncologists regarding sperm cryopreservation and assisted reproductive techniques for male cancer patients, *Cancer* 86(9):1812-1817, 1999.

71. Zelefsky MJ et al: High dose radiation delivered by intensity modulation conformal radiotherapy improves the outcome of localized prostate cancer, *J Urol* 166(3):876-881, 2001.

CHAPTER 19

THE FEMALE GENITAL/REPRODUCTIVE SYSTEM

WILLIAM G. BOISSONNAULT AND CATHERINE C. GOODMAN

The female genital or reproductive system is made up of the ovaries, fallopian tubes, uterus, vagina, and external genitalia (Figs. 19-1 and 19-2). The primary functions of this system are related to preparing the woman for conception and gestation and for gestation itself. The female hormonal system, including the ovarian hormones, estrogen and progesterone, plays a key role in these functions. Malfunctioning of this system can result in a multitude of local disorders, some benign and others life-threatening, as well as widespread systemic changes via the hormonal influences. The incidence of some of the disorders discussed in this chapter is quite high. For example, endometriosis is present in approximately 50% of women receiving treatment for infertility and in 10% to 15% of all premenopausal women. Further, breast cancer accounts for approximately one-third of all female cancers. Therefore therapists frequently encounter disorders of this system.

Therapists are now involved in the field of urogynecology with specific evaluation and assessment tools, treatment modalities, and therapeutic interventions. Increasingly, therapists are involved in the management of conditions such as vaginismus, dyspareunia, vulvodynia, sexual dysfunction, pelvic pain, levator ani syndrome, endometriosis, organ prolapse, and incontinence. Therapists' participation in women's health issues reflects the medical profession's changing view of women. The traditional allopathic emphasis on women's breasts and reproductive system (the "bikini view") is shifting focus to a more holistic view of women as unique individuals during their reproductive years and beyond, both in health and in disease.

AGING AND THE FEMALE REPRODUCTIVE SYSTEM

The most significant age-related change associated with the female reproductive system is menopause, which is the permanent cessation of menses. The average age at which this event occurs is 45 to 50 years, but changes begin as early as mid-30s for many women, a period of time leading up to complete menopause referred to as perimenopause. Menopause is caused by the gradual cessation of ovarian function with resultant reduced estrogen levels. During the reproductive years the primordial ovarian follicles, from which ova are expelled, steadily decrease in number. By middle age, the ovaries, which each held about 300,000 eggs at puberty, have resorbed or shed nearly all of them. Ovarian production of estrogen and progesterone decreases significantly when the number of these follicles approaches zero. The reduced level of hormones results in a cascade of events altering the physiology of multiple systems.

Symptomatically, women may experience hot flashes, vaginal dryness, fatigue, anxiety, sleep disturbances, reduced libido, mood swings, and irritability. Physiologic changes include endometrial, vaginal, and breast atrophy; decreased thyroid function; hyperparathyroidism; and decreased renal function, insulin release, and response to catecholamines. In addition, if not receiving hormonal replacement therapy (HRT),* postmenopausal women may be at greater risk of developing arteriovascular disease, including heart disease, hypertension, and cerebrovascular accidents, as well as osteoporosis and depression. Any of these conditions may account for the need for rehabilitation or complicate rehabilitative efforts if present as co-morbidities.

Local changes of the reproductive organs also occur secondary to decreased estrogen levels. The myometrium, endometrium, cervix, vagina, and labia all become atrophic to some degree. In addition, the pelvic floor musculature loses strength and tone, which can contribute to the development of cystocele, rectocele, uterine prolapse, and stress urinary incontinence. Although vaginal bleeding should stop with menopause, 80% of all gynecologic problems in women over age 60 years are related to postmenopausal bleeding (vaginal bleeding that occurs 1 year or more after the last period).† Such bleeding can be a symptom of a life-threatening problem (e.g., cancer) or a benign condition (e.g., polyps) but always requires a medical evaluation.

Although estrogen levels decline as women age, the ovaries continue to produce significant amounts of testosterone and androstenedione after menopause. As a result, levels of testosterone may not decline sharply at menopause for women whose ovaries are intact. Testosterone is a natural means of preserving bone and muscle mass and of alleviating menopausal symptoms, particularly the loss of libido.

---

*There is a difference between oral contraceptives and HRT. Contraceptives have more estrogen than standard hormone replacement with estrogen. The lowest dose of oral contraceptive available contains 20 μg of ethinyl estradiol. This is four times that in a standard hormone replacement regimen, which contains 5 μg of ethinyl estradiol (equivalent to 0.625 mg of conjugated equine estrogens).

†Women receiving continuous, combined HRT (estrogen in combination with progestin taken without a break) are likely to experience irregular spotting until the endometrium (vaginal lining) atrophies, which takes about 6 months. An evaluation is required only if bleeding persists or suddenly appears after 6 months. Those women taking sequential HRT (estrogen taken daily for 25 days each month with progestin taken for 10 or 12 days) normally bleed lightly each time the progestin is temporarily stopped.

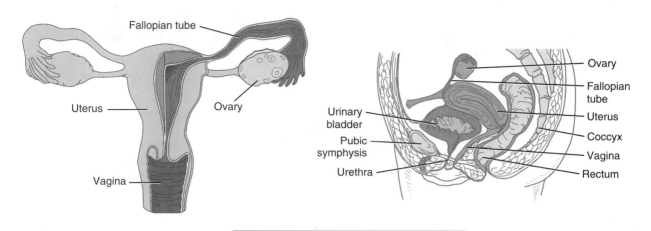

FIGURE   **19-1**   Female reproductive organs.

The diseases discussed in this chapter have several implications for therapists. Some conditions, for example, pelvic floor disorders or postsurgical rehabilitation following radical mastectomy, may be the primary reason the woman is seeing the therapist. Other conditions, such as endometriosis, may be manifested solely by pain, and the woman presents to the therapist with back or pelvic pain of unknown cause. Last, the presence of some of these conditions places the woman at higher risk of developing other diseases. For example, a history of endometriosis increases the risk of ectopic pregnancy, a potentially life-threatening disorder.

MENOPAUSE AND HORMONE REPLACEMENT THERAPY

Much has been written and debated about the need for HRT for menopausal women, and with nearly 80 million women currently approaching or going through menopause, this will remain an issue in the forefront of health care. Therapists do not evaluate the need for HRT or prescribe these medications, but clients frequently ask questions and seek additional educational information about this topic. Therapists themselves are often faced with making the decision about HRT use either personally or in relation to a close family member. Although an exhaustive discussion of this issue is not the focus of this text, a brief summary is warranted in today's health care environment.

The decision to use or not use HRT after menopause is based on a thorough understanding of the risks and benefits of HRT and how that understanding applies to each woman based on her individual risks. Much remains unknown about the long-term effects of HRT, but studies have been ongoing and new information is available daily. A decade ago, health experts were convinced that estrogen would be essential for reducing heart disease in women, and clinicians routinely offered it in HRT as part of a prevention plan. Now there is abundant evidence that HRT does not help women with heart disease and may even worsen their condition. As a result of this new information, cardiovascular protection is no longer included as a benefit of HRT although many questions remain unanswered.[72] Whatever decision a woman makes should be in conjunction with her health care provider keeping in mind that any decision made can be changed as new information becomes available.

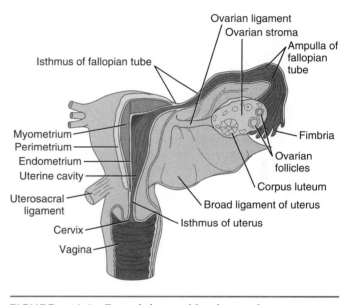

FIGURE   **19-2**   Expanded view of female reproductive organs.

Estrogen replacement therapy is used after menopause for two categories of reasons: (1) treatment of menopausal symptoms and (2) medical benefits (Table 19-1). The positive effects last only as long as therapy is continued; and in some cases, according to data from the Nurses' Health Study, excess risk of negative sequelae (e.g., breast cancer) disappears after hormone use is discontinued. Because of the increased risk of breast and uterine cancer with the use of estrogen alone, unopposed estrogen is now recommended only for women who have had a hysterectomy.

For the woman who prefers not to take long-term HRT, there are alternatives for preventing osteoporosis and heart disease and for modifying the transient and temporary symptoms of menopause. Drugs called *SERMs (selective estrogen receptor modulators)* are being tested to determine their effects in preventing bone loss, improving serum lipids, and reducing breast cancer risk. These pharmaceuticals stimulate estrogen receptors in some tissues but not in others. The importance of lifestyle measures such as exercising; maintaining a low-fat, calcium-rich diet; and not smoking has been clearly demonstrated. Natural substances such as black cohosh, dong quai,

TABLE   19-1

Advantages and Disadvantages of Hormone Replacement Therapy (HRT)

RISKS AND DISADVANTAGES	BENEFITS
Increased risk of endometrial cancer (estrogen alone with progestin)	Treats menopausal symptoms (e.g., hot flashes, night sweats, sleep disturbances, memory loss, fatigue, atrophic changes of vagina or urinary tract)
Increased risk of breast cancer with prolonged (>10 yr) use of HRT*	Maintains skin thickness and elasticity, prevents fine wrinkles
Side effects (e.g., vaginal bleeding, fluid retention, weight gain, bloating, breast swelling and tenderness, headaches, mood swings, depression, skin irritatin, constipation, loss of libidor†	Prevents accelerated bone loss; maintains bone density; reduces risk of fractures by 50%
Increased risk of gallstones, blood clots	Reduces risk of colon cancer and stroke
Increased breast density and reduced specificity and sensitivity of mammography	May improve blood pressure[95]
Contraindicated in women with the following:	Prevention or delay of Alzheimer's disease (preliminary data)
History of blood clots	Improves pain tolerance
Pancreatic or liver disease	Increases production or prolongs action of serotonin
Hormone-sensitive breast or uterine cancer	
Migraine headaches or hypertension that is aggravated by estrogen	
Other contraindications or precautions	
Recent heart attack	
History of uterine fibroids	
Endometriosis	
History of stroke or TIAs	
Fibrocystic breast disease	
Current breast or endometrial cancer	

TIA, Transient ischemic attack.
*New data suggest combined estrogen/progestin increases risk for breast cancer compared with estrogen alone.[86,91] These data run counter to previous studies that suggested the risks were similar for estrogen alone and combined therapy. Other epidemiologic reviews do not support this new finding.[10,13] Further research to clarify the effects of lowered dosage of HRT is warranted. This is just one exampe of the divergent and confusing information becoming available on this topic during this time of broad investigation. Again, each woman must assess her personal and family health history, lifestyle, and risks and make an individual decision regarding the use or continuation of HRT.
†Some side effects can be managed with a reduced dose, different schedule, or changing brands. Any woman experiencing intolerable side effects should see the prescribing physician for evaluation.

rose hips, soy products, flaxseed, and ginseng used in conjunction with alternative approaches (e.g., yoga, meditation, acupuncture) are becoming increasingly popular, but research results remain limited at this time.

For the therapist, knowing where a woman is in her life cycle and what medications, supplements, or other measures she is using is an important part of the personal medical history. Whether or not a woman is taking HRT postmenopausally (but especially if she is not), the therapist remains a key health care provider in risk assessment, assessment and prevention of falls, osteoporosis education, and a program of physical activity and exercise to minimize the effects of aging and estrogen deficiency.

EXERCISE AND THE REPRODUCTIVE SYSTEM

Exercise increases cardiovascular fitness, reduces adiposity, and aids in maintaining muscle mass and bone density in women of all ages from adolescents to frail older people. On the other hand, too much exercise can have negative effects on the reproductive and skeletal systems, including primary and secondary amenorrhea (absence of menstruation) caused by low body weight and improper nutrition (see further discussion in the section on Eating Disorders in Chapter 2).

The female athlete is at particular risk of reproductive system disruption with strenuous exercise. Hypothalamic dysfunction can result in delayed menarche (first menstruation) and disruption or cessation of menstrual cyclicity. When energy expenditure exceeds dietary intake, gonadotropin-releasing hormone (Gn-RH) is suppressed, resulting in hypoestrogenism and subsequent compromised bone density and infertility. Failure to attain peak bone mass combined with bone loss predisposes female athletes to osteopenia, osteoporosis, and stress reactions or fractures. Increasing caloric intake to offset high-energy demand may be sufficient to reverse menstrual dysfunction and stimulate bone growth.[113,114]

Obesity also has significant consequences for the reproductive system and contributes to menstrual disorders, infertility, miscarriage, poor pregnancy outcome, impaired fetal well-being, and diabetes mellitus. Weight loss has marked effects on improving the menstrual cycle, promoting ovulation, and fertility. Fertility is improved through exercise and balanced nutrition possibly through changes in sensitivity to insulin.[80]

Mood disorders, including depression and postpartum depression, anxiety, and vulnerability to autoimmune and inflammatory diseases seem to follow estradiol (one of three estrogen compounds present in the body) fluctuations.[21] Exercise has been shown effective in elevating mood, decreasing risk of cancer, and ameliorating some of these symptoms and conditions for most people (see individual discussions of these topics in this text).

SEXUAL DYSFUNCTION

The participation of a physical therapist in the management of sexual dysfunction is an increasing phenomenon. More and more adults (men and women) are experiencing altered sexual function and sexuality as a result of medical treatment and medications. For example, being able to enjoy sex after cancer treatment is a significant and necessary part of the recovery process. Altered body image and hormones affect both men and women after treatment (surgery, drugs, radiation) for cancer of the reproductive organs. Menopause may be triggered prematurely in some women. An excellent resource about the side effects of radiation and chemotherapy on sexual desire and performance along with helpful suggestions is available.[92]

Other medical problems, such as diabetes, arthritis, depression, pelvic floor disorders, menopause, prostate problems, and cardiovascular disease, can result in sexual dysfunction. Addressing these issues can have a positive effect on sexuality and quality of life. Most of these conditions can be managed with medications, lifestyle changes, and exercise. The therapist can be very instrumental in helping clients discuss sexual problems more readily and with less embarrassment and in helping them obtain the appropriate medical intervention, often including physical therapy intervention.

People who have been sexually victimized or traumatized are also seeking professional help for the first time. Sexual abuse occurs in approximately one of every three girls younger than 14 years and one of every seven boys; only a small proportion of these cases are ever reported. Sexual abuse, marital (or partner) rape, and assault occur in the adult population; the prevalence of these events remains unknown, but social scientists estimate that 20% to 25% of the U.S. population is affected. There is an increased incidence of obesity, incontinence (urinary and fecal), fibromyalgia, infertility, pelvic pain, and behavioral components (e.g., eating disorders, obsessive-compulsive disorders, learning difficulties) associated with sexual abuse.

DISORDERS OF THE UTERUS AND FALLOPIAN TUBES

◆ Endometriosis

Overview.   Endometriosis is marked by functioning endometrial tissue found outside the uterus. The disorder becomes apparent in the early teen years after menses have begun, and its symptoms continue until menopause. The most common sites of ectopic implantation include the ovaries, fallopian tubes, broad ligaments, pouch of Douglas, bladder, pelvic musculature, perineum, vulva, vagina, or intestines (Fig. 19-3). Although less common, endometrial tissue can also be found in the abdominal cavity, implanted on the kidneys, small bowel, appendix, diaphragm, pleura, and bony elements of the spine. Rarely, ectopic tissue has been found in joints, the nose, and the lungs.[109]

Wherever this tissue migrates, it is biochemically and endocrine active, behaving as if it were still under the control of the hormonal system. Every month during the menses, a woman with endometriosis develops a host of symptoms that depend on where the uterine tissue resides. During menstruation, the dislocated tissue is responding just as the uterine lining, but since it cannot shed as the endometrium does, it remains where it is, eventually forming scar tissue and irritating the affected area.

The American Society of Reproductive Medicine (ASRM) has classified endometriosis as I (minimal), II (mild), III (moderate), IV (severe), or V (extensive). Despite

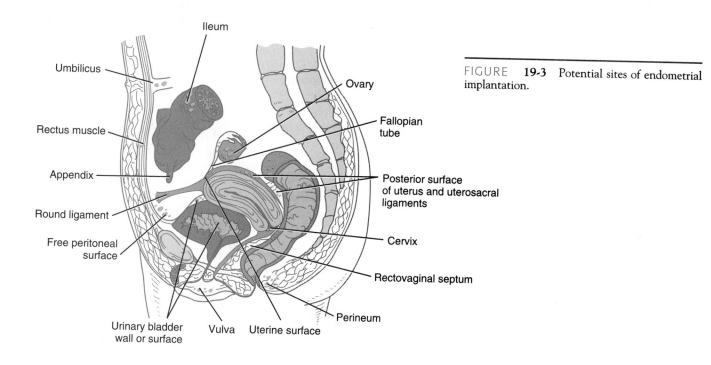

FIGURE   **19-3** Potential sites of endometrial implantation.

this classification system, a woman can have severe disease without symptoms or severe symptoms with minimal disease. This is most likely determined by the type of endometriosis and how biochemically active are the implants.

Incidence. The incidence of endometriosis has increased in the past 40 to 50 years in Western countries. Reports of incidence vary from as low as 7% to as high as 40% to 60% of all women. Endometriosis is found in 25% to 50% of all infertile women. Endometriosis affects women of all ethnic origins, socioeconomic backgrounds, and geographic locations.[109]

Etiologic and Risk Factors. Any woman of childbearing age is at risk of developing endometriosis, but it is more common in those who have postponed pregnancy. In addition, other risk factors include early menarche; regular menstruation, but of 27-day or shorter cycles; and menstrual periods lasting 7 days or longer.

The cause of endometriosis is unknown although the high prevalence among family members suggests a genetic predisposition. A daughter with a maternal history of endometriosis has twice the chance of developing endometriosis herself. The most widely espoused theory suggests that endometrial cells are flushed into the pelvic cavity through retrograde menstruation, a condition in which some of the menstrual flow backs up the fallopian tubes into the pelvic cavity. This retrograde menstruation has been shown to occur in up to 90% of women, but it is unclear why endometrial cells implant in some women and not in others. Since the fimbrial openings of the fallopian tubes are in the posterior aspect of the pelvis, more of the endometrial implants are found on posterior structures.

Another strongly held hypothesis is a dysregulation or dysfunction of the immune system that allows these cells to locate and survive where they do not belong. The cells from the uterine lining are resistant to the body's normal defense mechanisms and are not readily cleared away when they happen to stray outside the organ. Other theories include the (1) dissemination of endometrial cells through the lymphatics or vascular system (explains presence of tissue in lungs); (2) metaplasia of the mesothelium (Meyer's theory), that is, endometrial cells change from one type of cell to another whereby the endothelium undergoes transformation able to produce the same reproductive hormones (explains presence of tissue in joints); (3) intraoperative implantation associated with procedures such as hysterectomy and episiotomy; and (4) abnormal differentiation of precursor epithelial cells during early embryology whereby these cells are seeded before birth.

Pathogenesis. Once endometrial cells migrate to other parts of the body, they can form pockets of tissue referred to as implants. These implants swell in response to the cyclic surge of estrogen and progesterone-forming cysts on the underlying organs that contain a dark, syrupy fluid composed of old blood and menstrual debris, called "chocolate" cysts.

There are three primary pathologic types of endometriosis: (1) red or petechial implants: these are the most active with the greatest capacity to produce prostaglandins (inflammatory mediators) and also capable of producing endometrial protein and hormones; (2) brown or intermediate implants: these are moderately active and precursors to powder burns; and (3) black or brown powder burn implants: these are inactive with little cellular material but associated with adhesions that

stretch organs and cause direct nerve damage through devitalization and ischemia. The powder burn implants adhere structures together contributing to infertility, sometimes referred to as a "frozen pelvis." The severity of the disease depends on which one of these three types is present.

Clinical Manifestations. The symptoms and signs associated with endometriosis depend on the location of the implants, but pain and infertility are the two major symptoms. Abdominal pain, fatigue, and mood changes are common beginning 1 or 2 days before the onset of the menstrual flow and continuing for the duration. Dysmenorrhea (painful menstruation) will be the chief complaint if the implants are on the uterosacral ligaments. These lesions swell immediately before or during menstruation, resulting in pelvic pain. Dyspareunia (painful intercourse) is also associated with this condition because penile penetration during intercourse can aggravate the local adhesions.

Pain during defecation can occur when there are adhesions on the large bowel. The fecal material moves through the intestine, stretching and aggravating the scar tissue. Surprisingly, the extent of the disease does not always correlate with the intensity of the symptoms. A woman with widespread lesions may be asymptomatic, whereas a woman with few implants may have considerable pain. Other symptoms can include low-grade fever, diarrhea, constipation, rectal bleeding, and referred pain to the low back/sacral, groin, posterior leg, upper abdomen, or lower abdominal/suprapubic areas.

Medical Management
Diagnosis. Although the classic triad of dysmenorrhea, dyspareunia, and infertility strongly suggests the presence of endometriosis, accurate diagnosis requires direct visual examination by laparoscopy or laparotomy. One advantage of laparoscopy is that the technique is also therapeutic in that lesions can be removed immediately. Ultrasound and magnetic resonance imaging (MRI) are generally used to examine the pelvis, but MRI is more sensitive in detecting the implants. Researchers are trying to develop a radioimmune assay to measure endocrine protein associated or present with this disease toward the eventual development of a blood test.

Treatment. There is no cure for endometriosis; the goals of medical treatment are preservation of fertility (if fertility is an issue) and pain relief. Pregnancy does appear to suppress the disease, and in animal studies, the implants disappear during pregnancy.[109] Assisted reproduction may be recommended to stimulate ovulation and perform in vitro fertilization with transplantation of the embryo into the uterus.

Nonsteroidal antiinflammatory drugs may sufficiently relieve the pain, or other analgesics can be administered before or during menstruation. Other medications are used to inhibit ovulation and lower hormone levels to prevent the cyclic stimulation of the endometrial implants. Eventually, the implants will decrease in size. These medications include danazol,* a combination estrogen-progesterone acetate, leuprolide (Lupron; injectable once per month into the muscle), gosere-

---

*This synthetic male hormone inhibits the monthly surge of luteinizing hormone (LH), reduces estrogen production, and influences the way estrogen affects endometriosis. Primary adverse side effects include weight gain, edema, decreased breast size, acne, oily skin, headache, muscle cramps, and deepening of the voice. It can also adversely affect lipid metabolism and raise blood pressure.

lin (injectable under the skin), and nafarelin nasal spray, a Gn-RH (these analogs act on the hypothalamus-to-pituitary interface to shut down the ovaries by blocking the ability to produce gonadotropins such as follicle-stimulating hormone [FSH] and luteinizing hormone [LH]). Birth control pills may be used to reduce painful symptoms and inhibit menstrual periods, which stops the growth of endometriotic implants, but these do not cause complete regression of implants already present. Once the woman goes off the pill, these implants become active once again, sometimes with a rebound effect (symptoms are much worse).

Surgical intervention is another approach that is used less commonly than even 10 years ago because the etiology remains unchanged and regrowth occurs rather quickly. If the endometriosis is mild without extensive adhesions, laparoscopic cauterization or laser surgery may be indicated. If the woman is over 35 to 40 years of age, disabled by the pain, and childbearing is completed, a total hysterectomy, bilateral salpingo-oophorectomy (removal of ovaries and fallopian tubes), and implant removal are considered.

Nontraditional therapies, such as yoga, aromatherapy, reflexology, naturopathic medicine, and homeopathy, may be useful adjuncts to allopathic medicine. Many women are using this type of alternative/complementary intervention combined with diet and nutrition to self-treat without medications. Numerous resources are now available in this area.[4,24,31,75]

The future treatment of endometriosis may be based on the development of remodeling enzymes that work to remodel tissue at the cellular level. Understanding the mechanisms of growth factors for the growth and development of epithelial cells, the immune system, and implant physiology will help researchers develop more specific intervention techniques.

Prognosis As mentioned, there is no cure for endometriosis although pregnancy and menopause appear to arrest its continued development. Endometriosis has been linked with reproductive cancers and melanoma.[48,103] The link between endometriosis and these diseases remains unclear although a genetic predisposition or shared exposures to environmental toxins (especially dioxins) have been suggested, but the findings are inconsistent and inconclusive.[94,122]

Special Implications for the Therapist 19-1

ENDOMETRIOSIS

Preferred Practice Patterns:
4C: Impaired Muscle Performance
4D: Impaired Joint Mobility, Motor Function, Muscle Performance, and Range of Motion Associated With Connective Tissue Dysfunction

As common as this disease is, therapists often encounter endometriosis as a primary diagnosis, as co-morbidity, or as an undiagnosed condition. Many women note that their back or pelvic pain is cyclic. Therapists often justify this observation with an explanation that the hormonal changes associated with men-

struation can result in ligamentous laxity, thereby stressing the joints of the pelvis. This is only one possible scenario. Therapists need to consider all possibilities, including pelvic disease. Dyspareunia is a common complaint associated with sacroiliac, lumbar, or hip dysfunction. If the painful intercourse is related to endometriosis, the pain will be present regardless of position. If the pain is related to joint dysfunction, typically certain intercourse positions will be comfortable and others painful.

Endometriosis may account for false-positive findings during the therapist's physical examination. For example, if there are endometrial implants on the psoas major muscle, local palpation and length or strength testing of the psoas may be provocative. The therapist may be led to believe the psoas is the origin of the pain complaints. Endometrial implants on pelvic floor muscles and ligaments, sacroiliac ligaments, and abdominal wall muscle may lead to similar false-positive findings.

The medications commonly given to treat endometriosis can result in a variety of side effects that can account for a woman's symptoms. Gastrointestinal system complaints (dyspepsia, nausea, etc.) may be related to the pain or the antiinflammatory medication being taken. The Gn-RH medications can result in hot flashes and vaginal dryness. Danazol can cause weight gain, acne, decreased breast size, and hirsutism. ■

◆ Uterine Fibroids

Overview. Uterine fibroids (benign tumors of the uterus) are common, presenting in up to one-quarter of all women of childbearing age and constituting the primary reason women have hysterectomies.

Clinical Manifestations. Usually, uterine fibroids are asymptomatic, but in 10% to 20% of women with these tumors, pain and abnormally heavy bleeding during or between menstrual periods are common. Often these women become anemic, experiencing fatigue and weakness that contribute to an impaired lifestyle. Fibroids can and often do grow to the size of a grapefruit or larger, placing pressure on the bladder and resulting in urinary frequency and nocturia.

Medical Management
Treatment. Pharmacotherapy to control fibroid-related symptoms may include nonsteroidal antiinflammatories for pain control or hormonal agents that lighten or stop the period. Other options may include surgical removal through a procedure called *myomectomy*. One way to perform this operation is to pass a fiberoptic scope through the vagina into the uterus (called *hysteroscopy*) to remove the tumors. Fibroids embedded in the uterine wall usually require a laparoscopy or more invasive open abdominal surgery.

A new, less invasive technique (fibroid embolization) performed with the woman under local anesthesia and mild sedation involves the radiologist inserting a catheter into the femoral artery through a small incision in the thigh and then snaking the catheter into the uterus. Tiny plastic or small sponge particles (polyvinyl alcohol) are injected that block off the blood supply to the smaller arteries supplying the fibroids. Another alternative to hysterectomy is endometrial (or balloon) ablation in which the uterine lining is destroyed (but not the uterus) through electrical energy or heat from a balloon-tipped catheter inserted into the vagina, through the cervix, into the uterus. The balloon is then filled with a sterile solution until it conforms to the shape of the uterus and heated until the heat destroys the endometrial tissue.

Eliminating red meat and ham from the diet and eating green vegetables, fruit, and fish appear to have a protective effect. Presumably diet influences levels of the estrogen hormone, which is known to affect fibroid growth.[20]

◆ Endometrial Carcinoma (Uterine Cancer)

Overview. Cancer of the lining of the uterus (endometrium)* is the fourth most common cancer in women and the most common cancer of the female reproductive organs, accounting for approximately 6600 deaths per year in the United States. There is no apparent genetic component to endometrial cancer, but rather, environmental, social, and lifestyle factors are the most important.[106]

Risk Factors. Endometrial carcinoma is most common in women who are older (average age 60 years), white, affluent, obese, and of low parity. In fact, 75% of cases occur in postmenopausal women; the remaining 25% occur in premenopausal women, including 5% in women younger than 40 years. Hypertension and diabetes mellitus are also predisposing factors. Because any condition that increases exposure to unopposed estrogen increases the risk of endometrial cancer, tamoxifen (Nolvadex) therapy,† estrogen replacement therapy without progestin, and the presence of estrogen-secreting tumors are all risk factors. Cigarette smoking, physical activity and exercise, and the use of oral contraceptives appear to decrease the risk. In fact, women who exercise are 80% less likely to develop endometrial cancer than women who do not exercise at all.[106]

Clinical Manifestations. Unlike ovarian cancer, endometrial cancer has a major identifiable symptom in its early stages: abnormal bleeding (present in 80% of all cases). Irregular bleeding is a normal consequence of menopause, but the woman who is at least 12 months after menopause presenting with abnormal vaginal bleeding is the most typical presentation of endometrial cancer.

Metastases to the lymphatic system can result in abdominal or lower extremity swelling.

Medical Management

Diagnosis. Abnormal bleeding in any woman of any age must be medically evaluated. Women with increased risk and those with postmenopausal bleeding or vaginal discharge should be screened for endometrial cancer. When metastatic spread occurs, the most common sites are lymph nodes, lung, or liver. More rarely, bone metastases with isolated lesions to the femur, tibia, fibula, and calcaneus may occur.[70]

Endometrial sampling is currently the most accurate and widely used screening technique, but ultrasonographic measurement of endometrial thickness and hysteroscopy have also

been used. Staging has changed significantly over the last 25 years and is now determined surgically using the FIGO (International Federation of Gynecology and Obstetrics) classification. This classification system has a broad continuum from IA (tumor limited to endometrium), IB (invasion to less than one-half of the myometrium), and IC (invasion to more than one-half of the myometrium) to progression through IIA, IIB, IIIA, and IIIB (vaginal metastases), IIIC (metastases to pelvic or paraaortic lymph nodes), IVA (tumor invades bladder or bowel mucosa), and IVB (distant metastases, including intraabdominal or inguinal lymph nodes).

Other less invasive methods of staging are under consideration, such as laparoscopic assisted vaginal hysterectomy with lymphadenectomy.[6] Contrast-enhanced MRI may help decrease the number of unnecessary lymph node dissections.[36]

Treatment. Endometrial cancer is usually treated surgically with total abdominal hysterectomy and bilateral salpingo-oophorectomy. The plane of excision lies outside the pubocervical fascia and does not require unroofing of the ureters.[6] Progestin therapy may be used in those women who decline surgical intervention,[15] and hormonal therapy (including progestin and antiestrogen tamoxifen) has been used with recurrent disease. Most of these cancers are detected at an early stage when they are highly curable.

Women with advanced stages of endometrial cancer may not be candidates for operative intervention in the presence of tumor fixation or deeply invasive cancer. Medically inoperable cases may be treated with radiotherapy alone (external-beam pelvic radiotherapy or vaginal brachytherapy), and radiation may be used when the tumor spreads outside the uterus or in the case of advanced or recurrent disease after failed hormonal therapy. Cytotoxic combination chemotherapy also has been used with varying results.

Prognosis. Early detection makes this disease curable, but recurrences can occur; most recurrences occur within the first 3 years after surgery. Endometrial lining involvement of less than 50% is associated with 100% survival, but this drops precipitously when tumor growth involves more than one half of the endometrium, especially with local or distant metastases.[38]

Special Implications for the Therapist   19-2

ENDOMETRIAL CARCINOMA (UTERINE CANCER)

Preferred Practice Patterns:
4B: Impaired Posture
4C: Impaired Muscle Performance
6H: Impaired Circulation and Anthropometric Dimensions Associated With Lymphatic System Disorders

Physical activity and exercise are known to decrease the risk of endometrial cancer. This is yet another area of preventive medicine in which the therapist can be very instrumental in conducting a screening examination consisting of a few questions and prescribing an appropriate exercise program. Questions

---

*Endometrial carcinoma is commonly known as uterine cancer, but technically the term *uterine cancer* refers to all cancers found in the uterus body and the cervix.

†A great deal of attention has been paid to the possible induction of endometrial cancer by the antiestrogen tamoxifen, which has led to the development of new selective estrogen receptor modulators (SERMs). The National Cancer Institute's new STAR (study of tamoxifen and raloxifene) trials to compare these two drugs and their side effects are under way.

may include past personal or family history of endometrial (or other) cancer, presence of menses or menopause, use of HRT or neutraceutical supplements (e.g., rose hips, dong quai, soy), presence of osteoporosis or bone density testing results, and current exercise/physical activity levels. Any time a woman who is at least 12 months after menopause and not taking hormone replacements reports vaginal bleeding, a medical evaluation is required.

For the woman who has been treated for endometrial cancer with lymphadenectomy and/or radiation, posttreatment lymphedema and other potential side effects (see Chapter 4 and Table 8-8) may require physical therapy intervention. ■

◆ Cervical Cancer

Overview and Incidence.   Every year in the United States, approximately 13,000 women are diagnosed with cervical cancer and 4400 women die of this disease. Mortality has declined dramatically since the 1930s when the Papanicolaou (Pap) smear was introduced. It is now largely a preventable disease with preventive sexual practices, regular screening, and intervention at the precancerous stage. Twenty-five percent of new cases of cervical cancer develop in women 65 years and older.

Etiologic and Risk Factors.   Clinical studies have confirmed that the human papillomavirus (HPV; known as papillomas or genital warts) is the primary cause of cervical cancer. HPV is the most common sexually transmitted disease in the United States. More than 70 types of HPV have been identified: 23 of these infect the cervix, and 13 types are associated with cancer. Infection with one of these viruses does not necessarily predict cancer, but the risk of cancer is increased significantly and a link between HPV infection and female cervical cancer and male anal cancer has been demonstrated.[45]

Other risk factors include maternal use of diethylstilbestrol (DES), smoking (even passive smoking), oral contraceptive use, high parity, low socioeconomic status, ethnic background (black women experience a 72% higher incidence compared with whites),[82] young age at first intercourse (17 years or younger), multiple sexual partners (five or more), and other sexually transmitted diseases.[57] Women infected with human immunodeficiency virus (HIV) are at increased risk for cervical intraepithelial lesions (the precursors to invasive cervical cancer), presumably associated with a high rate of persistent HPV infection.[29] Other immunocompromised women (e.g., organ transplant recipients, women receiving immunosuppressants) are also at increased risk.

Pathogenesis.   The common unifying oncogenic feature of the vast majority of cervical cancers is the presence of HPV. The molecular basis for oncogenesis in cervical carcinoma can be explained to a large degree by the regulation and function of the two viral oncogenes E6 and E7. The ability of HPV to target the function of tumor suppressors is typical of DNA tumor viruses. The E6 gene product binds to the p53 tumor suppressor gene and induces p53 degradation. E7 targets another tumor suppressor that functions like p53 in cell cycle control and inactivates it.[56]

As a result of these molecular disruptions, dysplastic changes occur in the thin layer of cells known as the *epithe-*

lium that covers the cervix. The cells found covering the outer surface of the cervix are squamous (flat and scaly) whereas the cells lining the endocervical canal are columnar (column-like). About 75% of cervical cancer cases come from changes in the squamous cells (squamous cell carcinoma), 15% to 20% come from changes in squamous and columnar cells (adenosquamous carcinoma), and 5% to 10% arise from changes in just the columnar cells (adenocarcinomas).

Clinical Manifestations.   Early-stage cervical cancer, especially in the preinvasive stage, is usually asymptomatic. Often women have advanced disease before abnormal bleeding occurs. This can present as spotting between menstrual periods, longer and heavier periods, bleeding after menopause, or bleeding after sexual intercourse. Pelvic or low back pain can occur, but this is uncommon.

More advanced stages of cervical cancer may cause bowel and bladder problems because of pressure on the rectum or bladder or sexual difficulties because of the growth in the upper vagina, causing discomfort. Ureter blockage can lead to death because of uremia (the inability of the body to excrete waste), which causes uremic poisoning. The progression to this type of advanced cancer is relatively rare in developed countries.

The physical effects of cervical cancer after treatment are actually more significant. Women who have the conization procedure or loop electrosurgical excision procedure (LEEP) may experience cramping, bleeding, or a watery discharge. Hysterectomy, radiation therapy, surgery alone or combined with radiation, and/or chemotherapy may all cause significant side effects, which should improve over time with proper intervention.

The emotional effects of cervical cancer are often significant as well. Women treated with radiation almost always lose the benefits of estrogen because the ovaries are extremely sensitive to radiation. HRT is usually prescribed, and without this intervention, the emotional effects of cervical cancer can be compounded by hypoestrogenism and its emotional side effects. Sexuality after hysterectomy or other interventions for this cancer can be impaired; women may experience depression from no longer being able to have children; and some women may feel guilt and shame associated with feeling "unclean" because of genital tract disease.

Medical Management

Prevention.   HPV-related cases of cervical cancer are preventable using barrier contraceptives, engaging in monogamous sex with a likewise monogamous partner, or practicing sexual abstinence (see the section on Sexually Transmitted Disease in Chapter 7). Research is underway to develop a vaccine, but in the meantime, early detection is the key to a 100% cure rate for this cancer. Routine cervical screening is recommended for all women regardless of sexual orientation or practices from 18 years of age or on becoming sexually active (whichever comes first) throughout adulthood. Women with known HIV infection, HPV, or other sexually transmitted diseases must especially be screened for cervical cancer.[29]

Some experts advise that Pap screening can be performed at 3-year intervals in some women, discontinued in women over 65 years who have had normal findings on three consecutive tests, and discontinued in women who have had the cervix removed (e.g., in conjunction with hysterectomy). Others support annual testing for most women regardless of age and to detect vaginal cancer in women who have had the cervix removed.

Diagnosis.   Cervical cancer is detected using a Pap test, and the Pap test is credited with reducing the incidence of this cancer in the United States by 75% over the past 50 years. This test is used to detect changes in the cells of the cervix that may indicate a precancerous or cancerous condition. However, Pap tests have a 15% to 25% false-negative rate for detecting cervical dysplasia[97] and can be inconclusive, requiring further testing including HPV testing, colposcopy, conization (cone-shaped biopsy), or loop electrosurgical excision procedure (LEEP). New automated screening systems (PapNet, AutoNet) have been approved by the U.S. Food and Drug Administration (FDA) for computer review of negative Pap smears and for primary screening. These systems have the ability to reduce human error, but their cost effectiveness is under intense scrutiny. Numerous other cervical biomarkers are under investigation for possible diagnostic use.[56]

A new laparoscopic assessment of the sentinel lymph node* in early-stage cervical cancer is under investigation with excellent preliminary results.[23,71] Computed tomography (CT) scanning may be used in women who are not candidates for surgical staging.

Staging.   There are four stages of cervical cancer with intermediate steps within each one. *Stage 0* is the precancerous stage; there are no gross lesions, carcinoma is limited to the mucosa and is referred to as CIS (carcinoma in situ) or CINI to CINIII (cervical intraepithelial neoplasia). *Stage I* is strictly confined to the cervix, and lesions are measured as less than or greater than 4 cm in size. In *stage II*, the cancer extends beyond the cervix but has not extended to the pelvic wall. The vagina is minimally involved, and there may or may not be parametrial involvement. In *stage III* the carcinoma has extended to the pelvic wall and involves the lower one third of the vagina and there may be kidney involvement (spread via the ureters). *Stage IV* is characterized by carcinoma that has extended beyond the true pelvis or has infiltrated adjacent organs (e.g., mucosa of the bladder or rectum). There may be metastatic spread of the growth to distant organs.[57]

Treatment.   Precancerous stages (cervical intraepithelial neoplasia [CIN]) may be treated with cryotherapy, laser vaporization, excision (e.g., loop electrosurgical excision procedure [LEEP]), cone biopsies, and possibly indoles (phytochemicals found in cruciferous vegetables [e.g., broccoli, cauliflower, cabbage] when taken as a supplement).[8,119] More advanced cases are managed by surgery (i.e., hysterectomy) followed by radiation or chemoradiation therapy for high-risk or advanced stages.[56] In addition to a vaccine and chemopreventive agents, biologic response modifiers are under investigation for future treatment options.

Prognosis.   Cervical cancer is a slow-growing neoplasm with a good response rate to intervention. Almost all women with preinvasive cancer are cured. Reconstructive surgery and

ovary preservation may be able to preserve childbearing status in younger women. The majority of treated women who develop recurrences do so in the first 2 years following primary therapy. Women with more advanced-stage disease or with lymph node involvement have a significantly less favorable prognosis.

***Special Implications for the Therapist*   19-3**

CERVICAL CANCER

Preferred Practice Patterns:
4B: Impaired Posture
4C: Impaired Muscle Performance
6H: Impaired Circulation and Anthropometric Dimensions
Associated With Lymphatic System Disorders

The physical therapist can continue to function in the role of educator and prevention specialist when conducting a personal/family history that includes questions about the consistency of Pap testing and presence of sexually transmitted diseases (e.g., HPV, genital warts) since these relate to cervical cancer for women of all ages. Although new, more sensitive testing is available, the majority of medical specialists agree that being screened for cervical cancer on a regular basis is more important than the availability of the latest technology.

Any woman with a previous history of cervical cancer who presents with suspicious supraclavicular (or other) unusual lymph node presentation must be referred to her physician for medical evaluation. Reported symptoms of vaginal bleeding and gastrointestinal or genitourinary dysfunction must also be promptly investigated before initiating pelvic rehabilitation. ■

◆ **Ectopic Pregnancy**

Overview.   Ectopic pregnancy, also known as tubal pregnancy, is marked by the implantation of a fertilized ovum outside the uterine cavity (Fig. 19-4). The fallopian tube is the most common site of ectopic pregnancy with approximately 95% implanting there, but extrauterine pregnancies can occur anywhere outside the uterus (e.g., ovary, abdomen, pelvic peritoneum). Ectopic pregnancy is a true gynecologic emergency since accompanying complications are one of two primary causes of maternal death in the United States.

Incidence and Risk Factors.   The incidence of ectopic pregnancy is increasing in the United States and worldwide with approximately 100,000 ectopic pregnancies each year.[18] The reasons for this rise are unclear, although several risk factors have been identified, such as any condition that causes damage to the fallopian tubes that could impair transport of the ovum or impede the migration of the fertilized ovum to the uterus. Three risk factors have been traditionally associated with an increased risk of ectopic pregnancy: sexually transmitted diseases (especially chlamydia and gonorrhea), prior tubal surgery, and current intrauterine contraceptive device (IUD, IUCD).

---

*The sentinel node is the first node in the regional nodal basin that drains a primary tumor and reflects the tumor status of the entire nodal basin; see further discussion under Diagnosis in Chapter 8.

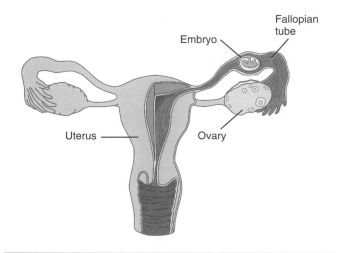

FIGURE   **19-4**   Ectopic pregnancy with implantation occurring in the fallopian tube.

Other risk factors include prior tubal surgery, ruptured appendix, endometriosis, pelvic inflammatory disease, douching,[60] and previous ectopic pregnancy. In addition, a history of infertility and the use of clomiphene citrate to induce ovulation are associated with an increased risk of this condition.

Etiologic Factors and Pathogenesis.   Ectopic pregnancy is caused by delayed ovum transport secondary to decreased fallopian tube motility or distorted tubule anatomy. During ectopic pregnancy, fertilization does not occur in the uterus. The sperm fertilizes the ovum soon after the ovum enters the ampulla of the fallopian tube. Three to four days are typically required for the ovum to travel through the fallopian tube to the uterus. The ovum is rapidly dividing and growing throughout the journey. If the journey is slowed sufficiently (tubule motility), the ovum becomes too large to complete the passage through the tubule. If the tubule anatomy has been affected by recurrent infection or endometriosis the same problem occurs. The trophoblasts that cover the surface of the ovum easily penetrate the mucosa and wall of the tubule, and implantation occurs.

Bleeding occurs during implantation with leakage into the pelvis and abdominal cavity. Vaginal bleeding that may be perceived as menstruation may occur. The pregnancy will typically outgrow its blood supply, terminating the pregnancy. If the pregnancy does not terminate, the thin-walled tubule will no longer support the growing fetus, and rupture can occur by the twelfth week of gestation. Tubal rupture is life-threatening because rapid intraabdominal hemorrhage can occur.

Clinical Manifestations.   The classic presentation of ectopic pregnancy is marked by amenorrhea or irregular bleeding and spotting, lower abdominal quadrant or back pain, and a pelvic mass. The woman may believe she had a menstrual period but when questioned will report the period was atypical for her. The pain reported can be diffuse and aching or localized and will progress to a sharper, lancinating type of pain. The pain can be sudden in onset and intermittent. The pain is thought to be primarily due to the leakage of blood into the pelvic and abdominal cavity. Pain referred to the shoulder area can occur if the blood comes in contact with the kidney or diaphragm.

Since the woman is pregnant, symptoms and signs associated with normal pregnancy may also be present. These findings include fatigue, nausea, breast tenderness, and urinary frequency.

Medical Management
Diagnosis.   Physical examination reveals a pelvic mass in approximately 50% of the cases. Pelvic ultrasound studies can reliably reveal a gestational sac by 5 to 6 weeks into the pregnancy. An empty uterine cavity with elevated (slight) human chorionic gonadotropin beta subunit (HCG-beta) and symptoms strongly implies an extrauterine pregnancy. Blood studies may show anemia while serum pregnancy tests (HCG-beta hormonal levels) will be positive but show levels lower than expected in the presence of a normal pregnancy (lack of doubling over 2 days). Definitive diagnosis requires laparoscopy.

Treatment.   Surgical intervention consisting of a laparoscopic salpingostomy to remove the ectopic pregnancy is performed if the fallopian tube has not ruptured. Laparotomy is indicated if there is internal bleeding or if the ectopic site cannot be adequately visualized with the laparoscope.

A chemotherapeutic agent, methotrexate, can be administered to remove residual ectopic tissue following laparoscopy. The drug is also used when the pregnancy is intact and surgery is contraindicated or the diagnosis is made early enough that the condition is not life-threatening and preserving fertility is desirable.

Special Implications for the Therapist   **19-4**

ECTOPIC PREGNANCY

An awareness of this potentially life-threatening condition is important for the therapist. This awareness should include knowledge of the preexisting conditions that increase the risk of ectopic pregnancy and of the symptoms associated with pregnancy. If a woman of childbearing age complains of an onset of lower abdominal, ipsilateral shoulder, or back pain, the therapist should ask questions regarding her menstrual cycle and if any of the symptoms of pregnancy are present. If the therapist suspects ectopic pregnancy, an immediate telephone call to the physician is warranted. ■

DISORDERS OF THE OVARIES

◆ Ovarian Cystic Disease
Overview.   Ovarian cysts, most of which are benign, are the most common form of ovarian tumor. The different types of cysts include functional cysts (follicular cysts, luteal cysts), endometrial cysts, neoplastic cysts, and polycystic ovary syndrome (PCOS). The follicle and corpus luteum are the source of most symptomatic ovarian cysts in premenopausal women. These cysts are called *functional cysts* and rarely produce symptoms (unless they rupture or hemorrhage) because they develop in the course of normal ovarian activity. A *follicular cyst* develops when an egg matures but does not erupt from the fol-

licle but rather continues to swell as it fills with fluid. A *luteal cyst* develops from a corpus luteum when the tissue that is left after the egg has been expelled fills with blood or other fluid.

Endometrial cysts develop when endometrial tissue migrates to the ovaries, forming blood-filled cysts called *endometriomas* or *chocolate cysts* because of the dark brown color of the contents. Endometrial cysts can grow large enough to impair ovulation and cause pain and cramping during menstrual periods.

Neoplastic cysts are "new growths" considered benign in the majority of cases; only a small percentage of neoplastic cysts are cancerous or have the capacity to invade neighboring tissues and metastasize to distant sites. Cystadenomas are the most common type of neoplastic cyst.

A disorder marked by the presence of multiple cysts is called *polycystic ovary syndrome (PCOS)*. This polycystic disorder is a hormonal disorder affecting premenopausal women and one of the most common causes of infertility. The disease gets its name from the many small cysts that build up inside the ovaries.

Incidence and Etiologic and Risk Factors.

Ovarian cysts are one of the most common endocrine disorders in women, affecting 3% to 7% of women of childbearing age. The exact etiology of ovarian cysts remains unknown, but intrinsic ovarian defect combined with factors outside the ovaries is suspected. In the case of PCOS, a series of central and peripheral mechanisms related to insulin resistance occurs that is determined genetically and inherited; PCOS is now considered a systemic metabolic disease.[28,62] About 20% of women in the United States have this disorder, and more than one half are obese. Among those women who seek treatment for infertility, more than 75% have some degree of PCOS.

Pathogenesis.

Two types of ovarian cysts (the follicle and corpus luteum) are a normal part of the reproductive cycle. At least one follicle (a sac containing an egg and fluid) matures in an ovary during each cycle. During ovulation, the follicle ruptures to release the egg. The follicular remnant, or corpus luteum, is a smaller sac containing a viscous yellow liquid. The corpus luteum releases progesterone, which promotes the development of the uterine lining in preparation for the implantation of a fertilized egg.

Ovarian cysts develop when excess circulating androgens are converted to estrone in the peripheral adipose tissue. The elevated levels of circulating estrogens stimulate the release of Gn-RH by the hypothalamus and inhibit the secretion of FSH by the pituitary. Gn-RH stimulates the pituitary, which produces LH. The increased secretion of LH stimulates the ovary to produce and secrete more androgens. This self-perpetuating cycle results in abnormal maturation of the ovarian follicles, the development of multiple follicular cysts, and a persistent anovulatory state.

Several genes have been implicated in the pathogenesis of PCOS. Researchers have discovered that many women are resistant to their own insulin. To counter this resistance, the pancreas makes extra insulin; over many years this may exhaust the pancreas's ability to make insulin and thus lead to diabetes and subsequent cardiovascular complications. In addition, high insulin levels boost the production of androgens that may induce muscular changes, leading to reduced insulin-mediated glucose uptake creating a repeated cycle and worsening condition.[47]

Clinical Manifestations.

The likelihood of symptoms developing often has more to do with the size and location than the type of ovarian cyst. As cysts grow, their weight often pulls the ovary out of its customary position, sometimes cutting off the blood supply to the ovary. Pressure from the ovary in its new position against the uterus, bladder, intestine, or vagina may result in a variety of symptoms, such as abdominal pressure; pain; abdominal bloating; or discomfort during urination, bowel movements, or sexual intercourse. Large cysts can impair ovarian function reducing ovulation and causing irregular periods or infertility in premenopausal women.

Depending on the type of cyst, if a cyst ruptures, the contents of the sac are usually absorbed by the body. When endometriomas rupture, the contents may be distributed on the uterus, bladder, and intestines. As the immune system moves in to clean up the debris, scar tissue develops forming adhesions with resultant chronic pelvic pain. In the case of neoplastic cyst rupture, the more toxic contents can result in peritonitis.

Pain can be a manifestation of cysts. A dull, aching sensation experienced in the lower abdominal, groin, low back, or buttock areas can occur. The sensation may also be described as a heaviness. This pain is associated with bleeding into the cyst or with quick enlargement of the cyst. Sudden or sharp pain can indicate a cyst rupturing or hemorrhaging or a torsion occurring.

PCOS is characterized by physical and metabolic changes, such as obesity, prominent facial or body hair, severe acne, thinning hair, infertility, and menstrual problems. Fifty percent of these women have amenorrhea, and another 30% have abnormal uterine bleeding. PCOS is associated with endometrial cancer because high levels of androgen interfere with ovulation so women with PCOS do not regularly shed the endometrium. Impaired glucose tolerance, a major risk factor for type 2 diabetes present in 40% of women with PCOS, and subsequent risk for heart disease have been documented.[73] Other symptoms or conditions associated with PCOS include obstructive sleep apnea and daytime sleepiness[110] and fibrocystic breasts.[22]

Medical Management
Diagnosis and Treatment.

The history and pelvic examination lead to suspicion of cystic disease. Confirmation is made by ultrasonography or laparoscopy. Ultrasound may be transvaginal (inserting a tampon-sized transducer into the vagina) or abdominal (moving a transducer across the lower abdomen) and can help identify the type of cyst and whether a cyst contains solid or liquid material. Laboratory tests include a complete blood count to identify infection or anemia (heavy bleeding) and a CA-125 test for ovarian cancer. All women with PCOS should be screened for glucose intolerance.[65]

The treatment of ovarian cysts depends on the results of the diagnostic tests and the age of the woman (preserving childbearing status). In premenopausal women, the decision whether or not to drain or remove the cyst depends on the problems the cyst is causing (e.g., follicular or luteal cysts resolve without treatment, endometriomas and neoplastic cysts may be removed surgically).

The treatment of PCOS is primarily hormonal with the goal being an interruption of the persistent elevated levels of androgens. Clomiphene citrate (Clomid) is often administered to induce ovulation. If medication is not effective, laser surgery can be instituted to puncture the multiple follicles. It is now known that the application of diabetes management techniques aimed at reducing insulin resistance and hyperinsulinemia (e.g., weight reduction, oral hypoglycemic agents, exercise) can reverse testosterone and LH abnormalities and infertility as well as improve glucose, insulin, and lipid profiles.

Special Implications for the Therapist   19-5

OVARIAN CYSTIC DISEASE

Depending on the clinical presentation, therapists may ask women if menstrual dysfunction is present. A history of ovarian cystic disease could account for a woman's low back or sacral pain, but usually there is some indication in the menstrual history to suggest a gynecologic link. In women with known PCOS, impaired glucose tolerance, or insulin resistance, elevated androgens with the associated muscular changes that further reduce glucose uptake and elevated cholesterol warrant the use of exercise and increased physical activity before the onset of macrovascular and microvascular symptoms.[47,62] See also the section on Diabetes Mellitus in Chapter 10.

Considering how common PCOS is, therapists need to be aware of the potential side effects of clomiphene citrate. These include insomnia, blurred vision, nausea, vomiting, urinary frequency, and polyuria. The onset of any of these symptoms warrants communication with the physician. ■

◆ Ovarian Cancer

Overview and Incidence.   Ovarian cancer is estimated to be the second most common female urogenital cancer and the most lethal of these cancers. An estimated 23,300 women in the United States were projected to develop ovarian cancer in 2002 with 13,900 deaths from ovarian cancer.[57] The poor outcome is based on the difficulty of diagnosing the disease, which results in 60% to 70% of the women having metastatic disease at the time of diagnosis.

Although there are a number of types of ovarian cancers, epithelial tumors make up approximately 90% of the cases. Although rare before puberty the incidence of epithelial tumors peaks in women during their 50s and 60s. The most common type of epithelial tumor, serous carcinoma, has a peak incidence between the ages of 40 and 60 years. In the United States white and Hawaiian women have the highest incidence of ovarian cancer, whereas Native American and black women have the lowest incidence.

The term *extraovarian primary peritoneal carcinoma* (*EOPPC*) is sometimes used interchangeably with *ovarian cancer.* This has been identified as a relatively newly defined disease that develops only in women, accounting for approximately 10% of cases with a presumed diagnosis of ovarian cancer. Characterized by abdominal carcinomatosis, uninvolved or minimally involved ovaries, and no identifiable primary form of cancer, EOPPC has been reported following bilateral oophorectomy performed for benign disease or prophylactically for ovarian cancer.[30] The occurrence of EOPPC may be explained by the common origin of the peritoneum and the ovaries from the coelomic epithelium. The various histologic differences of ovarian and peritoneal lesions are under investigation.

Etiologic and Risk Factors.   No single cause of ovarian cancer has been discovered, but a number of factors appear to influence the development of the disease (Box 19-1). None is as important as a family history of ovarian or breast cancer. The average woman has less than a 2% chance of developing ovarian cancer in her lifetime (1 in 57 versus 1 in 8 for breast cancer), whereas a woman with first-degree relatives with ovarian cancer or who has the *BRCA1* (*BRCA* stands for breast cancer) mutation has about a 45% lifetime chance, and for *BRCA2*, the risk is approximately 25%.[88] Loss of two tumor suppressor genes (*p53* and *BRCA1*) has been shown to occur early in ovarian carcinogenesis in women who are *BRCA1* mutation carriers.[115] Overall, more than 90% of all cases occur sporadically; only 10% of all women with ovarian cancer have a hereditary predisposition.

Nulliparous women are at increased risk of developing ovarian cancer. This factor may be related to the repeated epithelial surface disruption that occurs with cyclic ovulation. Since epithelial tumors make up approximately 90% of ovarian cancers, many of the risk factors described relate to this entity. A history of breast-feeding also is important since women who breast-feed are at decreased risk of developing this condition compared to nulliparous women and parous women who have not breast-fed.

Pathogenesis.   The development of ovarian cancer seems to correlate with the number of times a woman ovulates during her lifetime. Every time an egg is released, it ruptures the surface of one of the ovaries. Cells have to replicate to repair the damage, and the more times they do this, the greater the chances that a cancer-causing mutation will occur. This is why anything that interferes with ovulation (e.g., pregnancy, breast-feeding, oral contraceptives) diminishes the risk of developing ovarian cancer.

The classification of ovarian tumors is based on the tissue of origin. The most common tumors arise from the surface ep-

BOX   **19-1**
Risk Factors for Ovarian Cancer
Family history of breast, ovarian, or colon cancer Personal history of endometrial or breast cancer Increasing age (>40 years, most occur in women 55 to 75 years) Nulliparity (never pregnant or birthed children) Never breast-fed Presence of *BRCA1* or *BRCA2* mutation White race Exposure to talc Lives in an industrialized Western nation High dietary fat intake Prolonged use of estrogen (postmenopausal) Fertility drugs (under investigation; not yet confirmed) Never used oral contraceptives

ithelium or serosa of the ovary. As the ovary develops, the epithelium extends into the stroma of the ovary forming glands and cysts. In certain cases these inclusions become neoplastic. Other categories of tumor include germ cell tumors, sex cord and stromal tumors, and steroid cell tumors. Once present, ovarian cancer spreads to the pelvis, abdominal cavity, and bladder, whereas lymphatic metastasis carries the disease to the paraaortic lymph nodes and to a lesser extent the inguinal or external iliac lymph nodes. Hematogenous spread of the cancer can result in liver and lung involvement.

Clinical Manifestations.   Most ovarian cancers are asymptomatic or present with symptoms so vague that the disease is advanced in many cases by the time the woman seeks care. The vague complaints include abdominal bloating, flatulence, fatigue and malaise, gastritis, or general abdominal discomfort. Abnormal vaginal bleeding, leg pain, and low back pain are less common symptoms. Local pelvic pain also occurs late in the disease.

Symptoms associated with metastatic spread of the disease include unexplained weight loss, weakness, pleurisy, ascites,* and cachexia (general feebleness and wasting). Paraneoplastic cerebellar degeneration (PCD) is a type of paraneoplastic syndrome that primarily affects women with gynecologic cancers. Symptoms typically include ataxic gait, truncal and appendicular ataxia, nystagmus, and speech impairment (dysarthria).[67]

Medical Management
Prevention.   Women at high risk for ovarian cancer (e.g., those with a family history of ovarian cancer in a mother, sister, or daughter) and any woman with a personal history of breast, colon, or uterine cancer should receive annual screening with a combination of the CA-125 blood test, physical examination, and vaginal sonography. The CA-125 blood test measures CA-125, a protein produced by ovarian cancer cells, and is elevated in approximately 80% of women with advanced cancer and about 50% of those with early-stage ovarian cancer (normal range is between 0 and 35). This test is not adequate as a screening tool because it does not detect the disease early in women who are asymptomatic and it can be elevated in other conditions, such as pelvic infections, fibroids, endometriosis, and even during ovulation.

Researchers are continuing to evaluate CA-125 as a screening tool (e.g., rapidly rising CA-125 may be more predictive than elevation on a single test) and also investigating other substances, such as lysophosphatidic acid (LPA), a growth factor for ovarian cancer cells measured in the blood.[83] Routine ultrasound imaging is also under investigation as an effective screening tool when used to identify enlarged ovaries.[90]

Some women with a positive immediate family history of ovarian cancer choose to have prophylactic oophorectomies after completing childbearing to prevent development of this disease. This intervention is not 100% protective because the lining of the peritoneal cavity comprises the same cells as the lining of the ovaries and development of primary peritoneal cancer after prophylactic oophorectomy can occur.[88]

A history of one or more full-term pregnancies, a history of breast-feeding, and the use of oral contraceptives reduce the risk of ovarian cancer. Oral contraceptives (birth control pills) are recommended as chemoprevention for women with a family history of ovarian cancer, especially if the *BRCA* mutation is present. The mechanism of protection is unclear, but it is probably due to the inhibition of ovulation; there is a potential increased risk of cervical cancer with this treatment.[77,88] As a result of analgesics reducing the risk for colorectal cancer, studies of the effect of similar pharmacologic effects on ovarian cancer have been conducted. Regular use of acetaminophen (but not aspirin) may be associated with lower risk of ovarian cancer.[76]

Diagnosis and Staging.   Despite ovarian cancer's reputation as a silent killer, more than 90% of women with ovarian cancer (whether early or advanced) reported experiencing symptoms long before diagnosis.[44] However, these are often nonspecific and vague and frequently are misdiagnosed as irritable bowel syndrome or some other nongynecologic condition. A pelvic mass with ascites is usually indicative of ovarian cancer that is then confirmed by ultrasonography. A cervical smear may reveal malignant cells, and a biopsy will reveal whether the mass is benign or cancerous.

Staging of the disease is as follows: stage I—disease limited to the ovaries; stage II-extension to other pelvic organs; stage III—intraperitoneal metastasis (spread to other abdominal organs but not the liver); and stage IV—distant metastasis (spread to the liver or organs outside the abdominal cavity). The cancer is considered advanced at stages II to IV.

Treatment.   Treatment of ovarian cancer usually consists of cytoreductive surgery that includes total abdominal hysterectomy (TAH), bilateral salpingo-oophorectomy (BSO), omentectomy (removal of supportive tissue attached to organs in the abdominal cavity), and lymphadenectomy followed by adjuvant combination chemotherapy.[30] New cancer drugs are being developed to treat resistant or recurrent disease. Ovarian growth is angiogenesis-dependent, causing researchers to investigate the use of antiangiogenic treatment (e.g., angiostatin, endostatin) to inhibit tumor growth in this type of cancer.[118]

Other new interventions and approaches under investigation include the use of monoclonal antibodies (laboratory-produced substances that find and bind to cancer cells, delivering tumor-killing agents without harming normal cells); genetic techniques (e.g., gene therapy to supply a working copy of the tumor-suppressing gene *p53*); vaccines to boost a woman's immune response to ovarian tumor cells that emerge after treatment; and new combinations and sequences of currently used drug interventions.

Prognosis.   Ovarian cancer has a very poor prognosis because it is difficult to detect early and usually presents with advanced metastases (70% present in an advanced stage). If found early, the cancer is generally responsive to treatment, with a 90% 5-year survival rate. In most cases, clinical response to treatment is approximately 80%, but tumor recurrence within 3 years following treatment occurs in most women.[30] Return of the tumor within 6 months of therapy is a poor prognosticator because the cancer cells are often resistant to drug treatment. Five-year survival without recurrence is a good prognostic indicator.

---

*Ascites is an accumulation of fluid within the peritoneal cavity. This can occur when there is marked increased pressure within the liver sinusoids or portal hypertension that results in serum exuding through the superficial capillaries into the peritoneal cavity (see Fig. 16-4).

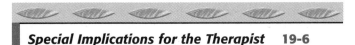

Special Implications for the Therapist 19-6

OVARIAN CANCER

Preferred Practice Patterns:
4B: Impaired Posture
4C: Impaired Muscle Performance
6H: Impaired Circulation and Anthropometric Dimensions
     Associated With Lymphatic System Disorders

Therapists treating women with a history of ovarian cancer need to be cognizant of the moderate to high risk of recurrence of the disease. Gait disturbance may be the first sign of a paraneoplastic syndrome associated with gynecologic cancer. Other symptoms associated with metastases may include thoracic or shoulder girdle pain secondary to lymphadenopathy; symptoms associated with lung (dyspnea; see Chapter 14) or liver (see Chapter 16) disease; and weight loss and fatigue. Onset of any of these complaints warrants communication with the physician. Oophorectomy induces menopause in women. Therefore an onset of the symptoms described in the beginning of this chapter may occur in addition to headaches, depression, and insomnia. ■

◆ Ovarian Varices

Incompetent and dilated ovarian veins (as well as other uterine and pelvic veins) are a known cause of abdominal and pelvic pain and contribute to pelvic congestion syndrome. This is only one of many possible causes of chronic pelvic pain and pelvic congestion syndrome (see the section on Pelvic Floor Disorders in this chapter). Ovarian varices may occur unilaterally or bilaterally, most often in women who have had children but occasionally in nonparous women.[87] Reported symptoms include pain that worsens toward the end of the day or after standing for a long time, pain that occurs premenstrually and after intercourse, sensations of heaviness in the pelvis, and prominent varicose veins elsewhere on the body.

This type of pelvic pain arises when blood pools in a distended ovarian vein rather than flowing back toward the heart and is more common among women with low blood pressure. This distention and pooling form a varicocele, a term traditionally applied to men to describe varicose veins in the testicles but varicoceles can also occur in the female counterparts of those organs. In fact, 10% of men experience pelvic varices of the gonadal veins presenting as varicoceles instead of the uteroovarian varices seen in women.[16]

Ovarian vein incompetence may be suspected from the presence of vulvar varicosities and can be diagnostically visualized with CT scanning, venogram, or transvaginal ultrasound. If observed during pregnancy, these may disappear after delivery but become more prominent with subsequent pregnancies. Treatment with embolization of the ovarian veins (see discussion of this technique in the section on Uterine Fibroids in this chapter) is relatively new but reportedly safe and effective in alleviating pain and symptoms, improving sexual functioning, and reducing anxiety and depression with subsequent improved quality of life reported.[69]

PELVIC FLOOR DISORDERS

◆ Pelvic Floor Dysfunction

Overview and Etiologic Factors.   Many diagnoses and symptoms are included under the heading of pelvic floor disorders resulting in dysfunction of the pelvic floor musculature or chronic pelvic pain (Box 19-2). Although men and women can both be affected by pelvic floor dysfunction, women are more often treated in a physical therapy practice. Only general concepts related to the multitude of causes and symptoms can be

---

BOX 19-2

Causes of Pelvic Floor Disorders

Pregnancy alone and/or birth-related trauma
Rectocele, cystocele, prolapsed uterus
Anorectal tumors or neoplasm anywhere in the pelvic cavity
Hypertonus dysfunctions
  Levator ani syndrome
  Tension myalgia
  Coccygodynia
  Dyspareunia
  Vaginismus
  Anismus
  Vulvodynia
  Vulvar vestibulitis
  Pudendal neuralgia
Ovarian varices, pelvic vein varicosities, congestion syndrome
Other vascular disorders (e.g., aortoiliac occlusion, claudication, arteriovenous malformations)
Dysmenorrhea, premenstrual syndrome (PMS)
Endometriosis
Uterine fibroids
Congenital malformation(s), uterine malposition
Musculoskeletal injury or trauma (back, sacrum, sacroiliac area, hip, pelvis)
Fibromyalgia, chronic fatigue syndrome
Nerve entrapment or injury, nerve root irritation
Spinal cord injury or other neurologic condition (e.g., stroke, Parkinson's disease, multiple sclerosis)
Myofascial pain syndrome, trigger points
Abdominal or pelvic surgery
Psychogenic origin
Sexual assault, sexual abuse, or negative sexual experiences
Sexually transmitted diseases
Pelvic inflammatory disease (PID); infection; postabortion syndrome (more common with multiple induced abortions)
Interstitial cystitis
Gastrointestinal disorders
  Diverticulitis
  Constipation
  Rectal hemorrhoids, rectal fissures
  Irritable bowel syndrome
  Regional enteritis (Crohn's disease)
  Appendicitis, peritonitis
Hernia (inguinal or femoral)
Unknown cause ("gynecalgia")

covered in this text. For more specific information related to each of these conditions, the reader is referred elsewhere.[101,116]

Chronic pelvic pain (continuous or intermittent pelvic pain lasting for 6 months or more) is a significant part of pelvic floor disorders. Any of the conditions listed in Box 19-2 can result in chronic pelvic pain, and, in turn, chronic pelvic pain can contribute to or result from hypertonus dysfunction of the pelvic floor muscles. Many of these conditions fall into several categories and are not strictly classified as one entity. For example, vulvodynia and vulvar vestibulitis are both hypertonus dysfunctions as well as neuropathic pain syndromes resulting in chronic pelvic pain (a third classification). Overall, there is considerable overlap of conditions in the categories listed.

Incidence.   The prevalence of pelvic floor dysfunction remains unknown, but it is considered a common problem among women of reproductive age, many of whom have never been diagnosed. The lack of a consensus on the definition of chronic pelvic pain and lack of a classification scheme hinder epidemiologic studies. Although the majority of these conditions affect women, men can also be affected.

Pathogenesis.   The pelvic floor muscles are a band of muscles sometimes referred to as the pubococcygeal (PC) muscles. These are actually made up of several muscle groups stretching like a sling from the pubic bone to the coccyx at the base of the spine that work together as a whole to support the internal and pelvic organs (Fig. 19-5). The pelvic floor muscles are voluntary, internal muscles surrounding the

vagina, urethra, and rectum and also function to help close off the urethra and rectum to maintain continence (Fig. 19-6).

Weakness or laxity in the endopelvic fascia or other structures of the pelvic floor results in partial or total prolapse of the organs it supports as described in the next section. Hypertonus dysfunction comprises a large portion of pelvic

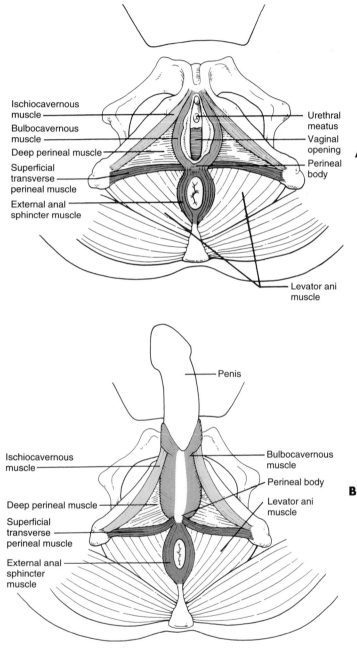

A

B

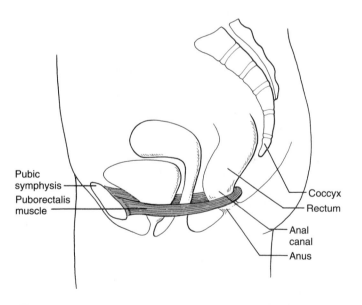

FIGURE   **19-5**   Pelvic floor sling. The first layer of the pelvic floor is made up of the endopelvic fascia, one continuous body of connective tissue surrounding and supporting the pelvic organs (not pictured). The levator ani muscles (pelvic floor muscles) make up the second layer, forming a sling across the pelvic cavity from the pubis to the coccyx with openings to allow passage of the urethra, lower vagina, and anus. The puborectalis muscle (part of the levator ani muscle) works together with cline pubococcygeus muscle (not shown, also part of the levator ani muscle) to support the pelvic viscera in both the male and female. (From Myers RS: *Saunders manual of physical therapy,* Philadelphia, 1995, Saunders, p 464.)

FIGURE   **19-6**   Pelvic floor muscles. Third layer of the pelvic floor, sometimes referred to as the urogenital diaphragm or deep perineum. The deep transverse perineal muscle, external urethral sphincter, and enveloping fascia of the third layer are overlaid by the fourth (superficial) layer (perineum), including the bulbocavernous, ischiocavernous, superficial transverse perineal muscles and the external anal sphincter and muscle. **A,** Female anatomy as described. **B,** Male anatomy is slightly different, but the urethral and rectal muscles remain the same as in the female. (From Myers RS: *Saunders manual of physical therapy,* Philadelphia, 1995, Saunders, p 465.)

floor dysfunctions and is characterized by an increase in pelvic floor muscle tension or active spasm causing musculoskeletal pain or dysfunction of the urogenital and/or colorectal system.[112] The pathogenesis of chronic pelvic pain remains poorly understood, and often laparoscopic investigation reveals no obvious cause for pain.

Clinical Manifestations.   Clinical manifestations of pelvic floor disorders are determined by the underlying etiologic factors and pathologic findings. For example, the primary presentation of someone with hypertonus is a pain, pressure, or ache, usually poorly localized in the perivaginal, perirectal, and lower abdominal quadrants and pelvis (suprapubic or coccyx regions) and sometimes radiating down the posterior aspect of the thigh. Symptoms are often reproduced by manual palpation and examination of the pelvic floor muscles.

Vulvar vestibulitis is characterized by a telltale patch of skin at the vaginal opening that is extremely sensitive to the gentlest tap with a cotton swab; and vulvodynia is marked by persistent pain and burning in the external genitalia, making it impossible for a woman to wear closely fitting pants or jeans, engage in sexual intercourse comfortably, or even sit comfortably. Signs and symptoms associated with prolapsed structures, ovarian or pelvic vein varices, and endometriosis are presented elsewhere in this chapter. Pelvic inflammatory disease, sexually transmitted diseases, hernia, and gastrointestinal disorders including hemorrhoids are presented in other chapters in this text.

Other symptoms of pelvic floor dysfunction may include low back pain that is intermittent and unpredictable, changing locations often and difficult to reproduce; groin pain with hip and knee flexion; sharp rectal pain; painful intercourse with penetration or inability to penetrate; extreme rectal pressure during intercourse; urinary or bowel incontinence; abnormal vaginal discharge; and pubic bone pain or tenderness.

Medical Management.   Diagnosis and diagnostic testing depend on history and clinical presentation. Ultrasonography is being used more often now that the technology has advanced. Previously, laparoscopic examination was used with poor results in more than one half of all cases. Specific medical intervention can be employed in cases of known and treatable causes, but more often, medical management has been limited to palliative use of pharmacologic and hormonal agents and surgical intervention with variable results. Physical therapy intervention is quickly becoming the first-line therapy of choice for many causes of pelvic floor dysfunction. Working with a counselor or other skilled professional is recommended when treating someone with a past (or current) history of abuse.

Special Implications for the Therapist   **19-7**

PELVIC FLOOR DYSFUNCTION

Preferred Practice Patterns:
4B: Impaired Posture
4C: Impaired Muscle Performance
4D: Impaired Joint Mobility, Motor Function, Muscle
    Performance, and Range of Motion Associated With
    Connective Tissue Dysfunction

It is imperative that women (including adolescent females) receive education about the functions and dysfunctions of the pelvic floor complex to promote preventive rather than restorative benefits of pelvic floor exercise. Exercises for the pelvic floor should be part of every woman's fitness regimen, either as prevention or specific to the type of pelvic floor muscle dysfunction and its causes.[111]

Therapists need to routinely ask women questions about pelvic floor function (e.g., presence of urinary incontinence, pain with sexual intercourse or other sexual dysfunction, presence of known reproductive organ or pelvic floor dysfunction, past history) and provide education and exercise programs for these muscles, making a medical referral when appropriate. Review of the normal pelvic floor function and the type of evaluation and intervention programs necessary for anyone with pelvic floor dysfunction is available.[111]

Intervention must be determined based on examination including external assessment and, in the case of those therapists with additional training, internal examination. Special considerations include cultural differences in modesty and the possibility of current substance use or abuse, and past (or present) sexual abuse or sexual dysfunction. Behavioral intervention options focus on physical therapy education, therapeutic exercise, physiologic quieting (e.g., relaxation exercises, hand or foot warming, diaphragmatic breathing), and the use of physical modalities that aid in pain relief and the restoration of muscle function.[111]

Intervention may also focus on postural education to place the pelvic floor in the most optimal position for relaxation and function and aerobic exercise to mobilize the pelvis; motor learning techniques (e.g., use of a Swiss ball); behavioral training; joint alignment (including craniosacral); soft tissue, scar, and/or visceral mobilization; trigger point therapy; strain-counterstrain; stretching for the adductors, iliopsoas, piriformis, internal obturator, abdominals, and other muscles as determined by the assessment. Principles of motor learning guide the therapist in incorporating pelvic muscle function with breathing (work of the diaphragm), the abdominals, and low back muscles. This is an important step in creating sensory awareness of the pelvic floor that takes time and repetition. ■

◆ Cystocele, Rectocele, and Uterine Prolapse

Overview.   Three types of pelvic floor disorders are discussed here: cystocele, rectocele, and uterine prolapse. A *cystocele* is a herniation of the urinary bladder into the vagina (Fig. 19-7, A and B). A *rectocele* is a herniation of the rectum into the vagina (Fig. 19-7, C and D); part of the rectum protrudes into the posterior wall of the vagina, forming a pouch in the intestine. A *uterine prolapse* is the bulging of the uterus into the vagina (Fig. 19-8). Other types of pelvic floor prolapse may include cystourethrocele: bladder and urethra prolapse into the vagina; urethrocele: bladder neck prolapses into the vagina; enterocele: part of the intestine and peritoneum prolapses into the vagina; and vaginal vault prolapse: the apex of the vagina prolapses, occurring sometimes after a hysterectomy.

Etiologic and Risk Factors.   Cystocele, rectocele, and uterine prolapse are a result of pelvic floor relaxation or structural overstretching of the pelvic musculature or ligamentous structures. Multiple pregnancies and deliveries combined with obesity increase the risk of these disorders developing. Prolonged labor, bearing down before full dilation, and force-

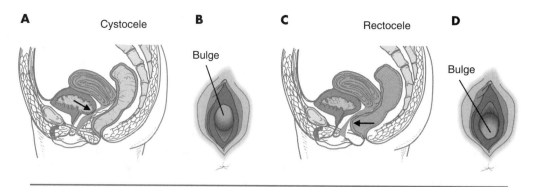

FIGURE   19-7   **A,** Cystocele (sagittal view). Note the bulging of the anterior vaginal wall. The urinary bladder is displaced downward. **B,** Lithotomy view: the bladder pushes the anterior vaginal wall downward into the vagina. **C,** Rectocele (sagittal view). **D,** Note the bulging of the posterior vaginal wall associated with rectocele (lithotomy view).

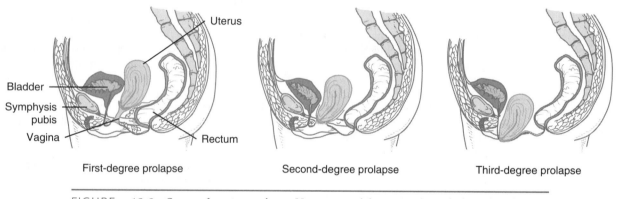

FIGURE   19-8   Stages of uterine prolapse. Herniation of the uterus through the pelvic floor resulting in protrusion into the vagina. *First-degree:* the cervix remains in the vagina. *Second-degree:* the cervix appears at the perineum or protrudes on straining. *Third-degree:* the entire uterus protrudes outside the body, and there is total inversion of the vagina.

ful delivery of the placenta are possible causes of prolapse. Trauma to the pudendal or sacral nerves during birth and delivery is an additional risk factor. Decreased muscle tone because of aging, complications of pelvic surgery, or excessive straining during bowel movements may also result in prolapse of some or all of these structures. Pelvic tumors and neurologic conditions such as spina bifida and diabetic neuropathy, which interrupt the innervation of pelvic muscles, can also increase the risk.

Pathogenesis.   The uterus and other pelvic structures are maintained in their proper position by the uterosacral, round, broad, and cardinal ligaments. The pelvic floor musculature forms a slinglike structure that supports the uterus, vagina, urinary bladder, and rectum (see Fig. 19-5). Multiple pregnancies and deliveries progressively stretch and potentially weaken or damage these important structures.

Cystocele occurs when the muscle support for the bladder is impaired. This allows the bladder to drop below the uterus. Over a period of time the vaginal wall will stretch and bulge downward. Eventually the bladder can herniate through the anterior vaginal wall and form a cystocele. A rectocele occurs when the posterior vaginal wall and underlying rectum bulge forward. Eventually protrusion occurs through the introitus as

the supporting structures continue to weaken. Uterine prolapse occurs when the supporting ligaments become overstretched.

Clinical Manifestations.   The symptoms associated with a *cystocele* include urinary frequency and urgency, difficulty in emptying the bladder, cystitis, and a painful bearing-down sensation in the perineal area. Urinary stress incontinence may also be associated with the presence of a cystocele.

The symptoms associated with a *rectocele* include perineal pain and difficulty with defecation. There may be a feeling of incomplete rectal emptying, constipation, painful intercourse, and aching or pressure after a bowel movement. If the rectocele becomes large enough to trap feces, manual pressure applied to the vaginal wall may be necessary in order to complete a bowel movement without excessive straining (a practice called *splinting* or *stenting,* usually an indication of the need for corrective surgery).

Primary symptoms resulting from *uterine prolapse* are backache, perineal pain, a sense of "heaviness" in the vaginal area, a perceived "lump" at the vaginal opening (third-degree prolapse), and irritation and excoriation of the exposed mucous membranes of the cervix and vagina, especially from sexual intercourse and from wiping after toileting. Symptoms may be relieved by lying down and are aggravated by prolonged standing, walking, coughing, or straining. Urinary incontinence is also a common problem as a result of uterine prolapse.

Medical Management

Diagnosis. The diagnosis of these disorders is primarily derived from observation and the pelvic examination. A uterine prolapse is graded as first, second, or third degree, depending on how far the uterus protrudes through the introitus. A first-degree prolapse is marked by some descent, but the cervix has not reached the introitus. A second-degree prolapse is marked by the cervix as part of the uterus having descended through the introitus. A third-degree prolapse is manifested by the entire uterus protruding through the vaginal opening.

Treatment. At one time, corrective surgery was the first treatment option, but pelvic floor rehabilitation has become the standard treatment of choice. Rehabilitation includes pelvic floor strengthening exercises and muscle reeducation, postural education, biofeedback, and electrical stimulation. Surgery remains a management tool for these disorders and may be required especially with second- and third-degree uterine prolapse. Vaginal hysterectomy, vesicourethral suspension, and abdominal hysterectomy are possible surgical approaches depending on the diagnosis. Strengthening of the pelvic floor should be incorporated into the postoperative rehabilitation program as well.

Lifestyle changes for constipation are often effective for rectocele, such as adequate hydration, fiber intake, developing regular bowel habits, and regular exercise. HRT may be used to help maintain the elasticity of the pelvic floor muscles.

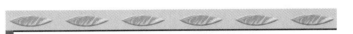

Special Implications for the Therapist   19-8

CYSTOCELE, RECTOCELE, AND UTERINE PROLAPSE

Preferred Practice Patterns:
4B: Impaired Posture
4C: Impaired Muscle Performance

As with urinary incontinence, physical therapists have a primary role in the treatment of pelvic floor disorders (see the section on Urinary Incontinence in Chapter 17). Therapists will also see people with pelvic floor disorders as a co-morbidity. In these cases, therapists must be vigilant that the woman does not hold her breath or perform Valsalva's maneuver because these could exacerbate the pelvic floor condition.

In addition, a woman with a second- or third-degree uterine prolapse will have difficulty tolerating extended periods of weight-bearing activities. Alternative positions for sexual intercourse should be discussed (e.g., pillow under the hips, avoiding being above the partner), and alternative positions for exercise will need to be incorporated into the rehabilitation program. Dabbing the vaginal/perineal area with soft toilet paper rather than wiping can help in reducing friction-related tissue injury. Women who leak urine when dabbing (applying pressure to the prolapsed bladder causes urine leakage) may be helped by a series of specific exercises to modulate the reflex responses of the urinary system. Sometimes, just rolling the legs in and out a series of four times before dabbing while sitting on the toilet is sufficient to prevent this from happening. Pelvic floor rehabilitation is recommended for eliminating this problem.[52] ■

BREAST DISEASE

Most breast lumps are benign or noncancerous and include fluid-filled cysts, fibrous tumors called *fibroadenomas*, fatty tumors called *lipomas*, and fibrocystic breast disease characterized by lumpy, tender breasts. Cancerous tumors of the breast cannot be distinguished from benign lesions so that all lumps of any kind must be medically evaluated.

◆ Fibrocystic Disease and Fibroadenoma

Overview. *Fibrocystic breast disease* or *mammary dysplasia* is a term used to describe a number of benign breast irregularities. The constellation of morphologic changes can include cystic dilation of terminal ducts, a relative increase in the fibrous stroma, and proliferation of the terminal duct epithelial elements. Fibroadenoma is the most common benign neoplasm of the breast. Epithelial and stromal elements that arise from the terminal duct lobular unit make up the tumor.

Incidence and Risk Factors. Fibrocystic disease and fibroadenomas make up the majority of benign breast neoplasms. Fibrocystic breast disease is the single most common breast disorder occurring in 89 per 100,000 woman-years and peaking between ages 40 and 44 years. This condition accounts for more than one-half of all surgical procedures on the female breast. The risk factors for developing breast cancer (see next section) also apply to the development of this condition. Fibroadenomas occur most commonly in premenopausal women (33 per 100,000 woman-years), with peak incidence between 20 to 29 years. Noncalcified fibroadenomas of the breast are not unusual in postmenopausal women and may simulate a carcinoma.[53]

Etiologic Factors and Pathogenesis. The cause of fibrocystic breast disease and fibroadenoma is unknown. Fibroadenomas appear to be estrogen-induced or estrogen-sensitive, stimulated by pregnancy and lactation, and usually regressing after menopause. The fibrocystic changes typically involve the terminal ducts and surrounding stroma and can be proliferative or nonproliferative. Nonproliferative fibrocystic changes are generalized, occurring in multiple areas of both breasts. A majority of the time these cystic changes are minimal and do not result in a discrete mass although cysts up to 5 cm can develop.

Clinical Manifestations. Fibroadenomas are typically solitary lesions and are 2 to 4 cm in size when first detected. A typical fibroadenoma is a nontender, round, firm, and discrete mass. This round and rubbery lesion is sharply demarcated from surrounding breast tissue and as a result moves freely within the surrounding tissue. These cysts can fluctuate in size with rapid appearance or disappearance. A fibrocystic breast mass may or may not be painful. The tenderness may become evident during the premenstrual phase of the cycle when the cysts tend to enlarge.

Medical Management

Diagnosis and Treatment.

Diagnosis of these benign lesions is based on physical examination, mammography, and biopsy. Because fibrocystic disease and fibroadenoma are often indistinguishable from carcinomas, biopsy is often used to confirm the diagnosis. More advanced ultrasonography now allows for the differentiation of cystic (fluid-filled) masses from solid masses.

Treatment for these conditions is often palliative and includes aspirin, mild analgesics, and local heat or cold. Dietary changes are often recommended, such as avoiding coffee, colas, chocolate, and tea (foods and drinks that contain xanthines). Women are encouraged to wear a brassiere that provides adequate support. For women in severe pain, danazol may be given. Surgery is performed if a suspicious mass that is deemed not to be malignant on cytologic examination does not resolve over several months.

◆ Breast Cancer

Overview. Breast cancer is the most common malignancy of females in the United States. Breast cancer begins in the lobules (20%) (milk-producing glands of the breast) or in the ducts (80%) that bring the milk to the nipple (Fig. 19-9). Most breast carcinomas are adenocarcinomas originating in the single layer of epithelial cells that line the ductal and lob-

ular systems of all milk ducts. There are six types of breast cancer: (1) ductal carcinoma in situ (DCIS); (2) invasive (infiltrating) ductal carcinoma (IDC); (3) invasive (infiltrating) lobular carcinoma; (4) medullary, tubular, and mucinous carcinoma; (5) inflammatory breast disease; and (6) Paget's disease of the breast.

Ductal carcinoma in situ (sometimes called *intraductal cancer*), the most common type of in situ cancer, occurs in 20% to 30% of newly diagnosed breast cancer cases and develops at several points along a duct, appearing as a cluster of calcifications or white flecks on a mammogram. This is a precancerous change in breast tissue (abnormal but not malignant cells and highly curable) with a broad continuum from slow-growing cells with little potential to be transformed into cancer to life-threatening aggressive types of cancer that will invade the duct wall and grow beyond it.

Infiltrative ductal carcinoma is the most common of the invasive breast cancers, beginning in a duct, breaking through the duct wall, and invading fatty tissue of the breast with further metastasis possible. IDC is usually detected as a mass on a mammogram or as a palpable lump during a breast exam.

Invasive lobular carcinoma comprises 10% to 15% of invasive cancers. This type grows through the wall of the lobule and spreads via the lymphatic or circulatory system.

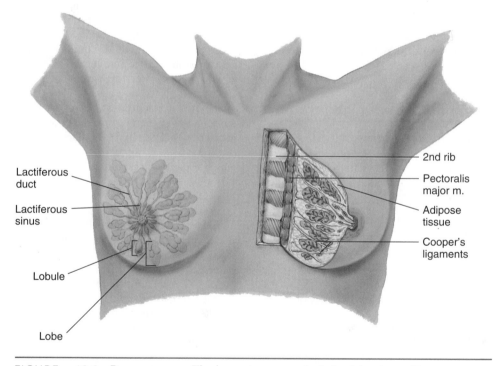

FIGURE **19-9** Breast anatomy. The breast is composed of glandular tissue, fibrous tissue including suspensory ligaments, and adipose tissue. Glandular tissue contains 15 to 20 lobes radiating from the nipple and composed of lobules. Within each lobe are clusters of alveoli that produce milk. Each lobe is embedded in adipose tissue and empties into a lactiferous duct. There are 15 to 20 lactiferous ducts that form a collecting duct system converging toward the nipple. These ducts form ampullae or lactiferous sinuses behind the nipple, which are reservoirs for storing milk. The lobules and ducts are surrounded by fatty and connective tissue, nerves, blood vessels, and lymphatic vessels. The suspensory ligaments (Cooper's ligaments) are fibrous bands extending vertically from the surface attaching to the chest wall muscle. These support the breast tissue and become contracted in cancer of the breast, producing pits or dimples in the overlying skin. (From Jarvis C: *Physical examination and health assessment,* ed 3, Philadelphia, 2000, Saunders, p 417.)

Medullary, tubular, and mucinous carcinomas are less common types of ductal carcinoma, together accounting for less than 10% of breast cancers. Medullary carcinoma and tubular carcinoma are both invasive but have better outcomes than invasive ductal or invasive lobular carcinomas.

Inflammatory breast disease is an unusual and aggressive form of breast cancer that presents much like an infection with warmth, redness of the skin, and lymphatic blockage.

Paget's disease of the breast is a rare form of ductal carcinoma arising in the ducts near the nipple with itching, redness and flaking of the nipple, and occasionally bleeding (Fig. 19-10).[43] This condition occurs in conjunction with a ductal adenocarcinoma of the breast, which has frequently metastasized to the axillary lymph nodes.

Breast cancer appears biologically similar in both genders, although it is often diagnosed at later stages in older men. Men and women develop the same types of breast cancer although lobular carcinoma is rare in men because of the absence of lobules in the male breast. Most breast cancers in men are carcinomas, most commonly infiltrating ductal carcinoma.

Incidence.   Breast carcinomas account for approximately 30% of all the female cancers in the United States. In addition, breast cancer is the number two cause of female cancer deaths in the United States, second only to lung cancer. Estimated new breast cancer cases in 2002 were 1500 for men and 203,500 for women, and approximately 400 men and 39,600 women died as a result of breast cancer in 2002.[57] The cumulative lifetime risk of developing breast cancer for white women in the United States is 1 in 8 based on a woman living 95+ years. A woman of average life expectancy has a 1 in 9 chance of developing breast cancer, but it should be kept in mind that a woman's risk at age 25 years is 1 in 21,441, with increasing risk as she ages.[34] Approximately 70% of all breast cancer occurs in women over age 50 years.

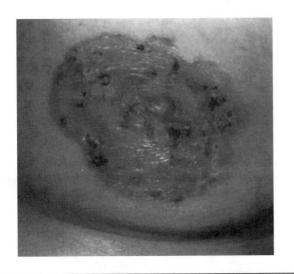

FIGURE   **19-10**   Paget's disease of the breast. An erythematous plaque surrounds the nipple in this female with ductal adenocarcinoma of the breast. (From Callen JP, Jorizzo J, Greer KE, et al: *Dermatological signs of internal disease*, Philadelphia, 1988, Saunders, p 105.)

Etiologic Factors.   The cause of breast cancer is unknown although there are some genetic bases, expression of which will vary in different ethnic groups. A known genetic mutation in two genes (*BRCA1, BRCA2*; the "breast cancer" genes) has been identified that may be responsible for most inherited cancers (account for 10% of all cases). *BRCA1* and *BRCA2* are tumor suppressor genes. Everyone has two copies of each gene, and when working properly, they produce proteins that keep cell growth in check. Mutations can render these genes inactive, increasing the risk for developing breast, ovarian, and certain other cancers.

Risk Factors.   Gender, age, ethnicity, family history, medical history, menstrual history (early onset of menstruation with greater exposure to estrogen), nulliparity or infertility (greater number of menstrual cycles with hormonal exposures), and geography are all factors linked to breast cancer (Box 19-3). Gender (female) is the most significant risk factor associated with this disease; fewer than 1% of breast cancers occur in males. In men, age (>60 years) and heredity are the most common risk factors, but more than one half have no known risk factors. Black men are at almost twice the risk of white men. Men and women who have several female relatives with breast cancer and those families with a *BRCA2* mutation on chromosome 13q are at greater risk. The associated lifetime risk for breast cancer in mutation carriers ranges from 40% to 90% depending on the extent of family history and other risk factors.[19]

Age is the second most significant factor; the incidence increases with advancing age. The median and mean ages of women with breast cancer are between 60 and 61 years. Women with a personal or family history (personal history of breast, ovarian, or uterine cancer; family history of breast cancer among first-degree relatives) have a significantly increased risk of developing breast cancer. Breast cancer in two or more first-degree relatives (mother, sister, daughter) increases the risk fivefold. In addition, a history of fibrocystic breast disease, when accompanied by proliferative changes, papillomatosis, or atypical epithelial hyperplasia, increases the risk of cancer. Even with all these potential risk factors, the majority of women with breast cancer do not have any apparent risk factors.

Scientists thus far have been unable to establish a direct link between breast cancer and tobacco smoke; electromagnetic fields; silicone breast implants; or the chemicals used in pesticides, plastics, herbicides, or hair colorings.[43,79] Likewise, studies of induced abortions (but not miscarriages, known as spontaneous abortions) in relation to breast cancer are inconclusive and inconsistent in their findings. There is a need for further clarification of induced abortion as a risk factor.[64,89,105]

Pathogenesis.   The pathogenesis of breast cancer is unknown, but estrogen is believed to be a key factor in promoting (rather than initiating) breast cancer. It may not trigger the series of genetic changes that are required to transform normal breast cells into malignant ones, but it may spur the proliferation of transformed cells, increasing the likelihood that they will develop into cancer. The development of invasive breast cancer involves epithelial hyperplasia, premalignant change, in situ carcinoma, and invasive carcinoma.

These progressive alterations in the structure of the mammary epithelium are accompanied by a reorganization in the composition of the epithelial, periductal, and stromal extra-

BOX 19-3

Risk Factors for Breast Cancer

Six Key Risk Factors

Age ≥ 60 years
Age at menarche (first menstruation <12 years = greater risk)
Age at first live birth (>35 years = greater risk)
Number of first-degree relatives (mother, sister or sisters, or daughter or daughters) with breast cancer
Number of previous breast biopsies (whether positive or negative)
At least one biopsy with atypical (ductal or lobular) hyperplasia or radial scars

Additional Risk Factors*

History of fibrocystic breast disease
Ethnicity (whites: greater incidence; blacks: more deaths)
Late menopause (>50 years)
Nulliparity, infertility
DES (diethylstilbestrol) exposure
Alcohol (≥2 drinks/day of beer, wine, hard liquor)
Postmenopausal weight gain (>45 lb since age 18 years); obesity
High doses of chest radiation before age 30 years (e.g., Hodgkin's disease)
Environmental exposures (under investigation)
High-fat diet
Long-term use of oral contraceptives or combined hormone replacement therapy
High bone density (postmenopausal women); circulating estrogen promotes bone formation

*These risk factors are not included in the National Cancer Institute's *Breast Cancer Risk Assessment* tool for two reasons: either (1) evidence is not conclusive or (2) researchers cannot accurately determine how much these factors contribute to the calculation of risk for an individual. Nevertheless, these additional risk factors are known to contribute to the increased risk of breast cancer. For more information about risk assessment see HYPERLINK "http://www.yourcancerrisk.harvard.edu" www.yourcancerrisk.harvard.edu or visit the National Cancer Institute's Breast Cancer Risk Assessment tool: HYPERLINK "http://bcra.nci.nih.gov/brc/learnmore.htm"

cellular matrix (ECM). This observation is important because ECM proteins (elastin, collagens, proteoglycans, glycoproteins) not only provide a physical support for cells within developing and mature tissues but also act as an informational system. These proteins detect and coordinate signals originating from the tissue microenvironment and adjacent cells. Networks of ECM interact with transmembrane receptors called *integrins* to transmit signals from the ECM to the cell interior. It is hypothesized that modifications in the mammary ECM that occur during tumor formation or a failure to respond appropriately to the preexisting ECM may result in aberrant cell behavior. Studies show that changes in cell adhesion play a major part in the development and progression of breast cancer.[59]

Biologists collecting and recording salivary estrogen levels have recognized patterns of low feminine fertility correlated with famine. Estrogen samples from the mouths of hungry women are found to be about one half of estrogen levels in the saliva of well-nourished women, a difference that can account for the drop in pregnancy rate in lean women. Improved nutrition in developed countries such as the United States has led to increased exposure to estrogen over a lifetime. This variable combined with the resulting earlier age of menarche, delayed and decreased childbearing, and the increase in exposure to environmental toxins, all of which contribute to more and prolonged estrogen exposure, may result in genetic mutations, loss of suppressor genes, and cell proliferation or cell growth.

An older but still unproved theory is the environmental exposure hypothesis that prolonged and cumulative exposure to hormonally active synthetic chemicals contributes to the rising incidence of breast cancer. Synthetic chemicals may do this directly by acting as estrogen, altering the way the body produces or metabolizes estrogen; they can work bifunctionally, through genetic or hormonal paths, depending on the periods and extent of exposure.[25] Prenatal exposure to estrogens may predispose a woman to breast cancer later in life through an "imprinting" process that sensitizes her to estrogen exposure. One way that synthetic chemicals may increase breast cancer risk is to alter the way the body processes its own estrogen. This theory is the basis for the use of indoles (phytochemicals found in vegetables) shown to reduce cancer risk.

Most carcinomas develop in the glandular epithelium of the terminal duct lobular unit. In the normal breast, the milk ducts and lobules are neatly lined with epithelial cells. Over time, some extra (noncancerous) cells may grow within the duct (hyperplasia) and begin to look odd (atypia). This condition is *atypical ductal hyperplasia*. When cancer cells multiply but remain contained within the duct, the condition is called *ductal carcinoma in situ*. A stromal invasion by malignant cells usually results in fibroblastic proliferation. A palpable mass within the breast tissue will typically develop. Invasive ductal carcinoma occurs when cancer cells break through the duct wall and enter other tissues.

Breast cancer has a propensity for metastases to the bone, possibly related to a small protein found in the bone marrow (osteonectin) that both attracts breast (and prostate) cancer cells to bone and once attracted, stimulates the cells to invade the bone. Researchers suggest that metastasis of breast cancer cells to the bone is mediated by the ability of osteonectin to promote migration, protease activity, and invasion.[55]

Clinical Manifestations. The most common initial presenting sign of breast cancer is a palpable lump or nodule. Approximately 90% of breast masses are discovered by the woman herself; for men, the lump is usually in the center behind the areola and for women, either centrally behind the areola or in the outer upper quadrant although neoplasm can occur anywhere in the breast tissue (Fig. 19-11). The mass tends to be firm and irregular if it is a carcinoma versus smooth and rubbery if it is benign. The mass is typically not painful if it is cancer.

Other manifestations include a change in breast contour or texture, nipple discharge and retraction or inversion, local skin dimpling, erythema, and a local rash or ulceration. Lymphadenopathy may also be the initial presentation of this disease. Symptoms associated with metastases can include upper extremity edema, bone pain, jaundice, or weight loss. These findings are rarely the initial complaint, however.

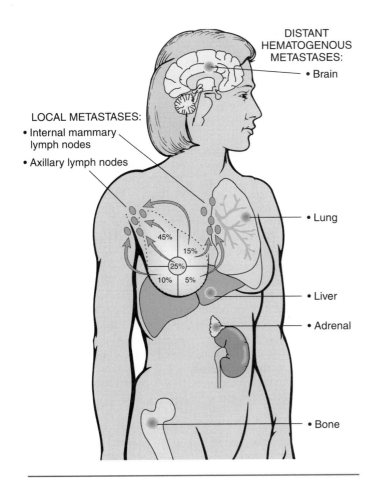

DISTANT
HEMATOGENOUS
METASTASES:
• Brain

LOCAL METASTASES:
• Internal mammary
  lymph nodes
• Axillary lymph nodes

• Lung

45%

15%

25%

10%   5%

• Liver

• Adrenal

• Bone

FIGURE **19-11** The distribution of breast carcinoma and the pathway of lymphatic metastases. Most tumors in women are found in the upper lateral quadrant and behind the nipple (areola) and for men, behind the nipple. (From Damjanov I: *Pathology for the health-related professions*, ed 2, Philadelphia, 2000, Saunders, p 397.)

If not diagnosed and treated early the cancer will spread to the regional lymph nodes, including the axillary, internal mammary, and supraclavicular nodes (see Fig. 12-7). As the disease progresses, the cancer commonly spreads to the lungs, liver, bone, adrenals, skin, and brain.

Medical Management

Prevention. *Healthy People 2010* has identified the reduction of the breast cancer death rate by 20% as its primary objective related to breast cancer. The American Cancer Society's 2015 Challenge Goals and Nationwide Objectives include a reduction of 15% in the age-adjusted incidence rate of the disease and a 45% reduction in the age-adjusted mortality rate. By the year 2008, the American Cancer Society hopes that 90% of women 40 year of age or older will undergo breast cancer screening that is consistent with their guidelines.[14,117]

The hallmark of effective intervention in cases of breast cancer is early detection using a combination of three tools: monthly self-breast examination (SBE),* clinical breast ex-

amination (CBE), and mammography. Women should start examining their breasts in their 20s so they are comfortable with doing it and familiar with the way their breasts feel from month to month. Monthly SBE should be performed 1 week after the cessation of bleeding from the menstrual cycle or in the postmenopausal woman consistently perhaps on the same day each month. CBE should be performed by a trained health care professional as follows.

The American Cancer Society makes the following screening recommendations for asymptomatic women at average risk: for women age 20 to 40 years, a monthly SBE and a CBE every 3 years; for women age 40 to 49 years, a monthly SBE, annual CBE, and screening mammogram* every 1 to 2 years; and for women age 50 years old and older,† a monthly SBE, annual mammogram, and CBE.

Tamoxifen is now used as a chemopreventive agent in women with a history of breast cancer or at increased risk for breast cancer based on results when administered postoperatively in stages I and II disease (>50% reduction of invasive and noninvasive breast cancer in all age-groups and all categories of estrogen-sensitive breast cancer). The major drawback to the use of tamoxifen is the increased rate of endometrial cancer. Giving the drug for more than 5 years failed to enhance its effect; more studies are under way to determine the optimal duration of tamoxifen administration, especially in relation to the concomitant development of endometrial cancer in some women. More information on the best candidates for tamoxifen is available.[35]

The use of raloxifene, a selective estrogen receptor modulator (SERM) drug approved for women at risk of osteoporosis that shows promise in breast cancer prevention, is also under investigation. A large number of other chemopreventive agents under investigation include other SERMs, cyclooxygenase-2 inhibitors, aromatase inactivators/inhibitors (a new class of endocrine agents that block an enzyme necessary to convert other hormones to estrogen in the breast; this group has also been approved for first-line treatment), Gn-RH agonists, isoflavones, and vitamin D derivatives.[33,66]

Controlling weight, especially in middle age, may help in preventing breast cancer, particularly in women who do not use postmenopausal hormones.[51] Fat tissue contains an enzyme that converts adrenal gland hormones to estrogen. The extra estrogen in overweight women acts as a nutrient and aids the growth of precancerous or abnormal cancerous cells in the breast. Restricting alcohol is a proven risk reducer. Excess risk of breast cancer associated with alcohol consumption may be reduced by adequate folate intake.[121] The effects of diet and nutrition (low fat, rich in fruits and vegetables) remain under investigation. Data from the Nurses' Health Study show a clear benefit for postmenopausal women from engaging in some

---

*Some discussion has centered on abandoning the SBE for women age 40 to 69 years, saying that studies on the topic suggest SBE and SBE education do not reduce deaths but increase unnecessary biopsies and anxiety.[7] The American Cancer Society continues to endorse the practice of SBE as one component of breast cancer screening understanding there are some limitations.[2]

*Screening mammography implies the mammogram is done when there is no palpable lump or anything else indicating cancer. Until 1997 the American Cancer Society recommended the first screening mammogram by age 40 years, whereas the National Cancer Institute stopped advocating routine mammograms for women between the ages of 40 and 50 years[78]; and in the rest of the world, screening mammograms were not recommended until age 50 years. Much controversy and debate centered around screening mammography for this particular age-group (40 to 49 years); but in 1997, based on data presented at a National Institutes of Health (NIH) conference on breast cancer screening establishing the effectiveness of mammography in women younger than 50 years, the NIH began recommending breast cancer screening to women in their 40s.[78,98]

†The cost effectiveness and efficacy of screening mammography in women age 70 years and older have come under examination. It has been suggested that the small gain in life expectancy is a variable that must be factored in when a woman is deciding about screening.[61]

form of exercise. Postmenopausal women who get at least 1 hour of physical activity per day are 15% to 20% less likely to develop breast cancer than sedentary women.[85]

Other preventive steps may include exposure to the sun needed by the skin to manufacture vitamin D and increased vitamin D intake (food or supplementation).[58] There is no scientific evidence to support a link between antiperspirants or deodorants and breast cancer so avoiding these products is not a means of preventing breast cancer.

Prophylactic mastectomy (also referred to as risk-reduction mastectomy) for women with a *BRCA1* or *BRCA2* mutation and positive family history has proven extremely effective, but there is a need for research to better guide high-risk women in the decision-making process.[66,102] Numerous reputable books are available on the trade market specifically addressing ways to reduce risk and prevent breast cancer.

Diagnosis. Clinical examination, mammography, and ultrasonography are all used to detect breast abnormalities. Tissue biopsy is the standard for a definitive diagnosis, and sentinel lymph node mapping to identify micrometastases has become standard practice to identify and remove only the first node or nodes that cancer cells reach after leaving the breast. This eliminates unnecessary dissection (see discussion of technique in the section on Diagnosis in Chapter 8). Only women whose sentinel nodes indicate the spread of cancer will need to undergo more extensive biopsy. Ultrasonography is primarily used to differentiate a cystic from a solid lesion. Mammography is an important tool for the detection of a lesion before the mass (cancerous or benign) is large enough to be palpable but is not a substitute for biopsy because by itself it is not diagnostic and it may not detect cancer in very dense breast tissue.

Updated technology, such as digital mammography (computerized x-rays), may improve early detection of breast cancer. With the added capability of transmitting results electronically to specialists worldwide for consultation, this technology may reduce further misdiagnosis and unnecessary surgery. Scientists are adapting MRI and positron emission tomography (PET) scanning, two imaging technologies that are good at distinguishing malignant from benign tissue, for use in breast cancer diagnosis, although these remain too costly to use in general screening programs.

Ductal lavage is another new method to detect early changes in ductal cells for women at high risk for developing breast cancer. Epithelial cells that line the ductal and lobular system of all milk ducts are collected using a microcatheter inserted into the milk ducts through the nipple surface. Results of this test may be able to diagnose abnormal ductal cells before cancer becomes evident on a mammogram or in a physical exam.[27,32]

The protein (oncogene) *c-erb B-2*, also known as HER-2/*neu*, is a prognostic breast cancer marker assayed in tissue biopsy specimens from women diagnosed with malignant tumors. Current studies suggest that soluble fragments of this oncogene may be released from the cell surface and become detectable in the saliva of men and women with the recurrence of breast cancer.[104] Other biomarkers are under investigation, including one ECM component called *tenascin-C.* Expression of this large glycoprotein is suppressed in the normal adult mammary gland but is induced in breast cancer and is present in preinvasive cancer as well as invasive breast cancer.[40] Researchers are investigating the use of mini-

mally invasive tests to seek out biologic markers in blood or other fluids before a tumor develops. Mammography does not detect all breast cancers, and it cannot distinguish well among the various kinds of breast cancer. A more precise, noninvasive screening technique that does not involve the use of radiation is the ultimate goal of investigators developing improved breast cancer screening.

Staging. Once the diagnosis is established the clinical stage is ascertained in order to determine optimal management, including selection of candidates for adjuvant systemic therapies. Staging is done in more than 90% of eligible breast cancer cases using intraoperative sentinel lymph node dissection. Preinvasive cancer referred to as *in situ* means that the cancer remains "in place" and has not spread from its point of origin. Stage I disease is marked by a tumor 2 cm in size or smaller. Stage II disease is marked by a tumor between 2 and 5 cm in size without nodal metastases or a tumor less than 5 cm with homolateral axillary lymphatic metastases (the nodes are movable). A tumor larger than 5 cm is classified as stage III, as is a tumor fixed to the pectoral muscle or fascia or if the diseased axillary lymph nodes are fixed to adjacent tissues. Stage IV disease is a tumor fixed to the chest wall or skin or any tumor with metastases to the homolateral infraclavicular or supraclavicular nodes, with upper extremity edema, or with any distant metastasis.

Treatment. Once the diagnosis of breast cancer is made the treatment is the same for men as for women and depends on the stage at diagnosis and hormonal sensitivity (estrogen or progesterone receptor-positive). Treatment options include surgery, chemotherapy, radiation therapy, and hormonal manipulation. Radical mastectomy was the most commonly employed procedure until the 1970s. This technique included removal of the entire breast, pectoral muscles, axillary lymph nodes, and some additional skin. Postsurgical problems included lymphedema, restricted shoulder mobility, impaired muscle function, and paresthesia. Likewise, axillary node dissection is no longer performed routinely since it has been shown that the therapeutic benefit of a complete dissection has no effect on survival rate or risk of metastasis but only local control of the tumor. Instead, intraoperative lymphatic mapping and sentinel lymph node dissection are replacing complete lymph node dissection as the preferred procedure for the management of early-stage disease.[50]

More recent treatment recommendations for women with stage I or II breast cancer include breast-conserving surgery (e.g., lumpectomy with wide excision of the tumor and preservation of the breast) and radiation therapy. Up to 50% of women with early breast cancer in the United States are now treated this way. In some geographic areas, modified radical mastectomy, which spares the pectoralis major muscle, is also a commonly used procedure with the primary advantage being avoidance of radiation therapy. However, radiotherapy, now an integral part of breast-conserving treatment, should not be withheld.[49]

Breast reconstruction with an implant is an option for women who have mastectomies. This is a two-stage process; first, a balloonlike tissue expander is placed under the chest wall muscle. Every 2 or 3 weeks for several months, saline is injected into the expander to gradually stretch the overlying chest wall muscles and skin. The expander is replaced in a second surgery with a permanent saline implant (silicone implants were banned in 1992). Alternately, muscle-flap procedures use tissue from the back or abdomen to either form a breast or create a pocket for an implant. The three most popular flap procedures are the latissimus dorsi (back) flap, the transverse rectus abdominis muscle (TRAM) flap, and the free flap.

Following surgery, radiation therapy, chemotherapy, hormone therapy, or a combination of these are often employed. Chemotherapy is used when a tumor is larger than 1 cm or when smaller tumors have spread to the lymph nodes. The primary objective of these treatments is to reduce the odds of occult metastases developing into disease. Increased disease-free survival times following combination chemotherapy have been noted consistently in premenopausal women with metastases to the axillary lymph nodes. Combination chemotherapy combines two or more drugs and is given in multiple courses over 3 to 6 months. The addition of hormone therapy (tamoxifen or ovarian ablation for premenopausal women) is more effective than chemotherapy alone in women whose tumors contain estrogen receptors.

In 1998, breast cancer was the most common indication for stem cell transplant in North America, accounting for nearly one third of all transplants. However, subsequent reports have concluded that high-dose chemotherapy plus autologous bone marrow transplantation does not improve survival in women with metastatic breast cancer.[9,100] Thus a gentler approach using trastuzumab (Herceptin) was developed with better outcomes and fewer side effects.

Trastuzumab (Herceptin), a humanized IgG monoclonal antibody,* is the first biologic therapy approved for use that attacks cancer at its genetic roots. It targets a defective growth-promoting oncogene known as HER-2/neu, found in about 30% of women with aggressive breast cancer. HER-2/neu is a protein that often appears on the surface of breast cancer cells. HER-2-positive tumors are like a car with the accelerator stuck to the floor with constant signaling to grow contributing to cell proliferation. After the antibody attaches to the protein, it is taken into the cell, where it interferes with basic cell function and eventually kills the cells but spares other fast-growing cells. HER-2-positive breast cancers are more aggressive and less likely to respond to conventional therapies. When administered to women with metastatic breast cancer along with standard chemotherapy, trastuzumab delayed the progression of the disease for several months and produced a greater regression in existing tumors without additional side effects.

Uncertainties remain about how to treat node-negative women, particularly when the tumor is small; how to treat DCIS; who should receive preoperative systemic therapy; and who should be given tamoxifen. Despite these unresolved issues, medical advances have saved the lives of many people and will continue to progress with further reduction in morbidity and mortality.

Prognosis.   If detected early before metastases, breast cancer is curable. There has been a reduction in mortality of 1% to 2% annually in the United States and other industrialized countries, possibly related to changes in lifestyle (e.g., diet, exercise, reproductive behavior), early diagnosis, and improved success of treatment.[26] More than one half of all cases reported are diagnosed as stage 0 or I disease. The status of the axillary nodes is the most important prognostic factor in breast cancer and determines the selection of treatment. Breast tumors that lack estrogen responsiveness have a poor prognosis because of estrogen's poor response to current treatment available.[63] The 5-year survival rate for localized tumors is 92%; survival rate drops considerably if there is nodal involvement; metastatic disease results in an overwhelming death rate.[41] Ten-year survival rate for stage I disease is 85%, for stage II 66%, for stage III 36%, and for stage IV 7%.[11]

Recurrence.   Breast cancer recurs in one fifth of women deemed by current tests to be at low risk. The probability of recurrence is higher with histologically positive axillary nodes and increases with each additional positive node. Patterns of recurrence and metastases are similar for men and women, usually occurring within 2 years of the initial diagnosis and treatment. Men are less likely than women to develop cancer in the opposite breast, but recurrence of cancer does happen. Local recurrence is treated with surgical excision or radiotherapy combined with chemotherapy, especially if hormonal therapy has failed.

A key to recognizing women whose cancer is most likely to recur might be a tumor-suppressing protein called *maspin*, produced by cells in the breast and an effective inhibitor of angiogenesis. Women who have high levels of maspin in the bone marrow tend to remain disease-free for 2 years, whereas those with low concentrations are more likely to have a recurrence.[68,120] The most powerful predictor of recurrence remains whether or not the cancer has spread to the lymph nodes although 20% of women whose nodes are clear still relapse.

Special Implications for the Therapist   19-9

BREAST CANCER

Preferred Practice Patterns:
4B: Impaired Posture
4C: Impaired Muscle Performance
6H: Impaired Circulation and Anthropometric Dimensions Associated With Lymphatic System Disorders

There are many considerations for the therapist working with men and women who report upper quadrant symptoms of unknown origin or who have been diagnosed with breast cancer, both before and after treatment. Besides the considerations discussed in this section, limited literature evaluating physical therapy and breast cancer is available.[42,54,74] See also the section on Lymphedema in Chapter 12.

Screening for Disease and Cancer Recurrence
Therapists examining the shoulder and shoulder girdle region need to be aware of the nonmusculature structures (including breast tissue and regional lymph nodes) located in these areas. The upper, outer quadrant of the breast can extend up toward the glenohumeral joint, and more cancerous masses occur in
Continued

---

*Monoclonal (mono = single cell) antibodies cloned from mice are "humanized" so that the human immune system will not reject them.

this area than in any other part of the breast. In addition, approximately 50% of women with breast cancer have metastasis to the axillary nodes at the time the diagnosis is made. When treating a woman with a history of breast cancer, an awareness of the symptoms and signs associated with breast cancer is important.

Approximately 10% of these women will develop cancer in the opposite breast. Local and distant metastases occur most frequently within 3 years of the initial diagnosis. Palpation of a lump or mass in these areas or new onset of edema or swelling in the upper quadrant should raise concern on the therapist's part and lead to further questioning regarding the clinical findings. If the mass lies in the pectoralis major muscle, the mass should change during palpation when the muscle is actively contracting. Metastases to the thorax are common in breast cancer, and pulmonary symptoms can be very similar to pulmonary abnormalities that occur after radiotherapy. If the therapist is in doubt regarding any reported or observed manifestations, the client should be evaluated by a physician (see the section on Lymphedema in Chapter 12).

Preoperative Considerations

Preoperative evaluation is recommended for all women undergoing surgical intervention for breast cancer whether the intervention is axillary node dissection, lumpectomy, or mastectomy of any kind. Upper quadrant motion, posture, joint range of motion (including accessory motions), flexibility, and soft tissue movement should be assessed. Identification of current physical activity level and exercise regimen is important. Preoperative education is included to teach safe movement and exercise techniques to be used in the early postoperative phase. Lymphedema precautions are also important (see Table 12-2).

Starting with the preoperative diagnosis and throughout the recovery process the therapist can guide women into physical activity and exercise routines that help them maintain endurance, function, flexibility, and strength; reduce pain and fatigue; and prevent musculoskeletal injury or debilitation, especially during adjuvant treatment such as chemotherapy or radiation. Helping women cope with the emotional challenges of living with a life-threatening and body-altering disease is integral to the healing and recovery process.

Side Effects of Treatment

Women receiving adjuvant therapy (chemotherapy, radiation therapy, or hormonal therapy) may experience numerous side effects that could interfere with rehabilitation (see Chapters 4 and 8; potential side effects of therapy are listed in Table 8-8; see Tables 4-9 and 4-10). Women receiving chemotherapy will likely be fatigued and experience flulike symptoms. Therefore the timing of scheduled therapy visits is important to maximize productivity during the session. Exercises and functional activities may have to be paced or therapy visits shortened to accommodate the woman's energy level. An exercise program to improve endurance in order to perform activities of daily living is important. Women who have undergone mastectomy should be instructed postoperatively and assisted with breathing and coughing exercises to prevent pulmonary complications. In addition, lower extremity exercises are also important to prevent thromboemboli. More specific rehabilitation recommendations based on specific oncologic treatment are available.[39]

There has been an increased frequency of rheumatoid symptoms reported following breast cancer treatment. Signifi-

cant joint pain and swelling of the upper extremity, morning stiffness lasting less than 1 hour (41%) or more than 1 hour (26%), and prolonged joint pain and stiffness have been documented.[3]

About 40% of women undergoing mastectomy experience a neuropathic pain phenomenon called *postmastectomy pain syndrome (PMPS)*. PMPS is thought to arise from damage to the axillary nerves during surgery, specifically the intercostobrachial nerve, a peripheral nerve with tributaries that branch into the armpit and upper arm. The pain occurs at the incision site, axilla, arm, or shoulder and is experienced as burning, numbness, tingling, or stabbing. Severity ranges from mild to extremely distressing; onset and frequency are highly variable (immediate to after 3 months; continuous, daily, weekly, monthly). Because PMPS seems to be on the rise, it is important to ask about postmastectomy pain. Prognostic risk factors that predispose an individual to PMPS are unknown with the possible exception of age (more common in women younger than 30 years).[17,99] In addition to medications for pain, a program to prevent loss of mobility and to prevent adhesive capsulitis must be initiated.

Women who receive breast implants for reconstruction after mastectomies may experience surgical complications caused by tissue damage from the cancer surgery and follow-up chemotherapy and radiation to the surrounding tissue. These alterations in tissue may prevent the implant from being fit in where the breast tissue was excised, thus affecting the way scar tissue forms around the implant. Scar-tissue formation that deforms or hardens the implant, called *capsular contraction,* is the most common complication followed by implant rupture or malfunction, bruising, infection, and chronic pain.[37] See further discussion in the section on Breast Implantation in Chapter 7.

The TRAM flap has an incision that runs laterally from hip to hip and may weaken the abdominal wall. Women with chronic back problems are usually not good candidates for this procedure without adequate preoperative rehabilitation. A postoperative strengthening program is essential to prevent further back-related musculoskeletal complications. Although uncommon (occurring in 1% to 5% of cases), the most serious complication of the flap procedure is a loss of blood circulation to the transferred tissue leading to necrosis and the loss of all or part of the reconstructed breast.

Exercise and Breast Cancer

A clear relationship between physical activity and exercise and breast cancer prevention has been established.[12,84,85,107]* Throughout this text, the benefits of exercise in relation to various diseases, disorders, and conditions have been discussed, including (pertinent to the diagnosis of breast cancer) exercise and immunology (see Chapter 6), exercise and cancer from a variety of viewpoints (see Chapter 8), exercise and the cardiovascular system (see Chapter 11), and exercise and the lymphatic system (see Chapter 12). For example, the impact of low- to moderate-intensity regular exercise is significant in maintaining functional ability and reducing fatigue in women with breast cancer receiving chemotherapy.[93] See also the sec-

---

*These studies have all been of white women; there are limited data on black women or women of other ethnic groups, but findings suggest that strenuous physical activity in early adulthood is associated with a reduced risk of breast cancer in black women as well.[1]

tion on Exercise During and After Chemotherapy in Chapter 8. Supervised exercise in women with breast cancer not receiving chemotherapy increases aerobic capacity and reduces body weight.[96]

Prescriptive exercise usually includes types, intensity, duration, and frequency since these parameters are carefully matched to the underlying pathologic process and clinical presentation. The association of physical activity and exercise to overall and site-specific cancer risk is under investigation, especially in relation to whether any dose-response correlation has been observed. Physical activity corresponding to 15 MET/wk or higher at age 10 to 24 years has been shown to significantly reduce breast cancer at age 51 to 60 years in a small number of women.[46] A review of 41 studies, including 108,031 breast cancer cases, identified an observed inverse association with a dose-response relationship between physical activity and breast cancer. Moderate activity (defined as >4.5 MET/wk) was shown to have a protective effect against breast cancer in premenopausal and postmenopausal women.[108] Other investigators reviewed number of hours per week, suggesting that breast cancer rates were 20% lower among women who exercise an average of 1 hour per day (or more), compared with those who exercised less than 1 hour per week.[85] Much more investigation in this area is both warranted and under way.

Even personality factors as these relate to exercise participation across the breast cancer experience have come under scrutiny. Personality may be an important determinant of exercise following breast cancer diagnosis. Women with outgoing personalities who are conscientious and have low scores of neuroticism were better able to discriminate when and how to exercise during and following cancer treatment as well as better able to recognize changes in exercise stage across the cancer experience (prediagnosis through treatment to posttreatment). Women with high scores of neuroticism especially engaged in maladaptive exercise patterns.[81] This type of information can be potentially helpful to the therapist when assessing the individual woman's needs and abilities as they relate to designing an effective interventional prescriptive program of exercise. ■

REFERENCES

1. Adams-Campbell LL, Rosenberg L, Rao RS, et al: Strenuous physical activity and breast cancer risk in African-American women, *J Natl Med Assoc* 93(7-8):267-275, 2001.
2. American Cancer Society: Breast self-exam is too valuable to discard, *CA Cancer J Clin* 51(5):265-270, 2001.
3. Androwski MA, Curran SL, Carpenter JS, et al: Rheumatoid symptoms following breast cancer treatment: a controlled comparison, *J Pain Symptom Manage* 18(2):85-94, 1999.
4. Ballweg ML, editor: *The endometriosis sourcebook: the definitive guide to current treatment options, the latest research, common myths about the disease and coping strategies*, New York, 1995, McGraw-Hill.
5. Banks E: Hormone replacement therapy and the sensitivity and specificity of breast cancer screening: a review, *J Med Screen* 8(1):29-34, 2001.
6. Barakat RR: Contemporary issues in the management of endometrial cancer, *CA Cancer J Clin* 48(5):299-314, 1998.
7. Baxter N: Preventive health care, 2001 update: should women be routinely taught breast self-examination to screen for breast cancer? *CMAJ* 164(13):1851-1852, 2001.
8. Bell MC, Crowley-Nowick P, Bradlow HL, et al: Placebo-controlled trial of indole-3-carbinol in the treatment of CIN, *Gynecol Oncol* 78(2):123-129, 2000.
9. Bergh J: Where next with stem-cell-supported high-dose therapy for breast cancer? *Lancet* 355(9308):944-945, 2000.
10. Bieber EJ, Barnes RB: Breast cancer and HRT-what are the data? *Int J Fertil Womens Med* 46(2):73-78, 2001.
11. Bland KI, Menck HR, Scott-Conner CE, et al: The National Cancer Data Base 10-year survey of breast cancer treatment at hospitals in the United States, *Cancer* 83:1262-1273, 1998.
12. Breslow RA, Ballard-Barbash R, Munoz K, et al: Long-term recreational physical activity and breast cancer in the National Health and Nutrition Examination Survey I epidemiologic follow-up study, *Cancer Epidemiol Biomarkers Prev* 10(7):805-808, 2001.
13. Bush TL, Whiteman M, Flaws JA: Hormone replacement therapy and breast cancer: a qualitative review, *Obstet Gynecol* 98(3):498-508, 2001.
14. Byers T, Mouchawar J, Marks J, et al: The American Cancer Society challenge goals. How far can cancer rates decline in the U.S. by the year 2015? *Cancer* 86:715-727, 1999.
15. Canavan TP, Doshi NR: Endometrial cancer, *Am Fam Physician* 59(11):3069-3077, 1999.
16. Capasso P: Endovascular treatment of varicoceles and utero-ovarian varices, *J Radiol* 81(9, suppl):1115-1124, 2000.
17. Carpenter JS, Sloan P, Andrykowski MA, et al: Risk factors after mastectomy/lumpectomy, *Cancer Pract* 7(2):66-70, 1999.
18. Centers for Disease Control and Prevention: Risk of ectopic pregnancy after tubal sterilization (on-line), 2001: HYPERLINK "http://www.cdc.gov/" www.cdc.gov/
19. Chang-Claude J: Inherited genetic susceptibility to breast cancer, *IARC Sci Publ* 154:177-190, 2001.
20. Chiaffarino F, Parazzini F, La Vecchia C, et al: Diet and uterine myomas, *Obstet Gynecol* 94(3):395-398, 1999.
21. Chrousos GP, Torpy DJ, Gold PW: Interactions between the hypothalamic-pituitary-adrenal axis and the female reproductive system: clinical implications, *Ann Intern Med* 129(3):229-240, 1998.
22. D'Amelio R, Farris M, Grande S, et al: Association between polycystic ovary and fibrocystic breast disease, *Gynecol Obstet Invest* 51(2):134-137, 2001.
23. Dargent D, Martin X, Mathevet P: Laparoscopic assessment of the sentinel lymph node in early stage cervical cancer, *Gynecol Oncol* 79(3):411-415, 2000.
24. Davis CM, editor: *Complementary therapies in rehabilitation: holistic approaches for prevention and wellness*, Thorofare, NJ, 1997, Slack, Inc.
25. Davis DL, Telang NT, Osborne MP, et al: Medical hypothesis: bifunctional genetic-hormonal pathways to breast cancer, *Environ Health Perspect* 105:571-576, 1997.
26. Del Turco MR: Breast cancer update: encouraging trends, *CA Cancer J Clin* 49(3):135-137, 1999.
27. Dooley WC, Veronesi U, Elledge R, et al: Detection of premalignant and malignant breast cells by ductal lavage, *Obstet Gynecol* 97(4, suppl 1): S2, 2001.
28. Dunaif A, Thomas A: Current concepts in polycystic ovary syndrome, *Annu Rev Med* 52:401-409, 2001.
29. Ellerbrock TV, Chiasson MA, Bush TJ, et al: Incidence of cervical squamous intraepithelial lesions in HIB-infected women, *JAMA* 283(8):1031-1037, 2000.
30. Eltabbakh GH, Awtrey CS: Current treatment for ovarian cancer, *Expert Opin Pharmacother* 2(1):109-124, 2001.
31. Endometriosis Association: Treatment options (on-line), 2001: HYPERLINK "http://www.endometriosisassn.org" www.endometriosisassn.org
32. Evron E, Dooley WC, Umbricht CB, et al: Detection of breast cancer cells in ductal lavage fluid by methylation-specific PCR, *Lancet* 357(9265):1335-1336, 2001.
33. Fabian CJ: Breast cancer chemoprevention: beyond tamoxifen, *Breast Cancer Res* 3(2):99-103, 2001.
34. Feuer EJ: The lifetime risk of developing breast cancer, *J Natl Cancer Inst* 85:892-896, 1993.
35. Fisher B, Costantino JP, Wickerham DL, et al: Tamoxifen for prevention of breast cancer: report of the National Surgical Adjuvant Breast and Bowel Project P-1 study, *J Natl Cancer Inst* 90:1371-1388, 1998.
36. Frei KA, Kinkel K: Staging endometrial cancer: role of magnetic resonance imaging, *J Magn Reson Imaging* 13(6):850-855, 2001.
37. Gabriel SE, Woods JE, O'Fallon WM, et al: Complications leading to surgery after breast implantation, *N Engl J Med* 336(10):718-719, 1997.

38. Garuti G, De Giorgi O, Sambruni I, et al: Prognostic significance of hysteroscopic imaging in endometrial adenocarcinoma, *Gynecol Oncol* 81(3):408-413, 2001.

39. Gerber L, Augustine E: Rehabilitation management: restoring fitness and return to functional activity. In Harris J, Lippman M, Morrow M, et al, editors: *Diseases of the breast*, Philadelphia, 2000, Lippincott, Williams & Wilkins, pp 1001-1007.

40. Goepeol C, Buchmann J, Schultka R, et al: Tenascin-a marker for the malignant potential of preinvasive breast cancers, *Gynecol Oncol* 79:372-378, 2000.

41. Greenberg PA, Hortobagyi GN, Smith TL, et al: Long-term follow-up of patients with complete remission following combination chemotherapy for metastatic breast cancer, *J Clin Oncol* 14:2197-2205, 1996.

42. Gutman H, Kersz T, Barzilai T, et al: Achievements of physical therapy in patients after modified radical mastectomy compared with quadrantectomy, axillary dissection, and radiation for carcinoma of the breast, *Arch Surg* 125(3):389-391, 1990.

43. Harvard Women's Health Watch: Breast cancer update, part I, *HWHW* 8(2):3-5, 2000.

44. Harvard Women's Health Watch: Progress report on ovarian cancer, *HWHW* 11(9):2-4, 2000.

45. Hemminki K, Dong C: Cancer in husbands of cervical cancer patients, *Epidemiology* 11(3):347-349, 2000.

46. Hofvind SS, Thoresen SO: Physical activity and breast cancer, *Tidsskr Nor Laegeforen* 121(16):1892-1895, 2001.

47. Holte J: Polycystic ovary syndrome and insulin resistance: thrifty genes struggling with over-feeding and sedentary life style? *J Endocrinol Invest* 21(9):589-601, 1998.

48. Hornstein MD, Thomas PP, Sober AJ, et al: Association between endometriosis, dysplastic nevi, and history of melanoma in women of reproductive age, *Hum Reprod* 12(1):143-145, 1997.

49. Hortobagyi GN: Treatment of breast cancer, *N Engl J Med* 339(14):974-984, 1998.

50. Hsueh EC, Hansen N, Giuliano AE: Intraoperative lymphatic mapping and sentinel lymph node dissection in breast cancer, *CA Cancer J Clin* 50(5):279-291, 2000.

51. Huang Z, Hankinson SE, Colditz GA, et al: Dual effects of weight and weight gain on breast cancer risk, *JAMA* 278(17):1407-1411, 1997.

52. Hulme J: *Beyond Kegel's*, Missoula, Montana, 1999, Phoenix Publishing.

53. Hunter TB, Roberts CC, Hunt KR, et al: Occurrence of fibroadenomas in postmenopausal women referred for breast biopsy, *J Am Geriatr Soc* 44(1):61-64, 1996.

54. Impello RF, Crane J: Musculoskeletal intervention for postmastectomy complications, *Phys Ther Case Rep* 3(1):22-25, 2000.

55. Jacob K, Webber M, Benayahu D, et al: Osteonectin promotes prostate cancer cell migration and invasion: a possible mechanism for metastasis to bone, *Cancer Res* 59(17):4453-4457, 1999.

56. Janicek MF, Averette HE: Cervical cancer: prevention, diagnosis, and therapeutics, *CA Cancer J Clin* 51(2):92-118, 2001.

57. Jemal A, Thomas MPH, Murray T, Thun M: Cancer statistics, 2002, *CA Cancer J Clin* 2: 23-47, 2002.

58. John EM, Schwartz GG, Dreon DM, et al: Vitamin D and breast cancer risk: NHANES I Epidemiologic follow-up study, 1971-1975 to 1992. National Health and Nutrition Examination Survey, *Cancer Epidemiol Biomarkers Prev* 8(5):399-406, 1999.

59. Jones PL: Extracellular matrix and tenascin-C in pathogenesis of breast cancer, *Lancet* 357:1992-1994, 2001.

60. Kendrick JS, Atrash HK, Strauss, LT, et al: Vaginal douching and the risk of ectopic pregnancy among black women, *Am J Obstet Gynecol* 176(5):991-997, 1997.

61. Kerlikowske K, Salzmann P, Phillips KA, et al: Continuing screening mammography in women aged 70 to 79 years: impact on life expectancy and cost-effectiveness, *JAMA* 282(22):2156-2163, 1999.

62. Kovacs G, Wood C: The current status of polycystic ovary syndrome, *Aust NZ J Obstet Gynaecol* 41(1):65-68, 2001.

63. Kuukasjarvi T, Kononen J, Helin H, et al: Loss of estrogen receptor in recurrent breast cancer is associated with poor response to endocrine therapy, *J Clin Oncol* 14:2584-2589, 1996.

64. Lazovich D, Thompson JA, Mink PJ, et al: Induced abortion and breast cancer risk, *Epidemiology* 11(1):76-80, 2000.

65. Legro RS: Diabetes prevalence and risk factors in polycystic ovary syndrome, *Obstet Gynecol Clin North Am* 28(1):99-109, 2001.

66. Leris C, Mokbel K: The prevention of breast cancer: an overview, *Curr Med Res Opin* 16(4):252-257, 2001.

67. Lin JT, Lachmann E, Nagler W: Paraneoplastic cerebellar degeneration as the first manifestation of cancer, *J Womens Health Gend Based Med* 10(5):495-502, 2001.

68. Maass N, Hojo T, Rosel F, et al: Down regulation of the tumor suppressor gene maspin in breast carcinoma is associated with a higher risk of distant metastasis, *Clin Biochem* 34(4):303-307, 2001.

69. Maleux G, Stockx L, Wilms G, et al: Ovarian vein embolization for the treatment of pelvic congestion syndrome: long-term technical and clinical results, *J Vasc Interv Radiol* 11(7):859-864, 2000.

70. Malicky ES, Kostic KJ, Jacob JH: Endometrial carcinoma presenting with an isolated osseous metastasis: a case report and review of the literature, *Eur J Gynaecol Oncol* 18(6):492-494, 1997.

71. Malur S, Krause N, Kohler C, et al: Sentinel lymph node detection in patients with cervical cancer, *Gynecol Oncol* 80(2):254-257, 2001.

72. Manson J, Martin K: Clinical practice: postmenopausal hormone-replacement therapy, *N Engl J Med* 345(1):34-40, 2001.

73. Marshall K: Polycystic ovary syndrome: clinical considerations, *Altern Med Rev* 6(3):272-292, 2001.

74. Megens A, Harris SR: Physical therapist management of lymphedema following treatment for breast cancer: a critical review of its effectiveness, *Phys Ther* 78(12):1302-1311, 1998.

75. Mills DS, Vernon MW: *Endometriosis: healing through nutrition*, New York, 1999, Element (Penguin Putnam).

76. Moysich KB, Mettlin C, Piver MS, et al: Regular use of analgesic drugs and ovarian cancer risk, *Cancer Epidemiol Biomarkers Prev* 10(8):903-906, 2001.

77. Narod SA, Risch H, Moslehi R, et al: Oral contraceptives and the risk of hereditary ovarian cancer, *N Engl J Med* 339(7):424-428, 1998.

78. National Institute of Health (NIH) Consensus Statement: Breast cancer screening for women ages 40-49, *NIH Consensus Statement* 15(1):1-35, 1997.

79. Nelson N: Institute of Medicine finds no link between breast implants and disease, *J Natl Cancer Inst* 91(14):1191, 1999.

80. Norman RJ, Clark AM: Obesity and reproductive disorders: a review, *Reprod Fertil Dev* 10(1):55-63, 1998.

81. Rhodes RE, Courneya KS, Bobick TM: Personality and exercise participation across the breast cancer experience, *Psychooncology* 10(5):380-388, 2001.

82. Ries LAG, Eisner MP, Kosary CL, et al: *SEER cancer statistics review, 1973-1997*, Bethesda, Md, 2000, National Cancer Institute.

83. Robb-Nicholson C: CA-125 for ovarian cancer screening, *Harvard Women's Health Watch* 11(8):8, 2001.

84. Rockhill B, Spiegelman D, Byrne C, et al: Validation of the Gail et al. model of breast cancer risk prediction and implications for chemoprevention, *J Natl Cancer Inst* 93(5):358-366, 2001.

85. Rockhill B, Willett WC, Hunter DJ, et al: A prospective study of recreational physical activity and breast cancer risk, *Arch Intern Med* 159(19):2290-2296, 1999.

86. Ross RK, Paganini-Hill A, Wan PC, et al: Effect of hormone replacement therapy on breast cancer risk: estrogen versus estrogen plus progestin, *J Natl Cancer Inst* 92(4):328-332, 2000.

87. Rozenblit AM, Ricci ZJ, Tuvia J, et al: Incompetent and dilated ovarian veins: a common CT finding in asymptomatic parous women, *AJR Am J Roentgenol* 176(1):119-122, 2001.

88. Rubin SC: Chemoprevention of hereditary ovarian cancer, *N Engl J Med* 339(7):469-471, 1998.

89. Sanderson M, Shu XO, Jin F, et al: Abortion history and breast cancer risk: results from the Shangai Breast Cancer Study, *Int J Cancer* 92(6):899-905, 2001.

90. Sato S, Yokoyama Y, Sakamoto T, et al: Usefulness of mass screening for ovarian carcinoma using transvaginal ultrasonography, *Cancer* 89(3):582-588, 2000.

91. Schairer C, Lubin J, Troisi R, et al: Menopausal estrogen and estrogen-progestin replacement therapy and breast cancer risk, *JAMA* 283(4):485-491, 2000.

92. Schover LR: *Sexuality and fertility after cancer*, New York, 1997, John Wiley & Sons.

93. Schwartz AL, Mori M, Gao R, et al: Exercise reduces daily fatigue in women with breast cancer receiving chemotherapy, *Med Sci Sports Exerc* 33(5):718-723, 2001.

94. Scialli AR: Tampons, dioxins, and endometriosis, *Reprod Toxicol* 15(3):231-238, 2001.

95. Scuteri A, Bos AJ, Brant LJ, et al: Hormone replacement therapy and longitudinal changes in blood pressure in postmenopausal women, *Ann Intern Med* 135:229-238, 2001.

96. Segal R, Evans W, Johnson D, et al: Structured exercise improves physical functioning in women with Stages I and II breast cancer: results of a randomized controlled trial, *J Clin Oncol* 19(3):657-665, 2001.

97. Shingleton HM, Patrick RL, Johnston WW, et al: Current status of the Papanicolaou smear, *CA Cancer J Clin* 45:305-320, 1995.

98. Smith RA: Breast cancer screening among women younger than age 50: a current assessment of the issues, *CA Cancer J Clin* 50(5): 312-336, 2000.

99. Smith WC, Bourne D, Squair J, et al: A retrospective cohort study of post mastectomy pain syndrome, *Pain* 83(1):91-95, 1999.

100. Staudtmauer EA, O'Neill A, Godlstein LJ, et al: Conventional-dose chemotherapy compared with high-dose chemotherapy plus autologous hematopoietic stem-cell transplantation for metastatic breast cancer: Philadelphia Bone Marrow Transplant Group, *N Engl J Med* 342(15):1069-1076, 2000.

101. Steege JF, Metzger DA, Levy BS: *Chronic pelvic pain: an integrated approach,* Philadelphia, 1998, Saunders.

102. Stefanek M, Nelson W: Risk-reduction mastectomy: clinical issues and research needs, *J Natl Cancer Inst* 93(17):1297, 2001.

103. Stern RC, Dash R, Bentley RC, et al: Malignancy in endometriosis: frequency and comparison of ovarian and extraovarian types, *Int J Gynecol Pathol* 20(2):133-139, 2001.

104. Streckfus C, Bigler L, Dellinger T, et al: Reliability assessment of soluble c-erb-2 concentrations in the saliva of healthy women and men, *Oral Surg Oral Med Oral Pathol Oral Radiol Endod* 91(2):174-179, 2001.

105. Tang MT, Weiss NS, Malone KE: Induced abortion in relation to breast cancer among parous women: a birth certificate registry study, *Epidemiology* 11(2):177-180, 2000.

106. Terry P, Baron JA, Weiderpass E, et al: Lifestyle and endometrial cancer risk: a cohort study from the Swedish Twin Registry, *Int J Cancer* 82(1):38-42, 1999.

107. Thune I, Brenn T, Lund E, et al: Physical activity and the risk of breast cancer, *N Engl J Med* 336(18):1269-1275, 1997.

108. Thune I, Furberg AS: Physical activity and cancer risk: dose-response and cancer, all sites and site-specific, *Med Sci Sports Exerc* 33(6, suppl):S530-S550, 2001.

109. Vernon MW: *What can we do for the pain and infertility of endometriosis?* Presentation at Combined Sections Meeting, New Orleans, Feb 3, 2000.

110. Vgontzas AN, Legro RS, Bixler EO, et al: Polycystic ovary syndrome is associated with obstructive sleep apnea and daytime sleepiness: role of insulin resistance, *J Clin Endocrinol Metab* 86(2):517-520, 2001.

111. Wallace K: Female pelvic floor functions, dysfunctions, and behavioral approaches to treatment, *Clin Sports Med* 13(2):459-481, 1994.

112. Wallace K: Hypertonus dysfunction of the pelvic floor. In Wilder E: *Gynecologic physical therapy manual,* Alexandria, Wash, 1997, Women's Health Section of the American Physical Therapy Association (APTA), pp 127-142.

113. Warren MP, Perlroth NE: The effects of intense exercise on the female reproductive system, *J Endocrinol* 170(1):3-11, 2001.

114. Warren MP, Stiehl AL: Exercise and female adolescents: effects on the reproductive and skeletal systems, *J Am Med Womens Assoc* 54(3): 115-120, 138, 1999.

115. Werness BA, Parvatiyar P, Ramus SJ, et al: Ovarian carcinoma in situ with germline BRCA1 mutation and loss of heterozygosity at BRCA1 and TP53, *J Natl Cancer Inst* 92(13):1088-1091, 2000.

116. Wilder E, editor: *Gynecologic physical therapy manual,* Alexandria, Wash, 1997, Women's Health Section of the American Physical Therapy Association (APTA). Contact (on-line): HYPERLINK "http://www.apta.org" www.apta.org

117. Woolam GL: Cancer: where we are now; goals for 2015, *J Surg Oncol* 75(3):155-156, 2000.

118. Yokoyama Y, Dhanabal M, Griffioen AW, et al: Synergy between angiostatin and endostatin: inhibition of ovarian cancer growth, *Cancer Res* 60(8):2190-2196, 2000.

119. Yuan F, Chen DZ, Liu K, et al: Anti-estrogenic activities of indole-3-carbinol in cervical cells: implication for prevention of cervical cancer, *Anticancer Res* 19(3A):1673-1680, 1999.

120. Zhang M, Volpert O, Shi YH, et al: Maspin is an angiogenesis inhibitor, *Nat Med* 6(2):196-199, 2000.

121. Zhang S, Hunter DJ, Hankinson SE, et al: A prospective study of folate intake and the risk of breast cancer, *JAMA* 281(17):1632-1637, 1999.

122. Zondervan KT, Cardon LR, Kennedy SH: The genetic basis of endometriosis, *Curr Opin Obstet Gynecol* 13(3):309-314, 2001.

CHAPTER 20

TRANSPLANTATION

CATHERINE C. GOODMAN AND CHRIS L. WELLS

Transplantation for the treatment of end-stage organ failure has been one of the major medical advances of the last 20 to 30 years.* The success of this form of treatment has improved dramatically with better understanding of the rejection process and the introduction of more effective immunosuppressive medications for infection control and management so that recipients of transplanted organs or cells live longer. A number of people have survived for well over 25 years, and survival rates at 5 years can be 70% or higher for many organ transplant programs.[127]

Although kidney transplants have been an established procedure since the 1950s, it was not until 1960, when a technique for heart transplantation was developed bringing with it the basis of standard clinical surgical transplant technique, that organ transplantation progressed. The first human heart procedure was performed in South Africa by Christiaan Barnard (1967), followed shortly by the first U.S. transplant by Norman Shumway at Stanford in 1968. Since that time, techniques to transplant other organs and to allow for early rejection detection and advances in immunotherapy have made treatment even more successful.

INCIDENCE

Transplantation remains limited by an acute worldwide shortage of available and suitable human organs. Each year, an estimated 12,000 to 15,000 deaths in the United States have the potential to yield suitable organs, yet there were only 6000 cadaveric organ donors in 2002. Each cadaveric donor can donate up to 25 organs and tissues to help as many as 50 recipients. This means up to 500,000 organs should be available for transplantation each year, but only approximately 24,000 transplantations are performed (Table 20-1). In the United States, 80,000 adults and children currently await a transplant; approximately 4000 people die every year while on the transplant waiting list.

TYPES OF TRANSPLANTATION

Many types of tissues and organs can be donated and therefore transplanted, including the heart, lungs, liver, pancreas, kidneys, intestines, skin, bone and bone marrow, umbilical cord blood, veins, soft tissues, heart valves, corneas, and eyes. The first ovarian reimplantation has been performed but is not yet available to the public. Spleen transplantation remains in the experimental phase using animal models at this time.

Many different terms are used to describe types of transplants (Box 20-1). *Allograft* (homograft) transplants are between individuals of the same species (e.g., human to human). *Autologous* transplants are within the same individual (e.g., skin graft from leg to hand; blood or bone marrow for own use later). *Xenogeneic* (heterograft) transplants are between individuals of different species (e.g., pig to human). *Allogeneic* transplantation is one in which the source comes from a human leukocytic antigen (HLA; see explanation of HLA in Chapter 6) matched donor (usually a sibling). *Syngeneic* transplants are between genetically identical members of the same species (identical twins); the syngeneic transplant is also called an *isograft*. *Orthotopic* homologous transplantation refers to the surgical placement (grafting) of the donor organ into the normal anatomic site. In the *heterotopic homologous* transplantation, the recipient's diseased organ is left intact and the donor organ is placed in parallel with anastomoses between the two organs.

◆ Combined-Organ Transplantation

Combined-organ transplants (Box 20-2) from a single donor are uncommon relative to single-organ transplants. Research to date generally suggests that organ rejection is decreased in cases of combined-organ transplantation compared to single-organ transplantation. Short-term survival in combined-organ transplantation seems to be acceptable, but long-term recipient and graft survival remains unknown at this time.[32]

◆ Organ Retransplantation

Occasionally, retransplantation is necessary because of graft rejection, mechanical failure, or, in the case of liver transplantation, recurrence of the primary disease. The organs most often involved include the kidney, liver, heart, and more rarely, the lung. When T cells cause chronic rejection in the heart, the result is accelerated atherosclerosis. This response cannot be treated with immunosuppressants and is a primary reason for heart retransplantation.

Transplant organ recipients in need of a retransplantation once again become organ candidates and must meet certain criteria, usually based on an increased level of risk for morbidity and/or mortality. A model to estimate sur-

---

*A comprehensive book encompassing a variety of information only discussed briefly in this text is available for interested clinicians and potential organ candidates.[59] See also the website: www.transweb.org/ for more information about transplantation.

TABLE 20-1

National Waiting List for Organ Transplants

ORGAN	YEAR 2002 WAITING LIST	YEAR 2001 ACTUAL TRANSPLANTS	YEAR 1998 ACTUAL TRANSPLANTS
Kidney	52,267	14,152	12,166
Liver	17,493	5177	4487
Heart	4146	2202	2345
Lung	3799	1054	862
Heart and lung	210	27	47
Kidney and pancreas	2526	884	973
Pancreas	1318	468	248
Pancreas and islet	292	Unavailable	Unavailable
Intestine	194	112	69
TOTALS	82,245	24,076	21,197

From: *The Bank Account* 24(2):4, Summer 2002. Published by The Living Bank, Houston.

BOX 20-1

Types of Transplants

Allogeneic: between individuals of the same species but of different genetic constitution (e.g., human to human)

Allograft (homograft; homologous; autologous): between individuals of the same species (e.g., human to human)

Autologous: within the same individual (e.g., transfer of skin from one site to another on the same body; donation of blood or bone marrow for own use later)

Heterologous (heterograft; xenogeneic): between individuals of different species (e.g., pig to human)

Heterotopic (autograft): transfer of organ or tissue from one part of a body of a donor to another area of the body of a recipient

Homologous (homogenous): corresponding or similar in structure, position, origin (e.g., pig heart, human heart)

Orthotopic: tissue transplant grafted into its normal anatomic position

Syngeneic (isograft): between genetically identical members of the same species (identical twins)

Xenogeneic (heterograft): between individuals of different species (e.g., pig to human)

vival after retransplantation is being developed to help identify individuals with a poor expected outcome; this information could be useful in further refining candidate selection criteria.[119]

Ethical issues centered on the availability (i.e., shortage) of organs are always a consideration with retransplantation. Graft survival after retransplantation is less than for primary transplants, both for immunologic (e.g., rejection) and non-immunologic (e.g., donor age, donor size, cadaver versus live donor) reasons, and requires more aggressive monitoring for rejection.

ORGAN PROCUREMENT AND ALLOCATION

◆ Organ Distribution

In 1984 a system for organ distribution was devised whereby people were ranked according to the severity of their sickness. The United States was divided into 62 local areas, ranging in population from 1 million to 12 million, and those areas were then divided into 11 regions (Fig. 20-1).

Each local area has a designated organ procurement organization (OPO) responsible for recovering and transporting organs to transplant hospitals in their territories. The United Network for Organ Sharing (UNOS; www.unos.org/) is the private, nonprofit organization that administers the national organ waiting list, allocates organs throughout the United States, tracks outcomes, and provides public education.[202]

In the past, determination of organ candidates has been a very difficult process with many inequities and seemingly unfair practices. An agreement made in 1999 between the Department of Health and Human Services (DHHS) and Congress (The National Organ Transplant Act) demanded resolution of the long-standing contention over the nation's method of distributing donated organs. A last-minute hold on the implementation of this regulation has been extended twice by Congress because of disagreements between the DHHS and some members of the transplant community.

The proposed system of organ procurement and allocation is designed to even out waiting times with distribution of donated organs proposed across regional lines. Under the current system, individuals waiting for an organ in certain parts of the United States may obtain an organ sooner than those in other areas, partly because donated organs are distributed to local candidates first, even if there is someone with a more immediate or urgent need in a neighboring community or region. Uneven donor acquisition occurs in the general population because the number and location of treatment centers are not evenly distributed across the United States. The proposed changes are to ensure that people who have the most urgent medical need will be given priority although this still may not eliminate the inequities for those who cannot financially afford to relocate near a treatment center.

◆ Organ Donation

Death is usually the circumstance under which organs are procured, either when complete and irreversible loss of all brain and brain stem activity occurs or when the heart stops in the case of cardiac death. The specific neurologic event that has resulted in brain death may include blunt traumatic injury to the head, intracranial hemorrhage, or penetrating traumatic injury.

Donor age is a consideration with the majority of donors being under 50 years of age, although this is being extended because of the need for donors. The cadaveric lung donor must be younger than 55 years (or 65 years if there is no history of smoking) with a clear chest x-ray, an absence of chest trauma, no thoracic surgery, clear bronchoscopic examination, and no aspiration or sepsis. Smoking history must be less than a 30 pack-year (see section on lung cancer in Chapter 14) with acceptable oxygenation measured as PO_2 greater than 300 mm Hg. A living-related donor must be ABO-compatible with the candidate without a history of lung disease and no previous thoracic surgeries and larger in size than the recipient (weight, height, chest size), the latter require-

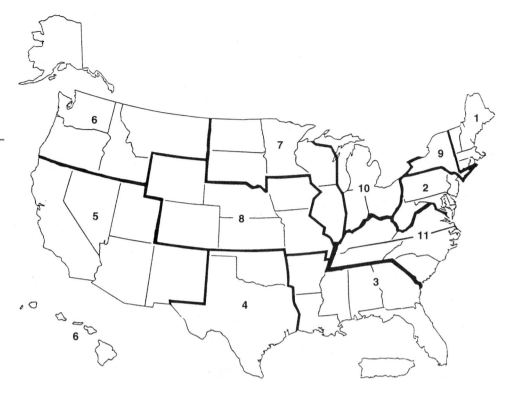

FIGURE 20-1 The United Network for Organ Sharing (UNOS) is divided into 11 geographic regions. (Courtesy United Network for Organ Sharing, Richmond, Va, 2000.)

ment because only two lung lobes are going to support the recipient's full pulmonary function.

Other criteria for donors vary according to the organ being harvested, but overall there must be no evidence of malignancy, human immunodeficiency virus (HIV) or hepatitis B, or sepsis (Box 20-3). Hepatitis C present in the donor is considered a precaution but not a contraindication. If the candidate already has hepatitis C or is critically ill, the risk of developing hepatitis C is considered a nonissue.* Body weight must be within 20% of the ideal (using the body mass index [BMI]; see discussion of BMI in Chapter 2) because of the ischemia-perfusion injury associated with obesity.[106] Biologically related donors are preferred with clear and altruistic motivation (as opposed to coerced by the family or guilt-driven).

Hearts and lungs can be preserved for up to 6 hours, livers up to 24 hours, and kidneys up to 72 hours. Lungs cannot be preserved outside the body for any extended period of time. This length of allowable ischemic time helps determine allowable distances between centers. Efforts are being made to improve organ harvest and preservation techniques and the number of organs harvested. For example, eliminating medical failures before donation through aggressive resuscitation, coagulopathy control, invasive monitoring, and dedicated intensive care unit (ICU) management while implementing a rapid brain death determination protocol has been documented as successfully increasing the number of donor organs available.[90] Technology to improve organ recovery, maintain organ perfusion, and recover normal cell metabolism is under investigation utilizing a kidney transporter, a portable organ preservation device. The ability to maintain and monitor organ viability over an extended period of time may allow live donors to avoid traveling to the recipient's location for explant surgery. Eventually, this type of technology may be extended to include transport devices for all other organs. Efforts to recover and maintain kidneys using this recovery technology have not yet been cleared by the U.S. Food and Drug Administration (FDA) or any foreign regulatory body for marketing in the United States or internationally.

---

*Organ transplantation carried a high risk of hepatitis C (HCV) transmission before 1990, but the use of organs and tissues from donors testing negative for HCV has virtually eliminated the risk of HCV transmission through transplantation except in cases such as this.

BOX **20-2**

Combined Organ Transplants

Heart-lung	Pancreas-liver
Heart-kidney	Pancreas-small intestine (rare)
Heart-liver	Liver-small intestine
Kidney-pancreas	Cluster operation: multiple organs
Kidney-liver	simultaneously (primarily pediatrics)

BOX **20-3**

Criteria for Organ Donor

Age <50 years, extended pool up to 60 years
No evidence of malignancy, human immunodeficiency virus (HIV), hepatitis B, sepsis
No evidence of other contraindicated illness or disease (e.g., cirrhosis for liver transplant, pulmonary hypertension for heart transplant, pulmonary diseases)
Within 20% of ideal body mass index (BMI)
Left ventricular ejection fraction (LVEF) >40% (heart donor)

Efforts to obtain consent for donation have also improved.* Public education now includes national donor awareness week and the choice to indicate organ donation on the driver's license. According to new Health Care Financing Administration (HCFA) regulations, hospitals are now required to report every death and impending death to their local OPO. Once a death has been reported, personnel from the OPO will determine who might be potential donors and initiate steps to procurement.

Early referral of all imminent deaths to OPOs can result in the OPO conferring with the physician and recommending continuation of medical treatment for a period of time. Early notification of the OPO is critical in order to ensure that care of potential organ donors continue without premature termination.[167] Donor evaluation by a medical specialist (e.g., cardiologist, pulmonologist, nephrologist, gastroenterologist, surgeon) is important so that the adequate function of the graft can be predicted before transplantation.

Living-related Donor.   Efforts to find a living donor are also on the rise, especially for kidney transplants. The number of living donor kidney transplants more than tripled from 1988 to 2002. The most significant increase in living donation has come from unrelated donors, such as spouses, friends, and in-laws. Kidneys from living donors last longer and function better than kidneys from deceased donors. Success with liver, lung, intestine, and pancreas islet cells from live donor transplants is also on the rise.[193]

◆ Criteria for Organ Candidates

People waiting for transplants (candidates) are listed at the transplant center where they plan to have surgery. A national, computerized waiting list of potential transplant candidates in the United States is maintained by UNOS with active input from treatment centers. UNOS maintains a 24-hour telephone service to aid in matching donor organs with people on the waiting list and to coordinate efforts with transplant centers.

Each individual on the waiting list to receive an organ has been classified by various key factors, such as blood type, body size, and medical urgency. Some candidates (e.g., heart, liver) are classified according to immediacy of need, referred to as UNOS status codes. These codes correspond to how medically urgent it is that the person receive a transplant and differ by organ (Table 20-2). When a donor becomes available, UNOS is notified and a list of potential organ candidates for that region is identified. UNOS notifies the OPO, who in turn notifies the treatment centers and the process of recipient selection begins.

Several factors are taken into consideration in identifying the best-matched candidate or candidates. In general, preference is given to candidates with the most critical status from the same geographic area as the donor because timing is a critical element in the organ procurement process. Waiting for combined-organ transplantation is much more complicated. Once the potential candidate is listed first for transplant (for either required organ) the second organ must be available and no other higher status candidate must be waiting for that second organ.

The transplant team bears the responsibility to conserve scarce resources for those who can benefit, requiring careful screening of potential candidates. Treatment centers follow UNOS guidelines, but criteria may vary from center to center; some centers adhere to a medical evaluation for the acceptance of applicants for transplant. Other teams have medical and nonmedical criteria with exclusion criteria for people with severely problematic behavior or other psychosocial factors (Box 20-4). There has been a recent trend to recognize the importance of nonmedical issues, such as psychologic stability, family support, and compliance history, when evaluating applicants.

Medical compatibility of the donor and candidate or candidates is determined based on characteristics such as blood type, weight, and age; urgency of need for some organs; and length of time on the waiting list. Any illness that cannot be treated or that will prevent the transplant success must be evaluated carefully. A transplant is usually not recommended if it is predictable that another illness will rapidly cause graft failure. For example, in the case of heart failure, it is likely that fixed pulmonary hypertension will result in destruction of the new donor heart. If the pulmonary artery cannot dilate, pulmonary artery pressure remains high and right-sided heart failure develops with subsequent death. A previous history of cancer or osteoporosis is considered carefully since postoperative medications can greatly advance these diseases.

A history of problematic behavior, such as noncompliance and psychiatric instability, leads to higher posttransplant mortality and morbidity.[44,171] Compliance issues associated with substance abuse usually include personality disorder, living arrangements, and/or global psychosocial factors. A history of substance abuse requires documentation of abstinence*; ongoing drug and/or alcohol abuse can potentially impair the success of the transplant and requires referral for treatment before placement on a transplant waiting list.

In the case of living donor transplants, psychosocial risk to donors must be taken into consideration. Most published reports have indicated an improved sense of well-being and a boost in self-esteem for living donors, but there have been some reports of depression and disrupted family relationships after donation, even suicide after a recipient's death.[93]

Pretransplant Evaluation.   Extensive medical testing is required before someone is placed on the transplant waiting list (Table 20-3). Blood typing including Rh factor analysis is used as one of the first eligibility criteria for donor-candidate matching. Predictor values for acute and chronic rejection are evaluated, such as the patent reactive antibody (PRA, a measure of the amount of antibodies circulating in the system), and offer some predictive value of hyperacute rejection.

Other serology testing determines exposure to cytomegalovirus (CMV), Epstein-Barr virus (EBV), herpes simplex viruses (HSVs), and hepatitis because complications can arise related to individual exposure to viral loading (i.e., the greater the viral replication, the higher the incidence of ac-

---

*It is estimated that of all the potential organ and tissue donors, only 32% agree to donate. Often potential donors are not identified, or families are not approached about donation. Aggressive public education remains an important key to improving the procurement rate.

---

*Each center will have individual criteria, but a general guideline includes abstinence from tobacco of at least 6 months and abstinence from alcohol and/or other illegal substances of more than 6 months with enrollment in rehabilitation.

TABLE 20-2

UNOS Organ Allocation Status List*

Organ	Status 1A	Status 1B	Status 2A	Status 2B	Status 3	Status 7
Kidney	Kidneys are allocated locally first, then regionally, and then nationally based on a point system. After matching donor and recipient by blood type, points are assigned according to age, time of waiting, quality of antigen mismatch, and level of panel reactive antibody. No points are assigned based on medical urgency for regional or national allocation of kidneys. Locally, issues of medical urgency are determined by the medical team.					
Liver	≥18 yr old Fulminant liver failure Life expectancy <7 days		Hospitalized with chronic liver failure Life expectancy <7 days Child-Turcotte-Pugh (CTP) score ≥10 Cirrhosis and a tumor <5 cm Meets one other medical criterion as listed by UNOS	CTP ≥10 or CTP ≥7 with one other medical criterion	Requires continuous medical care CTP score ≥7	Temporarily inactive
Heart	Hemodynamic instability Mechanical support <30 days (VAD or ventilatory) High inotropic support Life expectancy <7 days	VAD >30 days Low inotropic support	Active, stable candidate			Temporarily inactive
Lung	There are no status rankings in lung allocation. Individuals with a diagnosis of idiopathic pulmonary fibrosis are given 3-mo advancement in waiting time because of a high mortality rate. Donated lungs go first to local recipients with the identical blood type as the donor and then to local recipients with compatible blood types. If no local recipients are available, the same bloodmatching is carried out on a regional basis. Body size compatibility and length of time on the waiting list are also considered.					
Heart-lung	Candidates are listed on both heart and lung lists. Heart-lung allocation will occur when the candidate is eligible for either organ; the second organ will be allocated at that time.					
Pancreas	Two active status codes are used for the pancreas: Status 1 (urgent) and status 2 (nonurgent) Person who receives a clinical islet transplant becomes a status 1 for 3 wk; recipient needs islets from four or more donors within 3 wk		Anyone on the clinical islet list who does not meet the status 1 criteria			
Intestinal organ†	Abnormal liver function tests No longer has vascular access through subclavian, jugular, or femoral veins for intravenous feeding Other urgent medical indications		Waiting for transplant Does not meet criteria for status 1			Temporarily inactive

UNOS, United Network for Organ Sharing; *VAD*, ventricular assistive device.
*The assignment of allocation status is only one of many variables used in determining organ eligibility. Once an organ becomes available then this allocation status, geographic location, and other criteria (see Box 20-4) are assessed in the decision-making process.
†Intestinal organ may include stomach, small and/or large intestine, or any portion of the gastrointestinal tract as determined by the medical needs of the individual.

BOX 20-4

Criteria for Organ Candidate

Medical Considerations

Matched blood type required

Body weight (morbid obesity >20% of ideal body weight contraindicated; severe malnutrition <70% of ideal body weight contraindicated)

Presence of other illness or disease contraindicated

Other end-stage organ disease
- Irreversible renal insufficiency
- Irreversible hepatic insufficiency
- Severe pulmonary disease: FVC >50%, FEV₁ <60%
- Fixed pulmonary hypertension

At risk for cardiac problems (death, myocardial infarction, coronary angioplasty, bypass surgery, unstable angina)

Uncontrolled infection or acute sepsis

HIV

Malignancy with metastases

Malignancy with an expected 5-year survival <75%

Irreversible neuromuscular or neurologic disorder

Medical Considerations—cont'd

Severe PVD or cerebrovascular disease
- Abdominal aneurysm
- Peripheral ischemic ulceration
- Carotid disease

Decrease in chest wall mobility

Nonambulatory with poor rehabilitation potential

Nonmedical Considerations

History of noncompliance with medical therapy (last 5 years)

History of ongoing alcohol or drug dependence

Active or recent (within last 6 months) cigarette smoking (lung transplant)

History of psychologic instability

Financial resources available

Family and community support available

FVC, Forced vital capacity; FEV₁, forced expiratory volume in 1 second; HIV, human immunodeficiency virus; PVD, peripheral vascular disease.

TABLE 20-3

Referral to Transplant Center

BLOOD WORK	TESTING*	CONSULTATIONS*	OTHER
ABO blood type	Multigated acquisition scan (MUGA)	Surgeon	Urinalysis
Panel reactive antibodies (PRAs)	Echocardiogram (ECHO)	Pulmonologist	Sputum cultures
Serology	Transesophageal echo (TEE) or	Cardiologist	Creatinine clearance
Liver function tests (LFTs)	Transthoracic echocardiogram (TTE)	Nephrologist	Purified protein derivative (PPD)
Fasting lipids	Pulmonary function tests	Transplant coordinator	
Prostate specific antigen (PSA)	6-min walk test	Social service	
Prothrombin time (PT)	V/Q scan	Credit analysis	
Partial prothrombin time (PPT)	(ventilation-perfusion)	Neuropsychology	
Complete blood count (CBC)	Arterial blood gases (ABGs)	Physical therapy	
	Diffusion capacity of carbon monoxide (DLCO)	Rheumatologist	
	Organ catheterization (heart, kidney)	Gynecologist	
	X-ray	Dentist	
	Electrocardiogram (ECG)	Nutritionist	
	VO₂ max or VO₂ peak		
	Glucose testing (diabetes mellitus)		
	Peripheral vascular disease (PVD)		

*Specific consultants and the special tests orders are determined by the type of organ transplantation planned.

tive infection). CMV infection may contribute to an increased incidence of chronic rejection, HSV has been associated with an increased incidence of necrotizing pneumonitis and cervical cancer, and EBV has been associated with an increase in posttransplantation lymphoproliferative diseases. See further discussion of these infectious diseases in Chapter 7.

Transplant recipients are placed on appropriate medications to reduce the risk of infection and undergo repeated serologies if clinical signs and symptoms suggest infection or infectious disease (see Table 7-1). A candidate who is HBV- or HCV-positive and who is critically ill can receive a hepatitis-positive donor liver.

Fasting lipids, liver function studies, prostate-specific antigen (PSA) levels to determine prostate function, and then tests specific to the potential organ transplant are carried out. A person with isolated end-stage organ failure with no other complications has a better chance for selection than someone with other complicating factors. In addition to all the testing procedures, the organ candidate meets with a large team of professionals listed in Table 20-3 including, in some centers, rehabilitation staff such as physical and occupational therapists.

ADVANCES AND RESEARCH IN TRANSPLANTATION

Advances in understanding of immunology and organ preservation, surgical technique, pharmacology, and postoperative care have permitted the rapid development of organ transplantation other than heart and lungs (e.g., liver, pancreas, intestine). New transplantation is being developed for other organs, such as pancreatic islet cells for the treatment of diabetes or ovarian preservation for later use in cases of cancer requiring removal of the ovaries. The use of hepatic segments for transplantation (either from cadavers or from living-related donors) has decreased the number of people (especially children) awaiting liver transplantation.[159]

The first transplantation of skeletal muscle cells to test whether the cells can repair damaged heart muscle took place at Temple University's heart transplantation program in 2000. Muscle tissue taken from the individual's arm was transplanted into his own heart during a surgical procedure to implant an assistive device while waiting for a heart transplantation. Researchers will examine the heart after transplantation to determine whether the skeletal cells survived and whether they helped repair the damaged heart.[53] Research is under way to develop transplantable cells for the treatment of human diseases characterized by cell dysfunction or cell death and for which current treatment is inadequate or nonexistent. Additional products under investigation include porcine neural cells for stroke, focal epilepsy, and intractable pain; porcine spinal cord cells for spinal cord injury; neurologic cell transfer for Parkinson's disease or Huntington's disease; human liver cells for cirrhosis, and porcine retinal pigment epithelial cells for macular degeneration.[137]

The diverse research directions being undertaken around the world will continue to change the field of transplantation in the years to come. Gene therapy (including in utero), xenotransplantation, tissue engineering, chimerism, and new fields of study developing daily can only be presented briefly in this text but help represent the overall picture of rapid change in treatment approaches.

◆ Xenotransplantation
Allotransplantation remains the preferred treatment for human organ failure, but shortages of acceptable donor organs and the lack of success in developing suitable artificial organs have led researchers to investigate the use of organs from other species (xenotransplantation). Nonhuman primates are now considered an unethical and unsafe source of donor organs so that other species are being considered, in particular

the pig.* Researchers are now breeding pigs whose cells, tissues, and organs could be permanently transplanted into humans without being destroyed by the human immune system.

There are considerable risks and drawbacks to this approach at the present time. Hyperacute rejection (HAR) or acute vascular rejection can occur when circulation of recipient blood through the transplanted organ causes immediate graft failure. The binding of preexisting antipig antibodies to the vascular endothelium leads to a cascade of events causing massive intravascular coagulation and precipitating HAR.

Before the use of pig organs in humans can become a viable option, target antigens of human antipig antibodies must be identified and strategies developed that could either remove these antibodies from human candidates or eliminate target antigens on the donor organs, thus preventing HAR.

Considerable progress has been made in recent years, and experimental pig-to-primate organ xenotransplantation has resulted in transplant function for days and weeks rather than minutes. Researchers have successfully implanted pig organs as a short-term bridge (up to 10 hours) until a human donor organ could be found and implanted.[113] The first trial transplant of animal organs into humans is scheduled by a biotechnology company at this time.

Other hurdles to xenotransplantation include anatomic, physiologic, and biochemical differences. The upright position of humans is unique in nature. Gravity therefore exerts a different impact on the anatomic location of organs such as lung, heart, liver, and kidney. More pronounced are differences on the humoral and enzymatic basis. Complex interactions existing in allografts are totally disturbed in xenogeneic situations. Regaining physiologic function of the graft in the foreign environment may be prevented by molecular incompatibilities between the donor and recipient, and there is the possibility of transferring infectious diseases from the animal donor graft to the recipient. Virologists and molecular biologists are concerned about the serious potential for introduction of diseases foreign to the human immune system.[154]

◆ Tissue Engineering
Tissue engineering, the science of growing living human tissues for transplantation and other therapeutic applications, is a rapidly expanding industry. Tissue engineering applies the principles of biology and engineering toward the development of biologic substitutes that restore, maintain, or improve tissue function.

Tissue engineering, or the fabrication of functional living tissue, uses cells seeded on highly porous synthetic biodegradable polymer scaffolds as a new approach toward the development of biologic substitutes that may replace lost tissue function. Over the past decade, the fabrication of a wide variety of tissues has been investigated, including both structural and visceral organs.[102]

Bioengineered skin, bone, ligaments, tendons, and articular cartilage are already available in some clinical settings. Laboratory-grown organs are farther off with the hope for producing donor tissue and organs for transplants on demand and

---

*Baboon organs are too small to sustain humans for long periods. The risk of transmitting deadly infectious agents from nonhuman primates is greater than from other animal species. Physicians are already successfully using various pig components (e.g., heart valves, clotting factors, islet cells, brain cells) to treat human diseases.

developing living prosthetics (incorporating living tissue with electronics) for every organ system in the body.[111,204] Other examples of current progress in the area of bioengineering include implants filled with pig islets for people with diabetes to replace insulin injections, a method to generate natural breast tissue to replace saline implants, heart valves grown from blood vessel cells,[173,180] skeletal muscle tissue isolated from synthetic polymers,[164] formation of phalanges and small joints from bovine-cell sources (calves),[86] and bone substitutes made from synthetic substances[6,42] (see further discussion in Chapter 21).

◆ Medications

Tremendous advancement has been made in the pharmacologic management of transplant recipients. Medications are used with transplant recipients to prevent rejection and to treat rejection or infection. Research is ongoing to find ways to reduce or eliminate the long-term use of medications, especially immunosuppressants. New discoveries in cellular immunology have led to a greater understanding of the immune system and its implications for tissue transplantation. Immunosuppressive regimens continue to improve, and newer immunomodulatory strategies are evolving. In particular, new immunosuppressive drugs may allow the recipient to overcome or reduce the early antibody-mediated rejections.[22]

Cyclosporine (CsA, CYA, Sandimmune), the first effective immunosuppressive drug used as an antirejection drug, was approved for use in 1983. Although it selectively suppresses the proliferation and development of helper T cells, resulting in depressed cell-mediated immunity, it is difficult to administer in optimal doses because of tremendous variability in the way it is absorbed, distributed, metabolized, and eliminated by different individuals. Organ recipients whose CsA concentrations vary the most are most prone to chronic rejection or graft loss. This finding resulted in a more effective formulation of cyclosporine (Neoral) approved by the FDA in 1995. The new formulation improves drug absorption and reduces the risk of acute transplant rejection. The wide array of toxic side

effects of CsA has led to the combination of CsA with one or more other agents that act synergistically in order to allow CsA dose reduction and mitigation of drug-induced toxicity. For this reason, recipients will be given either cyclosporine or a more recent immunosuppressant, tacrolimus (Prograf, FK-506), now used widely in kidney transplants as well as other organ recipients (Fig. 20-2).

Two other classes of drugs with different mechanisms are also used, including azathioprine (Imuran), which works by suppressing the bone marrow (as exhibited by thrombocytopenia, leukopenia, anemia) and CellCept (mycophenolate), which inhibits inflammatory responses mediated by the immune system (Fig. 20-3). The third class of drugs includes prednisone, a corticosteroid with its effect at the level of the macrophages. Prednisone blocks the production of interleukin-2 in the presence of an antigen to stimulate a major histocompatible complex thus stimulating both B-cell and T-cell response (Fig. 20-4).

A new immunosuppressant, Rapamune (sirolimus [SRL], rapamycin), that inhibits cytokine-driven cell proliferation and maturation has been approved for use with renal transplants.[41,99] Preliminary studies have demonstrated that SRL in combination with CsA and steroids not only lowers the incidence of acute renal allograft rejection but also permits CsA sparing (reduced amounts or eventual elimination) without an increased risk of rejection.* One other way to reduce the amount of immunosuppression required is through the use of monoclonal antibodies, such as OKT$_3$, a mouse monoclonal antibody to human T cells. OKT$_3$ blocks the ability of the

---

*Among individuals who initially received rapamycin in combination with cyclosporine and steroids, steroid treatment stopped 1 month after transplant had significantly fewer rejection episodes and participants were spared the numerous toxic side effects associated with long-term steroids.[77] Withdrawal or marked reduction of corticosteroids is of particular benefit in the case of diabetes mellitus and in the presence of severe osteoporosis or aseptic necrosis of bone. Steroid withdrawal has been shown possible in up to 70% of pancreas transplant candidates who are otherwise maintained on tacrolimus-based immunosuppression.[83,94]

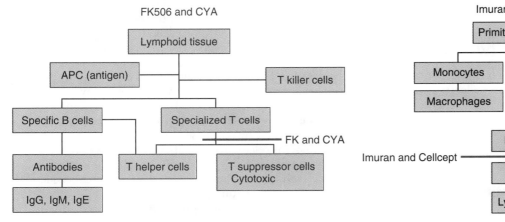

FIGURE 20-2 Cyclosporine (CsA, CYA; Neoral, Sandimmune) and a newer drug, FK506 (tacrolimus [Prograf]), block the sensitization of T cells. Cyclosporine blocks down to where the T cells are sensitized to begin the humoral cell-mediated response. (Courtesy Chris L. Wells, P.T., Ph.D., and James H. Dauber, M.D., University of Pittsburgh Medical Center-Health Systems, 2000.)

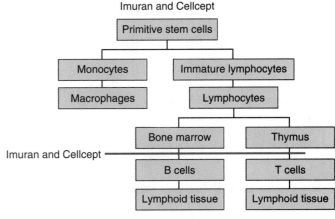
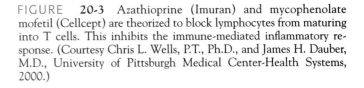

FIGURE 20-3 Azathioprine (Imuran) and mycophenolate mofetil (Cellcept) are theorized to block lymphocytes from maturing into T cells. This inhibits the immune-mediated inflammatory response. (Courtesy Chris L. Wells, P.T., Ph.D., and James H. Dauber, M.D., University of Pittsburgh Medical Center-Health Systems, 2000.)

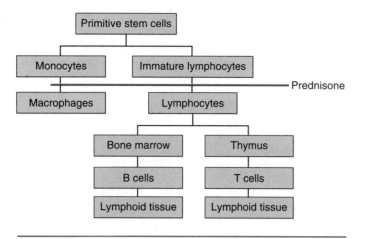

FIGURE 20-4 Prednisone works at the macrophage level and is theorized to block the production of interleukin-II, thus preventing the formation of major histocompatible complexes that normally stimulate both B- and T-cell response. (Courtesy Chris L. Wells, P.T., Ph.D., and James H. Dauber, M.D., University of Pittsburgh Medical Center-Health Systems, 2000.)

candidate's T cells to recognize foreign antigens, thus inhibiting both the generation and the function of cytotoxic T cells responsible for graft rejection. T cells are rapidly decreased in the circulation after the drug is given; by the third day there are usually no detectable circulating T cells.

Research groups are working toward identifying the critical components on particular grafts that are seen as foreign to modify them.[159] This will enable the graft to succeed while simultaneously allowing the host immune response to carry out its main tasks. Strategies that teach the immune system to accept the transplanted tissue rather than attack it, a process called chimerism,* are under investigation (see the section on Future Trends under Blood and Bone Marrow Transplantation in this chapter).[13,76] Researchers studying how the developing fetus avoids destruction may be able to identify protective biologic pathways and then use this model to develop drugs to interrupt the rejection process and promote tolerance of foreign tissue.[125,133]

BIOPSYCHOSOCIAL IMPLICATIONS

Many different ethical, social, moral, economic, and legal issues are associated with the procurement and allocation of living or bioengineered tissue. In addition, new information concerning the psychoneuroimmune responses (see the section on Psychoneuroimmunology in Chapter 1) in healthy tissues and organs has added new dimensions to understanding the emotional adjustment for recipients of living organ and tissue transplants.

◆ Legal and Ethical Considerations

Before alternate treatment methods can be fully implemented, scientific and medical communities and the general public will have to seriously consider and attempt to resolve legal and ethical issues.[39] For example, federal law prohibits

the sale of human organs in the United States and violators are subject to fines and imprisonment. Although Western opinion is almost universally against the practice of paid organ donation and the use of organs from judicially executed prisoners, similar laws are not in place worldwide. The ethics of both issues continue to be debated.

In other countries, such as Spain, organ donation is governed by "presumed consent" legislation. Unless legally designated otherwise, organ donation is presumed on the death of each individual. Interestingly, even this has not alleviated the problem of donor shortage because the success of allotransplantation as a treatment for end-stage organ failure has resulted in the need for an increasing number of organ donors.

◆ Bioethical Considerations

Another area of concern involves researchers growing human cells into tissues using stem cells derived from human embryos left over from attempts at artificial fertilization or following abortions.[197,209]* Unlike recombinant deoxyribonucleic acid (DNA) technology, embryonic stem cell research results in the destruction of living embryos but has the potential to cure diseases.

Until 1999, one major barrier to rapid development of these research findings was the uncertainty of federal funding for researchers using such embryo tissue. However, in January 1999, the director of the National Institutes of Health (NIH) announced that the NIH had concluded that the institutes may, under existing law, pursue and fund scientific research using derived human stem cells.[208] The NIH's conclusion about the legality of this decision was challenged by U.S. lawmakers on the grounds that federal laws passed in 1996 prohibit the use of federal funds for "research in which a human embryo or embryos are destroyed, discarded, or knowingly subjected to risk of injury or death."[23] NIH guidelines were subsequently changed to allow federally funded researchers to carry out stem cell research under carefully monitored conditions. For example, the stem cells must be derived from embryos that are "in excess of clinical need" (i.e., going to be discarded) and donors must be informed and consent to the research use of their embryos.

Many bioethicists and lawmakers still question the appropriateness of this research until the ethical issues and appropriate concerns can be voiced and resolved.[5,149] Questions about the nature of human life and its protection, the safeguard of human dignity, and the use of genetic material have been raised. However, new discoveries in the rapidly developing field of stem cell research, such as the discovery of master stem cells (see the section on Blood and Bone Marrow Transplantation in this chapter) replacing the use of embryonic tissue, may bypass these bioethical concerns.

Concerns related to animal-derived matrix proteins have also been raised. Some private bioengineering companies are proactively researching ways to develop human tissue with matrix proteins naturally secreted by the cells rather than developing tissue from animal-derived matrix proteins. In the area of animal organ transplantation (xenotransplantation), rules governing the welfare of animals bred for transplants are being formulated. Currently, a ban on having children has been placed for all people receiving an animal organ transplantation.

---

*Chimerism involves inducing the donor's immune system onto the candidate's so that the candidate's immune system no longer rejects the organ or tissue. In bone marrow transplantation (BMT), chimerism is achieved when bone marrow and host cells exist compatibly without signs of graft-versus-host disease (GVHD).

---

*The prohibition against producing embryos solely for research is currently being reconsidered in the regulation of embryo research in Europe.[112]

◆ Psychoemotional Considerations

Pretransplant. Transplant applicants face many challenges, including the obvious physical illness, complex assessment protocols, uncertainties about surgery and outcome, the possibility of relocation to obtain transplant services, and large expenses. Waiting for a transplant can be accompanied by a vast range of changing emotions, such as relief, despair, elation, depression, excitement, and apprehension. No single attitude is common or expected; each person's reaction is a valid expression of his or her experience. Most candidates find awaiting surgery a stressful time, and of course, the longer the wait, the greater the stress. The evaluation process itself and the wait for the results after tests and procedures require complex coping strategies especially if the person is denied for transplantation. Deciding whether to accept a donor organ or wait for a potentially better one can create considerable psychologic and emotional distress.

When death is a possibility, candidates may worry that negative thinking will harm their health. Others are distressed that someone else must die before an organ will be available for transplant or that receiving an available organ deprives someone else of life. Candidates are encouraged to focus on the desired outcome without completely ignoring the alternatives for themselves and outcomes for others. Counseling and support groups are often recommended.

Anxiety and depression are common complications of medical illness of any kind and may interfere with the candidate's or recipient's participation in rehabilitation. Clinical symptoms of anxiety or depression (see discussion in Chapter 2) can be subtle and mimic the individual's health condition, requiring candidate or recipient self-awareness and careful screening by all members of the transplant team to identify and treat early.

A condition severe enough to require organ transplant can sometimes impair concentration, memory, or ability to process thoughts. In particular, approximately one third of all liver transplant candidates have severe impairment of mental abilities (i.e., hepatic encephalopathy) and may be extremely confused or even delirious at the time of transplant. Similar mental impairment can occur with heart, lung, and kidney candidates although it is less common.

Posttransplant. Postoperatively, recipients face a long recovery period, the potential for graft rejection, reintegration into family and work roles, and lifelong changes, such as the need for drug compliance and changes in diet. Adaptation after a transplant is a lifelong process and depends on several factors, such as the success of the transplant, expectations before the transplant and perceived outcomes, postoperative complications or side effects of the antirejection drugs, permanent physical changes or changes in appearance, as well as other individual considerations. Identification of recipients most likely to have compliance and psychiatric problems early after transplant is important in focusing interventions that maximize recipients' psychosocial status in these areas and thus improve long-term physical health outcomes.[44,188]

Stress on the family and the need for family support and counseling also affect treatment outcomes. Health care staff may observe a deterioration of family relationships after transplantation (especially between husband and wife or between partners). Older children receiving organ transplantation may face the challenge of parents not allowing or unable to allow the child to grow into adulthood. Support groups can be extremely helpful in these types of situations and should be recommended early by the health care team.

Some recipients experience difficulty accepting the transplanted organ as their own. Others wonder if their new organ carries some donor characteristics. Typical literature available from transplant centers contains reassurances that a heart, liver, or kidney can be transplanted into another person without the transfer of personal characteristics. Changes reported are often attributed to the normal process associated with overcoming a serious life-threatening illness.

On the other hand, research pioneered by Candace Pert,[150] formerly a molecular biologist at the NIH, has discovered the biologic basis for emotions. The results of Dr. Pert's research have demonstrated that peptides and various other ligands (information carriers) and their receptors are the physiologic substrates of emotion. This work strongly helped establish the field of psychoneuroimmunology (see the section on Psychoneuroimmunology in Chapter 1) and supports the idea that emotions, personal characteristics, behaviors, and thoughts are biochemically derived, not only being actively present within our tissues but also making up a bodywide system carrying this type of information across cellular barriers.*

For example, many organ recipients report frequent dreams or nightmares. It is not uncommon to have dreams while they are half awake; sometimes, disorientation accompanies sleep disturbance or waking dreams commonly labeled delirium or confusion. Others report changes in temperament or mood, sexual libido, food preferences, and personal preferences. The exact etiology of these perceived changes remains unknown; previously, the dreams and dreamlike disturbances have been attributed to postoperative sleep disruption (e.g., anyone waking up often in the night is more likely to remember more dreams) or considered an unpleasant side effect of the medications (cyclosporine, prednisone). Other researchers suggest that it is reasonable to include the impact of depression, and possibly other psychologic states, among factors that may affect the net state of immunosuppression in transplant recipients.[104] New knowledge within the field of psychoneuroimmunology combined with many more case reports† of altered dreams, thought processes, memories, and behavior as the number of organ transplants increases may bring to light new understanding of transplantation psychoneuroimmunolgy in the decade ahead.

POSTTRANSPLANT COMPLICATIONS

With advances in technology and immunology, transplantation of almost any tissue is feasible, but the clinical use of transplantation to remedy disease is still limited for many organ systems because of the rejection reaction and other posttransplant complications. Complications following organ transplantation can be classified into three broad categories: (1) complications associated with the surgical procedure, (2)

---

*This is a very brief summary of Dr. Pert's research findings; the reader is referred to her book *Molecules of Emotion: the Science Behind Mind-Body Medicine*[150] for a more thorough treatise of her findings and similar organ-specific information presented by others.[141,147,206] The application of Dr. Pert's findings and their implications for transplantation are merely speculation at this time but raise some interesting and potentially serious psychosocial and legal issues.

†One of the first carefully documented and published reports to explore this type of phenomenon may be of interest to readers.[192]

complications of the transplantation, and (3) complications of the immunosuppressive agents used to prevent rejection. Each type of organ transplantation has its own accompanying surgical risks and complications (see discussion in each section). Ischemic-reperfusion injury may occur with any organ transplantation. The donated organ is very sensitive to the amount of time it is not being perfused or supplied with blood. After transplantation when the clamps are removed from the donated organ and the blood is once again allowed to circulate through the organ, pressures may be high and epithelial lining of blood vessels can be traumatized and damaged by the amount of pressure of a physiologically normal organ placed in a pathologic system. This is especially common in heart or lung transplantation in the presence of co-morbid pulmonary hypertension. Recovery from ischemia-perfusion injuries usually takes 3 to 5 days.

Following surgery, two main complications of organ transplantation remain infection and organ rejection. Both these complications are common and treatable, but prevention is the first step and for this reason, pretransplantation serologic testing is done to determine histocompatibility and to avoid transmitting infectious agents (e.g., cytomegalovirus [CMV], vancomycin-resistant enterococci [VRE], hepatitis virus [HBV, HCV]) from donor to recipient.

◆ Histocompatibility

In all cases of graft rejection, the cause is incompatibility of cell surface antigens. The rejection of foreign or transplanted tissue occurs because the recipient's immune system recognizes that the surface HLA proteins of the donor's tissue are different from the recipient's.

Certain antigens are more important than others for a successful transplant, including ABO and Rh antigens present on red blood cells and histocompatibility antigens, most importantly the HLA. As expected, there is a better chance of graft acceptance with syngeneic or autologous transplants because the cell surface antigens are identical. For all categories of transplants, minimizing HLA mismatches is associated with a significantly lower risk of graft loss.[33] Rh antigen is more important in heart and kidney transplants than in lung transplantation. In renal transplants HLA crossmatches are routinely performed whereas this is not commonly done in lungs (unless the candidate has a high panel reactive antibodies [PRA] count). Crossmatching policies may vary by institution.

The process of determining histocompatibility, that is, finding compatible donors and candidates, is called *tissue typing*. Before transplantation, testing in the laboratory is carried out to determine whether antibodies incompatible with the donor have been formed by the candidate (a positive crossmatch). If the crossmatch is positive, the transplant will fail; a negative test result is necessary for a successful transplant.

◆ Graft Rejection

Transplant rejection may occur for immunologic or nonimmunologic reasons. When the body recognizes the donor tissue as nonself and attempts to destroy the tissue shortly after transplantation, rejection occurs as an immunologic phenomenon primarily because of histocompatibility. Nonimmunologic factors can occur as a result of the draining-reperfusion process necessary in organ harvest and transplantation. Ischemic injury occurs when normal blood and oxygen supply to the donor organ is stopped at the time of organ harvest,

whereas reperfusion injury can occur when blood flow is returned to the organ after transplantation.

As residual blood is drained from the transplanted organ into the host's general circulation, the body recognizes the transplanted tissue cells as foreign invaders (antigens) and immediately sets up an immune response by producing antibodies. These antibodies are capable of inhibiting metabolism of the cells within the transplanted organ and eventually actively causing their destruction. Research to develop a reliable method to reduce the ischemic-reperfusion injury is currently ongoing. Eliminating the occurrence of poor early graft function and consequently reducing the chances for rejection episodes are the primary goal of these investigations.[34,49]

Types of Graft Rejection.   There are three types of transplant rejection-the hyperacute rejection, the acute or late acute rejection, and the chronic rejection-depending on the amount of time that passes between transplantation and rejection (Table 20-4).

Hyperacute rejection (rare with antibody screening and tissue typing) is dominantly mediated by humoral responses of the immune system (natural antibodies, complement cascade) and the activation of coagulation factors. There is an immediate rejection after transplantation when the recipient has preformed antibodies to donor tissue. This reaction necessitates prompt surgical removal of the transplanted tissue.

The *acute* or *late acute rejection* can appear days to years after the transplantation. This type of rejection involves a combination of cellular and humoral reactions. Clinically, there is sudden onset of organ-related symptoms, which may be associated with fever and graft tenderness. Graft rejection must be differentiated from immunosuppressive toxicity. This form of rejection can be reliably graded using a system of categories of mild, moderate, and severe rejection. Acute rejection, if detected in its early stages, can be reversed with immunosuppressive therapy.

Although *chronic rejection* can occur as early as 3 months, it is usually months to years before the chronic rejection occurs. This type of rejection develops as a function of the cell-mediated system and is characterized by slow, progressive organ failure. Growing evidence indicates that chronic rejection is the aggregate sum of irreversible immunologic and nonimmunologic injuries to the graft over time. A history of acute rejection episodes, either asymptomatic or clinically apparent, and inadequate immunosuppression likely attributable to inconsistent cyclosporine exposure or poor compliance are among the most recognizable immunologic risk factors for chronic rejection.[130]* Chronic rejection is an advanced state of damage and is not responsive to therapy.

◆ Graft-Versus-Host Disease

The discussion of graft rejection describes reactions in a transplant recipient with an intact immune system. The use of BMT to bone marrow-depleted or immunodeficient people has resulted in the complication of GVHD. People at highest risk include premature infants and others who are immuno-

---

*Adherence to immunosuppressive therapy is a key factor contributing to transplant failures that occur within 2 years after surgery. Financial barriers such as the lack of insurance coverage are the most common reason for noncompliance. The Immunosuppressive Medications Act supported by the National Kidney Foundation (NKF) would extend Medicare coverage of postoperative medications so that organs are not lost because of a lack of insurance coverage.[136]

TABLE 20-4

Clinical Manifestations of Organ Rejection

HYPERACUTE REJECTION	ACUTE (LATE) REJECTION		CHRONIC REJECTION
Immediate reaction Death	Occurs days to years after transplantation		Occurs 3 mo to years after transplantation
	May be asymptomatic in early stages		May be asympto- matic in early stages
	Fever; constitutional symptoms (flulike)		Organ-related symptoms
	Loss of appetite		Histologic changes
	Graft tenderness		
	Blood pressure changes		
	Dyspnea		
	Fatigue		
	Peripheral edema, weight gain		
	Inflamed skin lesions		
	Reduced exercise capacity		
	Organ-related symptoms		
	Kidney		
	Proteinuria		
	Uremia		
	Neurologic symptoms		
	Nausea and vomiting		
	Liver		
	Palpable liver		
	Jaundice		
	Hematemesis (vomiting blood)		
	Abdominal pain		
	Ascites		
	Neurologic symptoms (see Box 20-7)		
	Elevated transaminase		
	Elevated bilirubin		
	Heart		
	S_3 gallop		
	Arrhythmias		
	Jugular vein distention		
	Lung		
	Changes in respiratory status; breathlessness; prolonged need for ventilatory support		
	Fall in spirometric values (>10% change/reduction from baseline; <90% at rest)		
	Decreased FEV_1 >10%		
	Dry or productive cough		
	Change in sputum (color, amount)		
	Decreased oxygen saturation		
	Reduced vital capacity; decreased exercise tolerance		
	Radiographic changes		
	Pancreas:		
	Nausea		
	Vomiting		
	Anorexia		
	Other gastrointestinal symptoms		
	Urologic symptoms		

FEV₁, Forced expiratory volume in 1 sec.

suppressed as a result of either congenital or acquired disease or because of the administration of immunosuppressive therapy, as in the case of organ transplant recipients.

GVHD occurs when immunocompetent T-lymphocytes in the grafted material recognize foreign antigens in the recipient, initiating a cascade of events mediated by cellular and in-flammatory factors resulting in a reaction against the recipient's tissues.[58] GVHD may be acute, occurring in the first 1 to 2 months after transplantation, or chronic, developing at least 2 to 3 months after transplantation.

GVHD remains the major toxicity of BMT. It does not oc-cur in autologous BMT or peripheral blood stem cell transplantation but may occur in an allograft or syngeneic transplant, even with a perfect HLA match, because of unidentified and therefore unmatched antigens. Pretransplant immunologic and genetic manipulation using hematopoietic stem cells has minimized GVHD in individuals receiving high-dose chemotherapy.

Signs and symptoms of GVHD are fever, skin rash, hepatitis, diarrhea or abdominal pain, ileus, vomiting, and weight loss. Chronic GVHD is also characterized by hardening of organ tissues (connective tissue disorders such as scleroderma) and drying of mucous membranes (mucositis), especially in the gastrointestinal mucosa, liver, respiratory bronchioles (bronchiolitis), and skin (scleroderma or systemic lupus erythematosus) (Box 20-5).

A generalized polyneuropathy coincident with the occurrence of GVHD has been reported. The neuropathy affects proximal and distal muscles and demonstrates hyporeflexia or areflexia. Electrophysiologic studies do not meet strict criteria for demyelination. The signs of neuropathy improve after immunosuppressive treatment or simultaneously with the resolution of GVHD.

Untreated GVHD is often fatal as a result of hemorrhage and infection. Inhibition of cytotoxic T-lymphocyte-mediated tissue injury in the early stages of GVHD is recommended along with administration of agents to eliminate the donor's lymphocytes. Therapeutic strategies for treating acute GVHD using protease inhibitors and tumor necrosis factor to inhibit T-cell cytotoxicity are under investigation.[162,163] Present treatment with immunosuppressive therapy including prednisone, cyclosporine or tacrolimus (FK-506, Prograf), thalidomide, or a combination of these agents has improved the long-term outlook for people with chronic GVHD. Chronic GVHD may resolve slowly (sometimes taking years) with gradual restoration of cell-mediated and humoral immunity function.

◆ Immunosuppression

The fact that a primary role of the immune system is to distinguish between self and nonself presents a major problem for the transplant recipient: the immunologic response of the recipient to the donor's tissues. In the person with an intact immune system (immunocompetence), the recipient's immune system recognizes the transplanted tissue or organ as foreign (nonself) and produces antibodies and sensitized lymphocytes against it.

The ultimate objective of immunosuppressive therapy (see the section on Medications under Advances and Research in Transplantation) is to block transplant candidate reactivity to the donor's organ while sparing other responses. Since these drugs suppress all immunologic reactions, overwhelming infection is the leading cause of death in transplant recipients. However, increased understanding of rejection mechanisms has made it possible to suppress specific elements of the immune response.

Side Effects of Immunosuppressants.
Although lower amounts of immunosuppressive drugs are now prescribed, these drugs must be taken for the life of the recipient and physical changes (see Fig. 10-5 to 10-7) and other side effects remain a well-known problem (see Table 4-6, *Side Effects of Immunosuppressants*).

Organ recipients have three times the incidence of various cancers, and some specific cancers are 100 times more frequent in the immunosuppressed population after transplantation than in the general population. Cardiac transplant recipients have a higher incidence of cancer than do other transplant recipients, perhaps because of the higher levels of immunosuppression.

The most common tumors among transplant recipients are squamous cell cancers of the lips and skin owing to the enhanced photosensitivity,* Kaposi's sarcomas, non-Hodgkin's lymphomas and other posttransplant lymphoproliferative disorders, soft tissue sarcomas, carcinomas of the vulva and per-

---

BOX | **20-5**

Signs and Symptoms of Graft-Versus-Host Disease

Gastrointestinal

Mucositis
Esophageal inflammatory changes
Abdominal cramping
Diarrhea
Anorexia
Ileus
Hepatic injury (hepatitis)

Pulmonary

Bronchiolitis

Integument

Hypopigmentation or hyperpigmentation of the skin
Progressive maculopapular rash
Sclerodermatous changes
Pressure ulcer formation
Alopecia
Photosensitivity
Keratoconjunctival sicca

Neuromusculoskeletal

Generalized polyneuropathy
Muscle wasting and weakness
Joint contractures (chronic graft-versus-host disease)
Changes in deep tendon reflexes (hyporeflexia or areflexia)
Guillain-Barré syndrome (rare)
Polymyositis (rare)

Other

Hemorrhage
Infection

---

*Skin cancers involving papillomavirus are the most frequent cancers observed in transplant candidates, occurring in one half of the long-term survivors. Squamous cell carcinoma is often more aggressive than in nonimmunosuppressed people with multiple sites of presentation and frequent recurrence.[55]

ineum, carcinomas of the kidney, and hepatobiliary tumors.[43,198] Transplant recipients, however, have no increased risk of most cancers common in the general population, such as lung, breast, prostate, or cervical cancers. An increased risk for colon cancer remains controversial.[199]

Other effects of long-term immunosuppression have other serious consequences for the recipient, such as accelerated hyperlipidemia with the associated atherosclerosis and subsequent cardiovascular disease or the nonreversible paraplegia that occurs in approximately 4 out of 1000 cases associated with the immunosuppressant tacrolimus (FK-506).[177]

There is a high incidence of musculoskeletal effects that will concern the therapist, such as decreased bone density and osteoporosis,* steroid-induced myopathies, as well as avascular necrosis and musculoskeletal injuries. Neurotoxic reactions are manifested by a fine tremor, paresthesias, and occasionally seizures. The individual will report difficulty completing fine motor activities of daily living (ADLs), such as poor handwriting and difficulty eating. These changes may be significant enough to stop some people from going out publicly or dining out in restaurants. Reports of memory loss may not be secondary to actual alterations in memory but rather a decrease in executive function.[186] Most of these events are dose-related and reversible.

◆ Wound Healing

Chronic immunosuppressive drug therapy impairs and prolongs wound healing, especially common among those organ recipients with diabetic or neuropathic pedal ulcers. Therapists involved in wound therapy should inform their clients, members of the clients' families, employers of clients, and third-party payers to expect longer times in healing plantar ulcers because of long-term immunosuppressive therapy.[176]

Total-contact casting remains a highly effective and rapid method of healing neuropathic pedal ulcers in diabetic immunosuppressed clients and/or transplantation recipients although it may take several weeks longer than it would for those individuals who were not immunocompromised. Transplantation recipients who are immunocompromised appear to be no more at risk for wound failure complications when using total-contact casting as a treatment modality than those individuals without these additional variables.[176]

EXERCISE, ACTIVITY, SPORTS, AND ORGAN TRANSPLANTATION

Whereas some people will have a period of only a few days of physical inactivity before transplantation (e.g., toxic liver failure), the majority of organ candidates will live with their diseased organs for a prolonged period of time (often years). By the time of organ transplantation, candidates usually have experienced a period of long-term ill health leading to end-stage organ failure accompanied by severe deconditioning and exercise intolerance.

Complications of long-term immunosuppressive therapy and the kind of organ that has failed will determine some of

the problems an individual may face in relation to exercise, activities, and sports. Most transplantation candidates experience an impaired physical performance level that not only interferes with the ability to perform leisure-time exercise but also often limits the ability to perform even simple physical tasks, such as climbing stairs.[103] Weakness, dyspnea on exertion, and fatigue are often present, and there may be little motivation for exercise and sport. Finding an activity or exercise that the person can do successfully is the first step to initiating regular lifelong exercise.

Whether or not a potential candidate receives a transplant, therapy can be focused toward more function and improved quality of life. Exercise training increases work capacity as measured by increased oxygen consumption (VO_2), increases efficiency of oxygen utilization in the muscles, normalizes distribution of muscle fiber types, increases aerobic metabolism with delays in the onset of lactic acid buildup, and promotes modulation of the parasympathetic nervous system with more sensitive baroreceptors.[17] Exercise training also improves psychologic factors such as depression in pretransplant and posttransplant individuals.[30]

An assessment of transplant candidates must take into consideration daily life and daily activities including potential return to work requirements. For example, a job that requires lifting requires assessment of cardiovascular compliance and hemodynamic stability during lifting whereas someone at home must be safe in ADLs.

◆ Pretransplant Activity

It has been proposed that peripheral skeletal and respiratory (in the case of thoracic involvement) muscle work capacity is reduced before transplantation and contributes to the limitations of exercise seen in the posttransplantation population. Preservation of muscle strength before transplantation becomes impossible for some who are acutely ill. Muscular dysfunction attributable to detraining and deconditioning is common.[109]

For those individuals who can remain active, special emphasis should be placed on strengthening the long muscles of the lower extremities, especially the quadriceps. Weight training to build new muscle helps the candidate to counteract the steroid's targeting effects on muscle.[140] It has been reported by transplant centers around the United States that transplant candidates who do take part in an exercise program before surgery are likely to recover more rapidly following transplantation. As yet, little data exist on exercise performance before and after transplantation except with regard to 6-minute walk tests before and after thoracic transplantation.[166]

◆ Posttransplant Activity and Exercise

After organ transplantation the underlying pathophysiologic process returns toward normal. The extent of this recovery depends on the function of the transplanted organ, which in turn is determined by the quality of the organ donated, the quality of organ retrieval, the presence of any rejection or infection, and the development of other co-morbidities. Despite the pretransplant physical deconditioning and exercise limitations, transplant recipients can progressively return to a normal life with return to work and even safely participate in sporting activity and exercise.[103] National and International Transplant Games, a multidisciplinary sporting event started in 1978, illustrate the degree to which organ candidates can return to exercise and sports.

---

*Within the first 6 months after transplant, the organ candidate can lose more bone density than any woman during the postmenopausal period. Osteoporosis has become a silent contributor to mortality in organ transplantation.[181] Physical therapy intervention must address this concern.

Regular exercise enhances quality of life and lowers the risk of cardiovascular disease and diabetes. This is especially important in transplant recipients because many immunosuppressive drugs can be atherogenic and diabetogenic.[70,211] Standards for how soon after transplantation physical training can or should begin have not been uniformly established; some centers start as soon as the recipient is up and walking.

Ventilatory factors do not appear to limit exercise capacity in any transplant group, and despite the persistent limitations in aerobic capacity and work rate seen in many thoracic transplant candidates, cardiopulmonary performance is reasonably well-restored shortly after lung or heart-lung transplantation.[166]

Exercise training after transplantation increases exercise capacity, improves endurance, and increases muscle strength, contributing to higher quality of life after transplantation.[103,140,144*] However, effects of different training regimens remain unknown, and some individuals will be too fatigued to participate in regular exercise (especially liver and kidney recipients), making it impossible to determine the effect of regular training on the outcome of the transplantation.

Research shows that 6 months of specific resistance exercise training (weight training) restores fat-free mass to levels greater than before treatment and dramatically increases skeletal muscle strength. Resistance exercise, as part of a strategy to prevent steroid-induced myopathy, appears to be safe and should be initiated early after transplantation. Gaining density in the lumbar spine is especially important because up to 35% of transplant recipients develop lumbar spine bone fractures.[19]

◆ Guidelines for Activity and Exercise

Whether assessing aerobic exercise or ADLs (Table 20-5), measurements of blood pressure, rate pressure products (RRP = heart rate × systolic blood pressure), and myocardial oxygen consumption can provide valuable information and can be used as measurable outcomes of treatment intervention. As the intensity of activity increases, the heart rate and systolic blood pressure increase with a concomitant return to baseline with cessation of activity (see Appendix B). Reducing the time it takes for these measurements to return to baseline may be an objective measure of improvement. Consistent abnormal responses should be reported to the physician for further evaluation. Other considerations are determined according to the underlying pathologic condition (e.g., cardiomyopathy, congestive heart failure, renal failure, diabetes, cirrhosis) and pretransplant treatment (e.g., ventricular assistive devices, medications, dialysis). See Special Implications for the Therapist boxes for each specific diagnosis.

For all transplant candidates and recipients, the duration of beginning exercise should be until fatigue begins; then add 1 to 2 minutes per day. Until the duration is at least 20 minutes of continuous exercise, the person is best advised to exercise to the point of initial fatigue twice per day. The goal is to perform at least 30 minutes of nonstop activity daily before reducing exercise frequency to three to five times weekly. Individuals trying to control blood pressure or lose weight should work for a longer duration, 30 to 45 minutes, at a lower intensity (e.g.,

50% to 65% of predicted maximal heart rate). More specific exercise guidelines for ventilatory muscle training, ambulation, and use of the stationary bicycle are available.[26]

◆ Limitations on Activity and Exercise

Transplant trauma is a theoretic possibility so organ recipients are advised not to participate in contact sports. Except for this one general broad precaution, limitations on sporting and exercise must be evaluated on a case-by-case basis and may be determined by the course of the illness. For example, the person who undergoes emergency liver transplantation for acute liver failure will have relatively little secondary damage. On the other hand, someone with chronic renal failure can develop renal osteodystrophy (see Fig. 17-4 and the section on chronic renal failure in Chapter 17), decreased bone density, osteoporosis, reduced peak cardiac output (because of the arteriovenous fistula required for vascular access), and irreversible neuropathies and myopathies. Anyone experiencing renal failure secondary to diabetes will have multiple other secondary complications (see the section on Diabetes in Chapter 10).

Many other potential limitations on sporting and exercise must be recognized and evaluated, such as the condition of the recipient at the time of transplantation and the type of organ that has failed. For example, people with severe pulmonary disease necessitating heart-lung transplantation often experience malnutrition and muscle wasting before transplantation. Liver failure can cause abnormalities of lung function, including ventilation/perfusion mismatching and loss of oxygen-diffusing capacity.

Denervation of the transplanted heart, pancreas, liver, and kidneys results in a loss of sympathetic nerves to the organ (e.g., loss of vagal response in the heart, impaired insulin in the pancreas, and altered renin responses in the kidney) requiring some modifications in the exercise program. In contrast, surgical removal of sympathetic liver nerves does not inhibit hepatic glucose production during exercise and denervation of the lungs does not impair the ability to increase ventilation during physical exertion.[103] The denervated lung will experience reduced tidal volumes and decreased lung compliance. There is a delay in the bronchodilation response requiring an extended warm-up period in order to obtain the catecholamine response necessary for organ vasodilation and therefore increased tidal volume during exercise.

Besides the usual exercise-related risks anyone faces, recipients have additional medication-related risks associated with the long-term immunosuppressive therapy, including exaggerated hypertensive response, myopathies, neuropathies, and fractures. The muscle-wasting effects of glucocorticoids are well-known, and it is documented that quadriceps strength of renal transplant candidates is only 70% of normal, although this side effect can be counteracted by resistance exercise training.[78,79] Other potential side effects are listed in Table 4-6; see also the section on Immunosuppression under Posttransplant Complications in this chapter.

Finally, transplanted organs may be exposed to chronic rejection, limiting the function of the organ, especially during exercise for a transplanted heart when physiologic demand is high. In addition, chronic rejection of a donor heart results in accelerated atherosclerosis of the coronary arteries and myocardial necrosis, limiting cardiac function. However, despite all these

---

*For an excellent discussion of the positive effect of exercise conditioning on surgical success, see reference 26.

TABLE 20-5

Exercise Guidelines for Organ Candidates and Recipients*

Select an enjoyable activity or exercise and always have a goal! Some centers target a long-term goal by organizing an annual fun run/walk or join one already organized.

Include adequate warm-up, stretching, and cool-down periods.

Progress activity or exercise as described in text.

Include interval training, aerobic activity, strength training, and conditioning.

Combine activities and/or exercise program with energy conservation techniques (see Box 8-2).

Maintain a normal breathing pattern; breath holding my contribute to excessive elevation in blood pressure and produce associated symptoms, such as dyspnea and light headedness.

Exercise 3 days/week; allow 48 hours recovery time after moderate to high resistance training.

Follow guidelines for neuropathy and myopathy.

Endurance Training: High Repetitions/Low to Moderate Resistance
- Use weights that are 50%-60% of the one repetition maximum (RM).
- Perform 12-20 repetitions per set.
- Perform 2 or 3 sets of each exercise per workout.

Weight Training: Low Repetitions/More Resistance

Weight training must be approached very cautiously in this population, and it is recommended that endurance training precede weight training, progressing according to individual tolerance. When appropriate, pretransplant and posttransplant individuals must be cautiously progressed to low repetitions/increased resistance because of the incidence of hypertension (systemic and pulmonary); increased hemoptysis; overuse injuries; poorly regulated blood glucose, electrolyte, and nutritional imbalances; and surgical precautions (posttransplant). Low repetitions/high resistance is not part of the standard rehabilitation protocol. It should be avoided in the chronicalyl ill individual because of the secondary risk of injury, and it is contraindicated in the presence of documented pulmonary hypertension or signs and symptoms suggesting pulmonary hypertension (e.g. lightheadedness, dizziness, angina-like pain, decreased cardiac output with exercise). Medically documented right ventricular or right atrial dilation, tricuspid regurgitation, and symptoms of systolic murmur are also contraindications for this type of exercise.

Once all these criteria have been met, the therapist supervising weight training must determine a one RM taking into account any significant impairments present and the effects of long-term steroid use, especially muscle wasting, osteoporosis, and coagulopathy. Risk for injury is higher in this group when using one RM.
- Determine a one RM (i.e., the heaviest weight that can be lifted safely at the weakest position in the range of motion one time).
- Use weights that are 40%-60% of the one RM†.
- Perform 3-8 repetitions per set.
- Perform 3-5 sets of each exercise per workout.
- Perform each exercise through a functional range of motion.

For the Therapist

MAINTAIN OR MONITOR	TERMINATE EXERCISE IF
Allow only minimal dyspnea; respiratory rate should be <30 breaths/min with minimal rales heard on auscultation	Respiratory rate >40 breaths/min with increased rales
Allow only mild level of fatigue; use rate of perceived exertion (RPE, Borg scale; see Table 11-13)	(3/10 on Borg scale)
Maintain stable vital signs (heart rate [HR], blood pressure); maintain stable cardiac output (rate pressure product [RPP], pulse pressure [PP])	HR exceeds target zone; decrease in systolic blood pressure (SBP); pulse pressure (PP) narrows (SBP-diastolic blood pressure [DBP]); decrease in rate pressure product (RPP = HR × SBP)
Maintain stable electrocardiogram (ECG)	Increased incidence of arrhythmias or perceived palpitations
Maintain central venous pressure (CVP)	Monitor in the presence of right-sided heart failure; maintain CVP >20 mm Hg; terminate exercise relative to other symptoms
Maintain pulmonary arterial pressure (PAP)	Rest is indicated if PAP rises >5 mm Hg; terminate exercise if PAP rises and persists after rest and/or in the presence of other symptoms
Maintain oxygen saturation >90% (this is individually determined by each center according to each person's medical status)	Oxygen saturation <90% (or saturation below prescription)
Monitor for signs of bleeding	(See Tables 39-6 and 39-7)
Observe client response to exercise	Change in mental status (e.g., confusion, hostility); onset of pallor or diaphoresis; client request

*Guidelines for exercise are modified for the organ recipient but follow the ACSM's *Guidelines for Exercise Testing and Prescription*. These are only guidelines; each exercise program must be individually tailored to the organ recipient's condition and co-morbidities. Progression must be according to tolerance.
†Intensities of 80%-100% have been shown to produce the most rapid gain in muscle strength within the normal population. However, because of the possibility of overtraining or injury in the pretransplant or posttransplant population, caution must be used when overloading a muscle or muscle group.[21]

variables, the benefits of exercise in maintaining a healthy lifestyle and sense of well-being are much greater than the risks imposed by organ transplantation. Although it is assumed that transplant recipients will spontaneously increase their physical activity after transplantation, fear of harming the new organ or protective family members may discourage vigorous activity.

As a member of the transplant team, the therapist can encourage a program of regular activity immediately after transplantation and provide exercise guidelines as a part of the long-term transplant care plan. Vigorous exercise training for competition is not contraindicated for healthy transplant recipients. However, cardiorespiratory fitness and strength training should progress gradually first before the client engages in more strenuous sports participation. Exercise should be reduced in duration and intensity but not necessarily discontinued during rejection episodes.[144]

BLOOD AND BONE MARROW TRANSPLANTATION

◆ Definition and Overview

Hematopoietic stem cell transplant (HSCT) is defined as any transplantation of blood- or marrow-derived hematopoietic

stem cells, regardless of transplant type (i.e., allogeneic or autologous) or cell source (i.e., bone marrow, peripheral blood, or placental or umbilical cord blood).[131] HSCT, the collection and engraftment of hematopoietic stem cells from the bone marrow (and now also from the peripheral blood and umbilical cord blood) to cure a series of diseases previously considered incurable, is one of the most dramatic developments in the last 30 years. Initial attempts to transfer techniques derived from animal studies to humans failed until an understanding of human leukocyte antigen (HLA)* and tissue typing made it possible to select compatible sibling donors (and now unrelated donors).

Stem cell transplantation is an accepted form of treatment for people who require very high-dose chemotherapy or radiation therapy to treat their disease, usually a cancer. The chemotherapy and/or radiation therapy results in severe injury

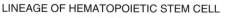

*The genes for the human leukocyte antigen (HLA), the human major histocompatibility complex, are located on the short arm of chromosome 6; siblings have a 25% chance of being a match. Nonrelated candidates have less than a 1 in 5000 chance of having identical HLA types. Graft rejection and graft-versus-host disease (GVHD) rates are inversely related to the degree of HLA compatibility. The National Bone Marrow Donor Registry types people as potential donors for unrelated people who require transplant.

LINEAGE OF HEMATOPOIETIC STEM CELL

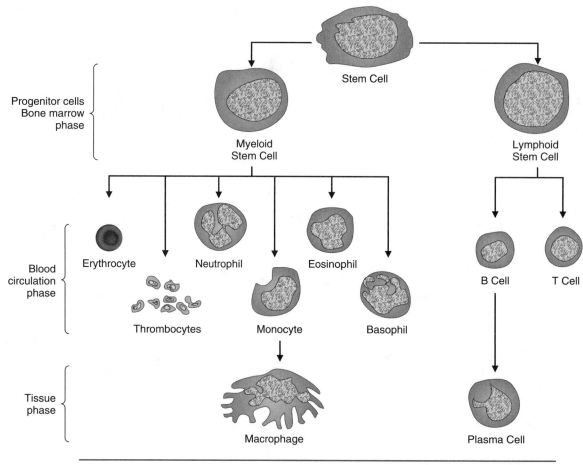

FIGURE   20-5   A stem cell is any precursor cell or "mother" cell that has the capacity for both replication and differentiation, giving rise to different blood cell lines. This figure shows the origin, development, and structure of thrombocytes, leukocytes, and erythrocytes from pluripotent (able to develop into different cells) stem cells. The process of hematopoiesis (formation and development of blood cells) usually takes place in the bone marrow.

to blood cells formed in the bone marrow (marrow ablation). In order to restore the person's ability to make blood and immune cells, stem cells from a compatible donor (or from the recipient) can be administered.

Stem cells are very immature cells that can develop into any of the three types of blood cells (red cells, white cells, platelets) (Fig. 20-5). Bone marrow is used for such transplants because it contains these "undifferentiated" stem cells. Blood also contains stem cells but in such small numbers that the cells cannot be counted or identified in ordinary blood tests. New procedures have made it possible to induce stem cells to leave the marrow and enter the blood from which they are collected or harvested for administration to a candidate in need of stem cell transplantation. Stem cells are also collected from umbilical cord and placental blood.

◆ Indications for Blood and Bone Marrow Transplantation

Today, transplantation of stem cells from peripheral blood, bone marrow, or cord blood is the treatment of choice for a variety of chemotherapy-sensitive hematologic malignancies, solid tumors, syndromes of bone marrow failure, genetic diseases, and more recently, autoimmune disorders. HSCT (i.e., peripheral blood stem cell transplantation [PBSCT] and bone marrow transplantation [BMT]) enables individuals to survive high-dose chemotherapy via "rescue" infusion of new, healthy bone marrow elements or stem cells.[66]

In 1998 breast cancer was the most common indication for stem cell transplant in North America, accounting for nearly one-third of all transplants. However, subsequent reports have concluded that high-dose chemotherapy plus autologous BMT does not improve survival in women with metastatic breast cancer.[8,182] Non-Hodgkin's lymphoma was the second most common indication, followed by acute myelogenous leukemia (AML), multiple myeloma, and chronic myelogenous leukemia (CML) (Fig. 20-6). Reduced transplant-related mortality has led to a widening of indications for stem cell transplantation, but based on the experience in the use of stem cell transplants with metastatic breast cancer, ongoing research is essential to verify the efficacy of this treatment modality for each individual disease entity.[124]

◆ Sources of Hematopoietic Stem Cell Transplant

The three types of peripheral blood or bone marrow transplantation are determined by the source of the donation: syngeneic, autologous, and allogeneic. As with all other transplantations, syngeneic involves peripheral blood or bone marrow from an identical twin with identical HLA antigens on the cell surfaces. Autologous transplants use the person's own stem cell sources and must be cancer-free by harvesting during remission or after cancer cells have been killed* (Fig. 20-7).

Allogeneic transplants require a donor with closely matched HLA antigens (usually a sibling); allogeneic sources

---

*The person who donates bone marrow for his or her own use does not have cancer in either the bone marrow or the blood cells. This autologous BMT greatly reduces the occurrence of side effects from the transplant.

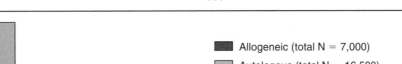
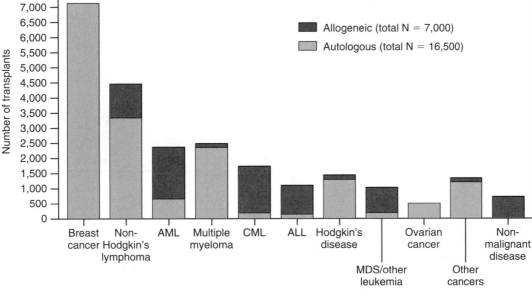

FIGURE **20-6** The most common indications for allogeneic and autologous transplants differ. *Allogeneic* transplant is the predominant approach for acute and chronic leukemias, myelodysplasia (MDS), and nonmalignant diseases such as aplastic anemia, immune deficiencies, and inherited metabolic disorders. *Autologous* transplant is used for ovarian and other solid malignancies, as well as Hodgkin's and non-Hodgkin's lymphomas and multiple myeloma. Routine use of this transplant for breast cancer has been discontinued and remains under investigation; see text discussion. (Courtesy International Bone Marrow Transplant Registry/Autologous Blood and Marrow Transplant Registry [IBMTR/ABMTR], Milwaukee, 2000.)

for stem cell transplantation are primarily derived from bone marrow with a smaller but steady increase in the number of allogeneic transplants from peripheral blood and cord blood (Fig. 20-8). Autologous blood stem cells are now widely used in place of allogeneic BMT, although allogeneic transplantation remains the only curative therapy for inherited disorders of metabolism and CML and the most effective treatment for severe aplastic anemia (Fig. 20-9).

Unlike allogeneic transplantation, autologous BMT can be performed in older people with relative safety owing to the freedom from GVHD as a complication. A primary concern with autologous BMT is the possible presence of viable tumor cells in the graft. Numerous methods have been developed to remove contaminating tumor cells from the graft in a process referred to as *purging*.

Peripheral blood has largely replaced bone marrow as a source of stem cells for autologous recipients. A benefit of harvesting such cells from the donor's peripheral blood instead of bone marrow is that it eliminates the need for general anesthesia associated with bone marrow aspiration. The most striking advantage of blood stem cell over bone marrow cell transplants is the shortened period of total aplasia of bone marrow after chemotherapy. This reduction in the period of aplasia may allow repeated marrow ablative treatment cycles in solid tumors, thereby reducing mortality. In addition, blood-derived grafts may contain fewer malignant cells than do the bone marrow cells.

Since the late 1980s umbilical cord blood has been harvested to assist people in need of stem cells previously only available through BMTs.* Like bone marrow, cord blood has been found to be a rich source of stem cells and may provide treatment advantages over bone marrow, especially if it comes from an immediate family member.† Cord blood banking is the process of collecting the blood immediately after delivery and freezing it for long-term cryogenic storage.

The potential advantages of cord blood stem cell transplantation over BMT include a large potential donor pool, rapid availability since the cord blood has been prescreened and tested, no risk or discomfort to the donor, rare contamination by viruses, and lower risk of GVHD. Potential disadvantages are primarily related to the many unknown variables with a new, experimental procedure, such as the possibility of genetic or congenital disease transmission by stem cells, uncertain long-term success using cord blood stem cells, and a longer period of time for treatment to be effective compared with cells from adult blood or bone marrow leaving the recip-

---

*Umbilical cord blood is the blood that remains in the umbilical cord and placenta after a baby is born. It is derived from the portion of the umbilical cord that has been cut and is usually thrown away.

†Family members wishing to store their newborn's cord blood for their own potential use can do so for a fee. However, anyone with a family member who has a condition for which stem cells may be a treatment option can store cord blood at no cost through the Cord Blood Registry's Designated Transplant Program. Contact the Cord Blood Registry at 1-888-267-3256 or www.cordblood.com to learn more about banking cord blood.

FIGURE 20-7 Approximately 90% of autologous transplants use only hematopoietic progenitor cells collected from blood. The remainder use bone marrow alone or in combination with cells collected from blood. (Courtesy International Bone Marrow Transplant Registry/Autologous Blood and Marrow Transplant Registry [IBMTR/ABMTR], Milwaukee, 2000.)

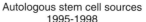

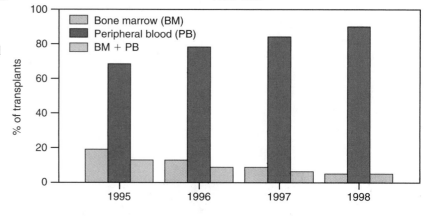

FIGURE 20-8 Most allogeneic transplants use bone marrow grafts. There has been a steady increase in the number of allogeneic transplants using cells collected from blood. Although use is increasing, there are still relatively few transplants using umbilical cord blood cells. (Courtesy International Bone Marrow Transplant Registry/Autologous Blood and Marrow Transplant Registry [IBMTR/ABMTR], Milwaukee, 2000.)

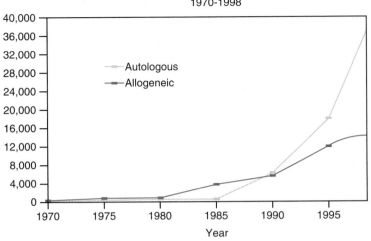

Annual number of blood and marrow transplants worldwide
1970-1998

FIGURE 20-9 Information for the annual number of blood and marrow transplants worldwide is based on data collected at more than 400 centers worldwide and represents approximately 40% of allogeneic bone marrow transplants done between 1970 and 1998 and 50% of autotransplants done in North and South America between 1989 and 1998. (Courtesy International Bone Marrow Transplant Registry/Autologous Blood and Marrow Transplant Registry [IBMTR/ABMTR], Milwaukee, 2000.)

ient at risk for infection. It remains unknown how long cord blood can be stored without losing its effectiveness.

Transplantation Procedure

Bone Marrow. The BMT process consists of several phases: conditioning, harvest, marrow infusion, preengraftment, and engraftment. Conditioning refers to the immunosuppression treatment regimen of chemotherapy, radiation therapy, or both used to eradicate all malignant cells, provide a state of immunosuppression, and create space in the bone marrow for the engraftment of the new marrow. Conditioning occurs 7 to 10 days before the actual BMT takes place.

Bone marrow is withdrawn from the donor by needle aspiration from the iliac crest or sternum on an outpatient basis and does not require surgical intervention. The donated marrow is usually infused through an intravenous (IV) line 48 to 72 hours after the last dose of chemotherapy or radiation therapy.

Peripheral Blood Stem Cells. PBSCT is harvested from the person's own stem cells through a process referred to as *leukapheresis*. Leukapheresis or hemapheresis is the process of removing a donor's blood to extract a specific component and returning the uneeded parts to the donor. The process uses continuous circulation of blood from a donor through an apparatus and back to the donor making it possible to remove desired elements from large volumes of blood. Besides stem cells, this process can harvest separately platelets, red blood cells, white blood cells, or plasma. The infused cells usually begin producing new blood cells in the marrow within a few weeks, and immune function returns within 1 to 2 years in successful transplants.

Cord Blood. Collection of cord blood takes place immediately after the umbilical cord is clamped after birth. After the baby is removed from the delivery area, a needle is inserted into the umbilical vein and blood is withdrawn and collected by gravity drainage. A standard blood collection bag is used containing nutrients and an anticoagulant solution to keep blood from clotting.

An alternate method involves collecting the cord blood after the child is delivered but before the placenta is delivered. This collection method may be advantageous because it allows earlier collection before the blood has a chance to clot and it uses the contractions of the uterus to enhance blood collection. This second technique is more intrusive and may potentially interfere with the mother's care after delivery.

After collection, the bag of cord blood is immediately transported to a facility for testing (e.g., HLA typing, identification of any viruses) and preservation. The blood is then frozen and held in liquid nitrogen at very low temperatures for future use. At the time of transplant, the cord blood is thawed and infused through a vein into the recipient.

Allogeneic transplant recipients remain hospitalized until their absolute neutrophil count exceeds 1500/mm³ for 48 hours (normal values = 3000 to 7000/mm³). Autologous transplant recipients may be managed as outpatients. All transplanted individuals are expected to remain geographically near during the first 100 days after transplant when the incidence of acute rejection is the greatest and to use reverse isolation (mask and glove wear) until they reach an acceptable neutrophil level.[66]

Complications of Blood and Bone Marrow Transplantation

Many people entering transplantation have already developed significant multisystem depletion, including cardiopulmonary, nutritional, musculoskeletal, and neurologic impairment related to the underlying disease. Bone metastasis, steroid myopathy, polyneuropathies, depleted protein stores, and impaired skin integrity are common co-morbidities before HSCT transplantation (Box 20-6).

The high-dose chemotherapy and radiation typically used as the preparative regimen for HSCT produces considerable morbidity and mortality. Virtually all HSCT recipients rapidly lose all T- and B-lymphocytes after conditioning, losing immune memory accumulated through lifetime exposure to infectious agents, environmental antigens, and vaccines. Transfer of donor immunity to HSCT recipients is variable and cannot be relied on to provide long-term immunity against infectious diseases. Cognitive slowing, impaired memory, and impaired executive functions are also seen in people following interferon-alpha treatments and whole-brain irradiation.[205]

Cardiac or pulmonary toxicity also may occur as a result of the irradiation and immunosuppressive drugs used to prepare candidates for the transplantation. Interstitial pneumonitis, an inflammation of the lungs, is a common complication,

Complications Associated with Hematopoietic Transplantation

Pretransplantation

Effects of immune suppression (see Table 4-6)
  Steroid myopathies, neuropathies
  Immobility
  Weakness
  Renal failure
Effects of chemotherapy and radiation therapy
  (see Tables 4-9 and 4-10)
  Cognitive impairment
  Neurologic impairment
  Neutropenia
  Thrombocytopenia
  Hemorrhage
  Anemia
  Cardiopulmonary toxicity
    Arrhythmias
    Cardiomyopathy
    Interstitial pneumonitis
    Obstructive or restrictive disease
  Nutritional deficits
  Bone metastasis
  Impaired skin integrity

Posttransplantation

Infection
Graft-versus-host disease (see Box 20-5)
Recurrence of malignancy
Sterility
Cystitis
Veno-occlusive liver disease
Fatigue
Hearing loss (ototoxic antibiotics)
Delayed effects of radiation
  Visual loss (cataract formation)

especially among allogeneic transplantations, which leaves the person susceptible to obstructive small airway disease. Arrhythmias may be the first sign that a chemotherapeutic agent is becoming cardiotoxic.

Infections and hemorrhagic complications during the period of bone marrow anaplasia and emerging immune competence and GVHD (see previous discussion of GVHD in this chapter) are the most life-threatening complications of BMT, and they may be fatal. Rejection of allogeneic transplantation resulting in infection, relapse, or GVHD is often fatal. Infections include early bacterial infections or later opportunistic infections, especially CMV interstitial lung disease. EBV-associated lymphoproliferative disorders (posttransplantation lymphoproliferative disorders) are a significant problem after stem cell transplantation from unrelated donors or mismatched family members.[73]

Recurrence of malignancy is always a possibility. Other complications of BMT include sterility, cystitis, cataract formation, cardiomyopathy, and veno-occlusive liver disease. Neuromuscular changes, such as peripheral neuropathies, muscle cramping, and steroid myopathies, may also develop.

The complications of PBSCT are essentially the same as those of BMT, but hematologic recovery after PBSCT is much more rapid (10 to 12 days, and as early as 7 days), thereby significantly shortening the period of postchemotherapy neutropenia (decreased neutrophils, a type of granular leukocyte used to fight infection) and thrombocytopenia (decreased platelets in peripheral blood). This in turn reduces platelet and red blood cell transfusion and facilitates earlier discharge from the hospital. In most cases, PBSCT can be performed on an outpatient basis.

◆ Prognosis

Enormous progress has been made in understanding the biology, therapy, and prophylaxis strategies of transplantation and in extending the range of potential bone marrow donors to include unrelated people. Dramatic advances have occurred in the prevention of serious infection, including CMV infection, formerly a cause of a high mortality rate.

One hundred-day mortality, defined as death before 100 days after transplant, is often used as a gauge of procedure-related toxicity. Allogeneic transplants are associated with relatively high risks of GVHD, failure of engraftment, infections, and liver toxicity resulting in high early mortality. Long-term survival rates are improved with BMT, but this type of transplantation does not confer a normal life span.[179,195] Unfortunately toxicities of conventional transplantation remain a major limitation to successful application of the procedure. Primary disease recurrence continues to account for the majority of deaths in autologous transplant recipients. New cancer, organ failure, and suicide are also cited as causes of death among long-term survivors after BMT. The incidence of suicide is higher among such survivors than among healthy subjects.[128]

Despite high morbidity and mortality after HSCT, recipients who survive long term are likely to enjoy good health. For those who survive more than 5 years after HSCT, 93% are in good health and 89% return to work or school full time. Eighty-eight percent of those who survive 10 years after HSCT report that the benefits of transplantation outweigh the side effects.[183] Although the success rates of transplantation have been improving over time, the prognosis still depends on the underlying disease, delays in transplantation, associated risk of relapse (e.g., leukemia) and current remission state, the development of GVHD based on the level of match between donor and recipient, and the age of the recipient. There is no effective therapy for severe GVHD, and people stricken with it rarely recover.

The success of allogeneic marrow grafting is inversely proportional to the age of the recipient. Most marrow transplant centers do not perform transplants in anyone older than 50 years, but some groups do make treatment decisions on the basis of a person's estimated physiologic age rather than chronologic age. These age restrictions do not apply to syngeneic or autologous transplants because these people will not develop GVHD. However, people older than 60 years do not tolerate intensive treatment as well as younger people.

◆ Future Trends

The development of techniques to achieve a state of chimerism and continued research efforts toward improved tolerance and elimination of malignant cells will lead to a wider application of hematopoietic cell transplantation in the coming decade.[194] Infusing donor bone marrow as an adjunct to solid-organ transplantation in order to prevent organ rejection is being investigated with animal studies.[152] This would open up an entirely new application of BMT and potentially alter the need for exogenous immunosuppression.

Efforts to reduce acute and long-term side effects of the high-dose conditioning regimens currently required to control the malignancy and prevent graft rejection may extend the use of allografts for people older than 55 years or for younger people with certain preexisting organ damage.[29] Transplantation using less toxic preparations may also make it possible to treat autoimmune diseases in the years ahead.

Researchers have located a master (stem) cell in the bone marrow of rats that will convert itself into functioning liver tissue cells under special conditions.[151] Preliminary studies from the same laboratory have also isolated a stem cell that converts into pancreatic cells. Other laboratory research has found in bone marrow the stem cells for bone, cartilage, tendon, muscle, and fat.[88,153] Although this work has been only demonstrated in laboratory animals it is a significant step toward learning how to regenerate human organs.

Swedish scientists isolated and identified for the first time the neural stem cell responsible for forming adult brain cells. This finding supports the idea that brain and other neural tissues regenerate despite conventional belief that these tissues do not regenerate.[91,92,129] Manipulation of these cells could open the door for replacing damaged neural tissues in spinal cord injuries and other neurologic conditions, such as multiple sclerosis, Huntington's disease, and Parkinson's disease.

Special Implications for the Therapist   20-1

HEMATOPOIETIC STEM CELL TRANSPLANTATION

Preferred Practice Patterns:
4A, 4B, 4C, 4G: One or more musculoskeletal patterns may be present depending on the complications present (e.g., bone metastasis, steroid myopathy, cancer-related surgery) (see previous discussion of complications associated with blood and bone marrow transplantation; see also Box 20-6)
5G: Impaired Motor Function and Sensory Integrity Associated With Acute or Chronic Polyneuropathies
6B: Impaired Aerobic Capacity/Endurance Associated With Deconditioning
6C: Impaired Ventilation, Respiration/Gas Exchange, and Aerobic Capacity/Endurance Associated With Airway Clearance Dysfunction
7A: Primary Prevention/Risk Reduction for Integumentary Disorders
7B: Impaired Integumentary Associated With Superficial Skin Involvement

The therapist's evaluation must include past medical history to assess other medical conditions, relevant past surgery, and prior level of exercise. Assessment of strength, skin condition, presence of neuropathy and myopathy, and balance impairment is necessary as part of the total evaluation with these individuals because of the specific medical treatment regimen associated with this type of transplantation. The combination of these factors puts the person at risk for immobility and subsequent pneumonia, pressure ulcers, muscle weakness, and overall deconditioning. In addition, long-term side effects of chemotherapy include peripheral neuropathy, and the prolonged use of steroids can induce steroid myopathy and osteoporosis. Any of these conditions places the individual at risk for falls and associated injuries.

Skin inspection and skin care are of primary importance to prevent pressure or shear injuries. The therapist must evaluate the need for turning schedules, specialized mattress surfaces, and wheelchair cushions. The client must be instructed in self-inspection especially when splinting is used to treat neuropathic weakness and proprioceptive loss.

Exercise After HSCT

Although initiating exercise after peripheral blood stem cell has been delayed up to 30 days, there is evidence that aerobic exercise can be safely carried out immediately after HSCT and can partially prevent loss of physical performance,[47] depending on the medical and physical condition both before the transplant and after transplant and chemotherapy. See the section on Exercise, Activity, Sports, and Organ Transplantation in this chapter. Exercise following BMT may be delayed longer owing to the intensity of the course of treatment required.

Exercise capacity in BMT recipients is low when transplantation is preceded by cardiotoxic chemotherapy or irradiation. Reduced exercise endurance, reduced maximal oxygen consumption, reduced rise in cardiac output during exercise, and reduced ventilatory anaerobic threshold are closely related to the chemotherapy.[87] Extremely abnormal responses require consultation with the physician before therapy is initiated or continued. These clients may need continuous monitoring over many therapy sessions rather than just using symptoms as a guide to exercise tolerance once a baseline is established.

Training studies of candidates before BMT to evaluate the impact of inactivity have not been performed. However, it has been demonstrated in individuals who have undergone BMT that a treadmill walking program started 18 to 42 days after transplantation results in significant improvement in maximal physical performance, walking distance, and lowered heart rate at a given workload.[48] Aerobic exercise improves the physical performance of peripheral stem cell recipients who have undergone high-dose chemotherapy. To reduce fatigue, this group of individuals should be counseled to increase physical activity rather than rest after treatment.[46]

During transplant induction and in the acute posttransplant phase, recipients must be encouraged to remain mobile and maintain ADLs despite the many unpleasant symptoms present. The loss of white blood cells exposes the individual to infection while the depletion of red blood cells reduces energy resulting in profound fatigue. Pulmonary conditioning with inspiratory muscle training, muscular strengthening, and endurance exercises is important to help maintain mobility but must be balanced with pacing, prioritizing, and other energy conservation techniques as an important part of treatment.

Continued

Range of motion, supervised or assisted ambulation, and resistive or endurance exercises can be utilized. Active assisted and passive range of motion is sometimes required for joint disuse and stiffness. Resistive exercises in the form of functional activities such as bridging, transfers, and walking are individually prescribed.[66]

Interval activity training (see Appendix B) combined with energy conservation techniques (see Box 8-2) is an important component of therapy since the client's blood counts drop (including hemoglobin count, resulting in anemia), thereby reducing the body's capacity for exertion or aerobic activity. Decreased platelet counts increase the person's susceptibility to bleeding from minor injuries. The amount of resistance and the use of equipment to provide resistance depend on platelet count. The therapist must monitor blood values to avoid causing joint hemorrhage (see Tables 39-6 and 39-7). Safety education is important, and assistive devices may be needed.

Infection

Myelosuppression as a result of specific chemotherapeutic agents or drug combinations is the number one factor that predisposes the person to infection (see Table 7-1). Until bone marrow function returns, the HSCT recipient is extremely susceptible to life-threatening infection, which requires all staff to practice interventions to minimize or prevent infection, such as good hand-washing technique. Preventing infections among HSCT recipients is preferable to treating infections. Any therapist working with this population is advised to obtain the guidelines for preventing opportunistic infections among HSCT recipients available from the Centers for Disease Control and Prevention (CDC).[131] See also Chapter 7.

Therapists and nursing staff must work closely together to prevent infection, recognize early signs of infection or rejection, and reinforce the educational program, which is complex and is often taught in a short time under less than ideal conditions. Expanding the lungs regularly during common movements, such as getting out of bed or turning, while coughing, and during exercise is an important part of minimizing infections.

Graft-Versus-Host Disease

Early symptoms of graft-versus-host reaction (see previous discussion in this chapter) usually appear within 10 to 30 days after transplant and may include rash, hepatomegaly, and diarrhea. Although some cardiopulmonary abnormalities can only be detected by echocardiography, early warning symptoms of cardiopulmonary complications, such as progressive dyspnea, sensation of heart palpitations, irregular heartbeats, chest pain or discomfort, or increasing fatigue, may be reported by the recipient or observed by the therapist. The physician must be notified of such changes and modifications made to the exercise program for mildly to moderately abnormal responses.

Monitoring Vital Signs

Vital signs must be monitored before, during, and after exercise to assess each HSCT recipient for an abnormal response. At this time, no data show the effects of drug interventions or the physiologic responses to transplant procedures in recovery or over the long term. Monitoring responses over time during the recovery process can alert the therapist to any developing cardiopulmonary compromise.

The concept of routine monitoring applies to anyone who is seemingly healthy after transplant and may provide helpful information about when to advance an exercise program. Knowledge of past medical history and preexisting conditions that could affect physical conditioning is essential. Preexisting conditions in the presence of extended periods of inactivity can contribute to further physical deconditioning.

Normal changes in vital signs include an increased heart rate and increased systolic blood pressure proportional to the workload, with minimal change in diastolic blood pressure (no more than $+/-10$ mm Hg). Hypertension or the use of antihypertensive medications (or other medications) can alter the normal response of blood pressure to exercise. Recipients may be deconditioned with a less than normal (sluggish) blood pressure response. (See Appendix B.)

Monitoring Laboratory Values

In addition to monitoring vital signs, the therapist must be aware of daily laboratory values for red blood cells, white blood cells, and platelets. Each facility will have its own guidelines for activity and exercise based on blood counts. Often, symptomatology is used as the primary measure of acceptable activity. Platelet levels must be evaluated (thrombocytopenia) before chest percussion is performed. See also the sections on Radiation Injuries and Chemotherapy in Chapter 4. ∎

ORGAN TRANSPLANTATION

◆ Kidney Transplantation

Overview. The first kidney transplant was done in 1954 by Joseph Murray, M.D., resulting in a successful graft and providing the recipient with an additional 8 years of life. It was the first organ transplantation of any kind ever performed, with the success credited to the live donor (adult twin brother). Kidney transplantation remains the most common type of solid-organ transplant (see Table 20-1).

As people over the age of 65 years become the fastest growing segment of our population, the number of cases of end-stage renal disease (ESRD) requiring kidney transplantation will continue to increase. Renal replacement remains the most successful form of treatment for ESRD and, in the case of diabetes, offers an opportunity to eliminate dependence on dialysis and exogenous insulin. Simultaneous kidney-pancreas transplantation has become a safe and effective method to treat advanced diabetic nephropathy and results in stable metabolic function, reduced cholesterol, and improved blood pressure control.[189]

Until recently, almost all candidates for renal transplantation had been treated for months or years with hemodialysis, but now it is possible to plan a kidney transplant before the complete shutdown of the kidney or kidneys, avoiding dialysis completely. Recent studies have shown that when dialysis is used, peritoneal dialysis* is associated with a lower incidence of delayed graft function and may be preferred over hemodialysis.[12,207]

---

*Continuous ambulatory peritoneal dialysis (CAPD) is a maintenance system of dialysis in which an indwelling catheter permits fluid to drain into and out of the peritoneal cavity by gravity. The individual remains able to complete this type of dialysis three or four times per day while at home rather than coming to a hemodialysis clinic three or four times per week for 3 or 4 hours at a time while the blood is filtered through a dialysis machine.

Receiving a kidney transplant without a prior history of hemodialysis or peritoneal dialysis presents some problems in adjustment for those people who, never having experienced the intrusion of dialysis, must now learn to live with the side effects of antirejection drugs and potential complications of surgery. Whereas the person on dialysis may see transplantation as a welcome relief, recipients who have never been treated with dialysis may be more likely to view the surgery and recovery as an ordeal and therefore experience more difficulties in adjustment.

Indications and Incidence.   The primary indication for renal transplantation is insulin-dependent diabetes with ESRD, which occurs in over one third of all cases of type 1 diabetes.[117] Cardiac autonomic neuropathy occurs as a result of uremia and diabetes with severe cardiac dysfunction when these conditions occur at the same time. Both kidney transplantation and kidney-pancreas transplantation result in improved cardiac autonomic function and modulation of heart rate.[31]

There are now more than 50,000 people on the waiting list for cadaveric kidney transplant, but only 14,000 of these procedures are performed yearly in the United States (see Table 20-1).[203] A more unusual indication would be polycystic kidney disease, especially when combined with polycystic liver disease.

Transplant Candidates.   As mentioned, people with type 1 diabetes and ESRD can choose dialysis or transplantation for renal replacement therapy. Those individuals with type 1 diabetes younger than 45 years with little or no atherosclerotic vascular disease are ideal candidates for a combined kidney and pancreas transplant. The addition of a pancreas transplant is associated with greater morbidity and may require higher levels of immunosuppression but can result in stabilization of neuropathy and improved quality of life.[117]

Some renal transplant candidates are at high risk for cardiac events, sometimes fatal. Analysis of these clinical risk factors (including age at least 50 years, insulin-requiring diabetes mellitus, and abnormal electrocardiogram [ECG]) may assist in identifying candidates who may be at risk for cardiac death.[114] For those choosing transplantation, a kidney from a living-related donor is associated with longer graft and individual survival.

Transplantation Procedure.   Kidney grafts may be positioned intraperitoneally, anastomosed to the iliac vessels, and then drained into the bladder; extraperitoneally in the iliac fossa through an oblique lower abdominal incision; or in small children, retroperitoneally with a midline abdominal incision.

Complications.   As with other solid-organ transplantation, renal recipients experience graft dysfunction, organ-related infection (nephrotoxicity), and graft rejection as the three most common complications. Surgical complications include renal artery thrombosis, urinary leak, and lymphocele although chronic rejection accounts for most renal allograft losses after the first year after transplantation. Donor organ quality, delayed graft function, and other donor and recipient variables leading to reduced nephron mass are nonimmunologic factors that contribute to the progressive deterioration of renal graft function.[130]

Cardiovascular and cerebrovascular diseases are major causes of morbidity and mortality after kidney transplanta-

tion. Extensive carotid vascular wall abnormalities increase significantly despite kidney and pancreas transplantation in those individuals with type 1 diabetes mellitus and progressive uremia. Although initiation of plaque development is related to systemic factors, progression of established plaque is largely influenced by local factors within the arterial wall and therefore unaffected by organ transplantation.[135] In fact, research has shown an association between CMV infection and atherosclerotic plaque formation in coronary heart disease, a finding that has also been found in posttransplant cardiac complications in kidney recipients with CMV.[82]

Other complications may include renal dysfunction with prolonged use of cyclosporine, hypertension, lipid disorders, hepatitis, cancer, and osteopenia. Hypertension occurs in up to 80% of renal graft recipients; approximately 15% of graft recipients develop chronic hepatitis. Basal cell and squamous cell carcinoma, Kaposi's sarcoma, lymphomas, and posttransplant lymphoproliperative disease are two to five times more frequent in this population.[148] There is a high degree of impaired bone formation associated with renal grafts resulting in severe osteoporosis when compared with other organ transplants.

Prognosis.   Long-term renal transplant survival has improved from 23% (graft) and 36% (recipient) for cadaveric donor in 1986 to 92% and 93% in 1996.[203] The long-term outcome of simultaneous kidney-pancreas transplant recipients is not well-established yet and ranges from 79% for a 1-year graft survival rate to 5-year survival rates for combined kidney-pancreas transplant, kidney transplant, and pancreas transplant reported as 95%, 85%, and 88%, respectively.[189]

Future Trends.   The renal research community has made great strides in improving client outcomes on dialysis and following organ transplantation. However, only a small fraction of individuals with ESRD are actually transplanted because of a lack of donor organs requiring continued research to find alternative methods of successful treatment. Alternately, preserving donor organs more effectively may ensure better graft survival rates. Since both glomerular and tubular functions are inhibited at temperatures below 18° C, efforts to develop organ preservation techniques at warmer temperatures are under way.[187]

Current research continues to examine the possibilities of reducing cyclosporine dosage through the concomitant use of rapamycin without increased infections or neoplasms developing and with the potential for reducing the incidence or progression of chronic rejection. Other efforts to reduce the incidence of acute rejection episodes include assessment of a chimeric monoclonal antibody.[95]

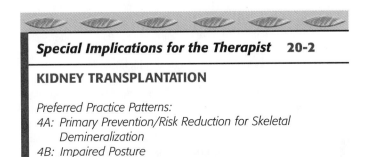

Special Implications for the Therapist   20-2

KIDNEY TRANSPLANTATION

Preferred Practice Patterns:
4A: Primary Prevention/Risk Reduction for Skeletal
     Demineralization
4B: Impaired Posture

4D: Impaired Joint Mobility, Motor Function, Muscle Performance, and Range of Motion Associated With Connective Tissue Dysfunction (ligament or tendon disorder)

5G: Impaired Motor Function and Sensory Integrity Associated With Polyneuropathies

6B: Impaired Aerobic Capacity/Endurance Associated With Deconditioning

6C: Impaired Ventilation, Respiration/Gas Exchange, and Aerobic Capacity/Endurance Associated With Airway Clearance Dysfunction

7A: Primary Prevention/Risk Reduction for Integumentary Disorders

As increasing studies document the effectiveness of exercise in disease prevention and prevention of transplant complications, timely and effective rehabilitation programs will be implemented. Physical and occupational therapy can offer a great deal to renal rehabilitation, especially to increase endurance and physical strength and to improve function and independence (see the section on Exercise, Activity, Sports, and Organ Transplantation in this chapter).

Acute Care Phase

Most kidney recipients are discharged about 5 days after surgery and are not seen by the therapist until later in the recovery process (or perhaps not at all) as an outpatient approximately 1 month postoperatively. At that time, the recipient will most likely still monitor both blood pressure and blood glucose levels. The therapist should pay close attention to both these measurements as the rehabilitation component is added.

Exercise

Kidney transplants have been performed longer than any other organ, providing a greater number of retrospective studies to assess the influence of exercise on kidney transplantation. It has been shown that pretransplant and posttransplant exercise training improves lipid profile, increases hematocrit level, normalizes insulin sensitivity, and lowers the requirement for antihypertensive medication.[67,68]

Although a kidney transplant recipient may be normotensive at rest, there is an elevated blood pressure response to exercise possibly caused by altered function of blood pressure control and by the effects of cyclosporine. This requires careful monitoring and documentation of vital signs in the exercise program planning and assessment.

Training effectively modifies factors known to be associated with atherogenesis and cardiac disease in hemodialysis clients. Before transplantation, clients with kidney disease, especially those receiving hemodialysis, are susceptible to bone loss as a result of altered vitamin D_3 function and its role in calcium absorption. Resistive exercises can help increase bone density (in the general population and in all organ transplantations) and should be initiated before transplantation or as early after transplantation as possible.[18,110,132]

Overuse tendon injuries occur at a high rate in kidney transplant recipients[1,134]; whether the mechanism for this is immunologic, metabolic, or medication-induced remains unclear although several reports have implicated the use of fluoroquinolones as a responsible factor.[120] Care should be taken to avoid overloading tendons since dramatic ruptures following even small trauma have been reported.[178] ■

◆ Liver Transplantation

Overview.   The first liver transplant in a human was performed in 1963. Since that time, the success of this procedure has improved so much that 1600 liver transplant operations were completed in the United States in 1990. In the following decade, a team of surgeons at the University of Chicago developed the living-related transplant that requires only a lobe of a liver or small pieces taken from living donors. This technique has also been applied to cadaveric donor livers by splitting the liver to expand the donor pool.[24]

Indications.   Orthotopic liver transplantation has become an established therapy for end-stage liver disease (e.g., cirrhosis caused by alcoholism, hepatitis C), acute liver failure, and primary biliary cirrhosis or primary sclerosing cholangitis, as well as for nonalcoholic cirrhosis and hepatic or biliary malignancy. Biliary atresia is the most common indication for pediatric liver transplantation. Theoretically, anyone with advanced, irreversible liver disease with certain mortality may be considered for a liver transplant provided the disease can be corrected by liver transplantation (Table 20-6).

Hepatitis B is not eliminated by transplantation, but its recurrence and the damage it can cause may be substantially reduced by giving the client hepatitis B globulin. Hepatitis recurs in the transplanted liver in 80% to 90% of cases, but the damage to the new liver is slow so that many years of symptom-free living can occur.

With the exception of metastatic malignancy and hepatic lymphoma, there are few absolute contraindications to liver transplantation. Liver transplantation for large primary liver cancers is very limited; transplantation remains the best treatment for small tumors (less than 5 cm) in a liver that is already cirrhotic.[214] People with metastatic disease that has spread to the liver are no longer treated with liver transplantation because of the poor outcome. The exception is a small

TABLE	20-6

Liver Transplantation

INDICATIONS	POSSIBLE CONTRAINDICATIONS
Primary biliary cirrhosis	Sepsis
Neoplasm (selected cases)	Hepatic lymphoma
Acute fulminant liver failure	AIDS
Inborn errors of metabolism	Poor client understanding
Alcoholic cirrhosis after documented treatment and recovery	Alcoholic cirrhosis (documented continued abuse)
Drug-induced liver disease	Cirrhosis secondary to drug abuse
Chronic active hepatitis (see text)	Chronic active (type B) hepatitis
Neonatal cholestasis (bile suppression)	Advanced cardiopulmonary disease
Biliary atresia	Inability to follow up with treatment
Sclerosing cholangitis	
Budd-Chiari syndrome	
Congenital hepatic fibrosis	
Cystic fibrosis	

AIDS, Acquired immunodeficiency syndrome.

group of people whose liver cancer is characterized by neuroendocrine tumors that are very slow-growing. The results of transplantation in this group are not as good as for those individuals with benign disease but acceptable enough to qualify for transplantation.

Some metabolic disorders (e.g., familial hypercholesterolemia) that arise in the liver but produce damage elsewhere in the body can be cured if the liver is replaced with a liver from a normal individual. Many inborn errors of liver metabolism are benign and are not associated with end-stage liver disease. Acute fulminant liver failure secondary to severe hepatitis owing to a virus, toxin, or poison can be life-threatening and requires liver transplantation to prevent death.

Transplant Candidates.   The decision to perform a transplant may be determined by how long the procedure will extend the candidate's life. In general, people with nonmalignant, nonalcoholic liver disease between ages 2 and 60 years are considered most suitable. A definite age cutoff has not been determined; although many transplant centers do not accept most people as candidates if they are older than 60 years, this limit is being expanded. Older people may be unable to survive the procedure, and clients with considerable damage to other major organs (e.g., heart, lungs) cannot handle the stress of the surgery. For technical reasons, with small-birth-weight infants, surgeons may prefer to wait until significant growth has occurred.

The potential candidate with an end-stage liver disease that is correctable by a liver transplant must also be a good operative candidate. Many potential risk factors have been reported to increase the risk of transplantation (Table 20-7). Clients with alcoholic cirrhosis may be required to remain abstinent 6 months before the transplant, although it has been suggested that liver transplantation itself contributes to recovery from alcoholism. The recidivism (relapse) rate following liver transplantation varies in reported studies from 4% to 32% although the majority of studies report a recidivism rate in the 4% to 9% range.[138,143] The use of the biologic marker carbohydrate-deficient transferrin to screen for alcoholic relapse has been used for the first time in liver graft candidates but remains controversial.[9,165]

Transplantation Procedure.   The liver from the cadaveric donor is removed through a midline incision from the jugular notch to the pubis including a median sternotomy with particular care to avoid hepatic injury or portal vein transection. The iliac artery and vein are also harvested in the event that vascular reconstruction is required. Living-related transplantation requires a much less extensive operative opening, and the reduced-size graft is usually taken from the donor's left lobe. In some situations (e.g., presence of metabolic abnormalities), the autologous graft is placed in an anatomically altered site, thereby preserving the orthotopic position for future use in the case of graft failure; this technique is not possible with disorders leading to portal hypertension.

Successful engraftment of the donor organ requires a recipient hepatectomy to remove the diseased liver, a procedure that can be difficult when there is severe portal hypertension and excessive collateral formation. In many centers, the recipient is placed on heart-lung bypass to avoid congestion of the portal circulation and improve venous return to the heart during implantation, thus improving hemodynamic stability. The implantation procedure begins with anastomoses, that is, surgical formation of a connection between the donor and the recipient's suprahepatic and then infrahepatic vena cava. Alternatively, the donor vena cava can be anastomosed side to side with the recipient vena cava if it is left in situ during the recipient hepatectomy (piggyback technique). The operation then proceeds to the portal anastomosis. After all venous connections, the liver is reperfused.

Complications.   Transplantation of the liver differs from renal, lung, or heart transplantation because there is no intervening assistance from an artificial liver; the technical aspects of liver transplantation require precise connection of the hepatic artery, hepatic and portal veins, and the bile duct. In the case of a living donor, there is a risk of hemorrhage and death if an artery is accidentally severed.

Rejection is the most common cause of liver dysfunction after transplantation, most likely after the first week and during the first 3 postoperative months. As with all organ transplantation procedures, the chance of organ rejection requires the use of immunosuppressants with their associated complications, especially suppression of the body's natural defenses, making infections a common complication and cause of graft dysfunction. Each person is also placed on prophylactic med-

TABLE   **20-7**

Liver Transplant Risk Factors

Low	Intermediate	High
Increasing age	Active extrahepatic infection	More than one other failing organ
Severity of liver dysfunction in otherwise stable person without encephalopathy	Hepatobiliary sepsis	Prolonge, severe coma
	Hepatorenal syndrome	Preoperative hemodynamic instability
	Small-sized infant	Extrahepatic malignancy
Previous abdominal surgery	Short-duration coma	Immunosuppressive disorders
Preexisting thrombotic disorder	Transplantation across ABO barrier	
	Previous portosystemic shunt	
	Portal vein thrombosis	
	Operative variable	

From Meyers WC, Jones RS: *Textbook of liver and biliary surgery,* Philadelphia, 1990, Lippincott, p 406.

ications for a period of time to decrease the risk of opportunistic infection. Cytomegalovirus (CMV), a common infectious process, occurs early after liver transplantation. CMV remains a major cause of morbidity but is no longer a major cause of mortality after liver transplantation.

Extrahepatic complications may include renal failure, neurologic disorders, and pulmonary involvement (e.g., pneumonia, atelectasis, respiratory distress syndrome, pleural effusion). Hepatocellular carcinoma, hepatitis B, and Budd-Chiari syndrome* may recur in the transplanted liver, but other chronic liver diseases do not recur.

Mechanical postoperative complications include biliary strictures, nonfunction of the graft (i.e., the transplanted liver does not function), hemorrhage, and vascular thrombosis of the hepatic artery, portal vein, or hepatic veins. Mononeuropathy of the ulnar nerve occurs in approximately 10% of orthotopic liver transplantation, primarily attributed to intraoperative compression or postoperative trauma. Other upper extremity mononeuropathies may occur as a result of vascular cannulations (flexible tube inserted to deliver medication or drain fluid).[28]

Other clinically significant neurologic events occur in a substantial percentage of adult liver transplant recipients. Central nervous system (CNS) complications after liver transplantation may be a consequence of liver disease itself, may be caused by the adrenergic effects of immunosuppressants (e.g., FK-506, CYA), or may result from a wide array of metabolic abnormalities or vascular insults occurring in the early postoperative period. The most common CNS lesions are listed in Box 20-7 (see also Table 4-6). The therapist is likely to be familiar with most of these terms, with the possible exception of central pontine myelinosis, which is demyelination of the central pons that causes a locked-in syndrome characterized by paralysis of the limbs and lower cranial nerves with intact consciousness.

Prognosis. Factors determining survival include the underlying cause of liver failure (e.g., poorer prognosis for advanced cirrhosis), the person's ability to stop the intake of alcohol in the case of alcoholic cirrhosis, and the presence of complications or symptoms of hematemesis, jaundice, and ascites. Continued advances in the use of immunosuppressant-steroid combinations have increased survival rates through effective immunosuppression with minimal toxicity.

In the case of liver transplantation, survival rates correlate with the number of liver transplant procedures performed in transplant centers. Overall 1-year survival rates have improved from 70% 10 years ago to more than 85% in many high-volume centers.[51] Survival after emergency liver transplantation for acute liver failure is less because such clients are seriously ill at the time of the operation.

The expected 1-year survival rate after a second or subsequent liver transplantation is about 50%. Two groups of people qualify for liver retransplantation: those with serious postoperative complications because of mechanical failure or rejection

---

*In Budd-Chiari syndrome, occlusion of the hepatic veins impairs blood flow out of the liver, producing massive ascites and hepatomegaly. It is associated with any condition that obstructs the hepatic vein (e.g., abdominal trauma, use of oral contraceptives, polycythemia vera, paroxysmal nocturnal hemoglobinuria, other hypercoagulable states, congenital webs of the vena cava).

BOX **20-7**

Central Nervous System Complications of Liver Transplantation

Focal seizures
Encephalopathy
Central pontine myelinolysis
Hemorrhages, infarcts, or both (intracranial, intracerebral, subarachnoid)
Confusion
Coma
Psychosis
Cortical blindness
Quadriplegia
Tremors
Alzheimer type II astrocytosis
CNS aspergillosis (fungal infection)
Cytomegalovirus (viral infection)

---

and those who have a slow progressive course of chronic hepatic dysfunction, usually caused by rejection or recurrence of primary disease. A model to estimate survival after retransplantation of the liver is being developed to help identify individuals with a poor expected outcome; this information could be useful in further refining candidate criteria selection.[119]

Future Trends. Current animal research is centered on identifying and harvesting specific stem cells from the bone marrow that under special conditions will convert into functioning liver tissue.[151] In human research, a new procedure called *hepatocyte transplantation* is being pioneered. In this procedure billions of donor liver cells are injected by IV infusion into the blood with the hope that the cells will correct life-threatening liver problems that would otherwise require a liver transplant.[71,160] Other research efforts are working toward the development of bioartificial devices for liver support. An effective temporary liver support system could improve the chance of survival with or without a transplant as the final treatment.[161]

Special Implications for the Therapist 20-3

LIVER TRANSPLANTATION

Preferred Practice Patterns:
4A, 4B: Prevention/Risk Reduction for Skeletal Demineralization Associated With Long-Term Use of Immunosuppressants; Impaired Posture is Especially Noted With Liver Transplantation
5C, 5D, 5E: Impaired Motor/Sensory Function Associated With Central Nervous System Involvement (see Box 20-7)
5F: Impaired Peripheral Nerve Integrity and Muscle Performance Associated With Peripheral Nerve Injury (ulnar nerve mononeuropathy is a common surgical complication in this population)
6A, 6B, 6C, 6F: Prevention/Risk Reduction for Cardiovascular/Pulmonary Disorders; Impaired Aerobic

Capacity/Endurance Associated With Deconditioning; Impaired Ventilation and Respiration (complications of treatment, especially pneumonia)

The majority of transplanted livers begin to function well within minutes to hours after the vascular clamps are released. The client must be closely monitored for signs of respiratory compromise, bleeding, infection, rejection, and fluid or electrolyte imbalance (see Chapter 4).Vital signs must be monitored as activities are slowly resumed with physician approval and according to the client's tolerance levels. (See Appendix B.)

Acute Care Phase

Postoperatively, the client will have multiple IV lines, drains, and a Foley catheter, as well as a painful abdomen with a large abdominal incision and a 4- to 5-inch left axillary incision (bypass procedure) restricted by staples and dressings. Standing postoperative orders are usually followed in the ICU. The large incisions are contraindications for resistive exercises; gradual low-resistance training can be introduced according to the physician's protocol. Upper extremity range of motion exercises and client education for prevention of adhesive capsulitis (i.e., frozen shoulder) are important concerns. Coughing and deep breathing with a pillow splint are taught early. These people do not want to cough, and respiratory infection is a hazard to avoid.

Often postoperative ascites is a significant problem, making functional training (e.g., bed mobility training, transfers) more difficult in the presence of an altered center of gravity. Hand, pedal, and, in men, scrotal edema from dependent positioning frequently develops, requiring active range of motion and bed mobility training as soon as possible. Assisted ambulation should occur as soon as the client is stable in the upright position; once the telemetry is removed, rehabilitation can progress rapidly. Ascites and associated edema usually resolve within 3 to 4 weeks, but if edema persists, comprehensive lymphedema therapy may be required (see discussion in Chapter 12).

Outpatient Phase

Outpatient therapy continues for approximately 8 weeks postoperatively. The liver transplant recipient with healthy heart and lungs can usually function well at home and resume independent ADLs. Rest and energy conservation balanced with nutrition, exercise, and correct, consistent, lifelong drug self-administration are all considered important features of the rehabilitation process. Pretransplant hepatic encephalopathy usually resolves slowly in the posttransplant period if the donor organ is functioning well; client and therapist will see a reduction or cessation of associated signs and symptoms.

The therapist must be alert to any self-medicating or use of over-the-counter drugs by the client; the client should be encouraged to check with the physician before continuing unmonitored drug use. Steroid usage in older women can cause posttransplant mental confusion; the woman may become uncooperative and disoriented to time and place and experience hallucinations.[177]

Exercise

Extreme weakness and fatigue reducing clients' activity level are common in many liver transplant candidates experiencing chronic liver disease. Low VO_2 max is common in pretransplant liver candidates with primary biliary or alcoholic cirrhosis along with alcohol-induced myopathy contributing to exercise limita-

tions. Improvement in exercise capacity with training before transplantation has been demonstrated, and new studies confirm the same outcome after liver transplantation on physical fitness, muscle strength, and functional performance in candidates treated for chronic liver disease (see also the section on Exercise, Activity, Sports, and Organ Transplantation in this chapter).[10,11]

The liver plays an important role in providing glucose for oxidation and the maintenance of glucose homeostasis during physical exercise. Denervation of the liver does not alter the release of glucose during physical activity. Consequently liver transplant candidates can perform quite heavy exercise and maintain acceptable glucose levels. ■

◆ Heart Transplantation

Overview. In 1960, Lower and Shumway developed the technique for heart transplantation that remains the basis of standard clinical surgical transplant technique worldwide. The first human heart procedure was performed in South Africa by Christiaan Barnard (1967), followed shortly by the first U.S. transplant by Norman Shumway at Stanford in 1968.

Heart transplantation has been *heterologous* (i.e., from a nonhuman primate, a procedure that is no longer performed) or more commonly, *homologous* (or allograft) (i.e., from another human). Future trends may develop the *heterologous* transplantation or xenograft (transplantation from other species, e.g., pig organs); see the previous section on Xenotransplantation.

Incidence. Two decades ago there were only a handful of heart transplant programs in the United States; today there are 141 programs that transplant hearts into approximately 2500 people each year. Unfortunately, 40,000 people under the age of 65 years die annually from heart failure and approximately 25,000 of those people could benefit from transplantation.

Indications. Potential candidates of cardiac transplants must have end-stage heart disease with severe or advanced heart failure (New York Heart Association class III or IV end-stage heart disease) to be considered for a donor heart. In the United States, the most common underlying cause of heart failure leading to cardiac transplantation is ischemic coronary heart disease.

The second most common disease leading to cardiac transplantation is idiopathic dilated cardiomyopathy. Other less common cardiac diseases that may be treated with heart transplantation include sarcoidosis, restrictive cardiomyopathy, hypertrophic cardiomyopathy, congenital heart disease untreatable by surgical correction or medical treatment, and valvular heart disease when the risk of cardiac surgery is prohibitively high.

Transplant Candidates. The selection of candidates for heart transplantation involves the use of multiple prognostic variables (Box 20-8; see also Box 20-4) in conjunction with medical urgency criteria established through UNOS status listings (see Table 20-2). People accepted as candidates for heart transplantation are expected to have a limited survival if they do not have surgery. Pediatric listings differ slightly. Status 1A characterizes a child less than 6 months of age with

BOX 20-8

Indications for Heart Transplantation

ESHD with NYHA class III or IV
Life expectancy <2 years
Cardiac index <2.0 L/min/m²
Age ≤65 years (combined procedures <55 years)
Peak exercise capacity: VO_2 <14 ml/min/kg with a respiratory exchange ratio (RER *; VCO_2/VO_2) >1.05
Wedge pressure >16 mm Hg
Cardiac index <2
Ejection fraction <20%

ESHD, End-stage heart disease; *NYHA,* New York Heart Association.
*RER gives information about substrate utilization at the cellular level. Ratios greater than 1.0 indicate carbohydrate oxidation.

pulmonary arterial pressure (PAP) greater than 50% of systolic pressure and life expectancy less than 14 days. Status 1B indicates growth failure in a child under 6 months of age with a PAP less than 50% of systolic pressure. Statuses 2 and 7 are the same for children as for adults.

Risk factors in the adult heart transplant candidate must be assessed to provide guidelines about the timing of placing a person on the UNOS waiting list and when to transplant. The measure of peak exercise oxygen consumption (peak VO_2) has become an indicator of prognosis in advanced heart failure and is currently being used as a major criterion in many centers for the selection of candidates for heart transplantation. Individuals with peak VO_2 less than 14 ml/min/kg have a lower survival rate unless treated successfully with transplantation. However, VO_2 can be affected by age, gender, muscle mass, and conditioning status. The multiple factors that affect peak exercise capacity may explain why some people with congestive heart failure and a peak VO_2 of less than 14 ml/kg/min have a favorable prognosis even when transplant is deferred.[7,155] Ejection fraction and capillary wedge pressures are also used to assess risk. Anyone with an ejection fraction* of less than 20% is also considered a potential candidate for transplantation.

Other selection criteria are being debated, such as the issue of transplantation in people with diabetes. Currently, most centers accept candidates with well-controlled diabetes who have no microvascular disease; some of the larger centers are treating people who have significant neuropathies or nephropathy. Age cutoff is also controversial; although the upper age limit for transplant candidates has been 55 to 65 years, some centers are now willing to transplant hearts or combined heart-kidney transplants into older people who are healthy in all other respects. Age limits for combined organ transplantation are more stringent, with a cutoff age at 55 years.

Complications may occur during the waiting period before the cardiac transplantation takes place. The supply of donor hearts is limited so that more than one half of people waiting die before an available heart can be transplanted; women die more often than men, possibly because of delayed diagnosis and more advanced heart disease at the time of diagnosis.

Transplantation Procedure. To perform a transplant, the heart is denervated and lacks autonomic neural control but has normal contractility (systolic function). Almost all heart transplantations done at this time are orthotopic; that is, the donor heart is grafted into the normal anatomic site. Current surgical technique for orthotopic heart transplantation involves removal of the recipient's heart except for the atrial wall, leaving a large portion of the posterior wall of the right and left atria in the recipient and implanting the donor heart in the atria, together with direct end-to-end anastomoses of the aorta and pulmonary artery.*

In the *heterotopic* cardiac transplantation, the recipient's diseased heart is left intact and the donor heart is placed in parallel with anastomoses between the two right atria, pulmonary arteries, left atria, and aorta. In the heterotopic transplantation, the donor heart assists the diseased heart. This type of procedure accounts for less than 1% of the transplant population and may be performed in an individual with fixed pulmonary hypertension or someone who is physically very large with a large thoracic cavity requiring a higher cardiac output than a smaller heart could provide.

Complications. The most common posttransplant complications are acute or chronic organ rejection and infections, especially pulmonary infections. Acute right ventricular failure is a frequent cause of early morbidity and mortality. The normal donor right ventricle may be unable to meet elevated pulmonary vascular resistance present in the recipient, especially during the early posttransplant period when there is a high degree of both pulmonary and tricuspid valve insufficiency.

Neuromusculoskeletal. Reports have also been made of generalized polyneuropathy accompanying solid organ rejection of the heart and kidneys. The neuropathy affects proximal and distal muscles and demonstrates hyporeflexia or areflexia.

Other complications occur as a result of long-term use of cyclosporine to prevent organ rejection (see the section on Immunosuppressants in Chapter 4). Specific to cardiac transplantation, cyclosporine- or tacrolimus (FK-506)-induced hyperuricemia may occur 3 to 4 years after initiation of these drugs, especially in people with a history of gout before transplantation. It is characterized by early symptoms of gout, including arthralgias and monoarthritis affecting the first metatarsophalangeal joint, knees, ankles, heels, and insteps. Over time, upper extremity joints become involved, progressing to polyarticular chronic arthritis. There is a greater occurrence of early involvement of atypical joints (other than knees and feet) in people taking cyclosporine with the development of tophi around the time of initial symptoms (Fig. 20-10). Treatment is as for primary gout (see Chapter 26).

A unique form of osteoporosis may develop in younger people who have their transplanted hearts longer. This condition is associated with long-term use of cyclosporine and is characterized by the most severe vertebral osteopenia. Significant osteopenia may already be present before cardiac transplantation in the presence of risk factors such as physical inactivity and dietary calcium deficiency.

---

*The amount of blood the ventricle ejects is called the *ejection fraction;* the normal ejection fraction is about 60% to 75%. A decreased ejection fraction is a hallmark finding of ventricular failure.

---

*Modifications of organ transplantation techniques are ongoing. This description provides the reader with a general concept; reading the operative report provides detailed individual information.

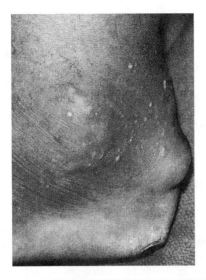

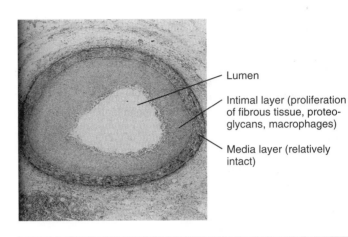

FIGURE 20-10 Tophus, a chalky deposit of sodium urate present in the Achilles tendon and foot, occurs in cardiac transplant recipients who have an associated history of gout. These tophi form most often around the joints in cartilage, bone, bursae, and subcutaneous tissue, producing a chronic foreign body inflammatory response. Tophi are not clinically significant for the therapist but indicate an underlying condition that requires medical attention. (From Howe S, Edwards NL: Controlling hyperuricemia and gout in cardiac transplant recipients, *Musculoskel Med* 12:15-24, 1995.)

FIGURE 20-11 Transplant coronary artery disease (TCAD). Proliferation of the intimal layer of the epicardial coronary artery from a 14-year-old cardiac transplant recipient 1 year after transplant. This condition produces a significant reduction in diameter of the arterial lumen that will compromise blood flow to the myocardium. (From Gajarski RJ: Update on pediatric heart transplant: long term complications, *Pediatr Cardiol* 24[4]:260-266, 1997.)

Transplant Coronary Artery Disease (TCAD; Allograft Vasculopathy).

Rapidly progressive TCAD may occur during the first year after transplant, although the cause remains unknown and is probably multifactorial. TCAD differs from typical coronary artery disease in that the lesions are diffuse and concentric throughout the vascular bed of the transplanted heart (Figs. 20-11 and 20-12) rather than asymmetric and focal as in the case of typical coronary artery disease. The small terminal branches of the myocardium are affected in the transplanted heart; they are rarely calcified, and the heart does not develop collateral circulation.

Because the heart has been denervated as a result of the surgical procedure, clients lack a consistent or predictable anginal warning system for myocardial ischemia. Some clients experience angina inconsistently and without clear explanation or predictability. More recent studies are suggesting angina experienced years after transplantation may indicate reinnervation of the autonomic nervous system in the donor heart in the presence of TCAD. Periodic exercise testing or coronary angiography is used to assess the development and progression of CAD in the transplanted heart.

Cancer.

As mentioned previously, cardiac transplant recipients have a higher incidence of posttransplant neoplasia, both solid and lymphoproliferative. Lymphoproliferative tumors occur early after transplantation, more frequently in younger recipients. Most of these tumors are thought to be the result of Epstein-Barr viral infection and occur because of T-cell suppression or depletion. The tumors typically arise in extranodal sites, such as lung, gut, or central nervous system.[146,191]

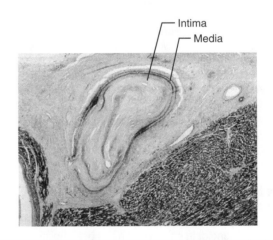

FIGURE 20-12 Transplant coronary artery disease (TCAD) resulting in complete occlusion of epicardial coronary artery in an 11-year-old heart transplant recipient 4 years after transplantation. The lumen is obstructed with dense fibrous tissue with thinning and fibrosis of the media layer. (From Gajarski RJ: Update on pediatric heart transplant: long term complications, *Pediatr Cardiol* 24[4]:260-266, 1997.)

Prognosis.

In general, people tolerate the transplant procedure well, and the graft resumes normal function promptly. Recipients are often extubated and out of bed into a chair 1 to 2 days after surgery. Survival times were short 30 years ago, but new immunosuppressive drugs developed in the mid-1980s and improved in the 1990s, more careful candidate selection, endomyocardial biopsy to allow for early rejection detection, and advanced medical-surgical techniques have contributed greatly to improved longevity.

Only a decade ago, infection and acute and/or chronic rejection were the major causes of death in heart transplant recipients. With improved longevity, chronic graft vasculopathy (accelerated atherosclerosis, TCAD) and malignancies are now the primary causes of death among heart transplant recipients. Infection, rejection, and sequelae of long-term immunosuppression (especially renal insufficiency or renal failure) remain the primary treatment issues.

Worldwide results of cardiac transplantation are excellent, with a 1-year survival rate of 87% owing to improved immunosuppression and more careful screening of donor hearts. Nearly one-half of all people with congestive heart failure who receive cardiac transplants survive at least 10 years with good exercise tolerance and acceptable side effects from immunosuppression. Although data are limited on the long-term success of heart transplantation, nursing homes are now receiving organ transplant recipients as residents.[60]

Special Implications for the Therapist   20-4

HEART TRANSPLANTATION

Preferred Practice Patterns:
4C: *Impaired Muscle Performance*
4G: *Impaired Joint Mobility, Muscle Performance, and Range of Motion Associated With Fracture (secondary to medications)*
5G: *Impaired Motor Function and Sensory Integrity Associated With Polyneuropathies (immunosuppressant-induced)*
6C: *Impaired Ventilation, Respiration/Gas Exchange, and Aerobic Capacity/Endurance Associated With Airway Clearance Dysfunction*
6D: *Impaired Aerobic Capacity/Endurance Associated With Cardiovascular Pump Dysfunction or Failure*
7A: *Primary Prevention/Risk Reduction for Integumentary Disorders*

Pretransplant
The therapist's role in transplantation varies from region to region. In some areas, the therapist is only involved with the pretransplant candidate if that person has been hospitalized. For all therapists working with individuals with heart disease, the 6-minute walk test provides a clinical assessment tool that is useful in developing an effective rehabilitation program and also offers the therapist some guidelines for recommending someone as a potential transplant candidate.[27]

Side effects of medications contribute to the high incidence of musculoskeletal injuries (e.g., steroid myopathies and neuropathies, avascular necrosis, osteoporosis). Prevention is an important component of the pretransplant habilitation and posttransplant rehabilitation programs. See specific recommendations in the section on Osteoporosis in Chapter 23.

Acute Care Phase
In the acute care setting, immediate postoperative considerations are important. Because most cardiac transplant candidates have experienced months of restricted activity before surgery, pulmonary hygiene and general strengthening are important

aspects of early treatment. Physical and occupational therapy initiated in the ICU focuses on restoring mobility and functional skills, increasing strength, and improving balance and reflexes; heel slides, ankle pumps, and bedside standing are included in the early postoperative protocol.

Pulmonary hygiene and breathing exercises are essential to prevent atelectasis (particularly left lower lobe atelectasis), especially in the case of implantation of an artificial heart because of the location of the device. Frequent, slow, rhythmic reaching, turning, bending, and stretching of the trunk and all extremities many times throughout the day help alleviate the surgical pain-tension cycle and facilitate pulmonary function.

Postoperative reports of chest pain may be due to the sternal incision and musculoskeletal manipulation during surgery. Chest pain secondary to myocardial ischemia or coronary insufficiency is not as likely in the early postoperative months because the heart has been denervated. Any other symptoms of ischemia, such as dyspnea, light-headedness, faintness, or increase in perceived exertion, should be attended to and reported.

Progressive ambulation can be initiated as soon as the client can transfer. Sternal precautions are standard postoperative orders but may vary from center to center (see Box 11-2); preventing separation of the sternum may require hand-held assistance in place of assistive devices such as a walker or quad cane initially. When the client can ambulate 1000 feet, the treadmill (1 mile/hr) or exercise cycle (0.5 RPEs [rating of perceived exertion]) can be used (see Table 11-13), usually around the fourth postoperative day, if there are no complications.[97]

Whether to use the treadmill or bicycle is generally an individual decision made by the client based on personal preference; presence of orthopedic problems must be taken into consideration. Resistive elastic or small weights and aerobic training are introduced between 4 and 6 weeks postoperatively. Pushing or pulling activities and lifting more than 10 lb are contraindicated in the first 4 to 6 weeks.

The primary physical therapy goals focus on increasing functional mobility and preparing for discharge and include a home exercise program, sternal precautions (see Box 11-2), and a plan for exercise progression (Table 20-8). Client education is a key component of the posttransplant program, and each member of the team must take this role seriously. It is important that the therapist have knowledge of medications and their potential side effects; monitor vital signs; encourage good nutrition, weight management, and good health; maintain pretransplant behavioral changes (including smoking cessation); and encourage the transplant recipient to continue exercising during the posttransplant period, even during episodes of rejection. By this time, the client is independent in pulse monitoring and scar management and can demonstrate knowledge of early signs and symptoms of rejection or infection, especially since these clinical manifestations may appear during exercise.

Other therapy program considerations may include balance assessment and falls prevention, spine care, osteoporosis prevention, weight-bearing exercises, and coordination and strengthening exercises, as well as a conditioning and aerobic program. Although assessing work capacity is important, performing an assessment of transplant recipients must take into consideration daily life and daily activities first. Assessing potential return to work and work requirements may not occur until 6 to 12 months after transplant (if at all). The team will assess hemodynamic status; the therapist will make objective assessments of the recipient's hemodynamic responses to activity and exercise. For example, a job that involves lifting requires assessment of cardiovascular compliance and hemodynamic stability during lifting whereas someone at home must be safe in ADLs.

Exercise

Individuals undergoing heart transplantation, like those undergoing coronary artery bypass surgery, are affected by preoperative inactivity and postoperative deconditioning and can benefit from exercise rehabilitation (see also the section on Exercise, Activity, Sports, and Organ Transplantation in this chapter). A major reason for low VO_2 max observed in heart transplant recipients is the low level of physical activity after transplantation. In addition to a reduced cardiac performance, it is likely that general fatigue and reduced muscle strength contribute to the relatively low exercise performance. Exercise can improve hemodynamics, normalize heart rate, improve oxygen uptake and delivery, and decrease diastolic blood pressure.[97]

Heart transplantation results in a denervated myocardium and an impaired ability by the autonomic nervous system to regulate cardiac function (Table 20-9). The resting heart rate after transplantation/denervation is higher than normal (usually in the range of 90 to 99 beats/min); an external pacemaker may be used if there is not an efficient heart rate to sustain cardiac output. Organ denervation and medications delay or blunt heart rate increase in response to exercise.

In the denervated myocardium, peak heart rate will (on average) only increase 20 to 30 beats/min from the resting level during submaximal exercise. Rate of exertion will be perceived as intense, and the recipient may feel very challenged despite this minimal heart rate increase. This is considered "within normal limits" for this posttransplant population. Individuals must be monitored for intensity and tolerance according to their symptoms and using an RPE scale while working within a range for heart rate response; the heart rate response should not exceed a peak range of 130 to 140 beats/min.

With the loss of fight or flight responses, over a period of time, the right ventricle hypertrophies and becomes stiff and noncompliant. This combined with the reduced cardiac output and therefore reduced reserve requires increased blood pressure to fill the ventricles (although blood pressure response may be blunted by medications or altered by kidney function complicating the clinical picture even more). This reduced reserve will be most evident during exercise, requiring close monitoring for increased diastolic blood pressure ($+/-10$ to 15 mm Hg). Other programs consider an increase or decrease greater than 20 mm Hg in diastolic blood pressure or a diastolic blood pressure greater than 120 mm Hg at rest to be significant. Each physician or center will have known protocols for these guidelines for the therapist to follow.

The loss of an immediate cardiac response to exercise can lead to an acute symptomatic clinical presentation. To counteract these influences, it is suggested that exercise in an upright position is preferred in order to increase venous return, improve heart compliance, increase heart rate, and improve cardiac performance.[14,126]

With the loss of vagal innervation, hypotension can be a problem, especially if there has not been an adequate warming-up or cooling-down period. The physiologic changes unique to heart transplant clients require a thorough warm-up before exercise to stimulate catecholamine release (epinephrine, norepinephrine) and to give the heart necessary time to prepare for peak activity. The warm-up period should be mild and long in order to prevent oxygen deficiency. Each step in the exercise protocol should be prolonged for up to 5 minutes to allow for a steady state of heart rate.[27] Likewise, a cool-down period is essential; after cessation of exercise the heart rate returns to normal over a much longer time in the transplanted versus the intact heart. This is most likely an effect of high levels of circulating catecholamines combined with an adrenergic hypersensitivity. Resting heart rate should be below 100 beats/min before leaving the clinic.

Although the denervation eliminates the sympathetic and parasympathetic nervous system input to the heart, the

Continued

TABLE	20-8

Physical Therapy Management

ACUTE	OUTPATIENT
Progression of functional mobility	Functional assessment
Sternal precautions	6-minute walking distance (6 MWD)
Assess hemodynamic stability; pulmonary clearance	Submaximal graded exercise test (GXT)
Monitor international normalized ration (INR):	Assess hemodynamic response
2.5-3.5	Monitor for hypertension
Monitor driveline site	Arrhythmias
Monitor volume/pressure	General strengthening and stretching
Assess for signs of rejection and infection	Assess for signs of rejection and infection
Assess for neurologic complications	Assess for neurologic complications
Education	Education and home exercise program
Side effects of medications	
Exercise response; pulse monitoring	
Signs of rejection and infection (see Tables 20-4 and 7-2, respectively)	

TABLE **20-9**

Effects of Cardiac Denervation

Heart rate
    Elevated at rest
    Blunted rise with exertion
Stroke volume: blunted rise with exertion
Cardiac output: 70%-75% of predicted
VO_2: 70%-80% of predicted
Pulmonary arterial pressure (PAP)
    Elevated at rest
    Marked rise with exertion
Anticipatory effect: lost
Abnormal diffusion capacity
Ventilation: increased response to exertion
Loss of anginal pain as a warning sign of myocardial ischemia
    during early years of denervation

Clinical Meaning
Need for extensive warm-up
Decrease in exercise capacity
Marked blood pressure response
Rely on other data to detect ischemia

Modified from Braith RW: Exercise training in patients with congestive heart failure and heart transplant recipients, *Med Sci Sports Exerc* 30(10):S367-S378, 1998.

Bainbridge reflex,* catecholamine response,† and Starling's law‡ allow for increased stroke volume. In other words, a strong initial increase in venous return associated with increased activity and large muscle contraction are responsible for early increases in heart rate; within 5 to 6 minutes after warm-up, catecholamines are activated and heart rate continues to increase. The heart rate may remain elevated after exercise secondary to remaining circulating catecholamines. A similar catecholamine response is not observed during isometric or isotonic contractions.

Isometric exercise puts a volume stress rather than a pressure stress on the heart and cannot be graduated. For this reason, isometric exercise may be considered contraindicated§; during the acute care phase, it should be initiated only with the physician's approval and performed with extreme caution only after considerable dynamic warm-up to raise the heart rate. Once the client has moved past the acute care phase, rehabilitation, including isometric exercise, can be utilized if indicated and progressed as tolerated. In addition, impaired skeletal mus-

*The Bainbridge reflex causes heart rate to increase as venous return to the heart stimulates volume receptors in the atria to trigger an increased heart rate.
†Catecholamines such as epinephrine and norepinephrine result in sympathetic stimulation to increase rate and force of muscular contraction of the heart, thereby increasing cardiac output, and to constrict peripheral blood vessels, resulting in elevated blood pressure.
‡Starling's law states that the greater the myocardial fiber length (or stretch), the greater will be its force of contraction. The more the left ventricle fills with blood, the greater will be the quantity of blood ejected into the aorta. This is like a rubber band: the more it is stretched, the stronger it recoils or snaps back. Thus a direct relationship exists between the volume of blood in the heart at the end of diastole (the length of the muscle fibers) and the force of contraction during the next systole.
§This contraindication is under consideration at this time; research for the transplanted population is ongoing, but no published studies are available regarding this issue.

cle metabolism and impaired vasodilation in skeletal muscle as a result of end-stage heart failure present before transplantation is reversed slowly after transplantation; these effects may persist 6 months after transplantation.

Following heart transplantation, there may be allograft vasculopathy, a manifestation of chronic rejection, which will cause increasing ischemia of the transplanted heart during increasing activity and exercise. This cardiac allograft vasculopathy can contribute to reduced oxygen uptake and a ventilation/perfusion mismatch limiting exercise capacity.[166] If the recipient has concomitant pulmonary involvement, abnormal diffusion capacities with altered ventilation responses may occur. These pulmonary components can cause a decrease in cardiac function with possible myocardial ischemia. Although there have been some documented cases of angina, most of these clients will not experience ischemia-induced angina as an early warning sign of cardiac impairment. This is another reason the therapist must follow appropriate exercise guidelines to stimulate a catecholamine response and monitor vital signs to assess cardiac function.

There is now some evidence that reinnervation (which is thought to be only partial) of the donor heart occurs as mentioned previously. This phenomenon does not happen until late after transplantation, and the magnitude of reinnervation is variable. Studies show a functional significance during exercise in people with marked reinnervation, including a higher maximal heart rate, increased peak oxygen uptake, increased oxygen pulse, and earlier heart rate peak after cessation of exercise (and falling more rapidly) than in the non-reinnervated cases.[98,200] Although exercise duration and maximal oxygen consumption do not appear to be related to reinnervation status, a longer exercise time in reinnervated hearts has been observed.[213]

When initiated early after cardiac transplantation, exercise training increases the capacity for physical work.[107] Exercise tolerance must be monitored closely during the early weeks after surgery. Ischemic damage during transport of the donor heart or subclinical damage associated with early rejection in combination with the denervated status of the heart may only become apparent during exercise. The therapist is encouraged to use perceived exertion scales such as the dyspnea index or Borg scale[15] (see Table 11-13), monitor changes in diastolic pressure, and rely on measurements of oxygen uptake to set exercise limits.

Despite denervation of the heart after transplantation, recipients have maintained a capacity to perform exercise and can return to vigorous sports activities. It is recommended that during endurance training in transplant recipients the therapist use 13 on the 0 to 20 Borg scale as a reasonable target to ensure that the client remains below the anaerobic threshold (i.e., at an exercise intensity that does not result in tachypnea). ■

Alternate Options: Mechanical Circulatory Support. Cardiac transplantation is a limited option because of the shortage of donor organs. For this reason, mechanical circulatory support has become an established procedure for bridging people to cardiac transplantation and is far more common than transplantation. Three options include the intraaortic balloon pump (IABP; see discussion in Chapter 11 and Fig. 11-14), extracorporeal membrane oxygenation (ECMO; see discussion under Lung Transplantation and Fig. 20-17), and mechanical or electric ventricular assistive devices.